Physical Management in Neurological Rehabilitation

Edited by

Maria Stokes PhD MCSP

Professor of Neuromuscular Rehabilitation, School of Health Professions and Rehabilitation Sciences, University of Southampton, Southampton, UK
Formerly Director of Research and Development, Institute of Complex Neuro-disability, Royal Hospital for Neuro-disability, London, UK

ELSEVIER
MOSBY

EDINBURGH LONDON NEW YORK OXFORD PHILADELPHIA ST LOUIS SYDNEY TORONTO 2004

ELSEVIER
MOSBY

The photo at the centre of the front cover and on the spine is from www.JohnBirdsall.co.uk.

First edition 1998
Second edition 2004

Coventry University

ISBN 0 7234 3285 6

British Library Cataloguing in Publication Data
A catalogue record for this book is available from the British Library

Library of Congress Cataloging in Publication Data
A catalog record for this book is available from the Library of Congress

Note
Medical knowledge is constantly changing. Standard safety precautions must be followed, but as new research and clinical experience broaden our knowledge, changes in treatment and drug therapy may become necessary or appropriate. Readers are advised to check the most current product information provided by the manufacturer of each drug to be administered to verify the recommended dose, the method and duration of administration, and contraindications. It is the responsibility of the practitioner, relying on experience and knowledge of the patient, to determine dosages and the best treatment for each individual patient. Neither the Publisher nor the editor and contributors assumes any liability for any injury and/or damage to persons or property arising from this publication.

The Publisher

 your source for books, journals and multimedia in the health sciences
www.elsevierhealth.com

The Publisher's policy is to use **paper manufactured from sustainable forests**

Printed in China

Contents

Contributors

Gillian Baer MSc MCSP ILTM
Senior Lecturer in Physiotherapy, Queen Margaret
University College, Edinburgh, UK

David Bates MA MB FRCP
Consultant Neurologist and Senior Lecturer, Department of
Neurology, Royal Victoria Infirmary, Newcastle upon Tyne, UK

J Graham Beaumont BA MPhil PhD CPsychol FBPsS
Head of Clinical Psychology, Royal Hospital for Neuro-
disability, London; Honorary Professor, University of Surrey,
Roehampton, UK

Rolfe Birch MChir FRCS FRCSEng
Consultant Orthopaedic Surgeon, Royal National
Orthopaedic Hospital NHS Trust, Middlesex, and
Visiting Professor at University College, London, UK

Thomas Britton MD FRCP
Consultant Neurologist, King's College Hospital,
London, UK

Maggie Campbell MCSP SRP
Brain Injury Coordinator, Sheffield West Primary Care Trust,
Sheffield, UK

Barbara Cook MCSP CertEd
Senior Physiotherapist, Richmond and Twickenham Primary
Care Trust, Teddington Memorial Hospital, Middlesex, UK

Lydia Dean DipCOT
Senior I Occupational Therapist, Royal National Orthopaedic
Hospital NHS Trust, Middlesex, UK

Carlos deSousa BSc MD MRCP
Consultant Paediatric Neurologist, Great Ormond Street
Hospital for Children NHS Trust, London, UK

Lorraine De Souza BSc MSc GradDipPhys PhD FCSP
Professor of Rehabilitation and Head of Department of
Health and Social Care, Brunel University College,
Middlesex, UK

Brian Durward MSc PhD MCSP
Dean, School of Health and Social Care, Glasgow Caledonian
University, Glasgow, UK

David Fitzgerald DipEng GradDipPhys GradDipManipTher MISCP
Private Practitioner/Lecturer, Dublin Physiotherapy Clinic,
Dublin, Ireland

Elizabeth Green BA(Hons) MD DCH DipHthMan FRCPCH
Consultant in Paediatric Rehabilitation, Chailey Heritage
Clinical Services, East Sussex, UK

Bernhard Haas BA(Hons) MSc ILTM MCSP
Head of Physiotherapy, University of Plymouth,
Plymouth, UK

Joanna Jackson EdD BSc(Hons) MSc CertEd(FE) MCSP DipTP
Principal Lecturer in Physiotherapy, Faculty of Health,
London South Bank University, London, UK

Anju Jaggi BSc(Hons) MCSP
Senior I Physiotherapist, Royal National Orthopaedic
Hospital NHS Trust, Middlesex, UK

Kathryn Johnson DipCOT
Senior I Occupational Therapist, Royal National Orthopaedic
Hospital NHS Trust, Middlesex, UK

Diana Jones PhD BA GradDipPhys MCSP
Principal Lecturer, School of Health, Community and
Education Studies, University of Northumbria, Newcastle
upon Tyne, UK

Fiona Jones MSc PGCertEd DipPhys ILTM MCSP
Senior Lecturer in Physiotherapy, St George's Hospital
Medical School – Physiotherapy, London, UK

Christopher Kennard PhD FRCP FRCOphth
Professor and Head of Division of Neuroscience and
Psychological Medicine, Imperial College School of Medicine,
Charing Cross Hospital, London, UK

Paula Kersten PhD BSc MSc
Lecturer in Health Services Research, Health Care Research Unit, School of Medicine, University of Southampton, Southampton General Hospital, Southampton, UK

Madhu Khanderia PhD BSc MRPharmS
Chief Pharmacist, Royal Hospital for Neuro-disability, London, UK

Cherry Kilbride MSc MCSP
Deputy Head of Therapy Services, The Royal Free Hampstead NHS Trust, London, UK

Dawn Langdon MA MPhil PhD CClin Psych
Senior Lecturer, Royal Holloway University of London, Surrey, UK

Nigel Lawes MBBS
Senior Lecturer, Department of Anatomy, St George's Hospital Medical School, London, UK

Sheila Lennon PhD BSc MSc MCSP
Lecturer in Physiotherapy, School of Rehabilitation Sciences, University of Ulster at Jordanstown, Northern Ireland, UK

Gillian McCarthy FRCP FRCPCH
Honorary Consultant Neuropaediatrician, Chailey Heritage Clinical Services, East Sussex, UK

Rory McConn Walsh MA MD FRCS(ORL)
Consultant Otolaryngologist, Beaumont Hospital, Dublin, Ireland

Dara Meldrum BSc MSc MISCP
Lecturer in Physiotherapy, Royal College of Surgeons in Ireland, Dublin, Ireland

Fred Middleton FRCP
Director, Spinal Injuries Unit, Royal National Orthopaedic Hospital NHS Trust, Middlesex, UK

Jane Nicklin MSc MCSP
AHP Clinical Development and Research Project Manager, Essex Workforce Developmental Confederation, UK

Caroline Nottle BSc(Hons) MCSP
Senior I Physiotherapist, King's College Hospital, London, UK

Betty O'Gorman MCSP
Superintendent Physiotherapist, St Christopher's Hospice, London, UK

David Oliver BSc FRCGP
Consultant in Palliative Medicine and Honorary Senior Lecturer in Palliative Care, Kent, Institute of Medicine and Health Sciences, University of Kent, Canterbury, UK

Sue Paddison GradDipPhys MCSP SRP
Superintendent III Physiotherapist/Clinical Specialist – Spinal Injuries Unit, Royal National Orthopaedic Hospital Trust, Middlesex, UK

Elia Panturin MEd RPT
Senior Instructor IBITA, Faculty of Physiotherapy, Tel Aviv University, Ramat Aviv, Israel

Jeremy Playfer MD FRCP
Consultant Physician in Geriatric Medicine, Royal Liverpool University Hospital, Liverpool, UK

Teresa Pountney PhD MA MCSP
Senior Paediatric Physiotherapist, Chailey Heritage Clinical Services, East Sussex, UK

Samantha Prisley BSc(Hons) MCSP
Senior I Physiotherapist, King's College Hospital, London, UK

Oliver Quarrell BSc MD FRCP
Consultant in Clinical Genetics, Sheffield Children's Hospital, Sheffield, UK

Ros Quinlivan BSc(Hons) MBBS DCH FRCPCH FRCP
Consultant in Paediatrics and Neuromuscular Disorders, Robert Jones and Agnes Hunt Orthopaedic Hospital, Shropshire, UK

Hillary Rattue MSc CertEd MCSP
Clinical Specialist in Paediatric Physiotherapy, St George's Hospital, London, UK

John C Rothwell PhD MA
Professor of Human Neurophysiology, Institute of Neurology, Queen Square, London, UK

Maria Stokes PhD MCSP
Professor of Neuromuscular Rehabilitation, School of Health Professions and Rehabilitation Sciences, University of Southampton, Southampton, UK

Nicola Thompson MSc MCSP SRCS
Clinical Specialist in Gait Analysis, Nuffield Orthopaedic Centre NHS Trust, Oxford, UK

Heather Thornton MBA MCSP PGCE
Senior Lecturer, Department of Physiotherapy, University of Hertfordshire, Hatfield, Herts, UK

Sue Tripp MSc CertPCAT RGN
Clinical Nurse Specialist, Royal National Orthopaedic Hospital NHS Trust, Middlesex, UK

Karen Whalley Hammell PhD MSc OT(C) DipCOT
Researcher and Writer, Oxbow, Saskatchewan, Canada.

Preface

This book is intended to provide undergraduate students in health professions, primarily physiotherapy, with a basic understanding of neurological conditions and their physical management. Qualified therapists may also find it a useful resource, particularly for conditions they only see rarely in routine clinical practice.

Since publication of the first edition in 1998 (previously entitled *Neurological Physiotherapy*), research has enabled neurological rehabilitation to advance considerably in certain areas. A survey of the views of clinical physiotherapists, lecturers and students on the first edition received extensive feedback, and their suggestions have produced three additional chapters, with other areas being incorporated into topics already covered. These include the specialist area of vestibular and balance rehabilitation (Ch. 24) and the controversial use of exercise in neurological rehabilitation (Ch. 29). Relatively new terms and concepts relating to clinical practice have been discussed in a new chapter 'The rehabilitation process' (Ch. 22).

All chapters are based on research and refer extensively to the scientific and clinical literature, to ensure clinical practice is evidence-based, although some areas still have a way to go.

Common themes throughout the book, the principles of which are discussed in the specific chapters indicated, include:

- a non-prescriptive, multidisciplinary, problem-solving approach to patient management (Ch. 22)
- involvement of the patient and carer in goal-setting (Ch. 3) and decision-making (client-centred practice; Ch. 22)
- an eclectic approach in the selection of treatments and consideration of their theoretical basis (Ch. 21)
- scientific evidence of treatment effectiveness (Ch. 22)
- use of outcome measures to evaluate the effects of treatment in everyday practice (Ch. 3)
- use of case studies to illustrate clinical practice (chapters on specific conditions).

An important area of care is to provide patients and carers with information and support, which includes directing them to appropriate specialist organisations (see Appendix).

SECTION 1: BASIC CONCEPTS IN NEUROLOGY

These chapters provide a basis for understanding subsequent sections and are referred to widely throughout the book. A degree of basic knowledge is assumed in Chapter 1, in which motor control mechanisms are discussed. Assessment by the neurologist (Ch. 2) and physiotherapist (Ch. 3) is then outlined, including outcome measures. Chapter 3 also reviews the revised classification system produced by the World Health Organization (WHO), which is now termed the *International Classification of Functioning, Disability and Health,* and referred to as ICF (WHO, 2001).

This section ends with discussion of abnormalities of muscle tone and movement (Ch. 4) and the adaptive changes in neural and muscle tissue involved in neuroplasticity (Ch. 5).

SECTION 2: NEUROLOGICAL AND NEUROMUSCULAR CONDITIONS

The neurological conditions in Chapters 6–12 are not presented in any particular order but the subsequent neuromuscular conditions are organised from proximal to distal parts of the motor unit. Disorders of nerves are presented in two sections: I, motor neurone disease (Ch. 13), which involves the anterior horn cell (but also upper motor neurones) and II, polyneuropathies (Ch. 14), which involve the motor nerves.

Disorders of muscle (Ch. 15) are then covered, including the neuromuscular junction (myasthenia gravis) and muscle fibres (muscular dystrophies). Post-polio syndrome is now included in this chapter but it is not strictly a muscle disorder, as it involves damage to motor neurones.

Muscle disorders of childhood onset are dealt with in Section 3 and mainly include muscular dystrophies and spinal muscular atrophy (the latter being a problem of the anterior horn cell, but so placed as the onset is in childhood).

Specific issues related to each disorder are given and, to avoid repetition of aspects common to all disorders, reference is made to chapters on general topics, such as assessment, treatment concepts and techniques and drugs. Case histories illustrate certain aspects of each condition, focusing on physical management, using a problem-solving approach.

SECTION 3: LIFETIME DISORDERS OF CHILDHOOD ONSET

This section is not simply termed paediatric conditions, since children with disorders such as muscular dystrophy and cerebral palsy are surviving more frequently into adulthood. The introduction to paediatric neurology discusses some of the rarer conditions which physiotherapists may come across (Ch. 16). The continuation of care into adulthood is stressed throughout Chapters 16–20.

SECTION 4: TREATMENT APPROACHES IN NEUROLOGICAL REHABILITATION

This section begins with a review of the theoretical basis of neurological physiotherapy (Ch. 21). Adequate evaluation has not been conducted of the different concepts and it is likely that no single approach has all the answers. An eclectic approach is being applied in all areas of physiotherapy, as rigid adherence to one school or another is progressively thought not to be in the best interest of patients.

The new chapter on 'The rehabilitation process' (Ch. 22) discusses: evidence-based practice; client-centred practice; the problem-solving process; and clinical reasoning.

Specific treatment techniques are discussed in Chapter 23, explaining the types of treatments available, their proposed mode of action (if known) and situations in which they might be applied. Limb casting and special seating are not discussed in detail, and are covered in depth by Edwards (2002).

Vestibular and balance rehabilitation is a recently recognised clinical specialty within physiotherapy and is included in a new chapter (24). This is followed by management of abnormal tone and movement in Chapter 25.

Pain (Ch. 26) and psychological issues (Ch. 27), which may influence physical management are then discussed. The final chapter in this section covers drug treatments used in neurology and provides a useful glossary, with details of effects and side-effects of drugs, some of which may influence physical management (Ch. 28).

SECTION 5: SKILL ACQUISITION AND NEUROLOGICAL ADAPTATIONS

This is a new section covering areas introduced relatively recently into clinical practice in neurology. Aerobic exercise and strength training in people with neurological conditions were traditionally avoided in case they exacerbated symptoms, particularly spasticity. Chapter 29 reviews the research emerging from different patient populations that suggests this fear of adverse effects is unfounded and that both forms of exercise are beneficial.

Two treatment concepts, originally developed in musculoskeletal conditions, are being applied increasingly in neurological rehabilitation and are discussed in the final two chapters: muscle imbalance (Ch. 30) and neurodynamics (Ch. 31).

CURRENT ISSUES AFFECTING CLINICAL AND RESEARCH PRACTICE

New initiatives, that are still evolving, relating to the management and conduct of practice include the following.

Clinical and research governance

Clinical governance was introduced in the UK by the Department of Health (DoH) in the late 1990s and is defined by the Chief Medical Officer as: 'A system through which NHS organisations are accountable for continuously improving the quality of their services and safeguarding high standards of care, by creating an environment in which clinical excellence will flourish' (DoH website for clinical governance). To achieve such excellence, systems need to be in place which: are patient-centred; monitor quality; assess risk and deal with problems early; have clear lines of accountability; are transparent; and provide information to professionals and the public. The clinical governance initiative recognises the importance of education and research being valued.

The *Research Governance Framework for Health and Social Care* was released by the DoH in 2002 and 'is intended to sustain a research culture that promotes excellence, with visible research leadership and expert management to help researchers, clinicians and managers apply standards correctly' (DoH website for research governance). The framework sets out targets for achieving compliance with national standards, developing and implementing research management systems covering general management arrangements, ethical and legal issues, scientific quality, information systems, finance systems and health and safety issues. In addition to closer monitoring of research activities, the new framework involves other requirements, such as involving consumers, informing the public and ownership of intellectual property. As well as reassuring the public by minimising fraud and misconduct, these robust, transparent management systems should also provide a healthy environment for all grades of researchers to be suitably supported and recognised, thus enhancing the quality and productivity of clinical research.

National standards and guidelines for clinical practice

Practice standards and guidelines have been produced by the DoH through NICE (National Institute for Clinical Excellence) and national service frameworks for different clinical conditions, e.g. cancer, coronary heart disease (DoH website for national service frameworks). Guidelines for the physical management of specific conditions are also produced by other organisations, such as the Stroke Association, the Intercollegiate Working Party on Stroke and the Association of Chartered Physiotherapists Interested in Neurology (ACPIN); these guidelines are referred to in relevant chapters throughout this book.

International Classification of Functioning, Disability and Health (ICF)

The revised ICF, which is discussed in Chapter 3, focuses on 'how people live with their health conditions and how these can be improved to achieve a productive, fulfilling life' (WHO, 2001).

A colourful illustration of how a young man has achieved such a fulfilling life, despite complex disabilities, is provided in an autobiography (Colchester, 2003). Jonathan Colchester's story is a prime example of how we can learn from patients, as alluded to by Professor Richard HT Edwards in the foreword of that book.

As professionals and society, it is not for us to dictate how people should live. We do, however, have an important contribution to make in creating optimal conditions for individuals to express their natural abilities and live as full a life as possible, within the limitations of their disabilities. This book aims to address some of the issues involved in achieving this objective, specifically relating to physical management.

Maria Stokes
London, 2004

References

Colchester J. *A Life Worth Living: Abilities, Interests and Travels of a Young Disabled Man*. Northwich, Cheshire: Greenridges Press; 2003.

Department of Health. *Clinical Governance*. Available online at: www.doh.gov.uk/clinicalgovernance.

Department of Health. *National Service Frameworks*. Available online at: www.doh.gov.uk/nsf.

Department of Health. *Research Governance Framework for Health and Social Care*. Available online at: www.doh.gov.uk/research.

Edwards S (ed.) *Neurological Physiotherapy*. London: Churchill Livingstone; 2002.

World Health Organization. *International Classification of Functioning, Disability and Health*: ICF. Geneva: World Health Organization, 2001. Available online at: http://www.who.int/classification/icf.

Acknowledgements

Firstly, I wish to acknowledge the major contribution to this book from Professor Ann Ashburn and to thank her for advising on its content, assisting with recruiting new authors, reviewing a number of chapters and for her constant support.

The revised format would not have been possible without suggestions for new topics from physiotherapists. Professor Ashburn and the following, who peer-reviewed this work by feeding back on the first edition and/or reviewing chapters for the current edition, can have a sense of ownership of the book: Maggie Bailey, Jane Burgneay, Monica Busse, Mary Cramp, Lousie Dunthorne, Phyllis Fletcher Cook, Nicola Hancock, Wendy Hendrie, Angela Johnson, Nicky Lamban, Anne McDonnell, Fiona Moffatt, Alex Morley, J Ramsay, Sue Richardson, Ros Wade, Martin Watson, Trish Westran, those who responded to the survey anonymously, and the Association of Chartered Physiotherapists Interested in Neurology (ACPIN) for distributing the survey to its members and encouraging them to respond.

My thanks go to the authors who generously shared their knowledge and expertise, as senior clinicians and academics, despite busy workloads. The time and effort they invested in this book are much appreciated. I am very grateful to Lilian Hughes, who has worked alongside me as research administrator for a number of years, for her hard work and dedication. I wish her well on her retirement and will always remember her kindness and sense of humour.

I thank the Royal Hospital for Neuro-disability in Putney, the Neuro-disability Research Trust, The Peacock Trust and the team at Elsevier, particularly Dinah Thom and Heidi Harrison for supporting me in this project. I also thank the following friends and colleagues for their help in various ways: Margaret Hegarty for administrative assistance (in the early days of her recovery from foot surgery!); Rosaleen Hegarty, George Kantrell and Gerard Cullen for IT support; Dr Keith Andrews, Jo Babic, Jo Lawrence and Professor Di Newham for helpful feedback on parts of the text; helpful discussions with fellow ex-London Hospital physiotherapy students at a reunion weekend in Bath in October 2003; and Dr Elaine Pierce for keeping life manageable in the day-job.

Special thanks go to Miss Anne Moore (Consultant Neurosurgeon) and Dr De Gaulle Chigbu (Optometrist) for making my involvement in this project possible, and to my family and friends who encouraged, entertained and supported me throughout.

Maria Stokes
London, 2004

Abbreviations

5HT	5-hydroxytryptamine	ART	applied relaxation training
ABI	acquired brain injury	ASBAH	Association for Spina Bifida and Hydrocephalus
ACA	anterior cerebral artery		
ACC	anterior cingulate cortex	ASCS	Advice Service Capability Scotland
ACE	angtiotensin-converting enzyme	ASIA	American Spinal Injury Association
Ach	acetylcholine	ASPIRE	Association of Spinal Injury Research, Rehabilitation and Reintegration
ACPIN	Association of Chartered Physiotherapists Interested in Neurology	ATNR	asymmetric tonic neck response
		ATP	adenosine triphosphate
ACPIVR	Association of Physiotherapists with an Interest in Vestibular Rehabilitation	ATPase	adenosine triphosphatase
		AVM	arteriovenous malformation
ACPOPC	Association of Chartered Physiotherapists in Oncology and Palliative Care	BAEP	brainstem auditory evoked potential
		BAN	British approved name
		BDNF	brain-derived nerve growth factor
ACTH	adrenocorticotrophic hormone	BIPAP	bivalent/bilevel intermittent positive airway pressure
ADEDMD	autosomal dominant Emery Dreifuss muscular dystrophy		
		BMD	Becker muscular dystrophy
ADEM	acute disseminated encephalomyelitides	BOT	Bruininks Oseretsky Test
ADHD	attention deficit–hyperactivity disorder	BP	blood pressure
		BPL	brachial plexus lesion
ADHD-MD	attention deficit-hyperactive disorder and motor dysfunction	BPPV	benign paroxysmal positional vertigo
		BSID	Bayley Scales of Infant Development
ADL	activities of daily living	BSRM	British Society of Rehabilitation Medicine
AFO	ankle–foot orthosis		
AGSD	Association for Glycogen Storage Disorders	Ca	calcium
		cAMP	cyclic adenosine monophosphate
AIDP	acute inflammatory demyelinating polyradiculopathy	CAOT	Canadian Association of Occupational Therapists
AIDS	acquired immune deficiency syndrome	CBIT	Children's Brain Injury Trust
AIMS	Alberta Infant Motor Scale	CDC	Child Development Centre
ALS	amyotrophic lateral sclerosis	CHART	Craig Handicap Assessment and Reporting Technique
AMPA	α-amino-3-hydroxy-5-methyl-4-isoxazole propionate		
		CIC	clean intermittent catheterisation
AMRC	Association of Medical Research Charities	CIDP	chronic inflammatory demyelinating polyradiculopathy/polyneuropathy
AMT	adverse mechanical tension	CIMT	constraint-induced movement therapy
ANT	adverse neural tension	CISC	clean intermittent self-catheterisation
ARGO	advanced reciprocal gait orthosis	CK	creatine kinase

CLA	Chailey Levels of Ability		FES	functional electrical stimulation
CMD	congenital muscular dystrophy		FET	forced expiratory technique
CMT	Charcot–Marie–Tooth		FIM	Functional Independence Measure
CNS	central nervous system		FLAIR	fluid-attenuated inversion recovery
CO_2	carbon dioxide		FMRP	fragile X-linked mental retardation protein
COMT	catechol-O-methyltransferase		FO	foot orthosis
COX2	cyclo-oxygenase 2		FSH	fascioscapulohumeral muscular dystrophy
CPG	central pattern generator		FVC	forced vital capacity
CPK	creatine phosphokinase		GABA	gamma-aminobutyric acid
CPM	continuous passive movement		GAP43	growth-associated protein
CPP	cerebral perfusion pressure		GAS	Goal Attainment Scaling
CPTII	carnitine palmitoyl transferase type II deficiency		GBS	Guillain–Barré syndrome
			GCS	Glasgow Coma Scale
CRPS	complex regional pain syndrome		GEF	guanine nucleotide exchange factor
CSF	cerebrospinal fluid		GFR	glomerular filtration rate
CSP	Chartered Society of Physiotherapy		GHJ	glenohumeral joint
CST	cranial sacral therapy		glu	glutamate
CT	computed tomography		GMCS	Gross Motor Classification Scale
CTSIB	Clinical Test of Sensory Interaction and Balance		GMFM	Gross Motor Function Measure
			GP	general practitioner
CVA	cerebrovascular accident		GPe	globus pallidus external nucleus
DA	dopamine		GPi	globus pallidus internal nucleus
DAG	diacylglycerol		GSDV	glycogen storage disease type V
DAI	diffuse axonal injury		H reflex	Hoffman reflex
DAMP	disorders of attention, motor and perception		HASO	hip and spinal orthoses
			HD	Huntington's disease
DCD	developmental co-ordination disorder		HGO	hip guidance orthosis
DEBRA	Dystrophic Epidermolysis Bullosa Research Association		Hist	histamine
			HIV	human immunodeficiency virus
DL	dorsolateral		HKAFO	hip–knee–ankle–foot orthosis
DLF	Disabled Living Foundation		HLA	human leukocyte antigen
DM	dermatomyositis		HMSN	hereditary motor and sensory neuropathy
DM1	dystrophic myotonica		HO	heterotopic ossification
DMD	Duchenne muscular dystrophy		HOT	hyperbaric oxygen therapy
DMSA	dimercaptosuccinic acid		IASP	International Association for the Study of Pain
DNA	deoxyribonucleic acid			
DoH	Department of Health		IBM	inclusion body myositis
DSD	detrusor sphincter dyssynergia		ICD-10	International Classification of Diseases
DTPA	diethylenetriamine penta-acid		ICF	International Classification of Functioning, Disability and Health
DVT	deep venous thrombosis			
ECG	electrocardiogram		ICIDH	International Classification of Impairments, Disabilities, and Handicaps
ECHO	echocardiogram			
EDMD	Emery Dreifuss muscular dystrophy		ICP	integrated care pathway (Ch. 3)
EEG	electroencephalography		ICP	intracranial pressure
EMG	electromyography		IgG	immunoglobulin G
enc	encephalin		IN	irradiation neuritis
ENG	electronystagmography		IP_3	inositol triphosphate
EP	evoked potentials		IPA	Impact on Participation and Autonomy
EPIOC	electric-powered indoor/outdoor chair		IPPB	intermittent positive-pressure breathing
ES	electrical stimulation		IPPV	intermittent positive-pressure ventilation
ESD	early supported discharge		KAFO	knee–ankle–foot orthosis
ESR	erythrocyte sedimentation rate		KP	knowledge of performance
FAM	Functional Assessment Measure		KR	knowledge of results
FCMD	Fukuyama congenital muscular dystrophy		LACI	lacunar infarcts

LCAD	long-chain acyl-CoA dehydrogenase deficiency	PCI	Physiological Cost Index
LEA	local education authority	PD	Parkinson's disease
LGMD	limb girdle muscular dystrophy	PDMS	Peabody Development Motor Scales
LHS	London Handicap Scale	PDS	Parkinson's Disease Society
LMN	lower motor neurone	PEDI	Pediatric Evaluation of Disability Index
LOC	loss of consciousness	PEG	percutaneous endoscopic gastrostomy
LSA	learning support assistant	PET	positron emission tomography
LSO	lumbar-sacral orthosis	PHAB	Physically Handicapped and Able Bodied
MABC	Movement Assessment Battery for Children	PKA	protein kinase A
MAI	Movement Assessment of Infants	PKB	prone knee bending
MAP	mean arterial blood pressure	PKC	protein kinase C
MAP	Miller Assessment for Preschoolers	PM	polymyositis
MAS	Modified Ashworth Scale	PNF	proprioceptic neuromuscular facilitation
MAS	Motor Assessment Scale	PO	parietal operculum
MBD	minimal brain dysfunction	PO_2	partial pressure of oxygen
MCA	middle cerebral artery	POCI	posterior circulation infarcts
MCS	minimally conscious state	POMR	problem-oriented medical records
MDT	multidisciplinary team	PP1	protein phosphatase 1
MELAS	mitochondrial encephalomyopathy, lactic acidosis and stroke	PPN	pedunculopontine nucleus
MHC	major histocompatibility	PPR	posterior parietal region
MMG	mechanomyography	PPS	post-polio syndrome
MND	motor neurone disease	PROM	passive range of movement
MNDA	Motor Neurone Disease Association	PSCC	posterior semicircular canal
MPTP	N-methyl-4-phenyl-1,2,3,6-tetrahydropyridine	PSP	progressive supranuclear palsy
MPVI	Motor Free Visual Perception Test	PTA	post-traumatic amnesia
MRC	Medical Research Council	QoL	quality of life
MRI	magnetic resonance imaging	RADAR	Royal Association for Disability and Rehabilitation
mRNA	messenger RNA	RCA	regional care adviser
MRP	motor relearning programme	RCT	randomised control trial
MS	multiple sclerosis	RDA	Riding for the Disabled Association
MSA	multiple system atrophy	RIG	radiological insertion of a gastrostomy
MTI	magnetisation transfer imaging	rINN	recommended international non-proprietary name
NA	noradrenaline (norepinephrine)	RNA	ribonucleic acid
NCAS	National Congenial Abnormality System	RNOH	Royal National Orthopaedic Hospital
NDT	neurodevelopmental therapy	ROM	range of movement
NGF	nerve growth factor	RSD	reflex sympathetic dystrophy
NGST	neuronal group selection theory	RSSI	rigid spine syndrome
NICE	National Institute for Clinical Excellence	SAH	subarachnoid haemorrhage
NICU	neonatal intensive care unit	SCC	semicircular canal
NIH	National Institutes of Health	SCI	spinal cord injury
NIPPV	non-invasive positive-pressure ventilation	SDR	selective dorsal rhizotomy
NMDA	N-methyl-D-aspartate	SEN	Special Educational Needs
NTD	neural tube defect	SHT	S-hydroxytryptamine (serotonin)
O_2	oxygen	SIGN	Scottish Intercollegiate Guidelines Network
OBPP	obstetric brachial plexus palsy	SF-36	Short Form-36
ODD	oppositional defiance disorder	SIP	Sickness Impact Profile
OLS	one-leg stance	SIU	spinal injuries unit
OSF	Oswestry Standing Frame	SLE	systemic lupus erythematosus
PACI	partial anterior circulation infarcts	SLR	straight-leg raising
PCA	posterior cerebral artery	SLT	speech and language therapist

SMA	spinal muscular atrophies		TNS	transcutaneous nerve stimulation
SMA	supplementary motor area (Ch. 1)		TORCH	toxoplasmosis, rubella, cytomegalovirus and herpes simplex virus
SMR	standardised mortality ratio		TVPS	Test of Visual Perceptual Skills
SN	substantia nigra		TVR	tonic vibration reflex
SNIP	sniff nasal pressure		UDS	urodynamic studies
SNpc	substantia nigra pars compacta		UKABIF	UK Acquired Brain Injury Foundation
SNpr	substantia nigra pars reticulata		ULNT	upper-limb neurodynamic test
SNR	substantia nigra reticulata		ULTT	upper-limb tension test
SOD	superoxide dismutase		UMN	upper motor neurone
SPKB	slump-prone knee-bending		VA	ventriculoatrial
SPOD	Sexual and Performance difficulties of the Disabled		VC	vital capacity
SRR	Society for Research in Rehabilitation		VEP	visual evoked potential
SSEP	somatosensory evoked potential		VL	ventrolateral
SSRI	selective serotonin reuptake inhibitor		VLCAD	very-long-chain acyl-CoA dehydrogenase deficiency
STN	subthalamic nucleus		VM	ventromedial
TA	tendo-achilles		VMI	Visual Motor Integration
TACI	total anterior circulation infarcts		VOR	vestibulo-ocular reflex
TBI	traumatic brain injury		VP	ventriculoperitoneal
TENS	transcutaneous electrical nerve stimulation		VS	vegetative state
TEV	talipes equinovarus		VSR	vestibulospinal reflex
TIA	transient ischaemic attack		WHO	World Health Organization
TLSO	thoracolumbosacral orthoses		WISCI	Walking Index for Spinal Cord Injury
TMS	transcranial magnetic stimulation		XLDC	X-linked dilated cardiomyopathy

SECTION 1

Basic concepts in neurology

Chapter 1

Motor control

JC Rothwell

INTRODUCTION

This chapter gives a brief summary of the basic principles used by the nervous system to control movement, together with the major central nervous structures involved.

MOVEMENT PLANS AND PROGRAMMES

A simple but fundamental observation about the control of movement can be made by anyone who has learned to write. A signature written small with a fine hard-tipped pencil on a sheet of paper will look virtually identical (if allowance is made for size) to the signature of the same person written using a blunt piece of chalk on a wall-mounted blackboard. Although the muscles used are different, ranging from the small muscles of the hand and forearm to the whole arm, shoulder and even legs when writing on the blackboard, the identity of the signature remains clear. The observation implies that within the motor system there is an idea of the signature and that this is transformed into the appropriate action irrespective of the precise combination of muscles and joints needed to achieve it. It is this transformation of an idea into a plan or programme of movement that is the fundamental task of the motor system.

Apraxia

Apraxia is a condition in which this transformation is compromised (Geschwind & Damasio, 1985). It occurs after lesions in several parts of the brain, and is particularly common in patients with damage to the left hemisphere or with lesions of the anterior part of the corpus callosum. There are many varieties of apraxia.

Ideomotor apraxia refers to the inability of patients to produce a correct movement in response to a simple external command. For example, if a patient is asked to hold out the tongue, he or she may be unable to do so, or will make an inappropriate movement such as chomping the teeth. However, although unable to use the tongue on command, the same patient may be able to move it quite normally in automatic movements such as licking the lips or speaking.

Careful testing shows that the patient understands what he or she should do, but simply cannot transform the command into an appropriate movement. Exactly where in the brain this transformation occurs is not clear. One idea is that apraxia can result from disconnection of areas of the brain which receive the instruction to move or which formulate the idea of the movement, from the final effector areas of the motor system.

Deafferentation

The production of any movement involves co-operation between plans or programmes of movements and feedback from sensory receptors in the periphery. Before discussing the role of the latter, it is useful to have some idea of the extent to which the central motor command system can store and replay sequences of movement without reference to sensory input. Studies of deafferented patients have shown that the central command system can store and execute an extraordinarily wide range of movement commands.

An example was seen in a patient with a severe peripheral sensory neuropathy affecting the hands and feet (Rothwell et al., 1982). This patient had no sense of movement, touch, temperature or pinprick in his hands, although his motor power was virtually unaffected. Despite an almost total lack of sensation, he could move his thumb to touch each finger in turn with his eyes closed, even though he could not feel the touch of each finger to the thumb. He could repeat this movement for several cycles quite well, but over the course of half a minute or so the movement would deteriorate and finally ended up with the fingers missing the thumb. What appeared to happen was that small errors crept into the performance of each cycle of the movement. They went uncorrected and gradually built up to produce severe disruption of movement.

The conclusion from such observations is that the central nervous system (CNS) can store a remarkably detailed set of movement commands which is quite sufficient in this example to orchestrate the timing and sequencing of the very many small muscles in the hand and forearm needed to produce finger and thumb movement.

Role of sensory feedback

Sensory feedback may involve interaction with reflexes during motor activity or adaptation after the movement, to update later motor commands.

Reflexes

It is now believed that sensory feedback interacts in two ways with these preformed movement commands. The most familiar way is in the reflex correction of movements (Carpenter, 1990; Shepherd, 1994). In the textbook example of a stretch reflex, if a subject holds a weight by flexing the biceps, then a sudden increase in the weight will cause elbow extension and stretch the biceps to recruit a stretch reflex that opposes the applied disturbance. Engineers refer to this as online correction of the central motor command. Under most circumstances, though, such reflex corrections are not very efficient. This is readily verified if we move from the textbook to the real world and note what happens to the angle of our elbow when someone unexpectedly places a heavy glass on to a light tray which we are holding in one hand. When the weight is added, the elbow extends and the tray moves downwards. Reflexes in the biceps may occur but they are insufficient to prevent movement of the tray and restore the angle of the elbow. In engineers' terms, the gain of the reflex is low. In fact, the rule for many reflexes is that they are relatively inefficient as compensatory mechanisms when the disturbance to movement is large, such as in the example of the glass on the tray, but in other conditions, when the disturbance is small, they may act very powerfully indeed.

In the example of the biceps, careful experiments have shown that very small disturbances of movement, at around the perceptual threshold of the subject, are almost totally compensated by reflex mechanisms, even though the disturbance itself may remain undetected by the subject. Under many conditions, this makes some sense. If a large disturbance occurs, it may be inappropriate to recruit the full strength of a muscle like the biceps in a reflex manner. Instead, it is more likely that we would wish to consider voluntarily whether a completely different movement strategy would be more appropriate (Marsden et al., 1983). Of course, this rule will not apply to all reflexes. Life-preserving or damage-limiting reflexes often operate at a very high gain in all conditions. Consider the enormous movements of the arms that we make if we begin to tip forward off balance when standing on the edge of a wall with the sea several metres below our feet. These arm movements are postural reflexes which try to force the body back to the safety of dry land (see below).

Adaptation

Sensory feedback is also used to update the instructions in the central motor command system so that subsequent movements are performed more accurately. The important distinction here is that the sensory correction is not online, but is used after the movement is complete to update the motor commands for the next time they are used. The information is used to adapt or improve an already formed set of movement commands. A good example of this way of using sensory feedback was noted during the study of the deafferented man referred to earlier. Despite the lack of sensation in his hands and feet, this man still drove a manual gear-change car. He considered himself to be safe, even though he could feel neither the gear stick nor the pedals. During the course of his illness, he bought a new car but found that he could not learn to drive it. Despite trying for several weeks, he ended up by selling the new car and buying back his old one. The interpretation was that, without sensory feedback from his arms and legs, he was unable to update his centrally stored commands for car driving and adapt them to the subtleties of the new driving position.

Another example of sensory adaptation of motor commands can be demonstrated in most normal subjects using prism spectacles (Thach et al., 1992). Such spectacles typically deviate gaze by, say, 30° to the right, so that objects which appear to be straight ahead to the subject are actually 30° to the left of the midline. If subjects are asked to point rapidly at objects in front of them, then their aim is to the right of the target. This effect is seen only on the first few trials after the spectacles are put on. Over the next 20 trials or so, subjects gradually become more accurate. Because the task is to point as fast as possible (the experiment works better if, rather than pointing, subjects throw an object at the target), it seems unlikely that visual feedback is used to correct the arm movement online. That is, it is unlikely that subjects see that their arm is moving in the wrong direction and immediately use that information to correct the movement as it is taking place. It is more likely that visual feedback of the error from one movement is used to update subsequent commands for the next attempt. After 20 or so trials, the improvement in accuracy means that subjects have reorganised the commands for arm movements to take account of the displacement of the visual field. When a subject points at an object which appears to be straight ahead, the arm movement control system points the arm 30° to the left of the midline.

We can show that this replanning occurs automatically by examining performance in the first few trials a subject makes after the spectacles are removed. In these trials a subject points to the left of the target as if the motor system was still assuming that the visual world was shifted to the right. Subjects have to relearn the new relation between a normal visual world and their arm-pointing movements as their motor systems recalibrate. Thach et al. (1992) contrast results of a prism experiment featuring dart-throwing in a normal subject with those of a patient with cerebellar disease. Whereas the normal subject showed the adaptations described above after putting on and removing the prism spectacles, the cerebellar patient was more inaccurate at the start of the experiment but, more importantly, did not show any adaptation to the prism spectacles or any after-effect on removing them. The implication is that cerebellar connections may be involved in this type of adaptation.

Finally, it is important to be aware that such adaptation is not an unusual phenomenon. For example, movement of a cursor on a computer screen rarely corresponds in distance to the amount by which the mouse is moved on the mouse-pad, but we can adjust quickly to the change in gain between mouse and cursor. Such adaptation is not the result of online reflex correction of movement, but the result of adapting our commands for arm movements to the new displacement that we see before us.

DESCENDING MOTOR PATHWAYS

Many parts of the brain are involved in the control of movement, but before we examine them in detail, it is useful to review briefly the descending pathways which convey the motor commands. The detailed anatomy of these pathways is dealt with by Nicholls et al. (1992), Shepherd (1994) and Rothwell (1994). In humans, the major motor pathways are:

- the corticospinal tract
- the reticulospinal tracts
- the vestibulospinal tracts.

Other descending motor pathways also exist but they are probably small compared with the three main systems. In particular, it should be noted that the rubrospinal tract, from the red nucleus to the spinal cord, is quite prominent in the cat; however, it is thought to be virtually non-existent in people.

Corticospinal tract

The corticospinal tract carries information from the cerebral cortex to the spinal cord. It is sometimes called the pyramidal tract because the only point at which all the fibres are collected together without contamination by other fibre tracts is in the medullary pyramids of the brainstem. The primary motor cortex is the main source of input to this tract, but other areas such as the premotor and supplementary motor cortex also contribute fibres. Its projections are primarily contralateral and have a strong influence on the activity of groups of spinal motoneurones which innervate distal muscles of the hands and feet. Like most other descending systems, the axons of the corticospinal tract usually synapse on to interneurones in the spinal cord. These interneurones then contact the motoneurones which innervate a muscle. However, particularly in higher primates and humans, the corticospinal system has developed many direct projections to motoneurones which omit the spinal interneurones. These monosynaptic connections are most prominent to motoneurones innervating distal muscles, and are termed the corticomotoneuronal component of the corticospinal tract. These direct connections are not present at birth but develop to the adult pattern over the first 2–4 years of life.

Reticulospinal tracts

The reticulospinal tracts arise in the pontine and medullary areas of the reticular formation. The fibres from the medullary portion descend in the dorsolateral funiculus of the cord near the corticospinal fibres, whereas the fibres from the pontine region travel in the ventromedial portion of the spinal cord. The former constitute the lateral reticulospinal tract whereas the latter are known as the medial reticulospinal tract. These pathways are predominantly bilateral and have the largest density of projections to axial and proximal muscles. There are no direct terminations on spinal motoneurones. The input to the reticulospinal tracts comes from many areas of the brain, including the motor areas of the cerebral cortex. This means that the motor areas have two ways of accessing the spinal cord: one through the direct corticospinal projection and the other via an indirect corticoreticulospinal route.

Vestibulospinal tracts

The vestibulospinal tracts arise in the vestibular nuclei, which receive input from the balance organs of the ear, with little input from cortical motor areas. Their projections to the spinal cord are mostly bilateral and to proximal and axial muscles.

Lesions of descending motor pathways

In the late 1960s Lawrence & Kuypers (1968) conducted a classic series of experiments in which they described the behavioural effects of lesions of various descending systems in monkeys. When the animals awoke from anaesthesia following bilateral section of the corticospinal tract at the level of the pyramids (pyramidotomy), their behaviour looked virtually indistinguishable from normal. They ran around the cage, climbed up the bars and fought with other animals as usual. However, they were noted to have problems in picking up small pieces of food from the floor of the cage.

When the monkeys were tested in a special apparatus that involved retrieving food from small wells drilled into a wooden board, Lawrence & Kuypers (1968) noted that the most persistent deficit was an inability to produce what they termed 'fractionated' movements of the fingers. When intact monkeys retrieved food pieces from each well they did it by forming a precision grip between the forefinger and thumb, flexing the other three fingers out of the way into the palm of the hand. Following pyramidotomy, animals could no longer perform a precision grip. They tried to retrieve the food by using all four fingers and the thumb in concert. The result was that they were mostly unsuccessful. The conclusion from these experiments was that in the monkey the corticospinal tract is particularly important for fine, fractionated control of distal arm muscles. (It should be noted that pyramidotomy produces relatively little muscle weakness and no detectable increase in muscle tone.)

Lawrence & Kuypers (1968) also examined how performance of the monkeys developed after birth. They found that (as in human babies) precision grip was not present in infant monkeys and developed only over the first 6 months to 1 year. Since the final monosynaptic connections of the corticospinal tract develop over the same period, it has been postulated that the precision grip is particularly dependent on the presence of the corticomotoneuronal component of the corticospinal tract (Porter & Lemon, 1994).

In a separate series of experiments, Lawrence & Kuypers (1968) also tried to evaluate the effect of transecting the brainstem–spinal pathways. Their experiments involved two stages. In the first stage the animals were given a pyramidotomy and allowed to recover. Later the brainstem pathways were also cut. The reason for the double lesion was that if the brainstem pathways alone were damaged, then part of their function could be taken over by the corticospinal system. Although recovery was good after the initial corticospinal lesion, the animals appeared to be very impaired after the second lesion involving the vestibulospinal and reticulospinal tracts. Even after some weeks' recovery, they had severe postural deficits and tended to slump forward when sitting. They had great difficulties in avoiding obstacles when walking, and an absence of righting reactions so that they could not readily stand up again if they fell. The conclusion was that these brainstem pathways are used chiefly in the control of gross postural movements. Although the corticospinal tract may also be involved to some extent in such movements, its most important role seems to be to superimpose upon them the ability to produce fractionated movements of the distal hand muscles.

Lawrence & Kuypers (1968) did not study whether the different brainstem–spinal pathways had different functions, nor did they comment extensively on the tone of their lesioned animals. However, earlier work on both cats and monkeys had suggested that reticulospinal pathways had a strong influence on muscle tone (reviewed by Brown, 1994). Lesions of these pathways, or the input to these pathways, were supposed to have a much larger influence on muscle tone than lesions of the corticospinal system. A model was developed in which it was proposed that the lateral reticulospinal system received excitatory input from the cortex and had the effect of reducing the excitability of both stretch and flexion reflexes. This system was opposed by the medial reticulospinal system that had no input from the cortex but excited stretch reflexes and inhibited flexion reflexes. Thus, if a capsular stroke, for example, destroyed the cortical input to the lateral system, the action of the medial system would be dominant and therefore stretch reflexes would be increased, whilst flexion reflexes would be only mildly affected. In contrast, a complete spinal section would destroy both tracts, and the main problem would be lack of reticulospinal suppression of flexion reflexes, with little change in stretch reflexes. However, it is now recognised that the reticulospinal systems are complex and that they are likely to play a role in normal movement as well as in regulating muscle tone and flexion reflexes.

AREAS OF THE CEREBRAL CORTEX INVOLVED IN CONTROL OF MOVEMENT

The motor areas of the cerebral cortex are defined as having: (1) a direct (corticospinal) projection to the spinal cord; and (2) corticocortical connections with the primary motor cortex. Three major areas are usually distinguished (Fig. 1.1):

- the primary motor cortex itself, lying anterior to the central sulcus
- the premotor cortex, which occupies an area in front of the primary motor cortex on the lateral surface of the brain
- the supplementary motor area, a region of the medial surface of the hemisphere anterior to the leg area of the primary motor cortex.

The primary motor cortex corresponds anatomically to Brodmann's area 4; the premotor cortex to the lateral part of area 6; and the supplementary motor area (SMA) to the medial part of area 6. In the monkey, both the premotor cortex and the SMA are subdivided into smaller parts. The premotor cortex is classified into a total of four dorsal/ventral and rostral/caudal sections, whilst the SMA has two divisions, rostral and caudal (Rizzolatti & Luppino, 2001). In addition, several other motor areas have recently been described that lie on the cingulate gyrus in the medial surface of the hemisphere. The function of these areas is still under investigation (He et al., 1995).

Primary motor cortex

The primary motor cortex is so called because it has the lowest threshold for production of movement after direct electrical stimulation of the cortex (see review by Porter & Lemon, 1994). Early mapping experiments in both primates and humans revealed the well-known motor homunculus. Stimulation of medial portions of the primary motor cortex produced movements of the legs, whilst stimulation of progressively more lateral regions produced movements of the trunk, arm, hand and then face on the opposite side of the body. Of all motor areas, the primary motor cortex has the largest number of corticospinal connections and it contributes some 40% of the total number of fibres in the

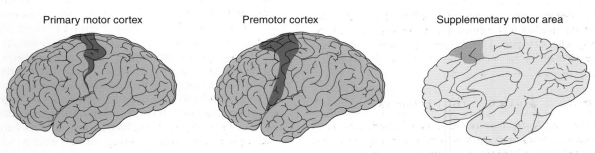

| Primary motor cortex | Premotor cortex | Supplementary motor area |

Figure 1.1 The three main motor areas of the cerebral cortex of the human brain. These locations are only approximate since the detailed neuroanatomical and neurophysiological studies that have been performed in monkeys have not been performed in humans.

corticospinal tract. This is one reason for its very low threshold to direct electrical stimulation or magnetic stimulation.

When a movement is made, the discharge of motoneurones in the spinal cord reflects the activity of all the inputs that they receive, both from local spinal circuits and from descending input in the corticospinal, vestibulospinal and reticulospinal pathways. Each input provides only part of the final motor command, and in different tasks the importance of each input may vary. In most voluntary movements, recording of single cell activity in the brains of conscious primates shows that primary motor cortex cells discharge in a manner very similar to that of spinal motoneurones. The cortical cells fire before the onset of movement, often at a rate proportional to the force exerted in the task. In these circumstances, the primary motor cortex probably provides a large proportion of the input to spinal motoneurones. In less voluntary tasks, such as swinging the arms when walking, the motor cortical contribution may be smaller.

Because such a large proportion of the corticospinal system originates in the primary motor cortex, lesions here can have very pronounced effects on movements. Such lesions also interrupt indirect output to the spinal cord via cortical projections to the reticular formation and the reticulospinal tracts. This explains why lesions of the motor cortex differ in their effects from the pure corticospinal lesions described above. Small lesions of the primary motor cortex result in weakness of a limited group of muscles on the contralateral side of the body. If the lesion is very small, recovery is good with little increase in muscle tone and little permanent deficit except in fine discrete movements (Hoffman & Strick, 1995).

Larger lesions produce greater weakness in more muscles, and there is less recovery of function. After an initial period of flaccid paresis, muscle tone may be permanently increased. Lesions in the internal capsule tend to affect a large number of descending (corticospinal as well as corticoreticulospinal) fibres because they are bundled together in a small volume. Thus, capsular lesions usually result in widespread and permanent deficits. It is as if the effect of small lesions can be compensated to a large extent by activity in remaining structures, but if the lesion is large then compensation is less likely.

Reorganisation in the primary motor cortex

Recently, there has been a good deal of interest in how motor cortical areas reorganise after injury (Donoghue & Sanes, 1994). The clearest effects are seen after injury to the peripheral motor system. Figure 1.2 shows an example of the changes which can occur. The upper part of the figure shows a map of the motor cortex of a rat indicating the forelimb area, the extraocular representation around the eyes, and a region in between, stimulation of which produces movement of the vibrissa (whiskers). After mapping the cortex (Fig. 1.2A), the experimenters cut the seventh cranial nerve which supplies the vibrissa, with the result that the rat could no longer move its whiskers. Figure 1.2B shows that preventing vibrissa movement leads to a substantial reorganisation of the cortex, such that when electrical stimuli are applied to what was previously the vibrissa area, they now produce movements of either the forelimb or of the extraocular muscles. It is as if the representation of these two muscle groups has expanded into the area previously occupied by the projection to the vibrissa.

These changes occur very quickly, and can be documented even in the space of 60 min or less. They appear to be due to changes in the activity of intrinsic cortical circuits rather than to reorganisation of the pattern of corticospinal projections. Figure 1.2C illustrates what is thought to happen. In the diagram, there are a number of corticocortical connections between the arm and the vibrissa area which are drawn as being excitatory. Under most conditions, the excitability of these connections is suppressed by the activity of local inhibitory interneurones. It is thought that these in turn are controlled by (amongst other things) sensory input from the periphery. When the nerve to the vibrissa is cut, sensory input from the whiskers is altered and this reduces the excitability of some of the inhibitory interneurones in the arm area. The effect is to open up the excitatory connections from the vibrissa to the arm area so that when the vibrissa area is stimulated electrically, activity in the corticocortical connections to the arm area can excite corticospinal output neurones which project to the arm. This change in the excitability of corticocortical connections can occur very rapidly indeed and explains why the effects on the motor cortex map occur after such a short time interval. It is possible that after a longer period of time such changes may become permanent through growth of new synaptic connections.

Similar changes have been demonstrated in patients with limb amputation or spinal cord injury using the new technique of transcranial magnetic stimulation (TMS) of the motor cortex (Cohen et al., 1991). Unfortunately, such reorganisation of the cortex does not seem to occur so readily after damage to central structures. Perhaps one reason for this is the dependence of the reorganisation on sensory input from the periphery. If this is disrupted in any way, or if the circuitry of the cortex itself is damaged, then this type of reorganisation may be compromised. This process of reorganisation, plasticity, is discussed in Chapter 5.

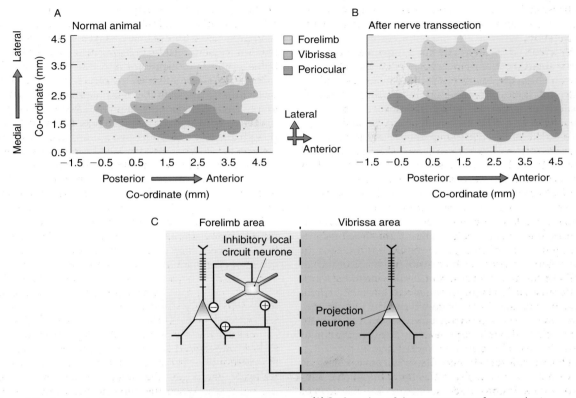

Figure 1.2 Reorganisation of motor map of the primary motor cortex. (A) Surface view of the motor cortex of a normal rat, illustrating the major functional regions. (B) Surface view of the motor cortex in a rat 123 days after transection of the buccal and mandibular branches of the facial (seventh cranial) nerve. Each dot indicates an electrode site at which movement occurred with small intracortical stimuli. Shading shows the periocular, vibrissa and forelimb areas of the cortex. Note that, after nerve transection, there is an apparent expansion of the forelimb and periocular sites into the vibrissa zone. (Redrawn from Sanes & Donoghue (1991), with permission.) (C) Hypothetical circuits to explain the reorganisation. Ordinarily, stimulation of the vibrissa area results only in vibrissa movement because spread of excitation (see branching axons from vibrissa output neurone to forelimb area) is limited by simultaneous activation of a local circuit inhibitory interneurone. It is thought that the activity of the inhibitory neurone is influenced by afferent input coming from the periphery. When the sensory input from the whiskers is altered by cutting the seventh cranial nerve, this reduces the excitability of some of the inhibitory interneurones in the forelimb area and opens up the excitatory connections from the vibrissa area.

Premotor and supplementary motor areas

The corticospinal projection from premotor and SMAs is smaller than that from primary motor cortex and the threshold for electrical stimulation is higher. These areas are thought to be more remote from the peripheral motor apparatus, and because of this they are often referred to as secondary motor areas. They both receive input from areas of parietal cortex involved in processing somatosensory and visual input; the most rostral portions of both areas also receive input from the prefrontal cortex. This type of connectivity puts them in a position where they may be involved in translating the aims of a movement, as defined in terms of its sensory consequences and the motivation of the subject, into the appropriate motor commands to achieve the task. There are subcortical inputs to both areas, but it is of note that the basal ganglia project (via thalamus) more strongly to the SMA than to the premotor cortex, whereas the situation is reversed for cerebellar projections.

When a movement is made, an appropriate plan or programme for the movement must be selected. It has been proposed that this selection occurs in one of two ways. In externally cued movements the instructions are retrieved on the basis of external signals in the environment. For example, a red traffic light means retrieve the programme for leg extension to press the brake to stop the car. In internally cued movements instructions are retrieved from memory without any external cues. It is thought that the supplementary motor area has a preferential role in internally cued movements, whereas the premotor cortex is preferentially involved in externally cued movements. Recent work suggests that this division of function is most prominent in the anterior parts of each area.

In the 1980s, Passingham in Oxford conducted several experiments which confirmed this idea (Passingham, 1995). Externally cued and internally cued tasks were used to train monkeys in which the premotor cortex or SMA were removed bilaterally. The implication of the findings of these lesion studies is that the premotor cortex is concerned with the retrieval of movements made on the basis of information provided by external cues, whereas the SMA is concerned with retrieval of movement on the basis of information within the animal's motor memory. Single cell recordings from these areas have confirmed the idea of internal and external cueing of movement. Neurones in the SMA may discharge when a monkey presses a series of buttons in a prelearned sequence (internally cued), but not when the same sequence is cued by illuminating a series of lights above each button in turn (externally cued). Premotor cortex neurones discharge in relation to the latter task, but not the former.

This subdivision of movements into two types has some important practical implications. In patients with Parkinson's disease the degeneration of dopaminergic cells, in the substantia nigra pars compacta, compromises the output of the basal ganglia. Such patients often have particular difficulty in performing internally cued movements, whereas their performance is often much better when external cues are provided. A typical example is the freezing which patients may experience when walking. Very often, walking can be improved if visual cues, such as lines or squares, are drawn on the floor, indicating to the patient where to place his or her feet next. Indeed, some patients who are particularly prone to freezing episodes may even go to the extent of always carrying an umbrella with them. If they experience a freezing episode, then they may be able to turn their umbrella upside down and place the handle in front of them so that they can use that as a visual cue to step over in order to initiate gait (see Ch. 11).

In the context of the theory outlined above, perhaps the disordered basal ganglia output in Parkinson's disease is primarily affecting the (internally cued) performance of an SMA, whilst externally cued movements mediated through the premotor system may be able to function relatively well.

An important question is how a visual cue can be used to select an appropriate pattern of muscle activity via the premotor system. In other words, how does the sight of the umbrella handle actually trigger release of

an appropriate movement? Single cell recordings show that some neurones in the (ventral) premotor cortex discharge when the monkey makes certain types of hand movement, such as grasping or holding an object. Some of the same neurones also discharge when the monkey is presented with an object that, if it were picked up by the animal, would require the same sort of movement. The important point is that the neurones discharge even though no movement is made. It is as though the sight of the object automatically calls up activity in neurones that can code for an appropriate movement. Indeed, a further class of these neurones is so specific that they are termed 'mirror neurones' (Rizzolatti & Luppino, 2001). These neurones fire both when the monkey makes a particular sort of movement and when it observes another animal or human making the same movement. It is an intriguing possibility that these neurones help us learn to do a task by watching others perform it.

SUBCORTICAL STRUCTURES INVOLVED IN CONTROL OF MOVEMENT

- Basal ganglia
- Cerebellum.

Anatomical and physiological features of these structures are discussed and clinical examples of dysfunction are given.

Basal ganglia

The basal ganglia have no direct connections either to or from the spinal cord, so that in order to understand their role in movement it is important first to understand their connections with other parts of the motor system (see Rothwell (1995), for review).

Anatomy

The basal ganglia consist of five main nuclei (Fig. 1.3) that lie deep within the cerebral hemispheres between the cortex and thalamus. The caudate nucleus and the putamen are two large nuclei, separated by white matter in humans, but in other animals they form one structure which is known as the striatum. The globus pallidus is placed medial to the striatum. Its name comes from the pale colour of the nucleus in fresh sections of the brain. It is divided into two parts, the external or lateral nucleus (GPe) and the internal or medial (GPi) nucleus, by a thin lamina. Although both subdivisions look similar, they have very different functions. The final two structures of the basal ganglia are the subthalamic nucleus (STN), which is a small lens-shaped

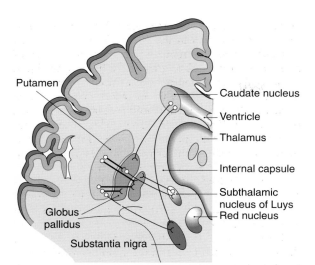

Figure 1.3 Location of the nuclei comprising the basal ganglia. This coronal section through the brain is slanted anteroposteriorly in order to show all the structures on one section. Note the two parts of the globus pallidus. The two subdivisions of the substantia nigra (pars reticulata and pars compacta) are not shown in this figure. The connections from the caudate nucleus and putamen to the substantia nigra are shown terminating in the pars reticulata. The dopaminergic connection from the pars compacta is not shown.

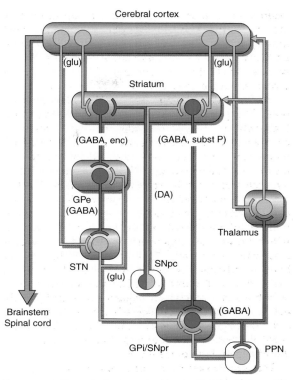

Figure 1.4 The main flow of information through the basal ganglia. The caudate nucleus and putamen are grouped together as the striatum in this diagram. The direct pathway from the striatum to the GPi is shown as the right-hand projection, whereas the indirect pathway is shown as the left-hand projection from the striatum. Filled neurones are inhibitory; pale connections are excitatory. Transmitters are shown in brackets. DA, dopamine; enc, encephalin; glu, glutamate; GABA, gamma-aminobutyric acid; Gpe, external nucleus; Gpi, internal nucleus; PPN, pedunculopontine nucleus; SNpc, substantia nigra pars compacta; SNpr, pars reticulata; STN, subthalamic nucleus; subst P, substance P. (Redrawn from Alexander & Crutcher (1990), with permission.)

nucleus underneath the thalamus, and the substantia nigra, which is readily visible in cut sections of the brain as a dark streak (due to the melanin pigment in the cells) in the midbrain. The substantia nigra is divided into two portions, the pars reticulata (SNpr) and the pars compacta (SNpc). As with the globus pallidus, the two subdivisions have very different functions.

The basal ganglia receive their main input from the cerebral cortex, and send the majority of their output back to the cortex via the thalamus. This circuit is known as a corticobasal ganglia–thalamocortical loop. A small proportion of the output also goes directly to structures in the brainstem rather than the thalamus. Two important targets are the superior colliculus, an area involved in the control of eye movement, and the pedunculopontine nucleus, an area known in the cat to be important in the control of locomotion.

Cortical input projects mainly to the caudate nucleus and putamen, which together constitute the receiving nuclei of the basal ganglia. The main output structures are the GPi and the SNpr. Although the latter two regions are separated by some distance anatomically, they are thought to form part of the same structure which has been split in the course of evolution by fibres of the internal capsule. The flow of information through the basal ganglia from input to output is shown in Figure 1.4. There are basically two main pathways

through the basal ganglia: the direct and indirect pathways. The direct pathway consists of direct projections from the striatum to the GPi or SNpr. The indirect pathway comprises projections from the striatum to the GPe, and thence to the STN, and finally to the GPi (or SNpr). It is now known which transmitters are released at each of the synapses in the pathway, and whether they are excitatory or inhibitory to the target cells.

The inhibitory and excitatory connections are shown in Figure 1.4; from tracing the two pathways it can be seen that the direct and indirect routes produce opposite effects on the final output nucleus. Activation of the direct pathway inhibits the output neurone, whereas activity in the indirect pathway produces final excitation of the output neurone. This opposite action is often likened to a neuronal brake and accelerator. It is not known whether the two pathways actually converge on to the same output cell, as shown in Figure 1.4, or whether the two pathways project to two separate populations of output cells.

A final important piece to add to the anatomical jigsaw is the dopaminergic pathway, which arises from cells in the SNpc and has axons that terminate in the striatum, where they release dopamine. Dopamine has opposite actions on the cells of the direct and indirect pathway, being excitatory to those involved in the direct pathway and inhibitory to those involved in the indirect pathway (Fig. 1.4).

It was once thought that the function of the basal ganglia was to integrate information from many cortical areas before relaying it back to the cortex for final use. Anatomically, this appears to be what might happen, since the cross-sectional area of the receiving nuclei is much larger than that of the final output nuclei, giving ample opportunity for anatomical compression of the information to occur. This idea is now thought to be incorrect, however. Information from different cortical areas appears to remain separate in its passage through the basal ganglia and flows through many independent parallel channels. For example, in the motor circuit, information from the somatomotor areas of cortex converges on to the putamen, which then sends information via the direct/indirect pathways back to the same areas of the cortex. Similarly, prefrontal areas of the cortex project on to the caudate nucleus, which then projects to particular subareas of the globus pallidus and back to the cortex. The oculomotor loop is one loop which will be referred to later. This receives input from frontal areas of the cerebral cortex, including frontal eye fields and supplementary eye fields, and sends output mainly to the superior colliculus in the brainstem.

Theories of basal ganglia function based on Figure 1.4

There are many theories about the possible role of the basal ganglia in control of movement. Many make use of an unexpected property of the final output neurones in the GPi and SNpr. These neurones are GABAergic (i.e. they produce gamma-aminobutyric acid) and are inhibitory to their target cells in the thalamus. In animals at rest, the firing rate of these cells is very high (50–150 Hz). The consequence is that, even when no movement is occurring, a large amount of inhibitory output leaves the basal ganglia. The simplest interpretation of this is that the output acts as a brake on movement and that when it is removed movement may occur (the thalamocortical projection is excitatory, so

that tonic inhibition of this projection would remove excitatory input to the cortex).

There is some evidence for this simple interpretation from studies of the eye movement control system. Just before the onset of a visually guided saccadic eye movement, cells in the SNpr that project to the superior colliculus reduce their firing rate. At about the same time, a burst of activity occurs in collicular neurones, which then starts the eyes moving. In the simple model it looks as if removal of the inhibitory output of the oculomotor loop of the basal ganglia 'allows' the eye movement to start. In fact, this interpretation is probably oversimplified. Removal of the tonic inhibitory output of the basal ganglia probably does not cause an obligatory eye movement. For the eyes to move, other excitatory inputs must probably converge upon the superior colliculus and other output centres in the brainstem. Removal of the inhibitory output from the basal ganglia is therefore regarded as being a facilitatory influence on the final movement.

Staying with this simple interpretation, we can use the anatomy of the basal ganglia to explain many of the movement disorders caused by basal ganglia disease (Wichmann & DeLong, 1993). These are considered in the following paragraphs and also discussed in Chapter 4.

Hemiballism

Hemiballism is caused by a lesion of the subthalamic nucleus on one side of the brain. It is characterised by wild involuntary movements of the contralateral side of the body which may be so large as to prevent patients from feeding or dressing themselves. This is usually caused by a vascular lesion, and often resolves within a few weeks. In the diagram of the basal ganglia circuit (Fig. 1.4), we see that removing the influence of the STN will reduce excitatory input to the GPi and SNpr. This will reduce the firing of the output nuclei, and therefore reduce inhibitory output to the thalamus. The final effect is similar to removing the brake of a car, and results in excessive motor output.

Huntington's disease

Huntington's disease is characterised by uncontrollable choreiform movements of the limbs and trunk, which often worsen with time (see Ch. 12). In the later stages of the disease the chorea may lessen and may be replaced by an akinetic–rigid state. Pathologically, Huntington's disease begins with preferential death of striatal neurones in the indirect pathway. Following the anatomy, we can see that reduction of inhibition from the striatum to the GPe will produce additional inhibitory activity in the pathway from the GPe to the STN (Fig. 1.4). This extra inhibition of the STN can be compared to a lesion of the STN, since it results in less excitatory output to the GPi and SNpr. The final result is less inhibitory input from the basal ganglia and an excess of movement.

Parkinson's disease

Parkinson's disease is due to a degeneration of the dopaminergic neurones in the midbrain, particularly those which project to the striatum. Following the model, we can see that this will result in overactivity in the indirect pathway and underactivity in the direct pathways through the basal ganglia (Bergman et al., 1990). The final result is excess inhibitory output from the basal ganglia and hence a reduction in the amount of movement (Fig. 1.5). Indeed, recent recordings taken from monkeys made parkinsonian by injection of the toxin MPTP (N-methyl-4-phenyl-1,2,3,6-tetrahydro-pyridine) show just this type of behaviour: neurones in GPi do indeed fire at a higher rate in parkinsonian monkeys than in normal monkeys. This has led to the idea that one way to treat Parkinson's disease may be to damage either the GPi (thereby decreasing the inhibitory output to the basal ganglia) or the STN (thereby removing some of the excitatory input to the output nuclei). Both approaches work very success-fully in the monkey model, and are now being used in people (see Ch. 11, p. 208).

Although the model of basal ganglia function is very successful in explaining many of the symptoms of basal ganglia disease, several questions are left unanswered. For example, the model predicts that lesions of the globus pallidus in normal subjects should produce a syndrome characterised by excess involuntary movement. In fact, bilateral lesions of the globus pal-lidus (as seen, for example, after carbon monoxide poi-soning) actually produce a condition which resembles mild Parkinson's disease rather than chorea. Similarly, we would also predict that lesions of the thalamus might sometimes produce a parkinsonian state (by removing the excitatory input to cortex). In fact, this is never seen. Thalamic lesions in the areas which receive input from basal ganglia normally produce a dystonic syndrome rather than a parkinsonian syndrome.

There have been many attempts to improve this model of basal ganglia function. In particular, the spa-tial pattern of the output to different cortical areas is likely to be important. Thus, basal ganglia projections to areas of the cortex which are involved in a movement might decrease their firing rate (thereby removing inhib-ition), whilst those cortical areas which are uninvolved in the movement might receive an increased output

A

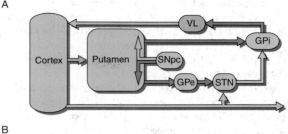

B

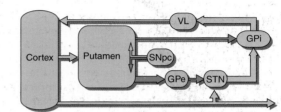

C

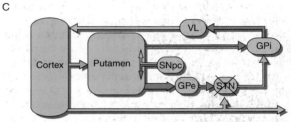

Figure 1.5 Basal ganglia circuitry changes in Parkinson's disease. (A) Normal activity in basal ganglia circuits; (B) changes in Parkinson's disease; and (C) reversal of these changes after lesion of the subthalamic nucleus (STN). Parkinson's disease causes underactivity in the direct pathway from the putamen to the internal nucleus (Gpi) and overactivity in the indirect pathway to the external nucleus (GPe). The result is excessive activity in the inhibitory output neurones of the GPi and a reduction in the final excitatory output from the thalamus to the cerebral cortex. This situation can be normalised by lesion of the STN. Less excitatory drive in the indirect pathway to the GPi leads to a reduction in the pallidal inhibition of the ventrolateral (VL) thalamus. SNpc, substantia nigra pars compacta.

from the basal ganglia. The effect would be that the pattern of basal ganglia output might help to focus excitation within the motor cortex.

Newer approaches to basal ganglia function

Although the circuit diagram of Figure 1.4 is an extraor-dinary achievement, it is unsatisfying in that there is no explanation of what sort of processing occurs at each synaptic relay in the circuit. For example, why does the indirect pathway have three synapses in it instead of there being just a direct excitatory connection from striatum to GPi? In an attempt to understand how signals are transformed at each relay station, attention has focused on the dopaminergic input to the striatum (Schultz, 1998). Ninety-five per cent of the striatum is composed of 'medium spiny' neurones. These receive the input from cortex on to the tips of small spines that cover their dendrites. Their axons form the output to GPe and GPi. The dopamine input from the SNpc also synapses on the same cells, at the base of the spines receiving cortical input. Such anatomy suggests that there may be an important interaction between the dopamine and cortical inputs.

One theory as to the nature of this interaction relies on the fact that each single neurone may be contacted by inputs from many thousand different cortical cells. It is then postulated that dopamine may be able selectively to strengthen the inputs from certain cortical cells, making the striatal neurone responsive to a particular pattern of inputs. Effectively the dopamine input is thought to 'teach' the medium spiny neurone to recognise particular combinations of cortical inputs, and pass this on to its projection targets. In terms of the motor loop of information flow through the basal ganglia, one might imagine that the striatum 'recognises' a particular pattern of cortical activity, such as the particular motor state of the animal, and uses this to select an output that would signal the most appropriate movement to make next. The rest of the circuitry of the basal ganglia would be needed to perform the translation of this recognised motor state into a pattern of inhibition and excitation that facilitates the most appropriate movement at a cortical level.

In terms of basal ganglia disease, one might then speculate that reduced dopamine levels would be associated with a state where no patterns of input are recognised by the striatum and therefore no signals are fed back to the cortex to indicate what movement to make next. Instead, such decisions would have to be taken by other areas of the brain, perhaps reflecting the increased mental effort of which patients complain when making voluntary movements.

Cerebellum

As with the basal ganglia, a great deal is known about the anatomy and synaptic connectivity of the cerebellum, but there is little consensus about its role in the control of movement (Stein, 1995).

Anatomy

In humans, the most conspicuous features of the cerebellum are the two lateral hemispheres which lie either side of a narrow ridge known as the vermis. Two main fissures divide the cerebellum transversely: the primary fissure divides the anterior from the posterior lobe, and the posterolateral fissure divides the much smaller flocculonodular lobe from the rest of the cerebellum (Fig. 1.6A). These structures form the cerebellar cortex, which sends its output to the cerebellar nuclei deep within the cerebellum (Fig. 1.6B).

Cerebellar cortex and nuclei

Three main longitudinal strips of cerebellar cortex project to the three main cerebellar nuclei. The medial zone (which is mainly equivalent to the vermis) projects to the fastigial nucleus; the intermediate zone projects to the interposed nuclei (globosus and embelliform nuclei in humans); and the lateral zone of the cerebellar hemispheres projects to the dentate nucleus. The vestibular nuclei also receive some direct output from the flocculonodular nodule lobe and parts of the vermis. The vestibular nucleus has a direct output to the spinal cord. The fastigial nucleus projects both to the vestibular nuclei and to other nuclei in the brainstem. However, the main output of the cerebellum arises in the interposed and dentate nuclei. They have projections to the red nucleus and (via the thalamus) to motor areas of the cerebral cortex, as well as direct outputs to brainstem structures.

All inputs to the cerebellum project to both the cerebellar nuclei and to the cerebellar cortex. Since the output of the cortex goes uniquely to the nuclei, it appears as if the cerebellar cortex is working as a side loop, modulating the main flow of information to the nuclei. However, the extent to which this is true physiologically is unknown.

Output neurones from the cerebellum

The Purkinje cells are the main, and largest, neurones of the cerebellar cortex (Fig. 1.7). They are the only output cells and their axons are inhibitory to the target neurones within the nuclei. The Purkinje cell dendrites stretch up to the surface of the cerebellar cortex, and the dendritic trees lie in a flat plane parallel to the axis of each cerebellar folium. The dendritic trees of adjacent Purkinje cells appear to stack on top of each other like plates.

Input neurones to the cerebellum

The cerebellar cortex receives two types of input fibre: climbing fibres and mossy fibres. Both are excitatory. Climbing fibres arise in the inferior olivary nucleus, and each forms 100–200 powerful synapses directly with one Purkinje cell. Mossy fibre input arises in cells of the pontine nuclei. The mossy fibre axons do not

A

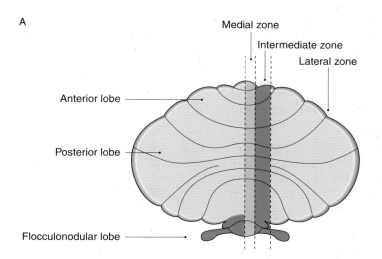

Medial zone

Intermediate zone

Lateral zone

Anterior lobe

Posterior lobe

Flocculonodular lobe

Figure 1.6 Subdivisions and connections of the cerebellum. (A) The transverse and longitudinal subdivisions of the cerebellum. (B) A highly simplified diagram of the input and output connections of the cerebellum. Note that all inputs go to both the cerebellar cortex and to the cerebellar nuclei.

B

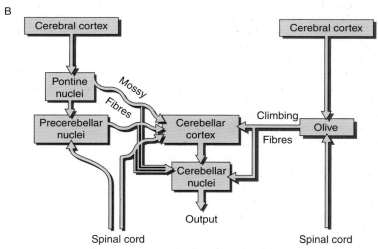

Cerebral cortex

Cerebral cortex

Pontine nuclei

Mossy Fibres

Precerebellar nuclei

Cerebellar cortex

Climbing

Olive

Fibres

Cerebellar nuclei

Output

Spinal cord

Spinal cord

synapse directly with Purkinje cells. They synapse with granule cells within the cerebellar cortex which have long axons that run perpendicular to the dendritic trees of Purkinje cells for several millimetres along the length of the cerebellar cortex. Each parallel fibre contacts very many Purkinje cells, but since the synapses are at the tip of the Purkinje dendrites each synapse is not very powerful. Thus the parallel fibre input is very diverse and weak compared with the very strong and focal input from the climbing fibres. Sensory input from the spinal cord may enter the cerebellar cortex directly in the mossy fibres, or travel via the olive to the climbing fibres. A similar arrangement applies to the input from motor areas of the cerebral cortex.

A special feature of the cerebellar circuitry is the adaptable synapse between the parallel fibre and the Purkinje cells. If the Purkinje cell is activated simultaneously by both parallel fibre and mossy fibre input, then the effectiveness of the synapse from parallel fibres to the Purkinje cell is decreased. This effect might allow the cerebellum to 'learn' or 'unlearn' associations between different inputs. Since the cerebellum has no direct motor output, it influences movement via projections to both brainstem–spinal and corticospinal motor systems. It is thought that the projection to vestibular nuclei and the reticular formation is important in the control of axial and proximal muscles, whereas the projection to the cerebral motor cortex is involved in the control of limb movements.

The role of the cerebellum

There are three main theories concerning the nature of the cerebellar contribution to movement control, all of

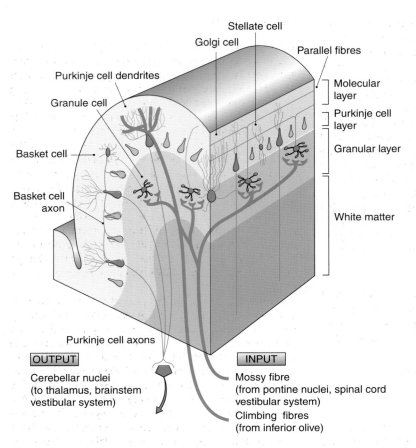

Figure 1.7 Three-dimensional diagram of the principal circuitry within the cerebellar cortex. Input enters via the mossy and climbing fibres; the only output is via Purkinje cell axons.

which are related to the symptoms of cerebellar disease:

1. timing
2. learning
3. co-ordination (Thach et al., 1992).

Timing Hypermetria (the tendency of cerebellar patients to overreach a target to which they are pointing) is usually caused by inappropriate timing of muscle activity such that antagonist force arises too late to stop a movement at the appropriate end point. It has been proposed that the time taken for impulses to travel along the long parallel fibre system to a particular group of Purkinje cells might be used to calculate times of muscle activation.

Learning A second deficit in cerebellar movement control is a failure to adapt motor commands to changes in the environment. An example of this in subjects wearing laterally deviating prism spectacles was given earlier. Experiments on animals have shown that such adaptation fails to occur if the cerebellar cortex is inactivated, and it has been suggested that changes in

the effectiveness of the parallel fibre-to-Purkinje cell synapse might underlie this type of adjustment.

Co-ordination The third function proposed for the cerebellum is that of co-ordination. Inco-ordination is one of the classical symptoms of cerebellar disease and is caused by a deficit in both timing of muscle activity and in the amount of activity in different joints.

POSTURE

The postural control system performs three main functions:

1. It supports the body, providing forces which bring form to the bony skeleton
2. It stabilises supporting portions of the body when other parts are moved
3. It balances the body on its base of support.

Like the rest of the movement control system, the postural system performs these functions in two different ways. It can act as an online feedback correction system, in which disturbances of posture are noted and corrected immediately by reflex mechanisms. Alternatively, it may predict that a postural disturbance will occur and provide anticipatory forces that will minimise the expected postural disturbance. For example, if we rapidly elevate our arms, then postural contractions occur simultaneously in muscles at the back of the leg and trunk. These contractions tend to pull the trunk backwards and compensate for the expected forward displacement which would be produced by holding the arms out in front of the body. Such anticipatory responses are often known as feed-forward corrections.

It is not known in which centres of the CNS these various functions are performed. They are likely to be distributed in many regions of the spinal cord, brainstem and even cerebral cortex (Horak & Woollacott, 1993).

Disturbances to posture are detected by three main sensory systems:

1. the somatosensory system (including muscle and joint receptors providing information on the position of body parts, as well as pressure receptors that provide an indication of the distribution of forces at points of contact)
2. the vestibular system (the semicircular canals and otolith organs)
3. the visual system.

In many circumstances, the same disturbance is signalled by all three inputs. For example, if the body falls forward, visual input indicates approach of the visual scene as the head moves forwards, vestibular input indicates a shift in the angle of the head relative to gravity and the somatosensory system signals rotation at the ankle and trunk as well as changes in the distribution of pressure on the soles of the feet.

All three of these inputs contribute to the corrective responses which may occur. However, in many cases things are not as simple as this, and discrepancies can arise between the different inputs. If we are standing upright in the cabin of a rocking boat, our bodies may sway together with the cabin. If the two movements are in phase, then there will be no apparent movement of the visual field, nor any change in angle of the ankle. Only the vestibular receptors will signal that the body is moving relative to gravity and this signal will conflict with the apparently stable signals coming through somatosensory and visual systems. One of the jobs of the postural system is to decide which inputs are providing the most useful information in different circumstances, so that if conflicts of information arise, more weight can be placed upon the most reliable input. Balance and vestibular disorders are discussed in Chapter 24.

Platform studies

The fact that the postural system can grade the importance of different sensory inputs means that at the limit, each type of input can on its own produce a postural response. This can be demonstrated in the following situation (see articles in Horak & Woollacott, 1993). Subjects stand on a special platform that can either rotate and tilt up and down (causing plantarflexion and dorsiflexion), or move backwards or forwards in the horizontal plane. The platform is placed within a special tent-like space which can, if necessary, sway backwards and forwards with the body so that the visual environment appears to be constant. In the situation when the platform is simply moved backwards, the subjects sway forwards, and all three channels of sensory input are activated: the visual field approaches, the ankle dorsiflexes and vestibular input signals a change in the direction of the pull of gravity with respect to the body.

Given the design of the platform, it is possible to arrange that the dorsiflexion of the ankle produced by backward translation is cancelled out by a simultaneous plantarflexion rotation of the platform around the ankles. In this situation, the subject is moved backwards, and the toes are rotated downwards, so that although the body tips forwards, the angle at the ankle remains constant. This therefore removes much of the somatosensory input to the postural system, but nevertheless postural responses are still generated by visual and vestibular input. It is also possible to remove the visual input, either by having subjects close their eyes, or by making the room around the subject move with the body. In this situation, vestibular input alone can generate corrective electromyographic responses in the leg and trunk. Although the pattern of response is very similar, the responses to different types of sensory inputs are not all the same. The latency of responses evoked by visual or vestibular input is longer than those produced when somatosensory inputs are available.

Moveable platforms can also be used to demonstrate how the postural system interacts with other local reflex circuits. If the platform is rotated toes-up, then subjects tend to fall backwards. However, a dorsiflexion of the ankle stretches the gastrocnemius/soleus muscles and tends to evoke a local stretch reflex, which if uncorrected would tend to pull the body further backwards off balance. Under these conditions the postural system rapidly learns, after only one or two trials, to reduce the stretch reflex in the gastrocnemius/soleus and increase the size of the corrective response in the anterior tibial muscles.

Finally, it is also possible to show that the postural system can modify its responses according to the way in which the body is supported. For example, when a moveable platform is moved backwards or forwards, subjects correct their posture by exerting torque around the ankle to oppose body sway. For this to work, the platform must be stable, so that the foot can exert pressure on the platform and move the body. If, instead, subjects are balanced on a seesaw then it is no longer possible to exert torque at that joint to oppose movement of the body. Balance in this condition is controlled by movements of the arm and trunk (rescue reactions). A change of postural strategy is produced by making the ankle muscle irrelevant to balance. It is an example of the postural system achieving the same end by different means.

Rescue reactions

The reactions that help to restore balance once the centre of gravity has fallen outside the postural base are perhaps most familiar. These rescue reactions involve obvious, gross movements of the whole body and may be classified as stepping, sweeping and protective reactions (Roberts, 1979).

If a standing subject is given a large unexpected push from behind, this will cause him or her to step forwards in order to capture the forward-moving centre of gravity. Often, the postural system does not wait until the centre of gravity has actually fallen outside the postural base before initiating the step; it predicts whether or not an initial displacement is likely to cause such a movement to occur and initiates a step before the point of no return is passed.

Under some conditions, stepping reactions are inappropriate and can be suppressed. For example, if a swimmer begins to overbalance when standing on the edge of the pool, he or she will rapidly swing the arms forwards in an attempt to use the reaction forces of the arm movements on the trunk to push the body back into equilibrium. In some circumstances, such reactions may also locate stable objects in the environment on to which the subject can hold to maintain balance (sweeping reactions). Finally, if all else fails and balance is lost, powerful protective reactions occur which are designed to protect the head and body during falls. The arms are thrown out, and the trunk rotated to break the fall. These reactions are not easily suppressed. The arms will be thrown out through panes of glass or into fire in order to fulfil their protective role. These reactions are not dependent on vestibular function; they are all present in vestibular-defective individuals. However, all rescue reactions are depressed in certain diseases of the basal ganglia.

References

Alexander GE, Crutcher MD. Functional architecture of basal ganglia circuits: neural substrates of parallel processing. *Trends Neurosci* 1990, **13**:266–271.

Bergman H, Wichmann T, DeLong MR. Reversal of experimental parkinsonism by lesions of the subthalamic nucleus. *Science* 1990, **249**:1436–1438.

Brown P. Pathophysiology of spasticity. *J Neurol Neurosurg Psychiatry* 1994, **57**:773–777.

Carpenter RHS. *Neurophysiology*. London: Edward Arnold; 1990.

Cohen LG, Bandinelli S, Findley TW, Hallett M. Motor reorganisation after upper limb amputation in man. *Brain* 1991, **114**:615–627.

Donoghue JP, Sanes JN. Motor areas of the cerebral cortex. *J Clin Neurophysiol* 1994, **11**:382–396.

Geschwind N, Damasio AR. Apraxia. In: Fredericks JAM, ed. *Handbook of Clinical Neurology*, vol. 1. Amsterdam: Elsevier; 1985:43–432.

He SQ, Dum RP, Strick PL. Topographic organisation of cortico-spinal projections from the frontal lobe: motor areas on the medial surface of the hemisphere. *J Neurosci* 1995, **15**:3284–3306.

Hoffman DS, Strick PL. The effects of a primary motor cortex lesion on the step/tracking movements of the wrist. *J Neurophysiol* 1995, **73**:891–895.

Horak FB, Woollacott M. [Editorial] In: Special issue on 'Vestibular control of posture in gait.' *J Vestib Res* 1993, **3**:1–2.

Lawrence DG, Kuypers HGJM. The functional organisation of the motor system in the monkey, parts 1 and 2. *Brain* 1968, **91**:1–14; 15–36.

Marsden CD, Rothwell JC, Day BL. Long latency automatic responses to muscle stretch in man, their origins and their function. In: Desmedt JE, ed. *Advances in Neurology*, vol. 39. New York: Raven Press; 1983:509–540.

Nicholls JG, Martin AR, Wallace BG. *From Neurone to Brain*. Sunderland, MA: Sinauer; 1992.

Passingham RE. The status of the premotor areas: evidence from PET scanning. In: Ferrell WR, Proske U, eds. *Neural Control of Movement*. New York: Plenum Press; 1995:167–178.

Porter RR, Lemon RN. *Corticospinal Function and Voluntary Movement*. Oxford: Oxford University Press; 1994.

Roberts TDN. *Neurophysiology of Postural Mechanisms*. London: Butterworth; 1979.

Rothwell J. *Control of Human Voluntary Movement*. London: Chapman & Hall; 1994.

Rothwell JC. The basal ganglia. In: Cody FWJ, ed. *Neural Control of Skilled Human Movement*. London: Portland Press; 1995:13–30.

Rothwell JC, Traub MM, Day BL et al., Manual motor performance in a deafferented man. *Brain* 1982, **105**:515–542.

Rizzolatti G, Luppino G. The cortical motor system. *Neuron* 2001, **31**:889–901.

Sanes JN, Donoghue JP. Organisation and adaptability of muscle representations in primary motor cortex. In: Caminiti P, Johnson PB, Burnod Y, eds. *Control of Arm Movement in Space*. Berlin: Springer; 1991: 103–127.

Schultz W. Predictive reward signal of dopamine neurons. *J Neurophysiol* 1998, **80**:1–27.

Shepherd GM. *Neurobiology*. New York: Oxford University Press; 1994.

Stein J. The posterior parietal cortex, the cerebellum and visual control of movement. In: Cody FWJ, ed. *Neural Control of Skilled Human Movement*. London: Portland Press; 1995:31–49.

Thach WT, Goodkin HP, Keating JG. The cerebellum and the adaptive coordination of movement. *Ann Rev Neurosci* 1992, **15**:403–442.

Wichmann T, DeLong MR. Pathophysiology of parkinsonian motor abnormalities. *Adv Neurol* 1993, **60**:53–61.

Chapter 2

Medical diagnosis of neurological conditions

C Kennard

INTRODUCTION

The diagnosis of neurological conditions is often viewed as complex, demanding a vast knowledge of neuroanatomy, neurophysiology and the large number of neurological diseases. It should, however, be remembered that in everyday neurological practice a relatively limited number of conditions are encountered. With a knowledge of these conditions and the manner of their presentation, and by taking a systematic history and carrying out an appropriately oriented neurological examination, it is usually possible to arrive at a correct diagnosis.

TAKING A NEUROLOGICAL CASE HISTORY

For the clinical neurologist, taking the patient's history is often more important than the clinical examination, which is simply confirmatory. Indeed, it is often claimed that about 80–90% of patients with neurological symptoms may be correctly diagnosed from the history alone. When taking a neurological history the examiner should always try to achieve two goals. The first is to try and localise along the neuraxis, from the cerebral hemispheres to the peripheral nerve and muscle, where the pathological process is taking place. For example, a patient complaining of weakness in both legs but none in the arms is most likely to have pathology in the peripheral nerves or muscles of the leg, or in the thoracic or lumbar spinal cord. The additional symptom of disturbed urinary function would strongly favour the spinal cord or cauda equina but not the peripheral nerves and muscle. The second goal is to identify the nature of the disease process from the description of the onset, evolution and course of the illness. For bilateral weakness in the legs, a gradual progression would suggest a chronic disorder of the peripheral nerves or muscles, whereas an acute onset with rapid progression would suggest either an acute peripheral neuropathy, such as the Guillain–Barré syndrome, or an acute spinal cord lesion. The sudden onset of a hemiplegia is likely to be due to infarction or haemorrhage in the contralateral cerebral hemisphere, whereas a progressive development would suggest a cerebral tumour.

The commonest neurological symptoms are headache, dizziness and blackouts. Patients complaining of headaches are often fearful of having a brain tumour, but in fact this is a rare presentation. Most will have either muscle contraction (tension) or migraine headaches. Dizziness is a very vague symptom which may indicate a rotatory illusion of movement, called vertigo. However, more commonly the patient describes a vague light-headed or 'swimmy' sensation. Whereas vertigo usually indicates a disturbance in the vestibular apparatus or more centrally in the brainstem, other symptoms of dizziness may be very difficult to diagnose accurately.

Blackouts or 'funny turns' indicate an epileptic seizure or a syncopal episode (faint), and careful questioning of the patient, as well as an eye witness, about events preceding, during and following the episode is absolutely crucial. There are many other symptoms which have neurological significance, including disorders of memory and consciousness, visual disturbances, speech and swallowing abnormalities, localised pain, sensory and motor symptoms, abnormal involuntary movements, problems with bladder control and walking difficulties. By elucidating the nature, location and timing of a particular symptom, and its association with other symptoms, it is often possible to reach either a single diagnosis or at least a reasonably limited set of differential diagnoses. These can then be further evaluated during the neurological examination and by appropriate investigations.

THE NEUROLOGICAL EXAMINATION

The neurological examination is primarily carried out to localise the site of the pathology in the neuraxis, and requires a knowledge of the course and innervation pattern of the cranial and peripheral nerves, and of the major fibre tracts in the brain and spinal cord. It commences as soon as the patient enters the consulting room, sits down and begins to relate the history of illness. Alertness, gait and speech may all provide important clues to the diagnosis. The manner in which the history is told may indicate impairments of judgement or memory, confusion or difficulties with comprehension or expression of ideas. After the history has been taken, before the patient is taken to the examining couch, a few moments should be spent in evaluating the mental state and some aspects of cognitive function. This should include determining whether the patient is oriented in time and place. Tests of attention, memory and clarity of thought include the immediate repetition of a series of digits forwards and backwards, serial subtraction of 7s from 100, and recall of an address or set of objects after an interval of 3 min. The ability of the patient to read, write, name objects, solve simple mathematical problems, copy diagrams and draw a clock face (for evidence of spatial neglect) should be noted.

The neurological examination should now proceed with the patient lying comfortably on the examination couch in a well-lit and warm room. It is preferable to examine the patient in undergarments. The examination should then proceed in a systematic manner, starting with the cranial nerves and then motor, reflex and sensory function in the trunk and limbs. Formal assessment of gait and balance should complete the examination.

The function of each cranial nerve is examined in turn: sense of smell (olfactory nerve); visual function including visual acuity, visual fields and examination of the optic fundi with an ophthalmoscope (optic nerve); examination of the pupils and eye movements (oculomotor, trochlear and abducens nerves); facial sensation, corneal sensation and reflex and jaw movement (trigeminal nerve); facial movement (facial nerve); hearing (auditory nerves); palatal sensation and movement, gag and cough reflex (glossopharyngeal and vagus nerves); movements of the sternomastoid and trapezius muscles (accessory nerve); and tongue movement (hypoglossal nerve) are all examined and any abnormalities noted.

Motor function should be examined next. This commences with observation of the patient's limbs and trunk, looking for wasting or fasciculation of the muscles (suggestive of damage to the anterior horn motor neurones), abnormal posture and involuntary movements such as tremor (usually indicating an extrapyramidal disorder). If the tremor is present only at rest then Parkinson's disease should be considered. If present only during maintained posture this may be physiological, due to stress or associated with thyrotoxicosis. The other likely diagnosis is of benign essential tremor, which may be hereditary. Tremors and other involuntary movements are discussed in Chapters 4 and 25.

The muscle tone in the limbs is then assessed. If increased, as in spasticity and rigidity, either an upper motor neurone (pyramidal tract) or an extrapyramidal disorder, respectively, is suggested. The strength and speed of movement in each muscle group are then systematically assessed, and any weakness should be graded according to the Medical Research Council

(MRC) scale from 0 to 5 (0 = absent contraction, 5 = full strength; see Box 3.2 on p. 33). In addition, it is useful to observe the patient's ability, in prone and supine positions, to maintain against gravity his or her arms outstretched, and then both legs; the weak arm or leg usually tires first and then sags. The ability to sit up from the lying position and the strength of neck flexion and extension should also be assessed.

Motor co-ordination, usually an indicator of cerebellar function, is then assessed by finger–nose and heel–shin movements, and asking the patient to perform rapid alternating movements of the limbs. To complete the motor examination the reflexes are tested, including the biceps, supinator, triceps, knee, ankle and cutaneous abdominal reflexes. Finally, the plantar responses (Babinski response) are assessed.

Testing sensory function is undoubtedly the most difficult part of the examination and should not be prolonged for more than a few minutes, since the patient will tire and the responses become inconsistent. All areas of the skin surface should be tested first for pain sensation with a pin, assessing whether there are differences between the two sides of the body, a level below which sensation is impaired or an area where sensation has been lost completely. Testing of other sensory modalities including light touch (cotton wool), joint position sense (by small movements of a finger or toe), vibration (tuning fork) and temperature is performed only if indicated by the history or other aspects of the examination which have been carried out earlier.

Finally, the patient should be asked to stand with eyes open and then closed (Rhomberg's test), and any unsteadiness noted. The patient's gait should then be tested, noting particularly posture, step amplitude and ability to turn. For further information on taking a neurological examination the reader is referred to Fuller (1993).

NEUROLOGICAL INVESTIGATIONS

After taking the history and completing the neurological examination, it should be possible to determine to what extent additional investigations are needed either to confirm a diagnosis or to differentiate between a range of possible diagnoses. However, it should always be remembered that neurological dysfunction may result from disease in another part of the body. It is also important to plan investigations which are going to provide the maximal amount of information about the patient's illness but which will result in the least possible discomfort and risk. The principal investigations for diagnosing brain and spinal cord disease are computer tomography (CT) scanning, magnetic resonance

imaging (MRI), evoked potentials (EP) and electro-encephalography (EEG), and for peripheral nerve and muscle disease electromyography (EMG) and nerve conduction studies.

Neuroimaging

The imaging technique used will depend on the quality of image required and the availability of the technique.

Plain radiology of the skull and spinal column

Following the introduction of CT scanning, the use of X-rays has declined. However, routine lateral and antero-posterior radiographs of the skull are still of use in the initial assesment of patients with head injuries, particularly those in whom there has been any alteration in the level of consciousness, when evidence of a skull fracture is an indication for hospital admission for observation. X-ray images of the skull also provide information about the integrity of the pituitary fossa, the presence or absence of intracranial calcification, and whether the frontal, maxillary and sphenoidal paranasal sinuses show opacification suggestive of infection or neoplasia.

Radiographs of the spine are taken to identify changes in the vertebrae themselves, the intervertebral discs and the intervertebral foramina. However, it should be appreciated that the intervertebral disc is not radiopaque, and a radiograph of the lumbosacral spine taken in a patient with a presumed acute disc prolapse is likely to be normal. It is only after a disc protrusion has been present for months or years that the margins of the prolapsed disc start to calcify, producing posterior osteophyte formation of the borders of the upper and lower vertebrae. Collapse of the vertebrae revealed by plain radiography may occur due to osteomyelitis, Paget's disease, fracture and neoplasia, either benign or malignant, which may result in cord compression.

CT scanning

This is a technique in which the transmission of photons across the head, through the brain, is recorded using crystals. The tissue density of the brain is measured across several tomographic horizontal levels, and computers construct images of slices of the brain (Latchaw, 1984). The differing densities of the grey and white matter, cerebrospinal fluid (CSF), blood and bone can be distinguished, as can abnormal tissue such as haemorrhage, tumour, oedema and abscess (Fig. 2.1A). Enhancement of the images, produced by the intravenous injection of a contrast medium, may add precision to diagnosis. Because of artefact from the surrounding bone, CT scanning is not ideal for examination of the posterior fossa and the spinal cord.

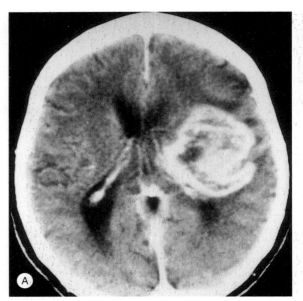 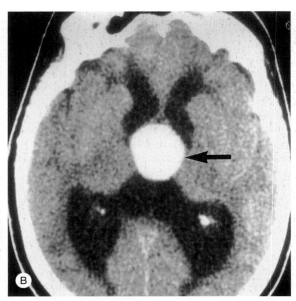

Figure 2.1 Computed tomography (CT) scans of the brain. (A) A malignant glioma in the right hemisphere. (B) Ventricular dilation (hydrocephalus) due to a colloid cyst (arrow) in the third ventricle, causing obstruction of cerebrospinal fluid flow from the third to the fourth ventricle through the aqueduct of Sylvius.

CT scanning is widely available, not only for the diagnosis and identification of focal cerebral lesions, but also to assess the presence or absence of ventricular dilation in cases of possible hydrocephalus (Fig. 2.1B), or of cortical atrophy resulting from ageing.

Magnetic resonance imaging

This relatively new technique produces, in a similar manner to CT scanning, 'slice' images of the brain in any plane, and has the great advantage of using non-ionising radiation (Moseley, 1988). The patient's head is placed in a powerful magnetic field that produces temporary physical changes in the atoms of the brain. This results in the production of radiofrequency energy, subjected to computer analysis, from which an image is constructed. This technique provides excellent visualisation of anatomical detail, particularly the difference between grey and white matter. Abnormalities in the white matter, as in multiple sclerosis (Fig. 2.2A), and the spinal cord with its cervical (Fig. 2.2B) and lumbar roots are clearly defined.

Vascular lesions, such as aneurysms, can also be visualised (Fig. 2.2C). The central location of the aneurysm seen in Figure 2.2C confirmed that the optic chiasm was being compressed, as indicated by the patient's symptoms of peripheral blurred vision and abnormalities (bitemporal hemianopia) found on

visual field testing (Chigbu, 2003). As this technique becomes more available, it is superseding CT scanning.

Angiography

In this technique a contrast medium opaque to X-rays is injected into the blood vessels leading to the brain to outline their intracranial course. It is extremely useful for the diagnosis of cerebral aneurysms (Fig. 2.3A, B), vascular malformations and occluded or stenosed arteries (Fig. 2.3C) and veins. Recent developments in MR angiography, which is non-invasive, suggest that it will eventually take over from X-ray angiography as the technique of choice (Sellar, 1995).

Positron emission tomography (PET)

Just as the transmission of X-rays through the head (transmission tomography) can be used to generate CT scans, so similar pictures can be obtained using positron-emitting radioisotopes (emission tomography; Sawle, 1995). These isotopes are produced in a cyclotron and are used to label various naturally occurring products, e.g. water and carbon dioxide are labelled with ^{15}O and glucose with ^{18}F. A variety of such ligands can be generated and delivered to the subject by inhalation or by injection. The isotopes produce positrons that, after a very short distance, collide with electrons, resulting in

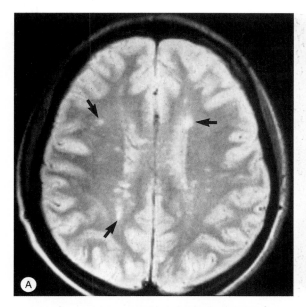

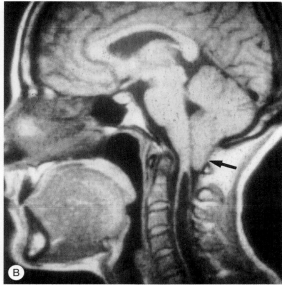

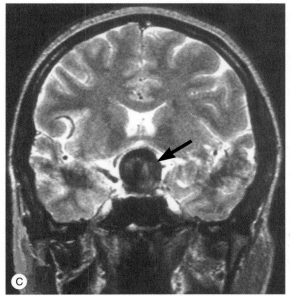

Figure 2.2 Magnetic resonance scans of the brain. (A) Axial section (T2-weighted) through the brain of a patient with multiple sclerosis. The plaques of demyelination appear as areas of high signal attenuation in the white matter (arrowed). (B) Sagittal section (T1) through the brain of a patient with cerebellar ectopia (Arnold–Chiari type 2 malformation) and syringomyelia. Note that the cerebellar vermis (arrowed) descends into the cervical canal well below a line drawn between the first cervical vertebra and the posterior margin of the foramen magnum. The spinal cord is expanded by the fluid–filled syrinx, which appears as a black core in the centre of the cord. (C) Coronal section (T2) through the brain of a patient with an aneurysm on the left internal carotid artery, lying centrally (arrowed) and compressing the optic chiasm.

annihilation and the release of photons. Multiple arrays of detectors are used to detect the photons and CT techniques allow maps of regional cerebral blood flow to be produced. In addition, cerebral blood volume and cerebral glucose uptake can be measured simultaneously, allowing the oxygen extraction ratio and cerebral metabolic rate for oxygen to be calculated. The density of neurotransmitter receptors can also be studied using appropriately labelled ligands, as can activation of the brain during specific neurobehavioural tasks. This technique is extremely costly and is available in relatively few centres throughout the world.

Electrodiagnostic tests

These tests involve the amplification and recording of the electrical activity of the brain and peripheral nerves, which may be either spontaneous or induced by appropriate stimulation. Details of these tests can be found in textbooks such as that by Misulis (1993).

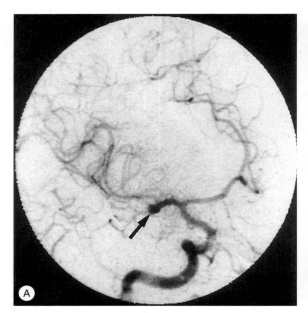

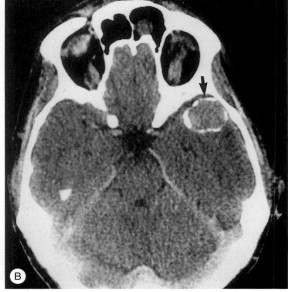

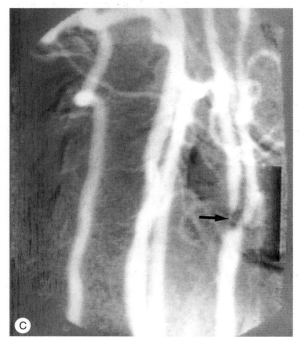

Figure 2.3 Imaging aneurysms and stenosis. (A) Cerebral angiogram showing a small aneurysm arising from the right middle cerebral artery (arrowed). (B) A contrast-enhanced computed tomographic scan of the same patient shows that the aneurysm (arrowed) located at the tip of the temporal lobe has a calcified wall and is in fact much larger than was shown on the angiogram. This indicates that the majority of the aneurysm is thrombosed. (C) A cerebral angiogram showing a tight stenosis of the right internal carotid artery (arrowed) at its origin from the common carotid artery. The patient presented with recurrent episodes of amaurosis fugax (monocular blindness) of the right eye.

Electroencephalography

EEG is a method of recording spontaneous cerebral electrical activity through the intact skull. A set of electrodes is attached to the scalp and the electrical activity is amplified to provide 16 or more channels of activity, usually displayed on a chart recorder. It is of use in the diagnosis of different types of epilepsy, in certain forms of encephalitis and in some cases of coma.

Evoked potentials

Sensory EPs are the time-locked electrical activations of specific parts of the brain in response to a stimulus that may be visual (flashed light or pattern such as an alternating checkerboard), auditory (click or tone) or somatosensory (electrical pulse) stimulus. The latency (the delay between the onset of the stimulus and the onset of the response) is measured and provides a measure of conduction along the sensory pathway, e.g. the optic nerve. These techniques have been used particularly to identify clinically silent lesions in sensory pathways due to multiple sclerosis and are of value in the differential diagnosis of a variety of cerebral metabolic disorders in infants and children.

Nerve conduction velocity

Conduction along the sensory or motor component of a peripheral nerve can be measured by recording the sensory or motor response downstream from a site of electrical stimulation. The time taken for the action potential to travel along a defined segment of nerve allows the conduction velocity to be calculated. This technique is used in the diagnosis of entrapment syndromes, such as the carpal tunnel syndrome due to compression of the median nerve at the wrist, and in diagnosing peripheral neuropathies that may be axonal or demyelinating.

EMG

EMG involves the insertion of recording electrodes into a variety of muscles in different parts of the body and recording spontaneous (at rest) and induced (by contraction of the muscle) electrical muscle activity. It can be used to differentiate between primary muscle disease and denervation of muscle due to lower motor neurone dysfunction. It is therefore useful in the diagnosis of neuromuscular diseases such as motor neurone disease, muscular dystrophies and polymyositis.

Lumbar puncture and examination of the cerebrospinal fluid

Examination of CSF is sometimes of great importance in the diagnosis of neurological disease, particularly in patients suspected of having meningitis, subarachnoid haemorrhage and suspected inflammatory brain disease (Thompson, 1995). Lumbar puncture carries a risk of tonsillar herniation, however, and possible death if the intracranial pressure is raised; if this is a possibility, a CT scan is required beforehand to exclude a mass lesion. A lumbar puncture is performed under sterile conditions; a local anaesthetic is given and then a fine-bore needle is inserted into the L3–L4 interspace until it enters the subarachnoid space and CSF is obtained. As well as obtaining CSF for analysis of its cellular, chemical and bacteriological constituents, the CSF pressure may be measured.

Muscle biopsy

Muscle biopsy can be extremely valuable in the diagnosis of neuromuscular diseases, particularly intrinsic pathology of the muscle as in inflammatory disorders such as polymyositis, or degenerative disorders such as the muscular dystrophies (Dubowitz & Brooke, 1973). The biopsy is taken from an affected muscle and then processed for light and electron microscopy. Special staining techniques are used to identify the different muscle fibre types and abnormalities in specific enzyme pathways. Recently, the introduction of immunocytochemical and immunohistochemical techniques has allowed the localisation of specific proteins. The interpretation of a muscle biopsy usually includes the description of a constellation of changes and then the association of these changes with a specific diagnosis (see Chs 15 and 20).

Other tests

Routine haematological, biochemical and serological analysis of blood may sometimes assist neurological diagnosis. In addition to analysis of red and white cells, haematological testing should include the platelet count in patients with cerebrovascular disease. Erythrocyte sedimentation rate (ESR) should be measured, especially in patients over the age of 50 years presenting with headache, to exclude temporal arteritis. In addition to the routine biochemical assessment of renal, liver and calcium function, measurement of creatine phosphokinase (CPK) is useful in the evaluation of neuromuscular disease, since raised levels indicate muscle damage. Patients with movement disorders should have the levels of serum copper and plasma caeruloplasmin (a copper transporter protein) checked to exclude Wilson's disease, which is treatable with chelating agents (Marsden, 1987).

Serological testing should include tests for syphilis and the human immunodeficiency virus (HIV) if the patient has specific risk factors. Tests for HIV can be performed only after the patient has received appropriate counselling.

CONCLUSIONS

This chapter has provided a brief overview of the clinical examination and investigative techniques which a neurological patient may undergo before being referred to the physiotherapist. Further details may be obtained from the recommended texts detailed below. Aspects of the medical examinations that are performed during the physiotherapy assessment are discussed in Chapter 3.

References

Chigbu de G. Visual field defect: a case of cerebral aneurysm. *Optom Today* 2003, July **11**:24–26.

Dubowitz V, Brooke MH. *Muscle Biopsy*. London: WB Saunders; 1973.

Fuller G. *Neurological Examination Made Easy*. Edinburgh: Churchill Livingstone; 1993.

Latchaw RE. *Computed Tomography of the Head, Neck and Spine*. Chicago: Mosby Year Book; 1984.

Marsden CD. Wilson's disease. *Q J Med* 1987, **65**:959–967.

Misulis KE. *Essentials of Clinical Neurology*. London: Butterworth Heinemann; 1993.

Moseley I. *Magnetic Resonance Imaging in Diseases of the Nervous System*. Oxford: Blackwell Scientific Publications; 1988.

Sawle GV. Imaging the head: functional imaging. *J Neurol Neurosurg Psychiatry* 1995, **58**:132–144.

Sellar RJ. Imaging blood vessels of the head and neck. *J Neurol Neurosurg Psychiatry* 1995, **59**:225–237.

Thompson EJ. Cerebrospinal fluid. *J Neurol Neurosurg Psychiatry* 1995, **59**:349–357.

General reading

Donaghy M. *Brain's Diseases of the Nervous System*, 11th edn. Oxford: Oxford University Press; 2001.

Perkin GD. *Neurology*, 2nd edn. Edinburgh: Mosby; 2002.

Warlow C. *Handbook of Neurology*. Oxford: Blackwell Scientific Publications; 1991.

Chapter 3

Principles of physiotherapy assessment and outcome measures

P Kersten

INTRODUCTION

Physiotherapy is 'a health care profession concerned with human function and movement, and maximising potential. It uses physical approaches to promote, maintain and restore physical, psychological and social well-being, taking account of variations in health status' (Chartered Society of Physiotherapy, 2002). The effectiveness of physiotherapy treatment depends on our ability to assess and analyse the main reasons behind patients' problems (Lennon & Hastings, 1996). Some might say that for too long, physiotherapy assessment has relied upon gut feeling, hunch and anecdotal stories where we may remember good clinical outcomes, conveniently forgetting poor outcomes. Fortunately, things have changed as now there are standardised tests for measuring functional tasks (to assist and challenge clinical skills). Currently, very few physiotherapists use outcome measures in their physiotherapy assessments or in the evaluation of physiotherapy outcomes. The opportunity and responsibility to improve our practice in this area are available.

This chapter will therefore be in two parts. The first part will deal with the principles of physiotherapy assessment and will utilise the context of the new World Health Organization (WHO) framework; the *International Classification of Functioning, Disability and Health* (ICF; World Health Organization, 2001). The second half of this chapter will be devoted to the use of outcome measures in relation to the physiotherapy assessment.

The role of assessment and outcome measures in the rehabilitation process, as well as problem-solving and clinical reasoning, is discussed in Chapter 22.

PRINCIPLES OF PHYSIOTHERAPY ASSESSMENT

It is important to establish the patient's difficulties and resulting problems in the physiotherapy assessment. However, assessment should also focus on the patient's abilities and aspirations. By focusing on abilities as well as difficulties, the treatment can be planned, the goals set and appropriate information provided.

HISTORY-TAKING

The physiotherapy assessment should begin by asking the patient, or when this is not possible a relative, friend or carer, about the history of the condition. There are several important aspects to the history-taking:

- Firstly, there is a need to find out details about the nature, severity, frequency and pattern of the problem, as well as the past medical history.

- Secondly, information about what precipitates or relieves symptoms, what previous treatments or examinations have been conducted and what other neurological symptoms are experienced needs to be collected. It is also paramount to find out about the difficulties patients may experience in daily life as a consequence of their movement problem, for example in terms of the home and community environment, the impact upon the social, school and work life and the impact upon social relationships.

- Finally, there is a need to enquire about what patients expect or hope the physiotherapy can help with and what outcomes they anticipate.

This dialogue of history-taking will set the focus for the subsequent physical assessment and will help the therapist and patient to understand more clearly what would be a meaningful outcome.

TYPES OF PHYSICAL ASSESSMENT

Physical assessments can be divided into those that use: (1) a clinical approach; (2) a checklist; or (3) a representational approach (Wade et al., 1985).

1. The **clinical approach** is easy to use and quick. In the UK, the use of problem-oriented medical records (POMRs) has aided this clinical approach since the late 1980s (King Edward's Fund for London, 1988).

   Using POMRs, the patient's main problems are identified by analysing the main reasons behind the movement dysfunction. The conduct of the clinical approach, however, is dependent upon the therapist's background, clinical judgement or expertise and time available. Subsequently, clinical assessments are difficult to repeat in a similar manner on separate occasions or by different therapists, which may result in missing important problems and bias in measuring levels of improvement or deterioration.

2. **Checklists**, which contain all possible problems, can overcome some of the problems with the clinical approach. Integrated care pathways (ICPs) often include various checklists. For example, ICPs for people with stroke (Jackson et al., 2002) and multiple sclerosis (Rossiter & Thompson, 1995) have been developed.

ICPs are comprehensive tools which set out procedures that should be followed in the clinical assessment of patients, over time, without making the error of missing things. For example, the ICP of hemiplegic shoulder pain sets out the time points at which the initial assessment should take place and what should be assessed (e.g. pain history, overall presentation), as well as subsequent assessments that should take place later (e.g. immediate multidisciplinary management of pain within 48 h of admission through medication, positioning and handling protocols and seating). However, checklists such as ICPs take a long time to develop, their length tends to be extensive and as a result they are often not completed in full (Jackson et al., 2002). This reduces their usefulness.

3. **Representational assessments** are outcome measures which contain fewer items (e.g. activities) to be examined and which are known to give an adequate representation of the overall functioning of the patient. The Rivermead Motor Assessment is an example of a frequently used representational scale in physiotherapy (Lincoln & Leadbitter, 1979). It quantifies the patient's ability on a number of motor tasks, which gives a good indication of the patient's overall level of motor function (Lincoln & Leadbitter, 1979; Collen et al., 1990). Thus, representational assessments are quicker to use than checklists, although without taking good histories from the patient they may miss some important problems.

Assessment and treatment must be seen as cyclical processes so that the therapist evaluates the outcome of the treatment, the achievement of the patient's goals, the changes that may occur within the patient's life or home situation and changes that occur as a result of the natural progression (which can be improvement or deterioration) of the condition. Also, in patients with acute complex neurological conditions, such as traumatic brain injury and stroke, it may take several weeks to complete an assessment and decide upon the best techniques to use (Lennon & Hastings, 1996).

PHYSIOTHERAPY ASSESSMENT IN THE CONTEXT OF THE ICF

Physiotherapy assessment can draw upon models or frameworks which enable the therapist to assess patients systematically, often extending to how one might conceptualise the consequences of a condition. One such framework is the new classification termed ICF (WHO, 2001). The ICF aims to provide a unified, standard language and framework for the description of health and health-related states. The ICF focuses on 'how people live with their health conditions and how these can be improved to achieve a productive, fulfilling life'.

As a clinical tool, the ICF is intended to help practitioners to assess needs, match treatments with specific conditions, vocational assessments and rehabilitation and outcome evaluation. The ICF takes into account and measures the social aspects of disability and provides a mechanism to document the impact of the social and physical environment on a person's functioning. The ICF has three main dimensions, which are body functions and structures, activities and participation. These will be described in brief before going on to talk about physiotherapy assessment using this framework.

Body functions and structures

Body functions refer to the physiological or psychological functions of body systems. Body structures refer to anatomical parts of the body such as organs, limbs and their components. Thus, positive aspects of this dimension relate to the person's functional and structural integrity.

Impairments

The negative aspects are classed as impairments. Impairments are 'problems in body function or structure such as a significant deviation or loss' (WHO, 2001). Impairments can involve anomaly, defect, loss or other significant deviation in body structures. Impairments can be temporary or permanent; progressive, regressive or static; intermittent or continuous.

Activities

Activity is defined as the execution or performance of a task or action by an individual. In other words, activities are concerned with positive aspects, such as what the person does.

Limitations in activity may arise as a result of impairments. This was formerly called 'disability' in the *International Classification of Impairments, Disabilities, and Handicaps* (ICIDH; WHO, 1980). The use of assistive devices or personal assistance does not eliminate impairments but may remove limitations on activities in specific domains.

Participation

Society is the level of functioning for this dimension. Participation (positive aspect) is an individual's involvement in life situations in relation to health conditions, body functions and structure, activities and contextual factors.

Participation restrictions (formerly 'handicap' in ICIDH; WHO, 1980) are problems an individual may have in the manner or extent of involvement in life situations.

The participation dimension codes the societal circumstances and the degree of involvement, including society's response to the individual's level of functioning. The involvement refers to the experience of people in the context in which they live, including environmental factors. Thus, environments with barriers, or without facilitators, will restrict participation, and environments that are more facilitating may increase participation.

Disability

The term 'disability', in the new ICF, is used as an 'umbrella term for impairments, activity limitations and participation restrictions'. As such it refers to the negative aspects of the interaction between an individual (with a health condition) and that individual's contextual factors (environmental and personal factors).

The ICF does not directly measure concepts of quality of life. However, it mentions that there is a conceptual comparability between quality of life and disability constructs. The distinction between the two is made by referring to the concepts of disease and disability as 'objective and exteriorized signs of the individual, whereas quality of life deals with what people feel about their health condition or its consequences and hence is a construct of well-being' (WHO, 2001, p. 251).

Physiotherapy assessment

During the assessment the therapist will examine the patient's impairments (whilst also noting what body functions and structure are intact), abilities and activity limitations, participation and participation limitations.

There will be times when the initial focus may be on impairments only, for example in patients with acute conditions. Other times, the history-taking can begin with the problems experienced, which could be largely in the arena of restricted participation. This can help to narrow the assessment to those areas that are most important to the patient to focus on and build the treatment around. In order to present this chapter in a logical structure, the outlining of physiotherapy assessment will be divided using the ICF framework.

Further, as discussed earlier in this chapter, clinical assessments can be used as a guide. However, they fail to quantify the activities observed. The physiotherapy assessment will be greatly enhanced if outcome measures are used. Useful outcome measures that can be incorporated in the physiotherapy assessment will therefore be suggested below. The second half of this chapter will go into more detail about the qualities outcome measures should have before using them.

ASSESSING IMPAIRMENTS

The initial assessment begins with a definition of the patient's impairment and the functional diagnosis placed in the context of neurological syndromes. It is important to consider the prognosis. This refers to the projection of the course and outcome probabilities in an estimated time frame based on the diagnosis, natural history, distribution, severity and type of the impairment, as well as other personal, social and environmental factors (Katz et al., 1997).

As neurological patients are usually referred with a diagnosis, physiotherapy assessment of body functions is focused on how the neurological impairments can be assessed in terms of their presence and severity, to establish the patient's baseline and subsequent reassessments (Fuller, 1999). Typical body functions that need to be assessed in the neurological patient are those related to functions of the:

- joints
- muscles
- movements
- sensation.

Joint function

The assessment of joint function includes the evaluation of the passive range of movement and, in particular, the presence of muscle shortening and contractures (see Chs 4 and 25). It is important to measure the passive range of movement in a reliable manner and this can be achieved using a goniometer (Macdermid et al., 2001).

Muscle function

The assessment of muscle function should include an examination of muscle strength, muscle tone and endurance, whilst considering different patterns of muscle tone and weakness that may occur in patients with neurological conditions (Box 3.1).

Muscle strength Oxford Scale

The assessment of muscle strength can be quantified with the Medical Research Council's (MRC) scale of muscle strength (MRC UK, 1978), which ranges from 0 to 5 (Box 3.2).

Another measure of muscle strength is that of the Motricity Index, which scores pinch grip, strength at

Box 3.1 Patterns of muscle tone and weakness (Fuller, 1999)

1 Upper motor neurone (UMN): increased tone, increased reflexes, pyramidal weakness (weak extensors in the arm, weak flexors in the leg)
2 Lower motor neurone (LMN): wasting, fasciculation, decreased tone and absent reflexes
3 Muscle disease: wasting, decreased tone, impaired or absent reflexes
4 Neuromuscular junction: fatiguable weakness, normal or decreased tone, normal reflexes
5 Functional weakness: normal tone, normal reflexes without wasting with erratic power
6 Mixed UMN and LMN: can occur for example in motor neurone disease, combined (see Ch. 13)

Box 3.2 Medical Research Council (MRC) scale of muscle strength (MRC UK, 1978)

0 No muscular activity
1 Minimal contraction of muscle but insufficient to move a joint
2 Contraction of muscle sufficient to move a joint but not to oppose gravity
3 Muscle contraction sufficient to move a joint against gravity but not against physical resistance
4 Muscle contraction sufficient to move a joint against gravity and against mild/moderate resistance
5 Normal power, that is, muscular contraction sufficient to resist firm resistance

(isokinetic) using strain-gauge dynamometry. Such equipment is costly and rarely available clinically but accurate, reliable and objective measures are essential for research.

Muscle size

The therapist will also need to look out for a decrease or increase in muscle bulk (atrophy or hypertrophy, respectively). Physiotherapists have traditionally used a tape measure to assess muscle size, e.g. by measuring limb circumference, but this is known seriously to underestimate muscle wasting (Young et al., 1980). Ultrasound imaging is being used increasingly in rehabilitation research, mainly for musculoskeletal conditions, and enables accurate and reliable measurement of muscle size (see Stokes et al. (1997) for a review).

Work continues to explore ultrasound imaging of different muscles and populations of normal subjects, to provide databases for comparison with patients to assess wasting. Such information could enable assessment with ultrasound imaging to become part of routine clinical practice, which would require appropriate training and awareness of the technical and safety aspects (Stokes et al., 1997). This application of the technique is distinct from diagnostic imaging of musculoskeletal pathology, performed by radiologists and sonographers.

Muscle tone

Observing the posture of the patient, position of the limbs, position of the trunk and shape of the hands and feet gives an indication of increased or decreased muscle tone.

Muscle tone is assessed by passively moving the limb(s) or trunk through the normal range of movement, whilst the patient remains relaxed. This enables the therapist to detect whether tone is normal, increased (hypertonic due to spasticity or rigidity) or decreased (hypotonic). These variations in tone are dealt with in further detail in Chapters 4 and 25. It is, however, worth mentioning some quantifiable means of measuring spasticity or rigidity.

Spasticity The severity, distribution and consequences of spasticity depend on the velocity of the movement, as well as the position of the patient (e.g. prone-lying may increase tone in the extensor muscles) and other factors such as tiredness, noxious stimuli (e.g. urinary infection), stress and medication. These factors are important to bear in mind in the assessment of spasticity. The most commonly used measure of spasticity in the clinical setting is the Modified Ashworth Scale

the elbow, shoulder, ankle, knee and hip on a six-point ordinal scale. The six scores are then summed to provide an overall score of muscle strength (Demeurisse et al., 1980). This index has been shown to be valid and reliable in people with a range of neurological conditions (Collin & Wade, 1990; Ozbudak-Demir et al., 1999; Donkervoort et al., 2002).

Grip strength and pinch strength are particularly useful tests of muscle function, as they can be used as a representational marker of recovery, for example after stroke (Sunderland et al., 1989). Grip strength is reliably tested using a hand dynamometer (Bohannon & Andrews, 1987).

More sophisticated equipment can be used to measure muscle strength (e.g. static or isometric) and power

Box 3.3   Modified Ashworth Scale of muscle spasticity (Bohannon & Smith, 1987)

0   No increase in muscle tone
1   Slight increase in muscle tone, manifested by a catch and release, or by minimal resistance at the end of the range of motion when the affected part is moved in flexion or extension
1+   Slight increase in muscle tone, manifested by a catch, followed by minimal resistance throughout the remainder (less than half) of the range of movement
2   More marked increase in muscle tone through most of the range of movement, but affected part easily moved
3   Considerable increase in muscle tone, passive movement difficult
4   Affected part rigid in flexion or extension

Box 3.4   Unified Parkinson's Disease Rating System scale (Lang & Fahn, 1989)

0 Rigidity absent
1 Rigidity slight or detectable only when activated by mirror or other movements
2 Mild to moderate rigidity
3 Marked rigidity, but full range of motion easily achieved
4 Severe rigidity, range of motion achieved with difficulty

(MAS; Bohannon & Smith, 1987). MAS scores range from 0 to 4 (Box 3.3).

Rigidity   Rigidity is felt as an increase in tone throughout the whole range of the passive movement (see Ch. 4). This has also been described a 'lead pipe' resulting from simultaneous contractions of the agonist and antagonist muscles. In cogwheel rigidity a regular intermittent break in tone is felt throughout the whole range of movement.

A commonly used quantitative measure of rigidity is the Unified Parkinson's Disease Rating System scale, which rates the level of rigidity from 0 to 4 (Box 3.4; Lang & Fahn, 1989). The scale is open to interpretation, however, due to the subjectivity of the words and as a result assessors do not always rate patients the same (poor interrater reliability; Richards et al., 1994).

Movement functions

Movement functions do not refer to the activities the patient can do, but rather to the co-ordination of the movement. This co-ordination requires the integration of sensory feedback with motor output of sufficient strength. Therefore, if the patient has significant weakness, tests of co-ordination are not that meaningful.

There are many movements that the therapist can examine in a neurological patient, such as involuntary contractions, involuntary movement reactions, control of voluntary movement functions and involuntary movement functions.

Involuntary contractions, or tendon reflexes, are increased in upper motor neurone lesions and decreased in lower motor neurone lesions and muscle abnormalities (Box 3.1). Quantification of reflexes ranges from 0 to 4+ (Box 3.5; Fuller, 1999). Six reflexes can be tested using this grading system: the ankle, knee, biceps, supinator, triceps and finger reflexes.

Involuntary movement reactions include those induced by body position (e.g. postural, righting and body adjustment reactions), balance and threatening stimuli.

Box 3.5   Grading of reflexes (Fuller, 1999)

0   Absent
±   Present but only with reinforcement
1+   Present but depressed
2+   Normal
3+   Increased
4+   Clonus

Balance

Balance disorders are discussed in Chapter 24. Well-validated measures of balance are the Berg Balance Scale (Berg et al., 1992) and the Functional Reach Test (Duncan et al., 1990). The Berg Balance Scale evaluates the patient's performance on 14 tasks which are common in daily activities. These tasks address the patient's ability to maintain positions of increasing difficulty. The full range of tasks is displayed in Box 3.6. This test takes about 15 min to complete and is a sensitive measure as it is able to discriminate between patients with various mobility aids (Berg et al., 1992).

The Functional Reach Test is shorter to complete, but less comprehensive than the Berg Balance Scale. The therapist will need to mark out a long ruler on a wall at the patient's shoulder height. When the patient stands comfortably, he or she should be asked to lift one arm

Box 3.6   Berg Balance Scale (Berg et al., 1992)

Tasks
1   Sitting to standing
2   Standing unsupported
3   Sitting unsupported
4   Standing to sitting
5   Transfers
6   Standing with eyes closed
7   Standing with feet together
8   Reaching forward with outstretched arm
9   Retrieving object from floor
10 Turning to look behind
11 Turning 360°
12 Placing alternate foot on stool
13 Standing with one foot in front
14 Standing on one foot

Each task is scored from 0 to 4. For each task, clear scoring instructions are provided. A lower score denotes poorer balance.

up at 90° and make a fist (start position). Then the patient is asked to reach forwards as far as possible (finishing position). Functional reach is defined by the distance between the start and finishing position (Duncan et al., 1990).

Co-ordination

Control of voluntary movement functions refers to the patient's ability to co-ordinate movements. Assessment of co-ordination should focus on the patient's ability to perform simple and more complex tasks, but also on functions, such as eye–hand co-ordination and right–left co-ordination. A specific co-ordination impairment is dysdiadochokinesia, which is the inability to tap and turn over the hand. This is tested by asking the patient to pat one hand on the back of the other quickly and regularly, to twist the hand as if opening a door, to tap the back of one hand alternately with the palm and back of the other hand. A lack of co-ordination of these movements or a lack of rhythm is caused by cerebellar lesions.

Involuntary movement functions are unintentional, non- or semipurposive involuntary contractions of a muscle or group of muscles. Ataxia is a common symptom that comes under this heading in patients with neurological conditions.

Finger–nose test   The presence of tremor and ataxia is examined with the finger–nose test, during which the patient is asked to touch the therapist's finger with the index finger and then touch his or her nose (Swaine et al., 1993; Desrosiers et al., 1995). If the patient is able to do this, he or she is then asked to make the movement faster. The therapist can increase the sensitivity of this test by moving the (target) finger. In this test, intention tremor is present when the patient's finger shows a tremor on approaching the target finger. Dysmetria is present if the patient overshoots the target and when the tremor is present during the entire action it is called an action tremor. There is no quantification of this test.

Heel–shin test   Another test of ataxia is the heel–shin test, in which the patient is asked to lie supine and run one heel from the knee down the sharp anterior edge of the shin. The inability to coordinate this movement suggests the presence of ataxia.

Ataxia can also be tested by asking the patient to lie supine with the knees bent at 90° and feet flat on the plinth. He or she then rolls both knees slowly from side to side, or moves one knee out to the side whilst keeping the other steady. Patients with ataxia at the hips will not be able to control this movement but those with mild ataxia may be able to. The test can be made more difficult by asking the patient to lie in the same starting position and slowly lift the buttocks off the plinth. Those with ataxia at the hips and/or trunk will wobble at the pelvis and/or trunk. Patients may try to increase their stability by fixing with the knees (pressing them together hard), the arms or the head (pushing them into the plinth).

Sensory functions

There are many sensory functions that may be impaired in patients with neurological conditions. Here those deemed most important in physiotherapy will be described (Fuller, 1999). When testing senses it is important that the patient understands the nature of the test; this is achieved by careful demonstration and explanation.

Proprioception

Joint position sense or proprioception is a sensory function for detecting and identifying the relative position of body parts and this is tested by moving joints whilst the patient has his or her eyes closed. Distal joints are tested before proximal joints. The patient is asked in what direction the joint is moved.

The Romberg's test is also a test of joint position sense, in which the patient is asked to stand with the feet together for a few seconds. The therapist will need to reassure patients that they will be caught if they fall. If the patient falls with the eyes closed then the test is positive and this indicates a loss of joint position sense.

Touch

The sensory function of touch involves sensing surfaces and their textures and qualities. It is tested with the pinprick test and the light touch test. Both tests should be demonstrated to the patient first. With the pinprick, the therapist gently touches the skin with the pin or back end and asks the patient whether it feels sharp or blunt. Light touch is tested by dabbing a piece of cotton wool on an area of skin. Both tests begin distally and then move proximally (aiming to test each dermatome and each main nerve).

Temperature

Temperature sense is tested using two tubes, one with cold and one with hot water. Again, this test needs to be demonstrated first and the patient will need to be told that the therapist will touch the skin with the hot or cold tube. As before, the test is carried out with the patient's eyes closed, and begins distally (aiming to test each dermatome and each main nerve).

Unfortunately, none of the above tests of sensation have been tested for their robustness, and the findings can be subjective and differ between therapists.

Other sensations the therapist will need to ask about or examine are dizziness and sense of falling (see Ch. 24 for both), and pain (see Ch. 26).

ASSESSING ACTIVITIES

There are many activities that can be investigated in the physical assessment. The ICF has divided these into nine domains (Table 3.1). The activities to be assessed will be guided by the purpose, time point in the rehabilitation process and, most importantly, the patient.

When examining patients' activities, the therapist will not only examine whether they can do the tasks but also the quality with which the task is performed. For example, the therapist will look for symmetry in movement, associated reactions or increase in tone, and the quality and the speed of the movement. For example, a stroke patient who is able to walk may be

Table 3.1 Activities as classified by the *International Classification of Functioning, Disability and Health* (ICF: World Health Organization, 2001)

Type of activities	Examples
Learning and applying knowledge	• Purposeful sensory experiences (e.g. watching, listening) • Basic learning (e.g. learning to write) • Applying knowledge (e.g. calculating)
General tasks and demands	• e.g. undertaking single or multiple tasks
Communication	• Communicating – receiving (e.g. spoken messages) • Communicating – producing (e.g. producing messages in formal sign language) • Conversation and use of communication devices and techniques (e.g. discussion)
Mobility	• Changing and maintaining body position (e.g. transferring) • Carrying, moving and handling object (e.g. fine hand use) • Walking and moving (e.g. walking) • Moving around using transportation (e.g. driving)
Self-care	• e.g. washing yourself
Domestic life	• Acquisition of necessities (e.g. acquisition of goods and services) • Household tasks (e.g. preparing meals) • Caring for household objects and assisting others
Interpersonal interactions and relationships	• General interpersonal interactions (e.g. appreciation in relationships) • Particular interpersonal relationships (e.g. family relationships)
Major life areas	• Education (e.g. school education) • Work and employment (e.g. acquiring, keeping and terminating a job) • Economic life (e.g. economic transactions)
Community, social and civic life	• e.g. recreation and leisure

found to lack active hip and knee extension, which could form a focus for physiotherapy treatment.

Observation of gait

Mobility, and in particular gait, is one activity that should be focused on. In gait assessment the therapist needs to look out for symmetry, duration of swing and stance phases, muscle activation around the ankles, knees, hips and trunk, arm swing, trunk rotation, balance and speed. Patients with extrapyramidal impairments (e.g. in Parkinson's disease) typically walk with small or shuffling steps, reduced or absent rotation and arm swing and a flexed posture (Parkinsonian gait; see Ch. 11). Patients with hemiplegia may present with a foot drop and subsequent lateral leg swing or high step, and hip hitch during the swing phase of the affected side (see Ch. 6). In the stance phase, the affected knee may overextend, there may be a lack of hip extension and a subsequent drop of the affected shoulder.

Patients with spastic paraparesis (e.g. in cerebral palsy, multiple sclerosis, spinal cord compression) can present with a scissoring gait with increased flexion and adduction of the hips, increased flexion of the knees and dragging of the toes.

The gait of patients with cerebellar ataxia (e.g. in multiple sclerosis, cerebrovascular accident (CVA), alcoholism) will be unsteady and often these patients veer towards the side of the lesion. Sensory ataxia (e.g. in peripheral neuropathy, compression of posterior column) will also result in an unsteady gait, but is caused by a loss of joint position sense. Gait which appears disjointed, as if the patient has forgotten how to walk, is present in patients with frontal lobe lesions (e.g. in CVA, normal-pressure hydrocephalus). Finally, waddling gait is characterised by marked rotation of the pelvis and shoulders and indicates proximal muscle weakness (e.g. in proximal myopathies). Thus, by observation the therapist can obtain a good impression of the quality of the gait.

Assessment of gait

More quantitative measures of gait include timing patients over a distance (Bohannon, 1989). These can test either short distances to examine speed or longer distances to examine endurance. Short-distance speed tests include the 5-m walk, the 10-m walk and the 20-m walk (10-m and return). To carry out these tests, a 5-m or 10-m straight course is marked out, allowing enough room for the patient to start and for chairs at the beginning and end of the course. During this test, the patient is asked to walk at his or her own preferred speed, using his or her usual walking aids (or personal assistance). If a turn is included in the test, the patient is instructed where to turn. The time it takes the patient to walk the set distance (in seconds) is measured with a stopwatch, as well as the number of steps the patient takes, to get an indication, over time, of increasing stride length. The type of aid or support the patient uses is also recorded.

Information about the patient's endurance is gathered by getting him or her to walk for 2, 6 or 12 min. These all provide similar information (Butland et al., 1982; Lipkin et al., 1986). Fixing this distance is important, as it will enable the distance walked in the specified time to be recorded, as well as the distance (and time) walked by those unable to walk for the required time.

These walking tests have been used extensively and are valid and reliable measures (Bohannon, 1989). They are also simple to use and can be used in the community (Collen et al., 1990). They have been shown to be responsive to change, or improvements over time, in patients with neurological conditions (Vaney et al., 1996; Mayo et al., 1999).

Hand and arm function

The nine-hole peg test is a commonly used representational measure of hand and arm function (Mathiowetz et al., 1985). The patient is asked to place nine wooden dowels, which are of a standard diameter and length, in nine holes in a wooden base. The time to complete the task is recorded, although the test should be stopped at 50 s if not all dowels are placed (the number of dowels placed is recorded). The strengths of this test are that it is simple, portable, quick, sensitive and normative values are available for comparison purposes. It is widely adopted and used in rehabilitation research and clinical practice.

Grip strength can also be used as a representative test of hand and arm function (Bohannon & Andrews, 1987), as discussed earlier in this chapter.

Global measures of activity limitations

Apart from the measures that have been introduced above, which measure very specific limitations in certain activities, there are also more global measures. These measures are designed to examine general limitations in activities (or the previous concept of disability). There are many outcome measures that could be introduced here, but a full description and appraisal would constitute a book on its own. Some texts which specifically review those types of measures include: Bowling (1991, 1995), McDowell & Newell (1996) and Wade (1992). Some commonly used outcome measures are:

- Barthel Index (Mahoney & Barthel, 1965)
- Functional Independence Measure (FIM; Granger et al., 1993)

- Rivermead Mobility Index (Collen et al., 1991)
- Frenchay Activities Index (Holbrook & Skilbeck, 1983).

The chapter will later provide some guidance in selecting the most appropriate measures for clinical practice.

ASSESSING PARTICIPATION

As explained earlier in this chapter, participation refers to the patient's involvement in life situations (in relation to health conditions, body functions and structure, activities and contextual factors). Participation is a more complex concept than impairments and activities but it is fundamental to understanding patients and their life, and help with planning treatment.

Physiotherapy assessment of participation therefore focuses on those activities or roles which:

- patients take part in
- patients are hindered in
- could be improved
- will inevitably deteriorate
- patients wish to work on.

The assessment also has to take into account the contextual factors which represent the complete background of the patient's life, including personal and environmental factors:

- The **personal factors** are composed of features that form an individual's background (e.g. age, race, gender, education) and are not part of his or her health condition or functional state.

- The **environmental factors** make up the physical, social and attitudinal environment in which the patient lives. These factors are external to the patient and can have a positive or negative influence on his or her participation as a member of society, on performance of activities or on body function or structure.

The ICF (WHO, 2001) groups participation into the same domains as activities (Table 3.1), which do not appear on their own as outcome measures. However, global measures of participation (or the previous concept of handicap) can be used.

One study reviewed all handicap scales up until 1999 (Cardol et al., 1999a) and found 20 outcome measures which addressed handicaps or life roles, environmental influences and social consequences of a disease. They encompassed different domains: the majority

assessed society-perceived handicap, and only six were to some extent person-perceived.

Two participation (or handicap) scales which could be used across different patient groups will be introduced here. The use of these outcome measures could be of assistance in focusing the treatment on areas of life which are most important to the patient, as opposed to those areas which other health professionals think are important (see Ch. 22 for discussion on a patient-centred approach).

1. **The London Handicap Scale** (LHS; Harwood et al., 1994). The LHS consists of six questions which measure handicaps in mobility, physical independence, occupation, social integration, orientation and economic self-sufficiency. It is easy to use and interpret, short and has been used in many studies, so comparative data are available.

2. **The Impact on Participation and Autonomy Scale** (IPA; Cardol et al., 1999b) is a global measure of participation and autonomy. The IPA assesses participation and as such not only looks at patients' involvement in life situations but also at the amount of choice or autonomy they have. So, in the context of patients' illnesses or activity limitations, it assesses what their chances are of doing certain activities or having certain roles and relationships in the way they wish, either independently or with help (Cardol et al., 2002). The IPA consists of five domains: autonomy indoors, family role, autonomy outdoors, social relations and work and educational opportunities.

GOAL-SETTING

Finally, part of the physiotherapy assessment is the determination of patients' expectations of the treatment. One way of eliciting this, as well as evaluating the efficacy of the treatment (Haas, 1993), is by enquiring after the goals patients wish to achieve.

The goal-setting process has been described as an active patient–therapist relationship incorporating opportunities for feedback, whereby patients take as much responsibility as possible for developing their own goals (Berquist & Jacket, 1993; also see Ch. 22).

Family members may also wish to be involved in the goal-setting process, as they often provide much of the support to the patient at home. Carers may have their own needs, which may need to be addressed, and these are not always recognised by the people they care for (Kersten et al., 2001). In this way, goal-setting can assist the treatment-planning process and ensure that this is relevant to the patient's needs and environment.

Differences between goals of the patient and therapist

Goal-setting has been described as one of the skills that specifically characterises professionals involved in rehabilitation (Wade, 1998). However, it has been shown that there are barriers to overcome as therapists and patients may have different goals and therapists may not be willing to accept patients' goals (Sumsion & Smyth, 2000; also see Ch. 22).

In a Canadian study of goal-setting with people after stroke, it was found that patients' defined goals were different from therapists' defined goals, patients did not actively participate in the goal-setting process, the goal formulation was vague and the goals were not measurable (Wressle et al., 1999).

In a study of information-giving during physiotherapy sessions with stroke patients, observations of the sessions and interviews showed that physiotherapists provided information about recovery and hence goals, but patients nevertheless had unrealistic expectations about their recovery (Wiles et al., 2002).

Conflicts between the patient's goals and the therapist's goals for the patient may arise if the patient pursues goals that the therapist believes to be impractical and unachievable. It could be that the therapist wishes 'the best' for the patient – in other words beneficence. This would have a significant impact on the patient's opportunities to make choices and be autonomous (Blackmer, 2000).

Guidelines for goal-setting

General guidelines in goal-setting (Haas, 1993) are:

- Involve the patient early in the process of goal-setting and goal-revising
- Respect the patient's preferences, as long as there are no safety concerns
- Inform the patient about possible anticipated needs
- Negotiate goals with the patient and restructure the goals when necessary
- Use clear and open communication
- Encourage the patient to consider the values of his or her social framework and the impact of the decisions upon family members.

Long-term goals

Long-term goals will need to be set with the patient first, whilst considering the:

- aetiology and clinical manifestations of the condition
- likely prognosis and anticipated recovery

- patient's objectives and perceived needs
- patient's personal circumstances.

Without this long-term strategic goal, the rehabilitation plan may turn into one that lacks focus for both the therapist and the patient. Thus, the long-term goals (Ward & McIntosh, 1993) should be:

- directly or indirectly beneficial to the patient
- agreed between the patient and the rehabilitation team or therapist
- feasible
- within the scope of the team.

Short-term goals

With clear long-term goals in mind, the rehabilitation team will be able to set short-term goals, which can be worked on across disciplines. Some, however, will be more specific to individual professional disciplines. Short-term goals (Ward & McIntosh, 1993) should be:

- relevant to the long-term goal
- functionally based
- not typically confined to a specific professional activity
- capable of objective confirmation
- agreed by the rehabilitation team and the patient
- feasible within the time-span of rehabilitation.

For example, a short-term goal 'improving sitting balance' is not specific enough, as it does not specify the outcome to be worked towards. By contrast, 'to be able to sit unsupported for up to 30 s on a plinth with feet supported' is a short-term goal which is specific and measurable.

Reviewing goals

Regular team meetings provide the opportunity to review whether short-term goals have been achieved and, if not, for what reasons. Methods of recording these have been proposed. For example, one coding system has been described which records up to 61 reasons for non-achievement that are related to the patient, the patient and carer, the therapists, nurses or clinicians, the external system or the rehabilitation unit systems (McLellan, 1995). Using their coding system, the developers found that not all patients were given the 'prescribed' treatment and that, although 95% of goals were achieved, only 60% were achieved on time, mainly due to inadequate resourcing of therapy time (Hanspal et al., 1994).

A difficulty with goal-setting is to anticipate the likelihood that the patient will be able to achieve it, as there is a dearth of information about long-term rehabilitation or physiotherapy outcomes. By setting the anticipated outcome in addition to the actual goal, it is possible to determine whether the goal has been met, or whether the goal posts have been moved.

One formal method of goal-setting is that of Goal Attainment Scaling (GAS), where the goal-setting process is made objective through discussion with the patient (Reid & Chesson, 1998). Importantly, when using GAS the expected outcome is projected and assigned zero on the GAS scale. If the outcome is somewhat better or much better than expected, the score assigned is +1 or +2, respectively. Similarly, if the score is somewhat or much worse than expected, the score assigned is −1 or −2, respectively. In a small study of stroke rehabilitation adopting this approach, it was found that the GAS method was acceptable to patients and physiotherapists and that it helped clarify the expectations of physiotherapy (Reid & Chesson, 1998). However, there were initial differences in the types of goals set, with those set by the patient being broader and hence more difficult to achieve. Also, the patients perceived the outcome differently from the physiotherapists.

SELECTING OUTCOME MEASURES FOR PHYSIOTHERAPY ASSESSMENT

Having read the above, the reader may still wonder:

- Why should therapists use outcome measures in physiotherapy assessment?
- Why did they come about?
- What constitutes a 'good' outcome measure?
- Are there different types of outcome measure?
- How should therapists go about choosing an outcome measure?
- Who are outcomes being measured for?

The next section of this chapter aims to answer these questions.

WHY USE OUTCOME MEASURES IN PHYSIOTHERAPY ASSESSMENT?

Outcome measures describe the results or effects of a number of possible health interventions by expressing the relative value or importance of each, so that outcomes can be expressed numerically. Why would we want to measure the importance or value of physiotherapy numerically? Why not ask patients simply whether they have improved following their physiotherapy treatment? This is because when people

are asked to respond to such a direct question, they first think about how they are feeling today, then they invoke an implicit theory about how they might have changed to reconstruct an estimate of their previous state (Ross, 1989). As this implicit theory is an unconscious introspection it will be difficult to control for this.

Also, medical diagnosis alone cannot predict service needs, length of hospitalisation, level of care, outcome of hospitalisation, receipt of disability benefits, work performance and social integration (WHO, 2001). Further, for the successful achievement of evidence-based physiotherapy practice, it is paramount that the achievements of desired and expected outcomes of the treatment or changes are measured and recorded (Greenhalgh et al., 1998; Greenhalgh & Meadows, 1999). So, in physiotherapy a systematic evaluation of its benefits is certainly of value.

Apart from looking at change, outcome measures can also assist departments and health organisations when comparing the benefits of health services and allocating resources between them. For example, accumulated data can be used to determine the prevalence of certain problems in the area on which service planning can be based. Data can be used to set priorities between different groups of patients, as well as determining work load between members of staff. However, there is also a danger that outcome measures can be used erroneously to determine funding levels for services. For example, a department that uses insensitive outcome measures may appear not to provide a beneficial service to patients, risking loss of funding. Choosing appropriate measures is therefore determined by their purpose.

WHAT IS THE HISTORY OF OUTCOME MEASURES?

Health indicators existed as far back as the eighteenth century, although the most commonly cited introduction of health indicators is that by Florence Nightingale in the nineteenth century (Rosser, 1983). Florence Nightingale was concerned with the quality of care in hospitals and was the first to develop systems for collecting hospital statistics; these were 'dead, relieved, and unrelieved.' As a result, she was the first person to apply health indicators in order to achieve change, for example in hospital designs.

In those early days the length of life was used as a sensible measure. However, with the increasing effectiveness of new treatments on the quantity of life, there needed to be a shift from measuring mortality rate to more sophisticated measures.

In the late 1960s and early 1970s more global health indicators were developed, in a response to the rise in demand for health care and the rise in cost of high-technology medicine. However, many of these global health indicators were still focused on physical morbidity and mental health.

In the 1980s and 1990s, more positive indicators of health were developed, such as degrees of well-being, ability, comfort and autonomy. As a result, treatment and care can now be evaluated in terms of whether they are more likely to lead to an outcome of a life worth living in social, psychological and physical terms. Using outcome measures also increases the profile of evidence-based practice.

WHAT CONSTITUTES A 'GOOD' OUTCOME MEASURE?

Outcome measures must fulfil certain criteria in order to measure the change that it is intended to measure. The key criteria are:

- validity
- reliability
- responsiveness to change
- sensitivity.

Validity

Validity is the extent to which an outcome instrument measures what is intended. In other words, what is the degree of confidence that can be placed on inferences made about patients, based on their scores from an outcome measure? For example, how do we know that the Barthel Index, which measures 10 activities of daily living, truly reflects anything to do with disability following stroke? There are different types of validity (Streiner & Norman, 1995).

Content validity

The items or questions on the scale should be relevant to the various objectives which are being measured. In other words, the outcome measure should measure aspects of the condition or life that are relevant to patients (content relevance). So, the higher the content validity of a measure, the broader the inferences we can draw about patients under a variety of conditions and in different situations.

Face validity

The questions should also be understandable and sound (face validity).

Criterion validity

One way to examine whether a new scale is valid is to compare it with other existing scales which have been used and accepted in the field – so-called 'gold standards'. This is termed criterion validity.

Construct validity

Construct validity refers to the power, adequacy and precision of the constructs or theories that underpin the actual outcome measure. For example, when mobility is measured, we would expect that those patients who are wheelchair-bound would score poorer on the scale than those who are able to walk with a walking aid.

There are further categories within these types of validity and the interested reader is referred to other textbooks e.g. Streiner & Norman (1995).

Reliability

Reliability is a concept used by all of us in our day-to-day lives. For example, when we look at a clock with hands but no numbers, we know that there is a likely measurement error of up to 5 min. If it also displays numbers, the error may be smaller, perhaps a minute. The measurement error that is allowable depends upon the situation in which the patient is assessed. For example, when timing a patient on a short walk of 5 m, a measurement error of 1 min would not be acceptable. Thus, in order to judge whether the degree of measurement error is acceptable, we need to know what the range of expected values is, i.e. the expected variation between individuals. The total variability between patients includes both any systematic variation between patients and measurement error (Wade, 1992).

Reliability also refers to evidence that the outcome measure is measuring something in a reproducible fashion, on different occasions, by different observers, by a similar or parallel test (stability of a measure).

Interrater reliability

The degree of agreement between different observers, raters or therapists (interobserver reliability) reflects the ability of two or more observers to score a patient the same on a particular measure. For example, if we take the same example of walking 5 m, how close are the timings of two observers who time the duration of the walk?

Intrarater reliability

The degree of agreement between observations made by the same observer on two or more different occasions is called intraobserver or test–retest reliability. This refers to the individual observer's ability to measure something accurately on repeated occasions. For example, if we ask a therapist to measure the range of knee flexion with a goniometer three times on the same patient, how close are the three measurements? Observations made on the same patient on two or more occasions separated by a time interval is called test–retest reliability.

Responsiveness to change

Health outcome has been defined as 'a change resulting from antecedent health care' (Donabedian, 1980). Thus, great emphasis is placed on the word 'change', which can imply improvement or deterioration. The responsiveness of an outcome measure we are usually interested in is its sensitivity to true, clinically meaningful change (Guyatt et al., 1987, 1992). The responsiveness of an outcome measure cannot be evaluated separately from its reliability, since changes in average scores on the measure can only be attributed to true clinical change if we can be confident that the outcome measure is stable, i.e. that it will not show change if there is no true clinical change (Guyatt et al., 1992).

Sensitivity

The measurement of change following treatment can be directed at different goals. Firstly, it is important to measure differences between individuals in the amount of change. In other words, outcome measures need to be able to distinguish between patients who show a large change and those who only change a little. The ability of an outcome measure to detect small changes within a patient is termed 'sensitivity'. The level of sensitivity required depends on the range of values we may expect and the goal of the assessment. For example, when measuring joint angles, to be 5° out in the fifth distal interphalangeal joint is more crucial than being 5° out in measuring hip flexion, as the latter range is much greater.

Increased sensitivity of an outcome measure is often achieved at the expense of reliability and simplicity. For example, the Barthel Index, a measure of activities of daily living, is a simple measure of 10 activities on which patients are scored on an ordinal scale (Mahoney & Barthel, 1965). It is sensitive after an acute stroke but it suffers from a ceiling effect, which is an inability to detect improvement beyond a certain point. For those people with severe impairments, which are unlikely to change quickly, it also suffers from a flooring effect, which is an inability to detect changes, or differences between patients, below a certain point. Using the FIM

(Granger et al., 1993) can overcome a degree of poor sensitivity, given its increased range of items and scoring range but more sensitive scales are still lacking, particularly for patients with severe, complex disabilities.

ARE THERE DIFFERENT TYPES OF OUTCOME MEASURES?

In outcome measurement, the best measures to use are those that:

- yield quantitative values for baseline and follow-up
- measure change in individuals
- make fine distinctions between individuals.

Quantification is the degree to which response categories can be accurately and meaningfully numbered. The degree of quantification is dependent upon the type of data gathered by using an outcome measure.

Different levels of data

For the purpose of quantification, we can distinguish between four levels of data – nominal, ordinal, interval and ratio data (Campbell & Machin, 1999).

Nominal data

Nominal data are data that one can 'name'. They are numbers assigned to categories, which are simply counted by their classification and are not ordered. For example, discharged home or discharged to a residential home is a simple nominal outcome following health care. Other commonly used examples in physiotherapy are goals achieved or not achieved, presence or non-presence of pain, types of pain (e.g. burning, aching, stinging). Whilst nominal data can be very useful in the measurement of pain relief, they do not reflect degrees of relief achieved.

Ordinal data

Ordinal data, also known as ordered categorical data, are presented as scale items, which relate to each other. For example, a pain-rating scale ranging from no pain through to severe pain could include two additional categories of pain severity, such as mild or moderate pain.

Ordinal scales are regularly used in rehabilitation. However, it is important to be aware that the distances between items on the ordinal scale are not necessarily a reflection of the ratio of the degree of severity. For example, on a four-item pain scale, a change from moderate to mild pain does not necessarily mean that the pain is halved, as the distances between the points on the scale do not have scaling properties.

Interval data

Interval scales have the characteristics of an ordinal scale, but the distances between any two numbers of the scale are of known size. For example, a deterioration of joint range of movement from 40° to 20° does truly represent a 50% reduction in range.

Ratio data

Finally, a ratio scale has the characteristics of an interval scale with the addition of a true, not arbitrary (as in an interval scale) zero point. For example, measurements of weight, in kilograms, have a true zero point and interval properties. The superiority of data (and its amenability to mathematics) is reflected in the above terminology, with ratio data being most superior.

Different types of measures

There are many ways in which outcome measures can be grouped. For example, there are measures that examine mortality rates, adverse outcomes and outcomes of care reflecting change in health status (Hopkins, 1990).

Mortality rates (e.g. population mortality or hospital mortality) are usually insensitive measure of outcome, and not very helpful in neurological physiotherapy. Adverse outcomes can be used as indicators of care of possible low quality. Examples of adverse outcomes could be at the extreme end, such as falls or other injury to the patient. Outcomes of care by changes in health status are of more interest to therapists as they can, if chosen wisely, reflect the benefits of physiotherapy to the patient.

Generic and disease-specific outcome measures

Outcomes of care can be measured across groups of people with different conditions (generic outcome measures), or within specific disease groups (disease-specific outcome measures).

Examples of generic measures are those that measure:

- patient satisfaction (e.g. with accessibility, technical aspects, interpersonal relationships with staff, continuity)
- discharge destination
- pain
- health status
- depression.

These are generic, so long as they are not specifically designed for use with people with a certain diagnosis.

Disease-specific measures are used to evaluate characteristics of people with a certain diagnosis. Examples include the National Institutes of Health (NIH) Stroke Scale (Goldstein et al., 1989) and the Expanded

Disability Severity Scale (Kurtzke, 1983), which are measures of disease severity in stroke and multiple sclerosis respectively (see Chs 6 and 10).

In deciding between generic or disease-specific measures, it is important to consider firstly the purpose of using an outcome measure. If the intention is to evaluate whether neurological outpatient physiotherapy results in an improvement in health status, and the patients attending the department have a range of diagnoses, then the choice would be to use a generic measure. However, generic scales cover a wide range of disorders and, as a result, many questions may be inappropriate or irrelevant for any one specific problem. By contrast, disease-specific scales include items which are by definition relevant for the patient and there should be no items which are not applicable or would not change with effective therapy.

HOW IS AN OUTCOME MEASURE SELECTED?

Therapists have to use valid, reliable and sensitive outcome measures (Cole et al., 1995) to determine the:

- effect of the overall treatment programme on patients
- impact of a specific treatment approach on patients
- overall impact of care on all patients within a programme
- relative outcome in a group of patients to identify those who benefit most and least from the services provided.

When selecting an outcome measure it is important, first of all, to consider what exactly should be measured. This may seem an overstatement. However, a common mistake is to select outcome measures that do not necessarily reflect the change that could be achieved with the given therapy. For example, a measure of activities of daily living, such as the FIM (Granger et al., 1993), may not show change over time if the physiotherapy treatment is specifically aimed at improving the ability to walk, although some patients may change on other parts of the scale. Secondly, a decision needs to be made whether a disease-specific or a generic outcome measure is more appropriate.

Some outcome measures have been developed in different countries and translated into English, without formal validation of the translation. When choosing these measures it is important to be confident that the translated items have retained their original meaning. This information should be published and the procedures that should have been followed are those of translation into the other language by someone who is: fluent in that language; knowledgeable about the content area; and aware of the intent of each item and of the scale as a whole. Thereafter, the items have to be translated back into the original language and if the meaning of an item seems to have been lost, then the item must go through the whole process again.

It can be useful if there are data available on the chosen outcome measure from other groups of patients or healthy people (termed 'reference ranges'). This will enable the scores to be interpreted with understanding. The method by which the overall score on an outcome measure is calculated and presented also needs to be considered. Some outcome measures require complicated computations before they can be interpreted (e.g. the SF-36; Ware et al., 1993) and this may not be practical in busy clinics. Similarly, some measures may be difficult to explain to other stakeholders. It may not always be appropriate to use the sum total of scores from different categories of function, although this might be the accepted way of using a scale. Such practice can reduce the sensitivity of a scale by masking significant improvement or deterioration in an important aspect of function, e.g. ability to communicate, if this category is not scored separately.

Some outcome measures require a substantial amount of skill from those who use it. For example, the FIM (Granger et al., 1993) is only reliably scored by a multidisciplinary team who have been trained in its use. The outcome measure should also be acceptable to the patient group, e.g. in terms of its length, types of questions and content, and the burden in terms of time it will take to complete.

WHO ARE OUTCOMES BEING MEASURED FOR?

Many outcome measures in rehabilitation are based on outcomes considered most important to funders of care and are 'expert'-defined. However, the perspective of an observer or a therapist does not necessarily capture the patient's perceptions, which are viewed against the unique background of his or her personal and social world (Peters, 1996). It is increasingly recognised that the subjective experience of patients is a vital basis for effective clinical care, as well as helping to guide policy,

technology development and resource allocation. Therefore, in selecting outcome measures it is important to include those that have meaning to patients.

CONCLUSIONS

This chapter has concentrated on the key principles of physiotherapy assessment and has set this in the context of the ICF. It emphasised the importance of history-taking and considering patients' abilities and participation, as well as their limitations in activities and participation.

The physiotherapy assessment has to be guided by the areas of activity and participation that are most important to patients, rather than therapists.

The assessment and subsequent planning of the treatment are strengthened and more focused if clear methods of goal-setting are used. Objective recording of the expected outcome of the goals and their actual outcomes is an important aspect of goal-setting, to ensure that goals are set at the right level.

Throughout this chapter, emphasis has been given on the use of standardised methods of measuring patients' problems. The use of outcome measures, which in physiotherapy is still minimal, will aid this systematic recording and reviewing of problems and progress, as well as the implementation of evidence-based practice. However, only outcome measures that have been shown to be valid, reliable, sensitive and responsive to change should be used. The choice of these measures will also depend on their administrative burden, the acceptability to patients and ease of interpretation.

ACKNOWLEDGEMENTS

The author wishes to thank Dr Kath McPherson, of the University of Southampton, School of Health Professions and Rehabilitation Sciences, who participated in discussions about this work and commented on an early draft of this chapter.

References

Berg KO, Maki BE, Williams JI, Holliday PJ, Wood-Dauphinee SL. Clinical and laboratory measures of postural balance in an elderly population. *Arch Phys Med Rehab* 1992, **73**:1073–1080.

Berquist TF, Jacket MP. Awareness and goal setting with the traumatically brain injured. *Brain Injury* 1993, **7**:272–282.

Blackmer J. Ethical issues in rehabilitation medicine. *Scand J Rehab Med* 2000, **32**:51–55.

Bohannon RW. Selected determinants of ambulatory capacity in patients with hemiplegia. *Clin Rehab* 1989, **3**:47–53.

Bohannon RW, Andrews AW. Interrater reliability of hand-held dynamometry. *Phys Ther* 1987, **67**:931–933.

Bohannon RW, Smith MB. Interrater reliability of a modified Ashworth scale of muscle spasticity. *Phys Ther* 1987, **67**:206–207.

Bowling A. Measuring Health. *A Review of Quality of Life Measurement Scales*. Buckingham: Open University Press; 1991.

Bowling A. Measuring Disease. *A Review of Disease-Specific Quality of Life Measurement Scales*. Buckingham: Open University Press; 1995.

Butland RJ, Pang J, Gross ER, Woodcock AA, Geddes DM. Two-, six-, and 12-minute walking tests in respiratory disease. *BMJ* 1982, **284**:1607–1608.

Campbell MJ, Machin D. *Medical Statistics. A Commonsense Approach*, 3rd edn. Chichester: John Wiley; 1999:49–66.

Cardol M, Brandsma JW, De Groot IJM, Van den Bos GAM, De Haan RJ, De Jong BA. Handicap questionnaires: what do they assess? *Disability Rehab* 1999a, **21**:97–105.

Cardol M, De Haan RJ, Van den Bos GAM, De Jong BA, De Groot IJM. The development of a handicap assessment questionnaire: the impact on participation and autonomy (IPA). *Clin Rehab* 1999b, **13**:411–419.

Cardol M, De Jong BA, Van den Bos GAM, Beelen A, De Groot IJM, De Haan RJ. Beyond disability: perceived participation in people with a chronic disabling condition. *Clin Rehab* 2002, **16**:27–35.

Chartered Society of Physiotherapy (CSP). *The Curriculum Framework for qualifying programmes in physiotherary*. London: Chartered Society of Physiotherapy; 2002.

Cole B, Finch E, Gowland C, Mayo N. Why am I reading this? In: Basmajian J, ed. *Physical Rehabilitation Outcome Measures*. Toronto: Williams & Wilkins; 1995: 7.

Collen FM, Wade DT, Bradshaw CM. Mobility after stroke: reliability of measures of impairment and disability. *Int Disabilities Studies* 1990, **12**:6–9.

Collen FM, Wade DT, Robb GF, Bradshaw CM. The Rivermead Mobility Index: a further development of the Rivermead Motor Assessment. *Int Disability Studies* 1991, **13**:50–54.

Collin C, Wade DT. Assessing motor impairment after stroke: a pilot reliability study. *J Neurol Neurosurg Psychiatry* 1990, **53**:576–579.

Demeurisse G, Demol O, Robaye E. Motor evaluation in vascular hemiplegia. *Eur Neurol* 1980, **19**:382–389.

Desrosiers J, Hebert R, Bravo G, Dutil E. Upper-extremity motor co-ordination of healthy elderly people. *Age Ageing* 1995, **24**:108–112.

Donabedian A. *Explorations in Quality Assessment and Monitoring. The Definition of Quality and Approaches to its Assessment*. Ann Arbor, MI: Health Administration Press; 1980.

Donkervoort M, Dekker J, Deelman BG. Sensitivity of different ADL measures to apraxia and motor impairments. *Clin Rehab* 2002, **16**:299–305.

Duncan PW, Horner RD, Reker DM et al. Functional reach: a new clinical measure of balance. *J Gerontol* 1990, **45**:M192–M197.

Fuller G. *Neurological Examination Made Easy*. Edinburgh: Churchill Livingstone; 1999.

Goldstein LB, Bertels C, Davis JN. Interrater reliability of the NIH stroke scale. *Arch Neurol* 1989, **46**:660–662.

Granger CV, Hamilton BB, Linacre JM, Heinemann AW, Wright BD. Performance profiles of the functional independence measure. *Am J Phys Med Rehab* 1993, **72**:84–89.

Greenhalgh J, Meadows K. The effectiveness of the use of patient-based measures of health in routine practice in improving the process and outcomes of patient care: a literature review. *J Evaluation Clin Pract* 1999, **5**:401–416.

Greenhalgh J, Long AF, Brettle AJ, Grant MJ. Reviewing and selecting outcome measures for use in routine practice. *J Evaluation Clin Pract* 1998, **4**:339–350.

Guyatt GH, Walter S, Norman G. Measuring change over time: assessing the usefulness of evaluative instruments. *J Chron Dis* 1987, **40**:171–178.

Guyatt GH, Kirschner B, Jaeschke R. Measuring health status: what are the necessary measurement properties? *J Clin Epidemiol* 1992, **45**:1341–1345.

Haas JF. Ethical considerations of goal setting for patient care in rehabilitation medicine. *Am J Phys Med Rehab* 1993, **72**:228–232.

Hanspal R, Wright M, Proctor D, Peggs S, Whitaker J, McLellan DL. Failure to deliver the formal therapy prescribed in an NHS rehabilitation unit. *Clin Rehab* 1994, **8**:161–165.

Harwood RH, Rogers A, Dickinson E, Ebrahim S. Measuring handicap: the London Handicap Scale, a new measure for chronic disease. *Qual Health Care* 1994, **3**:11–16.

Holbrook M, Skilbeck CE. An activities index for use with stroke patients. *Age Ageing* 1983, **12**:166–170.

Hopkins A. *Outcomes of Care*. London: Royal College of Physicians of London; 1990:33–60.

Jackson D, Turner-Stokes L, Khatoon A et al. Development of an integrated care pathway for the management of hemiplegic shoulder pain. *Disability Rehabil* 2002, **24**:390–398.

Katz DI, Mills VM, Cassidy JW. The Neurological Rehabilitation Model in clinical practice. In: Mills VM, Cassidy JW, Katz DI, eds. *Neurological Rehabilitation: A Guide to Diagnosis, Prognosis and Treatment Planning*. Oxford: Blackwell Science; 1997:1–27.

Kersten P, McLellan L, George S et al. Needs of carers of severely disabled people: are they identified and met adequately? *Health Social Care Commun* 2001, **9**:235–243.

King Edward's Fund for London. *Problem Orientated Medical Records (POMR): Guidelines for Therapists*. London: King's Fund; 1988.

Kurtzke JF. Rating neurological impairment in multiple sclerosis: an expanded disability status scale. *Neurology* 1983, **33**:1444–1452.

Lang AET, Fahn S. Assessment of Parkinson's disease. In: Musat TL, ed. *Quantification of Neurological Deficit*. Boston, MA: Butterworths; 1989:285–309.

Lennon S, Hastings M. Key physiotherapy indicators for quality of stroke care. *Physiotherapy* 1996, **82**:655–664.

Lincoln N, Leadbitter D. Assessment of motor function in stroke patients. *Physiotherapy* 1979, **65**:48–51.

Lipkin DP, Scriven AJ, Crake T, Poole-Wilson PA. Six minute walking test for assessing exercise capacity in chronic heart failure. *BMJ* 1986, **292**:653–655.

Macdermid JC, Fox E, Richards RS, Roth JH. Validity of pulp-to-palm distance as a measure of finger flexion. *J Hand Surg* 2001, **26B**:432–435.

Mahoney FI, Barthel DW. Functional evaluation: the Barthel Index. *Maryland State Med J* 1965, **14**:61–65.

Mathiowetz V, Volland G, Kashman N, Weber K. Adult norms for the box and block test of manual dexterity. *Am J Occup Ther* 1985, **39**:386–391.

Mayo NE, Wood-Dauphinee S, Ahmed S et al. Disablement following stroke. *Disabil Rehab* 1999, **21**:258–268.

McDowell I, Newell C. *Measuring Health. A Guide to Rating Scales and Questionnaires*, 2nd edn. Oxford: Oxford University Press; 1996.

McLellan DL. Neurorehabilitation. In: Wiles CM, ed. *Management of Neurological Disorders*. London: BMJ Publishing Group; 1995:301–328.

Medical Research Council (MRC) of the United Kingdom. *Aids to the Examination of the Peripheral Nervous System*. Eastbourne: Baillière-Tindall; 1978.

Ozbudak-Demir S, Akyuz M, Guler-Uysal F, Orkun S. Postacute predictors of functional and cognitive progress in traumatic brain injury: somatosensory evoked potentials. *Arch Phys Med Rehab* 1999, **80**:252–257.

Peters DJ. Disablement observed, addressed, and experienced: integrating subjective experience into disablement models. *Disabil Rehab* 1996, **18**:593–603.

Reid A, Chesson R. Goal attainment scaling: is it appropriate for stroke patients and their physiotherapists? *Physiotherapy* 1998, **84**:136–144.

Richards M, Marder K, Cote L, Mayeux R. Interrater reliability of the Unified Parkinson's Disease Rating Scale motor examination. *Move Disord* 1994, 9:89–91.

Ross M. Relation of implicit theories to the construction of personal histories. *Psychol Rev* 1989, **96**:341–357.

Rosser RM. A history of the development of health indicators. In: Smith GT, ed. *Measuring the Social Benefits of Medicine*. London: Office of Health Economics; 1983.

Rossiter D, Thompson AJ. Introduction of integrated care pathways for patients with multiple sclerosis in an inpatient neurorehabilitation setting. *Disabil Rehab* 1995, **17**:443–448.

Stokes M, Hides J, Nassiri DK. Musculoskeletal ultrasound imaging: diagnostic and treatment aid in rehabilitation. *Phys Ther Rev* 1997, **2**:73–92.

Streiner DL, Norman GR. *Health Measurement Scales. A Practical Guide to their Development and Use*, 2nd edn. Oxford: Oxford University Press; 1995.

Sumsion T, Smyth G. Barriers to client-centredness and their resolution. *Can J Occup Ther* 2000, **67**:15–21.

Sunderland A, Tinson D, Bradley L, Hewer RL. Arm function after stroke. An evaluation of grip strength as a measure of recovery and a prognostic indicator. *J Neurol Neurosurg Psychiatry* 1989, **52**:1267–1272.

Swaine BR, Sullivan SJ. Reliability of the scores for the finger-to-nose test in adults with traumatic brain injury. *Phys Ther* 1993, **73**:71–78.

Vaney C, Blaurock H, Gattlen B, Meisels C. Assessing mobility in multiple sclerosis using the Rivermead Mobility Index and gait speed. *Clin Rehab* 1996, **10**:216–226.

Wade DT. *Measurement in Neurological Rehabilitation*. Oxford: Oxford University Press; 1992.

Wade DT. Evidence relating to goal planning in rehabilitation. *Clin Rehab* 1998, **12**:273–275.

Wade DT, Langton Hewer R, Skilbeck CE, David RM. *Principles of Assessment*. London: Chapman and Hall; 1985:67–86.

Ward C, McIntosh S. The rehabilitation process: a neurological perspective. In: Greenwood R, Barnes MP, McMillan TM et al., eds. *Neurological Rehabilitation*. London: Churchill Livingstone; 1993:13–27.

Ware J Jr, Snow KK, Kosinski M, Gandek B. *SF-36 Health Survey. Manual and Interpretation Guide*. Boston, MA: Health Institute, New England Medical Center; 1993.

Wiles R, Ashburn A, Payne S, Murphy C. Patients' expectations of recovery following stroke: a qualitative study. *Disabil Rehab* 2002, **24**:841–850.

World Health Organization. *International Classification of Impairments, Disabilities, and Handicaps*. Geneva: World Health Organization; 1980.

World Health Organization. *International Classification of Functioning, Disability and Health: ICF*. Geneva: World Health Organization, 2001. Available online at: http://www.who.int/classification/icf.

Wressle E, Oberg B, Henriksson C. The rehabilitation process for the geriatric stroke patient – an exploratory study of goal setting and interventions. *Disabil Rehab* 1999, **21**:80–87.

Young A, Hughes I, Russell P et al. Measurement of quadriceps muscle wasting by ultrasonography. *Rheum Rehab* 1980, **19**:141–148.

Chapter 4

Abnormalities of muscle tone and movement

T Britton

CHAPTER CONTENTS

INTRODUCTION

This chapter presents an overview of the abnormalities of muscle tone and movement seen in patients with neurological disorders. The nature and proposed mechanisms of the abnormalities, the disorders in which they commonly occur and their medical treatment are outlined. Physical management is discussed in Chapter 25. Specialist texts in which further details can be found include those by Adams & Victor (2001), Weiner & Laing (1989) and Rothwell (1994).

MUSCLE TONE

Muscle tone can be defined clinically as the resistance that is encountered when the joint of a relaxed patient is moved passively. (This is the usual clinical definition of muscle tone, though there is no universally accepted definition. Physiologists, in particular, use 'tone' in a different way – to signify a state of muscle tension or continuous muscle activity.) In practice, the clinician (medical practitioner or physiotherapist) usually assesses muscle tone in one of two ways. He or she may grasp a patient's relaxed limb and try to move it, noting the amount of effort required to overcome the resistance – the muscle tone. Alternatively, the clinician may observe how a limb responds to being shaken or to being released suddenly: the greater the resistance to movement (i.e. the greater the muscle tone), the more rigidly the limb will behave.

The resistance encountered when moving the joint of a relaxed individual is a combination of the passive stiffness of the joint and its surrounding soft tissues plus any active muscle tension, especially that due to stretch reflex contraction. The passive stiffness is dependent upon the inherent viscoelastic properties of the tissues and varies with age and other physiological parameters (e.g. limb temperature, preceding exercise). The contribution of active stretch reflex contractions to overall muscle tone also varies considerably, even in normal individuals, being particularly influenced by the age and emotional state of the person, as well as whether tone is assessed at a proximal or distal joint.

All of the many factors that can affect normal muscle tone need to be taken into account before the clinician decides whether muscle tone is abnormal and this requires considerable skill. The assessment of muscle tone is an important and valuable part of the clinical examination and allows useful deductions to be made about the state of the nervous system.

Clinically, muscle tone may be abnormally increased (hypertonia) or decreased (hypotonia). In principle, hypertonia or hypotonia may arise either as a consequence of changes in the passive stiffness of the joint and its surrounding soft tissues or because of changes in the amount contributed by active muscle contractions. Most clinical and neurophysiological research has hitherto concentrated on the latter mechanism (in particular, muscle contractions reflexively evoked by muscle stretch), but there is increasing awareness of the potential importance of changes in passive joint stiffness.

Hypertonia

Two main types of hypertonia are recognised: spasticity and rigidity. These differ in their cause and clinical significance. Two rare types of hypertonia, gegenhalten and alpha-rigidity, are also discussed briefly.

Spasticity

Spasticity may be defined as a velocity-dependent increase in resistance to passive stretch of a muscle, with exaggerated tendon reflexes (Lance, 1990).

Clinical features   Spasticity is recognised clinically by:

1. the characteristic pattern of involvement of certain muscle groups
2. the increased responsiveness of muscles to stretch
3. the associated finding of markedly increased tendon reflexes.

Spasticity predominantly affects the antigravity muscles, i.e. the flexors of the arms and the extensors of the legs. As a result, the spastic upper limb tends to assume a flexed and pronated posture whilst a spastic lower limb is usually held extended and adducted, a posture that is characteristically seen (on the affected side) in hemiplegic patients following a stroke (see Ch. 6). However, spasticity is not always associated with such a posture. The actual posture adopted by any individual patient will depend upon the site of the neurological lesion (cerebral hemisphere, brainstem or spinal cord), the presence of internal (e.g. a full bladder) or external stimuli and on the patient's overall posture (i.e. sitting or lying).

Stretching the muscle of a patient with spasticity results in an abnormally large reflex contraction. The more rapidly the examiner moves the limb of a patient with spasticity, the greater the increase in muscle tone. Indeed, the resistance to movement may become so great as to stop all movement, the abrupt cessation of movement being described clinically as a 'catch'. If passive flexion of the arm or extension of the leg continues, the resistance to movement may then disappear rapidly. The catch, followed by the sudden melting away of resistance, is referred to clinically as the 'clasp-knife phenomenon'. In certain situations, sustained rhythmic contractions can be generated when a muscle is stretched rapidly and the tension maintained. The rhythmic contractions, which are usually at a frequency of 5–7 Hz, are termed 'clonus'. Clonus is most commonly seen at the ankle when the foot is dorsiflexed (ankle clonus). It can also be seen at the knee (patellar clonus) and occasionally at other sites in the body.

The pathologically brisk tendon reflexes that are typically associated with spasticity are further evidence of the increased responsiveness of muscle to stretch. The pathophysiological mechanisms involved in the response to brief phasic stretches almost certainly differ from those involved in the response to slower stretches discussed in the paragraph above (Sheean, 2002). Pathologically brisk tendon reflexes may spread or irradiate to other muscles or muscle groups (Adams & Victor, 2001). Thus, a tap on the Achilles tendon not only evokes a pathologically brisk ankle jerk but may also produce reflex contractions in the proximal muscles such as the hamstrings, quadriceps and hip adductor muscles.

Clinical significance   Spasticity is one of the cardinal features of an upper motor neurone syndrome. The presence of spasticity should therefore always lead to a search for lesions of the upper motor neurone anywhere from the motor cortex to the spinal motoneurones. Common causes of spasticity include cerebrovascular disease (Ch. 6), brain damage (Chs 7 and 18), spinal cord compression (Chs 8 and 19) and inflammatory lesions of the spinal cord such as those found in multiple sclerosis (Ch. 10).

Pathophysiological mechanisms of spasticity   The pathological basis of spasticity is the abnormal enhancement of spinal stretch reflexes. What causes the enhancement of spinal stretch reflexes is less certain. In principle, they could be enhanced by increased muscle spindle sensitivity (mediated via increased gamma-moto-neurone drive) or by increased excitability of central synapses involved in the reflex arc.

Microneurographic studies in humans and neuro-physiological studies in experimental animals have found no abnormality in the sensitivity of the muscle spindle in established spasticity (Burke, 1983; Pierrot-Deseilligny & Mazieres, 1985). Muscle spindle sensitivity may be increased in the early stages of an upper motor neurone lesion, but then return to normal. Increased excitability of central synapses involved in the reflex arc therefore appears to be the main factor determining the enhancement of spinal stretch reflexes (Thilmann et al., 1991; Dietz, 1992; Singer et al., 2001).

How does an upper motor neurone lesion alter the excitability of central synapses involved in the stretch reflex arc? In the short term, it seems that previously inactive (or silent) spinal synapses can become active following the disruption of descending motor inputs, thereby increasing the efficiency of the reflex arc (Pierrot-Deseilligny & Mazieres, 1985). In the longer term, the synapses of descending motor pathways on spinal motoneurones and interneurones degenerate and are replaced by sprouting of the remaining intraspinal synapses, again increasing the efficiency of the reflex arc (Tsukahara & Murakami, 1983; Noth, 1991).

Reading the preceding paragraphs might lead one to believe that spasticity was simply a release phenom-enon, caused by the removal of inhibitory descending influences on the spinal cord. Such an impression, however, would be wrong. The true situation is almost certainly more complicated. Removal of inhibitory descending influences is undoubtedly important but spasticity also occurs in the presence of facilitatory descending influences. The facilitatory descending path-ways may be responsible for the continuous muscle activity that can be seen in the upper motor neurone syn-drome and which is not dependent on the stretch reflex.

There are many descending pathways that arise in the brainstem and influence spinal cord excitability (see Ch. 1). For simplicity, these descending pathways can be divided into two main groups on the basis of their anatomy and physiology. One group, comprising the pontine and lateral bulbar reticulospinal pathways, along with the vestibulospinal pathways (although the functional contribution of the latter is probably limited in humans), descends in the ventral funiculus of the spinal cord and tends to facilitate muscle tone. The other group, comprising mainly the crossed reticulospinal pathways from the ventromedial bulbar reticular forma-tion, descends in the lateral funiculus (just behind the corticospinal tracts) and tends to inhibit muscle tone. Evidence from humans and experimental animals sug-gests that normal muscle tone depends on a balance between the facilitatory and inhibitory systems (Brown, 1994; Sheean, 2002). Spasticity may arise if the inhibitory pathways are interrupted or if there is increased activity in the facilitatory pathways.

Spasticity following lesions of the frontal cerebral cortex or internal capsule probably results from loss of cortical drive to the bulbar inhibitory centre (thereby reducing activity in the inhibitory crossed reticulospinal pathways and releasing the spinal stretch reflex). Such spasticity is often noted to be less severe than that asso-ciated with spinal cord disease. The usually severe spas-ticity associated with spinal cord disease may be due in part to the close proximity of the crossed reticulospinal pathways and the corticospinal pathways within the spinal cord.

The above discussion has concentrated on the neural and stretch reflex changes that accompany spasticity. Such changes are undoubtedly of prime importance. However, there is increasing awareness that established spasticity is also associated with significant changes in passive mechanical factors (Davidoff, 1992; Lin et al., 1994; Given et al., 1995; O'Dwyer et al., 1996). With weakness and disuse, muscles undergo shortening with a reduction in the number of sarcomeres and an increase in collagen content (Williams et al., 1988). They also tend to have a decreasing proportion of type II muscle fibres (Dattola et al., 1993). All of these changes lead to an increase in the passive stiffness of the joint and (to the cli-nician) a feeling of increased tone. The amount to which passive stiffness contributes to the feeling of increased tone varies from patient to patient, which may explain why it has proved so difficult to produce a device to measure spasticity automatically (Damiano et al., 2002).

The changes in the passive mechanical factors asso-ciated with spasticity are of practical importance. All clinicians know of the difficulty of dealing with estab-lished contractures in patients with spasticity. It has been proposed that such contractures are the result of a vicious circle. The increased gain of the stretch reflex loop causes the muscle to shorten. The shortened muscle then undergoes remodelling, losing some of its sarcomeres. Unless there is some intervention to stretch or lengthen the muscle, this process will continue, lead-ing to contracture (see Ch. 25). If this model were correct, then the most appropriate treatment would be regular stretching of affected muscles (e.g. stretching exercises). Such treatment might be assisted with the judicious use of muscle relaxants or botulinum toxin injections. In contrast, tendon-lengthening operations would not appear to be ideal, since the (released) muscle would continue to lose its sarcomeres and therefore shorten further. However, tendon-lengthening operations do allow the joint to assume a more natural position, thereby often increasing limb function and allowing

Table 4.1   Comparison of spasticity and rigidity

	Spasticity	Rigidity
Pattern of muscle involvement	Upper-limb flexors; lower-limb extensors	Flexors and extensors equally
Nature of tone	Velocity-dependent increase in tone; 'clasp-knife' phenomenon	Constant throughout movement; 'lead pipe'
Tendon reflexes	Increased	Normal
Pathophysiology	Increased spinal stretch reflex gain	Increased long-latency component of stretch reflex
Clinical significance	Upper motor neurone (pyramidal) sign	Extrapyramidal sign

the antagonist muscles to work at less mechanical disadvantage. A more recently proposed cause of shortening in pennate muscles is fibre atrophy, leading to shortening of the aponeurosis (Shortland et al., 2002). If this model were operating, strengthening exercises would be appropriate. The mechanism and clinical implications of this proposed phenomenon are discussed in Chapters 29 (p. 495) and 30 (p. 512).

The clinical and pathophysiological features of spasticity are summarised and contrasted with those of rigidity in Table 4.1.

Pharmacological treatment   Details of the drugs mentioned in this section are given in Chapter 28. The mainstay of treatment for spasticity is baclofen. Baclofen is believed to act on inhibitory GABA-B receptors within the spinal cord, reducing the gain of the stretch reflex loop. Like all drugs that are used in the treatment of spasticity, baclofen may uncover or exacerbate muscle weakness. Patients often rely on their spasticity for support and when it is reduced they find that their limbs are floppy and weak. Baclofen also causes drowsiness and tiredness, which can be lessened if the drug is given intrathecally by pump.

Benzodiazepines (e.g. diazepam, clonazepam) are also used in the treatment of spasticity, but are generally less favoured than baclofen because of their potential to produce addiction. They are believed to act on inhibitory GABA-A receptors within the spinal cord.

Dantrolene acts directly on muscle to produce weakness by inhibiting excitation–contraction coupling. It is rarely used on its own but may be used in conjunction with baclofen or benzodiazepines. Hepatotoxicity can be a problem with dantrolene.

Tizanidine is an alpha-2 agonist that decreases presynaptic activity in excitatory interneurones. It is claimed to cause (or uncover) less muscle weakness than baclofen, but hepatotoxicity may be a problem.

Botulinum toxin injections have been used to weaken muscles selectively. The results in adult patients with spasticity are mixed, but there may be a role for botulinum toxin in patients with severe adductor spasms (Hyman et al., 2000). More favourable results have been obtained in children with spastic cerebral palsy (Cosgrove et al., 1994). Experimental work in mice suggests that botulinum toxin injections may reduce the risk of developing contractures (Cosgrove & Graham, 1994).

Intrathecal phenol blocks are occasionally used in patients with severe lower-limb spasticity to help control pain or improve posture (Beckerman et al., 1996). The risk of non-specific damage to other neural structures is high, and such treatment is therefore usually restricted to patients who have no useful lower-limb function or sphincter control.

Rigidity

Rigidity is another cause of increased tone, which can occur in different forms. It should be noted that the terms 'decerebrate rigidity' and 'decorticate rigidity' describe abnormal posturing associated with coma rather than a specific type of hypertonia. The more correct terms would therefore be 'decerebrate and decorticate posturing'. Decerebrate posturing occurs with a variety of acute and subacute brainstem disorders and consists of opisthotonus, clenched jaws and stiffly extended limbs. The abnormal postures are characteristically triggered by passive movements of the limbs or neck or by any noxious stimulus. Decorticate posturing occurs with high or midbrain lesions (or above) and consists of flexion of the upper limb and extension of the legs similar to that of a spastic tetraplegia.

Clinical features   Rigidity is recognised clinically as an increased resistance to relatively slowly imposed passive movements. It is present in both extensor and flexor muscle groups. Typically the examiner will flex and extend the wrist slowly and may describe the resistance as being of 'lead pipe' type, reflecting the fact that the resistance is felt throughout the movement (in distinction to spasticity where the resistance initially increases rapidly and then melts away – the so-called clasp-knife phenomenon). It should be emphasised that the imposed movements must be slow: use of more rapid movements, that would be appropriate for examining spasticity, may result in the erroneous conclusion that the tone is normal. Tendon reflexes are normal, in contrast to the hyperreflexia associated with spasticity.

Many patients with rigidity have an additional tremor as part of their extrapyramidal disorder. When this is so, the tremor will be felt superimposed on the rigidity, giving rise to the clinical phenomenon of 'cogwheel rigidity'.

Rigidity may be appreciated in the limbs or axially. One of the best ways of demonstrating axial tone is to rotate the patient's shoulders while he or she stands relaxed. In normal individuals, the examiner will encounter little resistance and the arms will be seen to swing relatively freely. However, in patients with axial rigidity, the examiner has the feeling of trying to move a rigid structure and the arms fail to swing.

Clinical significance   Rigidity is one of the cardinal features of an extrapyramidal syndrome. The term 'parkinsonism' is synonymous with extrapyramidal syndrome; other synonyms used include parkinsonian syndrome and akinetic–rigid syndrome. Parkinson's disease (see Ch. 11) is a specific disease entity and is but one cause of parkinsonism. The other cardinal feature is hypokinesia/bradykinesia (reduced and slow movements, see below). Tremor is a frequent finding in parkinsonism, but is not always present. Extrapyramidal syndromes are caused by functional disturbances of the basal ganglia (caudate nucleus, putamen, globus pallidus and subthalamic nucleus).

Common causes of parkinsonism include Parkinson's disease itself, multiple system atrophy and a number of rarer conditions that are sometimes called 'Parkinson-plus syndromes' (e.g. progressive supranuclear palsy, corticobasal degeneration). Extrapyramidal syndromes are a not uncommon side-effect of drugs, especially the neuroleptic drugs and the so-called vestibular sedatives (e.g. metoclopramide, prochlorperazine, cinnarizine).

Cerebrovascular disease rarely gives rise to true parkinsonism. However, cerebrovascular disease affecting the frontal lobes may give rise to a superficially similar clinical syndrome, with gait dyspraxia (which can be mistaken for the shuffling gait of parkinsonism) and gegenhalten, mentioned below (which may be mistaken for rigidity). The condition can be distinguished from parkinsonism by the relative preservation of upper-limb and facial movement, the lack of a significant response to levodopa, and the frequent occurrence of urinary incontinence.

Pathophysiological mechanisms   The pathophysiological basis of rigidity appears to be enhancement of the long-latency component of the stretch reflex (Rothwell, 1994). The normal stretch reflex can be divided into a short-latency component and a long-latency component. In patients with parkinsonian rigidity, the short-latency (spinal) component is normal in size, reflecting

the fact that tendon reflexes in the condition are However, the long-latency component, which may take a transcortical route, is enlarged. Furthermore, the size of the long-latency component correlates with the clinical degree of rigidity: the greater the rigidity, the larger the size of the long-latency component.

Pharmacological treatment   Treatment is usually focused on the underlying extrapyramidal syndrome rather than the rigidity per se. It is always important to check whether the patient is taking any neuroleptic medication that could be causing or exacerbating the condition.

Parkinson's disease itself is usually treated with levodopa or a dopamine agonist drug (Ch. 11). Levodopa is generally given in conjunction with a peripheral dopa-decarboxylase inhibitor to prevent the drug's metabolism in the gut and to increase its availability to the brain. The initial response to levodopa is usually very gratifying. Unfortunately, longer-term treatment may be associated with a less satisfactory clinical response and the development of troublesome side effects, including involuntary movements and psychiatric disturbance. Dopamine agonist drugs are believed to produce fewer motor side-effects (i.e. involuntary movements) but are also probably less effective at relieving extrapyramidal symptoms and signs. Other drugs used in the treatment of Parkinson's disease include catechol-O-methyltransferase inhibitors, anticholinergics and selegiline. The same drugs are also frequently used in the treatment of other (non-Parkinson's disease) extrapyramidal syndromes, but the clinical response is generally less impressive.

Gegenhalten

Some elderly patients find it difficult to relax their limbs during examination. When attempting to examine tone, the patients appear to resist movement voluntarily but they are unable to prevent such movement and it is not therefore voluntary resistance. This phenomenon is usually termed 'gegenhalten' (Adams & Victor, 2001).

Gegenhalten is usually caused by damage to the frontal lobes of the brain, and may be seen in association with cerebrovascular disease or neurodegenerative conditions such as Alzheimer's disease. Cognitive impairment, grasp reflexes and other primitive reflexes are frequent accompaniments.

Alpha-rigidity

In some patients, tone may be increased in a rigid fashion (being present equally in both flexor and extensor muscles), but their tendon reflexes are absent or reduced. It is as though there is increased motor unit excitability in the absence of the spinal reflex arc. Such a condition may be seen in association with spinal cord lesions, particularly those affecting the central grey matter. Stiff-person syndrome, which is associated with antibodies against the enzyme glutamic acid decarboxylase, may produce a similar increase in muscle tone (Levy et al., 1999).

Hypotonia

In the normal individual, active stretch reflex contractions contribute little to resting muscle tone. Most of the tone arises from the passive viscoelastic properties of the joints and soft tissues. Reduced tone due to central nervous system (CNS) disorders is therefore often difficult to detect clinically (because the viscoelastic properties remain unchanged). Hypotonia due to central lesions may be apparent in certain situations, however. Patients with cerebellar hypotonia characteristically have pendular tendon reflexes because of limb underdamping. Children with hypotonia due to CNS disorders are often described as floppy. Hypotonia is also seen in the acute stage of spinal cord disease or trauma (see Ch. 8). With recovery from this spinal shock, the tone increases and the reflexes return to produce the characteristic upper motor neurone syndrome.

Reduced muscle tone due to peripheral nervous system disorders is usually easier to detect. This is mainly because the associated muscle wasting reduces the passive stiffness of the joint. The absence of stretch reflex contractions in lower motor neurone lesions probably contributes little to the reduction in muscle tone. When hypotonia is unequivocally present, it is usually indicative of a lower motor neurone lesion. Other features of a lower motor neurone lesion include weakness, areflexia and fasciculation.

MOVEMENT DISORDERS

Clinically distinctive patterns of involuntary movements occur in many diseases. Recognising these patterns may help to identify the underlying disorder. The aim of the remainder of the chapter is to give brief descriptions of the common movement disorders and their clinical significance. First, however, it may be helpful to define some general terms.

General terms for movement disorders

The terms discussed here describe the amount and speed of movement, as well as some involuntary movements.

Akinesia, hypokinesia and bradykinesia

Akinesia, hypokinesia and bradykinesia are often used loosely and inaccurately (Berardelli et al., 2001). Akinesia is the absence of movement while hypokinesia describes abnormally decreased movement. Bradykinesia refers to slowness of movement. Akinesia, hypokinesia and bradykinesia are cardinal features of extrapyramidal disease, to the extent that some neurologists refer to parkinsonism as an akinetic–rigid syndrome. It should be noted, however, that akinesia, hypokinesia and bradykinesia are not used when there is paresis (either upper or lower motor neurone) to account for the deficient or absent movements. Basal ganglia and frontal lobe dysfunction, particularly the supplementary motor area, are thought to underlie akinesia, hypokinesia and bradykinesia (Berardelli et al., 2001).

Clinically, patients with Parkinson's disease are slow in initiating movement (the patient may take longer than normal to respond) and also by slowness in carrying out a task. When such a patient is called from the outpatient waiting room, he or she will often take a long time to rise from the chair and then walk slowly from the waiting room into the clinic room itself. Part of the problem with walking is that people with parkinsonism tend to take shorter steps than is normal. Indeed, the amplitudes of all their movements tend to be smaller than required for optimal performance. In the upper limb, bradykinesia can most easily be demonstrated by asking the patient to open and close his or her fist as quickly as possible.

Dyskinesias and hyperkinesia

Some neurological diseases are associated with additional (involuntary) movements. Such involuntary movements are best termed dyskinesias and include myoclonus, chorea, ballism, dystonia, tic and tremor (Table 4.2). Some neurologists describe these conditions as hyperkinesias rather than dyskinesias in order to distinguish them from hypokinetic movement disorders (e.g. parkinsonism). However, confusion may then arise when a patient with (hypokinetic) Parkinson's disease develops (hyperkinetic) tremor or chorea. A further problem with the use of the term 'hyperkinesia' is that it is sometimes assumed that hyperkinetic movements are faster than normal. This is not the case (and hyperkinesia is not the converse of bradykinesia). Indeed, in most so-called hyperkinetic movement disorders, movement velocities are actually slower than normal. The term 'dyskinesia' is therefore preferred to hyperkinesia.

Hypometria and hypermetria

Movements that are smaller than intended are described as hypometric. Patients with Parkinson's

Table 4.2   Main causes of some dyskinetic movement disorders

Tremor

Rest tremor	Parkinson's disease
	Drug-induced parkinsonism
	Other extrapyramidal disease
Action tremor	Enhanced physiological tremor (e.g. anxiety, alcohol, hyperthyroidism)
	Essential tremor
	Cerebellar disease
	Wilson's disease
Intention tremor	Brainstem or cerebellar disease (e.g. multiple sclerosis, spinocerebellar degeneration)

Myoclonus

Without encephalopathy	Juvenile myoclonic epilepsy
	Myoclonic epilepsy
With encephalopathy	
Non-progressive	Postanoxic myoclonus
Progressive	Storage disorders (e.g. Lafora body disease)
	Unverricht–Lundborg disease
	Metabolic encephalopathies (e.g. respiratory, renal and liver failure)
	Creutzfeldt–Jakob disease

Chorea

Sydenham's chorea
Pregnancy-associated chorea
Contraceptive pill-associated chorea
Huntington's disease
Thyrotoxicosis
Systemic lupus erythematosus
Drug-induced chorea (e.g. neuroleptics, phenytoin)

Dystonia

Generalised	Idiopathic torsion dystonia
	Drug-induced
	Athetoid cerebral palsy
	Wilson's disease
	Metabolic storage disorders
	Dopa-responsive dystonia
Hemidystonia	Basal ganglia lesions (e.g. tumours, vascular, postthalamotomy)

disease often have hypometric movements. In contrast, patients with cerebellar disease may overshoot the target, producing so-called hypermetric movements.

Tremor

Tremor is best defined as any unwanted, rhythmic, approximately sinusoidal movement of a limb or body part (Elble & Koller, 1990). The fact that the movement is unwanted distinguishes tremor from voluntary oscillatory movements such as waving or writing. Its rhythmic and approximately sinusoidal character distinguishes it from myoclonus and chorea. The term 'myorhythmia' is occasionally used to signify a slow tremor of relatively large amplitude that affects the proximal part of a limb.

Clinically, tremor is usually classified according to the situation in which it occurs (Bain, 1993). Examples of types of tremor and the conditions in which they occur are given in Table 4.2. A tremor that is present when the limb is relaxed and fully supported is called a rest tremor. Action tremors occur when the patient attempts to maintain a posture (postural tremor) or to move (kinetic tremor). Tremor which gets worse at the end of a movement is called an intention or terminal tremor and is associated with cerebellar dysfunction.

There is no satisfactory pathological classification of tremor. A rest tremor almost always suggests parkinsonism. Postural tremors have many causes but are most commonly due to enhanced physiological tremor or essential tremor. All of us have a fine postural tremor (physiological tremor) of which we are usually completely unaware. Physiological tremor may become noticeable, however, in certain situations (e.g. anxiety, fear, thyrotoxicosis, fatigue, use of adrenergic drugs). This noticeable tremor is called enhanced physiological tremor. Essential tremor is suggested by the finding of a symmetrical postural upper-limb tremor that is absent at rest and is not made strikingly worse by movement (and in the absence of factors that might enhance physiological tremor). In a substantial proportion of patients with essential tremor, there is a family history of similarly affected relatives and up to half the patients may find temporary amelioration of their tremor with alcohol. For a discussion of other tremors the reader is referred to Elble & Koller (1990) and Bain (1993).

The pathophysiological mechanisms responsible for tremor are poorly understood. The nervous system, like all mechanical systems, has a natural tendency to oscillate. This tendency is due in part to the mechanical properties of the limbs and in part to neural feedback loops. Neuropathological studies have demonstrated physical and biochemical changes in brains from patients with different disorders involving tremor but have failed to elucidate the precise changes that can be attributed to the symptom of tremor (Bain, 1993). Recent evidence suggests that cerebellar mechanisms are of central importance to the maintenance and generation of essential tremor (Britton, 1995).

Myoclonus

Myoclonus describes brief shock-like jerks of a limb or body part. Myoclonic jerks may be restricted to one part of the body (focal myoclonus) or may be generalised (generalised myoclonus). Jerks can occur spontaneously or with movement, or they may be reflexly triggered by light, sound, touch or tendon taps. Following a myoclonic jerk there is a lapse of posture that is associated with electrical silence in the muscles, lasting for around 200 ms (Shibasaki, 1995). Lapses in posture can sometimes occur without a noticeable preceding jerk. Such postural lapses are called asterixis and typically occur with metabolic encephalopathies (e.g. in respiratory, renal or liver failure).

Neurophysiologically, there are three main types of myoclonus: cortical myoclonus, which arises from the cerebral cortex; reticular reflex myoclonus, which arises from the brainstem; and propriospinal myoclonus, which arises from the spinal cord. Neurophysiological studies are of special help in the assessment of patients with myoclonus (Shibasaki, 1995). Cortical myoclonus is preceded by an electrical 'spike' over the contralateral motor cortex (normal movements, even fast movements, are never preceded by an electrical spike). The jerks are focal and can often be triggered by touching the affected limb (cortical reflex myoclonus). The condition responds to anticonvulsants and piracetam. Occasionally, there may be repetitive bursts of cortical myoclonus. Such repetitive bursts are in essence a focal epileptic discharge.

Neurophysiological studies in reticular reflex myoclonus show that the abnormal electrical activity arises from the brainstem. Such jerks are symmetrical and generalised. They may be triggered by a startle (e.g. unexpected noise or light) and the jerks themselves have a number of similarities to an exaggerated startle response.

Some patients with spinal cord disease have abnormal jerks that begin at one segmental level and then spread to neighbouring segments. Such patients have spinal myoclonus.

Myoclonus is a feature of many neurological diseases. Most patients are found to have a progressive, usually degenerative, encephalopathy. Postanoxic myoclonus occurs, as its name suggests, after a respiratory arrest, especially in patients with chronic lung conditions. After recovery, such patients develop severe myoclonic jerking, especially in their legs, and they walk with a characteristic bouncy gait. There are often additional cerebellar signs and the condition is presumed to arise because of damage to the large (and hence oxygen-demanding) cerebellar Purkinje cells (see Ch. 1, p. 16). The condition is treated with valproate and 5-hydroxytryptamine.

Chorea

Patients with disease of the basal ganglia may develop frequent jerky movements that constantly flit from one part of the body to another. Such movements are termed 'chorea'. The movements flit randomly around the body, in contrast to myoclonus, which tends to affect the same part or parts of the body. The absence of sustained abnormal posturing distinguishes the condition from dystonia.

Chorea occurs in a range of basal ganglia diseases, including Wilson's disease, Huntington's disease (see Ch. 12), polycythaemia, thyrotoxicosis, systemic lupus erythematosus, cerebrovascular disease and several other rarer neurodegenerative conditions. Sydenham's chorea is still occasionally seen following streptococcal infection in the UK. Pregnancy and the oral contraceptive pill are also associated with chorea. Chorea can be a side-effect of chronic neuroleptic medication.

Where possible, the underlying cause of chorea should be treated. Chorea itself may respond to tetrabenazine, a drug that depletes presynaptic dopamine stores. Neuroleptic medication is also used.

Ballismus

Violent, large-amplitude, involuntary movements of the limbs are called ballismus, or, if they affect only one side of the body, hemiballismus. These movements are often so large that they throw the patient off balance. They are continuous and may lead to exhaustion and even death. The usual cause of ballismus is cerebrovascular disease (Berardelli, 1995). It can be treated with tetrabenazine.

Dystonia

Dystonia (previously known as athetosis) describes a condition where limbs or body parts are twisted into abnormal postures by sustained muscle activity. Typically, dystonia is brought out by attempted movement. However, despite the contorted posturing, such patients are often able to accomplish remarkably skilled tasks.

Dystonia may be generalised, affecting the whole body, or localised, affecting a single body part or segment. Dystonia affecting just one side of the body is termed 'hemidystonia' and is of clinical significance because its presence should lead to a search for a lesion in the contralateral basal ganglia.

Generalised dystonia is most commonly due to idiopathic torsion dystonia. The condition usually begins in childhood and affects the legs first. Most cases are inherited in an autosomal dominant fashion, most commonly being linked to the DYT1 gene (Misbahuddin & Warner, 2001). Dystonia is also seen following actual or presumed cerebral insults at or around the time of birth; a diagnosis of dystonic (athetoid) cerebral palsy may be made in such circumstances. More rarely, generalised dystonia may be a manifestation of a recognised metabolic disease or storage disorder. There is a rare type of familial dystonia called dopa-responsive dystonia with diurnal fluctuations. This condition responds exquisitely to levodopa. Dopa-responsive dystonia has recently been shown to result from an abnormality in the synthesis of tetrahydrobiopterin (Nygaard, 1995).

Focal dystonias usually begin in adult life and commonly affect the eyes (blepharospasm), neck (torticollis) or upper limb. The legs are rarely affected. Upper-limb dystonia may be task-specific and may be the cause of some occupational cramps. Standard investigations rarely identify an underlying cause, although some cases may have a genetic basis.

Electrophysiological recordings in dystonia show abnormal patterns of muscle activation with cocontraction of agonist and antagonist muscles (Rothwell, 1994). These abnormalities seem to be due to reduced reciprocal inhibition. When a muscle is activated voluntarily, its antagonist muscles normally relax. The relaxation of antagonist muscles depends in part upon reciprocal inhibition: afferent impulses from the activated muscle inhibit the firing of motoneurones subserving antagonists. In patients with dystonia, reciprocal inhibition is reduced and cocontraction occurs.

Various treatments have been used in dystonia, including drugs (especially anticholinergics, neuroleptics, tetrabenazine), botulinum toxin injections and surgery (section of nerves and roots). Botulinum toxin is the treatment of choice for blepharospasm (a focal dystonia of facial muscles causing involuntary eye closure) and is often very beneficial in torticollis.

Ataxia

Ataxia describes a disturbance in the co-ordination of movement. Movements are clumsy and the gait is unsteady with a wide base and reeling quality. Posture may also be affected, such that there are irregular jerky movements of the trunk when sitting (truncal ataxia or disequilibrium). In addition, there may be a limb tremor which generally gets worse towards the end of a goal-directed movement – so-called intention tremor. The latter can be brought out by asking the patient alternately to touch the examiner's finger and then his or her own nose: the task is one of accuracy and not speed and can be made more difficult by ensuring that the patient touches the examiner's finger as gently as possible.

Although it is relatively easy for an experienced clinician to recognise ataxia, it is much harder to analyse exactly what about the ataxic patient's movements is abnormal. Several features seem to contribute but none is pathognomonic. Patients tend to make hypermetric movements, i.e. their limbs move farther than the desired target. They also tend to use too much force. The mechanisms that normally bring a movement to a smooth halt are abnormal and tremor commonly results. The movements of ataxic patients are also slower than normal.

The significance of ataxia is that it is almost invariably associated with disease of the cerebellum or its brainstem connections (Adams & Victor, 2001). Common causes of ataxia include multiple sclerosis (see Ch. 10), Friedreich's ataxia, alcohol and posterior fossa tumours. Less common causes include paraneoplastic syndromes and a variety of neurodegenerative conditions, some of which are hereditary (e.g. the spinocerebellar ataxias and Friedreich's ataxia).

Other disorders of movement

The following are abnormal movements that are associated with different neurological disorders.

Hemifacial spasm

Hemifacial spasm describes unilateral twitching of facial muscles due to an irritative lesion of the facial nerve. The eye winks and the corner of the mouth on the affected side elevates. There may be mild facial weakness. It responds well to botulinum toxin injections. Some patients have neurosurgery to reposition blood vessels that impinge on the facial nerve.

Orofacial dyskinesias

Orofacial dyskinesias are commonly seen in the elderly as a complication of neuroleptic treatment. They consist of involuntary lip-smacking and chewing movements, occasionally associated with tongue protrusion. Neuroleptic medication should be avoided. Tetrabenazine may provide some benefit.

Palatal myoclonus (tremor)

Some patients develop involuntary rhythmical elevation of the soft palate, which produces an audible click and interferes with speech. Some cases are associated with hypertrophy of the inferior olivary nucleus in the brainstem.

Tics

Tics are involuntary movements or vocalisations that patients may be able to suppress temporarily at the expense of increasing inner tension. The movements can be simple, e.g. a twitch of the face or arm, or more complex, when they may appear semipurposeful. Tics are associated with obsessive–compulsive disorders and the Gilles de la Tourette syndrome. Neuroleptic medication may be required.

References

Adams RD, Victor M. *Principles of Neurology.* New York: McGraw-Hill; 2001.

Bain P. A combined clinical and neurophysiological approach to the study of patients with tremor. *J Neurol Neurosurg Psychiatry* 1993, **56**:839–844.

Beckerman H, Lankhorst GJ, Verbeek ALM, et al. The effects of phenol nerve and muscle blocks in treating spasticity: review of the literature. *Crit Rev Rehab* 1996, **8**:111–124.

Berardelli A. Symptomatic or secondary basal ganglia diseases and tardive dyskinesias. *Curr Opin Neurol* 1995, **8**:320–322.

Berardelli A, Rothwell JC, Thompson PD, Hallett M. Pathophysiology of bradykinesia in Parkinson's disease. *Brain* 2001, **124**:2131–2146.

Britton TC. Essential tremor and its variants. *Curr Opin Neurol* 1995, **8**:314–319.

Brown P. Spasticity. *J Neurol Neurosurg Psychiatry* 1994, **57**:773–777.

Burke D. Critical examination of the case for and against fusimotor involvement in disorders of muscle tone. *Adv Neurol* 1983, **39**:133–150.

Cosgrove AP, Corry IS, Graham HK. Botulinum toxin in the management of the lower limb in cerebral palsy. *Dev Med Child Neurol* 1994, **36**:386–396.

Cosgrove AP, Graham HK. Botulinum toxin A prevents the development of contractures in the hereditary spastic mouse. *Dev Med Child Neurol* 1994, **36**:379–385.

Damiano DL, Quinlivan JM, Owen BF et al. What does the Ashworth scale really measure and are instrumented measures more valid and precise? *Dev Med Child Neurol* 2002, **44**:112–118.

Dattola R, Girlanda P, Vita G et al. Muscle rearrangement in patients with hemiparesis after stroke: an electrophysiological and morphological study. *Eur Neurol* 1993, **33**:109–114.

Davidoff RA. Skeletal muscle tone and the misunderstood stretch reflex. *Neurology* 1992, **42**:951–963.

Dietz V. Human neuronal control of automatic functional movements: interaction between central programs and afferent input. *Physiol Rev* 1992, **72**:33–69.

Elble RJ, Koller WC. *Tremor.* Baltimore: Johns Hopkins University Press; 1990.

Given JD, Dewald JP, Rymer WZ. Joint dependent passive stiffness in paretic and contralateral limbs of spastic patients with hemiparetic stroke. *J Neurol Neurosurg Psychiatry* 1995, **59**:271–279.

Hyman N, Barnes M, Bhakta B et al. Botulinum toxin (Dysport) treatment of hip adductor spasticity in multiple sclerosis: a prospective, randomized, double-blind, placebo controlled, dose ranging study. *J Neurol Neurosurg Psychiatry* 2000, **68**:707–712.

Lance JW. What is spasticity? *Lancet* 1990, **335**:606.

Levy LM, Dalakas MC, Floeter MK. The stiff-person syndrome: an autoimmune disorder affecting neurotransmission of gamma-aminobutyric acid. *Ann Intern Med* 1999, **131**:523–524.

Lin JP, Brown JK, Brotherstone R. Assessment of spasticity in hemiplegic cerebral palsy. II: Distal lower-limb reflex excitability and function. *Dev Med Child Neurol* 1994, **36**:290–303.

Misbahuddin A, Warner TT. Dystonia: an update on genetics and treatment. *Curr Opin Neurol* 2001, **14**:471–475.

Noth J. Trends in the pathophysiology and pharmacology of spasticity. *J Neurol* 1991, **238**:131–139.

Nygaard TG. Dopa-responsive dystonia. *Curr Opin Neurol* 1995, **8**:310–313.

O'Dwyer NJ, Ada L, Neilson PD. Spasticity and muscle contracture following stroke. *Brain* 1996, **119**:1737–1749.

Pierrot-Deseilligny E, Mazieres L. Spinal mechanisms underlying spasticity. In: Delwaide PJ, Young RR, eds. *Clinical Neurophysiology in Spasticity.* Amsterdam: Elsevier; 1985:63–76.

Rothwell JC. *Control of Human Voluntary Movement*, 2nd edn. London: Chapman & Hall; 1994.

Sheean G. The pathophysiology of spasticity. *Eur J Neurol* 2002, **9** (Suppl. 1):3–9.

Shibasaki H. Myoclonus. *Curr Opin Neurol* 1995, **8**:331–334.

Shortland AP, Harris CA, Gough M et al. Architecture of the medial gastrocnemius in children with spastic diplegia. *Dev Med Child Neurol* 2002, **44**:158–163.

Singer B, Dunne J, Allison G. Reflex and non-reflex elements of hypertonia in triceps surae muscles following acquired brain injury: implications for rehabilitation. *Disabil Rehab* 2001, **23**:749–757.

Thilmann AF, Fellows SJ, Garms E. The mechanism of spastic muscle hypertonus. Variation in reflex gain over the time course of spasticity. *Brain* 1991, **114**:233–244.

Tsukahara N, Murakami F. Axonal sprouting and recovery of function after brain damage. *Adv Neurol* 1983, **39**:1073–1084.

Warner TT, Fletcher NA, Davis MB et al. Linkage analysis in British and French families with idiopathic torsion dystonia. *Brain* 1993, **116**:739–744.

Weiner WJ, Lang AE. *Movement Disorders: A Comprehensive Survey.* New York: Futura; 1989.

Williams PE, Catanese T, Lucey EG, Goldspink G. The importance of stretch and contractile activity in the prevention of connective tissue accumulation in muscle. *J Anat* 1988, **158**:109–114.

Chapter 5

Neuroplasticity

N Lawes

INTRODUCTION

Neuroplasticity is about changes in the connectivity of the nervous system and its relevance to clinical practice is now well established. While many of these changes are adaptive and allow us to cope with variation in the environment, some are maladaptive and contribute to clinical problems.

Although investigation of cellular mechanisms is still largely based on work on other animals, there are several papers dealing with plastic changes in the human central nervous system (CNS), many of which are clinical in context. This chapter is about how nerve cells:

- make contact with each other
- reinforce the connection when it is appropriate
- disconnect when the contact is inappropriate
- control the physiological use of anatomical connections.

The first section gives a brief overview of cellular neuroplasticity. The second section deals with plasticity in neural systems and its clinical relevance to rehabilitation. The third section gives a more detailed review of plasticity at the cellular level. Some of the material in the second section depends on familiarity with the content of the third section.

More detailed reviews can be found in Cramer & Bastings (2000), Barry & Ziff (2002), Chen et al. (2002), Fink & Meyer (2002), Gu (2002), Sjöström & Nelson (2002) and, in relation to physiotherapy, Shepherd (2001).

BRIEF OVERVIEW OF CONNECTIVITY OF THE NERVOUS SYSTEM

Nerve cells must first make contact with one another. This involves creating new neural processes, termed neurites, that will later form axons and dendrites. The neurites must then grow through the neuropil. To do this, an expansion at the distal end of the neurite, called the growth cone, must create new cell membrane (lamellipodia) and fill it with axoplasm. The growth cone must also find its way through the neuropil to target cells. To do this, the cone responds to guidance cues in its local environment. Some guidance cues attract the growth cone, while some repel it. On reaching the target, the cone must recognise the target cell, distinguishing it from non-target cells. On identifying an appropriate target, the cone has to differentiate into a mature synapse. The target cell now has to distinguish appropriate connections from inappropriate connections, retaining the former but shedding the latter.

Active and silent synapses

Once a connection has been established anatomically, cells have the option of allowing them to work physiologically, or of retaining them anatomically in a physiologically inert state. Non-functioning synapses are termed 'silent synapses'. Alternatively, a connection may be retained anatomically but presynaptically inhibited, so that it remains as a potential pathway only. The physiologically active connections of the nervous system are, therefore, a subset of the anatomical connections available.

Potentiation and depression of synapses

In an established connection that is working physiologically, cells have the option of increasing the effectiveness of the synapse, or of decreasing it. Increased effectiveness is termed 'potentiation' and if it lasts, 'long-term potentiation'. Major changes in the efficacy of a connection are achieved by the growth of new connections between cells. The number of synapses between cells alters in response to learning. Another way to increase traffic through a connection is to remove presynaptic inhibition. Some learning involves the reverse of long-term potentiation: an inhibitory pathway is made less effective. This is termed 'long-term depression'. It is particularly important in acquiring motor skills.

Detrimental and inhibitory connections

After injury resulting in denervation, cells alter their behaviour to attract new connections. Generally, cells reactivate the developmental processes that formed their connections in the first place. The cell is concerned with its own connectivity, not the functionality of the whole system to which it belongs. It follows that some of the new connections formed after injury are detrimental to the system as a whole and the task of physiotherapy is then to remove these inappropriate connections. It is also the unfortunate case that many of the cellular mechanisms enabling plasticity are, in excess, damaging to the nervous system. Activating repair mechanisms while pathological processes have already overactivated them could, in principle, do more harm than good. For example, treatment of rats within 1 week of an experimental stroke doubled the size of the lesion compared to not treating them or delaying treatment until the second week (Humm et al., 1998; Risedal et al., 1999). Many studies have shown that the molecules involved in neuronal plasticity are also neurotoxic if activated excessively during periods of cellular vulnerability (see, for example, McIntosh et al., 1997; Bazan, 1998; Dawson & Dawson, 1998; Mattson & Duan, 1999).

Once a nervous system has developed all the anatomical connections that it needs, further increases in connectivity could be maladaptive, scrambling the significance of a refined pathway. Mature nervous systems have mechanisms that prevent inappropriate new connections forming. These inhibitory mechanisms also prevent recovery from injury. Considerable effort is being made to find ways of overcoming these inhibitory mechanisms so that injured adult nervous systems can repair themselves. Generally, adult inhibitory mechanisms apply mainly to white matter, so regrowth of damaged tracts is currently very difficult without intervention. Grey matter, on the other hand, is largely free of these inhibitory mechanisms, so plasticity is more than just possible, it is probable throughout the whole of life, including old age.

PLASTICITY WITHIN NEURAL SYSTEMS

The principles outlined in the previous brief overview are expanded in the third section, which is on cellular plasticity. The current section moves up to the level of neural systems and focuses on clinically relevant changes to the nervous system.

Plasticity in muscle

There are many differing biomechanical tasks required of muscle. Two major tasks are to hold us in one position by preventing movement (postural, static activity) or to move us out of one position into another (phasic, dynamic activity). To meet the different demands, there are several types of muscle. These range from slow oxidative muscle with high endurance but not much strength at one end to fast glycolytic muscle with great strength but not much endurance at the other (see Ch. 30). In general, the neural control of these two extremes differs.

High-endurance fibre types are found in the postural and antigravity muscles controlled from the pontine reticular system and the utricular component of the vestibular system. These muscles hold a position dictated by the CNS because they are rich in muscle spindles and length-dependent group II stretch reflexes that correct any deviation from the required position. Fast glycolytic muscle fibres, by contrast, tend to be much less dominated by length-dependent spinal stretch reflexes. They are controlled by the cerebral cortex aided by the midbrain. They are more powerful because they move us from one position to another, which demands acceleration of the mass of the body part involved. Thus one set of muscle fibres prevents movement while the other produces it. How are the differing muscle types matched to the different neural pathways?

To a limited extent, the combinatorial codes of membrane proteins found elsewhere serve to identify different muscle types, predisposing them to innervation by the kinds of nerve terminal that recognise each type. This predisposition is insufficient to account for the high degree of matching actually found. As elsewhere, plasticity accounts for the bulk of the matching process. Motoneurones dependent on hindbrain and spinal afferent control have patterns of firing that differ from the patterns in motoneurones that depend on the cerebral cortex and midbrain. This is a result of their differing dendritic diameters and consequently on the ease of reaching the threshold necessary to excite them: small motoneurones have higher voltages for a given synaptic current than large motoneurones, so they are recruited earlier and more often.

> **Key point**
>
> Small motoneurones are recruited earlier and more often than large motoneurones

The muscle fibres they innervate therefore have a heavy energy demand imposed on them. This increases aerobic metabolism: capillary density, myoglobin levels and mitochondrial numbers all increase, to the detriment of the space available for contractile myofilaments. Cortically dependent muscle fibres, by contrast, are seldom activated but when they are, they reach higher intensities of contraction as they are required to produce movement, not prevent it. As they contract, fibroblasts in their tendons are compressed, causing the release of paracrine signals that diffuse into the muscle fibres. These paracrine signals upregulate the expression of genes for contractile filaments. The increase in actin and myosin causes an increase in the diameter of the muscle. These muscles have a type of myosin that hydrolyses adenosine triphosphate (ATP) rapidly. As ATP hydrolysis is the rate-limiting step in coupling contraction to excitation, these muscles have a fast twitch. The increase in force coupled with the high velocity of contraction (metres per second) combine to produce powerful contractions (joules per second). In this way muscle fibre type is very well matched to the neural demands imposed on the muscle. Such accurate matching would be miraculous were it not for the fine tuning afforded by plasticity.

Plasticity in adult humans after peripheral injury

Plasticity in adult human nervous systems has been revealed by stimulation and by imaging. Reorganisation occurs in response to loss of neural tissue centrally or peripherally.

After temporary blockade of human peripheral nerves with local anaesthetic or ischaemia (Corwell et al., 1997), there are several changes:

- Action potentials evoked by transcranial magnetic stimulation in muscles proximal to the block increase.
- The cortical area from which potentials can be evoked expands.
- The intensity of stimulation required to evoke a response decreases.

Amputation in humans has a similar effect. After amputation of an upper limb, the neighbouring cortical representation of the face expands (Flor et al., 1995). Conversely, after facial nerve injury, the representation of the hand expands. The face area can substitute for the hand and vice versa.

The change in representation of the amputated limbs provides an insight into at least one mechanism underlying chronic pain. Subjects who showed a change, with the face area expanding and the area representing the missing limb contracting, were more likely to experience phantom limb pain (Flor et al., 1995). Activation of the cerebral cortex with tasks that only the cortex can solve, such as the discrimination of tactile stimuli applied to the stump, reversed the change. As the area representing the stump expanded, so the phantom limb pain decreased. In contrast, the application of undiscriminated stimuli was unable to change the representation of the stump and did not improve the experience of phantom limb pain.

Subjects who go blind early in life, and learn to read Braille, show an increase in the motor area controlling the first dorsal interosseous muscle, which moves the index finger over the page. They also show a decrease in the representation of the abductor pollicis brevis, which would elevate their hand above the page. On the sensory side, they have larger auditory evoked potentials in the auditory cortex and expanded sensory representations of the fingers used to read Braille. They also have better sound localisation. These changes could, in principle, be nothing more than epiphenomena caused by loss of visual input but not contributing to any functional adaptation. That this is unlikely is suggested by the changes in the visual cortex. The occipital lobe, lacking any visual input, responds to somatosensory input during Braille reading. Transcranial magnetic stimulation of the occipital lobe disrupts the ability of these subjects to read Braille (Cohen et al., 1997). Interestingly, this implies that they are reading with the same cortex as sighted readers. It is only the modality of the input to this cortex that has changed.

Plasticity in adult humans after central injury

In the above studies, the injury is peripheral and intact neurones related to the injured part alter their behaviour. Intact neurones deprived of their usual role adopt the function of neighbouring areas whose functions have not been lost. After central injury, the opposite occurs: neurones whose functions have not been lost take on the role of neurones that are no longer present but whose peripheral targets are still intact.

Key point
Peripheral versus central injury
Peripheral — Intact neurones deprived of their usual role adopt the function of neighbouring areas whose functions have not been lost
Central — Neurones whose function has not been lost take on the role of neurones that are no longer present but whose peripheral targets still exist

After damage to the posterior limb of the internal capsule, for example, removing descending pathways for the upper limb, the cortical representation of the face is activated by recovering hand movements if the descending pathways for the face are still intact, but not otherwise. This implies that the descending pathways for the face are involved in the recovered hand movements. Given that white matter is not plastic in adults, this requires some explanation. Has the loss of descending pathways to the face destroyed the somata of cells that would otherwise participate in plasticity? Or is the plasticity at a subcortical site, perhaps where collaterals of the descending pathways enter the reticular formation?

Neuroplasticity and motor skills

The acquisition of a motor skill places different requirements on different parts of the nervous systems at different stages of the learning process. Critical systems involve the cerebral cortex, the basal ganglia and the cerebellum. The three systems involve the following structures:

- dorsolateral prefrontal cortex, caudate nucleus, globus pallidus, thalamus and supplementary motor cortex form one system
- sensorimotor cortex, putamen, globus pallidus, thalamus and premotor cortex form another
- cerebral cortex, pons, cerebellum, thalamus and motor cortex form a third.

The first of the above systems is concerned with learning sequences of movements, particularly the transition between components of a sequence. Many structures related to this system, such as the anterior cingulate gyrus, are active while acquiring the new sequence but become inactive once the sequence is learned. They are about learning new sequences, not about performance of what has been learned. This system has also been attributed with response selection, or deciding what to do.

More posterior structures, such as posterior parts of the striatum or the dorsal part of the dentate nucleus, are more involved in expressing what has been learned than in acquiring new learning.

The dorsolateral prefrontal cortex is also involved in explicit and declarative learning, whereas the cerebellum is more involved in implicit and procedural learning. The two forms of learning occur in parallel and one can to some extent substitute for the other. For example, when learning to respond to different cues with different fingers, learning can be measured by reaction times and by asking the subject. When there is a pattern in the cues, reaction times decrease before the subject is consciously aware that there is a pattern present. At this stage, the cerebral cortex is less active than the cerebellum. There follows a stage in which the subject is dimly aware of the presence of a pattern but cannot articulate what it is. The cortex and the cerebellum are now both active. Finally, the subject becomes explicitly conscious of the pattern and the cortex reverts to normal levels of activity. After damage to the cerebellum, implicit learning is lost and the subjects have to rely on declarative learning (Molinari et al., 1997). Educationalists who advocate learning skills from textbooks instead of by real practice need to rethink their approach.

It has been suggested that the cerebellum has an excitatory input to layers IV and V of the motor cortex via the thalamic nucleus ventralis lateralis, while a second inhibitory loop to layers I, V and VI of the sensory cortex travels via the intralaminar nuclei of the thalamus.

Site of plasticity: subcortical versus cortical

Whereas early changes in functional magnetic resonance imaging (MRI) are visible in the dorsolateral prefrontal cortex and the presupplementary motor areas, later changes are more prevalent in the intraparietal sulcus and the precuneus on the medial surface of the cerebral hemisphere (Sakai et al., 1998). Changes have been detected around the rim of an infarct, in supplementary motor areas and in the contralateral sensorimotor cortex. Positron emission tomography (PET) has revealed changes in the premotor cortex, sensorimotor cortex and the cerebellum. These studies have been extensively reviewed (Cramer & Bastings, 2000; Hikosaka et al.,

2002; Chen et al., 2002; Molinari et al., 2002; Rijntjes & Weiller, 2002).

Direct attempts to investigate the site of plastic change have been made. After both ischaemic nerve block and amputation, the excitability of the spinal cord and of descending pathways appears to be unaltered, whereas the excitability of cortical neurones increases. The assumption underlying these conclusions is that electrical stimulation accesses the axons of descending pathways directly, whereas transcranial magnetic stimulation acts on interneurones synapsing on the tract cells. The plasticity revealed in these studies thus appears to affect cortical interneurones rather than projection neurones (Nakamura et al., 1996).

Other studies, however, have shown that plasticity can occur in the spinal cord (Thompson et al., 1994; Kapfhammer, 1997). Deafferented dorsal column nuclei, for example, acquire connections from regions proximal to the amputation (Florence & Kaas, 1995). The H-reflex can be altered by reward in both humans and other primates. Transection of the spinal cord revealed that the alteration of the H-reflex, far from disappearing, generalised to the untrained side. Clearly, learning within the spinal cord was more widespread than its expression in the intact animal revealed. The role of descending pathways in this situation was to restrict the expression of learning to the rewarded limbs, rather than to mediate the learning directly. An early, small change in the H-reflex was attributed to supraspinal sites, whereas a larger, slower change was attributed to the spinal cord itself.

Site of plasticity: ipsilateral versus contralateral

The studies in the previous section considered cortical versus subcortical sites of plasticity. After damage in the cerebral hemispheres, two related issues are: what other areas in the same hemisphere can mediate recovery, and how much of the recovery depends on the contralateral hemisphere? Early animal work suggested that the recovery of lost function was restricted to the territory innervated by a single thalamocortical projection zone, or about 2000 μm. More recent work suggests that participation of areas as far away as 14 000 μm can adopt the functions of injured cells (Manger et al., 1996). Areas quite remote from damaged tissue also alter their activity. Areas as far away from motor cortex as the insula, inferior parietal cortex and the supplementary motor cortex are activated by finger movements after striatocapsular infarcts.

It is worth pointing out that after a cortical lesion, the cortex of the contralateral hemisphere has lost commissural input from the damaged hemisphere and also the target of its own commissural fibres, so that it is not actually intact. Changes in the contralateral hemisphere may therefore reflect responses to its own injury as well as responses to injury in the opposite, infarcted hemisphere.

Patients showing alterations in the hemisphere contralateral to a cerebral injury often also have mirror movements: as they attempt to move the paretic limb, movements appear in the non-paretic limb. Plasticity in the hemisphere contralateral to the main injury predicts poor recovery (Turton et al., 1996; Netz et al., 1997). Good recovery is associated with the absence of mirror movements and the development of an enlarged representation in the damaged hemisphere. On the other hand, there is a report of patients who made a recovery, but lost the recovery when the previously intact hemisphere was damaged by a second stroke (Fisher, 1992; Lee & van Donkalaar, 1995).

> ### Key point
>
> Good recovery from brain damage is associated with the absence of mirror movements

The significance of plastic changes

The changes shown by transcranial magnetic stimulation and by imaging studies are not direct visualisations of the stored information. Rather, they are expressions of altered metabolism and excitability during the process of acquiring the information. Once the information is fully acquired, the increased metabolism and excitability are no longer required so they revert to normal levels. Obviously, the new information is still stored in the nervous system but it is no longer directly visible to current methods of investigation; its presence can be verified only by indirect testing of its use. Six months after a fortnight of constraint-induced therapy, for instance, improvements in motor performance persisted, although the visible cortical changes brought about by the constraint therapy had reverted to normal (Liepert et al., 2000).

The inconsistencies between imaging studies and magnetic stimulation studies need interpretation. Transcranial magnetic stimulation indicates that recovery is associated with reorganisation of the damaged hemisphere and correlates negatively with responses being evoked from the undamaged hemisphere. Functional MRI and PET studies, in contrast, indicate that increased activation of the undamaged hemisphere predict good recovery. There are many speculative explanations for this discrepancy. High-intensity magnetic stimulation of the undamaged hemisphere could have excited the damaged hemisphere, or insufficient stimulation could have been subthreshold. Magnetic stimulation is a measure of excitability, not of activation. Increased activity in imaging studies may reflect increased inhibition rather than increased excitation, particularly in relation to the suppression of mirror movements.

Timing of therapeutic intervention

It is frequently claimed that most recovery after a stroke occurs in the first few months and that a plateau is reached within a year, after which further improvement is difficult to achieve. This claim is also cited as evidence that what recovery there is, is part of the natural history of the disease and not a result of therapeutic intervention. On the contrary, therapeutic intervention has been shown to be effective 6 years after a stroke (Liepert et al., 1998). After a stroke involving the upper limb, patients naturally tend to use the affected limb less than the normal one. This non-use reinforces and contributes to the lack of use. A study of constraint-induced therapy involved preventing the use of the unaffected hand while practising movement of the affected hand for a fortnight, 6 h a day. At the end of this period of intensive rehabilitation, the cortical area for the abductor pollicis brevis in the treated hand had increased, whereas that for the constrained hand had decreased (Liepert et al., 1998; also see Ch. 29). This correlated with an improvement in motor scores. Other studies of hand representation in humans have been conducted (Bastings & Good, 1997; Traversa et al., 1997) and the role of rehabilitation confirmed in animal studies (Nudo et al., 1996).

Age-dependent changes in plasticity

The age at which injury occurs has a profound effect on the type and extent of plasticity. Hemispherectomy, for example, is followed by extensive recovery if performed in early childhood, but little recovery in adulthood (Benecke et al., 1991). Subjects who are blinded in later life do not activate the visual cortex when reading Braille, nor is their reading of Braille disrupted by transcranial magnetic stimulation, in contrast to those who are blind from birth. Some of these age-dependent processes result from the closure of critical periods. Others depend on the type of central myelin being expressed.

One of the age-dependent changes that restricts the level and type of plasticity relates to the inhibition of regrowth of axons. The proteins found in adult, but not neonatal, myelin inhibit growth, as described in the section on growth cones below. Scar tissue also inhibits the growth of axons. In the immediate future, recovery in adults has to depend on plasticity restricted to grey matter, where there is significantly less adult myelin. In the context of research, regrowth in white matter has been achieved by neutralising the inhibitory effect of myelin and by avoiding scar tissue (Fouad et al., 2001).

Active participation by the patient

In some approaches to physiotherapy, much is made of the active participation of the patient. This is in line with the dominant viewpoint in educational theorising, to the effect that active learning is assumed to be better than passive learning. What mechanisms could justify this viewpoint?

Active participation of the patient (or student) involves modulatory systems in the core of the CNS. These systems mediate arousal, vigilance, sensory discrimination, focused attention, perception, learning, memory, emotions such as exhilaration, euphoria and anxiety, and feelings such as self-confidence and interest. They originate in a medial core of the brainstem and forebrain containing a number of relatively small nuclei that modulate plasticity in the nervous system. This section examines their contribution to neuroplasticity.

Cholinergic modulating system

One of the modulatory systems originates in cholinergic neurones. These reside in the medial basal forebrain and in the pons. They are particularly concerned with focused attention and sensory discrimination. As described above, after peripheral nerve injury the cortical representation of the denervated region shrinks and the neighbouring innervated representation expands. This change depends on the integrity of the medial basal forebrain whose cholinergic neurones innervate the cerebral cortex. Pairing of a stimulus with activation of cholinergic neurones leads to plastic changes. For example, if the basal nucleus of Meynart is electrically stimulated in synchrony with mechanical stimulation of the skin, cutaneous stimulation subsequently evokes larger responses. The same applies to the auditory system: pure tones paired with cholinergic stimulation are selectively enhanced. The mechanism involves enhancing the excitatory changes and reducing the inhibitory changes in a neurone. This is achieved by muscarinic receptors for acetylcholine, which reduce potassium conductance and increase the calcium conductance of the N-methyl-D-aspartate (NMDA) receptor channel (Gu, 2002). Activation of cholinergic neurones is known to delay the progression of dementia. For example, patients suffering from Alzheimer's disease who smoke deteriorate more slowly than non-smokers with the same condition.

Noradrenergic modulating system

Another modulatory system is noradrenergic. These cells reside in the locus ceruleus in the floor of the fourth

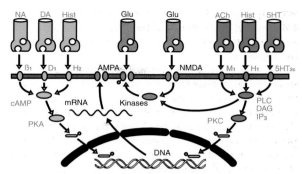

Figure 5.1 Modulatory transmitters and memory. Short-term memory depends on the activation of kinases that phosphorylate channels such as the α–amino-3-hydroxy-5-methyl-4-isoxazole propionate (AMPA) channel, so altering its dynamic characteristics. The N-methyl-D-aspartate (NMDA)–kinase–AMPA pathway represents this. Long-term memory depends on phosphorylating transcription factors that upregulate genes, represented by the DNA–mRNA–AMPA channel pathway in the figure. This can be activated either through the cAMP–protein kinase A (PKA) pathway or via the phospholipase C–protein kinase C (PKC) pathway. NA, noradrenaline (norepinephrine); DA, dopamine; Hist, histamine; glu, glutamate; Ach, acetylcholine; 5HT, 5-hydroxytryptamine (serotonin); cAMP, cyclic adenosine monophosphate; mRNA, messenger ribonucleic acid; DAG, diacylglycerol; IP$_3$, inositol triphosphate.

ventricle. The locus ceruleus is concerned with general arousal, vigilance and the response to interesting stimuli. It also generates anxiety. It has an important role in development. For example, the developmental plasticity of ocular dominance columns depends on noradrenergic systems. When one eye is closed during development, cells plastically increase their responses to the open eye, and then recover binocular responses when the closed eye is reopened. These changes are accelerated by noradrenaline (norepinephrine) and delayed by destruction of noradrenergic cells.

Serotonin is necessary for perception, emotion and mood. It is particularly notorious for its role in depression, being found at very low levels in the brains of people who successfully commit suicide. The plasticity of ocular dominance columns depends on serotonin.

Dopamine is involved in alertness, self-confidence, exhilaration and euphoria. It seems to be particularly important in learning that depends on reward.

Systems modulating memory

A summary of the actions of modulatory transmitters on short- and long-term learning is given in Figure 5.1.

Anything that increases activity in these modulatory systems will enhance neuroplasticity. It is therefore worth investing considerable time and energy in attempting to interest patients in their treatment, motivating them, influencing their emotional response to recovery and generally engaging them in the therapeutic process. Schoolteachers have traditionally activated these systems with rod and cane, or less traumatically, with the fear of exams. The gentler modern views on education have removed this option.

Prediction from neuroplasticity

Transcranial magnetic stimulation has been used to predict the outcome after a stroke (Cramer & Bastings, 2000), clearly of considerable importance where the provision of rehabilitation is insufficient to meet the needs of all patients. Magnetic fields are generated around a coil placed over the patient's head. As the magnetic field collapses, currents are induced in the brain. These excite neurones and evoke muscle action potentials in muscles controlled by the stimulated area.

Findings implying good recovery are the preservation of motor potentials in the affected hand evoked from the injured hemisphere and the early appearance of an expanded representation. Poor outcome is indicated by the appearance of motor potentials evoked from the undamaged hemisphere. This ipsilateral evoked response suggests that the undamaged hemisphere has acquired some control over the ipsilateral limb. Generally, mirror movements are evident when this happens. It implies that some compensatory strategies impede recovery. With midline structures, however, ipsilateral responses are a good indication of recovery from dysphagia.

Neuroplasticity as a cause of clinical problems

The recognition of neuroplasticity has justified therapeutic intervention after lesions of the CNS. By contrast, it is also becoming evident that neuroplasticity is sometimes a cause of clinical problems.

Cerebral palsy

If descending pathways are damaged in children before the myelin-associated inhibitory mechanisms develop, plasticity allows surviving axons to replace the damaged axons. This can result in a failure to differentiate the innervation of agonists and antagonists, which therefore are simultaneously activated, producing co-contraction. Patients must then struggle not only to activate their agonists, but also to contract against their own antagonists. This is a key issue in cerebral palsy, where therapy should be directed towards removal of inappropriate connections rather than towards creating new connections.

Experimental models

Similarly, in experimental adult animals, destruction of descending pathways reduces the number of synapses on motoneurones. Within 3 months, however, the number of synapses returns to normal. Since the descending pathways have not grown back, the additional synapses must be from local spinal neurones. It is at least plausible that some of these new synapses are maladaptive.

Chronic pain syndromes

Plasticity is particularly maladaptive in chronic pain syndromes. It affects peripheral nociceptors, mechanoceptors, dorsal horn neurones and cortical neurones (Coderre et al., 1993; Woolf & Doubell, 1994; Pockett, 1995; Baranauskas & Nistri, 1998; Mao, 1999; Vernon & Hu, 1999; Ramachandran & Rogers Ramachandran, 2000). In chronic pain attributable to peripheral nociceptors, synthesis and release of algesic proteins such as substance P increases, receptors with greater sensitivity to algesic signals are inserted into the cell membrane and potassium channels fail to open, preventing termination of the activation of pain pathways. These plastic changes are referred to as wind-up. They occur when a peripheral process sensitises C fibres, such as in chronic inflammatory conditions.

Low-threshold mechanoceptors have collaterals into pain pathways but do not normally evoke activity in them because they are presynaptically inhibited by gamma-aminobutyric acid (GABA) released from interneurones. Note that this is the exact opposite of the early versions of the gate-control theory of pain. After damage to peripheral mechanoceptors, they release nerve growth factor, causing aberrant innervation of the dorsal root ganglion cells by sympathetic neurones. They also turn on the expression of genes for noradrenergic receptors, so the sympathetic neurones form functioning synapses. They express growth-associated protein (GAP43), an indication of synaptic growth. This leads to sprouting of the mechanoceptors into the pain pathway. Finally, the GABA-mediated inhibition of the mechanoceptive terminals fails, so that low-intensity stimulation of the mechanoceptive afferents activates the spinothalamic tract cells. All this results in patients experiencing pain from low-intensity stimulation that would not normally be painful. In the past, many a patient with these plastic changes must have been dismissed as suffering from a functional condition.

In the dorsal horn, calcium entering through NMDA channels turns on enzymes that phosphorylate receptors, potentiating their responses to nociceptive input. The calcium activates enzymes that generate retrograde signals. Retrograde signals pass from dorsal horn neurones to afferent terminals, inducing an increase in the release of transmitters. These retrograde signals include prostaglandins as well as nitric oxide and carbon monoxide. Non-steroidal anti-inflammatory drugs help to prevent this plastic change (Dray et al., 1994). The calcium also activates enzymes that phosphorylate transcription factors controlling the expression of genes for receptors. The postsynaptic cell inserts additional receptors into its membrane, increasing its response to nociceptive input. All these plastic changes conspire to enhance the response of spinothalamic tract cells to peripheral input. Pain is therefore experienced even after resolution of the peripheral problem that originally evoked it.

Similar plastic changes responsible for phantom limb pain have been described above. The concept of neuroplasticity allows us to be more specific in targeting changes that were formerly attributed to an overactive imagination.

Failure to learn

One of the issues related to neural plasticity is the question of why it varies between people: if plasticity allows learning, why can't all people learn to the same extent? In the extreme, lack of the ability to learn leads to mental retardation, with an IQ of less than 70 and an inability to cope with the demands of daily life.

Among the findings associated with mental retardation are changes in the morphology of dendrites and synapses. Dendrites branch less often and they tend to have an excess of thinner spines to begin with, then a reduction in the number of spines later. The spines may be mushroom-shaped or stubby. The morphology of a synaptic spine is determined by actin, regulated by enzymes called Rho GTPases. Knowledge of the processes governing synaptic growth is becoming quite detailed, as outlined in the section on cellular plasticity below. Several genes related to failure to learn have now been identified (Boettner & van Aelst, 2002; Ramakers, 2002). Their products influence the conversion of extracellular signals into changes in connectivity, leading to development, learning and regeneration. Conversely, abnormalities of these proteins lead to morphological changes in synapses and to mental retardation.

For example, fragile X-linked mental retardation protein (FMRP) is a ribonucleic acid (RNA) binding protein that shuttles mRNA to the cytoplasm from the nucleus. As well as mental retardation, abnormalities of FMRP are associated with macro-orchidism, large ears, prominent jaws and high-pitched, jocular speech (Boettner & van Aelst, 2002).

The proteins of this signalling system also cause other pathological states apart from mental retardation. Alsin is an exchange factor for Rho GTPases (a guanine nucleotide exchange factor; GEF) and abnormalities cause the death of upper and lower motoneurones in amyotrophic lateral sclerosis. Intersectin is another Rho GEF, in this case linked to trisomy 21 or Down's syndrome. Clearly, these molecular details cannot be ignored if an understanding of abnormal-ities of the nervous system and of neuroplasticity is to be acquired.

CELLULAR CHANGES IN NEUROPLASTICITY

The growth cone

From the above overview, it is evident that the growth cone is a key structure in establishing the connections of the nervous system developmentally and also after injury. Ultimately, the adaptation of the nervous system to experience depends on neurites growing along a pathway, finding a target neurone, forming a synapse with it, and then modifying the synapse to increase or decrease its effectiveness as required. Experience leads to an alteration of synapses so that neural networks are optimised to the circumstances causing the change. This section examines the factors that induce the outgrowth of neurites, guide them to their destination, allow them to recognise a target and then alter in response to experience. In essence, an extracellular signal binds to an intramembranous receptor, which has an effect on intracellular enzymes leading to changes in the cytoskeleton.

Signalling proteins from outside the cell induce the formation of growth cones. These are called neurotrophins and they include a number of growth factors, such as nerve growth factor (NGF) and brain-derived nerve growth factor (BDNF). Attempts are being made to induce repair of damaged nervous systems by inserting grafts of cells carrying the genes for neurotrophins into the sites of damage (Blesch et al., 2002). Neurotrophins successfully induce neurite formation in several pathways. One problem, though, is that the regenerating axons tend to enter the graft instead of growing past it. A way of avoiding this is to attach a molecular switch to the DNA carrying the gene for the neurotrophic factor. The molecular switch can be turned on and off with an antibiotic such as tetracycline (Blesch et al., 2002). As the axon approaches the graft, the gene can be switched off, allowing the axon to grow past and connect to cells beyond the injury.

Mature nervous systems attempt to confine growing axons to a pathway and prevent the entry of aberrant connections. They do this with the type of myelin formed in the CNS by oligodendrocytes in adult mammals only.

This differs from the myelin found in the peripheral nervous system, in children and in non-mammals. Adult central myelin contains inhibitory factors variously known as myelin-associated glycoprotein, Nogo A to C, IN-35 and IN-250. When a growth cone comes into contact with such inhibitory factors it collapses, which stops further growth in that direction. Experimentally, it is possible to induce the growth of motor pathways across an injury by using antibodies to the inhibitory proteins (Fouad et al., 2001). Successful regrowth correlates with the acquisition or recovery of motor skills. Large molecules found in scar tissue, the chondroitin sulphate proteoglycans, also inhibit growth cones, so it is worth attempting to reduce the amount of neural scarring after injury.

A number of other signals are found either in the extracellular matrix or in the membranes of neighbouring cells (Kapfhammer, 1997). These signalling molecules control the formation of growth cones, their length and branching patterns, and whether they collapse or continue growing. They have related effects on adult synaptic spines.

The signalling molecules bind to receptors that act on enzymes within the growth cone. These enzymes, known as Rho GTPases, mediate effects on the cytoskeleton by influencing downstream enzymes, such as myosin light-chain kinase. For example, the shape of spines and growth cones is determined by polymerisation and depolymerisation of actin, controlled by Rho GTPases. Transport of vesicles to the growth cone and to active axon terminals depends on microtubules, the extension and retraction of which is controlled by these signalling molecules. Mechanical traction within the cone depends on actomyosin formation, contraction and disassembly. By controlling these cytoskeletal changes, the signalling molecules cause outgrowth, elongation, branching and retraction of nerve cell processes. They also control adhesion between cells and apoptosis, or planned cell death.

Once the growth cone reaches a suitable target cell it stops growing and differentiates into a synaptic bouton. Many of the cellular mechanisms involved in its initial growth then become available to regulate the shape and growth of the mature synapse.

Maintenance and refinement of connections

The pattern of connections achieved by guiding growth cones to appropriate targets is necessarily fairly crude. There are 10^{14} connections in the brain, but only about 15 000 proteins available to the entire nervous system. By combining proteins into combinatorial codes, analogous to combining just 10 numbers into the 10 000 different four-digit PIN numbers for cash machines, some increase in specificity is afforded. Target recognition is by a combination of a few molecules, just as the code to a security lock is a combination of a few numbers. It is a permissive code, so that loss of only one molecular type has little effect by itself. Despite this combinatorial coding, an ability to modify formed synapses is essential for any but the simplest invertebrate nervous systems. Such modification depends on the use of the synapse.

Aberrant or unhelpful axons tend to arrive at their target destination unaccompanied by other axons from the same source. Useful axons, on the other hand, tend to arrive with accomplices from the same neighbourhood. This is simply a result of mechanical jostling between axons growing together along a tract, as well as from a tendency of axons to bundle together under molecules that encourage fasciculation. When the synapse from an aberrant axon fires, it therefore tends to fire on its own, producing only a limited response from the target neurone. Synapses from coherent sources, on the other hand, tend to fire together. This results in spatial summation and strongly depolarises the postsynaptic cell. If a cell is sufficiently depolarised, it opens a special kind of channel, called the NMDA channel. The NMDA channel is a receptor to glutamate, which is the principal excitatory transmitter in the CNS. When open, it permits the entry of calcium into the cell. Normally, however, another similar ion, magnesium, prevents the channel from opening (Dudai, 2002).

Magnesium blocks the channel whenever the postsynaptic cell is not very depolarised. Only when the postsynaptic cell is already depolarised by other afferents will the magnesium be expelled from the channel, allowing it to open and increase calcium influx.

Spatial summation produces sufficient depolarisation to expel magnesium from the NMDA channel and cause an influx of calcium. Calcium then activates a number of enzymes. Some of these produce retrograde signals, which pass backwards from the postsynaptic cell to the presynaptic cell (Hawkins et al., 1998). They share the characteristic that they can penetrate cell membranes, either because they are small (NO and CO) or because they are lipids (prostaglandins). The retrograde signal encourages the presynaptic cell to remain connected.

Critical periods

In some neural systems, particularly sensory systems, the period of development and refinement of connections is limited. At the end of this critical period, the pathway has matured and further modification becomes very difficult. A well-known example is the refinement of binocular vision that allows us to develop stereoscopic vision. This gives us an indication of how far away objects are by comparing the disparity in viewpoint between the two eyes. If the two eyes are not properly aligned in early childhood, stereoscopic vision does not develop and correction of the squint after the end of the critical period is too late.

Systems with critical periods

There are a number of systems with critical periods. Language is an obvious one. If children do not learn a language before the end of the critical period, they are unable to acquire language later. Adults are well aware of the difficulty of learning a foreign language, yet young children do so effortlessly in a year or two. Learning to play music before the age of 9 induces an expansion of the auditory cortex devoted to musical notes. After the age of 9, this expansion does not take place.

Congenitally deaf people have enhanced visual detection of peripheral movement not found in people who become deaf later in life. They also have enhanced visual evoked responses in the striate cortex. Conversely, congenitally blind people have an enhancement of sound localisation that does not happen in people with visual impairment acquired later in life. There is some evidence that, depending on the sport, top-class athletes have to reach their high levels of skill by late adolescence or they never get to international standards.

Mechanisms for critical periods

There are two main mechanisms to account for critical periods (Chugani, 1998; Berardi et al., 2000). One relates to the subunits of the NMDA receptor. Early in life, subunit 2B predominates. This subunit promotes prolonged opening times, allowing the large influxes of calcium that result in plasticity. Later in life, the type 2B subunit is replaced by another type, 2A. This has a short opening time, restricting the entry of calcium and limiting the plastic changes produced.

A second mechanism is to do with the development of inhibitory interneurones. There is a temporal window between the development of excitatory and inhibitory synapses. The duration of window opening depends on the expression of neurotrophic genes such as BDNF. When this window is open, plastic changes can occur. Once inhibitory interneurones develop, the window closes and further change is difficult. If there is a long interval between the development of excitatory and inhibitory synapses, greater change can occur and higher levels of sophistication can be reached by the system. If, on the other hand, inhibitory synapses develop soon after the excitatory synapses, the window of opportunity for changing the system is too short to allow much

development and the level of sophistication reached is much lower. To the extent that this applies to any particular system, late developers may well develop further than precocious individuals who rapidly reach their peak and develop no further. The implications for the rearing and education of children need to be explored fairly carefully.

Critical windows can be held open by experimental techniques, such as keeping an animal in the dark, but these are too drastic to be of current therapeutic interest. Perhaps future approaches will involve reopening a critical window to allow redevelopment.

Removal of inhibition

There are many forms of plasticity extending over several different timescales. One form, which is very rapid, is the removal of inhibition. Within the forelimb representation in the motor cortex, there are axon terminals that originate from cells outside the forelimb area. These axon terminals are inhibited by GABA interneurones, so that they exist anatomically but make no contribution physiologically (Jacobs & Donaghue, 1991). Approximately a third of the neurones in the motor cortex release GABA. If these are blocked by injection of the antagonist bicuculline into the motor cortical representation of the forelimb, stimulation outside this area is able to evoke forelimb movements.

This implies that motor areas have dormant connections that are normally prevented by GABA interneurones from evoking the represented movement. A rapid form of plasticity simply involves removal of this inhibition, so enabling neighbouring areas to take on the disinhibited function. Similarly, loss of input to somatosensory cortex and visual cortex results in a reduction of the number of neurones that synthesise and release GABA, a major cortical inhibitory transmitter.

The NMDA channel

The NMDA channel responds to glutamate from the presynaptic cell only if the postsynaptic cell is already sufficiently depolarised. It opens only when both cells are sufficiently active at the same time, laying the foundations for the statement: 'if two cells fire together, they wire together'. When the NMDA channel opens, calcium enters the cell and activates enzyme systems that alter the cell's behaviour in the future. A previous section emphasises its role in refining the crude nervous system that developmental processes initially produce.

The NMDA channel continues in this process of adapting neural connections in response to variation in the environment throughout life. When calcium enters the postsynaptic cell through the NMDA channel, it activates an enzyme called calmodulin, which activates a calcium calmodulin-dependent kinase known as CaMKII. Calcium calmodulin kinase is weakly bound to actin until the entry of calcium disrupts this binding and allows it to translocate to the postsynaptic density for several minutes. The strength of binding to the postsynaptic density is increased by a stronger stimulus and by a priming stimulus. Binding to the postsynaptic density is terminated by protein phosphatase 1 (PP1). In the postsynaptic density, calmodulin acts on over 30 substrates, as a result of which existing α-amino-3-hydroxy-5-methyl-4-isoxazole propionate (AMPA) receptors increase their conductance and new AMPA receptors are delivered to silent synapses. The next time this pathway is used, the postsynaptic cell will respond with a larger postsynaptic potential. Calcium calmodulin kinase II also activates enzymes that change the cytoskeleton, so structural alterations occur as well. Animals deficient in this system can learn and retain information for up to 3 days, but after 10 days their memories are defective (Frankland et al., 2001).

Silent synapses

The main excitatory transmitter in the CNS is glutamate. Two important receptors to glutamate are the AMPA channel, which permits the entry of sodium into the cell, and the NMDA channel. Many synapses develop anatomically but remain dormant physiologically. Activating them so that they start to transmit is one of the mechanisms of inducing plastic change. These synapses have NMDA receptors to glutamate but they lack the conventional sodium receptor channel, known as the AMPA channel. When the pre- and postsynaptic cells are activated simultaneously, the NMDA channel opens to admit calcium, which causes the postsynaptic cell to turn on its genes for AMPA channels (upregulation). The newly synthesised proteins are inserted into the postsynaptic membrane. This potentiates the formerly silent synapse. Conversely, when the AMPA receptors of a previously active synapse are removed, synaptic depression has occurred. Removal of AMPA receptors follows phosphorylation at a site that disconnects the channel from its anchorage proteins. A protein, PICK1, binds protein kinase C to the GluR2 subunit, causing phosphorylation. The phosphorylated AMPA channel is then removed from the membrane by endocytocis. Long-term depression is particularly important in the cerebellum during the acquisition of new motor skills, for example.

The transition from silent synapse to active synapse, to potentiated synapse also involves a change in the specific components of the AMPA channel (Barry & Ziff, 2002).

Structural changes

Some synapses involve a postsynaptic protrusion known as the synaptic spine, while other synapses are on the dendritic shaft itself. Synaptic spines confine changes to that specific synapse, whereas synapses on dendritic shafts permit diffuse, non-specific changes to spread to distant synapses. New spines form very quickly: spines capable of neurotransmission have been seen to form in as little as 30 min (Friedman et al., 2000). This refutes any denial of neural plasticity based on the assumption that it is too slow to account for the changes obtained in learning. Spines form in the absence of calmodulin, but they will then degenerate within 3 days. Thus calmodulin is needed to maintain spine morphology. Spine morphology is abnormal in dementia and in mental retardation (Ramakers, 2002).

The shape of synapses alters with learning and development. After potentiation, synapses become concave towards the dendrite, whereas rapid synaptogenesis in development produces synapses that are convex away from the dendrite (concave towards the bouton). These changes relate to the cytoskeleton. Within a synaptic spine, there is a core of actin. High levels of activity and opening NMDA channels raise intracellular calcium, which leads to cytoskeletal assembly and concave synapses.

Low levels of activity cause a smaller rise in intracellular calcium, disassembly of the cytoskeleton and convex spines. Potentiation increases the number of synapses with incomplete postsynaptic densities, called 'perforated synapses'. Early interpretations suggested that perforation was a sign of a synapse about to split into two, but there are arguments against this interpretation (Marrone & Petit, 2002). An alternative explanation is that most of the release of transmitter occurs at the edge of the active zone. Perforations increase the edge of the active zone in proportion to its surface area and thereby increase the probability of releasing transmitter.

The timing of activity

When a pre- and postsynaptic cell fire, the relative timing of their action potentials is crucial. If the presynaptic cell fires less than 10–15 ms before the postsynaptic cell, potentiation occurs. If, on the other hand, the postsynaptic cell fires first, then long-term depression occurs instead (Sjöström & Nelson, 2002). In principle, knowledge of the relative times of activation of different pathways by different handling strategies could be important to physiotherapists wishing to modify pathways. Attempts to disconnect two groups of cells would involve activating the postsynaptic group before the presynaptic group. This section explores some of the cellular principles involved.

Action potentials generally begin in the axon hillock. An orthodromic potential propagates down the axon, but additionally, an antidromic potential can propagate backwards into the dendritic tree. The effectiveness of a synapse influences whether long-term potentiation occurs: effective synapses can induce potentiation without temporal summation, whereas less effective synapses have to summate temporally to have an effect. Thus weak synapses can potentiate only at high frequencies, whereas strong synapses can potentiate even at low frequencies.

The structure of the dendritic tree is also influential. Highly branched dendrites afford more opportunities for an action potential to fail, and the ratio of sodium to potassium conductance is less important. In less branched dendritic trees, on the other hand, there are fewer opportunities for failure and the ratio of ionic conductances becomes more important.

The rate of calcium influx is also important: small, slow influxes (180–450 nmol/L) induce long-term depression, whereas large fast influxes (>500 nmol/L) produce long-term potentiation. Intermediate levels of influx have neither effect.

Transcription and translation

The genome is encoded in double strands of DNA. Transcription is the copying of the DNA triplet codes into RNA triplet codes. A single strand of RNA, messenger RNA, leaves the cell nucleus and enters the cytoplasm. The triplet codes are then translated into amino acid sequences making up a protein. Some mRNA codes for general housekeeping proteins. These strands of RNA remain in the cell body. Other strands of mRNA code for the proteins used in synapses, particularly in relation to synaptic plasticity. These synapse-specific strands migrate retrogradely along the dendrites until they dock at a synapse, awaiting translation when the need arises.

Translation is then specific to the synapse that induces it. In this way, a single species of molecule can be distributed at several different synapses, but become activated at only one. This allows specific learning to occur, such that a single cell can learn about different inputs separately. For example, a neurone could learn to flex the lower limb in response to pinprick, but learn not to flex in response to innocuous contact with the floor. It is this synaptic specificity that ensures that information-rich therapies, such as physiotherapy, will always be more effective than information-poor therapies, such as drug therapy. Drugs will alter every synapse bearing the appropriate receptor, whereas physiotherapy activates specific pathways and depresses others.

Presynaptic mechanisms

In the presynaptic terminal, there is an active zone of readily releasable vesicles, and a reserve domain of less readily released vesicles. The vesicles in the readily releasable pool are docked to the presynaptic terminal. The vesicles in the reserve pool are tethered to the presynaptic cytoskeleton.

One form of plasticity involves moving vesicles from the reserve pool into the readily releasable pool so that they are more easily released the next time the synapse is used (Schneggenburger et al., 2002). Synapsins are actin-associated phosphoproteins that tether vesicles to the cytoskeleton. Vesicles move from the reserve domain to the readily releasable pool in response to large influxes of calcium through presynaptic voltage-gated channels, and the process involves the release of calmodulin from GAP43 by protein kinase C (PKC). Calcium calmodulin kinase phosphorylates synapsin, releasing vesicles from the reserve pool so that they are now available at docking sites. The next time the synapse is used, the probability of releasing a vesicle is higher.

The neuromuscular junction

Myogenic phase

In the myogenic phase of development, immature muscle fibres display behaviour that encourages innervation (Hannan & Zhong, 1999). They are capable of detecting the presence of approaching neurones because they have high-affinity acetylcholine receptors that can bind acetylcholine even in the low concentrations caused by diffusion from the approaching neurone. On receipt of the cholinergic signal, the muscle fibres secrete NGF. NGF alters the distribution of adhesion molecules on the surface of the growth cone in such a way that it can adhere only on the side nearest the muscle. This causes it to turn towards the muscle and the axon continues to grow until it reaches the muscle, which it identifies as a suitable target. The muscle fibre causes the growth cone to differentiate into a mature axon terminal.

Neurogenic phase

At this point, the beginning of the neurogenic phase, the axon terminal alters the muscle.

- Acetylcholine receptors are made to aggregate under the terminal.
- Extrajunctional receptors are removed from the sarcolemma by endocytosis so the muscle is less able to respond to extraneous acetylcholine from other neurones.

- At the same time, the genes for the high-affinity acetylcholine receptor are turned off and genes for the low-affinity adult form are upregulated.
- The muscle is now capable of responding only to the high concentrations of acetylcholine found at the neuromuscular junction.

For a time, muscle fibres are innervated by too many axon terminals, but in time the excess are pruned and only one terminal remains. Neurogenic domination of the muscle's phenotype is maintained by activity. Specific frequencies of excitation leading to pulses of intracellular calcium are involved. Subjunctional nuclei continue to make the proteins required by the axon terminal, while extrajunctional nuclei are inhibited from transcribing the genes suitable to the myogenic phase. For the physiotherapist, stimulation of a recovering muscle should attempt to imitate the specific patterns of neural activation that maintain the neurogenic phase. This is similar for musculoskeletal conditions, such as quadriceps weakness due to patellofemoral pain, where the effectiveness of electrical stimulation of the muscle is dependent on the stimulation frequency used (e.g. Callaghan et al., 2001).

> **Key point**
>
> Stimulation of a recovering muscle should attempt to imitate specific patterns of neural activation

Denervated muscle

If the muscle is denervated, the specific frequencies of excitation are no longer available. Suppression of extrajunctional muscle nuclei is terminated, so the genes of the myogenic phase are reactivated. The high-affinity form of the acetylcholine receptor is expressed. It is distributed all over the sarcolemma, instead of being confined to the neuromuscular junction. Consequently, the muscle fibre is able to respond to low levels of circulating acetylcholine, which cause it to fasciculate, a characteristic of lower motoneurone lesions. The genes for proteins that attract neurones back to the denervated muscle fibre and retain them are transcribed and translated. Thus denervated muscle fibres induce sprouting from neighbouring axons. Whereas the muscle fibres of a normally developed motor unit are scattered throughout the muscle, muscle fibres belonging to motor units formed by sprouting after denervation will tend to cluster in one place. The motor unit will also be larger than usual, decreasing the fine control of muscle contraction available. Such changes are also seen in old age.

CONCLUSIONS

From the evidence presented in this chapter, it is clear that the negative, pessimistic viewpoint of earlier decades was unjustified: considerable change can be made to the adult nervous system. By understanding the dynamics of the processes leading to such changes, physiotherapists can redesign less successful therapeutic strategies and defend more successful strategies. Techniques such as imaging the brain and transcranial magnetic stimulation can be used to monitor the progress of therapeutic intervention and predict outcomes during treatment, without waiting several months for a result. Eventually, perhaps, conventional therapeutic strategies may be combined with techniques derived from a cellular level of understanding to enhance the already considerable potency of the physiotherapist.

References

Baranauskas G, Nistri A. Sensitization of pain pathways in the spinal cord: cellular mechanisms. *Progr Neurobiol* 1998, **54**:349–365.

Barry MF, Ziff EB. Receptor trafficking and the plasticity of excitatory synapses. *Curr Opin Neurobiol* 2002, **12**:279–286.

Bastings E, Good DC. Changes in motor cortical representation after stroke: correlations between clinical observations and magnetic stimulation mapping studies. *Neurology* 1997, **48**(S2):A414.

Bazan NG. The neuromessenger platelet-activating factor in plasticity and neurodegeneration. *Progr Brain Res* 1998, **118**:281–291.

Benecke R, Meyer BU, Freund HJ. Reorganisation of descending motor pathways in patients after hemispherectomy and severe hemisphere lesions demonstrated by magnetic brain stimulation. *Exp Brain Res* 1991, **83**:419–426.

Berardi N, Pizzorusso T, Maffei L. Critical periods during sensory development. *Curr Opin Neurobiol* 2000, **10**:138–145.

Blesch A, Lu P, Tuszynski MH. Neurotrophic factors, gene therapy and neural stem cells for spinal cord repair. *Brain Res Bull* 2002, **57**:833–838.

Boettner B, van Aelst L. The role of Rho GTPases in disease and development. *Gene* 2002, **286**:155–174.

Callaghan MJ, Oldham JA, Winstanley J. A comparison of two types of electrical stimulation of the quadriceps in the treatment of patellofemoral pain syndrome. A pilot study. *Clin Rehab* 2001, **15**:637–646.

Chen R, Cohen LG, Hallett M. Nervous system reorganisation following injury. *Neuroscience* 2002, **111**:761–773.

Chugani HT. A critical period of brain development: studies of cerebral glucose utilization with PET. *Prev Med* 1998, **27**:184–188.

Coderre TJ, Katz J, Vaccarino AL, Melzack R. Contribution of central neuroplasticity to pathological pain. *Pain* 1993, **52**:259–285.

Cohen LG, Celnik P, Pascual-Leone A et al. (1997) Functional relevance of cross-modal plasticity in blind humans. *Nature* 1997, **389**:180–183.

Corwell BN, Chen R, Hallet M, Cohen LG. Mechanisms underlying plasticity of human motor cortex during transient deafferentation of the forearm. *Neurology* 1997, **48**:A345–A346.

Cramer SC, Bastings EP. Mapping clinically relevant plasticity after stroke. *Neuropharmacology* 2000, **39**:842–851.

Dawson VL, Dawson TM. Nitric oxide in neurodegeneration. *Progr Brain Res* 1998, **118**:215–229.

Dray A, Urban L, Dickenson A. Pharmacology of chronic pain. *Trends Pharmacol Sci* 1994, **15**:151–197.

Dudai Y. Molecular basis of long-term memories: a question of persistence. *Curr Opin Neurobiol* 2002, **12**:211–216.

Fink CC, Meyer T. Molecular mechanisms of CaMKII activation in neuronal plasticity. *Curr Opin Neurobiol* 2002, **12**:293–299.

Fisher CM. Concerning the mechanism of recovery in stroke hemiplegia. *Can J Neurol Sci* 1992, **19**:57–63.

Flor H, Elbert T, Knecht S et al. Phantom limb pain as a perceptual correlate of cortical reorganisation following arm amputation. *Nature* 1995, **375**:482–484.

Florence SL, Kaas JH. Large-scale reorganisation at multiple levels of the somatosensory pathway follows therapeutic amputation of the hand in monkeys. *J Neurosci* 1995, **15**:8083–8095.

Fouad K, Dietz V, Schwab ME. Improving axonal growth and functional recovery after experimental spinal cord injury by neutralising myelin associated inhibitors. *Brain Res Rev* 2001, **36**:204–212.

Frankland PW, O'Brian C, Ohno M, Kirkwood A, Silva AJ. α-CaMKII in experience-dependent plasticity in the cortex is required for permanent memory. *Nature* 2001, **411**:309–313.

Friedman HV, Bresler T, Garner CC, Ziv NE. Assembly of new individual excitatory synapses: time course and temporal order of synaptic molecule recruitment. *Neuron* 2000, **27**:57–69.

Gu Q. Neuromodulatory transmitter systems in the cortex and their role on cortical plasticity. *Neuroscience* 2002, **111**:815–835.

Hannan F, Zhong Y. Second messenger systems underlying plasticity at the neuromuscular junction. *Int Rev Neurobiol* 1999, **43**:119–138.

Hawkins RD, Son H, Arancio O. Nitric oxide as a retrograde messenger during long-term potentiation in hippocampus. *Progr Brain Res* 1998, **118**:155–172.

Hikosaka O, Nakamura K, Sakai K et al. Central mechanisms of motor skill learning. *Curr Opin Neurobiol* 2002, **12**:217–222.

Humm JL, Kozlowski DA, James DC et al. Use-dependent exacerbation of brain damage occurs during an early post-lesion vulnerable period. *Brian Res* 1998, **783**:286–292.

Jacobs K, Donaghue JP. Reshaping the cortical map by unmasking latent intracortical connections. *Science* 1991, **251**:944–947.

Kapfhammer JP. Axon sprouting in the spinal cord: growth promoting and growth inhibitory mechanisms. *Anatomy Embryol* 1997, **196**:417–426.

Lee RG, van Donkelaar P. Mechanisms underlying functional recovery following stroke. *Can J Neurol Sci* 1995, **22**:257–263.

Liepert J, Miltner WH, Bauder H et al. Motor cortex plasticity during constraint-induced movement therapy in stroke patients. *Neurosci Lett* 1998, **250**:5–8.

Liepert J, Bauder H, Wolfgang HR et al. Treatment-induced cortical reorganisation after stroke in humans. *Stroke* 2000, **31**:1206–1210.

Manger PR, Woods TM, Jones EG. Plasticity of the somatosensory cortical map in macaque monkeys after chronic partial amputation of a digit. *Proc R Soc Lond* B 1996, **263**:933–939.

Mao JR. NMDA and opioid receptors: their interactions in antinociception, tolerance and neuroplasticity. *Brain Res Rev* 1999, **30**:289–304.

Marrone DF, Petit TL. The role of synaptic morphology in neural plasticity: structural interactions underlying synaptic power. *Brain Res Rev* 2002, **38**:291–308.

Mattson MP, Duan WZ. 'Apoptotic' biochemical cascades in synaptic compartments: roles in adaptive plasticity and neurodegenerative disorders. *J Neurosci Res* 1999, **58**:152–166.

McIntosh TK, Saatman KE, Raghupathi R. Calcium and the pathogenesis of traumatic CNS injury: cellular and molecular mechanisms. *Neuroscientist* 1997, **3**:169–175.

Molinari M, Leggio MG, Solida A et al. Cerebellum and procedural learning: evidence from focal cerebellar lesions. *Brain* 1997, **120**:1753–1762.

Molinari M, Filippini V, Leggio MG. Neuronal plasticity of interrelated cerebellar and cortical networks. *Neuroscience* 2002, **111**:863–870.

Nakamura H, Kitagawa H, Kawaguchi Y et al. Direct and indirect activation of human corticospinal neurons by transcranial magnetic and electrical stimulation. *Neurosci Lett* 1996, **210**:45–48.

Netz J, Lammers T, Homberg V. Reorganisation of motor output in the non-affected hemisphere after a stroke. *Brain* 1997, **120**:1579–1586.

Nudo RJ, Wise BM, SiFuentes F et al. Neural substrates for the effects of rehabilitative training on motor recovery after ischaemic infarct. *Science* 1996, **272**:1791–1794.

Pockett S. Spinal cord synaptic plasticity and chronic pain. *Anesth Analg* 1995, **80**:173–179.

Ramachandran VS, Rogers Ramachandran D. Phantom limbs and neural plasticity. *Arch Neurol* 2000, **57**:317–320.

Ramakers GJA. Rho proteins, mental retardation and the cellular basis of cognition. *Trends Neurosci* 2002, **25**:191–199.

Rijntjes M, Weiller C. Recovery of motor and language abilities after stroke: the contribution of functional imaging. *Progr Neurobiol* 2002, **66**:109–122.

Risedal A, Zeng J, Johansson BB. Early training may exacerbate brain damage after stroke. *J Cerebral Blood Flow Metab* 1999, **19**:997–1003.

Sakai K, Hikosaka O, Miyauchi S et al. Transition of brain activation from frontal to parietal areas in visuo-motor sequence learning. *J Neurosci* 1998, **18**:1827–1840.

Schneggenburger R, Sakaba T, Neher E. Vesicle pools and short-term synaptic depression: lessons from a large synapse. *Trends Neurosci* 2002, **25**:206–212.

Shepherd RB. Exercise and training to optimise functional motor performance in stroke: driving neural reorganization? *Neural Plasticity* 2001, **8**:121–129.

Sjöström PJ, Nelson SB. Spike timing, calcium signals and synaptic plasticity. *Curr Opin Neurobiol* 2002, **12**:305–314.

Tang BL. Inhibitors of neuronal regeneration: mediators and signalling mechanisms. *Neurochem Int* 2002, **42**:189–203.

Thompson SWN, Dray A, Urban L. Injury-induced plasticity of spinal reflex activity. *J Neurosci* 1994, **14**:3672–3687.

Traversa R, Cicinelli P, Bassi A et al. Mapping of motor cortical reoganisation after stroke. A brain stimulation study with focal magnetic pulses. *Stroke* 1997, **28**:110–117.

Turton A, Wroe S, Trepte N et al. Contralateral and ipsilateral EMG responses to transcranial magnetic stimulation during recovery of arm and hand function after a stroke. *Electroencephal Clin Neurophysiol* 1996, **101**:316–328.

Vernon H, Hu J. Neuroplasticity of neck/craniofacial pain mechanisms: a review of basic science studies. *J Neuromusc Syst* 1999, **7**:51–64.

Woolf CJ, Doubell TP. The pathophysiology of chronic pain – increased sensitivity to low threshold A fibre inputs. *Curr Opin Neurobiol* 1994, **4**:525–534.

SECTION 2

Neurological and neuromuscular conditions

Chapter 6

Stroke

G Baer   B Durward

INTRODUCTION

The stroke patient presents the physiotherapist with a unique complex of physical, psychological and social problems. The onset of stroke is usually sudden, with maximum deficit at the outset, so the shock to patients and their families may be devastating. Stroke is the third leading cause of death in the western world (Khaw, 1996). Incidence of stroke varies slightly according to age and geographical location; however in the western world it is generally cited at 150–250:100 000. Prevalence data are more difficult to ascertain, but are generally estimated to be 5:1000 (Warlow, 2001). Outcome following stroke is death within the first 4 weeks in approximately 20% of first strokes, full recovery in 30% and residual disability in 40–50% (Langton Hewer, 1993; Warlow, 1998; Hacke et al., 2002). Stroke recurrence is about 5% per year.

DEFINITIONS

Stroke

The term 'stroke' is used synonymously with cerebrovascular accident (CVA). The World Health Organization definition of stroke is 'a rapidly developed clinical sign of focal disturbance of cerebral function of presumed vascular origin and of more than 24-hours' duration' (Aho et al., 1980).

Transient ischaemic attack

A transient ischaemic attack (TIA) is defined as 'a clinical syndrome characterised by an acute loss of focal cerebral or monocular function with symptoms lasting less than 24 hours' (Hankey & Warlow, 1994).

Hemiplegia

Hemiplegia is defined as the paralysis of muscles on one side of the body, contralateral to the side of the brain in which the CVA occurred.

ANATOMY AND PHYSIOLOGY

The central nervous system (CNS) requires a constant blood supply to ensure continuous provision of nutrients such as oxygen (O_2) and glucose, and removal of metabolic waste products, such as carbon dioxide (CO_2) and lactic acid. A disruption to the blood supply may result in loss of consciousness within seconds and irreversible neuronal damage, and subsequent neurological deficits if the disruption lasts for several minutes.

Evolution has ensured that the brain receives an abundant and anatomically diverse blood supply, together with mechanisms to regulate blood flow under changing physiological conditions. Normal cerebral blood flow occurs between mean arterial pressures of approximately 60–150 mmHg. Cerebral blood vessels respond to altered physiological circumstances by processes of autoregulation to protect the brain, to ensure O_2 delivery and removal of metabolites. One autoregulatory mechanism is the ability of arterioles to constrict in response to raised systolic blood pressure (BP) and to dilate when systolic BP falls. A second type of autoregulation allows brain arteriole vasodilation when arterial CO_2 rises and vasoconstriction when it falls (Kandel et al., 2000). These mechanisms ensure a stable blood supply over a range of arterial BP.

Cerebral circulation

The aerobic metabolism relies on a continuous supply of blood, a more detailed description of which can be found in anatomy texts (e.g. Williams, 1995). The brain is supplied with blood by two vertebral arteries and two internal carotid arteries. The right carotid artery arises from the innominate artery, and the left carotid artery directly from the aorta. Both arteries pass up the front of the neck, and then divide into two branches: the anterior and middle cerebral arteries. These important vessels supply the frontal, parietal and temporal lobes. The two anterior cerebral arteries join anteriorly, through the anterior communicating artery, to form the front section of the circle of Willis (Fig. 6.1). This anatomical configuration ensures that severe stenosis, or even occlusion, of one of the internal carotid arteries does not necessarily result in stroke, since blood can pass from right to left (or vice versa) via the anterior communicating artery.

The two vertebral arteries are smaller than the internal carotids and are branches of the subclavian vessels. Both arteries ascend the neck through the foramina in the transverse processes of the cervical vertebrae and anastomose in front of the brainstem to form the basilar artery. Branches of the basilar artery supply the medulla, pons, cerebellum and midbrain. At the top of the midbrain, the basilar artery divides into two posterior cerebral arteries that project backwards to supply the occipital lobes. These two arteries connect to the back of the circle of Willis by small posterior communicating arteries. Therefore an anastomosis occurs between the internal carotids and the vertebral circulation. This arrangement provides further protection, and it is not uncommon to see patients who appear well, despite having bilaterally occluded internal carotid arteries.

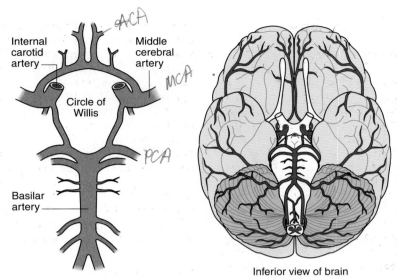

Figure 6.1 Blood supply to the brain, showing the circle of Willis. (Reproduced with permission from http://www.nlm.nih.gov/medlineplus/ency/images/ency/fullsize/18009.jpg.).

The anterior, middle and posterior cerebral arteries, which are branches of the major cerebral vessels, do not anastomose with each other and are therefore termed end arteries. The areas of the brain supplied by these vessels are relatively well designated and distinct, although anastomoses do occur at the peripheral margins of each region. If one of these vessels is blocked, then relatively predictable brain damage occurs in the area that it supplies. Systems for the classification of stroke are derived from the location and extent of brain damage (see below).

Mechanisms of neuronal cell damage

Neuronal damage after onset of stroke is progressive. There is a therapeutic window of opportunity during which stroke-specific therapy may reverse the effects of stroke or at least prevent further damage. Complex physiological, pathological and biochemical changes may cause ischaemia. Prolonged O_2 deprivation results in neuronal death; however damage can be more widespread than the specific O_2-deprived neurones. Both grey and white matter are involved. In the case of occlusion, if the infarct is not lethal, the dead tissue disintegrates and is removed by phagocytic action and replaced. The process commences at the edges of the infarct, which is gradually replaced over a period of 6 weeks or more and is eventually replaced by cerebrospinal fluid (Russell, 1983). Recent evidence also indicates that adjacent neurones may die due to the release of large quantities of an excitatory neurotransmitter, glutamate, from the axon terminals of the

O_2-deprived neurones. The excessive concentration of glutamate results in overexcitation of the neurone and subsequent excitotoxicity and cell death (Lundy-Ekman, 1998).

STROKE – TYPES, SIGNS AND SYMPTOMS

The classification of stroke types is based primarily on underlying pathology, e.g. ischaemia or haemorrhage. The extent and site of lesion can also classify types of ischaemic stroke (Bamford et al., 1991). The effects of stroke are determined by the anatomy of the brain affected, irrespective of the cause.

Ischaemic stroke

Approximately 80% of all strokes are due to occlusion, either as a result of atheroma in the artery itself or secondary to emboli (small clots of blood) being washed up from the heart or diseased neck vessels (Bamford et al., 1988). The most common cause of stroke is therefore obstruction of one of the major cerebral arteries (middle, posterior and anterior, MCA, PCA and ACA respectively, in descending order of frequency) or their smaller perforating branches to deeper parts of the brain. Brainstem strokes, arising from disease in the vertebral and basilar arteries, are less common. The patient does not usually lose consciousness but may complain of headache, and display symptoms of hemiparesis and/or dysphasia that develop rapidly. The muscles affected by hemiplegia exhibit low tone initially

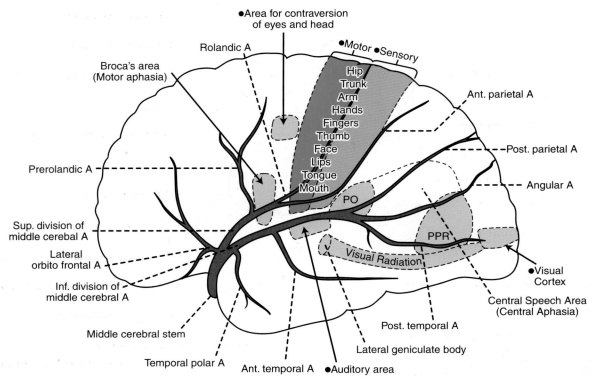

Figure 6.2   Middle cerebral artery: branches and distribution viewed from the lateral aspect of the brain. PO, parietal operculum (conduction aphasia); PPR, posterior parietal region (alexia with agraphia). (Reproduced from Adams et al. (1997) with permission, from the McGraw-Hill Companies.)

but within a few days may give way to a more mixed presentation of the muscles with high tone and soft-tissue changes (Carr & Shepherd, 1980).

The MCA supplies nearly all of the outer brain surface, most of the basal ganglia, and the posterior and anterior internal capsule via its cortical and penetrating branches (Fig. 6.2). Infarcts that occur within the vast distribution of this vessel lead to diverse neurological sequelae with a classic presentation of dense contralateral hemiplegia affecting the arm, trunk, face and leg. The optic radiation is typically affected, resulting in a contralateral homonymous hemianopia, and there may also be a cortical type of sensory loss. Cortical sensory loss is generally due to damage in the parietal cortex and refers to the paradoxical preservation of basic modalities of sensation like pain and light touch, whereas sensory modalities which require more extensive cortical processing (such as texture or sense of weight or two-point discrimination) are impaired.

Since the areas of the brain responsible for speech and language are on the left side of the brain, speech problems can be severe in left-hemisphere lesions. There may also be neglect of the contralateral side, where the patient behaves as if only perceiving information

from the unaffected side. In right-hemisphere lesions, parietal damage can lead to visuospatial disturbances, left-sided neglect and denial of weakness or other symptoms. If the main part of the MCA is not affected, but one of its distal branches is, the symptoms will be less extreme.

Posterior circulation disturbances lead to a more varied picture. Visual field defects are common and usually comprise a contralateral homonymous field deficit (Fig. 6.3). More complicated disturbances of visual interpretation or complete blindness can follow bilateral infarcts. The PCA also supplies much of the medial aspect of the temporal lobe and the thalamus, so strokes may involve impairment of memory and contralateral sensation. In addition, a thalamic syndrome with dysaesthesia may present, as may disorders of co-ordination of movement, such as tremor or ataxia.

The ACA supplies the anterior three-quarters of the medial aspect of the frontal lobe, a parasagittal strip of cortex extending back as far as the occipital lobe and most of the corpus callosum (Fig. 6.4). Occlusion of this artery may therefore cause a contralateral monoplegia affecting the leg, cortical sensory loss and sometimes the behavioural abnormalities associated with

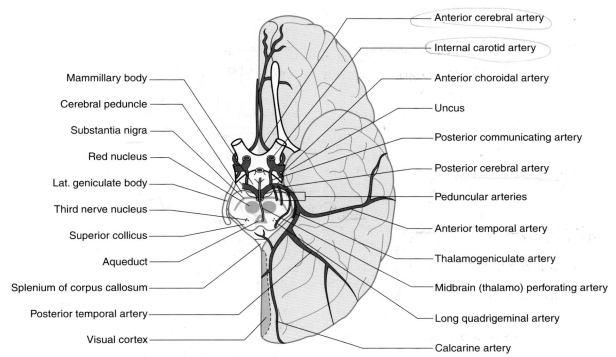

Figure 6.3 Posterior cerebral artery: branches and distribution viewed from the inferior aspect of the brain. (Reproduced from Adams et al. (1997), with permission from the McGraw–Hill Companies.)

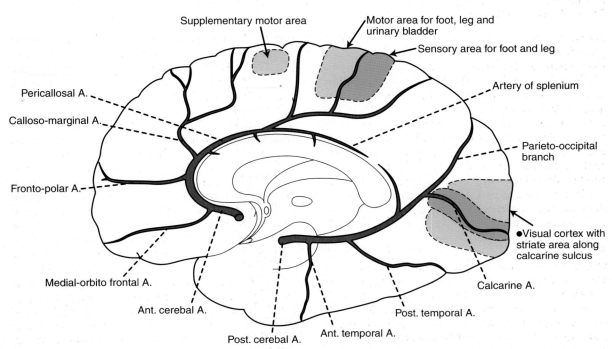

Figure 6.4 Anterior cerebral artery: branches and distribution viewed from the medial aspect of the brain. (Reproduced from Adams et al. (1997), with permission from McGraw–Hill Companies.)

frontal lobe damage. Urinary incontinence and a contralateral grasp reflex may also be apparent.

A more specific subclassification of cerebral infarct has been developed by Bamford et al. (1991). From an analysis of 543 patients with cerebral infarct, classifications were formed based on the areas of anatomical involvement. Seventeen per cent were found to have large anterior cerebral infarcts with both cortical and subcortical involvement; this group was classified as total anterior circulation infarcts (TACI). The largest group, 34%, presented with more restricted and predominantly cortical infarcts and were classified as partial anterior circulation infarcts (PACI). Twenty-four per cent had infarcts involving the brainstem, cerebellum or occipital lobes and these were called posterior circulation infarcts (POCI), and 25% had infarcts in the territory of the deep perforating arteries and these were called lacunar infarcts (LACI).

Noticeable differences have been identified in the natural history of these subtypes of infarct stroke. The TACI strokes tend to have a poor prognosis for independent functional outcome and a high mortality rate. Investigations of the different recovery patterns associated with each subtype of infarct have revealed differences that have implications for rehabilitation. Studies have indicated that patients with TACI strokes are less likely to regain an ability to walk and often walk slowly compared to those with other types of stroke (Smith & Baer, 1999; Baer & Smith, 2001). The growth of evidence related to type of stroke and recovery potential may lead to the development of more specific intervention strategies for individual patients.

Occlusion of the vertebral arteries, or the basilar artery and its branches, is potentially much more damaging, since the brainstem contains centres that control vital functions such as respiration and blood pressure. The nuclei of the cranial nerves are clustered in the brainstem and the pyramidal and sensory tracts project through it (Williams, 1995). Thus, ischaemic brain damage in the brainstem may be life-threatening and if the patient survives he or she may be severely incapacitated by cranial nerve palsies, spastic tetraplegia, ataxia and sensory loss.

Haemorrhagic stroke

Primary intracerebral haemorrhage is more frequent than subarachnoid haemorrhage. Of all first strokes, 9% are caused by haemorrhage into the deeper parts of the brain (Bamford et al., 1988). The patient is usually hypertensive, a condition that leads to a particular type of degeneration, known as lipohyalinosis or fibrohyalinosis, which results in necrotic lesions in the small penetrating arteries of the brain. The arterial walls weaken, are replaced by collagen, the wall thickens and the lumen narrows and it is thought that microaneurysms develop. These may rupture and lead to lacunar infarcts or small deep haemorrhages. The resultant haematoma may spread by splitting planes of white matter to form a substantial mass lesion. Haematomas usually occur in the deeper parts of the brain, often involving the thalamus, lentiform nucleus and external capsule, less often the cerebellum and the pons. If haemorrhage extends into the ventricular system, this is often rapidly fatal.

The onset of haemorrhagic stroke is usually dramatic, with severe headache, vomiting and, in about 50% of cases, loss of consciousness. Normal vascular autoregulation is lost in the vicinity of the haematoma and since the lesion itself may have considerable mass, intracranial pressure often rises abruptly. If the patient survives the initial haemorrhagic episode, then profound hemiplegic and hemisensory signs may appear. A homonymous visual field defect may also be apparent. The initial prognosis is poor due to the haemorrhagic lesion and the surrounding oedema. For those who survive the acute episode, recovery is often surprisingly good as the haematoma and surrounding oedema reabsorb, presumably because fewer neurones are destroyed than in severe ischaemic strokes. Occasionally, early surgical drainage can be remarkably successful, particularly when the haematoma is in the cerebellum.

Younger, normotensive patients sometimes suffer from spontaneous intracerebral haematoma from an underlying congenital defect of the blood vessels (see Ch. 7). Such abnormalities are commonly arteriovenous malformations (AVMs) – circumscribed areas of dilated and thin-walled vessels that can be demonstrated angiographically. Patients with AVMs are liable to subsequent rebleeding and surgical intervention or embolisation is undertaken when possible.

Subarachnoid haemorrhage

Subarachnoid haemorrhage (SAH) involves bleeding into the subarachnoid space, usually arising from rupture of an aneurysm situated at or near the circle of Willis (see Chs 7 and 16). The most common site is in the region of the ACA, with PCA and MCA locations almost as frequent. Congenital factors play some part in the aetiology of berry aneurysms but SAH is not predominantly a disease of the young. Hypertension and vascular disease lead to an increase in aneurysm size and subsequent rupture.

Onset generally follows a period of exertion and the patient almost always complains of sudden intense headache. Nausea and vomiting may occur, but these signs are slightly less common, as is neck stiffness. Consciousness may be lost in about 50% of cases and about 15% will die in the couple of hours prior to any medical intervention. Of those that survive, 50% will die within the first month and the survivors have a substantially increased risk of rebleeding for the next few weeks (Hijdra et al., 1988). A hemiplegia may be evident at the outset if the blood erupts into the deep parts of the brain, and other focal neurological signs may evolve over the first 2 weeks because there is a tendency for blood vessels, tracking through the bloody subarachnoid space, to go into spasm, leading to secondary ischaemic brain damage.

Early investigation by angiography, followed by either a competent neurosurgical procedure to clip the aneurysm or an endoplastic procedure to prevent rebleeding, offers the best hope for recovery (see Ch. 7).

Less frequent causes of stroke

In a small number of patients, stroke may occur due to generalised medical disorders which affect either the arteries or the blood going through them. Arteritis, or inflammation of the arteries, may be a secondary complication of meningitis, particularly tuberculous meningitis. The collagen vascular diseases, particularly systemic lupus erythematosus and polyarteritis nodosa, may affect medium and small cranial arteries which may result in stroke. Temporal arteritis, an inflammatory condition predominantly affecting the extracranial and retinal arteries in the elderly, may also give rise to stroke by intracranial involvement.

Conditions that may cause ischaemic stroke include bacterial infection of damaged heart valves (bacterial endocarditis) and atrial fibrillation (particularly if there is coincidental mitral stenosis) and mitral valve prolapse (floppy valve), which is a fairly common congenital abnormality. Echocardiography has demonstrated atrial shunts through which clots in the venous circulation can cross to the arterial supply.

Haematological diseases such as polycythaemia rubra vera, thrombocythaemia and sickle-cell disease can provoke stasis in the intracranial arteries, thus leading to ischaemic brain damage. Completed stroke occasionally complicates severe migraine if the vessel spasm which normally produces only temporary symptoms is of such intensity and such duration that ischaemic damage occurs. Leukaemia may, infrequently, cause intracranial haemorrhage due to the increased whole-blood viscosity.

There is a small but increasing number of strokes reported from drug abuse, with the most common association between cocaine and the onset of cerebral infarction, intracerebral or SAH within a short time-span.

Finally, there is evidence that women taking the contraceptive pill, particularly if it has a high oestrogen content, suffer a slightly higher incidence of stroke than those not on the pill (Hannaford et al., 1994); the absolute risk is small but is increased by cigarette smoking.

THE POPULATION AT RISK OF STROKE

Risk factors may indicate an association with increased likelihood of having a stroke but the presence of risk factors should not be taken to imply causality. Analysis of epidemiological studies indicates that the chance of having a stroke increases with age; however stroke is not a natural concomitant of increasing age (Kannel & Wolf, 1983; Warlow et al., 2001). The most significant risk factor is hypertension, either systolic (>160 mmHg) or diastolic (>95 mmHg), and there is evidence that prophylactic hypotensive therapy reduces this susceptibility but is not solely responsible for the decline in the incidence of stroke in the general population (Whisnant, 1996). A reduction of 5–6 mmHg in diastolic BP has shown a reduction of 42% in stroke in treated patients (Hacke et al., 2002). In a review, Whisnant (1996) summarised the results of 17 randomised controlled trials of treatment for hypertension, involving nearly 48 000 patients worldwide, which showed a 38% reduction in all types of stroke and a 40% reduction in fatal stroke, providing evidence which leaves no doubt about the effectiveness of treatment.

Other significant risk factors are ischaemic heart disease, high blood cholesterol, diabetes mellitus, a high-salt diet and smoking, which is a substantial independent risk factor (Whisnant, 1996; Warlow, 2001). The oestrogen-containing contraceptive pill also increases the risk of stroke (Hannaford et al., 1994).

The final common pathway for all these risk factors is the arterial disease atherosclerosis, a disease of the larger and medium-sized arteries, characterised by the deposition of cholesterol and other substances in the arterial wall. The irregular vessel wall provokes clot formation in the lumen of the artery, which may completely occlude the vessel or may dislodge to form emboli. Hypertension and other risk factors therefore predispose to ischaemic strokes, but it will be remembered that the most usual cause for intracerebral haematoma is also hypertension and the associated small-vessel disease (lipohyalinosis).

Prevention of stroke

Research evidence for strategies to reduce the lifetime risk of first stroke indicates that emphasis should be placed on reducing BP, lowering cholesterol levels, eating a diet rich in fresh fruit, vegetables and essential fats (fish oils) and low in salt and saturated fats, taking regular exercise and avoiding smoking (Gubitz & Sandercock, 2000). Such advice is available in the form of leaflets in hospitals and general practitioner (GP) surgeries and from the Stroke Association (see Appendix).

THREATENED STROKE

Threatened strokes include TIA, leaking aneurysm and asymptomatic carotid bruit, which are conditions that may predispose to stroke or may represent sub-clinical arterial disease that does not necessarily lead to a stroke.

Transient ischaemic attacks

A TIA refers to a stroke-like syndrome in which recovery is complete within 24 h. Approximately 10% of patients with TIA will go on to have a completed stroke. The symptoms depend on which part of the brain has been temporarily deprived of blood, e.g. hemisphere or brainstem. Thus, if the left MCA has been briefly occluded, symptoms may comprise weakness and clumsiness of the right side and difficulty making oneself understood (dysphasia). The symptoms evolve rapidly, and resolve more gradually, but it is unusual for the whole episode to last more than an hour and it is considered that there are no permanent sequelae. If the retinal artery is involved the patient complains of a unilateral visual field disturbance, or blindness, often descending like a curtain across the vision. Within half an hour or so (often much more rapidly) the problems resolve and vision is restored.

Virtually all patients with TIAs are put on anti-platelet therapy, such as aspirin, to reduce the chances of subsequent stroke. Risk factors may be amenable to modification (e.g. cessation of smoking, treatment of hypertension) and this can further reduce the risk of stroke (Whisnant, 1996; Intercollegiate Working Party for Stroke, 2002). A few patients will be identified as having severe stenosis (>70%) of the carotid artery and, provided this is considered symptomatic, they may be offered the operation of endarterectomy (Brown & Humphrey, 1992).

Leaking aneurysm

About 40% of patients who have an SAH have preceding symptoms of minor leaks, which usually occur within a month before the major bleed, and often go unrecognised. Symptoms are sudden headache, nausea, photophobia and sometimes neck stiffness which can resolve rapidly and may be incorrectly attributed to migraine.

Asymptomatic carotid bruit

An abnormal sound (or bruit) may be heard over the carotid artery during routine medical examination using a stethoscope. The bruit suggests turbulent blood flow due to underlying atherosclerosis and is an asymptomatic carotid bruit, if present in an otherwise healthy individual. Some 5% of patients with a bruit will go on to have a stroke, though not always in the distribution of the diseased artery.

MEDICAL EXAMINATION OF THE STROKE PATIENT

Initially, imaging and cardiac function tests are needed to differentiate between the different types of acute stroke, e.g. ischaemic, brain haemorrhage or SAH, to rule out other brain diseases, to obtain an impression about the underlying cause of brain ischaemia, to provide a basis for physiological monitoring of the stroke patient and to identify concurrent diseases or complications associated with stroke that may influence prognosis (Hacke et al., 2002). Brain imaging will differentiate between ischaemic and haemorrhagic lesions. These tests are of major importance in determining appropriate pharmacological management. The history and clinical examination are discussed in Chapter 2. Recent guidelines, produced by the Royal College of Physicians, advocate the routine imaging of all patients with suspected stroke within 48 h (Intercollegiate Working Party for Stroke, 2002, Section 6).

When tests indicate a SAH, examination of the cerebrospinal fluid (CSF) after lumbar puncture will assist confirmation of diagnosis. If the CSF is blood-stained, angiography should be undertaken to identify the source of bleeding.

Patients with small ischaemic strokes, who have made a good recovery, are investigated along the same lines as those with TIAs, to try to prevent further strokes. The cause may be immediately apparent, such as severe hypertension, in which case investigations will be limited to those indicated in the evaluation of hypertension. Assuming the patient is normotensive, routine blood tests may be helpful. An electrocardiogram (ECG) and echocardiogram should be performed if there is any chance that the heart is acting as a source of emboli. Patients with carotid-territory TIA or small completed stroke require carotid duplex (or magnetic resonance) angiography as a non-invasive technique to assess the presence and degree of carotid stenosis. Those with tight stenosis may have carotid angiography as a prelude to endarterectomy.

Integrated acute nursing, rehabilitation and medical mangement are important to (Warlow, 2001):

- maintain hygiene
- maintain hydration
- establish and maintain a clear airway
- prevent chest infection
- ensure safe swallowing
- provide appropriate positioning and regular turning.

MEDICAL MANAGEMENT

Recent recommendations for medical management based on research evidence indicate that stroke needs to be considered as a medical emergency that requires public education, specialist referral and fast management (Langhorne et al., 1993). Patients who have suffered a stroke remain at an increased risk of a further stroke (about 5% per annum). This risk is highest early after stroke or TIA. Therefore, high priority should be given to secondary prevention (Intercollegiate Working Party for Stroke, 2002).

Patients with SAH may either be treated surgically or by endoplastic procedures (see Ch. 7). Some patients with haematomas are also treated surgically. For the most part, however, the treatment of patients suffering stroke is conservative and is predominantly undertaken by GPs. There are no drugs that reduce infarct size convincingly. The neurological deficit is usually maximal at the outset and, if not severe, the patient can be managed at home satisfactorily, although recent evidence suggests that management in a specialist stroke unit has better outcomes (Kalra et al., 2000). The International Stroke Trialists Collaboration has shown that care in a stroke unit reduces mortality by 18% and reduces death or dependence by 29% (Langhorne et al., 1993). It is not clear, however, which aspects of stroke unit care contribute to improved outcomes. In practice, many patients are admitted to hospital for a short period of treatment and investigation. Patients with more severe strokes will require admission to hospital.

In some cases of ischaemic stroke, a secondary deterioration occurs 2 or 3 days after the initial event, usually due to evolving oedema around the infarct; this may respond to drug treatment. Severe hypertension should be treated cautiously and biochemical abnormalities corrected. The most rapid period of recovery occurs within the first 8–12 weeks and the time course is discussed below.

Almost all patients with ischaemic stroke are put on aspirin to prevent recurrence or extension. Those with dense hemiplegias should have antiembolic stockings and anticoagulants, such as warfarin, as prophylaxis against deep venous thrombosis (DVT). Pneumonia occurs in about 15–25% of stroke patients (Hacke et al., 2002), with the majority being caused by aspiration. Adverse outcomes may be reduced by appropriate nursing, chest physiotherapy and medication (Warlow, 2001). If the stroke is restricted and recovery good, or if the patient has suffered only from TIA and by definition has no residual deficit, then treatment aimed at preventing recurrence may be more aggressive, depending on the results of the investigations. If the heart is considered a likely source of emboli, then long-term treatment with anticoagulants may be indicated. Atherosclerosis, leading to tight stenosis of the internal carotid artery, can be confirmed angiographically and treated surgically by carotid endarterectomy (Brown & Humphrey, 1992).

RECOVERY FOLLOWING STROKE

The most common physical consequence of stroke is hemiplegia or hemiparesis, which is defined as 'paralysis (or weakness) of muscles of the arm, leg, trunk, and sometimes face on one side of the body' (Fredericks & Saladin, 1996). Other sequelae of stroke could include perceptual, cognitive, sensory and communication problems, all of which need to be considered in physiotherapy management. Good prognostic signs at approximately 2 weeks poststroke include youth, an initially mild deficit and speedy resolution of symptoms, no loss of consciousness, independent sitting balance, no cognitive impairment and urinary continence (Warlow, 2001).

Whatever the cause of the stroke, a proportion of patients will recover to some degree (Duncan et al., 1994). Recovery is related to the site, extent and nature of the lesion, the integrity of the collateral circulation and the premorbid status of the patient. Haemorrhagic and ischaemic strokes present with different patterns of initial recovery (see above). Characteristically, ischaemic infarct lesions present suddenly and the full extent of the initial insult is apparent. In contrast, with haemorrhagic strokes the extent of the impairment initially seems more extensive due to localised inflammation surrounding the site of the bleed. Some of the initial recovery in haemorrhagic stroke can be attributed to the resolution of inflammation (Allen et al., 1988).

Recovery after stroke can be attributed to different processes. Wade et al. (1985a) differentiated between spontaneous and adaptive recovery processes. It follows then that physiotherapy intervention should be designed to maximise functional activity during the weeks that follow the onset of stroke. More recent evidence from the field of neurophysiology indicates potential mechanisms of recovery based on cellular adaptation, neuronal growth or altered cortical function (see Ch. 5).

Some stroke patients fail to regain consciousness within the first 24 h following the CVA and it is widely considered that the majority will not regain consciousness. The physiotherapy management of these patients is similar to that after severe brain injury and will include regular chest care, turning and positioning (see Ch. 7).

In patients who regain consciousness within 24 h, the first 3 months are a critical period when greatest recovery is thought to occur (Wade et al., 1985b), although potential for improvement may exist for many months (Wade et al., 1992). Recent longitudinal studies of stroke recovery have indicated the ongoing capacity for improvement beyond the initial 3–6 month period (Dam et al., 1993; Widén-Holmqvist et al., 1993). From this evidence it is clear that physiotherapy during the initial period should aim to maximise all aspects of recovery in order to promote functional activity and potential for participation in the wider community. Therefore, physiotherapy commences as soon as the patient is admitted to hospital, or is stable, and should continue up to the time when the patient is able to return home either with support or to live an independent life. There is a lack of evidence supporting the benefits of ongoing physiotherapy intervention beyond 6 months but well-controlled studies in this area are required.

Hemiplegia as a consequence of stroke is considered by physiotherapists to be a recovering neurological condition (Carr & Shepherd, 1989; Bobath, 1990). Although the process of recovery remains unclear, it may be related to one or more of the following (Wade et al., 1985a; Jongbloed, 1986; Anderson, 1994; Duncan et al., 1994):

- the site and extent of the initial lesion
- the age of the patient
- the capacity to achieve a motor goal related to functional movement
- the capacity of the nervous system to reorganise (neuroplasticity; see Ch. 5)
- the premorbid status of the patient
- the motivation and attitude of the patient towards recovery.

Whilst the specific effects of physiotherapy during rehabilitation remain uncertain, there is increasing evidence that early physiotherapy can maximise physical recovery (Ernst, 1990; Anonymous, 1992; Ashburn et al., 1993; Indredavik et al., 1999).

A prospective study attempted to describe the time profile of some physical disabilities in 348 recovering stroke patients with weekly assessment of physical ability following referral for physiotherapy (Partridge et al., 1993). The results indicated that different milestones of recovery occur for different physical tasks (Table 6.1). Whilst nearly all patients (334/348; 96%) recovered an ability to maintain sitting balance by 6 weeks, the ability to walk inside independently at 6 weeks was achieved by only 195 patients (56%). Whilst the range of motor tasks investigated in this study was incomplete, the results indicated that specific gross movements may require either additional physiotherapy or more time during rehabilitation to ensure the restoration of ability.

Work undertaken to investigate recovery profiles of discrete subclassifications of stroke has identified that recovery profiles differ depending on the classification of stroke, such as partial or total (see above). For example, while the PACI group achieved 1 min sitting balance within a day, TACI patients took longer with a median time of 11 days. The ability to walk showed bigger discrepancies, with the PACI group achieving a 10-m walk in a median time of 7 days compared to a median time of 113 days taken by the TACI group (Smith & Baer, 1999). Emerging evidence shows that the capacity to recover is associated with the site and extent of the lesion.

The time history of recovery is discussed further in relation to rehabilitation below.

PHYSICAL MANAGEMENT OF STROKE

The physical management process aims to maximise functional ability and prevent secondary complications to enable the patient to resume all aspects of life in his or her own environment. Each stage involves integration of the patient's views and goals with those of the physiotherapist and multidisciplinary team (MDT; see Ch. 22).

The physiotherapist plays a major role in the physical management of stroke, using skills acquired during education and professional development, to identify and manage the problems of stroke using scientific principles (Durward & Baer, 1995). Operating as a clinical movement scientist, the physiotherapist is able to identify and measure the disorders of movement, and to design, implement and evaluate appropriate therapeutic strategies. This process includes dealing with the social and psychological factors which affect the stroke patient.

Table 6.1 Recovery from disability after a stroke. A total of 348 patients was studied: the numbers achieving each milestone are shown, with percentages in parantheses

Milestone items Gross body movements	On referral	Week 1	Week 2	Week 4	Week 6	Not at week 6
1. Lying supine, turn head to both left and right	302 (86.8)	323 (92.8)	331 (95.1)	335 (96.3)	341 (98.0)	7 (2.0)
2. Maintain sitting balance for 1 min	234 (67.2)	287 (82.5)	306 (87.9)	326 (93.7)	334 (96.0)	14 (4.0)
3. Lying supine, roll to both left and right side	149 (42.8)	208 (59.8)	240 (69.0)	273 (78.4)	294 (84.5)	54 (15.5)
4. Lying supine, get up to sitting from left to right	99 (28.4)	159 (45.7)	202 (58.0)	241 (69.3)	259 (74.4)	89 (25.6)
5. Stand up to free-standing	102 (29.3)	156 (44.8)	198 (56.9)	230 (66.1)	254 (73.0)	94 (27.0)
6. From sitting, transfer from bed to chair left and right side	84 (24.1)	138 (39.7)	174 (50.0)	217 (62.4)	241 (69.3)	107 (30.7)
7. From standing, take two steps forward	68 (19.5)	120 (34.5)	157 (45.1)	202 (58.0)	228 (65.5)	120 (34.5)
8. From standing, take two steps backwards	52 (14.9)	99 (28.4)	138 (39.7)	186 (53.4)	211 (60.6)	137 (39.4)
9. Independent walking inside	41 (11.8)	86 (24.7)	120 (34.5)	169 (48.6)	195 (56.0)	153 (44.0)

Data from Partridge et al. (1993), with permission.

Within the MDT of health care professionals, the main roles of the physiotherapist include:

- restoration of function
- prevention of secondary complications, such as shortening of soft tissues and the development of painful shoulder
- research: areas where research is required include development of scientific measurement and assessment techniques, evidence-based intervention strategies and valid and reliable outcome measures.

Typical time history for stroke rehabilitation

In the context of stroke rehabilitation, the management of the patient can be considered to take place in four distinct stages (Table 6.2), which are intended to be indicative; not all patients will adhere to these time-related stages and in some instances the stages may overlap.

Acute stage

In the acute stage the physiotherapist concentrates on basic problems such as respiratory function and the ability to cough and swallow. The patient may be unconscious and therefore require assistance to maintain normal respiratory function and removal of secretions from the upper airway (Carter & Edwards, 2002).

Communication with members of the MDT will be necessary to ascertain any complicating medical factors that may influence physiotherapy management. Routine skin, soft-tissue and joint care may be required, in conjunction with advice regarding positioning (Ada & Canning, 1990; Lynch & Grisogono, 1991). The physiotherapist should endeavour to communicate with the patient and carers regarding the nature of stroke, and provide an explanation of the aims and nature of rehabilitation.

A leading example of specialist stroke unit care comes from Trondheim, Norway, where significantly improved outcomes of acute stroke patients have been reported (Indredavik et al., 1999). Several factors were identified as contributing to this benefit: early systematic mobilisation and control of BP, glucose levels, dehydration and pyrexia. Early systematic mobilisation was identified as potentially the most important factor in acute stroke treatment and commenced on average within 8 h of stroke onset.

Intermediate stage

The intermediate stage may commence as early as 24 h following CVA, when it is important to complete a physiotherapeutic assessment that represents an extensive database comprising a range of details pertaining to the patient (see 'Assessment' below). The initial assessment serves as a baseline against which recovery or effectiveness of physiotherapeutic intervention can be gauged (see Ch. 3).

Where possible, the patient and carers should participate actively in the identification and agreement of realistic and achievable physiotherapy objectives, in collaboration with all members of the MDT (see 'Treatment planning' below).

Table 6.2 Typical time history for stroke rehabilitation

Stage	Definition	Typical management
Acute	The immediate period following the cerebrovascular accident	Initial assessment of basic systems, e.g. • Swallowing, coughing and respiration • Recognition of consciousness level • Skin and pressure areas • Muscle tone and soft-tissue shortening • Determination of medical stability Physiotherapy intervention for respiratory problems Initial dialogue with patient and carers regarding the nature of stroke Assessment of the patient's environment and social milieu
Intermediate	The period which commences once the patient is medically stable, conscious and actively engaged in the rehabilitation process	Regular identification and assessment of agreed rehabilitation objectives Active engagement in a physiotherapy intervention programme Formulation and adherence to self-treatment strategies
Discharge and transfer	The period immediately prior to, and following, discharge from formal rehabilitation	Assessment of residual disability Physiotherapy intervention for agreed discharge objectives Modifications to the patient's environment Management of transfer of skills between environments Review and monitoring of self-treatment strategies Determine the pattern of rehabilitation once the patient has returned home or when community physiotherapy stops
Long-term	The period following the cessation of formal regular rehabilitation	May include: • Regular review of patient status • Task-specific treatment sessions • Review and modification of self-treatment strategies

Tasks related to functional movements that the patient can practise independently should be identified to involve the patient as an active participant in his or her own rehabilitation (Ada & Canning, 1990), as discussed below (see 'Self-practice'). The home or ward may need to be adapted to enable the patient to participate safely in independent practice.

Intermediate care may now incorporate early supported discharge (ESD) schemes (Cochrane Review, 2001). The process involves a co-ordinated multidisciplinary approach to early discharge, with an emphasis on the delivery of rehabilitation services within the patient's own home. This approach is not suitable for all patients and selection criteria tend to include those with mild to moderate stroke. The benefits of this co-ordinated approach include a reduction in length of hospital stay and the potential for rehabilitation to meet personal needs closely.

Discharge and transfer stage

This is a critical period in the rehabilitation of the stroke patient and requires specific physiotherapy management. In the case of the patient in hospital or a Stroke Rehabilitation Unit, the decision is made to return him or her home or into residential care. For the patient in the community, this is the time when formal contact with physiotherapy ceases.

An important feature of this stage is the careful management of skill transference. Home visits should be carried out and discharge goals set to enable motor skills to be maintained when the patient is at home (see 'Transfer of learning' below). After leaving hospital, regular contact with the physiotherapist may continue on either an outpatient or community basis.

The self-treatment strategies devised during the intermediate stage should be reviewed. The physiotherapist should deliberately withdraw directed treatment and place emphasis on assisting the patient to adhere to an independent practice regimen. The patient and carers should also be guided in developing a record of self-practice strategies.

Long-term

Management issues in the long term will need to reflect the residual disability and handicap status of the patient. If resources allow, it may be desirable to plan regular but low-frequency reviews of the patient's status to confirm his or her continued independence or highlight the need for limited task-specific treatment sessions for certain functional disabilities. It will also allow the physiotherapist to review and modify self-treatment strategies if required.

Physiotherapy delivery for stroke patients

The location, mode and pattern of intervention need to be considered when planning the delivery of physiotherapy for stroke.

Location of treatment

Treatment may be given in a number of locations: home, Stroke Rehabilitation Unit, hospital ward, day hospital or nursing home.

The optimal environment for the physical management of stroke provides the patient with continuous stimulation and challenges directed towards maximising recovery. This environment should be organised to allow regular periods of activity under the direction of the physiotherapist and other health care professionals, regular periods for organised self-practice, periods of rest and relaxation and opportunity for social interaction. Observational studies of recovering stroke patients in hospital rehabilitation settings in the UK, however, have shown that the patient may be inactive for much of the day, with only 11–17% of the working day spent in therapy and around 40% spent in recreation (Tinson, 1989; Ellul et al., 1993; Lincoln et al., 1996).

The environment of the patient will affect the provision of physiotherapy. Evidence from a number of studies suggests that stroke patients treated in a specialist Stroke Rehabilitation Unit may live longer than those cared for in a hospital ward and that recovery may be greater in terms of mobility and return to independent living (Kalra, 1994).

The advocates for stroke units have proposed a number of specific benefits that may positively affect outcome (Kalra, 1994; Wood & Wade, 1995). A stroke unit provides highly trained staff with expertise and interest in stroke and a capacity to manipulate the environment to provide an appropriate challenge for each patient. Also, the physical organisation, daily timetables and the involvement of carers are more easily managed within a stroke unit.

The management of the patient in his or her own home offers some unique opportunities but also presents specific difficulties. Familiarity with the surroundings assists orientation and ensures that physiotherapy and self-practice tasks are specific to the functional demands of the home environment. Problems include co-ordination of the different rehabilitation professionals, the potential for less frequent physiotherapy, lack of access to specialised equipment and a less challenging environment.

Modes of intervention

Intervention may be given in a number of ways and by a variety of persons: physiotherapist alone; physiotherapist and carer; carer alone; organised self-practice; and physiotherapist with other professionals.

Assessment will enable selection of:

- treatment techniques to be administered directly by the physiotherapist
- strategies to enable the carer to participate in rehabilitation
- activities conducive to organised self-practice.

The nature of each mode of intervention will vary at different stages of rehabilitation. During the long-term stage, the emphasis should be on carer involvement and self-practice. Combined intervention from more than one professional may be appropriate. For example, the physiotherapist and occupational therapist may work together in re-educating the patient to be able to dress. While the occupational therapist teaches components of dressing tasks, the physiotherapist could re-educate the patient's balance (see Ch. 24) and prevent abnormal adaptive or compensatory activity.

Pattern of intervention delivery

The frequency of intervention refers to the number of interactions between a patient and physiotherapist over a prescribed time interval, such as a day or week. The duration of intervention indicates the length of time allocated to each interaction. Factors such as exercise tolerance and concentration, in terms of attention and memory, are likely to influence the pattern of intervention.

Factors leading to modification of intervention

Factors that may lead to the need to modify physiotherapy intervention need to be identified. These may be linked to the patient's age, other pathologies that can cause reduced exercise tolerance (cardiovascular fitness), and altered mental or cognitive states. When identifying these, it is important to separate true or chronological age from pathological age. Premorbid status and the presence of other pathologies are more likely than age to affect the final outcome and recovery from stroke. Modification of intervention is discussed below.

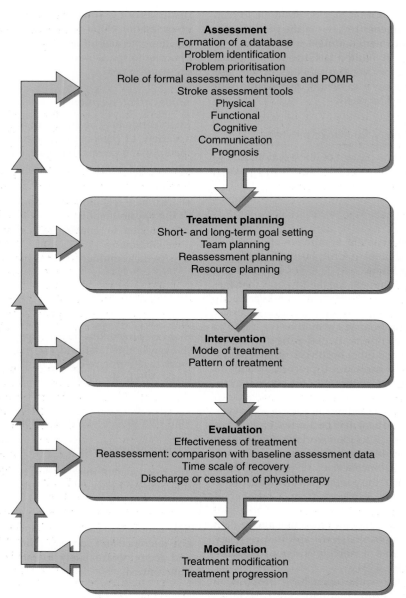

Figure 6.5 Problem-solving model for the physiotherapeutic management of patients after stroke. POMR, problem-oriented medical records.

Stroke management: a problem-solving process

Problem-solving is a process that provides the physiotherapist with a structured and efficient system of interlinked decision-making levels for the management of patients (see Ch. 22). Figure 6.5 represents a problem-solving model appropriate for the management of stroke (Salter & Ferguson, 1991).

The objectives of this model are to:

- establish physiotherapy objectives
- facilitate selection of therapeutic intervention strategies
- provide a decision-making algorithm that will lead the physiotherapist to determine whether intervention has been effective.

Assessment

The assessment process should be both formal and structured. It should include the collection of patient data, the formation of a documented record of the information, an analysis that will lead to the identification of physiotherapy objectives and the selection of appropriate therapeutic techniques. Initially, the assessment should be completed prior to any form of intervention and then repeated at regular and predetermined intervals thereafter. The provision of treatment before the initial assessment process could result in ineffective or possibly even harmful intervention.

An initial database should comprise personal details such as the age and address of the patient and the medical history, together with physical (functional and motor ability), psychological, family and social issues. The organisation and analysis of patient data and the identification of problems need to be documented in a systematic manner. Record systems such as problem oriented medical records (POMR) offer an appropriate method for structuring, retrieving and reviewing patient data (Kettenbach, 1990).

There are many assessment tools available for stroke and some examples are discussed in Chapter 3. Despite an extensive range, there is limited research evidence supporting the validity and reliability of these assessment tools. Most stroke assessment tools use ordinal scales to establish the status of the patient but measurement at this level may have inherent ceiling effects; at a certain point in recovery, the scale becomes insensitive to changes in the patient's status (Ashburn, 1986). The opposite may also be true, in that a floor effect may exist where the scale cannot reflect initial recovery.

Examples of commonly used stroke assessment tools that have been tested to establish levels of validity and reliability include the Rivermead Stroke Assessment (Lincoln & Leadbitter, 1979) and the Motor Assessment Scale (MAS) (Carr et al., 1985). Whilst both provide ordinal data derived using rating scales that can reflect the physical status of the patient, the MAS is directly linked to a specific physiotherapeutic approach for stroke (Carr & Shepherd, 1987). This close association between an assessment tool and a specific treatment approach may lead to bias in the data collected. This bias may be negative, i.e. the assessment tool may be insensitive to changes in the patient that are anticipated as part of the expectations of the treatment approach. Alternatively, bias may be positive; in this case the assessment tool may reflect the expectations of the treatment approach but be insensitive to other unexpected aspects of recovery or deterioration. In addition to functional assessment, there are new and emerging measurement tools for assessing quality of life specific to stroke (Williams et al., 1999; Duncan et al., 1999). These assessment tools attempt to discriminate levels of quality of life appropriate for stroke.

Treatment planning

Following assessment, short- and long-term physiotherapeutic objectives and the mode and pattern of intervention should be established, and appropriate therapeutic techniques selected. An example of where assessment data inform planning might be using the findings of measurement of impairments such as muscle strength and balance to plan re-education of gait. A systematic review of 24 studies found that certain impairments were highly correlated with gait performance and thus serve as appropriate targets for treatment and evaluation (Bohannon et al., 1995).

Communication between members of the MDT is central to the process of treatment planning and, whenever possible, the patient (and carers when appropriate) should also participate in this process (Draper et al., 1991; Ehrlich et al., 1992; see also Ch. 22). During planning, the MDT may function in both a retrospective and prospective manner. On a regular basis, the MDT will review the patient's progress in terms of achieving established short- and long-term objectives. The MDT should aim to establish common rehabilitation goals with short- and long-term treatment objectives. An example of a short-term objective might be 'achievement of independent sitting balance for a period of 30 s', which the patient might achieve within the next 7 days. This prospectively agreed objective will serve to unify the MDT and co-ordinate their separate interactions with the patient.

The planning process should also include strategic plans to prevent secondary complications such as painful shoulder or oedematous hand. Early identification of potential for secondary trauma, and the deliberate inclusion of plans to prevent its occurrence, can ensure that there is minimal disruption to the rehabilitation process.

A pattern for regular reassessment should be established during treatment planning to monitor the overall status at different stages during rehabilitation, concentrating on aspects of functional recovery that relate to current short-term objectives.

Resources that need to be considered include: the availability of staff; potential for involvement of carers; and resources for direct patient treatment and self-practice in the institutional setting, home and community. Availability and involvement of external agencies such as social workers, stroke support workers, carer support and stroke clubs may also need to be considered.

Intervention

Initial assessment data may indicate that some patients are more suitable for intensive rehabilitation whilst others, possibly the patient with complicating pathologies, may require less intensive intervention. The aims of intervention are to maximise functional ability and prevent secondary complications such as contractures and painful shoulder.

The modes of intervention may alter during rehabilitation in order to make the best use of available resources. For example, in striving to meet the short-term objective of holding a glass in order to drink, the patient may need to interact with the physiotherapist alone, the carer, or a combination of occupational therapist and physiotherapist. In addition, the patient will also have a task-specific programme of organised self-practice related to this short-term goal.

Different treatment approaches are discussed in Chapter 21 and actual physiotherapeutic intervention techniques are discussed in Chapter 23; the management of abnormal muscle tone is discussed in Chapter 25.

Evaluation

A central feature of the problem-solving model is the need to ensure that physiotherapeutic intervention is effective, both in immediate and long-term patient management.

A single physiotherapy treatment, irrespective of location, mode or pattern, should produce a positive therapeutic outcome. Effectiveness is determined either by testing patients with reference to time or performance criteria, or by observing their direct response to the treatment. This immediate evaluation may indicate that a specific therapeutic technique is effective, or may need to be either modified or replaced.

While day-to-day physiotherapy may appear to have an immediate effect, review of patient progress with regard to the specified short- and long-term physiotherapy objectives is necessary. This estimate of 'true' progress, or otherwise, can be established by comparing current assessment data with the initial baseline status of the patient. It follows that this process of evaluation may indicate the rate of progress during rehabilitation. An important aspect of evaluation is to determine whether the patient is capable of returning home and whether formal contact with a physiotherapist is no longer required.

Modification

Evaluation may reveal uncertainty regarding the effectiveness of intervention and should lead to the physiotherapist revisiting one or more levels of the problem-solving model. The section above on 'Factors leading to modification of intervention' is relevant to this process. Modification of treatment may include changing the mode or pattern of intervention, or the treatment techniques.

General management issues

This section will deal with a range of issues which need to be addressed in the overall management of stroke, and which may arise at any stage of recovery.

Respiratory care

Respiratory care includes both prophylactic and terminal care. Respiratory problems are most likely to occur in the acute and intermediate stages following stroke. Initial assessment should include the examination of rate, depth and pattern of respiration, in conjunction with chest auscultation, to prevent secondary complications such as atelectasis and pneumonia (Hough, 1991; Smith & Ball, 1998). The patient may be predisposed to these problems due to relative immobility, prolonged supine positioning and altered tone in the respiratory muscles. Also, the cough reflex may be suppressed or weak, resulting in difficulties with removal of secretions from the airways.

Altered breathing patterns may be characteristic of a stroke patient whose condition is considered to be terminal. A serious complication following a severe stroke with brainstem involvement may be the presence of Cheyne–Stokes breathing, in which periods of apnoea alternate with a series of respirations, which increase and decrease in amplitude. In the general management of stroke, the physiotherapist will aim to maintain a clear airway, stimulate the cough reflex, assist effective removal of secretions and encourage a normal respiratory pattern (Hough, 1991; Smith & Ball, 1998).

> **Key point**
>
> The physiotherapist may play a major role in maintaining respiration and clearing chest secretions

Positioning

Positioning of the patient needs to be considered with respect to the environment, as well as a suitable bed and chair.

The controlled orientation and position of the patient in the immediate environment can provide useful stimulation when problems of visual and perceptual dysfunction exist (see 'Perceptual problems' below). In these instances, effort should be made to ensure that the environment provides a challenging stimulus and the immediate surroundings should be organised so as to encourage the patient to look over his or her affected side (Davies, 1985; Riddoch et al., 1995).

The management of stimulation may be clarified if a distinction between visual and perceptual problems is established. During the acute stage, for a patient with visual and perceptual dysfunction, it may be reasonable to advise carers, relatives and members of the MDT to address the patient and provide stimulation from the midline (i.e. by standing directly in front of the patient). As the visual and perceptual problems start to resolve, stimulation may be provided from the affected side.

Strategies exist for positioning the hemiplegic patient when seated in a chair and lying on a bed (Lynch & Grisogono, 1991). These strategies are designed to optimise sensory stimulation and encourage the adoption of effective weight-bearing. In addition, these positions attempt to prevent secondary complications such as soft-tissue shortening and the development of a painful shoulder, and inhibit the development of abnormal muscle tone (Ada & Canning, 1990; Bobath, 1990). For further discussion of positioning strategies see Carr & Kenney (1992), as well as Chapter 25.

> **Key point**
>
> Appropriate positioning strategies may have a therapeutic effect

Continence

Physiotherapy intervention has a role to play in the management of urinary and faecal continence. Early encouragement and assistance to enable the patient to adopt weight-bearing standing and sitting positions may help overcome these problems. Special attention should be given to the patient with communication difficulties who may be unable to ask for either a bedpan or bottle. Regular offers to assist the patient to the toilet or to use a bedpan or bottle may help to preserve continence and maintain the patient's self-esteem.

Communication

Issues of communication include: the types of problems encountered; strategies for combatting them; and the roles of the patient, the MDT and carers.

The communication problems commonly associated with stroke include:

- dysarthria (problems of articulation)
- dysphasia (either a receptive or expressive problem which affects the understanding and use of correct words)
- aphasia (inability to express oneself in speech or writing or to understand written or spoken language)
- orofacial dysfunction
- loss of facial expression and gesture.

Dysphasia may result in the patient's being unable to understand what has happened or to ask questions regarding the stroke. The physiotherapist and the MDT should allow additional response times during verbal communication and use clear and simple speech. A designated member of the MDT should allocate time to give the patient information about the nature of the stroke, the recovery process and rehabilitation. The MDT, with guidance from a speech and language therapist, should determine clear and consistent approaches for communication with individual stroke patients. Use of communication aids may be appropriate (see Ch. 13, p. 243).

> **Key point**
>
> The physiotherapist should liaise with the speech and language therapist to ensure strategies to enhance communication are followed

Carer support

Carer support may involve education, counselling and access to support agencies.

The involvement of carers as active members of the MDT can facilitate the overall management of the stroke patient. Immediately following stroke, it is important to inform carers of the nature of stroke, the rehabilitation process and their involvement in it and the prospects of recovery. The carer may also require professional counselling.

The problems facing carers of the patient who remains at home may require quite different management strategies. Following discussion with the patient and carers, a designated member of the MDT, who is often the physiotherapist, should initiate access to appropriate support agencies. In the UK, many stroke services routinely involve agencies such as Meals on Wheels, Stroke Clubs, Crossroads (a carer respite agency), Chest, Heart and Stroke Association (Scotland) or the Stroke Association (England and Wales), and a designated Stroke Support Worker (see Appendix).

Re-education of movement

The physiotherapist should advise the MDT regarding the potential for recovery of functional movement, strategies for movement re-education, the extent to which each patient is susceptible to secondary trauma and intervention strategies to prevent their occurrence.

Patients with stroke are subject to the same effects of inactivity as the normal population, namely loss of cardiovascular fitness and muscle weakness. There is increasing evidence that exercise is beneficial after stroke and that both aerobic activities and strength-training can improve function without adverse effects (see Ch. 29). Recent advances in research in this area have led to a new section on resisted exercises being included in the National Clinical Guidelines for Stroke (Intercollegiate Working Party for Stroke, 2002). Specific activities and techniques are discussed in Chapters 23, 25 and 29, and include treadmill training, cycling and strength-training. A technique that has shown some of the most promising evidence so far, that motor recovery can be facilitated beyond the natural period of recovery after a stroke (Liepert et al., 2000), is constraint-induced movement therapy (CIMT) or forced use. This involves constraining the stronger limb to encourage use of the affected limb (see Ch. 29).

Learning strategies for the re-education of movement are selected for the individual patient and the variables that can be manipulated include aspects of practice, feedback, the self-practice programme and the environment.

Organised practice

Part or whole practice A decision should be made as to whether the patient should attempt to practise some components of a task as a pretraining for performance of the whole task (Winstein, 1991).

When the amount of practice time is greater than the rest period, this is termed massed practice. Conversely, when the rest period is greater than or equal to the time taken for the task, this is distributed practice (Shumway-Cook & Woollacott, 2001). Whilst massed practice may lead to greater fatigue, there is evidence that it may have a greater effect on learning. Blocked practice refers to consistent practice of a single task. Random practice is varying practice amongst distinctly different tasks (VanSant, 1991). One small study of 24 stroke patients has indicated that random practice of an upper-limb task produced greater learning of the task than blocked practice (Hanlon, 1996). More trials are required in this area before the optimal structure of task practice can be based on evidence.

Self-practice The patient should be considered to be an active learner during rehabilitation (Ada et al., 1990). It is the responsibility of the physiotherapist to devise and teach self-practice schedules that reflect the ability of the patient, the environment and the aims and objectives of rehabilitation. The physiotherapist should monitor performance to ensure that compensatory or adaptive strategies do not develop. Carers may play a crucial part in assisting with self-practice sessions.

Feedback

Information about the success of movement is a critical ingredient of motor learning, where the learner cannot establish this information independently (Schmidt, 1991). Feedback may be provided in many forms.

Knowledge of results (KR) normally entails providing verbal information, after the attempt to move, to augment other forms of feedback indicating whether the goal has been achieved. Knowledge of performance (KP) is feedback related to the patterns of actions that led to the achievement, or not, of the goal. The bandwidth of feedback is the acceptable margin of error (bandwidth) that may occur before feedback is provided. Decisions regarding bandwidth can relate to the strategic withdrawal of feedback during rehabilitation (Schmidt, 1991).

The frequency of feedback needs to be considered, as patients may become dependent upon continual verbal feedback (Schmidt, 1991). The physiotherapist should consider reducing the frequency of feedback to promote problem-solving by the patient and enhance learning.

Transfer of learning

When the patient is considered to be capable of living at home, motor skill acquisition must be maintained in that environment (Shumway-Cook & Woollacott, 2001). Strategies to assist in the transfer of learning include home visits involving the patient and carers, early involvement and education of carers themselves and ensuring self-practice strategies are well established prior to returning home. Task-specific training has been shown to be beneficial in stroke (Richards et al., 1993; Dean et al., 2000) and the home environment provides the ideal location for the practice of relevant and individualised tasks.

In addition to assessing the patient's living environment, home visits provide an opportunity for performance and practice of established functional skills, such as moving from a lying position to sitting up over the edge of the bed, standing up from a chair and walking. During a home visit the patient should be directed to attempt all self-practice programmes and, wherever possible, with the involvement of carers. Strategies for assisting the transfer of learning between environments should be planned well in advance of the patient's return home. This includes identifying the need for any modifications to the home.

> **Key point**
>
> Regular and varied task practice, both during and outwith physiotherapy treatment, is essential for recovery

A similar management strategy should be implemented when the decision has been reached that physiotherapy should stop for the patient in his or her own home. Treatment by the physiotherapist should be reduced, while the emphasis is placed on self-practice programmes.

Sexual dysfunction

Because of the sensitive nature of sexual dysfunction and the age of most stroke patients, these problems are seldom discussed or considered by the MDT. Sexual problems may be linked to physical disability and emotional factors in the patient, or fear and anxiety in the sexual partner. Counselling or referral to agencies such as SPOD (Sexual and Personal difficulties of the Disabled) may be appropriate (see Appendix).

Sociological issues

The patient's race and cultural background may affect how treatment can be given. The role of gender also needs consideration.

Direct physical contact from the physiotherapist or the need to undress the patient may be unacceptable to members of certain religious or ethnic groups. Effort should be made to identify these concerns at an early stage and to make appropriate modifications to physiotherapeutic intervention. These modifications may include physiotherapy outside the normal treatment area, inviting relatives to act as chaperones and alteration of the techniques used. Many hospitals employ representatives from ethnic groups to assist in communication between the patient and carers and health care professionals.

Within a pleuralistic society, religious, ethnic and gender issues that may influence the participation in rehabilitation must be considered. In some cultures, gender roles and responsibilities are quite distinct. It may be that the woman's role is to be a carer and the man to be the provider. These traditional roles may have a powerful influence on the individual following stroke with respect to motivation to become independent or to adopt a passive acceptance of the sick role.

Lifestyle

In forming a rehabilitation programme, full consideration should be given to important lifestyle factors such as the patient's hobbies, pastimes and leisure interests. It may be possible to relate specific components of directed treatment or self-practice to these activities, and therefore increase motivation. Modifications to the home, for example the construction of raised flower beds, may enable the patient to continue the pursuit of specific hobbies.

To determine if a patient can return to work a number of factors need to be considered, such as the nature of the occupation, the extent of physical handicap, the attitude of the employer, the capacity to travel to and from work and the potential to make adaptations to the work environment (see Ch. 22). It may be possible to alter the nature of the employment, with minimal retraining, to allow a return to work. In a longitudinal study of 183 patients, all of whom were under the age of 65 at the time they had a stroke, it was found that the most significant predictors of a return to work were normal muscle strength and the absence of dyspraxia (Saeki et al., 1995).

Problems influencing physical management

Various physical and psychological problems may affect physical management and the physiotherapist must be aware of these in order to modify the management programme. Psychological problems are discussed further in Chapter 27.

Soft-tissue complications

Soft-tissue problems may involve the skin, contractures or a painful shoulder.

Pressure sores or skin breakdown and contractures are avoidable secondary complications of stroke. Strategies for preventing skin breakdown include appropriate positioning of the patient in a bed or chair (Pope, 2002), regular assistance to enable the patient to alter position, the provision of appropriate equipment such as special seat cushions (see Ch. 7) and mattresses, and careful management of urinary and bowel incontinence.

The development of soft-tissue shortening and contractures due to disuse, immobility or spasticity will inevitably affect motor function. The effects of muscle length on sarcomere loss are well documented (see Ch. 30); the physiotherapist should ensure that the patient is positioned to avoid prolonged shortening of soft tissues and initiate a regimen of stretching for vulnerable tissues (see Ch. 25). Shoulder pain is common in patients with stroke and has been reported to affect rehabilitation (Van Langenberghe et al., 1988; Wanklyn et al., 1996). There is no clear picture of the scale or nature of the problem but shoulder pain has been reported as being present at least once during rehabilitation or follow-up in 72% of stroke patients (Van Ouwenaller et al., 1986), although more recent estimates cite the incidence at a much lower 30% (Intercollegiate Working Party for Stroke, 2002). A number of causes of shoulder pain in hemiplegia have been suggested and include trauma, altered muscle tone, glenohumeral subluxation, contracture of capsular structures and shoulder-hand syndrome (Van Langenberghe et al., 1988; Gamble et al., 2002). Prevention of a painful shoulder should be of prime concern to the physiotherapist. This may be achieved by careful assessment of the biomechanical integrity of the glenohumeral joint and shoulder girdle, and by ensuring careful positioning and handling of the patient by members of the MDT.

> **Key point**
>
> The physiotherapist has an active and educational role to prevent onset of soft-tissue complications and trauma

Feeding problems

Dysphagia Dysphagia is a problem with swallowing and may occur in approximately one-third of patients after stroke (Barer, 1989; Penington & Krutsch, 1990). Dysphagia can be caused by many pathologies, including stroke, when it is characterised by difficulty in safely moving a bolus from the mouth to the stomach without aspiration and may also involve difficulty in oral preparation for the swallow, e.g. chewing, tongue movement (Scottish Intercollegiate Guidelines Network, 1997). For most, dysphagia may resolve in the first few days after stroke. Initial attention should determine if the patient can eat and drink independently without fear of aspiration. Assessment by the MDT should include the integrity of the swallowing and cough reflexes and the ability to co-ordinate breathing with swallowing.

Effective management of dysphagia should involve the combined intervention of the speech and language therapist, nurse and physiotherapist. The physiotherapist should assist in the control of upright posture and

head position, and facilitate lip, tongue and jaw movements that may enable the patient to eat and drink.

Tube and parenteral feeding Feeding by means of a nasogastric tube may be required when a patient is unable to swallow, process food within the mouth or protect the airway with an effective cough reflex. If these patients are not fed via a tube, they may become dehydrated and/or malnourished. In the long term, if problems of dysphagia continue, feeding may be delivered via a gastrostomy tube.

Orofacial dysfunction

Orofacial dysfunction should be considered a major focus for physiotherapy following stroke. Muscle paralysis may lead to an inability to close the lips, move food in the mouth and swallow effectively, and the patient may also experience considerable embarrassment. Specific techniques to assist feeding may include stimulation of lip closure, activation of buccinator contractions and tongue movements and facilitation of the swallowing reflex. Attempts should be made to stimulate activity in the facial muscles, in particular those surrounding the eyes and mouth. The patient may be encouraged to practise these facial activities with a mirror. Problems such as hypersensitivity of the mouth or abnormal reflex activity, e.g. a positive bite reflex, may require desensitising techniques.

> **Key point**
>
> The physiotherapist should include orofacial re-education as part of rehabilitation and, where appropriate, work with other members of the multidisciplinary team to address problems with feeding and swallowing

Psychological problems

Psychological problems may include depression, unrealistic state, labile state and personality changes (see Ch. 27).

There is considerable evidence that a number of psychological problems may be associated with stroke. Mood disorders may affect intellectual capacity (Robinson et al., 1986) and adversely affect rehabilitation (Sinyor et al., 1986). The physiotherapist should be aware of any existing psychological problems and take them into account throughout the rehabilitation process. The direct management of psychological problems is the responsibility of the medical doctor and referral to a clinical psychologist may be required.

The incidence of depression may be greater in stroke patients admitted to hospital than in those who remain at home (House et al., 1991). This difference may be a function of severity of stroke and reflect the greater likelihood of being admitted to hospital with a severe stroke. Some patients may have had episodes of depression prior to the stroke (Gordon & Hibbard, 1997).

A patient may have unrealistic rehabilitation goals that are inappropriate for the stage of recovery. The physiotherapist should discuss realistic goals with the patient and encourage him or her to recognise successful achievements.

Depression is associated with slower progress in rehabilitation and a longer length of hospital stay (Scottish Intercollegiate Guidelines Network, 2002).

Emotional lability is a common problem following stroke (House et al., 1991) and there appears to be either a reduced threshold for, or inappropriate control of, emotions such as crying or laughing. The physiotherapist should discuss the problem sensitively with the patient.

Relatives or carers may notice personality changes – either aggressive or passive behaviour – in a person following a stroke. Carers and relatives may require counselling to help cope with feelings of fear, embarrassment, inadequacy and guilt.

Cognitive problems

Many forms of cognitive problems can arise following stroke and the initial physiotherapy assessment may identify difficulties that require further assessment by the clinical psychologist or occupational therapist. Reduced attention span may be a problem at any stage of rehabilitation and should be considered in the design of rehabilitation programmes.

The stroke patient may have difficulties with short-term memory recall (Wade et al., 1985a) that will affect the ability to relearn functional movement tasks. Repetitive simple instructions, visual and verbal cues, involvement of carers, part practice of tasks and the use of practice books or task performance diaries may be helpful (Ada et al., 1990).

Perceptual problems

Problems of perception are considered to be one of the main factors limiting functional motor recovery following stroke (Turnbull, 1986). Patients who have had a right-sided CVA, and therefore have left hemiplegia, have the most severe perceptual problems.

Visuospatial neglect

In visuospatial neglect the patient fails to respond appropriately to stimuli presented on the hemiplegic side. It is more common and often severe following right parietal lesions but may be present with damage to the left hemisphere. Clinical management strategies include addressing the patient from the affected side, deliberate placement of items such as tissues or drinks on that side, and advice to carers regarding the position they should adopt whilst talking to the patient (Riddoch et al., 1995; Robertson & North, 1992). There is currently limited evidence to suggest the above strategies are beneficial, although it has been suggested that some new approaches, including eye-patching techniques, video feedback during therapy, training in visual imagery and pharmacological therapy with dopamine agonists may be useful (Diamond, 2001).

> **Key point**
>
> Physiotherapy management strategies may need to be adapted to take account of cognitive and perceptual problems

Agnosia

Agnosia has been defined as loss of knowledge or inability to perceive objects through otherwise normally functioning sensory pathways (Kandel et al., 2000). This group of perceptual disorders, related to the inability to recognise previously familiar objects, may affect the patient in a number of ways. Patients may deny or disown the existence of their own affected arm or leg, and in severe instances they may exhibit an inability to recognise familiar faces (prosopagnosia). During any form of intervention, the patient should be assisted to observe his or her own limbs in an attempt to promote recognition.

Dyspraxia

Difficulty in executing volitional purposeful movements is termed 'dyspraxia'. This phenomenon may be exposed in the patient who appears to have good comprehension, normal sensation and some recovery of ability to move. Dyspraxia may influence the completion of any functional task. For example, a patient who is able to flex and extend the joints in a hand may be unable to grasp a cup when attempting to drink. Dressing dyspraxia is a recognised example of this perceptual impairment: the patient understands the purpose of dressing but is unable to complete the task appropriately. Typically, he or she may attempt to place the head in the sleeve of a shirt, or put a jacket on back-to-front. The literature provides little direction as to the management of these problems. The physiotherapist should reassure the patient and devise simple movement sequences that might facilitate the completion of functional tasks.

Summary of physical management

The main components of physiotherapeutic management for stroke have been reviewed and linked to current understanding of recovery. In the light of this knowledge, stages of physiotherapeutic management have been proposed, reflecting important episodes and processes inherent within physiotherapy management. Delivery of physiotherapy has been elaborated, with the intention of making appropriate use of finite resources. A problem-solving model, designed to facilitate decision-making and establish effectiveness of practice, has been detailed. Finally, key aspects of general management have been introduced and placed in the overall context of stroke rehabilitation.

CASE HISTORIES

CASE A

AB is a 64-year-old widower who lives alone in his terraced house with two flights of stairs. His hobbies are golf, gardening and chess. He has suffered from osteoarthritis in his right hip for 3 years, has a 10-year history of hypertension and smoked 20 cigarettes a day until 12 years ago.

Presenting history
He was found by his daughter collapsed on the bathroom floor, drowsy, uncommunicative and with a recent episode of vomiting. An ambulance was called and he was taken to the local district hospital, which did not have a stroke unit.

On arrival he was drowsy but appeared to understand basic commands, although he made no attempt to speak. A right-sided weakness, reduced tone and reflexes were found and he was noted to be pyrexial with a temperature of 39.2°C. A computed tomographic scan showed a primary intracranial haemorrhage in the left thalamic region. Chest X-ray showed patchy shadowing in the right base consistent with aspiration. On auscultation there was reduced air entry with bronchial breath sounds on the right. Immediate medical management was to commence

antibiotics, antihypertensive medication and the delivery of intravenous fluids.

Acute stage: key physiotherapy problems

- reduced level of consciousness
- reduced active movement
- altered muscle tone
- right basal aspiration and weak cough.

Acute-stage physiotherapy treatment plan

- clear chest secretions and maintain respiration – use modified postural drainage position for right base as tolerated. Assisted coughing techniques to aid expectoration
- positioning strategies in conjunction with nursing staff, taking cognisance of BP
- passive/assisted limb movements. Progress to sitting over edge of bed as BP stabilises.

After 72 h
AB's status had improved, BP had stabilised and he was less drowsy. Chest X-ray was clear and no added sounds were heard on auscultation. Some physical recovery was noted with detectable muscle activity in the flexors and extensor muscles of the right leg and some flickers of shoulder–shrugging and flexion noted. At this stage he was able to stand up from sitting with the assistance of two people, stand with the support of two but unable to take any steps. He had independent sitting balance, although he showed marked asymmetry, with his trunk slumped to the right and a tendency to hold on to the plinth with his left hand.

Key physiotherapy problems at 72 h

- reduced movement through right side
- altered tone
- altered posture
- reduced functional ability.

Physiotherapy treatment plan at 72 h
To attend daily rehabilitation with physiotherapist, occupational therapist and speech and language therapist, to have all key strategies reinforced by nursing staff:

- improve symmetry and body segment alignment
- improve active functional movement
- gradually increase task demands, e.g. by reducing supporting base to make tasks harder
- to ensure upright posture in wheelchair with extended lap table to reinforce symmetrical position and encourage bilateral upper-limb activities.

After 2 weeks

AB was transferred to the regional rehabilitation unit. At this stage he had independent sitting and standing balance, although his posture was asymmetrical. His right lower-limb control was improving and he was now able to take five steps with assistance from one person and a walking stick. His right upper limb showed mass flexion and extension movements at the shoulder and elbow with flickers of finger flexion. AB complained of intermittent shoulder pain but this reduced on assisted movement with correct alignment. A speech and language assessment indicated mild word-finding difficulties but his comprehension was not impaired.

Physiotherapy treatment plan at 2 weeks

- Improve symmetry and posture.
- Improve functional activities – especially transfers, gait and upper-limb tasks using random practice of tasks. Tasks practices both as part practice and whole practice.
- Create diary of simple exercises for AB to practise independently at bedside to improve sitting posture and weight transfer in sitting and upper-limb extension.
- Monitor and reduce shoulder pain – education rehandling and positioning to other staff.
- Continue close liaison with other members of MDT.

After 4 weeks in the rehabilitation unit

A case conference was held and AB had already achieved 10 steps independently with a stick. The team set the following goals:

1. Walk 10 m independently in 3 weeks.
2. Be able to undertake basic upper-limb activity tasks, e.g. washing, shaving, dressing and preparing light snack within 4–6 weeks.
3. Home visit after 6 weeks with occupational therapist and physiotherapist.

Post-home visit

The visit went well and appropriate aids and appliances were supplied after a further 2 weeks to ease independent living. Support services of home nursing and domiciliary physiotherapy were set up to support the discharge period and this was planned to be reviewed, initially on a monthly basis. Domiciliary physiotherapist provided home exercises to be undertaken independently to maintain functional level.

CASE B

JJ is a 55-year-old journalist who lives in a bungalow with his wife and two teenage sons. He has a history of hypertension and smokes heavily (30 cigarettes per day). He was having dinner when he developed sudden onset of drooling from the left side of his mouth, weakness in the left hand and some word-finding problems. Over the next 15 min his symptoms progressed. An ambulance was called and he was taken to the local district hospital.

Presenting history

On arrival he was drowsy. Dense sensorimotor signs were noted throughout the left arm, trunk and leg and a left facial weakness was evident. His head and eyes were deviated to the right. He appeared to understand basic commands but at this stage cognition and vision were unable to be fully assessed. He was diagnosed as having a probable total anterior circulation syndrome, was transferred to the stroke unit and referred for full assessment by the physiotherapist, occupational therapist, speech and language therapist and clinical psychologist.

Acute stage: key physiotherapy problems

- reduced level of consciousness
- no active movement in left arm and leg
- severe left-sided facial weakness
- altered muscle tone
- left-sided neglect
- no independent sitting balance or bed mobility.

Acute-stage physiotherapy treatment plan

- Maintain soft-tissue length and joint integrity through passive movement (assisted movement where possible).
- Positioning for soft-tissue viability and also to encourage awareness of left side of body and environment.
- Postural and balance re-education with two physiotherapists – sitting over edge of bed and progress to standing as able (or use tilt table).

After 1 week

JJ's drowsiness had resolved, although he tired quickly after physical activity. Further assessment by the MDT indicated he had a left homonymous hemianopia, perceptual difficulties and left-sided unilateral neglect. Physically there was minimal change in status, although it was noted that the neglect was compounded by a tendency to push away from his right side in sitting.

The treatment plan at this stage therefore remained the same, although the frequency of treatment sessions was increasing.

After 1 month

Progress was noted to be slow. Independent but asymmetrical sitting balance was achieved at 12 days poststroke. JJ was noted to have some activity around the left side of the trunk and around the left hip in sitting and standing. No activity was noted in the left arm. The left-sided neglect was improving but had not yet resolved.

Physiotherapy treatment plan at 1 month

- Maintain joint range of movement and soft-tissue integrity.
- Stimulate left-sided activity (and reduce tendency to push from right).
- Improve symmetry and posture.
- Practise balance and weight transfer activities in sitting and standing.
- Improve functional activities – especially transfers and stepping.
- Practise orofacial exercises and sounds.
- Ensure appropriate positioning of upper limb.

After 3 months

At this stage the left-sided neglect was noted to have virtually resolved. Physically, posture and body segment alignment had improved, although he had a tendency to slump when fatigued. JJ had achieved independent standing balance 6 weeks after his stroke and was now able to transfer weight and take 10 steps with a walking stick. He was able to get in and out of bed and a chair independently, and was managing some aspects of self-care, such as upper-body washing and dressing. A few flickers of left-sided trapezius and pectoral muscle activity were noted on attempting to shrug his shoulders, but JJ was now starting to complain of shoulder pain.

Physiotherapy treatment plan at 3 months
In addition to the treatment noted above:

- use of transcutaneous nerve stimulation was attempted for pain relief

- improve gait pattern and gait endurance
- patient and carers shown methods to undertake self-initiated stretches
- independent practice of standing up and sitting down.

At this stage it was decided that JJ could go home once walking ability had improved to 10 m and he was able to wash and dress himself, get in and out of a shower and make a light snack.

A home visit was undertaken at 5 months poststroke. Aids and equipment were ordered to enable a degree of independence around the home (e.g. rails in the bathroom and toilet, a shower stool and kitchen adaptations) and a wheelchair was ordered to allow greater independence due to restricted walking capacity. JJ was discharged home at 7 months poststroke.

9 months poststroke

JJ was reviewed at an outpatient clinic and, although he was coping reasonably well, he had fallen once getting out of bed and had only been outside twice in his wheelchair. With the exception of flickers of shoulder and elbow flexion activity, no active movement had returned to the left arm and there were soft-tissue contractures of the wrist and finger flexors.

At this stage he was referred to day hospital once a week for 6 weeks to try and improve confidence about walking indoors and undertaking daily functional tasks, such as getting in and out of bed. His wife was shown stretches to do daily and he was referred to the occupational therapist for a night splint. He was also shown how to get on and off the floor, with assistance from his wife.

On discharge from the day hospital he was seen by the domiciliary physiotherapist for three visits and then reviewed 3-monthly by the local stroke medicine clinic (including physiotherapy assessment). Long-term plans included trying CIMT or functional electrical stimulation to see if any more recovery in the arm was possible.

References

Ada L, Canning C, eds. *Key Issues in Neurological Physiotherapy*. Oxford: Butterworth Heinemann; 1990.

Ada L, Canning C, Westwood P. The patient as an active learner. In: Ada L, Canning C, eds. *Key Issues in Neurological Physiotherapy*. Oxford: Butterworth Heinemann; 1990:99–124.

Adams RD, Victor M, Ropper AH. *Principles of Neurology*, 6th edn. New York: McGraw-Hill; 1997.

Aho K, Harmsen P, Hatano S et al. Cerebrovascular disease in the community: results of a WHO collaborative study. *Bull WHO* 1980, **58**:113–130.

Allen CMC, Harrison MJG, Wade DT. *The Management of Acute Stroke*. Tunbridge Wells: Castle House; 1988.

Anderson C. Baseline measures and outcome predictors. *Neuroepidemiology* 1994, **13**:283–289.

Anonymous. *Stroke Rehabilitation*. Leeds: Leeds Evaluation Unit; 1992.

Ashburn A. Methods of assessing the physical disabilities of stroke patients. *Physiother Pract* 1986, **2**:59–62.

Ashburn A, Partridge CJ, DeSouza L. Physiotherapy in the rehabilitation of stroke: a review. *Clin Rehab* 1993, **7**:337–345.

Baer GD, Smith MT. The recovery of walking ability and subclassification of stroke. *Physiother Res Int* 2001, **6**:135–144.

Bamford J, Sandercock P, Dennis M et al. A prospective study of acute cerebrovascular disease in the community: the Oxfordshire Community Stroke Project 1981–1986. 1. Methodology, demography and incident cases of first-ever stroke. *J Neurol Neurosurg Psychiatry* 1988, **51**:1373–1380.

Bamford J, Sandercock P, Dennis M et al. Classification and natural history of clinically identifiable subtypes of cerebral infarction. *Lancet* 1991, **337**:1521–1526.

Barer DH. The natural history and functional consequences of dysphagia after hemispheric stroke. *J Neurol Neurosurg Psychiatry* 1989, **52**:236–241.

Bobath B. *Adult Hemiplegia: Evaluation and Treatment*, 3rd edn. London: Heinemann; 1990.

Bohannon RW, Andrews A. Relationship between impairments and gait performance after stroke: a summary of relevant research. *Gait Posture* 1995, **3**:236–240.

Brown MM, Humphrey PRD. Carotid endarterectomy: recommendations for the management of transient ischaemic attacks and ischaemic stroke. *Br Med J* 1992, **305**:1071–1074.

Carr EK, Kenney F. Positioning the stroke patient: a review of the literature. *Int J Nurs Stud* 1992, **29**:355–369.

Carr JH, Shepherd RB. *Physiotherapy in Disorders of the Brain*. Oxford: Butterworth Heinemann; 1980.

Carr JH, Shepherd RB. *A Motor Relearning Programme for Stroke*, 2nd edn. Oxford: Butterworth Heinemann; 1987.

Carr JH, Shepherd RB. A motor learning model for stroke rehabilitation. *Physiotherapy* 1989, **75**:372–380.

Carr JH, Shepherd RB, Nordholm L et al. Investigation of a new Motor Assessment Scale for stroke patients. *Phys Ther* 1985, **65**:175–180.

Carter P, Edwards S. General principles of treamtent. In: Edwards S, ed. *Neurological Physiotherapy: A Problem Solving Approach*. 2nd edn. London: Churchill Livingstone; 2002:121–153.

Cochrane Review. Early supported discharge trialists. Services for reducing duration of hospital care for stroke patients. In: *Cochrane Library*, issue 1. Oxford: Oxford Update Software; 2001.

Dam M, Tonin P, Casson S et al. The effects of long-term rehabilitation therapy on poststroke hemiplegic patients. *Stroke* 1993, **24**:1186–1191.

Davies P. *Steps to Follow*. Berlin: Springer Verlag; 1985.

Dean CM, Richards CL, Malouin F. Task-related circuit training improves performance of locomotor tasks in chronic stroke: a randomized, controlled pilot trial. *Arch Phys Med Rehab* 2000, **81**:409–417.

Diamond PT. Rehabilitative management of post-stroke visuospatial inattention. *Disabil Rehab* 2001; **23**:407–412.

Draper BM, Poulos CJ, Cole AM et al. Who cares for the carer of the old and ill? *Med J Aust* 1991, **154**:293.

Duncan PW, Goldstein LB, Horner RD et al. Similar motor recovery of upper and lower extremities after stroke. *Stroke* 1994, **25**:1181–1188.

Duncan PW, Wallace D, Lai SM et al. The stroke impact scale version 2.0. Evaluation of reliability, validity, and sensitivity to change. *Stroke* 1999 **30**:2131–2140.

Durward BR, Baer GD. Physiotherapy and neurology: towards research-based practice. *Physiotherapy* 1995, **81**:436–439.

Ehrlich F, Bowring G, Draper BM et al. Caring for carers – a rational problem. *Med J Aust* 1992, **156**:590–592.

Ellul J, Watkins C, Ferguson N et al. Increasing patient engagement in rehabilitation activities. *Clin Rehab* 1993, **7**:297–302.

Ernst E. A review of stroke rehabilitation and physiotherapy. *Stroke* 1990, **21**:1081–1085.

Fredericks CM, Saladin LK. *Pathophysiology of the Motor Systems: Principles and Clinical Presentations*. Philadelphia: FA Davis; 1996.

Gamble GE, Barbean E, Laasch HU, Bowsher D, Tyrrell PJ, Jones AK. Poststroke shoulder pain: a prospective study of the association and risk factors in 152 patients from a consecutive cohort of 205 patients presenting with stroke. *Eur J Pain* 2002, **6**:467–474.

Gordon WA, Hibbard MR. Post-stroke depression: an examination of the literature. *Arch Phys Med Rehab* 1997, **78**:658–663.

Gubitz G, Sandercock P. *Regular review: prevention of ischaemic stroke*. BMJ 2000, **321**:1455–1459.

Hacke W, Kaste M, Skyhoj Olsen T, Orgogozo J-M, Bogousslavsky J, European Stroke Initiative. *Recommendations for Stroke Management, European Stroke Initiative* 2002. Available at http://www.eusi-stroke.com/l3_pdf/Recommendations2002.pdf (accessed 5 February 2003).

Hankey GJ, Warlow CP. *Transient Ischaemic Attacks of the Brain and Eye*. London: WB Saunders; 1994.

Hanlon R. Motor learning following unilateral stroke. *Arch Phys Med Rehab* 1996, **77**: 811–815.

Hannaford PC, Croft PR, Kay CR. Oral contraception and stroke. *Stroke* 1994, **25**:935–942.

Hijdra A, van Gijn J, Nagelkerke N et al. Prediction of delayed cerebral ischaemia, rebleeding and outcome after aneurysmal subarachnoid haemorrhage. *Stroke* 1988, **19**:1250–1256.

Hough A. *Physiotherapy in Respiratory Care: A Problem Solving Approach*. London: Chapman & Hall; 1991.

House A, Dennis M, Morgridge L et al. Mood disorders in the year after first stroke. *Br J Psychiatry* 1991, **158**:83–92.

Indredavik B, Bakke F, Slørdahl SA et al. Treatment in a combined acute and rehabilitation stroke unit. Which aspects are most important? *Stroke* 1999, **30**:917–923.

Intercollegiate Working Party for Stroke. *National Clinical Guidelines for Stroke*, 2nd edn. London: Royal College of Physicians; 2002. Available at http://www.rcplondon.ac.uk/pubs/books/stroke/index.htm.

Jongbloed L. Prediction of function after stroke: a critical review. *Stroke* 1986, **17**:765–776.

Kalra L. The influence of stroke unit rehabilitation on functional recovery from stroke. *Stroke* 1994, **25**:821–825.

Kalra L, Evans A, Perez I et al. Alternative strategies for stroke care: a prospective randomized controlled trial *Lancet* 2000, **356**:894–899.

Kandel ER, Schwartz JH, Jessell TM. *Essentials of Neural Science and Behavior*. New York, USA: Appleton & Lange; 2000.

Kannel WB, Wolf PA. Epidemiology of cerebrovascular disease. In: Ross Rusell RW, ed. *Vascular Disease of the Central Nervous System*. Edinburgh: Churchill Livingstone; 1983:1–24.

Kettenbach G. *Writing SOAP notes*. Philadelphia: FA Davis; 1990.

Khaw KT. Epidemiology of stroke. *J Neurol Neurosurg Psychiatry* 1996, **61**:333–338.

Langhorne P, Williams B, Gilcrist B, Howie K. Do stroke units save lives? *Lancet* 1993, **342**:395–398.

Langton Hewer R. The epidemiology of disabling neurological disorders. In: Greenwood R, Barnes MP, McMillan TM et al., eds. *Neurological Rehabilitation*. London: Churchill Livingstone; 1993:3–12.

Liepert J, Bauder H, Miltner W et al. Treatment-induced cortical reorganisation after stroke in humans. *Stroke* 2000, **31**:1210–1216.

Lincoln NB, Leadbitter D. Assessment of motor function in stroke patients. *Physiotherapy* 1979, **65**:48–51.

Lincoln NB, Willis D, Philips SA et al. Comparison of rehabilitation practice on hospital wards for stroke patients. *Stroke* 1996, **27**:18–23.

Lundy-Ekman L. *Neuroscience: Fundamentals for Rehabilitation*. Philadelphia: WB Saunders; 1998.

Lynch M, Grisogono V. *Strokes and Head Injuries: A Guide for Patients, Families, Friends and Carers*. London: John Murray; 1991.

Partridge CJ, Morris LW, Edwards MS. Recovery from physical disability after stroke: profiles for different levels of starting severity. *Clin Rehab* 1993, **7**:210–217.

Pope PM. Postural management and special seating. In: Edwards S, ed. *Neurological Physiotherapy: A Problem Solving Approach*, 2nd edn. London: Churchill Livingstone; 2002:189–217.

Richards CL, Malouin F, Wood-Dauphinee S, Williams JI, Bouchard JP, Brunet D. Task-specific physical therapy for optimization of gait recovery in acute stroke patients. *Arch Phys Med Rehab* 1993, **74**:612–620.

Riddoch MJ, Humphreys GW, Bateman A. Cognitive deficits following stroke. *Physiotherapy* 1995, **81**:465–473.

Robertson IH, North N. Spatio-motor cueing in unilateral left neglect: the role of hemispace, hand and motor activation. *Neuropsychology* 1992, **30**:553–563.

Robinson R, Bolla Wilson K, Kaplan E et al. Depression influences intellectual impairment in stroke patients. *Br J Psychiatry* 1986, **148**:541–547.

Russell RW. *Vascular Disease of the Central Nervous System*, 2nd edn. Edinburgh: Churchill Livingstone; 1983.

Saeki S, Ogata H, Okubo T et al. Return to work after stroke: a follow-up study. *Stroke* 1995, **26**:399–401.

Salter PM, Ferguson RM. A process of physiotherapy: an analysis of the activities of the physiotherapist.

Proceedings of the World Confederation for Physical Therapy. London: 11th International Congress; 1991:1704–1706.

Schmidt RA. Motor learning principles for physical therapy. In: Lister MJ, ed. *Contemporary Management of Motor Control Problems. Proceedings of the II STEP Conference*. Alexandria, VA, USA: Foundation for Physical Therapy; 1991:49–63.

Scottish Intercollegiate Guidelines Network (SIGN). *Management of Patients with Stroke Part III: Identification and Management of Dysphagia*, 1997. Available at www.sign.ac.uk.

Shumway-Cook A, Woollacott M. *Motor Control, Theory and Practical Applications*, 2nd edn. Baltimore City: Williams and Wilkins; 2001.

Sinyor D, Amato P, Kaloupek DG et al. Post stroke depression: relationships to functional impairment, coping strategies and rehabilitation outcomes. *Stroke* 1986 **17**:1102–1107.

Smith MT, Baer GD. The achievement of simple mobility milestones following stroke. *Arch Phys Med Rehab* 1999, **80**:442–447

Smith M, Ball V. *Cardiovascular/Respiratory Physiotherapy*. London: Mosby; 1998.

Tinson DJ. How stroke patients spend their days. *Int Disabil Stud* 1989, **11**:45–49.

Turnbull GI. The application of motor learning theory. In: Banks M, ed. *Stroke*. Edinburgh: Churchill Livingstone; 1986.

Van Langenberghe HVK, Partridge CJ, Edwards MS et al. Shoulder pain in hemiplegia – a literature review. *Physiother Pract* 1988, **4**:155–162.

Van Ouwenaller C, LaPlace PM, Chantraine A. Painful shoulder in hemiplegia. *Arch Phys Med Rehab* 1986, **67**:23–26.

VanSant AF. Motor control, motor learning and motor development. In: Montgomery PC, Connolly BH, eds. *Motor Control and Physical Therapy: Theoretical Framework and Practical Applications*. Tennessee: Chattanooga Group; 1991:13–28.

Wade DT, Collen FM, Robb GF et al. Physiotherapy intervention late after stroke. *BMJ* 1992, **405**:609–613.

Wade DT, Langton Hewer L, Skilbech CE et al. *Stroke: A Critical Approach to Diagnosis, Treatment and Management*. London: Chapman Hall; 1985a.

Wade DT, Wood VA, Langton Hewer R. Recovery after stroke – the first 3 months. *J Neurol Neurosurg Psychiatry* 1985b, **48**:7–13.

Wanklyn P, Forster A, Young J. Hemiplegic shoulder pain (HSP); natural history and investigation of associated features. *Disabil Rehab* 1996; **18**:497–501.

Warlow CP. Epidemiology of stroke. *Lancet* 1998, **352** (Suppl III):1–4.

Warlow CP. Stroke, transient ischaemic attacks and intracranial venous thrombosis. In: Donaghy M, ed. *Brain's Diseases of the Nervous System*, 11th edn. Oxford: Oxford University Press; 2001, 775–896.

Warlow CP, Sandercock P, Dennis M et al. *Stroke: A Practical Guide to Management*, 2nd edn. Oxford: Blackwell Science; 2001.

Whisnant JP. Effectiveness versus efficacy of treatment of hypertension for stroke prevention. *Neurology* 1996, **46**:301–307.

Widén-Holmqvist L, de Pedro-Cuesta J, Holm M et al. Stroke rehabilitation in Stockholm. Basis for late intervention in patients living at home. *Scand J Rehab Med* 1993, **25**:173–181.

Williams P. *Gray's Anatomy*. London: Churchill Livingstone; 1995.

Williams LS, Weinberger M, Harris LE et al. Development of a stroke-specific quality of life scale. *Stroke* 1999 **30**:1362–1369.

Winstein CJ. Designing practice for motor learning: clinical implications. In: Lister MJ, ed. *Contemporary Management of Motor Control Problems. Proceedings of the II STEP Conference*. Alexandria, VA, USA: Foundation for Physical Therapy; 1991:65–76.

Wood J, Wade J. Setting up stroke services in district general hospitals. *Br J Ther Rehab* 1995, **2**:199–203.

Chapter 7

Acquired brain injury: trauma and pathology

M Campbell

INTRODUCTION

Acquired brain injury (ABI) is an overarching term applied to describe insults to the brain that are not congenital or perinatal in nature. Usually the term ABI is used to describe the outcome of a distinct traumatic injury or a single-event pathology, such as a subarachnoid haemorrhage or a cerebral abscess, but is not applied to the results of progressive disorders or degenerative disease. The most frequent cause of ABI in young adults and adolescents is trauma and this chapter, therefore, takes traumatic brain injury (TBI) as the primary focus for discussion.

Other common pathologies producing a similar scope of neural deficits to TBI, and that are amenable to a comparable approach in terms of physiotherapy management, are also included.

Discussion of physical management is confined to rehabilitation, recovery and adjustment. The management of ABI in the context of terminal illness is not addressed. Physiotherapists most commonly encounter individuals who have survived injuries at the more severe end of the spectrum: those who are admitted for extended periods of hospital care and those who continue to have significant impairments of motor performance following hospital discharge. However, the effects of brain injury extend far beyond overt physical disability (Table 7.1) and may impact on both family members and wider social networks. An adequate understanding of this extended effect is essential if physiotherapists are to work effectively with other health and social care professionals to assist a person's re-establishment within the community.

TRAUMATIC BRAIN INJURY

Different types of TBI and their general management are discussed here. The physiotherapist's role in the

Table 7.1 Definitions of traumatic brain injury

Organisation	Definition
Medical Disability Society, UK	Brain injury caused by trauma to the head (including the effects on the brain of other possible complications of injury, notably hypoxaemia and hypotension, and intracerebral haematoma)
National Head Injury Foundation, USA	Traumatic head injury is an insult to the brain, not of degenerative or congenital nature but caused by an external force, that may produce a diminished or altered state of consciousness, which results in impairment of cognitive abilities or physical functioning. It can also result in the disturbance of behaviour or emotional functioning. These impairments may be either temporary or permanent and cause partial or total functional disability or psychosocial maladjustment

rehabilitation of patients with ABI is discussed after the section on pathological conditions, as physical management is similar for patients regardless of the cause.

Mechanisms of injury

TBI occurs when there is a direct high-energy blow to the head or when the brain comes into contact with the inside of the skull as a result of a sudden acceleration or deceleration of the body as a whole. The brain is predisposed to certain types of injury by virtue of its structure and design, and because of irregularities on the inside of the skull. The type of brain injury sustained is a product of the circumstances generating the external force that reacts with the brain tissue, the amount of energy involved and how that energy is dissipated throughout the brain substance.

The brain has most of its mass in two large cerebral hemispheres, above the narrower brainstem and spinal cord (Nolte, 1999a). The brain and spinal cord are suspended within three layers of membranes known as the meninges and are further protected by a layer of cerebrospinal fluid between the inner two layers, the arachnoid and pia mater. The outer layer, the dura mater, is the most substantial layer and provides most of the

mechanical strength of the meninges (Nolte, 1999b). The dura mater is attached to the inner surface of the skull. During normal activities the brain is constrained to move with the head but as it is not directly anchored within the skull this does not apply during sudden, swift movements or high-energy impacts. The brain substance is composed of cells and axonal connections forming areas of different densities that move and respond to force in different ways. Thus, the brain is free to move independent of the skull and in the presence of high energy it does so in an irregular manner, causing stretching and shearing of brain tissue. Further damage is inflicted on the soft brain structure as it moves across the irregularities on the internal surface of the skull (Jennett & Teasdale, 1981).

Types of injury and associated damage

Primary damage

External forces are expressed via three main mechanisms of primary brain injury:

1. direct impact on the skull
2. penetration through the skull into the brain substance
3. collision between the brain substance and the internal skull structure.

TBI can occur without disruption of the skull and this is described as a **closed injury**. Alternatively, the skull may crack in a simple linear fracture, be depressed into the brain tissue or be pierced by a sharp or high-velocity missile. Such **penetrating injuries** may be complicated by fragments of bone, skin and hair being pushed into the brain tissue, increasing the damage and raising the risk of infection. In the case of high-velocity injuries, such as gunshot wounds, damage also occurs wide of the tract created by the course of the missile, as energy is dissipated within the brain substance.

Closed injuries can result in local impact, polar impact, shearing, laceration, axonal or blood vessel damage. Local impact damage occurs immediately below the site of impact and can affect the scalp and meninges, as well as the brain substance in different measure, depending on the velocity of the impact and the flexibility of the skull. The brain may collide with the skull at the opposite pole to the site of primary impact and oscillate between the two, producing additional shearing damage. Where shearing forces affect the long axonal tracts, such as in hyperextension or rotational injuries, axons may be stretched or severed within their myelin sheaths (Adams et al., 1977). This is known as **diffuse axonal injury** (DAI). When DAI is widespread it is associated with severe injury but has also been shown to occur in mild injuries (Povlishock et al., 1983).

Lacerations most commonly occur adjacent to the internal areas of the skull that are irregular, producing damage to the frontal and temporal lobes of the brain. Hyperextension injuries can cause damage to the carotid or vertebral arteries interrupting blood flow as a result of dissection or occlusion. Cerebral vessels can also be torn or ruptured and result in a local collection of blood. When this occurs in the immediate aftermath of an injury it is known as an *acute haematoma*. A slower accumulation of blood, known as a *chronic haematoma*, is most frequently found in the very young or in older adults.

Secondary damage

Secondary damage results from biochemical and mechanical factors. As soon as the injury occurs, the tissue damage and cell death that result spark a pathological process leading to chemical damage to adjacent but previously uninjured brain tissue and the development of oedema. The presence of oedema or a significant haematoma will result in displacement and distortion of other brain tissue. There is little internal capacity within the skull to accommodate the swelling or distorted brain and further damage occurs as the brain is pressed against the skull or pushed into adjacent intracranial compartments. As well as compression of brain substance, this can also result in occlusion of major arteries.

Secondary damage may be aggravated by infection or complications associated with systemic dysfunction, which may result from the effects of the brain injury or be caused by coexisting injuries. Around 40% of severely injured patients will have other significant injuries (Gentleman et al., 1986).

Epidemiology of TBI

Studies reporting the incidence of TBI in western developed countries produce a range of values of around 200–300 new cases presenting for medical evaluation per 100 000 population each year; for example, in the USA (Sorenson & Kraus, 1991), the UK (Jennett & MacMillan, 1981) and Australia (Hillier et al., 1997). The peak risk of injury is between the ages of 16 and 25, declining until late middle age before beginning to rise again around age 65 (Sorenson & Kraus, 1991). Males are almost three times more likely to be injured and to have more severe injuries, resulting in an injured survivor ratio of around 2:1 male to female (Kraus & McArthur, 1996). In 1998 the number of people living in the UK with significant disability after TBI was estimated to be between 50 000 and 75 000 (Centre for Health Service Studies, 1998).

Risk factors and preventive measures

Sporting accidents and falls are the primary causal factors for those under 20 years, with transport accidents accounting for less than 15% of injuries in one study focusing on an adolescent sample (Body & Leatham, 1996). In adult populations transport accidents are commonly responsible for around 50–60% of injuries, with falls and assaults being the other major causal factors. In older adults there is a very high level of falls and a more even level of occurrence across genders (Miller & Jones, 1990).

Injury prevention can be considered on three levels (Kraus & McArthur, 1996):

1. reduction of the frequency of any hazard, for example, games rule changes that reduce sporting collisions or improved vehicle design leading to the prevention of crashes, or the degree of exposure to that hazard, such as wearing protective clothing, physical restraints or the use of airbags
2. limitation of the immediate effects of an injury (see 'Principles of acute management of TBI', below)
3. limitation of the longer-term impact by preventing the development of additional problems; for example, by providing physical, psychological and vocational rehabilitation.

Positive effects have been reported for motorcyclists wearing helmets (Kraus & Sorenson, 1994; Gabella et al., 1995) and following the introduction of compulsory bicycle helmets in the USA (Thompson et al., 1989) and Australia (McDermott, 1995). Increasing awareness of the potential for enduring problems following minor brain injury and the cumulative effects of repeated minor trauma has led to the development of guidelines for the management of concussion injuries in sport (Fick, 1995; Leblanc, 1995). However, there remains a great deal to do in terms of educating health care providers, youth and sports organisations to ensure that guidelines are followed and the correct advice given (Genuardi & King, 1995).

The Pashby Sports Safety Fund Concussion website (Leclerc et al., 2002) gives definitions, explanations and advice, so that the effects of concussion can be recognised by those involved in sport at any level and to encourage return to participation to be appropriately paced.

In terms of individual risk factors, substance misuse and particularly exposure to alcohol are widely recognised as prominent contributory factors in accidental (Jennett, 1996) and violent injury (Drubach et al., 1993). However, although there is some evidence that withdrawal from chronic alcohol use may exacerbate toxic cell damage following trauma, the net effects of the presence of alcohol at the time of injury at an individual level have not yet been defined (Kelly, 1995).

Measures and diagnoses of severity

The severity of TBI ranges from mild concussion with transient symptoms to very severe injury resulting in death. The two domains most frequently taken as indicators of injury severity are coma (depth and duration) and posttraumatic amnesia (PTA).

Coma

Coma is defined as 'not obeying commands, not uttering words and not opening eyes' (Teasdale & Jennett, 1974). The Glasgow Coma Scale (GCS; Teasdale & Jennett, 1974, 1976) is the most widely used measure of depth and duration of coma. The GCS has three subscales, giving a summated score of 3–15:

- eye opening (rated 1–4)
- best motor response (rated 1–6)
- verbal response (rated 1–5).

Although a general impression of a person's conscious level can be gleaned from a summated score, retaining the scores at subscale level gives a more accurate clinical picture. For example, knowledge of the lowest motor response rating and the pattern of improvement over time can provide physiotherapists with a valuable insight into the initial severity of damage to brain tissue associated with physical performance. Regarding summated GCS scores the convention is to categorise injuries into mild, moderate or severe (Table 7.2) using the lowest score in the first 24 h.

Table 7.2   Traumatic brain injury severity: lowest summated Glasgow Coma Scale (GCS) in the first 24 h postinjury (Bond, 1986)

Grade	Summated GCS score
Mild	13–15
Moderate	9–12
Severe	3–8

Duration of coma is also used as an indicator of severity, where coma is generally numerically defined as a GCS score of 8 or less (Bond, 1990). This convention introduces a further grading of very severe (Table 7.3), reflecting the increasing knowledge that may be gained from longitudinal review.

Postcoma states (vegetative and minimally conscious states) are discussed below (see 'Loss of consciousness').

Table 7.3   Traumatic brain injury severity: duration of coma (Bond, 1986)

Grade	Duration of coma (GCS ≤ 8)
Mild	<15 min
Moderate	>15 min, <6 h
Severe	>6 h, <48 h
Very severe	>48 h

GCS, Glasgow Coma Scale.

Posttraumatic amnesia

The definition and assessment of PTA remain controversial. The original concept was developed by Russell and taken to be the period from injury until the return of day-to-day memory on a continuous basis (Russell, 1932). Most analyses now identify disturbances in three domains: orientation, memory and behaviour. For example, 'the patient is confused, amnesic for ongoing events and likely to evidence behavioural disturbance' (Levin et al., 1979, p. 675). However, Russell's categorisation of levels of severity is still used today (Table 7.4).

Tate and colleagues (2000) discussed the relative merits of currently available scales for prospective assessment of duration of PTA, addressing issues of orientation and memory, and highlighting in particular the difficulties in assessing the memory component. Retrospective assessment of PTA duration has been shown to be as reliable as prospective assessment in a severe population (McMillan et al., 1996), although Gronwall & Wrightson (1980) found that one-quarter of mildly injured patients changed their estimation at a second interview after 3 months.

In practice, severity, particularly after the acute period, is currently assessed with reference to all three factors discussed above and with additional consideration given to early computed tomographic (CT) scans and later magnetic resonance imaging (MRI) scans when available.

Table 7.4   Traumatic brain injury severity: duration of posttraumatic amnesia (PTA; Russell, 1932)

Grade	PTA
Mild	<1 h
Moderate	>1 h, <24 h
Severe	>1 day, <7 days
Very severe	>7 days

Service provision

Improvements in surgical techniques and medical management, particularly since the 1970s, have resulted in substantially improved survival rates, and there is clarity and consensus on many medical management issues. Precise guidelines for the early management of those who sustain a TBI are now available, for example, the Scottish national clinical guideline (Scottish Intercollegiate Guidelines Network, 2000). However, services beyond the acute phase have been very slow to develop in the UK (see Campbell (2000a, e) for discussion) and while there are areas of good practice, there is a growing recognition of the geographical inequalities and overall inadequacies of current provision (House of Commons, 2001).

Worldwide, a number of models of service provision have been proposed, based on clinical experience and available evidence (Burke, 1987; Eames & Wood, 1989; Oddy et al., 1989; McMillan & Greenwood, 1993b). Across these proposals there are a number of recurring themes, including: the need for organisational integration; interdisciplinary team work; professionals with advanced knowledge and skills; and a systematic programme of service evaluation and innovative research (Campbell, 2000e). Furthermore, there is acknowledgement of the need for multiple service components across health and social care, including options for supported living, and for services to be flexible in response, so that individuals may access them at a time of need and on more than one occasion, if appropriate.

Principles of acute management of TBI

The aims of initial emergency and early medical management are to limit the development of secondary brain damage, and to provide the best conditions for recovery from any reversible damage that has already occurred. This is achieved by establishing and maintaining a clear airway with adequate oxygenation and replacement fluids to ensure a good peripheral circulation with adequate blood volume. It is essential to achieve this before an accurate neurological assessment can be made.

During the initial evaluation, movement of the cervical spine is minimised until any fractures have been excluded. Where appropriate, prophylactic antibiotic therapy is commenced immediately (Bullock & Teasdale, 1990a, b). Except for the management of immediate seizures, the routine early use of anticonvulsant therapy is not now recommended (Hernandez & Naritoku, 1997).

Patients who exhibit breathing difficulties are assisted by intubation and ventilation (Bullock & Teasdale, 1990a). In addition, elective ventilation is often the treatment of choice in the presence of facial, chest or abdominal injuries, and for those with a summated GCS score of less than 9. Ventilation is usually achieved via endotracheal tube and tracheostomy is only performed where facial or spinal fractures determine this course of action or in the few cases when respiratory support is required over a more extended period. Even when ventilation is not indicated, oxygen therapy is recommended to help meet the injured brain's increased energy requirements (Frost, 1985).

Those with significant injuries are at risk of breakdown of the normal process of cerebral autoregulation that ensures blood flow to the brain is consistently maintained, independent of the normal fluctuations in systemic blood pressure (Aitkenhead, 1986). When this protective mechanism is lost, cerebral perfusion pressure (CPP) becomes directly related to the systemic mean arterial blood pressure (MAP) and the intracranial pressure (ICP). Breathing patterns and fluid volumes can be manipulated in a ventilated and sedated patient. With the prescription of appropriate drug therapy, optimum blood gas levels, systemic blood pressure and, as far as possible, cerebral blood flow can be achieved, minimising the development of additional brain damage.

The physical position and management of the patient are also important in the control of raised ICP and, in particular, the prevention of additional cerebral congestion due to obstruction of venous drainage. A slightly raised head position (avoiding neck flexion and compression of the jugular veins) is recommended (Feldman et al., 1992), although the maintenance of neutral alignment may be sufficient if raising the head threatens cerebral perfusion by lowering the systemic blood pressure (Rosner & Colley, 1986).

Activities that raise intrathoracic pressure also raise ICP and need to be minimised. This has particular relevance for respiratory care where the objective of preventing the organisation of secretions must be achieved, with minimal use of interventions likely to raise ICP, such as manual hyperinflation. When a problematic chest requires vigorous attention, pretreatment sedation may be indicated, allowing bronchial suction with minimal provocation of cough. There is some evidence that slow percussive techniques may help reduce ICP (Garrad & Bullock, 1986). The principles of intervention for respiratory health are considered in detail by Ada and colleagues (1990), Roberts (2002) and in brief below (see 'The role of the physiotherapist in the acute phase').

Neurosurgical intervention after TBI

In closed TBIs, surgery is undertaken as a matter of urgency to evacuate any significant haematoma and so decompress the injured brain (Jennett & Lindsay, 1994a). Where there is a depressed fracture or a penetrating wound, surgery will also be undertaken to remove any debris, clean the wound and restore the normal contour of the skull as far as possible. In some centres, minor procedures to insert an ICP-monitoring device will be performed, according to local protocols (Pickard & Czosnyka, 2000).

Physical management

Beyond intervention to save life and promote the ideal conditions for cerebral repair and recovery, the next most important issue is the prevention of secondary physical changes and the provision of optimum conditions to promote physical recovery. Patients may benefit from being cared for on a special pressure-relieving mattress (Moseley, 2002) and from intensive management of nutritional input (Taylor & Fettes, 1998). Sedated patients are paralysed and vulnerable to muscular and other soft-tissue changes associated with immobility and inactivity. They are also exposed to consistent environmental stimuli, which if left unmanaged will result in significant muscle length changes. For example, the combined effects of gravity and the weight of bedding over extended periods in lying can lead to the development of foot plantarflexion.

It is vital that physiotherapists are involved in developing a physical management plan to guide the management of physical factors over the full 24-h period and that this occurs at the earliest possible point following hospital admission. Common physical deficits and their management are described later in this chapter.

PATHOLOGICAL CONDITIONS

Cerebral aneurysms

A cerebral aneurysm is an abnormal dilation or ballooning of a cerebral artery, which is usually due to a congenital or acquired weakness in the wall of the vessel (Jennett & Lindsay, 1994b). It is not usually possible to identify a single cause for the development of an aneurysm, although hypertension and arteriosclerosis are seen as risk factors. A rare form, mycotic aneurysm, results from a blood-borne infection.

Presentation

Often the first indication of the presence of an aneurysm is when it ruptures and bleeds into or around the brain. Bleeding is most commonly into the subarachnoid space (subarachnoid haemorrhage) but rupture may also result in bleeding directly into brain tissue. Subarachnoid haemorrhage has an incidence of between 10 and 15 per 100 000 population per annum, with aneurysm rupture accounting for around 75% of cases (Lindsay & Bone, 1997). The mortality rate following aneurysm rupture is 1 in 4 and 30% of people who have a subarachnoid haemorrhage secondary to a ruptured aneurysm will have more than one aneurysm (Lindsay & Bone, 1997). Aneurysm rupture is most common between the ages of 40 and 60, a more mature population than the peak occurrence of TBI, but a younger age group than the mean age of 70 for stroke caused by cerebral infarct (Dombovy et al., 1998a).

Unruptured aneurysms may produce neurological symptoms due to their size or location and be diagnosed following medical investigation, including MRI brain scan (see Ch. 2). For example, a lesion on an internal carotid artery at the level of the optic chiasm can produce peripheral blurred vision (Chigbu, 2003). Some are discovered incidentally when investigations are performed for other reasons. The diagnosis of a cerebral aneurysm is usually confirmed by angiogram, a procedure that involves injecting a radiopaque substance into the blood vessels and taking X-rays of the head (Tavernas, 1996).

Complications

Before the advent of effective surgery, almost one-third of those with a ruptured aneurysm would bleed again within 1 month. The risk of a rebleed if surgery is not undertaken remains high for 6 months. Whether or not surgery is undertaken after subarachnoid haemorrhage, there is a risk of vasospasm causing ischaemia or infarction, with resultant additional neurological damage. This most frequently occurs between 4 and 12 days after the initial bleed.

Extracranial complications include cardiac arrhythmias, myocardial infarction, pulmonary oedema and stress ulcers. Hydrocephalus may occur in the early postbleed period but is also reported as a late complication in 10% of cases (Lindsay & Bone, 1997).

Medical management of aneurysms and subarachnoid haemorrhage (SAH)

Subarachnoid haemorrhage is graded into five levels of severity (Table 7.5). Until the mid-1980s surgery for all grades was routinely delayed for 1–2 weeks after a bleed for fear of provoking vasospasm. However, reappraisal of the risk of a rebleed within this period and improved surgical and non-surgical techniques has encouraged more aggressive management. In most centres, intervention will be undertaken for grades I and II within 3 days (Lindsay & Bone, 1997) and in

Table 7.5 Grades of subarachnoid haemorrhage (Teasdale et al., 1988)

Grade	Glasgow Coma Scale	Additional descriptors
I	15	No motor deficit
II	13–14	No motor deficit
III	13–14	With motor deficit
IV	7–12	With or without motor deficit
V	3–6	With or without motor deficit

some centres early intervention is becoming routine for the majority of cases (Dombovy et al., 1998a).

Intervention for subarachnoid haemorrhage or intact aneurysms will usually involve surgical clipping, that is, open brain surgery and the placing of a small metallic clip across the base of the aneurysm preventing blood flow into the weakened area, or embolisation (Jennett & Lindsay, 1994b). Embolisation is a more recent vascular technique whereby a metal coil or balloons are introduced into the artery to block off the aneurysm via the arterial system at the groin, under radiological guidance (Pile-Spellman, 1996). The choice of intervention is determined by the size and position of the aneurysm.

Physical management postintervention will vary, depending on the extent of damage caused by the prior SAH and the nature of the intervention. Endovascular treatment is usually followed by 24 h bed rest and then mobilisation. Following open surgery, management may be similar to that after surgery for TBI (see 'Rehabilitation after brain injury', below).

Arteriovenous malformations

An arteriovenous malformation (AVM) is an abnormal tangle of blood vessels lacking in capillary vessels and is thought to be a congenital abnormality. Within the central nervous system they can occur within the brain, associated with the dural layer of the meninges or within the spinal cord. As dural AVMs carry a low risk of haemorrhage and spinal AVMs produce symptoms more closely related to incomplete spinal lesions, we will only consider cerebral AVMs here.

A total of 40–60% of cerebral AVMs are discovered following haemorrhage, which produces symptoms such as seizures, neurological deficits or headache. Symptomatic AVMs present most frequently in the 20–40 age group and the mortality rate is lower than SAH at 10–20%. The risk of rebleed is also much less than following an aneurysmal haemorrhage and is

highest for small lesions (Lindsay & Bone, 1997). Haematomas associated with AVMs are often visible on CT or MRI scans. Otherwise diagnosis will be confirmed via angiography.

Medical management of AVM

If and when an AVM is thought to be amenable to direct intervention, there are a number of possible options. These include surgical resection, stereotactic radiosurgery and embolisation (Jennett & Lindsay, 1994b). Any one of these interventions may be regarded as the treatment of choice or, in some cases, a combination of these interventions may be used in a stepwise progression. Stereotactic radiosurgery is a method of precisely delivering radiation to a brain lesion while sparing the surrounding brain tissue (Pollock, 2002).

Infectious processes

Primary brain damage can result from meningitis, encephalitis or brain abscess.

Brain abscess

This condition is now relatively rare, with an incidence rate of 2–3 per 1 000 000 population per annum (Lindsay & Bone, 1997). The infection can have its source in such things as dental caries, sinusitis, mastoiditis, subacute endocarditis or pulmonary disease.

The abscess can accumulate in the extradural space or in the brain substance or in the subdural space, when it may be called empyema. With antibiotics and surgical drainage there is now a 90% survival rate, although around half of those who survive will experience subsequent seizures.

Meningitis

Meningitis has a range of bacterial and viral sources, and a variety of presentations, associated complications and outcomes (Kroll & Moxon, 1987; Johnson, 1998). Drug therapy is commenced immediately in any suspected case, even before the infective organism is identified, and continued up to 2 weeks after pyrexia has settled.

Encephalitis

The most common form of viral encephalitis results from the herpes simplex virus which selectively affects the inferior frontotemporal lobes of the brain. This can result in extremely amnesic survivors, although treatment with aciclovir has increased survival rates to 80% and lessened resultant deficits (Lindsay & Bone, 1997).

Cerebral tumours

Primary brain tumours have an incidence level of 6 per 100 000 population with slightly less than 10% of these occurring in children (Lindsay & Bone, 1997; see also Ch. 16). There are many different kinds of tumours with names reflecting the cells of origin and situation of growth. It is beyond the scope of this book to detail the treatment and prognostic factors for each kind but it is important to note that even large tumours can be benign, resulting in a stable neurological deficit. It is clearly important to understand the nature of the tumour involved and to have the best prediction of outcome in order to structure rehabilitative intervention appropriately (see Thomas, 1990, and Al-Mefty, 1991, for further reading).

DEFICITS ASSOCIATED WITH ACQUIRED BRAIN INJURY

There is a wide range of commonly occurring deficits after TBI that present in a variety of mixes and severities. These affect psychosocial domains, core cognitive and sensorimotor skills and specific integrative cognitive functions that, in the presence of adequate psychosocial function, allow the core skills to be used in the organisation, planning and implementation of functional activities. Recent work has begun to document a similar range of impairments between this population and those who survive a significant subarachnoid bleed (Dombovy et al., 1998a, b).

Impairments resulting from other sources of ABI may not necessarily encompass such a wide range of effects at an individual level but the same range of impairments will certainly be reflected across each population.

For the sake of clarity in this discussion, we will focus primarily on recovery following severe TBI and add further structure by considering rehabilitation as occurring in three consecutive phases as described by Mazaux & Richer (1998; Table 7.6).

Not all impairments are observable immediately following injury and the context within which assessment takes place will influence what residual impairments may be expected or detected at all stages of recovery. Time since onset is not on its own a guiding factor, even within the severe TBI subpopulation, and other potential influences to consider are injury mechanism, additional injuries, treatment received and the progress already made.

REHABILITATION AFTER BRAIN INJURY

Given the complex array of deficits that can occur, it should be apparent that physiotherapists do not have the knowledge or skills independently to address rehabilitation issues in this client group. Indeed, publications emanating from specialist provision advocate an interdisciplinary (Body et al., 1996; Children's Trust at Tadworth Rehabilitation Team, 1997; Powell et al., 1994; New Zealand National Health Committee, 1998) or transdisciplinary (Jackson & Davies, 1995) team approach. The role of the physiotherapist within an

Table 7.6 Objectives of three phases of rehabilitation after brain injury (compiled from information in Mazaux & Richer, 1998)

	Phase 1: acute	Phase 2: subacute	Phase 3: postacute
Objectives	● Prevent orthopaedic and visceral complications ● Provide appropriate sensory stimulation	● Accelerate recovery of impairments ● Compensate for disabilities	● Maximise independence ● Maximise community reintegration ● Maximise psychosocial adjustment and self-acceptance
Common domains of focus	● Global physical and sensory systems	● Mobility ● Cognition ● Behaviour ● Personality ● Affect	● Physical ● Domestic ● Social
Anticipated approach	● Supportive of medical management ● Preparatory for subsequent interventions	● Holistic ● Addressing physical independence ● Addressing psychological independence ● Addressing self-awareness	● Personalised

interdisciplinary team is described in detail by Campbell (2000f), setting the assessment approach described by Body and colleagues (1996) in a wider context, and adding further material to guide goal-setting and intervention planning.

Client- and family-centred approach

The particular interdisciplinary approach described by Campbell (2000f) includes a collaborative team assessment process that attempts to place the individual and close associates at the centre of that process. This is seen as crucial to effective service delivery and as an organisational mechanism to ensure a consistent standard of information-gathering.

The design of the assessment process, which includes a multiprofessional assessment case discussion, facilitates the development of agreed team goals that are feasible to deliver and relevant to the injured person as an individual. For each individual, as well as standard assessments to identify impairments and strengths (see Ch. 3), the preinjury cultural base, lifestyle and aspirations are acknowledged and incorporated into goal development. Psychosocial functioning, including the level of self-awareness and stage of adjustment to their new circumstance, is given prominent consideration and included in the discussion of assessment findings *by the whole team*.

Each team member, including the physiotherapist, contributes to the prioritisation of the intervention goals based on the global assessment findings. These recommendations are then fully discussed with the client and carer, and a plan of action is then agreed. This is an inclusive method of assessment, using multiple informants, both professional and personal, to the injured person. It uses professional expertise to synthesise and interpret assessment findings but there is also a formal process for referral back to, and discussion with, the client and family at the initial assessment stage and throughout the period of contact. In this way it is hoped to establish an effective collaborative relationship with all of those who have an interest in each case. Client-centred practice is discussed in Chapter 22.

Professional collaboration

The importance of professional collaboration in the development and delivery of services for this client group cannot be sufficiently stressed. It is important to address the range of deficits that occur, to avoid duplication of effort and ensure all aspects are addressed. Innovative ways of working have evolved, for example, to deal with those difficulties that clients encounter that are not seen as the traditional area of practice for any specific profession.

Many specialist centres use a *key worker system*, where one team member will take on some additional, mainly organisational, tasks to ensure that the wider needs of clients are met. Services for different phases of recovery are often provided on different hospital and community sites and the nature of the clients' and carers' needs demand the inclusion of specialist social work support for extended periods of time.

The complexities of health and social care services are challenging even for professionals involved in their delivery and cross-agency working, extending into other areas such as education, housing or vocational training, is required if effective service delivery is to be achieved. Currently, attempts are being made to link all of these service components and agencies by mechanisms such as *integrated care pathways*, *multiprofessional planning groups* and in some areas collaborative funding arrangements.

Physiotherapists have a unique body of knowledge to contribute to the team process but we have also much to learn from service users and from other professional groups. Learning for all is accelerated when knowledge is effectively shared and so we have a responsibility to be proactive in this regard to improve the delivery of care.

Impact on families and other social networks

At the beginning of this chapter reference was made to the wider impact of ABI on close relationships and wider social networks. These effects have been studied in reasonable depth since early work in the 1970s and 1980s first began to document carer distress and burden (Romano, 1974; Rosenbaum & Najenson, 1976; Brooks, 1984; Brooks et al., 1987). There is now little doubt of the intense early trauma, and for many the continuing stresses, that family and friends can endure.

Campbell (2000g) discussed the impact of this trauma in practical terms, using case examples and with reference to a model of response described by Douglas (1990; see Table 7.7). Not all families make it through this five-stage process (Ponsford, 1995) and not all family members are able to progress at the same speed (Campbell, 2000g). It is important to consider, along with other team members, where carers are in this process before making demands on them to actively contribute to the rehabilitation programme.

Treatment goals that presume active assistance from a family member who does not have either the physical or emotional resources to respond appropriately are unlikely to be achieved. It is also important to interpret carer behaviours in the light of the trauma they are experiencing and with reference to how they may be coping with the difficulties presented. Families have individual characteristics and coping styles before the

Table 7.7 Family response to traumatic brain injury: a five-stage model

Inpatient care	Shock	Confusion
		Anguish
		Frustration
		Helplessness
	Expectancy	Exaggerated optimism about recovery
		Denial
		Hope
Community-based care	Reality	Depression
		Anger
		Guilt
		Withdrawal from socialisation
		Disruption of family relationships and existing roles
	Mourning	Awareness of permanence of the situation
		Acceptance of changes in the injured family member
		Grieving for what might have been
	Adjustment	Readjusting expectations
		Redefining relationships and roles
		Restructuring the family environment

Reproduced from Douglas (1990), with permission.

advent of the brain injury; each family member has an established role within that family, and each family is at its own particular stage of progress with reference to normal life changes and developments (Turnbull & Turnbull, 1991). All of these factors will influence how, and how well, each will cope with the early trauma and the ongoing demands.

Physiotherapists do not have the role of assessing family systems or of providing intervention or support programmes to facilitate successful carer engagement. However, it is essential that they have a strong awareness of the issues involved so that they may function effectively within the wider team structure and understand the impact of the demands they make on carers as well as patients.

Issues emerging in the acute phase

Loss of consciousness

As described earlier, sudden neural dysfunction or significant damage is likely to result in loss of consciousness. This may be short-lived or may extend over weeks or months, and in some cases even years. There is often confusion about terminology of coma and postcoma:

- Coma is the state where there is no verbal response, no obeying commands and the patient does not open the eyes either spontaneously or to any stimulus (Jennett & Teasdale, 1977). Coma rarely lasts longer than a month; the patient either dies or emerges into the vegetative state.

- The vegetative state (VS; Jennett & Plum, 1972) is defined as 'a clinical condition of complete unawareness of the self and the environment, accompanied by sleep–wake cycles with either complete or partial preservation of hypothalamic and brainstem automatic functions' (Multi-Society Task Force, 1994, p. 1500).

- The minimally conscious state (MCS) is a condition that has been described more recently. This is 'a condition of severely altered consciousness in which minimal but definite behavioural evidence of self or environmental awareness is demonstrated' (Giacino et al., 2002, pp. 350–351). One or more of four diagnostic criteria confirm MCS and include: (1) following simple commands; (2) yes/no responses; (3) intelligible verbalisation; and (4) purposeful behaviour. Such meaningful interaction with the environment is not consistent but is reproducible or sustained enough to distinguish it from reflexive behaviour.

These three conditions are part of the continuum from coma through to emergence of awareness. The patient may remain in the VS or MCS as a transient phase or the condition may be permanent.

It is now recognised that patients may be misdiagnosed as being in VS when, in fact, they have significant levels of awareness. For example, Childs et al. (1993) reported that 37% of patients admitted more than 1 month postinjury with a diagnosis of coma or persistent VS had some level of awareness. In a group of longer-term patients in a nursing home, Tresch et al. (1991) found that 18% of long-term nursing home residents diagnosed as being in the persistent VS were aware of themselves or their environment.

Andrews et al. (1996) reviewed the records of 40 consecutive patients admitted to their specialist profound brain injury unit after 6 months following their brain injury and found that 43% had been misdiagnosed (41% of these for more than a year, including three for more than 5 years). The levels of cognitive functioning present in this misdiagnosed group at the time of discharge were such that 60% were oriented in time, place and person; 75% were able to recall a name after 15 min delay; 69% were able to carry out simple mental arithmetic; 75% were able to generate words to communicate their needs; and 86% were able to make choices about their daily social activities.

The implications of misdiagnosis involve legal as well as clinical aspects, given the practice of applying to the courts to withdraw nutrition and hydration from patients diagnosed as being in VS. Precise estimates of the incidence and prevalence of VS and MCS are not available and the relative rarity of the conditions means that most clinicians will have little or no experience in assessing such patients. It is recommended that the clinician contemplating a diagnosis of VS in any individual case should seek the views of two other doctors, one a neurologist, before confirming such a diagnosis (British Medical Association, 1996).

Increased muscle tone

Prior to sedation, during the period of emergence from coma or when sedation is withdrawn, abnormalities of motor behaviour may begin to be observed. In its most dramatic form this is seen as excessively raised muscle tone, producing rigid trunk and limbs. The quality and intensity of this raised muscle tone is strikingly different from that seen after stroke. In the lower limbs it is often highly organised across opposing muscle groups preventing hip and knee flexion and ankle dorsiflexion. In the upper limbs, there can be similar levels of extension or the same intensity of activity may be seen predominantly in the flexor muscle groups, resulting in a fixed flexed position with the limbs almost adhering to the chest wall. Another primary difference from stroke is that the increase in muscular tone can develop within a very short time of the injury, particularly in severe cases, unlike after stroke where there is often a period of low tone in the early stages.

When muscle tone is high there is usually a global effect involving the back and neck extensors as well as the limb muscles. One side of the body may be more affected than the other, but this may only become apparent when the overall level of tone begins to drop. At this stage, or in cases where the initial injury has not produced the dramatic high-tone picture described above, limb weakness will be observed, evidenced by lack of automatic movement. The use of elective ventilation has limited to some extent the frequency of occurrence of the severe tonal states described.

Experience of the speed of development of secondary soft-tissue changes has also led to the promotion of the use of preventive casting (Edwards & Charlton, 2002), applied before weaning off the ventilator. It is important to note, however, that although there may be very dramatic increases in tone in the acute phase and that without management this will result in hugely disabling secondary physical changes, the overall pattern of recovery often leads eventually to *low* levels of resting tone, sometimes complicated by contracture, giving the appearance of a continuing high-tone state. It is therefore important to limit early interventions to those with short-term or reversible effects and, in particular, to avoid radical orthopaedic surgical intervention.

Behavioural observation

In addition to motor performance, behavioural observation during this period may point to other transitory or potentially longer-lived deficits in cognition and communication and efforts are currently under way to develop a scale to formalise this type of observation and ultimately increase our understanding of patterns of recovery (Sheil et al., 2000).

The role of the physiotherapist in the acute phase

Mazaux & Richer (1998) identified the objectives of the acute phase of rehabilitation as the prevention of visceral and orthopaedic complications. This is clearly a multidisciplinary task but for physiotherapists it translates primarily into the promotion of respiratory and cardiovascular health and musculoskeletal integrity. Campbell (2000b) described a working model to guide intervention in the acute phase, as applied to a case example of severe TBI without additional injury. This discussion included reference to established clinical practice and supporting evidence. It is clear that, while much of established intervention techniques has not been tested at the level of clinical trials, many have been logically deduced from other knowledge areas such as pathophysiology and the basic sciences.

Treatment goals Common treatment goals and approaches for Campbell's (2000b) sample case were identified as:

- continuous assessment (Campbell, 2002d)
- respiratory care of the ventilated patient and the promotion of optimum blood oxygenation (Ada et al., 1990; Roberts, 2002)
- positioning and assisted movement (Gill-Body & Giorgetti, 1995), including proactive or reactive casting (Edwards & Charlton, 2002), to preserve the integrity of soft tissues, skin and range of motion (see Ch. 25)
- graded sensory stimulation (Wood, 1991)

- provision of information and education for family and friends
- the use of frequent, short-duration treatments with the gradual reintroduction of antigravity positioning and the experience of movement.

Physiotherapy assessment for respiratory and musculoskeletal health in the very acute period includes consideration of the level of intervention required and may result initially in an advisory-only role, for example, when there is no respiratory compromise in an electively ventilated patient (Roberts, 2002). However, the patient must be kept under direct review via routine auscultation, as well as by monitoring nursing and medical observations, so that advice is regularly updated and active intervention is commenced immediately if it is considered necessary. Careful monitoring of vital signs in this way will also provide the parameters within which interventions must take place. In any case, treatments should be well planned, of minimal duration and interspersed with adequate rest periods (Roberts, 2002).

Early observations focused on respiratory health also provide the opportunity to monitor physical status. It remains imperative within the limitations imposed by medical instability to identify any threats to soft-tissue extensibility and prevent venous stasis.

Movement through full range may be possible in a sedated and medically stable patient but access to all joints may not be possible. Some positions and movements may need to be avoided because of threats to medical status, for example, avoidance of neck flexion, a dependent head position or increased thoracic pressure to limit increases in ICP. Subtle alterations to classic nursing positions, for example, the use of foam wedges to modify supine (see Ch. 25), will help prevent the organisation of excess extensor activity. In those with moderately increased tone, the introduction of a degree of trunk flexion in side-lying has similar effects but this position is difficult to sustain in higher-tone states, when the judicious use of positioning supports to allow a semiprone position is effective in moderating tone and can have a positive impact on breathing patterns. In the severely injured, it is essential to consider proactive management of increased tone, which may potentially develop when sedation is decreased during the process of weaning from the ventilator.

The application of lower-limb casts with the feet in an appropriate plantargrade position is considerably easier before sedation is decreased than after, when tone is difficult to control, and the patient may be in a state of agitation or confusion. The ability to adopt plantargrade is an important factor in achieving stable sitting and standing positions, essential milestones in the reintroduction of the experience of normal movement and orientation within the wider environment.

The hospital environment is noisy and often lit throughout the 24-h period. A patient in intensive care or in a high-dependency unit also undergoes a plethora of interventions involving handling and movement. It may be necessary to *limit* rather than increase sensory stimulation to ensure periods of rest, for example, the use of eye-patching to promote normal diurnal rhythms (Ada et al., 1990). It is important that this concept of regulated sensory stimulation is imparted to friends and family members so that they may appropriately contribute to the promotion of recovery.

Feedback from families beyond the acute stage is that they appreciate accurate and timely information about the effects of the pathology, the rationale for interventions, what progress may be reasonably anticipated and what the next stage in the process is likely to be. Not many individuals want to read detailed information about long-term outcomes at this time, but they do want to understand what local services are available to them and to feel that everything possible is being done.

While formal treatment sessions may need to be short and paced throughout the day, the physiotherapist should provide direct advice and guidance to the whole team with regard to physical management objectives and strategies for the full 24-h period. Environmental controls need to be negotiated and agreed with other team members, for example, splints or casts with the occupational therapist, the use of T-rolls and the arrangement of positioning pillows with the nursing staff. Agreed plans should be clearly documented and easily accessible to all staff.

Key points

For the physiotherapist in acute care

- Initial treatment focuses on promoting respiratory health and preventing secondary adaptive changes in the musculoskeletal system
- The physiotherapist may provide direct treatment, specific advice to other team members or a combination of both to ensure effective 24-h management
- Treatments are of short duration with frequent review but allowing rest periods throughout the day
- In severe cases, proactive lower-limb casts should be considered to limit the negative effects of severe tonal states
- It is important to keep families informed of treatment objectives

Impact of early physical management on longitudinal outcome

There are no formal prospective studies comparing the effects of early active physical management against no intervention or comparing the relative merits of different types of physical management on long-term outcome. However, as pointed out by McMillan & Greenwood (1993a), there is a stark contrast between outcomes now and those reported by Rusk and colleagues on a series of 127 patients in the 1960s (Rusk et al., 1966, 1969), with 40 pressure sores, 200 joint contractures, 30 frozen shoulders and multiple urinary and respiratory complications. However, while it may be accepted that the convention for early active management of the effects of brain damage on the musculoskeletal system has improved the overall standard of physical outcomes, the need for a significant number of postacute remedial interventions, such as surgery (Marwitz et al., 2001), argues against any complacency in this area.

Similarly, we have to ensure that the potential for long-term negative effects of limited intervention, for those who carry an initially poor prognosis but go on to confound medical science, is fully taken into account and that optimum skeletal alignment and muscular balance are achieved wherever possible as the best basis for ongoing progress (Campbell, 2000d). With clinical experience extending over more than 20 years, the author can testify to the improved physical outcomes brought about by advances in medical care and changes in rehabilitation practice. Two significant factors can be singled out in the latter: the advent of proactive management of muscle length imbalance and postural alignment by way of casting to facilitate early anti-gravity activity, and the development of organised subacute rehabilitation programmes.

Issues emerging in the subacute phase

In this phase, the patient becomes medically stable and the period of disorientation and confusion begins to settle. It then becomes possible for all members of the team to undertake more extensive and accurate assessment across domains, and so begin to log specific impairments, and either observe or project their functional effects.

Time since injury

There are no hard and fast temporal indicators of when the subacute period begins or ends in any of the pathologies we have considered so far. It is also important to realise that what constitutes the subacute phase in each individual case, even within a pathology-specific population, can vary enormously and may, therefore, require a differential response from service provision.

Case histories

The different needs of two individuals at the same time after injury are illustrated by two comparative case histories, outlined in Table 7.8.

Julian and Angela were both 5 weeks postinjury but there were clear differences in the response they required from a service, the type of information that could be gathered from them and the scope of assessment that it was appropriate to undertake. There were also several differentiating factors concerning the impact of their residual impairments on function, and the potential for physiotherapy and other professional involvement. The comparison of the two cases illustrates some of the difficulties in focusing on time since injury as an indicator of likely progression. Julian's case also clearly illustrates the interdependent nature of cognitive and physical impairments in the early recovery period. Intervention to control for, or improve, his awareness and orientation would be of equal importance to work focused on preventing the development of additional complications (physical and behavioural) and ensuring optimal conditions to drive any potential recovery.

Physical impairments

Depending on the degree of co-operation that is feasible to elicit, it may be possible to detect limitations of cranial nerve function and to begin to document underlying motor performance difficulties, and to some degree disruption of sensory perception. The sense of smell is frequently lost following TBI, especially if there has been a fracture of the anterior fossa.

The visual system may be affected at the level of the optic nerve, or processing or interpretation of visual stimuli (Narayan et al., 1990). Eye movements and the control of binocular vision may be affected via damage to the oculomotor, trochlear or abducens nerves or to the cerebral areas involved in the processing of two images into one. Individuals may report double vision (diploplia) or a squint may be observed but not reported (strabismus). Oculomotor nerve damage may also affect pupillary reaction and result in difficulties with accommodation to light. The chances of some form of visual disturbance in diffuse injuries is high, since around one-third of the brain is involved in the processing of vision (Stein, 1995). This is an important observation for physiotherapists, given the role of vision in the guidance of movement and the maintenance of balance (see Ch. 24).

Facial bone fractures can result in damage to the trigeminal nerve, producing facial numbness or

Table 7.8 Case histories of traumatic brain injury

	Julian	Angela
Age	18	26
Time since onset	5 weeks	5 weeks
Summary	Road traffic accident	Fell from ladder at home
	GCS[a] 3 at the scene	LOC[b] unknown, presented as confused to
	Required neurosurgery to evacuate	husband in another room of the house
	a large subdural haematoma	GCS on arrival at hospital 14 (E = 4, M = 6, V = 4)
	Ventilated for 7 days	No skull fracture on X-ray, discharged
	Evidence of disturbed motor	Troublesome headache for 2–3 days, rested
	performance in all four limbs	in bed
	Normal sleep-and-wake cycle	Visited GP 5, 12 and 19 days post
	now re-established	Referred to follow-up clinic
	Only occasional vocalisation,	
	no recognisable words	
Place of residence	Subacute rehabilitation facility	Home
Self-report of current concerns	None verbal	Unable to return to work
	Grimaces	Poor concentration
	Fluctuating levels of muscle tone,	Feels unsteady
	? partly in response to discomfort	Intolerant of busy or noisy environments
Commentary	Julian is unable to express his own objectives or, indeed, give verbal direction to guide the scope of assessment. The professional team will have the full responsibility for deciding the scope and detail of his assessment and to set management objectives on his behalf	Initially, Angela was not regarded as having a significant injury and so did not expect to be away from work for so long. Work return is her key objective and she can easily express this within the assessment process. She is also aware, even within the context of home-based activities, that she has not fully recovered from the effects of her fall and can give clear direction towards at least some of the domains requiring analysis

[a]Glasgow Coma Scale summated score. GCS = E + M + V (E = eyes, M = motor, V = verbal).
[b]Loss of consciousness.

hypersensitivity. Facial nerve damage (facial palsy) may develop from temporal bone trauma (Narayan et al., 1990). Direct or indirect impacts in the temporal area can also cause vestibulocochlear nerve damage resulting in neural deafness. Direct damage to the bony chain or bleeding into the middle ear may produce conduction deafness. Trauma in and around the temporal bone region may also directly damage the vestibular apparatus or create a perilymph fistula, disrupting balance function and inducing dizziness (see Ch. 24). Occasionally damage to lower cranial nerves may occur, associated with basal skull fractures or neck trauma.

Symptoms more commonly associated with whiplash injuries may also be observed and, although rare, traumatic dissection of the carotid artery associated with neck trauma may also occur, producing a range of additional neurological symptoms relative to the level of ischaemia that results.

A variety of distinct or combined motor disorders may become apparent as sedation is withdrawn or as attempts are made to undertake functional activities. Presentations vary depending on the site and distribution of damage but may include:

- hypertonicity
- ataxia
- dyskinesia (involuntary movement)
- failure to initiate movement or sustain posture due to weakness
- dyspraxia (difficulty actioning purposeful movement despite having intact sensation and motor activity)
- sensory inattention.

Commonly after TBI, aspects of these disorders will be seen in complex mixtures, thus clearly differentiating this population from those with stroke or other more localised cerebral pathologies.

Heterotopic ossification (HO; extra periarticular bone growth) may be seen after severe TBI, more commonly in children and young adults (Hurvitz et al., 1992) and often associated with extended periods of coma (Anderson, 1989; also see Ch. 25, p. 433).

Cognitive and behavioural impairments

Structured observation across team members and the beginnings of formal assessment by occupational therapists, speech and language therapists and neuropsychologists will enable the development of a clearer picture of cognitive and communicative abilities. To some degree, the cognitive level, and therefore the ability to engage with formal assessment, will dictate the extent or limitations of assessment during the subacute phase. It is important for physiotherapists to appreciate this and, in particular, to note that even if cognitive limitations have not been identified via formal assessment they may still be present.

The frequent occurrence of lesions in the temporal and frontal lobes means that disorders of memory, attention and reasoning are common in this population along with many other cognitive and behavioural difficulties (Mazaux & Richer, 1998). All therapists working with patients at this stage need to develop excellent skills of behavioural observation and make allowances within their practice to accommodate for likely cognitive limitations.

The role of the physiotherapist in the subacute phase

The objectives for rehabilitation in the subacute phase as defined by Mazuax & Richer (1998) are to accelerate recovery of impairments and compensate for disabilities.

Case example

The physiotherapist's role can be illustrated by considering the case example of Jamie, an adolescent male with a TBI that resulted in a 2-h loss of consciousness. In addition to the TBI, he also sustained a left femoral fracture (surgically fixed) and an undisplaced pelvic fracture. His aftercare was provided on an orthopaedic ward. Initial assessment revealed that he had:

- no apparent difficulties in maintaining his own respiration
- minor limitation of left knee flexion and moderate limitation of left hip range associated with postoperative oedema and pain
- no other obvious restrictions of joint range or soft-tissue extensibility

- decreased muscle tone without loss of the ability to initiate movement in the limbs
- poor limb-girdle stability
- initial difficulty achieving and sustaining unsupported sitting
- distress in supported standing
- repeated eye-closure in antigravity positions.

Treatment goals   The goals for initial intervention were to:

- provide orientation and reassurance
- monitor respiratory function
- preserve the integrity of soft tissues, skin and range of motion
- assess further the factors provoking distress in standing
- promote active participation in meaningful tasks (to facilitate functional use of limbs and explore balance control)
- provide information and education to Jamie and his family and friends
- provide education for professional colleagues (particularly with regard to factors provoking distress in standing)
- ensure onward referral to a TBI-aware service.

Each contact session with Jamie included a reminder of the therapists' names until he began to use their names routinely. Similarly, a simple explanation of the objective of each part of each session was given immediately before proceeding. This applied particularly to those activities that had previously caused distress, such as movement into sitting and up into standing.

Jamie was encouraged to describe what he was experiencing at the time or soon afterwards, when that was not possible. From this process it became apparent that the eye-closure was an attempt to escape from a feeling of environmental movement (the world spinning around him). It also became clear that he experienced alignment in the primary upright position as being tipped forward so, even at times in standing when he was not dizzy, he felt on the verge of falling flat on his face.

Jamie had appeared unco-operative with nursing staff trying to encourage him to assist with personal care activities. This situation was improved when strategies to allow recovery from dizziness following positional change were introduced and physical support was provided to maintain upright sitting, allowing him free use of his arms. Jamie also required verbal reassurance of his safety, as he was initially fearful of attempting functional tasks without supervision.

This assessment and communication role again illustrates the extent to which the physiotherapist's role extends beyond direct therapy sessions. For Jamie it was important to ensure that seating arrangements and, in time, methods of assisted walking contributed positively to the physical management objectives of reinforcing correct alignment, providing the optimum environment to facilitate antigravity activity in the trunk and encouraging positional change to drive sensory recalibration (see Ch. 24). Collaborative working during formal sessions was also beneficial, for example, working with an occupational therapist at an early stage within the context of washing and dressing. This facilitated Jamie's engagement while he was still confused and increased the range of possible therapeutic activities that could be attempted with an extra pair of hands.

By the time of his transfer to the neurorehabilitation ward, almost 5 weeks postinjury Jamie had greatly improved hip mobility, was able to identify upright alignment in sitting during therapy sessions, but still preferred to rest in a backward-leaning position. He was beginning to attempt to use his arms functionally, away from his body, in unsupported sitting. Reports of dizziness were much decreased but anxiety during standing and walking was still a live issue. Jamie's preference was to have physical contact during walking but he had begun to master walking with two sticks, within the confines of the therapy space and to a lesser extent on the ward.

Key points

For the physiotherapist in subacute care

- Assessment of early residual sensorimotor deficits
- Treatment focuses on providing an appropriate environment to assist functional recovery and on assisted practice of meaningful tasks, relevant to ability
- A full range of treatment modalities may be used, including manual techniques, positioning and guided movement
- Collaborative sessions with other disciplines are often appropriate
- Effective communication with patient and family remains essential

---

Issues emerging in the postacute phase

Significant motor performance deficits will already be documented and interventions to manage or reduce their functional effects will be established within the subacute period. Cognitive deficits and limitations affecting social behaviour may not begin to be fully quantified until much later in the recovery process,

until the need to engage in social and community-based activities is encountered. This is true following any degree of injury and preinjury normality cannot be assumed until routine functional activities have been achieved and family and work roles are successfully re-established. It is also important to apply similar caution to considerations of normality in physical function, particularly concerning those who are in physically demanding employment, who like to engage in physical leisure pursuits or, as in the case of Angela, our second case history, those who bypass formal subacute provision.

Even at the minor or moderate end of the spectrum, complaints of fatigue and cognitive limitations are not uncommon (King et al., 1997). Information-processing and capacity problems may mean that, although individuals can successfully perform single tasks, they may experience problems where attention has to be given to more than one task simultaneously or when their lifestyle demands performance of a number of tasks in series without respite. Although it is not the only reason for balance difficulties after moderate or minor injuries, a parallel difficulty in dual-tasking may be observed during demanding physical tasks, such as carrying a squirming toddler while walking downstairs, or when physical and cognitive demands occur together, for example, maintaining balance or holding on to an object when required to respond to an unexpected verbal enquiry or a sudden change in the environment.

A subpopulation of individuals return to normal activity levels within a relatively short period of sustaining a brain injury and it is only after a period of return to full-scale activities that problems become apparent to themselves or to those around them. They may cope at work but growing levels of fatigue may interfere with their role and relationships at home. Alternately, they may cope with the demands made at home but encounter problems in the workplace. Work difficulties may only become apparent when they attempt to undertake new or more demanding duties and failure may not immediately be related to the brain injury. The development of late medical problems can include posttraumatic epilepsy, a 2.5–5% risk (Jennett, 1990), and hormonal imbalances as a result of hypothalamic or pituitary stalk damage. Some aspect of the latter may also be latent, emerging only when there is variance from normal age-related changes (Horn & Garland, 1990).

The role of the physiotherapist in the postacute phase

Mazaux & Richer's (1998) objectives for this phase are to maximise independence, community reintegration, psychosocial adjustment and self-acceptance. While on the face of it these objectives may seem to relate more to the skills of other professions, such as occupational therapy and psychology, the physiotherapist has much to contribute to the achievement of these objectives within the context of the interdisciplinary team.

The neurophysiotherapeutic role may be most easily recognised for those who continue to experience significant physical restrictions. Commonly these will be a mixture of limitations of primary motor skills and the impact of secondary musculoskeletal changes. Interventions are therefore targeted at reversing secondary changes and promoting improvement in specific motor skills. A third facet of treatment relates to translating the physical recovery already achieved into functionally oriented movement, with emphasis on improving performance for real-life functional goals.

The challenge for physiotherapists is that each individual presents with an almost unique mix of biomechanical and sensorimotor limiting factors and successful intervention is dependent on developing a clear hypothesis of the underlying and primary influencing factors in each case, so that intervention is focused. Therapists need to be able to apply a range of intervention strategies encompassing manual techniques (see Ch. 23), practice of isolated and task-specific movements (see Ch. 21) and the therapeutic use of functional activities requiring co-ordination of skilled movement, appropriately targeted to be demanding but achievable.

Intervention follows a cyclic pattern of movement analysis, work on subcomponents and skills and application to functional tasks. Work may be undertaken on a continuous basis over many months tackling several functional goals or may happen intermittently, prompted by the demands of new physical tasks or changes in personal circumstances, for example, a move to new accommodation or meeting the demands of getting about on a large educational campus. Even when there are regular intervention sessions, the limitation of direct contact time between therapist and client needs to be recognised and managed. It is important to empower individuals to contribute to their own physical progress (see Ch. 22) and to promote the development of a regular exercise habit, including the application of newly achieved or otherwise vulnerable motor skills. The strategies used will depend on clients' cognitive ability and the structure of their support network (Campbell, 2000c) but will always necessitate education sessions for clients and carers, clear and appropriate documentation (paper, electronic, audio, video) and regular review.

Demands for home practice need to be feasible (Campbell, 2000h) and supported by cognitive strategies for planning and actioning, if appropriate. Simple records of actual frequency of practice to be completed by the client provide a degree of motivation and aid programme evaluation.

For some the ultimate target may be functional mobility within the home, when intervention will focus on gait re-education. For others it may be to climb and work up a ladder, requiring work on speed of action, co-ordination and high-level balance skills. There is increasing recognition of the impact of sensory dysfunction in limiting physical recovery after brain injury (Campbell, 2004) and physiotherapy practice needs to develop to be more inclusive of the analysis of sensory dysfunction, including visual and vestibular factors (see Ch. 24).

In addition to developing our skills of recognition of more subtle disorders of motor performance that act as barriers to return to preinjury work or leisure pursuits, application of wider physiotherapeutic knowledge and skills should translate into work for the promotion of cardiovascular health. Successful community reintegration is a multifactorial process and there is clearly a physical dimension not only in terms of overcoming physical barriers but also in developing the client's skills, confidence and ability to undertake regular physical leisure activities. The role of exercise and strength-training in neurological disorders is discussed in Chapter 29.

Key points

For the physiotherapist in postacute care

- Physiotherapists may contribute to programmes for individuals with a range of residual sensorimotor deficits
- Treatment for those with significant physical restrictions may still focus on reversing secondary adaptive changes and improving specific motor skills
- Treatment includes helping to translate physical recovery into success with real–life functional goals
- Programme success is dependent on skilled sensorimotor assessment and the application of knowledge gleaned from a collaborative assessment process, which includes all disciplines, clients and carers
- Some individuals will require a lifelong physical management programme, some access to planned review and others an appropriate response at times of crisis

Provision for those not admitted for inpatient care

Physiotherapists have to date gained most experience in working with those with significant physical difficulties and in the early months after injury. Current services and referral patterns in the UK focus provision on those whose injuries are severe enough to require initial hospitalisation. However, in health care systems where service provision for those with moderate and minor injuries is better established, for example in New Zealand, work is beginning to develop on appropriate physiotherapy response (Quinn & Sullivan, 2000). In the second case described in Table 7.8, Angela had a physical component within her list of residual symptoms but it was unlikely that she would be seen by a physiotherapist, or given any physiotherapy-generated advice, within current UK provision. Although her residual impairments were significantly less than Julian's, they were sufficient to prevent her return to normal activity levels and are illustrative of the need in all cases to consider residual impairments as limiting factors to achieving immediate functional goals including, at the appropriate time, return to meaningful occupation.

Long-term management of established deficits over time

There is little published literature either documenting the need for long-term management of physical deficits or proposing effective management strategies (Watson, 1997). The author's experience of contributing to postacute services within the National Health Service and in the independent sector in the UK has identified a subpopulation of survivors where ongoing proactive management is required in order to prevent specific physical deterioration and/or declining levels of physical activity. This is one of the many areas of brain injury that warrants research and evaluation.

Within this subpopulation, a spectrum of needs exists. At the most severe end of the spectrum are those with complex disabilities, who remain very physically restricted (essentially confined to bed and chair) and who may be only minimally aware, or in some cases relatively well preserved from a cognitive point of view. In terms of the overall incidence of brain injury, the numbers of those who remain very severely affected are small and there is therefore limited expertise in their holistic management. Many will benefit from a period of assessment and management planning from a specialist centre, such as the Royal Hospital for Neuro-disability in London, where:

- the level of awareness can be ascertained (Gill-Thwaites & Munday, 1999)

- medical complications can be managed
- nutritional requirements and feeding can be assessed appropriately and managed
- potential to use environmental controls or communication systems can be assessed
- appropriate seating can be prescribed (Pope, 2002)
- methods of managing pressure areas and soft-tissue vulnerability can be identified.

Some people will continue to require specialist residential care for the remainder of their lives and their level of dependency will demand continuous proactive management to prevent the development of pressure sores and soft-tissue contracture.

An alternative, or secondary, approach is to establish specialist care, and rehabilitation if appropriate, in a suitable home environment. Such packages require a consistent source of funding and can be complex to manage but, under the direction of a skilled case manager, and with the aid of an appropriately trained care team, a high quality of life can be achieved. In addition, the personalised social contact and opportunities to pace care and activity appropriate to the individual, in a way that is not possible in any residential facility, provide an ideal environment to pursue any incremental progress that may be possible.

Ongoing physical management needs are not confined to the most severely disabled. In the presence of cognitive restrictions or behavioural difficulties, relatively minor physical deficits, such as a biomechanical imbalance from a residual weakness, can become incrementally more troublesome. This may show itself in the development of painful conditions or in diminishing levels of functional activity, contributing to increased behavioural problems or reduced social participation. Where there is an adequate support network, these factors can be proactively managed by including exercise or other forms of physical leisure within the weekly programme. Where this is not possible, or in cases when the client is unable to see the value in preventive measures, service provision that can respond quickly and appropriately at the time of crisis is required.

Challenges to the delivery of effective physical management after acquired brain injury

There are many challenges to effective physical management following brain injury but there are four key factors that are to some degree interdependent:

1. the high incidence of coexisting cognitive limitations and behavioural factors
2. fragmented services, across agencies and within service components
3. limitations of service provision

4. lack of detailed evidence to support the development of service provision.

The high incidence of coexisting deficits makes each case complex in its presentation. There are specific strategies that physiotherapists can adopt to help control for these confounding factors (Campbell, 2000c) but these are insufficient in the absence of action to link professional support for clients and carers at each rehabilitation phase and across all aspects of service delivery. Service provision and evaluation, particularly in the area of postacute care, need to develop further so that the service is both accessible and effective. There is great potential for physiotherapists to make a significant contribution to the development of services for this rewarding client group.

Support groups

There are a number of organisations (listed below), which provide support for individuals and carers across ABI pathology groups, many of which also provide information useful to professionals, as well as brain-injury survivors. For contact details, please see the Appendix.

- BASIC
- Brain and Spine Foundation
- British Epilepsy Association
- Children's Brain Injury Trust (CBIT)
- Encephalitis Support Group
- Headway: the brain injuries association
- Meningitis Trust
- UKABIF (UK Acquired Brain Injury Forum).

References

Ada L, Canning C, Paratz J. Care of the unconscious head-injured patient. In: Ada L, Canning C, eds. *Key Issues in Neurological Physiotherapy: Physiotherapy: Foundations for Practice*. London: Butterworth-Heinemann; 1990:249–287.

Adams J, Mitchell D, Graham D. 1977 Diffuse brain damage of the immediate impact type. *Brain* 1977, **100**:489–502.

Aitkenhead A. 1986 Cerebral protection. *Br J Hosp Med* 1986, **35**:290–298.

Al-Mefty O (ed.). *Meningiomas*. New York: Raven Press; 1991.

Anderson BJ. Heterotopic ossification: a review. *Rehab Nurs* 1989, **14**:89–91.

Andrews K, Murphy L, Munday R et al. Misdiagnosis of the vegetative state: retrospective study in a rehabilitation unit. *Br Med J* 1996, **131**:13–16.

Body C, Leatham J. Incidence and aetiology of head injury in a New Zealand adolescent sample. *Brain Inj* 1996, **10**:567–573.

Body R, Herbert C, Campbell M, Parker M, Usher A. An integrated approach to team assessment in head injury. *Brain Inj* 1996, **10**:311–318.

Bond MR. Neurobehavioural sequelae of closed head injury. In: Grant I, Adams KM, eds. *Neuropsychological Assessment of Neuropsychiatric Disorders*. New York: Oxford University Press; 1986:347–373.

Bond MR. Standardised methods for assessing and predicting outcome. In: Rosenthal M, Griffith E, Bond M, Miller J, eds. *Rehabilitation of the Adult and Child with Traumatic Brain Injury*. Philadelphia: FA Davis; 1990:59–74.

British Medical Association. *Treatment Decisions for Patients in Persistent Vegetative State*. London: British Medical Association; 1996.

Brooks D. *Closed Head Injury: Psychological, Social and Family Issues*. Oxford: Oxford University Press; 1984.

Brooks D, Campsie L, Symington C, Beattie A, McKinlay W. The effects of severe head injury on patient and relative within seven years of injury. *Head Trauma Rehab* 1987, **2**:1–13.

Bullock R, Teasdale G. Head injuries – 1. *BMJ* 1990a, **300**:1515–1518.

Bullock R, Teasdale G. Head injuries – 2. *BMJ* 1990b, **300**:1576–1579.

Burke D. Planning a system of care for head injuries. *Brain Inj* 1987, **1**:189–198.

Campbell M. About this book. In: Campbell M, ed. *Rehabilitation for Traumatic Brain Injury: Physical Therapy Practice in Context*. Edinburgh: Churchill Livingstone; 2000a:1–13.

Campbell M. Applying neurophysiotherapeutic principles. In: Campbell M, ed. *Rehabilitation for Traumatic Brain Injury: Physical Therapy Practice in Context*. Edinburgh: Churchill Livingstone; 2000b:169–205.

Campbell M. Cognitive, behavioural and individual influences in programme design. In: Campbell M, ed. *Rehabilitation for Traumatic Brain Injury: Physical Practice in Context*. Edinburgh: Churchill Livingstone; 2000c:207–230.

Campbell M. Initial considerations in the process of assessment. In: Campbell M, ed. *Rehabilitation for Traumatic Brain Injury: Physical Therapy Practice in Context*. Edinburgh: Churchill Livingstone; 2000d:75–100.

Campbell M. Policy, planning and proactive management. In: Campbell M, ed. *Rehabilitation for Traumatic Brain Injury: Physical Therapy Practice in Context*. Edinburgh: Churchill Livingstone; 2000e:233–251.

Campbell M. *Rehabilitation for Traumatic Brain Injury: Physical Therapy Practice in Context*. Edinburgh: Churchill Livingstone; 2000f.

Campbell M. Understanding the impact of the traumatic event and the influence of life context. In: Campbell M, ed. *Rehabilitation for Traumatic Brain Injury: Physical Therapy Practice in Context*. Edinburgh: Churchill Livingstone; 2000g:45–72.

Campbell M. Defining goals for intervention. In: Campbell M, ed. *Rehabilitation for Traumatic Brain Injury: Physical Therapy Practice in Context*. Edinburgh: Churchill Livingstone; 2000h:151–165.

Campbell M. Balance disorder and traumatic brain injury: preliminary findings of a mutifactorial observational study. *Brain Inj* 2004 (in press).

Centre for Health Service Studies. *National Traumatic Brain Injury Study*. Warwick, UK: Warwick University; 1998.

Chigbu de G. Visual field defect: a case of cerebral aneurysm. *Optom Today* 2003 July 11: 24–26.

Children's Trust at Tadworth Rehabilitation Team. Format and procedure for writing an interdisciplinary rehabilitation report. *Br J Ther Rehab* 1997, **4**:70–74.

Childs NL, Mercer WN, Childs HW. Accuracy of diagnosis of persistent vegetative state. *Neurology* 1993, **43**:1465–1467.

Dombovy ML, Drew-Cates J, Serdans R. Recovery and rehabilitation following subarachnoid haemorrhage. Part I: outcome after inpatient rehabilitation. *Brain Inj* 1998a, **12**:443–454.

Dombovy ML, Drew-Cates J, Serdans R. Recovery and rehabilitation following subarachnoid haemorrhage. Part II. Long-term follow-up. *Brain Inj* 1998b, **12**:887–894.

Douglas JM. Traumatic brain injury and the family. Paper presented at *Making Headway*. Christchurch, NZ: NZSTA Biennial Conference; 1990.

Drubach DA, Kelly MP, Winslow MM, Flynn JP. Substance abuse as a factor in the causality, severity and recurrence of traumatic brain injury. *Maryland Med J* 1993, **42**:989–993.

Eames P, Wood R. The structure and content of a head injury rehabilitation service. In: Wood RL, Eames P, eds. *Models of Brain Injury Rehabilitation*. London: Chapman & Hall; 1989:31–58.

Edwards S, Charlton P. Splinting and the use of orthoses in the management of patients with neurological disorders. In: Edwards S, ed. *Neurological Physiotherapy: A Problem Solving Approach*, 2nd edn. London: Churchill Livingstone; 2002:219–253.

Feldman Z, Kanter MJ, Robertson CS et al. Effects of head elevation on intra-cranial pressure, cerebral perfusion pressure and cerebral blood flow in head injury patients. *J Neurosurg* 1992, **76**:207–211.

Fick DS. Management of concussion in collision sports. Guidelines for the sidelines. *Postgrad Med* 1995, **97**:53–56, 59–60.

Frost EAM. Management of head injury. *Can Anaesth Soc J* 1985, **32**:532.

Gabella B, Reiner KL, Hoffman RE, Cook M, Stallones L. Relationship of helmet use and head injuries among motorcycle crash victims in El Paso County, Colorado, 1989–1990. *Accident Analy Prevent* 1995, **27**:363–369.

Garrad J, Bullock M. The effect of respiratory therapy on intracranial pressure in ventilated neurosurgical patients. *Aust J Physiother* 1986, **32**:107–111.

Gentleman D, Teasdale G, Murray L. Cause of severe head injury and risk of complications. *BMJ* 1986, **292**:449.

Genuardi FJ, King WD. Inappropriate discharge instructions for youth athletes hospitalised for concussion. *Pediatrics* 1995, **95**:216–218.

Giacino J, Ashwal S, Childs N et al. The minimally conscious state: definition and diagnostic criteria. *Neurology* 2002, **58**:349–353.

Gill-Body KM, Giorgetti MM. Acute care and prognostic outcome. In: Montgomery J, ed. *Physical Therapy for Traumatic Brain Injury*. New York: Churchill Livingstone; 1995:1–31.

Gill-Thwaites H, Munday R. The Sensory Modality Assessment and Rehabilitation Technique (SMART): a comprehensive and integrated assessment and treatment protocol for the vegetative state and minimally responsive patient. *Neuropsychol Rehab* 1999, **9**:305–320.

Gronwall D, Wrightson P. Duration of post-traumatic amnesia after mild head injury. *J Clin Neuropsychol* 1980, **2**:51–60.

Hernandez TD, Naritoku DK. Seizures, epilepsy, and functional recovery after traumatic brain injury: a reappraisal. *Neurology* 1997, **48**:803–806.

Hillier S, Hiller J, Metzer J. Epidemiology of traumatic brain injury in South Australia. *Brain Inj* 1997, **11**:649–659.

Horn LJ, Garland DE. Medical and orthopaedic complications associated with traumatic brain injury. In: Rosenthal M, Griffith ER, Bond MR, Miller JD, eds. *Rehabilitation of the Adult and Child with Traumatic Brain Injury*, 2nd edn. Philadelphia: FA Davis; 1990:107–126.

House of Commons. *Select Committee on Health Third Report: Head Injury Rehabilitation*. London: Parliamentary Publications; 2001.

Hurvitz EA, Mandac BR, Davidoff G et al. Risk factors for heterotopic ossification in children and adolescents with severe traumatic brain injury. *Arch Phys Med Rehab* 1992, **73**:459–462.

Jackson HF, Davies M. A transdisciplinary approach to brain injury rehabilitation. *Br J Ther Rehab* 1995, **2**:65–70.

Jennett B. Post-traumatic epilepsy. In: Rosenthal M, Griffith ER, Bond MR, Miller JD, eds. *Rehabilitation of the Adult and Child with Traumatic Brain Injury*. Philadelphia: FA Davis; 1990:89–93.

Jennett B. Epidemiology of head injury. *J Neurol Neurosurg Psychiatry* 1996, **60**:362–369.

Jennett B, Lindsay KW. Complications after head injury. In: Jennett B, Lindsay KW, eds. *An Introduction to Neurosurgery*, 5th edn. Oxford: Butterworth-Heinemann; 1994a:211–235.

Jennett B, Lindsay KW. Surgery for vascular lesions. In: Jennett B, Lindsay KW, eds. *An Introduction to Neurosurgery*, 5th edn. Oxford: Butterworth-Heinemann; 1994b:142–171.

Jennett B, MacMillan R. Epidemiology of head injury. *BMJ* 1981, **282**:101–104.

Jennett B, Plum F. Persistent vegetative state after brain damage: a syndrome in search of a name. *Lancet* 1972, **i**:734–737.

Jennett B, Teasdale G. Aspects of coma after severe head injury. *Lancet* 1977, **i**:878–881.

Jennett B, Teasdale G. Structural pathology. In: Jennett B, Teasdale G, eds. *Management of Head Injuries*. Philadelphia: FA Davies; 1981:19–43.

Johnson RT. Meningitis, encephalitis and poliomyelitis. In: Johnson RT, ed. *Viral Infections of the Nervous System*, 2nd edn. Philadelphia: Lippincott-Raven; 1998:87–132.

Kelly DF. Alcohol and head injury: an issue revisited. *J Neurotrauma* 1995, **12**:883–890.

King NS, Crawford S, Wenden FJ et al. Interventions and service needs following mild and moderate head injury: the Oxford Head Injury Service. *Clin Rehab* 1997, **11**:13–27.

Kraus J, Sorenson S. Epidemiology. In: Silver J, Yudofsky S, Hales R, eds. *Neuropsychiatry of Traumatic Brain Injury*. Washington: American Psychiatric Press; 1994:3–41.

Kraus JF, McArthur DL. Epidemiological aspects of brain injury. *Neurol Clin* 1996, **14**:435–450.

Kroll JS, Moxon ER. Acute bacterial meningitis. In: Kennedy PGE, Johnson RT, eds. *Infections of the Nervous System*. London: Butterworths; 1987:3–22.

Leblanc KE. Concussion in sports: guidelines for return to competition. *Am Family Phys* 1995, **50**:801–808.

Leclerc S, Shrier I, Johnston K. *Pashby Sports Fund Concussion Site*. 2002 Available online at http://www.concussionsafety.com.

Levin H, O'Donnell V, Grossman R. The Galveston Orientation and Amnesia Test: a practical scale to assess cognition after head injury. *J Nerv Ment Dis* 1979, **167**:675–684.

Lindsay KW, Bone I. *Neurology and Neurosurgery Illustrated*, 3rd edn. New York: Churchill Livingstone; 1997.

Marwitz JH, Cifu DX, Englander J, High WM. A multi-centre analysis of rehospitalizations five years after brain injury. *J Head Trauma Rehab* 2001, **16**:307–317.

Mazaux JM, Richer R. Rehabilitation after traumatic brain injury in adults. *Disabil Rehab* 1998, **20**:435–447.

McDermott FT. Bicyclist head injury prevention by helmets and mandatory wearing legislation in Victoria, Australia. *Ann R Coll Surg Engl* 1995, **77**:38–44.

McMillan T, Greenwood R. Head injury. In: Greenwood R, Barnes MP, McMillan TM, Ward CD, eds. *Neurological Rehabilitation*. Edinburgh: Churchill Livingstone, 1993a:437–450.

McMillan T, Greenwood R. Models of rehabilitation programmes for the brain-injured adult. II: Model services and suggestions for change in the UK. *Clin Rehab* 1993b, 7:346–355.

McMillan T, Jongen E, Greenwood R. Assessment of post-traumatic amnesia after severe closed head injury: retrospective or prospective? *J Neurol Neurosurg Psychiatry* 1996, **60**:422–427.

Miller J, Jones P. Minor head injury. In: Rosenthal M, Griffith E, Bond M, Miller J, eds. *Rehabilitation of the Adult and Child with Traumatic Brain Injury*. Philadelphia: FA Davis; 1990:236–247.

Moseley A. Physical management and rehabilitation of patients with traumatic head injury (2). In: Partridge CJ, ed. *Bases of Evidence for Practice: Neurological Physiotherapy*. London: Whurr; 2002:92–106.

Multi-Society Task Force. Medical aspects of the persistent vegetative state. *N Engl J Med* 1994, **330**:1499–1508.

Narayan RK, Gokaslan ZI, Bontke CF et al. Neurologic sequelae of head injury. In: Rosenthal M, Griffith ER, Bond MR, Miller JD, eds. *Rehabilitation of the Adult and Child with Traumatic Brain Injury*, 2nd edn. Philadelphia: FA Davis; 1990:94–106.

New Zealand National Health Committee. *Traumatic Brain Injury Rehabilitation Guidelines*. 1998. Available online at http://www.nzgg.org.nz/library/gl_complete/tbi/index.cfm.

Nolte J. Introduction to the nervous system. In: Nolte J, ed. *The Human Brain: An Introduction to its Functional Anatomy*. St Louis, MO: Mosby; 1990a:1–35.

Nolte J. Meningeal coverings of the brain and spinal cord. In: Nolte J, ed. *The Human Brain: An Introduction to its Functional Anatomy*. St Louis, MO: Mosby; 1999b:76–95.

Oddy M, Bonham E, McMillan TM, Stroud A, Rickard S. A comprehensive service for the rehabilitation and long-term care of head injury survivors. *Clin Rehab* 1989, **3**:253–259.

Pickard JD, Czosnyka M. Raised intracranial pressure. In: Hughes RAC, ed. *Neurological Emergencies*, 3rd edn. London: BMJ Publishing Group; 2000:173–218.

Pile-Spellman J 1996 Endovascular therapeutic neuroradiology. In Tavernas JM, ed. *Neuroradiology*, 3rd edn. Baltimore: Williams & Wilkins; 1996:1045–1179.

Pollock BE. *Contemporary Stereotactic Neurosurgery*. New York: Futura; 2002.

Ponsford J 1995 Working with families. In: Ponsford J, Sloan S, Snow P, eds. *Traumatic Brain Injury: Rehabilitation for Everyday Adaptive Living*. Hove: Lawrence Erlbaum; 1995:265–294.

Pope PM. Postural management and special seating. In: Edwards S, ed. *Neurological Physiotherapy: a Problem Solving Approach*, 2nd edn. London: Churchill Livingstone; 2002:189–217.

Povlishock JT, Becker DMP, Cheng CLY et al. Axonal change in minor head injury. *J Neuropathol Exp Neurol* 1983, **42**:225–242.

Powell T, Partridge T, Nicholls T et al. An interdisciplinary approach to the rehabilitation of people with brain injury. *Br J Ther Rehab* 1994, **1**:8–13.

Quinn B, Sullivan SJ. The identification by physiotherapists of the physical problems resulting from a mild traumatic brain injury. *Brain Inj* 2000, **14**:1063–1076.

Roberts S. Respiratory management of patient with traumatic head injury. In: Partridge CJ, ed. *Bases of Evidence for Practice: Neurological Physiotherapy*. London: Whurr; 2002:63–76.

Romano MD. Family response to traumatic head injury. *Scand J Rehab Med* 1974, **6**:1–4.

Rosenbaum M, Najenson T. Changes in life patterns and symptoms of low mood as reported by wives of severely brain injured soldiers. *J Consult Clin Psychol* 1976, **44**:881–888.

Rosner MJ, Colley IB. Cerebral perfusion pressure, intracranial pressure and head elevation. *J Neurosurg* 1986, **65**:636–641.

Rusk HA, Loman EW, Block JM. Rehabilitation of the patient with head injury. *Clin Neurosurg* 1966, **12**:312–323.

Rusk HA, Block JM, Loman EW. Rehabilitation following traumatic brain damage. *Med Clin North Am* 1969, **52**:677–684.

Russell W. Cerebral involvement in head injury. *Brain* 1932, **55**:549–603.

Scottish Intercollegiate Guidelines Network. *Early Management of Patients with a Head Injury*. 2000. Available online at http://www.sign.ac.uk.

Sheil A, Horn SA, Wilson B, Watson MJ, Campbell MJ, McLellan DL. The Wessex Head Injury Matrix (WHIM) main scale: a preliminary report on a scale to assess and monitor patient recovery after severe head injury. *Clin Rehab* 2000, **14**:408–416.

Sorenson SB, Kraus JF. Occurrence, severity, and outcomes of brain injury. *J Head Trauma Rehab* 1991, **6**:1–10.

Stein J. The posterior parietal cortex, the cerebellum and the visual guidance of movement. In: Cody FWJ, ed. *Neural Control of Skilled Human Movement*. Chichester: Portland Press; 1995:31–49.

Tate RL, Pfaff A, Jurjevic L. Resolution of disorientation and amnesia during post-traumatic amnesia. *J Neurol Neurosurg Psychiatry* 2000, **68**:178–185.

Tavernas JM. Angiography. In: Tavernas JM, ed. *Neuroradiology*, 3rd edn. Baltimore: Williams & Wilkins; 1996:909–1043.

Taylor SJ, Fettes SB. Enhanced enteral nutrition in head injury: effect on the efficacy of nutritional delivery, nitrogen balance, gastric residuals and risk of pneumonia. *J Hum Nutr Diet* 1998, **11**:391–401.

Teasdale G, Jennett B. Assessment of coma and impaired consciousness: a practical scale. *Lancet* 1974, **2**:81–84.

Teasdale G, Jennett B. Assessment and prognosis of coma after head injury. *Acta Neurochirurg* 1976, **34**:45–55.

Teasdale G, Drake CG, Hunt W et al. A universal subarachnoid haemorrhage scale: report of a committee of the World Federation of Neurological Societies. *J Neurol Neurosurg Psychiatry* 1988, **51**:1457.

Thomas DGT (ed.). 1990 *Neuro-oncology: Primary Malignant Brain Tumours*. London: Edward Arnold; 1990.

Thompson RS, Rivara FP, Thompson DC. A case control study of the effectiveness of bicycle safety helmets. *N Engl J Med* 1989, **32**:1361–1367.

Tresch DD, Farrol HS, Duthie EH et al. Clinical characteristics of patients in the persistent vegetative state. *Arch Intern Med* 1991, **151**:930–932.

Turnbull AP, Turnbull HR. Understanding families from a systems perspective. In: Williams JM, Kay T, eds. *Head Injury: A Family Matter*. Baltimore: Paul H Brooks; 1991:37–63.

Watson MJ. Evidence for 'significant' late stage motor recovery in patients with severe traumatic brain injury: a literature review with relevance to neurological physiotherapy. *Phys Ther Rev* 1997, **2**:93–106.

Wood RL. Critical analysis of the concept of sensory stimulation for patients in vegetative states. *Brain Inj* 1991, **5**:401–409.

Chapter 8

Spinal cord injury

S Paddison   F Middleton

INTRODUCTION

Traumatic spinal cord injury (SCI) is a life-transforming condition of sudden onset that can have devastating consequences. Clinical management involves the acute phase, rehabilitation to restore potential and subsequent interventions to restore function. The objectives of management are to produce a healthy person who can choose his or her own destiny.

Current research gives rise to the hope that in the near future clinicians will be actively intervening in an attempt to alter and augment natural recovery. As this comes to fruition, functional outcomes and quality of life for SCI patients should improve.

INCIDENCE AND AETIOLOGY

At the annual conference of the International Spinal Cord Society (2001) it was estimated that approximately 17.2 people per million of the population in Europe suffer a traumatic SCI per annum and 8.0 per million experience a non-traumatic SCI.

The ratio of male to female cases is approximately 5:1, and varies with age. The greatest incidence is in the age range of 20–39 years (45%), then 40–59 years (24%), and 0–19 years (20%), with those over 60 years showing the lowest incidence of 11% (Gardner et al., 1988). The incidence and aetiology vary greatly from country to country, with no clear data recorded in the UK.

Spinal cord damage can result from trauma (84% of cases) or non-traumatic causes (16%). The main causes of traumatic injury are shown in Figure 8.1. Gunshots and

stabbings also make small but increasing contributions (Whalley Hammell, 1995; Harrison, 2000). A significant number of patients with mental health problems will sustain injury from jumping from a height.

Non-traumatic causes include: developmental anomalies (e.g. spina bifida) and congenital anomalies (e.g. angiomatous malformations); inflammation (e.g. multiple sclerosis); ischaemia (e.g. cord stroke); pressure on the cord due to expanding lesions (e.g. abcess or tumour extrinsic or intrinsic to the spinal cord). Each condition has distinct management needs and features. Their management will benefit from the knowledge and skills derived from an understanding of traumatic SCI, which is the focus of this chapter.

TERMINOLOGY

Terms used to describe these patients indicate the general level of the spinal injury and loss of function (*International Classification of Functioning, Disability and Health*; World Health Organization, 2001).

Paraplegia

Paraplegia refers to the impairment or loss of motor, sensory and/or autonomic function in thoracic, lumbar or sacral segments of the spinal cord. Upper-limb function is spared but the trunk, legs and pelvic organs may be involved.

Tetraplegia

The term 'tetraplegia' is preferred to 'quadriplegia'. Tetraplegic patients have impairment or loss of motor, sensory and/or autonomic function in cervical segments of the spinal cord. The upper-limbs are affected as well as the trunk, legs and pelvic organs. In high cervical injuries the function of respiration will be affected. The term does not include the brachial plexus or injury to peripheral nerves (see Ch. 9). 'Quadraparesis' and 'paraparesis' were terms used previously to describe incomplete lesions and are now discouraged.

TYPES OF SPINAL CORD INJURY

SCI damages a complex neural network involved in transmitting, modifying and co-ordinating motor, sensory and autonomic control of organ systems. This dysfunction of the spinal cord causes loss of homeostatic and adaptive mechanisms which keep people naturally healthy. The American Spinal Injury Association (ASIA) motor and sensory assessments are used for establishing injury level (ASIA, 1992; Dittuno et al., 1994). The approximate incidence of levels of injury

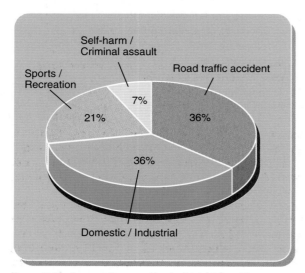

Figure 8.1 Causes of traumatic spinal cord injury. The percentages illustrated were obtained from the references cited in the text.

are: 51.6% cervical, 46.3% thoracic, lumbar and sacral and remaining percentage unrecorded. The ratio of incomplete SCI has now greatly increased compared to complete injuries in the UK; around 65% or more of patients admitted to a spinal injuries unit (SIU) now have an incomplete lesion. Accurate UK statistics are not available and so only a general consensus of agreement from each SIU can be quoted.

Changing trends towards incomplete lesions

There has been a significant reduction in mortality and preservation of neurology in new lesions (Whalley Hammell, 1995; Grundy & Swain, 2002). There are many reasons accounting for this:

- improved medical interventions: full-spectrum antibiotics, neuroprotective agents and advances in respiratory care
- better paramedical retrieval: improved accident and emergency resuscitation procedures and medical interventions to maintain blood pressure and oxygenation
- changes in vehicle design and usage, as well as greater public knowledge and awareness of the dangers of moving an injured person.

DIAGNOSIS

Incomplete versus complete injury classification

It is important to clarify these terms, depending on the context in which they are used. From a therapeutic point of view, a patient can be called functionally incomplete when he or she presents with some motor or sensory sparing below the level of the cord lesion. The therapist should acknowledge such sparing as potential activity, which may offer important functional benefits to the patient.

In terms of diagnosis and prognosis, the classification of SCI has important ramifications. The ASIA (1992) reviewed standards for assessing and classifying functional levels of SCI, including the definitions of complete and incomplete lesions. The criteria for these classifications will not be detailed here but the classification includes the zone of partial preservation and the modified Frankel classification of degree of incompleteness (Fig. 8.2).

The reason for this classification of incomplete versus complete lesions is that compelling evidence suggests the presence of sensation in the lowest sacral segments, or voluntary anal sphincter motor activity, as being significant prognostic indicators for neurological recovery. This implies the preservation of the long tracts through the lesion. The ASIA system defines

ASIA IMPAIRMENT SCALE

- **A= Complete:** No motor or sensory function is preserved in the sacral segments S4–S5

- **B= Incomplete:** Sensory but not motor function is preserved below the neurological level and extends through the sacral segments S4–S5

- **C= Incomplete:** Motor function is preserved below the neurological level, and the majority of key muscles below the neurological level have a muscle grade less than 3.

- **D= Incomplete:** Motor function is preserved below the neurological level, and the majority of key muscles below the neurological level have a muscle grade greater than or equal to 3.

- **E= Normal:** Motor and sensory function is normal.

CLINICAL SYNDROMES

- Central cord
- Brown-sequard
- Anterior cord
- Conus medullaris
- Cauda equina

Figure 8.2 The American Spinal Injury Association (ASIA) Impairment Scale. Reproduced with permission.

that a patient can have neurological sparing below the injury level but in the absence of the sacral sparing this is classified as a complete lesion ASIA A, with a zone of partial preservation. Where there is any S4–S5 sparing the patient is classified ASIA B–E.

It is important that physiotherapists understand the implications of this when undertaking the assessment of a new SCI patient. Often, as one of the first professionals to compile a thorough physical examination, the physiotherapist will be asked for information by the patient. Discussions of prognosis and hopeful signs should always be undertaken in the light of good assessment with evidence-based reasoning.

From a prognostic point of view, research suggests that 72 h postinjury (Maynard et al., 1979; Brown, 1994), and 1 month postinjury are good time points for this classification (Waters et al., 1994a, b).

Incomplete lesions and prognostic indicators

There are recognised patterns of incomplete cord injury which tend to present clinically as combinations of syndromes rather than in isolation. The signs and symptoms are related to the anatomical areas of the cord affected (Fig. 8.3). Clinically, incomplete lesions are referred to as either a syndrome or injury.

Anterior cord syndrome

Anterior cord syndrome describes the effects of ventral cord damage affecting spinothalamic and corticospinal tracts, there is complete motor loss caudal to the lesion, and loss of pain and temperature sensation as these sensory tracts are located anterolaterally in the spinal cord. Preservation of the posterior columns means that perception of vibration and proprioception on the ipsilateral side are intact. This syndrome can arise from anterior spinal artery embolisation. Motor recovery is thought to be less in these patients in comparison with other incomplete lesions (Foo, 1986; Crozier et al., 1991).

Brown–Séquard syndrome

Originally described by Galen, this syndrome describes sagittal hemicord damage with ipsilateral paralysis and dorsal column interruption with contralateral loss of temperature and pain sensation. The relatively normal pain and temperature sensation on the ipsilateral side is due to the spinothalamic tract crossing over to the opposite side of the cord. This hemisection injury of the cord is classically caused by stabbing. This syndrome has a favourable prognosis, with almost all patients ambulating successfully (Johnston, 2001). The theory for this is that, despite the loss of pinprick on the one side of the cord, axons in the contralateral cord may facilitate recovery (Little & Habur, 1985).

Central cord lesion

The upper-limbs are more profoundly affected than the lower limbs and the condition is typically seen in older patients with cervical spondylosis. Due to degenerative changes in the spinal column, there are osteophytes and possible disc bulges, combined with spondylitic joint changes in the anterior part of the vertebral column. Posteriorly, the ligamentum flavum is thickened. A hyperextension injury compresses the cord in the narrowed canal and leads to interference of the blood supply. This may be already compromised in an older person and so has less potential for recovery.

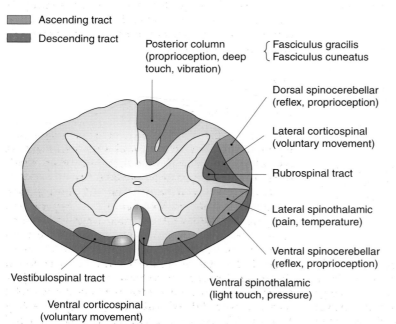

Ascending tract
Descending tract

Posterior column (proprioception, deep touch, vibration) { Fasciculus gracilis / Fasciculus cuneatus

Dorsal spinocerebellar (reflex, proprioception)

Lateral corticospinal (voluntary movement)

Rubrospinal tract

Lateral spinothalamic (pain, temperature)

Ventral spinocerebellar (reflex, proprioception)

Vestibulospinal tract

Ventral spinothalamic (light touch, pressure)

Ventral corticospinal (voluntary movement)

Figure 8.3 Cross-section of the spinal cord illustrating the main ascending and descending nerve tracts. The functions affected by damage to these tracts are indicated.

The central cervical tracts are predominantly affected. There is often flaccid weakness of the arms, due to lower motor neurone (LMN) lesions, and spastic patterning in the arms and legs due to upper motor neurone (UMN) injury. Bowel and bladder dysfunctions are common but only partial. Research findings vary, showing that 57–86% patients will ambulate, although 97% of younger patients under 50 years ambulate compared with 41% over 50 years (Foo, 1986).

Conus medullaris

Conus medullaris presents as either UMN or LMN lesions, with or without the sacral reflexes (anal/bulbocavernus), depending on the injury. There may be avulsion of the lumbar or sacral roots from the terminal part of the cord. Bladder and bowel dysfunctions occur with variable symmetrical lower-limb defecits.

Cauda equina lesion

This produces flaccid paralysis as there is peripheral nerve damage at this level of the spine, usually affecting several levels with variable sacral root interruption.

Posterior cord lesion

This rare condition produces damage to the dorsal columns (sensation of light touch, proprioception and vibration) with preservation of motor function and pain and temperature pathways. However, the patient presents with profound ataxia due to loss of proprioception.

PATHOGENESIS

A brief outline of the pathological changes that occur with SCI is now given; further details can be found in other texts such as Tator (1998).

Immediate/primary damage

Most traumatic injuries involve contusion or tearing of the underlying cord by displaced bony fragments, disc or ligaments. This results primarily in loss of axons due to damage of the white matter.

Secondary damage

Secondary damage, particularly loss of cells in the grey matter, results from a secondary process comprising changes in the cell membrane permeability, leakage of cell contents, release of chemical factors and arrival of blood cells and agents involved in the response to injury and subsequent repair. This process leads to swelling and increasing cord pressure, affecting the venous and arterial supply, and results in ischaemia, lack of necessary proteins and failure to remove the debris of injury.

Later problems

After some weeks, there is evidence of astroglial scarring with cyst formation producing distorted neural architecture. In some cases, months or years later, a syrinx, an expanding cavity within the spinal cord probably associated with disordered cerebrospinal fluid (CSF) flow, may extend rostrally to produce further spinal cord damage. This posttraumatic syringomyelia may require drainage by shunt to prevent further extension. In view of this possibility, the neurological status should be reassessed periodically (Illis, 1988) and appropriate magnetic resonance imaging (MRI) scanning performed at intervals to define those at risk before neurological loss occurs.

Spinal cord plasticity

When peripheral nerve is damaged, repair can lead to significant return of function (Ch. 9). It has been demonstrated that the central nervous system (CNS) has the capacity to regenerate and recover. It has similarly been hypothesised that there is capacity within the spinal cord to regenerate through a number of mechanisms. Theories of axonal budding, unmasking and interspinal spinal circuits (central pattern generators) are all being developed. Neuroplasticity is discussed in detail in Chapter 5. Current research to establish the management of spinal cord damage is discussed briefly below.

PROGNOSIS

Recovery of the incomplete SCI

It is essential to refer to the evidence of ongoing recovery in SCI and bear this in mind when treating these patients. Recovery will be at the forefront of a patient's mind when participating in rehabilitation.

Ninety per cent of incomplete SCI patients have some recovery of a motor level in their upper-limbs, compared to 70–85% of the complete injuries (Ditunno et al., 2000). Pinprick sparing in a dermatome is an excellent indicator of increased recovery of motor strength (Poynton et al., 1997) and it has been found that pinprick preservation below the level of the injury to the sacral dermatomes is the best indicator of useful recovery, with 75% of patients regaining the ability to walk. Fifty per cent of patients who had no sacral sparing regained some motor recovery but not of functional use (Katoh & El Masry, 1995).

Studies have found that incomplete SCI patients showed ongoing improvement in their motor activity, although this tended to slow during the second year postinjury, with the exception of incomplete tetraplegics who lacked sharp/blunt discrimination and failed to demonstrate any lower-limb motor recovery. In incomplete paraplegics, there was evidence of 85% of the muscles recovering from a flicker to an antigravity grade within the first year but if there was no activity initially, only 26% gained an antigravity grade (Waters et al., 1994a, b).

It is widely accepted that incomplete SCI patients will only make useful recovery within the first 2 years postinjury but from the authors' experiential observation, recovery can continue to occur slowly for at least 5 years or more, particularly in incomplete tetraplegics.

Ambulation recovery

Between 44 and 76% of people with incomplete SCI, with preserved sensation but no motor function, have been reported to achieve ambulation (Maynard et al., 1979; Waters et al., 1994a, b).

Crozier et al. (1991) reported, using ASIA assessment at 72 h, that 89% of ASIA B–E patients with pinprick preservation went on to ambulate, compared with 11% having preserved light touch but not pinprick.

The theory behind the significance of sacral preservation is the proximity of the spinothalamic tracts that mediate pinprick to the lateral corticospinal tracts. At 1 year postinjury, 76% incomplete paraplegics (ASIA B–E) become community ambulators by 2 years, compared to 46% of incomplete tetraplegics who ambulate, probably due to upper-extremity weakness compromising the ability to perform gait (Waters et al., 1994a, b). Age is a significant factor in indication of outcome (Ditunno et al., 1994; Burns & Ditunno, 2001).

ACUTE GENERAL MANAGEMENT

Although the primary damage is to the spinal cord, every organ system can be affected. Antecedent and posttraumatic psychological and social conditions must also be given full consideration as they play their inevitable parts in the success or failure of rehabilitation. Acute and rehabilitation specialities and disciplines are necessary to provide a holistic approach, in which all team members work towards common goals, agreed amongst the patient and team.

Trauma management

SCI presentation remains a key issue for all professionals, who should be vigilant about the risks of activities in which they may be involved, such as on rugby fields or at swimming pools.

Immediate management

When an accident occurs involving a SCI, other injuries should be suspected and the incident history recorded; pain, bruising and/or palpable spinal deformity are likely features. This is a crucial time for appropriate management to ensure the best chances possible for survival of the spinal cord fibres.

Proper handling will avoid unnecessary further damage, and the following simple advice can be immensely valuable:

- The patient should be advised not to move.
- The airway and breathing should be checked.
- If removal to another site is necessary, the transfer should be gentle, avoiding any twisting. Lifting should be performed by at least four people, with one acting as leader to co-ordinate the team.
- The patient should be placed in a supine position with the head and body kept strictly in alignment.
- If unconscious, the patient should be strapped to, and supported on, a board to allow tilt and avoid aspiration.
- Normal spinal curvature should be supported by a rolled-up cloth.
- The skin should be protected from pressure and ulceration by removing objects from pockets or by removing clothes.
- Point pressure from heels on hard surfaces, or 'knocking knees', should be avoided.
- Various spinal immobilisation boards, e.g. the scoop stretcher, and collars are available in ambulances for moving patients.
- Maintenance of oxygenation and blood pressure is essential.
- If possible, a motor and sensory charting should be performed for a baseline neuroassessment with diagrammatic recording.

Admission to hospital

Currently in the UK, after sustaining an SCI the person is admitted to the local accident and emergency or trauma unit. A full physical and neurological assessment is carried out and a decision is made about referral to a specialist unit. The decision for management (conservative or surgical) is made after the appropriate diagnostic testing. Spinal imaging can now provide reliable evidence of stability (X-ray, magnetic resonance imaging (MRI) and/or computed tomography (CT).

Research-based interventions for neuroprotection include the following managements (Tator, 1998; Johnston, 2001; Ramer et al., 2000):

- advanced trauma life support
- decompressive surgery
- steroids
- recent introduction of membrane-stabilising agents and neuroprotective agents.

Acute hospital management

Acute trauma management guidelines are well established (Moore et al., 1991). The ABCs, which are ensuring a patent airway, breathing and maintenance of circulation, are enshrined in all emergency practice, as is the importance of taking a history and performing an examination. Acute management of the patient with an SCI has special features resulting from spinal cord shock. Full details are described by Grundy & Swain (2002).

Breathing

Paralysis of respiratory muscles may be a feature. Patients with acute cervical cord injuries can fatigue in their breathing. Pulse oximetry is a crude indicator of respiratory distress because it measures only haemoglobin saturation and not partial pressure of oxygen (P_{O_2}) (Hough, 2001). Any evidence of desaturation or of falling saturation should be proactively addressed by the critical care team to maintain oxygenation and prevent further cord damage. Monitoring patients' breathing rate, pattern and colour, and noting agitation, drowsiness or distressed behaviour, is vital. Arterial blood-gas analysis may be the critical factor in deciding whether to provide ventilatory support.

Circulation

The sympathetic nerve supply to the heart is via cervical, cervical thoracic and upper thoracic branches of the sympathetic trunk. Cervical and upper thoracic injuries may produce sympathetic disruption, with impairment of tachycardia response. Therefore, pulse rate may mislead in the presence of circulatory shock. There is skin vasodilation within the dermatomes caudal to the injury. This causes a lowering of blood pressure. Injudicious fluid replacement to augment the blood pressure can cause pulmonary oedema. Pharyngeal suction, urethral catheterisation or simply repositioning of the patient can produce vagal overstimulation

and lead to bradycardia; intravenous atropine may be required to restore normal heart rate.

Spinal cord shock

This is the phenomenon of cessation of nervous system function below the level of damage to the cord and may be due to the loss of descending neural influences. After several seconds to months, the flaccid paralysis and areflexia of spinal shock are replaced by hyper-excitability, seen clinically as hyperreflexia, spasticity and spasms. Stauffer (1983) noted that it is rare to see patients in total spinal shock and totally areflexic. Strong spasticity almost immediately postinjury is indicative of an incomplete SCI. In these patients assessment of voluntary movement requires careful differentiation. In the authors' experience, development of increased muscle tone and involuntary movements may mislead patients to believe they have functional return of activity. It is important for the therapist to anticipate such reactions and to assess carefully in order to avoid confusion and disappointment.

Skin care

Denervated skin is at risk from pressure damage within 20–30 min of injury. If this occurs, it can cause distress and delay in the rehabilitation process. Clinical staff attending should be vigilant in monitoring the skin and should report red marks.

Gastrointestinal tract

SCI can produce ileus and gastric distension that can restrict movement of the diaphragm, further compromising breathing. A nasogastric tube should be placed for decompression if bowel sounds are absent. Gastric stress ulcers can occur and prophylactic treatment with mucosal protectors is recommended.

Bladder

Spinal shock causes retention of urine; the bladder should therefore be catheterised routinely in order to monitor fluid output and to protect it from overdistension damage.

Spinal stabilisation versus conservative management

Spinal fractures may be classified as stable, unstable or quasistable (i.e. currently stable but likely to become unstable in the course of everyday activity). Disagreement continues between protagonists and antagonists of surgical stabilisation of the spine but surgery is increasingly used (Collins, 1995).

Definition of instability or stability of a spinal lesion has now achieved substantial agreement based on the three column principles (Dennis, 1983). There is general agreement that restoration of the anatomy of the canal is sensible in terms of giving the cord the best opportunity for recovery.

It is debated whether neurological recovery or degree of spinal stability in the long term differs with surgical or conservative management. Surgery aims to minimise neurological deterioration, restore alignment and stabilisation, facilitate early mobilisation, reduce pain, minimise hospital stay and prevent secondary complications (Johnston, 2001).

From a physiotherapy and psychological point of view, the ability to mobilise a patient against gravity early seems to be a desirable outcome from surgery. This can be achieved by 7–10 days after surgery and results in a shorter inpatient stay.

Management of acute lesions at T4 and above

Surgical stabilisation may be achieved by anterior or posterior fixation, or a combination of the two (e.g. Collins, 1995). Patients managed conservatively are immobilised with bed rest; depending on the degree of instability, they may have to be maintained in spinal alignment by skull traction. Traction is applied usually by halo traction, Gardner–Wells or cone calipers (Grundy & Swain, 2002).

Early mobilisation may be indicated and can be achieved using a halo brace. Care in handling and positioning during physiotherapy is discussed below (see 'Acute physical management').

Length of immobilisation will vary depending on the extent of bony injury and ligamentous instability, and whether surgery has been performed. There may be several spinal segments affected and this will also influence the length of bed rest. Multiple-level fractures in the cervical spine are usually treated conservatively by halo traction and a period of immobilisation in a hard collar. Bed rest is usually for 3 months. On starting mobilisation, patients with all levels of injury will usually wear a collar of some type, depending on their stability.

Management of acute lesions at T4 and below

Thoracolumbar fractures are most common at the L1 level, this being the level of greatest mobility. Patients with unstable lesions at T9 and below must not have their hips flexed greater than 30° in order to avoid lumbar flexion.

Stable wedge fractures are usually treated conservatively with a brace or plaster of Paris (or similar) jacket. Unstable burst fractures, with cord compression, will justify surgical decompression and fixation. Generally, an anterior and posterior fixation technique will require a brace to be worn for 3 months postoperatively. If the spine is stable anteriorly, it may be sufficient to stabilise posteriorly. In this situation, a brace will be recommended for 6 months.

Bracing techniques vary greatly between institutions. A moulded hard plastic (subortholen) jacket can be made from an individual casting of plaster. Many braces are commercially available 'off the shelf' or other materials are used to form a brace, e.g. leather jackets or Neofract.

Special problems in SCI

Osteoporosis

Osteoporosis is a loss in bone mass without any alteration of the ratio between mineral and the organic matrix. A text by Riggs & Melton (1995) provides a comprehensive overview of osteoporosis. It is thought that immobilisation for long periods and a sedentary life lead to an increase in bone reabsorption, thus causing osteoporosis.

At 2 years after SCI, most patients will demonstrate a significant reduction in bone density in the lower-limbs, though the spine may be spared. The osteoporosis may cause fractures of long bones during relatively simple manoeuvres, such as transfer or passive movements.

It is not known how much effect weight-bearing has on reducing established osteoporosis (Goemaere et al., 1994). The question is frequently asked whether a patient who has not stood for several years should recommence standing. Currently the advice of the unit at Stanmore is to start the weight-bearing programme using a tilt table for 2 or 3 months, usually with bone-enhancing agents, and monitor using bone densitometry, before standing in a frame. Such advice is empirical and research is needed to provide informed guidelines.

Heterotopic ossification

Calcification in denervated or UMN-disordered muscle remains an ill-understood process and commonly occurs in patients with SCI (David et al., 1993). It may be confused in the early stages with deep venous thrombosis, when it presents as swelling, alteration in skin colour and increased heat, usually in relation to a joint. During the active process, analysis of plasma biochemistry shows a raised alkaline phosphatase. It can result in loss of range of movement (ROM) and difficulty in sitting. If ossification occurs around the hips it may lead to further skin pressure problems. Treatment of this condition is discussed by David et al. (1993). It must be emphasised that stretching should be gentle, as overstretching may be a predisposing factor for this condition (see Ch. 25, p. 433). Pharmacological treatment has not yet been fully evaluated.

The bladder

Urological complications of SCI are major mortal and morbid risks and the reader is referred to Fowler & Fowler (1993) for a review. Spinal cord damage disrupts the neural controls of bladder function. The objectives of bladder management are to provide a system ensuring safety, continence and least social disruption.

In the acute stage the bladder is catheterised to allow free drainage, to accommodate any fluid input and output fluctuations and to avoid bladder distension. Intermittent catheterisation is then established. After spinal shock passes, urodynamic studies are used to identify the emergent bladder behaviour.

Anterior sacral root electrical stimulation may be used, primarily for controlling urinary voiding but it may also facilitate defecation and penile erection separately. Reflex micturition (by tapping the abdominal wall or stroking the medial thigh) is not favoured because the bladder is unprotected from hyperreflexic complications.

The bowel

Although morbid complications rarely arise in the bowel, social embarrassment is common and often perceived by patients as more devastating than limb paralysis. Laxatives can achieve a bowel frequency within the normal range. For intractable constipation, occasional enemas can be useful. Increasing use of anterior sacral root stimulators and other surgical techniques may be beneficial. The mainstay of bowel care is to produce a predictable pattern, to minimise incontinence, impaction and interference with activities of daily living.

Fertility

Fertility is usually maintained in women, with the ovulatory cycle being normal within 9 months after injury. Fertility in men is, however, a problem (Brindley, 1984). Improvements in fertility rates for men after SCI have been made due to several important technical advances. These include improved methods in the retrieval and enhancement of sperm, such as electroejaculation, and improved means of achieving fertilisation with limited sperm quality and numbers through in vitro techniques.

Autonomic dysreflexia

Autonomic dysreflexia can be described as a sympathetic nervous system dysfunction producing hypertension, bradycardia and headache with piloerection and capillary dilation and sweating, above the level of the lesion. Some or all of these can result from any noxious stimulus such as bladder or rectal distension. If it occurs, the patient should be sat up, given appropriate medication and the underlying cause treated. Patients and therapists should be aware that the hypertension can rise sufficiently to induce cerebral haemorrhage, so this should be treated as an emergency. Mild autonomic dysreflexic symptoms act as signals to patients for toileting and induction of symptoms has been used foolishly, in the authors' view, to enhance sporting performance.

ACUTE PHYSICAL MANAGEMENT

In the early postinjury phase, physical management will mainly involve prevention of respiratory and circulatory complications, and care of pressure areas (Chartered Society of Physiotherapy Standards, 1997).

Principles of assessment

Assessment must be carried out as soon after admission as possible to obtain an objective baseline measurement of function, to identify where specific problems are likely to develop and to instigate prophylactic treatment. History of the injury is taken, including the results of relevant tests, e.g. lung function. Medical history is also noted. It is important to be aware of associated injuries, as these may influence management. The principles of assessment are discussed in Chapter 3.

The therapist needs to assess:

- respiratory state
- passive range of movement of all joints above and below the level of injury
- muscle function, i.e. strength using a muscle chart and the Oxford Grading System, Medical Research Council (MRC) scale or ASIA (1992) assessment (Fig. 8.2); and tone using the Ashworth Scale or another assessment tool (Bohannon & Smith, 1987)
- sensory and proprioceptive impairment, especially sharp/blunt sensation.

Treatment objectives in the acute phase

The main objectives are:

- to institute a prophylactic respiratory regimen and treat any complications
- to achieve independent respiratory status where possible
- to maintain full ROM of all joints within the limitations determined by fracture stability
- to monitor and manage neurological status as appropriate
- to maintain/strengthen all innervated muscle groups and facilitate functional patterns of activity
- to support/educate the patient, carers, family and staff.

Spasticity: a reminder!

Since the spinal cord is shorter than the vertebral column, lower-vertebral injuries will not involve damage to the cord, but there will be nerve root damage which will determine the presence of spasticity. The spinal cord usually extends to the first or second lumbar vertebra (Williams, 1995). Below this level, the nerve roots descend as the cauda equina and emerge from their respective vertebral levels. Injuries at these lower levels, therefore, are peripheral nerve (LMN) injuries.

A patient with a UMN injury, i.e. at the level of T12 or above, may present with a varied amount of spasticity. Weakness occurs but there may be preservation of muscle bulk to some extent due to the increased tone. A patient with an LMN injury, i.e. below the level of T12, will present with flaccid paralysis or weakness only. Obviously, this cut-off level of T12 is a general rule, as an individual's anatomy may vary from the usual.

Respiratory management

Effect of cord injury on the respiratory system

Respiration is a complex motor activity using muscles at various levels (see below). Patients with lesions of T1 and above will lose some 40–50% of their respiratory function but most patients with cervical injuries have an initial vital lung capacity of only 1.5 litres or less. Thus, all patients with cervical injuries should be fully evaluated for respiratory efficiency by monitoring spirometry and Po_2 in the initial weeks after injury. For an overview of respiratory physiology with an explanation of the tests mentioned here and normal values, the reader is referred to relevant textbooks (e.g. Hough, 2001; Smith & Ball, 1998).

Given the aetiology of SCI, many patients sustain associated injuries affecting respiration. Lung contusion or pneumo- or haemopneumothorax is common in patients with thoracic lesions, often associated with steering-wheel impact. They present at 24–48 h post-injury with deteriorating respiratory function, with a falling Po_2 and rising Pco_2. This is a serious development and mechanical ventilation may be required, occasionally for a number of weeks.

In other patients, deterioration of respiratory function in the first days after injury may be associated with an ascending cord lesion of two to three spinal levels, due to oedema or extending hypoxia in the cord or possibly due to fatigue. This again may lead to the need for mechanical ventilation for a period and then subsequent weaning from the ventilator as cord function returns. Occasionally the higher ascended level may become the permanent level. If significant hypoxia persists, particularly with associated low blood pressure, further damage to the cord may occur. These patients do improve their respiratory capacity with respiratory training (see below).

Atelectasis is common in patients with SCI. Subsequent infection and pneumonia still account for considerable morbidity and some mortality in tetraplegics. Prophylactic tracheostomy is often advised to assist in effective clearance of secretions. High cervical injuries are prone to bronchospasm due to disrupted sympathetic response and will require appropriate treatment with bronchodilators.

Extreme ventilatory compromise in spinal injury is caused by one or more of the following:

- inspiratory and expiratory muscle paralysis leading to decreased lung volume
- loss of effective cough
- diminished chest wall mobility
- reduced lung compliance
- increased energy cost of breathing and paradoxical chest wall movement.

Chest and head injuries are commonly associated with spinal injury and provide their own respiratory problems, which must also be assessed and treated appropriately.

Muscles affecting respiratory function

The abdominal muscles (innervated by T6–T12 spinal nerves) are essential for forced expiration and effective coughing. They also stabilise the lower ribs and assist the function of the diaphragm. The intercostal muscles (innervated by T1–T11 spinal nerves) have a predominantly inspiratory function as prime movers but also as fixators for the diaphragm. These muscle groups comprise about 40% of respiratory motor effort.

The diaphragm (innervation C3–C5, phrenic nerves) is the main inspiratory muscle but relies on other muscles to maximise efficiency. The accessory muscles (innervated by C1–C8 nerves and cranial nerve XI) include the trapezius, sternomastoid, levator scapulae and scalenii muscles; they can act as sole muscles of inspiration for short periods, but if the diaphragm is paralysed they cannot maintain prolonged adequate ventilation unassisted (see inspiratory muscle training in sections 'Acute respiratory care and management of complications' and 'Rehabilitation: Ongoing respiratory management', below).

Chest movement

The use of accessory muscles and diaphragm function can be assessed by palpation at the lower costal border. Muscle paralysis results in altered mechanics of respiration. In lesions involving paralysis of the abdominal and intercostal muscles, the lower ribs will be drawn in on inspiration in a paradoxical movement (Pryor & Webber, 1998). These abnormalities reduce the efficiency of the diaphragm in producing negative intrathoracic pressure, hence causing reductions in lung volume and efficiency of ventilation. Any asymmetry of movement, as well as respiratory rate, is noted.

Routine auscultation

This is as for any other patient. However, problems such as added breath sounds, pneumothorax or haemopneumothorax severely affect the patient's ability to maintain adequate ventilation and perfusion.

Forced vital capacity

The forced vital capacity (FVC) is a readily available objective measurement of respiratory muscle function, as is peak inspiratory flow rate. As mentioned earlier, it is used acutely to monitor respiratory status. If the FVC is <1 litre, the therapist may choose to instigate either intermittent positive-pressure breathing (IPPB), e.g. the Bird respirator, or bilevel intermittent positive airway pressure (BIPAP), as discussed by Hough (2001). This assisted ventilation can be used prophylactically to maintain and increase inspiratory volume and aid clearance of secretions. It is a useful adjunct to active manual techniques for patients with sputum retention and lung collapse, and can be used to administer bronchodilators (Pryor & Webber, 1998). Elective ventilation is normally undertaken if the FVC falls below 500 ml.

In cases of severe pain from rib fractures and associated soft-tissue injuries, a mixture of nitrous oxide and oxygen (Entonox) may be used and, if applicable, entrained into the IPPB circuit. Trancutaneous electrical nerve stimulation (TENS) has also been found to be effective in assisting pain management (see Ch. 23, p. 403). Breathing exercises and respiratory muscle training may also include the use of IPPB and incentive spirometry, in the acute phase.

Cough

A patient with a lesion above T6 will not have an effective cough as he or she will have lost the action of the abdominal muscles. The physiotherapist can compensate for this loss by the use of assisted coughing, in order that the patient can clear secretions (Bromley, 1998).

Acute respiratory care and management of complications

If no other respiratory complications are present, the physiotherapist will teach prophylactic breathing exercises to encourage chest expansion and improve ventilation. Incentive spirometry is useful for patients with mid thoracic lesions and above, to give the patient and family positive feedback of breathing function and strengthen recovering muscles. Care is necessary to maintain the stability of the spine. It is advised that shoulders are held for patients with unstable lesions of T4 and above when performing an assisted cough. In these circumstances, bilateral techniques should always be used in order to maintain spinal alignment. Adapted postural drainage for an unstable lesion is performed using specialised turning beds that allow spinal alignment to be maintained.

Ventilation Assisted ventilation may be necessary. Proactive intervention before the patient becomes exhausted will make subsequent management easier. Elective intubation is potentially less damaging to the spinal cord than intubation following cardiac arrest. Respiratory therapy for the spinal-injured ventilated patient is similar to that for other ventilated patients (Smith & Ball, 1998; Hough, 2001), apart from added vigilance to protect the fracture site.

Weaning from the ventilator should start as soon as the patient's condition stabilises. It is important to avoid fatigue whilst weaning, so careful monitoring ensures that FVC does not fall by more than 20%, or respiratory rate rise above 25–30 breaths/min. Patients who fail to wean – usually those with a greater degree of diaphragm paralysis – require long-term ventilation (see 'The long-term ventilated patient', below).

Suctioning This should always be undertaken with care in patients with SCI and is not recommended in the cervical non-intubated patient, as the neck cannot be extended to open the airway. It is important to assist the cough when stimulating the cough reflex, as merely stimulating the reflex will not produce an effective cough.

In patients with lesions above T6, the thoracolumbar sympathetic outflow is interrupted. During suction the vagus nerve is unopposed and the patient may become hypotensive and bradycardiac, possibly resulting in cardiac arrest. Endotracheal intubation may produce a similar response. Suction causes vagal stimulation via the carotid bodies, which pass impulses to the brain via the glossopharyngeal nerves and are sensitive to lack of oxygen (Williams, 1995). It is therefore wise to pre-oxygenate the patient, monitor heart rate and have atropine on standby.

Active assisted facilitation of movement and passive movements

As the majority of SCI patients present as incomplete, it is important to facilitate and utilise any active movement available. During the acute phase, whilst the patient is immobilised in bed, the physiotherapist can assist in exploiting the potential for functional return. Where patients have any active movement they should be encouraged to participate in activity and it should be purposeful if possible.

Functional electrical stimulation (FES) is a useful adjunct to improve a movement where only a flicker is first available (see Ch. 23). Similarly, electromyographic (EMG) biofeedback can assist the patient to move in the absence of full sensation (see Ch. 23). More recently, cortical mapping has demonstrated change, by the performance of passive movements with the patient visualising the movement and in the presence of some sensory feedback (Reddy et al., 2001).

The aims of all such movements, as discussed in Chapter 25, are to:

- assist circulation
- maintain muscle length, preventing soft-tissue shortening and contracture
- maintain full ROM of all joints
- maintain movement patterns.

Movements are commenced immediately after injury and features specifically important for SCI patients are now discussed. Shoulder movements are usually performed at least twice a day and leg movements once a day, in order to monitor any return of movement. For lumbar and low thoracic fractures, hip flexion should be kept to below 30°, to avoid lumbar flexion, until stability is established. Knee flexion must, therefore, be performed in Tailor's position, i.e. 'frogging' (Fig. 8.4).

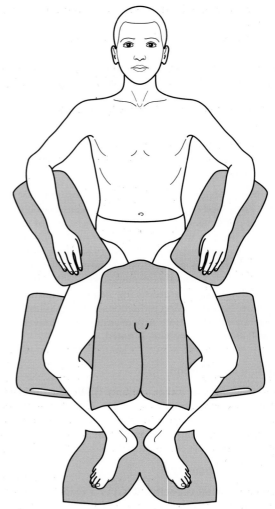

Figure 8.4 The 'frogging' or Tailor's position. This position is used to prevent movement of the lumbar spine during passive movements of the knees. It is also used to prevent mass extensor tone.

Special emphasis should be put on the following:

- stretch finger flexors with wrist in neutral to preserve tenodesis grip (Bromley, 1998)
- ensure a full fist can be attained with wrist extension
- pronation and supination in elbow flexion and extension
- full elevation and lateral rotation of the shoulder from day 1
- stretch long head of triceps – arm in elevation with elbow flexion

- stretch rhomboids bilaterally – avoid twisting cervical spine
- stretch upper fibres of trapezius muscle.

Key points

Movements commence from the first day after injury:

- To monitor any return of movement
  Shoulder movements performed at least twice a day
  Leg movements performed once a day
- For lumbar and low thoracic fractures (prestabilisation)
  Hip flexion maintained below 30°
- Knee flexion performed in Tailor's 'frogging' position
- Special emphasis placed on specific stretches to tissues of upper-limbs (see text)
- Extreme range of movement must be avoided

Where there is no active flexion of the fingers and thumb, it is appropriate to allow shortening of the long flexors. The ROM of individual joints at the wrist, fingers and thumb must be maintained. When the wrist is actively extended, the fingers and thumb are pulled into flexion to produce a functional 'key-type' grip, the tenodesis grip. If this contracture does not occur naturally, it can be encouraged by splinting whilst in the acute phase.

During recovery, the handling principles apply to facilitate normal movement and not to elicit spasm and reinforce the spastic pattern. Extreme ROM must be avoided, especially at the hip and knee, as microtrauma may be a predisposing factor in the formation of periarticular ossification (see above). Passive movements of paralysed limbs are continued until the patient is mobile and thus capable of ensuring full mobility through his or her own activities, unless there are complications, such as excessive spasm or stiffness.

A complication that may occur over the few days after injury and remain a risk for some months is the development of pulmonary emboli associated with deep venous thrombosis (DVT). Prophylactic measures, including frequent passive movement, wearing pressure stockings and early mobilisation, are important. The use of antithrombolytic agents has become mandatory. Extreme vigilance with regard to leg size and other signs of DVT by all team members is important, as there is a 1–2% incidence of mortality from massive pulmonary embolus each year.

Turning and positioning

Whilst managed on bed rest patients will require frequent turning. Turning charts can be used to assist staff with a regimen over each 24-h period, to avoid pressure-marking of anaesthetic skin and offering an opportunity to check skin tolerance. This regimen can be used in conjunction with postural drainage positions. Turning beds can be used to reposition a patient, and the choice of bed depends on the individual unit's policy.

Upper-limb positioning of the tetraplegic patient is very important during bed rest. Incomplete cervical lesions are particularly prone to shortening of soft tissues due to muscle imbalance, resulting in partial shoulder subluxation and pain.

Waring & Maynard (1991) reported that 75% of tetraplegics had shoulder pain, 60% lasting 2 weeks or more. Of the patients with pain, 39% had unilateral and 61% bilateral symptoms. In over a third, onset was within the first 3 days postinjury and 52% within the first 2 weeks postinjury. The reasons for pain are diverse but not least due to the muscle imbalance, spasticity and direct trauma to the shoulder girdle. This combines with the joint immobilisation, central and peripheral sources of nerve pain.

Patients who are delayed in the initiation of shoulder exercises beyond 2 weeks postinjury are significantly at risk of shoulder pain. The Spinal Injuries Unit at Stanmore advocates early intervention of consistent shoulder ROM exercises.

Scott & Donovan (1981) described special positioning to prevent loss of range: 90° abduction, combined with other positioning techniques, leads to decreased frequency and severity of shoulder pain.

Positioning is used to minimise spasticity similarly to patients with other conditions. When the patient is exhibiting mass muscle tone in flexion or extension, the limbs and trunk may be placed into reflex-inhibiting positions. Some examples of positioning are shown in Figures 8.4–8.7. Positioning is also discussed in Chapter 25 and by Pope (2002).

Preparation for and initiation of mobilisation

Patient education begins during the acute phase, and with explanation of treatment interventions, patients are encouraged to take control of their rehabilitation.

Once radiographs have confirmed spinal stability, mobilisation is initiated by progressively sitting the patient up in bed. Postural hypotension will be the main problem and patients with lesions at T6 and above will require an elasticated abdominal binder. This helps to maintain intrathoracic pressure and reduce pooling of the blood, from lack of abdominal

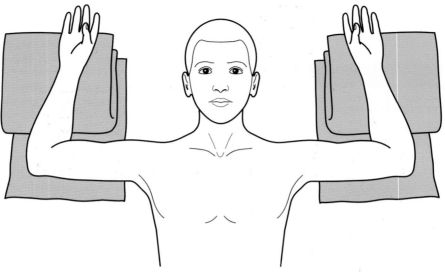

Figure 8.5 Upper-limb positioning in the tetraplegic patient. This position is used to maintain full external rotation with abduction of the shoulders, in patients with unopposed activity of the internal rotators and adductors.

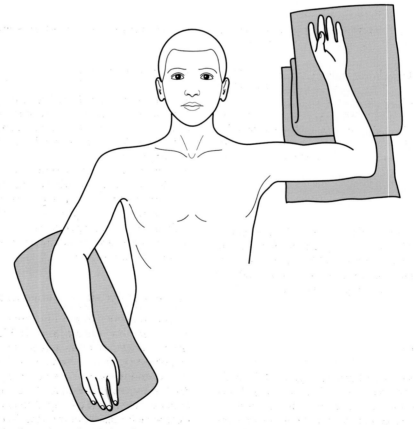

Figure 8.6 This position is an alternative to that shown in Figure 8.5. It provides a more gentle position to maintain abduction and external rotation and can be alternated from arm to arm as comfort allows.

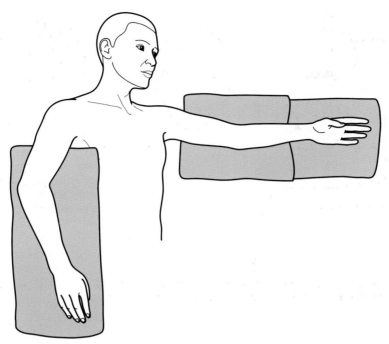

Figure 8.7 Side–lying. This position provides a comfortable resting position for the shoulders in side–lying, whilst still maintaining abduction of the shoulder and a supported biceps stretch.

action. Once the patient starts to sit up, he or she will be supported in a hard or soft collar, or a brace. Antithrombotic stockings will still be worn. Special adaptations to wheelchairs can help to reduce hypotensive fainting, e.g. reclining back and raised-leg supports. When patients can sit up for an hour they can initiate rehabilitation for the restoration of functional activities.

Pressure lifting

This is a technique in which patients lift themselves in their wheelchairs to relieve pressure. It is recommended that they lift every half-hour, for approximately 30 s. Where a patient cannot lift, a modified position in forward-leaning or side-to-side tilt is used.

REHABILITATION

The following section outlines management from the start of mobilisation phase through to discharge. Much of this information has been gained from the authors' experience; procedures may vary between centres but the principles are similar (Bromley, 1998; Whalley Hammell, 1995).

Aims of rehabilitation

- to establish an interdisciplinary process which is patient-focused, comprehensive and co-ordinated
- physical motor functional activities with early intervention and prophylaxis to prevent further complications
- to learn new information to equip the individual with knowledge to achieve independence
- to achieve functional independence, whether physical or verbal, and equipment provision in order to facilitate this independence
- to achieve and maintain successful reintegration into the community.

Goal–planning and outcome measures

Evaluation of progress by review of goal achievement is advised. The goals can be divided into achievable targets and should be patient-focused, appropriate and objective. It is recommended that they are created in a team environment, led by the patient, with interdisciplinary co-operation. It is at this point that patients are fully encouraged to take the locus of control for their rehabilitation. This theme is extended into the philosophy of their future reintegration. Chapter 22 discusses these issues of patient-centred practice in goal-setting and treatment, using a problem-solving approach.

There are several local measures used to evaluate patient progress, some applicable to an intervention or management technique. In general the World Health Organization recognises Functional Independence Measures (FIM; Hamilton & Granger, 1991), and Craig Handicap Assessment and Reporting Technique (CHART; Whiteneck et al., 1992) as appropriate validated measures. Other outcome measures are discussed in Chapter 3.

Objectives of rehabilitation

The progression of objectives as the patient gains more ability is outlined below. These objectives need to be set in relation to the level of spinal injury and the appropriate functional goals (Table 8.1). These expectations for function, depending on level of SCI, can only be a guide, especially in the light of the prevalence of incomplete lesions.

Increased muscle tone

This is an important issue in the management of patients with SCI (Young & Shahani, 1986; Priebe et al., 1996); it is a very large subject and requires more consideration than this chapter allows (see Ch. 4 and 25). Spasticity is a motor disorder characterised by an increase in muscle tone in response to stretch of relaxed muscle and the response is velocity-dependent.

Table 8.1 Functional goals of rehabilitation in relation to the level of the spinal cord lesion

Level	Key muscle control	Movement	Functional goals
C1–C3	Sternocleidomastoid Upper trapezius Levator	Neck control	Ventilator-dependent Electric wheelchair Verbally independent
C4	C3 plus diaphragm	Shoulder shrug	Electric wheelchair Verbally independent
C5	Biceps Deltoid Rotator cuff Supinator	Elbow flexion, supination Shoulder flexion, abduction	Manual wheelchair with capstans Electric wheelchair for long distance Independent brushing Teeth/hair/feeding with feeding strap
C6	Extensor carpi radialis longus, extensor carpi radialis brevis Pronator teres	Wrist extension, pronation	Tenodesis grip Manual wheelchair ($\pm$capstans) Independent feeding, grooming, dressing top half, simple cooking Same-height transfers
C7	Triceps Latissimus dorsi Flexor digitorum, flexor carpi radialis, extensor digitorum	Elbow extension Finger flexion/extension	Manual wheelchair Independent activities of daily living, simple transfers, i.e. bed, car, toilet, may drive with hand controls
C8	All upper-limbs except lumbricals, interossei	Limited fine finger movements	Manual wheelchair Full dexterity
T1–T5	Varying intercostals and back muscles	Trunk support No lower-limb movements	Full wheelchair independence Orthotic ambulation
T6–T12	Abdominals	Trunk control	Orthotic/caliper ambulation
L1–L2	Psoas major Iliacus	Hip flexion	Caliper ambulation
L3–L4	Quadriceps Tibialis anterior	Knee extension Ankle dorsiflexion	Ambulation with orthoses and crutches/sticks
L5	Peronei	Eversion	Ambulation with relevant orthoses
S1–S5	Glutei, gastrocnemius Bladder, bowel, sexual function	Hip extension Ankle plantarflexion	Normal gait

In incomplete cord lesions, depending on the pattern, spasticity tends to occur earlier and may present immediately. When severe, it will inhibit any underlying voluntary movement. In complete spinal cord lesions, it most commonly becomes apparent about 3 months after the injury. It tends to reach a maximum between 6 and 12 months after injury and then to diminish and become manageable. However, in a minority it remains at a high level and presents a major problem of management, affecting function, posture and joint movement (Sheean, 1998).

A moderate amount of spasticity will assist with standing transfers, maintain muscle bulk, protect the skin to some extent and may contribute to prevention of osteoporosis. It is when the spasticity is excessive that problems occur.

Spasticity management

The management of spasticity should be undertaken by a co-ordinated multidisciplinary team rather than by clinicians in isolation (Barnes et al., 2001). Spinal cord spasticity presents in different patterns to that usually seen in stroke patients.

The best management is prevention in the first few months after injury. These strategies have been discussed earlier (see Ch. 25).

It is also important to avoid triggering factors, such as urinary tract infection, constipation or skin breakdown. A collaborative assessment and evaluation tool to determine the best management of spasticity in SCI patients is currently being developed to accompany the document by Barnes et al. (2001).

The main medical approach is through pharmacology, although none of the drugs commonly used (baclofen, dantrolene and tizanidine) is universally effective or indeed predictable in its effect. Nerve blocks have been used for many years, usually using either phenol or alcohol. All of the above drugs have significant and numerous side-effects (see Ch. 28). As the use of intramuscular botulinum toxin increases, the use of other nerve blocks will diminish.

Surgery has some place in treatment, in the form of tendon release and nerve divisions, e.g. obturator neurectomy. These techniques can be successful, particularly where the procedure has been carried out for hygiene and posture reasons.

Psychological aspects

Management of psychological and social issues must take place in parallel with early medical and rehabilitation aspects. It is recognised that patients will experience symptoms of stress and anxiety, and these should be treated specifically. In the early weeks and months after injury, the patient may present with rapid and dramatic changes in mood state and may express denial of his or her situation, anger at what has happened and depression, which may include stating the desire to die.

Although all the members of the MDT will play a role in supporting a patient, advice and guidance from a qualified psychologist are essential and, at times, one-to-one direct patient therapy by the psychologist is necessary. The process of adaptation to spinal paralysis, reflected as integration back into the community, is a gradual one. Maintaining a positive approach with realistic expectations is essential for the patient's well-being (see Ch. 27).

Pain management

Pain can be a problem initially during movements, notably due to neurodynamics (see Ch. 31). There may be more than one origin of pain present in the SCI patient. Common syndromes include mechanical instability, muscle spasm pain, visceral pain, nerve root entrapment, syringomyelia, transitional zone pain and central dysaesthesia syndrome. There are many modalities available to physiotherapists to contribute to the management of pain, such as electrotherapy, movement re-education, positioning, TENS and acupuncture (see Chs 23 and 26).

Skin care

Common sites of pressure sores are ischial (from prolonged sitting), sacral (from sheer loading), trochanteric, malleolar, calcaneal and plantar surfaces from prolonged loading or direct trauma. Spasticity producing contractures and postural deformity are potential risk factors. Although poor nutrition, incontinence and comorbid factors increase the risk of decubitus ulceration, without ischaemia the ulcers do not arise. Therefore, patients are taught about risk management and provided with pressure redistributing mattresses and cushions.

Bed mobility

Rolling from side to side is taught first, then lying to sitting, and sitting to lying. Function is achieved dependent upon the level of the lesion, e.g. C5, rolling side to side; C6, rolling, lying to sitting and sitting to lying; C7, independent in all aspects of bed mobility.

Sitting balance

Sitting supported in the wheelchair is progressed to sitting on a plinth supported, unsupported, static and then dynamic. Balance is practised in short and long sitting, hamstring length determining the ability to long sit independently.

Lifting

Lifting starts with partial pressure lifts in the wheelchair, and progresses to lifts on blocks on a plinth and then unaided without blocks.

Wheelchair mobility

Wheelchair mobility and safety are taught. Adaptations, such as extended brakes and a modular supportive backrest, are required for higher lesions.

Transfers

Depending on the level of the lesion and functional ability, a sliding board may be used for legs-up and legs-down transfers on to the bed. This is progressed without a board where possible. Transfers then progress to lifting from various levels for functional activities: high to low; low to high; between two plinths; floor to plinth; floor to chair; chair to car, bath and to easy chair.

Standing programme

Care must be taken when initiating standing. The autonomic disturbance present in patients with cervical and thoracic injuries can result in significant problems with hypotension. Blood pressure studies and monitoring of pressures in sitting and gradual tilt table standing have been suggested. These problems usually resolve as the venous return improves.

Tilt table standing is commenced as soon as possible. This has many benefits: respiratory and psychological, maintenance of bone density, and improved systemic body functions. Standing is of great value in preventing soft-tissue contracture and in reduction of spasticity (Bohannon & Larkin, 1985; Goemaere et al., 1994; Golding, 1994).

An abdominal binder is recommended for patients with lesions of T6 and above. Once the patient can stand with no ill effect, progression is made to a standing frame e.g. Oswestry Standing Frame (OSF), working up to standing for 1 h, three times a week. Patients with lesions of C5 and below should be capable of standing into a hoist-assisted OSF. There are many standing systems commercially available which will lift the patient into a standing posture. Some wheelchairs also offer this facility. Whilst standing, trunk balance work can be re-educated, for example, removing hand support, throwing and catching a ball. Once good balance is achieved, the patient may go on to develop gait with orthoses or actively.

Upper-limb strengthening

This activity is continued from the acute phase using a variety of techniques (see Chs 23 and 29). Once the patient mobilises in the wheelchair, there are many options for strengthening during functional activities.

The evidence of shoulder pain in wheelchair users is undeniable – 78% of tetraplegics and 59% of paraplegics, although studies vary in numbers. Specific exercises to address muscle imbalance and maintenance of full range have been shown to reduce this incidence (Curtis et al., 1999).

Other specific exercises can be useful, e.g. assisted/resisted arm bike, resistance circuits and sporting activities. This is an enjoyable adjunct to rehabilitation and encourages reintegration.

Hydrotherapy is used for strengthening and as preparation for swimming. Patients are taught how to roll in the water and to swim. If the patient is wearing a brace, this will limit activities in the water. Anyone with an FVC of <1 litre will need careful consideration before swimming is introduced.

Ongoing respiratory management

Tetraplegic and some high thoracic paraplegic patients will require ongoing respiratory monitoring and will benefit from respiratory training. Respiratory capacity is impaired by motor weakness, spasticity and pain. Inspiratory muscle-training devices are of great benefit for improving FVC. The reader is encouraged to read the appropriate chapter in Hough (2001).

Motivation, endurance and cardiovascular fitness

Patients are motivated to achieve their physical goals in a variety of ways. Fitness training using adapted equipment is useful, e.g. an arm-powered ergonomic bike may be used for endurance. Wheelchair circuits and advanced skills are encouraged. Hydrotherapy can lead on to swimming, an enjoyable activity that can improve cardiovascular fitness.

Sports activities cannot be underestimated even for those people who did not enjoy sports previously. The known benefits of group or sports activities translate into the rehabilitation process. Patients will often sustain an activity for much longer when engaged in a sport.

There are many charities and organisations available to promote these opportunities and support equipment funding for SCI individuals (Spinal Injuries Association, 2002). Activities can eventually progress to more competitive sports and clubs, as well as encouraging attendance at the many fully integrated fitness centres available. Cardiovascular fitness after SCI has been reviewed (Jacobs & Nash, 2001) and in general for neurological conditions in Chapter 29.

Education/advice to carers/family

Carers are actively involved in the rehabilitation process and are taught how to assist with normal daily activities, to support the patient's ongoing health needs. Assisted exercises, standing programme and chest care are taught in addition to moving and handling the patient, whilst paying attention to skin care and their own safety and back care.

Wheelchairs

The variety of wheelchairs available increases each year, including some that enable the patient to rise into standing. Initially, patients are mobilised in a standard wheelchair offering greatest support and stability, following a comprehensive assessment to ensure it is correctly fitted and adjusted. Adaptations are made to provide a well-supported, evenly balanced seating position (Pope, 2002).

The key to good stability is achieved by support and alignment at the pelvis. The cushion is equally important and should be assessed in a similar way, also taking into account the need for protection of pressure areas. Various pressure assessment tools are used to evaluate skin viability when sitting and these aid cushion prescription (Barbenel et al., 1983). Later in rehabilitation, it will be appropriate to try a variety of wheelchairs to offer greater mobility and independence according to an individual's needs. In view of the incidence of shoulder pain in wheelchair users (Ballinger et al., 2000), it is appropriate to consider adaptations and weight of the wheelchairs. There are many light-weight wheelchairs available and the use of assisted wheeling systems can ease the effort of wheeling.

Powered chairs

All tetraplegic patients should always be provided with a powered chair, even if they chose a manual light-weight chair initially. This should also be considered for some paraplegics, depending on their age and expected functional activities.

Functional electrical stimulation in restoration of function and gait

Research and technologies have influenced our clinical practice, e.g. body weight support treadmill gait training is based around the central pattern generator (CPG) theory (see below). Research to incorporate FES with this training is underway. In future methods that use the concept of activity-dependent neuroplasticity will most likely play an increasing role in the rehabilitation of SCI.

FES and its role in functional activities and gait requires further evaluation (see Ch. 23). Currently it is used as a neuroprosthesis in activities of daily living (ADL) to restore upper-limb function, e.g. the Freehand system (Neurocontrol Systems, Cleveland, OH, USA). Surface FES systems that aim to assist paraplegic patients to walk are already approved in the USA – Parastep System (Sigmedics, Inc., IL, USA) and for incomplete injuries the Odstock Drop Foot Stimulator is widely used. Other systems are still at an experimental stage and implanted devices are being developed (Chae et al., 2000).

Despite promising advances in technology, the physiological limitations of the neuromuscular system prohibit the clinical use of FES alone to achieve a realistic and successful functional outcome. Principles of the technique are discussed in Chapter 23. Gait remains inefficient, needing high energy levels. It has been demonstrated that function achieved through an external locus of control will always be of limited value to patients (Bradley, 1994). The recent research is seeking to provide cortical patterns of activity to trigger the stimulation for movement (Grill et al., 2001).

Some patients choose to use FES to maintain muscle bulk for cosmesis and others to maintain bulk or circulation for reduction of pressure over bony areas. Patients who are very slim, with bony prominences, are predisposed to pressure marking and the maintenance of muscle bulk by FES can help to reduce this problem and allow them to sit for longer in their wheelchair.

Rehabilitation of incomplete lesions

The management of the incomplete patient presents many challenges, not least because experience has shown that the expected outcomes are unknown. This can affect the psychological adjustment of the patient and, as physical changes extend over many years, may delay patients in moving on with their life.

Emphasis is placed on managing muscle imbalance, spasticity and tone, and sensory loss. As incomplete lesions present with a wide range of loss of functional activity, treatment will depend on the level of disability and specific physical problems.

Treatment may include: facilitation of normal movement; muscle strengthening (see Ch. 29); reduction of muscle imbalance (see Ch. 30); and inhibition of spasticity (see Ch. 25). Balance re-education may include: use of the gymnastic ball; mat and plinth work; and use of a wobble board or balance performance monitor (see Ch. 24). Gait re-education, wheelchair skills and functional activities are performed as appropriate to the patient's level of ability.

Recent research has led to the exploration of gait facilitation using a partial weight-bearing system on the treadmill. This approach is based on the principles of CPGs and repeated exercise of gait motion to increase strength, co-ordination and endurance. There is evidence from animal studies that neural networks in the isolated spinal cord are capable of generating rhythmic output (reciprocally organised between agonists and antagonists) in the absence of efferent descending and movement-related afferent sources (Duysens & Van de Crommert, 1998). This is postulated to be similar in humans. Spinal systems contribute to the control of locomotion by local segmental and intersegmental spinal circuits (Grillner & Wallen, 1985).

In normal walking, it has been shown that muscle activity patterns are not centrally generated by reflex-induced activity, e.g. through stretch reflexes (Prochazka et al., 1979). The gait facilitation on the treadmill system is thought to be influenced by three main sensory sources acting on the CPGs:

1. load/proprioceptive feedback from the extensor muscles
2. exteroceptive afferents from the mechanreceptors of the foot
3. joint position and muscle stretch from the hip flexors and ankle plantarflexors.

Some outcome measures being assessed as evaluation tools for this work in the national spinal injuries units are: Walking Index for Spinal Cord Injury (WISCI). (Ditunno et al., 2000) and WISCI II (Ditunno et al., 2001).

There have been concerns from physiotherapists against gait exercise too early, causing the development of 'wrong patterns'. The motion of the hip is helped by the harness so as to move almost entirely within normal range limits. Therapists helping to guide foot placement manually found this an effective way of controlling motion and blocking abnormal harmful patterns. FES has been introduced as an adjunct to assist with the gait pattern (see Ch. 23). The advantages of this gait training would be to improve systemic functions and stimulate the vegetative nervous sequelae. Early training with some weight-bearing may help reduce osteoporosis and patients have been shown to need less support after training (Abel et al., 2002).

Questions remain if this treatment is effective: is progress due to other factors, e.g. muscle plasticity or spontaneous recovery, or can the cord learn from the increased demands of loading the limbs? The supraspinal and afferent influences on the cord are not yet understood in humans.

Patients with LMN damage require early diagnosis and may benefit from acute surgical and later restorative interventions, and also provision of orthoses to accommodate for the weakness (see Ch. 9).

Assisted gait, calipers and orthoses

During rehabilitation, the patient may be assessed for suitability for walking with orthoses. Depending on the fracture, gait training will normally commence about a year after surgery, or earlier if no fixation surgery was indicated or if the patient is incomplete. There should be surgical review on an individual basis. Some patients may require a temporary orthosis during their recovery.

It should be recognised that, even if a patient has the ability to walk with calipers, he or she may not choose to or may be advised not to try. Techniques used for gait training have been discussed in detail by Bromley (1998) and an outline of the progression of training is given below.

The gait-training process is physically demanding and requires commitment. Criteria which should be considered include:

- appropriate risk assessment
- sufficient upper-limb strength to lift body weight
- full ROM of hips and knees, and no contracture
- cardiovascular fitness sufficient to sustain walking activity
- assessment of spinal deformity, e.g. scoliosis, that may hinder standing balance
- motivation of the patient
- assessment of spasticity that may make walking unsafe.

Experience has shown that many patients complete their training with calipers, only to discard them a few months or years later as walking has become too much effort. Wheelchair use may be preferable, as the hands are free for functional activities whereas they are not when walking with calipers.

Orthoses

The ability to walk with calipers and the degree of support required depend on the functional level of injury. The following are examples of orthoses used for different levels of injury:

- C7–L1: hip guidance orthosis (HGO), advanced reciprocal gait orthosis (ARGO), RGO, Walkabout
- T6–T12: caliper walk/Walkabout with rollator; progress to crutches depends on patient's function
- T9–L3: caliper walk with comfortable handle crutches
- L3 and below: appropriate orthoses or walking aid.

Initial gait work

Caliper training is commenced in backslabs of Dynacast or similar light-weight casting material. The backslabs are bandaged on and toe springs applied. For all orthotic gait training adjustable training orthoses are used. Standing balance is achieved in the parallel bars, in front of a mirror, by standing in extension and resting back on the tension of the iliofemoral ligaments. The lifting technique is taught in the standing position, lifting the whole body weight with full control. Lift from sitting to standing and back to sitting is also taught.

Once the patient has achieved standing balance and the appropriate degree of support required, dynamic balance work is started. This includes turning safely, swing-to and swing-through gait patterns, and the four-point gait technique for stepping practice.

Transfers

Transferring in backslabs is then practised, from plinth to chair, chair to plinth, and from chair to standing.

Middle stage of gait work

Progression to a rollator or crutches is begun at this stage. Balance is achieved using one parallel bar and one crutch, or with a rollator and one person to assist. Gait patterns and transfers (described above) are then practised. Depending on the functional level, four-point gait with crutches is taught, then kerbs, slopes and stairs. Video assessment for problem-solving and improvement of gait techniques may be useful at this stage.

Late stage of gait work

On completion of training, the patient is measured for the definitive othoses. For patients using reciprocal gait orthoses, gait re-education is practised in the parallel bars then progressed to a rollator and possibly crutches, as outlined above.

A home standing programme for caliper patients is devised to improve confidence. This entails using backslabs daily to maintain strength and cardiovascular fitness and to improve mobility. Goals are decided mutually as to how calipers and walking aids will be used at home and at work, to achieve optimum function.

The long–term ventilated patient

Increased survival of patients with high lesions is now expected, especially in the young. Resettlement into the community requires domiciliary ventilation and a complex care package.

Once past the acute phase, their individual needs are ascertained. Specialised wheelchairs are available which can be mouth- or head-controlled. Prophylactic chest management is vital, with tracheostomy, regular bagging and suction to reduce atelectasis and prevent infection. FES for the abdominal muscles has been evaluated as a method to assist coughing (Linder, 1993).

Non-invasive ventilation may be appropriate for some patients and some others may be candidates for diaphragmatic pacing. Usually those with lesions above C3 are most successful. Lesions of C4 segmental level tend to have involvement of the anterior horn and cannot be stimulated, as stimulation relies on an intact lower motor system.

Assessment involves nerve conduction studies and may include fluoroscopic examination to visualise diaphragmatic excursion (Zejdlik, 1992). Electrodes are placed around the phrenic nerve either in the thorax or neck. An external pacing box is attached to external transmitter antennae; these are placed over the implanted receivers and when stimulated provide diaphragmatic contraction (Buchanan & Nawoezenski, 1987). There is no set regime for training but some patients have managed to achieve 24-h pacing. Others use the ventilator part-time.

Initially, physiotherapy will aim to maximise strength in all innervated muscles to assist in head control and strengthen accessory respiratory muscles. Glossopharyngeal breathing techniques and use of a biofeedback training system can allow the patient to manage for short periods off the ventilator. Regular tilt table standing is recommended in addition to passive movements. Management of spasticity is also an important consideration (see Ch. 25) and may involve medication (see Ch. 28, p. 471).

The aim for these patients is to achieve verbal independence and control of their environment. Technology offers systems linked to computerised environmental controls, operated by a head or mouth control, or is voice-activated.

Children with spinal cord injury

The number of children with spinal cord damage which is non-congenital is thankfully quite low. Numbers vary between studies but a study gives an example that less than 2% of children admitted with all forms of traumatic injury have an SCI (Brown et al., 2001). Traumatic causes are mostly from traffic accidents and falls.

In very young children, the head is proportionally larger and heavier and therefore injuries are commonly cervical. The range of maximum flexion of the cervical spine tends to move lower as the child gets older (Grundy & Swain, 2002). The review provided by Flett (1992) offers a comprehensive overview of the management of children with SCI. Other texts include Osenback & Menezes (1992) and Short et al. (1992).

Special considerations for children with SCI include the following:

- Children are very sensitive to hypotension, autonomic dysfunction and thermoregulatory dysfunction. There is potential for damage of the immature brain from chronic hypotension when first mobilising.
- Children have a high metabolism and therefore have high calorific needs for healing and recovery.
- Paralytic ileus is a very common problem in cervical and thoracic lesions.
- Standing is a priority in rehabilitating children. It is important for social skills and development of curiosity, and is essential in preventing osteoporosis and facilitates the development of the epiphyseal growth plates. A number of methods can be employed to maintain standing using many mobile standing systems. Spinal support braces, calipers or other orthotic supports are used to allow supported standing and walking. The child can stay in the brace for 90% of the day and remain ambulant for 80% of the day.
- The child must be closely monitored during growth spurts for the development of spinal deformity, e.g. scoliosis. Soft-tissue shortening is caused by altered posture and muscle imbalance, leading to further deformity.
- Support and education of the parents about the implications of the SCI will enable them to educate their child and family, and monitor the child for any complications. Schooling should be continued during rehabilitation, in liaison with the education authorities. Ongoing communication with the local education teams will ensure a smooth discharge and aid reintegration.

Discharge plan, reintegration and follow-up

The process of rehabilitation and reintegration is complex, involving many agencies and resources. In the last 5 years many spinal injuries units in the UK have found that the development of the case management process has helped to co-ordinate the complex process of discharge into the community. The patient thus has an advocate to complement the core rehabilitation team, who provide support in overcoming functional difficulties and liaise with the various organisations and authorities throughout rehabilitation.

On discharge, all patients will require further close follow-up and reassessment, which may involve the community teams. Ideally this will be a multidisciplinary review to maintain continued support, monitor physical well-being and facilitate reintegration into society. During rehabilitation, patients are introduced to groups who can offer social and leisure activities, whilst others have a support and advisory role, to assist in the reintegration process (see Appendix).

A home visit is made by the occupational therapist and community team and may include school or workplace. The physiotherapist may be involved to assess mobility issues. If home adaptations or rehousing are not completed but the patient is ready for discharge, transfer to an interim placement may be necessary. Return to work is discussed in Chapter 22.

Preparation for discharge is described well in the Chartered Society of Physiotherapy Standards (1997). From the authors' experience, we know that many incomplete patients with UMN and LMN lesions go on to make functional recovery past the quoted time of 2 years. As physiotherapists, we can ensure this opportunity is not lost and real qualitative changes can be made. The economic implications are strongly argued when someone can be kept mobile and carer input reduced. We must encourage utilisation of all treatment modalities and equipment available.

Patients will need ongoing follow-up and may require later-stage interventions, such as tendon transfer and implant surgery to restore function (mentioned previously). The spinal injuries unit should be available as a resource back-up when any complications or problems arise.

CONCLUSION

The management of the person with SCI is complex and lifelong. A functional, goal-oriented, interdisciplinary, rehabilitation programme should enable the patient with SCI to live as full and independent a life as possible. Evidence-based therapeutic interventions are already altering our expectations and the development of technology and pharmacology offers exciting prospects for the management of SCI individuals.

CASE HISTORIES

Patient A

C4 incomplete spinal cord injury – central cord syndrome
The patient sustained a hyperextension injury at C3–C4 level during a rugby tackle.

- male, aged 25 years
- no bony injury
- he was managed in a Philadelphia collar for 4 weeks. He was ASIA muscle-charted on admission and found to have flickers of activity in quadriceps, and left biceps and triceps (Table 8.2)
- managed on bed rest for 2 weeks.

Main problems

1. ↓ selectivity of movement around pelvis and trunk
2. ↓ selective movement of upper-limbs – dominant upper fibres of trapezius
3. ↑ Extensor tone throughout
4. ↓ selective movement of lower-limbs right > left
5. general stiffness throughout thoracic and lumbar spine – premorbidly
6. premorbid anterior instability of the right shoulder girdle
7. overactive hamstrings and hip flexors.

Table 8.2 American Spinal Injuries Association (ASIA) scoring for patient A on admission

	On admission	
Key ASIA muscle	Left	Right
C5 – Elbow flexors	1	0
C6 – Wrist extensors	0	0
C7 – Elbow extensors	1	0
C8 – Finger flexors	0	0
T1 – Finger abductors	0	0
L2 – Hip flexors	0	0
L3 – Knee extensors	1	1
L4 – Ankle dorsiflexors	0	0
L5 – Long toe extensors	0	0
S1 – Ankle plantarflexors	1	1

Goal-setting
Goals were set on a 2-weekly basis in a multidisciplinary meeting and were agreed by both patient and staff.

Treatment aims

- to facilitate selective movement of the pelvis
- to improve weight-bearing over an extended right hip and leg
- progress left single-leg stance to produce selectivity in swing phase of right lower-limb, in preparation for gait
- to address soft-tissue tightness of the trunk and lower-limbs
- lengthen left hip flexors by use of reciprocal inhibition, by facilitation of active extension patterns
- recruit stability around the shoulder girdle
- facilitate selectivity of the right rotator cuff, serratus anterior and lower fibres of trapezius.

Treatment progression

- initial treatment – gaining trunk control and selective upper- and lower-limb movements in lying and sitting. Achieved through facilitation of lateral pelvic tilt to left and rotation of trunk to the left and right, with facilitation of anterior pelvic tilt
- hamstring overactivity was treated with specific inhibitory mobilisations in supine and side-lying
- upper-limb activity was facilitated through propping with trunk rotation, as well as reaching activities
- progressed to prone standing (forward leaning standing, with knees extended but trunk flexed forward and supported on a high plinth), standing and step standing. Standing treatment was aimed at soleus and gasrocnemius lengthening in preparation for stepping. Progressed into facilitation of swing-through by working on release of pelvis with knee flexion and toe-off
- improved to walk with a posture walker to promote trunk extension and then on to elbow crutches
- shoulder girdle stability: in four-point kneeling (Fig. 8.8), propped sitting and forwards lean-sitting. FES, biofeedback and strapping were used in conjunction with this to obtain selective scapular setting. His upper-limb tone responded well to a course of acupuncture to his right upper-limb. His hand function was tapped into with specific mobilisations, lumbrical activity facilitation and lengthening
- late-stage rehabilitation consisted of balance work in single-leg stance (Fig. 8.9), trampette, wobble board, gym ball with hands-on facilitation at pelvis and hips to encourage righting and equilibrium reactions.

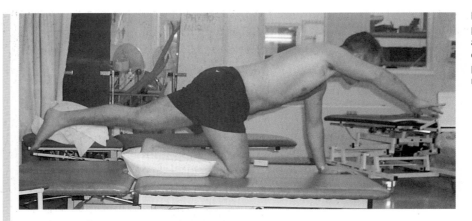

Figure 8.8 Patient A: four-point kneeling progressed to alternate arm and leg lift, to challenge shoulder and pelvic girdle stability, whilst maintaining a stable trunk.

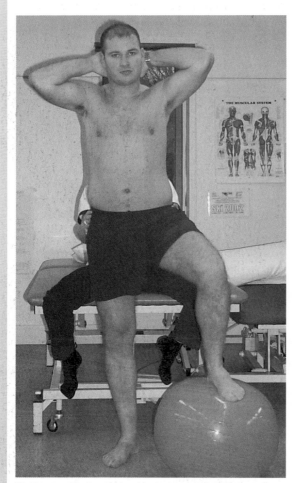

Figure 8.9 Patient A: late-stage progression of single-leg dynamic balance; placing the upper-limbs out of the way to reduce fixing the trunk and stabilising, in order selectively to lift the left leg.

Summary
On discharge, 7 months after injury, the patient:

- mobilised independently with elbow crutches
- was independent on stairs, slopes, rough ground and walking outside
- mobilised for short distances indoors without crutches
- continued to have problems with increased tone throughout, especially on exertion, as a compromise for weakness
- still had poor upper-limb control, with limited dexterity of hands and poor shoulder-girdle control
- was independent in all areas of daily living except for buttons.

Patient B

C6 incomplete spinal cord injury
Patient sustained a C5–C6 fracture dislocation following a road traffic accident.

- male, aged 17 years
- surgical management with anterior stabilisation of C5–C7
- managed in a Philadelphia collar for 4 weeks following surgery
- transferred to a specialist spinal injuries unit 2 months postinjury. Motor and sensory function were assessed on admission using the ASIA scale (Table 8.3)
- managed on bed rest for 3 months following transfer due to sacral pressure sores.

Main problems
Once attending the gym, a full neurological and functional assessment identified the following main problems:

1. ↓ selectivity of movement of pelvis
2. ↓ activity in abdominal muscles

Table 8.3 American Spinal Injuries Association (ASIA) scoring for patient B on admission and discharge

Key ASIA muscle	On admission		On discharge	
	Left	Right	Left	Right
C5 – Elbow flexors	4	3	4	4
C6 – Wrist extensors	3	3	4	3
C7 – Elbow extensors	1	0	2	1
C8 – Finger flexors	1	0	0	0
T1 – Finger abductors	0	0	1	1
L2 – Hip flexors	2	0	4	2
L3 – Knee extensors	2	0	4	4
L4 – Ankle dorsiflexors	2	0	4	2
L5 – Long toe extensors	2	0	5	2
S1 – Ankle plantarflexors	1	0	5	4

3. ↓ selective extensor activity throughout trunk and lower-limbs
4. overactivity of lumbar extensors in standing → anterior pelvic tilt + +
5. shortening of hip flexors right > left
6. positive support reaction of the right lower-limb
7. associated reaction of right upper-limb into internal rotation and depression on effort → stereotypical patterning – exaggerated by use of manual wheelchair and use of upper-limbs for function, i.e. transfers
8. ↓ selectivity of cervical spine movement/ overactivity of upper cervical extensors
9. overactivity of pectoral muscles and latissimus dorsi → instability shoulder girdles right > left
10. ineffective tenodesis grip.

Goal-setting

Goals were agreed with the patient at weekly multidisciplinary goal-planning sessions, which focused on gaining maximal functional independence with minimal compromise of normal movement. His main goal was to walk independently with elbow crutches.

Treatment aims

- facilitate graded selective pelvic movement
- facilitate graded selective extension of trunk
- facilitate activity of abdominal muscles
- facilitate stability around shoulder girdles and reduce overactivity of pectoral muscles, upper fibres of trapezius and latissimus dorsi
- facilitate extensor activity in lower-limbs
- re-education of selective trunk activity to facilitate
- reciprocal inhibition and normalise tone, giving a background for selective movement

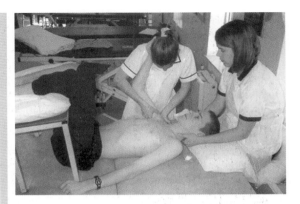

Figure 8.10 Patient B: facilitation of normal alignment of the shoulder girdle, via facilitation of eccentric lengthening of the pectoral and latissimus dorsi muscles. Stability and feedback are provided by the second physiotherapist.

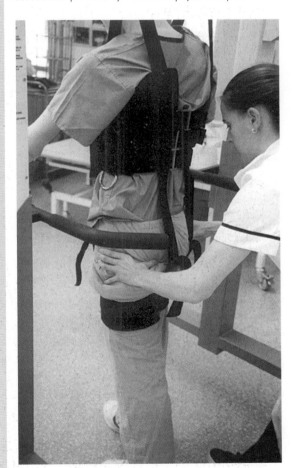

Figure 8.11 Patient B: gait re-education using a body support harness system. This mobile gantry allows the patient to walk freely with the trunk and weight supported, and facilitation is provided by the physiotherapist.

Treatment progression
Treatment included the following:

- using an electric wheelchair to reduce habitual use of associated reactions around right shoulder and reinforcement of malalignment when self-propelling
- facilitation of cervical selective movement in both sitting and supine to enable the patient to dissociate neck from trunk, including the use of specific soft-tissue mobilisation to encourage lengthening of shortened muscles (Fig. 8.10)
- facilitation of activity around pelvis in sitting, kneeling, prone standing and standing to increase antigravity extensor activity in trunk and lower-limbs
- facilitation of normal alignment of shoulder girdles in supine, sitting and standing, via facilitation of eccentric lengthening of pectoral muscles and latissimus dorsi, taping techniques; specific strengthening and muscle imbalance work; and biofeedback
- re-education of sit to stand from a variety of surfaces with facilitation
- work in kneeling, standing and one-leg stance to challenge balance, righting reactions and equilibrium reactions and facilitate reciprocal innervation

- gait re-education including use of body weight support and treadmill system (Fig. 8.11)
- progression of gait from rollator frame to elbow crutches
- FES for functional strengthening of hands, alongside specific soft-tissue mobilisations.

Summary
On discharge home after 10 months the patient was:

- mobilising with elbow crutches inside and outside
- able to climb a small step
- independent in all activities of daily living
- re-charted using the ASIA scale on discharge, which showed significant improvement (see Table 8.3). Other outcome measures used throughout rehabilitation included the Berg Balance Scale (see Ch. 3, p. 35), photography and video
- continuing outpatient physiotherapy to optimise functional gains in the home environment.

ACKNOWLEDGEMENTS

The authors would like to acknowledge the contributions by Miss E Roberts and Mrs S Bulpitt, Senior Physiotherapists at Royal National Orthopaedic Hospital, Stanmore, for providing the case histories.

References

Abel R, Schablowski M, Rupp R, Gemer HJ. Gait analysis on the treadmill – monitoring exercise in the treatment of paraplegia. *Spinal Cord* 2002, **40**:17–22.

American Spinal Injuries Association (ASIA). *International Standards for Neurological and Functional Classification of Spinal Cord Injury*. Chicago: ASIA; 1992.

Ballinger DA, Rintala DH, Hart KA. The relation of shoulder pain and range of motion problems to functional limitations, disability and perceived health of men with spinal cord injury: a multifaceted longitudinal study. *Arch Phys Med Rehab* 2000, **81**:1575–1581.

Barbenel JC, Forbes CD, Lowe GDO. *Pressure Sores*. London: Macmillan Press; 1983.

Barnes M, Bhakta B, Moore P et al. *The Management of Adults with Spasticity using Botulinum Toxin. A Guide to Clinical Practice*. Byfleet: Harvard Health; 2001.

Bohannon RW, Larkin PA. Passive ankle dorsiflexion increases in patients after a regime of tilt table-wedge board standing. A clinical report. *Phys Ther* 1985, **65**:1676–1678.

Bohannon RW, Smith MB. Interrater reliability of a modified Ashworth scale of muscle spasticity. *Phys Ther* 1987, **67**:206–207.

Bradley M. The effects of participating in a functional electrical stimulation exercise programme on affect in people with FES. *Arch Phys Med Rehab* 1994, **75**: 676–679.

Brindley GS. The fertility of men with spinal injury. *Paraplegia* 1984, **22**:337–348.

Bromley I. *Tetraplegia and Paraplegia*, 5th edn. London: Churchill Livingstone; 1998.

Brown P. Pathophysiology of spasticity. *J Neurol Neurosurg Psychiatry* 1994, **57**:773–777.

Brown RL, Brunn MA, Garcia VF. Cervical spine injuries in children: a review of 103 patients treated consecutively at a level 1 pediatric trauma center. *J Pediatr Surg* 2001, **36**:1107–1114.

Buchanan LE, Nawoezenski DA. *Spinal Cord Injury Concepts and Management Approaches*. London: Williams & Wilkins; 1987.

Burns AS, Ditunno JF. Establishing prognosis and maximizing functional outcomes after spinal cord injury. *Spine* 2001, **26**:S137–S145.

Chae J, Kilgore K, Triolo R et al. Functional neuromuscular stimulation in spinal cord injury. *Phys Med Rehab Clin North Am* 2000, **11**:209–226.

Chartered Society of Physiotherapy (CSP). *Standards of Physiotherapy Practice for People with Spinal Cord Lesions*. London: CSP; 1997.

Crozier KS, Groziani V, Ditunno JF et al. Spinal cord injury, prognosis for ambulation based on sensory examination in patients who are initially motor complete. *Arch Phys Med Rehab* 1991, **72**:119–121.

Collins W. Surgery in the acute treatment of spinal cord injury: a review of the past forty years. *J Spinal Cord Med* 1995, **18**:3–8.

Curtis KA, Tyner TM, Zachary L et al. Effect of a standard exercise protocol on shoulder pain in long term wheelchair users. *Spinal Cord* 1999, **37**:421–429.

David O, Sett P, Burr RG et al. The relationship of heterotopic ossification to passive movements in paraplegic patients. *Disabil Rehab* 1993, **15**:114–118.

Dennis F. Three column spine and its significance in the classification of acute thoracolumbar spinal injuries. *Spine* 1983, **8**:817–831.

Ditunno JF, Young W, Donovan WH. The International Standards booklet for neurological and functional classification of spinal cord injury. *Paraplegia* 1994, **32**:70–80.

Ditunno JF, Ditunno PL, Graziani V et al. Walking index for spinal cord injury (WISCI). An international multi centre validity and reliability study, *Spinal Cord* 2000, **38**:234–243. Revision: (WISCI II) *Spinal Cord* 2001, **39**:654–656.

Duysens J, Van de Crommert HWAA. Neural control of locomotion: Part 1: The central pattern generator from cats to humans. *Gait Posture* 1998:131–141.

Flett PJ. Review article. The rehabilitation of children with spinal cord injury. *J Paediatr Child Care* 1992, **28**:141–146.

Foo D. Spinal cord injury in forty four patients with cervical spondylosis. *Paraplegia* 1986, **24**:301–306.

Fowler CJ, Fowler CG. Neurogenic bladder dysfunction and its management. In: Greenwood R, Barnes MP, McMillian TM et al., eds. *Neurological Rehabilitation*. London: Churchill Livingstone; 1993:269–277.

Gardner BP, Theocleous F, Krishnan KR. Outcome following acute spinal cord injury: a review of 198 patients. *Paraplegia* 1988, **26**:94–98.

Goemaere S, Van Laere M, De Nerve P et al. Bone mineral status in paralegics patients who do not perform standing. *Osteoporosis Int* 1994, **4**:138–143.

Golding JS. The mechanical factors which influence bone growth. *Eur J Clin Nutr* 1994, 48 (Suppl 1): S178–S185.

Grill WM, McDonald JW, Peckham PH et al. At the interface: convergence of neural regeneration and neuroprostheses for restoration of function. *J Rehab Res Dev* 2001, **38**:633–639.

Grillner S, Wallen P. Central pattern generators for locomotion, with special reference to vertebrates. *Annu Rev Neurosci* 1985, **8**:233–261.

Grundy D, Swain A. *ABC of Spinal Cord Injury*, 4th edn. London: British Medical Journal Publications; 2002.

Hamilton BB, Granger CV. *A Rehabilitation Uniform Data System*. New York: Buffalo Publications; 1991.

Harrison P. *The First 48 Hours*. London: Spinal Injuries Association; 2000.

Hough A. *Physiotherapy in Respiratory Care: An Evidence Based Approach to Respiratory Management and Cardiac Conditions*, 3rd edn. Cheltenham: Nelson Thornes; 2001.

Illis LS. *Spinal Cord Dysfunction Assessment*. Oxford: Oxford University Press; 1988.

Jacobs PL, Nash MS. Modes, benefits and risks of voluntary and electrically induced exercise in persons with spinal cord injury. *J Spinal Cord Med* 2001, **24**:10–18.

Johnston L. Human spinal cord injury: new and emerging approaches to treatment. *Spinal Cord* 2001, **39**:609–613.

Katoh S, El Masry WS. Motor recovery of patients presenting with motor paralysis and sensory sparing following cervical spinal cord injury. *Paraplegia* 1995, **33**:506–509.

Linder SH. Functional electrical stimulation to enhance cough in spinal cord injury. *Chest* 1993, **103**:166–169.

Little JW, Habur E. Temporal course of motor recovery after Brown Séquard spinal cord injury. *Paraplegia* 1985, **23**:39–46.

Maynard FM, Reynolds GG, Fountain S et al. Neurological prognosis after traumatic quadraplegia, three years experience of California Regional Spinal Cord Injury Care System. *J Neurosurg* 1979, **50**:611–616.

Moore EE, Mattox KL, Feliciano DV. *Trauma*, 2nd edn. Connecticut: Appleton & Lange; 1991.

Osenback RK, Menezes AM. Paediatric spinal cord and vertebral column injury. *Neurosurgery* 1992, **30**:385–390.

Pope PM. Postural management and special seating. In: Edwards S, ed. *Neurological Physiotherapy: A Problem Solving Approach*, 2nd edn. London: Churchill Livingstone; 2002:189–217.

Poynton AR, O'Farrel DA, Shannon F et al. Sparing of sensation to pinprick predicts motor recovery of a motor segment after injury to the spinal cord. *J Bone Joint Surg Br* 1997, **79**:952–954.

Priebe MM, Sherwood AM, Thornby JI et al. Clinical assessment of spasticity in spinal cord injury: a multidimensional problem. *Arch Phys Med Rehab* 1996, **77**:713–716.

Prochazka A, Stephens JA, Wand P. Muscle spindle discharge in normal and obstructed movements. *J Physiol* 1979, **287**:57–66.

Pryor JA, Webber BA. *Physiotherapy for Respiratory and Cardiac Problems*, 2nd edn. Edinburgh: Churchill Livingstone; 1998.

Ramer MS, Harper GP, Bradbury EJ. Progress in spinal cord research. A refined strategy for the International Spinal Research Trust. *Spinal Cord* 2000, **38**:449–472.

Reddy H, Floyer A, Donaghy M et al. Altered cortical activation with finger movements after peripheral denervation: comparison of active and passive tasks. *Exp Brain Res* 2001, **138**(4):484–491.

Riggs BL, Melton LJ III. *Osteoporosis: Etiology, Diagnosis and Management*. Philadelphia: Lippincott–Raven; 1995.

Scott JA, Donovan WH. The prevention of shoulder pain and contracture in the acute tetraplegia patient. *Paraplegia* 1981, **19**:313–319.

Sheean G. (ed.) *Spasticity Rehabilitation*. London: Churchill Communications Europe; 1998.

Short DJ, Frankel HL, Bergström EMK. *Injuries of the Spinal Cord in Children*. London: Elsevier Science; 1992.

Smith M, Ball V. *Cardiovascular/Respiratory Physiotherapy*. London: Mosby; 1998.

Spinal Injuries Association (SIA). *Moving Forward 3*. London: SIA; 2002.

Stauffer ES. Rehabilitation of posttraumatic cervical spinal cord quadraplegia and pentaplegia. In: *The Cervical Spine*. Philadelphia: Lippincott; 1983.

Tator CH. Biology of neurological recovery and functional restoration after spinal cord injury. *Neurosurgery* 1998, **42**:696–707.

Waring WP, Maynard FM. Shoulder pain in acute traumatic quadraplegia. *Paraplegia* 1991, **29**:37–42.

Waters RL, Adkins RH, Yakura JS et al. Motor and sensory recovery following incomplete paraplegia. *Arch Phys Med Rehab* 1994a, **75**:67–72.

Waters RL, Adkins RH, Yakura JS et al. Motor and sensory recovery following incomplete tetraplegia. *Arch Phys Med Rehab* 1994b, **75**:306–311.

Whalley Hammell K. *Spinal Cord Injury Rehabilitation*. Canada: Chapman & Hall; 1995.

Whiteneck GG, Charlifue SW, Gerhart KA et al. Quantifying handicap: a new measure of long-term rehabilitation outcomes. *Arch Phys Med Rehab* 1992, **73**:519–526.

Williams P. *Gray's anatomy*, 38th edn. Edinburgh: Churchill Livingstone; 1995.

World Health Organization. *International Classification of Functioning, Disability and Health*. 2001. Geneva: World Health Organization. Available online at: http://www.who.int/classification/icf.

Young RR, Shahani BT. Spasticity in spinal cord injured patients. In: Block RF, Basbaum M, eds. *Management of Spinal Cord Injuries*. Baltimore: Williams & Wilkins; 1986:241–283.

Zejdlik CP. *Management of Spinal Cord Injury*, 2nd edn. Boston: Jones & Bartlett; 1992.

Chapter 9

Peripheral nerve injuries

A Jaggi   R Birch   L Dean   K Johnson   S Tripp

CHAPTER CONTENTS

INTRODUCTION

The nervous system is the mechanism through which the organism is kept in touch with its internal structures and external environments, and reacts to changes in them. The peripheral nervous system connects the brain and the spinal cord to the periphery and it includes the cranial nerves, the spinal nerves, the peripheral nerves and the peripheral extension of the autonomic nervous system (Brown, 1991; Shepherd, 1994; Williams, 1995). Within peripheral nerves are motor fibres to skeletal muscle; sensory or afferent fibres from skin, muscle, tendon and joint; and autonomic fibres to the blood vessels, sweat glands and muscles controlling hair. The concentration of functional capacity is great, so that severance of an adult's arm, for example of a median nerve, perhaps 5 mm in diameter, effectively ruins the function of the hand and the forearm.

The consequence of injury to a peripheral nerve may include: loss of sensation with risk of damage to skin and joint; paralysis leading to atrophy, not only of muscle but also of skin and, in the neglected case, to fixed deformity. A particularly severe consequence of injury to a peripheral nerve is pain.

Historical background

Pioneering work by Robert Jones with the wounded during World War I resulted in principles of treating peripheral nerve injuries being established. Jones' fundamental principle was continuity of treatment. He said: 'the treatment of those cases in the early part of the war was deplorable. I heard frequently "we cannot follow up our cases". During the first twelve months of war no provision of any sort was made for cases crippled and deformed and this became a focus of seething discontent' (Jones, 1917). Robert Jones founded the great military hospital at Shepherd's Bush and it existed to provide cohesion between compartments of treatment. At its zenith, in 1916, there were 800 patients at Shepherd's Bush, 500 of whom were employed in regular physical work and, as he said, 'the difference in the atmosphere and morale in hospitals where patients have nothing to do but smoke, play cards or be entertained from that found in those where, for part of the day, they have regular useful and productive work, is striking'. By 1917 this principle of structured rehabilitation had been extended to 14 other centres (Jones, 1921).

Robert Jones' work from the First World War was extended in the Second World War, when the Medical Research Council set up specialist hospitals and units to treat service men and women with injuries to nerves. The Peripheral Nerve Injury Unit at the Royal National Orthopaedic Hospital (RNOH) was one of these and the Rehabilitation Unit was established there 40 years ago. This chapter draws on the experience of the RNOH and outlines the work of the multidisciplinary team (MDT), in particular in the treatment of brachial plexus injuries in adults and in children. There is a lack of literature and research on this subject but comprehensive references include Wynn Parry's book of 1981, Wynn Parry et al. (1987) and Barsby (1998).

SOME ANATOMICAL AND FUNCTIONAL FEATURES

Peripheral nerves

The peripheral nerves consist of bundles or fascicles of nerve fibres embedded in connective tissue and a rich longitudinally oriented network of blood vessels. The axons are cytoplasmic extensions of cells lying within the dorsal root ganglia, the autonomic ganglia or the spinal cord itself. Axons are enveloped by satellite Schwann cells. This composite structure of the axon and a sheath of Schwann cells is the nerve fibre. The axons range in diameter from <1 to 20 μm. The smallest axons, surrounded by columns of Schwann cell processes, are the non-myelinated nerve fibres and are the most common. Larger axons are surrounded by a sheath of myelin, a lamellar condensation of the Schwann cell cytoplasm and are hence termed myelinated nerve fibres. The characteristics of nerve fibres and the transmission of neural impulses are described in physiology textbooks, e.g. by Brown (1991) and Shepherd (1994).

The connective tissues

Numbers of nerve fibres are surrounded by the endoneurium, a tightly packed tissue containing collagen, fibroblasts and capillary blood vessels. Surrounding these clusters of nerve fibres is an envelope termed the perineurium, a sheath of flattened cells. This is the most discrete of the connective tissue envelopes of a peripheral nerve. The perineurium together with its contents is called a fascicle or bundle. Numbers of fascicles are grouped together by the epineurium, a condensation of areolar connective tissue. There is a rich network of blood vessels within this tissue, which forms the greater part of the cross-sectional area of a peripheral nerve. One of the functions of the epineurium is to protect nerve fibres from pressure and its smooth glistening structure permits gliding of the nerve across joints. Scarring or entrapment inhibits nerve gliding by tethering of the epineurium and this is a common source of pain and disturbance of function. Physiotherapists commonly encounter examples of this, such as entrapment of spinal nerves by an osteophyte encroaching within the intervertebral foramen.

CAUSES AND INCIDENCE OF NERVE INJURIES

The causes of peripheral nerve injuries are summarised in Table 9.1. Most open wounds, in civilian practice, are caused by sharp objects such as knives or glass, and in the majority of these early repair of the nerve is preferred. Injury to a nerve from a missile or from an open fracture is much more severe. Closed traction injury is usually the result of a high-energy injury and the patient may have suffered multiple and even life-threatening injuries. The main cause is road traffic accidents, typically in young motor cyclists who sustain a brachial plexus injury (Rosson, 1987). Another type of brachial plexus damage is irradiation neuritis (IN), a condition caused by radiotherapy for cancer of the neck and axilla (Birch, 1993). Birth injuries occur, leading to a condition termed obstetric brachial plexus palsy (OBPP). The incidence of brachial plexus injuries in the UK is reported to be 1000 cases per year (Birch, 1993); over 500 cases are closed traction injuries, and there are about 200 cases of IN and at least 100 cases of OBPP.

Tables 9.2 and 9.3 set out the numbers of patients treated at the RNOH over a 25-year period. Nerve injuries in the upper limb greatly exceed those in the lower limb. There is a high incidence of damage to the adjacent axial artery. The most serious cases, of complete injury to the brachial and to the lumbosacral plexus, were usually caused by high-energy transfer closed traction lesions, and most of these followed high-energy transfer road traffic accidents. In these cases potentially life-threatening injuries to head, chest, spine or viscera occurred in about 10% of patients; fractures of long bones were seen in over 30% of cases. The treatment and rehabilitation of such cases are of particular concern.

Table 9.1 Causes of peripheral nerve injuries

Lesion	Characteristic	Agent
Open	Tidy	Knife, glass or scalpel
	Untidy	Missile, burn, open fracture–dislocation
Closed	Compression–ischaemia	Pressure neuropathy in the anaesthetised patient
		Compartment syndrome
	Traction–ischaemia	Fracture–dislocation
	Thermal	Acrylic cement, electrical burn
	Irradiation	Irradiation neuritis
	Injection	Regional anaesthetic block, intravenous or intra–arterial catheterisation

Table 9.2 Repairs of major (mixed) peripheral nerves in adults and children at the Royal National Orthopaedic Hospital 1979–2001

Nerve repaired	No. of cases
Upper limb	
Spinal accessory	98
Nerve to serratus anterior (excluding brachial plexus injuries)	22
Circumflex nerve	148
Suprascapular nerve	48
Musculocutaneous nerve	160
Radial nerve	285
Median and ulnar nerves in infraclavicular brachial plexus	65
Median and ulnar nerves in axilla or arm	165
Median and ulnar nerves in forearm and wrist	282
Total	1253
Lower limb	
Lumbosacral plexus	11
Common peroneal division of sciatic nerve or common peroneal nerve	94
Tibial division of sciatic nerve or posterior tibial nerve	65
Femoral nerve	13
Total	183

Table 9.3 Operations for injuries of the brachial plexus, showing incidence of open and vascular injuries in adults and children treated at the Royal National Orthopaedic Hospital 1976–2001

Injury	Total	Vascular
Supraclavicular	1360	142
Infraclavicular	510	108
Penetrating missile injury	63	31
Stab or knife, including iatropathic	121	24
Postirradiation neuropathy	54	2
Total	2308	307

CLINICAL PRESENTATION AND GENERAL MANAGEMENT

The cause and severity of damage will determine the type of injury, which can be classified as described below. Various nerves which are commonly injured are also outlined below. The principles of management apply to all nerves, although the brachial plexus is generally used as an example in the following sections.

Classification of nerve injuries

The most clinically useful classification of nerve injuries is that described by Seddon (1975) and is based on the behaviour of the axon after different types of injury (Table 9.4). In neurapraxia, a conduction block, there is no interruption of the axon and the architecture of the nerve is more or less undisturbed. It is relatively uncommon in clinical practice and most cases rapidly recover if the cause has been removed. In axonotmesis and neurotmesis, the axon is cut across. The distal part undergoes a process called Wallerian degeneration in which the axoplasm fragments and disappears and myelin gradually disintegrates (Lundborg, 1993). In axonotmesis, the connective tissues of the nerve are more or less intact and there is a high chance of spontaneous recovery. For details on the process of neural regeneration, see Mitchell & Osterman (1991). In neurotmesis the whole nerve trunk is cut and there is separation of the stumps. Spontaneous recovery does not occur in humans, and surgical repair is necessary.

Neurapraxia is characterised by absence of pain, preservation of sweating and normal vasomotor tone in the extremities, preservation of some modalities of sensation such as deep pressure sense, and by rapid recovery. In the degenerative lesions, axonotmesis and neurotmesis, there is complete loss of all nerve function distal to the level of the injury. The distinction

Table 9.4 Classification of nerve injuries

Seddon (1975)	Sunderland	Functional loss	Anatomical lesion	Neurophysiological
Neurapraxia (non-degenerative)	Grade I	Muscle power, gnosis	Axon and nerve fibre sheath intact	Distal conduction maintained – no fibrillation
Axonotmesis (degenerative)	Grade II, III	All modalities	Interruption of axon and distal Wallerian degeneration	Conduction lost; fibrillation
Neurotmesis (degenerative)	Grade IV, V	All modalities	Interruption of the nerve trunk; Wallerian degeneration	Conduction lost; fibrillation

between these two lesions can be made only by waiting for recovery, which may not occur, or by surgical exploration of the injured nerves (Seddon, 1975).

Common sites of peripheral nerve injury

Injury to the brachial plexus is the most severe of upper-limb nerve injuries since it affects the innervation to the whole limb. The reader should refer to an anatomy text for a reminder of the structure of the brachial plexus (e.g. Williams, 1995). Briefly, the plexus is formed by the anterior branches of the fifth to eighth cervical nerves and the first thoracic nerve. It extends from the lower lateral aspect of the neck to the axilla and then divides into numerous branches to form the nerves of the upper limb.

The axillary nerve may be injured in association with fractures of the neck of the humerus and shoulder dislocation. Injuries to the ulnar and median nerves commonly occur at the wrist, as a result of putting a hand through a window, or from elbow injuries. The ulnar nerve can also be damaged in fractures of the medial epicondyle of the humerus. The median nerve can become damaged in carpal tunnel syndrome.

The radial nerve is most often damaged in fractures of the humerus, at the point where it wraps around the humerus. It is also damaged in the axilla by pressure from axillary crutches or by the arm being left hanging over the edge of a chair for a long period (i.e. 'Saturday-night palsy', when a person falls asleep after drinking alcohol).

In the lower limb, common nerve injuries include: the sciatic nerve, from pelvic and thigh wounds or dislocation of the hip; the common peroneal nerve, from fractures of the neck of the fibula or pressure from a plaster cast; and the posterior tibial nerve, from supracondylar fractures of the femur. Many of these occur in sporting injuries (Lorei & Hershman, 1993).

Diagnosis, signs and symptoms

A reasonable knowledge of anatomy contributes to accurate diagnosis in most clinical situations and the Medical Research Council (MRC) *Atlas* (MRC, 1982) is an invaluable aid. The motor and sensory loss which occurs with specific nerve injuries will not be discussed in detail here.

Muscle function and sensation

The extent of paralysis is described using the MRC system for measuring muscle strength (see Ch. 3, p. 33). One deficiency of the MRC system is that it does not record endurance and stamina, which is a significant defect when one is choosing muscles for transfer or when assessing a patient's ability to do certain types of work. Recording loss of sensation is best achieved by the examiner working with the patient; the complete area of anaesthesia is marked out by a skin marker pen and then, using a different colour, the surrounding area of impaired sensation is similarly marked. The sensory loss can be recorded by a standard chart, photographed or both.

Differential diagnosis

There are three features which enable the examiner to distinguish between neurapraxia and the degenerative lesions of axonotmesis and neurotmesis. The first of these is sympathetic paralysis. The sympathetic fibres controlling sweating and the tone of the smooth muscles within the skin blood vessels pass with the trunk nerves of the limbs. The median, ulnar and tibial nerves are richly endowed with such nerve fibres and they pass into the nerves of cutaneous sensation in the hand and foot. Loss of sweating and vasomotor tone after wounding of a nerve is indicative of a degenerative lesion. A diagnosis of neurapraxia cannot be made in the face of this evidence.

Neuropathic pain states

Neuropathic pain is caused by a lesion of the nervous system, usually of the peripheral nerves. Some neuropathic pain states are exceptionally severe and the different types have been reviewed by Birch (1993). They are characterised by: persistence, intractability; disproportion between the extent of lesion and the severity of the pain; and by the fact that it is no longer necessary for the survival of the organism. There is associated sensory or motor disturbance and often sympathetic dysfunction. The positive sensory symptoms described by patients are sometimes so clear that diagnosis of cause and some understanding of the subsequent pathophysiological events are possible from the history alone.

In the present authors' opinion, the vogue for measuring pain by visual analogue scales is to be deprecated for neuropathic pain; it offers a spurious sense of objectivity. Explanations of neuropathic pain which predicate a structural change within the central nervous system do not account for the instantaneous onset of pain in most cases of causalgia, nor in the frequent instances of central pain in many cases of brachial plexus lesion.

Growing dissatisfaction with the concept of the role of the sympathetic nervous system in maintaining many neuropathic pain states (such as reflex sympathetic dystrophy (RSD)) led to proposals for a new classification of pain states adopted by the International Association for the Study of Pain.

There is some debate as to the relevance of this classification to the analysis of the different states of pain that may follow injury to the peripheral nerves. For example, it appears inappropriate to: abandon the term causalgia, since the characteristics are so clear; discard all the evidence demonstrating the role of the sympathetic nerves on mechanoreceptors, damaged or regenerating nerve fibres, or their parent neurones; or discard the evidence concerning the role of visceral afferents (Birch et al., 1998). Furthermore, success has followed the application of the principles underlying the pain gate theory in the treatment of peripheral nerve lesions (Melzack & Wall, 1965; Wall, 1978).

The RNOH has classed pain after nerve injury as follows (Birch et al., 1998, pp 373–404):

1. Causalgia (complex regional pain syndrome; CRPS type 2)
2. RSD (CRPS type 1)
3. Posttraumatic neuralgia, which can be divided between that following major injury to a major trunk nerve and that following injury to a nerve of cutaneous sensation

4. Pain due to persistent compression, distortion or ischaemia. This pain is termed neurostenalgia (Wall & Melzack, 1996).
5. Central pain. This can be divided between that following rupture of spinal nerves at the level of the transitional zone leading to pure deafferentation and that following avulsion of roots of the plexus from the spinal cord itself, a lesion which is in truth an injury to the central nervous system (Schenker & Birch, 2001).
6. Pain maintained either deliberately or subconsciously by a patient in response to a challenge, such as a wish to obtain compensation or resentment against a public body such as insurance company or other provocation.

Causalgia   Causalgia is one of the most clearly defined of neuropathic pain states and diagnosis can be made from the history alone. There has been a wound to the proximal part of the limb, there has been partial damage to major nerve trunks. Pain is intense, spontaneous, persistent and often of a burning nature. Whilst localised principally in the distribution of the nerve or nerves affected, pain spreads beyond that distribution and is particularly aggravated by physical and emotional stimuli.

The skin is hypersensitive, to the extent that patients cannot tolerate light touch. Intense allodynia is seen, in which normal sensations are perceived as painful ones. Hyperpathia is a severe example of abnormal pain following nerve injury. There is also disturbance of circulation and sweating. Sympathetic blockade is valuable both in diagnosis and in treatment, and the core of treatment is operative, directed towards diagnosis and rectification of the prime cause of the injured nerves and vessels. Causalgia can occur rarely in children. Stewart & Birch (2001) described 58 consecutive patients treated for penetrating missile injuries of the brachial plexus. Thirty-three of these patients presented with severe pain, 10 with causalgia. Most of these cases displayed arterial rupture, false aneurysm or arteriovenous fistula. Significant and lasting relief of pain followed repair of nerve and vascular lesions in 31 of the 33 patients.

Reflex sympathetic dystrophy   The syndrome of RSD (CRPS type 1) has been ascribed various terms, including Sudeck's atrophy, causalgia, shoulder–hand syndrome and algoneurodystrophy (van Laere & Claessens, 1992; Veldman et al., 1993). Its cause and pathogenesis are poorly understood but it is often associated with fractures or crush injuries of the wrist and hand or foot. The syndrome also presents after injuries or operations at the shoulder, elbow and knee. There is usually an injury in which no major nerve trunk is damaged but this is followed by spontaneous pain that spreads.

Characteristic symptoms are inflammation (oedema, which increases after exercise), pain, limited range of movement, vasomotor and pseudomotor instability, sweating, allodynia, trophic skin changes and discoloration and patchy bone demineralisation. Later, there are changes in the nails and hair, and stiffness of the joints.

The initial stages are characteristic. The pain is diffuse and disturbs sleep; the hand is swollen and stiff; it is often wet and warm but it may be cold and blue. If untreated, fibrosis follows and the part becomes a dysfunctional, stiff appendage.

Most cases in orthopaedic practice can and should be prevented by early treatment, and this calls for alertness in detection of the early stages of the syndrome. It is an error to label every painful, stiff and swollen hand or foot presenting in a fracture clinic as RSD, so consigning that patient to a pain clinic. More often these are examples of inadequate primary treatment. In most early cases, the cause will be found by those who look: a splint or bandage which is too tight; a limb improperly supported in a sling; a patient who is too frightened to keep the part elevated and functioning. Those treating this disorder must be alert for an underlying lesion of compression or irritation of a nerve trunk, either from swelling or a displaced bone fragment.

The mainstay of treatment is use of the part. Making such a diagnosis of 'RSD' or 'CRPS type 1' is highly questionable. Again it is emphasised that no patient should be sent to a pain clinic unless and until a diagnosis has been made.

Neurostenalgia This is, with causalgia, the most rewarding neuropathic pain state to treat by operation. Chronic compression, distortion or chronic ischaemia of the nerve will produce pain but in most cases the nerve trunk is intact. The lesion is one of conduction block (neurapraxia) or, if it is degenerative, it is a lesion of potentially favourable prognosis (axonotmesis). The nerve is in some way irritated, tethered, compressed or ischaemic and treatment of the cause relieves the pain. Neurostenalgia is frequently seen in children where the nerves are trapped in fractures or in dislocations, or are compressed in the swollen ischaemic limb.

Central pain in brachial plexus injury Frazier & Skillern (1911) set out the description of pain given them by their patient, a physician, who had sustained a closed traction lesion of the brachial plexus: 'the pain is continuous, it does not stop a minute, either by day or night. It is either burning or compressing ... in addition,

there is, every few minutes, a jerking sensation similar to that obtained by touching ... a Leyden jar. It is like a zig-zag made in the sky by a stroke of lightning. The upper part of the arm is mostly free of pain; the lower part, from a little above the elbow to the tips of the fingers, never'.

It is all here. The pain is severe, it has two components, one constant, the other intermittent and it is worst in the hand and forearm. Frazier & Skillern's (1911) patient described how his pain developed within hours of his injury, a fact stated to us by about one-half of our patients with severe closed traction lesion. Although recent published work does show that reinnervation of the limb and the restoration of muscular function go some way to mitigating pain (Berman et al., 1996, 1998), none the less distraction, by engagement in the normal activities of life, is by far the most effective measure in relief of pain (Wynn Parry et al., 1987). Potentially, the most effective drug is cannabis but the results of controlled clinical trials have yet to be released (e.g. work led by Dr J Berman at the RNOH, by personal communication, with permission). This at times terrible pain is the greatest challenge for those of us working with a sufferer towards rehabilitation. Assisting their re-entry into work and normal life is the central purpose of a rehabilitation unit. It is a remarkable fact that this central pain is not seen in children who have suffered the most severe lesions in obstetrical brachial plexus palsy (Anand & Birch, 2002).

Special investigations

Neurophysiological investigations, measuring nerve action potentials and detecting the response of muscle to the insertion of concentric needles, distinguish between conduction block (neurapraxia) and the degenerative lesions axonotmesis and neurotmesis (Misulis, 1993). Recording nerve action potentials from electrodes attached to the skin of the scalp or neck after stimulation of the nerve trunk in the neck or arm establishes whether there is continuity of the rootlets within the spinal canal. These investigations are particularly important in the accurate diagnosis of injuries of the brachial plexus in adults and in babies. However, such neurophysiological work can be applied only after allowing time for degeneration, i.e. after about 3 weeks from the injury (Friedman, 1991).

Radiological investigations are particularly useful in demonstrating the state of the spinal nerves within the spinal canal. Myelography is certainly useful and accuracy is increased when it is combined with computed tomographic (CT) scanning (Marshall & de Silva, 1986). Magnetic resonance imaging (MRI) gives valuable information about the state of the spinal cord but as yet it does not provide precise information about the situation of the spinal nerves themselves. These investigations are often necessary in the analysis of cases of injury to the brachial and lumbosacral plexuses.

MEDICAL AND SURGICAL MANAGEMENT

Early repair of damaged nerves and prompt and adequate treatment of the associated injuries to blood vessels, skeleton, muscle and skin are essential. Injuries of the brachial plexus are the most serious of all peripheral nerve lesions. In many cases the damage lies within the spinal canal, and spinal nerves are either ruptured or torn directly from the spinal cord. A Brown–Séquard syndrome is found in 2–5% of complete lesions (see Ch. 8, p. 128) and rupture of the subclavian or axillary arteries is found in about 20% of cases (Birch, 1993). Life-threatening associated injuries to the head, chest and viscera are common, and associated fractures of long bones are almost the rule.

The treatment of life-threatening injuries must take priority but urgent surgical exploration to confirm diagnosis and to repair damaged nerves, which may involve grafting, is advocated. Results of repair of the fifth, sixth and seventh cervical nerves are a great deal better than they were 20 years ago but restoration of function of the hand in a complete lesion remains exceptional in rare cases of urgent repair in the younger patient or the stab wound.

Later surgical procedures include sympathectomy or deafferentation for severe pain, reconstructive surgery such as tendon transfers to restore function (postoperative treatment for which is discussed below) and amputation in cases where other means of treatment have failed and the limb is a hazard to the patient during daily activities (Birch, 1993). Surgery is only one step in the rehabilitation of the patient.

The introduction of new drugs for neuropathic pain provides a more effective analgesic ladder for sufferers. These agents include opioids, anticonvulsants, low-dose tricyclic antidepressants and other membrane-stabilisers (see Ch. 28). Some patients find that relaxation and visualisation techniques are helpful in providing pain relief and in assisting sleep, and they can be taught quick and discreet techniques they can utilise whenever necessary. This approach enables patients to take charge of their situation and to learn methods of controlling their pain from within their own resources.

Prognosis after repair of nerve injuries

There are two main factors which govern the prognosis of repair of damaged peripheral nerves: firstly, the severity of injury, i.e. the extent of damage to the nerve, and adjacent tissues, most especially to the vascular system; and secondly, delay between the nerve injury and repair. Other factors are relevant, such as age of the patient, the particular nerve injured and the level of lesion.

Repair of a transected major trunk nerve is an urgent matter. When the adjacent axial artery is severed, the case must be taken as an emergency. Fixed deformity from postischaemic fibrosis is invariably seen after neglect of injury to the axial artery or as a consequence of untreated compartment syndrome. Shergill et al. (2001) described the results of 260 repairs of the radial nerve. Useful results were seen in over 70% of open 'tidy' wounds; 36% of cases with arterial injury reached this level. Few effective outcomes followed repair of a defect exceeding 10 cm. Forty-nine per cent of repairs performed within 14 days of injury achieved a good result, but only 28% of later repairs. All repairs undertaken after 12 months failed. The harmful effect of delay is perhaps most clearly demonstrated in severe traction lesions of the brachial plexus.

Birch & Achan (2000) reviewed over 400 cases of nerve injuries in children aged between 6 months and 15 years. Results were better than those seen following equivalent injuries in adults but children are not immune from the effects of postischaemic fibrosis. The outcome in 18 cases of severe Volkmann's ischaemic contracture showed severe and permanent loss of function. Muscle imbalance is a potent cause of severe and progressive deformity in the growing child and this, with postischaemic fibrosis, presents an inevitable and serious problem in reconstruction and rehabilitation.

The multidisciplinary team in rehabilitation

The rehabilitation unit at the RNOH is headed by a physician. For those patients with injuries to brachial plexus and peripheral nerves it is the responsibility of the treating surgeon to oversee the conduct of care from beginning to end. The ward is low-dependency in nature and the role of the senior nurse is described briefly below. There is considerable integration of the work of the physiotherapy and occupational therapy departments, which is discussed in more detail in the section on 'Principles of physical management'.

Orthotists provide functional splints for the paralysed upper limb. Social workers are important in advising about family and community issues. The employment advisor/benefit advisor assists with work-related problems. A clinical psychologist or psychiatrist will contribute to making a diagnosis and then assist the patient in dealing with any emotional and psychological difficulties, as well as aid the patient to explore beliefs about illness and disability. Advice about driving is particularly useful. The disablement resettlement officer is an essential member of the team in guiding patients back to their original occupation or in helping them retrain for another occupation. The treatment team must recognise when they are unable to go further and be prepared to call on other specialist services, particularly in the treatment of intractable pain.

The nursing role

Suitably experienced nursing staff are in a unique position to reinforce the aims of rehabilitation. The role of the nurse within the multidisciplinary rehabilitation programme may be summarised as:

- developing the patient's own communication skills
- increasing the patient's knowledge of peripheral nerve injury and neuropathic pain mechanisms
- seeking to understand the implications of the injury for the patient and family
- caring for the physical and emotional needs of the patient
- providing education and advice for both patient and family
- identifying the need to refer on for other specialist help when necessary.

An urgent concern is to help the patient manage the pain, which may prove to be extremely debilitating. Tripp (1999) discussed the role of nursing staff in psychological support and their potential contribution in chronic pain management. Carers must have a basic understanding of pain mechanisms, without which they are unable to empathise with, and assist, the patient in achieving as full a return as possible to normal life.

In the first weeks after injury, many patients will see the end of their working life, especially if they were manual workers. The rehabilitation nurse has an important role with other members of the MDT in assisting patients to explore all options, encouraging them to think laterally, which may indeed involve a complete rethinking of their life and possibly retraining. A broad range of disciplines is necessary, as outlined above.

The severe impact of the injury is not confined to the patient; it also involves their family. The rehabilitation nurse fulfils an important role in communicating with family and friends, enabling them to offer support, encouragement, understanding and reinforcement of the aims of treatment. The family should be actively encouraged to assist the patient towards regaining independence as soon as possible, and not to allow him or her to maintain a sick role. Patients will be left with a lifelong disability and will need to make major adaptations to self-image and to a view of themselves and their future.

It is appropriate for the rehabilitation nurse to reinforce, with other members of the team, the patient's duty of care for the affected limb because of loss of sensation. The patient is regularly reminded to check the condition of the limb, look for inadvertent injury and unnoted infection, and to maintain healthy skin with moisturising creams. The hazards of extreme cold or heat must be explained and care of nails is important. The monitoring of postoperative bandages and splints, and then later of fabricated orthoses, is an element of this work.

The senior nursing staff are in a particularly good position to detect significant psychological problems or they become alert to the financial implications of injury and so point the way to retraining or to further education.

Psychological support

Patients with lesions of the brachial plexus will present not only with upper-limb sensory and motor deficits but also with needs relating to the associated effects of the injury on independence, employment and lifestyle. Patients may become self-conscious about physical appearance and will require reassurance to assist in coping with their injury. They may suffer cognitive defects from an associated head injury and may require help from a clinical psychologist (see Ch. 27).

Role of the physiotherapist and the occupational therapist

In the rehabilitation unit within the RNOH, the work of the physiotherapy and occupational therapy departments is integrated. The majority of patients with peripheral nerve injuries, other than those sustaining multiple injuries, do not require complex nursing care, although they may need physical and emotional support. The physical problems will be dealt with by appropriately trained therapists but there may be difficulties in coming to terms with the consequences and implications of the injury. Nursing and occupational therapy staff with suitable experience can give appropriate support and counselling. The role of the therapist is elaborated in the sections below.

PRINCIPLES OF PHYSICAL MANAGEMENT

The aims of rehabilitation are:

- objective measurement of disability and the accurate measurement of treatment outcome

- reduction of disability by physical and other therapies
- return of the patient to his or her original work, the original work modified, or to suitable other work
- restoration of the patient's ability to live in his or her own home, to enjoy recreation and social life, and to be independently mobile.

As mentioned above, brachial plexus injuries are the most serious of peripheral nerve injuries and this section will concentrate on their management in adults and children. The principles of treatment can be applied to other nerve injuries and treatment of fixed deformities is a major priority.

Management of the adult brachial plexus lesion

The patient with a brachial plexus lesion (BPL) presents with a wide variety of problems and challenges for the therapist. The consequences of the injury will usually last for the rest of the individual's life, and the patient may present to a physiotherapist at any time following injury (Frampton, 1984).

Early management

Since BPLs are usually caused by high-energy injuries, the damage to the brachial plexus is commonly accompanied by damage to the head, chest and viscera. Initial assessment and management are therefore as varied as the patient's medical condition, and brachial plexus damage cannot be considered in isolation.

Treatment after repair of the brachial plexus After repair of the brachial plexus by nerve grafting, the patient's arm is immobilised in a Hunter sling for up to 6 weeks. The Hunter sling holds the affected arm securely against the trunk, maintaining the shoulder in adduction and medial rotation, with the elbow flexed. Movements of the shoulder are restricted during this time but movements of all other joints are encouraged to diminish stiffness. These movements should be performed at least daily, using the other hand or calling on the aid of a relative to maintain range of movement (ROM), or more frequently if improving ROM or controlling oedema is necessary. These movements are performed actively in cases where the eighth cervical and first thoracic nerves are spared; otherwise they must be carried out as passive movements, using the other hand or assisted by a relative or friend (assistance being more effective).

Slings Slings/upper-limb supports are usually provided by the occupational therapist. At 6 weeks after a repair the Hunter sling may be replaced with a Ministry of Pensions sling. This assists reducing oedema and, by supporting the weight of the affected limb, prevents further glenohumeral joint subluxation. When there is some shoulder control and no subluxation, the patient is encouraged not to wear the sling, so allowing the elbow to regain further extension. In those lesions where C5 and C6 function has been damaged it is usual to observe subluxation of the glenohumeral joint; this is due to paralysis of the rotator cuff, where there is an inability for the cuff to stabilise the humeral head on the glenoid. Stretching the limb will not be detrimental to this. However, in situations where the patient experiences pain from the subluxation, resting in a sling can be of benefit. For patients wishing to return to active sports, a poly sling is recommended. This sling holds the arm firmly against the body with the aid of a waist strap, preventing any uncontrolled movement of the shoulder, which would impede function or aggravate pain.

Assessment The initial physiotherapeutic assessment is ideally carried out together with the occupational therapist. Specific aspects of assessment are discussed in Chapter 3. Areas which require particular attention when assessing patients with nerve injuries are: pain (including night pain); sensation; oedema; active and passive ROM; muscle power and activities of daily living. Horner's (or Bernard–Horner's) sign is a common feature of BPL and indicates a preganglionic injury of T1. The signs are constriction of the pupil and ptosis (drooping of the eyelid) on the affected side, and these inform the therapist that the lesion is severe and that pain may be a major problem.

Evaluation of sensation to light touch should include all of the upper quadrant. Areas of hypersensitivity are recorded; cutaneous sensitivity without pain may be a sign of reinnervation. It is difficult to distinguish this from the hypersensitivity of partial denervated skin where there is an abnormal pain response to light touch (Frampton, 1982) which can be disabling. Pain distribution can be recorded on a body chart. Subjective assessment can be made with a visual analogue scale (0–10). Questions are asked about the pattern of pain, and aggravating and mitigating factors. Night pain is a useful indication of both the type and severity of pain experience.

Early treatment aims The aims of early treatment cover several areas:

- pain control
- oedema control
- maintain/increase ROM of the affected limb
- maintain/increase muscle power
- teach management of the affected limb

- teach postural awareness
- prevent/correct deformity
- address muscle imbalance as recovery occurs
- encourage functional independence.

Pain control   Adequate control of pain with drugs is vital in the early stages and analgesia should be timed to be effective during therapy sessions. If adequate analgesia cannot be achieved, transcutaneous nerve stimulation (TNS; see below under 'Treatment of the late case: Pain') or acupuncture can be used. Whilst healing is taking place, pain caused by stretching to soft tissues to regain ROM slowly eases over time. Relaxation techniques and distraction through activity may also be effective.

Oedema   Oedema of the limb can be a problem in the initial stages following injury and may lead to joint stiffness or contractures if not addressed. If accompanying bone and soft-tissue injuries permit, elevation in a roller towel with active or passive exercises of the wrist, hand and fingers can be carried out. Compression garments must be used with caution because of the already altered circulation and sensation of the limb. Massage, both manual and mechanical, may be used to assist in the management of oedema.

Maintain/increase ROM of the affected limb   The patient should be shown self-assisted movements for all joints of the affected limb. Active exercises should be encouraged. The patient should attempt to stretch and to do exercises hourly. Self-assisted abduction and lateral rotation of the shoulder are awkward to carry out effectively, and it is therefore important to involve the family members and friends in the treatment programme and to teach them the passive stretches if this is indicated. The ethos from the start must be to encourage patients to be as independent as possible in maintenance of their limb and that stretching becomes part of a routine to their day.

Scar massage should be carried out, especially where a scar lies across a joint, as it may further restrict the movement at the joint.

ROM should be monitored at regular intervals as cocontraction can become a problem, as can muscle imbalance. This is also important as a preoperative measure to enhance the outcome of surgical intervention.

Maintain/increase muscle function   The early exercise programme should include active exercises for all intact muscle groups, including the shoulder girdle. Adapting the exercises to match the grade of muscle power may be required, e.g. gravity-eliminated/gravity-assisted work using hydrotherapy, sling suspension or resistive work with weights as appropriate.

Postural awareness   Correction of the abnormal posture, commonly seen in these patients (Fig. 9.1), should begin as soon as possible by raising awareness in the patient and his or her family. The initiation of active correction as part of the early exercise programme focusing primarily on the core stability of the patient is vital for successful management. Many of these patients can go on to develop muscle imbalances in the trunk, as well as of the upper quadrant, e.g postural scoliosis. It is therefore important to teach the patient exercises to maintain good core stability to prevent further stress on the spine.

Care of the limb   Early advice and education in care of a limb with no, or reduced, sensation is important. The patient and the family must be involved. It is important to note that the patients may self-mutilate to check for sensory recovery and this must be monitored closely.

Prevent and manage deformity   Splinting may be used to manage oedema, maintain soft-tissue length, address muscle imbalance, prevent or correct deformity, protect postsurgery, strengthen muscle groups, prepare for surgery and to enhance functional use (Figs 9.2 and 9.3). Splinting, combined with passive stretches, should be started as soon as possible. The patient should be taught about skin care with splints to prevent pressure areas developing.

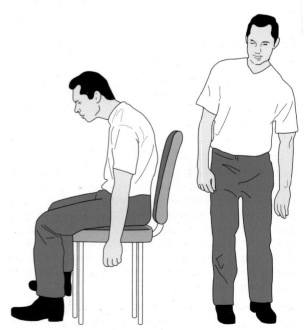

Figure 9.1   The typical posture of a patient with a lesion of the brachial plexus.

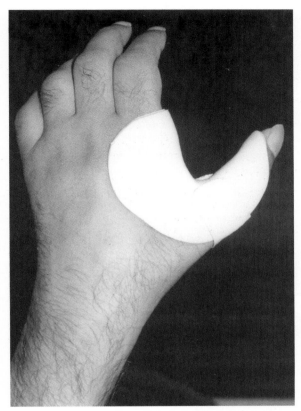

Figure 9.2 Static spacer to maintain thumb web space in a patient with brachial plexus lesion.

Later rehabilitation

The principles of treatment are the same for each individual but, since patients may present at any time following injury, the therapist should be familiar with regeneration times of nerves repaired (Salter & Cheshire, 2000). This will provide an indication of the expected outcome so that the patient can be approached with reasonably accurate expectations of final recovery.

Assessment   In addition to the assessment principles discussed in Chapter 3, specific aspects relating to nerve injuries are outlined here. It is important to know details of the injury, any repair performed and how long after the repair the patient is presenting. Examination should include posture, deformity, appearance of the limb (including oedema, colour and skin condition), presence of Horner's sign, pain, sensation, ROM, muscle power and functional use of the limb.

Posture   Many of these patients adopt a typically flexed posture, as shown in Figure 9.1. This is particularly obvious in those recently injured. Patients with long-standing injuries are often found to have shortening

and reduced flexibility in the side flexors of the trunk on the affected side. The posture should be observed in sitting and standing, and from anterior, posterior and lateral aspects. The degree of active and passive correction should be noted to establish whether the problem is largely that of changes in trunk tone or whether there are established associated soft-tissue changes.

The posture of the limb should be examined while standing. Muscle wasting occurs rapidly after injury and the extent of loss of muscle bulk in upper limb and shoulder girdle is noted. Depending on the extent and level of injury, subluxation of the shoulder may be observed. The arm commonly hangs in medial rotation and forearm pronation.

Deformity   The most common fixed deformities are medial rotation of the shoulder and extension of the metacarpophalangeal joints, with flexion of the proximal interphalangeal joints.

Deformity is also seen at the elbow as a flexion deformity, as well as in the wrist. Damage to the eighth cervical and first thoracic nerves can produce deformities similar to those seen in other peripheral nerve injuries, such as the claw hand of the ulnar nerve lesion. Prevention of deformity is mentioned below when discussing complications.

Treatment of the late case

Later treatment concentrates on regaining ROM, muscle power and good posture, as well as controlling pain, which may still be a significant problem. The treatment techniques mentioned below are discussed in Chapter 23.

Range of movement   Stretches should be performed as soon as possible if there is limitation in ROM in the upper limb. It is important to stress to the patient that, even if there is no recovery in the hand, for example, maintaining range in the joints is important for cosmetic and hygienic reasons. Stretches are taught for all joints of the shoulder girdle and upper limb, in all directions of movement.

After removal of the Hunter sling at 6 weeks after exploration and repair, stretches every 2 h are suggested to regain range as quickly as possible. Once ROM is achieved, a daily stretching session will maintain passive range. Family or friends should be involved with the programme and be taught the necessary exercises; ideally they should assist with abduction and lateral rotation of the shoulder, since these are the most awkward to perform independently. Lateral rotation is the movement that is most frequently lost and the most difficult to regain. If the patient is particularly

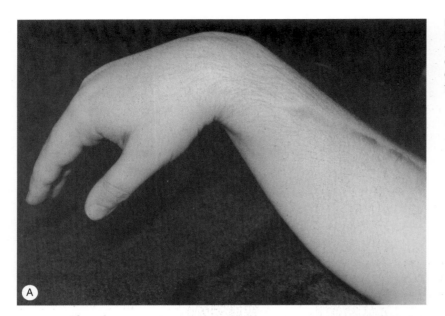

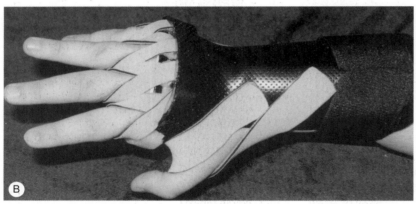

Figure 9.3 A C5–C7 brachial plexus lesion showing: (A) paralysis of forearm extensors; (B) a dynamic extension splint (low profile) to correct the deformity and enable function.

stiff and unable to cope with independent stretches, the hydrotherapy pool can be a useful environment from which to start the patient and hence make a land stretching programme easier.

Following exploration and repair, the patient will have surgical scars which can become tethered to the soft tissue below and contribute to loss of movement, or can become hypersensitive and painful. Scars can be present in several areas, depending where the grafts were taken, most commonly: along the forearm; inside the upper arm running up into the axilla; across the clavicle; and, if the sural nerve has been used as a donor nerve, the back of the calf. Patients are taught scar massage techniques while they are still inpatients and they have use of the Niagra hand unit (a mechanical massager using multidirectional vibration) and silicone gel for particularly hypertrophic scarring.

Muscle function   An exercise programme should be devised to strengthen the functioning muscles. As each presentation is different, the programme has to be individually designed. Each muscle group will have to be strengthened within the limitations of its grade, i.e. gravity-assisted, neutral or resisted. Electromyographic (EMG) biofeedback can be very useful when starting to strengthen muscles and it can provide an objective method for monitoring progress. Functional electrical stimulation (FES) can be useful in situations where muscle reinnervation is occurring but no research has been conducted specifically in patients with BPLs. Furthermore, the motor end plate must be intact for FES to produce a contraction. It may be useful when signs of recovery begin.

Facilitation techniques, such as proprioceptive neuromuscular facilitation (PNF), are particularly useful for upper-limb and single-joint strengthening (see Ch. 23). The patient should be encouraged to use the limb as functionally as possible. Introduction to the flail arm splint can augment the strengthening programme.

General strengthening and fitness are important (see Ch. 29). This can involve specific exercises (shoulder-girdle exercises, trunk-strengthening), as well as a general fitness programme. Swimming is an ideal sport for these patients; it is quite possible for the patient who was a competent swimmer prior to injury to return to a good level of swimming, even with a complete BPL. For the first session after injury, patients ought to be accompanied and encouraged to start swimming on their back while they get used to their altered weight in the water.

Oedema This is a problem in the early stages and is best managed by elevation of the limb at night, use of a sling during the day, active exercises, massage and careful use of a compression bandage. The pressure garment can be worn long-term for persistent oedema. If compression is to be used, then regular checks on skin condition and monitoring of sudden onset of new pain, or even oedema, must be performed.

Pain Pain in the postacute stage is caused by the nerve injury (see above) and may persist as an extremely disabling problem. Many patients respond to TNS, and specific placement of electrodes has been described by Frampton (1982). Barsby (Birch et al., 1998, p. 256), with physiotherapy colleagues, studied 281 inpatient episodes from 1995 to 1998. High-intensity, low-frequency stimulation was found to be preferable, in bursts or continuously for stretching pain; low-intensity, high-frequency stimulation, again in bursts or continuously, was preferable for neuralgic pains.

Transcutaneous stimulation was not useful in the treatment of hyperaesthesia. About 80% of patients gained relief, but the results deteriorated after 3–6 months in more than half the patients. Acupuncture has been used over the past 4 years; it has been helpful in a few cases only. When hypersensitivity is a serious problem, the Niagra hand unit may be used for sensory bombardment as part of a desensitising programme.

Sometimes compression of the limb eases pain and a pressure garment can be tried. A shoulder subluxation support may be used if subluxation at the glenohumeral joint is increasing pain levels. It is important to be fully aware of the nature and behaviour of the patient's pain. Patients often notice that the pain is worse when they have little else to think about but that it improves when they are busy or distracted. Activities, such as taking up a new hobby, sports such as

swimming, or resuming or taking up new employment are important. As well as being central to the overall restoration of a normal lifestyle, these activities can act as an effective means of pain control.

Postural awareness The rehabilitation programme should include some form of balance and proprioceptive work in the form of wobble-board and gym ball stretches, and stability exercises for deep postural muscles. The extreme example of the typical BPL-related posture has already been shown (Fig. 9.1). Postural education should be supplemented with visual feedback. Poor ability to extend laterally and poor control of trunk or pelvis should be addressed using general trunk re-education exercises.

Care of the limb As with any area of the body with reduced or no sensation, the principles of skin care must be taught (Salter & Cheshire, 2000). Patients should check their skin regularly and become 'limb-aware'. They must get into the habit of knowing where the arm is, because the normal withdrawal response to pain, or extremes of heat or cold, is lost. The patient should be taught about the consequences of not taking care of the limb, such as prolonged healing time, and the increased risk of sores from reduced circulation.

Deformity Splints are useful, particularly in the early stages for the management of soft-tissue length and joint alignment. Night splints are required for the hand and wrist, and serial splinting is a valuable component of an active programme to treat deformities that have already occurred. The provision of splints is usually accompanied by an upper-limb and hand therapy programme, and followed up at regular intervals to address progress and any changes in the recovery status. An example of a static splint to place the hand in a functional position is shown in Figure 9.4.

Activities of daily living Patients are encouraged to utilise any available function in their affected limb in their daily activities. As well as promoting independence, this provides exercise to the weak muscles and stimulation for sensory-impaired areas. When an injury occurs to the dominant upper limb, it is important for the therapist to work on increasing strength, stamina and manual dexterity of the non-dominant limb prior to attempting functional activities. Patients with no functional use in the affected arm are trained in one-handed techniques and, when appropriate, assistive appliances are used, e.g. the flail arm splint (Fig. 9.5). Leisure pursuits need to be addressed, including the feasibility of returning to previous sports.

Use of splints or assistive equipment may be an option and often specific appliances for participating in the sport will need to be constructed if they are not

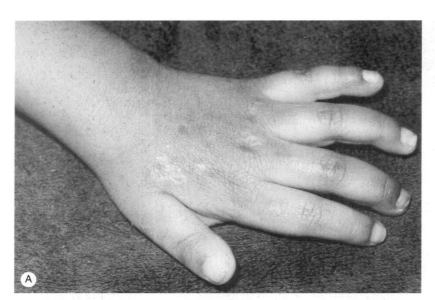

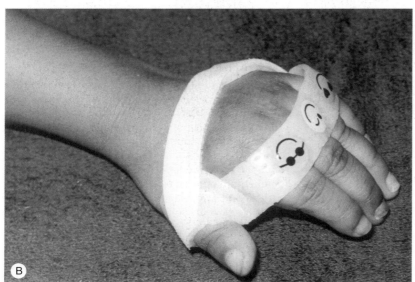

Figure 9.4 Severe obstetrical brachial plexus palsy showing: (A) persisting paralysis of small muscles of hand; (B) a static splint providing improved posture and function.

commercially available. Return to employment is discussed and the patient must be reassured that the loss of arm function does not necessarily lead to loss of employment and financial security. Referral to an employment advisor provides the patient with the necessary support.

Monitoring recovery

The nature of this injury means that it is inappropriate and unnecessary to have long-standing and constant physiotherapy. Indeed, this may be counterproductive. The ultimate aim of rehabilitation for these patients is a return to maximum function within the limitations of

the injury. Therapeutic intervention should always include realistic treatment goals that empower patients to take responsibility for their rehabilitation. Intervention should not be continued once these goals have been achieved. Monitoring progress at intervals and reviewing management if the situation changes is the most appropriate method of long-term care for these patients.

Treatment after muscle and tendon transfers

Restoration of function often requires surgical transfer of musculotendinous units to provide or augment poor

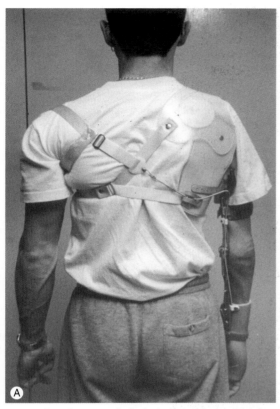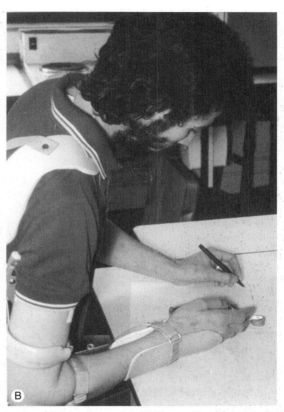

Figure 9.5   Complete supraclavicular lesion of the brachial plexus showing: (A) the position of the flail arm splint; (B) a patient using this device for his work.

active movement. Figures for operations performed over a 24-year period at the RNOH are shown in Table 9.5. Some common transfers include pectoralis major-to-biceps and flexor-to-extensor transfer in the forearm. The transferred muscle should be at least grade 4 on the MRC Scale (since it will lose a grade in transfer) and have flexibility.

Preoperatively, appropriate therapy intervention needs to be provided to enhance the result of surgical intervention and ultimate functional movement. It is vital that there is an assessment of joint mobility and strength; the affected limb should be mobile, without contractures of relevant joints. Dynamic splintage may be considered to assist in strengthening the transferred muscle and may assist in proprioceptive feedback (see below). Postoperatively, maintaining ROM in the free joints during the period of immobilisation is vital to the overall success of the transfer. Dynamic splintage may be considered at 2 weeks postoperatively (in liaison with the surgeon) to allow functional movement whilst protecting the surgery (i.e flexor-to-extensor transfer in the forearm).

Table 9.5   Operations performed at the Royal National Orthopaedic Hospital (1977–2001) for reconstruction of function in adults and children (excluding obstetric brachial plexus palsy)

	Brachial plexus lesions			Peripheral nerve lesions
Shoulder	148		Forearm and wrist	196
Arm	398		Hand	162
Forearm and wrist	326		Thumb	192
Hand	285		Hip and knee; ankle and foot	238
Total	1152[a]		Total	788[a]

[a] These figures include 298 operations for release of deformity and 62 amputations.

The aims of treatment after transfer include increasing ROM, re-educating muscle to perform new functions and management of adherent scars using scar management techniques.

Increase ROM   Active work may commence 3 weeks after the operation, but passive stretching at the transfer site must be avoided for a further 3 weeks, sometimes longer, dependent on the surgical procedure. Patients continue to wear a splint for at least 6 weeks after transfer.

Facilitation of muscle action   The transferred muscle must now learn to work in a different way; the patient must understand the original action of the muscle, transferred and the new desired action. PNF techniques using minimal resistance at first, and within the range of the muscle, can provide an effective way of initiating this. Active work, initially in the gravity-eliminated positions, and with the arm supported, using EMG biofeedback, and introducing functional use of the limb is a useful method of treatment and can be adapted as the active power and ROM improve. It is always important to remember the patient's social and occupational background and, if this is relevant, focus rehabilitation with this in mind. Functional and recreational activities are ideal for spontaneous use of the hand.

With lower-limb transfers, such as transfer of tibialis posterior to tibialis anterior, rehabilitation must include gait and balance re-education with a graduated weight-bearing regimen, as well as re-education similar to that in the upper limb.

Splintage   Thermoplastic splints are provided by the occupational therapist, after thorough upper-limb assessment. The purpose of splinting is to:

- position the limb correctly and thus prevent secondary complications
- increase functional use of the affected limb
- protect surgical intervention
- prevent or correct deformity
- address muscle imbalance and strengthen muscles
- maintain soft-tissue length and ROM

The design of the splint must take into consideration the individual patient's needs, and available function should be utilised to maintain muscle strength and avoid dependency on a splint. Splintage is always used in conjunction with a therapy programme. Dynamic splints may be required for exercise purposes, as well as for functional use, to enhance function without restricting movement. Advice is given regarding the wearing regime and great care is taken when sensation is impaired. Examples of dynamic, semidynamic and static splints to enable function are shown in Figures 9.6–9.8 respectively.

At the RNOH, patients with loss of shoulder/elbow function or a complete brachial plexus lesion will be given the option of having a Stanmore flail arm splint, which is a dynamic splint to which assistive devices can be attached (Fig. 9.5).

The splint is basically a skeleton of an upper-limb prosthesis, fitting around the paralysed arm and consists of:

- a shoulder support allowing flexion and abduction
- an elbow-locking device
- forearm shelf or gutter with wrist support
- removable terminal appliances
- a cable which allows operation of the hand appliance by protraction and retraction of the unaffected shoulder.

Any combination of these parts may be appropriate and encouragement is given to utilise any available function in the affected limb (Birch, 1993).

Appropriate splintage of the hand may be considered in place of the terminal appliances. A thorough assessment, including a discussion regarding potential functional benefits to the individual of providing the splint, is completed by the occupational therapist. If suitable, the splint is then fitted by the orthotist and subsequent training in its use given by the occupational therapist.

In a long-term review of 200 patients fitted with these splints, Wynn Parry et al. (1987) found that 70% used them for work or recreation. The most useful devices are the tool holder, the split hook and the appliance for steadying a sheet of paper. 'True success' is measured by continuing use of the splint but they are also justified if they help carry a patient through a period of recovery, if they serve to distract patients from pain and if they provide motivation to start rehabilitation.

Probert (Birch et al., 1998, p. 460) analysed prospective data from over 400 patients (between 1980 and 1996) and found that about one-third of patients supplied with the splint used them. Schuette (Birch et al., 1998, p. 461) confirmed a relatively low rate of continued use.

Return to work

Taggart (Birch et al., 1998, p. 461) prospectively studied 324 patients who underwent operations of supraclavicular injury of the brachial plexus. They were entered into the study between 1986 and 1993 and were followed for at least 13 months. All had at least one period of admission for rehabilitation. A relatively high rate of return to work was an important finding,

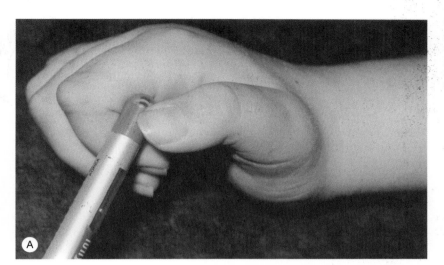

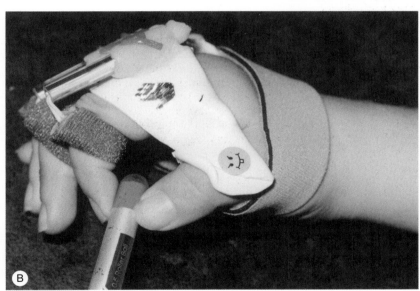

Figure 9.6 Obstetrical brachial plexus palsy showing: (A) weakness of intrinsic muscles of the hand with poor posture of the thumb; (B) improvement in posture and function with a dynamic splint.

with 60% entering a different occupation and only 17% returning to the same occupation as before the injury. It was also found that the majority of patients spent 7–12 months off work.

This rate of return to work after serious injury to the brachial plexus is encouraging but the high rate of those returning to a different job indicates the importance of retraining, and of systems of information about employment.

Apart from the physical disability, other factors militate against an early return to work. When compensation is at stake, early return to work may be perceived by the patient and his or her solicitor as financial loss. Recent changes in the benefits system are a potent

inhibition against returning to work. Evidently, these two factors are becoming more and more important. Close liaison with the family practitioner is necessary at all stages of rehabilitation, most especially when that process falters. The patient's views and circumstances need to be considered when setting goals for returning to work (see section on 'Participating in the process' in Ch. 22, p. 384).

Management of complications

The most common complication of peripheral nerve injuries is fixed deformity. RSD can also occur after fractures and is difficult to manage.

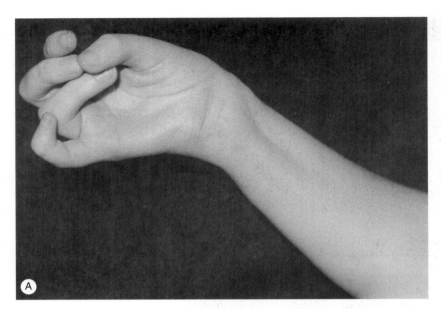

Figure 9.7 Ten years after severe injury of the brachial plexus in an adult, with limited recovery in the middle and lower trunks, having had an opposition tendon transfer, showing: (A) posture of the hand; (B) a semidynamic splint improved posture of the thumb and provided a degree of pronation.

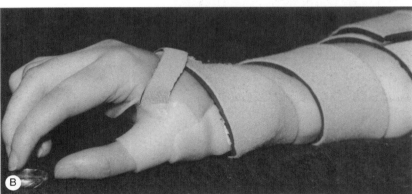

Fixed deformity

The prevention of fixed deformity is one of the first priorities in treatment. Many cases of fixed deformity are a reflection of neglect of elementary principles in the treatment of paralysed limbs. Pain is an important cause of fixed deformity; in the upper limb it leads to severe flexion deformity of the wrist with extension of the metacarpophalangeal joints. Fixed deformity can occur with postischaemic fibrosis of muscle and this is seen particularly involving flexor muscles of the forearm, the small muscles of the hand and the deep flexor compartment of the leg. In children, the unopposed action of muscles during growth is an important cause; the effect on the posture of the foot after irreparable tibial or common peroneal lesion in the growing child

is severe. Serial splinting is very useful in the treatment of many of these deformities.

Serial splinting of fixed deformity   This technique can be used to correct flexion deformity of the elbow, wrist, fingers, knee and ankle, and is discussed in Chapters 23 and 25. The skin should be healthy and radiographs taken to ensure that the skeleton is sound. Splinting is applied in collaboration with the physiotherapist who will achieve a few more degrees of correction before the new splint is applied each time, and the technique is continued in this way until the required extension is gained. It is important to avoid trying to gain too much correction at one time. Splints are worn at night and in some cases for an hour or two during the day. The technique depends entirely on the

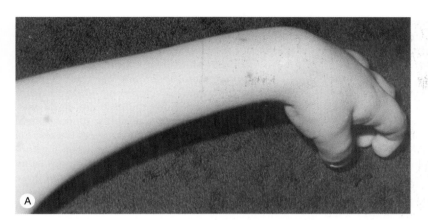

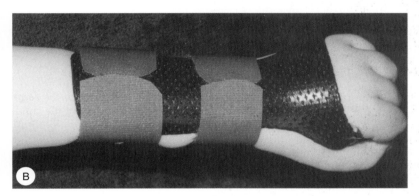

Figure 9.8 Obstetric brachial plexus palsy showing: (A) poor recovery at the wrist extensors; (B) a static dorsal wrist extension splint which greatly enhanced function and confirmed indication for appropriate muscle transfer.

co-operation of the patient, who should maintain flexion and gentle stretching of the joint during the day when the splint is not worn.

Reflex sympathetic dystrophy

This disorder has been described above. The foundation of treatment in these difficult cases is encouragement towards functional activity. In some cases, guanethidine blocks and/or other drugs are helpful. Forceful manipulation of the part is damaging.

Birth injury of the brachial plexus

Obstetric brachial plexus palsy (OBPP) is a serious complication of childbirth, which appears to be increasing in incidence. Although accurate figures are not available in the UK, the centre at the RNOH now sees over 150 new cases a year (the majority of cases seen in the UK). There are two significant risk factors. Injuries in children born by breech delivery are serious and may be bilateral. Disproportion in the birth canal is a much more common cause; we have found that shoulder dystocia was a complication in 70% of our

cases. The weight of the child is the single most significant risk factor and heavy babies are at risk.

A relatively simple classification of OBPP has evolved amongst surgeons in the field and consists of four groups (Narakas, 1987):

1. Group 1: the fifth and sixth cervical nerves are damaged, and the shoulder and elbow flexor muscles are paralysed. About 90% of these babies make a full spontaneous recovery; this usually begins within 3 months of birth and is complete by 6 months.
2. Group 2: the fifth, sixth and seventh cervical nerves are damaged. There is paralysis of the shoulder, elbow flexors and extensor muscles of the wrist and digits. About two-thirds of these children make a full spontaneous recovery, though serious defects of the shoulder persist in the remainder. Recovery is slower than in group 1, with activity in the deltoid and biceps muscles becoming clinically apparent at 3–6 months.
3. Group 3: paralysis is virtually complete; there is some flexion of the fingers at or shortly after birth. Full spontaneous recovery occurs in <50% of these

children. Most are left with substantial impairment of function at the shoulder and elbow, with deficient rotation of the forearm, and wrist and finger extension does not recover in about 25% of cases.

4. Group 4: the whole plexus is damaged; paralysis is complete. The limb is atonic and Bernard–Horner syndrome is present. No child makes a full recovery, the spinal nerves have either been ruptured or avulsed from the spinal cord, and there is permanent and serious defect within the limb.

Operations to repair the plexus are indicated in severe cases where there is no clinical evidence of recovery, or operation is necessary to overcome secondary fixed deformities. The most serious of all these secondary deformities is medial rotation contracture of the shoulder which, if untreated, progresses to posterior dislocation of the shoulder.

Of 78 patients assessed in the unit at the RNOH in a 12-month period in 1995–1996, there were 6 patients with group 1 injuries (8%), 36 with group 2 (46%), 23 with group 3 (29%) and 13 with group 4 (17%).

Physical management of OBPP

The information in this section is original and has evolved from the experience gained at the authors' centre. Since there is a lack of literature to draw from, more detail is given in this section than is generally presented in this book.

The therapist may become involved at any stage in the life of a child with OBPP. The therapeutic needs of the child will change with growth but the approach must be holistic and acknowledge the key role played by the family.

Assessment   *In the baby.*   The assessment is most relevant at 2–3 weeks after birth, since mild cases can improve within a matter of days. The following should be assessed: asymmetry of posture; normal active spontaneous movements of the limb as appropriate to the developmental level of the baby (see Ch. 17); range of movement of the upper limb; and muscle power, though this cannot be performed very accurately in the newborn.

In the older child.   The birth history and operative procedure should be noted to obtain an idea of predicted recovery. The therapist should evaluate how the child is performing functionally in relation to the stage of development; this includes activities ranging from clapping, eating and dressing to participation in sports. Any limb deformity should be noted.

Formal assessment of sensation is difficult in toddlers, but a child who chews, burns or traps his or her fingers without noticing and cannot handle objects without looking is likely to have a considerable deficit. Occasionally hypersensitive areas occur; they usually resolve with time. Pain is not usually a problem in OBPP.

The scapulohumeral angles are important to record because of the rapid development of contractures within this complex. Three of these are significant: medial rotation contracture; posterior glenohumeral contracture, which is shown by winging of the scapula when the child protracts the arm; and inferior glenohumeral contracture so that the scapula moves away from the chest when the arm is elevated. Most of these deformities are caused by contractures of soft tissue rather than bony deformity. Posterior dislocation is, on the whole, developmental and is preventable in the majority of cases.

Observation of function is a more useful assessment tool than trying to grade the strength of specific muscles. Activities such as crawling, reaching out, throwing and catching provide a good guide to muscle power.

Treatment   The principles of treatment are the same as those for adults. Regardless of the age of the child, the aims of therapy are to:

- educate and involve the child and family in the management of the lesion
- prevent deformity
- maintain and increase the range of movement
- encourage function along with the normal development of the child.

It is essential to ensure full involvement of the family to achieve the child's full potential. Formal physiotherapy is only given for short periods, to educate the parents who carry out most of the treatment.

In all cases, stretching to prevent deformity is the most important aspect of treatment. In the newborn baby, stretches should be encouraged at every nappy change; in older children they are usually performed 3–5 times a day. The parents should be guided about the sensation of the end feeling of the movement but they can be reassured that their baby will also be able to tell them!

Exercise to improve ROM and strength can be incorporated into play activities. The child should be encouraged to use the limb as normally as possible and when of school age to take part in swimming, gym and games activities. The child's teacher may need to be involved with the rehabilitation at this stage. Independence in normal functional tasks (washing, eating) should be promoted. Splinting may be appropriate at night for the child with the more severe lesion with limited recovery or if contracture develops (see Figs 9.4, 9.6 and 9.8).

Maximising function Parents often need to be reminded that children are very adaptable and will use their unaffected hand quite spontaneously, even if it is their non-dominant hand. It is not until the child needs to perform bilateral activities, at the age of 4 or 5 years, that he or she will fully utilise what function there is. The more the affected arm and hand can be used, the better, but parents need to find the right balance between encouragement and frustration. Dressing presented the greatest functional problem for the 78 children reviewed. Dressing can be practised, away from the early-morning rush, using large dressing-up clothes. Feeding activities can also be simulated through play. A problem-solving approach to overcoming functional difficulties should be encouraged (see Ch. 22). Use of the imagination can be very helpful, so parents and children should be encouraged to think of alternative approaches and be assured that if it works for them, it is all right.

Continuing care For those patients diagnosed with lesions of groups 1 and 2, follow-up should continue until they have regained full function. For the child with the more severe injury, in groups 3 and 4, review should be regular in the initial stages but may become less frequent as recovery plateaus. Intermittent checks that the parents are performing the appropriate stretches effectively should be made and, if required, short bursts of treatment carried out should a contracture develop.

Parents can be put in touch with a self-help group for parents of children with OBPP so that they do not feel so isolated. (These groups exist locally and a national contact address cannot be given.) Parents can also be reassured that their child's function will improve over time, or in a more severely affected child that surgery is available and may increase function. They also need reassuring that by allowing a child to struggle, they are encouraging independence even though they may find this difficult.

Encourage a positive self-image If parents are encouraged to refer to the affected arm as 'special' as opposed to 'bad', the child should grow up with a more positive self-image. These children may require support in dealing appropriately with other children's curiosity or remarks about their arm once they start school, and again in adolescence when the appearance of the arm will be increasingly important. Encouragement from therapists and parents is essential to help these children maintain a positive view of themselves and maximise their potential so that they are able to lead full and active lives.

CONCLUSION

Rehabilitation of the patient with a peripheral nerve injury requires a multidisciplinary approach. The focus is on function, assessing and managing the patient's problems with the long-term goal of facilitating a return to the home, work and social environment.

CASE HISTORY

Patient with a right brachial plexus injury
A 28-year-old female sustained lacerations to the right side of her neck when she fell from a table about 2 m from the ground on to broken glass. She sustained lacerations to her subclavian, vertebral and internal jugular veins and ruptured C5 and C6.

The injuries to the veins were successfully tied and treated. The nerves of C5 and C6 level were repaired by nerve grafts. Her arm was immobilised in a Hunter sling for 4 weeks. Active hand, wrist and finger movements were encouraged. After 4 weeks the patient was admitted for a week of rehabilitation.

Main problems

- reduced grip strength in right hand
- adhered scar on right side of neck and volar side of elbow which restricted neck and elbow ROM
- reduced function and ROM in shoulder and elbow
- not currently able to drive
- not able to carry out job tasks as a nurse
- difficulty putting on bra
- difficulty cutting food
- numbness on the dorsal and volar side of thumb, tingling sensation on the volar side of index finger
- experiencing 'rubbing' pain across and front of shoulder and shooting pain along the forearm
- difficulty writing with right hand due to instability in elbow and shoulder
- poor postural awareness of shoulder/arm alignment
- reduced balance and core stability.

Goal-setting
Joint therapy goals were set with the patient:

- to increase functional independence
- to give education and advice about management and recovery of the right arm
- to discuss and give advice on how to return to driving and work
- to increase and maintain passive ROM at shoulder and elbow

- to improve balance and core control
- to improve posture.

Treatment progress

1. Muscle strengthening and dexterity exercises were given to the patient. She was encouraged regularly to use and incorporate right hand in functional activities.

2. Scar massage to the neck and elbow. Treatment given daily for 30 min with the aim to loosen up scar from the soft tissue to increase ROM. Plus myofascial scar release (form of massage) in physiotherapy.

3. Demonstration and advice given regarding shoulder–elbow lock splint to support shoulder and externally lock elbow in different flexion positions (30°, 70°, 90°) to enable increased functional use of right hand.

4. Advice given to patient on how to return to driving; legal information and information about adaptations provided.

5. Sling suspension (gravity-eliminated) for MRC grade 2 triceps.

6. Passive range of movement (PROM) stretches using gym ball, pulleys, wall bars, etc. therefore using trunk to help mobilise shoulder girdle.

7. Posture re-education using mirror for feedback and scapula-setting exercises.

8. Core stability, including gym ball and wobble-board work.

9. Discussion around what plans patient has to return to work. Work options discussed. Support and encouragement given to patient to explore work options.

10. Advice and adaptations suggested for patient to put bra on independently.

11. Equipment, adaptations and techniques discussed and demonstrated to enable patient to cut food independently.

12. Education and advice given with regard to diminished sensation. Visual compensation when gripping and manipulating items, check out for whiteness or redness around thumb if grip too hard. Also compensate visually when handling sharp and hot items.

13. Education given jointly with physiotherapist and medical team about neuropathic pain, symptoms, treatment and progress of injury, anatomy of nervous system and brachial plexus injuries.

14. Assessed writing position and posture. With correct posture and support of forearm on table patient was able to write well. Discussion regarding importance of posture and support of arm in activities.

Conclusions

The patient felt independent with personal and domestic activities by the end of the week. She reported gaining more self-confidence and knowledge about how to manage the injury both from a physical and psychological point of view.

She also gained knowledge and confidence in how to use her right arm in functional activities.

The intense work on her scars resulted in a smoother, more mobile scar tissue which facilitated an increase in active neck movement and passive elbow extension, for her to continue scar management and a hand exercise programme at home.

She reported that her future short-term goals were (in 6 months' time) to get back to driving and pick up academic studies for specialised nursing.

Shoulder–elbow splint was planned to be moulded in a few weeks' time through Orthotics Department, to encourage functional use of the right arm and hand.

The patient felt her arm had become a part of her again and was more aware of gaining stability around the shoulder-girdle and trunk.

References

Anand P, Birch R. Restoration of sensory function and lack of long-term chronic pain syndromes after brachial plexus injury in human neonates. *Brain* 2002, **125**:113–122.

Berman J, Birch R, Anand P, Chen L, Taggart M. Pain relief from preganglionic injury to the brachial plexus by late intercostal transfer. *J Bone Joint Surg* 1996, **78B**:759–760.

Berman JS, Birch R, Anand P. Pain following human brachial plexus injury with spinal cord root avulsion and the effect of surgery. *Pain* 1998, **75**:199–207.

Birch R. Management of brachial plexus injuries. In: Greenwood R, Barnes MP, McMillan TM et al., eds. *Neurological Rehabilitation*. London: Churchill Livingstone; 1993:587–606.

Birch R, Achan P. Peripheral nerve repairs and their results in children. *Hand Clinics* 2000, **16**:579–597.

Birch R, Bonney G, Wynn Parry C. 1998 *Surgical Disorders of the Peripheral Nerves*, 1st edn. London: Churchill Livingstone; 1998.

Brown AG. *Nerve Cells and Nervous Systems. An Introduction to Neuroscience*. London: Springer Verlag; 1991.

Frampton V. Pain control with the aid of transcutaneous nerve stimulation. *Physiotherapy* 1982, **68**:77–81.

Frampton V. Management of brachial plexus lesions. *Physiotherapy* 1984, **70**:388.

Frazier CH, Skillern PG. Supraclavicular subcutaneous lesions of the brachial plexus not associated with skeletal injuries. *JAMA* 1911, **57**:1957–1963.

Friedman WA. The electrophysiology of peripheral nerve injuries. *Neurosurg Clin N Am* 1991, **2**:43–56.

International Association for the Study of Pain. Available online at www.iasp-pain.org.

Jones R. *Notes on Military Orthopaedics*. (Introductory note by Surgeon General Sir Alfred Keough GCB.) London: Casell; 1917.

Jones R. *Orthopaedic Surgery of Injuries*. London: Hodder/Oxford University Press; 1921.

Lorei MP, Hershman EB. Peripheral nerve injuries in athletes: treatment and prevention. *Sports Med* 1993, **16**:130–147.

Lundborg G. Peripheral nerve injuries: pathophysiology and strategies for treatment. *J Hand Ther* 1993, **6**:179–188.

Marshall RW, de Silva RD. Computerised tomography in traction lesions of the brachial plexus. *J Bone Joint Surg* 1986, **68B**:734–738.

Medical Research Council. *MRC Atlas: Aids to the Examination of the Peripheral Nervous System*. London: HMSO; 1982.

Melzack R, Wall PD. Pain mechanisms: a new theory. *Science* 1965; **150**:971–979.

Misulis KE. *Essentials of Clinical Neurophysiology*. London: Butterworth Heinemann; 1993.

Mitchell JR, Osterman AL. Physiology of nerve repair: a research update. *Hand Clin* 1991, **7**:481–490.

Narakas A. Obstetrical brachial plexus injuries. In: Lamb DW, ed. *TheParalysed Hand*. Edinburgh: Churchill Livingstone; 1987:116–135.

Rosson JW. Disability following closed traction lesions of the brachial plexus – an epidemic among young motor cyclists. *Injury* 1987, **19**:4–6.

Salter M, Cheshire L. *Hand Therapy: Principles and Practice*, 1st edn. Oxford: Butterworth Heinemann; 2000:181–195.

Schenker M, Birch R. Diagnosis of level of intradural ruptures of the rootlets in traction lesions of the brachial plexus. *J Bone Joint Surg (Br)* 2001; **83B**:916–920.

Seddon HJ. *Surgical Disorders of the Peripheral Nerves*, 2nd edn. Edinburgh: Churchill Livingstone; 1975.

Shepherd GM. *Neurobiology*. New York: Oxford University Press; 1994.

Shergill G, Birch R, Bonney G et al. The radial and posterior interosseous nerves: results of 260 repairs. *J Bone Joint Surg* 2001;**83B**:646–649.

Stewart M, Birch R. Penetrating missile injuries. *J Bone Joint Surg* 2001; **83B**:517–524.

Tripp S. Providing psychological support. In: Smith M, ed. *Rehabilitation in Adult Nursing Practice*. Edinburgh: Churchill Livingstone; 1999: 105–123.

van Laere M, Claessens M. The treatment of reflex sympathetic dystrophy syndrome: current concepts. *Acta Orthop Belg* 1992, **58**:259–261.

Veldman PH, Reynen HM, Arntz IE et al. Signs and symptoms of reflex sympathetic dystrophy: prospective study of 829 patients. *Lancet* 1993, **342**:1012–1016.

Wall PD 1978. The gate control theory of pain mechanisms. A re-examination and re-statement. *Brain* **101**:1–18.

Wall PD, Melzack R. *The Challenge of Pain*, 2nd edn. London: Penguin; 1996.

Williams P. *Gray's Anatomy*, 38th edn. Edinburgh: Churchill Livingstone; 1995.

Wynn Parry CB. *Rehabilitation of the Hand*, 4th edn. London: Butterworth; 1981.

Wynn Parry C, Frampton V, Monteith A. Rehabilitation following traction injuries of the brachial plexus. In: Terzis JK, ed. *Microreconstruction of Nerve Injuries*. Philadelphia: WB Saunders; 1987: 483–498.

Chapter 10

Multiple sclerosis

L De Souza   D Bates

INTRODUCTION

Multiple sclerosis (MS) is the major cause of neurological disability in young and middle-aged adults. It is almost twice as common in women as in men, and though it can present at any age from childhood to the elderly, it has a peak incidence between the ages of 25 and 35 years. The impact of MS upon the lives of those affected can be enormous, partly because the course of the illness is unpredictable and partly because its effects and symptoms are so protean.

The course of the disease ranges from a single transient neurological deficit with full recovery to, in its most severe form, permanent disability being established within weeks or months of onset. Many people remain mobile and can live a near-normal life but physiotherapists tend to see those whose lives are more seriously affected.

PATHOLOGY

MS is the principal member of a group of disorders known as 'demyelinating diseases'. Many conditions involve the process of demyelination as part of their disease pathology but the term 'demyelinating disease' is reserved for those conditions which have the immune-mediated destruction of myelin as the primary pathological finding, with relative sparing of other elements of central nervous system (CNS) tissue.

The other conditions that are part of this group are rare and may be variants of MS. They include:

- diffuse cerebral sclerosis of Schilder
- concentric sclerosis of Balo
- neuromyelitis optica of Devic
- the acute disseminated encephalomyelitides (ADEM), which may be postinfective or postvaccinal
- acute necrotising haemorrhagic encephalomyelitis, which is probably due to herpes infection
- other demyelinating diseases with a known underlying infective or metabolic cause are now classified according to their specific pathology (Scolding, 2001).

Demyelination of nerve fibres

In the CNS, myelin is produced by oligodendrocytes (Shepherd, 1994). Each oligodendrocyte gives off a number of processes to ensheath surrounding axons. These processes, which envelope the axon, form a specialised membranous organelle – the myelin segment. A myelinated nerve fibre has many such myelin segments, all of a similar size, arranged along its length. Between the myelinated segments there is an area of

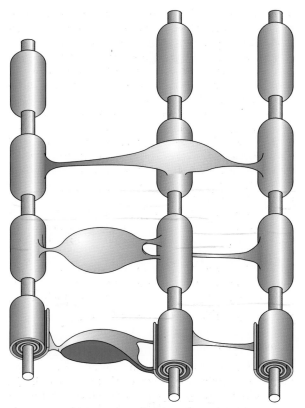

Figure 10.1 Myelinated nerve fibres in the central nervous system.

exposed axon known as the node of Ranvier. The myelin segment is termed the 'internode' (Fig. 10.1). When an action potential is conducted along the axon, ionic transfer predominantly occurs across the axonal membrane at the node of Ranvier. The lipid-rich myelin of the internode insulates the axon and inhibits ionic transfer at the internode. This arrangement of segmental myelination allows rapid and efficient axonal conduction by the process of saltatory conduction where the signal spreads rapidly from one node of Ranvier to the next.

When myelin is lost the insulation fails and the action potential cannot be conducted normally and at speed along the nerve, the function of which thereby effectively ceases, even though the axon remains intact.

Distribution of plaques

Pathological examination of the brain and spinal cord reveals characteristic plaques of MS which are predominantly, though not exclusively, in the white matter where most myelin is deposited around the axons of the fibre tracts. The lesions are random throughout the cerebral hemispheres, the brainstem, the cerebellum and the spinal cord, but there is a proponderance of lesions in the periventricular white matter, particularly at the anterior and posterior horns of the lateral ventricles, within the optic nerves and chiasm and in the long tracts of the spinal cord.

The microscopic appearance of a plaque depends upon its age. An acute lesion consists of a marked inflammatory reaction with perivenous infiltration of mononuclear cells and lymphocytes (Lucchinetti et al., 1996). There is destruction of myelin and degeneration of oligodendrocytes with relative sparing of the nerve cell body (neurone) and the axon. Axonal integrity may be disrupted early in the inflammatory process and may be the most important determinant of residual damage and disability (Trapp et al., 1998). In older lesions there is infiltration with macrophages (microglial phagocytes), proliferation of astrocytes and laying down of fibrous tissue. Ultimately this results in the production of an acellular scar of fibrosis which has no potential for remyelination or recovery.

Remyelination

Remyelination can occur following an acute inflammatory demyelinating episode. There are, within the brain, oligodendroglial precursors which can mature into oligodendrocytes, infiltrate the demyelinated area and provide partial remyelination of axons (Prineas & Connell, 1978). This can be demonstrated in postmortem tissue and, though remyelination always appears thinner than the original myelin, it may allow functional recovery.

Axonal damage

In addition to the scarring at the site of the inflammatory plaques, later stages of the disease are associated with damage to the axons which may occur both at the site of the original inflammation and separate from the evident inflammatory areas. It is likely that this axonal damage is an important part of the pathology of MS and, though less well-recognised and researched than demyelination, is probably responsible for the more progressive and chronic forms of the illness. This axonal loss can be demonstrated on magnetic resonance imaging (MRI) scans as atrophy of the brain white matter, ventricular dilatation, 'black holes' and degeneration of the long ascending and descending tracts of the brainstem and spinal cord. Brain atrophy is also the main morphological counterpart of psychological deficits and dementia occurring in people with MS (Loseff et al., 1996).

AETIOLOGY AND EPIDEMIOLOGY

Geographical prevalence

Epidemiological research into MS has been bedevilled by problems with ascertainment, identification of the baseline population to estimate prevalence, and the difficulty in interpreting minor changes in small numbers of patients identified. None the less, there appears to be a reproducible finding that the prevalence of MS varies with latitude (see Langton Hewer, 1993, for a review). In equatorial regions the disease is rare, with a prevalence of less than 1 per 100 000, whereas in the temperate climates of northern Europe and North America this figure increases to about 120 per 100 000 and in some areas as high as 200 per 100 000. In the UK it has a prevalence of about 80 000, affecting approximately 120 in every 100 000 of the population (O'Brien, 1987).

There is a similar, but less clearly defined relationship of increasing prevalence with latitude in the southern hemisphere. Some regions with the same latitude have widely differing prevalence of MS; Japan has a relatively lower incidence, whereas Israel has an unexpectedly high level; the two Mediterranean islands of Malta and Sicily have a 10-fold difference in prevalence. Studies within the USA appear to confirm this variation with latitude but may in part reflect genetic differences in the origin of the populations, predominantly derived from European Caucasians (Page et al., 1993).

Genetic influences

Migration studies have lent support to the possibility of incomers adopting the risk and prevalence of MS closer to their host population. Studies have suggested that when migration occurs in childhood, the child assumes the risk of the country of destination but these studies rely upon relatively small numbers of defined cases and interpretation is difficult (Dean & Kurtzke, 1971).

A familial tendency towards MS is now well established but no clear pattern of Mendelian inheritance has been found. Between 10 and 15% of people with MS have an affected relative, which is higher than expected from population prevalence. The highest concordance rate is for identical twins – about 30%; non-identical twins and siblings are affected in 3–5% of cases. Children of people with MS are affected in about 0.5% of cases (Ebers et al., 1986).

A genetic factor is supported by the excess of certain major histocompatibility (MHC) antigens in people with MS. Human leukocyte antigen (HLA) DR_2, DR_3, B_7, and A_3 are all overrepresented and have been suggested as markers for an MS 'susceptibility gene'. Systematic genome screening to attempt to define the number and location of susceptibility genes has been undertaken and identified several regions of linkage and disease association but the probability is that, as in the case of diabetes mellitus, any genetic cause of MS is likely to involve several different genes and be complex (Compston, 2000).

Viral 'epidemic' theory

One other intriguing aspect of epidemiology of MS is the so-called 'epidemics' of MS occurring in the Faroes, the Orkney and Shetland Islands and Iceland in the decades following the Second World War (Kurtzke & Hyllested, 1986). It was suggested that the occupation troops may have introduced an infective agent which, with an assumed incubation period of 2–20 years, resulted in the postwar 'epidemic'. It should be emphasised that, despite extensive research, no such infective agent has ever been isolated. Several factors influence the accuracy of such research and one or two errors in the numerator, when defining the base population, would make huge differences in the interpretation of the data.

Summary

It is highly likely that MS is the product of both environmental and genetic factors. Exposure to some external agent, possibly viral, during childhood in those who are genetically susceptible results in the development of an autoimmune response against native myelin. When the blood–brain barrier is subsequently injured, often in the context of an infective illness, the autoimmunity can manifest, the myelin is attacked and the symptoms develop. Many autoimmune diseases are more common in women than men but whereas some commonly coexist, there is no evidence that other autoimmune diseases are more prevalent in people with MS than in general.

CLINICAL MANIFESTATIONS

There are different types of MS, which are classified in Table 10.1. The disease can run a benign course, with many people able to lead a near-normal life with either mild or moderate disability.

The fundamental clinical characteristic of MS is that episodes of acute neurological disturbance, affecting non-contiguous parts of the CNS, are separated by periods of remission; attacks are disseminated in time and place. The disease can be progressive in nature and initially, resolution following a relapse is usually complete. Some attacks, however, do not recover completely, there remains some continuing disability and further attacks can leave the individual with increasing and permanent neurological disability.

Table 10.1 Classification of multiple sclerosis (MS)

Classification	Definition
Benign MS	One or two relapses, separated by some considerable time, allowing full recovery and not resulting in any disability
Relapsing remitting MS	Characterised by a course of recurrent discrete relapses, interspersed by periods of remission when recovery is either complete or partial
Secondary progressive MS	Having begun with relapses and remissions, the disease enters a phase of progressive deterioration, with or without identifiable relapses, where disability increases even when no relapse is apparent
Primary progressive MS	Typified by progressive and cumulative neurological deficit without remission or evident exacerbation

The disease can enter a phase of secondary progression, in which deterioration occurs without evident exacerbations.

Rarely, particularly with the presentation of paraparesis in older males, the disease may be steadily progressive from the outset. This is termed 'primary progressive' multiple sclerosis.

Multiple sclerosis can also be classified according to the certainty of diagnosis (Table 10.2). It should always be remembered that the diagnosis is one of exclusion; haematological and biochemical investigations are essential to rule out other confounding diseases and, during the course of the disease, the physician must always be willing to reconsider the possibility of differential diagnosis. The classification of disease by the certainty of the diagnosis is of predominant importance for the inclusion of patients into drug trials and for epidemiological studies (Poser et al., 1983; McDonald et al., 2001). Recently an updated classification of disease certainty has been produced by McDonald et al. (2001) and this is currently being assessed.

Early signs and symptoms

It is a common misconception that the first attack of MS strikes as a 'bolt out of the blue', in a young adult previously in good health. In fact, a careful history will often reveal vague feelings of ill health over the preceding months or years, often taking the form of sensory disturbances, aches, pains and lethargy. Not uncommonly

Table 10.2 Classification of multiple sclerosis (MS) according to certainty of diagnosis

Clinically definite MS	Two attacks and clinical evidence of two separate lesions Two attacks; clinical evidence of one lesion and paraclinical evidence of another separate lesion
Laboratory-supported definite MS	Two attacks; either clinical or paraclinical evidence of one lesion and CSF oligoclonal bands One attack; clinical evidence of two separate lesions and CSF oligoclonal bands One attack; clinical evidence of one lesion and paraclinical evidence of another, separate lesion and CSF oligoclonal bands
Clinically probable MS	Two attacks and clinical evidence of one lesion One attack and clinical evidence of two separate lesions One attack; clinical evidence of one lesion and paraclinical evidence of another, separate lesion
Laboratory-supported probable MS	Two attacks and CSF oligoclonal bands

Paraclinical evidence is derived from magnetic resonance imaging, computed tomographic scanning or evoked potentials measurement. CSF, cerebrospinal fluid.

there is a history which clearly suggests a previous episode of demyelination, such as the symptom of double vision, blurring of vision or blindness, rotational vertigo or weakness. Such episodes have often been dismissed as trivial by the patient and, as such, are poorly remembered and may not have caused the person to seek advice from the general practitioner. Demyelination can occur anywhere throughout the white matter of the CNS and therefore the initial presentation of MS is enormously variable.

Visual symptoms

- visual loss
- double vision. (diplopia)

The most common single symptom in presentation is of acute or subacute visual loss in one, or rarely both, eyes. Twenty-five per cent of patients will present in this way, often with pain or discomfort in the eye and the classical symptom of a lesion in an optic nerve (optic neuritis or retrobulbar neuritis) is of loss of colour vision of the eye followed by blurring and ultimately by a central scotoma (blind spot) and visual loss. Improvement usually begins spontaneously within days to weeks; in about 30% of cases recovery will be complete but the remainder will be aware of some reduction in visual acuity or of the brightness of their vision. Following an episode of optic neuritis, the optic disc becomes pale and atrophic (optic atrophy). More than a half of those presenting with optic neuritis will go on to develop other signs of MS. Those who do not may have had a single episode of inflammatory demyelination or they may have some other disease entity.

Double vision (diplopia) is a particularly common presenting complaint and may be due to weakness of muscles innervated by the third, fourth or sixth cranial nerves, or the connections between their nuclei in the brainstem. A very characteristic abnormality is an internuclear ophthalmoplegia due to a lesion of the medial longitudinal fasciculus, in which there is failure of adduction of the adducting eye on lateral gaze with nystagmus in the abducting eye. When a bilateral internuclear ophthalmoplegia is seen in the young adult this is virtually diagnostic of MS.

Neurological deficit

The second most common presenting symptom is a clearly defined episode of neurological deficit, that may occur alone or with others, such as:

- weakness
- numbness
- unsteadiness, imbalance, clumsiness
- slurred speech
- nystagmus
- intention tremor
- trigeminal neuralgia.

Weakness, numbness or tingling can affect one or more limbs. Symptoms may develop acutely over minutes or chronically over weeks to months but more typically they evolve over hours or days. Such a presentation, with or without sphincter involvement, usually indicates an area of spinal demyelination. Lhermitte's phenomenon, which is the sensation of shooting, electric-shock-like sensations radiating down the back and into the legs when the neck is flexed, is a symptom of cervical cord irritation and is commonly described when there is demyelination within the cervical spinal cord.

Not infrequently the disease may begin with the signs and symptoms of cerebellar dysfunction causing unsteadiness, imbalance, clumsiness and dysarthria (slurring of speech). Examination may reveal the patient to have nystagmus (a jerky movement of the eyes), an intention tremor (see Ch. 4) and a cerebellar dysarthria, the combination of which is termed Charcot's triad and is one of the classical features of MS. These symptoms are due to demyelination occurring within the brainstem and there are a wide variety of brainstem syndromes causing cranial nerve disturbances and long tract signs. Other clues are the development of trigeminal neuralgia, or tic douloureux (sharp facial pains), in young adults suggesting the presence of a lesion within the brainstem.

Possible signs and symptoms in the course of MS

A number of symptoms and signs can become established and can be severe, although many can occur at any stage of the disease. These include:

- fatigue
- optic atrophy – with associated visual symptoms
- ophthalmoplegia – with facial sensory and motor symptoms
- cerebellar disease causing nystagmus, ataxia and tremor
- muscle hypertonia
- muscle weakness
- brisk reflexes
- impaired walking ability
- sphincter disturbances
- sexual dysfunction
- psychiatric and psychological disturbances
- symptoms are exacerbated by heat and cold.

General weakness and fatigue are almost invariable symptoms and fatigue may indeed be the presenting symptom in people with MS. There is often optic atrophy with associated decreased visual acuity, a central scotoma or large blind spot and pupillary abnormalities. There may be bilateral internuclear ophthalmoplegia with facial sensory disturbance, or weakness, and a brisk jaw jerk, with slurring speech. There is usually evidence of cerebellar disease with nystagmus, ataxia and tremor which, in its most severe form (dentatorubral) can be incapacitating such that any attempt to move the limbs precipitates violent uncontrollable movements and prevents mobility and feeding. In the limbs there is usually increased tone and weakness in a pyramidal distribution. The reflexes are pathologically brisk; the plantar responses are extensor. Walking is usually affected due to progressive weakness, spasticity and ataxia, and the combination of spasticity and ataxia is suggestive of inflammatory demyelination. Many people will rely on walking aids and a significant proportion will need a wheelchair.

When there is disease affecting the spinal cord, symptoms of sphincter disturbances are common. These range from mild urgency and frequency of micturition to acute retention of urine, constipation and incontinence. Sexual dysfunction is common with erectile and ejaculatory difficulties in men and loss of libido in women. Modern prospective studies of the effect of pregnancy in MS are reassuring and there is no reason to suggest that families should be limited. During pregnancy, the patient has a statistically lower likelihood of relapse, though this may be counterbalanced by a slight increase early in the puerperium.

Psychiatric and psychological disturbances are common (see Ch. 27). Depression is the most common affective disturbance in MS and may compound the underlying physical problems, exaggerating symptoms of lethargy and reduced mobility. With diffuse disease some people develop frank dementia, a few become psychotic and epileptic seizures are seen in 2–3% of cases, an increase of four to five times over that of the normal population. Patients can show evidence of emotional instability or affective disturbance. Euphoria, or inappropriate cheerfulness, was said to be a classical feature of the disease but this is now considered a myth. It is, in practice, quite rare and probably occurs when lesions affect the subcortical white matter of the frontal lobes, resulting in an effective leucotomy.

Patients will frequently record an increase in their symptoms with exercise and with a rise in body temperature. The physiology behind these symptoms is probably the same, due to the fact that the propagation of an action potential along a neurone is greatly affected by temperature. Nerve conduction in an area of demyelination can be critical and paradoxically an increase in temperature, which normally improves conduction, may, in the demyelinated axon, result in a complete conduction block. This phenomenon of worsening of symptoms with exercise and increased temperature is Uhthoff's phenomenon and is most dramatically manifest when patients describe how they are able to get into a hot bath but not able to extricate themselves. Patients should be warned to avoid extremes of temperature and overexertion to avoid this increase in symptoms (Costello et al., 1996).

DIAGNOSIS

To make a clinical definitive diagnosis of MS there has to be a history of two attacks and evidence, clinically, of two separate lesions (Poser et al., 1983). It is also important to remember that other diagnoses should be excluded and, since at presentation all these criteria may not be fulfilled, corroborative paraclinical, laboratory and radiological evidence is usually sought (see O'Connor, 2002, for a review).

Magnetic resonance imaging

MRI of the head and spinal cord is extremely useful in demonstrating the lesions of MS (see Fig. 2.2 in Ch. 2). Typically, high signal lesions on T2-weighted sequences are seen throughout the white matter. Gadolinium enhancement demonstrates areas of active inflammation with breakdown in the blood–brain barrier, which are associated with an acute relapse (Paty et al., 1988). In particular circumstances, as with acute optic neuritis or cervical myelopathy, the demonstration on an MRI scan of disseminated asymptomatic lesions is particularly helpful in confirming the diagnosis and there are rigid criteria for interpreting the MRI scan changes. Newer techniques, such as fluid-attentuated inversion recovery (FLAIR) and magnetisation transfer imaging (MTI), improve the sensitivity and selectivity of MRI in MS (Filippi et al., 1998).

Lumbar puncture

Analysis of the cerebrospinal fluid (CSF) in a patient suspected of having MS is valuable diagnostically. There is production of immunoglobulin (mainly IgG) within the CNS and these antibodies are detected by biochemical analysis of the CSF. Electrophoresis of the CSF allows the immunoglobulin fraction to separate into a few discrete bands (oligoclonal bands) and simultaneous analysis of the immunoglobulin from the blood can demonstrate that these antibodies are confined to the CNS and therefore provide confirmatory evidence of inflammatory CNS disease (Tourtellotte & Booe, 1978).

The antigens that provoke this antibody response have not been identified, nor is it known whether the response is integral to the underlying pathogenic process or a 'bystander reaction'. The CSF normally contains very few cells but during an acute exacerbation of MS there may be an increase in the lymphocytes in the CSF. The level of protein in the CSF is slightly raised but the level of sugar is normal. CSF examination is important in helping to differentiate other diseases from MS and is one of the prerequisites to making a diagnosis of primary progressive MS.

Evoked potentials

A typical history, the signs of more than one lesion affecting the CNS, together with disseminated white-matter lesions shown on MRI and the presence of unmatched oligoclonal bands in the CSF, puts the diagnosis beyond reasonable doubt. However, when one or more of these findings are inconclusive, further

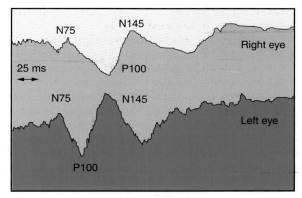

Figure 10.2 Evoked potentials (EP). A visual EP study showing the typical prolonged latency and poor waveform in a lesion of the right optic nerve, such as optic neuritis, in a patient with multiple sclerosis.

support for the diagnosis may be obtained by evoked potential (EP) testing (Misulis, 1993) (Fig. 10.2). These tests, which include visual, brainstem auditory and somatosensory evoked potentials (VEP, BAEP, SSEP) may provide evidence of a subclinical lesion, which has previously been undetected (Halliday & McDonald, 1977). For example, the finding of abnormal SSEPs from both legs, in a patient presenting with blindness in an eye, strongly suggest a lesion in the spinal cord and raises the possibility of MS. The demonstration of more than one lesion is essential in making a secure diagnosis of MS.

THE MANAGEMENT OF MULTIPLE SCLEROSIS

Not all MS patients require active intervention but even those with mild symptoms should be given support and advice from appropriate professionals, relevant to the patient's condition and circumstances. Interventions available for those with moderate to severe disabilities mainly involve drug therapy and physiotherapy. For a recent review of the management of MS, see O'Connor (2002).

There is no proven benefit from any dietary restrictions, though there is suggestive evidence that diets low in animal fat and high in vegetable oil and fish-body oil have potential benefits (Klaus, 1997; Payne, 2001).

Breaking the news

The neurology outpatient clinic is full of people with a history of episodic neurological symptoms, particularly sensory disturbances. The decision to investigate depends upon the individual presentation, consideration of the evidence for relapses, the clinical and objective evidence for multiple sites of disease and the suspicion of the physician. Anxious, polysymptomatic patients with normal neurological examination would not usually be investigated for the possibility of MS and, although the symptom of fatigue is common in MS, it may also be a physiological symptom which is heightened by the presence of depression.

At present many neurologists, jointly with their patients, prefer not to investigate a single resolved attack, especially when there are no objective signs. However, if early treatment with disease-modifying therapies can reduce long-term disability, then the threshold for investigating such patients will be lowered.

The diagnosis of MS is in part the exclusion of other diagnoses, but when the clinical conditions and the laboratory and imaging tests support the diagnosis, then such should be discussed with the patient with the aim of reducing the initial shock and giving an optimistic picture of the prognosis. Once the diagnosis of MS has been intimated, it is important that individuals have time to ask questions and be given the necessary information, often in the form of literature or videos, to enable them to formulate their questions. It is here that the role of an MS specialist nurse is so vital; he or she can visit the patient at home, provide more time than is possible for the physician and hopefully answer many of the relevant questions.

Drug therapy

Many patients with MS do not require drug therapy but when they do, the treatment options are threefold (see Ch. 28):

1. drug management of an acute exacerbation, e.g. steroids
2. symptomatic drug therapy to alleviate individual problems, e.g. antispasticity drugs
3. use of disease-modifying therapies to reduce the underlying pathological process, e.g. interferons.

Since MS is an incurable condition, drug treatments aim primarily to manage acute episodes and specific symptoms. The disease-modifying therapies are, at best, only partially effective to date.

The management of the acute exacerbation

Corticosteroids hasten recovery from an acute exacerbation of MS and improve rehabilitation. The most commonly used agent is intravenous methylprednisolone (see Ch. 28).

Steroids have many significant and potentially serious side-effects, including aseptic necrosis of the femoral head, immunosuppression, sugar intolerance, osteoporosis, weakness of muscles and even psychosis,

all of which may be deleterious to the patient with MS. The most important side-effects are dose-related and guidelines for frequency should be followed.

There is some evidence that the use of steroids in early acute symptoms of MS, specifically optic neuritis, may retard the development of MS during the next 2 years (Beck et al., 1993). However, the use of long-term steroids has no effect on the natural history of the disease and the risks outweigh any benefit.

Symptomatic drug therapy

The effective use of symptomatic agents is intended to make the life of the person with MS more tolerable (Thompson, 2001).

Spasticity One of the most common symptoms of MS is spasticity, often in association with painful cramps and spasms. There are a number of effective agents available, some working at a central level, others peripherally. Baclofen is a GABA-receptor agonist and acts centrally by inhibiting transmission at the spinal level. It reduces tone but may thereby reveal weakness and always needs to be titrated in the individual patient. Its most common side-effects are those of more widespread depression of the CNS, such as drowsiness and sedation. It should always be remembered that legs with hypertonic muscles are weak and a degree of spasticity may have a beneficial splinting action, which aids mobility. The use of baclofen, together with physiotherapy, is often most beneficial. When more intractable spasticity is present, baclofen may be given intrathecally via an implanted subcutaneous pump and the smaller dose thereby required has the advantage of reducing side-effects.

Tizanidine (Zanaflex) is another centrally acting agent which is less sedating and has less of an underlying effect on muscle than baclofen but is potentially hepatotoxic (see Ch. 28). Again it must be used by titration against the symptoms and spasticity in the individual patient and is used together with physiotherapy to improve mobility.

Dantrolene sodium reduces contraction of skeletal muscles by a direct action on excitation–contraction coupling, decreasing the amount of calcium released from the sarcoplasmic reticulum. Its action is more pronounced on the fast fibres in the muscle, which results in a diminution of reflex activity and spasticity rather than voluntary contraction. It is therefore theoretically less likely to cause the side-effect of weakness but its major side-effect is of generalised fatigue.

Benzodiazepines, such as diazepam and clonazepam, may have a role to play in the management of spasticity, though they are more likely than other agents to result in drowsiness and are therefore most useful for night-time spasms and cramps when their sedation is advantageous.

In severe painful spasticity, where the aim is to alleviate the distressing symptoms or to aid nursing care rather than to restore function, there are a number of more invasive procedures which may be useful. Local injection of botulinum toxin causes a flaccid paralysis in the muscles injected, with minimal systemic side-effects. The effect usually lasts for 3 months and may be repeated indefinitely (Snow et al., 1990). More graduated doses of the toxin can improve mobility in people with less severe spasticity. The more destructive techniques of intrathecal or peripheral nerve chemical blocks, or surgery, are now rarely required.

When treating the symptom of spasticity it is important to remember that it may often be worsened by triggers such as constipation or underlying infection, particularly urinary tract infection or decubitus ulceration. Infective causes should be sought and treated whenever spasticity appears unexpectedly or worsens.

Pain People with MS develop pain for a variety of reasons, some of which are central and some peripheral. Plaques affecting the ascending sensory pathways frequently cause unpleasant dysaesthesiae, or allodynia, on the skin, often with paraesthesiae. Such central pain is most responsive to centrally acting analgesics, such as the antiepileptics carbamazepine, sodium valproate or gabapentin. It may also respond to tricyclic antidepressants, such as amitriptyline or dothiepin. Alternatively, electrostimulation with cutaneous nerve stimulation (see Ch. 23) or dorsal column stimulation (Tallis et al., 1983) can be effective.

The second cause of pain is the spasms described as part of spasticity in the previous section. The third is that the abnormal posture, so often adopted by people using walking aids or in wheelchairs, itself results in pain and discomfort in the back and limbs. These symptoms are often best helped with physiotherapy and simple analgesics.

The lancinating neuralgic pains, such as trigeminal neuralgia, may respond to antiepileptic therapy with carbamazepine or gabapentin but they can also be helped by steroids, particularly if occurring in the course of an acute exacerbation. If these agents are not effective, then trigeminal neuralgia may respond to surgical intervention; a lesion is placed within the Gasserian ganglion.

Cannabis is thought to be helpful for MS patients but is not used widely and is currently under investigation. Principles of pain management are discussed in Chapter 26.

Bladder, bowel and sexual dysfunction These symptoms, which often occur in combination, are due to spinal cord disease and have a major impact upon the patient (see Barnes, 1993, for a review).

Bladder disturbance Pelvic floor exercises may help in women and the combination of clean intermittent self-catheterisation (CISC) and the use of anticholinergic agents, such as oxybutinin or tolterodine, usually helps to overcome the problem of incomplete emptying and hyperreflexia, which are the common causes of this syndrome. The most appropriate approach to bladder management is to recognise the common symptoms of urgency and frequency, to measure a residual urine by ultrasound after the patient has passed urine and if this is greater than 100 ml, educate the patient in CISC and prescribe a bladder relaxant. If there is less than 100 ml residual then the use of a bladder relaxant alone is probably sufficient.

When nocturnal frequency and enuresis cause a problem, the synthetic diuretic desmopressin (DDAVP) may be used but care should be taken to avoid hyponatraemia (low serum sodium), particularly in the elderly.

When there is severe bladder spasticity, the intravesical installation of the neurotoxic agent capsiacin may reduce detrusor hyperreflexia.

It is rare now to require permanent catheterisation but, when necessary, this is better provided by the suprapubic route and ultimately urinary diversion may be necessary.

Bowel disturbances Constipation is the most common symptom but it may be complicated by faecal incontinence intermittently. A bowel-training programme is usually most successful with the use of iso-osmotic laxatives and ensuring adequate fibre intake.

Sexual dysfunction Erectile dysfunction in men is a common problem and is now helped by the use of sildenafil, which has been demonstrated, in a randomised placebo controlled trial, to be effective (DasGupta & Fowler, 2003). Alternative methods are still available but the use of intracorporeal papaverine has now been replaced by prostaglandin.

In women there are many factors which may affect the expression of sexuality, including neurological symptoms from sacral segments, such as diminished genital sensitivity, reduced orgasmic capacity and decreased lubrication (Hulter & Lundberg, 1995).

Both sexes are affected by leg spasticity, ataxia, vertigo and fatigue. Counselling may be appropriate in some cases and referral to a specialist counselling service, such as SPOD, may be useful (see Appendix).

Fatigue Almost all patients with MS will, at some time, complain of fatigue and in the majority of cases it is regarded as being the most disabling symptom. Pharmacological treatment is disappointing, though amantidine and pemoline have been suggested to be beneficial. Other agents used in the past have now been replaced by the less addictive modafinil. Reassurance and graded exercise programmes are considered to be at least as effective (see 'Physical management', below).

Tremor The treatment of tremor in MS, as in most other situations, is difficult (see Ch. 4). Minor action tremors may be helped by the use of beta-blockers, such as propranolol, or low-dose barbiturates such as primidone. The more disabling intention tremor of cerebellar disease and the most disabling dentato-rubral thalamic tremor, which prevents any form of movement or activity, is refractory to treatment. There have been reports of agents such as clonazepam, carbamazepine and choline chloride helping individuals, and by serendipity, the antituberculous agent isoniazid has been shown to be effective but should be given with a vitamin B_6 supplement. None of these treatments are particularly effective and the possibility of deep brain stimulation is now being increasingly considered. Surgical treatments are most effective for unilateral tremor; bilateral treatment is associated with significant morbidity and mortality.

Psychological symptoms Depression is the most common symptom and, if clinically significant, requires treatment with antidepressant medication, either a tricyclic agent or a selective serotonin reuptake inhibitor (see Ch. 28). Cognitive dysfunction is reported to occur in up to 60% of patients. Psychological issues and behavioural management are discussed in Chapter 27.

Epilepsy Epilepsy is rare in MS but more common than in a peer group. It is treated with anticonvulsants (see Ch. 28). Electroencephalography (EEG) will identify unrelated primary generalised epilepsy, but most seizures in MS are focal and may cause secondary generalisation.

Disease-modifying therapies

During the past decade, two forms of immunomodulatory therapy, beta-interferon and glatiramer acetate, have been shown in large controlled, randomised clinical trials to be effective in reducing the frequency and severity of relapses and delaying the development of disability in people with relapsing remitting MS. Immunosuppressive therapy has also received much attention. For a review of disease-modifying therapies, see Corboy et al. (2003).

Interferon-β Interferons are naturally occurring polypeptides produced by the body in response to viral infection and inflammation. There are three types, alpha (α), beta (β) and gamma (γ), all of which have antiviral, antiproliferative and immunomodulatory properties. All have been tried in MS because of the postulation that the disease might have a viral origin. Interferon-α may have some effect, but requires further study; interferon-γ has been shown to be deleterious. Interferon-β, however, has been shown to be beneficial.

An initial trial, giving interferon-β by intrathecal route, showed a reduction in attack rate and was followed by a large trial in North America using the bacterially derived product interferon β-1b (IFBN Multiple Sclerosis Study Group, 1993). This showed that high doses of interferon β-1b, given subcutaneously on alternate days, reduced clinical relapses by one-third over 2 years as compared to placebo. There was a dramatic reduction in the changes seen on the MRI scans in the treated group but the study was not powered to show an effect upon progression of disability (Paty & Li, 1993).

Subsequent studies using a mammalian cell-line-derived interferon β-1a have shown benefit, in both frequency of attack and in development of disability (Jacobs et al., 1996; PRISMS Study Group, 1998), and three agents are now available:

1. the original interferon β-1b (Betaferon),
2. the subcutaneous interferon β-1a given thrice-weekly (Rebif),
3. the intramuscular form of interferon β-1a (Avonex), given once-weekly.

These agents are licensed for use in relapsing remitting MS and a national trial is underway in the UK to compare the different agents in a novel 'risk-sharing scheme', in which the proof of efficiency in reducing attack rate and disability, as well as in cost-effectiveness, is being studied.

There are common side-effects of injection site reactions and flu-like symptoms; the latter are ameliorated by the use of non-steroidal anti-inflammatory agents. A variable number of patients, between 4 and 40%, may develop antibodies to the interferon, though the effect of these antibodies is still under review.

The effect of the agents in people with secondary progressive disease only appears to be beneficial in those who have acute exacerbations occurring in addition to their progressing disease (European Study Group on Interferon β-1b in Secondary Progressive Multiple Sclerosis, 1998) and to date there has been no benefit shown in people with primary progressive illness. The use of these immunosuppressive agents may be effective only in that phase of the disease proven to be inflammatory and immune-mediated, and not in the phase of more prolonged axonal injury to the CNS.

Glatiramer acetate The synthetic polypeptide glatiramer acetate made to imitate part of the antigenic area of myelin basic protein, and therefore to block the effect of putative antibodies upon the disease process, has been shown to be effective in reducing relapse rate and improving disability in a randomised controlled clinical trial (Johnson et al., 1995). It has to be taken parenterally (see Ch. 28). It is well tolerated, freer from side-effects than the interferons and is now widely licensed for use in relapsing remitting MS. There is less evidence about its effectiveness in secondary progressive disease and none about its effectiveness in primary progressive disease, though a large trial is underway.

Immunosuppression Despite our incomplete understanding of the pathogenesis of MS, there is strong circumstantial evidence of an autoimmune process. There is increasing interest in treating MS with immunosuppression and cytotoxic agents ranging from azathioprine, methotrexate and cyclophosphamide to cyclosporin A and total lymphoid irradiation. There is even a trial of bone marrow transplantation but it remains a research tool (Fassas et al., 2002). With each of these agents, some claims of initial success have been encouraging but have not generally stood up to more rigorous trials. A great difficulty in assessing the effectiveness of such treatments in MS is the unpredictable progression of the disease and the possibility of a placebo effect (Goodin et al., 2002).

Despite such reservations, immunosuppressive agents are used worldwide and a recent meta-analysis suggested that the use of azathioprine shows a modest reduction in both attack rate and in the rate of progression of the disease (Yudkin et al., 1991). It is recognised that 6 months is necessary for the agent to show its therapeutic effect. These agents are usually reserved for patients with a particularly malignant form of MS and in whom other treatments have not prevented relentless progression.

Cyclophosphamide has been commonly used in some parts of Europe and North America but it is difficult to evaluate in a double-blind fashion because of its marked side-effects (Weiner et al., 1993) and it is not used widely in the UK because of its toxicity.

Methotrexate has also been used and shown to have some effect on retarding the rate of progression in patients with progressive disease (Goodkin et al., 1995), but further corroborative evidence should be obtained.

The most recent arrival in the field of treatment of progressing disease is mitoxantrone (Hartung et al., 2002). This potentially cardiotoxic drug (Ghalie et al., 2002a) is given in boluses at intervals over a period of years. Again, it is necessary to monitor carefully white cells, since it significantly suppresses the T cells (Ghalie et al., 2002b), but it does have some beneficial effect and is probably the most used aggressive agent at this time.

Trials have been undertaken with other aggressive therapies, such as Campath 1H, and shown to have some effect in control of the disease. There are, however, significant problems with thyroid dysfunction after this agent and further work is required (Moreau et al., 1994).

PHYSICAL MANAGEMENT

People with MS are often referred for physiotherapy, or request it for themselves, when they experience loss of movement skill or the ability to perform functional activities. Not all patients deteriorate to this degree but if they reach this stage, the disease has caused irreversible damage to the CNS and created a level of impairment which results in noticeable and persistent disability. This section focuses on progressive conditions but the MS Healthcare Standards (Freeman et al., 1997a, 2001) recommend early intervention for those with mild impairment (see below).

The attitude of the physiotherapist towards the person with MS during their initial encounters is crucial, as it will set the scene for the therapist–patient relationship and any ensuing programme of physiotherapy. The patient may fear that the therapist could expose further physical weaknesses and insufficiencies. Physiotherapists need to be aware that the same professional skills that can help the patient can also undermine self-confidence.

The success of treatment should not be determined by whether or not the patient improves, but rather by whether he or she achieves the best level of activity, relevant to lifestyle, at each stage of the disease (De Souza, 1990) and whether the patient's own goals have been reached (see Ch. 22). In order to achieve this, the treatment of those with MS is best approached with a philosophy of care (Ashburn & De Souza, 1988).

Approaches to physiotherapy

Physiotherapy for those with MS acts mainly at the level of disability and is unlikely to modify the lesions or change the progression of the disease. For the majority of people with MS, it is likely that physiotherapy will be one of several treatments and should, therefore, address the issues of disability within the context of the aims of other treatments and the needs of the individual. In addition, people with MS are likely to be engaged in several self-help activities they value and therapy should build on this motivation (O'Hara et al., 2000; see also Ch. 22).

An approach to physiotherapy that views the individual in his or her social, family, work and cultural roles informs the physiotherapist about the impact of disablement on the individual's lifestyle. This is important in the case of MS as it mostly affects young adults who, when diagnosed, will face an average of 35–42 years living with this disease (Poser et al., 1989). A shift in focus away from problems and towards a more positive attitude, which considers disablement as just one of a variety of ways in which a normal life may be pursued, has been called for (Oliver, 1983). An understanding of the priorities of individuals with disability, the value they attach to different activities and their choices for conducting their lives should have a profound influence on the physiotherapy provided (Williams, 1987; see also Ch. 22).

The approach to physiotherapy should therefore be patient-centred, with the patient taking an active participatory role in treatment. This will include consultation for joint decision-making and goal-setting, the opportunity to exercise choice and the provision of information so that the patient has feedback on progress and knowledge of his or her level of ability.

Principles of physiotherapy

Treatment plans should be flexible and responsive to the needs of the patient as they change over time. Although each patient should be considered as an individual, Ingle et al. (2002) have determined what deterioration might be expected over a 2-year period in progressive MS, in terms of the Kurtzke Scale (Kurtzke, 1983), walking ability (10-m timed walk), and upper-limb ability (nine-hole peg-test). Therapy should encompass not only the changes due to progression of MS, but also life changes such as employment, pregnancy and childbirth, parenthood and ageing. The principles of physiotherapy have been described by Ashburn & De Souza (1988) and further by De Souza (1990). These include:

- Encourage development of strategies of movement
- Encourage learning of motor skills
- Improve the quality of patterns of movement
- Minimise abnormalities of muscle tone
- Emphasise the functional application of physiotherapy
- Provide support to maintain motivation and co-operation, and reinforce therapy
- Implement preventive therapy
- Educate the person towards a greater understanding of the symptoms of MS and how they affect daily living.

Four primary aims of physiotherapy were also identified:

1. Maintain and increase range of movement (ROM)
2. Encourage postural stability
3. Prevent contractures
4. Maintain and encourage weight-bearing.

The underlying principle for all the above is one of building on, and extending, the patient's abilities. Emphasis during assessment and treatment should be on what the individual can and does achieve, rather than on what he or she fails to achieve.

> **Key point**
>
> Emphasis during assessment and treatment should be on what the patient achieves, rather than on what he or she fails to achieve

Assessment

Assessment is discussed in Chapter 3 but aspects of specific importance to MS will be addressed here.

Fatigue

As mentioned above, fatigue is a well-documented symptom of MS; it is reported to occur in 78% of patients (Freal et al., 1984). It is related to neither the amount of disability nor to mood state (Krupp et al., 1988). The assessment of fatigue should include:

- the daily pattern of fatigue
- times of the day when energy is high, reasonable and low
- activities or occurrences (e.g. hot weather) which worsen or alleviate fatigue
- the functional impact of fatigue on everyday activities
- whether fatigue is localised to specific muscle groups (e.g. ankle dorsiflexors), a body part (e.g. hand or leg), or functional system (e.g. vision or speech)
- whether central fatigue is causing overall excessive tiredness.

Formal, standardised assessment of fatigue can be carried out, if appropriate, for reports, audit or research, using the Fatigue Severity Scale (Krupp et al., 1989). The results of any physical assessments carried out on people with MS can easily be influenced by their fatigue. It is not unusual for MS patients to have a worse outcome when undergoing a battery of tests and a better one when tests are distributed over time or rest periods are given. Excessive fatigue, in association with poor physical fitness, has a deleterious effect on activities of daily living (ADL: Fisk et al., 1994).

Activities of daily living

It is important to know exactly what information is required from an assessment of ADL. If the information needed concerns what the MS person can do overall, then the assessment requirement is one of the physical capacity of the individual to complete the tasks in the ADL instrument. However, if the information needed is about what the person does on a daily basis, it will require an exploration of the person's social, family and cultural roles. Once again, the effects of fatigue may have a profound influence on how choices are made. For example, a person may choose to have help to wash and dress in the morning in order to save energy for the journey to work, or may elect to have shopping done so as to have sufficient time and energy to collect the children from school.

It should be noted that many of the domestic (e.g. changing and bathing the baby, or playing with children) and social (e.g. talking on the telephone, or surfing the internet) activities carried out by young adults are not reflected in the available standardised ADL assessments.

Cognitive assessment

The importance of cognitive dysfunction and its assessment in MS has been brought to the attention of research and clinical readership (Rao, 1990). Detailed cognitive assessment is best carried out by a health care professional with expertise in the field (e.g. clinical psychologist). The physiotherapist should ensure that he or she accesses such assessments when available, as limitations identified will inform the provision of therapy (see Ch. 27). Where expert cognitive assessment and diagnosis is unavailable, the physiotherapist may find simple, generic assessments for memory, mood and visuomotor action helpful.

Patient self-assessment

Participation of the patient in assessment should be encouraged by the physiotherapist so that self-evaluation is instrumental to the process. This evaluation should address the following issues:

- the individual's perception of his or her abilities and limitations
- ability to cope
- willingness to change
- personal priorities and expectations of physiotherapy.

The self-assessment should be formally documented, dated, and form part of the assessment record in the physiotherapy and/or medical notes.

Planning treatment

The assessment forms the basis for developing a plan of treatment, deciding the goals and priorities and formulating a process which will put the plan into action. All these issues must be negotiated with the patient, who provides the context within which physiotherapy must operate from his or her experience of living with the disease and preferred lifestyle. A scheme for negotiating a goal-directed plan of physiotherapy has been suggested by De Souza (1997). It highlights the active roles played by both the physiotherapist and the patient and advocates shared responsibility for the actions to be taken in order for the plan to be operational.

A guided self-care programme suitable for people with MS living in the community has recently been demonstrated to have beneficial effects (O'Hara et al., 2002). It facilitates the priorities of the MS person to be central to the planning and execution of the programme, and promotes client empowerment to help those with MS pursue strategies which are beneficial to their health.

In order to have a good chance of succeeding, a plan of physiotherapy should have the following features:

- meets the patient's needs
- provides a focus on agreed goals
- is a feasible and negotiated plan of action
- is progressive in nature
- harmonises with other concurrent treatments
- is acceptable to the individual and carers, as appropriate
- is flexible to changing circumstances.

The need for good communication and interpersonal skills employed throughout the process of therapy cannot be overemphasised.

Physiotherapy interventions

Physiotherapy is a widely used treatment for MS patients, who often demand it and have high expectations of its value. As Matthews (1985) stated: 'Every account of the rehabilitation of patients with multiple sclerosis includes physiotherapy and every physician uses it.' However, research evidence of the specific benefits of physiotherapy is scarce despite widespread recommendations for its use. This is not surprising as the majority of physiotherapy treatments for a wide range of conditions, including MS, have developed ad hoc from an empirical base rather than from a scientific research base. None the less, all have the underlying aim of reducing disability and increasing ability. Two issues are pertinent in planning physiotherapy: (1) timing – when should therapy be given? and (2) content – what therapy should be given?

Timing of intervention

The issues here concern:

- when therapy should be given in the course of the disease
- how long it should continue
- how often it should be given.

Early intervention was seen by some authors as desirable, though not always possible (Todd, 1986; Ashburn & De Souza, 1988). However, there were few suggestions advocating therapy on the basis of disease duration; rather, patients are referred for physiotherapy, or seek it for themselves, when MS has resulted in a noticeable disability rather than at the time of diagnosis (De Souza, 1990).

Recently published MS health care standards describe appropriate support at diagnosis (Freeman et al., 1997a, 2001). Although specific physiotherapy treatment is not recommended at this stage, the physiotherapist should be appraised of the standards and be able to participate as part of the care team. General exercises, tone management, posture and fatigue management are recommended for those with minimal impairment (Freeman et al., 1997a, 2001), while, based on research evidence, inpatient and outpatient rehabilitation is recommended for those with moderate disability (Solari et al., 1999; Wiles et al., 2001; Freeman et al., 1997b, 1999; Di Fabio et al., 1997, 1998).

It is not known whether rest or exercise is more appropriate during a relapse and the lack of research in this area may be due to the random nature of attacks and the wide fluctuations in symptoms seen in relapsing patients. Despite this, some authors have recommended therapy during recovery from relapse and considered it effective (Alexander & Costello, 1987), but evidence of effectiveness was not provided. Another argument could be that maintenance of ability during relapse might enable the patient to maximise the benefit of remission.

Several authors have favoured long-term intervention (Greenspun et al., 1987; Ashburn & De Souza, 1988; Sibley, 1988) but optimum frequency of treatment was not examined. One study reported significant benefits of long-term intervention in a prospective group study of non-relapsing MS subjects (De Souza & Worthington, 1987). Those gaining benefit received on average 8 h of physiotherapy a month for 18 consecutive months. Patients receiving less physiotherapy did not show significant improvements in function. On the basis of the scant information available, the issue remains open regarding frequency and timing of treatment.

Key points	
Timing of intervention	
• Support at diagnosis	No specific physiotherapy treatment but the physiotherapist has a role as part of the care team
• Minimal impairment	General exercise; management of tone, posture and fatigue
• Moderate disability	Inpatient and outpatient rehabilitation, as appropriate
• Long-term intervention	Frequency and timing of treatment require further study

Type of intervention

Very little research is available to indicate what type of physiotherapy should constitute the content of a treatment programme, although many opinions have been expressed.

Stretching A clear consensus, and some experimental evidence, exists in favour of muscle stretching (see Ch. 25). Research on a small number of patients has shown that muscle hypertonus can be reduced, and voluntary range of lower-limb movement increased, by muscle stretching (Odeen, 1981). In addition, muscle stretching was considered valuable by many authors (e.g. Alexander & Costello, 1987; Sibley, 1988; De Souza, 1990; Arndt et al., 1991) and no reports have so far come to light which counsel against its use.

Active exercise Active exercises have been advocated in the treatment of MS but for varying reasons. They have been suggested for retraining function (De Souza, 1984), muscle strengthening (Alexander & Costello, 1987), retraining of balance and co-ordination (De Souza, 1990; Arndt et al., 1991) and maintaining ROM (Ashburn & De Souza, 1988).

Despite the support for active exercises for MS, only a few studies have investigated their use. One reason for such general agreement may be the predilection of physiotherapists for exercise regimens for a wide variety of conditions. However, it has been shown that chronic disuse of muscles in MS causes not only weakness but also extreme fatiguability (Lenman et al., 1989) as it does in normal muscle. This could imply that active exercises are beneficial for maintaining and increasing strength and endurance, but this needs to be examined in MS patients.

A physiotherapy programme utilising both muscle stretching and free active exercise was evaluated in a prospective long-term study of MS patients (De Souza & Worthington, 1987) which showed that, whilst the motor impairments worsened, subjects who had an intensive physiotherapy programme deteriorated significantly less than those who had had less treatment. In addition, functional, balance and daily living activities were also significantly improved in the group receiving more treatment. This study is one of the few which has provided research-based evidence for the efficacy of a physiotherapy programme for MS.

Therapeutic exercises causing fatigue were widely thought to be damaging and the consensus is that moderate exercise is appropriate but that too much, which precipitates fatigue, is inappropriate. However, few studies have been carried out to determine the appropriate quantities of active exercises (see 'Aerobic exercises', below), and fatigue thresholds may differ between individuals.

Weight-resisted exercises Weight-resisted exercises were advocated by Alexander & Costello (1987) for MS, despite an earlier finding that a large proportion of patients deteriorated (Russell & Palfrey, 1969). This type of treatment would seem to be inappropriate for inclusion in a physiotherapy programme.

Aerobic exercises Aerobic exercise is a relatively new approach to treatment for MS, as it is for other neurological disorders (see Ch. 29 for a review). Current available evidence indicates that there are benefits for patients, particularly those with mild disability. This approach to treatment aims to increase overall physical activity and cardiovascular effort, prevent general muscular weakness and reduce health risks due to deconditioning and disuse.

Aerobic exercise programmes for MS of up to 6 months have been shown significantly to increase physical fitness, improve mood and enhance cardiovascular demand (Petajan et al., 1996; Tantacci et al., 1996; Ponichtera-Mulcare et al., 1997). Benefits to gait have also been reported (Rodgers et al., 1999). Increases in activity level, reduced fatigue and improvement in health perception have recently been reported for an aerobic exercise training programme (5×30 min per week of bicycle exercise) for people with mild to moderate MS (Kurtze scores 2.5–6.5; mean 4.6, SD 1.2) over a period of only 4 weeks (Mostert & Kesselring, 2002). Adverse reactions to aerobic exercises are reported to be low in the above studies. For example, Mostert & Kesselring (2002) reported symptom exacerbations in the form of increased spasticity, paraesthesia and vertigo in 10% of 63 graded maximal exercise tests, and in only 6% of 180 training sessions. Such effects were not reported for other conditions and could have been due to heat sensitivity (Ch. 29).

Walking aids Physiotherapy to maintain ambulation has been considered beneficial by many authors (e.g. Burnfield & Frank, 1988) but no agreement on the use of lower-limb bracing could be determined (Alexander & Costello, 1987; Arndt et al., 1991). Walking aids were also widely recommended by the above authors but care must be taken to avoid postural instability and deformity with long-term use (Todd, 1982). It would seem, therefore, that opinion is generally in favour of patients using aids if required, but warns against overreliance. Walking aids are discussed further below.

Hydrotherapy, heat and cold Many anecdotal reports exist as to the usefulness or otherwise of hydrotherapy and heat or cold therapy. Burnfield (1985), as both a doctor and an MS patient, recommended avoiding hydrotherapy as 'it may make things worse and bring on fatigue'. Conversely, Alexander & Costello (1987) stated that exercises in a pool could be beneficial. However, these reports lack specificity as they do not refer to any particular symptoms or signs being affected by the treatment.

With respect to heat and cold, Forsythe (1988), another doctor with MS, reported that warm baths aided muscle-stretching exercises. Burnfield (1985), however, found that cool baths were beneficial, but also described one case where this treatment had a 'disastrous' result. Descriptions were not given as to what constituted either the benefit or the disaster, but these anecdotal reports serve to highlight the individual nature of responses to intervention experienced by some MS patients.

Clear warnings against heat therapy in MS were given by Block & Kester (1970), who thought that it caused severe exacerbation of clinical and subclinical deficits, while De Souza (1990) warned against the use of ice, or ice-cold water, in patients with compromised circulation, as this can cause vasoconstriction and further reduce the circulation.

Electrical stimulation Low-frequency neuromuscular electrical stimulation can be beneficial for some MS patients (Worthington & De Souza, 1990) but the need for careful selection of patients for this form of treatment is emphasised as it does not benefit all MS patients. In addition, neuromuscular stimulation is recommended as an adjunct to other physiotherapy, mainly active exercise and muscle stretching (see Ch. 23).

Conclusions In the absence of any sound evidence, and no consensus of clinical opinion regarding hydrotherapy, heat or cold therapy, and the small amount of evidence available on muscle stimulation, these treatments may not be appropriate for general application in MS, but may prove helpful to some individuals. On the basis of available evidence, the two components of physiotherapy likely to be the most useful in MS are muscle stretching and active exercises. It is further suggested that the exercises should incorporate training to improve ambulation, and also be paced so as to account for fatigue. These treatment components may be appropriate for a physiotherapy intervention programme for the majority of people with MS, and are further described by De Souza (1984, 1990), and Ashburn & De Souza (1988), and are summarised below.

A physiotherapy treatment programme

The programme proposed by Ashburn & De Souza (1988) consisted of active and active-assisted free exercises based upon 12 core exercises, and a simple muscle-stretching regimen. The emphasis of the active exercise programme was on functional activities, and the use of the exercises to achieve a functional goal was taught. For example, a sequence which incorporated knee rolling, side sitting (stretch exercise), low kneeling, high kneeling, half kneeling and standing would achieve the functional activity of rising up from the floor. Other gross body motor skills, such as transferring, may be retrained in a similar way. Benefits to MS patients from facilitation (impairment-based) and task-oriented (disability-focused) physiotherapy were observed, with no differences between the two approaches (Lord et al., 1998).

The active exercise programme could also be adjusted to emphasise balance activities. These incorporated 'hold' techniques into the basic exercise programme to encourage postural stabilisation and stimulate balance reactions. Patients were required to hold certain positions and postures for a few seconds to begin with and subsequently gradually to increase the period. For example, the position of high kneeling was required to be held for a 10-s period without the patient using any upper-limb support, while an upright standing posture utilising a narrow base of support and no upper-limb aid was required to be held for 30 s. Patients could self-monitor their progress and were encouraged to note their levels of achievement.

The programme may be adjusted to individual levels of ability, e.g. by diversifying exercises in a variety of sitting or kneeling positions if the individual is unable to stand. The emphasis of the different exercises may also be adjusted according to the needs of individuals. Those whose major problems are spasticity, and muscle and joint stiffness, require an emphasis on stretching and increasing active and passive ROM. Those with problems of ataxia and instability need more emphasis on the smooth co-ordination of movements, and on balance and postural stability. The majority of MS patients will have a combination of different motor symptoms, and a balanced programme will need to be constructed.

Management of the MS person with mainly hypertonic symptoms

Physiotherapy for an MS patient with predominantly symptoms of spasticity is generally similar to that for other neurological patients with the same problem (see Ch. 25). However, some specific issues need to be attended to in MS, and the progressive nature of the disease borne in mind. Most importantly, any decision to reduce the level of muscle tone must have a clear objective, and an identifiable and achievable functional benefit. A high level of tone is useful for some MS patients, e.g. those who use their spasticity for standing, transferring or for utilising a swing-to or swing-through gait pattern for crutch-walking (De Souza, 1990; Ko Ko, 1999). For these people, spasticity should not be reduced at the expense of their mobility.

For other MS patients, spasticity will hinder their ability, masking movement and adding to the effort of voluntary actions, so reduction of muscle tone may be appropriate for these patients. However, careful monitoring of any movement is required during the reduction of tone, as in MS the spasticity often overlies other symptoms, such as weakness or ataxia, which are more difficult for the patient to cope with than the spasticity (De Souza, 1990).

Some MS patients exhibit an extremely changeable distribution of tone in different positions, e.g. lower-limb extensor hypertonus in standing and flexor hypertonus in lying. These features are probably due to lesions disrupting CNS pathways which control limb and trunk postural responses to muscular information. Irrespective of the variability of spasticity in MS patients, there are certain muscle groups which tend to exhibit the symptom more than others. It should be recalled that, where there is a hypertonic muscle group, there is also generally another muscle group, often the antagonists, which exhibits low tone. These imbalances, if allowed to become permanent, will result in contractures and deformity. The muscle groups most often developing contracture in people with MS are:

- trunk rotators
- trunk lateral flexors
- hip flexors
- hip adductors
- knee flexors
- ankle plantarflexors
- inverters of the foot.

Spasticity in the upper limbs is less common than in the lower limbs; the muscle groups most often affected are the wrist and finger flexors, and the shoulder adductors and internal rotators. Occasionally, the forearm pronators and elbow flexors are affected, but the full flexion pattern of spasticity, as seen in the hemiplegic arm, is rare, though not unknown, in MS.

Physiotherapy for spasticity is described in Chapter 25. With MS, simple strategies to alleviate spasticity, which patients can carry out for themselves, are preferable. The techniques of choice are muscle stretching and the use of positions which retain prolonged muscle stretch (Ashburn & De Souza, 1988; De Souza, 1990).

The effectiveness of physiotherapy on reducing spasticity in MS has been demonstrated using F-wave amplitude as a measure of motor neurone excitability (Rosche et al., 1996).

Management of the MS person with ataxia

Ataxia is one of the major motor symptoms affecting people with MS. It rarely occurs in isolation, and is most commonly seen with other motor symptoms, notably spasticity. It is a disturbance that, independently of motor weakness, alters the direction and extent of a voluntary movement and impairs the sustained voluntary and reflex muscle contraction necessary for maintaining posture and equilibrium.

The main problem that ataxic MS patients show is an inability to make movements which require groups of muscles to act together in varying degrees of co-contraction. The difficulty is easily observed during gait as the single-stance phase requires the cocontraction of leg muscles in order to support body weight, whilst at the same time a co-ordinated change in the relative activity of the muscles is needed to move the body weight forward (e.g. from a flexed hip position at heel strike to an extended hip position at toe-off). The ataxic patient has greatest difficulty with this phase of gait and either uses the stance leg as a rigid strut, or staggers as co-ordination is lost. Compensation is often afforded by walking aids which reduce the need for weight support through stance, whilst providing at least two (one upper- and one lower-limb) points of

Table 10.3 Types of ataxia and associated motor disorders

Sensory ataxia
- A high-stepping gait pattern
- More reliance on visual or auditory
- information about leg or foot position

Vestibular ataxia
- Disturbed equilibrium in standing and walking
- Loss of equilibrium reactions
- A wide-based, staggering gait pattern

Cerebellar ataxia
- Disturbance in the rate, regularity and force of movement
- Loss of movement co-ordination
- Overshooting of target (dysmetria)
- Decomposition of movement (dyssynergia)
- Loss of speed and rhythm of alternating movements (dysdiadochokinesia)
- Inco-ordination of agonist–antagonist muscles and loss of the continuity of muscle contraction (tremor, e.g. intention tremor)

---

support in all phases of gait. The reduction of upper-limb weight-bearing has been considered an essential component for retaining functional gait in ataxic patients (Brandt et al., 1981). Using walking aids, the ataxic patient can ambulate with the hips remaining in flexion, thus eliminating the need to effect a co-ordinated change from hip flexion to extension while bearing weight through the stance leg.

The aim of physiotherapy is to counteract the postural and movement adjustments made by the ataxic patient in order to encourage postural stability and dynamic weight-shifting, and to increase the smooth co-ordination of movement. It is also to prevent the preferred postures of ataxic patients, adopted to eliminate their instability, from becoming functional or fixed contractures (De Souza, 1990). The features of postural abnormality are:

- an exaggerated lumbar lordosis
- an anterior pelvic tilt
- flexion at the hips
- hyperextension of the knees
- weight towards the heel parts of the feet
- clawed toes (as they grip the ground).

The different types of ataxia have been reviewed by Morgan (1980) and are summarised in Table 10.3 with the main features of motor dysfunction. In MS there may be a mixture of cerebellar, vestibular and sensory components depending on the sites of the lesions.

Ataxia is a very complex movement disorder and there is little research evidence to inform the content of

Table 10.4 Assessment and treatment approaches for patients with ataxia

Predominant problem	Dysfunction expressed in	Primary aims of treatment
Maintaining equilibrium	Weight-bearing and weight transference	Increase postural stability Enhance control of the centre of gravity in weight-shifting Encourage maintenance of the control of the centre of gravity in movement from one position to another Progress from a wide to a narrow base of support
Co-ordination of dynamic movement	Patterns of movement	Enhance smoothness of control of movement patterns Progress from simple to complex patterns Progress from fast to slow movements
Located in body axis and trunk	Gross body movements (e.g. transfers)	Independent and free head movement Increase control of movement to, from and around the midline (body axis) Encourage movement of limb girdles in relation to body axis (especially rotation)
Located in limbs	Voluntary body movements	Enhance proximal limb stabilisation Encourage co-ordinated activity of agonist and antagonist muscle groups Progress from large-range to small-range movements Reduce the requirement for visual guidance of movement

physiotherapy programmes to treat this symptom. However, there are some indications that physiotherapy can help (Brandt et al., 1986; Armutlu et al., 2001) and indeed may be essential for preventing unnecessary inactivity and dependency, and for reducing the risk of falls. The key issue in the treatment of ataxia is to identify the predominant problem to guide the primary aims of treatment. This should be achieved by careful observational assessment of the ataxic patient carrying out a range of activities. Generally, patients should progress from simple movements to more complex ones as they master the ability to co-ordinate muscle groups.

Assessment and treatment strategies for the ataxic MS patient are summarised in Table 10.4. As there is little research evidence to indicate the most useful way forwards for treatment, however, physiotherapy for ataxia must by necessity take a pragmatic approach.

Therapy techniques that could be used to good effect include:

- weight-shifting in different positions (e.g. kneel walking, step stride and side stride standing)
- lowering and raising the centre of gravity (e.g. by knee bending and straightening in standing; or moving from high kneeling to side sitting and back to high kneeling)
- proprioceptive neuromuscular facilitation techniques (see Ch. 23)

- the use of slow reversals, rhythmic movements and stabilisations.

Whichever techniques are employed, due attention must be given to fatigue. Within a therapy session, frequent periods of rest are generally required and the work performed in a session may be wasted if the patient has been exhausted by the treatment.

Aids for mobility

Mobility is perhaps the major functional disability in MS. Scheinberg (1987) stated that when patients are asked about their main problem with MS, 90% will cite a walking difficulty. In addition, those with more severe mobility problems incur a greater individual, state and health services cost burden (Holmes et al., 1995). Therefore maintaining walking ability for as long as possible is a priority and should form a primary aim of physiotherapy.

Walking aids have both advantages and disadvantages (Table 10.5) and therapists need to be aware of both in order to discuss the issues with their patients (De Souza, 1990). The main detrimental effects of using a walking aid and the ways by which physiotherapy can reduce the disadvantages have been identified by Todd (1982). Once a mobility aid has been provided, regular review is essential, as the fluctuating and

Table 10.5 Advantages and disadvantages of aids to mobility

Advantages	Disadvantages
Increased safety and stability	Less lower-limb weight-bearing
Reduced risk of falls	Loss of lower-limb muscle strength
Increased walking distance	Reduced head and trunk movements
Increased walking speed	Reduction of balance reactions
Increased gait efficiency	Alteration of muscle tone
Improved quality of gait pattern	Postural abnormality (e.g. hip flexion, trunk lateral flexion)
Reduced fatigue	Upper-limb function may be compromised

Table 10.6 Preventive and maintenance physiotherapy for immobile patients with multiple sclerosis

Prevent	Treatment
Respiratory inadequacy Partial lung collapse Chest infections Accumulation of sputum	Establish correct breathing pattern Teach deep breathing exercise in recumbent and sitting positions Promote effective cough
Cyanosis	Ensure air entry to all areas of lung
Circulatory stasis	Active rhythmic contraction and relaxation of lower-limb muscles
Deep vein thrombosis	Massage, passive movement or use of mechanical aids if no activation of muscles possible
Contractures	Ensure full passive range of movement at all joints Correction and support of posture in lying and sitting Prolonged stretch of hypertonic muscles
Pressure sores	Distribute loading over weight-bearing body surfaces Avoid pressure points Change position frequently and regularly Support correct posture Implement moving and handling techniques that protect skin integrity
Muscle atrophy	Encourage active contraction in all able muscle groups Use passive and assisted movements as appropriate Implement assisted or aided standing when safe and within patient tolerance

progressive nature of MS may indicate a need to change the type of aid used or the type of gait pattern employed. Follow-up is also essential if a mobility aid has been provided for a patient during a relapse, as any recovery of movement must be maximised and not compromised by the patient retaining an inappropriate aid or gait pattern for his or her level of recovery (De Souza, 1990).

Regular use of mobility aids may have a detrimental effect on the upper limbs and the physiotherapist should include an examination of them in the review process. The major issues to be addressed are:

- loss of upper-limb function
- injury to soft tissue, particularly of the shoulders
- joint and muscle pain, including neck pain
- loss of joint ROM
- compromised skin integrity, especially of the palmar surfaces of the hands.

This section has focused primarily on the physical aspects of walking and the need for aids. However, walking is not only a physical function but also has social, emotional and cultural meanings. For some, the personal disadvantages outweigh the physical advantages, and they decide not to use recommended mobility aids. This could be interpreted, mistakenly, as non-compliance with professional advice, or non-acceptance of the disability if the physiotherapist has not explored and understood the social, cultural and emotional needs of the patient.

Management of the immobile person with MS

People with MS may become immobile, either due to progression of the disease causing severe disablement or during a relapse. It is essential that, when immobile in relapse, the patient is managed in a way that will not disadvantage functional ability after relapse, or prolong unnecessarily the duration of immobility and dependency. Physiotherapy should provide preventive treatment, maintenance regimens and appropriate, staged active exercises when recovery first becomes apparent. Table 10.6 illustrates a typical preventive and maintenance physiotherapy programme.

Attention should also be directed to the general good health and well-being of the patient. For example, if immobility lasts over several days or weeks, help may be needed to retain a sound level of nutrition, a social support network or for continence management.

For those who are immobile due to the severity of the MS, a symptom management approach involving all members of the care team is advised (Cornish & Mattison, 2000). The *MS Healthcare Standards* (Freeman et al., 2001) have recommended appropriate provision under key issues, such as information access, expertise, communication and co-ordination, community care and mobility, respite care and long-term and palliative care. The physiotherapist is likely to be a part of the professional care team for those with very severe MS and should be knowledgeable and fully appraised of the current recommended standards.

Helping carers

People with MS generally have a number of family members and friends who also have to learn to live with MS. As Soderburg (1992) stated, 'the diagnosis of MS will affect every aspect of family life. Its impact will extend to work roles, economic status, relationships within the family, and relationships between the family and the larger community'. Professional carers, such as physiotherapists, have an important role in helping the informal carers. Teaching safe and efficient moving and handling techniques is a major area where direct physiotherapeutic intervention can bring substantial benefits.

Carers should be valued participants of the health care team, and be part of the decision-making process (McQueen Davis & Niskala, 1992). Tasks that may be required of carers should not compromise their long-term support in order to achieve a short-term goal. Just as the person with MS is identified and treated as an individual with specific needs, so should the uniqueness of the carer's needs be acknowledged. Recognition must also be given to the social and family role of the carer, and the environmental and emotional settings within which caring takes place. It should be remembered that care-giving takes place throughout the day and night (Spackman et al., 1989).

The co-operation of carers cannot be assumed, but must be negotiated. When a carer consents to carry out a task, it is inappropriate to assume that a blanket consent has been obtained for all tasks. The carer should have the opportunity to exercise choice, discretion and judgement about what is best for him or her. Even in situations where carers consent, their willingness to help must be consonant with their apparent physical, psychological and emotional abilities to do so. This issue deserves particular attention where the main carer is an elderly parent, and even more so when the carer is a child (Blackford, 1992; Segal & Simpkins, 1993). Physiotherapists must be aware of the current local and national recommendations, and demonstrate that they have executed their duty of care to both patient and carer.

CONCLUSIONS

MS is probably one of the most complex and variable conditions encountered by physiotherapists. There is no 'typical' MS patient or presentation of the disease. People with MS require comprehensive management that incorporates the expertise appropriate to their symptoms, yet is flexible and able to respond rapidly to their changing pattern of need.

An interdisciplinary team approach to the management of MS will improve the quality, continuity and comprehensiveness of care, with the patient and carer being integral to the team. Patients require information and support to enable their own involvement in the management of the condition, retain a sense of control and achieve maximal independence.

As a team member, the physiotherapist will be required to have high levels of assessment, treatment and interpersonal skills, and knowledge of MS. In general terms, patients should be advised to enjoy as full and as active a life as possible. Whilst excessive exercise should probably be avoided, regular exercise is to be encouraged, though patients should be warned at times of acute infective illness that they should rest and control fever. Best practice does not consist of a series of interventions, but embodies a cohesive care plan, which allows the patient to develop skills for living.

The importance of a sympathetic and understanding medical adviser, whether physician, nurse or therapist, who has the trust and confidence of the patient cannot be overstated. There are many support groups, such as the MS Society, to which people with MS can be directed and most regional centres now run new diagnostic clinics to inform and enable people newly diagnosed with the condition.

A philosophy of care encompasses an understanding that functions, such as walking and transferring, reach far beyond the physical issues, and extend to social, cultural, psychological and emotional effects of loss and limitation. The physiotherapist, therefore, cannot just offer treatment, but must also offer care and support to all those who need to learn to live with MS.

CASE HISTORY

Presenting history and diagnosis

Mrs H is 47 years old and experienced her first symptoms attributed to MS in 1981 at the age of 21. She suffered weakness and sensory disturbance in both legs for 2 weeks and recovered without any residual disability. In 1983, she experienced a relapse following her second pregnancy and did not recover fully, being left with some residual loss of movements in her lower limbs and intermittent spasms. Her doctor referred her for investigations. Although MS was suspected, it was not confirmed at this stage.

In 1984, Mrs H complained of generalised tiredness, closely followed by sensory deficits in both legs. She was admitted to hospital and, while under investigation, experienced a sudden onset of partial paralysis in her legs. Her history, the results of a lumbar puncture and evidence from an MRI brain scan clearly indicated that she had a definite diagnosis of relapsing remitting MS.

Once her diagnosis was made, Mrs H was treated with adrenocorticotrophic hormone (ACTH), the medication of first choice to alleviate relapses of MS. However, she was left with some residual loss of sensation and movement in her lower limbs, and was referred to a neurological rehabilitation team with special expertise in MS. Mrs H attended with her husband, who was concerned for her and supportive.

Commentary

It became clear that Mr and Mrs H were a team and had a strong relationship. As a team, they were willing to work with the professional staff, participating in decisions and in planning of treatment. With the agreement of Mrs H, both she and her husband were always seen together, and would be allowed the time and privacy within appointments with the professional care team to discuss issues between themselves.

Initial assessment by specialist team

Mrs H was judged to have mild disability due to her MS. However, her major concerns focused on her fatigue, loss of sensation and anxiety about being able to care for her new baby and meet the demands of her first child, who was 3 years old. Mr and Mrs H also wanted to know more about MS and were provided with information booklets and given the contact address and telephone number of the MS Society. Mrs H was given a simple 3-day diary to use as a self-assessment of her fatigue. She was asked to note her worst times of fatigue, the best times when fatigue was low/non-existent, and times when she needed a lot of effort to manage, or could manage with a bit of effort. Her general practitioner and health visitor were informed of her neurological management programme and asked to contact the professional care team with any queries or concerns about her progress.

Initial treatment programme

From her self-management of fatigue, a distinct pattern emerged. The physiotherapist, together with Mrs H and her health visitor, worked out a daily routine where most activity occurred in the morning. Mrs H was given a 15-min active exercise programme to do in the morning and a 10-min stretching exercise programme to do mid-afternoon. She and the children would take a nap in the early afternoon. Mrs H was provided with information about how to cradle her baby in a large scarf used as a sling across her shoulder and how to breast-feed in side-lying, in order to reduce the fatigue of having to hold the baby for feeding.

Four years after diagnosis

On formal assessment in 1987, there was increasing spasticity in her legs, the left being worse than the right. She remained mobile, but began to rely on holding on to walls and furniture, and struggled to remain independent in ADL.

Treatment

Mrs H attended for 6 weeks of outpatient physiotherapy, twice a week, which focused on functional and balance activities, lower-limb ROM exercises and gait re-education. This required Mr H to drive her to the hospital 22 miles each way, and to take time off. They also had to arrange paid child care for their younger child and be back to pick up the older child from school at 3 p.m.

Mrs H gained important benefits from her treatment. She improved her mobility so that she was walking indoors without the support of walls and furniture, and chose to have a walking stick to help, should she need it. Her upper-limb function and ROM were checked during her attendance at outpatient physiotherapy and found to be functionally normal. Her home exercise regimen was updated, and it was decided to seek more local physiotherapy support from community services or MS therapy centre.

She had no further treatment for 6 months, until the local NHS community physiotherapy service was able to offer 1 month's (once a week) treatment at home. The community physiotherapist continued the functional activities and gait re-education programme, and carried out a reassessment.

Reassessment

The reassessment demonstrated that Mrs H had lost some voluntary ROM in her left lower limb, but could walk 12 m unaided at a rate of 1.2 m/s. Thereafter, she needed to use her walking stick, and could then manage another 15 m. She had full function and range of movement in her upper limbs and continued to be independent in ADL. The community physiotherapy services agreed to continue to see Mrs H once a month.

11 years after diagnosis

In 1995, Mrs H suffered a significant relapse of MS, lasting 1 month. Initially, her legs 'gave way' and she was admitted to hospital with sudden onset of flaccid paralysis of her lower limbs and urinary incontinence. She received intravenous steroids, and was referred for urodynamic tests to assess her bladder dysfunction. The consultant neurourologist decided that adequate bladder management should be achieved with medication (desmopressin), but would review Mrs H on a 3-monthly basis.

Mrs H was anxious, depressed and tearful about her condition and requested help. She was referred to a counsellor specialising in MS, and provided with the number of the MS Society's 24-h counselling helpline service, which she reported that she and her husband had subsequently used.

Commentary

Relapses of MS are unpredictable, and people with the disease and their family are, understandably, completely unprepared for what might happen due to a relapse.

The counsellor helped Mrs H refocus on what she could do, rather than what she could not do, and, following counselling, Mr and Mrs H were motivated to attend again for further physiotherapy assessment and treatment.

On physiotherapy assessment, Mrs H was found to have severe loss of ROM in the lower limbs with hypertonus in the extensor muscle groups. She could stand independently, but needed upper-limb support to walk. Her posture and balance were abnormal, which caused problems with transfers. However, she retained independent transferring ability and had bladder control with the help of medication. Her walking ability had been reduced to 15 m with the aid of a triwheel delta walker. She was referred to a local MS therapy centre for physiotherapy which comprised:

- free active exercises, or active-assisted exercises for the lower limbs, aimed at reducing tone and increasing voluntary range of movement
- stretching regimen, aimed at maintaining muscle and joint flexibility and reducing tone

- static and dynamic muscle contractions of the lower-limb muscle groups aimed at preventing disuse atrophy
- weight-bearing, standing and gait re-education, aimed to facilitate transfers and mobility
- postural re-education, aimed at normalising tone and strengthening trunk muscles
- upper-limb and respiratory exercises, aimed at maintaining arm/hand function and lung capacity
- information and advice about aids and appliances to help with everyday tasks
- options for referral to community occupational therapy services, counselling, the disablement assessment centre, aimed at opening up the network of care available to people with MS
- reassessment at 6-monthly intervals, aimed at retaining contact with Mrs H, monitoring progress, and continuing to provide advice and support.

18 years after diagnosis

Mrs H made progress since her major relapse. She regained the ability to walk 20 m with a triwheel delta walker, was independent in transfers and retained upper-trunk and upper-limb strength and function. She elected to use a wheelchair for outings. On assessment by the community occupational therapist, Mrs H now uses a perching stool in the kitchen, a seat in the shower and has taken up embroidery, which she used to do before she had her first child. She is also learning computer skills alongside her elder child, and has just set up the family's first web-page.

Commentary

The case of Mrs H illustrates the ups and downs of living with MS. She shows great determination to do her best to live with MS. It is thought that Mrs H has now reached the secondary progressive stage of the disease. Although the absence of relapses cannot be guaranteed, further deterioration is likely to be slowly progressive. Mrs H has taken up activities which use her upper-limb functions, and which she enjoys. She considers that her quality of life is 'quite good – all things considered'.

The case of Mrs H illustrates that the role of the physiotherapist includes, not only one of providing assessment and treatment, but also roles for supporting people and their families, providing information, and referring on to allow access to the network of care. It also illustrates that successful management of MS focuses not only on the physical impact of the disease, but also on the whole person and context of his or her personal and family life.

References

Alexander J, Costello E. Physical and surgical therapy. In: Scheinberg LC, Holland NJ, eds. *Multiple Sclerosis: A Guide for Patients and their Families*, 2nd edn. New York: Raven Press; 1987:79–107.

Armutlu K, Karabudak R, Nurlu G. Physiotherapy approaches in the treatment of ataxic multiple sclerosis: a pilot study. *Neurorehab Neural Repair* 2001, **15**:203–211.

Arndt J, Bhasin C, Brar SP et al. Physical therapy. In: Schapiro RT, ed. *Multiple Sclerosis: A Rehabilitation Approach to Management*. New York: Demos; 1991:17–66.

Ashburn A, De Souza LH. An approach to the management of multiple sclerosis. *Physiother Pract* 1988, **4**:139–145.

Barnes M. Multiple sclerosis. In: Greenwood R, Barnes MP, McMillan TM, et al., eds. *Neurological Rehabilitation*. London: Churchill Livingstone; 1993:485–504.

Beck RW, Cleary PA, Trobe JD et al. The effect of corticosteroids for acute optic neuritis on the subsequent development of multiple sclerosis. *N Engl J Med* 1993, **329**:1764–1769.

Blackford KA. Strategies for intervention and research with children or adolescents who have a parent with multiple sclerosis. *Axon* 1992, **Dec**:50–55.

Block JM, Kester NC. The role of rehabilitation in the management of multiple sclerosis. *Modern Treat* 1970, **7**: No. 5.

Brandt T, Krafczyk S, Malsbenden J. Postural imbalance with head extension: improvement by training as a model for ataxia therapy. *Ann NY Acad Sci* 1981, **374**:636–649.

Brandt T, Buchele W, Krafczyk S. Training effects on experimental postural instability: a model for clinical ataxia therapy. In: Bles W, Brandt T, eds. *Disorders of Posture and Gait*. Amsterdam: Elsevier, 1986:353–365.

Burnfield A. *Multiple Sclerosis: A Personal Exploration*. London: Souvenir Press; 1985.

Burnfield A, Frank A. Multiple sclerosis. In: Frank A, Maguire P, eds. *Disabling Diseases – Physical, Environmental and Psychosocial Management*. London: Heinemann Medical; 1988.

Compston DAS. Distribution of multiple sclerosis. In: Compston A, Ebers G, Lussmann H et al. eds. *McAlpine's Multiple Sclerosis*, 3rd edn. New York: Churchill Livingstone; 2000: 63–100.

Corboy JR, Goodin DS, Frohman EM. Disease-modifying therapies for multiple sclerosis. *Curr Treat Options Neurol* 2003, **5**:35–54.

Cornish CJ, Mattision PG. Symptom management in advanced multiple sclerosis. *CME Bull Palliative Med* 2000, **2**:11–16.

Costello E, Curtis CL, Sandel IB et al. Exercise prescription for individuals with multiple sclerosis. *Neurol Rep* 1996, **20**:24–30.

DasGupta R, Fowler CJ. Bladder, bowel and sexual dysfunction in multiple sclerosis: management strategies. *Drugs* 2003, **63**:153–166.

De Souza LH. A different approach to physiotherapy for multiple sclerosis patients. *Physiotherapy* 1984, **70**:429–432.

De Souza LH. *Multiple Sclerosis: Approaches to Management*. London: Chapman & Hall; 1990.

De Souza LH. Physiotherapy. In: Goodwill J, Chamberlain MA, Evans C, eds. *Rehabilitation of the Physically Disabled Adult*, 2nd edn. London: Chapman & Hall; 1997:560–575.

De Souza LH, Worthington JA. The effect of long-term physiotherapy on disability in multiple sclerosis patients. In: Clifford Rose F, Jones R, eds. *Multiple Sclerosis: Immunological, Diagnostic and Therapeutic Aspects*. London: John Libbey; 1987:155–164.

Dean G, Kurtzke JF. On the risk of multiple sclerosis according to the age at immigration to South Africa. *Br Med J* 1971, **3**:725–729.

Di Fabio RP, Choi T, Soderberg J et al. Health related quality of life for patients with progressive multiple sclerosis: influence of rehabilitation. *Phys Ther* 1997, **77**:1704–1716.

Di Fabio RP, Soderberg J, Choi T et al. Extended outpatient rehabilitation: its influence on symptoms frequency, fatigue and functional status for persons with progressive multiple sclerosis. *Arch Phys Med Rehab* 1998, **79**:141–146.

Ebers GC, Bulman DE, Sadovnick AD. A population-based study of multiple sclerosis in twins. *N Engl J Med* 1986, **315**:1638–1642.

European Study Group on Interferon β-1b in Secondary Progressive Multiple Sclerosis. Placebo controlled multi-centre randomised trial of interferon β-1b in the treatment of secondary progressive multiple sclerosis. *Lancet* 1998, **352**:1491–1497.

Fassas A, Deconinck E, Musso M et al. Haematopoietic stem cell transplantation for multiple sclerosis; a retrospective multi centre study. *J Neurol* 2002, **249**:1088–1094.

Filippi M, Horsefield MA, Ader HJ et al. Guidelines for using quantitative measures of brain magnetic resonance imaging abnormalities in monitoring the treatment of multiple sclerosis. *Ann Neurol* 1998, **43**:499–506.

Fisk JD, Pontefract A, Ritvo PG et al. The impact of fatigue on multiple sclerosis. *Can J Neurol Sci* 1994, **21**:9–14.

Forsythe E. *Multiple Sclerosis: Exploring Sickness and Health*. London: Faber & Faber; 1988.

Freal JE, Kraft GH, Coryell JK. Symptomatic fatigue in multiple sclerosis. *Arch Phys Med Rehab* 1984, **65**:135–138.

Freeman J, Johnson J, Rollinson S et al. (eds). *Standards of Healthcare for People with MS*. London: Multiple Sclerosis Society; 1997a.

Freeman JA, Lagndon DW, Hobart JC et al. The impact of inpatient rehabilitation on progressive multiple sclerosis. *Ann Neurol* 1997b, **42**:236–244.

Freeman JA, Lagndon DW, Hobart JC et al. Inpatient rehabilitation: do the benefits carry over into the community? *Neurology* 1999, **52**:50–56.

Freeman J, Ford H, Mattison P et al. (eds). *Developing MS Healthcare Standards*. The MS Society, London: Multiple Sclerosis Society; 2001.

Ghalie RG, Edan G, Laurent M et al. Cardiac adverse effects associated with mitoxantrone (Novantrone) therapy in patients with MS. *Neurology* 2002a, **59**:909–913.

Ghalie RG, Mauch E, Edan G et al. A study of therapy-realted acute leukaemia after mitoxantrone therapy for multiple sclerosis. *Mult Scler* 2002b, **8**:441–445.

Goodin DS, Frohman EM, Garmany GP. Disease modifying therapies in multiple sclerosis: report of the therapeutics and technology assessments sub-committee of the American Academy of Neurology and the MS Council for Clinical Practice Guidelines. *Neurology* 2002, **58**:169–178.

Goodkin DE, Rudick PS, Vanderbrug Medendorp S et al. Low dose (7.5 mg) oral methotrexate reduces the rate of progression of chronic progressive multiple sclerosis. *Ann Neurol* 1995, **37**:30–40.

Greenspun B, Stineman M, Agri R. Multiple sclerosis and rehabilitation outcome. *Arch Phys Med Rehab* 1987, **68**:434–437.

Halliday AM, McDonald WI. Pathophysiology of demyelinating disease. *Br Med Bull* 1977, **33**:21–27.

Hartung HP, Gonsette R, Konig N et al. Mitoxantrone in progressive multiple sclerosis: a placebo-controlled, double-blind, randomised, multicentre trial. *Lancet* 2002, **360**:2018–2025.

Holmes J, Madgwick T, Bates D. The cost of multiple sclerosis. *Br J Med Economics* 1995; **8**:181–193.

Hulter BM, Lundberg OL. Sexual function in women with advanced multiple sclerosis. *J Neurol Neurosurg Psychiatry* 1995, **59**:83–86.

IFBN Multiple Sclerosis Study Group. Interferon β-1b is effective in relapsing-remitting multiple sclerosis. I. Clinical results of multicentre, randomised, double-blind, placebo-controlled trial. *Neurology* 1993, **43**:655–661.

Ingle GT, Stevenson VL, Miller DH et al. Two year follow-up study of primary and transitional progressive multiple sclerosis. *Multiple Sclerosis* 2002, **8**:108–114.

Jacobs LD, Cookfair DL, Rudick RA et al. Intramuscular interferon β-1a for disease progression in relapsing multiple sclerosis. *Ann Neurol* 1996, **39**:285–294.

Johnson KP, Brooks BR, Cohen JA et al. Copolymer-1 reduces relapse rate and improves disability in relapsing-remitting multiple sclerosis: results of a phase III multi-centre, double blind, placebo controlled trial. *Neurology* 1995, **45**:1268–1276.

Klaus L. Diet and multiple sclerosis. *Neurology* 1997, **49** (Suppl. 2):S55–S61.

Ko Ko C. Effectiveness of rehabilitation for multiple sclerosis. *Clin Rehab* 1999, **13** (Suppl. 1):33–41.

Krupp LB, Alvarez LA, LaRocca NG et al. Fatigue in multiple sclerosis. *Arch Neurol* 1988, **45**:435–437.

Krupp LB, La Rocca NG, Muir-Nash J et al. The fatigue severity scale. Application to patients with multiple sclerosis and systemic lupus erythematosus. *Arch Neurol* 1989, **46**:1121–1123.

Kurtzke JF. Rating neurological impairment in multiple sclerosis: an expanded disability scale (EDSS). *Neurology* 1983, **33**:1444–1452.

Kurtzke JF, Hyllested K. Multiple sclerosis in the Faroe Islands: II. Clinical update, transmission and the nature of MS. *Neurology* 1986, **36**:307–312.

Langton Hewer R. The epidemiology of disabling neurological disorders. In: Greenwood R, Barnes MP, McMillan TM et al., eds. *Neurological Rehabilitation.* London: Churchill Livingstone; 1993:3–12.

Lenman JAR, Tulley FM, Vrbová G et al. Muscle fatigue in some neurological conditions. *Muscle Nerve* 1989, **12**:938–942.

Lord SE, Wade DT, Halligan PW. A comparison of two physiotherapy treatment approaches to improve walking in multiple sclerosis: a pilot randomised controlled study. *Clin Rehab* 1998, **12**:477–486.

Loseff NA, Wang L, Lai HM et al. Progressive cerebral atrophy in multiple sclerosis. A serial MRI study. *Brain* 1996, **19**: 2009–2019.

Lucchinetti CF, Bruek W, Rodriguez M et al. Distinct patterns of multiple sclerosis pathology indicates heterogeneity in pathogenesis. *Brain Pathol* 1996, **66**:259–274.

Matthews WB. Symptoms and signs in multiple sclerosis. In: Matthews WB, Acheson ED, Batchelor JR, Weller RO, eds. *McAlpine's Multiple Sclerosis.* Edinburgh: Churchill Livingstone; 1985.

Matthews WB, Acheson ED, Batchelor JR et al. *McAlpine's Multiple Sclerosis*, 2nd edn. Edinburgh: Churchill Livingstone; 1991.

McDonald WI, Compston A, Edan G et al. Recommended diagnostic criteria for multiple sclerosis: guidelines from the International Panel for the Diagnosis of Multiple Sclerosis. *Ann Neurol* 2001, **50**:121–127.

McQueen Davis ME, Niskala H. Nurturing a valuable resource: family caregivers in multiple sclerosis. *Axon* 1992, **March**:87–91.

Misulis KE. *Essentials of Clinical Neurophysiology.* London: Butterworth Heinemann; 1993.

Moreau T, Thorpe J, Miller D et al. Reduction in new lesion formation in multiple sclerosis following lymphocyte depletion with CAMPATH-1H. *Lancet* 1994, **344**:298–301.

Morgan MH. Ataxia – its causes, measurement and management. *Int Rehab Med* 1980, **2**:126–132.

Mostert S, Kesselring J. Effects of a short-term exercise training program on aerobic fitness, fatigue, health perception and activity level of subjects with multiple sclerosis. *Multiple Sclerosis* 2002; **8**:161–168.

O'Brien B. *Multiple Sclerosis.* Office of Health Economics Publications no 87. London: 1987.

O'Connor P. Key issues in the diagnosis and treatment of multiple sclerosis. An overview. *Neurology* 2002, **59** (Suppl. 3):S1–S33.

Odeen I. Reduction of muscular hypertonus by long-term muscle stretch. *Scand J Rehab Med* 1981, **13**:93–99.

O'Hara L, De Souza LH, Ide L. A delphi study of self-care in a community population of people with multiple sclerosis. *Clin Rehab* 2000, **14**:62–71.

O'Hara L, Cadbury H, De Souza L et al. Evaluation of the effectiveness of professionally guided self-care for people with multiple sclerosis living in the community: a randomised controlled trial. *Clin Rehab.* 2002, **16**:119–128.

Oliver MJ. *Social Work with Disabled People.* London: Macmillan Press; 1983.

Page WF, Kurtzke JF, Murphy FM et al. Epidemiology of multiple sclerosis in US veterans: ancestry and the risk of multiple sclerosis. *Ann Neurol* 1993, **33**:632–639.

Paty DW, Li DKB. The UCB MS/MRI study group and the IFNB multiple sclerosis study group. Interferon β-1b is effective in relapsing remitting multiple sclerosis II MRI results in a multi-centre randomised, double blind, placebo controlled trial. *Neurology* 1993, **43**:663–667.

Paty DW, Oger JJF, Kastrukoff LF, et al. MRI in the diagnosis of MS: a prospective study with comparison of clinical evaluation, evoked potentials, oligoclonal banding and CT. *Neurology* 1988, **38**:180–185.

Payne A. Nutrition and diet in the clinical management of multiple sclerosis. *J Hum Nutr Dietet* 2001, **14**:349–357.

Petajan JH, Gappmaier E, White AT et al. Impact of aerobic fitness and quality of life in multiple sclerosis. *Ann Neurol* 1996, **39**:432–441.

Ponichtera-Mulcare JA, Matthews T, Barrett G et al. Change in aerobic fitness of patients with multiple sclerosis during 6-month training program. *Sports Med Train Rehab* 1997, **7**:265–272.

Poser CM, Paty DW, Scheinberg L et al. New diagnostic criteria for multiple sclerosis: guidelines for research protocols. *Ann Neurol* 1983, **13**:227–231.

Poser S, Kurtzke JF, Schaff G. Survival in multiple sclerosis. *J Clin Epidemiol* 1989, **42**:159–168.

Prineas JW, Connell F. The fine structure of chronically active multiple sclerosis plaques. *Neurology* 1978, **28**:68–75.

PRISMS study group. Randomised double blind, placebo controlled study of interferon β-1a in relapsing/remitting multiple sclerosis. *Lancet* 1998, **352**:1498–1504.

Rao SM and Cognitive Function Study Group. *A Manual for the Brief Repeatable Battery of Neuropsychological Tests in Multiple Sclerosis.* New York: National MS Society; 1990.

Rodgers MM, Mulcare JA, King DL et al. Gait characteristics of individuals with multiple sclerosis before and after a 6-month aerobic training program. *J Rehab Res Dev* 1999, **36**:183–188.

Rosche J, Rub K, Niemann-Delius B et al. Effects of physiotherapy on F-wave amplitudes in spasticity. *Electromyogr Clin Neurophysiol* 1996, **36**:509–511.

Russell WR, Palfrey G. Disseminated sclerosis: rest-exercise therapy – a progress report. *Physiotherapy* 1969, **55**:306–310.

Scheinberg LC. Introduction. In: Scheinberg LC, Holland NJ, eds. *Multiple Sclerosis: A Guide for Patients and their Families,* 2nd edn. New York: Raven Press; 1987:1–2.

Scolding N. The differential diagnosis of multiple sclerosis. *J Neurol Neurosurg Psychiatry* 2001, **71** (Suppl.):9–15.

Segal J, Simpkins J. *'My Mum Needs Me': Helping Children with Ill or Disabled Parents.* London: Penguin Books; 1993.

Shepherd GM. *Neurobiology.* New York: Oxford University Press; 1994.

Sibley W. *Therapeutic Claims in Multiple Sclerosis.* New York: Demos; 1988:104.

Snow BJ, Tsui JKC, Bhatt MH, et al. Treatment of spasticity with botulinum toxin: a double blind study. *Ann Neurol* 1990, **28**:512–515.

Soderberg J. MS and the family system. In: Kalb R, Scheinberg LC, eds. *Multiple Sclerosis and the Family.* New York: Demos; 1992:1–7.

Solari A, Filipini G, Gasro P et al. Physical rehabilitation has a positive effect on disability in multiple sclerosis patients. *Neurology* 1999, **52**:57–69.

Spackman AJ, Doulton DC, Roberts MHW et al. Caring at night for people with multiple sclerosis. *BMJ* 1989, **299**:1433.

Tallis RC, Illis LS, Sedgwick EM. The quantitative assessment of the influence of spinal cord stimulation on motor function in patients with multiple sclerosis. *Int J Rehab Med* 1983, **5**:10–16.

Tantacci G, Massucci M, Piperno R et al. Energy cost of exercise in multiple sclerosis patients with low degree of disability. *Multiple Sclerosis* 1996, **2**:161–167.

Thompson AJ. Symptomatic management and rehabilitation in multiple sclerosis. *J Neurol Neurosurg Psychiatry* 2001, **71** (Suppl. 2):ii22–ii27.

Todd J. Physiotherapy in multiple sclerosis. In: Capildeo R, Maxwell A, eds. *Progress in Rehabilitation: Multiple Sclerosis.* London: Macmillan Press; 1982:31–44.

Todd J. Multiple sclerosis – management. In: Downie PA, ed. *Cash's Textbook of Neurology for Physiotherapists,* 4th edn. London: Faber & Faber; 1986:398–416.

Tourtellotte WW, Booe IM. Multiple sclerosis: the blood–brain barrier and the measurement of *de novo* central nervous system IgG synthesis. *Neurology* 1978, **28** (Suppl.):76–82.

Trapp PD, Peterson J, Ransohoff RM, et al. Axonal transection in the lesions of multiple sclerosis. *N Engl J Med* 1998, **338**:278–285.

Wiles C, Newcombe RG, Fuller KJ et al. A controlled randomised crossover trial of the effects of physiotherapy on mobility in chronic multiple sclerosis. *J Neurol Neurosurg Psychiatry* 2001, **70**:174–179.

Williams G. Disablement and the social context of daily activity. *Int Disabil Stud* 1987, **9**:97–102.

Worthington JA, De Souza LH. The use of clinical measures in the evaluation of neuromuscular stimulation in multiple sclerosis patients. In: Wientholter H, Dichgans J, Mertin J, eds. *Current Concepts in Multiple Sclerosis.* London: Elsevier; 1990:213–218.

General reading

Compston A, Ebers G, Lassman H et al. (eds) *McAlpine's Multiple Sclerosis,* 3rd edn. London: Churchill Livingstone; 1998.

Paty DW, Ebers GC (eds) *Multiple Sclerosis.* Philadelphia: EA Davis; 1997.

Chapter 11

Parkinson's disease

D Jones   J Playfer

INTRODUCTION

Parkinson's disease (PD) is a chronic progressive neurodegenerative disorder and is the second most common cause of chronic neurological disability in the UK (Schoenberg, 1987). Although PD is usually classified as a movement disorder, it also causes disorders of cognitive function, emotional expression and autonomic function. The Global Parkinson's Disease survey (Findley et al., 2000) reported that depression contributed more to disability than purely motor symptoms.

Idiopathic, or primary, PD accounts for over 70% of all cases of the more general syndrome of parkinsonism (Macphee, 2001). Secondary parkinsonism may result from a variety of pathological processes including infection, drugs, toxins, trauma and vascular disease. Parkinsonism is a clinical syndrome characterised by slowness of movement (bradykinesia) accompanied by increased muscle tone (rigidity), usually with the additional feature of a resting tremor (Calne et al., 1992). Later in the disease postural abnormalities occur. The usual definitions do not include psychological features but these are almost inevitably present at the early stages of the disease, reflecting impairment of frontal lobe executive function (Poewe & Wenning, 1998).

EPIDEMIOLOGY

The incidence of PD is 18 per 100 000 of population per year, amounting to approximately 10 000 new cases per year in the UK. Because patients with PD are long-lived, the prevalence of the disease, the total number of cases in the population, is much higher than the incidence, amounting to 164 per 100 000 of population. There are approximately 120 000 people with PD in the UK (Meara & Hobson, 2000).

PD becomes more common with increasing age (2% of the population over 65 have PD). Although PD is more likely to occur in males, because females survive longer there is a fairly even distribution of overall cases between the sexes. Although PD is age-related with the commonest onset in the seventh decade, the disease does occur in younger patients (Ben Shlomo, 1997). Onset below the age of 20 is known as juvenile PD and always raises the possibility of genetic variants of PD.

Studies of mortality in PD are limited by the accuracy of death certification and diagnostic confusion between PD and other neurodegenerative conditions. If the standardised mortality ratio (SMR), derived from cohort and case-matched studies that compare mortality in PD with that of the general population, is greater than one, decreased life expectancy is indicated. The SMR for PD before the introduction of levodopa was 2.9 (Hoehn & Yahr, 1967). With the introduction of levodopa this initially fell to 1.3, giving patients with PD a near-normal life expectancy. However, a systematic review of the effect of levodopa in changing life expectancy (Clarke, 2000) demonstrated that the improvement with drug treatment was more modest, estimating the SMR in the last decade at 2.1. Patients with PD are less likely to die of cardiovascular disease or cancer than the general population but have an increased risk of dying of chest infections.

AETIOLOGY

The cause of PD remains obscure; however it is likely that parkinsonism results from many different pathological processes, with ageing, environmental and genetic factors playing variable roles.

Ageing is not a cause of PD. Although the number of dopamine-producing neurones in the substania nigra declines with age, it is estimated that with normal ageing one would need to live to be 400 years old before developing symptoms of parkinsonism. There is no evidence of accelerated ageing of these cells, although an environmental insult or infection earlier in life might reduce the population of cells, allowing ageing to push the population beyond the threshold for developing symptoms (Samii & Calne, 1999).

A variety of environmental factors have been implicated in the development of PD. The most dramatic example is the neurotoxin N-methyl-4-phenyl-1,2,3,6-tetrahydropyridine (MPTP). This substance is chemically related to common pesticides such as paraquat. It was a contaminant of illicit recreational drugs, which led to a miniepidemic of drug-induced parkinsonism in the early 1980s in California. Patients exposed to MPTP presented with a sudden dramatic onset of PD

features and were particularly liable to develop complications such as dyskinesias and cognitive failure (Langston et al., 1983, 1999).

MPTP when given to primates produced a valuable experimental model of PD, although the pathology in the basal ganglia was distinctive, without the characteristic Lewy bodies of the naturally occurring disease. Experiments demonstrate damage to mitochondrial function from free radicals produced as a result of oxidation of MPTP catalysed by the enzyme monoamino oxidase type B. Similar changes in mitochondrial function are present in the natural disease. It is therefore speculated that idiopathic PD may result from chronic damage to mitochondrial function due to exposure to toxins in the environment, resulting in oxidative stress in dopamine-producing neurones (Schapira 1997).

Potential environmental toxins include pesticides, manganese and copper. Cigarette smoking and drinking large amounts of caffeine have weak protective effects, reducing the risks of PD (Ben-Shlomo & Marnot, 1995). A related disorder to PD in which features of parkinsonism are associated with dementia and motor neurone disease has been described on the Pacific island of Guam and is linked to the ingestion of cycad flour (Steele & Guzman, 1987). A similar neurotoxin to MPTP has been postulated.

Increased familial association in PD was postulated over 100 years ago by Gowers. Mjones (1949), in a study of Scandinavian families, inferred autosomal dominant inheritance with partial penetration. In a study of a set of twins using the technique of PET scanning, preclinical changes were found which when analysed showed increased hereditability (Ward et al., 1983; Burn et al., 1992). The younger the age at onset of the disease, the more likely genetic factors play a role in aetiology.

Genetic studies are reinforcing the impression that PD does not have a single cause. There are now eight genes that have been identified as being associated with rare forms of the disease. The first gene in a familial form of PD was determined in the Italian–American Contursi kindred and was a point mutation in a gene that produces a protein called alpha-synuclein (Polymeropoulos et al., 1996). This protein accumulated in the Lewy body (the hallmark pathological sign of PD). The gene demonstrates autosomal dominance.

A rare form of juvenile PD found in Japan was found to be associated with a mutation in the parkin gene (Lansbury & Brice, 2002). This gene codes for an enzyme associated with the protein ubiquitin found in the Lewy body. Both the abnormalities in the alpha-synuclein and parkin genes affect the ability of the neurone to destroy abnormal proteins. Accumulation of abnormal proteins is a feature of many neurodegenerative conditions, including most notably Alzheimer's disease.

It is likely that genetic mutations interact with environmental factors that are unique in each individual patient, but trigger a similar pattern of degeneration of cells in the basal ganglia. The way protein aggregation occurs in affected cells resulting in the formulation of Lewy bodies is analogous to the accumulation of amyloid protein in Alzheimer's disease. Understanding of the molecular processes involved in neurodegeneration is rapidly expanding and with it the promise of future drug treatments.

PATHOPHYSIOLOGY

The pathology responsible for PD occurs in a group of grey-matter structures in the subcortical region of the cerebrum and in the ventral midbrain, the basal ganglia (Flaherty & Grabiel, 1994). They consist of the striatum (caudate nucleus and putamen), the globus pallidus (internal and external parts), the subthalamic nucleus and the substantia nigra (compact and reticular parts). In PD neurodegeneration occurs mainly in the pars compacta of the substantia nigra. This area is rich in neuromelanin-containing cells, which give the region its characteristic pigmented appearance. In PD there is less of the pigment as a result of the loss of more than 70% of the neuromelanin-containing neurones. The death of these cells appears to result from programmed cell death (apoptosis) as opposed to necrosis (accidental cell death). Apoptosis is a sequential process initiated by the cell itself in which the genetic material of the cell is enzymatically degraded. Immune cells remove the dying cells. Destruction of this population of cells results in neurochemical changes, the most important of which is dopamine depletion. The substantia nigra is the main source of the neurotransmitter dopamine and projects on to the striatal region. Dopamine is synthesised from the amino acid L-tyrosine. In PD, as the amount of dopamine available falls, compensatory changes occur in the circuitry of the basal ganglia, and these changes are responsible for most of the features we observe in PD.

The basal ganglia are part of a series of parallel loops linking with the thalamus and the cerebral cortex (particularly the motor cortex and frontal cortex). Whilst there is considerable debate about the circuitry of the basal ganglia, the classic model proposes two principal pathways concerned with movement – the direct and the indirect pathways (Flaherty & Grabiel, 1994).

The direct pathway flows from the putamen and inhibits the internal part of the global pallidus (GPi) and the substantia nigra reticulata (SNR). These two nuclei project to the thalamus. The indirect pathway, as its name suggests, is longer and links the putamen and the external segment of the global pallidus (GPe) via the subthalamic nucleus (STN) to the GPi and the SNR. The two pathways have opposite effects on basal ganglia output to the thalamus. In PD the decreased production of dopamine leads to an increased inhibitory output to the thalamus so that the rest of the circuit from the thalamus to the cortex suppresses movement, causing bradykinesia. Dopamine is a modulatory neurotransmitter and its deficiency results in a change in the setting of background tone, resulting in rigidity and releasing the inhibition of tremor. The medical treatment of PD is concentrated on replacing the deficient dopamine.

Dopamine is stored in presynaptic vesicles. Action potentials release dopamine across the synaptic cleft. The action on the postsynaptic cell depends on the interaction with dopamine receptors. There are at least six different types of dopamine receptors. These consist of two families, D1-like and D2-like (Strange, 1992). The distribution of dopamine receptors varies throughout the brain depending on the functions undertaken. D2 receptors are most important in mediating motor effects. Both levodopa and dopamine agonists used in the treatment of PD are capable of increasing the stimulation of D2 receptors.

CLINICAL FEATURES

The diagnosis of PD depends on the recognition of characteristic clinical signs. At least two of three cardinal features need to be present to make the diagnosis. These are bradykinesia, rigidity and tremor at rest.

Bradykinesia (also termed akinesia or hypokinesia) is a poverty of voluntary movement with a slower initiation of movement and a progressive reduction in the speed and amplitude of repetitive actions. Bradykinesia is a mandatory sign; the diagnosis of PD cannot be made in its absence. The sign is established firstly by general observation, notably the lack or slowness of spontaneous facial expression and absent arm swing on walking, and then established by getting the patient to undertake a repetitive opposition with the thumb and each of the other fingers in turn. This is the sign which most improves on treatment.

Rigidity is experienced by the patient as stiffness, and sometimes muscular pain. The physical sign of rigidity is an experience of resistance to passive movement, usually tested by flexion and extension of the wrist or elbow. It can be equally elicited in the lower limbs and trunk. The distribution and severity of rigidity vary between patients and at different times in the same patient. There is a background increase in tone, which gives rise to a resistance, which is constant throughout the whole range of movement; this is termed 'lead pipe' rigidity. Most characteristically, PD patients exhibit 'cog-wheel' rigidity where the resistance has a ratchet quality. This is due to the combination of increased background tone and tremor and is pathognomonic of parkinsonism.

Tremor is the presenting sign in 70% of patients with PD. PD tremor is defined as an alternating movement most commonly seen in the upper limb as a reciprocal movement of thumb and forefinger, so-called 'pill-rolling' tremor. The frequency is 4–6 Hz. Importantly, PD tremor is present at rest and diminishes or is abolished by active movement. The tremor is asymmetrical at the onset of PD, spreading to the other limb later in the disease.

Postural instability, the fourth cardinal sign of PD, develops later in the disease. The characteristic stooped posture is the result of a dominance of flexor tone over extensor tone (Fig. 11.1). Patients may fall backwards (retropulsion) or forwards (propulsion) on examination.

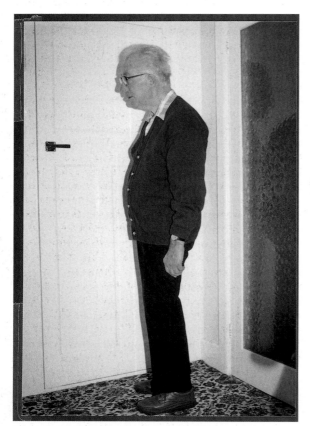

Figure 11.1 Typical posture in a patient with Parkinson's disease. He shows slight flexion at the knees and hips, with rounded shoulders, and holds his head forward.

Shuffling gait is in part a compensatory change, with the shortening of the stride reducing postural instability, and slowness of moving forward (festinating) is a result. Patients' ability to initiate or sustain movement may be affected by transient loss of voluntary movement of the feet. Such freezing episodes usually occur late in the disease and are often related to 'off' periods due to failure of medication. Postural factors are the major reason for increased falls in PD.

There is a range of other clinical features in PD. Speech is affected, with the voice becoming monotonous, exhibiting reduced volume and a lack of rhythm and variety of emphasis. Speech impairment is often associated with problems of swallowing leading to drooling. It is not unusual for patients to complain of muscle pain and this can be due to dystonia, which is an abnormal pattern of muscle contraction, most characteristically toe curling, associated with wearing off of drug effects. A number of patients with PD present with a frozen shoulder due to the immobility and rigidity. Autonomic nervous system signs include an increased tendency to constipation, bladder hyperreflexia, postural hypotension and sexual dysfunction. Sleep disorders are increasingly recognised as a feature of PD, sometimes associated with drug treatment. The lack of movement and ability to turn at night can adversely affect sleep.

Several cognitive changes can be determined early in the disease, particularly frontal lobe executive dysfunction. As the disease develops psychiatric problems can dominate the clinical picture. Depression is the most common of these, with about a third of patients suffering from depression at some stage in the course of their illness. About 25% of patients develop dementia, with psychiatric complications triggered by drug treatment, particularly hallucinations, often visual, involving people, animals or illusions (Hindle, 2001).

Making a clinical diagnosis

When the accuracy of clinical diagnosis of PD was studied and correlated with postmortem findings in PD brain-bank studies, it was found that there was a 25% diagnostic error rate (Hughes et al., 1992a, b). This is very significant as all the patients had been seen by either neurologists or geriatricians who are experts in the field of PD and applied the strictest diagnostic criteria. This research was repeated 10 years later and the error rate had gone down to 10% (Hughes et al., 2001). Nevertheless, in ordinary practice it is likely that some of the patients who have been labelled with PD actually have other related conditions. The commonest differential diagnoses are essential tremor; drug-induced PD; Parkinson-plus syndromes such as multiple system atrophy (MSA), progressive supranuclear palsy (PSP) and Shy–Drager syndrome; arteriosclerotic parkinsonism; viral infections such as postencephalic parkinsonism; repeated head trauma as experienced by sportsmen such as boxers (dementia pugilistica); rare metabolic diseases such as Wilson's disease; rare genetic disorders such as Hallervorden–Spatz syndrome; normal-pressure hydrocephalus; diffuse Lewy body disease; cortical basal ganglionic degeneration; and tumours (Quinn, 1989; Lennox & Lowe, 1997; Litvan, 1997).

Physiotherapists must always be alert for atypical cases of PD. In particular, patients who present with bilateral signs who have a disproportion of postural instability at an early stage in the disease should be suspected of having atypical parkinsonism.

PHARMACOLOGICAL MANAGEMENT

Two crucial areas of decision-making in relation to medication can be identified:

1. which treatment to initiate in the early stages of the disease
2. how to prevent or reduce the motor complications of drug treatment (abnormal involuntary movements, dyskinesias and dystonias).

Patients often need complex combinations of drugs (Bhatia et al., 1998; Olanow & Koller, 1998). Apart from anticholinergic drugs (benzhexol, procyclidine), the symptoms of PD are treated by replacing lost dopaminergic function. The anticholinergic drugs are now only used in younger patients with tremulous disease as in the longer term they can affect cognitive function and are best avoided in the older patient. They have a range of unpleasant side-effects, including dry mouth, postural hypotension and bladder problems and have low efficacy (Playfer, 2001).

Levodopa (Madopar or Sinemet) is the most widely used drug for Parkinson's patients. In these drugs levodopa is combined with a decarboxylase inhibitor which prevents peripheral metabolism of levodopa to dopamine. Levodopa is the most effective drug at relieving parkinsonian symptoms; however its use is associated with two major long-term complications – fluctuations in motor performance and abnormal voluntary movements. Levodopa has a short half-life and its effects can wear off. Once this occurs, increasing dosage of drugs causes involuntary movements affecting the face and tongue or choreoathetoid movements of the limbs. The response to levodopa can become unpredictable and patients can exhibit rapid switches from being 'on', where motor performance is well maintained, to being 'off', where they are immobile or frozen. Moments of freezing (gait blocks), which are more common in the later stages and after long-term levodopa treatment, can occur in both the on and off state (Nieuwboer et al., 1997). On–off syndrome becomes so unpredictable that it is extremely disabling to patients and drug strategies are needed to cope with this problem (Clarke & Sampaio, 1997).

The half-life of levodopa can be increased by the use of adjunct therapy. These are enzyme inhibitors, which slow the breakdown of levodopa. Catechol-*O*-methyltransferase (COMT) inhibitors inhibit the enzyme catechol-*O*-methyltransferase, which is responsible for inactivating levodopa by methylation. Two such agents have been available. Entacapone, a reversible peripheral COMT inhibitor, is given together with each dose of levodopa. The drug is well tolerated and has been shown effectively to increase on time and reduce wearing-off (Poewe & Granata, 1997). The second agent, tolcapone, has been withdrawn in Europe because of toxicity to the liver.

Monoamine oxidase type B inhibitors, exemplified by selegiline, inhibit the oxidative metabolism of dopamine. In addition to making levodopa more efficient, selegiline has been claimed to be neuroprotective. The DATATOP study in the USA showed that use of selegiline before the introduction of levodopa delayed the necessity to start levodopa therapy (Parkinson Study Group, 1989). Although these results were originally interpreted as the drug being neuroprotective, the debate on this continues. A larger study on this drug, undertaken by the UK Parkinson's Disease Research Group, indicated that the side-effects of levodopa were increased and that there was increased mortality (Lees, 1995). Since this finding selegiline has been much less widely used. Selegiline has a mild antidepressant and mood-elevating effect. However, it also tends to increase hallucinations and other psychiatric problems.

An alternative to initial therapy with levodopa is to use dopamine agonists. These drugs act directly on the postsynaptic receptor and, unlike levodopa, are not dependent on the dopaminergic neurones. There has been increased use of these drugs because they have fewer long-term motor complications. In addition it is recognised that, if the turnover of dopamine is reduced, there is the potential to protect neurones from oxidative stress. It is seen to be desirable from a pharmacological view that the dopamine receptor has continuous stimulation. The short half-life of levodopa gives rise to a pulsatile stimulation, which may be responsible for dyskinesias.

Many of the dopamine agonists have long half-lives and therefore can approach continuous dopaminergic stimulation. There are currently six available orally acting dopamine agonists and one parenteral drug. Two of these drugs are now not widely used: bromocriptine because of poor patient toleration and lisuride because of increased psychiatric side-effects. Pergolide, ropinirole, cabergoline and pramipexole have all been shown to reduce long-term motor complications and are selected for individual patient use on varying pharmacological characteristics (Clarke, 2001a).

Apomorphine is possibly the most potent and effective dopamine agonist in the treatment of Parkinson's disease but can only be used parenterally together with a drug blocking its major side-effect of nausea. Apomorphine can be used by means of a pen injection to rescue patients in an 'off' state. Continuous subcutaneous infusion of apomorphine has proved an effective treatment for patients with severe motor complications. Use of such drugs depends on availability of PD nurse specialists.

SURGICAL APPROACHES TO PARKINSON'S DISEASE

With the introduction of levodopa, the need for surgery, widely used prior to the 1970s, diminished. However the emergence of long-term complications has led to renewed interest. The success of surgery depends on carefully defined indications and patient selection. Two types of surgical approaches are available.

Implantation

Transplanted fetal mesoencephalic cells harvested from aborted fetuses, grown in cell culture and injected into the brain in a form of cell suspension, have been shown to survive in the brain and replace the production of dopamine (Hauser et al., 1999). This type of surgery remains experimental and controversial and disabling dyskinetic movements following such transplants have been reported in the USA. Fetal transplants were pioneered in Sweden where successful long-term follow-up has been demonstrated (Lindvall, 1998). Manipulation of the patient's own cells by genetic therapy is an active area of research. The number of transplants undertaken is minuscule compared with the number of patients with PD and the procedure is never likely to be a mass treatment.

Stereotactic surgery and implantation of stimulators

Better understanding of pathophysiology of Parkinson's disease has helped to identify areas in the brain that may either be targets for stereotactic surgery or the implantation of stimulators. The original target for such surgery was the thalamus. This has been replaced in recent years by targeting either the globus pallidus or, more recently, the STN. The target area of the brain may be lesioned to reduce its output to benefit the movement disorder or it may be stimulated in order to inhibit output with similar effect (see Ch.1 p. 13). Use of stimulators to the STN can demonstrate dramatic improvements in patients' motor abilities; however these procedures are only in the initial stages of being subjected to double-blind controlled trials (Limousin et al., 1998). Unfortunately, cognitive and psychiatric problems with PD can be made worse by surgery and great caution has to be applied to the selection of patients.

TEAM MANAGEMENT OF PARKINSON'S DISEASE

PD affects all aspects of life for both patients and carers. The only way of effectively managing these challenges for both individuals and professionals is within an interdisciplinary rehabilitative framework. Clinical stages (Thomas et al., 1999) can provide a starting point for considering professional involvement. Criteria for entry into the clinical staging categories of diagnosis, maintenance, complex and palliative relate to the increasing challenges involved in maintaining optimal medication regimes and management in response to increasing signs and symptoms, and loss of efficacy of drug therapy.

The core team which should be accessible in the diagnostic/maintenance phases for assessment, treatment and advice include the consultant, nurse specialist, physiotherapist, occupational therapist, speech and language therapist, social worker and dietician. Neuropsychiatry and neurosurgical expertise may be required in the complex stage, with specialist medical and nursing input, e.g. in relation to continence in the palliative stage. Teams should be able to access chiropody and psychology services. They should have links with primary, secondary and tertiary services, together with the long-stay, respite, residential and nursing home sector, and the voluntary sector. Information should be available on a wide range of topics such as employment, driving, benefits and support groups (Guidelines Group, 2001).

The development of the PD nurse specialist role has been promoted by the Parkinson's Disease Society and the pharmaceutical industry. Nurse specialists co-ordinate packages of care, often acting as key workers linking patients and professionals. They provide advice on all aspects of care, including supervision of apomorphine injections or infusions. The effect of community-based nurses specialising in PD on health outcome and costs was investigated in a randomised control trial (RCT; Jarman et al., 2002). Results showed that nurses improved their patients' sense of well-being at no extra health care cost but there was little effect on clinical condition. Cochrane systematic reviews have identified the need for high-quality research into the effectiveness of physiotherapy, occupational therapy and speech and language therapy in the treatment of PD (Deane et al., 2001a, b). The evidence base for physiotherapy will be examined in the following sections.

PHYSICAL MANAGEMENT OF PARKINSON'S DISEASE

Reviewing the evidence

Two systematic reviews of randomised or quasi-randomised controlled trials of physiotherapy and PD have been undertaken by the Cochrane Collaboration. In a review focusing on the comparison of physiotherapy with placebo or no treatment (Deane et al., 2001a), literature searches identified 11 trials involving a total of 280 patients. Seven trials that had compared two forms of physiotherapy in 142 patients were identified (Deane et al., 2001b). Treatment techniques used in the trials included strengthening, mobilising and balance exercises; Bobath, Peto and proprioceptive neuromuscular facilitation (PNF) approaches; gait re-education; and cueing techniques.

In the studies comparing physiotherapy with placebo or control intervention there was some limited evidence of efficacy, particularly in relation to specific gait characteristics such as walking velocity and stride length, and activities of daily living. The technique of using visual, auditory and tactile cues was employed in four trials comparing two forms of physiotherapy (Mohr et al., 1996; Thaut et al., 1996; Shiba et al., 1999; Marchese et al., 2000), with two trials comparing physiotherapy techniques with and without cues (Thaut et al., 1996; Marchese et al., 2000). The efficacy of physiotherapy was improved by the addition of cueing techniques in both trials.

Another systematic review using different inclusion criteria evaluated the effect of physiotherapy on neurological signs, activities of daily living and walking ability (de Goede et al., 2001). A meta-analysis was performed on a total of 12 studies involving 419 patients. Significant results were achieved for activities of daily living, stride length and walking speed, but not for neurological signs.

Methodological flaws in the trials and heterogeneity in relation to physiotherapy techniques, lengths of treatment episode, locations for therapy, outcome measures, together with the inclusion of multidisciplinary elements, led the Cochrane reviewers to conclude that there was insufficient evidence to support or refute the efficacy of physiotherapy in PD or the use of one form of physiotherapy over another. However, this did not imply lack of effect. Detailed suggestions were made to improve the quality of future trials based on the CONSORT guidelines (Begg et al., 1996).

Using best evidence

Whilst there is currently insufficient gold-standard RCT evidence to guide referrers on whether or when to refer to physiotherapy (Rascol et al., 2002), there are ongoing initiatives which aim to help referrers and physiotherapists themselves to take informed decisions in the light of the available best evidence. The Guidelines Group (2001) used the full range of evidence to develop answers to a range of questions about physiotherapy and PD articulated by therapists themselves. The evidence base was also reviewed in the *Neurology Physiotherapy Effectiveness Bulletin* (CSP, 2001).

Models of physiotherapy management

The tendency to late referral (Clarke, 2001b) is illustrated in the models for physical therapy management of PD (Turnbull, 1992) (see Fig. 11.2).

The 'cure' paradigm is inappropriate in a long-term condition. The 'current' paradigm charts the prevailing approach to the physiotherapeutic management of PD, with referral for therapy taking place, if at all, only when the pharmacological approach begins to fail. The 'progressive' paradigm aims to maintain optimal function over time by early and continuing targeted therapy. However only 27% of members had been referred to a physiotherapist in the most recent Parkinson's Disease Society survey (Yarrow, 1999). This figure was only 10% higher than the previous survey almost 20 years earlier (Oxtoby, 1982), despite reported difficulties for individuals in core areas of physiotherapy practice such as walking and turning in bed (Yarrow, 1999).

As part of an evaluation of best-practice physiotherapy in PD in the UK (Plant et al., 2000), a model linking core areas of physiotherapy practice (gait, balance, posture and transfers); physiotherapy treatment concept (movement enablement through exercise regimes and strategies) and optimal level of measurement of effects (functional performance) was proposed. Morris (2000) also places functional performance centrally in a model of physical therapy intervention for PD. Analysis of functional task performance is used as a basis for designing task-specific training programmes, which incorporate current knowledge of basal ganglia pathology and its effect on motor and cognitive processes. Box 11.1 sets out the principles of physiotherapy management of PD based on the management and

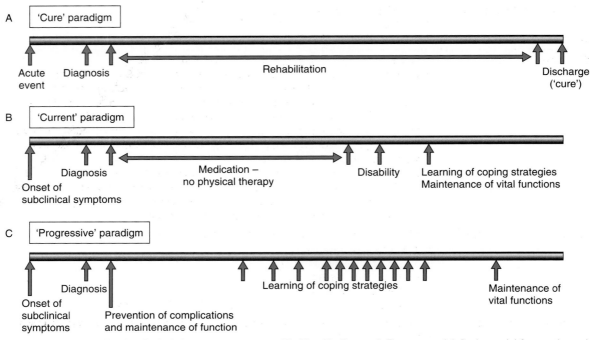

Figure 11.2 Three models for physical therapy management of Parkinson's disease. A: The cure model; B: the model frequently used; C: the progressive model. (Redrawn from Turnbull 1992, with permission from WB Saunders.)

Box 11.1 Principles of physiotherapy management

- Early referral to encourage participation in regular physical activities to prevent muscle weakness, restricted range of movement, reduced exercise capacity and social isolation
- Ongoing assessment and review, incorporating patient-centred goals and meaningful outcome measures in the core areas of physiotherapy practice, to monitor progress and jointly identify management priorities
- Targeted intervention for movement difficulties, based on current knowledge of basal ganglia pathology, in the context of functional tasks of everyday living
- Training in the home and community setting or a simulated home/community environment

- Modification of treatment and home exercise regime to take account of levels of cognitive impairment, medication, ageing and multiple pathology
- Provision of a forum, such as a regular group session, to share information and identify continuing needs of both individuals and carers[a]
- Physical management within the context of a multidisciplinary team to ensure co-ordination and integration of professional input around patient-centred goals

Based on Turnbull (1992), Plant et al. (2000), Morris (2000).
[a]Carers include both family and formal carers from a range of organisations and agencies.

---

treatment models proposed by Turnbull (1992), Plant et al. (2000) and Morris (2000). These principles can be adapted for physiotherapy service delivery across the full range of settings from hospital to home.

The following sections will explore these principles in the context of referral related to disease stage, assessment and outcomes, and physiotherapy management. An illustrative case history will be presented.

Referral related to disease stage

It is important for physiotherapists to educate potential referrers if appropriate referrals are to be encouraged and the low referral rate to physiotherapy (Yarrow, 1999) is to be overturned. Table 11.1 presents the Guideline Group's (2001) answer to the question 'When should people be referred for physiotherapy?' in the

Table 11.1 When should people be referred for physiotherapy?

Clinical stage [a]	Potential reasons for referral for physiotherapy
Diagnosis – maintenance	Individuals may benefit from early referral to physiotherapy: • to address concerns about differential diagnosis, e.g. early onset of postural instability [b] • for assessment and monitoring to allow early identification of movement problems [c] • to encourage participation in programmes designed to encourage general fitness through optimal condition of cardiovascular, musculoskeletal and neuromuscular systems [c, d, e] • for preventive management of the typical secondary complications such as learned non-use of affected parts of the body; postural, gait and transfer deficits; muscle weakness; joint stiffness; orofacial and respiratory dysfunction [c, d, e] • to introduce movement strategies for use over the course of the condition [e] • for education of individuals and carers about the physical management of Parkinson's disease, ideally within the context of a support group run with multidisciplinary colleagues [c, d] • for monitoring of drug efficacy to optimise motor performance [f]
Maintenance – early complex	In addition, specific physiotherapy intervention may be required for: • musculoskeletal impairment • gait, falls and transfer difficulties • environmental assessment • provision of aids and equipment • advice for carers about promoting movement and effective handling [c, d, e]
Late complex – palliative	In addition, work with family and formal carers may be required to ensure optimal movement, positioning and handling to: • prevent falls • promote nutrition, skin care, chest care [c, d, e]

Based on Guidelines Group (2001).
References (see reference list at end of chapter for full details): [a]Thomas et al. (1999). [b]Quinn (1995); [c]Turnbull (1992); [d]Cutson et al. (1995); [e]Morris (2000); [f] Morris et al. (1998).

context of the clinical staging categories for PD proposed by the Parkinson's Disease Primary Care Task Force (Thomas et al., 1999). The increasing complexity of management over time is reflected in Table 11.1 in relation to the potential reasons for referral for physiotherapy at different stages. The monitoring, prevention, advice, education and support roles of the diagnosis/maintenance stages provide the background for a more active rehabilitation role in the maintenance/early complex stages, with a palliative role emerging in the late complex/palliative stage. This is congruent with the 'progressive paradigm' for physical therapy (Fig. 11.2).

Assessment and outcomes

Physiotherapists may contribute to multiprofessional record keeping which can assist in limiting the repetition of background history individuals and carers need to provide to individual professionals. Multidisciplinary records may include a staging of PD using e.g. the Hoehn & Yahr (1967) stages, results of global PD outcome measures such as the Unified Parkinson's Disease Rating Scale (Wade, 1992), in addition to assessments of cognition, vision, hearing, speech and swallowing, and continence.

The emphasis in physiotherapy-specific assessment is on evaluating the difficulties associated with functional performance identified by the individual, carer and therapist. Ideally, functional assessment should take place in the individual's familiar surroundings as this environment offers the best opportunity for understanding movement problems (Ashburn et al., 2001a, b). Box 11.2 summarises the main areas of functional performance that may be assessed, in addition to other potentially relevant domains of assessment. Findings can be recorded by means of description and scoring of observed movement parameters, strategies and aids, timed tests and video recording (Suteerawattananon & Protas, 2000). Interview prompts and a checklist have been proposed to maximise recall about falls in people with PD (Stack & Ashburn, 1999).

Standardised outcome measures that are expected to change as a result of intervention with an individual can be used at the beginning and end of a course of

Box 11.2 Domains of physiotherapy assessment in Parkinson's disease

Functional performance:
- Walking (indoors and outdoors)
- Turning and changing direction
- Standing up
- Sitting down
- Turning in bed
- Getting up from the floor
- Stairs
- Car transfers
- Reaching, grasping and manipulating objects
- Writing

Posture
Balance
Falls
Freezing
Range of movement
Muscle strength
Muscle tone
Sensation
Pain
Respiratory function
Feet and footwear
Walking aids
Wheelchairs
Aids and equipment
Home environment

Based on Guidelines Group (2001).

Table 11.2 Potential outcome measures for physiotherapy assessment domains in Parkinson's disease

If focusing on:	Potential outcome measure
Walking	Clinical gait assessment [a]
	10-m timed walk [b]
Balance	Clinical balance assessment [c]
	Performance-oriented balance assessment [d]
	Berg balance scale [e] (see Ch.3 p. 35)
	180° turn step number [f]
	Distance between the feet [f]
	Falls diary [g]
Turning in bed	Checklist for rating turning in bed [h]
Combined aspects of functional performance	Timed up-and-go test [i]
	Rivermead mobility index [j]
	Parkinson activity scale [k]
	Elderly mobility scale [l]
Dexterity	Nine-hole peg test [b]
Endurance	6-min walk test [b]
Respiratory function	Respiratory tests [m]
Quality of life	Parkinson's disease questionnaire –39 [n]
Perception of change with therapy	Visual analogue scale [m]

Based on Guidelines Group (2001).
References (see reference list at end of chapter for full details):
[a] Turnbull (1992); [b] Wade (1992); [c] Smithson et al. (1998); [d] Tinetti (1986); [e] Berg et al. (1989); [f] Ashburn et al. (2001a); [g] Yekutiel (1993); [h] Ashburn et al. (2001b); [i] Podsialdo & Richardson (1991); [j] Collen et al. (1991); [k] Nieuwboer et al. (2000); [l] Smith (1994); [m] Carr & Shepherd (1998); [n] Jenkinson et al. (1998).

therapy to evaluate effectiveness (Cole et al., 1994), and for monitoring over time (see 'Case history', below). Whilst work is needed to establish and validate a battery of relevant measures which could constitute a minimum data set for clinical physiotherapists working with people with PD, the Guidelines Group (2001) highlighted a number of measures more commonly used in research and clinical practice (Table 11.2).

Measurement in PD is complicated by clinical fluctuations (Morris et al., 1998). However, recording current medication, the time of day, time since last dose, and on or off status can guide the taking of comparable measurements. Health care professionals should ensure that the needs of carers are assessed (Thomas et al., 1999), and the incorporation of the Caregiver Strain Index could be considered (Wade, 1992).

The importance of sharing the outcomes of multi-professional assessment can be illustrated by focusing on falls. Previous falls, disease duration, dementia and loss of arm swing have been shown to be independent predictors of falling, and significant associations have been found between disease severity, balance impairment, depression and falling (Wood et al., 2002). Only if this information is brought together with the perceptions of individuals and carers (CSP, 2000) can intervention for modifiable risk factors be formulated. A multidisciplinary pathway of care and a care programme approach can facilitate this process (Bilclough, 1999).

Physiotherapy management

Physiotherapists draw on techniques from a range of approaches, e.g. theories of learning, neurophysiological and biomechanical approaches, to manage individuals with PD (Plant et al., 2000). The following sections will review the current best evidence in relation to exercise regimes and movement strategies, and will consider issues in relation to individual and group therapy and hospital and home contexts.

Exercise regimes

Whilst further research is recommended in relation to exercise and PD (Protas et al., 1996), evidence is available in the areas of general physical activity, specific and general exercise programmes.

General physical activity

Individuals with PD who were active in sport prior to diagnosis are more likely to retain their interest for longer. However there is an overall tendency to reduce physical activity compared to older people generally, and specific difficulties are experienced with a number of common activities, e.g. swimming and walking (Fertl et al., 1993). Support to maintain an active lifestyle is therefore important, especially as regular physical exercise has been shown to influence the survival rate in PD by preventing decline from disuse (Kuroda et al., 1992). It has been demonstrated that individuals with mild to moderate PD can maintain normal exercise capacity with regular aerobic exercise such as walking and cycling (Canning et al., 1997).

Specific exercise programmes

A number of studies have focused on specific exercise programmes designed to promote strength, increase flexibility, re-educate balance and improve function. The incorporation of strengthening exercises specific to the trunk into a course of aerobic exercise classes held twice a week over 12 weeks improved trunk muscle performance in individuals with early PD (Bridgewater & Sharpe, 1997). Strengthening exercise in different neurological conditions is discussed in Chapter 29.

A 10-week exercise programme designed to promote spinal flexibility, delivered on an individual basis three times a week, improved spinal flexibility as measured by functional axial rotation and functional reach in people with early and mid-stage PD (Schenkman et al., 1998). Improvements in equilibrium (Forkink et al., 1996) and reduction in falls (Hirsch, 1996) were the outcome of balance and lower-limb strength training programmes held three times a week for 10 weeks.

General exercise programmes

The aims of most general exercise programmes for individuals with PD, whether delivered individually (Hurwitz, 1989; Formisano et al., 1992; Comella et al., 1994; Patti et al., 1996) or in a group setting (Pederson et al., 1990; Viliani et al., 1999) relate to promoting function through improvements in strength, flexibility, co-ordination, balance and the use of relaxation.

Components of a typical programme include: exercises for the trunk, upper and lower limbs and face in lying, sitting and standing; speech and breathing exercises; gait, balance and transfer training; and relaxation. Largely positive results were reported in relation to the outcome measures selected for these studies. However, the difficulty of continuing an exercise regime alone after a period of supported physiotherapy was highlighted. Home visiting on a regular basis supports the continuation of exercise behaviour (Hurwitz, 1989), and the opportunity to take part in top-up exercise programmes on an ongoing basis has been proposed to aid carry-over of effect (Banks & Caird 1989; Yekutiel et al., 1991).

Strategies

The basal ganglia play a pivotal role in running complex motor sequences that make up skilled, largely automatic, movement such as walking and turning in bed. Phasic neural activity acts as a cue to initiate movement and release linked submovements of a movement sequence (Morris & Iansek, 1997). The rehabilitation of gross motor skills in PD requires compensatory (Kamsma et al., 1995) as opposed to normal movement strategies. Compensatory strategies are atypical approaches to meeting the sensory and motor requirements of a task (Shumway-Cook & Woollacott, 1995) which address ongoing motor control difficulties, such as processing sequential tasks and undertaking motor and cognitive tasks concurrently (Bloem et al., 2001). Box 11.3 highlights the principles underlying the development of compensatory movement strategies, which can be applied to activities such as getting out of a chair, turning in bed and getting into a car.

Box 11.3 Principles underlying compensatory movement strategies

- Break down complex movement sequences into simple component parts
- Arrange parts in a logical, sequential order
- Utilise prior mental rehearsal of the whole movement sequence
- Perform each part separately, ideally ending in a stable resting position from which the next step can be initiated
- Execute each part under conscious control
- Avoid simultaneous motor or cognitive tasks
- Use appropriate visual, auditory and somatosensory cues to initiate and maintain movement

Based on Kamsma et al. (1995), Morris & Iansek (1997), Morris (2000).

Table 11.3   Examples of strategies used to cue movement

Cue category	Cue mechanism	Specific strategy to cue movement
External		
• Visual	Spatial	Practice of walking with visual cues, e.g. stripes on floor [a]
	Spatial	Stepping over lines placed on the floor to aid initiation where freezing/falls can occur [b]
	Spatial	Strategically placed cue cards containing key words or phrase to prompt optimal movement performance [c]
• Auditory	Rhythm	Listening to a beat provided by a metronome or music to initiate movement and maintain walking cadence [d]
	Spatial/rhythm	Using verbal instructions from another person to normalise gait variables [e]
• Auditory/visual	Spatial	Verbal prompt to a visual cue to focus attention on large steps [f]
• Somatosensory	Rhythm	Using a small current pulse as a single cutaneous cue to provide a 'go' signal to initiate a step [g]
Internal		
• Somatosensory and vestibular	Rhythm	Taking a step back before starting to walk; rocking gently from side to side to overcome freezing [h]
• Mental rehearsal	Spatial	Visualisation of walking with appropriate step length [a]
	Spatial	Memorising the separate parts of a movement sequence, e.g. sit–stand–walk, and rehearsing them mentally [i]
• Mental focus	Rhythm	Focusing on a component of movement such as heel strike ('heel' … 'heel'); counting in head whilst walking [h]
	Spatial	Focusing on the changed components of a turn – moving in one curved arc as opposed to two linear trajectories to avoid falls [j]

References (see reference list at end of chapter for full details): [a] Morris et al. (1996); [b] Morris et al. (1999); [c] Morris & Iansek (1997); [d] Thaut et al. (1996); [e] Behrman et al. (1998); [f] Weissenborn (1993); [g] Burleigh-Jacobs et al. (1997); [h] Nieuwboer et al. (1997); [i] Kamsma et al. (1995); [j] Yekutiel (1993).

The inability of the basal ganglia to cue movement can be compensated for by the use of alternative cues, which activate and sustain movement via pathways that bypass the defective circuit in the basal ganglia–supplementary motor area (Morris, 2000). Cues, which provide both a prompt for movement and information about how a movement should be undertaken, can be divided into two main categories. External cues use visual, auditory or somatosensory information to trigger movement or provide spatial or rhythmic information to improve the quality of movement. For example, stripes on the floor at the optimal step length for an individual's age, sex and height (Morris & Iansek, 1997) provide visuospatial information to guide movement. Internal cues utilise somatosensory and vestibular stimuli, together with mental rehearsal and mental focus, to raise awareness of spatial and rhythmic components of movement. The mechanism by which cues are effective may relate to the focusing of attention on the task in hand (Morris et al., 1996). Table 11.3 gives examples of cue categories and the information they provide, together with examples of specific strategies to cue movement.

Longer-lasting retention of gains in performance has been recorded in programmes using compensatory movement strategies and the full range of sensory cues (Kamsma et al., 1995; Dam et al., 1996; Marchese et al., 2000) compared to programmes centred on exercise and functional activities alone. The rehabilitation strategy of cueing is currently under investigation in a multicentre international study, which will develop and test the effectiveness of a rehabilitation strategy utilising cues in an RCT (Plant, Nieuwboer & Kwakkel, 2002 by personal communication, with permission).

Individual/group therapy, hospital/home therapy

Individual sessions supplemented by group work was the model of service delivery favoured by specialist physiotherapists in an evaluation of best practice (Plant et al., 2000). In the same study, individuals identified as the main benefit of individual sessions, having their personal needs met, whilst the social contact and motivation provided by group work were valued. Most groups were run on a multidisciplinary basis with monitoring, exercise, advice, the sharing of information and an

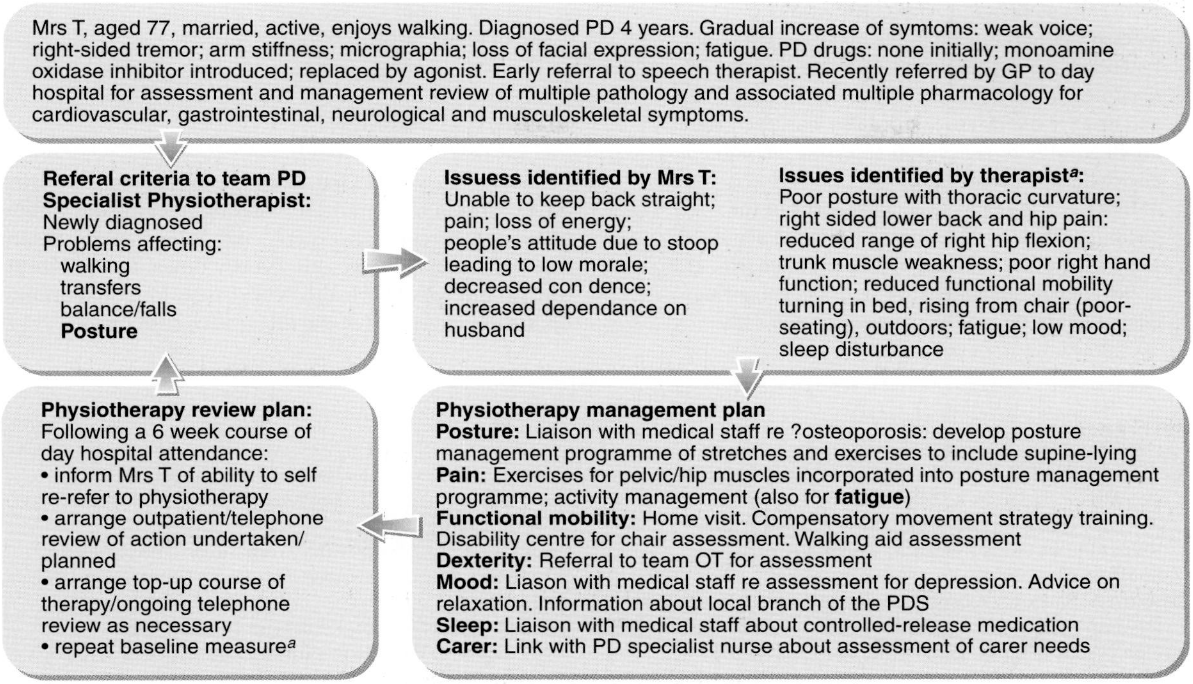

Mrs T, aged 77, married, active, enjoys walking. Diagnosed PD 4 years. Gradual increase of symtoms: weak voice; right-sided tremor; arm stiffness; micrographia; loss of facial expression; fatigue. PD drugs: none initially; monoamine oxidase inhibitor introduced; replaced by agonist. Early referral to speech therapist. Recently referred by GP to day hospital for assessment and management review of multiple pathology and associated multiple pharmacology for cardiovascular, gastrointestinal, neurological and musculoskeletal symptoms.

Referal criteria to team PD Specialist Physiotherapist:
Newly diagnosed
Problems affecting:
  walking
  transfers
  balance/falls
  Posture

Issuess identified by Mrs T:
Unable to keep back straight; pain; loss of energy; people's attitude due to stoop leading to low morale; decreased con dence; increased dependance on husband

Issues identified by therapist[a]:
Poor posture with thoracic curvature; right sided lower back and hip pain; reduced range of right hip flexion; trunk muscle weakness; poor right hand function; reduced functional mobility turning in bed, rising from chair (poor-seating), outdoors; fatigue; low mood; sleep disturbance

Physiotherapy review plan:
Following a 6 week course of day hospital attendance:
• inform Mrs T of ability to self re-refer to physiotherapy
• arrange outpatient/telephone review of action undertaken/planned
• arrange top-up course of therapy/ongoing telephone review as necessary
• repeat baseline measure[a]

Physiotherapy management plan
Posture: Liaison with medical staff re ?osteoporosis: develop posture management programme of stretches and exercises to include supine-lying
Pain: Exercises for pelvic/hip muscles incorporated into posture management programme; activity management (also for **fatigue**)
Functional mobility: Home visit. Compensatory movement strategy training. Disability centre for chair assessment. Walking aid assessment
Dexterity: Referral to team OT for assessment
Mood: Liaison with medical staff re assessment for depression. Advice on relaxation. Information about local branch of the PDS
Sleep: Liaison with medical staff about controlled-release medication
Carer: Link with PD specialist nurse about assessment of carer needs

[a]Baseline measures for monitoring – 10 m timed walk (Wade, 1992), Berg Balance Scale (Berg et al., 1989).

Figure 11.3   Illustrative physiotherapy case history. PD, Parkinson's disease; OT, occupational therapist; PDS, Parkinson's Disease Society.

emphasis on self-management as the key components. De Goede (2001) evaluated a 6-week group programme, undertaken twice a week for 1½h, which focused on gait training, simulation of everyday activities, general physical activity and relaxation. Improvements in gait parameters were recorded but not in activities of daily living or quality of life outcome measures.

The importance of context of therapy was highlighted in a study of a home physiotherapy programme undertaken by Nieuwboer et al. (2001). Functional activity was measured in both the hospital and home contexts, with improvement of functional activity scores assessed at home more than twice those observed in hospital. The researchers postulate that this was due to better retention of treatment strategies within the actual learning context. This has implications for carers who offer high levels of support in core areas of physiotherapy practice, particularly when cognitive impairment is present. A comprehensive understanding of both the home environment and support mechanisms is essential when assessment and treatment are taking place in the hospital context. These issues are explored within an illustrative case history outlining a physiotherapy intervention with an individual with PD in the context of a day hospital for older people.

CASE HISTORY (Fig 11.3)

Diagnosed and initially treated by her general practitioner, one of Mrs T's first symptoms was a weak voice, and she had had an early referral to a speech therapist. However, since diagnosis 4 years previously she had not been under the care of a multidisciplinary team and had developed a range of physical, functional and psychological problems which were impacting on her quality of life. Criteria had been developed to guide appropriate referral to physiotherapy of individuals with PD, referred to the day hospital team. In Mrs T's case it was her poor posture with pain that prompted referral.

Physiotherapy assessment identified a range of other issues which would benefit from liaison within the team: with medical staff in relation to further diagnostic assessment and drugs management; with occupational therapy colleagues in relation to upper-limb function; and with specialist nursing staff in relation to carer issues. In addition, links were made with the Parkinson's Disease Society for support and advice, and with the local disability centre. Physiotherapy intervention incorporated both a specific exercise programme to address posture and pain, and compensatory movement strategy assessment and training in the home setting to aid functional mobility problems. Baseline outcome measures would allow subsequent monitoring of gait and balance on review. Information was given about arrangements for review and accessing physiotherapy advice between planned contacts.

Mrs T was in the early complex stage of the condition (Table 11.1). Evidence is needed about the role of targeted physiotherapy intervention (Fig. 11.2) in the diagnosis/maintenance stages in enhancing quality of life through the prevention and early management of the secondary complications which Mrs T's case history illustrate.

ACKNOWLEDGEMENTS

Diana Jones would like to thank Dr Lynn Rochester, Northumbria University, for sharing insights into strategies used to cue movement, and Julie Easton, Senior Physiotherapist, Newcastle, North Tyneside and Northumberland Mental Health NHS Trust, for collaborating on the development of the illustrative case history.

References

Ashburn A, Stack E, Jupp K. *Movement Strategies Used by People with Parkinson's Disease During Fall-related Activities*. Final report. Southampton: Health and Rehabilitation Research Unit, University of Southampton; 2001a.

Ashburn A, Stack E, Dobson J. *Strategies Used by People with Parkinson's Disease when Turning Over in Bed: Associations with Disease Severity, Fatigue, Function and Mood*. Southampton: Health and Rehabilitation Research Unit, University of Southampton; 2001b.

Banks M, Caird F. Physiotherapy benefits patients with Parkinson's disease. *Clin Rehab* 1989, **3**:11–16.

Begg C, Cho M, Eastwood S et al. Improving the quality of reporting of randomized controlled trials. The CONSORT statement. *JAMA* 1996, **276**:637–639.

Ben-Shlomo Y. The epidemiology of Parkinson's disease. In: Quinn NP, ed. *Parkinsonism*. London: Baillière-Tindall; 1997:55–68.

Ben-Shlomo Y, Marnot MV. Survival and cause of death in a cohort of patients with parkinsonism: possible clues to etiology? *J Neurol Neurosurg Psychiatry* 1995, **58**:293–299.

Behrman AL, Teitelbaum P, Cauraugh JH. Verbal instructional sets to normalise the temporal and spatial gait variables in Parkinson's disease., *J Neurol Neurosurg Psychiatry* 1998, **65**:580–582.

Berg KO, Wood-Dauphinee S, Williams JI et al. Measuring balance in the elderly: preliminary development of an instrument. *Physiother Can* 1989, **41**:304–310.

Bhatia K, Brooks D, Burn D et al., 1998 Guidelines for the management of Parkinson's disease. *Hosp Med* **59**: 469–480.

Bilclough J. Managed care: evaluating the impact of a multidisciplinary pathway of care and the care programme approach in Parkinson's disease. In: *Proceedings of the Science and Practice of Multidisciplinary Care in Parkinson's Disease and Parkinsonism*. London: 1999: 22–23.

Bloem BR, Valkenburg VV, Slabbekoorn M et al. The multiple tasks test. Strategies in Parkinson's disease. *Exp Brain Res*, 2001. Available online at: http://link. springer.de/link/service/journals/00221/contents/00/00672/papers/s002210000672ch000.html 25 July 2002.

Bridgewater KJ, Sharpe MH. Trunk muscle training and early Parkinson's disease. *Physiother Theory Pract* 1997, **13**:139–153.

Burleigh-Jacobs A, Horak FB, Nutt FB et al. Step initiation in Parkinson's disease: influence of levodopa and external sensory triggers. *Move Disord* 1997, **12**:206–215.

Burn DJ, Mark MH, Playford ED et al. Parkinson's disease in twin studies with 18F-DOPA and positron emission tomography. *Neurology* 1992, **42**:1894–1900.

Calne D, Snow BJ, Lee C. Criteria for diagnosing Parkinson's disease. *Ann Neurol* 1992, **32**:125–127.

Canning CG, Alison JA, Allen NE et al. Parkinson's disease: an investigation of exercise capacity, respiratory function, and gait. *Arch Phys Med Rehab* 1997, **78**:199–207.

Carr J, Shepherd R. *Neurological Rehabilitation. Optimizing Motor Performance*. Oxford: Butterworth Heinemann; 1998.

Chartered Society of Physiotherapy. *Standards of Physiotherapy Practice*. Chartered Society of Physiotherapy; London: 2000.

Chartered Society of Physiotherapy. Neurology: Parkinson's disease, multiple sclerosis and severe traumatic brain injury. *Physiother Effect Bull* 2001, **3**:2–3.

Clarke CE. Mortality from Parkinson's disease. *J Neurol Neurosurg Psychiatry* 2000, **68**:254–255.

Clarke C. Medical management – dopamine agents. In: Clarke C, ed. *Parkinson's Disease in Practice*. London: Royal Society of Medicine; 2001a:51–60.

Clarke CE. *Parkinson's Disease in Practice*. London: Royal Society of Medicine Press; 2001b.

Clarke CE, Sampaio C. Movement Disorders Cochrane Collaborative Review Group. *Move Disord* 1997, **12**:477–482.

Cole B, Finch E, Gowland C et al. *Physical Rehabilitation Outcome Measures*. Toronto: Canadian Physiotherapy Association; 1994.

Collen FM, Wade DT, Robb DF et al. The Rivermead Mobility Index: a further development of the Rivermead Motor Assessment. *Int Disabil Studies* 1991, **13**:50–54.

Comella CL, Stebbins GT, Brown-Toms N et al. Physical therapy and Parkinson's disease: a controlled clinical trial. *Neurology* 1994, **44**:376–378.

Cutson TM, Cotter Laub K, Schenkman M. Pharmacological and nonpharmacological interventions in the treatment of Parkinson's disease. *Phys Ther* 1995, **75**:363–372.

Dam M, Tonin P, Casson S et al. Effects of conventional and sensory-enhanced physiotherapy on disability of Parkinson's disease patients. In: Battistin L, Scarlato G, Caraceni T et al., eds. *Advances in Neurology*, vol. 69. Philadelphia: Lippincott-Raven; 1996:551–555.

de Goede CJT. *The Effects of a Physical Therapy Group Training Program for Patients Suffering from Parkinson's Disease: A Randomized Crossover Trial.* Masters thesis. Amsterdam: Faculty of Human Movement Scences, Vrije Universiteit; 2001.

de Goede CJT, Keus SHJ, Kwakkel G et al. The effects of physical therapy in Parkinson's disease: a research synthesis. *Arch Phys Med Rehab* 2001, **82**:509–515.

Deane KHO, Jones D, Playford ED et al. *Physiotherapy for Patients with Parkinson's Disease (Cochrane Review).* I The Cochrane Library 3. Oxford: Update Software; 2001a.

Deane KHO, Jones D, Ellis-Hill C et al. *A Comparison of Physiotherapy Techniques for Patients with Parkinson's Disease (Cochrane Review).* I The Cochrane Library 1. Oxford: Update Software; 2001b.

Fertl E, Doppelbauer A, Auff E. Physical activity and sports in patients suffering from Parkinson's disease in comparison with health seniors. *J Neural Transm* 1993, **5**:157–161.

Findley L, Peto V, Pugner K et al. The impact of Parkinson's disease on quality of life: results of a research survey in the UK. *Move Disord* 2000, 15(Suppl. 3):179.

Flaherty AW, Grabiel AM. Anatomy of the basal ganglia. In: Marsden CD, Fahn S, eds. *Movement Disorders 3.* New York: Butterworth-Heinemann; 1994:3–27.

Forkink A, Toole T, Hirsch MA et al. *The Effects of a Balance and Strengthening Program on Equilibrium in Parkinsonism.* Florida: Pepper Institute on Aging and Public Policy, Florida State University; 1996.

Formisano R, Pratesi L, Modarelli FT et al. Rehabilitation in Parkinson's disease. *Scand J Rehab Med* 1992, **24**:157–160.

Guidelines Group. *Guidelines for Physiotherapy Practice in Parkinson's Disease.* Newcastle upon Tyne: Institute of Rehabilitation; 2001. Available online at: http://online.unn.ac.uk/faculties/hswe/research/Rehab/Rehab.htm (accessed 13 June 2002).

Hauser RA, Freeman TB, Snow BJ et al. Long-term evaluation of bilateral fetal nigral transplantation in Parkinson's disease. *Arch Neurol* 1999, **56**:179–187.

Hindle JV. Neuropsychiatry. In: Playfer JR, Hindle J, eds. *Parkinson's Disease in the Older Patient.* London: Arnold; 2001:106–107.

Hirsch M. *Activity Dependent Enhancement of Balance Following Strength and Balance Training.* PhD thesis. Florida: Florida State University; 1996.

Hoehn MM, Yahr MD. Parkinsonism: onset, progression and mortality. *Neurology* 1967, **17**:427–442.

Hughes AJ, Daniel SE, Kilford L, Lees AJ. Accuracy of clinical diagnosis of idiopathic Parkinson's disease: a clinicopathologic study of 100 cases. *J Neurol Neurosurg Psychiatry* 1992a, **55**:181–184.

Hughes AJ, Ben-Shlomo Y, Daniel SE, Lees AJ. What features improve the accuracy of clinical diagnosis in Parkinson's disease: a clinicopathologic study. *Neurology* 1992b, **42**:1142–1146.

Hughes AJ, Daniel SE, Lees AJ. Improved accuracy of clinical diagnosis of Lewy body Parkinson's disease. *Neurology* 2001, **57**:1497–1499.

Hurwitz A. The benefit of a home exercise regimen for ambulatory Parkinson's disease patients. *J Neurosci Nurs* 1989, **21**:180–181.

Jarman B, Hurwitz B, Cook A et al. Effects of community based nurses specialising in Parkinson's disease on health outcome and costs: randomised controlled trial. *BMJ* 2002, **324**:1072–1075.

Jenkinson C, Fitzpatrick R, Peto V. *The Parkinson's Disease Questionnaire.* Oxford: Health Services Research Unit, University of Oxford; 1998.

Kamsma YPT, Brouwer WH, Lakke JPWF. Training of compensational strategies for impaired gross motor skills in Parkinson's disease. *Physiother Theory Pract* 1995, **11**:209–229.

Kuroda K, Tarara K, Takatorige T et al. Effect of physical exercise on mortality in patients with Parkinson's disease. *Acta Neurol Scand* 1992, **86**:55–59.

Langston JW, Ballard PA, Tetrud JW, Irwin I. Chronic parkinsonism in humans due to a product of meperidine-analog synthesis. *Science* 1983, **219**:979–980.

Langston JW, Forno LS, Tetrud J et al. Evidence for active nerve cell degeneration in the substantia nigra of humans years after 1-methyl-4-phenyl-1,2,3,6-tetrahydrophyridine exposure. *Ann Neurol* 1999, **46**:598–605.

Lansbury P, Brice A. Genetics of Parkinson's disease and biochemical studies of implicated gene products: commentary. *Curr Opin Cell Biol* 2002, **14**:653.

Lees AJ. Comparison of therapeutic effects and mortality data of levodopa and levodopa combined with selegiline in patients with early, mild Parkinson's disease. Parkinson's Disease Research Group of the United Kingdom. *BMJ* 1995, **311**:1602–1607.

Lennox GG, Lowe JS. Dementia with Lewy bodies. In: Quinn NP, ed. *Parkinsonism.* London: Baillière-Tindall; 1997:147–166.

Limousin P, Krack P, Pollok P et al. Electrical stimulation of the subthalamic nucleus in advanced Parkinson's disease. *N Engl J Med* 1998, **339**:1105–1111.

Lindvall O. Update on fetal transplantation: the Swedish experience. *Move Disord* 1998, 13 (Suppl. 1):83–87.

Litvan I. Progressive supranuclear palsy and corticobasal degeneration. In: Quinn NP, ed. *Parkinsonism.* London: Baillière-Tindall; 1997:167–185.

Macphee GJA. Diagnosis and differential diagnosis of Parkinson's disease. In: Playfer JR, Hindle J, eds.

Parkinson's Disease in the Older Patient. London: Arnold; 2001:43–77.

Marchese R, Diverio M, Zucchi F et al. The role of sensory cues in the rehabilitation of Parkinsonian patients: a comparison of two physical therapy protocols. *Move Disord* 2000, **15**:879–883.

Meara J, Hobson P. Epidemiology of Parkinson's disease and parkinsonism in elderly subjects. In: Meara J, Koller W, eds. *Parkinson's Disease and Parkinsonsim in the Elderly*. Cambridge: Cambridge University Press; 2000:111–122.

Mjones H. Paralysis agitans. A clinical genetic study. *Acta Psychiatr Neurol* 1949, 25 (Suppl. 54):1–195.

Mohr B, Muller V, Mattes R et al. Behavioral treatment of Parkinson's disease leads to improvement of motor skills and to tremor reduction. *Behav Ther* 1996, **27**:235–255.

Morris ME. Movement disorders in people with Parkinson disease: a model for physical therapy. *Phys Ther* 2000, **80**:578–597.

Morris M, Iansek R. *Parkinson's Disease: A Team Approach*. Cheltenham, Australia. Southern Healthcare Network; 1997. Available online at: http://www.quartec.com.au/parkinsons/public.html (accessed 2 September 2002).

Morris ME, Iansek R, Matyas TA et al. Stride length regulation in Parkinson's disease. Normalization strategies and underlying mechanism. *Brain* 1996, **119**:551–568.

Morris M, Iansek R, Churchyard A. The role of the physiotherapist in quantifying movement fluctuations in Parkinson's disease. *Aust J Physiother* 1998, **44**:105–114.

Morris M, Huxham F, McGinley J. Strategies to prevent falls in people with Parkinson's disease. *Physiother Singapore* 1999, **2**:135–141.

Nieuwboer A, Feys P, de Weerdt W et al. Is using a cue the clue to the treatment of freezing in Parkinson's disease? *Physiother Res Int* 1997, **2**:125–134.

Nieuwboer A, de Weerdt W, Dom R et al. Development of an activity scale for individuals with advanced Parkinson disease: reliability and "on-off" variability. *Phys Ther* 2000, **80**:1087–1096.

Nieuwboer A, De Weerdt W, Dom R et al. The effect of a home physiotherapy program for persons with Parkinson's disease. *J Rehab Med* 2001, **33**:266–272.

Olanow CW, Koller WC. An algorithm (decision tree) for the management of Parkinson's disease. *Neurology* 1998, **50**(suppl. 3):S1–S57.

Oxtoby M. *Parkinson's Disease Patients and their Social Needs*. London: Parkinson's Disease Society; 1982.

Parkinson Study Group. Effect of deprenyl on the progression of disability in early Parkinson's disease. *N Engl J Med* 1989, **321**:1364–1371.

Patti F, Reggio A, Nicoletti F et al. Effects of rehabilitation therapy on Parkinsonians' disability and functional independence. *J Neurol Rehab* 1996, **10**:223–231.

Pederson S, Oberg B, Insulander A et al. Group training in parkinsonism: quantitative measurements of treatment. *Scand J Rehab Med* 1990, **22**:207–211.

Plant R, Jones D, Ashburn A et al. *Physiotherapy for People with Parkinson's Disease: UK Best Practice*. Newcastle upon Tyne: Institute of Rehabilitation; 2000.

Playfer JR. Drug therapy. In: Playfer JR, Hindle J, eds. *Parkinson's Disease in the Older Patient*. London: Arnold; 2001:283–309.

Podsialdo D, Richardson S. The timed "Up & Go": a test of basic functional mobility for frail elderly persons. *J Am Geriatr Soc* 1991, **39**:142–148.

Poewe W, Granata R. Pharmacological treatment of Parkinson's disease. In: Watts RL, Koller WC, eds. *Movement Disorders: Neurologic Principles and Practice*. New York: McGraw-Hill; 1997:201–209.

Poewe WH, Wenning GK. The natural history of Parkinson's disease. *Ann Neurol* 1998, **44**:S1–S9.

Polymeropoulos MH, Higgins JJ, Golbe LI et al. Mapping of a gene for Parkinson's disease in the Contursi kindred. *Ann Neurol* 1996, **40**:767–775.

Protas E, Stanley RK, Jankovic J. Exercise and Parkinson's disease. *Crit Rev Phys Rehab Med* 1996, **8**:253–266.

Quinn N. Multiple system atrophy – the nature of the beast. *J Neurol Neurosurg Psychiatry* 1989, **June** (Suppl.): 78–89.

Quinn N. Parkinsonism – recognition and differential diagnosis. *Br Med J* 1995, **310**:447–452.

Rascol O, Coetz C, Koller W et al. Treatment interventions for Parkinson's disease: an evidence based assessment. *Lancet* 2002, **359**:1589–1598.

Samii A, Calne DB. 1999 Research into the etiology of Parkinson's disease. In: LeWitt PA, Oertel WH, eds. *Parkinson's Disease. The Treatment Options*. London: Martin Dunitz; 1999:229–243.

Schapira AHV. Pathogenesis of Parkinson's disease. In: Quinn NP, ed. *Parkinsonism*. London: Baillière-Tindall; 1997:15–36.

Schenkman M, Cutson TM, Kuchibhatla M et al. Exercise to improve spinal flexibility and function for people with Parkinson's disease: a randomized, controlled trial. *J Am Geriatr Soc* 1998, **46**:1207–1216.

Schoenberg BS. Epidemiology of movement disorders. In: Marsden CD, ed. *Movement Disorders 2*. London: Butterworths; 1987:17–32.

Shiba Y, Obuchi S, Toshima A et al. Comparison between visual and auditory stimulation in gait training of patients with idiopathic Parkinson's disease. In: *Proceedings of the 13th International Congress of the World Confederation for Physical Therapy*, Japan, May 1999, p. 458.

Shumway-Cook A, Woollacott MH. *Motor Control. Theory and Practical Applications*. Baltimore: Williams & Wilkins; 1995.

Smith R. Validation and reliability of the Elderly Mobility Scale. *Physiotherapy* 1994, **80**:744–747.

Smithson F, Morris ME, Iansek R. Performance of clinical tests of balance in Parkinson's disease. *Phys Ther* 1998, **78**:577–592.

Stack E, Ashburn A. Fall events described by people with Parkinson's disease: implications for clinical interviewing and the research agenda. *Physiother Res Int* 1999, **4**:190–199.

Steele JC, Guzman T. Observations about amyotrophic lateral sclerosis and the parkinsonism dementia complex of Guam with regard to epidemiology and etiology. *Can J Neurol Sci* 1987, 14 (Suppl. 3):358–362.

Strange PC. Dopamine receptors in the basal ganglia. *Movement Disorders* 1992, **8**:263–270.

Suteerawattananon M, Protas EJ. Reliability of outcome measures in individuals with Parkinson's disease. *Physiother Ther Pract* 2000, **16**:211–218.

Thaut MH, McIntosh GC, Rice RR et al. Rhythmic auditory stimulation in gait training for Parkinson's disease patients. *Move Disord* 1996, **11**:193–200.

Thomas S, MacMahon D, Henry S. *Moving and Shaping – The Future. Commissioning Services for People with Parkinson's Disease*. London: Parkinson's Disease Society; 1999.

Tinetti M. Performance-oriented assessment of mobility problems in elderly patients. *J Am Geriatr Soc* 1986, **34**:119–126.

Turnbull G. *Physical Therapy Management of Parkinson's Disease*. New York: Churchill Livingstone; 1992.

Viliani T, Pasquetti P, Magnolfi S et al. Effects of physical training on straightening-up processes in patients with Parkinson's disease. *Disabil Rehab* 1999, **21**:68–73.

Wade D. *Measurement in Neurological Rehabilitation*. Oxford: Oxford University Press; 1992.

Ward CD, Duvoisin RC, Ince SE et al. Parkinson's disease in 65 pairs of twins and in a set of quadruplets. *Neurology* 1983, **33**:815–824.

Weissenborn S. The effect of using a two-step verbal cue to a visual target above eye level on the parkinsonian gait: a case study. *Physiotherapy* 1993, **79**:26–31.

Wood BH, Bilclough JA, Bowron A et al. Incidence and prediction of falls in Parkinson's disease: a prospective multidisciplinary study. *J Neurol Neurosurg Psychiatry* 2002, **72**:721–725.

Yarrow S. *Survey of Members of the Parkinson's Disease Society*. London: Parkinson's Disease Society; 1999.

Yekutiel MP. Patients' fall records as an aid in designing and assessing therapy in Parkinsonism. *Disabil Rehab* 1993, **15**:189–193.

Yekutiel MP, Pinhasov A, Shahar G et al. A clinical trial of the re-education of movement in patients with Parkinson's disease. *Clin Rehab* 1991, **5**:207–214.

Chapter 12

Huntington's disease

O Quarrell   B Cook

INTRODUCTION

George Huntington may not have been the first to describe this condition but he gave a clear and concise account of its clinical and genetic features in 1872. In the early literature, the condition was called 'Huntington's chorea', which denotes emphasis on the most obvious clinical sign. However, not all patients have chorea, so focusing on this one sign may detract from other important aspects. The term 'Huntington's disease' (HD) seems more appropriate and is now widely accepted.

The major features of HD may be considered as a triad of a movement disorder, often choreic in nature; an affective disturbance; and cognitive impairment. The condition is inherited as an autosomal dominant, so on average half the offspring of an affected person will be similarly affected. The recent identification of the mutation causing HD means that laboratory diagnostic and presymptomatic tests are now much easier. Despite this, there is no treatment that will effectively prevent or ameliorate the progressive neurodegeneration. Current treatment is, at best, supportive and symptomatic, requiring input from different professionals at different stages of the disease. Ideally, needs should be anticipated and continuity of care maintained throughout all stages of the disease so that a relationship builds up between professionals, patients and their families.

This chapter will describe the genetic and pathological aspects of the disease before describing the major clinical features and general management. Physical management strategies will be considered under broad categories of early, mid and late stages of the disease. Other useful texts, which discuss this condition, include those by Ward et al. (1993) and Bates et al. (2002).

PREVALENCE

There have been a number of studies of the prevalence of HD in different areas of the UK but there is a problem obtaining a picture from a large population (see Harper, 1992, for review). Most UK studies quote the range of 4–10 per 100 000 and most European countries, the USA, Australia and South Africa have also given prevalence figures within this range. Low prevalence has been documented in Finland and Japan. The low prevalence in Finland may indicate that the population has been relatively isolated from the rest of Europe. The low prevalence in Japan cannot be due to poor ascertainment and requires a separate explanation. It is difficult to be sure of prevalence in parts of the world in which there have not been extensive surveys.

Whilst HD may be considered a rare disorder, it should be remembered that the burden will be great for the patient, the immediate carers and the offspring, half of whom will, on average, develop the condition.

GENETICS

Since HD is inherited in an autosomal dominant fashion, a mutation on one copy of a pair of genes is sufficient to cause the disorder. The gene for HD was localised to chromosome 4 in 1983 (Gusella et al., 1983) but it was not until 10 years later that the mutation was identified (Huntington's Disease Collaborative Research Group, 1993). The gene has been called IT15 and the protein encoded by that gene termed huntingtin. The 3-basepair DNA sequence, CAG, which codes for the amino acid glutamine, is repeated a number of times on the normal gene but there is a marked expansion in the number of repeats on HD genes. The abnormal huntingtin protein can therefore be said to contain an expanded polyglutamine tract.

Normal chromosomes have an HD gene with fewer than 35 CAG repeats, whereas HD chromosomes have a gene with more than 36 repeats. The mutation is said to be dynamic in that the number of repeats on the HD gene varies between generations. The increase in the number of repeats is specific for HD and does not occur in patients with Parkinson's disease, schizophrenia or other movement disorders (Kremer et al., 1994; Rubinsztein et al., 1994, 1995).

It is relatively easy to determine the number of CAG repeats from a sample of venous blood. This has made confirmation of diagnosis reliable in the vast majority of cases. It also means that a simple laboratory test is now available for anyone at risk of HD, to determine whether or not they have inherited the mutation. Given that there is no effective treatment to delay or alter the nature of the progressive degeneration, presymptomatic predictive testing should be undertaken in the context of skilled genetic counselling. There is an inverse correlation between the number of CAG repeats and age of onset; the higher the number of repeats, the lower the age of onset. Very broad categorisation is possible: people with 36–39 repeats may develop HD late in life or even not at all; people with 40–60 repeats usually develop HD in adult life; and people with over 60 repeats develop juvenile-onset HD. It should be emphasised that approximately 50% of the variability in age of onset is attributed to the number of repeats; this degree of correlation is insufficient to give useful information to an individual who has been identified as having the gene presymptomatically.

Whilst identifying the gene has simplified diagnostic tests and facilitated presymptomatic predictive testing, this was not an end in itself. Cloning the gene was considered an essential prerequisite to understanding the pathophysiology, which is essential if effective treatments are to be developed.

NEUROPATHOLOGY

The most striking neuronal cell loss occurs in the basal ganglia, especially the caudate and putamen nuclei, which together are termed the striatum (see Ch. 1, Figs 1.3 and 1.4). However, it should be noted that neuronal cell loss occurs in other areas of the brain, including the cortex, particularly layers III, V and VI (Roos, 1986). To emphasise this point, the brain of a patient with HD will be smaller and weigh less than that of an age-matched control.

Perry et al. (1973) demonstrated loss of the inhibitory neurotransmitter gamma-aminobutyric acid (GABA) in the basal ganglia. It has since been shown that there is selective loss of the efferent medium spiny neurones in the striatum, with relative sparing of the large aspiny interneurones.

The striatum receives excitatory neurones from the cortex and has efferent neurones containing the neurotransmitters GABA and substance P or GABA and metencephalin. These neurones project to the internal globus pallidus and substantia nigra via direct and indirect pathways. The pathways damaged in HD are shown in Figure 12.1. Loss of neurones from the indirect pathway results in loss of inhibition of the external globus pallidus, which produces more inhibition of the subthalamus, less stimulation of the internal globus pallidus, less inhibition of the thalamus and overstimulation of the thalamocortical feedback, resulting in chorea.

Loss of neurones from the direct pathway results in increased inhibition of the thalamus and less activity

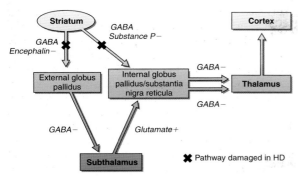

Figure 12.1 Connections of the basal ganglia, showing the pathways damaged in Huntington's disease (HD). GABA, gamma-aminobutyric acid.

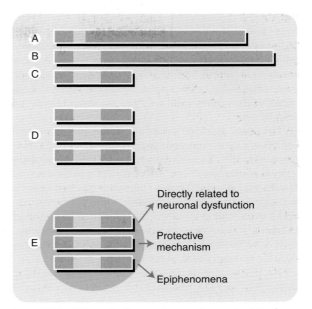

Figure 12.2 Schematic diagram showing the mechanism of inclusion formation. The normal huntingtin protein is labelled A and the polyglutamine repeat is shaded. The abnormal huntingtin is illustrated as B, showing the expanded polyglutamine repeat. The first part of the protein is cleaved and translocates to the nucleus, shown as C. Within the nucleus, the cleaved protein product can form aggregates, as in D. Other proteins can also become trapped in the inclusions, as shown in E. It is not clear if the inclusions are directly related to the pathology; it is possible that the inclusions represent a defence mechanism by the cell to remove the cleaved huntingtin fragment. The final possibility is that the inclusions are epiphenomena and the cellular pathology is related to another aspect of the abnormal huntingtin.

of the thalamocortical feedback, producing bradykinesia and rigidity. The exact distribution of motor signs seen in a patient will, in part, depend on the degree of degeneration between these two pathways. Hedreen & Folstein (1995) have suggested that both pathways degenerate at a similar rate but that excess dopamine from the substantia nigra produces an inhibitory effect on the indirect pathway and a stimulatory effect on the direct pathway, thus giving an apparent appearance of a different rate of degeneration. This theory is consistent with the observation that medical treatment with dopa-blocking drugs or dopa-depleting drugs can modify the physical sign of chorea.

A clear understanding of the neuropathophysiology of HD requires an explanation of how the abnormal huntingtin protein results in late-onset selective neuronal dysfunction and eventually neurodegeneration, together with a detailed description of how the cognitive, affective and physical signs and symptoms of the disorder are related to the observed changes within the brain. It is not possible to present such a detailed account of the neuropathophysiology of HD here. The huntingtin protein is present in a wide variety of neurones (Landwehrmeyer et al., 1995); therefore, it is unclear why a huntingtin protein with an expanded polyglutamine tract should result in selective neuronal dysfunction and degeneration.

Since the identification of the gene there have been a number of different approaches to understanding basic pathology. It is clear that the expanded huntingtin protein exerts its effect from gaining a new function within the cell. A range of experiments have shown that abnormal huntingtin binds to other proteins but this still does not explain the selective dysfunction and degeneration. A different approach was to insert the first part of the abnormal gene into mice (Mangiarini et al., 1996). This greatly accelerated the disease process and allowed the observation that this shortened protein

formed insoluble inclusions in the nuclei of neurones (Davies et al., 1997). A similar process occurs in humans (see Vonsattel & DiFiglia, 1998, for a review). Huntingtin is normally found in the cytoplasm of neurones. Abnormal huntingtin is cleaved and the smaller protein moves to the nucleus. It does form aggregates and other proteins get sequestered in these inclusions. It is not clear if the inclusions are directly related to the basic pathology, a defence mechanism by the cell or an epiphenomenon and the main pathology relates to another function of the abnormal huntingtin protein. This is summarised in Figure 12.2 and a comprehensive review of these issues is provided by Tolbin & Singer (2000).

SIGNS AND SYMPTOMS AND THEIR GENERAL MANAGEMENT

Onset of HD is most frequently between the ages of 35 and 55, which is after the usual years of reproduction, although it can develop at almost any age. Onset may occur before the age of 20, which is arbitrarily defined as 'juvenile onset', and may also occur after the age of 60. Patients with juvenile onset tend to have more bradykinesia and rigidity than chorea. Those with onset after the age of 60 appear to have an illness which subjectively appears milder than those with onset in middle age.

The onset of HD is insidious. Patients may present with frank neurological or psychiatric signs and symptoms and either they or their relatives have some difficulty in dating the onset. Alternatively, a patient with a family history of HD may present with non-specific complaints of feeling depressed, forgetful or clumsy, and it is difficult to be sure if these features are the onset of HD or have another cause. Under these circumstances it may be prudent to wait a year or so to see if more definite features of HD develop.

Movement disorders

It has been emphasised that HD patients have a mixture of movement abnormalities, but chorea is seen most frequently. Lakke (1981) defined chorea as 'A state of excessive, spontaneous movement, irregularly timed, randomly distributed and abrupt. Severity may vary from restlessness with mild intermittent exaggeration of gesture, fidgeting movements of the hands, unstable dance-like gait to a continuous flow of disabling violent movements'.

In the early stages of the disease the chorea may be barely perceptible, although those who see HD patients on a regular basis will be aware of the movements even if the patient and his or her relatives are unaware of them. All parts of the body may be affected. As the disease develops, the chorea may become progressively more obvious and then reach a plateau (Folstein et al., 1983). In the later stages of the disease, other movement disorders may become more prominent, such as dystonia, bradykinesia and rigidity (see Ch. 4); these are important features of HD.

Dystonia implies sustained slow muscle contractions that may result in twisting movements of the trunk or abnormal postures of the limbs. This sign may be more obvious in the later stages of the disease. The bradykinesia and rigidity may also worsen as the disease progresses, but early in the course of the disease there may be impairment in the rhythm and speed of rapid alternating movements, e.g. finger taps, movement of the tongue between the corners of the mouth or alternating pronation and supination of the forearm (Folstein et al., 1986). A useful early sign may be impaired saccadic eye movements, i.e. an impaired ability to flick the eyes from side to side without undue blinks, delay or head

movements. As the disease progresses, the patient may become unable to perform this test.

Patients with a very early age of onset, or those in the later stages, may have little in the way of chorea. At one time the phrase 'rigid variant' was used, but this is not a helpful term as patients with rigidity do not truly have a different variety of HD; it is just that one particular movement disorder predominates over another.

Abnormalities of heel-to-toe walking may occur in the early stages but as the disease progresses the gait is wide-based and staggering. Patients with HD do fall; however, it is surprising that falls are not more frequent given the abnormal posture of the trunk and limbs. As the disease progresses, patients may become chair- or bed-bound and require considerable nursing care and physiotherapy. Other aspects of the motor disturbance include dysarthria and dysphagia (see below). Motor disorders in HD were discussed in relation to electrophysiological findings by Yanagisawa (1992).

Dysarthria

The rate and rhythm of speech may be disturbed early in the course of HD (Folstein et al., 1986), progressing to become unintelligible; occasionally patients become mute. Abnormalities in phonation have been noted with the movement abnormality affecting the laryngeal and respiratory muscles (Ramig, 1976). The neuronal loss causes a cognitive impairment (see below) and may disrupt linguistic ability (Gordon & Illes, 1987). A speech and language therapist can advise on methods of communication and provide technological aids (see Ch. 13, p. 243).

Dysphagia and cachexia

Dysphagia, particularly for liquids, is a common complaint in middle to late stages of the disease, with abnormalities occurring in all aspects of the swallowing process (Kagel & Leopold, 1992). Indeed, aspiration and choking may ultimately be the cause of death. Advice from a speech and language therapist will help with feeding, and assessment of swallowing problems will indicate the risk of choking.

Advice needs to be given regarding seating the patient in an upright position and encouraging him or her to eat slowly with bite-sized pieces. It is useful to consider whether a dry mouth is a known side-effect of any medication prescribed for the patient. As the disease progresses, consideration needs to be given to practical issues such as non-slip plates and utensils with large grips. Carers need to be instructed in the use of the Heimlich manoeuvre. Over time patients may become unable to feed themselves and the dietician may recommend that the texture of the food be altered so that it is soft and smooth (Ramen et al., 1993).

Weight loss is an integral part of the disease process for the majority of patients; the neuropathological aetiology of this is unclear. Patients may be offered high-calorie diets. For some patients with significant cachexia, it may be appropriate to discuss the use of a gastrostomy feeding tube with the affected patient, if possible, and the family. The objective is to provide nourishment and comfort but the decision has to be tempered by a consideration of the patient's general mobility, ability to communicate and quality of life (Bates et al., 2002). This subject should be approached before the patient is unable to communicate or take an active part in this decision.

Incontinence

Urinary and faecal incontinence occur in the late stage and may be due partly to dementia rather than a specific neurological cause. However, in a small study of 6 patients, Wheeler et al. (1985) found some evidence of detrusor hyperreflexia. Nursing care involving regular changing and cleaning will help to prevent skin breakdown and pressure sores, as well as maintain dignity.

Psychiatric features and behavioural management

For many of the carers of HD patients, disturbances of affect (depression, temper tantrums and apathy) and the cognitive impairment may be as difficult to manage as the movement disorder (or more difficult). The management of psychiatric and behavioural problems is discussed in Chapter 27.

Depression is said to be very common in patients with HD and may precede the onset of a variety of neurological disorders. Morris & Scourfield (1996) summarised the prevalence of depression from eight surveys and found rates of 9–44%. There may be difficulties in comparing diagnostic criteria between surveys. However, further surveys have reported high prevalence rates of 39–44% (Folstein et al., 1983; Mindham et al., 1985; Shiwach, 1994). Frank psychosis with schizophrenia-like symptoms is much less frequent but known to occur in HD. Specific psychiatric syndromes or diagnoses should be sought in patients with HD, as they may respond to therapy with modern antidepressants or dopa-blockers as appropriate.

Carers of patients with HD may also complain about apathy, irritability and temper tantrums. Whilst these may not be seen as a problem by the patient, they can pose difficult management problems for the family. In addition, disturbance of sleep patterns may be a particularly difficult management issue for the family.

Although behavioural problems are accepted and recognised symptoms of the disease, they may sometimes result from inadequate support and crisis management. Patients may be forced into unfamiliar situations that cause anger, fear and non-compliance. Carers need to learn to deal with outbursts of aggression, and behavioural psychotherapy for the patient may be necessary (Marks, 1986).

The older literature commented on anecdotes of increased libido and abnormal sexual behaviour. Whilst this may occur, it is likely that decreased libido is more common. A systematic study of sexual disorders in HD was conducted by Federoff et al. (1994).

In his original description, George Huntington commented on the tendency to suicide. There is an increased rate of suicide amongst HD patients, mainly occurring around the time of onset or early in the course of the disease, possibly associated with depression (Shoenfeld et al., 1984; Di Maio et al., 1993).

Cognitive impairment

This is the third in the triad of characteristic abnormalities seen in HD. There is general decline in intellectual function during the course of HD but it is qualitatively different from the more global dementia of Alzheimer's disease, as aphasia, agnosia and apraxia are not prominent features (for a review see Brandt, 1991). Patients with either Alzheimer's disease or HD have been compared over the course of the two disorders using brief tests of mental state, the mini-mental state exam or the dementia rating scale, and different cognitive profiles were obtained (Brandt et al., 1988; Rosser & Hodges, 1994; Paulsen et al., 1995). This supports the concept of qualitative differences in the nature of cognitive impairment in a disease which mainly affects the cortex, as in Alzheimer's, and a disorder which affects the subcortex (basal ganglia), as in HD. Patients with HD have difficulty with concentration (especially if there are distractions), forward planning and cognitive flexibility. These deficits in executive function may contribute to the behavioural problems seen in HD.

Despite slowness of thinking and dysarthria, it should be remembered that the patient retains the ability to comprehend throughout most of the course of the illness. Therefore, care should be taken when talking about patients in their presence.

Duration of illness

The average duration of illness is difficult to estimate. Whilst the age of death may be recorded accurately, the age of onset is of necessity inexact. There is considerable variation of the duration of the disease from patient to patient but estimates from a number of studies

Table 12.1 Symptoms and secondary complications in Huntington's disease

Symptoms	Complications
Choreiform movements	Asymmetry
	Injury
	Loss of range
	Loss of function
Rigidity	Loss of range
	Immobility
	Contracture/deformity
	Pain
Spasms	Exaggerated head and neck movements
	Pain at end-of-range movements
Speech abnormalities	Communication breakdown
Swallowing problems	Aspiration
	Chest infections
Weight loss	Infections
	Pressure problems
	Poor healing of injury
	Fatigue
	General debilitation
Incontinence	Discomfort
	Indignity

have varied between an average of 10 and 17 years (Bates et al., 2002). Our experience would suggest that the average is towards the higher end of that range. The average duration is similar for HD of juvenile and adult onset; those with a late age of onset have a lower duration, perhaps because of other unrelated causes of death (Bates et al., 2002; Roos et al., 1993).

Secondary complications

Complications that may occur are shown in Table 12.1. All these complications will give rise to pain or discomfort and therefore result in diminished performance. In order to correct or control these complications, more input is required from the physiotherapist and there is also an increased care load on all clinical staff. Continuous physical management is therefore necessary to reduce the risk of these complications (see below).

GENERAL ASPECTS OF MANAGEMENT

Given the slowly progressive nature of the disease, the wide spread in age of onset and the variations in relative importance of motor, cognitive and affective dysfunction between individual patients, it is difficult to describe a comprehensive management suitable for all patients. At best some general guidance may be attempted. A useful overview of management which contains many practical suggestions has been given by Ramen et al. (1993).

The multidisciplinary team

The complexity of physical, social and behavioural aspects of HD requires considerable efforts from all professionals involved to achieve appropriate management of the patient and family. The secondary complications listed in Table 12.1 indicate the range of disciplines needed to care for the HD patient. The main disciplines include social work, dietetics, speech therapy, medicine, physiotherapy, occupational therapy, psychology and nursing.

The roles of the team members overlap in places and the degree of input required varies for the different stages of the disease. For example, the speech therapist will help with speech and swallowing problems in the middle stage to cope with current problems and also prepare the patient and team for the late stage when communication aids may need to be provided. The physiotherapy input (see 'Physical management', below) essentially concerns maintenance of function in the early/middle stages, safety and prevention of secondary complications in the middle stage and management of complications to minimise discomfort in the terminal stage. The social worker is the key person at every stage to co-ordinate services and ensure that respite care, transition into residential care and other milestones are managed with minimal trauma to the patient and family. This involves liaison with funding authorities and the different support services. Forward planning is essential; deterioration can occur, so placement must be available and the multidisciplinary team must be able to respond when help is needed.

Medical management

This can best be divided into pharmacological and non-pharmacological care.

Non-pharmacological management

As discussed above, the behavioural aspects of HD may be more of a problem to the carers than the movement disorder. It is important for carers to understand that someone with HD can be more easily overwhelmed by tasks, less able to adapt to changing situations, and respond with seemingly unreasonable outbursts of temper. A direct confrontation should be avoided and emphasis placed on devising strategies to side-step precipitating factors, avoiding the need to concentrate on several tasks at once, having some structure to the day and encouraging the person to participate in joint activities for as long as possible. In general, it is better to try these tactics rather than immediately turning to drugs.

Pharmacological management

In the past there has been a tendency to treat the movement disorder using dopamine-blocking or dopamine-depleting drugs. Chorea may be the focus of pharmacological treatment if it is of large amplitude or causing distress to the patient, in which case a dopa-blocking agent (such as haloperidol or sulpiride) is used. Otherwise, the focus of pharmacological management should be on depression and irritability and this involves the use of modern antidepressants (selective serotonin reuptake inhibitors, SSRIs), together with other drugs such as propranolol, sodium valproate or carbamazepine. There are problems with focusing therapy on the physical sign of chorea; firstly, it is often not a problem to the patient; and secondly, overmedication can lead to worsening bradykinesia and dystonia.

A complaint by some patients and their carers is that, after a diagnosis has been made, nothing specific is done for years. General practitioners and hospital clinics have a role in being generally supportive to families over a prolonged period of time.

Genetic counselling

The genetic counselling clinic has a role to play in supporting the family, especially the extended family, due to the implications of this inherited disease (Bates et al., 2002). Some members of the family may seek predictive testing and, depending on the outcome, may need support for some time afterwards.

Social management

In the early stages of the disease the movement disorder and the intellectual decline may be minimal, enabling the patient to continue in employment for some time. As the disease progresses, a social worker may advise on disability payments. The principal carer will need help, support and an opportunity to take a break, even if that involves someone else looking after the patient for a few hours per week.

Many of the behavioural problems of the patient are difficult to manage but, where possible, practical solutions should be considered to provide a safe and calm environment. Given the selective cognitive deficits, a non-confrontational approach should be adopted, with a routine established if possible.

Patients with HD do fall; therefore physiotherapists and occupational therapists have a role in suggesting modifications to the home, such as the provision of additional handrails so as to maintain mobility and independence with reduced risk.

The carer may need advice on the management of incontinence, following the exclusion of a urinary tract infection. Practical advice may focus on regular toileting, depending on mobility, or the use of incontinence pads.

Respite care

As the disease progresses further, the degree of physical dependence will increase so that the social worker has a role in organising home help and, depending on the degree of co-operation of the patient, respite care. Placement into residential care in the later stages is made easier if periods of respite have been taken in the same establishment. Such periods prior to admission enable the patient and family to become familiar with the environment and make the transition less traumatic. They may also avoid crisis placement for terminal care, a situation which is far from satisfactory.

Support in the community

In the later stages of the disease, a significant proportion of patients need residential care. The main reasons are the inability of the family to cope, often because of unreasonable behaviour, or because patients who are living alone are unable to manage and home conditions may become too unkempt. Patients may become a danger and health hazard to themselves and to others.

Local authority services can be very important in enabling the affected person to remain in the community for as long as possible. The support and quality of care will depend on the resources of the authority and the co-operation of the patient. The multidisciplinary team should be involved at this stage to provide the best package of care.

PHYSICAL MANAGEMENT

As patients progress through the stages of the disease, careful management can ease the impact of change by anticipating the patient's needs before each functional loss occurs.

The physical management of HD is similar to that of motor neurone disease (see Ch. 13) but certain features of HD due to the movement disorders require specific attention.

Principles of physiotherapy

At present there is no means of allaying the progression of the disease but physiotherapy can be valuable in preventing secondary complications and maintaining independence for as long as possible. Principles of physiotherapy are based on clinical experience since research into this area of HD is lacking.

The specific approaches to treatment and techniques used are not discussed in detail here but can be found in Chapters 21 and 23, respectively. In the early and middle stages, physiotherapy aims to maintain balance and mobility, and in the middle to late stages to achieve optimal positioning and comfort. Mobility aids may be prescribed where appropriate. Physiotherapists can also teach patients relaxation techniques and instruct carers in movement and handling techniques. Literature on physiotherapy for patients with HD is sparse but an exercise programme was suggested by Peacock (1987).

Early, middle and late management stage are not definite categories into which signs and symptoms can be easily placed or for which timescales can be given. This is due to the variability of the disease in different patients.

Early stage

This is the time from diagnosis to the stage of decreasing independence. Active physiotherapy is not necessary at this stage but it is beneficial to make contact with the patients and their families and encourage the patients to participate in their own management. The benefits of functional activity, and how to identify any postural changes, can be explained. The physiotherapist can give advice at this stage on stretching exercises to prevent contracture and deformity from soft-tissue shortening (see Ch. 25 and below).

HD can have such a devastating effect on patients and their families that the postural problems may be considered insignificant and ignored. Physical problems can therefore become established and escape notice until they cause functional disability.

Middle stage

At this stage, patients still have some independence and are usually managed in their own home. The main aims of physiotherapy are to maintain functional ability and prevent contractures and deformity. The disorder of posture, balance and movement is apparent and manifests itself with increased chorea, dystonia, a weaving gait and bradykinesia (see Ch. 4). These contribute to a decline in functional activity which can result in apathy. This may defeat any attempt at physical intervention; support of families and care teams may be the only possibility. Physiotherapists and occupational therapists can advise on equipment and furniture, and health and safety issues, particularly those relating to moving and handling.

Continuous assessment and re-evaluation of the physical ability of the patients, which can change quite dramatically, is important to maintain a safe environment for both patients and carers. An occupational therapist may provide adaptations to the home to help with safety, e.g. stair rails, poles for transferring in and out of the bath.

Many people mistakenly presume that involuntary movements and walking will maintain range of movement (ROM). With such a bizarre disorder of posture, balance and movement (in spite of the activity), there is misalignment of body segments and patients lose the ability to rotate. Alignment and rotation are essential for postural control and efficient movement and functional ability. Specific exercises are required to maintain ROM (see Chs 23 and 25).

Preventive care is beneficial and a routine of physical management must be devised and be practical and cost-effective. The overall approach to treatment is to help patients organise and regulate their movements in order to function more effectively and to have the opportunity to remain independent for as long as possible. In this intermediate stage, a daily physiotherapy programme that is useful for identifying problems before they become too established might include prone lying for 20 min, exercise to maintain ROM, walking for endurance and posture control (see below). The physical management in the middle stage of HD was discussed by Imbriglio (1992).

Late stage

As the disease progresses, specially adapted padded chairs may need to be suggested to control posture whilst seated and to minimise damage from the effects of chorea or progressive dystonia. Further progression of the disease may mean that wheelchairs have to be considered if patients are to be taken for an appreciable distance outside the home. In the later stages of the disease, chorea may be less troublesome but stiffness and dystonia more marked. These symptoms may predominate throughout the course of the disease in those patients with an early onset. Patients are at risk of developing the complications listed in Table 12.1. Physical management at this stage is aimed at aiding nursing care and comfort. It has been suggested that treatment of specific disabilities may not be effective and that a general programme may be more appropriate (Mason et al., 1991).

Assessment

There are a number of rating scales which have been used to quantify clinical aspects of HD; a useful, simple and practical one is the functional disability scale of Shoulson & Fahn (1979). Examples of functional and motor assessment forms were described by Imbriglio (1992).

The principles of physiotherapy assessment are discussed in Chapter 3; the main aspects applicable to HD include assessment of co-ordination, mobility, functional abilities and safety in activities of daily living.

Maintaining joint range and mobility

Physiotherapy plays an important part in maintaining movement and mobility. The bizarre movements that patients may have contribute to asymmetry and the development of preferred postures. This may lead to secondary complications such as deformities and contractures, which will cause seating and management problems.

Positioning and posture should be controlled at all times, i.e. lying, sitting and standing. Standing frames, standing risers and tilt tables may be useful in the later stage when patients are no longer able to stand. Posture in sitting and lying is discussed below.

Prone lying and stretching exercises

Prone lying should be encouraged as part of a daily routine, e.g. 20 min each day, to help maintain ROM, and is particularly useful for identifying any asymmetry or preferred postural pattern.

Full-range movements of all joints can be incorporated into daily activities such as dressing or, if preferred, a suitable programme of self-assisted exercises (see Ch. 25). In the later stages, passive/assisted and passive stretching will be required to maintain joint ROM.

A variety of techniques may be used to reduce rigidity and facilitate movement and functional activity: trunk mobilisations, proprioceptive neuromuscular facilitation (PNF), joint approximation, gym ball activities and relaxation techniques. These techniques are discussed in Chapter 23.

Walking and functional activities

Walking should be encouraged to maintain stamina and ability for as long as possible. The tendency is to offer too much support, thus inhibiting locomotion and denying the patient the opportunity to walk (Gardham, 1982). Walking may become physically impossible or too dangerous for patients and their carers. Whatever the reason, a multidisciplinary decision must be made which includes the patients and carers. The quality of gait can be analysed and abnormalities identified and modified if possible.

Many HD patients are severely disabled, largely due to disuse. Skilled handling can facilitate efficient movement and enable patients to participate actively and thus become more independent. Functional activity is the most effective way of maximising their remaining ability.

Head control is important, as stability of the head is vital for communication, eating, visual fixation, manual activities and all activities requiring balance, including walking. Patients should be encouraged to look at what they are doing, and practice eye–hand co-ordination activities.

All functional activities involve patterns of movement and have an element of rotation, which plays an important role in postural adjustment and normal postural activity. Rotation is vital for balance and activities should include rotation of the trunk.

Patients can be stimulated through exercise, sport and the provision of an element of competition for those who need it. Hydrotherapy can provide recreation and enjoyment (see Ch. 23). Gym group activities can include skittles, balloon badminton, archery and throwing games.

Experience has shown that regular activities such as hydrotherapy and gym groups are looked forward to, and that with familiarity and regularity, participation is increased. This is also the case with music therapy and occupational therapy and reinforces the reasoning behind many claims that the majority of patients are cognitively aware, in spite of their dementia and reduced ability to communicate.

Transfers

Independent transfers should be maintained for as long as possible. Standing transfers may require only one person to facilitate movement but it is important to maintain the safety of both patients and carers (National Back Pain Association in collaboration with the Royal College of Nursing, 1998). The wearing of transfer belts can assist safe transfers and enable patients to continue walking for as long as possible. Transfers may be assisted by means of equipment, and hoists are a necessity in the later stages for some people. The type of hoist and sling must be assessed for each individual patient.

Safety

In all stages of the disease it is a great challenge to everyone concerned to match the needs of patients with health and safety needs. Many patients apparently have no fear and seem unaware of danger, and this can put them and their carers at risk. Many of the minor injuries that are sustained can be caused by restraining devices that are provided in the interest of safety. Special seating and beds are discussed below. A balance must be found between function, freedom, risk, challenge and health and safety.

Carers may be at risk from injury when managing patients. Guidance on the European Community Directives for Manual Handling Operations Regulations (1990, 1992) requires risk assessments to be made if the need for manual handling involves a risk of injury. The assessment takes an ergonomic approach and looks at the task, the patient, the environment and the carer's ability. Carers need to be informed about the disease and need support from appropriate people to help them to cope with the patient's personality changes and bizarre behavior.

Posture and seating

Awareness of posture and signs of developing abnormalities must be taught in the early stages and include posture in standing, sitting and lying. Posture and special seating for neurological patients were discussed in detail by Pope (2002).

Positioning in the early and middle stages

Posture and seating should be addressed in the early stage and a suitable seating regimen for everyday activities agreed upon, e.g. a comfortable easy chair for some activities and a change of chair for sitting at a table. Long periods of poor positioning or habitual postures may lead to deformity and reduced ability and independence later on, so seating needs to be monitored from the outset of HD.

The choice of chair aims to achieve the optimal position to suit the individual person's needs, and adaptations will be necessary as disability increases.

Symmetry of posture and movement should be sought, as this helps patients to organise themselves and provides a more natural position from which to initiate movement.

Special seating in the middle to late stages

When it is no longer possible or safe to walk independently, a wheelchair may be appropriate, though not always acceptable, for some patients. On the whole, the standard wheelchair is adequate and patients may be able to propel themselves with their arms or 'paddle' with their feet. Trays and footplates are not always appropriate or desirable; the floor can act as a stable footrest and the chair can be parked at a table for mealtimes or reading. While patients are still reasonably able, functional independence is of vital importance.

If a patient is seated in a chair for several hours each day, a firm base is essential as well as an appropriate seat cushion and a pelvic strap. Extra padding may be needed to protect patients from knocks. Because of the progression of the disease and the nature of the symptoms, it is unlikely that a powered wheelchair would be appropriate; there may, however, be exceptions to this.

If wheelchairs are not acceptable to the patient, ordinary upright chairs or suitable armchairs can be adequate and maintain normality for as long as postural stability allows.

When the movements become so exaggerated that the patient is endangering himself or herself, then it is time for some other form of seating (Pope, 2002).

Patients with high tone and rigidity will need a very supportive seating system. This could be a recliner chair with adaptations, or a more custom-made system such as a full matrix support system (Sharman & Ponton, 1990). There are many chairs on the market that can be used as the support base for the special seating systems, e.g. the Kirton chair that was developed for the HD patient. Some of these special chairs can provide safety but they do nothing to maintain function or ability.

Because of the variation in range and velocity of movement, it is not ethical or possible to provide physical restraint against such movements; restraint may be more injurious than actually falling out of the chair.

Positioning in bed in the middle and late stages

Special beds, log rolls, T-rolls and bed wedges can help maintain alignment and stability of posture, but obviously uncontrolled movements will limit their effectiveness. Positioning strategies are also discussed elsewhere in relation to patients with brain injury (see Ch. 7) and motor neurone disease (see Ch. 13).

The choreiform movements place the patient at risk of injury and falling out of bed. Net beds may be chosen for safety reasons since they conform to the body and spread the load, thus reducing pressure; the patient can be turned without handling, thereby reducing injury to carers, and the bed does not have to be made. The disadvantages of these hammock-like net beds are:

- They maintain a flexed unfunctional posture.
- They are difficult for transfers.
- It is not possible to sit the patient up.
- There is no stability for functional movement.
- It is difficult to protect the sides without awkward gaps.
- Patients' fingers can get caught in the netting.
- Patients are deprived of human contact.

- Patients are not able to use equipment which promotes stability and alignment.

Net beds provide a supposedly safe environment but should only be used as a last resort as they increase disability.

Profile beds can provide some stability and enable the patient to have changes of position, i.e. sit up in bed. They have good cot sides which can be protected by cushions and have air-filled mattresses. The bed can be used with log rolls, T-rolls and bed wedges, though ideally these are better placed on a firm mattress.

If a patient's movements are so violent that they are damaged by hitting the cot sides, even when padded, it may be appropriate to place a mattress on the floor. A pelvic strap may have to be used to maintain safety.

ASPECTS OF

Management involves keepi supporting the and describing was published Ethics and Hur also a very diffi who have com Imbriglio (1992) between team m lar to that for mo to allow patient with dignity and minimal discomfort.

References

American Academy of Neurology Ethics and Humanities Subcommittee. Palliative care in neurology. *Neurology* 1996, **46**:870–872.

Bates G, Harper PS, Jones L. *Huntington's Disease*, 3rd edn. Oxford: Oxford University Press; 2002.

Brandt J. Cognitive impairments in Huntington's disease: insight into the neuropsychology of the striatum. In: Boller F, Grofman J, eds. *Handbook of Neuropsychology*, vol. 5. Amsterdam: Elsevier; 1991:241–263.

Brandt J, Folstein SE, Folstein MF. Differential cognitive impairment in Alzheimer's disease and Huntington's disease. *Ann Neurol* 1988, **23**:555–561.

Davies SW, Turmaine M, Cozens BA et al. Formation of neuronal intranuclear inclusions underlies the neurological dysfunction in mice transgenic for the HD mutation. *Cell* 1997, **90**:537–548.

Di Maio L, Squitieri F, Napolitano G et al. Suicide risk in Huntington's disease. *J Med Genet* 1993, **30**:293–295.

EEC Council Directive May 1990. Article 16 (1) of Directive 89/391 (90/269/EEC) 29 Journal of the European Communities, No. L156/9-13, Brussels. Official Commission of European Communities, Department of Health, 1992. *Manual Handling Operations Regulations, Guidance on Regulations*, L23. London: HMSO; 1990.

European Community Directive. *Manual Handling Operations Regulations*. London: Health and Safety Executive; 1992.

Federoff JP, Peyser C, Franz ML et al. Sexual disorders in Huntington's disease. *J Neuropsych* 1994, **6**:147–153.

Folstein SE, Jensen B, Leigh RJ et al. The measurement of abnormal movement: methods developed for Huntington's disease. *Neurobehav Toxicol Teratol* 1983, **5**:605–609.

Folstein SE, Leigh RJ, Parhad IM et al. The diagnosis of Huntington's disease. *Neurology* 1986, **36**:1279–1283.

Gardham F. *On Nursing Huntington's Disease*. London: Huntington's Disease Association; 1982:28–30.

Gordon WP, Illes J. Neurolinguistic characteristics of language production in Huntington's disease: a preliminary report. *Brain Lang* 1987, **31**:1–10.

Gusella JF, Wexler NS, Conneally PM et al. A polymorphic DNA marker genetically linked to Huntington's disease. *Nature* 1983, **306**:234–238.

Harper PS. The epidemiology of Huntington's disease. *Hum Genet* 1992, **89**:365–376.

Hedreen JC, Folstein SE. Early loss of neostriatal neurones in Huntington's disease. *J Neuropathol Exp Neurol* 1995, **54**:105–120.

Huntington G. On chorea. *Med Surg Report* 1872, **26**:317–321. Republished in *Adv Neurol* 1973, **1**:33–35.

Huntington's Disease Collaborative Research Group. A novel gene containing a trinucleotide repeat that is expanded and unstable on Huntington's disease chromosomes. *Cell* 1993, **72**:971–983.

Imbriglio S. Huntington's disease at mid-stage. *Clin Manage* 1992, **12**:63–72.

Kagel MC, Leopold NA. Dysphagia in Huntington's disease: a 16 year perspective. *Dysphagia* 1992, **7**:106–114.

Kremer B, Goldberg P, Andrew SE et al. A worldwide study of the Huntington's disease mutation. *N Engl J Med* 1994, **330**:1401–1406.

Lakke PWF. Classification of extrapyramidal disorders. Proposal for an international classification and glossary of terms. *J Neurol Sci* 1981, **51**:313–327.

Landwehrmeyer GB, McNeil SM, Dure LS et al. Huntington's disease gene: regional and cellular expression in brain of normal and affected individuals. *Ann Neurol* 1995, **37**:218–230.

Mangiarini L, Sathasivam K, Seller M et al. Exon1 of the HD gene with an expanded CAG repeat is sufficient to cause a progressive neurological phenotype in transgenic mice. *Cell* 1996, **87**:493–506.

Marks IM. *Behavioural Psychotherapy: Maudsley Pocket Book of Clinical Management*. Bristol: Wright; 1986.

Mason J, Andrews K, Wilson E. Late stage Huntington's disease – effect of treating specific disabilities. *Br J Occ Ther* 1991, **54**:4–7.

Mindham RHS, Steele C, Folstein MF et al. A comparison of the frequency of major affective disorder in Huntington's

...d in families. *Psychol Med* 1985,

... Psychiatric aspects of Huntington's
...per PS, ed. *Huntington's Disease*, 2nd edn.
...Saunders; 1996:73–122.

... Pain Association (NBPA) in collaboration with
...yal College of Nursing (RCN). *The Guide to the
...ndling of Patients: Introducing a Safer Handling Policy*,
...4th edn. London: NBPA/RCN; 1998.

Paulsen JS, Butters N, Sadek JR et al. Distinct cognitive
profiles of cortical and subcortical dementia in advanced
illness. *Neurology* 1995, **45**:951–956.

Peacock IW. A physical therapy program for Huntington's
disease patients. *Clin Manage* 1987, **7**:22–23, 34.

Perry TL, Hansen S, Kloster M. Huntington's chorea:
deficiency of gamma-aminobutyric acid in brain. *N Engl J
Med* 1973, **288**:337–342.

Pope PM. Postural management and special seating.
In: Edwards S, ed. *Neurological Physiotherapy: A Problem
Solving Approach*, 2nd edn. London: Churchill
Livingstone; 2002:189–217.

Ramen NG, Peyser CE, Folstein SE. *A Physician's Guide to the
Management of Huntington's Disease*. London:
Huntington's Disease Association; 1993.

Ramig LA. Acoustic analyses of phonation in patients with
Huntington's disease. *Ann Otol Rhinol Laryngol* 1976,
95:288–293.

Roos RAC. Neuropathology of Huntington's chorea. In:
Vinken PJ, Klawans HL, eds. *Extrapyramidal Disorders*.
Amsterdam: Elsevier Science; 1986:315–326.

Roos RAC, Hermans J, Vegter-van der Vlis M et al. Duration
of illness in Huntington's disease is not related to age of
onset. *J Neurol Neurosurg Psychiatry* 1993, **56**:98–100.

Rosser AE, Hodges JR. The dementia rating scale in
Alzheimer's disease, Huntington's disease and

progressive supranuclear palsy. *J Neurol* 1994,
241:531–536.

Rubinsztein DC, Leggo J, Goodbarn S et al. Study of the
Huntington's disease (HD) gene CAG repeats in
schizophrenic patients shows overlap of the normal and
HD affected ranges but absence of correlation with
schizophrenia. *J Med Genet* 1994, **31**:690–695.

Rubinsztein DC, Leggo J, Goodbarn S et al. Normal CAG
and CGG repeats in the Huntington's disease gene of
Parkinson's disease patients. *Am J Med Genet
(Neuropsychiatr Genet)* 1995, **60**:109–110.

Sharman A, Ponton T. The social, functional and
physiological benefits of intimately-contoured
customized seating; the Matrix body support.
Physiotherapy 1990, **76**:187–192.

Shiwach R. Psychopathology in Huntington's disease
patients. *Acta Psychiatr Scand* 1994, **90**:241–246.

Shoenfeld M, Myers RH, Cupples LA et al. Increased rate
of suicide among patients with Huntington's disease.
J Neurol Neurosurg Psychiatry 1984, **47**:1283–1287.

Shoulson I, Fahn S. Huntington's disease: clinical care and
evaluation. *Neurology* 1979, **29**:1–3.

Tolbin AJ, Singer ER. Huntington's disease: the challenge
for cell biologists. *Trends Cell Biol* 2000, **10**:531–536.

Vonsattel JPG, DiFiglia M. Huntington disease. *J Neuropathol
Exp Neurol* 1998, **57**:369–384.

Ward C, Dennis N, McMillan T. Huntington's disease.
In: Greenwood R, Barnes MP, McMillan TM et al., eds.
Neurological Rehabilitation. London: Churchill Livingstone;
1993:505–516.

Wheeler JS, Sax DS, Krane RJ et al. Vesico-urethral function
in Huntington's chorea. *Br J Neurol* 1985, **57**:63–66.

Yanagisawa N. The spectrum of motor disorders in
Huntington's disease. *Clin Neurol Neurosurg* 1992, **94**
(Suppl.):S182–S184.

Chapter **13**

Disorders of nerve I: Motor neurone disease

B O'Gorman   D Oliver   C Nottle   S Prisley

INTRODUCTION

Motor neurone disease (MND) is characterised by the progressive degeneration of: anterior horn cells of the spinal cord, causing lower motor neurone lesions; the corticospinal tracts, causing upper motor neurone lesions: and certain motor nuclei of the brainstem, leading to bulbar palsy.

The aetiology of the disease is unknown, although many theories for its cause have been suggested. About 5% of patients have a familial form; they often present earlier in life and with the spinal form of the disease (Figlewicz & Rouleau, 1994). As with other degenerative neurological disorders (e.g. Huntington's disease, see Ch. 12), the impact on the family can be devastating and care must take into account the needs of the family as well as the patient.

GENETICS AND PREVALENCE

Recently, in a small number of families with the familial form of the disease, a mutation of the superoxide dismutase (SOD) gene has been found (Rosen et al., 1993). This mutation accounts for about 20% of familial cases – i.e. 1% of all MND patients.

The incidence is around 2 per 100 000 and the prevalence varies across the world from 6 to 8 per 100 000 (Borasio & Miller, 2001). There is a slightly higher occurrence in males. It is a disease of later middle life, most patients being between 50 and 70 years, with a mean age of onset of 58 years (Borasio & Miller, 2001), although younger people may be affected. The mean duration of survival from the onset of symptoms is 3–4 years, although some patients live for much longer (Borasio & Miller, 2001). In one large study, the overall 5-year survival rate was 40% (Rosen, 1978) and about 10% of patients survive for over 10 years (Borasio & Miller, 2001). Younger patients survive for longer periodsand the worst prognosis is for patients with bulbar onset – a median survival of only 2.5 years (Borasio & Miller, 2001).

CLINICAL PRESENTATION

The clinical presentation of MND tends to be insidious and depends on the extent and distribution of the central nervous system (CNS) affected. Progressive degeneration of both upper and lower motor neurones occurs. If lower motor neurone degeneration is predominant, the main features are weakness, wasting and fasciculation of the muscles supplied by the nerves undergoing degeneration. Upper motor neurone degeneration also leads to weakness and often to muscle wasting

Table 13.1 Lesions in motor neurone disease and their related signs and symptoms

Site of lesion	Type of lesion	Signs and symptoms
	Upper motor neurone lesion Pseudobulbar palsy	• Tongue – spastic, no fasciculation • Speech – spastic and explosive dysarthria • Dysphagia • Increased reflexes (hyperreflexia) • Emotional lability and decreased control of expression
Medulla	Upper and lower motor neurone lesions	• Dysarthria • Dysphagia • Wasting of tongue • Jaw jerk increased
	Lower motor neurone lesion Bulbar palsy	• Tongue – shrunken, wrinkled, fasciculation • Speech – slurred • Dysphagia • Paralysis of diaphragm
Corticospinal tracts	Upper motor neurone lesion	• Spastic weakness • Hyperreflexia • Stiffness • Extensor plantar responses • Clonus • Slowed repetitive movements
Anterior horn cells	Lower motor neurone lesion	• Flaccid weakness • Muscle wasting (atrophy) • Muscle fasciculation • Hyporeflexia

Adapted from Oliver (1994) with permission.

but the muscles become hypertonic (Table 13.1). Due to plasticity, involving enlargement of surviving motor neurones, up to 50% of motor neurones can be lost before weakness becomes apparent (see Ch. 5).

Three main forms of the disease are recognised: amyotrophic lateral sclerosis (ALS); progressive bulbar palsy; and progressive muscular atrophy.

Amyotrophic lateral sclerosis

ALS accounts for about 66% of all patients with MND and is commoner in older men. There are both lower motor neurone changes, such as muscle fasciculation, weakness and flaccidity, together with upper motor neurone changes, such as spasticity and weakness. There may also be a mixture of bulbar signs, including dysarthria and dysphagia, and emotional lability.

Most commonly ALS first affects the hands, with symptoms of clumsiness and weakness and evidence of wasting of the thenar eminences. The shoulders may also be affected early in the disease. If there is bulbar involvement the tongue becomes wasted and fasciculates, and speech and swallowing are affected because of muscle weakness.

Progressive bulbar palsy

About 25% of patients with MND present with progressive bulbar palsy, which affects the bulbar region and causes dysarthria and dysphagia. When lower motor neurones are affected, the tongue is atrophied, fasciculates and has reduced mobility, and there is nasal speech and dysphagia. If the upper motor neurones are affected, the tongue is spastic and causes dysarthria. Emotional lability may occur, with only a small or no obvious stimulus. Although the limbs may be affected little early in the disease, as it progresses there may be weakness of the arms and legs (Tandan, 1994).

Progressive muscular atrophy

About 10% of patients with MND present with progressive muscular atrophy; it develops earlier in life, affecting predominantly men under 50 years. Initially, only the lower motor neurones are affected and there is wasting and weakness of the arms. There may be progression to the legs, but bulbar involvement is rare until late in the disease. The rate of progression is slower than in the other forms and the majority of patients live more than 5 years, often more than 10 years.

Although these three main forms of the disease are described, many patients present, or develop, a mixed picture of symptoms and signs. Every patient is different and the development of the disease varies greatly. The sphincter control of bladder and bowels is rarely affected. Mental deterioration and dementia are found in less than 5% of patients (Tandan, 1994), although there is increasing evidence of frontal lobe involvement which may be found on testing and may lead to emotional lability and other subtle mental changes (Abrahams et al., 1996). Anxiety and depression, understandably associated with a progressive, seriously disabling disease, may be seen.

Other variants less commonly seen include Kennedy's disease, Guam variant MND and primary lateral sclerosis.

DIAGNOSIS

The clinical diagnosis is confirmed by electromyography (EMG). The motor neurone conduction velocity is normal until late in the disease. The motor action potentials are of increased amplitude and duration, but are reduced in number, whereas the sensory action potential is normal. On mechanical stimulation of the needle, fibrillation and fasciculation potentials are seen (Schwartz & Swash, 1995).

Other investigations may be necessary to exclude other conditions leading to muscle wasting and bulbar palsy, such as syringomyelia or cervical spondylosis (Swash & Schwartz, 1995).

The diagnosis is confirmed when certain criteria are found – in particular, evidence of progression of upper and lower motor neurone deterioration at different levels (Brooks et al., 1998).

SYMPTOMS AND THEIR CONTROL

Control of the following problems involves the multidisciplinary team (MDT); the specific role of the physiotherapist is elaborated in 'Physical management', below. Drug treatments mentioned are covered in detail in Chapter 28. From the time of diagnosis there should be a palliative care approach, aiming for the assessment and management of the problems and concerns of patients and their family – considering the physical, psychological, social and spiritual aspects (Oliver, 2000).

Pain

Pain is a common problem in MND, with up to 73% of patients complaining of pain (Oliver, 1996). In a study by Newrick & Langton Hewer (1985), 27 out of 42 patients reported significant pain of varying origin. Weak muscles can create abnormal stresses on the musculoskeletal system, leading to an imbalance, especially around the shoulder joint, causing pain. Pain can be caused by muscle cramps, spasticity or spasms. If a patient is unable to change position, then mechanical stress and areas of pressure can lead to pain. Chronic pain, especially in the back, is a commonly reported problem.

Management should be preventive (Francis et al., 1999). Early education to carers regarding safe moving and handling techniques is advocated, and advice given on positioning and adequate support for the patient over a 24 h period. For the immobile patient, frequent repositioning may help to reduce any discomfort from pressure on the skin and prevent pressure sores. Pressure relief systems must be adequate, i.e. mattress and seat cushions. An opoid, such as regular morphine, can be very effective in reducing this discomfort (Oliver, 1998).

Maintenance of soft-tissue length by active or passive stretches may alleviate pain (Peruzzi & Potts, 1996). When exercising, adequate rest periods to prevent overuse are advised. Various medications can be useful, including analgesics, non-steroidal anti-inflammatory drugs and muscle relaxants. Intra-articular injection of steroids and local anaesthetic may also be helpful, especially if a shoulder is very painful. Pain secondary to muscle cramp may occur early in the disease and can be alleviated by medication, such as diazepam or quinine sulphate at night, and muscle stretches. Similarly, pain due to spasticity can be relieved by antispasmodic medication, e.g. baclofen, and physiotherapy (see 'Tone management', below). Acupuncture may also be considered. Often an opioid analgesic may be the most effective treatment for this pain (Oliver, 1998).

Dyspnoea

The dysfunction of respiratory muscles caused dyspnoea in 47% of the patients in one series (O'Brien et al., 1992). A calm and confident approach is necessary as dyspnoea may be exacerbated by anxiety. Careful positioning is important, especially of the neck when there is neck weakness, and the body and shoulder-girdle need to be stabilised to ease breathing. Antibiotics may be considered if there is evidence of infection in the early stages of the disease (Oliver, 1993). The use of non-invasive ventilation may reduce the symptoms of ventilatory insufficiency, such as morning headache, sleeplessness, feeling unwell and anorexia, as well as reducing the feelings of dyspnoea (Lyall et al., 2000).

In the later stages of disease, an episode of acute breathlessness may be treated effectively by an injection of an opioid (such as diamorphine) with hyoscine hydrobromide or glycopyrronium bromide, to reduce secretions and midazolam to act as a sedative (Oliver, 1994).

Morphine, or other opioid analgesics, when used in carefully selected doses, effectively controls distressing symptoms such as pain, dyspnoea, restlessness and cough (Oliver, 1998). In a series of patients in a hospice, 89% of patients received parenteral opioids that were effective in controlling acute breathlessness or choking and the symptoms of terminal illness (O'Brien et al., 1992).

Dysphagia

Impaired swallowing is a troublesome symptom in over 75% of patients, and is due to involvement of the motor nuclei of the medulla. There is not only muscle weakness but spasticity and inco-ordination. Careful, slow feeding is essential and referral to a speech and language therapist for a swallowing assessment and advice on feeding should be sought. Postural modifications such as chin tuck may assist with airway protection.

Dribbling salivation can be controlled by hyoscine, sublingually or as a transdermal patch. Botulinum toxin injections into the salivary glands have also been found to be helpful. Choking and respiratory distress is a great fear of patients but if the symptoms are well controlled it is rarely a cause of death. Only one patient died in a choking attack in two large series (Saunders et al., 1981; O'Brien et al., 1992) and no evidence of obstruction of the respiratory tract was found on autopsy (O'Brien et al., 1992). By careful positioning of the patient, providing appropriately textured nutrition and liquids, and by controlling salivation, choking attacks may be prevented. Assessment and advice on swallowing safety can be provided by the speech and language therapist. For a choking attack in the later stages of the disease, (dia)morphine (to reduce the cough reflex and lessen anxiety), hyoscine hydrobromide or glycopyrronium bromide (to dry up secretions and relax smooth muscles) and midazolam (to reduce anxiety) may be given as an injection.

If feeding becomes more difficult and the patient becomes very tired during meals, he or she may start to lose weight. Assessment and advice from a speech and language therapist and dietician should be sought at the first signs of swallowing difficulty.

Alternative enteral feeding systems may be necessary to supplement or replace the oral diet. Nasogastric feeding may increase the oropharyngeal secretions (Scott & Austin, 1994) and long-term management is not advised but may be used in the short term. Some people find nasogastric feeding unpleasant and unsightly. A percutaneous endoscopic gastrostomy (PEG) may be very helpful in maintaining nutritional status (Wagner-Sonntag et al., 2000). The PEG tube is inserted under local anaesthesia and sedation in a relatively simple procedure but the risks are increased if respiratory function is compromised. It is suggested that the procedure should be performed when forced vital capacity (FVC) is over 50% of expected (Miller et al., 1999). Radiological insertion of a gastrostomy feeding tube (RIG) has been proposed as a safer option if FVC is below 60% (Strand et al., 1996).

Dysarthria

Difficulties with speech are experienced by 80% of patients with MND and on admission to a hospice 36% had no intelligible speech (O'Brien et al., 1992). Initially assistance may be required on strategies to optimise the intelligibility of speech. Great patience and concentration are necessary to understand the patient. Assessment by a speech and language therapist will allow the most to be made of the remaining speech, and carers may spend much time aiding communication. As dysarthria increases, speech will need to be supplemented by alternative means, such as writing using a mechanical communication aid or computers (Unsworth, 1994; Langton Hewer, 1995). Aids for writing and typing may be helpful and very sensitive switches allow a patient with minimal movement to summon help, thus aiding confidence (Scott & Foulsum, 2000). Technological advances are constantly providing new solutions in this area and therefore referrals to specialist organisations will assist independence. Communication aids are discussed further below.

Sore eyes

Eye blinking may be reduced as a result of muscle weakness and the eyes may then become sore and secondarily infected. Lubricating eye drops are helpful and antibiotic eye drops may be necessary if infection occurs.

Constipation

Any patient who is inactive, debilitated and taking a low-roughage diet may become constipated. If the abdominal muscles weaken it may be difficult to raise the intra-abdominal pressure sufficiently to open the bowels. A regular aperient prevents this but local rectal measures such as suppositories, enemas or manual evacuation may become necessary in some patients.

Insomnia

Insomnia may be due to insecurity, fear and pain, and was reported in 48% of patients admitted to a hospice (O'Brien et al., 1992). Insomnia may also be due to breathlessness, which is a sign of respiratory dysfunction (see 'Respiratory management', below). Attention to detail and regular positioning will aid confidence and, therefore, sleep. A sensitive switch that allows the patient to call for help may enable him or her to relax and sleep at night. Sedatives, antidepressants and opioid analgesics should also be considered (see Ch. 28).

Fatigue

Patients with MND frequently experience generalised fatigue, which can be one of the most disabling features of the condition. However, with good advice, they can learn how to minimise the effect of this problem. Activity should be encouraged but not so as to exhaust the patient (see 'Exercise and maintaining range of movement', below).

Management strategies should include organising the environment to minimise unnecessary energy expenditure, leading a healthy lifestyle, adopting good posture and positioning and employing relaxation techniques. Activity modification can be very effective. This encour-

ages patients to eliminate unnecessary tasks from their day, plan ahead and divide the tasks into manageable sections, allowing rest periods in between. Adapted equipment and appropriate packages of care should also be considered.

Corticosteroids may aid appetite and increase the feeling of well-being, but if they are used for long periods, weakness may be increased and other side-effects encountered.

Pressure sores

Pressure sores are uncommon, as sensation is retained. Prevention by regular turning and the use of pressure-relieving cushions and mattresses is important (see 'Positioning and seating', below). The treatment of established sores is by the preferred methods of the nursing team.

Urinary problems

Weakness of the abdominal wall musculature may lead to urinary retention in some patients but urinary incontinence is always due to other pathological processes, e.g. benign prostatic hypertrophy in men. Urinary catheterisation may be necessary in some cases for the convenience of nursing care.

PHYSICAL MANAGEMENT

The physical management will depend on the physical symptoms present as well as the rate of progression, which may be gained from the history. It is important that the onset of the symptoms is known rather than the date of diagnosis, as it is from the onset that the rate of deterioration of the disease can be gauged.

There are no clearly defined stages of progression in MND and patients do not follow a set pattern. The distribution of weakness and clinical course of the condition are variable, so that management must be specific to the individual, but general guidelines to rehabilitation can be given (Francis et al., 1999; Miller et al., 1999).

The multidisciplinary team approach

Optimal management of patients with MND requires a team approach, with early referral for clinical assessment and prompt intervention (Corr et al., 1998). Patients with MND are often seen by several different teams, i.e. community teams, hospice care teams, wheelchair services and social services. Good communication is essential to provide appropriate care for this client group.

There are six specialist MND centres in the UK (London (King's), Newcastle, Nottingham, Cardiff, Birmingham and Liverpool; see Appendix for details).

The primary responsibility of the team at these MND care and research centres is to ensure that care is co-ordinated across the range of health, social care and voluntary agencies. The teams are also involved in research in partnership with people affected by MND.

Role of the physiotherapist

The physiotherapist is a core member of the team and part of the role is to liaise with the patient and other members of the MDT in the decision-making, treatment-planning and goal-setting process. Much of the physiotherapist's role involves teaching and advising the other team members, as well as the patient and family (O'Gorman, 2000).

The physiotherapist's overall aim is to maintain optimal function and quality of life for the patient throughout the course of the disease. This may include:

1. providing a baseline assessment and ensure monitoring throughout the course of the disease
2. maintaining muscle strength, muscle length and joint range of motion, and managing muscle tone to maximise function
3. promoting mobility and independence by provision of aids and adaptations
4. advice about exercise
5. providing information, education and support to the patient and carer
6. pain management
7. fatigue management
8. treating and monitoring any respiratory dysfunction.

General aspects of progression

Some patients experience a rapid decline in their abilities with continual losses – at times weekly. Others will have a slow decline and not notice much loss over a period of months or years. If the early presentation is of weakness in one foot or one hand, referral to an outpatient physiotherapy department will help. Ideally, review appointments should be set up to monitor abilities, power and any early signs of joint stiffness.

If bulbar signs present first, with dysarthria or dysphagia becoming an escalating early problem, referral to a speech and language therapist will be the first priority.

Eventually the general weakness is so profound as to confine the patient to bed or a wheelchair. Some may need admission to a unit caring for the terminally ill. Many patients and their families can be supported successfully in their own home by a co-ordinated team approach in the community. The overall aim of physical management is the maintenance of independence, however small.

Exercise and maintaining range of movement

The role of exercise in the treatment of patients with MND is a contentious issue. The commonly held belief is that exercise is ineffective and may cause further muscle damage but recent evidence presents a strong case for its use (see below). This situation is also true for other neurological conditions and new approaches, based on emerging research, are discussed in Chapter 29.

Damage to both the upper and lower motor neurones is seen in MND. A summary of the changes in motor neurone activation from each type of damage is presented in Table 13.1. When the motor neurones are damaged by the disease process, the muscle tissue that they innervate can no longer be activated and, therefore, atrophies. These motor units are permanently damaged and cannot be changed by exercise (Peruzzi & Potts, 1996). Other parts of the muscle, however, may have an intact motor neurone and still be functioning. As the patient becomes less mobile and less active due to, for example, fatigue, these otherwise healthy fibres may start to show some signs of disuse atrophy. These disused fibres will respond to exercise and may allow the patient to develop a small reserve of healthy, usable muscle.

Other factors may affect the muscles of a patient with MND, including increased likelihood of fatigue, impaired respiratory function (resulting in poor delivery of oxygen to the tissues), impaired nutritional intake and hypertonicity.

Benefits of low-resistance submaximal exercise

The benefits of exercise that are seen in the healthy population can also apply to people with MND (see Ch. 29 for review). The primary effect of exercise training is to improve the neural control of the muscle, which will allow more effective recruitment and, therefore, stronger contractions (Sanjak et al., 1987). Since it is only the disused muscle tissue and not the diseased parts that can be strengthened in MND patients, the best results are seen in the least affected muscles.

Studies in other neuromuscular conditions show that exercise at a submaximal level can be safe and effective (see Ch. 29; Aitkens et al., 1993; Kilmer et al., 1994). High-resistance work is thought to be unnecessary and can be damaging to the muscles, particularly with eccentric (muscle-lengthening) contractions, which can cause delayed-onset muscle soreness (Lieber & Friden, 1999). Normal muscle recovers from such damage but repair in diseased muscle may not be possible. Although eccentric contractions are difficult to avoid within an exercise programme, consideration should be given to how eccentric activity is used to avoid unnecessary strain.

Muscles in patients with MND will fatigue more rapidly than those in healthy individuals. It has not been established whether this is due to impaired central control (Kent-Braun & Miller, 2000) or to impaired activation at a muscular level (Sharma et al., 1995). For this reason, short but frequent exercise sessions may be preferable to prolonged activity.

Muscle length

Optimal tissue length is essential if muscle activation and the resultant function are to be maximised (see Ch. 30 for effects of length changes on muscle function). Due to the weakness that results from MND, muscle imbalance causes changes in muscle length. Muscle shortening is especially likely where upper motor neurone involvement leads to increased muscle tone. Therefore, it is imperative that steps are taken early on to prevent changes in tissue length. These may include preventive splinting, stretching programmes and active exercise, positioning, appropriate seating and antispasmodic medication (see other sections of this chapter and Chs 4 and 25).

Where muscle imbalance is seen, joints are at risk of being held in malalignment. This may be due to high muscle tone pulling them out of line or weakness and low muscle tone allowing the joints to be hypermobile. In either case, splinting may be necessary to prevent further malalignment and the risk of damage.

It is important to make a differential diagnosis to ascertain whether limb stiffness is due to joint stiffness, muscle inelasticity or, indeed, predisposing factors such as osteoarthritis, as the physical management and medication are different depending on the cause.

Recommendations for exercise

In light of the above evidence, the recommendations for using exercise in the management of patients with MND are:

1. Allow patients to continue with sports or activities that they participated in prior to diagnosis, for as long as they are safely able to do so.

2. Encourage low-stress, low-impact activities such as walking or swimming, in preference to high-impact or contact sports.

3. Encourage an active lifestyle when sport and other exercise activities become impracticable.

4. Avoid high-resistance exercises that increase the risk of muscle damage, without providing any additional benefits above a moderate-resistance programme.

5. Advise patients to build up their programme slowly and to monitor the effects of their exercise on fatigue and pain. Teach patients to recognise delayed-onset muscle soreness as a sign of overuse.

6. Advise patients to exercise little and often to maintain activity but to avoid fatigue. Attempt to schedule exercise when there is time available to rest afterwards.

7. Advise patients that their exercises should not make them too tired to do anything else in their day. Having energy left to play with the children or grandchildren or go out for a meal with their partner is much more important than rigidly adhering to an exercise regime.

8. Exercise programmes should incorporate cardiovascular exercise, stretches and strengthening work.

9. Educate patients about exercise. They should be made aware that it will not cure their condition or prevent deterioration but may enhance the activity they have and provide them with the general benefits that we all experience from exercise.

Tone management

The clinical features of MND were summarised in Table 13.1. Hypertonia, a feature of upper motor neurone syndrome, is defined as an increase in resistance to passive stretch and has both a neural (spasticity) and non-neural component (inherent viscoelastic properties of the muscle) which provides resistance to movement and contributes to muscle tone (see Chs 4 and 25). The result of tonal changes can lead to inappropriate movement, discomfort, decreased mobility, reduced function and difficulty with positioning. Spasticity is managed in the same way as for other neurological patients (e.g stroke, brain injury and multiple sclerosis) and there needs to be a multidisciplinary approach to treatment.

Medical management includes the use of oral medication to reduce tone, such as baclofen, diazepam, dantrolene and tizanadine (see Chs 4 and 28). Careful monitoring of the effects of medication is needed, as excessive weakness caused by the medication can lead to flaccidity and a reduction in the patient's functional ability. Intramuscular botulinum toxin injection can be used to reduce focal spasticity (Richardson & Thompson, 1999). The drug weakens the muscle by inhibiting the release of acetylcholine at the neuromuscular junction, preventing muscle contraction.

Physical management of tone includes careful positioning and the interventions outlined below. Massage and aromatherapy can be used to assist relaxation but their effectiveness at reducing muscle tone has not been demonstrated. The physiotherapist aims to maximise a patient's functional ability and comfort. A comprehensive assessment of the patient's main problems needs to be completed (see 'Assessment and outcome measures', below).

Physiotherapy interventions for tone management

Stretching programme   A home exercise programme can be devised for the patient, incorporating stretches to maintain muscle length. As the patient becomes less active, passive stretches can be taught to the carer. Splinting may also be used as a means of imposing a sustained stretch (Edwards & Charlton, 2002). Guidelines have been prepared by the Association of Chartered Physiotherapists Interested in Neurology (ACPIN) in 1998, and these provide information regarding the assessment, procedure, risk factors and protocols for casting. Guidelines for casting patients with complex neurological conditions have also been produced (Young & Nicklin, 2000). Adequate training in splinting techniques is essential.

Standing   The theory behind weight-bearing activities is to maintain joint range and stimulate antigravity muscle activity (Brown, 1994). Standing exercises can be performed independently by the patient, with assistance, or with the use of specialised equipment such as a tilt table or Oswestry standing frame.

The use of muscle-relaxant drugs needs to be carefully monitored, as some patients use their muscle tone to stand. Reducing this tone may thus limit their functional ability.

Positioning/seating   Different postures and positions have an influence on tone and movement. If a patient is uncomfortable, then this may lead to an increase in muscle tone. Therefore, correct positioning over a 24-h period is vital. Liaison with the local wheelchair team is important to provide the patient with a suitable wheelchair (see 'Positioning and seating' section, below).

Activity modification   If a task is very effortful for a patient, then this may increase muscle tone and lead to difficulties completing the task. Therefore, activity modification is advised. Decreasing the effort of the task by either activity modification or the use of aids and adaptations may assist with reducing tone.

Other factors that may exacerbate spasticity   A noxious stimulus such as constipation or ingrowing toe nail may lead to an increase in tone. Poor positioning or an ill-fitting orthotic appliance may also increase tone unnecessarily. Therefore, it is important to identify any cause and make adjustments or withdraw the cause when managing patients with hypertonia.

Positioning and seating

Positioning is an essential part of the management of the patient with MND. Good positioning will help to maintain joint range and soft-tissue length, prevent deformity, improve comfort, prevent pressure areas and maximise function (Pope, 2002). Positioning is a 24-h approach that includes lying and standing positions, as well as static and mobile seating. The combined resources of nurses, physiotherapists and family are needed to achieve this.

When the antigravity muscles, which maintain an erect head, neck and trunk, become weakened, it becomes increasingly difficult to maintain the upright position. This applies whether the patient is standing, sitting in a wheelchair or sitting in bed. It is not sufficient to place more and more pillows behind and around the patient. In order to minimise the effect of gravity on the body, the patient should be reclined back from the vertical at the hips, so that the line of gravity passes in front of the head and neck through the thorax. This position also enables the diaphragm to work more efficiently and so aid breathing (see 'Respiratory management', below).

Equipment used for positioning can range from the simple use of pillows and wedges to complex seating systems (see 'Wheelchairs', below). Electric adjustable beds, pressure-relieving mattresses and cushions plus one-way glide sheets will all assist comfort as well as facilitating easy adjustment of the patient's position. Small neck or support pillows could also be used. The patient's positioning in the environment must also be considered to allow the greatest degree of function, social interaction and stimulation.

Table 13.2 presents some of the problems associated with MND and their possible positioning solutions.

Mobility

Although maintaining ambulation is a priority for many patients, the physiotherapist has a responsibility to ensure that this does not become too energy-inefficient and fatiguing or unsafe. This may necessitate the use of walking aids such as sticks, crutches, zimmer or delta frames, or wheelchairs. It is important to gauge the patient's feelings on this subject before issuing an aid. It is not unusual for patients to refuse aids on grounds of cosmesis, and wheelchairs and crutches are often perceived as socially unacceptable symbols of disability. Mobility and independence are clearly linked with self-esteem and it is sometimes difficult for a patient to acknowledge that he or she has deteriorated enough to require a stick or a chair.

Table 13.2 Some of the problems associated with motor neurone disease and their possible positioning solutions

Problem	Solution
Patient experiences breathlessness at night, especially when lying flat	Back rest and pillows to provide comfortable upright sleeping position. Call bell/alarm within reach to reduce anxiety
Patient experiences pain in neck/shoulders/back when rolled on to side in lying	Wedges/pillows placed behind back and under uppermost arm and leg to support the patient in the side-lying position and prevent arms and legs falling into adduction. A roll placed in the space under the patient's neck gives support
Patient experiences shoulder pain in flail arms when upright (either sitting or standing)	Collar and cuff bands across body (from opposite shoulder to near hip) to support arm within. Clothes with pouch pockets at front can also provide this support
Decreased head control	Tilt-in-space wheelchairs can offload the head. Upper-limb support, e.g. trays or tables, can provide improved support for the upper body and, in turn, the head. Head rest/lateral head supports can be added to wheelchairs. Collars may support the head in upright positions

If a patient is unable to stand from sitting unaided, but can still walk, then a chair with an electric seat raise may overcome this problem.

It is necessary to consider arm function as well as lower-limb activity when selecting an aid, as poor grip, for example, will preclude the use of many walking aids. Patients who fatigue may prefer wheeled frames that have an integral seat, so that they can rest at stages in their journey.

Transfers may become difficult and advice from the physiotherapist on safe and effective technique may help to maintain independence in this activity. Many devices are commercially available to improve transfers, such as sliding boards, transfer belts and hoists. Transfer belts placed around the lower thorax/pelvis can be particularly useful where the patient has flail arms or painful shoulders, allowing the carer to have a firm hold on the patient without the risk of trauma to the limbs. However, this requires the patient to be able to maintain an upright posture and therefore may not be appropriate in the late stages of the disease. Consideration of comfort, type of transfer and environment should be made when selecting a hoist. Manual handling legislation must be part of the reasoning process when selecting transfer techniques.

Orthoses

Orthoses may also be necessary to maximise mobility. Lively or rigid splints and light-weight orthoses can be of use but careful assessment of their value must be made frequently. An ankle-foot orthosis is often provided where the patient presents with foot drop (Fig. 13.1).

Insoles, calipers and knee braces can all improve the efficiency of gait and protect the soft tissues from the trauma of repeated malalignment.

Wheelchairs

Due to the progressive nature of MND, early referral for wheelchair provision is essential. Patients' local wheelchair service should be able to provide a chair that meets their mobility and postural needs but if the patient desires something beyond this remit, there is a large selection of wheelchairs available commercially which have other features. If a wheelchair is being bought privately, it is worthwhile seeking advice from the wheelchair service to ensure it fully meets the patient's requirements and to investigate voucher scheme funding. The wheelchair may be manually propelled by the patient or attendant, or powered for indoor and/or outdoor use. Scooters will not be provided by the National Health Service but may provide another mobility option. Consideration must be given to postural requirements, function and pressure care when providing a wheelchair and seating system.

Assistive devices

In order to maximise both function and quality of life it is necessary to provide patients with knowledge of the various types of aids and equipment available to them. Again, such aids may be seen as a sign of deterioration and not readily accepted by the patient. Careful consideration when introducing these devices is important to assist acceptance, as they serve a number of purposes.

Management of neck weakness

Neck weakness causes many problems for the patient with MND. It causes stress on the muscles and ligaments of the neck, resulting in pain, impaired breathing and

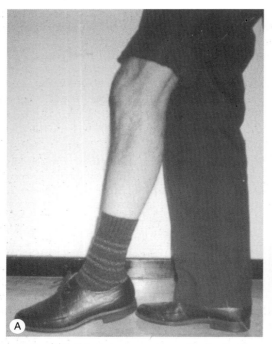 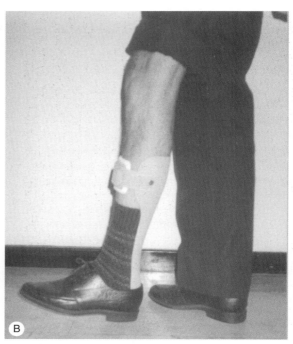

Figure 13.1 (A) Left foot drop – weakness of ankle dorsiflexors. (B) Use of ankle–foot orthosis to correct foot drop.

swallowing, increased drooling, decreased interaction with the environment and is cosmetically unpleasant.

There are several specially designed collars available that may offer a solution to these problems. These include two specifically designed rigid head supports, the Headmaster and the MNDA (Mary Marlborough Lodge) collar. Both provide a flexible platform for the chin that allows a small amount of anteroposterior movement for speaking and chewing but prevents the head falling forwards, and are open at the front to avoid throat compression.

Patients who side-flex as well as fall forwards often prefer a soft foam collar, such as the Adams collar (Johnson & Johnson), that feels supportive in all directions. These need to be replaced frequently to maintain good support and patients who drool can be given lengths of stockingette to cover the collar; these may be removed and washed. Sometimes a collar cut from block foam to act as a wedge on which the chin can rest may help.

Wheelchairs can be adapted to minimise the effects of neck weakness. A chair with a tilt-in-space arrangement will allow the neck to be relieved of load, whilst a good seated position is maintained. Head supports can be made integral to the chair and there is a wide range of available head rests. The patient's local wheelchair service should be able to advise on this. Positioning the upper limbs on a tray or pillows may allow the patient

better control of the neck and decrease the pull on the muscles.

Upper-limb function

The seating position has a significant effect on ability to use the upper limbs functionally. It is, therefore, advisable to position the patient well, prior to attempting any upper-limb activities. Patients with decreased activity may find that leaning their elbows on a table or wheelchair tray allows them more hand function or that mobile arm supports help them with activities such as feeding. Splints, such as thumb spicas, may improve alignment and give better ability to grip.

There are a multitude of adapted devices that will allow patients to participate in or be independent in activities of daily living, such as feeding, washing, writing and domestic tasks. For patients with marked bulbar signs, hot plates and heated food dishes make slow eating more palatable. Anti-slip table mats and thickened handles on cutlery, pens and toothbrushes aid independence. Anti-slip floor mats and the Rotastand aid transfers, and the use of Velcro and zip fasteners will help dressing.

Referral to the occupational therapist early after diagnosis will mean that the patient has access to these devices and the necessary advice as the need arises.

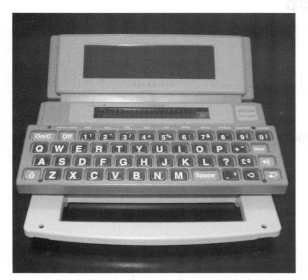

Figure 13.2 Lightwriter communication device (Toby Churchill Ltd) for people with impaired intelligibility. (Courtesy of G Derwent, Compass, Electronic Assistive Technology Service, Royal Hospital for Neuro-disability, London).

Communication

Various devices can be used to allow the patient a means of communication. These range from simple pointer charts (which can be used with eye movements or head pointers, as well as finger pointing) to high-technology solutions, such as lightwriters (Fig. 13.2) and computers. Information technology equipment, training and advice may be accessed through charities or organisations such as Ability Net. Communication aids, including POSSUM, can be combined with environmental control units and may be set up to activate alarm-call systems for when the patient is alone, or to respond to the telephone (Unsworth, 1994; Langton Hewer, 1995). Call systems sensitive to light touch can be operated by head, hands or feet, enabling the patient to signal for help.

A variety of communication systems are available; some connect to the telephone and can speak recorded phrases, including emergency messages, activated by pressing buttons on a keypad. Some also have a memory capacity which allows the speech-impaired person to answer an incoming telephone call by using recorded phrases instead of speech. Telephone answer machines may allow those with impaired speech to receive messages; the response is made by family or carer.

The Royal National Institution for Deaf People operates Typetalk, which allows a person with speech difficulties to type in a message; a trained operator then speaks the message to the caller, who is then able to reply. The service operates 24 h a day (see Appendix).

Answer machines, faxes and e-mail give great scope for communicating with people outside the patient's immediate vicinity.

Respiratory management

Failure of the respiratory system is the most common cause of death in patients with MND (Francis et al., 1999; Lyall et al., 2001a). Ventilatory failure occurs when the load placed on the respiratory muscle pump exceeds the capacity of the respiratory muscles. The family needs to be fully informed of a failing chest expansion and the implications of this, in order that they are as prepared as possible.

Signs and symptoms of inspiratory muscle weakness (diaphragm and accessory muscles) include dyspnoea, orthopnoea, disturbed sleep and day-time somnolence. Morning headaches can be a sign of carbon dioxide retention overnight. Difficulty coughing is a sign of expiratory muscle weakness, or loss of abdominal muscle tone. Paradoxical abdominal motion during respiration indicates substantial diaphragm weakness (Polkey et al., 1999).

Patients with bulbar involvement may present with reduced control and strength of laryngeal and pharyngeal muscles, decreasing the effectiveness of the swallow and leading to a higher risk of aspiration pneumonia and added respiratory complications. In addition, the indirect effects of reduced activity levels as the disease progresses may lead to increased areas of lung atelectasis and secretion retention.

Pulmonary function tests are recommended to test respiratory muscle strength, guide management and determine prognosis. Vital capacity (VC) is the volume of gas that can be exhaled after full inspiration (normal value 3–6 litre) and can detect diaphragmatic weakness. A VC of 1 litre (or 25% of predicted) indicates significant risk of impending respiratory failure or death (Miller et al., 1999). Other respiratory tests include blood-gas analysis to detect day-time hypercapnia or a raised bicarbonate level, suggesting hypoventilation (Lyall et al., 2001a). Overnight oximetry is often used to highlight hypoventilation as reflected by desaturations. Mustfa & Moxham (2001) discuss different respiratory muscle assessments in MND. One specific test is the sniff nasal pressure (SNIP). Sniff is a natural manoeuvre and patients find it easier to perform than static mouth pressures (especially patients with orofacial muscle weakness). A value of less than 70 cm H_2O for men and less than 60 cm H_2O for women indicates respiratory muscle weakness. The patient should be referred for respiratory assessment. In addition, the use of auscultation and checking the effectiveness of a patient's cough are important inclusions to the respiratory assessment.

Close monitoring of the respiratory status of a patient with MND is an important role of the physiotherapist, who should inform the MDT of any reduction in chest expansion, as this may be a sign of the rate of deterioration. Increased activity of the accessory muscles of respiration, especially if the patient is at rest, and the development of morning headaches, due to a high level of carbon dioxide at night, are often other signs of deterioration.

The main aims of physiotherapy intervention are to maximise ventilation and gas exchange, aid in the removal of secretions and provide education and support to the patient and carer.

Treatment of respiratory complications is symptomatic and best managed with a well co-ordinated team approach by physical methods (including non-invasive ventilation), drug therapy and advice and education.

Physiotherapy interventions for respiratory management

Maintaining chest wall compliance In the early stages, active exercises may be advocated to maintain trunk mobility, as well as deep-breathing exercises, including diaphragmatic breathing, to increase chest expansion and prevent atelectasis (Peruzzi & Potts, 1996).

As a patient becomes less active, the use of active assisted and passive movements of the trunk can be used. These are aimed at reducing stiffness of the joints and soft tissues, aiming to minimise a reduction in chest wall compliance.

Active cycle of breathing techniques Breathing exercises can be useful in maintaining lung expansion in all areas. Used in conjunction with manual techniques, they can improve expansion and mobilise secretions in the presence of a chest infection (Pryor & Webber, 1998). These techniques are more appropriate in the early stages of MND, as the majority of patients are unable to cough or even huff in the later stages. Similarly, the forced expiratory technique (FET) is less effective in the later stages (Hough, 1991) and assisted cough should be used in this situation.

Postural drainage Postural drainage may be used, if appropriate, to aid drainage of secretions using gravity and a modified position may be required if orthopnoea is present (Peruzzi & Potts, 1996). However, this is often difficult for patients to tolerate in the late stages.

Positioning Advice to the patient and carer on positioning is important to optimise ventilation perfusion matching and prevent development of atelectasis and retention of secretions (Ross & Dean, 1989). Advice on modified posture and seating may be of value when orthopnoea or dyspnoea is a problem.

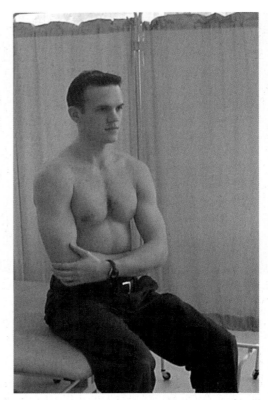

Figure 13.3 Self-assisted cough. Start with a good upright position. Place one forearm under the ribcage and support with the other arm. As cough is initiated, use the forearm to apply pressure inwards and upwards (bucket-handle action). If the cough is effective it will sound stronger and louder.

Assisted–cough technique Often patients with MND find the clearance of secretions difficult due to an ineffective cough. An assisted cough can be taught to the patient and/or carer (Polkey et al., 1999). The aim of the assisted cough is to replace the function of the paralysed or weak abdominal muscles. Indications for the use of the assisted cough include weakness of the abdominal or respiratory muscles leading to an ineffective cough and difficulty clearing secretions. Contraindications include a paralytic ileus, internal abdominal damage, bleeding gastric ulcer and rib fractures (Bromley, 1998). Vibration on expiration may be used to mobilise secretions (Sutton et al., 1985).

It is recommended that the physiotherapist liaises with nursing/medical staff regarding contraindications prior to teaching the techniques. It is important to inform and explain the procedure to the patient and carer, and obtain consent.

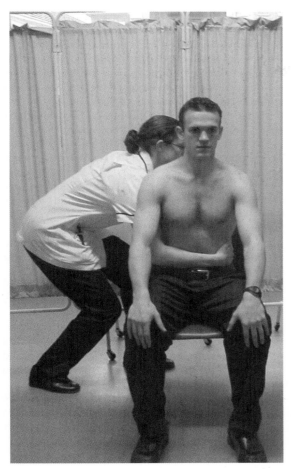

Figure 13.4 Assisted cough in sitting. The assistor brings one arm in front, just below the ribcage, and one arm behind to support the trunk. As cough is initiated, pressure is applied by the front arm (bucket-handle action). Co-ordination between the patient and assistor is important.

Self-assisted cough (Fig. 13.3)

● Start with a good upright position.

● Place the patient's forearm under the ribcage and support with the other arm.

● As the patient coughs, he or she uses the forearm and applies pressure in and upwards (bucket-handle action).

● The patient's cough should sound strong and loud.

Assisted cough in sitting (Fig. 13.4)

● Start with a good upright position.

● The assistant brings one arm in front and one arm behind to support the trunk.

● The front arm is placed just below the ribcage with hand curved around the opposite side of the chest.

● Pressure is applied in an inwards and upwards direction (bucket handle).

● Co-ordination between the patient and assistant is important.

● The patient's cough should sound strong and loud.

Removal of secretions

Suction may be used if pooled secretions in the upper airway are causing distress and the patient cannot clear them independently. In the late stages, patients find this distressing but suction of secretions from the mouth can be tolerated. Alternatively, hyoscine can be used to help dry secretions, whilst at the same time sedating the patient, so alleviating the distress. In a choking attack the patient must not be left alone; if the attack does not subside naturally, medication detailed above ('Dysphagia') can be given.

Prevention of aspiration and recognising infection

Education on the prevention of aspiration is advised, when appropriate. Liaison with the speech and language therapist is essential. Recommendations such as the chin-tuck position when upright may be appropriate when the patient is still oral feeding. A full speech and language therapy assessment is required at this stage. It is important to give advice on the signs and symptoms of pulmonary infection to the patient and carer.

Non-invasive positive-pressure ventilation (NIPPV)
NIPPV can be used for symptomatic chronic hypoventilation to reduce the work of breathing by supporting the respiratory muscles via positive pressure. NIPPV can enhance the quality of life when used to treat sleep-disordered breathing in patients with MND (Lyall et al., 2001b). It has also been shown to prolong survival in some patients with MND by several months (Pinto et al., 1995), and Polkey et al. (1999) warned that this increased longevity was at the cost of increased disability.

When the respiratory function deteriorates further, it is essential that all are prepared and a treatment plan is ready, to allow the symptoms to be relieved effectively. Ventilatory support with tracheostomy needs to be discussed very carefully, with all implications fully explained to the patient and family. The institution of full ventilatory support may occur in a crisis situation and later be regretted by patient and family (Gelinas, 2000). They also need to be made aware that a few people (up to 10%) on tracheostomy ventilation may become 'locked-in' and unable to communicate (Hayashi, 2000).

Medication The general practitioner, neurologist or palliative care service provides medication advice to relieve symptoms of breathlessness. The MND Association provides the Breathing Space Kit. This kit comprises a medication storage box, the necessary injections for use in emergency, together with a leaflet on their use and advice sheets on management of respiratory problems.

Assessment and outcome measures

The general principles of outcome measurement are discussed in Chapter 3. In patients with neurodegenerative conditions, outcome measures are used to assess the effectiveness of treatment intervention and the extent to which physiotherapy input prevents the complications that may arise as a consequence of the disease.

When treating a patient with MND it is important to have a clear baseline assessment so that progression can be easily monitored. Appropriate impairment measures include the use of goniometry to measure joint range of motion. Muscle strength can be measured using the Medical Research Council (MRC) scale. Activity measures, i.e. the 10-m timed walk, can also be used. Selection of appropriate measures is vital.

There are several subjective measures specific to MND. The ALS Severity Scale was devised in 1989 by Hillel and colleagues, as a measure of functional status in patients with ALS/MND. It is split up into four sections that describe speech, swallowing, lower-extremity and upper-extremity abilities. It has good interrater reliability and in a small sample of patients indicated an accurate assessment of a patient's disease status (Hillel et al., 1989). Further research is needed to test its effectiveness as an outcome measure. More recently, in 1996, another subjective rating scale, the Amyotrophic Lateral Sclerosis Functional Rating Scale, was devised (Brooks, 1996). It is used to demonstrate functional change in patients with MND. It is commonly used as a screening measure for entry into clinical trials and to chart disease progression. Quality of life is frequently assessed using the Short Form 36 (SF-36; e.g. Brazier et al., 1992) and the Sickness Impact Profile (SIP; Bergner et al., 1976).

PSYCHOSOCIAL ASPECTS

The emotional and spiritual needs of the patient and family require attention, and counselling is part of the care given by all team members.

Emotional problems

The moods of patients seriously disabled by a progressive illness will vary. Moreover, communication and the expression of emotion may be restricted by dysarthria, and, due to reduced facial movements, the control of expression may be lost and lead to an inability to control laughing or tears. These changes may frighten both the patient and the family and it is important to stress the physiological causes, and that mental deterioration is unlikely in the illness so that patients are not treated as if they are lacking intelligence.

How the news of the diagnosis is broken to the patient and family can profoundly affect how they cope with the later course of the disease. There is the need for the diagnosis to be given sympathetically and accurately (Borasio et al., 1998). All professionals involved with the patient and family should be well informed about the disease and be able to discuss the likely progression themselves or to involve other members of the MDT as necessary.

Every person will have his or her own particular fears and concerns. It is essential to allow patients the opportunity to share these concerns with members of the caring team and to address them if possible. Fears may be of the disease itself, of the future, of disability and dependence, or of death and dying.

Anxiety may be reduced by a calm and confident approach from the caring team and by careful control of the other symptoms. Sedatives may be helpful, and in an emergency situation of severe panic an injection will promptly control the anxiety.

It is often very difficult to differentiate a depressive illness from the natural sadness of a severely disabled patient. Careful listening and explanation are important and antidepressants may be helpful.

Cognition

Although unusual, recent research has provided evidence that cognitive deficits can arise from MND. Radiological studies confirm that the frontotemporal region is affected (Ellis et al., 2001; Neary et al., 2000), which may lead to executive dysfunction and social interaction problems (Barson et al., 2000). Cognitive difficulties are associated most commonly, although not exclusively, with bulbar-onset MND. Assessment and advice from a neuropsychologist may benefit these patients.

Family care

The family of someone with MND will face their own challenges and fears. They may fear the disease, or the future deterioration, or the death of the patient (Gallagher & Monroe, 2000). These fears need to be shared and, if possible, the patient and the family should be able to be open and share their concerns together. There may also be the need to discuss the sexual needs of the patient and spouse. Although the disease may not affect sexual drive, the disability may affect performance. Help and advice on movement and sexual positions, or the consideration of other ways of expressing sexuality, such as mutual masturbation, may be necessary.

There may also be wider family issues. If there are young children, the help of a social worker may be very helpful in talking with the children about their understanding and fears of the disease. There may also be financial issues to be addressed.

Listening to, and supporting, the family is essential to management. The family needs to be closely involved in the care of the patient and in the formulation of any plans for care.

Spiritual aspects

Many people with a serious illness may start to think about the more profound aspects of life, even if they are not religious. There are no easy answers to these questions, such as 'Why me?', but listening and sharing the concerns may be very helpful. Local religious leaders may be of help.

Counselling

The patient may seek more knowledge or advice about the condition from the physiotherapist. As part of the MDT, the physiotherapist must feel able to seek help from the appropriate person to suit the patient's needs. When the physiotherapist provides the relevant information, he or she must ensure that not only the family and patient receive it but also the rest of the team. One must not give too much information at one session, or too soon, as it may not be absorbed.

The physiotherapist needs to be aware of the process of grief and loss, not only for a life that is coming to an end, but for the ongoing losses that the patient and indeed the family are experiencing (McAteer, 1990; Oliver, 1995). 'Physiotherapists can, and must be prepared to, step out of their more traditional role as purely physical therapists and be available to offer their patients, not only physical treatment, but a counselling relationship as well' (McAteer, 1989).

The multidisciplinary approach is vitally important, not only for the ongoing support of the professional carers but in order that management problems are addressed as early as possible. O'Gorman & O'Brien (1990) stated:

> ...care of the patient may become difficult because natural preferences occur for different team members and their way of working. With continuing losses it is understandable that the patient may feel insecure, angry and become demanding in his/her behaviour. These problems have the potential of splitting the team. It could become necessary to address these problems with team members and the patient, to define boundaries. (p. 45)

Ted Holden, an inpatient at St Christopher's Hospice for nearly 6 years, wrote (Holden, 1980):

> Obviously and naturally my wife's visits have the greatest impact, but our very closeness means that we can more easily hurt each other and so we do have our problems, but we keep trying and considering the strains and tensions we manage pretty well. I believe that the main problem is simply to expect too much. One spends hours in eager anticipation which creates an oversensitive reaction to anything which falls short of expectation. The disappointment leads to poor communication and misunderstanding and as one realises that the mood is set and one is fully aware of the fundamental stupidity of it all, frustration, anger and remorse ensure that there is little prospect of recovery. What is sad is that you can do nothing until the next meeting which can be a long, long time. It needs the skill of the interdisciplinary team to attempt to stay alongside such feelings ... (p. 44)

Another patient's view can be found in a paper by Henke, published in 1980.

Not all patients with MND will be found in special units, and the physiotherapist may not have the back-up of a committed team. In such instances, the therapist must apply the principles which are outlined not only in this chapter but throughout this book. Continual assessment is necessary as MND follows no rules and what suits one patient may be useless for another. Individual gadgets, aids and appliances are essential.

At times, a family meeting to include family, appropriate professionals (not necessarily the whole team) and/or the patient will help to discuss problems, ongoing care and overall management. As many members of the family as appropriate should be included so that issues can be discussed with everybody hearing the same information at the same time. This minimises misinterpretation of the facts. The physiotherapist can play a useful part in such meetings.

TERMINAL MANAGEMENT

The palliative care of a patient with MND starts at the time of diagnosis (Oliver, 2000). As the patient deteriorates, there is an even greater need to ensure that the symptoms are well controlled and the patient and family are supported. The final deterioration may be short; of the hospice patients studied, 40% deteriorated over a period of <12 h (O'Brien et al., 1992). The commonest course of the disease is development of a respiratory infection with increased secretions and increasing respiratory distress (if untreated), and death from respiratory failure (Neudert et al., 2001). A smaller proportion of patients have acute respiratory failure, with a sudden deterioration in respiration and death occurring within minutes.

Anticipation of any potential problems is essential. It is important to ensure that all the team caring for the patient are aware of the changes and that medication is easily available for any emergency. Oral medication may be possible until close to death, but if swallowing deteriorates, parenteral medication may be necessary. The Motor Neurone Disease Association has developed the Breathing Space Programme to help patients at this time. The patient and family can discuss the use of the Breathing Space Kit (see 'Medication', above) with their own doctor, who can then prescribe the medication so that it is immediately available at home if there is an episode of pain, breathlessness or choking.

The majority of specialist palliative care units and teams are involved in the care of people with MND (Oliver & Webb, 2000). This may be in the provision of respite care (Hicks & Corcoran, 1993) and care in the terminal stages, and only a minority (17%) are involved from soon after the diagnosis (Oliver & Webb, 2000).

The Motor Neurone Disease Association

The MND Association acts as a support and information service as well as funding research. It publishes a number of leaflets for the patient and the family, as well as for professionals involved in care. Regional support groups for patients and carers are available throughout the UK. There is also a 24-h help line and the Association is able to loan equipment (see Appendix).

CASE HISTORY 1

Mr G was a 74-year-old married man who had noticed weakness of his left arm while doing DIY in December 1994. The diagnosis of MND was made in May 1995 and he was first visited at home by a doctor and physiotherapist from the hospice in September 1995.

A full assessment showed a very disabled person whose wife was finding the situation very difficult. The power in Mr G's arms ranged from 0 to 2 on the Oxford Scale, the best strength being in the right elbow. All joint movements were restricted by pain. The legs were also weak; the left hip flexors had only a flicker of movement but the right leg was stronger. There was some oedema of the right hand and lower legs. He required assistance from two people to stand and walking was impossible. Chest expansion was reduced and he needed help for all

personal care, feeding, transfers and even wiping his nose. He was unable to change his position in bed at night. His main carer was his 75-year-old wife who was 'desperate'. The district nurse visited weekly and carers came twice a day to help him out of and into bed.

It was agreed that he would be admitted to the hospice for 2 weeks for respite care and assessment. A reclining wheelchair was provided and a regular programme of active and passive movements started as a daily exercise regimen to mobilise joints and maximise ability. A page turner allowed him to read unassisted. He talked about his deterioration and manner of death with the physiotherapist during one of these treatments. After a meeting of the family it was decided that he would remain at the hospice.

A lumbar cushion and head support cushion were necessary in the wheelchair and a non-slip mat prevented his feet slipping from the foot rests. As he tended to fall forwards it was suggested that the wheelchair should be reclined further but he refused this. By October the chair was reclined twice a day for rest periods, but as it was difficult to drink and eat in the reclined position, it could not be reclined for longer. Throughout this time he continued to have regular physiotherapy with a regular exercise programme.

Joint pain was a problem, so a non-steroidal anti-inflammatory drug was commenced. This helped initially but the pain became more pronounced and on 19 October morphine elixir 2.5 mg was started at night. After further difficult nights, morphine sulphate modified-release tablets were started at night. The nights improved but he continued to deteriorate, and swallowing and speech became more difficult. The exercise programme continued.

By 6 December a hoist was tried as this would soon be necessary to move him but he did not like it. His voice was very weak and there was severe oedema of the legs and Tubigrip bandages were used. On 13 December his chest expansion was very poor and morphine was increased due to increasing pain. He continued to deteriorate: his speech was very difficult to understand and chest expansion was hardly perceptible; the accessory muscles of respiration were being used. On 6 January a communication chart was supplied. He was tearful at times. However, the exercise programme continued.

On 9 January the physiotherapist was asked by the nursing staff for help as Mr G could not transfer due to his knees giving way. After discussion with Mr G, he agreed reluctantly to the use of the hoist, as he preferred to be in the chair. He was unable to swallow and said he was not hungry and did not feel the need to eat. His wife needed increasing support and was seen by a social worker.

On 11 January he was very weak but still insisted on getting up and having exercises. He eventually returned to bed. He was only able to take a little fluid by syringe. A subcutaneous infusion, using a syringe driver, was used for analgesia. Mr G died peacefully during the night.

This case history illustrates the rapid decline in power and function, and the many measures needed to assist in comfort and positioning. It also shows the involvement of the physiotherapist in the daily management of a person with advancing MND and how one patient was committed to his daily exercise regimen.

CASE HISTORY 2

First clinic visit

A 33-year-old man, recently diagnosed with MND, presented to clinic with proximal upper-limb weakness. On assessment, he was unable to reach above his head or to dress himself but was independently mobile and still working full-time. Interventions at this stage included:

- stretches to maintain range of motion at the shoulder joint complex
- advice on exercise
- advice on positioning upper limbs
- liaison with occupational therapist regarding limitations in activities of daily living
- MNDA contact number given.

Second clinic visit

Six months later, the patient showed increasing weakness in the upper limbs, with no activity proximally but some persisting in the hands. He was experiencing some pain in his shoulders and had to reduce his working hours, as he was fatiguing and struggling to use his keyboard.

Interventions included:

- advice on 24-h positioning of upper limbs, including use of collar and cuff support whilst mobilising and supporting his arms on a table to facilitate keyboard use
- advice on activity modification for fatigue
- referral back to medical team for analgesia.

Third clinic visit

A year after diagnosis, there was minimal change since the previous visit. Ongoing input was given for maintaining level of function.

Prior to the fourth clinic appointment, the patient telephoned to report increasing neck weakness. The physiotherapist referred him to the local physiotherapy service for assessment.

Fourth clinic visit

When seen 18 months after diagnosis, the patient had been issued with an MNDA collar by the local physiotherapist who reviewed him regularly. On respiratory testing, the patient's VC was 75% of predicted value and the consultant referred him to the physiotherapist for assessment of his cough, which proved to be ineffective. As the patient was unable to self-assist due to upper-limb weakness, the assisted-cough technique was taught to his wife.

Fifth clinic visit

Two years after diagnosis, the patient reported disturbed sleep and orthopnoea. The team recommended a trial of NIPPV at night and the patient was brought in as an inpatient for this. Liaison with the inpatient team identified that he was concerned about mobilising outdoors due to breathlessness and fatigue. Referral was made by the inpatient team to the local wheelchair service and hospice team, with the patient's consent.

Sixth clinic visit

The patient reported that attending clinic was very fatiguing. The physiotherapist ensured that the hospice team continued with regular reviews and input. The patient was reassured that clinic appointments were available to him on request but no further routine appointments were made at this stage. He continued to be reviewed regularly by the hospice team.

This patient's case demonstrates that the physiotherapist has an essential role in the management of patients with MND. It is vital that the physiotherapist understands the course of the disease and its possible consequences in order to provide timely and appropriate input. It is also important for the physiotherapist to appreciate the balance between therapeutic input and quality of life issues in order to organise the patient's care in the most appropriate manner.

References

Abrahams S, Goldstein LH, Kew JJM et al. Frontal lobe dysfunction in amyotrophic lateral sclerosis. A PET study. *Brain* 1996, **119**:2105–2120.

Aitkens S, McCrory M, Kilmer D, Bernauer E. Moderate resistance exercise program: its effect in slowly progressive neuromuscular disease. *Arch Phys Med Rehab* 1993, **74**:711–715.

Barson FP, Kinsella GJ, Ong B, Mathers SE. A neuropsychological investigation of dementia in motor neurone disease. *J Neurol Sci* 2000, **180**:107–113.

Bergner M, Bobbitt RA, Pollard WE et al. The sickness impact profile: validation of a health status measure. *Med Care* 1976, **14**:57–67.

Borasio GD, Miller RG. Clinical characteristics and management of ALS. *Semin Neurol* 2001, **21**:155–166.

Borasio GD, Sloan R, Pongratz D. Breaking the news in amyotrophic lateral sclerosis. *J Neurol Sci* 1998, **160** (**suppl.1**):S127–S133.

Brazier JE, Harper R, Jones NM et al. Validating the SF-36 health survey questionnaire: new outcome measure for primary care. *Br Med J* 1992, **305**:160–164.

Bromley I. *Tetraplegia and Paraplegia – A Guide for Physiotherapists*, 5th edn. Edinburgh: Churchill Livingstone; 1998.

Brooks BR. The ALSCNTF Study Group. The amyotrophic lateral sclerosis functional rating scale. *Arch Neurol* 1996, **53**:141–147.

Brooks BR, Miller RG, Swash M et al. *El Escorial Revisited: Revised Criteria for the Diagnosis of Amyotrophic Lateral Sclerosis.* World Federation of Neurology Research Group on Motor Neuron Diseases. 1998. Available online at: www.wfals.org/Articles/elescorial1998.htm.

Brown P. Pathophysiology of spasticity. *J Neurol Neurosurg Psychiatry* 1994, **57**:773–777.

Corr B, Frost E, Traynor BJ, Hardiman, O. Service provision for patients with ALS/MND: a cost effective multidisciplinary approach. *J Neurol Sci* 1998, **160**:141–145.

Edwards S, Charlton P. Splinting and the use of orthoses in the management of patients with neurological disorder. In: Edwards S, ed. *Neurological Physiotherapy: A Problem-solving Approach,* 2nd edn. London: Churchill Livingstone; 2002:219–253.

Ellis CM, Suckling J, Amaro E et al. Volumetric analysis reveals corticospinal tract degeneration and extramotor involvement in ALS. *Neurology* 2001, **57**:1571–1578.

Figlewicz DA, Rouleau GA. Familial disease. In: Williams AC, ed. *Motor Neuron Disease.* London: Chapman & Hall; 1994:427–450.

Francis K, Bach JR, DeLisa JA. Evaluation and rehabilitation of patients with adult motor neurone disease. *Arch Phys Med Rehab* 1999, **80**:951–963.

Gallagher D, Monroe B. Psychosocial care. In: Oliver D, Borasio GD, Walsh D, eds. *Palliative Care in Amyotrophic Lateral Sclerosis.* Oxford: Oxford University Press, 2000:83–103.

Gelinas D. Amyotrophic lateral sclerosis and invasive ventilation. In: Oliver D, Borasio GD, Walsh D, eds. *Palliative Care in Amyotrophic Lateral Sclerosis.* Oxford: Oxford University Press, 2000:56–62.

Hayashi H. ALS care in Japan. In: Oliver D, Borasio GD, Walsh D, eds. *Palliative Care in Amyotrophic Lateral Sclerosis.* Oxford: Oxford University Press, 2000: 152–154.

Henke E. Motor neurone disease – a patient's view. *Br Med J* 1980, **4**:765–766.

Hicks F, Corcoran G. Should hospices offer respite admissions to patients with motor neurone disease? *Palliat Med* 1993, **7**:145–150.

Hillel AD, Miller RM, Yorkston K et al. Amyotrophic lateral sclerosis severity scale. *Neuroepidemiology* 1989, **8**:142–150.

Holden T. Patiently speaking. *Nurs Times* 1980, **76**:1035–1036.

Hough A. *Physiotherapy in Respiratory Care.* London: Chapman & Hall; 1991.

Kent-Braun JA, Miller RG. Central fatigue during isometric exercise in amyotrophic lateral sclerosis. *Muscle Nerve* 2000, **23**:909–914.

Kilmer D, McCrory M, Wright N et al. The effect of a high resistance exercise program in slowly progressive neuromuscular disease. *Arch Phys Med Rehab* 1994, **75**:560–563.

Langton Hewer R. The management of motor neurone disease. In: Leigh PN, Swash M, eds. *Motor Neurone Disease: Biology and Management.* London: Springer Verlag; 1995:391–393.

Lieber RL, Friden J. Mechanisms of muscle injury after eccentric contraction. *J Sci Med Sport* 1999, **2**:253–265.

Lyall R, Moxham J, Leigh N. Dyspnoea. In: Oliver D, Borasio GD, Walsh D, eds. *Palliative Care in Amyotrophic Lateral Sclerosis.* Oxford: Oxford University Press, 2000:43–56.

Lyall RA, Donaldson N, Polkey MI et al. Respiratory muscle strength and ventilatory failure in amyotrophic lateral sclerosis. *Brain* 2001a, **124**:2000–2013.

Lyall RA, Donaldson N, Fleming T et al. A prospective study of quality of life in ALS patients treated with non-invasive ventilation. *Neurology* 2001b, **57**:153–156.

McAteer MF. Some aspects of grief in physiotherapy. *Physiotherapy* 1989, **75**:55–58.

McAteer MF. Reactions to terminal illness. *Physiotherapy* 1990, **76**:9–12.

Miller RG, Rosenberg JA, Gelinas DF et al. Practice parameter: The care of the patient with amyotrophic lateral sclerosis (an evidence-based review). *Neurology* 1999, **52**:1311–1323.

Mustfa N, Moxham J. Respiratory muscle assessment in motor neurone disease. *Q J Med* 2001, **94**:497–502.

Neary D, Snowden JS, Mann DMA. Cognitive changes in motor neurone disease/amyotrophic lateral sclerosis. *J Neurol Sci* 2000, **180**:15–20.

Neudert C, Oliver D, Wasner M et al. The course of the terminal phase in patients with amyotrophic lateral sclerosis. *J Neurol* 2001, **248**:612–616.

Newrick PG, Langton Hewer R. Pain in motor neurone disease. *J Neurol Neurosurg Psychiatry* 1985, **48**:838–840.

O'Brien T, Kelly M, Saunders C. Motor neurone disease – a hospice perspective. *Br Med J* 1992, **304**:471–473.

O'Gorman B. Physiotherapy. In: Oliver D, Borasio GD, Walsh D, eds. *Palliative Care in Amyotrophic Lateral Sclerosis.* Oxford: Oxford University Press, 2000: 105–111.

O'Gorman B, O'Brien T. Motor neurone disease. In: Saunders C, ed. *Hospice and Palliative Care: An Interdisciplinary Approach.* London: Edward Arnold; 1990:41–45.

Oliver D. Ethical issues in palliative care – an overview. *Palliat Med* 1993, **7** (Suppl. 2):15–20.

Oliver D. *Motor Neurone Disease*, 2nd edn. Exeter: Royal College of General Practitioners; 1994.

Oliver D. *Motor Neurone Disease: A Family Affair*. London: Sheldon Press; 1995.

Oliver D. The quality of care and symptom control – the effects on the terminal phase of MND/ALS. *J Neurol Sci* 1996, **139** (Suppl.):134–136.

Oliver D. Opioid medication in the palliative care of motor neurone disease. *Palliat Med* 1998, **12**:113–115.

Oliver D. Palliative care. In: Oliver D, Borasio GD, Walsh D, eds. *Palliative Care in Amyotrophic Lateral Sclerosis*. Oxford: Oxford University Press, 2000:23–28.

Oliver D, Webb S. The involvement of specialist palliative care in the care of people with motor neurone disease. *Palliat Med* 2000, **14**:427–428.

Peruzzi AC, Potts AF. Physical therapy intervention for persons with amyotrophic lateral sclerosis. *Physiother Can* 1996, **48**:119–126.

Pinto AC, Evangelista T, Carvalho M. Respiratory assistance with a non-invasive ventilator (Bipap) in MND/ALS patients: survival rates in a controlled trial. *J Neurol Sci* 1995, **129**:19–26.

Polkey MI, Lyall RA, Davidson AC et al. Ethical and clinical issues in the use of home non-invasive mechanical ventilation for the palliation of breathlessness in motor neurone disease. *Thorax* 1999, **54**:367–371.

Pope PM. Postural management and special seating. In: Edwards S, ed. *Neurological Physiotherapy: A Problem Solving Approach*, 2nd edn. London: Churchill Livingstone; 2002:189–217.

Pryor J, Webber B. *Physiotherapy for Respiratory and Cardiac Problems*. London: Churchill Livingstone; 1998.

Richardson D, Thompson AJ. Botulinum toxin: its use in the treatment of acquired spasticity in adults. *Physiotherapy* 1999, **85**:541–551.

Rosen AD. Amyotrophic lateral sclerosis. *Arch Neurol* 1978, **35**:638–642.

Rosen DR, Siddique T, Patterson D et al. Mutations in Cu/Zn superoxide dismutase gene are associated with familial amyotrophic lateral sclerosis. *Nature* 1993, **362**:59–62.

Ross J, Dean E. Integrating physiological principles into the comprehensive management of cardiopulmonary dysfunction. *Phys Ther* 1989, **69**:255–259.

Sanjak M, Reddan W, Rix Brooks B. Role of muscular exercise in amyotrophic lateral sclerosis. *Neurol Clin* 1987, **5**:251–267.

Saunders C, Walsh TD, Smith M. Hospice care in motor neurone disease. In: Saunders C, Summers DH, Teller N, eds. *Hospice: The Living Idea*. London: Edward Arnold; 1981:126–147.

Schwartz MS, Swash M. Neurophysiological changes in motor neurone disease. In: Leigh PN, Swash M, eds. *Motor Neurone Disease: Biology and Management*. London: Springer Verlag; 1995:331–344.

Scott AG, Austin HE. Nasogastric feeding in the management of severe dysphagia in motor neurone disease. *Palliat Med* 1994, **8**:45–49.

Scott A, Foulsom M. Speech and language therapy. In: Oliver D, Borasio GD, Walsh D, eds. *Palliative Care in Amyotrophic Lateral Sclerosis*. Oxford: Oxford University Press, 2000:117–125.

Sharma KR, Kent-Braun JA, Majumdar S et al. Physiology of fatigue in amyotrophic lateral sclerosis. *Neurology* 1995, **45**:733–740.

Strand EA, Miller RM, Yorkston KM et al. Management of oral–pharyngeal dysphagia symptoms in amyotrophic lateral sclerosis. *Dysphagia* 1996, **11**:129–139.

Sutton P, Lopez Vidriero M, Paria D et al. Assessment of percussion, vibratory shaking and breathing exercises in chest physiotherapy. *Eur J Resp Dis* 1985, **66**:147–152.

Swash M, Schwartz MS. Motor neurone disease: the clinical syndrome. In: Leigh PN, Swash M, eds. *Motor Neurone Disease: Biology and Management*. London: Springer Verlag; 1995:1–17.

Tandan R. Clinical features and differential diagnosis of classical motor neurone disease. In: Williams AC, ed. *Motor Neurone Disease*. London: Chapman & Hall; 1994:3–27.

Unsworth J. Coping with the disability of established disease. In: Williams AC, ed. *Motor Neurone Disease*. London: Chapman & Hall; 1994:231–234.

Wagner-Sonntag E, Allison S, Oliver D, Proseigel M, Rawlings J, Scott A. Dysphagia. In: Oliver D, Borasio GD, Walsh D, eds. *Palliative Care in Amyotrophic Lateral Sclerosis*. Oxford: Oxford University Press, 2000:62–72.

Young T, Nicklin C. *Lower Limb Casting in Neurology: Practical Guidelines*, 1st edn. London: Royal Hospital for Neuro-disability; 2000.

Chapter 14

Disorders of nerve II: Polyneuropathies

J Nicklin

INTRODUCTION

The term 'polyneuropathies' refers to the group of disorders where the peripheral nerves are affected by one or more pathological processes, resulting in motor, sensory and/or autonomic symptoms. Generally these symptoms are diffuse, symmetrical and predominantly distal. Muscle weakness may be confined distally or may be more extensive in chronic cases. The range of sensory symptoms covers the spectrum from complete loss of sensation to mild tingling to unbearable painful dysaesthesia.

Autonomic dysfunction, such as disturbances of blood pressure, can be present in some of the polyneuropathies, e.g. diabetic neuropathy. Most neuropathies are slowly progressive, the deterioration occurring in a stepwise fashion, or as a continuous downward progression.

For the physiotherapist, patients with a polyneuropathy present a challenge best managed using a problem-solving approach. In this chapter, the range of polyneuropathies will be described and a case presentation given to illustrate some of the issues confronted in these conditions. Mononeuropathies and neuropathies due to trauma are not included.

PATHOLOGICAL PROCESSES AFFECTING PERIPHERAL NERVES

Pathological processes affecting the peripheral nerves are defined according to which structures are involved: the axon (axonopathy); the Schwann cell that produces the myelin sheath (myelinopathy); or the nerve cell body (neuronopathy).

Axonopathies

Interruption to the axon results in axonopathy. All metabolic processes occur in the cell body, which supports the axon, and if axonal transport of nutrition fails, the axon dies back from the distal end. Surviving axons will conduct at a normal rate but, because of the reduced number, will be less effective in producing a muscle contraction. Early loss of the ankle jerk is seen because the longest, large-diameter fibres, such as those to the leg muscles of the posterior compartment, are the most vulnerable to axonopathy. This process underlies most metabolic and hereditary neuropathies and leads to long-term disability. Regeneration is slow, at 2–3 mm/day (Schaumburg et al., 1992).

Myelinopathies

When the Schwann cell that produces myelin is damaged, nerve conduction is slowed. Normally the impulse is conducted by jumping from node to node (saltatory conduction), which is extremely fast. The internodes (area between nodes) become longer where myelin has been destroyed and the impulse is conducted comparatively slowly along this part of the nerve fibre. If several adjacent segments of nerve become demyelinated, the effect is magnified and this can result in complete block of nerve conduction in that particular axon (Hopkins, 1993). This leads to the clinical manifestations of weakness and fatigue. Remyelination can occur, producing shorter sections of myelination.

Neuronopathies

Once the cell body is damaged, recovery is unlikely. Either the sensory or motor nerves can be affected. Motor neurone disease is one example of a neuronopathy (see Ch. 13).

Once the nerve is affected by one of the above processes, it is at greater risk of entrapment or pressure. Severe disability may predispose to prolonged pressure, e.g. at the fibula head, but entrapment neuropathies occur despite adequate cushioning, suggesting other processes (deJager & Minderhoud, 1991). Focal neuropathies (Table 14.1) affecting one nerve may be replicated in several nerves over time and come to resemble a polyneuropathy. This picture is seen where ischaemia occurs to the nerve, as in polyarteritis.

CLASSIFICATION OF POLYNEUROPATHIES

The neuropathies are broadly divided into acquired and inherited types. Many of the named neuropathies are rare and will not be discussed in great detail in this chapter. However, the principles of assessment and treatment remain the same. For greater detail, consult the definitive reference book by Dyck & Thomas (1993).

Acquired neuropathies

Table 14.1 shows the classification of acquired neuropathies, which may be generalised or focal.

Metabolic neuropathies

The peripheral nerves are vulnerable to disorders affecting their metabolism and this gives rise to the largest group of neuropathies.

Diabetic neuropathy

This is the commonest form of neuropathy in developed countries and is becoming more common with an increase in the ageing population and hence in the prevalence of diabetes (Mitchell, 1991). The prevalence of neuropathy rises from 7.5% at diagnosis of diabetes to 50% after 25 years (Pirart, 1978). The patterns of

Table 14.1 Classification of acquired neuropathies

Symmetrical generalised neuropathies	
Metabolic	Diabetes
	In renal disease
	In alcoholism
	Vitamin deficiencies
Inflammatory	Guillain–Barré syndrome (acute)
	Chronic inflammatory demyelinating polyneuropathy
Drug/toxin-induced	Antineoplastic
	Antirheumatic
	n-Hexane
	Acrylamide
	Tri-orthocresyl Phosphate
Associated with malignant disease	Carcinoma of the breast, lung, colon
Associated with monoclonal disease	Paraproteinaemias
Infection	Leprosy
	Human immunodeficiency virus (HIV)
	Diphtheria
Focal or multifocal neuropathies	
Collagen vascular disease	Polyarteritis nodosa
	Systemic lupus erythematosus
	Rheumatoid arthritis

neuropathy seen are distal symmetrical sensory neuropathy and proximal motor neuropathy.

Distal symmetrical sensory neuropathy This is the most common presentation, producing weakness and sensory impairment in the feet. These sensory symptoms range from numbness to an aching pain. The discomfort is often worse at night (Thomas & Thomlinson, 1993). Occasionally, the loss of joint positional sense can be severe, leading to sensory ataxia. Loss of deep pain sense and ischaemia increases the risk of chronic foot ulceration. Weakness of intrinsic foot muscles produces changes in foot alignment and distribution of pressure when weight-bearing. Diabetic ulcers can be prevented with careful checking of the skin and attention to footwear. Where necessary, footwear may need to be individually tailored to prevent pressure (see 'Orthoses', below). Charcot arthropathies of the foot are seen in a subgroup but they can also develop in the absence of a sensory neuropathy. Here it is suggested that an autonomic neuropathy affects regulation of blood flow leading to damage to joints following minor trauma (Sinacore, 2001).

Proximal motor neuropathy This is seen predominantly in elderly diabetics. The weakness and wasting are asymmetrical and affect most often the iliopsoas, quadriceps and hip adductor muscles. Pain can be severe, especially at night. Recovery normally follows better control of the diabetes but may take months and may not be complete. Pain is the most distressing symptom for the patient. Drugs such as phenytoin and antidepressants have been used with varying success (Thomas & Thomlinson, 1993).

Renal disease

A symmetrical distal motor and sensory neuropathy that affects the legs more than the arms is associated with chronic renal failure. Uraemic patients often complain of 'restless legs', i.e. their legs are continuously moving and uncomfortable in bed. Dialysis or transplantation causes the neuropathy to stabilise or improve (Hopkins, 1993).

Alcoholism

Neuropathy can occur as a result of long-term alcohol abuse. Weakness of the lower limbs progresses from the feet proximally but can usually be detected in all the lower-limb muscles to a variable degree. Muscle pain (myalgia) and unpleasant dysaesthesiae are common. The major reason for the neuropathy is thought to be nutritional deficiencies, and possibly the effect of alcohol on the nerve (Asbury & Bird, 1992). However,

Monforte et al. (1995) demonstrated a significant correlation between the total time a patient had been drinking excessively and the presence of a neuropathy, and no correlation with nutritional status. The risk of an autonomic neuropathy also increased with duration of alcoholism, leading to changes in heart responses to exercise. Ataxia is seen in people with chronic alcoholism but this can be attributed to specific cerebellar damage as much as to sensory loss (Thompson & Day, 1993).

Vitamin deficiencies

Neuropathies can appear with a poorly balanced diet without starvation. Nutritional deficiency in western countries is seen in some forms of dieting, malabsorption and anorexia nervosa. In the Third World, nutritional polyneuropathy is commonly a result of dietary deprivation. Beriberi is one example still common in countries where people live mainly on a diet of highly milled rice. This is due to the specific lack of thiamine in the diet.

The motor sensory neuropathy starts distally but progresses to affect more proximal musculature. Cardiac involvement is common. It is often difficult to define exactly which vitamins are lacking in the diet. Treatment generally consists of multivitamin supplements in a balanced diet (Windebank, 1993). Foot drop may persist for many months following initiation of treatment (Schaumburg et al., 1992).

Inflammatory demyelinating polyneuropathies

Demyelination is the primary pathological process in this group. Axonal degeneration can be a feature and, if it occurs, it results in the more serious clinical manifestations sometimes seen in Guillain–Barré syndrome (GBS) (Feasby, 1992). There are two forms of these neuropathies, one acute and the other chronic. Both are considered autoimmune disorders.

Acute inflammatory demyelinating polyneuropathy: Guillain–Barré syndrome

The prevalence of GBS has been reported as 0.5–4.0 per 100 000 (Sridharan et al., 1993). Most commonly, leg weakness is noted first (Ropper et al., 1991). Often this progresses proximally and can involve all muscle groups, including those of the upper limb, trunk and face.

Many patients will have experienced a respiratory tract or gastric infection in the weeks preceding muscle weakness. Immunisation and surgery have also been cited as precipitating factors (Hartung et al., 1995).

In order to be classified as GBS, the time from onset to peak disability (i.e. nadir) should be less than 4 weeks. Studies have shown that 50% of patients will reach nadir within 2 weeks (Asbury & Cornblath, 1990).

Some patients become fully paralysed at the height of the illness. Nearly 50% of patients have facial weakness. Frequently the bulbar muscle groups are sufficiently affected to require nasogastric feeding to avoid aspiration. Paralysis of the respiratory muscles, causing the vital capacity to fall to <15 mm/kg, occurs in 30% of patients. Elective ventilation is indicated in this situation (Ng et al., 1995). Autonomic dysfunction occurs in some more severe cases and can lead to sudden unexpected mortalities, normally because of cardiac arrhythmias (McLeod, 1992).

GBS is predominantly a motor neuropathy but 42–75% of patients have some alteration in sensation (Pentland & Donald, 1994). Winer et al. (1988) found that joint positional sense was absent in the toes of 52% of patients. Pain is a frequent feature that appears very early in the disorder (Asbury, 1990). It has been postulated that the inflamed and tightened neural structures that occur in the acute stage may be the source of the pain (Simionato et al., 1988). During recovery, it is suggested that pain may be due to abnormal forces on joints poorly protected by weakened muscles (Pentland & Donald, 1994).

Recovery generally begins within a month of nadir and has the potential to be complete, provided secondary complications, such as contractures, are avoided. However, a percentage of patients with GBS do not make a full recovery. deJager & Minderhoud (1991) found that 37% of patients with GBS could not perform at the same physical level as prior to their illness at least 2 years after the nadir.

Periarticular contractures are one major cause of residual disability but there are few studies of their incidence, cause and prevention (Soryal et al., 1992). Physiotherapy is noted as important to prevent contractures (Ropper et al., 1991; Soryal et al., 1992), but this has not been researched. A case history of a GBS patient is given at the end of this chapter.

The Miller Fisher syndrome is a variant of GBS. The classic features are ataxia, ophthalmoplegia (causing double vision) and areflexia (Berlit & Rakicky, 1992). Diplopia and ataxia are the commonest first symptoms. Severe weakness is less common in Miller Fisher syndrome but when evident it may mask the ataxia.

Chronic inflammatory demyelinating polyneuropathy (CIDP)

This chronic form of polyneuropathy occurs mainly in the fifth or sixth decade of life. Sensory loss is more apparent in CIDP than in GBS. It is also differentiated from GBS by a longer time course to nadir, more than 4 weeks, developing over longer time periods in the majority of cases. Most patients have foot drop severe enough to require ankle–foot orthoses (AFOs). Fine hand control and grip may also be impaired. Fatigue unrelated to the degree of weakness or sensory change is a significant disability in a high proportion of patients with immune-mediated neuropathies (Merkies et al., 1999). Autonomic dysfunction is uncommon (McLeod, 1992). Most cases are slowly progressive but some follow a relapsing remitting course (Albers & Kelly, 1989); patients tend to have a more favourable prognosis if in the latter group (Ropper et al., 1991). Most will remain able to walk with aids but a few become dependent on a wheelchair.

Toxin- or drug-induced polyneuropathies

There are many industrial and agricultural chemicals which can produce neuropathies. Adhesives and their solvents can cause an axonal neuropathy which may be seen in industrial or agricultural workers and in solvent-abusers.

Adulterated rapeseed oil caused a notorious epidemic of peripheral neuropathy in Spain in 1981. Ingestion of the oil resulted in severe axonopathy, and there were a number of deaths (Schaumburg et al., 1992). Organophosphates used in agriculture have been implicated in cases of peripheral neuropathies. The effect of a toxin does not arrest once the cause is removed; rather, the symptoms progress over weeks or months due to continuing axonal degeneration (Schaumburg et al., 1992). Because the damage is generally axonal, the symptoms are often severe and only partially reversible.

Drug groups that are known to carry the risk of neuropathic side-effects include antirheumatic, antineoplastic, antimicrobial and anticonvulsant medication. Ceasing the drug has variable results.

Neuropathies associated with malignant disease

Compression and infiltration of nerve roots by neoplasms is common. Less frequently, polyneuropathies may occur as a remote effect of carcinoma of the lung, stomach or breast (Schaumburg et al., 1992). Sensory symptoms predominate, with motor symptoms developing much later. The features can appear between 6 months and 3 years prior to the detection of a tumour. Tumours of the peripheral nerve do occur, the majority of which are benign. In schwannomas (tumours arising from the Schwann cell), pain is always the predominant feature. Sensory or motor loss is rarely seen.

Neuropathies associated with monoclonal disease

Gamma-globulins are plasma proteins associated with antibody activity in the immune system. In paraproteinaemias, excessive amounts of gamma-globulins are present in the blood, often associated with reduced immune activity. They act to attack the myelin sheath (Albers & Kelly, 1989). Immunoglobulin M (IgM) is the most common gamma-globulin; excess IgM produces a mixed sensorimotor neuropathy which appears in the sixth decade or later in life. Tremor and ataxia are frequently seen. These are distressing symptoms, which greatly affect hand function, particularly as tremor is worse on activity. Other gamma-globulins present in neuropathies are IgG and IgA.

Neuropathies associated with infection and infestation

Neuropathy occurs with infections of the nervous system, and can involve both sensory and motor nerves.

Leprosy   Leprosy is the most common cause of peripheral neuropathy in the world and is caused by infection with *Mycobacterium leprae* (Hopkins, 1993). Sensory loss is a cardinal feature. Nerves become enlarged in response to invasion by bacteria and eventually, in addition to widespread sensory loss, motor loss becomes evident. Weakness of the intrinsic hand muscles is often noted first.

Human immunodeficiency virus (HIV)   A distal symmetrical polyneuropathy is detectable in over a third of patients infected with HIV who have developed acquired immune deficiency syndrome (AIDS). Most complain of a burning sensation in their feet, particularly at night (Simpson & Olney, 1992). A motor neuropathy is also seen and can look like GBS (Schaumburg et al., 1992). A multidisciplinary approach to managing this patient group is recommended (McClure, 1993).

Neuropathies associated with collagen vascular disease

Single or multifocal ischaemia of nerves may follow occlusion of small blood vessels to the nerves. The symptoms – pain, loss of strength and sensation – occur suddenly. Repeated episodes lead to a symmetrical and predominantly distal polyneuropathy. Two-thirds of all patients with polyarteritis will develop a mononeuropathy that may proceed as detailed above (Schaumburg et al., 1992). In rheumatoid arthritis, compression neuropathies are common. A mild sensory polyneuropathy is sometimes seen. Systemic lupus erythematosus (SLE) may be associated with neuropathy of variable presentation.

Table 14.2   Classification of inherited neuropathies

Unknown metabolic defect	Known metabolic deficit
Hereditary motor sensory neuropathy	Porphyria
Type I (Charcot–Marie–Tooth disease)	
Type II	Refsum disease
Type III (Dejerine–Sottas)	Leucodystrophy
Hereditary sensory neuropathy	
Types I–IV	
Amyloidoses	

Inherited neuropathies

The inherited neuropathies are listed in Table 14.2 and the metabolic abnormality, where known, is given.

Hereditary motor and sensory neuropathy

This is also known as Charcot–Marie–Tooth (CMT) disease or peroneal muscular atrophy. Most hereditary motor and sensory neuropathies (HMSNs) are inherited in an autosomal dominant fashion. The abnormal gene is located on chromosome 17 and the disorder results from a duplication of part of it. The most common forms are type I, a predominantly demyelinating form, and type II, an axonal disorder. The symptoms are similar for the two forms but they generally appear at a younger age in type I (Harding, 1993).

Initial symptoms are pes cavus, loss of tendon reflexes and clumsiness of gait. This clumsiness is partly due to increasing weakness of the muscles in the peroneal compartment and sensory changes in the feet (also seen in the hands). This muscle imbalance leads to the characteristic high-stepping gait and increasing foot deformities seen in this group. If sensory loss is severe, patients rely on visual information for regulation of postural control. When standing, they show more postural sway in the fore–aft direction than normal, which is due to distal weakness and deformities affecting the ankle strategy of controlling sway (Geurts et al., 1992). The lower leg takes on a stalk-like appearance because of peroneal wasting. Cramps and paraesthesiae are common early symptoms. The combination of deformity of the foot and changes in sensation predisposes patients with HMSN to tissue damage, which may lead to ulceration.

Surgical intervention to correct the deformity of high arches and/or very flexed toes with hyperextension of the metatarsophalangeal joints includes arthrodesis. However, early and appropriate provision of orthoses may make surgery unnecessary (Edwards & Charlton, 2002). Generally, patients with HMSN remain walking, albeit with orthoses and aids such as sticks. In some patients, particularly with type II HMSN, the disorder is more progressive and wheelchairs are needed.

The diaphragm is involved in some cases. Vital capacity should be measured in lying and sitting and will be much lower in the reclining position where the diaphragm is involved. Other symptoms may include orthopnoea, morning headaches and general fatigue. These need to be investigated further because nocturnal ventilatory support may be necessary to alleviate the symptoms (Hardie et al., 1990).

With the discovery of the genetic defect in these types of neuropathies, genetic counselling is possible and very important. Prenatal testing is available in some specialist centres but its use remains controversial.

Hereditary sensory neuropathy

Hereditary sensory neuropathies are inherited in a dominant fashion and affect the sensory nerves. Trophic changes occur in the hands and feet and may lead to severe ulcers and loss of digits. In another form, there is additional loss of unmyelinated fibres that produces insensitivity to pain. There may also be involvement of the autonomic system and this condition is termed 'sensory autonomic neuropathy'.

Other forms of inherited neuropathy

Most other forms are very rare. In acute episodes of porphyria, a proximal motor neuropathy appears with rapid wasting of affected muscle groups; the neuropathy can be severe enough to warrant ventilation.

ASSESSMENT AND DIAGNOSTIC INVESTIGATIONS

Principles of clinical examination by the neurologist and physiotherapist are described in Chapters 2 and 3. Features of assessment that are particularly important for the polyneuropathies are discussed below.

Electrophysiological tests

Electromyography (EMG) is important for differentiating between a demyelinating and an axonal process. The effect of an axonopathy is permanent because of the greater difficulty in repair of the axon. The presence of axonal changes in GBS is considered a poor prognostic indicator, although there are cases that confound this axiom (Feasby, 1994).

Genetic testing and counselling

Genes for the inherited neuropathies can be identified by deoxyribonucleic acid (DNA) testing (Harding, 1995). Once a patient is shown to have the gene, counselling can be offered and the implications for other family members discussed. Prenatal testing can identify a fetus at risk of developing an inherited neuropathy and give the parents the option of termination. However, testing does not predict the severity of the neuropathy as an adult, and approximately 20% of patients will be asymptomatic.

Observation

Analysis of movement, and observation of the condition and shape of muscle contours, are essential as part of the problem-solving approach. Wasting of the intrinsic hand muscles may be noted (Fig. 14.1), leading to clumsiness in gripping a cup or difficulty manipulating small items such as bottle tops. If the patient displays this kind of functional difficulty, the therapist should also consider what role sensory changes play in the problem.

Muscle imbalance will lead to shortening of unopposed muscle groups (Mann & Missirian, 1988). The intrinsic foot and the anterior leg compartment musculature are most commonly affected and foot deformities may result.

Gait assessment

Distal weakness, more marked in the dorsiflexors than the plantarflexors, will lead to a tendency to trip and a compensatory high-stepping gait. As the quadriceps muscles weaken, hyperextension occurs at the knees to produce a rigid structure when weight-bearing.

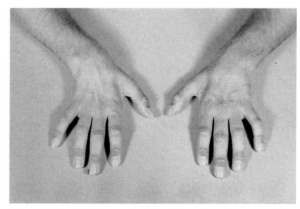

Figure 14.1 Typical wasting of small hand muscles as seen in chronic neuropathies.

Proximal muscle weakness, especially in the hip abductors, gives rise to a positive Trendelenburg sign in more severely affected patients. Gait analysis laboratories, pressure transducers coupled with EMG, and video recordings (Mueller et al., 1994) are all useful for analysing movement and for objective comparison over time. However, little research has been published on the neuropathic gait.

Muscle strength testing

Grading strength 0–5, using an ordinal scale such as the Medical Research Council (MRC) scale, is inadequate (see Ch. 3). Whilst this semiquantitative scale will give a global clinical picture, it does not allow for accurate comparisons over time. Measurement is recommended using an interval scale such as that produced by isokinetic or isometric equipment (see Ch. 3). These approaches are sensitive enough to detect changes where the strength may not change in grade on the manual testing scale, although improving or deteriorating. This is particularly relevant for muscles measuring grade 4. For instance, 90% of the range of muscle strength available in the biceps muscle falls in grade 4 (Munsat, 1990). Change is not recorded in the most relevant part of the range if one relies solely on the MRC scale. A hand-held myometer has been shown to be sensitive and reliable in assessing neuropathies (Wiles et al., 1990), in particular GBS (Bohannon & Dubuc, 1984; Karni et al., 1984). Positions for testing, commands and techniques must be standardised. Some authors have pointed out the need for frequent testing of interexaminer reliability and have shown that one examiner performing repeated tests is more desirable than having several different examiners (Lennon & Ashburn, 1993).

Weakness of the hand muscles can best be assessed and monitored using a grip dynamometer. This is often a very sensitive measure in the distal motor neuropathies. Reference values are available for many muscle groups, including hand grip and pinch grip (Wiles et al., 1990; van de Ploeg et al., 1991). This allows the degree of weakness to be compared to the normal range and expressed as a percentage of the lower limit of normal. The most sensitive measure of strength change is achieved if the assessment method mirrors the type of exercise used in a regimen, e.g. measurements of isokinetically gained strength should be made using an isokinetic device.

Fatigue testing

There is a subgroup of patients with neuropathies who have difficulties with fatigue. The fatigue may be of a global nature, i.e. getting tired writing letters or walking distances; there is also a more specific variety that affects the actual contraction of a muscle. Timed tests give the best indication of endurance and are most appropriate to physiotherapy practice (Cook & Glass, 1987). These are discussed under 'Functional assessment', below and in Chapter 3. However, endurance tests are dependent on motivation, and feedback is essential. The Fatigue Severity Scale has been demonstrated to be a reliable measure in neuropathies (Merkies et al., 1999).

Fatigue diaries are a good way of analysing more generalised fatigue where overwork is suspected. The patient is asked to keep a diary documenting activities and length of time performing each one. In addition, symptoms of fatigue are noted. The diary may then be analysed, to try and develop a structure to the patient's activities that prevents severe fatigue, but does not lead to the opposite problem of weakness from disuse by cutting out all activity that causes any degree of fatigue.

Sensory testing

Although subjective sensory testing is unreliable, it is important to note the extent and distribution of sensory loss or impairment. Some attempts have been made to devise grading scales which combine motor and sensory changes, but they have not yet been validated (Dellon, 1993).

Functional assessment

In the majority of neuropathies functional changes are subtle and gradual, such that a very sensitive objective measure is required. Appropriate timed tests are a useful indicator of change (Moxley, 1990), particularly up and down a standardised set of stairs or a timed 10-m (Watson & Wilson, 1992) or 30-m walk (Nicklin, unpublished data). The longer distance is preferred because it is only over this extended walk that change is shown, probably due to fatigue (Cook & Glass, 1987). In the case of GBS, the possible changes in performance cover many varied areas, e.g. ability to breathe independently through to ability to run. A performance indicator must be employed that can demonstrate these large changes but also capture more subtle changes (Karni et al., 1984). Dyck et al. (1995) used ability to rise from a chair and standing on heels in their study of diabetic neuropathy.

Whilst the use of an outcome measure involving function is both desirable and necessary to assess disability, the therapist must be aware that changes in the score may occur as a result of compensation as opposed to changes in strength, and that a change in sensation may have a significant effect, particularly on fine hand function. Another factor may be increasing body weight, particularly affecting activities such as rising from the floor or climbing stairs.

TREATMENT

A multidisciplinary problem-solving approach is recommended in the management of disability in order to maximise function, and an example of this approach is illustrated in the case history below. A proposed structure for a problem-solving approach is given in Chapter 22. Where a problem-solving approach is taken, many members of the MDT may be involved. However, it must be recognised that the number of health workers involved in a patient's care may be bewildering. For this reason, the use of a key-worker system is recommended to improve communication and reduce anxiety.

The involvement and information from well-organised support groups, such as the GBS Support Group UK and CMT UK, is important to empower individuals to manage their own disability (see Appendix). A practical guide on managing Charcot–Marie–Tooth (Northern, 2000) is particularly recommended.

Principles of physiotherapy intervention

A scientific basis for much of physiotherapy in this specialty has not been demonstrated and there is a paucity of research in this field. Therapy can be management of problems that cannot be reversed or treatment where improvement is possible, but should always address specific problems identified during assessment.

Acute neuropathies

Important aspects of physical management in acute neuropathies include prevention of contractures; control of pain; and respiratory care.

Stretching to prevent contractures

Neuropathy may result in severe disability whereby the patient is bed-bound. Prevention of contractures and musculoskeletal stiffness is a priority if maximum potential is to be achieved. When muscles are not stretched adequately but are left in a shortened position, structural changes, involving loss of sarcomeres, occurs and compromises potential recovery (see Ch. 25). The therapist should ensure that all structures, including the nervous system, are moved through their full range. Adverse neural tension signs can occur if neural tissues are not stretched and this concept is discussed in Chapter 31. Wherever possible, the patient should be encouraged to join in with the movement and use what is still available. Using a continuous passive motion machine has been suggested (Mays, 1990) as a means to maintain range of movement. Tightening of the posterior crural muscle group develops rapidly. This is nearly always preventable in neuropathy. In the bed-bound patient, foot drop splints should be provided and gentle stretches performed. More able patients should be taught self stretches in a weight-bearing position.

Positioning

Frequent changes in position are also necessary to prevent selective muscle shortening and pressure sores. Truncal weakness can cause the patient to lie with scapulae retracted, unless a wedge is positioned under the thoracic region as well as the head and shoulders. The pelvis should be supported in a position of posterior tilt with the hip flexors stretched, to prevent shortening. Positioning by nurses and physiotherapists can help prevent pressure neuropathies, e.g. at the medial epicondyle or fibula head (Watson & Wilson, 1989), though these can occur spontaneously.

Pain

The therapist should be aware of the existence of pain and liaise with the medical team to provide effective management (see Ch. 26). Pain is an early symptom in acute neuropathy such as GBS (Ropper et al., 1991) but has never been satisfactorily explained, although it is suggested this is due to spontaneous discharge in demyelinated sensory neuropathies (Ropper, 1992). Many patients demonstrate pain from adverse neural tension (see Ch. 31) and respond to treatment to manage this (Fearnhead & Fritz, 1996). Some therapists, including Freeman (1992), have suggested that the reason why patients with acute GBS enjoy large-amplitude mid-range movements is because of their pain-relieving properties. This accords with the findings of Butler, who gives two examples of mobilising the nervous system in GBS (Butler, 1991). In other neuropathies, massage and ice packs have been found to be helpful.

Respiratory care

In some instances the patient may be ventilated and the role of the physiotherapist is to help prevent atelectasis when breathing is compromised (Smith & Ball, 1998). Where there is facial muscle weakness, care must be taken to ensure there is lip seal around the mouth piece when measuring vital capacity (Fearnhead & Fritz, 1996).

Where the autonomic system is affected, disturbed blood pressure is of particular relevance to the physiotherapist, especially when using suction (Ng et al., 1995) or when attempting early sitting (Ropper et al., 1991). It is therefore essential to monitor vulnerable patients.

Chronic neuropathies

The role of the physiotherapist is largely one of management in chronic cases. Early referrals are important to advise on activities to maintain ambulation and prevent avoidable complications such as foot deformities (see 'Orthoses', below).

Strengthening exercises

Historically, there has always been a wariness of giving muscle-strengthening exercises to patients with neuromuscular diseases. This arose out of several anecdotal papers (e.g. Bennett & Knowlton, 1958). More recently there have been papers supporting the use of exercise to improve strength or endurance (Aitkens et al., 1993; Lindeman et al., 1995; Ruhland & Shields, 1997). Kilmer et al. (1994) found that high-resistance exercise was no better than low-resistance exercise for strengthening muscle and there was some evidence of damage when tested eccentrically. There is some limited evidence that endurance training can improve cardiopulmonary fitness in established neuropathies (Pitetti et al., 1993). Physical training in neurological conditions, for strengthening and endurance, is discussed in more detail in Chapter 29.

Most research on exercise in neuromuscular disorders has used a heterogeneous group and it is difficult to generalise results to specific polyneuropathies (Aitkens et al., 1993; Milner Brown & Miller, 1988). However Ruhland & Shields (1997) used a sample of 28 subjects, of whom 21 had CIDP. They demonstrated that a 6-week home programme of strengthening, stretching and aerobic conditioning increased strength and also led to an improved score on a health-related quality of life measure of physical role limitation.

Some authors have suggested concentrating on exercising the hip and knee, not the more severely affected distal muscle groups, in order to compensate and produce a more stable gait pattern (Mueller et al., 1994). The addition of an AFO would also increase stability by allowing the development of plantarflexor movement, despite very weak muscles, as well as preventing tripping. Compliance with an exercise regimen is variable and improvement is often gradual. A successful adjunct to face-to-face sessions with the physiotherapist is an exercise diary for recording both changing symptoms and amount and quality of exercise (Lindeman et al.,

1995). Of particular relevance is the noting of abnormally prolonged muscle ache following exercise, or sudden loss of functional ability. This may indicate damage from overuse. These symptoms should be noted and exercise modified to allow recovery.

The effect of exercise should be explained to the patient, including the possibility that the rate of deterioration may be reduced or recovery hastened but without affecting the underlying disorder (Cowan et al., 1993). The degree of weakness will have an effect on the final outcome. Where muscles are severely weakened, below 10% of the lower limit of normal for that group, the chance of strengthening is slim and exercise could cause further damage to the motor unit (Milner Brown & Miller, 1988).

Anecdotally, patients have been known to lose strength permanently following a bout of unaccustomed exercise such as decorating a room. In contrast, someone with a stable neuropathy may become less active, perhaps due to surgery, and then lose a former ability to perform an everyday function, primarily due to disuse and resulting weakness. Whenever the neuropathic patient becomes bed-bound, for whatever reason, physiotherapy is essential to facilitate functional recovery. Atrophy following disuse is preventable by specific exercises for identified muscle groups (see Ch. 29).

Where weakness is severe, it may be necessary to explore ways of maximising function through compensatory techniques. Generally, those with the slower progressive disorders develop strategies for themselves.

Stretches

Particularly in HMSN, gentle stretches for muscle groups that are liable to shorten are advocated. However, if real shortening has already occurred, attempts to stretch are more likely to cause damage to other related structures, e.g. attempting to stretch shortened Achilles tendon can lead to medial arch collapse.

Pain relief

Malalignment of joints due to muscle imbalance often leads to pain. Ice, massage and vibration are suggested as means of diminishing painful chronic sensory neuropathies, particularly in patients with HIV infection. Transcutaneous electrical nerve stimulation may also be helpful. These treatment techniques are discussed in Chapter 23.

Functional and mobility aids

Equipment used to aid function and mobility includes a range of orthoses and wheelchairs.

Orthoses

Where there is an abnormal gait pattern, mainly due to weakness of the dorsiflexors and/or the intrinsic muscles of the feet, the use of orthoses should be considered. Often, by the time a patient is referred to the physiotherapist or orthotist, foot deformities have become irreversible and insoles are necessary to allow the foot to sit comfortably in a standard shoe and to redistribute the weight across the total surface of the sole. Custom-made shoes may be necessary. In the first instance, insoles should be tried prior to using AFOs (Edwards & Charlton, 2002). Where foot drop exists, the option of a light-weight polypropylene splint should be discussed with the patient. Ready-made AFOs can be experimented with first to establish their usefulness. The permanent orthosis should mould to the calf and support the foot at 90°, extending as far as the toes. Where there is poor fit around the leg, there is the risk of chafing and skin damage, and the splint will also be less effective at maintaining the foot at 90°. Unless the forefoot is supported, the long flexors will be able to tighten where they are unopposed and may become contracted.

It is essential to discuss skin care with the patient. Many of those requiring splints will have sensory problems and there is always a risk of pressure areas developing. The patient should take responsibility for daily vigilance of the state of his or her skin. Where there is progressive weakness, muscle wasting will also occur and will lead to the need for remoulding of the splint. The use of any orthoses is an emotive subject and women, in particular, may not like their appearance. Careful explanation and, where possible, video recording of the improved gait attained whilst wearing a splint may help guide the patient's decision. However, there are disadvantages to wearing bilateral AFOs, such as negotiating stairs, and these should be considered when assessing the patient (Edwards & Charlton, 2002).

Hand function is often compromised through weakness or paralysis of intrinsic muscles of the thumb and fingers. The patient notices particular difficulties with the pincer grip. The introduction of a simple thumb opposition splint may allow a patient to produce legible writing for a longer time, or to grip a cup or knife. However, the difficulties of fitting and using a splint must be weighed against the benefits derived from wearing one. Where the thenar eminence becomes severely weak and wasted, a night splint cast in a functional position will help prevent severe contracture.

Wheelchairs

In a minority of cases the neuropathy progresses to render the patient dependent on a wheelchair. Assessment by specialists in posture and seating will lead to provision of appropriate wheelchairs (Pope, 2002). In the early stages of rehabilitating a patient with GBS, a reclining wheelchair is valuable to help cope with possible fluctuations in blood pressure and to allow gradual accommodation to the upright position.

Drug therapy

For the majority of the inflammatory and immune-based neuropathies, the mainstay of drug therapy is steroids and immunosuppressants. Deviations from this have already been mentioned above, as have drugs for pain management (see also Chs 26 and 28). Immunosuppressants, such as azathioprine, carry the risk of neoplasms but are effective in combination with prednisolone.

Plasmapheresis and immunoglobulin therapy

There are two treatments used for polyneuropathies which have a likely immunological basis. Plasmapheresis (plasma exchange) is an invasive technique whereby the patient's plasma is removed from the blood and treated to remove the antibodies attacking the myelin sheath, before being replaced (Hartung et al., 1995). Several controlled trials have demonstrated the benefits of plasma exchange, particularly in GBS where recovery time was shown to be shortened (Winer et al., 1988).

Immunoglobulin therapy is an alternative treatment to plasmapheresis and is less invasive. Among other effects, it is thought to help remyelination (Dalakas, 1999). The patient is given a booster of immunoglobulin over a period of 1–5 days. In pure motor GBS this has been shown to be possibly more effective in reducing recovery time (Visser et al., 1995). A percentage of patients with CIDP respond to immunoglobulin therapy (van-Doom, 1994) but the effect gradually fades and patients require repeated treatments to maintain functional level and prevent significant deterioration (Dalakas, 1999).

CASE HISTORY

A 31-year-old woman was admitted with a 3-day history of increasing weakness in the legs and paraesthesiae in the hands and feet, following an upper respiratory tract infection. A provisional diagnosis of GBS was made. The problems identified were:

Impairments

1. generalised motor impairment
2. impaired respiratory function

3. pain
4. reduced distal sensation
5. autonomic disturbance.

Disabilities

6. difficulty in swallowing
7. dependent for activities of daily living
8. inability to communicate effectively
9. anxiety.

The time course for these events is illustrated in Figure 14.2; nadir was reached at 12 days.

A multidisciplinary co-ordinated plan was agreed to address the above problems, and was modified as new problems appeared and others became inactive. At all stages, the patient was encouraged to be fully involved in the planning that incorporated rest periods to counteract the fatigue induced by interaction with many different professionals and the condition itself. Short-term realistic goals with functional significance were used to motivate the patient and provide structure to the problem-solving process. This approach enabled rehabilitation to continue throughout 24 h with the support of the nurses. Management of each of the problems is discussed below.

Generalised motor impairment
The motor impairment was the primary cause of problems 2, 6, 7 and 8. Where weakness was profound, especially at nadir, only passive movements were possible. Stretches were included to mobilise the nervous tissue, as well as the muscles and supportive tissues. The nurses and physiotherapist positioned the

patient to prevent shortening of muscles and relieve pressure areas, using wedges.

Together, the occupational therapist and physiotherapist made splints to support the feet in a plantigrade position and the hands in flexion at the metacarpophalangeal joints, with abduction of the thumb.

As muscle power began to recover, assisted active movements were performed by the physiotherapist with the patient. Encouragement was given to concentrate on the feeling of movement and join in as possible. Where an imbalance of returning muscle strength around a joint was identified, the physiotherapist encouraged the patient to relax the dominant group and facilitated the weaker group (see Ch. 30).

As soon as some recovery occurred in the trunk muscles (3 weeks after onset), while still ventilated, the patient worked on trunk control in sitting, to improve endurance in postural muscles and truncal alignment. Antigravity muscles were strengthened in standing, initially requiring two physiotherapists. Later, backslabs were used to support the lower limbs in extension. To supplement rehabilitation sessions, a regimen of low-resistance strengthening exercises for the elbow extensors, hip extensors/abductors and quadriceps muscles was used by the patient. Relatives were involved in helping the patient perform her exercises.

As trunk and pelvic control was gained, the emphasis shifted to improving lower-limb power and co-ordination. Knee control was refined standing at a table and then the patient progressed to practising control of the weight-bearing leg when stepping. Muscle strength was monitored using a hand-held

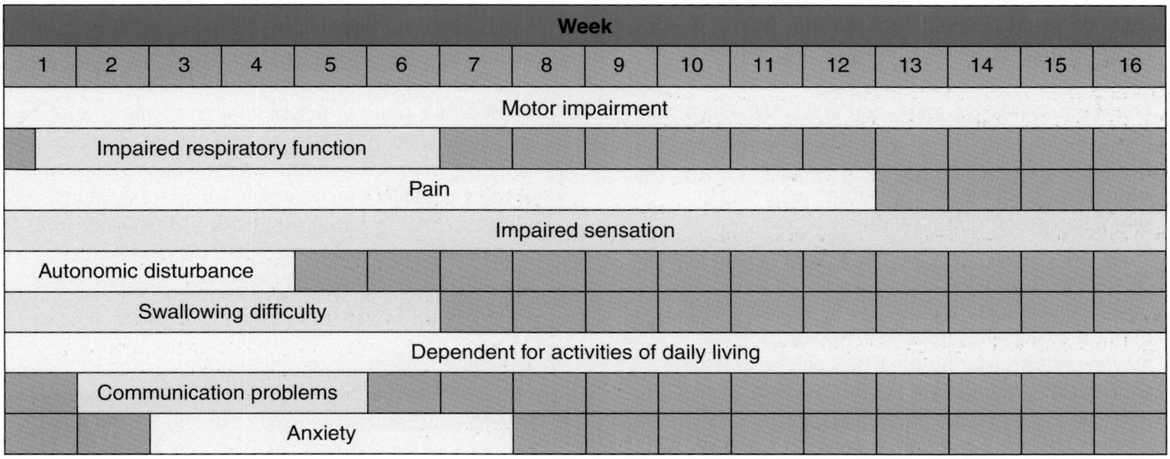

								Week								
1	2	3	4	5	6	7	8	9	10	11	12	13	14	15	16	
Motor impairment																
	Impaired respiratory function															
Pain																
Impaired sensation																
Autonomic disturbance																
	Swallowing difficulty															
Dependent for activities of daily living																
	Communication problems															
	Anxiety															

Figure 14.2 Time course of problems presenting in a patient with Guillain–Barré syndrome over a 16-week period. The case history of this patient is described in the text.

myometer. At the patient's weakest, recordings could be obtained only in the neck side flexors and right elbow pronators. Demonstrating objective strength improvements during the first 3 weeks, when the patient could not perform any activity, was encouraging for her.

Impaired respiratory function

Following admission, respiratory status was monitored regularly. Forced vital capacity (FVC) readings dropped rapidly because of respiratory muscle weakness, necessitating intubation and ventilation. Nurses and physiotherapists provided appropriate respiratory care, ensuring blood pressure was monitored when using suction. Ventilation was necessary for 4 weeks, after which the patient was gradually weaned off the ventilator.

Pain

Pain appeared as an early symptom. The physiotherapists and nurses positioned the patient to alleviate discomfort as far as possible, e.g. the 'frogging position' (legs flexed, abducted and laterally rotated over a pillow, taking care to avoid pressure to the common peroneal nerve; see Fig. 8.4, p. 136). Massage of affected muscles and large-amplitude passive movements gave temporary relief but medication was required, particularly at night. Later, increasing pain and the resulting disturbance to sleep limited more active physiotherapy. Treatment had to be co-ordinated with effective analgesia. Pain remained the limiting factor for rehabilitation during the acute phase.

Reduced distal sensation

Impaired sensation occurred in a glove–stocking distribution, and there was impairment of joint position sense below the knees. This reduction in sensation caused considerable difficulties with positioning the feet on initial standing and walking (10 weeks after onset). Air-cast splints were used to increase sensory input and mirrors provided visual feedback. Stairs were particularly difficult. Two weeks working on compensatory strategies enabled the patient to be safely discharged to her two-storey house.

Autonomic disturbance

Tachycardia and profound sweating occurred each time the patient was moved from lying to sitting (however slowly) during the first 3 weeks. Gradual adjustment to the upright position was one of the goals set by nurses and physiotherapists. Use of a reclining chair and a tilt table allowed graded movement into the upright position. At all times, blood pressure and cardiac trace were monitored.

Difficulty in swallowing (dysphagia)

Assessment by the speech and language therapist demonstrated a poor ability to swallow that placed the patient at risk of aspiration, therefore a nasogastric tube was inserted. Nurses and a dietician monitored her nutritional intake. Five weeks later, the patient was able to commence a soft diet under the guidance of the speech therapist. Concurrently, the physiotherapist worked with the patient on an effective cough to prevent aspiration.

Dependent for activities of daily living

The interaction of impairments led to dependency in all aspects of care. Throughout rehabilitation, functional goals were set. This allowed the patient to measure her improvement in terms of regaining useful activities rather than gradual improvement of an impairment. The patient's sudden loss of functional independence and dignity was handled sensitively by all team members. Wherever possible, remaining functional ability was maximised by assisting the patient rather than taking over the task, e.g. allowing time for the patient to initiate rolling and then assisting as directed by the patient.

Wheelchair assessment occurred whilst the patient was still being ventilated. This allowed the patient to regain a more normal view of the world as well as being an adjunct to coping with autonomic disturbance (see above). As some recovery began, the physiotherapist aimed to improve trunk control so that the patient had a stable base of support to perform activities of daily living. Once achieved, movements over the base of support were incorporated. Sitting to standing from a high plinth allowed work on pelvic and trunk control (essential for gait) and enabled the patient to transfer independently. The physiotherapist and occupational therapist worked together to improve posture and hand control to regain independence in feeding.

Independence in the wheelchair was achieved by week 8, as a result of better trunk and hand control. Backslabs were made to allow the patient to practise standing when knee control was still poor. Stepping became possible after 10 weeks but air-cast splints were essential to prevent inversion of the ankle. Gait re-education progressed over the next 4 weeks. Crutches were used initially, progressing to two sticks and finally one stick.

Inability to communicate effectively

Intubation and ventilation prevented speaking and increasing weakness hindered gesturing. At nadir, communication was only possible using eye blinks. At all times staff would make every effort to understand the patient and in turn spend time talking to her.

The speech therapist provided a communication aid, which was used for 5 weeks until bulbar muscles recovered.

Anxiety

The patient's anxiety increased the longer she remained on the ventilator. Close relatives also needed to be reassured about the prognosis. A visitor from the GBS Support Group with personal experience of GBS was helpful in allaying both the patient's and relatives' fears (see Appendix). Five weeks after onset, the patient started becoming agitated if her daily routine was disturbed. Maximum effort was made to adhere to a timetable drawn up with the patient.

At discharge

Sixteen weeks after admission most problems had resolved and the patient was discharged. The remaining problems were:

Impairments

1. weakness of specific muscle groups, e.g. the dorsiflexors bilaterally, right elbow extensors, left thenar eminence and the quadriceps

2. reduced proprioception below the knees, right worse than left.

Disabilities

3. requiring one stick and an air-cast splint on the right ankle to walk
4. requiring bath aids and grab rail (fitted in the home before discharge) to bathe independently.

The patient was discharged with a scheme of exercises to strengthen the major groups, which still fell below the normal range. A home exercise programme was drawn up with the patient to further her recovery. Arrangements were made for continuing physiotherapy in the community.

The problems encountered by this patient are typical of those in GBS, although the time scale can vary. The wide range, and constantly changing nature of the problems, highlights the need for an integrated and co-ordinated multidisciplinary intervention for the successful management of this syndrome.

References

Aitkens SG, McCory MA, Kilmer DD et al. Moderate resistance exercise program: its effect in slowly progressive neuromuscular disease. *Arch Phys Med Rehab* 1993, **74**:711–715.

Albers JW, Kelly JJ. Acquired inflammatory demyelinating polyneuropathies: clinical and electrodiagnostic features. *Muscle Nerve* 1989, **12**:435–451.

Asbury AK. Pain in generalised neuropathies. In: Fields HL, ed. *Pain Syndromes in Neurology*. London: Butterworth; 1990:131–141.

Asbury AK, Bird SJ. Disorders of peripheral nerve. In: Asbury AK, McKhann GM, McDonald IW, eds. *Diseases of the Nervous System: Clinical Neurobiology*, 2nd edn. Philadelphia: WB Saunders; 1992:252–269.

Asbury AK, Cornblath DR. Assessment of current diagnostic criteria for Guillain–Barré syndrome. *Ann Neurol* 1990, **27** (Suppl.):21–24.

Bennett RL, Knowlton GC. Overwork weakness in partially denervated skeletal muscle. *Clin Orthop* 1958, **12**:22–29.

Berlit P, Rakicky J. The Miller Fisher syndrome: review of the literature. *J Clin Neuro-Ophthalmol* 1992, **12**:57–63.

Bohannon RW, Dubuc WE. Documentation of the resolution of weakness in a patient with Guillain–Barré syndrome: a case report. *Phys Ther* 1984, **64**:1388–1389.

Butler DS. *Mobilisation of the Nervous System*. Melbourne: Churchill Livingstone; 1991.

Cook JD, Glass DS. Strength evaluation in neuromuscular disease. *Neurol Clin* 1987, **5**:101–123.

Cowan J, Greenwood R, Fletcher N. Disorders of peripheral nerve. In: Greenwood R, Barnes MP, McMillan TM et al., eds. *Neurological Rehabilitation*. Edinburgh: Churchill Livingstone; 1993:607–613.

Dalakas MC. Intravenous immunoglobulin in the treatment of autoimmune neuromuscular diseases: present status and practical therapeutic guidelines. *Muscle Nerve* 1999, **22**:1479–1497.

deJager AEJ, Minderhoud JM. Residual signs in severe Guillain–Barré syndrome. *J Neurol Sci* 1991, **104**:151–156.

Dellon AL. A numerical grading scale for peripheral nerve function. *J Hand Ther* 1993, **6**:152–160.

Dyck PJ, Thomas PK. *Peripheral Neuropathy*, 3rd edn. Philadelphia: WB Saunders; 1993.

Dyck PJ, Litchy WJ, Lehman KA et al. Variables influencing neuropathic endpoints. *Neurology* 1995, **45**:1115–1121.

Edwards S, Charlton P. Splinting and the use of orthoses in the management of patients with neurological disorders. In: Edwards S, ed. *Neurological Physiotherapy: A Problem Solving Approach*, 2nd edn. London: Churchill Livingstone; 2002:219–253.

Feasby TE. Inflammatory demyelinating polyneuropathies. In: Dyck PJ, ed. *Neurologic Clinics: Peripheral Neuropathy: New Concepts and Treatments*, Vol. 10. Philadelphia: WB Saunders; 1992.

Feasby TE. Axonal Guillain–Barré syndrome. *Muscle Nerve* 1994, **17**:678–679.

Fernhead L, Fritz VU. Guillain–Barré syndrome: rationale for physiotherapy management of the acute severe patient. *S Afr J Physiother* 1996, **52**:85–87.

Freeman J. Clinical notes of physiotherapy management of the patient with Guillain–Barré syndrome. *Synapse* 1992, April.

Geurts ACH, Mulder TW, Neinhuis B et al. Postural organisation in patients with hereditary motor and sensory neuropathy. *Arch Phys Med Rehab* 1992, **73**:569–572.

Hardie R, Harding AE, Hirsch N et al. Diaphragmatic weakness in hereditary motor and sensory neuropathy. *J Neurol Neurosurg Psychiatry* 1990, **53**:348–350.

Harding AE. *Hereditary Motor and Sensory Neuropathies (HMSN)*. London: Muscular Dystrophy Group of Great Britain and Northern Ireland; 1993.

Harding AE. From the syndrome of Charcot, Marie and Tooth to disorders of peripheral myelin proteins. *Brain* 1995, **118**:809–818.

Hartung HP, Pollard JD, Harvey GK. Immunopathogenesis and treatment of the Guillain–Barré syndrome. Part II. *Muscle Nerve* 1995, **18**:154–164.

Hopkins A. *Clinical Neurology: A Modern Approach*. Oxford: Oxford University Press; 1993.

Karni Y, Archdeacon L, Mills KR et al. Clinical assessment and physiotherapy in Guillain–Barré syndrome. *Physiotherapy* 1984, **70**:288–292.

Kilmer DD, McCory MA, Wright NC et al. The effect of a high resistance exercise program in slowly progressive neuromuscular disease. *Arch Phys Med Rehab* 1994, **75**:560–563.

Lennon SM, Ashburn A. Use of myometry in the assessment of neuropathic weakness: testing for reliability in clinical practice. *Clin Rehab* 1993, **7**:125–133.

Lindeman E, Leffers P, Spaans F et al. Strength training in patients with myotonic dystrophy and hereditary motor and sensory neuropathy: a randomised clinical trial. *Arch Phys Med Rehab* 1995, **76**:612–620.

Mann RA, Missirian J. Pathophysiology of Charcot–Marie–Tooth disease. *Clin Orthop* 1988, **234**:221–228.

Mays ML. Incorporating continuous passive motion in the rehabilitation of a patient with Guillain–Barré syndrome. *Am J Occup Ther* 1990, **44**:750–753.

McClure J. The role of physiotherapy in HIV and AIDS. *Physiotherapy* 1993, **79**:388–393.

McLeod JG. Autonomic dysfunction in peripheral nerve disease. In: Bannister R, Mathias C, eds. *Autonomic Failure*, 3rd edn. Oxford: Oxford Medical Publications; 1992:659–681.

Merkies IS, Schmitz PI, Samijn JP et al. Fatigue in immune-mediated polyneuropathies. *Neurology* 1999, **53**:1648–1654.

Milner-Brown HS, Miller RG. Muscle strengthening through high-resistance weight training in patients with neuromuscular disorders. *Arch Phys Med Rehab* 1988, **69**:14–19.

Mitchell S. Neuropathies. *Rev Clin Gerontol* 1991, **1**:347–357.

Monforte R, Estruch R, Valls-Sole J et al. Autonomic and peripheral neuropathies in patients with chronic alcoholism. *Arch Neurol* 1995, **52**:45–51.

Moxley RT. Functional testing. *Muscle Nerve* 1990, **13**:26–29.

Mueller MJ, Minor SD, Sahrmann SA et al. Difference in gait characteristics of patients with diabetes and peripheral neuropathy compared with age-matched controls. *Phys Ther* 1994, **74**:299–308.

Munsat TL. Clinical trials in neuromuscular disease. *Muscle Nerve* 1990, **13**:3–6.

Ng KPP, Howard RS, Fish DR et al. Management and outcome of severe Guillain–Barré syndrome. *Q J Med* 1995, **88**:243–250.

Northern A (ed.). *Charcot–Marie–Tooth Disease: A Practical Guide*. Dorset: CMT International; 2000.

Pentland B, Donald SM. Pain in Guillain–Barré syndrome: a clinical review. *Pain* 1994, **59**:159–164.

Pirart J. Diabetes mellitus and its degenerative complications: a prospective study of 4400 patients observed between 1947 and 1973. *Diabetes Care* 1978, **1**:168–188.

Pitetti KH, Barrett PJ, Abbas D. Endurance exercise training in Guillain–Barré syndrome. *Arch Phys Med Rehab* 1993, **74**:761–765.

Pope PM. Postural management and special seating. In: Edwards S, ed. *Neurological Physiotherapy: A Problem Solving Approach*, 2nd edn. London: Churchill Livingstone; 2002:189–217.

Ropper AH. The Guillain–Barré syndrome. *N Engl J Med* 1992, **326**:1130–1136.

Ropper AH, Wijdicks EFM, Truax BT. *Guillain–Barré Syndrome*. Philadelphia: FA Davis; 1991.

Ruhland JL, Shields RK. The effects of a home exercise program on impairment and health-related quality of life in persons with chronic peripheral neuropathies. *Phys Ther* 1997, **77**:1026–1039.

Schaumburg HH, Berger AR, Thomas PK. *Disorders of Peripheral Nerves*, 2nd edn. Philadelphia: FA Davis; 1992.

Simionato R, Stiller K, Butler D. Neural tension signs in Guillain–Barré syndrome: two case reports. *Aust J Physiother* 1988, **34**:257–259.

Simpson DM, Olney RK. Peripheral neuropathies associated with human immunodeficiency virus infection. In: Dyck PJ, ed. *Neurologic Clinics: Peripheral Neuropathy: New Concepts and Treatments*, Vol. 10. Philadelphia: WB Saunders; 1992:685–711.

Sinacore DR. Severe sensory neuropathy need not precede Charcot arthropathies of the foot or ankle: implications for the rehabilitation specialist. *Physiother Theory Pract* 2001, **17**:39–50.

Smith M, Ball V. *Cardiovascular/Respiratory Physiotherapy*. London: Mosby; 1998.

Soryal I, Sinclair E, Hornby J et al. Impaired joint mobility in Guillain–Barré syndrome: a primary or a secondary phenomenon? *J Neurol Neurosurg Psychiatry* 1992, **55**:1014–1017.

Sridharan GV, Tallis RC, Gautam PC. Guillain–Barré syndrome in the elderly. *Gerontology* 1993, **39**:170–175.

Thomas PK, Thomlinson DR. Diabetic and hypoglycaemic neuropathy. In: Dyck PJ, Thomas PK, eds. *Peripheral Neuropathy*, 3rd edn. Philadelphia: WB Saunders; 1993:1219–1250.

Thompson PD, Day BL. The anatomy and physiology of cerebellar disease. *Adv Neurol* 1993, **61**:15–30.

van de Ploeg RJO, Fidler V, Oosterhuis HJGH. Handheld myometry: reference values. *J Neurol Neurosurg Psychiatry* 1991, **54**:244–247.

van-Doom PA. Intravenous immunoglobulin treatment in patients with chronic inflammatory demyelinating polyneuropathy. *J Neurol Neurosurg Psychiatry* 1994, **57** (Suppl.):38–42.

Visser LH, Van-der-Meche FG, Van-doorn PA et al. Guillain–Barré syndrome without sensory loss (acute motor neuropathy): a sub group with specific clinical diagnostic and laboratory features. *Brain* 1995, **118**:841–847.

Watson GR, Wilson FM. Guillain–Barré syndrome: an update. *NZ J Physiother* 1989, **17**:17–24.

Wiles CM, Karni Y, Nicklin J. Laboratory testing of muscle function in the management of neuromuscular disease. *J Neurol Neurosurg Psychiatry* 1990, **53**:384–387.

Windebank AJ. Polyneuropathy due to nutritional deficit and alcoholism. In: Dyck PJ, Thomas PK, eds. *Peripheral Neuropathy*, 3rd edn. Philadelphia: WB Saunders; 1993:1310–1321.

Winer JB, Hughes RAC, Osmond C. A prospective study of acute idiopathic neuropathy, clinical features and their prognostic value. *J Neurol Neurosurg Psychiatry* 1988, **51**:605–612.

Chapter 15

Disorders of muscle and post–polio syndrome

R Quinlivan   N Thompson

INTRODUCTION

Muscle diseases include a number of rare, often progressive conditions leading to physical disability and frequently reduced life expectancy. Individual disorders tend to present at around the same age, although there may be a wide range. Those conditions which present in childhood are discussed in Chapter 20, but increased life expectancy due to improved care means that a greater number of patients are presenting for physiotherapy as young adults, while knowledge of these conditions tends to be poor outside the specialist area of paediatric physiotherapy. This chapter describes some muscle disorders presenting in adulthood and an overview of the disorders is given so that the physiotherapist is aware of the different diagnoses, since these can influence overall management. For a comprehensive text on muscle disorders the reader is referred to Karpati et al. (2001).

The principles of physical management of muscle disorders are discussed in general in this chapter and in more detail in Chapter 20. This arrangement is to avoid repetition and to show the continuum of management from childhood to adulthood. Where special consideration is required for a particular disorder, due to specific clinical features, these are discussed where relevant in both chapters.

CLASSIFICATION AND DIAGNOSTIC INVESTIGATIONS

Muscle disorders are inherited or acquired and include a wide range of rare conditions, which can be classified according to the site of the defect in the motor unit (Table 15.1). Since the 1980s tremendous advances in genetics and molecular biology have enhanced our understanding of the pathogenesis of these disorders.

Table 15.1 Classification of neuromuscular diseases according to the site of defect in the motor unit

Site of defect	Diagnosis
Anterior horn cell	Spinal muscular atrophy (SMA) (proximal and distal)
	Poliomyelitis
	Motor neurone disease[a]
Nerve fibre	Peroneal muscular atrophies (CMT)
	Inflammatory polyradiculo-neuropathies (AIDP, CIDP)
	Toxic neuropathy (e.g. organophosphates, mercury)
	Metabolic neuropathy (e.g. metachromatic leucodystrophy, Refsum's disease)
Neuromuscular junction	Myasthenia gravis
	Congenital myasthenic syndromes
	Lambert–Eaton syndrome
	Botulism
Muscle fibre	Muscular dystrophies
	Congenital myopathies, e.g. central core disease
	Collagen disorders (Bethlem myopathy)
	Mitochondrial myopathies
	Glycogen storage diseases affecting muscle (e.g. acid maltase deficiency, McArdle's disease)
	Disorders of lipid metabolism and fatty acid
	Oxidation (carnitine and CPT11 deficiencies, LCAD and VLCAD)
	Inflammatory myopathies (polymyositis, dermatomyositis and inclusion body myositis)
	Endocrine myopathies (thyroid dysfunction and hyperparathyroidism)
	Muscle channelopathies (e.g. sodium channel and muscle chloride channel diseases)

[a] Motor neurone disease involves not only the motor unit but also upper motoneurones (see Ch. 13).
CMT, Charcot–Marie–Tooth; AIDP, acute inflammatory demyelinating polyradiculopathy; CIDP, chronic inflammatory demyelinating polyradiculopathy; CPT11, carnitine palmitoyl transferase type 11 deficiency; LCAD, long-chain acyl-CoA dehydrogenase deficiency; VLCAD, very-long-chain acyl-CoA dehydrogenase deficiency.

Table 15.2 Classification of the limb girdle and sex-linked muscular dystrophies in relation to the genetic defect

Type	Gene locus	Gene product
Autosomal dominant		
LGMD1A	5q22–q34	Myotilin
LGMD1B	1q11–21	Lamin A/C
ADEDMD		
LGMD1C	3p25	Caveolin 3
Autosomal recessive		
LGMD2A	15q15.1–q21.1	Calpain 3
LGMD2B	2p13	Dysferlin
LGMD2C	13q12	γ Sarcoglycan
LGMD2D	17q21	α Sarcoglycan
LGMD2E	4q12	β Sarcoglycan
LGMD2F	5q33–q34	δ sarcoglycan
LGMD2G	17q11–12	Telethonin
LGMD2H	9q31–34.1	Not yet known
LGMD2I	19q13.3	FKRP
LGMD2J	2q31	Titin
Sex-linked		
Dystrophinopathy (DMD, BMD)	Xp21	Dystrophin
EDMD	Xq28	Emerin

LGMD, limb girdle muscular dystrophy; ADEDMD, autosomal dominant Emery Dreifuss muscular dystrophy; DMD, Duchenne muscular dystrophy; BMD, Becker muscular dystrophy; EDMD, Emery Dreifuss muscular dystrophy.

The availability of genetic testing for many conditions has broadened our concept of the classical phenotype of many disorders to include milder, even subclinical presentations. Becker muscular dystrophy (BMD) is a good example, whereby the disorder can result in loss of mobility as early as 16 years of age or as late as the sixth decade (Bradley et al., 1978), and the same condition can also present with exertional cramps and myoglobinuria (Gospe et al., 1989).

The limb girdle muscular dystrophies (LGMD) are a diverse group of disorders classified according to age of onset, mode of inheritance and genetic defect, as shown in Table 15.2.

The classification of congenital muscular dystrophies (CMD), based on clinical and/or pathological features, is also expanding as a consequence of genetic and molecular advances. Other conditions included within this diagnostic category of congenital disorders are the congenital myopathies, myotonic disorders, hereditary peripheral neuropathies (Charcot–Marie–Tooth), spinal muscular atrophies (SMA), mitochondrial and metabolic

myopathies, as well as disorders affecting the neuro-muscular junction, which can be inherited or acquired. Despite many advances in the field, a definitive diagnosis will still be lacking for some individuals other than the finding of clinical and pathological features of a myopathy or neuropathy.

Acquired neuromuscular disorders are more common in adults than children. Polymyositis and dermatomyositis are inflammatory conditions presenting with weakness and pain. The onset is either acute or subacute and may be precipitated by infections in children or malignancy in adults. Myasthenia gravis is an autoimmune disorder presenting in adults or older children, frequently associated with a thymoma (a benign enlargement of the thymus); there may be a history of diplopia (double vision), ptosis (droopy eyelids), bulbar symptoms and weakness precipitated by repetitive tasks. In adults, endocrine disorders, especially hypothyroidism, can present as a myopathy.

The history will most often elicit muscle weakness which is predominantly axial, proximal, distal or global, depending on the disorder. Exercise-induced myalgia is more likely to be the presenting complaint of a metabolic or mitochondrial myopathy. Sometimes the development of a systemic complication, such as early-onset cataracts, cardiac rhythm disorder or dilated cardiomyopathy, is the presenting feature of a muscle disorder. Examination may demonstrate muscle hypertrophy or atrophy (wasting) and nearly always elicits muscle weakness. Some disorders, such as Bethlem myopathy, may present with more prominent joint contractures than weakness.

Respiratory muscle involvement does not necessarily correlate with the severity of skeletal weakness and it is, therefore, essential that all patients with neuromuscular disorders are monitored regularly for forced vial capacity (FVC: Griggs & Donohue, 1985; Hough, 1991). Symptoms of incipient respiratory failure include recurrent chest infections, weight loss, early-morning headaches, sweating, disturbed nights and day-time somnolence. A sleep study will confirm nocturnal hypoventilation and non-invasive respiratory support can be life-saving.

Diagnostic investigations include the serum concentration of creatine kinase (CK). This enzyme is the most reliable biochemical indicator of muscle disease; however, in many muscle disorders the CK level will be normal. Where appropriate, biochemical analysis for metabolic disorders will include lactate, carnitine and acyl carnitine levels together with exercise testing. Electromyography (EMG) and nerve conduction studies may be useful in some cases but this is by no means universal. Muscle biopsy is the definitive diagnostic test for most of the muscular dystrophies and myopathies.

In many cases, however, a blood test to undertake DNA analysis is sufficient to confirm a diagnosis (Mastaglia & Laing, 1996). A good example is the demyelinating form of Charcot–Marie–Tooth disease (CMT1a), in which 75% of patients will possess a duplication in the PMP22 gene on chromosome 17q (Ionasesco, 1995).

PRINCIPLES OF MANAGEMENT

A great deal of research is being targeted towards finding a means of replacing or repairing the abnormal protein so as to develop effective new treatments. Those individuals with fewer secondary complications of their disorder (e.g. contractures and spinal deformity) will almost certainly derive the greatest benefit from such treatment when it becomes available.

The management of patients with neuromuscular disease is based upon the recognition of the patient's specific needs, together with monitoring for other complications of the disorder, e.g. 24-h cardiac monitoring in Emery Dreifuss muscular dystrophy (EDMD) and respiratory monitoring in rigid spine syndrome (RSSI). Recently, steroids have been shown to improve muscle power in Duchenne muscular dystrophy (DMD), thus prolonging independent walking (Dubowitz, 2000).

Generally, an approach to managing the family rather than the individual is an important factor which influences an integrated multidisciplinary and multispecialty approach (medical rehabilitation, neurology, clinical genetics, physiotherapy, paediatrics, orthopaedics, dietetics, orthotics). Close liaison with community therapists to provide care, support and adaptations to school and home is an essential element in enabling independence and quality of life for the patient and family.

MUSCLE DISORDERS AND THEIR CLINICAL FEATURES

A small selection of disorders, which predominantly manifest in adulthood, are discussed here and some of those which present in childhood are discussed in Chapter 20. Although this is a fairly arbitrary differentiation, many childhood myopathies present in young adulthood and vice versa, and increasing numbers of affected children survive into adulthood.

Fascioscapulohumeral muscular dystrophy (FSH)

This condition follows an autosomal dominant pattern of inheritance with a high degree of penetrance but variable expression. The clinical features are always present by 30 years of age. As many as 30% of cases present sporadically and are due to germ line

271

quence of their abnormal bulbar function. Several drugs, such as phenytoin, can be used to relieve the myotonia, although in practice the side-effects often outweigh any benefit (see Ch. 28, p. 471).

Muscle sodium channel and muscle chloride channel diseases

The muscle channelopathies comprise two groups of disorders – those where the muscle is hyperexcitable,

often lead to a precise diagnosis.

Dilated cardiomyopathy is a relatively frequent complication of the LGMDs: routine ECG and, where appropriate, echocardiogram (ECHO) are recommended. In autosomal dominant Emery Dreifuss muscular dystrophy (ADEDMD, allelic to LGMD1B), cardiac conduction block requiring a pacemaker is almost universal by the third decade and can be life-saving. Respiratory failure from diaphragmatic weakness, leading to sleep hypoventilation syndrome, occurs in most

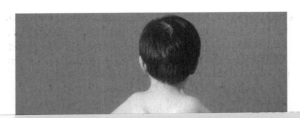

progress to loss of ambulation, which occurs in approximately 20% of cases. Joint contractures are rare and mild.

Cardiac involvement is uncommon and reported to occur in about 5% of cases; atrial arrhythmias are the most usual manifestation (Laforet et al., 1998). Sometimes the severe facial weakness may be mistaken for Moebius syndrome (Miura et al., 1998). The serum CK

of the muscular dystrophies and must be screened for regularly. Generally, if the FVC is less than 50% of that expected for height, or if there is a greater than 20% drop in FVC when the patient lies flat, sleep hypoventilation should be suspected and a sleep study should be arranged. Treatment with non-invasive mask ventilation is highly effective in alleviating symptoms. Scoliosis may occur in adolescents, necessitating spinal fusion. While skeletal contractures can occur in all patients once they become wheelchair-dependent, they are a particular problem in ambulant ADEDMD and calpain-deficient muscular dystrophy (LGMD2A). Severe lower-limb contractures may compromise mobility.

General management

As with other disabling neuromuscular diseases, patients with LGMD need help and support to adapt their environment to suit their needs. A self-raising chair or pneumatic cushion can be invaluable in assisting rising to standing. Adaptations to the patient's home may be required to ensure appropriate bathroom facilities, hoists or stair lifts. Adaptations to the patient's vehicle may also be required to maintain independence. Weight gain can be a major problem for some individuals, especially when they are confined to a wheelchair, and may compromise respiration. Encouraging exercise is important for general health and wellbeing; swimming is an excellent example which also helps maintain strength and reduce contractures (see Chs 25 and 29). Many patients appreciate the benefit of regular passive stretching exercises and the opportunity to stand using either a tilt table or standing frame. Prevention of chest infections with pneumococcal vaccination and yearly flu vaccines is important for any patient with evidence of respiratory muscle weakness.

Mitochondrial myopathies

These are rare myopathies with a wide range of clinical presentation, from extraocular weakness to severe fatal infantile encephalomyopathies (see Mastaglia & Laing, 1996, for classification of types). This diverse group of disorders may be confined to the muscles, causing weakness or myalgia, or may present with a variety of neurological and multisystem disorders, e.g. dementia, convulsions, ataxia, stroke-like episodes, extrapyramidal syndromes, deafness and peripheral neuropathy. Muscle biopsy reveals an absence of cytochrome oxidase activity, reduced respiratory chain enzyme levels or ragged red fibres seen on a trichrome stain, caused by an accumulation of mitochondria at the periphery of the muscle fibres.

The onset can occur at any age and the management will depend on the presenting symptoms and their severity. Riboflavin and coenzyme Q10 have been reported to help anecdotally, although there are no large-scale controlled studies because of the rarity of these disorders.

Glycogen storage diseases

The glycogen storage diseases (GSDs) are characterised by abnormal glycogen metabolism.

Acid maltase deficiency

Acid maltase deficiency (GSD11) is, in fact, a lysosomal storage disorder. The condition can present in infancy as Pompes disease with a severe phenotype, resulting in progressive muscle weakness and cardiomyopathy. Death usually occurs by 2 years of age from cardiac and respiratory failure. Clinical trials are in progress using a genetically modified enzyme replacement, genzyme, but the results are yet to be published; however, early reports are encouraging (Di Mauro et al., 1997). Less severe forms of GSD11 present during childhood (juvenile-onset) and adulthood. The condition is milder with a slower progression, causing limb girdle weakness, which closely resembles LGMD or mild SMA. Respiratory failure due to both diaphragmatic involvement and cardiomyopathy occurs and can be disproportionate to the skeletal weakness. Regular cardiorespiratory monitoring is therefore recommended.

McArdle's disease

McArdle's disease (glycogen storage disorder type V; GSDV) is caused by a deficiency of the enzyme muscle phosphorylase, resulting in impaired utilisation of muscle glucose during anaerobic exercise. Muscle pain and fatigue occurring early during exercise are the cardinal symptoms. Often the patient will describe a second wind, whereby muscle pain occurs within the first few minutes of exercise, but when the patient slows down or stops, pain-free exercise can be resumed. This phenomenon is probably due to a switch from glycolytic metabolism to aerobic oxidative phosphorylation.

If exercise is continued despite pain, an electrically silent contracture occurs where the muscle seizes and later becomes swollen. This is followed by myoglobinuria, a dark red/brown or black discoloration of the urine caused by rhabdomyolysis (muscle damage), which, if severe, can cause acute renal failure.

The serum CK is invariably raised at rest and there is a lack of rise in venous lactate during an ischaemic forearm exercise test. Muscle biopsy demonstrates a subsarcolemmal accumulation of glycogen and absent

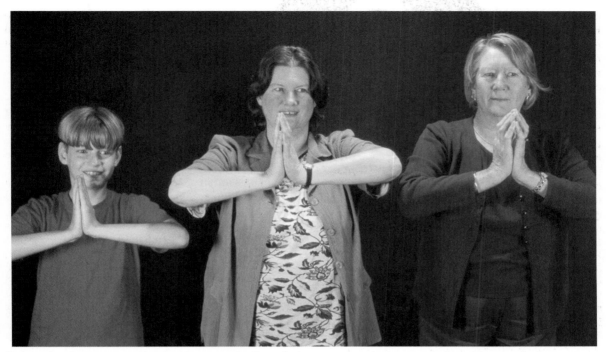

Figure 15.2   Bethlem myopathy: note the progressive finger flexion contractures in three generations of the same family.

muscle phosphorylase activity. The condition is caused by mutations in the muscle phosphorylase gene on chromosome 11q13 (Beynon et al., 2002). Strenuous anaerobic exercise should be avoided to prevent muscle damage; however, regular gentle aerobic exercise is recommended, to upregulate fatty acid oxidation, thus conditioning the muscles and improving performance.

Bethlem myopathy

This autosomal dominant condition is caused by a defect in the alpha 1 and 2 subunits of collagen VI. Mutations affecting COL6A1 or COL6A2 on chromosome 21q22.3, or COL6A3 on chromosome 2q37, have been described in a small number of families (Jobsis et al., 1999). The condition is probably relatively common. The clinical presentation includes a neonatal presentation with joint contractures, torticollis, congenital hip dislocation and hypotonia with motor delay, or prominent joint contractures and muscle weakness presenting in late childhood or adulthood.

Muscle weakness preferentially affects the extensor muscles. Prominent flexion contractures of the elbows, wrists, knees and ankles are relatively common. Progressive flexion contractures affecting the distal interphalangeal joints of the last four fingers are a characteristic feature (Fig. 15.2). Muscle weakness is slowly progressive, with about one-half of the patients

losing ambulation in the fifth and sixth decades. Cardiac complications do not seem to occur but there are reports of diaphragmatic weakness necessitating non-invasive respiratory support.

The CK may be normal, mildly or moderately elevated (up to 10 times normal). Muscle biopsy may show only mild, non-specific changes or can even look dystrophic. In older patients, the muscle biopsy may show reduced labelling of beta 1 laminin; however, collagen VI staining will appear normal.

It is important to exclude mutations in the lamin A/C gene responsible for ADEDMD, as part of the differential diagnosis. Management is aimed at reducing or preventing contractures.

Myasthenia gravis

Myasthenia gravis is a condition affecting acetylcholinesterase receptors at the neuromuscular junction. The disorder can be inherited (in young children) or acquired (in adolescents and adults). The condition causes muscle fatiguability so that the symptoms are variable and often more noticeable towards the end of the day. Patients may experience ptosis and ophthalmoplegia (squint), which often results in double vision. There may be bulbar symptoms with a weak voice, stridor and swallowing difficulty, and there may be proximal muscle weakness. The acquired form of the condition is caused by the development of antibodies to the acetylcholinesterase receptors and is more common in women than men. An abnormal response to repetitive nerve stimulation is seen in 60% of patients; single-fibre EMG shows increased jitter in almost all cases (Sanders, 2002). A tensilon test confirms the diagnosis; edrophonium, an anticholinesterase drug, is injected intravenously and an almost immediate improvement in the patient's signs is demonstrated, which lasts for a few minutes. Other investigations include acetylcholinesterase antibodies, which are frequently elevated in young adults; a chest X-ray and computed tomographic scan of the chest should be undertaken to exclude a thymoma. Treatment involves oral anticholinesterase drugs to alleviate the symptoms, together with steroids, immunosuppresssion and thymectomy.

Inflammatory myopathies

Inflammatory myopathies can be divided into three distinct groups:

- dermatomyositis (DM)
- polymyositis (PM)
- inclusion body myositis (IBM).

DM and PM have an autoimmune etiology, while IBM does not always respond to steroids and may be hereditary in some cases (see Dalakas, 1995, for a fuller text).

DM is an inflammatory muscle condition associated with a characteristic facial rash occurring around the eyes (heliotrope rash). The condition affects children between the ages of 5 and 15 years. A second peak in incidence occurs in middle and old age, and is frequently associated with an underlying malignancy (Callen, 1988). The disease is characterised by muscle pain and proximal weakness. Joint contractures can develop rapidly. The serum CK and erythrocyte sedimentation rate may be elevated, and a muscle biopsy confirms the inflammatory process. Treatment includes immune suppression and physiotherapy to minimise contractures.

PM presents with subacute proximal weakness, without myalgia and rash. The condition may occur as part of a more generalised autoimmune connective tissue disease and can also be precipitated by some drugs, including penicillamine and zidovudine (AZT). Muscle biopsy confirms an inflammatory myopathy and patients respond to steroids and immune suppression.

Inclusion body myositis occurs more commonly in males than females and tends to occur over the age of 50. IBM should be suspected when a patient with an inflammatory myopathy fails to respond to steroids. Unlike DM and PM, there may be facial weakness and there is frequently distal weakness, especially of the finger flexors and foot extensors, in addition to proximal weakness. About 20% of cases will be associated with an underlying autoimmune connective tissue disorder.

Endocrine myopathies

Muscle weakness and myalgia may be the presenting complaints of an underlying endocrinopathy, especially hypothyroidism and hyperparathyroidism. Confirming the diagnosis is most gratifying because hormone replacement or correction of the metabolic abnormalities will result in resolution of the symptoms.

Post-polio syndrome

Poliomyelitis epidemics came to a dramatic end in most countries with the introduction of the Salk polio vaccination in 1955, although acute polio remains a threat in many parts of the Third World. Recent research shows that over one-half of the survivors of paralytic polio experience new health problems related to their original illness (Windebank et al., 1995).

In the acute stage of infection, the poliovirus attacks the motor neurones in the spinal cord and brainstem nuclei. In most cases the disease remains subclinical. In other instances the disease leads to weakness or paralysis, depending on the number and distribution of motor neurones affected and the number of nerve cells that survive viral attack. After the initial illness, muscle strength may partially recover as a result of several physiological adaptive mechanisms, including terminal sprouting and reinnervation, myofibre hypertrophy and possibly myofibre-type transformation.

Survivors of polio who have exhibited stable, permanent impairments and loss of function begin to experience an onset of new neuromuscular problems around 30 years after acute polio. The most prevalent of these new complaints are:

- weakness
- fatigue
- muscle or joint pain
- functional loss, particularly related to walking and stair climbing.

Since there is little objective research data to indicate progressive atrophy or a rapid decline in strength, the term 'post-polio syndrome' (PPS) best describes the complaints and findings of polio survivors. It is essentially a diagnosis by exclusion and Halstead & Rossi (1987) provide a definition based on five criteria:

1. a confirmed history of paralytic polio
2. partial to fairly complete neurological and functional recovery

3. a period of neurological and functional stability of at least 15 years' duration
4. the onset of two or more of the following health problems since achieving a period of stability: unaccustomed fatigue, muscle and/or joint pain, new weakness in muscles previously affected and/or unaffected, functional loss, cold intolerance, new atrophy
5. no other medical diagnosis to explain these health problems.

There are a number of hypotheses concerning the possible causes of these muscle changes. Among the suggested causes are: premature ageing of motor neurones damaged by the poliovirus; premature ageing of the motor neurones due to increased metabolic demand; loss of muscle fibres within the surviving motor units; death of motor neurones due to the ageing process; disuse weakness; overuse weakness; or weight gain (Agre et al., 1991). The physical management of PPS is discussed below.

PHYSICAL MANAGEMENT OF NEURO-MUSCULAR DISORDERS

Physical management is aimed at preventing deformity from contractures, respiratory complications and pressure sores, as well as maintaining function and mobility for as long as possible. Assessment is not required as regularly in adults as it is in children, but contact should be maintained with a physiotherapist and care team.

Key points

Aims of physical management of muscle disorders are to:

- Maintain/improve muscle strength
- Prevent deformity from contractures
- Maintain function and mobility for as long as possible
- Prevent respiratory complications
- Prevent pressure sores

Management depends on the presenting signs and symptoms as well as the prognosis. A multidisciplinary problem-solving approach is preferable, with the patient being actively involved in goal-setting and decision-making (see Ch. 22).

To avoid repetition, the principles of physical management are discussed in Chapter 20. Specific aspects of management in FSH, myotonic syndromes and PPS are discussed below.

Fascioscapulohumeral dystrophy

Clinically, fatigue and/or muscle pain may be seen in patients with FSH and concerns have been raised whether exercise may cause overwork weakness. There is, however, no evidence to support this, and indeed strength has been shown to improve with high-resistance training in muscles that are not already severely weak (Milner Brown & Miller, 1988). Similar benefits have been reported for other neurological disorders (Ch. 29).

Postoperative management after scapular fixation requires the shoulder to be managed in a shoulder spica, with the arm abducted in the salute position, for 2–3 months. Isometric deltoid exercises should be encouraged with the spica cast in place. The likely occurrence of some muscle atrophy from disuse during the period of immobilisation, over and above any dystrophic process, implies that those with mild to moderate, rather than severe, weakness are more likely to benefit from surgical intervention. All parties need to be clear that the patient will be able to cope with this both practically and psychologically. Bunch & Siegel (1993) reported one patient who was so self-conscious in the shoulder spica he refused to leave his home and subsequently lost the ability to climb the stairs due to exacerbation of lower-limb weakness.

Despite the name given to this condition, it is important not to overlook trunk and lower-extremity involvement. Pelvic girdle weakness, and specifically hip extensor weakness, may give rise to a compensatory lordosis. This is sometimes so severe that the sacrum assumes a horizontal plane and it can lead to back pain and spondylosis that may jeopardise the patient's ambulatory status. Targetting strengthening exercises to the hip and trunk extensors should be considered before this stage is reached. A flexible spinal support may relieve the back symptoms without destroying the necessary functional lordosis, although the two are difficult to reconcile. The therapist should be vigilant for the development of hip flexor contractures which would exacerbate the problem.

Myotonic syndromes

Prevention of contractures due to muscle weakness is managed as in other muscle disorders (see Chs 20 and 25). In myotonic dystrophy there is evidence to suggest that patients can benefit from muscle strengthening and aerobic training (Lindeman et al., 1995; Tollback et al., 1999). However, the beneficial effects may be limited by other manifestations of the disease, such as cardiac problems, reduced respiratory volume, short attention span, memory loss and particularly poor motivation.

The myotonia, which is less of a problem than weakness, can be overcome by utilising the 'warm-up' effect (Cooper et al., 1988). Prior to an activity, the patient contracts the muscles several times, so that relaxation in between the contractions becomes faster and the contractions themselves become stronger. This enables the activity to be carried out more effectively. Examples include strategies which patients may have worked out for themselves, such as chewing gum before an interview so that speech is fluent, arm exercises prior to playing golf, or opening and closing the fist prior to a handshake. Appropriate strategies could be worked out for different functional activities.

Post-polio syndrome

Since the pathophysiology of PPS remains unclear, there has been controversy about the management of weakness. A review of the literature indicates that, overall, patients can improve both muscle strength and cardiovascular endurance from a well-planned training programme. There appear to be positive benefits, regardless of whether the muscle group is with or without new weakness but the programme must be tailored to the individual to avoid problems of overuse or excessive fatigue (Carrington-Gawne & Halstead, 1995).

An isometric programme is of benefit in those who have less than antigravity strength or a painful joint. An isotonic programme is more appropriate for a home exercise programme for a non-painful joint with greater than antigravity strength. An isokinetic programme can be used when equipment is available and the muscles have greater than antigravity strength.

Secondary symptoms, such as generalised fatigue, may be reduced as cardiovascular fitness improves. An ideal cardiovascular programme should exercise the muscles least affected by polio in order to maximise the cardiovascular benefits. This may mean, for example, a more strenuous programme for the arms if the legs are more involved. The role of physical activity in the management of neurological disorders is discussed in Chapter 29 and other strategies are illustrated in the case history below.

CASE HISTORY: POST-POLIO SYNDROME

PB is a 53-year-old man who was diagnosed with paralytic poliomyelitis at the age of 5 months. He was left with residual weakness of the lower limbs, right > left, and since childhood has been a limited independent community ambulator wearing a right knee–ankle–foot orthosis (KAFO).

Presenting history

Over the previous 3 years he had become concerned by increasing weakness of the left leg with instability of the

left knee. When walking he had to brace the left knee with the left hand to prevent its collapse into flexion and could walk only short distances with difficulty. He tired easily and had difficulty keeping up with the demands of his job as a senior manager in a large company.

Problems identified on examination

He was seen by a consultant orthopaedic surgeon for an opinion on his deteriorating walking ability. Investigations included a magnetic resonance imaging (MRI) scan of the spine, which ruled out spinal stenosis. He was diagnosed with PPS and referred to the physiotherapy department for advice on management.

On clinical examination PB had marked weakness and wasting of both legs and a leg-length discrepancy of 3 cm, the right leg being the shorter. Grades of muscle strength on the Medical Research Council (MRC) scale were as follows:

- Pelvic girdle strength was generally grade 2 but only grade 1 in the hip abductors.
- There was severe weakness of both quadriceps, with a flicker of activity on the right side (grade 1) but complete paralysis (grade 0) on the left.
- The left hamstrings were strong at grade 4, but were grade 0 on the right.
- Ankle dorsiflexors were grade 2 bilaterally.
- Ankle plantarflexors were stronger on the left (grade 3) than the right (grade 2).

There were no fixed hip flexion contractures but the hips were windswept, with excessive external rotation of the left hip and excessive internal rotation of the right hip. PB had a 20° fixed flexion contracture of the left knee and 15° fixed equinus of the left ankle.

Sagittal and coronal video analysis when walking with the right KAFO revealed:

1. an anterior pelvic tilt and forward trunk lean in stance, as a result of hip extensor weakness and also having to brace the left knee with the left hand
2. increased range of pelvic obliquity and rotation to aid forward progression, due to weakness of the pelvic girdle
3. increased left hip abduction and external rotation throughout the gait cycle to aid clearance of this longer leg (it is both truly longer and also functionally longer due to equinus in swing). This resulted in an external left foot progression angle
4. persistent ankle equinus and knee flexion throughout stance phase.

Goals and treatment options

Specifically, PB had inadequate left quadriceps strength, combined with a knee flexion contracture preventing stance-phase knee extension. A strengthening programme for the quadriceps was not an option due to the severity of weakness. In an attempt to stabilise the knee and reduce the considerable effort of walking, the following alternatives were considered:

1. If the left knee flexion contracture could be reduced, an anterior ground reaction AFO to help extend the knee was a possible option. The degree of proximal weakness and marked external foot progression angle might limit its effectiveness.

2. Fitting of a left KAFO to stabilise the left knee. This would necessitate a percutanous tenotomy of the left tendo achilles to achieve a plantigrade foot to facilitate fitting of the orthosis. (Accommodating the equinus contracture would make this leg functionally even longer and increase the clearance problem on this side.) It may be difficult for PB to cope with bilateral KAFOs in the presence of severe pelvic girdle weakness, even with the use of walking aids. In this case there is the risk that following tenotomy the knee would collapse completely without orthotic support and he would therefore not be able to revert to his current walking ability.

Intervention and outcome

PB wished to proceed with the first option. Serial casting of the left knee and ankle to reduce contractures was undertaken prior to fitting an anterior ground reaction AFO, and a period of gait re-education. Slight equinus was accommodated in the orthosis, in part to facilitate the plantarflexor/knee extensor couple as a compensation for left quadriceps weakness, i.e. flat-foot contact and plantarflexion in early stance results in delayed tibial advancement and knee hyperextension to assist knee stability. A small shoe raise was provided on the right side to facilitate clearance in swing on the left. His wife was taught passive stretching exercises to maintain the position of the left knee.

Combined with the existing right KAFO and also the use of a stick in the right hand, stability of the left knee improved. He was then able to walk reasonable distances indoors, and had one hand free to facilitate function at work. He walked short distances outdoors and his car was adapted to incorporate hand controls.

Long-term compensations for muscular weakness places increased demands on joints and muscles, and can lead to joint deformity and pain (Fig. 15.3). Early recognition of the patterns of weakness, to optimise function and minimise compensatory strategies, is preferable (Perry et al., 1995). Orthoses have a role to play in supporting unstable or painful joints, minimising deformity and promoting function. However, when compensatory strategies have been long-standing,

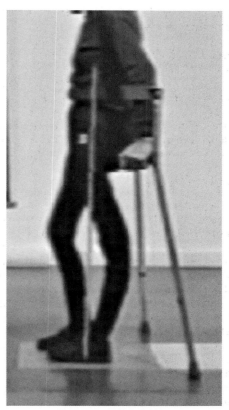

Figure 15.3 Poliomyelitis: prolonged compensation for quadriceps paralysis has resulted in excessive knee hyperextension and knee pain.

orthoses may not always be well tolerated and will need to be monitored carefully.

CONCLUSIONS

While awaiting a successful cure for patients with neuromuscular disease, there should be a clear recognition that much can be done to improve function, quality of life and life expectancy of these patients. Physiotherapy, as part of an integrated multidisciplinary management approach, has a major contribution to offer, particularly in relation to preserving posture, physical fitness and muscle strength, and preventing contractures.

ACKNOWLEDGEMENTS

Dr Quinlivan gratefully acknowledges support in her clinical work from the Muscular Dystrophy Campaign and the Association for Glycogen Storage Disorders UK (AGSD).

References

Agre JC, Rodriquez AA, Tafel JA. Late effects of polio: critical review of the literature on neuromuscular function. *Arch Phys Med Rehab* 1991, **72**:923–931.

Beynon R, Quinlivan RCM, Sewry CA. Selected disorders of carbohydrate metabolism. In: Karpati G, ed. *Structural and Molecular Basis of Skeletal Muscle Diseases*. Basel: ISN Neuropath Press; 2002:182–188.

Bradley WG, Jones MZ, Fawcett PRW. Becker type muscular dystrophy. *Muscle Nerve* 1978, **1**:111–132.

Bunch WH, Siegel IM. Scapulothoracic arthrodesis in fascioscapulohumeral muscular dystrophy. *J Bone Joint Surg* 1993, **75A**:372–376.

Callen JP. Malignancy in polymyositis/dermatomyositis. *Clin Dermatol* 1988, **2**:55–63.

Carrington-Gawne A, Halstead LS. Post-polio syndrome: pathophysiology and clinical management. *Crit Rev Phys Rehab Med* 1995, **7**:147–188.

Cooper RG, Stokes MJ, Edwards RHT. Physiological characterisation of the 'warm up' effect of activity in patients with myotonic dystrophy. *J Neurol Neurosurg Psychiatry* 1988, **51**:1134–1141.

Dalakas MC. How to diagnose and treat the inflammatory myopathies. *Semin Neurol* 1995, **14**:137–145.

DiMauro S, Servidei S, Tsujino S. Disorders of carbohydrate metabolism: glycogen storage disease. In: Rosenberg RN, Prusiner SB, DiMauro S, Barohn RJ, eds. *The Molecular and Genetic Basis of Neurological Disease*, 2nd edn. Boston, MA: Butterworth-Heinemann; 1997:1067–1097.

Dubowitz V. Treatment of muscular dystrophy: *75th ENMC International Workshop*, Baarn, 10–12 Dec 1999. *Neuromusc Dis* 2000, **10**:313–320.

Eagle M, Peacock CK, Bushby K, Major R, Clements P. Fascioscapulohumeral muscular dystrophy: gait analysis and effectiveness of ankle foot orthoses (AFOs) (abstract). *Neuromuscular Dis* 2001, **11**:631.

Fawcett PRW, Barwick DD. The clinical neurophysiology of neuromuscular disease. In: Walton JN, Karpati G, Hilton-Jones D, eds. *Disorders of Voluntary Muscle*, 6th edn. Edinburgh: Churchill Livingstone; 1994:1033–1104.

Friedrich U, Brunner H, Smeets D et al. Three points linkage analysis employing C3 and 19cen markers assign the myotonic dystrophy gene to 19q. *Hum Genet* 1987, **75**:291–293.

Gospe SM, Lazaro RP, Lava NS, Grootscholten PM, Scott MO, Fischbeck KH. Familial X linked myalgia and cramps: a non-progressive myopathy associated with a deletion in the dystrophin gene. *Neurology* 1989, **39**:1277–1280.

Griggs RC, Donohue KM. Emergency management of neuromuscular disease. In: Henninng RJ, Jackson DL, eds. *Handbook of Critical Care Neurology and Neurosurgery*. New York: Praeger; 1985:9–12.

Halstead LS, Rossi CD. Post polio syndrome: clinical experience with 132 consecutive out-patients. In: Halstead LS, Wiechers DO, eds. *Research and Clinical Aspects of the Late Effects of Poliomyelitis*. White Plains, NY: March of Dimes Birth Defects Foundation; 1987:13–26.

Harper PS. *Myotonic Dystrophy*, 2nd edn. Philadelphia: WB Saunders; 1989.

Hough A. *Physiotherapy in Respiratory Care*. London: Chapman & Hall; 1991.

Illarioshkin SN, Ivanova-Smolenskala IA, Tanaka H. Refined genetic location of the chromosome 2p linked progressive muscular dystrophy gene. *Genomics* 1997, **42**:345–348.

Ionasesco VV. Charcot–Marie–Tooth neuropathies: from clinical description to molecular genetics. *Muscle Nerve* 1995, **18**:267–275.

Jobsis GJ, Boers JM, Barth PG, de Visser M. Bethlem myopathy a slowly progressive congenital muscular dystrophy with contractures. *Brain* 1999, **122**:649–655.

Karpati G, Hilton-Jones D, Griggs RC. *Disorders of Voluntary Muscle*, 7th edn. Cambridge: Cambridge University Press; 2001.

Kissell JT. Fascioscapulohumeral dystrophy. *Semin Neurol* 1999, **19**:35–43.

Laforet P, De Toma C, Eymard B et al. Cardiac involvement in genetically confirmed fascioscapulohumeral muscular dystrophy. *Neurology* 1998, **51**:1454–1456.

Letournel E, Fardeau M, Lytle JO et al. Scapulothoracic arthrodesis for patients who have fascioscapulohumeral muscular dystrophy. *J Bone Joint Surg* 1990, **72A**:78–84.

Lindeman E, Leffers P, Spaans F et al. Strength training in patients with myotonic dystropy and hereditary and motor sensory neuropathy: a randomised clinical trial. *Arch Phys Med Rehab* 1995, **76**:612–620.

Mastaglia FL, Laing NG. Investigation of muscle disease. *J Neurol Neurosurg Psychiatry* 1996, **60**:256–274.

Milner-Brown HS, Miller RG. Muscle strengthening through high resistance weight training in patients with neuro-muscular disorders. *Arch Phys Med Rehab* 1988, **69**:14–19.

Miura K, Kumagai T, Matsumoto A et al. Two cases of chromosome 4q35-linked early onset fascioscapulo-humeral muscular dystrophy with mental retardation and epilepsy. *Neuropaediatrics* 1998, **29**:239–241.

Moore JK, Moore AP. Postoperative complications of dystrophia myotonica. *Anaesthesia* 1987, **42**:529–533.

Orrell RW, Forrester JD, Tawil R et al. Definitive molecular diagnosis of fascioscapulohumeral muscular dystrophy. *Neurology* 1999, **52**:1822–1826.

Perry J, Fontaine JD, Mulroy S. Findings in post-poliomyelitis syndrome. Weakness of muscles of the calf as a source of late pain and fatigue of muscles of the thigh after poliomyelitis. *J Bone Joint Surg* 1995, **77A**:1148–1153.

Sanders DB. Diseases associated with disorders of neuromuscular transmission In: *Neuromuscular Function and Disease: Basic, Clinical and Electrodiagnostic Aspects*. WF Brown, CF Bolton, M Aminoff, Pub WB Saunders; 2002:1345–1353.

Siegel IM. *Everybody's Different, Nobody's Perfect*. London: Muscular Dystrophy Group of Great Britain; 1982:1–13.

Tollback A, Ericksson S, Wredenburg A, Jenner G, Vargas R, Ansved T. Effects of high resistance training in patients with myotonic dystrophy. *Scand J Rehab Med* 1999, **31**:9–16.

Wijmenga C, Padberg GW, Moerer P et al. Mapping of fascioscapulohumeral gene to chromosome 4q35-qter by multipoint linkage analysis and *in situ* hybridization. *Genomics* 1991, **9**:570–575.

Windebank AJ, Lichty WJ, Daube JR et al. Late effects of paralytic poliomyelitis in Olmstead County, Minnesota. *Neurology* 1991, **41**:501–507.

SECTION 3

Lifetime disorders of childhood onset

General introduction to paediatric neurology

C deSousa   H Rattue

NEUROLOGICAL DISORDERS OF CHILDHOOD

There is a continuum of neurological illness from infancy to adulthood. Most disorders that occur in adults also occur in children – this includes common adult disorders such as stroke, multiple sclerosis and Parkinson's disease. The prevalence of these disorders in childhood is often much less than in adults and prevalence also varies in children of different ages. There may be different underlying causes for some disorders that also occur in adults: cerebrovascular disease in children is seldom due to atherosclerosis; the most frequently encountered childhood cause of bacterial meningitis is *Haemophilus influenzae*, which is a less common pathogen in older people; and cerebral tumours in children occur more commonly in the posterior fossa than at other sites, unlike in adults.

A pathological process, such as cerebral ischaemia or demyelination, may exert a very different effect on the developing nervous system compared to its effect in the fully mature individual. The developing nervous system is at risk from any process that permanently alters development at critical stages, as occurs with congenital infections such as rubella or cytomegalovirus. Despite this, the plasticity of the infant brain often means that extensive recovery of function can take place following surgery, ischaemia or damage to one cerebral hemisphere (see Ch. 5).

Neurological disorders are a major cause of illness in childhood (Kurtz & Stanley, 1995). Approximately 7% of all children have some form of moderate handicap and 0.7% have a severe handicap; there is neurological dysfunction in a high proportion of such children. One-fifth of children admitted to hospital have a neurological problem, either as their principal complaint or in association with it. Three categories of neurological disorder predominate in children: cerebral palsy, epilepsy

Table 16.1 Prevalence of neurological disorders in childhood

Neurological disorder	Prevalence
Epilepsy	8 per 1000
Complex mental handicap	5 per 1000
Cerebral palsy	2 per 1000
Duchenne muscular dystrophy	3 per 10 000 boys
Spina bifida	6 per 10 000
Hydrocephalus	5 per 10 000
All neurodegenerative disorders	5 per 10 000
Meningitis	4 per 10 000 per year (incidence)
Neurofibromatosis	3 per 10 000
Rett syndrome	1 per 10 000 girls
Central nervous system tumours	0.5 per 10 000

Table constructed from various sources cited in the text and reflecting worldwide prevalence. Values for some disorders are changing with time.

and complex mental handicap. Each of these categories includes individual disorders with a variety of aetiologies and outcomes, and many affected individuals will suffer from more than one of these. The prevalences of these and some other neurological disorders are given in Table 16.1. The prevalence of some of these neurological disorders of childhood is changing with time. There is an increase in the prevalence of cerebral palsy (see Ch. 18) and cerebral tumours. There is a decrease in the prevalence of neural tube defects (see Ch. 19), epilepsy, serious head injury and *Haemophilus* meningitis. Some of these changes are due to changing medical practice, but the reasons for others are not well understood.

Many of the neurological disorders of childhood are congenital and occur because of maldevelopment of the nervous system or as a result of adverse factors during pregnancy and birth. Many genetic disorders give rise to neurological dysfunction from birth but others, such as Duchenne muscular dystrophy (see Ch. 20) or some inborn errors of metabolism, do not manifest symptoms for months or years. Acquired neurological disorders of childhood include important treatable and sometimes preventable conditions such as central nervous system (CNS) infection (particularly in infancy), serious head injury (most commonly in older children and teenagers) and brain tumours (in all age groups). In some disorders there is considerable improvement during childhood, but many neurological disorders arising in childhood have implications for later life. It is important for therapists who treat adults with disorders of childhood onset to be familiar with how these conditions present in childhood.

PHYSIOTHERAPY FOR CHILDREN WITH NEUROLOGICAL DISORDERS

All aspects of the management of childhood neurological illness require familiarity with normal development (see Ch. 17) and the ability to work effectively and sympathetically with children and families. The child is an integral part of a family. The parents of the child newly diagnosed as having a neurological disorder undergo a period of adaptation which is not dissimilar to a grief response. There may be denial, anger and sadness at the loss of the child they expected. The assessment and treatment of such a child will require the therapist to balance the expectations of parents with the abilities and requirements of the child.

It is important to be able to engage and communicate with children, some of whom have severe cognitive, communication and behavioural problems. Therapy techniques need to be adapted to children of different ages, and active participation is difficult to obtain in the younger child. Medical and physical management must be integrated into the whole life of the child, including education, play and family and social life. Parents and carers should be made to feel involved in the assessment and treatment of the child. Parents are often the best therapists the child has. The therapist and the family achieve the best for the child by sharing their skills and by developing a working relationship in which each is sensitive to the other's needs. Some families like to be very involved in the child's care whilst others require support to feel confident in their abilities with the child. It is important that the therapist assesses the individual child's and family's needs and plans intervention that is appropriate to that particular situation. There will be some children with neurological disorders for whom physiotherapy is not appropriate or in whom therapy should be postponed or discontinued temporarily for a variety of reasons.

Aspects of physiotherapy management

There are four aspects to the work of physiotherapy in children with neurological disorders:

1. Assessment of the child's abilities and difficulties is carried out to define whether a problem exists and what the nature of the problem is. This assessment may also be part of the medical diagnosis of underlying causes.
2. The treatment of the child is intended to enhance function, improve quality of life and alter outcome in the face of neurological deficits.

3. Measurement of change in function with time is necessary to evaluate the effects of intervention and plan further treatment.
4. The physiotherapist is involved in linking specialist knowledge about the child's physical development to the overall treatment of the child, including other aspects of development (cognitive, communication, social and emotional).

The multidisciplinary team (MDT)

The child with a neurological disorder may have differing areas of need and will benefit from a holistic approach to treatment. The physiotherapist works as part of the MDT. There are many examples of problems which can be dealt with most effectively by professionals from different backgrounds working together. These include the feeding disorders of children with motor impairments, which can be addressed by a feeding disorders team comprising a speech and language therapist, physiotherapist and dietician; and the 'clumsy' school-age child who can be helped by a joint approach from occupational and physiotherapy. The physiotherapist is also a key member of the multidisciplinary assessment team of the child with suspected neurodevelopmental abnormalities, and of the team planning orthopaedic and non-surgical treatments for children with gait and postural disorders.

Assessment and observing change

The assessment of children with static or progressive neurological disorders can be difficult, especially in the early stages. It is always important to listen carefully to what parents are describing, as in many cases such a description is more valuable than a 'hands-on' assessment with an uncooperative child. The observation of children at play, in the home or at school, is invaluable. The process of assessment needs to make allowance for many factors, which can influence the individual's performance. These include:

- cultural and family norms
- the effects of prematurity
- coexisting systemic disease in infancy (cardiac, renal or gastrointestinal) that may cause significant changes in function
- the effects of drugs such as antiepileptics.

Regression, or the loss of previously acquired skills, is a hallmark of degenerative disorders of the CNS, such as metachromatic leucodystrophy. At an early stage, however, there will be only a slowdown in the acquisition of skills, which is then followed by plateauing and eventually a loss of skills. Loss of function is also sometimes seen in children with non-progressive disorders. The child with a congenital spastic hemiplegia, for instance, may develop increasing gait abnormality in later childhood due to progressive shortening of the Achilles tendon in the absence of progression of the underlying neurological disorder. For assessment and goal-setting, a problem-solving approach is preferable, actively involving the child and parents (see Chs 3 and 22).

Physical activity

The role of exercise and strength training is becoming recognised as an important aspect of managing different neurological disorders. The emerging evidence from research and the clinical implications are discussed in Chapter 29.

Transition from paediatric to adult services

The time of transition from children's services to the adult services can be unsettling for the adolescent with a neurological disorder as well as for the family. It may come at a time of upheaval in the life of a young person who is seeking greater independence in the face of continuing limitations due to the neurological condition. One way to facilitate a smooth transition from paediatric to adult services is for therapists from both services to meet, jointly with patients, in order to plan in advance for the move from one service to another. This often provides an opportunity to review the objectives, goals and methods of therapy.

CHROMOSOMAL DISORDERS AND RECOGNISABLE PATTERNS OF MALFORMATION

Chromosomal disorders are caused by an abnormality in an individual's complement of chromosomes. The normal situation is to possess 23 pairs of chromosomes, of which one pair are sex chromosomes (two X chromosomes in females and an X and a Y in males). Individuals with Down's syndrome have an additional chromosome 21, with most having a total of 47 chromosomes. This disorder occurs in approximately 1 in 800 births and is more common with advancing maternal age (Jones, 1988). Children with Down's syndrome have an increased likelihood of a variety of congenital abnormalities, including cardiac malformations, intestinal atresias and cataracts. The intellectual development of children with Down's syndrome is slower than normal and the average IQ is around 50. Other specific neurological problems include hypotonia, an increased incidence of epilepsy and the occurrence of dementia from 40 years onwards in many individuals.

Physiotherapy alone or as part of a multidisciplinary programme has been used in the management of children with Down's syndrome. There is evidence for improvement in motor skills, particularly following early-intervention programmes that include a series of individualised therapy objectives (Harris, 1981; Connolly et al., 1984). Physiotherapy includes management of low muscle tone (see Ch. 25) and strategies to improve strength, co-ordination, general fitness and functional activities. Many children with Down's syndrome have asymptomatic atlantoaxial instability and around 1% are at increased risk of atlantoaxial subluxation, which may cause quadriplegia. Cervical spine radiographs are not carried out routinely in children with Down's syndrome, but should be taken if there is head tilt or the emergence of neurological signs, or if participation in tumbling or contact sports is planned (American Academy of Pediatrics, 1995).

Other trisomies include Edward's syndrome (trisomy 18) and Pattau's syndrome (trisomy 13), both of which cause profound retardation and usually death in early infancy.

Some chromosomal anomalies can be detected only by high-resolution chromosomal studies or by analysis of dioxyribonucleic acid (DNA). Prader–Willi syndrome, for instance, is due to a deletion of part of chromosome 15. Most affected infants are extremely hypotonic in the neonatal period, often with marked feeding difficulties that require tube feeding. Later they have excessive appetites and obesity, short stature, and moderate learning difficulties. Because of the hypotonia there is an increased risk of scoliosis in early infancy and the role of physiotherapy includes providing advice about positioning and seating to promote good postures and reduce the risk of deformity developing.

MALFORMATIONS OF THE CNS

The development of the CNS in the fetus and embryo is a complex process and it is not surprising that abnormalities may occur at any stage (see Ch. 17). Malformations that result from such abnormal development are an important cause of neurological illness in childhood (Aicardi, 1992). Between one-third and a half of all infants who die in the first year of life have a serious CNS malformation. The survivors may have a range of neurological disorders including motor deficits, mental retardation, epilepsy and impairments of the special senses.

In those malformations that arise before about 20 weeks of gestation there is usually a disturbance of CNS morphology (Table 16.2). This is a time of intense change in the structure of the nervous system, including neural tube closure (by 29 days), formation of the forebrain and diencephalon (by 6 weeks) and migration of cortical neurones (by 20 weeks). Abnormal development may occur because of a faulty genetic code (e.g. in Miller–Dieker syndrome, in which there is a deletion of chromosome 17 and lissencephaly) or there may be external abnormalities that interfere with CNS development. Well-recognised causes include: fetal infections (such as rubella, which causes microcephaly, and cytomegalovirus, which can cause abnormal neuronal migration); drugs (such as sodium valproate, which can cause spina bifida); and drug abuse (alcohol causing microcephaly and crack cocaine, causing early vascular destruction). No cause can be identified in about two-thirds of children with CNS malformations of early onset.

By about 20 weeks of gestation all the major components of the nervous system are in place and most malformations arising after this time do so because of destructive processes. One example is periventricular leucomalacia, in which there is destruction of white matter adjacent to the lateral ventricles of the brain. This usually arises between 20 and 30 weeks of gestation, and is the neuropathological change seen most often in children with diplegic cerebral palsy who were born prematurely.

The physiotherapeutic needs of children with cerebral malformations depend upon the nature of the motor and other neurodevelopmental deficits as well as other individual and family factors. This group includes some children with the most severe impairments. Although the malformations themselves are not progressive, there is a high morbidity and mortality related to intercurrent infection, epilepsy and feeding disorders. In many cases, malformations of the nervous system coexist with abnormalities of other organ systems, including congenital heart disease and limb abnormalities. It is important to be aware of these when these children are undergoing physiotherapy.

NEUROCUTANEOUS SYNDROMES

The neurocutaneous syndromes are a group of disorders in which abnormalities of the skin and brain coexist (Gomez, 1987). Both the skin and the nervous system are derived from the ectodermal layer of the developing embryo. Many of these disorders are genetic and arise because of faulty chromosomal regulation of cell growth and proliferation. Other body organs may also be involved.

Table 16.2 Some important malformations of the central nervous system

Malformation	Description	Clinical features
Cerebral malformations		
Microcephaly	Abnormally small brain	Usually learning difficulties, may also have motor deficits
Lissencephaly	Smooth brain without normal central gyri	Severe learning difficulties, epilepsy, hypotonia and pyramidal motor deficits
Hydrocephalus	Enlargement of cerebral ventricles due to impaired CSF drainage	May be normal; often specific learning deficits and language disorders
Holoprosencephaly	Undivided forebrain, often with fused lateral ventricles	Severe learning difficulties, midline facial clefts, hypopituitarism
Porencephaly	Destructive change in one cerebral hemisphere	Often hemiplegia; may have epilepsy, learning difficulties and hemianopia
Cerebellar malformations		
Cerebellar hypoplasia	Maldevelopment of cerebellar hemispheres or vermis	Ataxia, hypotonia, disordered eye movements
Dandy–Walker syndrome	Posterior fossa cyst and cerebellar vermis hypoplasia	Symptoms of hydrocephalus and may have learning difficulties
Chiari malformation	Cerebellar tonsils project through foramen magnum	Type I – rarely symptomatic Type II – occurs with spina bifida
Neural tube defects		
Encephalocele	Skull defect with protrusion of meninges with or without brain	Anterior: meningitis, CSF leak Posterior: high mortality and disability
Myelomenigocele	Vertebral defect with exposed meninges and spinal cord	Paraplegia, neuropathic bowel and bladder, hydrocephalus
Spina bifida occulta	Maldevelopment of lower spinal cord and vertebrae covered by skin	Progressive unilateral foot deformity and weakness, neuropathic bladder

CSF, cerebrospinal fluid.

Neurofibromatosis type 1 (von Recklinghausen disease)

This is the commonest neurocutaneous syndrome with a prevalence of 1 in 3000 (Huson et al., 1988). It is inherited as an autosomal dominant trait, with those affected having a 50% chance of passing on the condition to their children. About a third of cases are new mutations. The skin abnormalities are multiple café-au-lait patches, axillary freckles and firm subcutaneous neurofibromas. The most frequent neurological abnormalities are mild learning difficulties, attention deficit disorders and poor co-ordination. There is an increased risk of developing CNS tumours, especially gliomas of the optic pathway. Although many children with neurofibromatosis type 1 will not need physiotherapy, some will benefit from therapy if they have motor deficits resulting from brain tumours, spinal cord and root compression or bony deformity of the limbs. See Appendix for a support group.

Tuberous sclerosis

Tuberous sclerosis is also inherited in a dominant fashion but it is both rarer (1 in 10 000) and more severe than neurofibromatosis. The skin changes include hypopigmented skin patches and red papules (angiofibromata) over the nose and cheeks. The neurological abnormalities include epilepsy in 80% and learning difficulties (which may be severe) in 50%. Motor deficits are not common. Brain scans demonstrate tubers, which are benign growths in the cortex. Cerebral tumours can also occur and may cause hydrocephalus.

Sturge–Weber syndrome

This is another, rarer neurocutaneous syndrome that is frequently associated with motor deficits. These children have a 'port wine' haemangioma over the upper face, in the area innervated by the first division of the trigeminal nerve. They may have congenital glaucoma. They also have an angioma on the meninges on one or both sides of the brain, usually extending over the occipital cortex. Although most such children are normal at birth, many have debilitating focal epileptic seizures and a progressive hemiplegia, often together with progressively more apparent learning difficulties. Physiotherapy is often required for the hemiplegia and associated abnormalities.

GENETIC METABOLIC AND NEURODEGENERATIVE DISORDERS

There are a large number of individually rare genetic metabolic disorders that cause neurological symptoms in childhood (Holton, 1994). Some important disorders are listed in Table 16.3. Some may cause symptoms from birth, for instance phenylketonuria and hypothyroidism. Others may not present until after months or years of normal development, as occurs with some of the leucodystrophies. Some may cause intermittently severe symptoms such as coma, ataxia and seizures, as occurs in children with organic acidaemias. In others there is a progressive deterioration in motor and cognitive abilities, resulting eventually in death, as occurs with the gangliosidoses. Specific and effective treatments are available for some disorders. In phenylketonuria and hypothyroidism, screening for the defect at birth allows treatment to be commenced immediately and minimises the risk of neurological sequelae. Even in those disorders for which a specific treatment is not available it is important to make a diagnosis. Most of these disorders are inherited in an autosomal recessive fashion with a 1 in 4 risk of siblings being affected. Prenatal diagnosis can be offered to many

couples (by chorionic villous biopsy), allowing for the termination of an affected fetus at an early stage of the pregnancy.

There are some disorders of childhood that share features in common with these neurometabolic disorders, but for which no cause is known. One such disorder is Rett syndrome, which occurs in 1 in 10 000 girls and is one of the most important causes of progressive neurological handicap in girls (Hagberg, 1993). The gene for this disorder has recently been discovered, and the full spectrum of disorders caused by this gene abnormality is now evident (Percy, 2001). Girls with Rett syndrome appear normal or only slightly slow in their development until 6–18 months of age. At around this time they undergo a period of regression in development, followed by many years of almost developmental standstill. At the same time new features appear, including stereotyped hand-wringing movements, tachypnoea and breath-holding, progressive gait apraxia, scoliosis and epilepsy. Ambulation is usually lost and feeding difficulties are often severe. Despite these considerable difficulties most girls survive into adulthood. Physiotherapy has an important part to play in the management of girls with Rett syndrome. It is important that the therapist is familiar with the natural history and particular features of this singular disorder. The maintenance of optimum function and prevention of deformity are very difficult in the face of a changing series of neurodevelopmental abnormalities, often combined with periods of agitation and misery on the part of these girls. Important aspects include the provision of adequate aids to seating and mobility, as well as surveillance and early intervention for the scoliosis which is common in this condition.

Table 16.3 Important genetic, metabolic and degenerative disorders of childhood

Group of disorders	Examples	Clinical symptoms
Amino acidurias	Phenylketonuria[a]	Microcephaly, severe learning difficulties, quadriplegia and epilepsy
Organic acidurias	Glutaric aciduria	Encephalopathy, dystonia, seizures
Leucodystrophies	Metachromatic leucodystrophy	Progressive spasticity, ataxia and peripheral neuropathy
Batten's disease	Juvenile Batten's disease	Progressive visual impairment, seizures and dementia
Mucopolysaccharidoses	Hurler's syndrome	Coarse features, learning difficulties, kyphosis
Gangliosidoses	Tay–Sachs disease	Dementia and progressive spasticity and blindness in infancy
Hypothyroidism	Congenital hypothyrodism[a]	Learning difficulties ('cretinism')
Copper metabolism	Wilson's disease[a]	Progressive dystonia, ataxia and behavioural changes in adolescence
Mitochondrial disorders	MELAS	Encephalopathy, lactic acidosis and stroke-like episodes

[a]These disorders can be treated successfully.
MELAS, mitochondrial encephalomyopathy, lactic acidosis and stroke.

CNS INFECTION AND INFLAMMATORY DISORDERS IN CHILDHOOD

Infections of the CNS are amongst the most frequent causes of injury to this system in childhood. The likelihood of permanent sequelae following CNS infections is related to the age of the child, the site of infection, the nature of the organism, the rapidity with which effective treatments are commenced and the need for intensive care support. Most children with viral meningitis due to an organism such as the mumps virus make an excellent recovery, whereas viral encephalitis due to herpesvirus often leads to permanent sequelae, including seizures, hemiparesis and memory impairments. Bacterial meningitis due to *Haemophilus influenzae* is largely preventable by immunisation and much less likely to cause permanent damage than is tuberculous meningitis, which often causes hydrocephalus, cranial nerve palsies, hemiparesis and visual loss. If recognised and treated early, a cerebral abscess resulting from extension from sinus infection often has a very good outcome. However, the neonate who develops abscesses as a result of infection with an organism such as *Citrobacter* is often left with severe damage, resulting in quadriplegia, seizures and blindness.

Physiotherapy for children with such infections may start during the period of hospital treatment, at which stage it may still be difficult to predict the eventual outcome. Early interventions are intended to prevent deformity and encourage rehabilitation. Regular review and assessment are necessary to monitor how the child is recovering function.

The amount and type of physiotherapy input can be reviewed regularly as the child's recovery indicates, and in response to each family's needs.

Some viruses may cause chronic CNS infection, resulting in relentlessly progressive and severe neurological disorders. Measles virus causes subacute sclerosing panencephalitis in about 1 in 100000 infected children, with an onset of symptoms 5–15 years after the original infection. Neurological deficits include myoclonus, dementia and dystonia, with death occurring within months to years from onset.

The human immunodeficiency virus (HIV) is neurotropic and frequently causes neurological symptoms in affected children (Epstein et al., 1986). These include a slowing in the acquisition of developmental skills followed by a loss of previously acquired milestones. A progressive paraparesis is common. Opportunistic CNS infections in children with acquired immune deficiency syndrome (AIDS) may cause severe sequelae.

Head injury in childhood

Head injury becomes an increasingly important cause of neurological morbidity or death as children get older, especially boys. Serious head injury in older children is usually the result of accidents outside the home. Certain children are more vulnerable, including those from poorer homes or living in deprived areas, as well as those with pre-existing behavioural or neurodevelopmental problems. When rehabilitating a child following a head injury, it is important to know about problems that were present before the accident.

Non-accidental head injury occurs especially in children less than 1 year of age (Duhaime et al., 1998). Parents or other carers are the usual perpetrators. They may themselves have been the victims of violent abuse in childhood. Some children, including those with pre-existing neurological handicaps, are more at risk of being abused. The mechanism of injury includes shaking (infantile whiplash injury), blows to the head or throwing the child against a hard surface. Injury is often repeated and associated with other evidence of abuse including fractures of the limbs and ribs. Intracranial injury includes subdural haematomas (often of differing ages) with contusion of the underlying brain (Fig. 16.1). There may be more widespread

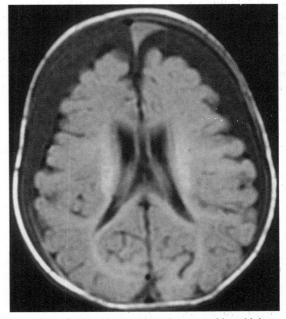

Figure 16.1 Subdural haemorrhage in non-accidental injury. Magnetic resonance brain scan (T1-weighted) shows bilateral subdural collections with layering of the fluid, suggesting haemorrhage on two or three separate occasions.

brain injury than at first suspected, with shearing injuries of the white matter of the brain. Retinal haemorrhages are a frequent finding. Surgical treatment may be required for the subdural haemorrhage. Over half these children have permanent neurological handicaps, including hemiplegia or quadriplegia, seizures and visual impairments.

The physiotherapist will often be involved from an early stage in the management of a child who has suffered a head injury (see Ch. 7). Early involvement will include the maintenance of good respiratory function, whilst ensuring that the techniques used have no detrimental effects on the injured brain. During the acute stages it is important to maintain the range of movement in all joints. Splinting is often necessary to maintain good joint position, although this will depend upon the nature of the underlying neurological deficit. The rehabilitation of the child with a serious head injury involves close working with parents, nursing staff, doctors, speech therapists, occupational therapists, psychologists and school teachers (Scott-Jump et al., 1992). Reintegration into schooling and the successful provision of support from community-based professionals (including physiotherapists and doctors) are essential following severe head injuries.

CNS TUMOURS IN CHILDHOOD

Brain tumours are the commonest solid tumours of childhood and second only to leukaemia as a cause of malignancy in this age group (Deutsch, 1990). Certain types of brain tumour are more common in children than in adults (Table 16.4), particularly medulloblastomas (primitive neuroectodermal tumours; Fig. 16.2) and craniopharyngiomas, whereas secondary brain tumours are rarer. About half of brain tumours in children arise in the posterior fossa, a much higher rate than in adults. Presenting symptoms include progressive ataxia (in children with posterior fossa tumours), headaches due to raised intracranial pressure, seizures due to some tumours of the cerebral hemispheres and cranial nerve palsies due to brainstem tumours.

Most brain tumours are treated by surgery and in many cases the outcome correlates most closely with the extent of surgical resection. Surgery can sometimes produce deficits where none existed previously, in an attempt at radical treatment of a potentially fatal tumour such as a medulloblastoma. Malignant and partially resected tumours are often treated with radiotherapy, sometimes in combination with chemotherapy to reduce the chance of relapse (Deutsch, 1990). These treatments, especially radiotherapy, can also produce neurological deficits. Radiotherapy particularly affects

Table 16.4 Tumours of the central nervous system in childhood

Site	Type	Frequency (%)
Brain		
Cerebral hemispheres	Glioma	20
	Ependymoma	3
	Primitive neuroectodermal tumour	5
	Meningioma	2
	Pineal germinomas and teratomas	4
	Choroid plexus papilloma	1
Pituitary region	Craniopharyngioma	7
	Pituitary adenoma	2
Cerebellum	Medulloblastoma	20
	Astrocytoma	17
	Ependymoma	5
Brainstem	Glioma	7
	Other types	7
Total		100
Spinal cord		
Extradural	Neuroblastoma	40
	Rhabdomyosarcoma	
	Histiocytosis X	
Intradural and extramedullary	Meningioma	25
	Schwannoma	
Intradural and intramedullary	Astrocytoma	35
	Ependymoma	
Total		100

the growing brain, causing intellectual loss and occasionally more severe neurological disorders such as radionecrosis. For this reason radiotherapy is not now given to children under 3 years of age.

The outcomes of treatment depend upon the site and type of tumour. The worst prognosis is in children with brainstem gliomas, <20% of whom will be alive 5 years after treatment. The best prognosis is in children with benign gliomas, >80% of whom survive for longer than 5 years (Duffner et al., 1986).

Spinal cord tumours are much less common than brain tumours (Table 16.4). They are often diagnosed very late, with intervals of sometimes months or even years between the onset of symptoms and diagnosis. This is because the significance of changes in gait or sphincter control and the onset of back pain may be overlooked, especially in young children. Diagnosis

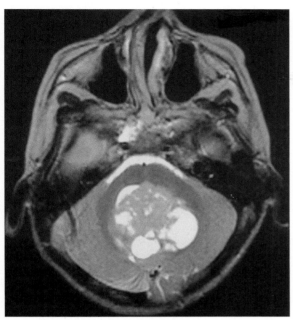

Figure 16.2 Medulloblastoma. Magnetic resonance brain scan (T2-weighted) shows a large mixed solid and cystic mass arising from the middle of the cerebellum.

Table 16.5 Cause of stroke in childhood

Type	Cause
Haemorrhagic (50%)	Arteriovenous malformation Aneurysm Unidentified
Ischaemic (50%) Thrombotic	Postinfectious (e.g. chickenpox, bacterial meningitis) Sickle cell disease Hypercoagulation (e.g. protein C deficiency) Moyamoya disease Cerebral vasculitis (e.g. lupus) Metabolic (e.g. homocystinuria) Migraine
Embolic	Endocarditis Myocarditis Congenital heart disease Dissecting aneurysm

by magnetic resonance imaging is much more rapid and less invasive than myelography, which was used in the past. Treatment of these tumours is with surgery, radiotherapy and chemotherapy; again, a high risk exists of worsening neurological deficits with treatment.

Children with brain and spinal tumours have a high incidence of motor deficits, especially ataxia and hemiplegia with brain tumours and paraplegia with spinal tumours. Some of these may worsen with time, either as a result of tumour progression or as a side-effect of treatment. They require skilled physiotherapy from a person who understands the nature of the underlying disorder, the often long-drawn-out treatment that may be necessary and the impact on the child and family.

CEREBROVASCULAR DISORDERS IN CHILDHOOD

Stroke occurs much less commonly in children than in adults (see Ch. 6), affecting 1 child in 40 000 per year. About half of childhood strokes are due to haemorrhage (subarachnoid and/or intracerebral) and half to ischaemia (Table 16.5; deVeber, 2002). Most haemorrhages are from arteriovenous malformations (see Ch. 7). Aneurysms affect the vertebrobasilar circulation more often in children than in adults. In 15% of cases

no cause is found for cerebral haemorrhage. Most ischaemic strokes occur during or following infections, including meningitis. Atherosclerosis is very unusual in young children.

Children, and especially young infants, can recover impressively following strokes. In part this may be due to plasticity of the nervous system, which is particularly evident in the developing brain (see Ch. 5). A good example is the transference of language function from the dominant to the non-dominant hemisphere that occurs during the recovery from middle cerebral artery infarction (Fig. 16.3) in early childhood.

PERIPHERAL NERVE INJURIES

Nerve injuries are discussed in detail in Chapter 9, but obstetric brachial plexus injuries deserve special mention here. These occur in 1 in 4000 births and are associated with shoulder dystocia in two-thirds of cases and with breech delivery in a further 15% (Sandmire & De Mott, 2002). Most are Erb's palsies involving the C5 and C6 roots of the brachial plexus and only rarely is there involvement of C8 and T1. Around 75% recover, although recovery may take many months and can continue for some years. Nerve grafting is indicated for the most severe lesions (Laurent & Lee, 1994). The failure to develop active elbow flexion in the affected limb by 3–6 months of age may be one indicator of poor outcome in a lesion, and grafting should be considered.

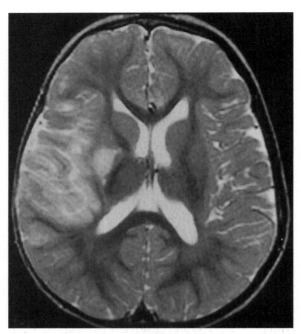

Figure 16.3 Middle cerebral artery infarction. Magnetic resonance brain scan (T2-weighted) shows a signal change in the distribution of the right middle cerebral artery (left side of image) as a result of ischaemia and reperfusion.

Table 16.6 Important causes of progressive ataxia in childhood

Group of disorders	Examples
Structural lesions	Cerebellar tumour
Parainfectious and paraneoplastic	Dancing-eye syndrome
Demyelinating	Multiple sclerosis
DNA repair abnormalities	Ataxia telangiectasia
Metabolic diseases	Wilson's disease
Spinocerebellar degenerations	Friedreich's ataxia

and their skin is excessively sensitive to exposure to sunlight. They have a tendency to develop malignancies, especially leukaemias and lymphomas, from adolescence onwards. In neither of these disorders is dementia a feature.

CHILDREN WHO RAISE CONCERNS

Most children acquire motor developmental milestones in a predictable pattern and at similar ages. When children deviate from these it may serve as a warning that there is a significant underlying disorder. For instance, the boy who does not walk until after 18 months of age could have Duchenne muscular dystrophy (see Ch. 20). However, there are some children who have an unusual pattern of early motor development for which no cause can be found. In some cases this may be a familial pattern. An example is children who 'bottom-shuffle' rather than crawl and who often do not walk independently until well after their first birthday and often closer to their second.

Hypotonia

Hypotonia in infancy may be due to neuromuscular disorders or to central causes (including neurological disorders, chromosomal abnormalities and metabolic disorders). There are some children who are hypotonic in infancy in the absence of discernible underlying disease and who can be markedly delayed in their early motor development, but with normal acquisition of other developmental skills. After infancy many such children often have little residual abnormality, if any. The term 'benign congenital hypotonia' has been applied to this group, which probably includes more than one cause for this striking variation in early development. A similar group of children often have a familial tendency to joint hypermobility, in the absence of a definable disorder of connective tissue, and many of them are also often delayed in their early gross motor

SPINOCEREBELLAR DEGENERATIONS AND HEREDITARY ATAXIAS

Congenital ataxia may be due to structural abnormalities of developing cerebellum, principally affecting either the cerebellar hemispheres or vermis (Aicardi, 1998). Some of these disorders are genetic, for instance Joubert syndrome, an autosomal recessive disorder in which, in addition to the ataxia, there are learning difficulties, retinal abnormalities and abnormalities of respiratory pattern.

Acquired ataxia in childhood may be due to progressive disorders (Table 16.6). As well as structural lesions, such as cerebellar tumours, there are genetic disorders. Friedreich's ataxia is inherited as an autosomal recessive disorder and has its onset usually between 5 and 15 years (see Ch. 4, p. 55). As well as a progressive ataxia, affected people develop pes cavus and scoliosis. Cardiomyopathy and diabetes mellitus are other frequent findings. Most patients lose the ability to walk by about 15 years after the onset of symptoms. Ataxia telangiectasia is another disorder inherited in an autosomal recessive fashion with its onset in early childhood. Affected children have an increased susceptibility to sinopulmonary infections

development. Hypotonia and other abnormalities of tone and movement are discussed in Chapters 4 and 25.

The role of physiotherapy includes the assessment of such children and the differentiation of patterns which are normal variants from those due to underlying disease. This requires familiarity with the range of normal development (see Ch. 17).

The 'clumsy' child

There is a further group of children who present to the medical and therapy services with increasing frequency. These are children with the label of 'clumsiness'. The description covers a variety of different problems. Some children demonstrate particular difficulties with acquisition of fine motor skills such as pencil skills, using utensils and tying laces or doing up buttons. Others have greater difficulties with tasks requiring good hand–eye co-ordination and balance, such as ball-throwing or learning to ride a bicycle. Some children have problems in several of these areas, others in only a few. What they have in common is the absence of definable neurological deficits, such as ataxia, spasticity or dystonia. Often there is a family history of a parent or sibling with similar difficulties.

Many such clumsy children suffer from poor self-esteem. They can be helped by occupational therapists and physiotherapists to learn strategies to overcome areas of particular difficulty (Schoemaker et al., 1994). The majority grow up to be normal adults, often choosing in their adolescent years to shun physical activities which they find hard to succeed at. A number of descriptions have been applied to these children, including 'minimal brain damage', 'dyspraxia' and 'cerebral palsy' (Peters et al., 2001). None of these terms is accurate for all of this group and 'developmental co-ordination disorders' is the preferred term (see Ch. 18).

NON-ORGANIC NEUROLOGICAL DISORDERS IN CHILDHOOD

Some children adopt a 'sick' role as a means of avoiding intolerable life situations. Such illness behaviour is not often seen in children under 10 years of age but occurs with increasing frequency in young teenagers. The presenting problem may be an abnormal gait, a paralysed limb, or pain or sensory loss in one part of the body. The onset is often after a minor illness or accident, for which the child may have received medical attention. The symptom frequently causes the child to withdraw from normal activities and absence from school can be prolonged, despite attempts at encouraging a return.

Many of these children have had some personal experience of illness, either in themselves or in a close relative. One or other parent may have experienced a similar period of illness in the past. The parents, or one parent, will often closely identify with the child and may find it very difficult to accept that there is not a serious illness underlying the symptoms. Health professionals may unwittingly collude in perpetuating the child's symptoms by expressing concern and uncertainty about an undiagnosed disease process. Children may be referred from one specialist to another for opinions and tests which serve only to reinforce the worry the child has about his or her own health. Many of these children are academically or athletically very able, sometimes setting themselves very high standards that they may find hard to achieve. Others may be the victims of bullying at school or of physical or sexual abuse at home. In our experience, many children presenting with chronic fatigue syndrome and some with reflex sympathetic dystrophy are indistinguishable from this group with non-organic neurological disorders.

These children need an assessment of their condition which reaches a definite conclusion, and this can then be confidently and sympathetically discussed with the child and parents. This is followed by a goal-oriented rehabilitation programme. It is important that there is good teamwork between the disciplines involved, as opportunity exists to play professionals off against one another. Physiotherapy has a key role in the physical rehabilitation of these children, but therapists will often need the support of doctors and psychologists if they are going to succeed. It can be helpful to have a child draw up his or her own list of goals for a coming week, which can then be renegotiated each week on an ongoing basis. It is important to reintegrate the child into education, beginning for instance with the hospital school and gradually building up to a return to full-time school. If there are underlying issues within the home or school these also need to be tackled, usually by child psychiatrists or clinical psychologists working with the whole family.

MEASURING OUTCOMES

Some parents will express satisfaction with the care and interest shown in their child's condition. They may feel more confident and in control of the situation when there is someone to guide them as to how to manage their child's physical problems. Others may embark on a search for new therapies for their child, often in the belief that what is readily available is never enough and that exceptional treatments exist that may unlock their child's potential. Sometimes they are right and some children will benefit from forms of therapy which are more intensive or use novel techniques. Too often, however, this search for novel remedies or additional therapy places undue emphasis on the motor disorder at the expense of education, play, emotional and social development. It can also distort the care that other children in the family receive (which may already be considerably affected by having a sibling with a neurological disorder).

Any form of therapy requires evaluation. However, assessing the effectiveness of interventions can be particularly difficult when working with children with neurological disorders. It requires validated measures, which are responsive to clinically important functional change. Unfortunately there are too few such measures designed for this purpose in children with neurological disorders (Rosenbaum et al., 1990) and some are mentioned in Chapter 3. Although there have been a number of studies which have sought to evaluate physiotherapy for children with neurological disorders such as cerebral palsy, it is difficult not to make the focus of such studies a too narrow set of goals (Sommerfeld et al., 1981). Some assessments used in adults (see Ch. 3) may be applicable to children but require evaluation and perhaps modification. Some simple practical measures can be used, such as range of movement, photography and video recording, to monitor changes in functional abilities and deformity.

Change in motor function is not the only clinical change that requires evaluation. The goals of a therapy programme should also include patient comfort, prevention of deformity, integration into schooling, ability to participate in leisure activities and family satisfaction. Measures of quality of life are also lacking but developments are being made in this area (see Chs 3 and 27).

IMPORTANT MOTOR DISORDERS IN CHILDHOOD

The remaining chapters of this section, on disorders of childhood onset, deal with the most common motor disorders in which physiotherapy plays an important role. These include the cerebral palsies (see Ch. 18), neural tube defects such as spina bifida (see Ch. 19) and muscle disorders, including the muscular dystrophies and spinal muscular atrophy (see Ch. 20). As mentioned previously, an understanding of normal development is essential when treating children with such disorders and this topic is outlined in Chapter 17. With more children surviving further into adulthood with these disorders, the need for those involved in adult services to understand these conditions is stressed throughout the subsequent chapters.

THE PREMATURE CHILD

Advancing technology and changes in neonatal care have led to an increased survival rate among infants born early. The immaturity of their neurological systems makes them more vulnerable to neurodevelopmental difficulties in later life (Stewart et al., 1989; Roth et al., 1994). Some of these children will present with a picture of emerging cerebral palsy; however, there is an ever-increasing group of children who suffer some difficulties with gaining appropriate developmental skills.

An increasing number of studies are being undertaken to investigate and evaluate this specific group of children's needs in an attempt to minimise the effects of their early birth. Some studies report that the majority of premature and low-birth-weight infants survive with little or no disability. In studies undertaken on neonates weighing less than 1500 g, 62–80% have been reported as normal, 16–21% as having mild to moderate disability, and 5–12% as having severe disability (Agostino, 1998). It is generally accepted that the lower the gestational age, the higher the incidence of major disability.

These children may well be referred for some form of physiotherapy in order to try and promote their motor skill development. Studies have shown that one-third of children with birth weight less than 1500 g demonstrate poor gross motor skills in standardised testing (Stewart et al., 1989). These children display difficulty with balance, control, co-ordination and postural control and present as less athletic than their full-term classmates do (Stewart et al., 1989; Roth et al., 1994).

The therapy needs of this particular group of children depend on careful assessment of their primary needs. All too often the lack of gross motor skills is the most easily observed and every effort is made to address that particular area of deficit. However, often the child and carers need to have a programme of activities to influence many of the other aspects that might be affecting the development (Barb & Lemons, 1989). An holistic approach is needed, which attempts to minimise the detrimental effects and promote the experience of positive effects the infant has been denied. Many of the stimuli of a modern neonatal intensive care unit are inappropriate for optimal sensory/motor development. The least mature sensory systems of the premature infant, visual and auditory, receive the most random stimulation, whereas the more developed systems of tactile, gustatory and vestibular receive the least amount of stimulation (White-Taut et al., 1994).

Early intervention, advice and activity programmes can be of benefit for these children and their families, in order to optimise their ultimate outcomes. A family-centred and MDT approach is indicated in the assessment and management of these children (see Ch. 22).

References

Agostino D. Neurodevelopmental consequences associated with the premature neonate. *AACN Clin Issues: Adv Pract Acute Crit Care* 1998, **9**:11–24.

Aicardi J. *Diseases of the Nervous System in Childhood*, 2nd edn. Oxford: MacKeith Press/Blackwell Scientific Publications; 1998.

American Academy of Pediatrics Committee on Sports Medicine and Fitness. Atlantoaxial instability in Down syndrome: subject review. *Pediatrics* 1995, **96**:151–154.

Barb S, Lemons P. The premature infant: toward improving neurodevelopmental outcome. *Neonatal Network* 1989, 7:7–15.

Connolly B, Morgan S, Russell F. Evaluation of children with Down syndrome who participated in an early intervention program. *Phys Ther* 1984, **64**:151–155.

Deutsch M. *Management of Childhood Brain Tumours*. Boston: Kluwer; 1990.

deVeber G. Stroke and the child's brain: an overview of epidemiology, syndromes and risk factors. *Curr Opin Neurol* 2002; **15(2)**:133–138.

Duffner PK, Cohen ME, Myers MH, et al. Survival of children with brain tumours: SEER program 1973–1980. *Neurology* 1986, **36**:597–601.

Duhaime AC, Christian CW, Rorke LB et al. Nonaccidental head injury in infants – the 'shaken-baby syndrome'. *N Engl J Med* 1998, **338**:1822–1829.

Epstein LG, Sharer LR, Oleske JM et al. Neurologic manifestations of human immunodeficiency virus infection in children. *Paediatrics* 1986, **78**:678–687.

Gomez MG. *Neurocutaneous Diseases – A Practical Approach*. Boston: Butterworth; 1987.

Hagberg B. *Rett Syndrome – Clinical and Biological Aspects*. London: MacKeith Press; 1993.

Harris SR. Effects of neurodevelopmental therapy on motor performance of infants with Down's syndrome. *Dev Med Child Neurol* 1981, **23**:477–483.

Holton J. *The Inherited Metabolic Diseases*. London: Churchill Livingstone; 1994.

Huson SM, Harper PS, Compston DAS. Von Recklinghausen neurofibromatosis: a clinical and population study in south-east Wales. *Brain* 1988, **111**:1355–1381.

Jones KL. *Recognisable Patterns of Human Malformation*. Philadelphia: WB Saunders; 1988.

Kurtz Z, Stanley F. Epidemiology. In: Harvey D, Miles M, Smyth D, eds. *Community Child Health and Paediatrics*. Oxford: Butterworth Heinemann; 1995:3–22.

Laurent JP, Lee RT. Birth-related upper brachial plexus injuries in infants: operative and non-operative approaches. *J Child Neurol* 1994, **9**:111–117.

Percy AK. Rett syndrome: clinical correlates of the newly discovered gene. *Brain Dev* 2001; **23** (Suppl. 1):S202–S205.

Peters JM, Barnett AL, Henderson SE. Clumsiness, dyspraxia and developmental co-ordination disorder: how do health and educational professionals in the UK define the terms? *Child Care Health Dev* 2001, **27**:399–412.

Rosenbaum PL, Russell DJ, Cadman DT et al. Issues in measuring change in motor function in children with cerebral palsy – a special communication. *Phys Ther* 1990, **70**:125–131.

Roth SC, Baudin J, Pezzani-Goldsmith M et al. Relation between neurodevelopmental status of very preterm infants at 1 and 8 years. *Dev Med Child Neurol* 1994, **36**:1049–1062.

Sandmire HF, DeMott RK. Erb's palsy causation: a historical perspective. *Birth* 2002, **29**:52–54.

Schoemaker MM, Hijlkema MGJ, Kalverboer AF. Physiotherapy for clumsy children: an evaluation study. *Dev Med Child Neurol* 1994, **36**:143–155.

Scott-Jump R, Marlow N, Seddon N et al. Rehabilitation and outcome after severe head injury. *Arch Dis Child* 1992, **67**:222–226.

Sommerfeld D, Fraser B, Hensinger RN. Evaluation of physical therapy service for severely mentally impaired students with cerebral palsy. *Phys Ther* 1981, **61**:338–344.

Stewart AL, Costello AM, Hamilton PA et al. Relationship between neurodevelopmental status of very preterm infants at 1 and 4 years. *Dev Med Child Neurol* 1989, **31**:756–765.

White-Taut R, Nelson M, Burns K, Cunningham N. Environmental influences on the developing premature infant: theoretical issues and application to practice. *J Obstet Gynaecol Neonatal Nurs* 1994, **23**:393–401.

Chapter 17

Developmental neurology

E Green

PRENATAL DEVELOPMENT OF THE BRAIN AND SPINAL CORD

The brain develops from a single cell into a very complex structure containing billions of neurones. This chapter describes brain development. The brain's life cycle can be studied in greater detail in Thompson (1993).

Structural development

There are many unanswered questions about how the human brain develops its precise, detailed and extremely complicated neuronal circuits. The answers will probably be found at the level of individual nerve cells (neurones) and their interactions, their processes of growth and migration, as well as the physical or chemical events responsible for those processes.

Induction

Induction is the general principle believed to underlie the development of the nervous system. Neurones are first formed from the embryo's outer ectodermal layer, similar to the cells of the epidermis covering the outer body surface. They are formed by interaction with the cells beneath them, which will become the vertebral column and other tissues constituting the mesoderm. Before the ectodermal cells interact with the mesodermal cells, the epidermal cells can become either nerve cells or skin cells. It is presumed that the mesodermal cells release a substance that causes certain ectodermal cells to change into neurones.

Neural plate and neural tube

About 3 weeks after conception, the neural plate is formed by a thickening of the ectodermal cells on the dorsal surface of the embryo (Fig. 17.1A). This is the start of the process called neurulation, in which the first phase of neural tube formation occurs with the development of a neural groove with a neural fold along each side. By the end of the third week the neural folds have begun to fuse with one another, so converting the neural groove into a neural tube (Fig. 17.1B, C). This is the forerunner of the brain and spinal cord.

Neural crests

Neuroectodermal cells not incorporated into the tube form neural crests running dorsolaterally along each side of the neural tube (Fig. 17.1C). From the neural crests are derived the dorsal root ganglia of spinal nerves, some of the neurones in sensory ganglia of cranial nerves, autonomic ganglia, the non-neuronal cells (neuroglia) of the peripheral nerves, and the secretory

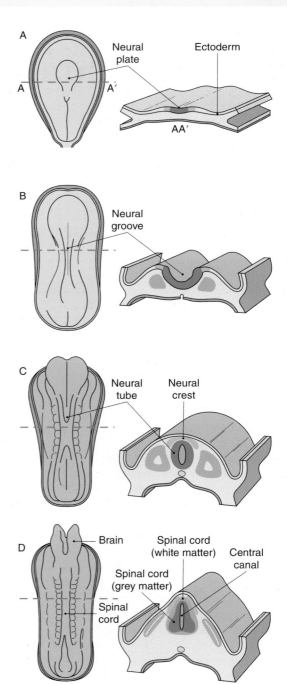

Figure 17.1 Early development of the human nervous system. Drawings on the left are external views; cross-sections are shown on the right. (A) Neural cells develop from ectoderm (skin-to-be) cells to form the neural plate. (B) The plate folds in to form the neural groove. (C) Further folding inwards forms the neural tube. (D) As the developing neurones send out axons, the basic form of the grey matter (cell bodies) and white matter (axons) of the spinal cord develops.

nerves of the adrenal medulla. Others differentiate into cells of non-neural tissue, such as the melanocytes of the skin and some of the bones, muscles and other structures of the head that are of dermal origin. The target tissues determine the fate of the neural crest cells, though it is not yet clear how. This stage of migration is practically complete by 24 weeks after conception. It is thought that the time of migration of different cells is controlled by the neurones losing their capacity to synthesise deoxyribonucleic acid (DNA) and therefore ceasing to divide and form new cells.

Neuroblasts – precursors of neurones

The first population of cells produced in the neural tube are neuroblasts, the precursors of neurones. The number of neuroblasts formed in the neural tube far exceeds the number of neurones in the adult brain and spinal cord. Outgrowth of axons and dendrites from the cells occurs and neuroblasts that fail to make synaptic connections die as part of the normal course of development (see Ch. 5). This happens particularly in the spinal cord. As the developing neurones send out axons, the basic form of the grey matter (cell bodies) and white matter (axons) of the spinal cord develops (Fig. 17.1D).

Formation of the brain

Growth and differentiation are greatest at the end of the neural tube where the brain develops; the rest of the neural tube becomes the spinal cord. Three distinct regions are formed at the end of the fourth week: the forebrain, the midbrain and the hindbrain. Within each of these three regions and within the embryonic spinal cord, neuroblasts multiply and migrate to form the characteristic structures of the brain as aggregates of neurones. These neurones send their axons in fibre tracts to other brain regions and also receive synaptic input from axons migrating from other brain regions. The forebrain and the hindbrain both divide further during the fifth week to form a structure with five regions. During this expansion, the neural tube takes on a number of flexures, or bends, to accommodate its length within the skull. The parts of the brain derived from the five regions are shown in Figure 17.2. The development of the human brain in stages from 25 days until birth can be seen in Figure 17.3.

Neuronal and synapse production

Myelination and transmitter production take place in parallel with the axonal growth and synapse formation, and continue postnatally. The structural layers of the cerebral cortex are completed during the last months of pregnancy and the first postnatal months. Synapse production and network formation continue to a considerable extent through the first years of life. At the end of the first year synapse density is greatest, decreasing to adult densities at about 7 years of age. The reduction in the number of neurones seems to be an active, genetically determined process.

Development of the spinal cord

As the brain is developing, there is a parallel development of spinal cord structures and of the connections between them. Spinal cord neurones form two discrete regions of grey matter, which become the posterior

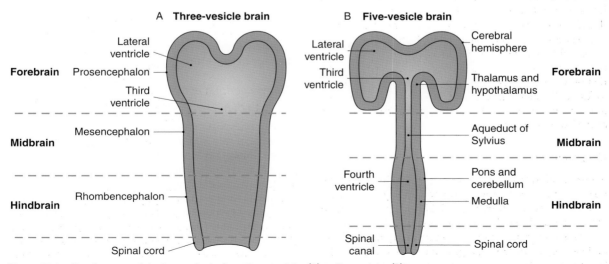

A Three-vesicle brain

- Lateral ventricle
- **Forebrain** Prosencephalon
- Third ventricle
- **Midbrain** Mesencephalon
- **Hindbrain** Rhombencephalon
- Spinal cord

B Five-vesicle brain

- Lateral ventricle
- Third ventricle
- Cerebral hemisphere
- Thalamus and hypothalamus — **Forebrain**
- Aqueduct of Sylvius — **Midbrain**
- Fourth ventricle
- Pons and cerebellum
- Medulla — **Hindbrain**
- Spinal canal
- Spinal cord

Figure 17.2   Development of the human brain from three vesicles (A) to five vesicles (B).

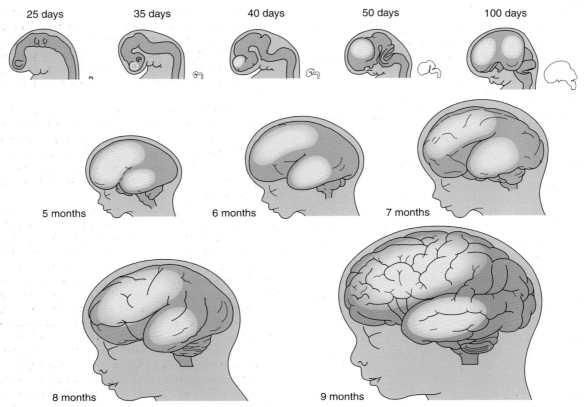

Figure 17.3 Development of the human brain in stages from 25 days until birth. The drawings from 5 to 9 months are about one-third life size. Those from 25 to 100 days are much enlarged. The actual sizes are shown to the right of each (note the little speck at 25 days). The three major parts of the brain – forebrain, midbrain and hindbrain – begin as swellings in the neural tube. As the human brain grows, the cerebral hemispheres (forebrain) expand enormously and cover most of the rest of the brain.

(sensory) and the anterior (motor) regions respectively. Some motoneurones in the anterior horn send their axons to innervate the sympathetic ganglia, part of the autonomic nervous system. In the peripheral nervous system the neural crest cells migrate along pathways which do not have organised glial structures.

Mechanisms of brain development

The three different ways that the specific pathways and patterns of connections are hard-wired in the brain are chemical signals, cell and terminal competition and fibre-guided cell movements.

Chemical signals or trophic growth

Chemical gradients of some substances encourage the growth of the axon in a particular direction and to a particular set of target cells. Nerve growth factor (NGF) was the first chemical signal to be discovered by Levi-Montalcini & Hamburger in 1951 (Levi-Montalcini, 1982)

and it is specific to the neurones of the sympathetic ganglia. Injection of NGF into chickens triggers a large increase in cell division in the sympathetic ganglia (Thompson, 1993). Several other growth factors have been identified and offer some hope of repair of brain damage in the future.

Cell competition and death

Neuronal death is probably regulated by competition for trophic substances released by the target tissue. An example of this is in the innervation of skeletal muscle fibres. Initially a motoneurone connects with several muscle fibres by sending out motor axons, usually several to one muscle fibre. As development proceeds, the terminal branches of most of the motor axons retract so that one motoneurone comes to dominate a given muscle fibre completely (see Ch. 5, p. 59). The process of retraction and cell loss appears to be general in the development of the nervous system, allowing modification of the anatomical organisation of synaptic connections.

Fibre-guided cell movement

Fibre-guided cell movement is thought to result from a growing neurone sending out a fibre alongside radially oriented glial cells. The neurone eventually reaches a boundary, such as the surface of the brain, and cannot grow any further. The cell body then travels up the fibre to the boundary. Glial cell proliferation starts very early in pregnancy and continues through the postnatal years.

Development of the cerebral cortex

The cerebral cortex begins as one layer a few cells thick, known as the germinal zone. As the cells proliferate, some stop dividing and move up to another layer. From here, some cells move up to form the next layer and so on, forming a columnar organisation superimposed on the horizontally arranged cellular layers. A particular type of neurone (subplate neurone) lies under the developing cortex in the white matter. The subplate neurones send their axons up into the cortex and appear to be physiologically active, forming synapses with the developing neurones in the cortex. They may play an important role in the guidance of the growth of the cortical neurones and the incoming fibres which die out as the cortex becomes established.

Plasticity in development

Experience also plays an important part in the ultimate growth and fine-tuning of the neural circuits in the brain. The role of experience is discussed further below in 'Innate versus learned behaviour' and plasticity is discussed in detail in Chapter 5.

Times of vulnerability to damage

The central nervous system (CNS) is most vulnerable to damage during periods of rapid change, for example when the constituents of the neural networks are being formed. Teratogenic substances (i.e. those which produce physical defects in the developing embryo), such as drugs, are particularly damaging during the early weeks of pregnancy. The anticonvulsant medication, sodium valproate, can cause neural tube defects if taken in the third week after conception, during neurulation. Viruses such as hepatitis B and rubella, as well as irradiation, have their most damaging effects during neuronal proliferation in the first trimester of pregnancy. Maternal alcoholism appears to have a teratogenic effect at, and following, the second and third months of gestation.

Infections with organisms such as cytomegalovirus and *Toxoplasma* may damage the neural developmental processes over a much longer time interval, sometimes throughout pregnancy. Cytomegalovirus transmission through the placenta has most clinical effect during the first two trimesters of pregnancy, whereas toxoplasmosis is most devastating in early pregnancy, even though the protection against maternofetal transmission is also greatest at that time.

The placenta has a protective effect and some damage to the developing nervous system may occur from maternal or fetal metabolic disease when the protection has ended after birth. Migration failures, which are thought to be responsible for some types of epilepsy and dyslexia, occur during the second trimester (Touwen, 1995).

Disturbances of circulation have varying effects according to the timing of their occurrence. Reduced blood flow carries the risk of impairing the blood supply to the fetus, especially to the most metabolically active parts of the nervous system. These areas are notably the germinal matrix around the central canal and ventricles during the phase of cell proliferation and initial migration, and, at later fetal ages, those areas to which the cells have migrated and where axonal and synapse formation are taking place, such as the cortex and basal ganglia. Hypoxic and ischaemic episodes have different effects depending on the stage of neural development. In young preterm babies, periventricular leucomalacia (softening of the white matter) and haemorrhage result, with cortical and basal ganglia involvement in term babies.

Functional development of the nervous system in utero

The first signs of movement in utero have been picked up by ultrasound scanning at about 7–8 weeks after conception, with a fast increase in the repertoire of movement. By 20 weeks of gestation, all types of movement seen in the term fetus are present. They consist of well-organised and complex patterns, with no craniocaudal or proximal–distal sequence in the development of these types of subcortically mediated movements (Prechtl, 1984).

The time of the first discernible fetal movements coincides with the time of direct contact between the motoneurones and muscle fibres and the afferent and efferent cells in the spinal cord. However, the wide range of movement develops before the time of most of the major morphological processes in the brain, suggesting that the immature brain can still generate active motor patterns in spite of limited structural development. It is likely that the increase of structural development of the brain allows the quality of the movement to develop postnatally.

POSTNATAL DEVELOPMENT

Changes that occur postnatally include maturation of the CNS, and the development of learning and perception.

Physiological maturation of the CNS

Maturation of the CNS involves myelination and changes in synaptic density. These occur at different rates in the different areas of the brain.

Myelination and regional brain maturation

The rate of myelination varies with both site and age. Some neural tracts are myelinated early and rapidly, others early and slowly. In general, those which function first tend to be myelinated first and those with long phases of myelination are particularly at risk of damage. Myelination begins earliest in the lower brainstem and spinal cord, starting in mid-gestation, and there is heavy myelination here by birth. Myelination reaches the cerebral hemispheres by birth and cortical myelination shows an anatomical sequence. It begins in the sensorimotor systems, followed by the secondary cortical areas. It occurs last in the frontal, parietal and temporal association cortex and myelination of the association fibres continues throughout adulthood. Myelination principally affects the speed of transmission of neural impulses and therefore cannot be taken as a direct marker of functional significance. Some myelination is not complete until adolescence.

Synaptic density in the striate cortex (an early-maturing sensory region) is maximal at about 8 months of age, whereas that in the prefrontal cortex (one of the latest-maturing regions) is maximal at about 2 years of age. In both areas, synaptic density declines during the first decade to reach adult values during adolescence. Total brain size reaches adult values at about 2 years of age but specific patterning of synapses presumably occurs later, leading to emerging psychological processes. Induction of brain structure also occurs by experience (see below).

Innate versus learned behaviour

The double influence of experience and learning on one hand, and of biological inheritance on the other, has led to the argument called the 'nature–nurture controversy'. The focus of the argument is the extent to which human behaviour is determined by genetic inheritance and how much it can be modified by experience.

Whenever skills and habits are acquired, whether these are manipulative, motor, intellectual or social, learning takes place.

Innate learning

Knowledge of biological or innate inheritance has increased greatly over the past century. Mendel discovered that, for simple physical traits such as eye colour, there are statistically valid relationships between the traits of the parents and those of their offspring.

Later biological and chemical research has identified chromosomes with genes carrying genetic information occupying specific sites on the chromosomes. The term 'genotype' is used to describe this genetic inheritance. The term 'phenotype' describes the characteristics the person displays. Genetic inheritance is increasingly proving to be complex as the interactions of the different genes become more fully understood. For example, it is now known that some genes may alter the effect of other genes.

Learning through experience

Even if the genetic material is laid down without mishap, experience by the individual has been shown to be necessary to ensure that the appropriate neuronal architecture develops. The most researched example of this is in the growth and development of the visual system. Hubel & Wiesel's experiments on the developing visual system of kittens in the early 1960s led to the concept that a clear visual stimulus is necessary for normal physiological and morphological development of previously immature visual pathways and that there is a critical period of time during which this development can take place. Kittens who had one eye occluded from birth to the age of 3 months showed histological evidence of small shrunken cells in the lateral geniculate body, the part of the visual pathway which should have been receiving stimulation from the occluded eye. Kittens who had one eye occluded from birth for only 2 months produced similar but less severe histological changes. No changes were seen at all in adult cats deprived of vision. A similar picture has been found in experiments on other animals.

Movement of the eyes during this critical period has also been found to be essential to enable the development of cells in the visual cortex that will give information about orientation. Immobilisation of all movements of the animal apart from those of the eyes does not impair neurones in the visual cortex becoming selective for orientation (Buisseret et al., 1978). However, if the eye movements are prevented, even selectively, there is a corresponding effect on the development of the visual cortex. The visual experience necessary for the development of the visual cortex includes information about eye movements and head movements (Gary-Bobo et al., 1986). It is likely that children developing with impairment of kinaesthetic sensation and limitation of eye movements consequently develop an impairment of the structural formation of the visual cortex.

Development of perception

Perception involves visual and spatial aspects that are obviously related.

Development of visual perception

The neuroanatomy of the eye and the visual system is described in Thompson (1993). The optic nerve transmits information to the various parts of the brain where analysis of visual sensations occurs. When a person moves through the environment or the environment moves relative to the person, a moving pattern of light falls on the retina. The resulting optical flow field provides useful information about the person's movement as well as the three-dimensional layers of the scene. Sensitivity to optic flow develops early in life.

Bower (1977), in experiments with young babies, some only a few days old, has shown that visual events such as the sight of an object looming up and appearing to be on a path to hit the person ('hit path') are just as likely to be interpreted by the baby as they would by an adult. The baby moves its head back and raises its arms as if to defend itself against an impending contact.

The role of visual proprioception (feedback) in the development of postural stability in normal infancy has been studied using a moving-room technique. Lee & Aronson (1974) found that in standing infants, when the end of the room moved away from or towards them, balance was lost in a direction specific to the movement of the room. Butterworth & Hicks (1977) replicated the experiment on two groups of infants. The first group could both sit and stand unsupported whilst the second group could sit unsupported but could not stand. The proprioceptive effect of vision influenced both sitting and standing postures. In another study the role of postural experience on the proprioceptive effects of vision was examined (Butterworth & Cicchetti, 1978). A group of infants who could both sit and stand were compared with a group who were only able to sit. It was found that the effect of partial visual feedback was greatest in the first 3 months after acquiring the ability to sit or stand and declined thereafter. This was true for normal babies and for those with motor delay such as Down's syndrome. The same effect is seen when adults stand on a narrow beam inside a moving room. They can fall off the beam even after the walls shift by as little as 1 or 2 cm.

Gibson & Walk (1960) performed the 'visual cliff' experiment in which visual cues for the height of the cliff were achieved by a texture change and parallax (Fig. 17.4). Babies aged 8 months were allowed to crawl

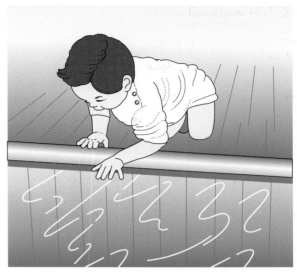

Figure 17.4 The visual cliff: the baby will not cross a drop, despite a strong glass cover.

over a flat surface that appeared to have a deep step or 'cliff' in the floor surface. The babies, and the young of other species, avoided the deep side of the cliff. The same effect was seen in rats reared in the dark, suggesting that the tendency to avoid the cliff is independent of experience.

Perception of space: learned or innate?

In learned perception, the retina transfers information about space in a two-dimensional form to the brain. The brain, however, is able to convert that to a three-dimensional experience by associating aspects of visual experience simultaneously with previous experiences giving direct spatial knowledge. An example of this inference using experience can be seen in Figure 17.5. In (A) the brain suggests that the square is nearer since it appears to be in front of the circle; in (B) the brain suggests that the pencil is nearer because of the familiar relative sizes of a pencil and a car; and in (C), the line grid suggests that the triangle is further away.

Innate perception of space is achieved by a combination of convergence of the eyes, accommodation and stereopsis. As each eye sees the world from a slightly different angle, there are minute differences between right and left retinal images.

Link between appreciation of spatial relations and mobility

Benson & Uzgiris (1985) demonstrated a relationship between appreciation of spatial relations and infants'

A **Interposition:**
   Which is nearer, the circle or the square?

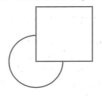

B **Familiar size:**
   Which is nearer, the car or the pencil?

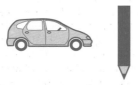

C **Position in visual field:**
   Which is nearer, the triangle or the square?

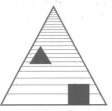

Figure 17.5. Distance cues in perception. (A) Interposition. (B) Familiar size. (C) Position in visual field.

mobility. The infants were placed behind a plastic barrier and then watched someone place a toy under one of two tablecloths. The infants were then allowed to walk or crawl round, or were carried if immobile. It was found that those who were carried round were not as successful at retrieving the object as those who crawled or walked.

POSTNATAL LANDMARKS IN THE DEVELOPMENT OF POSTURAL CONTROL, REFLEXES, BALANCE AND MOVEMENT

Classically, children's development has been viewed from a neurological perspective, particularly looking at the changing neurological reflexes during the first year of life. However, there are also changes in the relative positions of the bony structures of the body, such as the pelvis and shoulder girdle, which play an important role in the child's increasing developmental ability.

Neurological perspective/reflexes and responses

Detailed neurological observations of children during the first 2 years of life have led to a number of classic studies (Andre-Thomas & Saint-Anne Dargassies, 1960; Prechtl & Beintema, 1964; Touwen, 1976; Prechtl, 1977). Brazelton (1973) provided further information about the newborn infant, particularly from a behavioural perspective.

Neonatal or 'primitive' reflexes

These are present even in babies with a severe neurological abnormality, but asymmetry, absence of a response at the normal stage and persistence of the response after the normal stage are all important neurological signs. The term 'primitive reflex' was coined during a period when it was thought that all infant behaviour resulted from reflex function of the brain rather than from cortically controlled voluntary activity. However, evidence of early function such as perceptual function, and of individual movement patterns in the fetus that do not change much during the course of gestation, has discounted this notion of solely reflex activity. There are striking similarities between prenatal and postnatal patterns of movement, the only differences being in the quality of movement, probably because of the increased influence of gravity after birth. There is a noticeable continuum of neural function from prenatal to postnatal life (Prechtl, 1984).

Reflexes and responses remain a useful part of neurological examination of infants and will be discussed below. Assessment of muscle tone is also very important; exaggerated or marked hypotonia suggests abnormality (see Ch. 4). Interpretation of most of these tests requires experience and the presence of abnormality should not rely on one negative test result. Further evidence from other neurological tests is required to substantiate abnormality.

Moro response

This is usually elicited by allowing the baby's head to fall backwards by about 10° when supported in the supine position, particularly behind the chest and head. The response is abduction of the shoulders and arms and extension of the elbows followed by the 'embrace' adduction and flexion of the arms. The legs extend and flex during the sequence. The Moro response is well-developed in the newborn infant and gradually disappears during the first 4 months of life.

Palmar grasp

With the child lying supine, a finger put transversely across the palm elicits a strong sustained flexion of the fingers for several seconds. This grasp reflex normally lasts for the first 2 months of life.

Plantar grasp

Stimulation of the plantar surface of the root of the toes elicits active flexion. A clear developmental range of expression for this sign has not been found.

Rooting response

Both corners of the child's mouth are stroked in turn. The response consists of a head turn towards the side which has been stroked, together with mouth opening and apparent reaching with the lips. It is seen before feeding in babies up to 6 months of age.

Sucking response

The index finger is placed in the child's mouth with the finger pad uppermost. A normal sucking response is a strong sustained sucking action. The sucking response is variable and inconsistent.

Walking response

The child is held in a standing position with chin and head well supported. A normal response is discernible steps, with knee and hip flexion. The response has usually disappeared by about 4–6 weeks of age.

Asymmetric tonic neck response (ATNR)

In this response, when the child's head is turned to the side, the arm and leg extend on that side and flex on the opposite side. Although this posture is seen in normal babies up to the age of about 3 months, an ATNR is not seen as an obligatory response in neurologically normal babies.

Forward parachute reaction

This appears at about 7 months and consists of extension of the arms and hands with spreading and slight hyperextension of the fingers when the child is held in the prone position and moved downwards towards the ground. It is an important test as it demonstrates asymmetry of function well, and its absence at the appropriate age suggests abnormality.

Downward parachute reaction

This also appears at about 7 months and consists of extension of the legs and feet as the child is lowered in an upright position towards the ground.

Sideways saving reaction

Tilting the child sideways whilst in a sitting position elicits an arm movement to that side. The reaction starts at about 7 months and should always be present by 15 months.

Development of early postural control

Modern models of motor development are based on systems theory (see below and Ch. 21) and take account of the fact that emergent motor behaviour depends on the organism, the environment and the motor task involved. An outline of the developmental changes of movement of the trunk, head and limbs, as well as of the changes in load-bearing, biomechanics and function, provides a useful model on which to base assessment of early postural control and more information than assessment of neurological responses alone. The latter are also unreliable, being dependent particularly on the state of the child (e.g. relaxed, anxious) and the environment. Levels of postural ability in the supine and prone positions, and of sitting ability, are described in full in Green et al. (1995) and in summary in Figures 17.6–17.8. The child progresses from an asymmetric non-conforming position, through a symmetrical fairly static position, to a variety of mobile, active and voluntary positions.

Development of lying ability

This is shown in Figure 17.6 for supine and Figure 17.7 for prone ability. At levels 1 and 2, the child lies asymmetrically with the pelvis posteriorly tilted and shoulder girdle retracted. In supine the pelvis, trunk, shoulder girdle and head are all load-bearing, although very momentarily at level 1. Dissociation of head movement from the trunk and pelvic movement is very difficult, causing an inability to move the head without concomitant pelvic movement. In the prone position, the posterior pelvic tilt prevents load-bearing through the pelvis and most of the load-bearing is through the upper trunk and head, making lifting of the head very difficult.

Progression to levels 3 and 4 results in a symmetrical posture as the shoulder girdle becomes more protracted and the pelvis more anteriorly tilted. Load-bearing in the supine position is through the shoulder girdle and pelvis. In the prone position it is through the abdomen and thighs, with hands or arms used to prop the upper trunk. This increase in girdle control allows dissociation of movement between the upper and lower trunk and the beginning of arm movement independent from that of the trunk. The ability to vary the position of the pelvis and shoulder girdle begins at level 4.

When the child reaches levels 5 and 6, no predominant positions are displayed. A full range of movement in the shoulder girdle and the pelvis allows the child to adopt a variety of positions. As this is achieved, the child can move in the position, such as pivoting or moving backwards, as well as into and out of the lying position.

Supine

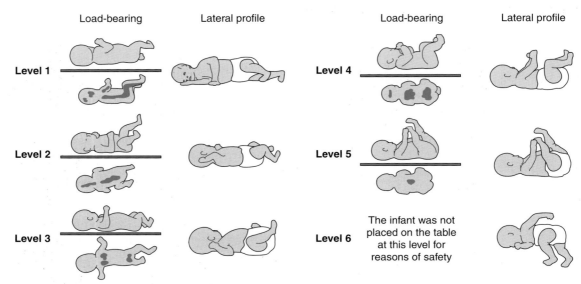

Figure 17.6 Levels of supine lying ability. For reflected images showing load-bearing, the child was placed on a clear acrylic-topped table with a mirror angled at 45° beneath it. (Redrawn from Green et al. (1995), with permission.)

Prone

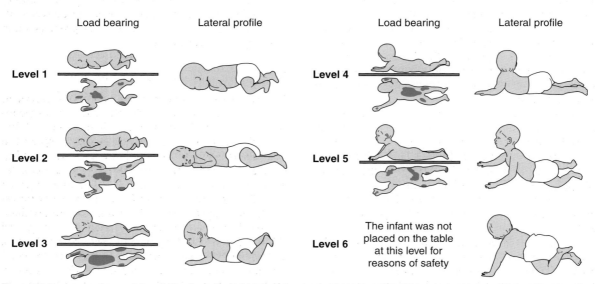

Figure 17.7 Levels of prone lying ability. For reflected images showing load-bearing, the child was placed on a clear acrylic-topped table with a mirror angled at 45° beneath it. (Redrawn from Green et al. (1995), with permission.)

Age ranges for the different levels of ability are not available but level 3 is usually achieved soon after 6 weeks, with level 6 starting at about 4 months, and present in all infants with normal development by 15 months.

Development of sitting ability

Levels of sitting ability are shown in Figure 17.8. From early infancy (level 1 lying ability) a child can be supported in a sitting position as well as anchoring his or

Sitting

Level 1   This level is not observed in normal infants

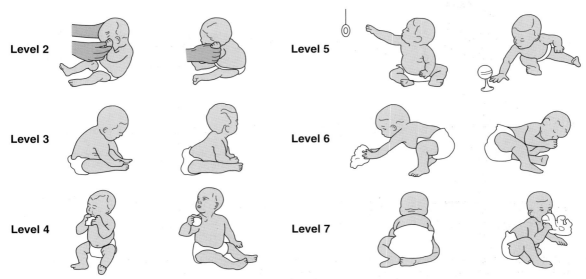

Figure 17.8   Levels of sitting ability. (Redrawn from Green et al. (1995), with permission.)

her bottom when pulled to a sitting position. Anchoring means that the child can bear weight through the pelvis sufficiently to enable the trunk to be brought forwards over it and to be maintained upright (level 2 sitting ability). The lateral profile at this level has a rounded spinal curvature with a posteriorly tilted pelvis and the shoulders maintained forwards over the sitting base in order to balance.

Independent sitting is achieved only after the child is able to tilt the pelvis anteriorly and protract the shoulder girdle and, when lying, to transfer weight efficiently and longitudinally (level 4 lying ability). This begins at about 6 months of age. In sitting the child has adequate pelvic and shoulder girdle stability to bear weight through the ischial tuberosities and through the arms in a forward prop position (level 3 sitting ability).

As the child masters the ability to shift weight laterally when lying (level 5 lying ability), he or she becomes able to move outside the area of the sitting base and to continue to maintain balance (level 5 sitting ability). The ability to counterpoise laterally is seen before the ability to recover sitting balance when the trunk weight is behind the sitting base.

As the interplay between pelvic and upper-trunk stability and movement becomes efficient, the child gains increasing ability to transfer weight in an upright position. He or she becomes efficient at counterpoising in

a variety of sitting postures, including long sitting, eventually gaining control of movement between sitting and lying, and movement from the prone position to sitting in a variety of ways.

Development of reach and hand function

There is a close relationship between the development of postural control and the development of independent arm and hand movement. At level 3 lying ability the child starts to have unilateral hand grasp and to be able to take toys to the mouth. By level 4 lying ability, increased protraction of the shoulder girdle enables midline play above the chest with the hands together. Level 5 lying ability means a full range of pelvic movement, allowing efficient limb movements with prehensile feet. Hand play is well established at this stage. All children reach level 4 lying ability before level 3 sitting ability, the start of independent sitting when the child can sit momentarily, often using the hands for support. By level 4 sitting ability, the arms can be raised to shoulder height and by level 5 the child can reach sideways outside the base of support and recover balance.

There is a developmental progression in the arc of movement as a child reaches for an object, in both lateral and vertical deviation (Fig. 17.9), and a progression in the position of the object grasped (distally and radially) with respect to the palm (Fig. 17.10).

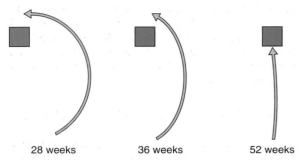

Figure 17.9 Developmental progression in arc of movement taken by a child when reaching for an object.

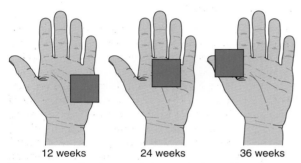

Figure 17.10 Developmental changes in the position of a grasped cube on the palm of the hand.

Development of standing

There is a similar developmental sequence in the standing posture, which is currently under evaluation. During the prestanding levels of ability, the infant is able to make either no or minimal movements against gravity. During the levels of supported early standing, the height of support needed changes from waist-height to shoulder-height as the level of ability improves. This change coincides with an increase in controlled weight shift and leg movements. At low levels of standing ability, the standing base is narrow, with weight-bearing taken particularly through tiptoes. At higher levels of ability, the standing base widens, using flattened feet, before narrowing again later as standing balance improves. The appearance of standing with support shows a wide range of variation from 9 to 18 months. The median age for standing free is about 15 months of age.

Development of more complex motor skills

Once an independent standing posture is achieved, it becomes increasingly necessary to assess the way that a motor skill is performed, i.e. a qualitative assessment rather than simply whether it is performed, which is a quantitative score. Standardised measures of motor ability are listed in Chapter 18, p. 319. Noller & Ingrisano

(1984) suggest that it is important to measure both the emergence and achievement of a motor skill. These may vary in different skills in both time interval and performance pattern. For example, the ability to stand up from the floor without support shows emergence at 12–17 months with achievement by 18–23 months. However, standing up from the floor without trunk rotation is likely to be achieved only between 66 and 71 months. Walking with arms at low guard has a much quicker development, with emergence at 12–17 months and achievement at 18–23 months.

THEORIES OF SENSORIMOTOR SKILL DEVELOPMENT

Some of the theories outlined here relate to theories of motor control, discussed in Chapters 1 and 21.

Neuromaturational model

This is the traditional model of motor development (e.g. Gesell & Armatruda, 1947) and provides the framework for many therapeutic techniques. Neuromaturational theory proposes that changes in gross motor skills during infancy result solely from the neurological maturation of the CNS. Increased myelination of the CNS is accompanied by concurrent inhibition of the lower subcortical nuclei of the brain by the higher functioning cerebral cortex. This is seen as the organisational centre for controlled movement, with the instructions for the emergence of motor skills encoded in the brain and little influence from the environment. Piper & Darrah (1994) challenge the assumptions of this model, which was influenced by the early embryologists demonstrating that the embryo developed in a symmetrical manner, beginning in cephalocaudal and proximal–distal directions.

Central executive

The development and execution of movements are entirely dependent on commands from a 'central executive' in the brain (situation unspecified).

Open–loop model

Input from the environment, such as environmental conditions and posture, passes to a central process or programme that arranges the output as movement.

Closed–loop model

This has a feedback loop in addition to the arrangement noted under the open-loop model. There are a number of feedback loops proposed according to the model, such as sensory feedback and kinaesthesis. Laszlo & Bairstow (1985) explain this model in greater detail.

Dynamic systems theory

Rather than considering functional activity as simply the result of a set of neural commands generated hierarchically as part of a motor programme, the dynamic systems theory of motor activity involves many subsystems. Systems theory arises from the natural sciences, where it was observed that when elements of a system work together, certain behaviours or properties emerge that cannot be predicted from the elements separately. A new behaviour is constructed that is dependent on input from all the parts of the system. This is called 'emergent behaviour' (Thelen et al., 1987; Shepherd & Carr, 1991).

Neuronal group selection theory

This theory may bridge the gap between the neuro-maturational model and dynamic systems theory. It is based on the work of Sporns & Edelman (1993). Hadders-Algra (2000) proposed that the structure and function of the nervous system are dependent on function and behaviour. The process of neuronal selection is divided into three phases: primary variability, selection and secondary variability. During the initial phase the neural system explores all possible variations of movement. In the second phase, the most effective patterns are selected. Finally, secondary neural repertoires are created with a wide variety of mature movements, which are task-specific.

DEVELOPMENT OF VISION

Detailed information about the development of vision is given in Grounds (1996). From birth, babies are capable of searching out detail, thus ensuring that the visual system develops satisfactorily. Cortical awakening generally occurs between 3 and 6 months postnatally. It is shortly after that period that any restricted input to one eye causes reduction of acuity to begin. Colour vision is normal by about 2 months. Visual acuity and contrast sensitivity have a long timescale of development, taking up to 6–12 years to become truly adult-like. Infants' eyes tend to be long-sighted for some months but appear short-sighted because of the lack of cortical development.

DEVELOPMENT OF HEARING

Babies should have normal levels of hearing from birth, although this may not be easy to demonstrate (Yeates, 1980). Early hearing responses are measured by the child becoming still on hearing a sound. Once head and upper-trunk control has started to develop, the child is able to turn towards a sound at the level of the ear. Localisation of a sound above and below the ear is present by about 1 year.

LANDMARKS OF INTELLECTUAL DEVELOPMENT

Important aspects of the intellectual development of the child are outlined below. Further details can be found in Illingworth (1983) and Eysenck (1984).

Learning and memory

The simplest forms of learning, habituation and sensitisation are non-associative. Habituation is simply a decrease in a response to a stimulus with repeated stimulation. Sensitisation is an increase in a response to a stimulus as a result of stimulation. A human presented with a sudden loud sound usually jumps but if the sound is repeated with no other consequence, jumping will cease at the sound (habituation). If, however, a painful shock is given just before the loud sound, jumping will be greater than after a sound without a shock (sensitisation).

Associative learning is a very broad category that includes much of learning, such as learning to be afraid, learning a foreign language and learning the piano. It involves the formation of associations amongst stimuli and/or responses or movement sequences. It is generally divided into classical and operant conditioning or learning.

In classical conditioning, a reflex response is conditioned so that it may be elicited by a new stimulus. Pavlov's experiments showed that a dog's salivation at the sight of food could be conditioned to occur at the sound of a bell if this was rung just before, or as, the food was presented. Eventually the dog salivated at the sound of the bell.

In operant conditioning, the animal's own behaviour plays a part in what happens. The behaviour is instrumental in obtaining a particular outcome and therefore in the learning process itself. The subject's behaviour can lead to either the gain or the loss of something, e.g. a rat receives food each time it presses a lever.

Positive reinforcement refers to the gain of something after a particular response is made, e.g. food being given to the rat. Negative reinforcement occurs if there is loss of something unpleasant once a particular response is made, such as an electric shock stopping when a lever is pressed. The hypothalamus, the amygdala and the cerebellum appear to be the parts of the brain where the memory traces are formed.

Visual learning

There are two visual memory systems in the monkey brain and this is also assumed to be the case in the human brain. One of these systems extends from the primary visual cortex in the occipital lobe through visual association areas to the temporal lobe. The other projects from the primary visual cortex to the parietal cortex.

Memory and the hippocampus

Studies on humans, particularly those with damage to brain structures, have identified at least three different types of long-term memory formation: declarative (learning what), procedural (skill or learning how) and implicit (memory without awareness). Declarative and procedural memory are based in the hippocampus; the brain circuits for implicit memory are not yet known.

Mechanisms of long-term memory storage

There is overwhelming evidence that experience results in structural changes at synapses (see Ch. 5). This is particularly true of experience early in life. A wide variety of early experiences cause an increase in the extent of the dendritic branching in output neurones, especially in the cortex.

Human memory sequence

After an initial sensory information storage stage, the memory passes through a temporary storage stage (short-term memory) before transfer to long-term storage. Children's memory ability increases up to about the age of 18 years, with a particular increase of memory ability at around 7 years.

Language acquisition

Babies are born as competent, active beings capable of complex, organised behavioural sequences. Initially communications are expressed non-verbally, then by co-ordinating behaviour with vocalisation and, finally, verbal expression. Communication is the exchange of thought and messages by speech, signals or writing. Language is the basis of communication and may be verbal or non-verbal.

Non-verbal communication

Early in life a baby can signal by crying, smiling, vocalising and chuckling and can show orientation by watching and listening. Smiling is elicited by human voices during the first month and by faces by 3 months.

Crying has identifiable characteristics for causes such as hunger and pain. Over the first 2–3 months, babies show a gradual increase in their ability to interact with other people.

Co-ordination of behaviour with vocalisation

Vocalisations start from the age of 7–8 weeks and progress into babbling at around 4 months. Neither vocalisation nor babbling is dependent on adequate hearing. By 4 months, babies can associate the tape-recorded speech of a parent with the appropriate parent. Babies lead communication at this stage, timing their movements and attention in a way that supports and strengthens the interaction. By 6 months, awareness of strangers begins.

Verbal communication

By 9 months babies use more complex vocalisations and early words. Children learn the meaning of words by associating them with objects but further development of language depends on simultaneously increasing cognitive skills. From the age of 9 months, babies develop knowledge that objects and events still exist when not being directly seen or experienced, of cause and effect and of yes/no understanding. This development of both spoken language and comprehension takes time to develop, comprehension often preceding speech by some months. For example, around the age of 18 months, a baby can often indicate the parts of the body such as the nose and mouth, not only on him- or herself but also on a doll of reasonable size. Naming of the body parts comes much later.

Situational understanding

Between 8 and 12 months the child understands familiar phrases as part of a sequence of events without the individual words having meaning.

Symbolic understanding

Approximate age levels for the levels of symbolic understanding are shown in Table 17.1.

Cognitive development

Piaget organised the growth of a child's mind into four periods (Piaget, 1967). In the sensorimotor period the child is preoccupied with co-ordinating his or her sensory and motor abilities (birth to 2 years). During the preoperational period (2–6 years), perception and language are the dominant areas of development. In

Table 17.1 Levels of symbolic understanding during a child's development

Concrete objects Understanding is shown by using objects appropriately, i.e. brushes hair with a hairbrush	12–18 months
Object representation Understanding of representational objects, e.g. in Wendy house play, small doll play and use of miniature toys, e.g. dolls' house furniture and dolls	18–21 months
Picture by name Understanding of two-dimensional representation	18–24 months
Picture by function	24–30 months
Matching symbol to symbol Matching small toys to non-identical pictures	24–30 months
Meaningful symbol	36–42 months
Alphabet/abstract symbol	4–5 years

the concrete operational period (7–11 years) the child acquires the ability to think intuitively, and during the period of formal operations (12 years plus) the ability to think logically and to understand the scientific method.

Personal, social and emotional development

The basic biological drives of a young infant change into the complex goals of childhood such as achievement and curiosity. Parents also influence their children, both through the genes passed to their offspring and through the family atmosphere in which the child grows. The first major social interactions occur within the family but after about 6 years of age both peers and educators come to exert increasingly more control over the child's social behaviour.

Nutritional needs of the developing CNS

The infant's developing brain has high nutritional needs. The findings from several authors confirm that undernutrition at an early age affects brain growth and intellectual quotient (Leiva Plaza et al., 2001). An increasing body of research is clarifying the essential fatty acids that are necessary, particularly for the formation of myelin (Brown, 1995). Brain lipids in the human infant are known to change according to dietary lipid intake and there are concerns that fatty acid deficiency may be partly related to the failure of myelination seen in some types of cerebral palsy. Myelin produced by inadequate means may be unstable and responsible for demyelination in later life. It is also known that certain nutritional deficiencies, such as that of folate, cause neural tube defects (see Ch. 19). Deficiency of iodine causes mental impairment and diplegia, and the role of zinc deficiency is under investigation.

References

Andre-Thomas YC, Saint-Anne Dargassies S. *The Neurological Examination of the Infant*. London: William Heinemann Medical Books Ltd; 1960.

Benson JB, Uzgiris IC. Effect of self-initiated locomotion on infant search activity. *Dev Psychol* 1985, **21**:923–931.

Bower TGR. *The Perceptual World of the Child*. London: Fontana; 1977.

Brazelton TB. *Neonatal Behavioural Assessment Scale*, 2nd edn. London: William Heinemann Medical Books; 1973.

Brown JK. Food for thought. *Dev Med Child Neurol* 1995, **37**:189–190.

Buisseret P, Gary-Bobo E, Imbert M. Ocular motility and recovery of orientation properties of visual cortical neurones in dark-reared kittens. *Nature (Lond)* 1978, **272**:816–817.

Butterworth G, Cicchetti D. Visual calibration of posture in normal and motor retarded Down's syndrome infants. *Perception* 1978, **7**:513–525.

Butterworth G, Hicks L. Visual proprioception and postural stability in infancy. A developmental study. *Perception* 1977, **6**:255–262.

Cowan WM. The development of the brain. In: *The Brain*. San Francisco: WH Freeman; 1979:298.

Eysenck MW. Cognitive development. In: Eysenck MW, ed. *A Handbook of Cognitive Psychology*. London: Lawrence Erlbaum; 1984:231–245.

Gary-Bobo E, Milleret C, Buisseret P. Role of eye movements in the developmental processes of orientation selectivity in the kitten's visual cortex. *Vision Res* 1986, **26**:557–567.

Gesell A, Armatruda C. *Developmental Diagnosis*, 2nd edn. New York: Harper & Row; 1947.

Gibson EJ, Walk PD. The 'visual cliff'. *Sci Am* 1960, **202**:64.

Green EM, Mulcahy CM, Pountney TE. An investigation into the development of early postural control. *Dev Med Child Neurol* 1995, **37**:437–448.

Grounds A. Child visual development. In: Barnard S, Edgar D, eds. *Pediatric Eye Care*. Oxford: Blackwell Science; 1996:43–74.

Hadders-Algra M. The Neuronal Group selection theory: a framework to explain variation in normal motor development. *Dev Med Child Neurol* 2000, **42**:566–572.

Hubel TH, Wiesel TN. Part 4, The Visual Pathways SD285, Module B3; Open University Press, 1985:36–55.

Illingworth RS. *The Development of the Young Child, Normal and Abnormal*, 8th edn. Edinburgh: Churchill Livingstone; 1983.

Laszlo JI, Bairstow PJ. *Perceptual–Motor Behaviour: Developmental Assessment and Therapy*. London: Holt, Rinehart & Winston; 1985.

Lee DN, Aronson E. Visual proprioceptive control of standing in human infants. *Percep Psychophys* 1974, **15**:529–532.

Leiva Plaza B, Inzunza Brito N, Perez Torrejon H et al. The impact of malnutrition on brain development, intelligence and school work performance. *Arch Latinoamer Nutr* 2001, **51**:64–71.

Levi-Montalcini R. Developmental neurobiology and the natural history of nerve growth factor. *Annu Rev Neurosci* 1982, **5**:341–362.

Noller K, Ingrisano D. Cross-sectional study of gross and fine motor development: birth to 6 years of age. *Phys Ther* 1984, **64**:308–316.

Piaget J. *The Child's Conception of the World*. Totowa, NJ: Littlefield, Adams; 1967.

Piper MC, Darrah J. *Motor Assessment of the Developing Infant*. Philadelphia: WB Saunders; 1994.

Prechtl HFR. *The Neurological Development of the Full Term Newborn Infant*, 2nd edn. London: William Heinemann Medical Books; 1977.

Prechtl HFR. *Continuity of Neural Functions from Prenatal to Postnatal Life*. London: Spastics International Medical Publications; 1984.

Prechtl HFR, Beintema DJ. *The Neurological Development of the Full Term Newborn Infant*. London: William Heinemann Medical Books; 1964.

Shepherd R, Carr J. An emergent or dynamical systems view of movement dysfunction. *Aust J Physio* 1991, **37**:4–5, 17.

Sporns O, Edelman GM. Solving Bernstein's problem: a proposal for the development of coordinated movement by selection. *Child Dev* 1993, **64**:960–981.

Thelen E, Kelso JAS, Fogel A. Self-organising systems and motor development. *Dev Rev* 1987, **7**:39–65.

Thompson RF. *The Brain*, 2nd edn. New York: WH Freeman; 1993.

Touwen B. *Neurological Development in Infancy*. London: William Heinemann Medical Books; 1976.

Touwen B. Development of the central nervous system. In: Harvey D, Miles M, Smyth D, eds. *Community Child Health*. Oxford: Butterworth Heinemann; 1995:396–400.

Yeates S. *The Development of Hearing*. Lancaster: MTP Press; 1980.

Chapter 18

The cerebral palsies and motor learning disorders

T Pountney   E Green

INTRODUCTION

In 1862, Little described spastic diplegia resulting from birth asphyxia and brain damage. However, Sigmund Freud suggested that infantile cerebral paralysis was caused by prenatal abnormalities, birth asphyxia being a marker for, rather than a cause of, brain dysfunction (Pellegrino, 1995). Little's views were widely accepted until the last 25 years, during which epidemiological studies have refuted the causation of cerebral palsy by birth trauma and asphyxia.

Greater understanding of genetic and other constitutional disorders has led to a change in the 'brain damage' model. This had been applied to a wide range of developmental disabilities ranging from cerebral palsy to mental retardation, learning disabilities and attention deficit-hyperactivity disorder (ADHD). Although there was little proof of actual brain damage, there was an assumption that a milder degree of birth asphyxia or other brain-damaging event had resulted in a milder form of impairment. Cerebral palsy is now more commonly used as a description of the disability suffered due to an unspecified deficit rather than of the impairment itself (see World Health Organization, 2001; and Ch. 3, p. 31).

A similar situation occurs with the less severe motor impairments seen as part of a generalised neurological dysfunction, such as in disorders of learning motor control and attention. These are now classified in the *Diagnostic and Statistical Manual of Mental Disorders* (American Psychiatric Association, 1994) by descriptions of observable behaviour rather than by aetiology.

The lifestyle and opportunities available to people with cerebral palsy have improved remarkably and many adults live independent, though supported, lives and contribute to society through employment and further education. Children with cerebral palsy have a right to mainstream education; they are accepted by their peers, included in holidays and outings, and can take part in competitive games. Advances in technology have also made a significant contribution, particularly in the area of communication.

Since cerebral palsy and motor learning disorders have different aetiologies, manifestations and management, they will be addressed in separate sections in this chapter.

CEREBRAL PALSY

Definition and diagnosis

'Cerebral palsy' is an umbrella term encompassing a wide range of different causative factors and describing an evolving disorder of motor function secondary to a non-progressive pathology of the immature brain. A definition by the World Commission for Cerebral Palsy in 1988 was: 'a persistent but not unchanging disorder of posture and movement, caused by damage to the developing nervous system, before or during birth or in the early months of infancy' (Griffiths & Clegg, 1988).

A diagnosis of cerebral palsy should not be made unless the motor disorder is obvious in comparison to other findings, such as developmental delay. This excludes most children with clumsiness and also children with a severe degree of mental retardation and motor signs such as mild spasticity or mild hypotonia.

Aetiology and incidence

Mutch et al. (1992) reported on a number of international meetings devoted to the epidemiology of cerebral palsy. There have been consistent reports of recent rises in the prevalence amongst live births of cerebral palsy and of its severity, particularly amongst preterm infants. The rises can be accounted for largely by improvements in survival rate, since the incidence of low birth weight and the birth weight-specific prevalence rates of cerebral palsy amongst birth weights of 2500 g or more seem to be remaining largely stable. Data are documented from the UK, Western Australia and Sweden, showing a consistent trend from low to high cerebral palsy rates as birth weight falls. Within countries in the low-birth-weight populations, there is a trend to higher rates of cerebral palsy as mortality falls. The birth weight-specific prevalence of cerebral palsy in the highest weight groups seems to remain stable within each population, despite falling mortality levels.

Some speculation still exists regarding the causes of cerebral palsy, largely because the expected drop in cases as obstetric care improved has not occurred. This has led to investigations that indicate there is a greater correlation between abnormalities during pregnancy and cerebral palsy than abnormalities during labour with cerebral palsy (Hagberg & Hagberg, 1996). Birth asphyxia accounts for approximately 10% of all cases with cerebral palsy and only a small number of these are due to poor obstetric care (Rosenbloom, 1995; Stanley et al., 2000). Infrared and magnetic resonance imaging indicate that the normal infant withstands considerable hypoxia during a normal labour and delivery without ill effect, suggesting that infants who suffer damage may have a pre-existing condition making them vulnerable to hypoxia (Stanley et al., 2000).

Two five-year studies of the changing epidemiology of cerebral palsy have shown a startling rise in the incidence of cerebral palsy amongst low- and very-low-birth-weight infants (Hagberg & Hagberg, 1996; Pharoah & Cooke, 1996). Such preterm infants now account for 50% of all cases of cerebral palsy compared to 32% at the start of the studies and this is now considered to be the strongest predictor of cerebral palsy in newborn infants, with a 30-fold increase in risk.

The developing brain of the fetus is a vulnerable organ; damage to it prior to birth is often dependent on the timing and type of insult, as well as the predilection of certain brain areas to certain types of insult (Stanley et al., 2000). These include hypoxia, vascular accidents, infections and toxicity. Pre- and periconceptional causes include familial or genetic influences, teratogens, such as the viral infections of toxoplasmosis, rubella, cytomegalovirus and herpes simplex virus (TORCH); fetal malformation syndromes; iodine deficiency and consanguinity (Stanley et al., 2000).

Multiple pregnancies are increasing within the developed countries and the higher rates of cerebral palsy reflect this increase (Pharoah et al., 1996; Stanley et al., 2000). Multiple pregnancy increases the risk of cerebral palsy to 4.5 times in a twin and to 18.2 times in a triplet pregnancy compared to singleton births (Stanley et al., 2000). The reasons for this increase include placental malformations, fetal growth and birth weight, intrapartum factors and co-fetal death. A proportion of affected children have lost a twin perinatally or in utero (Pharoah et al., 1996).

Cerebral palsy is also acquired postnatally in a significant number of cases, usually within the first year of life, the primary causes being cerebral infection and infantile spasms.

The changing aetiology of cerebral palsy has resulted in a changing pattern in the presentation of the condition, including increasing levels of visual impairment, eating and drinking difficulties, sleep disturbance and types of epilepsy.

Classification

It is traditional and clinically useful to classify cerebral palsy according to its type, distribution and severity. Type is categorised according to the impairment: spastic, dyskinetic, ataxic and hypotonic. Where a mixture of types is seen in one child, the classification will be made on the predominating form (McCarthy, 1992). Approximately 70% of children with cerebral palsy have spasticity, 20–25% have dyskinesia and the remaining 5–10% have ataxia (McCarthy, 1992).

The classical distribution of symptoms is:

- hemiplegia – one side of the body primarily involved
- diplegia – the lower half of the body primarily involved
- quadriplegia – the entire body is involved.

Common presentations include:

- Spastic quadriplegia – where a child has all four limbs involved with a mixture of spasticity and dyskinesia. Individuals in this group are usually at the severe end of motor disability and cannot sit or walk independently, and have little co-ordinated movement of their arms and hands

- Spastic diplegia – where there is increased tone in the legs but little or no involvement in the arms. This group can usually walk with or without aids but tend to adopt a 'W' kneeling posture in preference to long sitting

- Spastic hemiplegia is characterised by spasticity in the arm, leg and trunk on one side of the body, and most walk independently but there is a wide variation in the function of the affected arm and hand.

Severity of cerebral palsy can be classified according to the Gross Motor Classification Scale (GMCS). It is a five-level system, which ranks children according to the severity of motor involvement based on age, motor ability and use of assistive technology (Palisano et al., 1997).

Natural history

The natural history of cerebral palsy has been documented by several authors, including Crothers & Paine (1988) and Freud (1968), who present a picture of a child generally below normal size, with poor motor and cognitive skills and beset by deformities of joints and bones. The initial neurological lesion the child sustains, which causes the cerebral palsy, in fact remains by definition unchanged throughout life (Griffiths & Clegg, 1988). However, the effects of this lesion on other systems, including musculoskeletal and digestive systems, can be more debilitating than the original insult if left untreated.

There are associated complications of cerebral palsy, which include epilepsy, visual impairment, musculoskeletal deformities, growth delay, sleep disturbance and reduced life expectancy.

Epilepsy occurs frequently in children with cerebral palsy, with a higher incidence in children with quadriplegia than those with dyskinesia and spastic diplegia, especially preterm infants. Epilepsy is linked with an increased risk of sensory impairment and cognitive impairment. Damage to the brain only occurs if seizures are prolonged or as a result of infantile spasms in the first year of life (Aicardi, 1990). Seizures of this nature are often accompanied by developmental regression. Epilepsy is not necessarily a long-term condition and treatment with anticonvulsant therapy, such as carbamazepine or sodium valproate, is usually effective and many add-on medications are available to improve control. Surgical treatment is now an option for intractable seizures (Aicardi, 1990).

Most children with cerebral palsy experience some disorder of their sensory system, the most common of which is visual impairment (see below). Sensory deficits, which have a profound impact on movement co-ordination, are also found in the proprioceptive and tactile systems. Diminished anticipatory control and impaired tactile regulation in reaching and grasping objects have been demonstrated in children with cerebral palsy (Eliasson et al., 1995). These studies suggest that children with cerebral palsy have a diminished ability to build internal models of objects and movement patterns, and may require additional environmental cues to execute movement successfully. This is reflected in the improved performance of children who are asked to undertake concrete rather than abstract tasks, e.g. raising the arm to shoulder height or reaching for a ball (van der Weel et al., 1991).

Visual impairment in children with cerebral palsy is estimated at between 7 and 9%. Visual impairments can result from abnormalities of the eye but are more commonly a result of lesions in the retrochiasmatic visual pathway or the perceptual and processing areas of the brain responsible for visual stimuli (Guzzetta et al., 2001). Visual impairment has an important role in motor development, particularly the acquisition of trunk and head control (Sonksen et al., 1984).

It is commonly recognised that, as a group, children with severe cerebral palsy are considerably below the normal growth curves for height and weight. Nutritional problems in children with cerebral palsy are well recognised and can result in a failure to thrive and chronic ill health (Stallings et al., 1993; Krick et al., 1996). Nutritional factors and ability to walk have been shown to be significant factors in decreased bone mineral density in these children, making bones vulnerable to fracture (Henderson et al., 1995).

The main causes of this growth delay are problems with the facial and bulbar muscles making chewing and swallowing difficult, often requiring extended periods for eating amounting to several hours daily. Reflux may also occur, which can result in aspiration and consequent chest infection (Rogers et al., 1994). Gastrostomy insertions to provide enteral feeding have improved the nutritional status of many children and relieved carers and children of the time-consuming task of eating (Bachlet et al., 2002).

There is a high frequency of sleep disturbance in children with cerebral palsy and this has been attributed to a number of causes, including sleep hypoxaemia, upper-airway obstruction, decreased melatonin levels, nocturnal seizures, reflux and positional discomfort (Khan et al., 1996). Hypoxaemia is probably due to brainstem dysfunction and upper-airway obstruction from hypertrophy of the tonsils and adenoids, and both are implicated in night-wakening (Khan et al., 1996). Children with visual impairment due to malformation of the eyes or abnormalities and malformations of the sleep centres in the brain may experience dysfunction of melatonin release, which regulates sleep patterns and can in some cases be treated by melatonin (Hung et al., 1998).

The life expectancy of children with cerebral palsy has been investigated in two well-researched studies (Evans et al., 1990; Crichton et al., 1995): both found high survival rates of around 90% into their teens and 20s. Immobility and severe learning difficulties were cited as the main factors influencing survival. Evans et al.'s study (1990) concluded that 'cerebral palsy is a condition with which one lives rather than a condition from which one dies' and that long-term planning is realistic to meet the needs of this group as adults.

Musculoskeletal deformities in different types of cerebral palsy

The neurological lesion will slow the development of normal patterns of movement, often resulting in the adoption of asymmetrical postures and limited ranges of movement. This will cause muscle and bone to develop in different ways, resulting in imbalances in muscle groups, deformities of joints and bones, and often osteoporosis in children unable to walk independently. The development of deformity is largely related to the child's motor activity, and consequently different distributions and type of cerebral palsy result in different patterns of deformities. The treatment and management of these deformities are through the use of hands-on therapy, postural management equipment, orthotics, botulinum toxin and surgery. These approaches and their use and efficacy will be described later in this chapter.

Hemiplegia

Children with hemiplegia often experience underdevelopment of the affected side, which results in smaller limbs on this side and leg-shortening. Equinus of the foot and ankle, flexion of the elbow, wrist and fingers, and adducted thumb are classical deformities of the child with hemiplegia.

Spastic diplegia

The deformities most commonly associated with spastic diplegia are contractures of the hip flexors and adductors, the hamstrings and internal rotation of the hip and femoral anteversion. Most of this group of children walk independently and these deformities develop as a result of the crouch gait adopted by many children with spastic diplegia due to spasticity in the hip adductors and flexors, hamstrings and calf muscles. Children in this group may alternatively develop hyperextension of the knee to compensate for tight tendo-achilles (Fig. 18.1). Kyphosis may develop as a sequela to tight hamstrings or hyperlordosis as a compensatory balance mechanism.

Quadriplegia

The deformities seen in children and adults with quadriplegic cerebral palsy include the deformities described above but, in addition, many develop dislocation of their hip joints and spinal curvature. Hip subluxation or dislocation can cause significant morbidity in terms of pain, and difficulty with postural control, causing limitations in sitting, standing and walking, and hygiene and personal care considerations. An association between hip dislocation and spinal curvature is well documented and children with a windswept deformity of the hip and pelvis, where the hip is subluxated or dislocated and the pelvis is in obliquity, present a precursor to spinal curvature.

In the group of children who do not walk independently, approximately 60% of this group will have one or both hips dislocated by the age of 5 years. It is recognised that dislocation continues to occur well into adolescence (Miller & Bagg, 1992). Scrutton & Baird (1997) offered a protocol for the surveillance of hips in young children, which recommends a baseline X-ray at 30 months to determine risk (Figs 18.2 and 18.3).

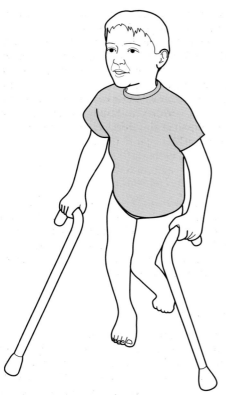

Figure 18.1 Diplegic gait with internal rotation, excessive hip and knee flexion and lack of heel strike. (Reproduced from McCarthy (2002), with permission.)

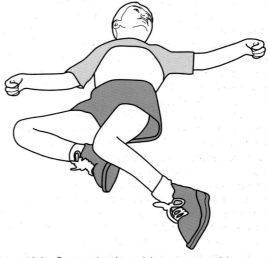

Figure 18.2 Posture showing pelvic asymmetry with subluxation of the left hip.

Figure 18.3 Hip and pelvic X-ray showing dislocation of the right hip.

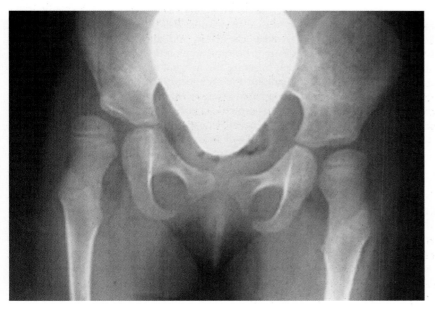

Spinal curvatures

Spinal curvature occurs in up to 70% of children with bilateral cerebral palsy, being most prevalent in those with quadriplegia. Scoliosis is the most common curve seen but kyphosis and hyperlordosis are also common. Rotatory elements are present in many spinal curves and combinations of curve patterns, such as kyphoscoliosis, are frequently present. Spinal curvature can occur from a very young age and continue to progress well into adulthood, with individuals with the spastic form of cerebral palsy at greatest risk (Lonstein, 1995; Saito et al., 1998).

Joint pain

Many of these musculoskeletal deformities will cause joint pain in adults with cerebral palsy and a study by Schwartz et al. (1999) reported that 67% of their subjects had pain in one or more areas for durations greater than 3 months. The lower limb and back were the most common areas where pain was experienced. Strategies need to be implemented to avoid deformities where possible and also to help individuals control the frequency and duration of painful episodes.

Medications

Medications are frequently used in children with bilateral cerebral palsy to control epilepsy, reflux and high muscle tone. The use of anticonvulsants is a complex balance between controlling seizures and causing adverse side-effects. Antiemetics are used to control gastric reflux and are considered the first line of control for this problem. Baclofen, which can be taken orally or intrathecally, is one of the main pharmacological treatments for spasticity and acts to inhibit the gamma-aminobutyric acid (GABA)-B receptors in the spinal cord by blocking the excitatory effect of sensory input (Ivanhoe et al., 2001). Intrathecal baclofen is increasing in popularity as it is thought to be more effective, as baclofen does not cross the blood–brain barrier well and side-effects are limited.

Botulinum toxin

Botulinum toxins are protein products of the *Clostridium botulinum* bacterium, which are taken up by endocytosis at the cholinergic nerve terminals, blocking release of synaptic vesicles. This effectively blocks the action of the synapse at the neuromuscular junction. The effect lasts for several months until a new neuromuscular junction is established (Cosgrove et al., 1994). Botulinum toxin in children with bilateral cerebral palsy is used to reduce increased tone for a period of time in selected muscles, to enable the establishment of new movement patterns and the reduction of contractures (Cosgrove et al., 1994). Carr et al. (1998) recommend criteria for patient selection, dosage, administration and likely long-term effects. This approach is rapidly gaining popularity as a method of improving gait in children with spastic hemiplegia and diplegia, with several studies showing encouraging results (Koman et al., 2000; Ubhi et al., 2000; Metaxiotis et al., 2002).

The effectiveness of botulinum toxin is known to decrease with age and there are some limited side-effects, usually related to administration, such as incontinence.

SURGICAL AND ORTHOPAEDIC MANAGEMENT

The musculoskeletal deformities which can result from different types of cerebral palsy have been mentioned earlier and every effort should be made to prevent the development of these deformities by conservative methods but in many cases orthopaedic surgery is required at some point to alleviate deformities.

Orthopaedic surgery needs to be undertaken in full consultation with the individual, family and/or carers so that they have an understanding of postoperative care and the long-term management required to prevent recurrence of the deformity. The surgery should form part of the individual's overall physical management programme.

Soft-tissue surgery involves the release of tendon, muscle or connective tissue and usually aims to equalise the muscle length balance across joints. By lengthening a muscle or tendon it is theorised that it effectively weakens its action and allows the opposing muscle group to become dominant. In the hip joint it will aim to help recentre the femoral head. Bony surgery involves changing the architecture of the bone and sometimes the joint to alter the biomechanics of movement and improve muscle action. In many cases a combination of soft tissue and bony surgery will be performed.

Multilevel surgery at the hip, knee and ankle is used in children with diplegia to improve their gait and can be extremely successful if the postoperative exercise programme is followed. This type of surgical intervention can prevent the 'birthday syndrome', where surgery at one level results in muscle contracture developing in the proximal muscles, which then requires surgery the following year.

There have been a number of studies undertaken to determine the outcome of different types of surgical interventions but many compounding variables, such as postoperative management, use of different surgical techniques, the measurement of outcome, the length of follow-up and heterogeneity of the sample in terms of age and physical ability, make analysis of the findings difficult (Reimers, 1980; Moreau et al., 1995; Cottalorda et al., 1998; Song & Carroll, 1998; Abel et al., 1999; Turker & Lee, 2000). However, for hip surgery some criteria have been established, including indications that soft-tissue surgery is unlikely when the hip is migrated over 40% and that bony surgery is indicated at this level (Barrie & Galasko, 1996).

Surgical correction of spinal curvature is considered when a curve is greater than 35–40° and there is an increasing difficulty in positioning.

Selective dorsal rhizotomy

Selective dorsal rhizotomy (SDR) is a neurosurgical technique to divide the posterior nerve rootlets in the lumbosacral region to reduce the level of spasticity, in particular muscle groups of the lower limb. The roots are selected by stimulation to determine which are responsible for innervating each muscle. Results are dependent on the skill of the surgeon and pre- and postoperative physiotherapy (Hare et al., 1998). The technique is only used rarely in the UK but is quite widespread in the USA (Heim et al., 1995; Chicoine et al., 1997). Several studies have reviewed the outcomes of SDR, with little definitive evidence of its effectiveness and a possible risk of spinal deformity (Turi & Kalen, 2000).

PHYSICAL MANAGEMENT

Motor assessment

Assessment of motor ability can be made by using the positive signs of the neurological lesion; tone, spasticity and reflex activity; or the negative signs of muscle weakness, fatigue and co-ordination. Some physiotherapists will use a combination of these factors. Assessment needs to be objective, relevant and act as a guide to intervention. Many of the positive signs are subjective, due to the variability of the examiner's interpretation and dependent on the position. Assessment of the biomechanical aspects of ability, e.g. position of head, shoulder and pelvis, and co-ordination are more likely to guide prescription of treatment. The normal model of motor activity provides our only consistent model and is therefore used as a basis for general motor assessments and gait analysis.

Commonly used tests

There exists a wealth of measures for assessing functional and motor skills in children with cerebral palsy.

Some of the most commonly used tests include:

- Gross Motor Function Measure – GMFM (Russell et al., 2002)
- Chailey Levels of Ability – CLA (Pountney et al., 2000)
- Movement Assessment of Infants – MAI (Chandler et al., 1980)
- Bayley Scales of Infant Development – BSID (Bayley, 1983)
- Pediatric Evaluation of Disability Index – PEDI (Haley et al., 1992, 1993)
- Alberta Infant Motor Scale – AIMS (Piper & Darrah, 1994)
- Peabody Development Motor Scales – PDMS (Folio & Fewell, 1983)
- gait analysis.

The approach to assessment and the structure of the tests are variable, and selection of the appropriate test is made according to the child's age and level of physical and cognitive ability.

The AIMS, MAI and PDMS are screening tools for identification of children at risk. The AIMS is a naturalistic, norm-referenced test based on age- and sex-stratified normative data, which is capable of differentiating infants' development into abnormal, suspicious or normal. The MAI and PDMS offer a more structured approach with more emphasis on tone and reflexes.

The GMFM is a structured test which consists of 88 items in five sections. It is scored according to how much of each specified skill the child achieves. It does not evaluate how the movement is achieved but is a measure of the quality of the movement and is currently under development. The sensitivity of this test at the severe end of motor ability is limited.

The CLA offers a scale which is sensitive at low levels of ability up to independent standing (see 'Positioning and postural management', below). It does not include assessment of walking. This scale is a naturalistic assessment based on developmental biomechanics and assesses ability in lying, sitting and standing. Components of the levels clearly identify which aspect of postural development is hindering achievement of higher ability levels. The scale is widely used as a prescription for postural management equipment.

In adults with cerebral palsy there are fewer options, particularly for the more severely affected. The GMFM and CLA can continue to be used into adulthood, as well as functional measures such as the Barthel Index (Mahoney & Barthel, 1965) and the Functional Independence Measure or FIM (Granger et al., 1986).

Assessment of walking is now increasingly undertaken in sophisticated gait laboratories. This method of assessment has led to a better analysis of the cause of gait abnormalities by distinguishing between the primary factors of motor control abnormalities and the secondary factors of inadequate muscle growth and bony deformity. Appropriate aspects of the abnormality can thus be corrected (Gage & Novacheck, 2001). Simplified assessment using observation and video analysis can be useful for less complex gait problems.

The PEDI is a useful measure of a child's level of function with or without the use of assistive technology. It evaluates the areas of self-care, mobility and transfers, and social function (Haley et al., 1992).

Treatment approaches

The treatment of children with bilateral cerebral palsy has seen the development of many treatment methods: Winthrop Phelps, Vojta, Conductive Education, Bobath and Doman Delacato (Scrutton, 1984). In the mid-part of the twentieth century, treatment was largely orthopaedic in emphasis, concentrating on surgery and splinting. The late 1950s and early 1960s saw a swing towards a neurological emphasis (Bobath and Vojta), followed by a functional approach (Conductive Education) and finally a synthesis of all these methods, with the Chailey approach (Pountney et al., 1990, 2000) and Hare approach (Hare et al., 1998).

As yet, there is no evidence that any one method is superior to another (see Ch. 21). Hur (1995) reviewed 37 studies of therapeutic interventions for children with cerebral palsy and concluded that, although some studies showed some improvements, these were rarely sustained and for most the sample size or methodology was not rigorous enough to demand a change in practice. A more recent randomised controlled trial of intensities of treatment, goal-setting and current levels of physiotherapy found no significant differences between the groups (Bower et al., 2001). Below are described some orthodox physiotherapy approaches and some alternative therapies now available.

Neurodevelopmental therapy

The most widely used form of neurodevelopmental therapy (NDT) is the Bobath approach. Bobath, who originally devised this approach in the 1940s, suggested that moving and handling patients in a certain way could inhibit spastic patterns of movement, allowing the emergence of more normal patterns. The treatment techniques involve specialised handling, with control being given at key points to inhibit spasticity and guide movements. Such techniques are taught to the parents of the child in order that they may be continued at home. A rationale to support these practical

findings was developed around the idea that brain lesions result in the release of abnormal movement patterns of co-ordination, abnormal postural tone and disordered reciprocal innervation (Bobath, 1980).

This theoretical hierarchical rationale for this approach has been refuted by more recent studies on the nervous system. Bobath methods of handling continue to provide a cornerstone for physiotherapeutic treatment but a review of the evidence on NDT by Butler & Darrah (2001) concluded that there was no consistent evidence that it facilitated more normal motor development or functional activity, or changed the amount of abnormal movement. Butler & Darrah (2001) suggested that not all therapists have 'kept pace with the evolution of the approach', which recognises the importance of the interaction between biomechanical and neurological aspects of motor development (Neilson & McCaughey, 1982; Carr et al., 1995; Mayston, 1995).

Conductive Education

Conductive Education, also known as the Peto method, is an approach to the treatment of children with cerebral palsy which was brought to the UK from Hungary. Users of this approach describe it as a system of education which encompasses motor development and aims to engage children in active learning (Hari & Tillemans, 1984). Conductive Education programmes are provided in structured groups led by a conductor, who combines the roles of a teacher and therapist. In younger children, songs and rhythmic intention are used to encourage movement. Older children use task analysis. Studies in Australia and the UK have found little difference between the progress of children using traditional approaches and those involved in Conductive Education (Bairstow et al., 1993; Reddihough et al., 1998). There have been some criticisms of this approach because of its intensive nature with little evidence of improved outcomes (Oliver, 1990; Pountney et al., 2000).

Hare approach

The Hare approach to assessment and treatment focuses on the underlying disorder of posture and movement rather than neurological signs. Assessment is made in all positions, with attention paid to the relationship between the trunk and body parts, and the supporting surface. Levels of ability are identified on fundamental postural skills. Treatment techniques involve the use of arm and leg gaiters, below-knee plaster boots, aids and adapted furniture. The approach is applicable for all ages (Hare et al., 1998).

Eclectic approach

Limitations imposed by time restraints and service delivery options mean in reality that most therapists select from the variety of treatments available, which best meet the child's and family's situation. Elements of the Bobath approach are used in individual sessions, whereas Conductive Education ideas may be used in group work. Children react in different ways to different approaches and play often provides the vehicle for delivering treatment to maintain interest and motivation.

Parental ability to continue treatment programmes outside sessions is variable and strict adherence to specific treatment methods can therefore be limited. Bower et al. (2001) found little difference between the type or intensity of treatment in the change of GMFM score, suggesting that eclectic approaches, which fit into family lifestyles, are appropriate.

Key points

- There is no evidence that any one treatment method is superior to another
- Therapists select, from the variety of treatments available, those which best meet the child's and family's needs

Strength-training

There is growing evidence of the benefits of strength-training programmes in improving functional ability in individuals with cerebral palsy and this needs to be considered as part of physiotherapy interventions. Concerns regarding the increase of spasticity with muscle strengthening have been refuted (see Ch. 29). Damiano et al. (2002) stressed the importance of differentiating between repetitive practice and specific training programmes designed to increase muscle strength.

Recent work on the gastrocnemius muscles suggests that muscle strength may have an important role to play in the maintenance of muscle length (Shortland et al., 2002). The study of children with spastic diplegia found that muscle fibre length was not reduced and it was suggested that decreased fibre diameter may shorten the aponeuroses to cause contracture (see also Ch. 29).

Alternative therapies

There is a burgeoning number of alternative therapies available to parents, often at great personal expense. The most widely used of these are hyperbaric oxygen therapy (HOT), acupuncture and cranial sacral therapy (CST). Very few studies have been undertaken to establish the effectiveness of these approaches. A randomised multicentre trial of HOT in Canada found no differences in GMFM scores between children receiving minimal air pressures and those receiving HOT (Collet et al., 2001).

Conclusion

With lack of firm evidence for the efficacy of any one current therapy approach, there is a need to look more closely at theories of motor development and motor learning, and compare outcomes of other rehabilitation approaches, such as muscle-strengthening and assistive technologies.

Management strategies

Management strategies differ from treatment approaches, as they reflect the need for ongoing interventions which support the individual beyond the confines of physiotherapy treatment. Examples of these strategies will be orthotics, postural management, positioning programmes, medications, botulinum toxin and orthopaedic management. These management strategies often require multiprofessional collaboration, which includes clients and often their families along with a pooling of resources to achieve the desired outcomes. Many of these strategies will begin early in life and continue through child- and adulthood to meet the individual's changing needs.

Positioning and postural management

The role of positioning and management of posture begins in the neonatal unit. Grenier (1988) described the early effects of muscle shortening and bony malformation, which can be aggravated in the neonatal period by the 'frog-lying' position commonly adopted by premature infants. This posture results in shortening of the iliopsoas and adductor muscles, and exerts a rotational force leading to excessive anteversion. Protocols for positioning infants at this stage are available (Harrison, 1998).

From the earliest possible age, parents should be taught and encouraged to carry, position and move their child in a way which promotes normal movement and discourages abnormal, stereotypical patterns (see Ch. 5, p. 64). This type of approach should be incorporated into the child's normal activities and not occur as an isolated daily activity. This should also become a lifelong approach and be complemented by postural management equipment.

Postural management forms an essential element of a physiotherapy programme for children and adults with cerebral palsy who are unable to maintain the lying, sitting or standing posture independently, cannot change position or require extra support to maintain their postural stability when active. Without appropriate support, these individuals are unable to participate in many activities or do so in postures which are likely to lead to deformity.

At Chailey Heritage Clinical Services, a 24-h approach to postural management has been developed to prevent musculoskeletal deformities, whilst improving the ability of individuals with low motor abilities to participate more actively in life, with the use of powered mobility and communication aids (Pountney et al., 2000). The approach combines postural control in the positions of lying, sitting and standing with hands-on therapy, active exercise programmes, such as cycling, horseriding and swimming, and is supported by education programmes for users, parents and professionals.

The postures simulate a higher level of physical ability by changing the load-bearing surface and positioning the head, shoulder girdle, trunk, pelvis and legs. The postures adopted within the Chailey postural management equipment are based on a scheme of assessment, the Chailey Levels of Ability (Green et al., 1995). The levels detail the position of the head, shoulder and pelvic girdles and limbs, and the load-bearing pattern of infants from birth through lying and sitting to achieving independent standing.

These biomechanical data have informed the design of this equipment. Lying, sitting and standing supports provide a starting position for movement and allow a range of movement within which the child can move and recover balance. With a stable base, the child's use of his or her head, arms and legs can be more controlled. Control of the hip, pelvis and spine is achieved by applying corrective forces via the supporting surface, lateral thoracic and pelvic control and kneeblocks. Figures 18.4 and 18.5 illustrate the effect of seating on balance and movement (Pountney et al., 2000). The use of the Chailey 24-h postural management approach prior to hip subluxation has been shown to reduce the level of hip subluxation significantly (Pountney et al., 2002).

The neuronal group selection theory (NGST; see Ch. 17, p. 309) suggests that the selection of motor patterns is dependent on behaviour and experience. The use of positioning through equipment and hands-on activities, which promote the experience of normal movement, should logically improve movement pattern selection in young children (Hadders-Algra,

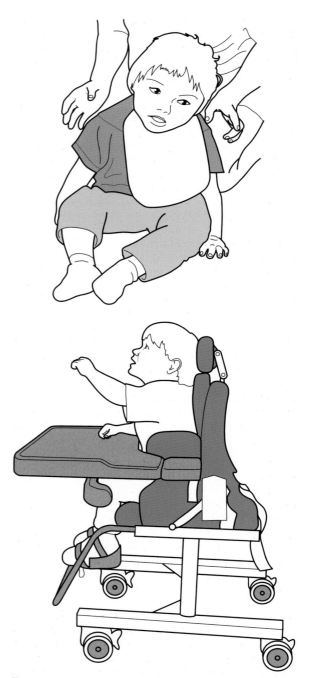

Figures 18.4 and 18.5 Impact on posture and functional ability of placing the patient in special seating.

2000). These effects occur early in development and intervention should begin as soon as motor impairments are identified. A symmetrical lying position is achieved at approximately 3 months in the normal infant and persistence beyond this age should alert clinicians to possible motor impairment. In the older population, neuroplastic adaptation can occur at a peripheral level. In both instances, more time needs to be spent in the postures which promote the desired movement than those that do not. The effect of postural management in improving functional ability may be explained by the theory of reducing the degrees of freedom during skill acquisition. This has been a long-recognised method of achieving motor skills (Turvey et al., 1982; Vereijken et al., 1992). Higher levels of function are possible within postural management equipment, as the number of motor tasks requiring attention at any one time is reduced and concentration can be focused on specific motor or cognitive tasks.

Night positioning   Night positioning for sleep appears to be a crucial element of the programme, possibly because it offers a substantial time period of gentle muscle stretch while muscle activity is quiet. Several studies indicate that periods of between 5 and 7 h are required to change muscle length (Tardieu et al., 1988; Lespargot et al., 1994). Postural support at night must promote good-quality sleep, which can be compromised by a number of factors, such as nocturnal seizures, reflux oesophagitis and nocturnal hypoxaemia. Supine positioning can aggravate some of these conditions, and investigation and observation of these conditions must be carried out prior to allowing a child to sleep unattended in a postural support (Cartwright, 1984; Martin et al., 1995).

Seating   A variety of seating options are available, including corner seats, forward-lean seats and 90/90 systems, and evaluation of these products needs to be made to ensure appropriate posture is achieved (Pope, 2002). Older children and adults who have fixed deformities may require more complex systems which are contoured to the body's shape to accommodate the deformities. Every effort should be made to prevent further deterioration of posture and this may include the use of sleep systems (Fig. 18.6).

Standing   The opportunity to stand has long been cited as important in the development of bone joint development but there is limited evidence to support this. Stuberg (1992) recommended that children should weight-bear for an hour four to five times a week in order to enhance bone and joint development (Fig. 18.7).

Assistive technology

Assistive technology is an umbrella term for a wide range of equipment, which ranges from simple devices

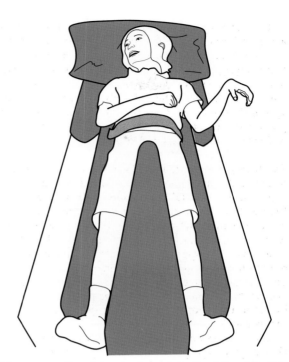

Figure 18.6   Use of sleep support to correct existing deformity of the spine and hips.

such as walking sticks to complex electronic equipment, such as environmental control equipment or communication aids (Cook & Hussey, 1995). Assistive technology offers individuals an opportunity to achieve a level of independence in a number of areas, including play, environmental controls, mobility and communication.

From a very young age children can start to learn basic switch skills, cause and effect, momentary versus press-and-hold operation through battery-operated toys. These skills can be transferred to the use of environmental, mobility and communication systems.

Mobility options for individuals include powered wheelchairs, which are available for small children upwards, and driver-assist modules which offer protection from obstacles and prevent the driver from hurting others or themselves while learning to control the powered mobility. Advice should always be sought when choosing assistive technology and this is available from a number of sources. Occupational therapists are traditionally the group who hold knowledge about a wide range of assistive technology and there are a number of centres nationally which give advice on this type of equipment (see Appendix). Centres include the

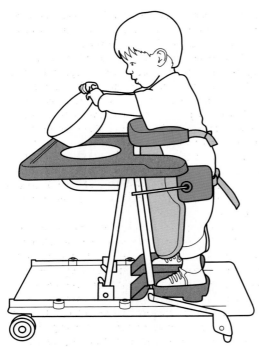

Figure 18.7 Use of standing support enabling functional activity.

Ace Centre (www.ace-centre.org.uk), Ability net (www.abilitynet.org.uk) and the Disabled Living Foundation (www.dlf.org.uk).

Orthotics

Orthotic management offers a conservative approach to prevent deformity, improve joint alignment and biomechanics and improve function. Orthoses provide intimate control of joints, which is not possible in positioning equipment. Evidence is available of the immediate impact of orthotics on gait but very little rigorous evidence exists on the long-term effect of orthotics (Morris, 2002).

Lower-limb orthotics can be used to provide stability in standing transfers, clearance in swing and support for children with limited walking ability. Orthoses need to be used with care, as excessive use can lead to immobility and consequent muscle weakness and atrophy (Shortland et al., 2002). Prescription for orthoses needs to be made in the light of the theories of muscle and bone adaptation, and joint biomechanics to ensure that satisfactory outcomes are achieved.

Hip and spinal orthoses (HASO) are prescribed to control hip and spine position but there is no literature to support their effectiveness. Thoracolumbosacral orthoses (TLSO) are used to control spinal curvature during growth. The construction of these jackets varies widely between orthotists and includes front or side opening, complete shells or shells with selected areas cut away. There is no evidence that spinal orthoses can reduce the rate of progression in scoliosis but studies have only introduced bracing when the degree of spinal curvature exceeded 25°. A clinical benefit of improved sitting balance has been cited (Miller et al., 1996).

MULTIPROFESSIONAL AND MULTIAGENCY WORKING

Cerebral palsy is a condition which requires multiprofessional and multiagency involvement to meet the needs of individuals and their families. Children and adults with cerebral palsy are likely to be involved with a variety of health professionals, possibly from more than one centre, social services and education. Local health commissioners are responsible for ensuring that clear methods for collaboration exist between social services and the local education authority (LEA) to fulfil their joint responsibilities of meeting children's needs.

This form of collaborative working requires liaison between agencies, both at senior organisational levels and at operational levels to ensure frameworks and resources are in place, including pooling of budgets and integration of commissioning which can best support services for individuals with cerebral palsy. For children, the current *Special Educational Needs (SEN) Code of Practice* (2001) aims to increase the number of children with disabilities in mainstream education and, as such, necessitates much closer working between agencies.

The transition to adult services often results in a reduction of medical and therapy input, and therefore preparation in terms of equipment provision and therapy needs to be put in place before leaving children's services.

CASE HISTORY

Cerebral palsy

SA was one of twins born at 28 weeks' gestation at his local maternity unit where he was ventilated at 3 min for respiratory distress. After 3 days he was weaned off the ventilator but reintubated due to increasing apnoeas and desaturations. At 10 days he was transferred to a tertiary unit for neonatal care. He continued to be ventilated until day 14, when his condition became more stable. He had a stormy neonatal period during which he developed periventricular leukomalacia. At 7 weeks of age he returned home and came under the care of his local team.

Initial involvement included physiotherapy on a weekly basis at the local child development centre. Physiotherapy included parental advice on handling the child to promote normal motor development; positioning for play, sleep and feeding; and stretches to maintain muscle length. At 7 months of age he was able to achieve symmetry in supine and prone but unable to sit independently. When held in sitting he had a rounded spinal profile and a tendency to push back into extension. At this time concerns were raised regarding his level of useful vision. At home he had a simple contoured seat which was used for play, eating and drinking.

At 12 months of age there was little change in his physical ability and it was decided to prescribe a modular seating system, which maintained hip and pelvic position, and provided good position for hand control and a standing support.

From 2 years he used an adapted trike and began to attend a swimming group, using a head flotation aid. He tried a variety of walkers, none of which were found to be useful in terms of mobility or exploratory activities.

SA continued to have difficulty with eating and drinking, and mealtimes were prolonged. He gained weight slowly but steadily and had high-calorie supplements to help with weight gain.

At this age he still did not have an established sleep pattern. Investigation of sleeping habits revealed some behavioural issues but also the possibility of upper-airway obstruction. His adenoids were removed and consequently his sleep pattern improved.

At 2½ years he joined a mulitdisciplinary therapy group at the Child Development Centre (CDC) with input from occupational therapist, physiotherapist and speech and language therapist to work on physical, play and communication skills. A simple picture-based communication system was devised to enable him to make choices.

At 30 months he had a routine X-ray to screen for hip and spinal problems. His hips showed only limited migration and were deemed not to be at risk. Clinically he had a postural scoliosis with a curve to the left from the lumbar region. This was completely correctable and therefore no intervention was taken at this time but annual monitoring was implemented.

At 3½ years he joined a nursery attached to a special school and his medical and therapy care were transferred there. He was beginning to show

decreased range of movement at his ankles and stood on his tiptoes. Ankle–foot orthoses were prescribed to maintain the length of the tendo-achilles.

He continued to use his seating and standing supports, and was introduced at this stage to assistive technology to facilitate his ability to play with toys, access a computer and begin independent mobility.

At school age he joined the mainstream primary school with a specialist unit for children with SEN where his twin was attending. He had a full-time learning support assistant (LSA) who enabled him to access most of the curriculum with the help of assistive technology. He received weekly physiotherapy sessions at school and a daily programme of stretches by the LSA.

At home, adaptations were made to his house to provide a downstairs bathroom and bedroom. Doors and corridors were made wide enough to manoeuvre a wheelchair. Respite care with a local family was introduced for one weekend a month to relieve family stresses, and because a new baby was due.

At age 11 he transferred to a residential school for weekly boarding. His parents were struggling with his full-time care and his mother had a back problem and was unable to help with lifting. At 13 his spinal curve increased to about 25° and a TLSO was prescribed. He was also exhibiting equinus deformity of the foot and some mild contractures of the upper limb. None of these has an impact on functional activity and therefore only the stretching programme was increased. He continued to use his ankle–foot orthoses.

He used a powered chair and computer with specialised switches. At 15 years, the standing programme was stopped due to manual handling issues and a reluctance on the part of SA to stand.

At 19 years he left school and returned home with care assistance. He attended local tertiary college for a course in computing skills. Employment prospects were limited. He moved into a small unit for adults with disabilities with carer support. At this stage, physiotherapy input was on a needs-led basis with intervention on request. No regular treatment was available and his carers were encouraged to do passive movements. SA was encouraged to take part in some active exercise, such as swimming, if possible.

MOTOR LEARNING DISORDERS (DEVELOPMENTAL CO-ORDINATION DISORDER)

Introduction

In the 1960s minimal brain dysfunction (MBD) used to be a definition describing a group of children who had combinations of perception, language, attention, impulse control and motor control impairments. The term 'disorders of attention, motor and perception' or DAMP was used, particularly in Scandinavia. These umbrella terms fell into disrepute and, as explained at the start of this chapter, different areas of dysfunction were identified and given separate diagnostic categories. At least four separate areas of dysfunction have emerged (Kadesco & Gillberg, 1998):

1. **behavioural problems**, such as hyperactivity disorder, ADHD, oppositional defiance disorder (ODD) and conduct disorder
2. **motor-control problems** (clumsy child syndrome, motor perception dysfunction, specific disorder of motor development, motor learning difficulties or developmental co-ordination disorder (DCD))
3. **specific learning disorders** such as dyslexia and dyscalculia
4. **other cognitive disturbances** such as language disorder.

However, it has become clear that these areas of dysfunction are not isolated but that there are a number of comorbidities or other areas of dysfunction. For example, children with ADHD often have comorbid learning problems or motor control difficulties (Reeves & Werry, 1987). Children with DCD or clumsiness often have associated behavioural problems and specific learning disorder (Bax & Whitmore, 1987)

and visual–perceptual problems (Lord & Hulme, 1987). Children who have specific language impairment may be clumsy and have perceptual problems as well. One way of illustrating this is shown in Figure 18.8.

Incidence

Much of the data on incidence has come from Scandinavia, where there have been a number of longitudinal studies. Using the terminology at the start of the studies, DAMP has been shown to be a common childhood symptom combination, occurring about 1 in 20 in Swedish children aged 6 years (Gillberg et al., 1982; Landgren et al., 1996). Using the modern terminology, Kadesco & Gillberg (1998) conducted a population study in a Swedish town of 409 children. The rate of the combination of ADHD and DCD was 6.1%, with boys being affected more frequently than girls. There was considerable overlap between ADHD and DCD, with about half of each diagnostic group meeting the criteria for the other diagnosis. Clumsiness showed striking stability over time. Kadesco & Gillberg (2001) examined patterns of comorbid or associated diagnoses in a population sample of children with ADHD. Eighty-seven per cent of this group had one or more and 67% at least two comorbid diagnoses. The most common comorbidities were oppositional defiance disorder and DCD.

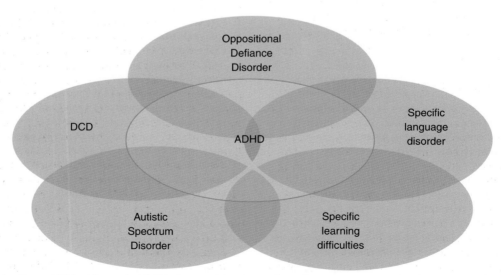

Figure 18.8 Co-morbidities of attention deficit–hyperactivity disorder (ADHD), developmental co-ordination disorder (DCD), specific learning difficulties, autistic spectrum disorder, specific language disorder and oppositional defiance disorder.

Aetiology

The majority of children in this group do not have a medical diagnosis and their problems are thought to be constitutional, often genetically based, in origin. A large number of potential diagnoses must be excluded by medical examination before a diagnosis of developmental co-ordination disorder is made by exclusion. Some important ones include: cerebral palsy, neuromuscular diseases such as early Duchenne muscular dystrophy (see Ch. 20), epilepsy, congenital hypothyroidism and hydrocephalus.

Landgren et al. (1998) performed a population-based case–control study analysing the contribution of background factors in the pathogenesis of DAMP. They found that low socioeconomic class was common in the DAMP group. Familial language disorder and familial motor clumsiness were found at higher rates in the DAMP group. Neuropathic risk factors in utero were also more common in the children with DAMP. Maternal smoking during pregnancy appeared to be an important risk factor. Language problems were present in two-thirds of the DAMP children and sleep problems and gastrointestinal disorders, but not atopy or otitis media, were significantly more common in the DAMP group.

Although little is known about the nature of the underlying cause of the motor control difficulties of children with co-ordination problems, there is some evidence to suggest that the construction of the central motor programme may be problematic for this group (Williams et al., 1992). For example, the sequence and timing of muscle responses involved in correcting for anterior or posterior sway are significantly more variable in children with co-ordination problems than in normal children. Response latencies are also longer in the former group.

Natural history of DAMP or ADHD/DCD

In Sweden, a number of short, intermediate and long-term studies of population-based groups of children with and without DAMP, diagnosed at 6–7 years, confirmed the long-term chronic nature of these difficulties (Gillberg & Gillberg, 1989). However the nature of the difficulties may change over the years.

Follow-up for behavioural problems in this group at age 10 years confirmed a high rate in the children with DAMP (Gillberg et al., 1983). School achievement problems were examined in the same group and age-matched controls, demonstrating a level of 80% compared with 16% in the control group (Gillberg, 1983). In this study, examination of the neurological and neurodevelopmental problems at 10 years confirmed the disappearance of the neurological deficit (Gillberg, 1985).

The cohort of children was re-examined at age 13 years to compare behaviour and school achievements. The DAMP group had persisting high levels of severe behavioural problems (Gillberg & Gillberg, 1989). However the neurodevelopmental profiles at age 13 years did show change, with more than two-thirds of the DAMP children no longer having detectable motor problems. They did continue to have prolonged complex reaction times (Gillberg et al., 1989). Christiansen (2000), however, did not confirm improvement in motor control with age.

The general health of a group of children with DAMP at 16 years showed a significant excess of substance abuse, fractures and other accidents in addition to increased motor problems, clumsiness and height and weight problems (Hellgren et al., 1993). They also showed more psychiatric disorders, especially affective disorders (Hellgren et al., 1993).

In a longitudinal cohort of Dutch children, the frequency of minor neurological dysfunction amongst all the children rose with increasing age, but especially so for a group which had been found to be neurologically impaired neonatally (Lunsing et al., 1992). The same authors studied behavioural and cognitive development at 12 years of age in children with and without minor neurological dysfunction (Soorani-Lunsing, 1993). Fine manipulative disability related significantly to problems of cognition and behaviour; co-ordination problems related to cognitive problems and hypotonia and dyskinesia related to behavioural problems, the former more than the latter.

Losse (1991) re-examined a group of children who had been shown to be clumsy at the age of 6 years. At 16 years they continued to have substantial motor difficulties as well as a variety of educational, social and emotional problems. Skinner & Piek (2001) compared a group of children aged 8–10 years and a group of adolescents aged 12–14 years with significant movement problems (DCD) to a control group. Overall, DCD groups had lower self-worth and higher levels of anxiety than the control groups.

The natural outcome of ADHD with DCD at age 22 years has been investigated by Rasmussen & Gillberg (2000). In the ADHD/DCD group, 58% had a poor outcome compared with 13% in the comparison group. Remaining symptoms of ADHD, antisocial personality disorder, alcohol abuse, criminal offending, reading disorders and low educational level were overrepresented in the ADDH/DCD groups. The combination of ADHD and DCD appeared to carry a particularly gloomy outlook.

Evidence-based treatments for ADHD aspects of DCD

There is little evidence base for treatment methods apart from medication treatment of the attentional aspects of the dysfunction. Tervo et al. (2002) evaluated the medication responsiveness of ADHD–MD (attention deficit hyperactivity disorder and motor dysfunction) and ADHD only. Both groups responded to methylphenidate (Ritalin). Santosh & Taylor (2000) found that fine motor function improved on stimulant drugs.

Nyden et al. (2000) found that the neuropsychiatric problems of the children were significantly underdiagnosed and that intervention programmes resulted in better and less expensive care. Mandich (2001) reviewed the treatment literature for DCD over the past 15 years and found little evidence. They noted that a movement towards interventions based on functional outcomes is recommended to add to the evidence base.

The need for behavioural therapy depends on the particular combination of difficulties in a child. Motor learning disorder unaccompanied by other difficulties will not need behavioural therapy but associated problems, such as conduct disorder and ADHD, may benefit from this type of therapy.

Assessment

The assessment of children with motor learning disorders needs to be multiprofessional to ensure that all aspects of the child's difficulties can be established and addressed appropriately, involving a paediatric neurologist and all the therapies. Joint physiotherapy and occupational therapy assessments will address the gross and fine motor and visual–perceptual skills. Children with cognitive and behavioural difficulties will require referral to a psychologist and speech and language difficulties to a speech and language therapist.

Neurological examination will involve a detailed history of the child's birth, developmental and educational history, along with that of the family. Observation will reveal signs of a motor learning disorder which may include inability to sit still, constant fidgeting, inability to attend to one activity and constant interrupting. Soft neurological signs which appear during activities include tremor and associated movements of the hand or face; mirror movements may be used as an indicator of minor neurological dysfunction in conjunction with other signs. Useful subjective tests to observe the presence of soft neurological signs include: screwing together a nut and bolt; asking the child to place the tip of his or her finger on his or her nose repeatedly; checking of laterality of eye, hand and foot by offering the child a tube to look through on repeated occasions; observing catching and kicking activities.

Several standardised tests are available to assess gross and fine motor skills. For young children, the Miller Assessment for Preschoolers (MAP) offers a norm-referenced screening test, which includes fine and gross motor, language, memory, visual perception and complex task skills (Miller, 1988). It is designed to be conducted by any member of the child development team to identify areas of difficulty. The Movement Assessment Battery for Children (MABC) and the Bruininks Oseretsky Test of motor impairment (BOT) are designed for older children between 5.5 and 14 years and assess fine and gross motor, visual motor skills and balance skills (Bruininks, 1978; Henderson & Sugden, 1992).

Tests of visual perception skills include:

- Motor Free Visual Perception Test – MPVI (Colarusso & Hammill, 1996)
- Test of Visual Perceptual Skills – TVPS (Gardner, 1988)
- Beery test of Visual Motor Integration – VMI (Beery, 1989).

Non-standardised assessments of clinical and general observation and parent and school questionnaires are useful to place the standardised testing into the context of how a child behaves and functions within different environments.

Physical treatment and management

A number of theoretical frameworks for intervention are used to guide treatment, including sensory integration, perceptual motor and motor. These frameworks have been reflected in the evolution of different treatment approaches.

Sensory integration therapy involves stimulation of the vestibular (see Ch. 24), proprioceptive and tactile systems, as a means of exploring new skills to help with co-ordination and body image (Bundy & Fisher, 1991). Activities involved in this type of approach include use of swings, hammocks, scooter boards and soft play. The activities need to be pitched at a level which stimulates and challenges but is within the child's capabilities.

Perceptual motor approaches are often education-based programmes which involve training of tasks stepwise from simple activities to more complex movements (Lazlo & Bairstow, 1985). These types of programme are useful for activities to be undertaken by children supported in school and should be part of group sessions. Skill acquisition works on children learning specific tasks which they find difficult, e.g. hopping, ball catching, and is often used for children with specific difficulties with gross motor skills. Group sessions, which combine different aspects of treatment and offer positive feedback, can be useful in building children's confidence and self-esteem.

It is now recognised that children do not grow out of motor learning disorders and, although some improvements can be made through treatment, many continue to have difficulties into adult life. During the teenage and early adult years it is important that strategies to combat these problems are learnt and this may include simple things like maintaining a diary, list writing, engaging in physical activities which do not require good hand–eye co-ordination and using a computer for written work.

CASE HISTORY

Child with motor learning difficulties

JA was the first-born child in his family, after an uneventful pregnancy, labour and delivery, and was of average weight. He thrived postnatally and appeared to be developing normally through the first year of his life. He learnt to walk unaided at the age of 14 months but continued to walk with a wide-based gait, would walk into furniture in his path and frequently fell. By the age of 2 years he could point at objects he wanted but did not have many spoken words. His understanding was age-appropriate. His walking was still unsteady and he continued to crawl up and downstairs.

JA started nursery school at 3 years and staff noticed he missed the chair when sitting down, had difficulty pulling up his trousers and tended to eat with his fingers and spill his drink. The nursery staff alerted his parents to their concerns and recommended they arrange to see their general practitioner, who referred JA to a paediatrician. The paediatrician suggested a diagnosis of DCD and referred him for speech and language therapy and physiotherapy.

The physiotherapy assessment found specific difficulties in motor planning and poor fine motor skills. An individual programme of activities was devised which could be carried out at school and home. Activities included: practising motor skills as part of play; encouraging parents and nursery staff to modify tasks, such as using a two-handled cup and a thick pencil and Velcro on his shoes instead of laces.

When JA began school the physiotherapist referred him on to the occupational therapist who further assessed his visual, perceptual and fine motor skills. A joint visit by the therapists was made to JA's school and his difficulties were explained to the staff. LSAs worked on a programme of fine motor activities and physical education sessions were differentiated to enable him to join in.

A joint occupational therapy and physiotherapy group offered 6-week blocks of therapy which aimed to increase JA's confidence by allowing him to experiment with new physical skills in a safe environment and build interpersonal skills.

References

Abel MF, Blanco JS, Pavlovich L et al. Asymmetric hip deformity and subluxation in cerebral palsy: an analysis of surgical treatment. *J Pediatr Orthop* 1999, **19**:479–485.

Aicardi J. Epilepsy in brain injured children. *Dev Med Child Neurol* 1990, **32**:191–202.

American Psychiatric Association. *Diagnostic and Statistical Manual*. Arlington, VA, USA: American Psychiatric Publishing; 1994.

Bachlet A, Thomas AG, Eltumi M et al. A 12 month prospective study of gastrostomy feeding in children with disabilities. *Dev Med Child Neurol* 2002, **44** (Suppl. 92):12–13.

Bairstow P, Cochrane R, Hur JJ. *Evaluation of Conductive Education for Children with Cerebral Palsy*. London: HMSO; 1993.

Barrie JL, Galasko CSB. Surgery for unstable hips in cerebral palsy. *J Pediatr Orthop* 1996, **5**:225–231.

Bax M, Whitmore K. The medical examination of children on entry to school. The results and use of neurodevelopmental assessment. *Dev Med Child Neurol* 1987, **29**:40–55.

Bayley N. *Bayley Scales of Infant Development*. San Antonio: Therapy Skill Builders; 1983.

Beery KE. *The Developmental Test of Visual Motor Integration (3R)*. Cleveland, Toronto: Modern Curriculum Press; 1989.

Bobath K. *A Neurological Basis for the Treatment of Cerebral Palsy*. Clinics in Developmental Medicine, London: Heinemann; 1980.

Bower E, Michell D, Burnett M et al. Randomized controlled trial of physiotherapy in 56 children with cerebral palsy followed for 18 months. *Dev Med Child Neurol* 2001, **43**:4–15.

Bruininks RH. *Bruininks–Oseretsky Test of Motor Proficiency Examiner's Manual*. Circle Pines, MN: American Guidance Service; 1978.

Bundy A, Fisher AG. *Sensory Integration Theory and Practice*. Philadelphia: Davies; 1991.

Butler C, Darrah J. Effects of neurodevelopmental treatment (NDT) for cerebral palsy: an AACPDM evidence report. *Dev Med Child Neurol* 2001, **43**:778–790.

Carr J, Shepherd R, Ada L. Spasticity: research findings and implications for intervention. *Physiotherapy* 1995, **81**:421–429.

Carr LJ, Cosgrove AP, Gringras P et al. Position paper on the use of botulinum toxin in cerebral palsy. *Arch Dis Child* 1998, **79**:271–273.

Cartwight RD. Effect of sleep position on sleep apnea severity. *Sleep* 1984, **7**:110–114.

Chandler LS, Andrews MS, Swanson MW. *Movement Assessment of Infants – A Manual*. Rolling Bay Washington, USA: Child Development and Mental Retardation Center, 1980.

Chicoine MR, Park TS, Kaufmann BA. Selective dorsal rhizotomy and rates of orthopaedic surgery in children with spastic cerebral palsy. *J Neurosurg* 1997, **86**:43–49.

Christiansen AS. Persisting motor control problems in 11–12 year old boys previously diagnosed with deficits in attention, motor control and perception (DAMP). *Dev Med Child Neurol* 2000, **27**:3–16.

Colarusso RP, Hammill DD. *Motor Free Visual Perception Test – Revised*. Novato, CA, USA: Academy Therapy Publications; 1996.

Collet J-P, Vanasse M, Marois P et al. Hyperbaric oxygen for children with cerebral palsy: a randomised multicentre trial. *Lancet* 2001, **357**:582–586.

Cook A, Hussey S. *Assistive Technologies: Principles and Practice*. London: Mosby; 1995.

Cosgrove AP, Corry IS, Graham HK. Botulinum toxin in the management of the lower limb in cerebral palsy. *Dev Med Child Neurol* 1994, **36**:386–396.

Cottalorda J, Gautheron V, Metton G et al. Predicting the outcome of adductor tenotomy. *Int Orthop* 1998, **22**:374–379.

Crichton JU, Mackinnon M, White CP. The life expectancy of persons with cerebral palsy. *Dev Med Child Neurol* 1995, **37**:833.

Crothers B, Paine R. *The Natural History of Cerebral Palsy*. London: MacKeith Press; 1988.

Damiano DL, Dodd K, Taylor NF. Should we be testing and training muscle strength in cerebral palsy? *Dev Med Child Neurol* 2002, **44**:68–72.

Eliasson A, Gordon AM, Forssberg H. Tactile control of isometric fingertip forces during grasping in children with cerebral palsy. *Dev Med Child Neurol* 1995, **37**:72–84.

Evans P, Evans SJW, Alberman E. Cerebral palsy: why we must plan for survival. *Arch Dis Child* 1990, **65**:1329–1333.

Folio MR, Fewell RR. *Peabody Developmental Motor Scales and Activity Cards*. Austin, TX: PRO-ED; 1983.

Freud S. *Infantile Cerebral Palsies*. Coral Gables: University of Miami Press; 1968.

Gage J, Novacheck TF. An update on the treatment of gait problems in cerebral palsy. *J Orthop* 2001, **10**:265–274.

Gardner MF. *The Test of Visual Perceptual Skills (Non-motor)*. Northern California, USA: Health Publishing; 1988.

Gillberg C. Three year follow up at age of 10 of children with minor neurodevelopmental disorders II. School achievement problems. *Dev Med Child Neurol* 1983, **25**:566–573.

Gillberg C. Children with preschool minor developmental disorders III. Neurological and neurodevelopmental problems at age 10. *Dev Med Child Neurol* 1985, **27**:3–16.

Gillberg IC, Gillberg C. Children with preschool minor neurodevelopmental disorders. IV: Behavior and school achievement at age 13. *Dev Med Child Neurol* 1989, **31**:3–13.

Gillberg C, Rasmussen P, Carlstrom G et al. Perceptual, motor and attentional deficits in 6 year old children. Epidemiological aspects. *J Child Psychol Psychiatry* 1982, **23**:131–144.

Gillberg IC, Gillberg C, Rasmussen P. Three year follow up at age of 10 of children with minor neurodevelopmental disorders I. Behavioral problems. *Dev Med Child Neurol* 1983, **25**:483–499.

Gillberg IC, Gillberg C, Groth J. Children with preschool minor developmental disorders. V: Neurodevelopmental profiles at age 13. *Dev Med Child Neurol* 1989, **31**:14–24.

Granger CV, Hamilton BB, Keith RA. Advances in functional assessment for medical rehabilitation. *Topics Geriatr Rehab* 1986, **1**:59–74.

Green EM, Mulcahy CM, Pountney TE. An investigation into the development of early postural control. *Dev Med Child Neurol* 1995, **37**:437–448.

Grenier A. Prevention of early deformation of the hip in brain-damaged neonatals (in French). *Ann Pediatr* 1988, **35**:423–427.

Griffiths M, Clegg M. *Cerebral Palsy: Problems and Practice*. London: Souvenir Press; 1988.

Guzzetta A, Mercuri E, Cioni G. Visual impairment associated with cerebral palsy. *Eur J Paediatr Neurol* 2001, **5**:115–119.

Hadders-Algra M. The neuronal group selection theory: promising principles for understanding and treating developmental motor disorders. *Dev Med Child Neurol* 2000, **42**:707–715.

Hagberg B, Hagberg G. The changing panorama of cerebral palsy – bilateral spastic forms in particular. *Acta Paediatr* 1996 (Suppl. 416).

Haley SM, Coster WJ, Ludlow LH et al. *Pediatric Evaluation of Disability Inventory*. Boston: New England Medical Center Hospital; 1992.

Hayley SM, Ludlow LH, Coster WJ. Paediatric Evaluation of Disability Inventory: clinical interpretation of summary scores using Rasch Rating Scale Methodology. *Phys Med Rehab Clin North Am* 1993, **4**:529–540.

Hare NS, Durham S, Green EM. The cerebral palsies and motor learning disorders. In: Stokes M, ed. *Neurological Physiotherapy*. London: Mosby; 1998:229–241.

Hari M, Tillemans T. Conductive education. In: Scrutton D, ed. *Management of the Motor Disorders of Children with Cerebral Palsy*. London: Spastics International Medical Publications; 1984:19–35.

Harrison M. *Positioning the Neonate*. 10th Annual Meeting of the European Academy of Childhood Disability, Helsinki, 1998. Available from Physiotherapy Dept, St James University Hospital, Leeds.

Heim RC, Park TS, Vogler GP et al. Changes in hip migration after selective dorsal rhizotomy for spastic quadriplegia in cerebral palsy. *J Neurosurg* 1995, **82**:567–571.

Hellgren L, Gillberg C, Gillberg IC et al. Children with deficits in attention, motor control and perception (DAMP) almost grown up: general health. *Dev Med Child Neurol* 1993, **35**:881–892.

Henderson SE, Sugden DA. *Movement Assessment Battery for Children*. Sidcup: Therapy Skill Builders; 1992.

Henderson RC, Lin PP, Greene WB. Bone-mineral density in children and adolescents who have spastic cerebral palsy. *J Bone Joint Surg* 1995, **77**:1671–1681.

Hung JCC, Appleton RE, Nunn AJ et al. The use of melatonin in the treatment of sleep disturbances in children with neurological or behavioural disorders. *J Pediatr Pharmacy Pract* 1998, **3**:250–256.

Hur JJ. Review of research on therapeutic interventions for children with cerebral palsy. *Acta Neurol Scand* 1995, **91**:423–432.

Ivanhoe CB, Tilton AH, Francisco GE. Intrathecal baclofen therapy for spastic hypertonia. *Phys Med Rehab Clin North Am* 2001, **12**:923–937.

Kadesco B, Gillberg C. Attention deficits and clumsiness in 7-year-old Swedish children. *Dev Med Child Neurol* 1998, **40**:796–804.

Kadesco B, Gillberg C. The co-morbidity of ADHD in the general population of Swedish school age children. *J Child Psychol Psychiatry* 2001, **42**:487–492.

Khan Y, Kuenzle C, Green EM et al. Sleep problems and overnight oxygen saturation in children with cerebral palsy. *Eur Acad Child Disab* 1996, **69**.

Koman LA, Mooney JF, Paterson-Smith BP et al. Botulinum toxin type A neuromuscular blockade in the treatment of lower extremity spasticity in cerebral palsy: a randomised, double blind, placebo-controlled trial. *J Pediatr Othop* 2000, **20**:108–115.

Krick J, Murphy-Miller P, Zeger S et al. Pattern of growth in children with cerebral palsy. *J Am Diet Assoc* 1996, **96**:680–685.

Landgren M, Pettersson R, Kjellman B et al. ADHD, DAMP and other neurodevelopmental/psychiatric disorders in 6-year-old children: epidemiology and co-morbidity. *Dev Med Child Neurol* 1996, **38**:891–906.

Landgren M, Kjellman B, Gillberg C. Attention deficit disorder with developmental coordination disorders. *Arch Dis Child* 1998, **79**:207–212.

Lazlo J, Bairstow P. *Perceptual–Motor Behaviour: Development and Assessment*. London: Holt Publications; 1985.

Lespargot A, Renaudin E, Khouri M et al. Extensibilitiy of hip adductors in children with cerebral palsy. *Dev Med Child Neurol* 1994, **36**:980–988.

Lonstein JE. The spine in cerebral palsy. *Curr Orthop* 1995, **9**:164–177.

Lord R, Hulme C. Perceptual judgements of normal and clumsy children. *Dev Med Child Neurol* 1987, **29**:250–257.

Losse A. Clumsiness in children – do they grow out of it? A 10 year follow up study. *Dev Med Child Neurol* 1991, **33**:55–68.

Lunsing RJ, Hadders-Algra M, Huisjes HJ et al. Minor neurological dysfunction from birth to 12 years. Increase during late school age. *Dev Med Child Neurol* 1992, **34**:399–403.

Mahoney F, Barthel D. Functional evaluation: the Barthel index. *Maryland State Med J* 1965, **14**:61–65.

Mandich AD. Treatment of children with developmental coordination disorder: what is the evidence? *Phys Occup Ther Paediatr* 2001, **20**:51–68.

Martin SE, Marshall I, Douglas NJ. The effect of posture on airway caliber with the sleep apnea/hypopnea syndrome. *Am J Resp Care Med* 1995, **152**:721–724.

Mayston MJ. Developments in neurology – some aspects of the physiological basis for intervention techniques. *APCP J* 1995, 15–21.

McCarthy GT. Cerebral palsy: definition, epidemiology, development and neurological aspects. In: McCarthy GT, ed. *Physical Disability in Childhood – An Interdisciplinary Approach*. London: Churchill Livingstone; 1992.

McCarthy GT. Cerebral palsy: the clinical problem. In: Squier W, ed. *Acquired Damage to the Developing Brain: Timing and Causation*. London: Arnold; 2002:14.

Metaxiotis D, Siebel A, Doederlein L. Repeated botulinum toxin A injections in the treatment of spastic equinus foot. *Clin Orthop Rel Res* 2002, **394**:175–185.

Miller LJ. *Miller Assessment for Preschoolers*. San Antonio: Therapy Skill Builders; 1988.

Miller F, Bagg MR. Age and migration percentage as risk factors for progression in spastic hip disease. *Dev Med Child Neurol* 1992, **37**:449–455.

Miller A, Temple T, Miller F. Impact of othoses on the rate of scoliosis progression in children with cerebral palsy. *J Pediatr Orthop* 1996, **16**:332–335.

Moreau M, Cook PC, Ashton B. Adductor and psoas release for subluxation of the hip children with spastic cerebral palsy. *J Pediatr Orthop* 1995, **15**:672–676.

Morris C. A review of the efficacy of lower-limb orthoses used for cerebral palsy. *Dev Med Child Neurol* 2002, **44**:205–211.

Mutch L, Alberman E, Hagedorn R et al. Cerebral palsy epidemiology: where are we now and where are we going? *Dev Med Child Neurol* 1992, **34**:547–555.

Neilson PD, McCaughey J. Self regulation of spasm and spasticity in cerebral palsy. *J Neurol Neurosurg Psychiatry* 1982, **45**:320–330.

Nyden A, Paananen M, Gillberg C. Neuropsychiatric problems among children are significantly underdiagnosed. Intervention programs result in better and less expensive care. *Lakartidningen* 2000, **97**:5634–5639, 5641 (in Swedish).

Oliver M. *The Politics of Disablement*. London: MacMillan; 1990.

Palisano R, Rosenbaum P, Walter S et al. Gross motor function classification system for cerebral palsy. *Dev Med Child Neurol* 1997, **39**:214–223.

Pellegrino L. Cerebral palsy: a paradigm for developmental disabilities. *Dev Med Child Neurol* 1995, **37**:834–839.

Pharoah POD, Cooke T. Cerebral palsy and multiple births. *Arch Dis Child* 1996, **75F**:169–173.

Pharoah POD, Platt MJ, Cooke T. The changing epidemiology of cerebral palsy. *Arch Dis Child* 1996, **75F**:169–173.

Piper MC, Darrah J. *Motor Assessment of the Developing Infant*. London: WB Saunders; 1994.

Pope PM. Postural management and special seating. In: Edwards S, ed. *Neurological Physiotherapy: A Problem*

Solving Approach, 2nd edn. London: Churchill Livingstone; 2002:189–217.

Pountney TE, Mulcahy CM, Green EM. Early development of postural control. *Physiotherapy* 1990, **76**:799–802.

Pountney TE, Mulcahy CM, Clarke S et al. *Chailey Approach to Postural Management*. Birmingham: Active Design; 2000.

Pountney TE, Mandy A, Green EM et al. Management of hip dislocation with postural management. *Child: Care, Health Dev* 2002, **28**:179–185.

Rasmussen P, Gillberg C. Natural outcome of ADHD with developmental coordination disorder at age 22 years: a controlled, longitudinal, community based study. *J Am Acad Child Adolesc Psychiatry* 2000, **39**:1424–1431.

Reddihough DS, King J, Coleman G et al. Efficacy of programmes based on Conductive Education for young children with cerebral palsy. *Dev Med Child Neurol* 1998, **40**:763–770.

Reeves JC, Werry JS. Soft signs in hyperactivity. In: Thupper DE, ed. *Soft Neurological Signs*. Orlando: Grune and Stratton; 1987:224–245.

Reimers J. The stability of the hip in children. *Acta Orthop Scand* 1980 (Suppl. 184).

Rogers B, Arvesdon J, Buck G et al. Characteristics of dysphagia in children with cerebral palsy. *Dysphagia* 1994, **9**:69–73.

Rosenbloom L. Diagnosis and management of cerebral palsy. *Arch Dis Child* 1995, **72**:350–353.

Russell DJ, Rosenbaum PL, Avery LM et al. The *Gross Motor Function Measure*. London: Mackeith Press; 2002.

Saito N, Ebara S, Ohotsuka K et al. Natural history of scoliosis in spastic cerebral palsy. *Lancet* 1998, **351**:1687–1692.

Santosh PJ, Taylor E. Stimulant drugs. *Eur Child Adolesc Psychiatry* 2000, **9**:127–I43.

Schwartz L, Engel JM, Jensen MP. Pain in persons with cerebral palsy. *Arch Med Rehab* 1999, **80**:1243–1246.

Scrutton D. *Management of Motor Disorders of Children with Cerebral Palsy*. London: Spastics International Medical Publications; 1984.

Scrutton D, Baird G. Surveillance measures of the hips of children with bilateral cerebral palsy. *Arch Dis Child* 1997, **56**:381–384.

Shortland AP, Harris CA, Gough M et al. Architecture of the medial gastrocnemius in children with spastic diplegia. *Dev Med Child Neurol* 2002, **44**:158–163.

Skinner RA, Piek JP. Psychosocial implications of poor motor coordination in children and adolescents. *Hum Move Sci* 2001, **20**:73–94.

Song H-R, Carroll NC. Femoral varus derotation osteotomy with or without acetabuloplasty for unstable hips in cerebral palsy. *J Pediatr Orthop* 1998, **18**:62–68.

Sonksen PM, Levitt S, Kitsinger M. Constraints acting on motor development in young visually disabled children and principles of remediation. *Child: Care, Health Dev* 1984, **10**:273–286.

Soorani-Lunsing RJ. Is minor neurological dysfunction at 12 years related to behaviour and cognition? *Dev Med Child Neurol* 1993, **35**:321–330.

Special Educational Needs (SEN) Code of Practice. 2001. London: Department of Education and Skills: Available by email from dfes@prolog.uk.com.

Stallings VA, Charney EB, Davies JC et al. Nutrition-related growth failure of children with quadriplegic cerebral palsy. *Dev Med Child Neurol* 1993, **35**:126–138.

Stanley F, Blair E, Alberman E. *Cerebral Palsies: Epidemiology and Causal Pathways*. London: Mac Keith Press; 2000.

Stuberg W. Considerations to weight bearing programs in children with developmental disabilities. *Phys Ther* 1992, **72**:35–40.

Tardieu CA, Lespargot A, Tabary C et al. For how long must the soleus be stretched each day to prevent contracture? *Dev Med Child Neurol* 1988, **30**:3–10.

Tervo RC, Azuma S, Fogas B et al. Children with ADHD and motor dysfunction compared with children with ADHD only. *Dev Med Child Neurol* 2002, **44**:383–390.

Turi M, Kalen V. The risk of spinal deformity after selective dorsal rhizotomy. *J Paediatr Orthop* 2000, **20**:104–107.

Turker RJ, Lee R. Adductor tenotomies in children with quadriplegic cerebral palsy: longer term follow-up. *J Pediatr Orthop* 2000, **20**:370–374.

Turvey MT, Fitch HL, Tuller B. The Bernstein perspective: the problems of degrees of freedom and context conditioned variability. In: Kelso JAS, ed. *Human Behaviour*. Hillsdale, NJ: Erlbaum; 1982:239–252.

Ubhi T, Bhakta BB, Ives Hl et al. Randomised double blind placebo controlled trial of the effect of botulinum toxin on walking in cerebral palsy. *Arch Dis Child* 2000, **83**:481–487.

van der Weel FR, van der Meer ALH, Lee DN. Effect of task on movement control in cerebral palsy: implications for assessment and therapy. *Dev Med Child Neurol* 1991, **33**:419–426.

Vereijken B, Whiting HTA, Newell KM. Free(z)ing degrees of freedom. *J Motor Behav* 1992, **24**:133–142.

World Health Organization. International classification of functioning, disability and health (ICF). Geneva: World Health Organisation; 2001. Online. Available: http://www.who.int/classification/icf.

Williams GW, Woollacott H, Ivry R. Timing and motor control in clumsy children. *J Motor Behav* 1992, **24**:165–172.

Chapter 19

Neural tube defects: spina bifida and hydrocephalus

T Pountney   G McCarthy

CHAPTER CONTENTS

INTRODUCTION

Neural tube defects (NTDs) are a group of developmental abnormalities in which the neural tube fails to fuse somewhere along its length from the spinal cord to the brain (McCarthy et al., 1992). Spina bifida is the commonest NTD, where the lesion occurs in the spine. Hydrocephalus commonly occurs in association with spina bifida and is the condition where excess cerebrospinal fluid (CSF) circulates in and around the brain. This chapter describes the different NTDs and then focuses on the management of patients with spina bifida.

MECHANISM OF NEURAL TUBE DEFECTS

The neural tube develops from the neural plate early in embryonic development. Fusion normally occurs smoothly so that only the ends of the tube remain open. This means that the central canal remains in communication with the amniotic fluid. The upper (head) end of the tube develops into the brain and the lower end into the spinal cord (see Ch. 17). The lower end of the cord normally closes at 26 days of embryonic life (Levene, 1988).

The tube can fail to fuse anywhere along its length but this occurs most commonly at the lower end (McCarthy et al., 1992). The vertebrae develop from ectodermal tissue and normally close over the cord at 11 weeks of embryonic life. In spina bifida there may be associated abnormality of the skin, bone, meninges and neural tissue. If only skin, bone and dura meninges are involved, a meningocele occurs (Fig. 19.1A). This is relatively uncommon and may be associated with hair or a naevus. In spina bifida cystica the skin, dura and spinal cord are involved, and this is termed a myelomeningocele (Fig. 19.1B); this occurs in 80% of spina bifida

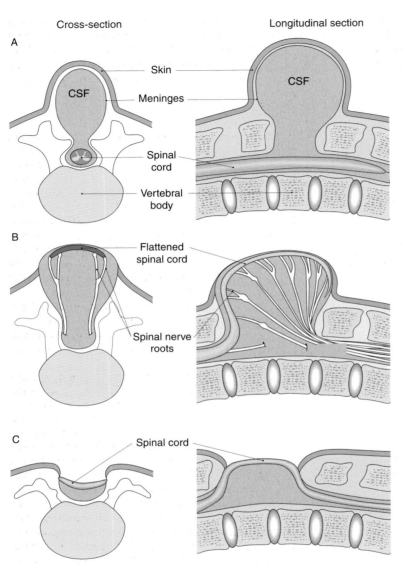

Cross-section   Longitudinal section

A

Skin

CSF

CSF

Meninges

Spinal cord

Vertebral body

B

Flattened spinal cord

Spinal nerve roots

C

Spinal cord

Figure 19.1   Types of spinal lesion in spina bifida. (A) Meningocele: no neural tissue outside the vertebral canal. (B) Myelomeningocele: neural tissue and nerve roots may be outside the vertebral canal. There may be fatty tissue or a bony spur present. (C) Rachischisis: there is no sac and the neural tissue lies open on the surface as a flattened plaque. CSF, cerebrospinal fluid. (Redrawn from McCarthy et al. (1992), with permission.)

lesions. When the neural tissue of the spinal cord is displaced and exposed on the surface of the lesion, the term rachischisis is used (Fig. 19.1C). In some cases the defect of the spinal cord and vertebrae may be covered by skin and hidden from sight, producing spina bifida occulta, which is a more minor abnormality.

At a higher level in the neural tube, the posterior part of the brain may fail to develop and fuse normally, producing an encephalocele. Of these lesions, 75–80% occur in the occipital region; however, lesions can be anterior, including over the bridge of the nose. If the whole of the anterior aspect of the neural tube fails to develop, anencephaly occurs, when there is complete absence of

the cerebral hemispheres; this is incompatible with life after birth.

It is possible for both major and subtle abnormalities of the central nervous system (CNS) to accompany the spinal manifestations of spina bifida. The commonest problem is hydrocephalus, caused by obstruction of the outflow of CSF from the cerebral ventricles through the narrow canal or aqueduct, or the small exit foramina that allow the passage of CSF to the surface of the brain (Fig. 19.2).

Another common problem is the Arnold–Chiari abnormality, in which the brainstem and cerebellar vermis are herniated through the foramen magnum. This can be associated with cysts, or dilation of the central canal of the spinal cord, syringomyelia, which may present with neurological abnormalities affecting swallowing, phonation, and power and sensation in the arms.

GENETIC ASPECTS OF NTDs

There is known to be a genetic element to the occurrence of NTDs, with a risk of recurrence of spina bifida of 1 in 20 following the birth of a first affected child. The risk of recurrence increases to around 1 in 10 if a second affected child is born. Thereafter, risk increases to 1 in 4. There is known to be a racial bias in the occurrence of NTDs. The Welsh and Irish have a higher incidence than the English, and Europeans a higher incidence than Asians.

PREVALENCE OF NTDs

In the UK the prevalence of NTDs has been falling steadily over the past 30 years. Since it was unclear what part prenatal screening played in the reduced prevalence, a survey was carried out to clarify the position in relation to practice in 1985 (Cuckle et al., 1989). The available information in 1985 showed that only 36% of the decline in prevalence of spina bifida could be accounted for by terminations of pregnancy. It was concluded that an NTD register should be set up to monitor the situation accurately. Figures from the National Congenital Abnormality System (NCAS; Botting, 2001) show a continuing decline in the UK (Table 19.1).

In the mid-1970s, next to Ireland, the UK had the highest birth prevalence of NTDs in the world; now it has one of the lowest rates. Prenatal screening and diagnosis have been largely responsible for this but do not give the whole answer.

Folic acid has been shown to have a beneficial effect in preventing the occurrence of NTDs in a population of women at risk of producing further affected babies. An intake of folic acid of 4 mg/day before conception and for the first 3 months of pregnancy was sufficient to reduce the risk of recurrence of NTDs if there was a history of NTDs in the parents or first-degree relatives (Expert Advisory Group, 1992). Since at least 30% of pregnancies are unplanned, there is an argument for the fortification of flour with folic acid (Wald & Bower, 1995). In the USA, fortification of all enriched grain products, such as flour, has resulted in a population-wide increase in the concentration of serum folate (Lawrence et al., 1999). It has been suggested that an increased intake of folic acid by the population in the UK of 0.4 mg/day could be sufficient to reduce the incidence of NTDs by approximately 1000 per year. However, there is still delay in implementing the proposal in the UK and Europe (Oakley, 2002).

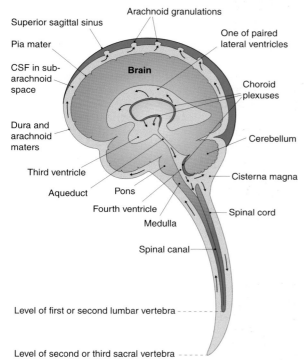

Figure 19.2 Cerebrospinal fluid (CSF) pathways. CSF is made by the choroid plexus in the lateral ventricles and flows through the third ventricle, aqueduct, fourth ventricle and, via the foramina of Magendie and Luschka and basal cisterns, over the surface of the brain, where it is absorbed by the arachnoid granulations. It also passes through the cisterna magna and spinal canal to circulate around the spinal cord. (Redrawn from McCarthy et al. (1992), with permission.)

Table 19.1 The incidence of anencephaly and spina bifida in the UK

	Rates per 10 000 births				
	1975–1979	1980–1984	1985–1989	1990–1994	1995–1999
Anencephaly	9.8	3.0	0.6	0.3	0.4
Spina bifida	15.1	8.5	3.3	1.3	1.0

Data from the National Congenital Anomaly System, cited in Botting (2001).

MANAGEMENT OF THE SPINAL LESION AFTER BIRTH

The neonate with open spina bifida needs to be assessed carefully after birth but it is not necessary to rush into rapid surgical intervention. Experience has shown that full assessment of the neurological, orthopaedic and medical problems should be carried out, together with social and emotional aspects of the family. The parents should be fully involved with decision-making, including when not to treat babies with severe problems (Charney, 1990).

The higher the neural lesion and hence the level of paralysis, the worse the prognosis for morbidity and mortality. The outlook is poor if severe hydrocephalus is present at birth, or there is marked spinal deformity or additional birth injury. Active surgical treatment of myelomeningocele consists of closure of the lesion on the first or second day of life. The sac is opened, the neural placode mobilised, and the dura then closed over the placode to form a watertight cover that is then covered by skin. Early closure reduces the risk of infection but the back can be covered by a sterile moist dressing and the sac will eventually epithelialise over. It is important to treat hydrocephalus at the same time as the closure of the back lesion, as pressure in the system rises and the back incision may leak CSF and fail to heal (see below).

HYDROCEPHALUS

The hydrocephalus associated with spina bifida is caused by obstruction to the normal pathways of flow of CSF in the brain, usually at the aqueduct, although it can occur at any point in the CSF circulation (Fig. 19.2).

The CSF is produced by the choroid plexuses in the ventricles and normally circulates through the ventricular system and around the surface of the brain, where it is absorbed by the arachnoid granulations into the sagittal sinus. CSF also circulates around the spinal cord and down the central canal (Fig. 19.2). If circulation of CSF is blocked, the fluid cannot be absorbed and pressure builds up.

Hydrocephalus develops in about 80% of children with spina bifida but is less likely to occur in those with lower spinal lesions (McCarthy & Land, 1992). Hydrocephalus often develops after birth when the lesion on the back is closed (see above). This is caused by the rise in pressure caused by closure of the fluid-filled sac, which was previously able to absorb pressure rises. In addition, the Arnold–Chiari malformation may be displaced downwards by rising pressure in the cranium, obstructing the outflow of the foramen magnum and the posterior cisterns.

In the infant, pressure rises are more easily absorbed because the cranium is more flexible, the bones of the skull can be stretched and the head size increases rapidly. In the older child the skull becomes more rigid and the pressure is transmitted to the brain. The ventricular system dilates in three dimensions, stretching the brain and disrupting the architecture. The lateral ventricles themselves can increase the obstruction at the aqueduct by curling round and pressing directly on it.

There was no effective treatment for hydrocephalus until 1956 when John Holter, an engineer who had a son with hydrocephalus, working with Eugene Spitz, a neurosurgeon, perfected a valve and shunt system. This system was designed to provide a bypass for CSF from the cerebral ventricles to the right atrium of the heart, the ventriculoatrial (VA) shunt. Since that time many other types of shunts have been developed with the same principle of providing a bypass for the excess CSF. The most common route now used is from the cerebral ventricle to the peritoneum, a ventriculoperitoneal (VP) shunt, but shunts can also be drained into the lumbar theca, the pleura, or even into a gastric pouch.

In addition to bypasses for CSF, efforts have been made to place a tube into the aqueduct, using neuroendoscopy, or to reduce production of CSF by cauterising the choroid plexus. The use of neuroendoscopy to make a window in the third ventricle to bypass the aqueduct, third ventriculostomy, has been successful in avoiding shunts in some children. This technique can also be used to make windows in cyst walls, or between the ventricles through the septum pellucidum, which is helpful if there is an uneven CSF flow between the two lateral ventricles. This is an exciting way of avoiding long-term shunts but is possible only if the ventricular system is very dilated at the time of neuroendoscopy.

MECHANISMS OF ASSOCIATED NEUROLOGICAL PROBLEMS

If hydrocephalus is treated effectively from birth, neurological problems are likely to be reduced. However, some problems are undoubtedly caused by structural neurological abnormalities occurring during brain development and can be identified with magnetic resonance imaging (MRI). The effects of disruption of the immature brain can be inferred from the commonly encountered learning difficulties and problems of attention seen in children with hydrocephalus.

Vision

Pressure on the optic nerve can cause optic atrophy, which reduces visual acuity and can cause blindness. The optic pathways can be disrupted and the visual cortex may be damaged by huge dilatation of the ventricles, causing visual field defects or more subtle visual association difficulties. Eye movements can be affected by pressure on the oculomotor nerves, especially the sixth nerve, which has a long intracranial route, producing a convergent squint. Upward gaze can also be affected, causing the 'setting-sun' appearance. Cognitive visual problems are common in children with shunted hydrocephalus and should be sought by taking a structured history (Houliston, 1999).

Muscle power and sensation

The spinal lesion can affect innervation of the skin, muscles, bladder and bowel in many ways. Since MRI scanning became widely available it has become clear that spinal cord abnormalities are very common. The cord may be divided by a bony spur or surrounded by fatty tissue. There may be a cystic swelling of the central canal, a syrinx, which occurs most commonly in the cervical or lumbar regions. The cord may be adherent to the dural sac or stuck down by abnormally sited tissue. This tethering can cause gradual neurological damage and changes in neurological signs as the child grows, for example, loss of muscle power, altered skin sensation, or changes in bladder and bowel control.

SPINAL LEVEL OF THE LESION IN SPINA BIFIDA

The spinal level of neurological damage determines the functional abnormality, e.g. which muscles are affected and whether the bladder or bowel function is involved, although it is rare to get the precise cut-off level seen in spinal injury (Fig. 19.3).

Neurological basis of orthopaedic problems

The spinal cord function may be impaired at a certain level or, more commonly, there may be interruption of the corticospinal tracts with isolated reflex activity present. A spastic paraplegia may occur, with some preservation of voluntary movements and sensation. Some children have a hemimyelomeningocele, with one leg affected and usually some bladder and bowel involvement.

Occult spinal dysraphism occurs when there is disordered closure of the neural tube or its coverings but the lesion is covered by skin. There may be external clues such as a fatty swelling or hairy tuft or haemangioma, a dermoid or dermal sinus. There is usually no neurological abnormality at birth but the lesion should be fully investigated with MRI as neurological complications develop with growth.

Low lesions – sacral (10% of cases) or lumbosacral (20%)

With low lesions, there may appear to be very good neurological function at birth and the legs may look normal. It is important to examine the hips for instability and look at movement of the feet. The weakness of plantarflexion, small muscles of the feet and hip extension may not be immediately obvious. Sensory testing is also difficult but should be attempted in the neonatal

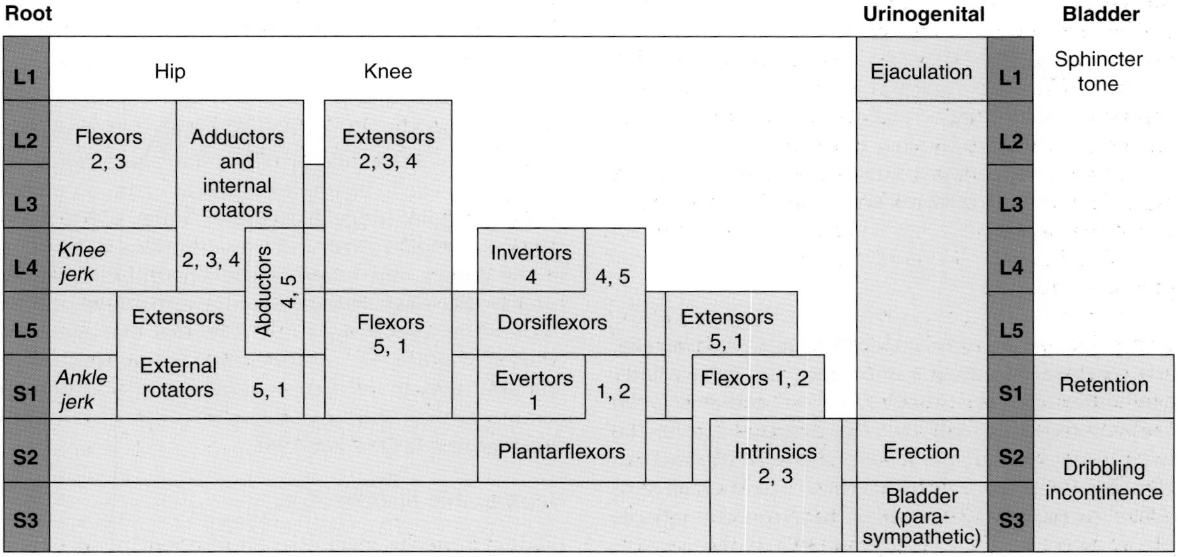

Root	Hip			Knee								Urinogenital		Bladder
L1	Hip			Knee								Ejaculation	**L1**	Sphincter tone
L2	Flexors 2, 3	Adductors and internal rotators		Extensors 2, 3, 4									**L2**	
L3													**L3**	
L4	Knee jerk	2, 3, 4	Abductors 4, 5			Invertors 4	4, 5						**L4**	
L5		Extensors 5, 1		Flexors 5, 1		Dorsiflexors		Extensors 5, 1					**L5**	
S1	Ankle jerk	External rotators 5, 1				Evertors 1	1, 2	Flexors 1, 2					**S1**	Retention
S2				Plantarflexors				Intrinsics 2, 3		Erection			**S2**	Dribbling incontinence
S3										Bladder (parasympathetic)			**S3**	

Figure 19.3 Segmental nerve supply of the lumbar (L1–L5) and sacral (S1–S3) nerve roots. Reading across from the nerve roots listed on the left of the diagram, the associated muscles of the lower limbs and bladder, bowel and sexual function can be seen.

period in order to get an idea of the level of lesion. Testing is performed using a firm pinprick from the toes upwards until a pain reaction is elicited. This indicates the spinal level of involvement.

Talipes equinovarus deformities of the feet may be present at birth and it is important to initiate strapping or splinting to maintain a good position. The knees may be either flexed or hyperextended and there may be instability of the hips or frank dislocation, which requires immediate treatment (conservative management) in this group of children who have a good prognosis for walking independently.

Lumbar lesions (20%)

In higher lesions muscle activity may be limited to hip flexion and adduction with some knee extension. The hips may be dislocated at birth but surgery in these circumstances is not indicated (Fixsen, 1992).

High lesions – thoracolumbar (50%)

If the lesion is above L1 there is usually no useful muscle activity in the legs. Isolated reflex activity may be present, causing flexion contractures and flexor spasms that are difficult to manage and interfere with postural management and the use of orthoses.

Spinal deformity

Spinal curvature may be congenital or may occur as the child develops; the principles of management are similar for both.

Congenital curve

Spinal deformity may be present at birth, particularly in children with high lesions. There may be a kyphosis with a prominent forward curve. This is usually caused by the underlying vertebral, and sometimes rib, fusion abnormalities.

Paralytic curves

Paralytic curves are often associated with syringomyelia; they are related to muscle imbalance and appear later than other curves. About 75% of patients with myelomeningocele will develop a spinal curve; the majority of curves are paralytic or mixed, with less than one-third being entirely congenital. The incidence of scoliosis is related to the level of the lesion. All patients with a defect at T12 or above have a scoliosis, with the incidence reducing steadily to around 25% at L5 (Morley, 1992).

Management of spinal deformity

During growth it is important to hold the spine as straight as possible, using a thoracolumbar spinal orthosis (TLSO). The anaesthetic skin can make bracing difficult, especially in the presence of kyphosis.

Conservative management of spinal deformity is, wherever possible, the best treatment. For this to be effective, the curve must be detected early and referred for specialist management. Bracing is the most commonly used treatment for curves which are flexible and less than 40°, and for children with remaining growth potential (Morley, 1992).

Where surgery is indicated it is usual to carry out an MRI scan of the spinal cord preoperatively to exclude any underlying abnormalities, including tethering of the cord. Assessment of respiratory function is important, especially in curves involving the chest, which may cause reduction of ventilatory capacity. Spinal fusion is carried out at the optimum time, usually between 10 and 13 years, carrying out anterior release, distracting the spine with a Harrington rod and fusing the spine posteriorly by excising the posterior joints and laying on bone grafts (Morley, 1992).

Postoperative physiotherapy is vital to ensure that a child returns to full function as quickly as possible. Immediately postoperatively, no form of spinal brace is worn but when the child resumes sitting a removable polypropylene brace must be worn at all times for about 6 months to provide stability. When the child is sitting, care must be taken to prevent traction of the spine during lifting and transferring. Support must be given under the bottom during these procedures, either by the lifter or by the use of transfer boards. There is a risk of pressure sores developing on anaesthetic skin and the child must be positioned and lifted to relieve pressure regularly (see below).

The child can usually begin sitting 4–7 days after surgery. While the child is in hospital, a programme of exercises needs to be implemented to maintain muscle length and joint range in the lower limbs, and to maintain the strength of arm and trunk muscles. Positioning of the ankles and knees to prevent muscle contractures is necessary, with passive movements to prevent decrease in joint ranges (see 'Physical management', below). Significant postoperative complications of spinal surgery in children with spina bifida occur more commonly than with any other type of spinal deformity (Leatherman & Dickson, 1988).

Neuropathic bladder

Bladder function may also be affected by the spinal lesion depending on its anatomical site. If the sphincter is unable to relax during the normal sequence of micturition, there may be incomplete emptying of the bladder. This is often associated with high-pressure contractions of the bladder muscle, the detrusor, which can lead to back-pressure on the kidneys, detrusor sphincter dyssynergia (DSD). The combination of high pressure and infection can cause kidney damage, which may occur silently, eventually leading to renal failure.

Bladder activity can be monitored with urodynamic studies (UDS), which can be repeated at intervals. Renal function can also be monitored using different types of scan, e.g. dimercaptosuccinic acid (DMSA) nuclear scan, radionucleotide diethylenetriamine penta-acid (DTPA) scan or glomerular filtration rate (GFR) scanning.

In general there are three types of bladder behaviour: contractile, intermediate and acontractile. The contractile problem of DSD, which causes obstruction to outflow at the level of the distal sphincter, is recognised as the commonest cause of impaired renal function in children with congenital spinal cord problems. The most vulnerable times for renal function are in the first 5 years of life and the late teens (McCarthy et al., 1992).

Management of the neuropathic bladder

The aims of management are to achieve continence and preserve renal function. Continence management depends on bladder function. Clean intermittent catheterisation (CIC) is an effective method of management for some children, particularly with the use of medication to reduce bladder contractions and increase sphincter tone. Children can be taught to catheterise themselves from the age of about 6 years. If the bladder is small and contracts continuously, CIC is not helpful. If medication is not successful in reducing contractions (see Ch. 28), surgery may be necessary to increase bladder size or correct sphincter weakness.

Neuropathic bowel

Management of bowel incontinence can be a major problem, particularly for children with low spinal lesions who have poor anal sphincter tone and are active on their feet. The importance of early toileting to develop a pattern of bowel emptying, even if it is through an incompetent sphincter, cannot be overemphasised. Other basic areas such as appropriate diet, high fluid intake and the use of laxatives to aid the programme need to be addressed.

The anocutaneous reflex, which has been used in planning bowel movement, is seen in 40% of children with spina bifida regardless of the level of the spinal lesion (Agnarsson et al., 1993). Biofeedback has been used in the treatment of faecal incontinence in myelomeningocele (Whitehead et al., 1986), and relies

on the presence of some rectal sensation and a capacity to squeeze the external anal sphincter. Motivation and intelligence are also important for patient selection.

PHYSICAL MANAGEMENT

The physical management of a child with an NTD, as with any disability, requires that the parents and therapists work in partnership to help the child achieve his or her full potential. Ultimately the parents' day-to-day care will have the greatest impact on the child's development and it is therefore vital that they are presented with a positive approach that puts value on their child's life and their ability to influence it. Professionals can give negative attitudes to disability that can be highly influential in shaping parental attitudes (French, 1994). The physiotherapist needs to develop a lasting relationship with the child and family, and recognise the valuable role the parents play in this, by working with them to develop management programmes that can become part of their lifestyle.

The overall objective of physiotherapy in a child with a neural tube lesion is to promote normal development within the limits of the neurological constraints and achieve as much independence as possible.

The main aims of physiotherapy at all stages of an individual's life will include:

- development of physical skills leading to independence
- achievement of independent mobility, either walking or in a wheelchair
- prevention of the development of deformity.

Management at different stages from birth to adulthood will now be considered.

Neonatal physiotherapy

Assessment

An initial assessment should be made to determine the likely severity of the child's disability. Assessment of the baby's sensation and movement can be the responsibility of either the paediatrician or the physiotherapist. This assessment will give a fairly accurate picture of the child's future physical ability.

The assessment needs to be performed quickly and efficiently, as the child will be in an incubator and unable to tolerate excessive handling. The physiotherapist should first record the baby's resting posture, any active movements and any abnormalities or deformities. Reflexes and muscle groups, rather than individual muscles, are then tested. A definite movement of the tendon or joint must be seen as an indication of the muscle's activity. The examiner should work from the toes upwards, as once normal activity is seen the areas above this should be normal.

The test of sensation needs to be of protopathic (deep) feeling, as testing epicritic feeling (light touch) is not conclusive at this stage. Movements may be elicited due to uncontrolled reflex activity and a reaction to pain is a much more definite sign of sensation. This testing is best performed using a firm pinprick.

Physiotherapy interventions

Once the assessment is completed, a programme of passive movements and stretching exercises can be implemented to maintain and improve muscle length and joint range.

The most common deformities in the neonate with spina bifida are talipes equinovarus (TEV) and congenital dislocation of the hip. The management of TEV follows the same protocol as for idiopathic TEV and varies according to the severity of the deformity and between orthopaedic consultants. The most frequently adopted treatments are strapping with zinc oxide tape, the application of a corrective splint and serial plastering. Great care must be taken during these techniques as there may be impaired skin sensation and circulation that can lead to the development of pressure sores (see below).

The management of the baby with a congenital dislocation of the hips is conservative, unless the lesion is low and the child will be an active independent walker (Fixsen, 1992). The use of abduction splints is thought (from clinical observation) to lead to contractures of the abductors, causing later difficulties, and is not recommended.

During the neonatal period, early positive involvement by parents in their baby's care can aid acceptance of the disability. The main priorities will be the daily programme of stretching exercises and passive movements (see Chs 23 and 25) and care of the skin.

Preschool physiotherapy

The physiotherapist will often provide an ongoing link between home and hospital. Following the child's discharge from hospital, the parents will need regular support as the realities of the child's disability become evident. Visiting the family at home will reduce the unnecessary travelling and allow the child to be treated in a familiar environment. It also enables the physiotherapist to make a clearer assessment of the child's needs in the context of the family.

The physiotherapy programme started in hospital will need to continue and, as the child begins to develop, be updated. Between the ages of 6 and 12 months it is useful to update the muscle chart so that preparations can be made to provide the necessary orthotic equipment.

Passive movements to all lower-limb joints should be performed at each nappy change to maintain joint range and stimulate the circulation. Once the child begins active arm and upper-body movements, these should be encouraged and strengthened. Children with spina bifida are often reliant on their arms for ambulation with sticks or crutches so they need to be strong. The child should be positioned as any normal infant in prone, supine and sitting positions to promote the normal developmental milestones of rolling and sitting (see Ch. 17) and maintain muscle length. The physiotherapist should educate parents in strategies to help their child develop, and this is more successful through play and stimulation rather than rigid exercise programmes.

Children with high lesions may find developing sitting balance difficult and may require help with positioning so that they can free their hands for play. Trunk support or a wider sitting base may aid balance.

The normal child begins to explore the environment towards the end of the first year and it is important that the child with spina bifida is offered this opportunity, even if he or she cannot do it independently. Various items of equipment, such as prone trolleys and small carts, enable the child to propel him- or herself.

Children with spina bifida and hydrocephalus often experience difficulties with perception (Dunning, 1994), including spatial difficulties, impaired hand function, and poor lateralisation and figure–ground discrimination (the ability to identify details from a background and ignore irrelevant information). They may also have poor visual tracking skills so that they cannot track horizontally across the midline and converge and diverge rapidly. The combination of motor and perceptual deficits may result in the child having difficulty with walking, as these skills are all needed to manoeuvre in relation to a stable and moving environment. An early opportunity to move about in the environment and experiment with movement may help to reduce these difficulties in later life.

A thorough occupational and physiotherapy assessment should be made to assess the level of the child's perceptual and motor skills, so that the necessary strategies can be implemented to overcome any deficits. Such tests are difficult to perform in detail in the preschool child but activities involving spatial awareness, e.g. moving over and under objects without touching them, judging speed of moving objects and general ability to move around in the environment, should be observed and any difficulties noted. Occupational therapists use a range of tests from the age of 4 years.

The child is usually ready to begin standing between the ages of 18 months and 2 years. An assessment of the degree of support needed can be made and the type of orthoses required discussed with parents. There are many benefits to standing, even if functional walking is not achieved. Mazur et al. (1989) suggested that early mobility and the upright posture are valuable in promoting independence and mobility, decreasing the occurrence of pressure sores, reducing obesity and contractures, and beneficial to the child's psychosocial well-being.

Children with a more severe disability who cannot walk will use a wheelchair and will be at high risk of developing postural deformities, so it is important that an assessment of their posture is made. The assessment should consider the child's needs in lying, sitting and standing. For a child who is sitting most of the day, there is a risk of hip flexion deformities developing alongside windswept hips and scoliosis. The child should be controlled in a variety of symmetrical postures during the day and night to reduce the risk of developing deformity (see below), and sitting should be limited.

Before the child starts school, an assessment of his or her physical and educational needs is made. The physical environment needs to be adapted to allow children with disabilities to move around freely and access all areas of the school. The addition of ramps, wider doorways and improved toilet facilities may be required. Consideration of the specific learning difficulties experienced by a child with hydrocephalus, such as perceptual difficulties that involve figure–ground discrimination, spatial awareness, motor organisational skills, poor lateralisation of skills, reasoning ability, and number work may necessitate different learning strategies and the teacher needs to be made aware of these problems.

The 2001 *Special Educational Needs (SEN) Code of Practice* reinforces the 'stronger rights of children with SEN to be educated in mainstream school'. Following assessment, parents and professionals will consider the available educational options based on the child's needs.

School–aged child

Once the child is in school, the physiotherapist will need to provide ongoing support to the parents and teaching staff. In many instances physiotherapists provide the link between the medical, home and school environments.

All staff working with children with hydrocephalus must be made aware of the signs that indicate shunt problems; these may include headache, vomiting, weakness or loss of dexterity, decreased levels of consciousness, irritability, slowing of performance, visual problems and worsening of any squint.

During the school years children develop their independence and begin to branch out from their families. This is a worrying time for parents and they need support in allowing their children opportunities to do this within safe boundaries. Teaching staff also need to recognise that a child with spina bifida experiences the same feelings and expectations as other children and should not allow the disability to interfere with the child's development. A child's attitude to his or her disability is likely to reflect the attitude of the adults encountered. If adults perceive the child as a difficulty to be endured, the child's self-esteem will plummet. Imagination is often needed to enable the child to participate in all activities, but solutions can usually be found.

The school environment is much larger than home and the choice of walking or using a wheelchair for different activities may need to be made. Many children find that a wheelchair provides a speed and freedom they do not have when walking. For physical education and games, a wheelchair can be a real asset, as the child's hands are free. Physiotherapists or occupational therapists are responsible for teaching basic wheelchair skills.

During the school years, as a child is expected to take on more daily living and educational tasks, any difficulties with learning will become evident. Dressing and putting on orthoses, intermittent catheterisation, learning the way to and around the school, as well as school work, may prove arduous for children with perceptual, concentration or organisational difficulties. Tasks need to be broken down into manageable units and the use of visual cues introduced. Classroom assistants are invaluable in implementing such programmes. The physiotherapist needs to visit the school and/or home regularly to update these programmes.

A child's independence rests to a large extent on mobility – both moving around and transferring. Children need to develop strength and stamina in their arm muscles whether they wish to walk or use a wheelchair as their main form of mobility. To maintain this strength, children should be encouraged to do a regular programme of strengthening exercises, such as push-ups in prone or sitting positions, alongside an active sporting programme, which could include activities such as swimming, cycling with a hand-propelled or low-geared tricycle and wheelchair basketball. Not only do these activities strengthen muscles, they also increase the circulation and help with weight control, which are both contributory factors in the development of pressure sores.

Children should be taught to transfer safely to and from surfaces at different heights, e.g. from floor to chair, from wheelchair to toilet. It is important that the child is careful not to damage anaesthetic skin during transfers by clearing the surface over which they are moving and not dragging the skin. When a child is not wearing orthoses, he or she needs to make sure the legs are supported during the transfer.

Children who are walking with sticks or crutches need to practise how to fall safely and be able to regain the upright position. They must learn to release their crutches quickly and use their arms to protect themselves. Practice should begin on a soft crash mat and gradually move towards firmer surfaces. Reducing fear of falling is an important confidence booster for entering busy environments.

As the child grows, there is a risk of developing deformity and this must be monitored carefully. The most common deformities seen are hip dislocation and kyphoscoliosis. For children who have high lesions and spend most of their time in a wheelchair, it is essential that they are seated to maintain a symmetrical posture with an even distribution over the weight-bearing surfaces. Although seating cannot correct an existing deformity it can contain postures and decrease the rate of progression (see below).

Muscle contractures of the hip flexors, hamstrings and calf muscles can develop due to spasticity if the child does not continue with a programme of stretching activities (see Chs 23 and 25). The child needs to stand or lie prone for at least half an hour daily to stretch the hip flexors, to sit in the long sitting position, preferably with orthoses to stretch the hamstrings and to position the feet in the plantigrade position when sitting or standing.

During the years at primary school, most children with hydrocephalus will undergo a revision of the shunt to lengthen the drainage tube. If a total revision is needed there may be some deterioration in physical skills. Intensive physiotherapy will be needed during these periods to restore the children to their previous levels of function.

Adolescence

The onset of puberty in children with spina bifida is often early and this can cause problems, as they can be socially and emotionally immature. Parents and teachers need to be aware of the conflict this creates within children and help them through this confusing period.

By the time children are in their teens, they should be able to take responsibility for much of their day-to-day care. They should also have an understanding of their disability and the implications of leading an independent lifestyle. Time should be spent on educating children in all self-management skills: physical management, catheterisation, application of orthoses and skin care. They should also know where to seek help.

As children grow they need to take more responsibility for their health and fitness. They should learn to check their skin for signs of pressure, using inspection mirrors, when putting their orthoses on and off, and know the likely danger spots, i.e. toes, heels, behind the knees, buttocks and hips. If they are in wheelchairs for long periods they must do regular lifts, e.g. half-hourly, to relieve the pressure on the buttocks.

During the teenage years, many children will decide to increase the amount of time they use a wheelchair or opt to become a full-time wheelchair-user. A wheelchair can be liberating in terms of increasing speed and distance covered. This change can be a difficult decision to make and the child should ultimately make this decision.

The growth spurt experienced in adolescence will accelerate the progression of spinal deformities. Orthopaedic surgery of the spine and hips is often undertaken when the growth period is almost over. Preoperative physiotherapy is important to prepare a child physically for surgery. He or she must be prepared for a change in posture and the need to develop a different sense of balance. Some activities, such as moving the legs for transfers and putting on socks and shoes, may be limited after surgery.

With the decreasing incidence of NTDs and increasing inclusion in mainstream education, many children and teenagers lack the opportunity to socialise with others with similar disabilities. Such opportunities can be beneficial in terms of sharing experiences and learning more about practical management of their condition. In the USA, summer camps have proved a popular way of achieving this.

Adulthood

Transition to adulthood can prove difficult as the level of physiotherapy advice decreases and responsibility for care transfers to the young adult. Education can go some way towards enabling a young adult to be capable of caring for him- or herself, or of seeking care. Technological advances mean that adults can often achieve a high level of independence (Fig. 19.4). However, where hydrocephalus has caused specific difficulties, such as short-term memory loss, the ability to cope may be severely compromised. In these cases appropriate care plans should be put in place for young adults who wish to live independent lives.

The young adult should be introduced to an adult physiotherapy team before leaving paediatric services so that there is a clear understanding of when and where to seek help. It may be useful for the physiotherapist to undertake an annual review to maintain contact (see Ch. 16, p. 285).

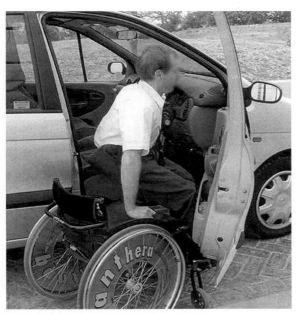

Figure 19.4 Independent young adult preparing to go to work in his adapted car.

Table 19.2 Ambulatory support according to level of paralysis

Level of paralysis	Equipment required
Above L1	Thoracolumbar spinal orthosis (TLSO) with knee–ankle–foot orthoses (KAFOs) and hip guidance orthosis (HGO)
Below L2	TLSO with KAFOs and lumbar–sacral orthosis (LSO) LSO with KAFOs
Below L3–L4	LSO with KAFOs KAFOs alone
Below L5	KAFOs or ankle–foot orthoses (AFOs)
Below S1	AFOs

Obesity and pressure sores are the main problems encountered in adults and it is important that opportunities to keep fit are offered via sports clubs for their active participation.

Orthoses

Orthoses that enable the child to achieve independent walking need to become an integral part of the child's life and should be introduced to the child and family in a positive, enthusiastic manner. The child should be encouraged, but not forced, to wear them and a gradual increase in their use advised. Edwards & Charlton (2002) reviewed orthotic devices used in adult neurological patients. Table 19.2 outlines the level of orthotic support required for different levels of lesion.

Children who require support above the pelvis frequently opt to use a wheelchair as an adult and it is important to be realistic in terms of walking for these children. The support required for a high lesion will include thoracic, lumbar, sacral and lower-limb orthoses. The child usually begins walking with a swivel movement, transferring weight from leg to leg, but progresses to a swing-through gait as strength and balance improve. Initially a rollator is used for support but the aim is to move to quadruped sticks and eventually to crutches. The rate of progress will depend on the child's motivation to walk, parental input and physical limitations. The hip guidance orthosis (HGO)

was developed for children with high lesions who experience difficulty with walking (Rose et al., 1991). It enables the child to walk at a reasonable speed with a low energy output. The brace consists of a rigid body and leg brace with a fixed hip abduction of 5° that allows hip articulation during walking of between 5° and 10° on a shoe rocker (Fig. 19.5).

Swivel walking plates may also aid the development of walking by enabling the child to move in an upright position before walking is possible.

The provision of orthoses to a child adds another very important dimension to the parental care already in place. It is important that parents understand how to apply the orthoses correctly and the need to make regular checks on the child's skin. Anaesthetic skin can easily develop pressure sores and care must be taken to prevent this.

The following guidelines should be implemented:

- a daily check of all anaesthetic skin areas
- smooth clothing must be worn under orthoses and cover the whole area of skin contact; vest and socks should fit well and be worn with seams out
- toes need to be uncurled when putting shoes on by running a finger underneath them
- regular checks on the fit of orthoses and boots should be made.

A more definitive method is needed to assess the energy consumption of children with spina bifida who are walking, in order to assess their prognosis for long-term ambulation and as an indicator as to when ambulation should cease. Reliable predictive factors could reduce unnecessary surgery for children who will not be ambulant as adults. The Cosmed K2 system is a reliable

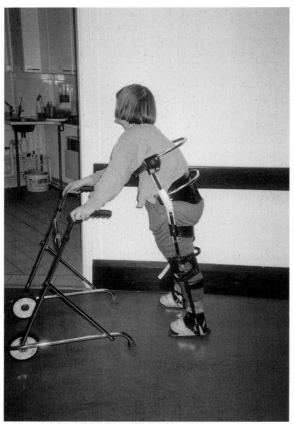

Figure 19.5 Hip guidance orthosis (HGO) in use with a rollator. The HGO is available under various brand names.

method that can be used to measure energy cost in children with spina bifida (Duffy et al., 1996).

Pressure care, posture and seating

The main factors in the development of tissue trauma are:

- excessive force, causing tissue deformation and restriction of the blood supply
- shear forces from friction of retaining a position or changing position
- low temperature of tissues should be avoided – warm tissues have a better blood supply and therefore are at less risk of developing pressure sores
- humidity – wet skin is more vulnerable to damage.

Children with spina bifida are at great risk of developing pressure sores, as most of the above factors are applicable, and where there is anaesthetic skin they are unaware of them. From birth the parents, and later the individual, must be vigilant in reducing these factors. Daily inspection is vital to spot areas that are developing

redness. If reddened areas do not subside within 20 min of removing the pressure, then there is a real risk of sores developing and the pressure should not be reapplied.

Excessive force can arise from uneven distribution of weight in sitting, failure to relieve pressure, poorly fitting orthoses and creased clothing. Relieving pressure during long periods of sitting needs to become a habit alongside frequent orthotic checks.

Shear forces can be created when the person's sitting position does not maintain him or her in a stable posture and there is a tendency to slide down the chair or bed. Postural control systems that distribute pressure evenly and provide sufficient support are needed to prevent this (Pountney et al., 1999). Seating systems for enhancing good posture in wheelchairs are discussed in Chapters 7 and 25, and have been reviewed by Pope (2002). Light-weight, high-performance wheelchairs are now available that are more functional and aesthetically pleasing than older models. Transfers by the child or carer can cause friction if the surface across which he or she is moving is not adequately cleared.

Temperature is difficult to assess where there is no sensation and is likely to fall in non-moving muscles and joints. The child should always be kept warm and learn to feel the skin regularly to check its temperature. Massage can be beneficial in warming the tissues and increasing blood flow. Sheepskin-lined boots can be worn in the winter.

Wet skin can be a danger area in children and adults who are incontinent. This, combined with excessive pressure or shearing forces, can be disastrous for anaesthetic skin. Skin hygiene in susceptible areas must be meticulous and, for later independence, wash-and-dry toilets are recommended.

Conservative management of pressure sores is achieved by relieving pressure on the affected area. For buttocks, contoured cushions and/or use of a self-propelled trolley is indicated. For legs, plaster of Paris or Baycast splinting, changed weekly, can be effective. Minor or plastic surgery is indicated for sores that do not respond to conservative management. Measures must be taken following healing to prevent pressure redeveloping in the same area.

CASE HISTORY

JF was born in April 1989 with a myelomeningocele in the sacral region, L5–S1. The myelomeningocele was closed at 2 days and a shunt to control hydrocephalus inserted at 4 days.

An assessment of her muscle power at 10 days indicated that she would be an active walker with the help of orthoses. To maintain muscle length and joint range, a daily regimen of passive movements to the lower limbs was implemented.

Physiotherapy assessment at 2 months showed an infant with general low muscle tone and poor prone extension. There was no fixed calcaneus deformity; active dorsiflexion was present but no plantarflexion. Stretching of the ankles was recommended at each nappy change. Parents were advised to place JF in the prone position once a day to stretch hip flexors and to encourage active movement with stimulating play activities.

Equinus deformities were seen to be developing at 8 months and night splints to control ankle inversion were fitted. Parents were taught to check her skin regularly for marked areas.

At 12 months JF could roll, sit unaided and take weight in standing. She was attending a specialist nursery once a week and developing into a happy and sociable little girl.

At 17 months she was beginning to pull to standing and at 21 months ankle–foot orthoses were prescribed but she disliked them and preferred walks without them, exhibiting an asymmetrical gait with hip-hitch and inverted feet. At 22 months knee–ankle–foot orthoses (KAFOS) were prescribed and gait education begun. Although able to walk without a rollator, she was encouraged to use it to develop a more symmetrical gait pattern.

At 2 years 8 months, JF suffered major shunt problems with infection and disconnection that lasted 4 months and included a bout of peritonitis. This was a very stressful period for her parents and left JF very weak. An intensive period of physiotherapy followed to regain lost muscle strength and mobility. Her left foot had developed an equinus deformity due to lack of splinting while she was ill, so splinting and frequent passive movements were encouraged.

At 4 years 3 months, JF was able to walk independently with KAFOs and a rollator but needed to hip-hitch to gain swing-through and later implications for

her spine were noted. A Physiological Cost Index (PCI) of 1.92 (normal 0.4) indicated that a great deal of effort was required to walk at this stage.

During this year preparations for JF to enter a mainstream school were made and she was awarded a statement of educational needs with ancillary help for 15 hours a week. This time was for educational support for specific learning difficulties related to hydrocephalus and physical support for moving around the school and toiletting. At 5 years, JF began mainstream first school where staff were very concerned about accepting JF, and the specialist health visitor and physiotherapist spent a great deal of time liaising to support her entry into school.

Poor bladder function was successfully controlled with intermittent catheterisation and JF was taught to perform the technique herself. This was a combined gradual approach, led by the specialist health visitor, with the parents and JF's non-teaching assistant.

JF had learnt to use quadruped sticks by the age of 6 years. She was managing well in school, walking independently and beginning to introduce crutches. She could walk independently but the asymmetry of her gait was reduced with sticks. She used a self-propelled wheelchair for long distances and games, rode a low-geared tricycle and swam weekly. These activities contributed to the promotion of specific muscle strength, general fitness and weight control.

At 6 years 6 months, problems with her shunt recurred. This was evident due to a loss of dexterity and general fatigue. She had a shunt revision, which was unsuccessful, followed by 2 weeks' exteriorisation of the shunt due to infection. Another very stressful period with a long hospitalisation occurred. Following this there was a considerable loss of balance and strength. JF returned to using a rollator for several weeks and increased her wheelchair use. Physiotherapeutic intervention was aimed at maintaining independent mobility whilst rebuilding muscle strength and fitness to previous levels.

References

Agnarsson U, Warde C, McCarthy G et al. Anorectal function of children with neurological problems. *Dev Med Child Neurol* 1993, **35**:893–902.

Botting B. Trends in neural tube defects. *Health Statistics Q* 2001, **10**:5–13.

Charney EB. Parental attitudes toward management of newborns with myelomeningocele. *Dev Med Child Neurol* 1990, **35**:14–19.

Cuckle HS, Wald NJ, Cuckle PM. Prenatal screening and diagnosis of neural tube defects in England and Wales in 1985. *Prenat Diag* 1989, **9**:393–400.

Duffy CM, Hill AE, Cosgrove AP, Corry IS, Graham HK. Energy consumption in children with spina bifida and

cerebral palsy: a comparative study. *Dev Med Child Neurol* 1996, **38**:238–243.

Dunning D. *Children with Spina Bifida and/or Hydrocephalus at School*. Peterborough: Association for Spina Bifida and Hydrocephalus; 1994.

Edwards S, Charlton P. Splinting and the use of orthoses in the management of patients with neurological disorders. In: Edwards S, ed. *Neurological Physiotherapy: A Problem Solving Approach*, 2nd edn. London: Churchill Livingstone; 2002:219–253.

Expert Advisory Group. *Report on Folic Acid and the Prevention of Neural Tube Defects*. London: Department of Health; 1992.

Fixsen JA. Orthopaedic management. In: McCarthy GT, ed. *Physical Disability in Childhood*. Edinburgh: Churchill Livingstone; 1992:198–201.

French S. Attitudes of health professionals towards disabled people. A discussion and review of the literature. *Physiotherapy* 1994, **80**:687–693.

Houliston MJ, Taguri AH, Dutton GN et al. Evidence of cognitive visual problems in children with hydrocephalus: a structural clinical history taking strategy. *Dev Med Child Neurol* 1999; **41**:298–306.

Lawrence JM, Pettiti DB, Watkins M, Umekubo MA. *Lancet* 1999, **354**:915–916.

Leatherman KD, Dickson RA. *The Management of Spinal Deformities*. London: Wright; 1988:191.

Levene MI. The spectrum of neural tube defects. In: Levene MI, Bennett MJ, Punt J, eds. *Fetal and Neonatal Neurology and Neurosurgery*. Edinburgh: Churchill Livingstone; 1988:267.

Mazur JM, Shurtleff D, Menelaus MB, Colliver JJ. Orthopaedic management of high level spina bifida. *J Bone Joint Surg* 1989, **71A**:5661.

McCarthy GT, Land R. Hydrocephalus. In: McCarthy GT, ed. *Physical Disability in Childhood*. Edinburgh: Churchill Livingstone; 1992:213–221.

McCarthy GT, Cartwright RD, Jones M et al. Spina bifida. In: McCarthy GT, ed. *Physical Disability in Childhood*. Edinburgh: Churchill Livingstone; 1992:189–212.

Morley TM. Spinal deformity in the physically handicapped child. In: McCarthy GT, ed. *Physical Disability in Childhood*. Edinbugh: Churchill Livingstone; 1992:356–365.

Oakley GP. Delaying folic acid fortification of flour. *BMJ* 2002, **324**:1348–1349.

Pope PM. Postural management and special seating. In: Edwards S, ed. *Neurological Physiotherapy: A Problem Solving Approach*, 2nd edn. London: Churchill Livingstone; 2002:189–217.

Pountney TE, Green EM, Mulcahy CM, Nelham RL. The Chailey approach to postural management. *J Assoc Paediatr Chartered Physiother* 1999, **March**:15–33.

Rose J, Gamble JG, Lee J et al. Energy expenditure index: a method to quantitate and compare walking energy expenditure for children and adolescents. *J Paed Orthop* 1991, **11**:571–578.

Special Education Needs (SEN) Code of Practice. London: Department for Education and Skills, HMSO; 2001.

Wald NJ, Bower C. Folic acid and the prevention of neural tube defects. *BMJ* 1995, **310**:1019–1020.

Whitehead WE, Parker L, Basmajian L et al. Treatment of faecal incontinence in children with spina bifida: comparison of biofeedback and behaviour modification. *Arch Phys Med Rehab* 1986, **67**:218–224.

Chapter 20

Muscle disorders of childhood onset

N Thompson   R Quinlivan

CHAPTER CONTENTS

INTRODUCTION

This chapter deals with the muscular dystrophies of childhood onset as well as the spinal muscular atrophies. Muscle disorders of adult onset were described in Chapter 15. Details of investigations and general management issues are discussed under the section on Duchenne muscular dystrophy (DMD) but most of these also apply to the other disorders. The physical management section applies to all the conditions but prognosis must be taken into account. For a more comprehensive discussion of differential diagnosis and prognosis, clinical features and general management, the reader is referred to Karpati et al. (2001) and Dubowitz (1995).

THE MUSCULAR DYSTROPHIES

The muscular dystrophies are a group of genetically determined disorders associated with progressive degeneration of skeletal muscle. They can be subdivided into a number of different disorders based upon mode of inheritance, protein, enzyme and/or genetic defect (see Ch. 15, Tables 15.1 and 15.2).

The Xp21.2 myopathies or dystrophinopathies are progressive disorders of muscle resulting in a wide spectrum of disease severity, with DMD at the most severe end and Becker muscular dystrophy (BMD) at the milder end of the spectrum. X-linked dilated cardiomyopathy (XLDC) is also caused by a deletion in the same gene and results in a severe life-limiting cardiomyopathy but little, if any, muscle weakness. All of these disorders are caused by a defect of the protein dystrophin and are characterised by X-linked inheritance, in which males are affected and females are carriers, although up to 10% of carriers manifest muscle weakness. There is a normal appearance at birth (though the level of plasma creatine kinase (CK) is very high), and an early hypertrophy of muscle, but also weakness, followed by progressive wasting and disability.

Duchenne muscular dystrophy

DMD was first described by Meryon in 1852 and later by Guillaume Duchenne. It is rapidly progressive and is the most severe of all the muscular dystrophies; it is inherited in an X-linked recessive fashion. It occurs in 18–30 per 100 000 males at birth with a prevalence in the population of 1.9–4.8 per 100 000 (Emery, 1991).

Clinical and diagnostic features

The first clinical manifestations of DMD appear when the child shows delayed motor milestones at 3–5 years. The child may be late in sitting, standing and walking and when he does begin to walk, he often falls. If there is no family history the diagnosis is often not suspected. By the age of 5 there is obvious muscle weakness; the child is unable to run or jump. Physical examination reveals enlarged calf muscles due to compensatory hypertrophy but this will develop later into pseudohypertrophy since the muscle is replaced by fat and connective tissue.

Hip and knee extensor weakness results in difficulty getting up from the floor. Initially, in order to rise from the floor, the child must give some assistance to hip and knee extension by pushing off from the thigh with the hand or forearm. With increasing weakness, the child climbs up his legs using both arms, and this is the classic Gowers' manoeuvre which is associated with, though not confined to, DMD. As muscles become weaker the corresponding tendon reflexes become depressed and are eventually lost, but there is no sensory loss.

An abnormal 'waddling' gait is a well-recognised presenting symptom (Emery, 1987). Owing to early weakness of the hip abductors, the child is unable to maintain a level pelvis when lifting one leg off the ground. He therefore inclines towards the other leg to bring the centre of gravity of the body over that leg, and as he moves forward this action is continually repeated and accounts for the Trendelenburg sign. This is accompanied by widening of the base of support for increased stability, which contributes to the evolution of hip abduction contractures (iliotibial band tightness).

By 7–8 years of age, contractures of heel cords and iliotibial bands lead to toe-walking. Between 8 and 9 years, walking usually requires the use of braces (Fig. 20.1) and by the age of 13 years independent ambulation is lost in 100% of patients (Bertorini et al., 2002). Prolonged sitting leads to further flexion contractures of the elbows, hips and knees.

In the early ambulatory phase of DMD, an equinus foot posture is precipitated by relative weakness of the ankle dorsiflexors compared with the better-preserved plantarflexors. Gait analysis has shown that a dynamic equinus is a necessary biomechanical adaptation to maintain knee stability in the presence of gross quadriceps muscle weakness. Forceful action of the ankle plantarflexors provides a torque which opposes knee flexion (Khodadadeh et al., 1986). Thus, contracture of the Achilles tendon, which eventually accompanies disease progression, is secondary to dynamic equinus.

Muscle involvement is bilateral and symmetrical and the proximal muscles are more affected than the distal groups. In the ambulatory stage, the pelvic girdle is slightly more affected than the shoulder girdle. There is more severe weakness in the extensor groups than in the flexors although this differential muscle involvement becomes less clear as the disease progresses, so that ultimately such patterns of weakness are no longer obvious. Finally, contractures become fixed and a progressive scoliosis develops. Scoliosis exacerbates existing respiratory muscle weakness, and in severe cases may render the child bed-bound. Scoliosis occurs in 50–80% of patients and causes additional respiratory problems (Kurz et al., 1983).

Muscle imbalance (caused by the specific pattern of developing weakness) and postural malalignment (resulting from compensatory adjustments to maintain standing equilibrium) are factors precipitating the eventual development of contractures about weight-bearing joints. These are relatively mild while the child remains ambulant but progress rapidly once there is dependence on a wheelchair. These postures combine lumbar lordosis, hip flexion and abduction, and ankle equinus.

The first alteration of body alignment in DMD is a lumbar lordosis due to early weakness of the hip extensors, so that active stabilisation of the hip joint is compromised. In order to maintain the line of force behind the hip joint and prevent collapse into hip flexion, there is an initial posterior alignment of the upper trunk resulting in a compensatory lumbar lordosis. As weakness progresses this is accompanied by an exaggerated anterior tilt of the pelvis which predisposes to contractures of the hip flexors.

It is important to realise that DMD is a multisystem disease and not only a problem of skeletal muscle. Gastrointestinal problems can be evident clinically through oropharyngeal, oesophageal and gastric dysfunction (Jaffe et al., 1990), and constipation is common, especially once ambulation is lost. About 59% of patients have lower than normal intelligence (IQ 70–85; Billard et al., 1992). Others have normal or above-normal intelligence. The mental retardation does not increase with age. Thus, DMD is an incurable and ultimately fatal disease characterised by muscle weakness, contracture, deformity and progressive disability. However,

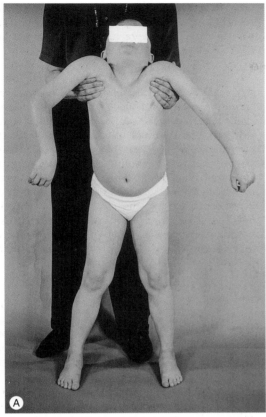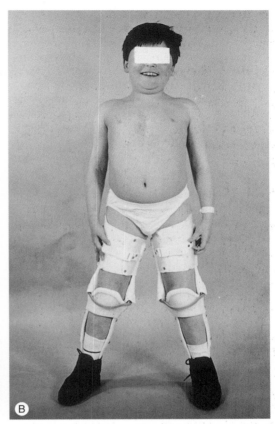

Figure 20.1   Boy with Duchenne muscular dystrophy. (A) At the point of loss of independent walking. (B) Following percutaneous Achilles tenotomies and rehabilitation in light-weight ischial weight-bearing knee–ankle–foot orthoses (KAFOs).

'incurable' is not synonymous with 'untreatable'. A variety of therapeutic and surgical measures are available that can help to minimise deformity, prolong independent ambulation and maximise functional capabilities. There is also evidence that improved management strategies are resulting in increased survival rates (Galasko et al., 1992). Most boys will die from respiratory or cardiac failure, but the introduction of nocturnal nasal ventilation has improved survival figures, such that the average life expectancy is now 25 years with non-invasive ventilation, compared with 19 years without this treatment (Eagle et al., 2002).

The principles of successful management are based on an understanding of the natural evolution of patterns of weakness, contracture and deformity, so that intervention can be staged appropriately.

Pathology

Muscle weakness in DMD primarily arises due to the gradual loss of functional muscle fibres, which are replaced by fat and connective tissue; this is evident on muscle biopsy (Fig. 20.2). The clinical manifestation of this proliferation of fat and connective tissue is pseudohypertrophy of certain muscle groups, particularly the calf.

Failure to produce dystrophin, a protein encoded by the DMD gene, is the primary biochemical defect (Hoffman et al., 1988). Dystrophin is an integral protein within a complex of proteins which stabilizes the integrity of the sarcolemmal membrane, particularly during the stress associated with repeated cycles of contraction and relaxation. Absence of dystrophin production may explain a reduction in permeability of the muscle cell membrane, so allowing excessive quantities of calcium to accumulate within the muscle fibre, leading to myofibrillar overcontracture, breakdown of myofibrils and various metabolic disturbances that culminate in the death of the muscle fibre (Dubowitz, 1985). Although the precise function of this cytoskeletal protein is not understood, its complete or virtual absence is associated with a worse prognosis, whereas in BMD, in which there is a capability to produce (albeit abnormal) dystrophin, the prognosis is less severe.

Questions have been raised as to whether the absence of dystrophin is merely an early trigger in the pathogenesis of the dystrophy, with subsequent secondary mechanisms being more important (Dubowitz, 1989). Edwards et al. (1984) theorised that the pathogenesis may be related to the largely postural antigravity role of the proximal muscles, rendering them more susceptible to damaging eccentric contractions.

Confirmation of diagnosis

The tests mentioned in this section are discussed in Chapter 2 and the features relevant to DMD are outlined here and discussed further by Karpati et al. (2001) and Mastaglia & Laing (1996).

Biochemical blood tests

The serum CK is a useful marker pointing towards the diagnosis and is markedly elevated, even at birth when there are no other clinical signs. In DMD and BMD the enzyme is raised up to 50 times greater than normal (normal range 33–194 IU/l) but the levels drop once ambulation is lost (Karpati et al., 2001).

Electromyography (EMG)

In practice EMG is no longer required to make a diagnosis of DMD and is rarely undertaken; however, a myopathic pattern would be expected.

Muscle biopsy

A muscle biopsy is usually required to confirm the diagnosis (Bertorini et al., 2002). This can be undertaken either as a percutaneous technique using a biopsy needle or as an open procedure, depending on the practice of the investigating unit. Muscle histology demonstrates dystrophic features which include an increased variation of fibre size, evidence of necrosis with phagocytosis, an increase in central nuclei, hypercontracted eosinophillic hyaline fibres and an increase in fat and connective tissue (Fig. 20.2). Histochemical staining using antibodies to N, C and rod domain epitopes of dystrophin usually show complete absence of the protein, except for occasional revertent fibres (these are fibres which label normally with antibodies to dystrophin; their origin is not understood; Fig. 20.2F).

Weak or uneven labelling of dystrophin may be seen in BMD and intermediate phenotypes. In manifesting carriers, dystrophin immunolabelling demonstrates a mosaic appearance with positive and negative fibres. Immunolabelling with other antibodies in both DMD and BMD shows a reduction of membrane proteins associated with dystrophin, and overexpression of utrophin, an autosomal protein very similar to dystrophin.

Deoxyribonucleic acid (DNA) probes

DNA testing from a blood sample will demonstrate a frame-shift deletion within the dystrophin gene in approximately 60% of DMD cases. The remaining cases will result from duplications and point mutations (Mastaglia & Laing, 1996). The finding of a DNA deletion, duplication or point mutation allows carrier detection and prenatal diagnosis in the affected boy's mother and female relatives. In some cases DNA analysis is the only test required to confirm the diagnosis of DMD. In BMD the same proportion of patients will have deletions but the reading frame of the gene is preserved (in-frame). Exceptions to the frame-shift rule occur and thus a muscle biopsy is usually recommended.

General management of DMD

There is no cure for DMD but much can be done to improve the boy's quality of life and increase life expectancy. The key milestones in the disease progress that require sensitive management, particularly of the parents, are:

- suspicion of abnormality
- diagnosis
- loss of ambulation
- consideration of spinal surgery
- leaving school and transition from paediatric to adult services
- final illness
- bereavement.

Informing parents that their child has DMD causes extreme distress and should only be undertaken by the most senior member of the team in an appropriate environment with a support worker present who can maintain contact with the family once they have left the hospital. The information given to the parents must be factual and honest, but delivered with sensitivity and empathy.

The long-term care of the child will require a specialist multidisciplinary team liaising closely with community medical, educational and social agencies. As soon as the diagnosis is confirmed the child's paediatrician will ensure that developmental or IQ assessments are made to ensure that appropriate educational support is put in place for the child at the start of his educational career. Social services will be required to become involved to ensure the family receives the correct state financial entitlements and will be paramount in

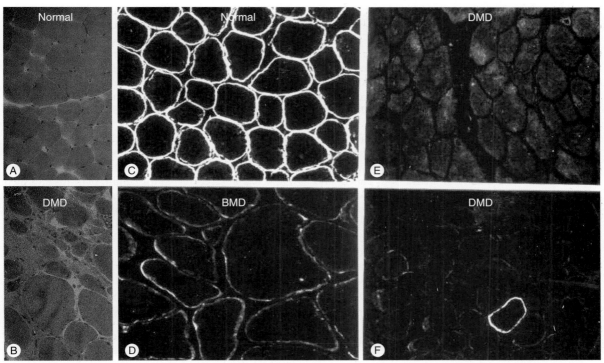

Figure 20.2 Biopsies of normal (A, C) and dystrophic muscle (B, D–F). Note the abnormal histology of the dystrophic muscle (B) with a wide variation in fibre size, fibrous tissue surrounding the fibres and nuclei within the fibres. An antibody to dystrophin has been used to label the muscle in panels (C–F). Note the normal intense sarcolemmal localisation on all fibres in (C), the reduced patchy labelling of dystrophin in a case of Becker muscular dystrophy (BMD) in panel (D), and the absence of dystrophin in a case of Duchenne muscular dystrophy (DMD) in (E). One revertent fibre with apparently normal dystrophin is shown in (F). (Courtesy of Professor Caroline Sewry.)

arranging home adaptations, which are usually necessary by the time the child is 7 or 8 years of age, at which time climbing stairs will be impossible.

Management of disability

From an early age, tightness and subsequently contractures of the tendo-achilles (TA) develop. Daily passive stretching of the TA and provision of night splints are recommended as soon as any tightening of the TA is demonstrated. Later on, when significant pelvic girdle weakness is manifest by a waddling gait, the iliotibial bands and hip flexors may start to tighten. Care must be taken to ensure assessment at each outpatient visit with advice to undertake stretching exercises. The priority of physical management is to prolong ambulation for as long as possible, since once ambulation is lost, scoliosis and joint contractures develop rapidly. As soon as ambulation is lost, light-weight ischial weight-bearing long leg calipers can be used to prolong walking. This usually involves a minor surgical procedure to release any lower-limb contractures percutaneously, together

with an intensive rehabilitation programme. The parents and child must be strongly motivated for this form of rehabilitation to be successful.

In recent years, there is growing evidence that treatment with steroids (prednisolone or deflazacort) will stabilise muscle function for some time, therefore delaying the loss of ambulation by up to 2 years (Dubowitz, 2000). Careful monitoring for side-effects is essential, especially weight gain, which may potentially have a negative effect on function. The potential benefit of longer-term steroid treatment has yet to be evaluated. Premature loss of ambulation can follow lower-limb fractures or ligament strains unless active management, such as internal fixation, is instigated to promote early mobility. Immobilising any joint beyond the initial painful phase should be actively discouraged. Likewise, careful monitoring of growth is essential, since rapid weight gain will have a deleterious effect on ambulation. Growth charts specifically produced for DMD may be useful (Griffiths & Edwards, 1988).

Once independent ambulation is lost, regular standing in a standing frame is essential to maintain good posture and reduce contracture development. Rigid ankle–foot orthoses (AFOs) are recommended for day-time use to maintain a good foot position. Likewise it is essential to ensure that the wheelchair provides good back and neck support (Pope, 2002) and ideally the controls of an electric wheelchair should be centrally placed. Swimming and hydrotherapy are particularly useful and enjoyed by the boys who find they can make more movement in the water.

A rapidly progressive scoliosis requiring stabilisation will develop in up to 95% of boys. The Luque procedure is highly successful in correcting the deformity, improving posture and the quality of life for both patient and carer (Mehdian et al., 1989). The timing of operation is crucial because a decline in vital capacity occurs at about the same time as scoliosis. To avoid undue anaesthetic risks the procedure must be undertaken before the vital capacity falls below 40% of that expected for height (Galasko et al., 1992; Miller et al., 1992). The consequence is that surgical correction is often recommended when the degree of spinal curvature is still relatively mild.

Management of restricted participation

Restricted participation has replaced the term 'handicap' in the revised *International Classification of Functioning, Disability and Health* by the World Health Organization (WHO, 2001; see Ch. 3) and its management must take into account psychosocial issues, mobility and education. Providing an electric wheelchair is essential to providing a degree of independence, but this requires appropriate home adaptations, including widened doors and indoor/outdoor wheelchair access. A hoist is required for lifting in and out of the wheelchair, and the child will require a ground-floor bedroom and bathroom with disabled shower and toilet facilities. An electric bed enables the child to alter his position and saves the parents many sleepless nights. An adapted motor vehicle is required for transport to enable the child to drive his own wheelchair in and out of the vehicle.

The revolution in computer technology and its application to assistive devices has transformed the lives of many disabled people, e.g. the possum system enables the child to open and close doors, windows, curtains and turn on and off lights. Access to the internet allows friendships to develop and provides a source of information and various services. Electronic games enable the boys to play competitively alongside their able-bodied companions and probably have a major effect on building self-esteem and reducing boredom.

Respiratory problems

With advancing age, respiratory impairment becomes inevitable and if not recognised is an important cause of unpleasant symptoms and death (Vignos, 1976). Characteristically there is a restrictive defect, with a reduction in total lung capacity caused by a combination of diaphragmatic and intercostal muscle weakness. Chest wall stiffness, recurrent aspiration and an inability to cough effectively compound the respiratory insufficiency leading to an increased frequency of chest infections (Smith et al., 1991a). The forced vital capacity is a reliable measure of respiratory function, provided the boy is able to undertake a good technique (in some boys with learning difficulty this may be a problem; Griggs et al., 1981). The forced vital capacity, when corrected for height, plateaus and then falls progressively on average between 12 and 14 years of age. Once the vital capacity falls below 1 litre, in a boy who has reached skeletal maturity, the average life expectancy without treatment is 3 years (Phillips et al., 2001).

Sleep-related respiratory abnormalities play a major role in ventilatory failure, resulting in symptoms of hypercapnia, which include early-morning headache, nausea and sweating, day-time somnolence and a loss of respiratory drive (resulting in rapid deterioration into coma if a high concentration of oxygen is administered). Chronic nocturnal hypoxaemia leads to cor pulmonale (right heart failure); the electrocardiogram (ECG) may show evidence of pulmonary hypertension and right heart strain (Carroll et al., 1991). Once the vital capacity falls below 1 litre, or if there are symptoms to suggest nocturnal hypoventilation, sleep studies should be undertaken at regular intervals to confirm the diagnosis. Treatment by non-invasive nasal ventilation is effective in alleviating symptoms and prolongs survival (Simonds, 2000; Eagle et al., 2002).

Cardiac problems

Postmortem studies show that all boys with DMD have evidence of cardiomyopathy. In practice, however, symptomatic cardiomyopathy is less common than might be expected. It has been assumed that the sedentary lifestyle of these boys contributes to the lack of symptoms (Hunsaker et al., 1982). Abnormalities of the ECG are evident from an early age and will be present in all boys by 18 years of age (Nigro et al., 1990); the most common abnormality is a resting tachycardia, which is almost universal. Cardiac arrhythmias occur and may be a cause of early sudden death. When congestive cardiac failure does occur, the progression is rapid and relentless. Monitoring with cardiac echo is recommended once ambulation is lost. Early treatment with angiotensin-converting enzyme (ACE) inhibitors may be beneficial, although published evidence is currently lacking.

The final illness

Close monitoring and liaison with the general practitioner and palliative care services are paramount. Children's hospices play a vital role in supporting families and boys during this difficult time. Patient support groups, such as the Muscular Dystrophy Campaign, frequently fund care workers to support families (see Appendix).

Becker muscular dystrophy

BMD is the milder form of X-linked recessive muscular dystrophy (see Table 15.2) and has a prevalence of 1 in 30 000. It is caused by a partial deficiency of the protein dystrophin (Karpati et al., 2001).

Clinical and diagnostic features

BMD has a wide spectrum of severity; at the severest end, ambulation may be lost by 16 years of age, compared with the mildest form with non-progressive cramps and myoglobinuria (Gospe et al., 1989). Distribution of weakness is similar to DMD but progression of the disease is much slower and contractures are often less severe than in DMD. As with DMD, muscle hypertrophy, especially of the calves occurs. Up to 40% of patients will lose ambulation; prolonging ambulation with long leg calipers is more difficult than in DMD because of adult height.

In some patients an unexpected malignant hyperthermia reaction following anaesthesia may be the first manifestation of the disease. Cardiomyopathy is common and more likely to be symptomatic than in DMD. ECG and echocardiogram abnormalities may be evident in up to 50% of cases (Steare et al., 1992) and many patients have successfully undergone cardiac transplantation (Quinlivan & Dubowitz, 1992).

Because the life expectancy is much better than for DMD, genetic implications are more important for the patient who will not father affected sons, but will pass the faulty gene to all daughters who will be carriers for the disorder. The diagnosis is confirmed by finding a DNA mutation in the dystrophin gene and/or abnormal dystrophin staining on a muscle biopsy.

General management of BMD

The management of BMD involves prevention of contractures and prolonging ambulation, as with DMD. In addition, the patient requires support to continue working in an adapted environment if he desires. Home adaptations again are essential in promoting independence. For those patients who are wheelchair-dependent, regular standing, preventing excessive weight gain and constipation are important. Prevention of respiratory infections by vaccination against influenza and *Pneumococcus*, together with prompt antibiotic treatment of infection, are necessary. Monitoring of respiratory function and sleep hypoxaemia are necessary. Symptoms of chronic ventilatory failure should be managed with non-invasive ventilation, as for the DMD group. Regular cardiac monitoring with yearly ECGs and cardiac echos every 2 or 3 years is necessary. Early intervention with ACE inhibitors for ventricular dysfunction may be helpful but as yet has to be fully evaluated. If cardiac symptoms fail to respond to medical treatment, assessment for cardiac transplantation is warranted (Quinlivan & Dubowitz, 1992).

Emery Dreifuss muscular dystrophy

This is a rare but clinically distinct form of MD. Two modes of inheritance exist; firstly, a sex-linked form (EDMD) in which the defective gene is located at Xq28 and the defective protein is emerin, a nuclear envelope protein (Mastaglia & Laing, 1996). Secondly, there is an autosomal dominant form (ADEDMD) in which the defective gene is at 1q11-q23 encoding for another nuclear envelope protein, lamin A/C (Bonne et al., 1999).

Clinical and diagnostic features

The main feature of the nuclear envelope dystrophies is the predominance of joint contractures and muscle weakness. Contractures predominantly affect the neck and spine, elbows and TA. Disturbances of cardiac rhythm are universal by the second or third decades and may result in sudden death unless detected and cardiac pacing instituted (Bialer et al., 1991). Thus, regular ECG and 24-h ECG monitoring are essential. Muscle weakness is slowly progressive and involves the humeroperoneal groups of muscles. Many patients retain some ambulation throughout adult life.

General management

Management of contractures involves stretching exercises and night splints, as discussed below. Provided the diagnosis is made sufficiently early, the insertion of a cardiac pacemaker may be life-saving. In the case of ADEDMD a defibrillator pacemaker is recommended.

The associated weakness is usually mild. However, due to rigidity of the spine throughout its length, the patient is unable to compensate for any hip extensor weakness with a lumbar lordosis, as is commonly seen in many of the other neuromuscular diseases. Instead, the patient maintains the centre of mass with increasing equinus at the ankles, leading to secondary contracture of the TA. If these contractures become severe, they may in themselves jeopardise mobility and require

Table 20.1 The congenital muscular dystrophies (CMD)

Type	Gene	Protein	Disease
MDC1A (LAMA2)	6q2	Laminin α-2 chain of merosin	Merosin-deficient CMD
FCMD	9q31–33	Fukutin	Fukuyama CMD
ITGA7	12q	Integrin α-deficiency	
MEB	1p3	POMGnTI	Muscle–eye–brain disease
WWS	9q34	POMT1	Walker–Warburg syndrome
RSMD1	1p36	SEPN1	Rigid spine syndrome
MDC1B	1q42	Secondary merosin deficiency	CMD with secondary merosin deficiency 1
MDC1C	19q1	FKRP	CMD with secondary merosin deficiency 2
UCMD	21q32 21q2 2q	COL6A2 COL6A3 COL6A3	Ullrich CMD

percutaneous surgical correction. Management should be aimed at controlling the progression of deformity by appropriate strengthening, passive stretching and splinting techniques (see Chs 23 and 25).

Congenital muscular dystrophies

There are several recognised forms of congenital muscular dystrophy depending upon the protein/gene defect and/or the association of central abnormalities (Table 20.1). They are all caused by autosomal recessive genes and present at birth or in infancy with hypotonia and joint contractures, often involving the spine. The serum CK may be normal in some groups and elevated in others; intellect may be normal or impaired depending upon the presence of neuronal migration defects. White-matter changes may be seen on magnetic resonance imaging in cases with merosin deficiency, although there is normal intellect. Muscle biopsy shows dystrophic features and in some types specific protein abnormalities.

Clinical and diagnostic features

Reduced fetal movements during pregnancy suggest that signs are already present before birth. Features in early infancy consist of muscle weakness and generalised hypotonia, 'floppiness', poor suck and respiratory difficulty (Kobayashi et al., 1996). In childhood, motor milestones are delayed, with severe and early contractures and often joint deformities (arthrogryposis). Weakness is greater in the pelvic girdle and upper-leg muscles than in the shoulder girdle and upper-arm muscles. On the whole, with the exception of Fukuyama congenital muscular dystrophy (FCMD), these conditions are relatively slowly progressive and functional ability can improve over time. Contractures at birth are common and may restrict function to a greater degree than weakness if not controlled. It is particularly important to be vigilant for the insidious development of contractures and to treat them promptly.

Other features of the disease are hip dislocation, pes cavus and kyphoscoliosis. The motor development is slow, leading to late sitting, standing and walking. Intelligence is normal. Serum CK activity is usually very high in the early stages. The EMG shows short-duration, small-amplitude and polyphasic motor potentials. There may be variable respiratory difficulties due to associated diaphragmatic involvement, at both presentation and later in adolescence.

General management

Attention to feeding and breathing is important in the neonatal period. Some patients will require percutaneous endoscopic gastrostomy (PEG) feeding due to bulbar involvement. Later on, useful mobility should be maintained for as long as possible. Regular exercise should be encouraged and obesity avoided. Regular gentle stretching is required to avoid or control contractures (see below). Nocturnal hypoventilation may develop in the second decade and is a particular feature of the rigid-spine phenotype, which responds well to nocturnal nasal ventilation.

THE SPINAL MUSCULAR ATROPHIES

The spinal muscular atrophies (SMAs) are a group of neurogenic disorders in which there is degeneration of the anterior horn cells of the spinal cord, resulting in muscle weakness. They are the most common neuromuscular disease in childhood after DMD and affect both sexes. The mode of inheritance is mainly autosomal recessive but can vary, with dominant or X-linked traits (Emery, 1971). The genetic defect lies on the long arm of chromosome 5 (Brzustowicz et al., 1990). Weakness is symmetrical, is greater proximally than distally, and the pelvic girdle is usually slightly more affected than the shoulder girdle. Weakness is generally non-progressive, although as a result of increasing height and weight there may be some loss of functional activities over time. There is no facial weakness and intellectual development is normal. Classification of SMAs is most usefully based on clinical severity (Dubowitz, 1995):

- severe: unable to sit unsupported
- intermediate: able to sit unsupported; unable to stand or walk unaided
- mild: able to stand and walk.

The clinical and diagnostic characteristics, as well as general management, are now discussed for each type of SMA.

Severe SMA (type 1 or Werdnig–Hoffmann disease)

This is a progressive infantile type of SMA that is inherited in an autosomal recessive manner. Children with severe SMA present neonatally as 'floppy' babies with progressive, severe, generalised weakness in the first few months of life. There is marked respiratory involvement and as a result they rarely survive beyond 2 years of age. Treatment will be mainly supportive.

The infant is unable to move out of a lying position and the upper limbs adopt an internally rotated 'jug-handle' position and the lower limbs a flexed and abducted 'frog position'. Limb contractures may develop related to these positions and, if untreated, activities such as dressing and lifting will become uncomfortable. Regular passive stretching techniques can become part of the daily routine at bathtimes and nappy changes. Moulding of the ribs can occur if the infant is always positioned on one particular side. This will further compromise respiratory capacity, and so alternation of sleeping positions is recommended.

The child will not achieve a sitting position unaided and is best supported in a slightly reclined, rather than upright, sitting position so that the diaphragm is not restricted and the head is supported. A supportive spinal jacket with a diaphragmatic aperture may be useful in helping to maintain a sitting position. The child is unlikely to have any antigravity strength and toys need to be small and light-weight.

The intercostal muscles are severely affected and breathing is almost entirely diaphragmatic, giving a characteristic bell-shaped chest. Cough is weak and bulbar weakness may give rise to sucking and swallowing difficulties. The child will be prone to recurrent respiratory infections, which should be treated promptly with antibiotics and chest physiotherapy.

Intermediate SMA (type 2)

Weakness usually develops between 6 and 12 months and the child presents with inability to stand or walk.

Long-term prognosis is dependent on respiratory function, and rapidly progressive scoliosis is a common complication associated with this group. Early spinal bracing will help to control the rate of progression, but spinal fusion may be necessary. Limb joints are often hyperextendable, particularly at the elbow and hands, but are prone to contractures related to positioning.

A major aim of management would be to promote standing and/or walking and the ability to achieve this will be dependent on residual muscle strength, particularly in the trunk and pelvic girdle, which should be carefully assessed. Some children show functional improvement and, with appropriate training, progression from standing in a frame to walking with calipers is possible. Since muscle weakness is not generally progressive, the ability to walk using ischial weight-bearing knee–ankle–foot orthoses (KAFOs) may be maintained over many years, helping to control both joint contractures and scoliosis. It should be noted that spinal bracing and spinal fusion are not normally compatible with continued mobility in calipers, since they limit compensatory trunk side flexion which aids weight transference when the hip abductors are weak.

Mild SMA (type 3 or Kugelberg–Welander disease)

Mild SMA is inherited as an autosomal recessive gene at 5q11-q13. The ability to walk is achieved at the normal age or slightly late and the child often presents with difficulty hopping, running and jumping. Proximal weakness, which is slightly more marked in the lower limbs, may give rise to a Gowers'-type manoeuvre when getting up off the floor. Strengthening programmes should be targetted to functional difficulties. Joint contractures and progressive scoliosis are rare in this group (Carter et al., 1995). Weakness is generally relatively static, but rapid periods of growth may result in loss of ambulation, and rehabilitation can be achieved in light-weight calipers.

PHYSICAL MANAGEMENT OF NEURO-MUSCULAR DISORDERS

This section highlights the areas of management which are specific to muscle disorders, in both adulthood and childhood. Details of treatment concepts and techniques are found in Chapters 21 and 23, respectively. A problem-solving approach is preferable and this is discussed in Chapter 22. Treatment planning should involve the multidisciplinary team (MDT), the patient, parents and preferably a carer at school.

Assessment

Thorough, standardised and regular assessment of children is essential because they change rapidly. Assessment is important both for guiding clinical management and for evaluating therapeutic outcome for research purposes. Aspects of assessment pertinent to muscle disorders are measurement of muscle strength, performance and lung function, and principles of assessment are discussed in Chapter 3.

Measurement of muscle strength

Strength assessments provide information for the planning and monitoring of intervention as well as diagnostic information.

Manual muscle testing   Manual muscle testing is the most widely used means of assessing muscle strength in clinical practice and has been recommended as an outcome measure for therapeutic trials in neuromuscular disease (Brooke et al., 1981). The Medical Research Council (MRC) scale of grading muscle strength is probably the most widely known grading system and is based on an ordinal scale of 0–5 (see Ch. 3, p. 33).

Whilst no special equipment is needed, and manual muscle testing is a rapid method of determining the distribution and severity of weakness over a large number of muscle groups, the major criticism of this method is the subjectivity in grading strengths. There are no standardised joint positions at which testing should be performed and the point at which counterforce is administered is also self-selected. The proportion of maximum strength required to overcome gravity is markedly different between muscle groups (Wiles et al., 1990), and a loss of strength in excess of 50% may develop before weakness can be detected by manual muscle testing (Fisher et al., 1990).

Dynamometry   Force can be measured directly with dynamometers; these quantitative measurements of muscle force are superior to manual muscle testing and provide the most direct method of assessing a particular muscle group. The design of the dynamometer has been gradually refined to produce a simple hand-held electrodynamometer which can measure maximal isometric strength of many different muscle groups as both a research and clinical tool (Hyde et al., 1983).

Myometry readings are highly reproducible, provided standardised techniques are used and the same observer performs the measurement on each occasion (Bohannon, 1986; Lennon & Ashburn, 1993). Serial measurements of a single patient will be the most useful means of evaluating the distribution and rate of change of muscle weakness, whilst the degree of weakness can be established by comparison with published normal values of muscle strength (Wiles et al., 1990). Muscle strength is a valid measure in that force is related to functional performance (Bohannon, 1989).

Hand-held dynamometers are only useful when muscles are weak, since their use is restricted by the strength of the operator to oppose the patient's efforts. Strain gauges attached to rigs, and also commercially available isometric and isokinetic machines, are available.

Measurement of joint range

The development of joint contractures should be monitored carefully and joint range of movement can be measured using a goniometer. However, caution must be taken with this method as it shows variable interrater reliability and measurements should be made by the same assessor where possible (Pandya et al., 1985).

Measurement of functional performance

The quantification of muscle strength has proved to be of value in the assessment and management of many muscle diseases, but it can be seen that this is a measure of impairment and is incomplete without concomitant measures of disability and ultimately the handicap to the patient. Measures of functional performance range from simple tests, such as the ability to rise from the floor (Rideau, 1984), to more detailed measures of motor ability and gait (Sutherland et al., 1981; Khodadadeh et al., 1986). These measurements are susceptible to the effects of impairments other than strength, but it is important in terms of patient management to determine whether a change in disability can properly be attributed to a change in the strength of the muscles measured.

There may be disparities between strength and disability in muscle for a variety of reasons. These include: a failure to assess the relevant muscle groups that cause disability; a failure to note progressing severe weakness in an important group, perhaps because of the averaging of many groups; or the intrusion of other relevant factors, such as the development of compensatory biomechanical manoeuvres or a gain in weight or height. It is of paramount importance that the measure of physical performance is both valid and reliable and these factors need to be recognised.

Table 20.2 Hammersmith score of motor ability

Motor ability	Score: 2, 1 or 0[a]
Lifts head	
Supine to prone over right	
Supine to prone over left	
Prone to supine over right	
Prone to supine over left	
Gets to sitting	
Sitting	
Gets to standing	
Standing	
Standing on heels	
Standing on toes	
Stands on right leg	
Stands on left leg	
Hops on right leg	
Hops on left leg	
Gets off chair	
Climbing step, right leg	
Descending step, right leg	
Climbing step, left leg	
Descending step, left leg	
Total score out of 40	

[a]Scoring: 2 for every completed movement; 1 for help and/or reinforcement; 0 if unable to achieve the movement. All movements are attempted and scored. (Adapted from Scott et al. (1982), with permission from John Wiley & Sons Inc.)

Motor ability tests

Whilst the Vignos scale was associated with the assessment of functional ability, particularly in DMD, it was originally designed as a functional classification and its sensitivity as an objective measure of function is doubtful. The Hammersmith motor ability score (Table 20.2) is a measure of disability that was developed and validated to measure functional ability in progressive neuromuscular conditions and has been shown to correlate closely with changes in muscle strength (Thompson et al., 1996). Its 20 motor activities are biased towards activities involving the lower limbs, making it a more suitable assessment for ambulant patients. The patient sequentially performs a succession of movements that are scored on a three-point scale, and the motor ability score is a numerical value obtained out of a possible maximum of 40 points. The method of scoring had high interrater reliability (Smith et al., 1991b).

Timed tests

Timed performance tests are commonly recommended as supplementary measures of physical performance (Brooke et al., 1981). The most common tests, chosen to reflect progressive weakness in children with DMD, are walking speed over a set distance and the time taken to get up from the floor, i.e. using Gowers' manoeuvre. In the latter, supine lying is a more reproducible starting position than is sitting.

Lung function

Spirometry forms part of the regular assessment to monitor changes in lung function. Inspiratory and expiratory mouth pressures can also be measured to assess the strength of the respiratory muscles. Details of lung function tests can be found elsewhere, e.g. in the chest, heart and vascular disorders book in this series (Connellan, 1998), and in Griggs et al. (1981) and Hough (1991).

Treatment principles

The benefits of an active approach to the physical management of neuromuscular disease are increasingly recognised. These include not only minimising complications in order to maximise abilities but also maintaining the patient in the best possible physical condition so that he or she could benefit from new treatments. Exciting developments in molecular genetics make the latter suggestion a possibility.

The main principles of treatment are:

- to maintain muscle strength and retard contracture progression to maximise function
- to promote or prolong ambulation with appropriate orthoses
- to delay or control the development of scoliosis
- to treat promptly any respiratory complications.

Treatment concepts (see Ch. 21) and details of techniques (see Ch. 23) are not discussed here but the principles relevant to patients with muscle disorders are outlined.

Maintenance of muscle strength

The results of resistance exercise programmes in progressive muscular dystrophies have shown limited increases in strength, with no negative effect on muscle function (e.g. Milner-Brown & Miller, 1988). Greatest effects occur in patients with mild to moderate weakness and in the more slowly progressive myopathies, whilst patients with severely weak muscles do not generally benefit from strengthening programmes. It appears in normal subjects that a prerequisite for successful strength-training is a high content of type II fibres (Jones et al., 1989). The relative deficiency of type II fibres in DMD (Dubowitz, 1985) may contribute to the poor force-generating capacity of dystrophic muscle and could also be a limiting factor in the eventual benefit of a strengthening programme.

Eccentric muscle training is increasingly being used in the training of athletes to facilitate the development of muscle power, i.e. the rate of force generation. Eccentric exercise can cause appreciable morphological damage to muscle fibres (Newham et al., 1986) and damage of this nature is commonly seen in the muscles of patients with myopathic diseases. Whilst normal muscle recovers from this damage, eccentric exercise would seem best avoided in muscle disease, in favour of more traditional concentric protocols.

Edwards et al. (1987) documented important differences in the rate of progression of various muscle groups and highlighted a particularly rapid loss of force in the hip and knee extensors. Insufficiency of these muscle groups has been shown to be the key deficit in functional decline and gait deterioration in DMD (Sutherland et al., 1981). Whilst maximising muscle strength to achieve optimal or improved functional ability is a primary objective of treatment, the effect of specific muscle-strengthening programmes on function in neuromuscular disorders awaits objective evaluation. To devise a strengthening programme, the required functional gain should be considered, and appropriate muscle groups targeted.

It is well accepted that in normal individuals physical exercise increases muscle strength, whilst inactivity causes deconditioning, and there is also widespread observation amongst clinicians that severe restriction of activity causes rapid weakening of muscle in dystrophic conditions and should be avoided. It is therefore important that the duration of enforced immobilisation during any acute illness, and after surgery, should be kept to a minimum so that the patient's return to mobility is not compromised by muscle atrophy. Exercise and strength training in patients with neuromuscular disorders are discussed in Chapter 29.

Weakness occurs when a muscle is held in a shortened position due to joint deformity, and also when it is contracting over a reduced range (Gossman et al., 1982; see also Ch. 30). The establishment of compensatory postures long before the development of fixed contracture means that the muscle is biomechanically disadvantaged earlier than is obvious, since it is continually contracting over a shortened range. This could be a major factor in further progression of the disease as optimal function of the muscle is prevented. Joint positioning during strengthening may therefore be important but research in these patients is required.

Electrical stimulation of normal muscle can improve strength and fatiguability but evidence that the technique is safe, as well as beneficial, in muscle disorders has yet to be produced (see Ch. 23).

Of the many drugs tested in the treatment of DMD, prednisolone has been shown to have a beneficial effect on muscle force. Research continues to find the optimum age to start therapy and the optimum dosage regimen associated with fewest side-effects (Sansome et al., 1994).

Gene therapy using myoblast transfer, in which the gene for dystrophin is inserted into the muscle, is a possible method for preventing loss of muscle tissue but is only at the experimental stage (Partridge et al., 1989). The technique has been successful in animal models but clinical trials in humans have so far been negative.

Retarding contracture progression

The management of contractures is one of the major contributions of physiotherapy in neuromuscular disease. The aim is not only to retard the progression of contracture but, more importantly, to promote or prolong independent ambulation and functional ability. Impairment of mobility caused by contractures compromises the strength of the muscles working across the involved joint or joints. The force-generating ability of a muscle is influenced by the length at which it contracts (Jones & Round, 1990) and thus the strength of a muscle held in a shortened position is reduced. In the presence of profound weakness, the maintenance of full joint range of motion is essential for optimal muscle function. The possible role of strength training in the management of contractures is discussed in Chapter 29.

A sustained programme of splinting and passive stretching in the early stages of DMD can retard the development of lower-limb contractures. Various types of splints may be used to maintain the joints in position and ankle–foot orthosis (AFO) night splints are recommended. Two studies have specifically evaluated the effect of passive stretching and the use of orthoses on the development of contractures. Both concluded that the combination of passive stretching and night splints is more effective than passive stretching alone at delaying contractures and prolonging independent ambulation (Scott et al., 1981; Hyde et al., 2000).

Whilst independently ambulant, the provision of AFOs for control of TA contracture should be confined to night use only. Gait analysis has shown that an equinus position of the foot is used as a compensatory manoeuvre to increase knee stability during walking. Khodadadeh et al. (1986) observed that boys with DMD necessarily adopt a dynamic equinus during gait in order to maintain a knee-extending moment in the presence of gross quadriceps weakness. AFOs intended to correct the foot position by reducing the equinus during walking will have biomechanical effects which will destabilise the knee. If there is significant quadriceps weakness the knee will buckle. Thus AFOs used in this way reduce the available compensatory manoeuvres and can result in premature loss of ambulation.

Promoting or prolonging ambulation

Following the cessation of independent walking, the duration of useful ambulation in children can be prolonged with an immediate programme of percutaneous achilles tenotomy and rehabilitation in light-weight ischial weight-bearing KAFOs and intensive physiotherapy. The gains in additional walking time have varied in different centres but on average an extra 2 years of walking can be achieved and sometimes up to 4 years (Bakker et al., 2000). This approach is now generally accepted as a means of maintaining mobility after independent walking ceases and has been shown to impede the development of both lower-limb contractures (Vignos et al., 1996) and scoliosis (Rodillo et al., 1988).

The accurate timing of intervention and prompt provision of orthoses are crucial to the success of prolonging ambulation. The optimal time for the provision of the orthoses is when the child has lost useful walking but is still able to stand or walk a few steps. There is no advantage in providing orthoses earlier than this. Two of the important factors used to predict successful outcome are the absence of severe hip and knee contractures, and the percentage of residual muscle strength (Hyde et al., 1982). Swivel walkers may be appropriate to allow walking over short distances at home or school. Once the child has been wheelchair-bound for even a short time, fixed lower-limb deformities and muscle weakness rapidly progress, and therefore any delay in undertaking this programme may compromise a successful outcome.

Maintenance of activities

A positive management strategy is to introduce a variety of aids to sustain a broad range of normal activities for as long as possible, as outlined above. In children, calipers are initially used to prevent contractures and sustain upright standing posture as well as for walking (Fig. 20.1). Later, a standing frame allows patients to stand for several hours a day with a view to delaying spinal curvature and contractures of hips, knees and ankles. Lastly, a wheelchair can be introduced as a means of improving mobility and independence. Adults should be encouraged to perform exercise to reduce contractures and thus be able to enjoy physical leisure activities.

Management of scoliosis

Scoliosis is a serious complication of DMD and intermediate SMA. Whilst scoliosis is also associated with other neuromuscular disorders, it is rapidly progressive in these two conditions unless treated.

In DMD, scoliosis may become clinically apparent as ambulation becomes increasingly limited. The period of most rapid deterioration is once the child has become dependent on a wheelchair and corresponds most closely with the adolescent growth spurt between the ages of 12 and 15 years (McDonald et al., 1995). Progressive scoliosis is also a threat in the adolescent years of patients with SMA, but due to the profound weakness that is present from early infancy it may become a problem at a much earlier age.

The curve often develops in a paralytic long C pattern in the thoracolumbar areas and is associated with increasing pelvic obliquity. It further compromises respiratory capacity, which is already restricted by involvement of the respiratory muscles. Kurz et al. (1983) reported that for each 10° of thoracic scoliosis, the forced vital capacity is decreased by approximately 4%, in addition to the 4% loss per year due to progressive muscle weakness in DMD. An increasing scoliosis also leads to difficulty in sitting and maintaining head control, and can cause discomfort and pressure areas. Patients will often need to use their elbows for support in maintaining an upright position, so preventing them from using the arms for other functions. Untreated, the scoliosis may cause patients to become bed-ridden.

One of the major benefits of treatment aimed at maintaining an upright posture is that it will help to delay the progression of scoliosis significantly. Once the patient is dependent on a wheelchair, the main means of managing scoliosis are conservative, using a spinal orthosis, or surgical spinal stabilisation (see below).

The spine should be monitored carefully where scoliosis is a likely complication of the disease, in conjunction with the respiratory capacity using simple spirometry (see above). Once a curve is clinically apparent, any progression is most accurately measured from radiographs using Cobb's angle. Prompt provision of a spinal orthosis is advisable, to be worn during the day whilst the patient is upright. The orthosis should be corrective rather than supportive; ideally, radiographs should be taken during the fitting process to evaluate the degree of correction achieved. It is recognised that spinal bracing is not the definitive treatment in curves that are known to be rapidly progressive, but it is important in slowing the rate of progression of the curvature (Seeger et al., 1990) and can be used effectively for skeletally immature patients in whom spinal fusion is not yet indicated.

Close monitoring continues whilst the patient is wearing a spinal orthosis, so that surgery can be offered before cardiopulmonary function deteriorates to a point where anaesthesia presents an unacceptably high risk. Spinal bracing in a patient with established severe scoliosis may cause appreciable respiratory impairment when there is respiratory muscle involvement, and is less likely to be tolerated than early prophylactic bracing (Noble-Jamieson et al., 1986).

Although there is continuing debate regarding the ideal type of spinal instrumentation, the segmental spinal instrumentation was a major advance in the treatment of paralytic scoliosis (Luque, 1982). Luque instrumentation provides rigid internal fixation without the need for postoperative immobilisation or orthoses. Early surgery has been shown to be beneficial in achieving maximum curve correction and minimising respiratory complications. It is recommended that surgery should be offered when the patient still has adequate respiratory and cardiac function to allow him or her to undergo the procedure safely. In DMD, vital capacity increases with age and growth in the early years, then reaches a plateau, and then declines in the early teens, so there is a window of opportunity when surgery can be performed safely. Surgery is recommended soon after the child has ceased to walk, while the curve is >20% and the forced vital capacity is >40% (Galasko et al., 1992; Miller et al., 1992).

In the immediate postoperative period, respiratory therapy to aid removal of secretions will be necessary in patients who are unable to achieve this unaided. It is possible for a lumbar lordosis and dorsal kyphosis to be moulded into the rods (Galasko et al., 1992), which helps prevent loss of head control in sitting when weakness of the neck and trunk musculature is likely to be advanced. However, seating requirements will need to be reassessed postoperatively. For example, due to significant upper-limb weakness the child is likely to utilise upper-trunk flexion to help get his mouth down to his hands for feeding purposes. Following surgery the height of wheelchair arm supports or table height will need to substitute for a fused spine.

Management of respiratory complications

Chest infections are a serious complication to vulnerable patients with respiratory muscle weakness and a poor cough. Long-standing weakness may lead to more serious secondary problems, including widespread microatelectasis with reduced lung compliance, a ventilation–perfusion imbalance and nocturnal hypoxaemia (Smith et al., 1991a). Vaccines for influenza and *Pneumococcus* are recommended for the non-ambulant child with a falling vital capacity.

Chest infections should be promptly treated with physiotherapy, postural drainage, antibiotics and, when appropriate, assisted ventilation. Spinal orthoses that control scoliosis may reduce respiratory capacity and should be temporarily removed if causing distress or interfering with treatment. The aim of treatment is to help clear the lungs of secretions effectively in the shortest possible time without causing fatigue. Thoracic expansion exercises will allow increased air flow through small airways and the loosening of secretions, while forced expiration techniques, the use of intermittent positive-pressure breathing (IPPB) and assisted coughing will aid removal of secretions (Webber, 1988). If this approach is insufficient to clear secretions adequately, an alternative approach is the use of mechanical insufflation–exsufflation delivered via a facial mask. This uses positive pressure to promote maximal lung inflation followed by a rapid change to apply negative pressure to the upper airway. This aims to simulate the flow changes that occur with a cough and thus assist sputum clearance. Diaphragmatic weakness may limit the use of supine or tipped positions for postural drainage. Parents of children prone to recurrent chest infections can become competent at administering chest physiotherapy but will require support that is readily accessible if children become distressed.

The results of respiratory muscle training are difficult to evaluate due to inclusion of patients with a variety of diagnoses and disease severity, as well as differences in periods of training and methodology. Overall there is some evidence of improvement in respiratory force and endurance in more mildly affected patients or more slowly progressive diseases, without side-effects (McCool & Tzelepis, 1995). There is, however, little evidence that improvements are clinically relevant and insufficient to advocate an exercise regime. It is possible that a short-term respiratory training programme may be of benefit prior to surgery but this awaits evaluation.

Respiratory failure may be precipitated by chest infection or it may occur as a result of increasing nocturnal hypoventilation and hypoxia. The onset is often insidious but symptoms include morning drowsiness, headache or confusion and night-time restlessness, and can be confirmed by sleep study. Life expectancy is less than 1 year once diurnal hypercapnia develops. Symptoms, quality of life and survival can be improved by non-invasive nasal ventilation (Simonds, 2000; Eagle et al., 2002).

SOCIAL AND PSYCHOLOGICAL ISSUES IN NEUROMUSCULAR DISORDERS

A complexity of factors influence management at different stages of the patient's life. For lifelong disorders, these influences pose similar problems as in other disabling conditions, as discussed, for e.g. in Chapter 18 in relation to cerebral palsy. The need for more training and support for professionals managing these patients was highlighted in a survey by Heap et al. (1996).

Preschool years

The time of diagnosis will be traumatic for the parents and sensitive support will be needed. If not already known to the family, the genetic implications will need to be discussed and family members offered genetic counseling. A realistic picture of the future should be given, with appropriate information to prepare for each stage as it comes. Precise details of the end stages would not be appropriate, for obvious psychological reasons; also, they may not apply 20 years ahead as medical advances may have occurred by that time.

The school years

Optimal management can be achieved only if there is good communication between the medical team, parents and carers at school. Facilities at school and integration with able-bodied children are important. Physical management programmes should involve realistic goals and take into account other aspects of life which may demand the child's time, particularly, for e.g. at exam times. The timing of surgery should also consider such issues and not just the medical considerations.

Preparation for leaving school should include organisation for continuation of support services as well as careers advice.

Transition from childhood to adulthood

There is a lack of provision of services for the young disabled adult. On leaving school, the support system often ceases and, apart from occasional visits to the hospital consultant, physiotherapy and other services are not always offered. Patients whose disorder begins in adulthood may never be offered any services or treatment, or even referred to a specialist, despite having a significant disability.

There is a need for centres that provide specialist advice and treatment from therapists, and offer an environment for social interaction and training for vocational and leisure activities. This would enable children to continue with their physical management programmes as adults, taking responsibility for their own treatment but receiving help for monitoring and modifying treatment. Those with disorders of adult onset could be educated in physical management strategies by therapists and other patients, and learn how to maximise their abilities and remain functional for as long as possible. Other areas, such as weight control and sexual counselling, could also be dealt with or referral made where appropriate.

Patients with neuromuscular disorders, particularly adults, often feel isolated in the community and some do not lead as full a life as they have the potential for because of lack of support and education about their condition. Some give up employment or even going out of the house. Specialist centres could provide an important function and fill a major gap in care and support.

In the terminal stage of illness, support from the care team, particularly the general practitioner, is essential and bereavement counselling may be required. The Muscular Dystrophy Campaign Family Care Officers (see Appendix) play a very important role at all stages, particularly during the final illness in guiding and supporting families.

Living with disability

People with disabilities, their carers and professionals can take inspiration from the example set by individuals who overcome difficulties to live a fulfilling life. The autobiography of Johnathan Colchester gives an account of an exceptional young man living with muscular dystrophy and provides some practical advice (Colchester, 2003).

ACKNOWLEDGEMENT

Dr Quinlivan wishes to thank the Muscular Dystrophy Campaign for supporting her clinical work.

References

Bakker JPJ, De Groot IJM, Beckerman H, de Jong BA, Lankhorst GJ. The effects of knee–ankle–foot orthoses in the treatment of Duchenne muscular dystrophy: review of the literature. *Clin Rehab* 2000, **14**:343–359.

Bertorini TE, Narayanaswami P, Senthilkumar K. Important neuromusuclar disorder diagnostic criteria. In: Tulio E, Bertorini TE, eds *Clinical Evaluation and Diagnostic Tests for Neuromuscular Disorders*. Oxford: Butterworth-Heinemann Press; 2002:763–798.

Bialer MG, McDaniel NL, Kelly TE. Progression of cardiac disease in Emery–Dreifuss muscular dystrophy. *Clin Cardiol* 1991, **14**:411–416.

Billard C, Gillet P, Signovet JL. Cognitive functions in Duchenne muscular dystrophy: a reappraisal and comparison with spinal muscular atrophy. *Neuromusc Dis* 1992, **2**:371–378.

Bohannon RW. Test–retest reliability of hand-held dynamometry during a single session of strength assessment. *Phys Ther* 1986, **66**:206–209.

Bohannon RW. Correlation of lower limb strengths and other variables with standing performance in stroke patients. *Physiother Can* 1989, **41**:198–202.

Bonne G, Di Barletta MR, Varnous S et al. Mutations in the gene encoding lamin A/C cause autosomal dominant Emery–Dreifuss muscular dystrophy. *Nat Genet* 1999, **21**:285–288.

Brooke MH, Griggs MD, Mendell JR et al. Clinical trial in Duchenne dystrophy. 1. The design of the protocol. *Muscle Nerve* 1981, **4**:186–197.

Brzustowicz LM, Lehner T, Castilla LH et al. Genetic mapping of chronic childhood-onset spinal muscular atrophy. *Nature* 1990, **344**:540.

Carroll N, Bain RJI, Smith PEM et al. Domiciliary investigation of sleep-related hypoxaemia in Duchenne muscular dystrophy. *Eur Resp J* 1991, **4**:434–440.

Carter GT, Abresch RT, Fowler WM et al. Profiles of neuromuscular disease: Spinal muscular atrophy. *Am J Phys Med Rehab* 1995, **74**:150–159.

Colchester J. *A Life Worth Living: Abilities, Interests and Travels of a Young Disabled Man*. Northwich, Cheshire: Greenridges Press; 2003.

Connellan SJ. Lung function testing/chest assessment. In: Smith M, Ball V, eds. *Cardiovascular Respiratory Physiotherapy*. London: Mosby; 1998:21–38.

Dubowitz V. *Muscle Biopsy: A Practical Approach*, 2nd edn. London: Baillière Tindall; 1985.

Dubowitz V. The Duchenne dystrophy story: from phenotype to gene and potential treatment. *J Child Neurol* 1989, **4**:240–249.

Dubowitz V. *Muscle Disorders in Childhood*, 2nd edn. London: WB Saunders; 1995.

Dubowitz V. Treatment of muscular dystrophy. 75th ENMC International workshop, Baarn 10–12 Dec, 1999. *Neuromusc Disord* 2000, **10**:313–320.

Eagle M, Baudouin SV, Chandler C et al. Survival in Duchenne muscular dystrophy: improvements in life expectancy since 1967 and the impact of home nocturnal ventilation. *Neuromusc Disord* 2002, **12**:926–930.

Edwards RHT, Chapman SJ, Newham DJ et al. Practical analysis of variability of muscle function measurements in Duchenne muscular dystrophy. *Muscle Nerve* 1987, **10**:6–14.

Edwards RHT, Newham DJ, Jones DA et al. Role of mechanical damage in pathogenesis of proximal myopathy in man. *Lancet* 1984, March **10**:548–552.

Emery AEH. The nosology of the spinal muscular atrophies. *J Med Genet* 1971, **8**:481–495.

Emery AEH. *Duchenne Muscular Dystrophy*. Oxford: Oxford University Press; 1987.

Emery AEH. Population frequencies of inherited neuromuscular diseases – a world survey. *Neuromusc Dis* 1991, **1**:19–29.

Fisher NM, Pendergast DR, Calkins EC. Maximal isometric torque of knee extension as a function of muscle length in

subjects of advancing age. *Arch Phys Med Rehab* 1990, **71**:729–734.

Galasko CSB, Delaney C, Morris P. Spinal stabilisation in Duchenne muscular dystrophy. *J Bone Joint Surg* 1992, **74B**:210–214.

Gospe SM, Lazaro RP, Lava NS et al. Familial X linked myalgia and cramps: a non-progressive myopathy associated with a deletion in the dystrophin gene. *Neurology* 1989, **39**:1277–1280.

Gossman MR, Sahrmann SA, Rose SJ. Review of length associated changes in muscle. *Phys Ther* 1982, **62**:1799–1808.

Griffiths RD, Edwards RHT. A new chart for weight control in Duchenne muscular dystrophy. *Arch Dis Child* 1988, **63**:1256–1258.

Griggs RC, Donohoe KM, Utell MJ et al. Evaluation of pulmonary function in neuromuscular disease. *Arch Neurol* 1981, **38**:9–12.

Heap RM, Mander M, Bond J et al. Management of Duchenne muscular dystrophy in the community: views of physiotherapists, GPs and school teachers. *Physiotherapy* 1996, **82**:258–263.

Hoffman EP, Fischbeck KH, Brown RH. Characterisation of dystrophin in muscle-biopsy specimens from patients with Duchenne's or Becker's muscular dystrophy. *N Engl J Med* 1988, **318**:1363–1368.

Hough A. *Physiotherapy in Respiratory Care*. London: Chapman & Hall; 1991.

Hunsaker RH, Fulkerson PK, Barry FJ et al. Cardiac function in Duchenne's muscular dystrophy. Results of 10-year follow up study and noninvasive tests. *Am J Med* 1982, **73**:235–238.

Hyde SA, Scott OM, Goddard CM et al. Prolongation of ambulation in Duchenne muscular dystrophy. *Physiotherapy* 1982, **68**:105–108.

Hyde SA, Scott OM, Goddard CM. The myometer: the development of a clinical tool. *Physiotherapy* 1983, **69**:424–427.

Hyde SA, Fløytrup I, Glent S et al. A randomised comparative study of two methods of controlling tendo achilles contracture in Duchenne muscular dystrophy. *Neuromusc Disord* 2000, **10**:257–263.

Jaffe KM, McDonald CM, Ingman E et al. Symptoms of upper gastrointestinal dysfunction in Duchenne muscular dystrophy: case-control study. *Arch Phys Med Rehab* 1990, **71**:742–744.

Jones DA, Rutherford OM, Parker DF. Physiological changes in skeletal muscle as a result of strength training. *Q J Exp Physiol* 1989, **74**:233–256.

Jones DA, Round JM. *Skeletal Muscle in Health and Disease*. Manchester: Manchester University Press; 1990.

Karpati G, Hilton-Jones D, Griggs RC. *Disorders of Voluntary Muscle*, 7th edn. Cambridge: Cambridge University Press; 2001.

Khodadadeh S, McClelland MR, Patrick JH et al. Knee moments in Duchenne muscular dystrophy. *Lancet* 1986, September **6**:544–555.

Kobayashi O, Hayashi Y, Arahata K et al. Congenital muscular dystrophy. *Neurology* 1996, **46**:815–818.

Kurz LT, Mubarek SJ, Schultz P. Correlation of scoliosis and pulmonary function in Duchenne muscular dystrophy. *J Paediatr Orthop* 1983, **3**:347–353.

Lennon SM, Ashburn A. Use of myometry in the assessment of neuropathic weakness: testing for reliability in clinical practice. *Clin Rehab* 1993, **7**:125–133.

Luque ER. Segmental spinal instrumentation for correction of scoliosis. *Clin Orthop* 1982, **163**:192–198.

Mastaglia FL, Laing NG. Investigation of muscle disease. *J Neurol Neurosurg Psychiatry* 1996, **60**:256–274.

McCool FD, Tzelepis GE. Inspiratory muscle training in the patient with neuromuscular disease. *Phys Ther* 1995, **75**:1006–1014.

McDonald CM, Abresch RT, Carter GT et al. Profiles of neuromuscular disease. Duchenne muscular dystrophy. *Am J Phys Med Rehab* 1995, **74**:70–92.

Mehdian H, Shimizu N, Draycott V et al. Spinal stabilisation for scoliosis in Duchenne muscular dystrophy. Experience with various sublaminar instrumentation systems. *Neor Orthop* 1989, **7**:74–82.

Miller F, Moseley LF, Koreska J. Spinal fusion in Duchenne muscular dystrophy. *Dev Med Child Neurol* 1992, **34**:775–786.

Milner-Brown HS, Miller RG. Muscle strengthening through high-resistance weight training in patients with neuromuscular disorders. *Arch Phys Med Rehab* 1988, **69**:14–19.

Newham DJ, Jones DA, Edwards RHT. Plasma creatinine kinase changes after eccentric and concentric contractions. *Muscle Nerve* 1986, **9**:59–63.

Nigro G, Comi LI, Politano L et al. The incidence and evaluation of cardiomyopathy in Duchenne muscular dystrophy. *Int J Cardiol* 1990, **26**:271–277.

Noble-Jamieson CM, Heckmatt JZ, Dubowitz V et al. Effects of posture and spinal bracing on respiratory function in neuromuscular disease. *Arch Dis Child* 1986, **61**:178–181.

Pandya S, Florence JM, King WM et al. Reliability of goniometric measurements in patients with Duchenne muscular dystrophy. *Phys Ther* 1985, **65**:1339–1342.

Partridge TA, Morgan JE, Coulton GR et al. Conversion of mdx myofibres from dystrophin-negative to positive by injection of normal myoblasts. *Nature* 1989, **337**:176–179.

Phillips MF, Quinlivan RCM, Edwards RHT et al. Changes in spirometry over time as a prognostic marker in patients with Duchenne muscular dystrophy. *Am J Crit Care Med* 2001, **164**:2191–2194.

Pope PM. Postural management and special seating. In: Edwards S, ed. *Neurological Physiotherapy: A Problem Solving Approach*, 2nd edn. London: Churchill Livingstone; 2002:189–217.

Quinlivan RM, Dubowitz V. Cardiac transplantation in Becker muscular dystrophy. *Neuromusc Disord* 1992, **2**:165–167.

Rideau Y. Treatment of orthopaedic deformity uring the ambulatory stage of Duchenne muscular dystrophy. In: Serratrice G, Cros D, Desnuelle C et al., eds.

Neuromuscular Diseases. New York: Raven Press; 1984:557–564.

Rodillo EB, Fernandez-Bermejo E, Heckmatt JZ et al. Prevention of rapidly progressive scoliosis in Duchenne muscular dystrophy by prolonging walking with orthoses. *J Child Neurol* 1988, **3**:269–274.

Sansome A, Royston P, Dubowitz V. Steroids in Duchenne muscular dystrophy: a pilot study of a new low-dosage schedule. *Neuromusc Disord* 1994, **3**:567–569.

Scott OM, Hyde SA, Goddard C et al. Prevention of deformity in Duchenne muscular dystrophy. *Physiotherapy* 1981, **67**:177–180.

Scott OM, Hyde SA, Goddard C et al. Quantitation of muscle function in children: a prospective study in Duchenne muscular dystrophy. *Muscle Nerve* 1982, **5**:291–301.

Seeger BR, Sutherland A, Clark MS. Management of scoliosis in Duchenne muscular dystrophy. *Arch Phys Med Rehab* 1990, **65**:83–86.

Simonds AK. Nasal ventilation in progressive neuromuscular disease: experience in adults and adolescents. *Monaldi Arch Chest Dis* 2000, **55**:237–241.

Smith PEM, Edwards RHT, Calverley PMA. Mechanisms of sleep-disordered breathing in chronic neuromuscular disease: implications for management. *Q J Med* 1991a, **296**:961–973.

Smith RA, Newcombe RG, Sibert JR et al. Assessment of locomotor function in young boys with Duchenne muscular dystrophy. *Muscle Nerve* 1991b, **14**:462–469.

Steare SE, Benatar A, Dubowitz V. Subclinical cardiomyopathy in Becker muscular dystrophy. *Br Heart J* 1992, **68**:304–308.

Sutherland DH, Olshen R, Cooper L et al. The pathomechanics of gait in Duchenne muscular dystrophy. *Dev Med Child Neurol* 1981, **23**:3–22.

Thompson N, Choudhary P, Hughes RAC et al. A novel trial design to study the effects of intravenous immunoglobulin in chronic inflammatory demyelinating polyradiculoneuropathy. *J Neurol* 1996, **243**:280–285.

Vignos PJ. Respiratory function and pulmonary infection in Duchenne muscular dystrophy. In: Robin GC, Falewski de Leon G, eds. *Muscular Dystrophy*. Basel: Karger; 1976:123–130.

Vignos PJ, Wagner MB, Karlinchak B et al. Evaluation of a program for long-term treatment of Duchenne muscular dystrophy: experience at the University Hospitals of Cleveland. *J Bone Joint Surg Am* 1996, **78**:1844–1852.

Webber BA. *The Brompton Hospital Guide to Chest Physiotherapy*. Oxford: Blackwell Scientific Publications; 1988.

Wiles CM, Karni Y, Nicklin J. Laboratory testing of muscle function in the management of neuromuscular disease. *J Neurol Neurosurg Psychiatry* 1990, **53**:384–387.

WHO. *International Classification of Functioning, Disability and Health* (ICF). Geneva: World Health Organization; 2001. Available online at http://www.who.int/classification/icf.

SECTION 4

Treatment approaches in neurological rehabilitation

SECTION CONTENTS

Chapter 21

The theoretical basis of neurological physiotherapy

S Lennon

INTRODUCTION

This chapter aims to explain the theoretical framework underlying current practice in neurological physiotherapy for adults with central nervous system (CNS) damage. The World Health Organization (WHO) has developed an international classification, which provides a systematic way of understanding the problems faced by patients, illustrating the multiple levels at which therapy may act. This classification, originally developed in 1980 to explain the consequences of disease, has been revised as the *International Classification of Functioning, Disability and Health* (WHO, 2001).

The ICF organises information according to three dimensions:

1. a body level
2. an individual level
3. a society level.

The body dimension comprises both body structure and function. The activities dimension covers the range of activities performed by an individual. The participation dimension classifies the areas of life in which for each individual there are societal opportunities or barriers. This revised framework provides a mechanism to document the impact of the environment on a person's functioning. It now deals with functional states associated with health.

Terminology within the new ICF has been modified. The definition of 'impairment' remains similar – a deficit in body structure or function. In other words, for example, the signs and symptoms associated with a cerebrovascular accident (CVA). 'Disability' is now described as a restriction in activity, whereas handicap has been replaced as a 'restriction in participation'. The ICF is discussed further in Chapter 3.

Following a CVA, an example of impairment would be weakness, with a restriction in the activity of walking thus requiring the use of a wheelchair for mobility. Being in a wheelchair may limit that individual from resuming his or her job, a restriction in participating in that individual's previous role in society.

Within the ICF framework, neurological physiotherapy targets both impairment (a loss or abnormality of body structure) and activity (performance in functional activities). It is important to stress that physiotherapy takes place within the wider context of rehabilitation; recent guidelines have summarised the basic principles of rehabilitation as interdisciplinary care, patient assessment, continuity of care, and patient and family involvement (Gresham et al., 1995). Although the application of these principles greatly influences the potential outcome of care, and these principles are common to all professions involved in rehabilitation, the focus of this chapter will be solely on the physiotherapy component of care. Elements of optimal rehabilitation practice, which are common to the health care team, are discussed in Chapter 22 on the rehabilitation process.

Plant (1998) suggested that physiotherapy practice was derived from three broad treatment approaches, which targeted specific conditions: neurophysiological, motor learning and eclectic (using aspects of different approaches). These approaches have traditionally been named after the therapist who developed them. While acknowledging the outstanding contributions of these pioneering therapists, is it now time to leave the named treatment approaches in the past?

Recent reviews confirm that there is little evidence to support the superiority of one approach over another; there are indications that it is the content of the therapy delivered which influences outcome (Kwakkel et al., 1999a, b; Parry et al., 1999; Pomeroy & Tallis, 2000). There appears to be a need to move away from labelled approaches to treatment because within many treatment approaches there are common components of potentially successful interventions (Pomeroy & Tallis, 2000; Foster & Young, 2002).

It will be argued in this chapter that neurotherapists should use a problem-solving approach to rehabilitation based on a systems theory of movement control, integrating evidence from neurophysiology, biomechanics and motor learning. A historical overview will be followed by a comparison of the similarities and differences between two major treatment approaches, the Bobath concept (Bobath, 1990; known as neurodevelopmental treatment in the USA) and the motor relearning programme (MRP: Carr & Shepherd, 1987, 1998), ending with a consensus of the key theoretical concepts underlying the evidence base for current practice.

HISTORICAL OVERVIEW

Prior to the introduction of neurophysiological approaches to rehabilitation in the 1950s, patients with neurological damage were re-educated using a compensatory approach consisting of using the unaffected body parts to become as independent as possible (Ashburn, 1997). At that time there was little evidence to support the view that the CNS could recover from damage and therefore recovery of movement was not expected (Lennon, 1996; Hallett et al., 1998). Pioneers of neurofacilitation approaches, e.g. Bobath, Knott and Voss, Rood, Brunnstrom, had observed from clinical observation and experience that muscle tone and movement patterns could be changed using muscle stimulation and specialised handling techniques.

An explosion of neuroscience research in the 1980s confirmed that the CNS is plastic; in other words, the CNS could be reshaped by environmental needs and demands, and training (Stephenson, 1993; Pomeroy & Tallis, 2000; also see Ch. 5). These findings thus substantiated the beliefs of therapists using these new neurophysiological treatment approaches; rehabilitation had the potential to restore movement and function following brain damage.

However several issues for debate were raised in the late 1980s, leading to the emergence notably of the MRP, advocated by two Australian physiotherapists (Carr & Shepherd, 1987), who had initially acquired training and used one of the main neurophysiological approaches, the Bobath concept. The MRP incorporated musculoskeletal and motor learning considerations into neurological physiotherapy. The main drivers for change in thinking were a concern for carryover between therapy sessions and everyday life; an overemphasis of therapy on impairments rather than functional tasks; a professional debate about the non-neural component to tone and skill acquisition; and experimental evidence on motor control suggesting that movement was controlled via systems theory as opposed to a hierarchical model (Carr & Shepherd, 1987).

In the 1990s, the government-driven agenda in the UK required clinical governance, meaning that each organisation must take responsibility for the delivery of a quality service using tools such as audit, evidence-based practice, guidelines and care pathways (Wade, 2000). There is a shift in resources away from the acute hospital sector towards primary care in the community, with an emphasis on patient-centred care. Thus, the manner in which neurological physiotherapy services are delivered is under scrutiny; therapists must subject their practice to systematic evaluation.

WHY IS THEORY IMPORTANT?

Theory is dynamic, integrating new knowledge and innovative ideas. Several authors have emphasised the importance of identifying the theoretical assumptions underlying practice for several reasons (Shephard, 1991; Carr et al., 1994; Partridge & De Weerdt, 1995; Lennon, 1996). Theory provides the explanation not only for the behaviour of people following CNS damage, but also for the actions of therapists in clinical practice (Shephard, 1991). Physiotherapists assess and treat patients according to these beliefs, which are influenced by experience and their preferred treatment approaches (Ballinger et al., 1999; Lennon, 2000; Lennon et al., 2001; Van Vliet et al., 2001). Therefore the theoretical framework to which therapists aspire determines therapy input in neurorehabilitation (Shephard, 1991; Partridge & Edwards, 1996). However it must be remembered that having a plausible theory to explain how and why therapy is structured and delivered in a specific way is only the first step. Having a theory does not constitute evidence; it is necessary to set up research trials to put these theories to the test! Research provides the data to support or reject the theoretical assumptions underlying treatment.

A major problem for neurological physiotherapy is the fact that what is done under the guise of a named approach can vary widely, as therapists may vary in terms of their knowledge, experience, clinical skills and patient interaction skills (Partridge & Edwards, 1996). Patients and their carers do not necessarily have a say in which treatment approach is used in their care; individual therapists tend to interpret their preferred approach in their own way. Further research is required to identify the theory that clinicians use to inform their clinical decisions (Lennon & Hastings, 1996; Kwakkel et al., 1999b).

Key points

- No single treatment approach has been shown to be the best
- Therapists need to stop referring to named approaches and investigate the actual content of therapy
- Having a plausible theoretical rationale for intervention is not the same as having evidence!
- Research is essential to provide the data to support or reject therapists' beliefs

WHICH TREATMENT APPROACH?

Therapists use their theoretical knowledge and clinical experience to analyse and interpret patient assessment findings in order to explain the patient's movement problems and to develop a treatment plan (Freeman, 2002, p. 24). Where does this theory come from?

Therapists tend to rely on their preferred treatment approach and their clinical experience to justify the theory and knowledge they use to treat patients (Nilsson & Nordolm, 1992; Carr et al., 1994). Several surveys in the field of stroke rehabilitation, with the exception of Carr et al. (1994), have confirmed the dominance of the Bobath concept as the preferred treatment approach (Nilsson & Nordolm, 1992; De Gangi & Royeen, 1994; Sackley & Lincoln, 1996; Davidson & Waters, 2000; Lennon et al, 2001); interest in using the other neurophysiological approaches presented by Plant (1998) has waned.

Currently there is much debate about which therapy approach should be adopted in stroke rehabilitation, in particular comparing the Bobath concept and the MRP (Carr & Shepherd, 1998, pp. 16–17; Kwakkel et al., 1999b; Langhammer & Stanghelle, 2000; Barrett et al., 2001), yet there appear to be more similarities than differences between the two treatment approaches (Table 21.1; Lettinga et al., 1999; Lennon, 2000; Van Vliet et al., 2001).

Using gait re-education as an example, both treatment approaches support the need for task-specific practice; both work on re-educating essential movement components; both analyse abnormal gait in relation to normal gait; both practice limb loading and stepping in different directions and both actually practise walking (Lennon, 2000).

There are three main differences between the two approaches relating to:

1. the amount of time spent on task-specific activities
2. the incorporation of strength training
3. the use of hands-on techniques during all types of activities.

Carr & Shepherd (1998) focus on strength training and skill acquisition in actions critical to everyday life, with the therapist in the role of a coach rather than manually guiding the patients' movements and activities; they are firm proponents of strength training and organising practice outside therapy sessions.

Bobath therapists have reservations about allowing the patient to practise independently outside therapy and the use of resisted exercise as they are concerned that the effort of working either without the therapist's handling skills or against resistance will exacerbate abnormal tone and reinforce abnormal movement patterns (Bobath, 1990; Lennon, 2000; Ng & Shepherd, 2000). However, few strength-training studies to date have documented any adverse effects on tone (see Ch. 29). Bobath therapists do not reject all types of

Table 21.1 A comparison of the Bobath concept and the motor re-learning programme (adapted from Plant (1998), with permission)

Treatment approach	The Bobath concept (Lennon, 2000)	The motor re-learning programme (Carr & Shepherd, 1998)
Conditions	All CNS disorders	All CNS disorders
Basis of approach	Neurophysiological	Motor learning, biomechanics
Key aim	Restoration of normal movement	Re-education of everyday activities
Treatment concepts	• Neuroplasticity • Systems model of motor control • Recovery of damaged systems • Avoidance of compensation • Normalisation of tone • Facilitation of normal movement components • Task-specific practice • Strategies to maintain muscle length and joint alignment • Emphasis on manual handling (hands-on) • Avoidance of strength training • Restriction of practice outside therapy (if abnormal movement is reinforced)	• Neuroplasticity • Systems model of motor control • Recovery of damaged systems • Avoidance of compensation • Abnormal tone is not an issue • Training of missing components of a task • Task-specific practice • Strategies to maintain muscle length and joint alignment • Emphasis on cognitive guidance (hands-off) • Advocates of strength training • Promotion of practice outside therapy (patients learn from their mistakes)

CNS, central nervous system.

strength training; for example, they strengthen muscle groups by using the patient's body weight within a functional activity such as sitting to standing (Ryerson & Levitt, 1997; Lennon et al., 2001). Bobath therapists prefer to use manual rather than cognitive guidance to re-educate everyday movement patterns (Lennon & Ashburn, 2000); they avoid using progressive resisted exercise of specific muscle groups in treatment (Lennon et al., 2001).

Both facilitation of normal movement components (which includes strategies to maintain muscle and joint alignment) and task-specific practice, using specific manual guidance, would appear to be critical elements of the Bobath concept (Lennon & Ashburn, 2000; Lennon, 2001; Lennon et al., 2001). Carr & Shepherd (1998, p. 16) advocate an emphasis on training control of muscles, promoting learning of relevant actions and tasks, and the preservation of muscle length.

It seems that both these approaches use task-specific practice. Task-specific training, a concept of motor learning, should be viewed as a training method that can be applied within any treatment approach rather than a treatment approach in its own right. As it is, the actual content of therapy that appears to influence the outcome (Kwakkel et al., 1999a; Parry et al., 1999), and what is done under the guise of a named approach, can vary widely (Partridge & Edwards, 1996); the evidence suggests that the components of the therapy administered needs to be evaluated rather than the label attached to the programme (Partridge & Edwards, 1996; Pomeroy & Tallis, 2000; Foster & Young, 2002). Therapists need to stop referring to named approaches, and start referring to the theoretical evidence base for their practice (Ashburn, 1997). Is there a consensus within neurological physiotherapy about the theoretical basis underpinning practice?

KEY THEORETICAL CONCEPTS

This section discusses the assumptions that physiotherapists working in the clinic subscribe to, in relation to the current evidence base. The work related to stroke rehabilitation will be presented, as this area has been the main focus for the investigation of the theoretical basis of physiotherapy practice. Guidelines for physiotherapy practice within the health care team have now been published for people with Parkinson's disease (Plant et al, 2000; Guidelines Group, 2001); whereas multidisciplinary guidelines for people with multiple sclerosis are currently under development (CSP, 2001). Although further research is required in relation to patient populations other than stroke, it is realistic to assume that these assumptions could apply in other conditions, as physiotherapy management is problem-based, not condition-based; patients with brain damage present with a range of common problems across conditions. Physiotherapy management specific to common neurological conditions is discussed in Chapters 6–15 and 18–20.

Six postal-based surveys have been undertaken to determine current clinical practice in stroke rehabilitation (Nilsson & Nordolm, 1992; Carr et al., 1994; De Gangi & Royeen, 1994; Sackley & Lincoln, 1996; Davidson & Waters, 2000; Lennon et al., 2001).

Three surveys, by De Gangi & Royeen (1994), Davidson & Waters (2000) and Lennon et al. (2001), have confirmed four key theoretical themes to varying degrees:

1. promotion of normal movement
2. control of tone
3. promotion of function
4. recovery of movement with optimisation of compensation.

These themes will be discussed in turn by extracting data from Lennon (2000, 2003), who asked all Senior 1 level physiotherapists working in stroke care in the UK ($n = 1022$; response rate = 78%) to rate a series of theoretical assumptions related to these themes. Only the statements where the consensus reached a level of 90% or more, and the level of uncertainty and disagreement combined surpassed 40%, are presented (Lennon, 2003).

Key points

- Neurological physiotherapy is problem-based, not condition-based
- There are many similarities, as well as some differences, between the Bobath concept and the motor re-learning programme (see Table 21.1)
- Expert consensus confirms that there are four theoretical themes underlying practice:
  1. Normal movement
  2. Tone
  3. Function
  4. Recovery with optimisation of compensation

Therapists have several sources of evidence at their fingertips in order to verify their assumptions. The Cochrane library has several systematic reviews in various stages of preparation, e.g. Pollock et al. (2003), which can be accessed on their database; access is available to all members of the Chartered Society of Physiotherapy (CSP) on their website (www.csphysio.org.uk). The CSP publishes effectiveness bulletins on a regular basis (*Physiotherapy Effectiveness Bulletin*, 2001). The *National*

Clinical Guidelines for Stroke (2000, 2002) provide a comprehensive review of all the available evidence to date. These guidelines, developed by a multidisciplinary panel and subjected to peer review, are based on the best available evidence. It is important to realise that there are still many key areas of clinical practice where there is no evidence available. The expert consensus views of all senior-level physiotherapists working in stroke care in the UK will now be examined in relation to this evidence (Lennon, 2003).

The promotion of normal movement

The expert consensus identifies the analysis of normal movement as the basis of assessment in neurological physiotherapy. Table 21.2 confirms that physiotherapists use the analysis of normal movement to plan treatment, including alignment of the musculoskeletal system. It also highlights some debate about evidence from biomechanical and motor-learning literature, and the use of the unaffected side following stroke.

Normal movement appears to be a logical model for therapy, provided that the patient has the potential to recover movement, for several reasons. Firstly, these movement patterns, used in everyday life, are already well engrained in each individual's motor system, as they have been practised throughout an individual's motor development at an early stage, and secondly, they are more energy-efficient. There is strong evidence to support the effects of rehabilitation (remembering that physiotherapy is only one component of rehabilitation) on improving functional independence, but limited evidence to support the effects of therapy on restoring normal movement (*National Clinical Guidelines for Stroke*, 2000; Pomeroy & Tallis, 2000). Therapists favour using bilateral movements to re-educate movement and getting the patient to follow the therapist's guided movements with the unaffected side, yet they seem unsure about the theoretical basis for these interventions. There is some evidence to suggest that ipsilateral pathways play a role in recovery following stroke; this accords credence to the practice of activating movements bilaterally and also teaching the patient to follow movements with the unaffected side (Lee & Van Donkelaar, 1995).

Consensus favours the re-education of more normal movement but how this is achieved may differ according to the individual therapist's approach to treatment. For example, Bobath therapists place great store on re-educating normal movement components which are common to functional activities (Lennon et al., 2001), whereas proponents of Carr & Shepherd (1987, 1998) focus on the critical biomechanical requirements of everyday activities. Emerging evidence supports the

Table 21.2 The promotion of normal movement, based on the expert consensus views of senior-level stroke care physiotherapists in the UK

Theoretical assumption	Unsure (%)	Agree (%)	Disagree (%)
The therapist's role is to facilitate normal movement components	3	94	3
Assessing the alignment of key points and the interaction of the patient's base of support with gravity in different postural sets lays the foundation for current practice	5	92	3
A well-aligned musculoskeletal system is important, i.e. alignment of joints and muscles	5	91	4
Concepts from biomechanical literature are incorporated into current Bobath theory	51	42	7
Concepts from motor-learning literature are incorporated into current Bobath theory	51	36	13
Activating movements bilaterally makes use of ipsilateral movements to promote recovery of the affected side	43	48	9
Getting the patients to follow movements with the unaffected side makes use of ipsilateral pathways to promote recovery of the affected side	55	24	21

Adapted from Lennon (2003), with permission.

Table 21.3 The control of tone, based on the expert consensus survey

Theoretical assumption	Unsure (%)	Agree (%)	Disagree (%)
In patients where tone is considered to be a major problem, normalising tone is important when facilitating movement	2.5	96.5	1
Inhibition of spasticity does not necessarily result in movement; movement needs to be facilitated	4	94	2

Adapted from Lennon (2003), with permission.

advantages of task-specific practice over impairment-focused intervention in improving outcomes (Kwakkel et al., 1999b; *National Clinical Guidelines for Stroke*, 2002). Judgements about appropriate therapeutic goals should not always be made solely on the basis of quality of movement, as the solutions to patient problems change according to the interaction between the individual, the task and the environment (Shumway-Cook & Woollacott, 1995, p. 4).

Textbooks recommend that a systems model of motor control be adopted, integrating evidence from neurophysiology, biomechanics and motor learning (Shumway-Cook & Woollacott, 1995; Ryerson & Levitt, 1997; Carr & Shepherd, 1998; Edwards, 2002). This survey confirmed that therapists incorporate musculoskeletal considerations into patient management; however, evidence from motor learning and the musculoskeletal systems is not explicitly integrated into current theory.

However, is aiming for more normal movement realistic in all patients with brain damage? Normal movement is not achievable for all patients; this depends to some extent on whether or not the patient has a progressive condition (Edwards, 2002, p. 256). Currently there is very little evidence to support the way in which neurological physiotherapy should be provided to people with progressive conditions. Further research is required to evaluate physiotherapy intervention along with the organisation and delivery of services to these patient groups (*Physiotherapy Effectiveness Bulletin*, 2001).

The control of tone

Control of tone is a key theoretical belief of current practice (see Ch. 25). However, therapists confirm that changing tone does not automatically unmask the ability to move, and that movement needs to be actively promoted (Table 21.3). Abnormal tone is viewed as an important target of physiotherapeutic intervention, because it can exacerbate patient problems and lead to complications; this is in line with expert consensus of multidisciplinary teams (*National Clinical Guidelines for Stroke*, 2000; Barnes et al., 2000).

In current practice the normalisation of tone remains a contentious issue (Carr et al., 1995). The main thrust of research has focused on the evaluation of medication and botulinum toxin on spasticity; there is minimal evidence concerning the effects of physiotherapy on the control of tone (*National Clinical Guidelines for Stroke*, 2000; Mayston, 2002, p. 12). One train of thought suggests that therapists can change hypertonia at a non-neural level by influencing muscle length and range; this enables improved alignment for more efficient muscle activation, thus allowing patients to experience more effective movement (Mayston, 2000a, b).

Impaired movement performance is multifactorial in nature, with abnormal movement patterns, weakness and inco-ordination all contributing to the disorder of movement following brain damage (Edwards, 2002, p. 93). It is likely that weakness and altered viscoelastic properties of muscle are a more likely explanation of the movement problems experienced by patients than increased tone (Mayston, 2002, p. 15). It must be emphasised, in relation to stroke, that therapists do not focus treatment only on reducing hypertonus. Bobath therapists view low proximal tone as the key problem rather than the more obvious distal increases in tone (Lennon & Ashburn, 2000). More research is required to determine the impact of physiotherapy on abnormal tone. In any case, therapists agree that the main emphasis in treatment should be on the facilitation of movement, not the normalisation of tone.

The promotion of function

Recent research confirms that experienced therapists accord a high priority to task practice (Lennon & Ashburn, 2000; Lennon et al., 2001). However, the degree of task and context specificity within current practice is subject to debate (Carr & Shepherd, 1998; Kwakkel et al., 1999a, b). Table 21.4 highlights therapists' views on task versus component practice, practice outside therapy and carryover as well as the need for preparation for movement and function.

There is confusion in current practice about the automatic translation of improved movement performance into the performance of functional tasks; 79% of therapists do not believe that improved movement patterns transfer automatically into task performance, yet 58% confirm that this does occur, when the statement is phrased differently (see statement 2, Table 21.4). Recent surveys have identified that between 28 and 58% of therapists are concerned about the problem of carryover from activities practised in therapy to everyday activities (Davidson & Waters, 2000; Lennon et al., 2001). Ninety-one per cent of therapists confirm that patients need to practise activities outside therapy. However, they are concerned that practice without therapy supervision may promote abnormal tone and movement. These are all issues related to task and context specificity. Which activities should be practised in therapy, and how should practice be structured?

According to Bobath (1990, p. 60), treatment is designed to prepare the affected side for functional use; treatment should be done in real-life situations. According to Ryerson & Levitt (1997, p. iv), patients need both hands-on therapy to re-educate muscles and, later in recovery, they may benefit from task-oriented, functional practice. Several reviews have highlighted

Table 21.4 The promotion of function, based on the expert consensus survey

Theoretical assumption	Unsure (%)	Agree (%)	Disagree (%)
Changing a patient's ability to move does not necessarily improve the patient's ability to perform functional tasks	8	79	13
Facilitating normal movement components such as pelvic tilt will automatically lead to an improvement in functional tasks	13	58	29
Carryover from therapy sessions into everyday activities is problematic	12	58	30
Generalisation of treatment effects should be sought by giving the patient activities to practise outside therapy as long as the patient is able to perform these activities with optimal movement patterns	0	91	9
Stroke patients need both hands-on and task-oriented functional practice	6	92	2

Adapted from Lennon (2003), with permission.

that therapy effects are limited to the skills being trained, showing minimal transfer effects to related tasks that are not directly trained; e.g. a technique may improve activity in a muscle group without transfer to functional tasks in everyday life (Wagenaar & Meijer, 1991a, b; Duncan, 1997; Kwakkel et al., 1999a, b). Current evidence suggests that the practice of motor skills needs to be both task- and context-specific (Carr & Shepherd, 1998, pp. 37–38; Kwakkel et al., 1999a, b; *National Clinical Guidelines for Stroke*, 2000, 2002), but does this mean that preparation for functional task practice is a waste of time? Evidence from motor learning and skill acquisition can provide some guiding principles.

Therapists in the clinic interpret preparation as the use of treatment strategies to normalise tone to lengthen muscles, and to facilitate core elements of movement (Lennon, 2001; Mayston, 2002). Motor-learning literature also differentiates between whole and part practice of a task. Current evidence does not suggest that whole task practice is more effective at regaining function than activities aimed at preparation or facilitation of movement (Schmidt, 1991; Shumway-Cook & Woollacott, 1995, Ch. 2; Majsak, 1996; Leonard, 1998, Ch. 7). Research has highlighted practice and feedback as two crucial issues for therapists (Lennon, 2000). The type of practice used may depend on the task at hand; for example, part practice of fast, discrete tasks or tasks with interdependent parts is less effective than practising the whole task. It has also been suggested that patients need to rely on both intrinsic and extrinsic information to learn new skills (Leonard, 1998, Ch. 7).

Motor skill learning can be divided into three phases: an early cognitive phase, an intermediate associative phase and an autonomous phase (Leonard, 1998, Ch. 7). Certain types of feedback should be used at different points in skill acquisition. For example, manual guidance should mainly be used at the early cognitive stage of motor learning, whereas physical and verbal guidance may actually interfere with motor learning in the later associative and autonomous stages of skill acquisition (Schmidt, 1991).

It may not be necessary to spend time preparing and practising components of movement before practising functional tasks; the practise of the task itself may normalise tone and access normal movement patterns (Lennon & Ashburn, 2000; Lennon et al., 2001). Different techniques may work better with different patients; sometimes it will be necessary to practise the components of normal movement that comprise an activity such as pelvic tilting. Sometimes it will work best to break tasks down into the different parts before getting the patient to practise the whole sequence of activity in a functional task. On other occasions it will work best to practise the functional task. The majority of motor learning research is based on normal patient populations; much more research is required in patients with neurological impairments to determine the most effective ways in which to structure practice and provide feedback.

In any case, expert consensus suggests that preparation is of no value in itself; it must be incorporated into functional activity (Lennon, 2000; Lennon et al., 2001; Mayston, 2002, p. 16). Changes in tone and improvements in movement must be transferred into functional activity (Lennon, 2000; Lennon et al., 2001). It would appear that many therapists may restrict the activities that patients practise outside therapy, as this may make their movement patterns more abnormal (Davidson & Waters, 2000; Lennon & Ashburn, 2000; Pomeroy & Tallis, 2000; Lennon et al., 2001). This assumption requires further investigation, as it concerns the issue of promoting carryover outside therapy and also, perhaps more importantly, because it may not take patient and carer wishes into account (Pound et al., 1994a, b; Kelson et al., 1998). For example, patients may associate recovery in terms of the resumption of previously valued activities; they may not be overly concerned about how they perform an activity (Hafsteindottir & Grypdonck, 1997). Although therapists voice concern about patients using abnormal tone and movement patterns, there is currently no evidence to suggest that preventing or delaying a patient from moving will worsen abnormal tone and movement (*National Clinical Guidelines for Stroke*, 2000; Pomeroy & Tallis, 2000; Mayston, 2000, p. 15).

Recovery and compensation

Therapists were questioned about neuroplasticity, the need to work on trunk and limb movements and the use of the neurodevelopmental sequence in the management of patients following stroke (Table 21.5).

Therapists (94%) believe that recovery of movement should be encouraged; they believe that physiotherapy can influence neuroplastic change. They confirmed that both proximal activity at the level of the trunk and the pelvis and distal movement need to be practised in therapy. Therapists believe that recovery can occur either proximally and/or distally. Therapists (76%) no longer believe that recovery following brain damage mimics the neurodevelopmental sequence followed during child development.

There is strong evidence that the CNS is plastic (see Ch. 5); however, evidence for specific therapy-induced changes in brain recovery remains sparse (Pomeroy & Tallis, 2000). Therapists aim to promote neuroplasticity of the CNS by targeting different pathways in the CNS (Kidd et al., 1992).

Table 21.5 Recovery and compensation, based on the expert consensus survey

Theoretical assumption	Unsure (%)	Agree (%)	Disagree (%)
Physiotherapy can enhance motor recovery following stroke because of the central nervous system's neuroplasticity	4	94	2
Treating proximal instability will not necessarily result in recovery of distal movement in the limbs; distal movement needs to be facilitated	5	91	4
Recovery from stroke follows a predictable sequence that mimics the normal development of movement during infancy	14	10	76

Adapted from Lennon (2003), with permission.

Kidd et al. (1992) discussed three main systems which contribute to the control of movement:

1. the ventromedial (VM) descending system which controls postural adjustments and proximal muscles
2. the dorsolateral (DL) descending system which controls selective movements
3. the afferent ascending system.

In addition, brain areas such as the basal ganglia, the cerebellum and the premotor area probably store learned motor programmes and direct automatic postural adjustments via the brainstem. The descending information can be initiated through afferent inputs accompanied by feedforward and feedback information to other levels, such as the spinal cord and cerebellum. Therapists aim to manipulate afferent information from the periphery in order to activate these different routes, thus initiating descending information to produce motor output. There is sound neurophysiological evidence to support the use of afferent information, in particular from the proximal regions, such as the trunk and the hip, as well as the foot, to trigger both postural adjustments and planned sequences of muscle activation during goal-directed movements (Allum et al., 1995; Park et al., 1999; Bloem et al., 2000).

This belief in neuroplastic change implies that recovery of movement and function should be the main aims of therapy rather than the promotion of independence using the unaffected side, e.g. compensation. This therefore implies that compensation is undesirable and should be prevented, as it is detrimental to recovery. This assumption has not been investigated in research trials. Compensation is not well defined in the literature; it refers to the use of alternative strategies to complete a task (Shumway-Cook & Woollacott, 1995, p. 38; Carr & Shepherd, 1998, p. 12). It can be viewed as both a negative and a positive contributor to movement dysfunction following brain damage (Edwards, 2002, p. 2; Rogerson, 2002).

Some experts suggest that compensation is not always detrimental for the patient; therapists need to focus on promoting compensatory strategies necessary for function and discouraging those that may be detrimental to the patient (Edwards, 2002, p. 2; Rogerson, 2002). The damaged CNS must function in some way, which will be different from before. Currently the evidence suggests that no therapist should stop a patient from moving unless an alternative strategy can be substituted to achieve the same goal (Mayston, 2000b, p. 14). There should be a balance between the re-education of more normal movement patterns and both the acceptance and the promotion of necessary and desirable compensation (Shumway-Cook & Woollacott, 1995, p. 113; Ryerson & Levit, 1997, pp. 47–49; Edwards, 2002, p. 2).

Key points

- Aiming for the restoration of normal movement is unrealistic for most patients with central nervous system damage
- The main emphasis in treatment is on the facilitation of movement, not the normalisation of tone
- Current evidence suggests that the practice of motor skills needs to be task- and context-specific, i.e. therapists need to practise functional tasks in meaningful contexts with patients
- There is no evidence to suggest that delaying a patient from moving will promote abnormal tone and movement
- Compensation is not always detrimental. It may actually be desirable and necessary for the patient

SERVICE DELIVERY

Although further research is required in relation to patient populations other than stroke, it is realistic to assume that these theoretical assumptions could apply in other conditions, as physiotherapy management is

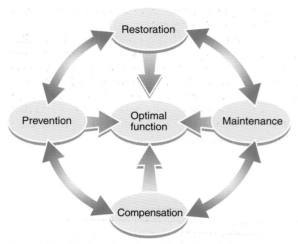

Figure 21.1 The key aims of neurological physiotherapy.

problem-based, not condition-based. Therapists assess patients in a similar fashion, using the same repertoire of treatment techniques depending on the aims of intervention.

These aims of neurological physiotherapy (Fig. 21.1) are focused on:

- restoration (recovery or correction of a complication, such as contracture)
- maintenance
- prevention of complications
- compensation.

The frequency with which each aim is incorporated into a patient's management plan essentially depends upon a number of considerations, such as: the nature of each patient's problems stemming from a static pathology, such as a stroke, or a progressive disorder, such as multiple sclerosis; the timing of the intervention; the patient's needs and preferences; and the therapist's philosophy of care (Edwards, 2002, Ch. 11). There are different stages in patient management, where these aims have differential priorities:

- early recovery phase (medical stabilisation/ maintenance/prevention)
- rehabilitation phase (restoration/prevention/ compensation)
- ongoing management phase (maintenance/ prevention).

Textbooks advocate that all patients with movement dysfunction that interferes with their participation in everyday activity should be assessed and monitored by a physiotherapist on a regular basis with a view to maintaining optimal function and preventing complications (Ryerson & Levitt, 1997; Carr & Shepherd, 1998; Edwards, 2002). There is some evidence to support this view as improvements in disability have been demonstrated, despite unchanging or even deteriorating impairments (*Physiotherapy Effectiveness Bulletin*, 2001).

CONCLUSIONS

Mayston (2002) suggested that the therapist should act as a problem-solver using knowledge derived from understanding motor control, the effects of brain damage, neuroplasticity and skill acquisition. In the past there had been an overemphasis on understanding the neurophysiology underlying movement. Mayston (2002, p. 11) stated that more importance needs to be explicitly awarded to the musculoskeletal system and behavioural psychology, in particular motor learning. These points have been argued and published by Carr & Shepherd since 1987, yet have only started to become an integral part of current practice in the UK since the 1990s.

It is clear that changes in the musculoskeletal constraints of movement alter neural response. Therapists have taken this knowledge on board by incorporating biomechanical constraints into practice, for example using splinting not only as a means of reducing contracture, but also as a means of substituting for impaired activity or preventing contracture developing in the first place (Edwards, 2002, Ch. 10). However, therapists have been less explicit in their application of motor learning research. Actions are influenced and modified by experience, repetition, patient activity and participation (Leonard, 1998, pp. 171, 218, 227–229); these areas have also been well studied in the psychology literature. Thus neurophysiological, musculoskeletal and motor learning principles need to be taken into account in the theoretical framework underlying neurological physiotherapy. This view is supported by many textbooks (Shumway-Cook & Woollacott, 1995; Ryerson & Levitt, 1997; Carr & Shepherd, 1998; Edwards, 2002).

This chapter has identified four key theoretical themes underlying current practice in neurological physiotherapy: the promotion of normal movement, the control of tone, the promotion of function, and the recovery of movement with optimisation of compensation. Current evidence suggests that physiotherapy does play a role in the recovery of movement and function; however, the content of therapy is critical in determining the outcome of treatment (Kwakkel et al., 1999a, b; Parry et al., 1999). The majority of these studies contain methodological flaws, such as a wide range in age, or in time of stroke onset, small sample sizes and a lack of control groups (Olney & Richards, 1996; Richards & Olney, 1996; Duncan, 1997; Kwakkel et al., 1999a). Although in many cases valid outcome measures have been used, the content of therapy has not been presented, and few studies have looked at long-term effects. Evidence-based practice is still in its infancy in relation to neurological physiotherapy; it is important to clarify that the contribution of physiotherapy within the rehabilitation package over

and above spontaneous recovery remains to be determined (Foster & Young, 2002).

It is crucial to link clinical practice to quality research; it is proposed in this chapter that it is now time to move away from allegiance to named treatment approaches (Foster & Young, 2002). The evidence confirms that the components of the therapy programme administered need to be evaluated rather than the label attached to the programme (Pomeroy & Tallis, 2000).

References

Allum A, Honegger F, Acuna H. Differential control of leg and trunk muscle activity by vestibulo-spinal and proprioceptive signals during human balance corrections. *Acta Otolaryngol (Stockh)* 1995, **115**:124–129.

Ashburn A. Physical recovery following stroke. *Physiotherapy* 1997, **83**:480–490

Ballinger C, Ashburn A, Low J et al. Unpacking the black box of therapy – a pilot study to describe occupational and physiotherapy interventions for people with stroke. *Clin Rehab* 1999, **13**:301–309.

Barnes M, Bassett L, Broughton S et al. Guidelines for the management of spasticity in primary care. *Progr Neurol Psychiatry* 2000, March/April: 2–7.

Barrett JA, Evans L, Chappell J et al. Bobath or motor relearning programme: a continuing debate (letter to the editor). *Clin Rehab* 2001, **15**:445–446.

Bloem BR, Allum JH, Carpenter MG et al. Triggering of balance corrections in a patient with total loss proprioceptive loss. *Exp Brain Res* 2002, **142**:91–107.

Bobath B. *Adult Hemiplegia: Evaluation and Treatment*. Oxford: Heinemann; 1990.

Carr JH, Shepherd RB. *A Motor Relearning Programme for Stroke*, 2nd edn. Oxford: Butterworth Heinemann; 1987.

Carr JH, Shepherd RB. *Neurological Rehabilitation: Optimising Motor Performance*. Oxford: Butterworth Heinemann; 1998.

Carr JH, Mungovan SF, Shepherd RB et al. Physiotherapy in stroke rehabilitation: bases for Australian physiotherapists choice of treatment. *Physiother Theory Pract* 1994, **10**:201–209.

Carr JH, Shepherd RB, Ada L. Spasticity: research findings and implications for intervention. *Physiotherapy* 1995, **81**:421–429.

Chartered Society of Physiotherapy (CSP). *Physiotherapy Effectiveness Bulletin*: Neurology 2001:3(2). London.

Davidson I, Waters K. Physiotherapists working with stroke patients. *Physiotherapy* 2000, **86**:69–80.

De Gangi GA, Royeen CB. Current practice among neurodevelopmental treatment association members. *Am J Occup Ther* 1994, **48**:803–809.

Duncan P. Synthesis of intervention trials to improve motor recovery following stroke. *Topics Stroke Rehab* 1997, **3**:1–20.

Edwards S. *Neurological Physiotherapy*. Edinburgh: Churchill Livingstone; 2002.

Foster A, Young J. *The Clinical and Cost Effectiveness of Physiotherapy in the Management of Elderly People Following Stroke*. London: Chartered Society of Physiotherapy; 2002.

Freeman J. Assessment, outcome measurement and goal setting in physiotherapy practice. In: Edwards S, ed. *Neurological Physiotherapy*. Edinburgh: Churchill Livingstone; 2002:21–34.

Gresham GE, Duncan PW, Stason WB et al. *Post Stroke Rehabilitation: Clinical Practice Guidelines*. Rockville, Maryland: AHCPR;1995.

Guidelines Group. *Guidelines for Physiotherapy Practice in Parkinson's Disease*. Newcastle upon Tyne: Institute of Rehabilitation; 2001.

Hafesteindottir TB, Grypdonck M. Being a stroke patient: a review of the literature. *J Adv Nurs* 1997, **26**:580–588.

Hallett M, Wassermann EM, Cohen LG et al. Cortical mechanisms of recovery of function after stroke. *Neurorehabilitation* 1998, **10**:131–142.

Kelson M, Ford C, Rigge M. *Stroke Rehabilitation: Patient and Carers' Views*. London: Royal College of Physicians; 1998.

Kidd G, Lawes N, Musa I. *Understanding Neuromuscular Plasticity*, pp. 57–68. London: Edward Arnold; 1992.

Kwakkel G, Wagenaar RC, Twisk JWR et al. Intensity of leg and arm training after primary middle-cerebral-artery stroke: a randomised trial. *Lancet* 1999a, **354**:191–196.

Kwakkel G, Kollen BJ, Wagenaar RC. Therapy impact on functional recovery in stroke rehabilitation. *Physiotherapy* 1999b, **85**:377–391.

Langhammer B, Stanghelle JK. Bobath or motor relearning programme? A comparison of two different approaches of physiotherapy in stroke rehabilitation: a randomised controlled study. *Clin Rehab* 2000, **14**:361–369.

Lee RG, Van Donkelaar P. Mechanisms underlying functional recovery following stroke. *Can J Neurol Sci* 1995, **22**:257–263.

Lennon S. The Bobath concept: a critical review of the theoretical assumptions that guide physiotherapy practice in stroke rehabilitation. *Phys Ther Rev* 1996, **1**:35–45.

Lennon S. *Gait Re-education Based on the Bobath Concept in Adult Patients with Hemiplegia Following Stroke*. PhD thesis. Northern Ireland: University of Ulster at Jordanstown; 2000.

Lennon S. Gait re-education based on the Bobath concept in two patients with hemiplegia following stroke. *Phys Ther* 2001, **81**:924–934.

Lennon S. Physiotherapy practice in stroke rehabilitation: a survey. *Disabil Rehab* 2003 **25**:455–461.

Lennon S, Ashburn A. The Bobath concept in stroke rehabilitation: a focus group design of the experienced physiotherapists' perspective. *Disabil Rehab* 2000, **22**:665–674.

Lennon S, Hastings M. Key physiotherapy indicators for quality of stroke care. *Physiotherapy* 1996, **82**:655–664.

Lennon S, Baxter GD, Ashburn A. Physiotherapy based on the Bobath concept in stroke rehabilitation: a survey within the United Kingdom. *Disabil Rehab* 2001, **23**:254–262.

Leonard CT. *The Neuroscience of Human Movement*. St Louis: Mosby; 1998.

Lettinga AT, Siemonsma PC, Van Veen M. Entwinement of theory and practice in physiotherapy: a comparative analysis of two approaches to hemiplegia in physiotherapy. *Physiotherapy* 1999, **85**:476–490.

Majsak MJ. Application of motor learning principles to the stroke population. *Topics Stroke Rehab* 1996, **3**:27–59.

Mayston M. Handling and spasticity (letter to the editor). *Physiotherapy* 2000a, **86**:559.

Mayston M. Compensating for CNS dysfunction (letter to the editor). *Physiotherapy* 2000b, **86**:612.

Mayston M. Problem solving in neurological physiotherapy– setting the scene. In: Edwards S, ed. *Neurological Physiotherapy*. Edinburgh: Churchill Livingstone; 2002:3–19.

National Clinical Guidelines for Stroke. London: Royal College of Physicians. 2000, Update 2002. Available online at: http://www.rcplondon.ac.uk/pubs/books/stroke.

National Clinical Guidelines for Stroke. An update. London: Royal College of Physicians; 2002. Available online at: http://www.rcplondon.ac.uk/pubs/books/stroke.

Ng SM, Shepherd RB. Weakness in patients following stroke: implications for strength training. *Phys Ther Rev* 2000, **5**:227–238.

Nilsson L, Nordholm L. Physical therapy in stroke rehabilitation: bases for Swedish physiotherapist's choice of treatment. *Physiother Theory Pract* 1992, **8**:49–55.

Olney SJ, Richards C. Hemiparetic gait following stroke. Part 1: characteristics. *Gait Posture* 1996, **4**:136–148.

Park S, Toole T, Lee S. Functional roles of the proprioceptive system in the control of goal-directed movement. *Percept Motor Skills* 1999, **88**:631–647.

Parry RH, Lincoln NB, Appleyard MA. Physiotherapy for the arm and hand after stroke. *Physiotherapy* 1999, **85**:417–425.

Partridge CJ, De Weerdt W. Different approaches to physiotherapy in stroke. *Rev Clin Gerontol* 1995, **5**:199–209.

Partridge CJ, Edwards S. The basis of practice: neurological physiotherapy. *Physiother Res Int* 1996, **1**:205–208.

Physiotherapy Effectiveness Bulletin. Neurology: Parkinson's disease, multiple sclerosis, and severe traumatic brain injury. London: Chartered Society of Physiotherapy; 2001: vol. 3, issue 2.

Plant R. The theoretical basis of treatment concepts. In: Stokes M, ed. *Neurological Physiotherapy*. London: Mosby; 1998:271–286.

Plant R, Walton G, Ashburn A et al. *Physiotherapy for People with Parkinson's Disease: UK Best Practice*. Newcastle upon Tyne: Institute of Rehabilitation; 2000.

Pollock A, Langhorne P, Baer G et al. *Physiotherapy for the Recovery of Postural Control and Lower Limb Function Following Stroke (Protocol)*. Cochrane Library, Issue 4. Oxford: Update Software; 2003.

Pomeroy V, Tallis R. Physical therapy to improve movement performance and functional ability post stroke. Part 1: existing evidence. *Rev Clin Gerontol* 2000, **10**:261–290.

Pound P, Bury M, Gompertz P, Ebrahim S. Views of survivors of stroke on benefits of physiotherapy. *Q Health Care* 1994a, **3**:69–74.

Pound P, Gompertz P, Ebrahim S. Patient's satisfaction with stroke services. *Clin Rehab* 1994b, **8**:7–17.

Richards CL, Olney SJ. Hemiparetic gait following stroke. Part 2: recovery and physical therapy. *Gait Posture* 1996, **4**:149–162.

Rogerson L. How does the Bobath concept view the relationship between low tone, associated reactions and compensatory strategies? *Synapse* 2002, Spring:10–15.

Ryerson S, Levitt K. *Functional Movement Re-education*. Edinburgh: Churchill Livingstone; 1997.

Sackley CM, Lincoln NB. Physiotherapy treatment for stroke patients: a survey of current practice. *Physiother Theory Pract* 1996, **12**:87–96.

Schmidt RA. Motor learning principles for physical therapy. In: *Proceedings of the 2nd STEP Conference on Contemporary Management of Motor Control Problems*. Virginia: Foundation for Physical Therapy; 1991:49–63.

Shepard K. Theory: criteria, importance and impact. In: *Proceedings of the 2nd STEP Conference on Contemporary Management of Motor Control Problems*. Virginia: Foundation for Physical Therapy; 1991:5–10.

Shumway-Cook A, Woollacott M. *Motor Control: Theory and Practical Applications*. Baltimore: Williams & Wilkins, 1995.

Stephenson R. A review of neuroplasticity: some implications for physiotherapy in the treatment of lesions of the brain. *Physiotherapy* 1993, **79**:699–704.

Van Vliet P, Lincoln NB, Robinson E. Comparison of the content of two physiotherapy approaches for stroke. *Clin Rehab* 2001, **15**:398–414.

Wade DT. Clinical governance and rehabilitation services. *Clin Rehab* 2000, **14**:1–4.

Wagenaar RC, Meijer OG. Effects of stroke rehabilitation (1). *J Rehab Sci* 1991a, **4**:61–73.

Wagenaar RC, Meijer OG. Effects of stroke rehabilitation (2). *J Rehab Sci* 1991b, **4**:97–109.

WHO. *International Classification of Functioning, Disability and Health* (ICF). Geneva: World Health Organization; 2001. Available online at: http://www.who.int/ classification/icf.

Chapter 22

The rehabilitation process

K Whalley Hammell

INTRODUCTION

People who have a neurological condition such as a brain injury, stroke, spinal cord injury or multiple sclerosis experience not only physical sequelae but disruptions to their ways of life, encountering long-term problems that change over time and are experienced and given meaning within the context of their individual lives. This chapter will explore the process of rehabilitation for people with chronic neurological conditions with a predominant emphasis on meaning and context. Acknowledging that some of the arguments in this chapter challenge both traditional rehabilitation dogma and professional dominance, research literature will be used to demonstrate the evidence base that supports its contentions.

The aim of the chapter is to challenge therapists to embrace a mode of practice that places clients' perspectives, values and priorities at its centre; promotes clients' rights to self-determination; and strives to achieve a rehabilitation process that is both useful and relevant. To this end, therapists are encouraged to engage in a dynamic rehabilitation process that fosters communication, endeavours to negate power differentials and promotes autonomy. Such a mode of practice is informed by *meaning* – individuals' perceptions of the consequences of impaired functioning within their own lives – and by *context* – the circumstances of individuals within physical, social, cultural, economic, political and legal environments.

THE CONTEXT OF REHABILITATION

It has been claimed that:

> *Rehabilitation is user and community centred, with an emphasis on the rights of individuals to make*

choices and control their own lives from a range of options (NHS Executive 1997, p. 7).

Given the propensity for rehabilitation researchers to emulate the methods of medicine, few qualitative studies have been undertaken to explore the experience of rehabilitation from clients' perspectives. These few studies suggest, however, that the statement from the NHS Executive might best be regarded as a goal rather than a reality, with changes in rehabilitation practice lagging behind changes in political rhetoric. Research that has sought clients' perspectives of rehabilitation demonstrates that this process is frequently experienced as being meaningless, irrelevant to clients' lives, inappropriate to their roles and values and incongruent with their goals; and is perceived to reinforce powerlessness and dependency rather than fostering choice and control (Morris, 1991; Johnson, 1993; Abberley, 1995; Dalley, 1999). Research evidence also reveals clients' perceptions of physiotherapy as 'problem-centred' rather than 'client-centred' (Johnson, 1993) and as focused on the implementation of standard treatment regimens rather than upon the client as a person (Jorgensen, 2000).

This first section examines the social context in which rehabilitation services are currently located, reviewing the assumptions that have traditionally underpinned the rehabilitation endeavour as well as the political, legal, social policy and ethical contexts that inform both the mandate and framework for contemporary practice.

The historical context

Rehabilitation has traditionally been viewed as: (1) a process of restoring individuals to their optimal level of physical function and of (2) promoting physical independence, thereby (3) enhancing quality of life among those affected by illness or injury. These are core assumptions that have underpinned service provision, yet they are challenged by research evidence.

For example, while the philosophy of (1) maximising physical function through specific treatment regimens might be effective for people with minor, short-term problems (e.g. Pott's fractures), it is clearly inadequate for people with chronic or deteriorating neurological conditions for whom restoration of maximum physical function is an insufficient goal. Someone who has sustained a stroke, brain injury or spinal cord injury (for example) has disrupted not just a body but an entire life (Mattingly, 1991), thus dysfunction alone cannot determine the priorities for intervention (Hammell, 1995a).

Further, the idea that (2) rehabilitation is a process of teaching those skills that will enable the highest level of independence suggests that this is a goal to which all clients aspire, irrespective of culture, role demands or personal values. Indeed, therapists and their clients do not appear to have a common understanding of *independence*. For rehabilitation practitioners, independence tends to be construed as the ability to perform self-care activities without assistance, while for disabled people it implies control over their lives and the opportunity to enact choices (Oliver, 1990). With support from research evidence (Fuhrer et al., 1992; Draper, 1997; Hammell, 1998a), independence could be usefully redefined 'not as the ability to perform necessary tasks but as the freedom to control one's own life and determine its course' (Williams & Wood, 1988, p. 132).

By focusing predominantly on reteaching the skills that most 4-year-olds have attained – self-care and mobility – rehabilitation services have both limited and demeaned their adult clients (Hammell, 1995b). Outcome studies have demonstrated, moreover, that clients often choose to live interdependently, preferring to use their time and energies in those activities that have personal meaning and relevance rather than in performing self-care activities without assistance (Yerxa & Locker, 1990; Holcomb, 2000). Clearly, these findings have implications for an evidence-based approach to rehabilitation practice.

Finally, rehabilitation practitioners often claim (3) to be working towards enhancement of their clients' quality of life by improving physical functioning and physical independence. This is a worthy goal. However, research has demonstrated, counterintuitively, that perceptions of quality in living do not correlate with degree of physical function, level of neurological impairment or extent of physical independence (Lindberg, 1995; Fuhrer, 1996; Vogel et al., 1998; Dijkers, 1999; Kemp & Krause, 1999). Further, neither level and severity of neurological impairment nor degree of physical independence is predictive of psychological distress (Daverat et al., 1995; Hartkopp et al., 1998; Post et al., 1998; Krause et al., 2000).

Although it appears that rehabilitation's claim to be enhancing the quality of lives through maximising physical function and physical independence is not evidence-based, this belief persists among the rehabilitation professions. This confirms, perhaps, that the more powerful a professional idea becomes and the greater its longevity, the greater its ability to survive contact with contesting evidence (Childs & Williams, 1997).

The social, political and policy context

Rehabilitation practitioners undertake their work in an evolving context of consumer demands and government policies. These constitute part of the social, political and policy environment that both informs the operational framework and determines the mandate of rehabilitation practice.

Government policies are responding to consumer demands for health care services that are accountable, responsive to the needs of users and appropriate to their individual circumstances (Department of Health, 1997, 1999). Health care practitioners are exhorted to embrace client-focused care (Ritchie, 1999) and to empower people living with chronic long-term medical conditions to become key decision-makers in their own care (Chief Medical Officer, 2001). Such innovations prompted Hughes (2002, p. 12) to observe: 'the decision about whether to involve clients actively in their own care is no longer optional'.

Evidence-based practice

Recent government policy and subsequent professional initiatives demand that professional practice be 'evidence-based'. There is pressure to justify both the choices made for particular clients and patterns of practice 'by reference to a body of evidence about efficiency and effectiveness' (Gomm & Davies, 2000). Consequently, evidence-based practice has become a preoccupation for those therapists who seek to inform their interventions with a sound knowledge base (Hammell, 2001).

Evidence-based practice incorporates the judicious use of relevant and current research evidence, clinical expertise and the 'thoughtful identification and compassionate use of individual patients' predicaments, rights, and preferences in making clinical decisions' (Sackett et al., 1996, p. 71).

Unfortunately, the rehabilitation professions have subjected relatively few of their interventions to rigorous research (Banja, 1997), providing an unstable basis for their claims to knowledge. In the absence of an extensive evidence base with which to inform practice, clients are reliant upon the therapist's 'best guess' or 'whim' (Banja, 1997, p. 53) to guide practice, or upon increasingly out-of-date primary training or the over-interpretation of experiences with individual clients (Rosenberg & Donald, 1995).

The ethical and legal context

Clinical ethics constitute a further part of the context within which rehabilitation is undertaken and are informed by four principles (nonmaleficence, beneficence, justice and autonomy). The ethical principle of *autonomy* (and the associated respect for client preferences) is concerned with the moral right of clients to make choices and to follow their own plans of action and of life, in so far as these do not infringe upon someone else's rights or welfare (Jonsen et al., 1998). If the client's values and aspirations are not

unreasonable, health care ethics insist that their values 'trump' those of the service providers (Banja, 1997). The principle of autonomy constitutes an ethical requirement for contemporary health care practice and is not an optional modus operandi.

Key points

Autonomy

- The capacity to act on particular desires and choices
- The capacity to be self-determining
- The capacity to be in control of one's own life
- The power or right of self-government

In addition, the ethical and legal principle of informed consent (which arises from respect for autonomy) implies at least a minimum of shared decision-making. Indeed, governments in Canada and the USA currently endorse the principle of informed choice rather than mere consent (Charles et al., 1997).

Although physical function does not have a demonstrable effect upon quality of life, researchers have found that perceptions of choice and control are positive contributors to perceptions of quality of life following neurological injury (Crisp, 1992; Fuhrer et al., 1992; Krause, 1992; Draper, 1997; Hammell, 1998a). Conversely, studies have indicated an association between perceptions of reduced control and low perceptions of life satisfaction (Krause & Kjorsvig, 1992; Krause, 1997). Thus it may be said that ethical practice – respecting client autonomy – is evidence-based practice.

Key points

Research review

- Positive perceptions of quality of life are not correlated with physical function, degree of physical independence or proximity to 'normality'
- Positive perceptions of quality of life are associated with the opportunity to make choices and control one's life
- Governments have determined that rehabilitation services should be client-focused and interventions should be evidence-based
- Clinical ethics demand respect for client autonomy
- Rehabilitation services are not currently perceived to be user-centred or focused on clients' rights to make choices and control their own lives, but are claimed to be problem-oriented and focused on standard treatment regimens

---

MANAGEMENT OF CHRONIC AND DETERIORATING CONDITIONS

Having briefly highlighted the historical, political, legal, social policy and ethical contexts in which rehabilitation is undertaken, it is pertinent to consider the provision of rehabilitation in the context of chronic and deteriorating neurological conditions: how might this differ from the management of those acute conditions that share the goal of cure?

Rehabilitation following an orthopaedic injury, for example, often adheres to a mechanistic, medical model of care: following diagnosis, various treatment approaches are employed at the discretion of the therapist; the therapist assumes a paternalistic or maternalistic, 'expert' stance (determining the treatment goals) while the client adopts a deferential and compliant role. While it has been argued that 'it is never sufficient to work within a traditional medical model in a profession such as physiotherapy' (Jorgensen, 2000, pp. 105–106), this model is particularly inappropriate for the management of chronic disability.

Although clients may share a diagnosis with other clients, interventions must be applicable to the unique environment, life stage and goals of each individual and must consider the meaning that disability holds for them in the context of their lives (Hammell, 1998b). Thus, Leavitt (1999, p. x) observed: 'it may be less important to teach a patient exercises than it is to understand what having an impairment … means to the patient'.

> **Key point**
>
> A rehabilitation process that enables each client to live a meaningful life in his or her chosen environment will be a dynamic process – one that is as concerned with teaching the therapist about the meaning and consequences of disability for the individual's life as it is about teaching the client about how to live with a functional impairment (Hammell, 1995a)

THE COMMUNICATION PROCESS BETWEEN CLIENT AND THERAPIST

Client–therapist relationships are the cornerstone of client-centred practice and communication is therefore the most important contributor to effective and accountable rehabilitation. Researchers who explored the experience of hospitalisation following a stroke found that the feeling of being valued and respected by hospital staff had an important impact on patients'
self-esteem, leading to better self-management of their conditions on discharge (Pound et al., 1995). How might therapists attempt to enhance the quality of client–therapist interaction?

Adopting roles

Peloquin (1990) provided a useful summary of three roles typically assumed by (occupational) therapists in their relationships with clients. The 'technician' confuses efficiency and skill with caring, valuing techniques over relationships and appearing to the client as cold and aloof. Former clients claim these detached 'technical' relationships provoke resentment, indignity and demoralisation (Johnson, 1993). The 'parent' strives for a more personal rapport with the client, but, by adopting a nurturing and paternalistic or maternalistic role, fosters dependency and undermines autonomy. The 'covenantor' achieves an interaction founded on reciprocity and characterised by respect (Peloquin, 1990). In this relationship the client is encouraged to use the therapist as a resource while the therapist strives to understand the concerns and priorities of the client. This results in a more personal approach in which clients feel that their needs as a person are being met. By being treated as equals they feel involved in their treatment (Johnson, 1993).

Relationships based on acceptance and respect are found to inspire and motivate (Johnson, 1993). Such relationships are dependent upon a conscious realignment of power and require that the therapist reject the posture of detached and objective expert.

The dynamics of difference

Leavitt (1999) suggests that one component of competent practice is a consciousness of the dynamics of difference, that is, an awareness of how cultural assumptions, power differentials and the various social positions of people will affect communication between them. Variables that contribute to personal and cultural differences include: professional status and education, gender, 'race', ethnicity, age, social class, sexual orientation, (dis)ability, religion, income and language (Hammell, 2001). Although physiotherapists reflect homogeneity on many of these variables, their clients are likely to be more diverse and thus unlikely to share their therapists' value systems. Indeed, an early study of women with spinal cord injuries found that their values and interests least resembled those of physiotherapists, occupational therapists, nurses, social workers and psychologists (Rohe & Athelstan, 1982). This suggests the futility and irrelevance of interventions informed by therapists' values.

Different values: divergent perspectives

Research evidence demonstrates that clients' and therapists' perspectives differ in many critical areas. The two groups differ, for example, on the meaning of 'rehabilitation', the relevance and value of treatment services, preferred approaches to service delivery, priorities of treatment goals and desired treatment outcomes (Yerxa & Locker, 1990; McGrath & Davis, 1992; Clark et al., 1993; Corring, 1999). In fact, it seems to be more difficult to identify points of commonality than difference between the values and visions of clients and their therapists (Hammell, 2001).

Compliance or collaboration?

Rehabilitation professionals have traditionally favoured patient behaviours that reflect compliance, co-operation, deference to 'expert' knowledge and submissiveness to the goals established by those holding more power. Indeed, clients who fail to assume these behaviours have often been subjected to pseudodiagnostic and derogatory labelling, such as 'unmotivated', 'non-compliant' or 'unrealistic', or have been referred for psychiatric assessment (Steinglass et al., 1982; Caplan & Shechter, 1993). Thus, clients are blamed for deficient client–therapist collaboration. If clients are neither permitted to define their own problems nor to engage actively in a problem-solving process, the consequent sense of powerlessness and loss of autonomy may, indeed, appear as non-compliance (Pollock, 1993).

Although therapists purportedly strive to foster independent behaviour among their clients, this is not compatible with the traditional roles of 'expert' (superior) therapist and compliant (inferior) client. Indeed, an early study found that rehabilitation clients exhibited the most independent behaviours in hallways and cafeterias and the least in occupational therapy or physiotherapy (Willems, 1972). While compliance may be rewarding to therapists, it is difficult to imagine how it might serve the interests of clients. Compliant behaviour does not foster the problem-solving abilities required to live well with a neurological impairment (Tucker, 1984; Trieschmann, 1986).

Learned powerlessness: taught helplessness

The theory of learned helplessness states that unless people feel able to exert control over their circumstances, they will cease making the effort to try to do so (Seligman, 1975). If rehabilitation practitioners require deference, compliance and submissiveness from clients, then the dependent behaviour that ensues could appropriately be termed 'taught helplessness' (Hammell, 1995a).

It is suggested that those people who believe they have both abilities and opportunities to control their lives have an 'internal locus of control'. Conversely, those who believe that their life circumstances are the result of luck, fate or powerful people have an 'external locus of control' (Rotter, 1966). Studies have indicated that, while people with an internal locus of control assume more responsibility for self-care and enlargement of life opportunities, those with an external locus of control experience more distress following neurological injury and exhibit less adaptive behaviours (Frank & Elliott, 1989). External expectancy of control is closely affiliated with learned helplessness; this is a learned expectation. Johnston et al. (1992) demonstrated that internal control could be increased simply by providing additional information to clients about their own role and potential impact upon treatment outcomes.

Clients who have been taught that those with more power will determine their problems, establish goals, dictate interventions and assess outcomes (informed by their own values and priorities) cannot be expected to assume self-directive, independent behaviours.

> **Key points**
>
> **Research review**
>
> - Positive relationships between therapists and clients inspire, motivate and lead to increased self-esteem, self-management and involvement in the rehabilitation process
> - Positive relationships are characterised by reciprocity, respect and a realigning of power
> - Positive relationships are fostered when therapists understand the dynamics of difference and seek to understand perspectives and priorities that are informed by different values
> - Relationships that require compliance and deference produce powerlessness, helplessness and dependency

THE PROCESS OF EDUCATING TO ENABLE

Rehabilitation has been defined as the process of learning to live with a functional impairment in the context of one's own environment (Trieschmann, 1986) and education has been described as the key to rehabilitation (Brillhart & Stewart, 1989), yet few rehabilitation professionals have received explicit education to enable them to be effective educators (Hammell, 1995a). Education philosophers have defined the process of education as enabling people to achieve autonomy by equipping them with the problem-solving skills required to gain greater control over their lives (Hammell, 1995a). It has been observed that adults learn best when they are enabled to define their own problems, decide on a course of action and, most importantly, evaluate the consequences of their decisions (Coles, 1989). Perversely, rehabilitation clients who assess their own needs, decide on their goals and implement strategies to meet these goals are often labelled 'demanding' or 'difficult' (Tucker, 1984; Oliver et al., 1988).

Adult education requires the learner to be an active participant in an interactive process, not the passive recipient of a list of information (Hammell, 1995b). Research indicates that a teaching process characterised by the presentation of facts and skills deemed important by the teacher may actively inhibit the very attributes desired of the learners, namely analytic thinking and problem-solving abilities (Sadlo et al., 1994). This teacher-centred approach focuses on informational content rather than the use to which the information might be put. Service providers are urged to encourage a reflective dialogue with a client in order to place information and skills into the framework of the individual's life and experiences – placing knowledge into context (Schön, 1983).

Traditionally, knowledge claimed to be objective or scientific ('ours') has been accorded privilege over expertise derived from lived experience ('theirs'). Thus, while health care professionals consider themselves to have knowledge, patients are deemed to have beliefs: 'Knowledge requires both certitude and correctness; belief implies uncertainty, error, or both' (Good, 1994, p. 17).

Peer learning

Informal support groups may provide the opportunity to learn both from the experience of others who have similar neurological impairments and their families. In addition, the use of peers in the rehabilitation process enables both the client and therapist to learn from the experiences of someone who already lives with a specific neurological problem, thus enabling them to place knowledge into context. Clients with neurological impairments have complained that their therapists knew very little about what it means to live with a disability in the community, thereby providing little real-life experiential knowledge (Hammell, 1991). Lack of involvement of peers during the rehabilitation process has been lamented by people with high spinal cord injuries, who felt unable to envision what kind of life opportunities might be possible for them in the absence of role models (Hammell, 1998a). Therapists who forge links with support groups provide their clients with the opportunities for both peer learning and long-term support.

Key points

Optimal learning outcomes

- Autonomy
- Problem-solving abilities
- Analytic thinking

Optimal learning conditions

- Defining own problems
- Decide on action
- Evaluate consequences
- Reflective dialogue to place knowledge in context
- Active participant in interactive process

Outcome cannot be assessed in terms of a list of skills and information that have been taught but by the autonomy and problem-solving abilities demonstrated by the client (Hammell, 1995b).

PARTICIPATING IN THE PROCESS

The consequences of a neurological impairment depend not solely upon specific dysfunctions but upon the context in which the impairment is experienced and the meaning of dysfunction within individuals' lives (Oliver et al., 1988). The experience of living with a stroke, for example, will be determined by a range of environmental variables (such as income, social support, physical access to the home and community and social policies and services), personal variables, for example, one's age, role expectations (such as worker, wife, mother), interests and beliefs (such as fate or divine will) and the meanings or values that the person attributes to all these factors. These meanings and values will determine the priorities and hence the goals of rehabilitation for each individual and cannot, therefore, be addressed by a generic, prescriptive approach to stroke management. Clearly, the objective is not to 'manage the stroke' but to assist someone to manage his or her life, given the occurrence of a stroke.

Evidence presented in this chapter has demonstrated that therapists' value systems, informed by their personal and cultural backgrounds, are not necessarily compatible with those of their clients; neither are their priorities, goals or visions of desirable outcomes (see Box 21.1). Rather than encouraging an approach to practice that tailors interventions to meet the expressed goals of clients, research has identified a rehabilitation culture which equates competence with 'patient miles': the number of patients treated over many years (Richardson, 1999). This is problematic in light of further

Box 22.1   Diverging values: the example of return to work

Some critics contend that the rehabilitation process frequently focuses on mobility and self-care skills to the neglect of adult roles, such as assisting return to paid employment. In contrast, some disability theorists would argue that by often proclaiming 'return to work' as the optimal measure of rehabilitation success, therapists act as agents of the state, actively perpetuating specific ideologies that devalue those deemed 'unproductive'. Clearly, the opportunity for paid employment should be a person's right but this may not be a valued goal for every client.

Erik and Beth are pseudonyms for two young adults who both sustained complete C3 or C4 spinal cord injuries more than a decade ago. Formerly a labourer, since his injury Erik has trained as a stockbroker and accountant. He lives alone in his own home, making use of a government programme that enables him to hire his own care assistants. He works full-time in paid employment and is also his local union representative.

Reliant upon financial support from the state, Beth also lives alone in a social housing unit and has care assistants. Formerly a librarian, she has chosen to devote her time and energies to full-time volunteer activities for a disability advocacy group (Hammell, 1998a).

Erik and Beth both report high degrees of satisfaction with their lives, and fulfilment in using their time in ways they find meaningful. Time use and goals reflect values. Our job as therapists is to support clients' goals, not dictate them.

research demonstrating that misperceptions of clients' problems actually worsen with the length of clinical experience (Bach et al., 1991; Gerhart et al., 1994).

Respect for clients and their values, and support for their rights to autonomy, requires an approach to practice which enables clients to identify their needs and strives to ensure the relevance of interventions (Hammell, 1998b). This is client-centred practice.

Client–centred practice

Client-centred practice is characterised by collaborative and partnership approaches to practice that encourage and respect clients' autonomy, control and choice and support their right to enact these choices (Law et al., 1995). 'Clients' may be individuals, couples, families or others. A client-centred approach to practice enables clients to identify their own priorities and needs. This requires the therapist to respect the client's values (having determined what these are), work collaboratively towards the client's goals and assess the achievement of outcomes that matter to the client. Fundamentally, client-centred practice is concerned with a realignment of power and with ensuring that the rehabilitation process is useful and relevant to the client's life (Law et al., 1995, Canadian Association of Occupational Therapists (CAOT) 1997).

Law (1998) examined research literature to determine whether client-centred practice could be considered an effective mode of service delivery. Evidence gleaned from diverse client groups demonstrated that a client-centred approach to health service delivery led to both improved client satisfaction and to improved outcomes. Law noted that time and resources were maximised when attention was focused on those issues of greatest importance to the client/family. Because research evidence supports client-centred service delivery, it can be claimed that client-centred practice is an evidence-based mode of practice (Hammell, 2001).

Being client-centred does not mean that therapists abandon legal and ethical responsibilities for identifying and seeking to avoid harm. While clients have the same rights as other citizens to pursue actions that place themselves at risk, therapists have the obligation to identify and examine risk, enabling clients to understand the implications of their decisions and to deal with possible consequences. Therapists who respect clients and therefore aspire to client-centred practice will not tell a client that he or she *must not* get into the bath, but rather will acknowledge the client's expressed wish to do so, state their concerns about safety and assist the client to consider how any problems might be dealt with, should these arise. Rehabilitation practitioners can refuse to cooperate with clients' requests if these are believed to be unethical or would constitute malpractice (CAOT, 1997).

People who have spinal cord injuries, strokes and multiple sclerosis have all identified a loss of autonomy and sense of being in control that occurred following injury or diagnosis (Toombs, 1987; Kaufman, 1988; Becker, 1993; Carpenter, 1994). Toombs (1987) claimed that this perception of helplessness and dependency was exacerbated by having one's activities and plans determined by 'powerful others', an argument supported by the theory of learned helplessness (Seligman, 1975). In light of these observations it is argued that a client-centred approach to goal-planning and decision-making may be intrinsically therapeutic, irrespective of the intervention that ensues (Hammell, 1998a).

Client-oriented service delivery

Much has been written about the need for an interdisciplinary approach to rehabilitation. It would seem redundant to note that when teams are involved in goal-planning or collaborative decision-making, this process should be focused on the client's goals and that the client/family should be a part of every meeting or decision, as an active and not a token team member.

Members of an interdisciplinary team can work towards complex goals identified by the client through co-ordinated action (McGrath & Davis, 1992). Davis et al. (1992) and McGrath & Davis (1992) described changes in working practices implemented at a neurological rehabilitation centre to incorporate client-oriented goal-planning and an interdisciplinary approach to problem-solving.

Client-oriented service provision will enable access to rehabilitation services in local areas when needs are identified and at times that suit clients (Hammell, 1998b). Physiotherapists, for example, have traditionally worked only on weekdays, and then only during social hours. While working social hours may be viewed as a privilege (and congruent with professional power), it does not fit well with a philosophy of client-centredness (Hammell, 1995a).

Working in a client-centred mode of practice is both challenging and complex. 'The process of giving more power/control to the client threatens the traditional view of the therapist as expert' (Law et al., 1995, p. 255). This is a mode of practice that *accords* respect.

Key points

Values inform priorities, which inform goals. These should be the client's.

Features of client–centred practice

- Collaborative and partnership approaches to service delivery
- Individualised service delivery
- Facilitation of client participation in the rehabilitation process
- Provision of client-oriented information to inform choices
- Respect for the client
- Respect for clients' values
- Respect for clients' autonomy, and right to choose and enact choices
- Realigns power
- Results in service provision that is useful and relevant

THE PROBLEM-SOLVING PROCESS

'Rehabilitation, like many aspects of human behaviour, can be thought of as a purposive problem solving activity' (McGrath & Davis, 1992, p. 226). The following exploration draws upon the problem-solving process delineated in Chapter 6, examining this process from a client-centred perspective (Fearing et al., 1997).

Assessment

The purpose of assessment is to enable clients to identify and prioritise their problems and catalogue their resources (Ch. 3). This analysis becomes the foundation for establishing goals and initiating interventions that will be relevant to the client's life (Stratford et al., 1995). Clients who are actively involved in identifying priorities for intervention not only become more knowledgeable about their conditions but express more faith in the competence of those providing care (Steele et al., 1987).

Clearly, client-centred assessment requires client-focused tools for evaluation (Dalley, 1999). 'The use of a set protocol of assessments and interventions for diagnostically defined types of clients is not supported within client-centred practice' (Law et al., 1995, p. 253). Unfortunately, few assessments are designed to reflect the perspectives of the client (although see Stratford et al., 1995; Law et al., 1998; Bodiam, 1999), yet listening to clients' perceptions and life goals 'offers an optimal condition for therapeutic success' (van Bennekom et al., 1996).

Once the client's issues have been identified and prioritised, decisions can be made concerning which standardised assessment should now be used (Fearing et al., 1997).

Intervention planning

(The term 'intervention' is chosen instead of 'treatment', not solely because 'treatment' implies client passivity but also to reflect a mode of practice that might focus upon environmental changes – such as bathroom modifications – rather than attempts to modify the individual.)

This is a process in which the therapist provides information to facilitate client choice in establishing meaningful and achievable goals and identifying skills and resources (Law et al., 1995). The client-centred therapist shifts from a role as prescriber/dictator to that of enabler. Research has demonstrated a link between shared decision-making and positive patient outcomes (Charles et al., 1997) and indicates that client–therapist collaboration on intervention goals results in both shorter hospital stays and better goal attainment (Neistadt, 1995).

Further studies have indicated 'that people whose expectations are higher than the judgements made by clinicians do substantially better than people whose expectations accord with or are less than those of the treating clinicians' (Batterham et al., 1996, p. 1222). Yet researchers have found that physiotherapists and occupational therapists frequently strive to change clients' goals and perceptions to match their own (Johnson, 1993; Abberley, 1995). This process is deemed by therapists to be 'educational' and justified by their claims to superior knowledge (Abberley, 1995). However, a treatment environment that overrides clients' goals and superimposes goals informed by therapist-centred values results in ineffective rehabilitation (Cook, 1981).

Intervention

This is the process of implementing plans. In physiotherapy, for example, this might be through enabling clients to relearn balance so they can engage in activities that have personal value and importance. This is the phase in which therapists maximise both their own skills and resources and those of the client in striving to achieve the goals the clients have established (Law et al., 1995).

Motivation

It is pertinent to add a note concerning motivation. A rehabilitation goal which has a low value to a client and to his or her evaluation of its importance to his or her life will be likely to elicit low motivation and poor outcomes (Jordan et al., 1991) or antisocial behaviour, such as verbal or physical aggression among people with brain injuries or other difficulties with communication (McGrath & Davis, 1992). Clients who are disparagingly labelled 'unmotivated' may be those for whom a rehabilitation process dictated by therapist-designated goals offers no personally meaningful rewards for which they choose to strive (Mattingly, 1991; Caplan & Shechter, 1993).

Evaluating the process: counting outcomes or outcomes that count?

This is the phase in which the client and therapist evaluate the effectiveness of intervention. Reassessment will enable comparisons to be made and may identify further issues for change (Fearing et al., 1997). A client-centred orientation to practice requires that outcome assessments reflect the values, priorities and goals of the client. Clearly, the impact and outcome of rehabilitation cannot only be considered from the viewpoints of service providers. Appraising the quality of care must have two dimensions: 'the objective, technical one derived from the research evidence and the subjective,

personal one as experienced by the individual' (Ritchie, 1999, p. 253).

While outcome assessments have traditionally focused on functional achievements, these constitute superficial outcome indicators, at best. As Woolsey (1985, p. 119) observed: 'Some functionally independent patients are happy, productive and socially active following spinal cord injury. Others are not'. Assessment of physical function is an insufficient gauge of the usefulness or value of rehabilitation services.

In light of considerable evidence showing that disabled people do not share the same priorities, preoccupations or perceptions of problems as their health care providers (Clark et al., 1993; Corring, 1999), it has been queried whether the purpose of judging successful outcomes by measuring those skills prioritised by therapists is simply a means of justifying and validating customary rehabilitation practice (Eisenberg & Saltz, 1991).

Modification

Modification may be required if evaluation suggests the need to change the focus, mode or pattern of intervention (see Ch. 6).

Key points

The problem–solving process: a client–centred approach

Assessment

- Enabling clients to identify and prioritise their problems

Intervention-planning

- Using assessment as a guide for establishing relevant goals and meaningful interventions
- Shared decision-making; provision of information to enable informed choices

Intervention

- Therapist and client work in collaboration to achieve client's goals, drawing upon their combined skills, abilities and resources

Evaluation

- Client and therapist together evaluate the effectiveness of intervention, using outcome assessment tools that reflect the values, priorities and goals of the client

Modification

- Client and therapist determine whether modification to the process is required

THE PROCESS OF CLINICAL REASONING

During the past decade there has been considerable interest in clinical reasoning among the rehabilitation professions. It is not possible within the confines of this chapter to review the plethora of analyses of reasoning that have been spawned by researchers with diverse academic orientations. This section will therefore provide a brief overview of the process of clinical reasoning as this pertains to everyday practice.

Clinical reasoning is more than the application of theory to practice, it is a cognitive process of critical analysis and reflection that underpins decision-making and guides practice. The purpose of rehabilitation is to tailor interventions to suit the skills, needs and priorities of the client. Clinicians who apply theories and techniques to clients on the basis of diagnosis might best be termed 'technicians', while those who engage in critical reflection and seek to make techniques relevant to clients' lives could be designated 'professionals' (Richardson, 1999). Clinical reasoning blends theoretical knowledge, research evidence and experiential knowledge with the client's knowledge, to provide meaning and context.

Theoretical knowledge

Theories are conceptual frameworks that encapsulate specific professional knowledge. 'Theory, although understated (or even unstated) is what guides all clinical practice and every research inquiry: informing what we believe should be done in various situations' (Hammell & Carpenter, 2000, p. 10). Clinical reasoning requires the therapist to decide: which theoretical approach or approaches is appropriate to understanding and addressing this client's situation?

Research evidence

Relevant current research is identified and critically evaluated for its relevance and usefulness, given the specific circumstances of an individual client (Hammell, 2001). Without recourse to research evidence, the reasoning process is dependent upon intuition, trial and error and perpetuation of formerly fashionable routines (Ritchie, 1999).

Experience

Practical knowledge is derived from clinical experience and from the lived experience of the client and others from the client's peer group.

Context

Consideration of context is necessary to ensure the relevance of reasoning. For example, physiotherapists and occupational therapists acknowledge the importance of environmental context (physical, social, cultural, economic, political, legal) in their theories of movement (Cott et al., 1995) and of occupational performance (CAOT, 1997).

Meaning

The reasoning process solicits and respects the client's knowledge, considering the client's values and priorities (Sackett et al., 1996) and the meaning of disability within individual lives (Mattingly, 1991).

Studies investigating 'expert' practice in physiotherapy (Jensen et al., 2000) and occupational therapy (Strong et al., 1995) have demonstrated that 'expert' clinicians are those who strive to understand clients, the context of their lives and how these are affected by illness or impairment. Because clients are key sources of knowledge, collaboration and communication are central to the process of clinical reasoning (Jensen et al., 2000).

Key points

Applying clinical reasoning
Clinical reasoning

Theoretical knowledge (specific professional concepts)
Research evidence – current and relevant (a component of evidence-based practice)
Experience – of therapists, clients and their peers (a component of evidence-based practice)
Context – social, cultural, physical, political, economic, legal (a component of evidence-based practice)
Meaning – impact of impairment and clients' values, goals (a component of evidence-based practice)

The problem-solving process

Assessment
Intervention planning

Intervention

Evaluation

Modification

Therapists clearly need to communicate their reasoning to the client to illuminate the links between their interventions and the client's goals (Peloquin, 1990).

CONCLUSIONS

This chapter briefly explored the social, political and ethical imperatives for a client-centred orientation to the rehabilitation process. Clearly, for the rehabilitation process to be useful, meaningful and relevant it must be congruent with the values and goals of the client. Research demonstrates that positive rehabilitation outcomes are attained by collaborative partnerships between therapists and clients.

It is claimed that professional competence depends upon a sound grasp of the techniques and formal knowledge of the profession as well as 'the ability to enter the patient's life-world so that the techniques are tailored to meet the patient's needs' (Crepeau, 1991, p. 1024). This is the hallmark of client-centred practice. This client-centred rehabilitation process maximises the skills of therapists in tailoring interventions to each individual's context (social, cultural, physical, legal, economic and political) and to the meaning of the consequences of disability in his or her life.

Client-centred practice respects clients' rights to self-determination, to control their own lives and enact choices, and is consistent with a vision of independence: 'not as the ability to perform necessary tasks but as the freedom to control one's own life and determine its course' (Williams & Wood, 1988, p. 132).

CASE HISTORIES

ACUTE MANAGEMENT: EXAMPLE

Mike is 20 years old and has sustained a complete spinal cord injury at C6. In describing the impact (meaning and consequences) of the injury on his life he expresses his fears that he will be unable to complete his university degree and that girls will no longer be interested in him. His physiotherapist establishes contact with the Spinal Injuries Association, enabling Mike to meet and learn from others who are already living well with similar injuries. These peers provide role models and reassurance that intimate relationships and children remain real possibilities for Mike. The physiotherapist works with Mike to improve his balance, sitting tolerance and upper-body strength so that he can transfer, dress and manoeuvre his light-weight wheelchair. However, because the university campus is large, they decide that a power wheelchair will be most appropriate for his everyday life, enabling him to conserve energy for activities he values.

LONG-TERM MANAGEMENT: EXAMPLE

Tanya is a 36-year-old teacher, married and with two children. She has been living with multiple sclerosis for almost a decade. Recently her balance has deteriorated and she finds walking increasingly difficult. She contacts her community physiotherapist, Jane, for help. Jane and Tanya are both well informed about multiple sclerosis, its management and its consequences. Tanya is the expert in terms of its manifestations and impact on her life, and Jane has specialised knowledge and skills to assist her. Tanya experiences problems that change over time and the community physiotherapists have maintained an open-door policy, enabling Tanya to initiate contact and use them as sources of information and practical assistance whenever she feels the need. Together, Tanya and Jane examine the problems Tanya faces in her everyday life, and her resources – the context of her life. These include social/cultural factors (a supportive family and neighbours), physical (the accessibility of her home, community and school) and political/legal/economic factors (social policies dictating the availability of mobility aids, support for home accessibility, requirements for workplace access and community transportation). Interventions will be focused on both Tanya (balance, exercise and mobility aids) and the environment (assuring access).

References

Abberley P. Disabling ideology in health and welfare: the case of occupational therapy. *Disabil Soc* 1995, **10**:221–232.

Bach JR, Campagnolo D, Hoeman S. Life satisfaction of individuals with Duchenne muscular dystrophy using long-term mechanical ventilatory support. *Am J Phys Med Rehab* 1991, **70**:129–135.

Banja JD. Values and outcomes: the ethical implications of multiple meanings. *Topics Stroke Rehab* 1997, **4**:59–70.

Batterham RW, Dunt D, Disler P. Can we achieve accountability for long-term outcomes? *Arch Phys Med Rehab* 1996, **77**:1219–1225.

Becker G. Continuity after a stroke: implications of life-course disruption in old age. *Gerontologist* 1993, **33**:148–158.

Bodiam C. The use of the Canadian Occupational Performance Measure for the assessment of outcome on a neurorehabilitation unit. *Br J Occup Ther* 1999, **62**:123–126.

Brillhart B, Stewart A. Education as the key to rehabilitation. *Nurs Clin North Am* 1989, **24**:675–680.

Canadian Association of Occupational Therapists. *Enabling Occupation. An Occupational Therapy Perspective.* Ottawa: CAOT; 1997.

Caplan B, Shechter J. Reflections on the 'depressed', 'unrealistic', 'inappropriate', 'manipulative', 'unmotivated', 'non-compliant', 'denying', 'maladjusted', 'regressed', etc patient. *Arch Phys Med Rehab* 1993, **74**:1123–1124.

Carpenter C. The experience of spinal cord injury: the individual's perspective – implications for rehabilitation practice. *Phys Ther* 1994, **74**:614–629.

Charles C, Gafni A, Whelan T. Shared clinical decision-making in the medical encounter: what does it mean? (Or it takes at least two to tango). *Soc Sci Med* 1997, **44**:681–692.

Chief Medical Officer. The expert patient – a new approach to chronic disease management for the 21st century. 2001 Cited in: More control for patients. *Occupational Therapy News* 2002, February:16.

Childs P, Williams P. *An Introduction to Post-colonial Theory.* London: Prentice-Hall; 1997.

Clark C, Scott E, Krupa T. Involving clients in programme evaluation and research: a new methodology. *Can J Occup Ther* 1993, **60**:192–199.

Coles C. Self-assessment and medical audit: an educational approach. *BMJ* 1989, **299**:807–808.

Cook DW. A multivariate analysis of motivational attributes among spinal cord injured rehabilitation clients. *Int J Rehab Res* **4**:5–15.

Corring DJ. The missing perspective on client-centred care. *OT Now* Jan–Feb:8–10.

Cott CA, Finch E, Gasner D, Yoshida K, Thomas S, Verrier M. The movement continuum theory of physical therapy. *Physiother Can* 1995, **47**:87–95.

Crepeau EB. Achieving intersubjective understanding: examples from an occupational therapy treatment session. *Am J Occup Ther* 1991, **45**:1016–1025.

Crisp R. The long term adjustment of 60 persons with spinal cord injury. *Aust Psychol* 1992, **27**:43–47.

Dalley J. Evaluation of clinical practice: is a client-centred approach compatible with professional issues? *Physiotherapy* 1999, **85**:491–497.

Daverat P, Petit H, Kemoun G, Dartigues J, Barat M. The long term outcome in 149 patients with spinal cord injury. *Paraplegia* 1995, **33**:665–668.

Davis A, Davis S, Moss N et al. First steps towards an interdisciplinary approach to rehabilitation. *Clin Rehab* 1992, **6**:237–244.

Department of Health. *The New NHS: Modern, Dependable.* London: Stationery Office; 1997.

Department of Health. *National Service Framework for Mental Health, Modern Standards and Service Models.* London: Department of Health; 1999.

Dijkers M. Correlates of quality of life in a spinal cord injured sample. *SCI Psychosoc Proc* 1999, **12**:30–31.

Draper P. *Nursing Perspectives on Quality of Life.* London: Routledge; 1997.

Eisenberg M, Saltz C. Quality of life among aging spinal cord injured persons: long term rehabilitation outcomes. *Paraplegia* 1991, **29**:514–520.

Fearing V, Law M, Clark J. An occupational performance process model: fostering client and therapist alliances. *Can J Occup Ther* 1997, **64**:7–15.

Frank RG, Elliott T. Spinal cord injury and health locus of control beliefs. *Paraplegia* 1989, **27**:250–256.

Fuhrer MJ. The subjective well-being of people with spinal cord injury: relationships to impairment, disability and handicap. *Topics Spinal Cord Inj Rehab* 1996, **1**:56–71.

Fuhrer MJ, Rintala D, Hart K, Clearman R, Young M. Relationship of life satisfaction to impairment, disability and handicap among persons with spinal cord injury living in the community. *Arch Phys Med Rehab* 1992, **73**:552–557.

Gerhart KA, Koziol-McLain J, Lowenstein S, Whiteneck G. Quality of life following spinal cord injury: knowledge and attitudes of emergency care providers. *Ann Emerg Med* 1994, **23**:801–812.

Gomm R, Davies C. *Using Evidence in Health and Social Care.* London: Open University/Sage; 2000:x.

Good B. *Medicine, Rationality and Experience.* Cambridge: University of Cambridge Press; 1994.

Hammell KW. *An Investigation into the Availability and Adequacy of Social Relationships Following Head Injury and Spinal Cord Injury: A Study of Injured Men and their Partners.* Unpublished Master of Science thesis. Southampton: University of Southampton; 1991.

Hammell KW *Spinal Cord Injury Rehabilitation.* London: Chapman and Hall; 1995a.

Hammell KW. Application of learning theory in spinal cord injury rehabilitation: client-centred occupational therapy. *Scand J Occup Ther* 1995b, **2**:34–39.

Hammell KW. *From the Neck Up: Quality in Life Following High Spinal Cord Injury.* Unpublished doctoral thesis. Vancouver: University of British Columbia; 1998a.

Hammell KW. Client-centred occupational therapy: collaborative planning, accountable intervention. In: Law M, ed. *Client-centered Occupational Therapy.* Thorofare, NJ: Slack; 1998b:123–143.

Hammell KW. Using qualitative research to inform the client-centred evidence-based practice of occupational therapy. *Br J Occup Ther* 2001, **64**:228–234.

Hammell KW, Carpenter C. Introduction to qualitative research in occupational and physical therapy. In: Hammell KW, Carpenter C, Dyck I, eds. *Using Qualitative Research: A Practical Introduction for Occupational and Physical Therapists.* Edinburgh: Churchill Livingstone; 2000:1–12.

Hartkopp A, Brónnum-Hansen H, Seidenschnur A-M, Biering-Sorensen F. Suicide in a spinal cord injured population: its relation to functional status. *Arch Phys Med Rehab* 1998, **79**:1356–1361.

Holcomb LO. Community reintegration and chronic spinal cord injury. *SCI Nurs* 2000, **17**:52–58.

Hughes JL. Illness narrative and chronic fatigue syndrome/myalgic encephalomyelitis: a review. *Br J Occup Ther* 2002, **65**:9–14.

Jensen GM, Gwyer J, Shepard K, Hack L. Expert practice in physical therapy. *Phys Ther* 2000, **80**:28–43.

Johnson R. 'Attitudes don't just hang in the air …': disabled people's perceptions of physiotherapists. *Physiotherapy* 1993, **79**:619–627.

Johnston M, Gilbert P, Partridge C, Collins J. Changing perceived control in patients with physical disabilities: an intervention study with patients receiving rehabilitation. *Br J Clin Psychol* 1992, **31**:89–94.

Jonsen AR, Siegler M, Winslade W. *Clinical Ethics*, 4th edn. New York: McGraw Hill; 1998.

Jordan SA, Wellborn W, Kovnik J, Saltzstein R. Understanding and treating motivational difficulties in ventilator dependent SCI patients. *Paraplegia* 1991, **29**:431–442.

Jorgensen P. Concepts of body and health in physiotherapy: the meaning of the social/cultural aspects of life. *Physiother Theory Pract* 2000, **16**:105–115.

Kaufman S. Illness, biography and the interpretation of self following a stroke. *J Aging Stud* 1988, **2**:217–227.

Kemp BJ, Krause J. Depression and life satisfaction among people ageing with post-polio and spinal cord injury. *Disabil Rehab* 1999, **21**:241–249.

Krause JS. Life satisfaction after spinal cord injury: a descriptive study. *Rehab Psychol* 1992, **37**:61–70.

Krause JS. Adjustment after spinal cord injury: a 9 year longitudinal study. *Arch Phys Med Rehab* 1997, **78**: 651–657.

Krause JS, Kjorsvig J. Mortality after spinal cord injury: a four year prospective study. *Arch Phys Med Rehab* 1992, **73**:558–563.

Krause JS, Coker J, Charlifue S, Whiteneck G. Health outcomes among American Indians with spinal cord injury. *Arch Phys Med Rehab* 2000, **81**:924–931.

Law M. Does client-centred practice make a difference? In: Law M, ed. *Client-centered Occupational Therapy*. Thorofare, NJ: Slack; 1998:19–27.

Law M, Baptiste S, Mills J. Client-centred practice: what does it mean and does it make a difference? *Can J Occup Ther* 1995, **62**:250–257.

Law M, Baptiste S, Carswell A, McColl MA, Polatajko H, Pollock N. *The Canadian Occupational Performance Measure*, 3rd edn. Ottawa, ON: CAOT Publications; 1998.

Leavitt RL. *Cross-cultural Rehabilitation: An International Perspective*. London: WB Saunders; 1999:x.

Lindberg M. Quality of life after subarachnoid haemorrhage, and its relationship to impairments, disabilities and depression. *Scand J Occup Ther* 1995, **2**:105–112.

Mattingly C. What is clinical reasoning? *Am J Occup Ther* 1991, **45**:979–986.

McGrath JR, Davis A. Rehabilitation, where are we going and how do we get there? *Clin Rehab* 1992, **6**:225–235.

Morris J. *Pride against Prejudice. Transforming Attitudes to Disability*. London: The Women's Press; 1991.

Neistadt M. Methods of assessing clients' priorities: a survey of adult physical dysfunction. *Am J Occup Ther* 1995, **49**:428–436.

NHS Executive. *Rehabilitation: A Guide*. Leeds: Department of Health; 1997.

Oliver M. *The Politics of Disablement*. Basingstoke: Macmillan; 1990.

Oliver M, Zarb G, Silver J, Moore M, Salisbury V. *Walking into Darkness: The Experience of Spinal Cord Injury*. Basingstoke: Macmillan; 1988.

Peloquin SM. The patient–therapist relationship in occupational therapy: understanding visions and images. *Am J Occup Ther* 1990, **44**:13–21.

Pollock N. Client-centred assessment. *Am J Occup Ther* 1993, **47**:298–301.

Post M, de Witte L, vanAsbek F, van Dijk A, Schrijvers A. Predictors of health status and life satisfaction in spinal cord injury. *Arch Phys Med Rehab* 1998, **78**: 395–402.

Pound P, Bury M, Gompertz P, Ebrahim S. Stoke patients' views on their admission to hospital. *BMJ* 1995, **311**:18–22.

Richardson B. Professional development. 2. Professional knowledge and situated learning in the workplace. *Physiotherapy* 1999, **85**:467–474.

Ritchie JE. Using qualitative research to enhance the evidence-based practice of health care providers. *Aus J Physiother* 1999, **45**:251–256.

Rohe DE, Athelstan G. Vocational interests of persons with spinal cord injury. *J Counsel Psychol* 1982, **29**:283–291.

Rosenberg W, Donald A. Evidence-based medicine: an approach to clinical problem-solving. *BMJ* 1995, **310**:1122–1126.

Rotter JB. Generalised expectancies for internal versus external control of reinforcement. *Psychol Monograph* 1966, **80**:1–28.

Sackett DL, Rosenberg W, Gray J, Haynes R, Richardson W. Evidence-based medicine: what it is and what it isn't. *BMJ* 1996, **312**:71–72.

Sadlo G, Piper D, Agnew P. Problem-based learning in the development of an occupational therapy curriculum. Part I: The process of problem-based learning. *Br J Occup Ther* 1994, **57**:49–54.

Schön DA. *The Reflective Practitioner: How Professionals Think in Action*. San Francisco, CA: Jossey-Bass; 1983.

Seligman M. *Helplessness, on Depression, Development and Death*. San Francisco, CA: WH Freeman; 1975.

Steele DJ, Blackwell B, Guttman M, Jackson T. The activated patient: dogma, dream or desideratum? *Patient Educ Counsel* 1987, **10**:3–23.

Steinglass P, Temple S, Lisman S, Reiss D. Coping with spinal cord injury: the family perspective. *Gen Hosp Psychiatry* 1982, **4**:259–264.

Stratford P, Gill C, Westaway M, Binkley J. Assessing disability and change on individual patients: a report of a patient-specific measure. *Physiother Can* 1995, **47**:258–262.

Strong J, Gilbert J, Cassidy S, Bennet S. Expert clinicians' and students' views on clinical reasoning in occupational therapy. *Br J Occup Ther* 1995, **58**:119–123.

Toombs SK. The meaning of illness: a phenomenological approach to the patient–provider relationship. *J Med Phil* 1987, **12**:219–240.

Trieschmann R. The psychosocial adjustment to spinal cord injury. In: Bloch RF, Basbaum M, eds. *Management of Spinal Cord Injuries*. Baltimore, MD: Williams & Wilkins; 1986:302–319.

Tucker SJ. Patient–staff interaction with the spinal cord patient. In: Krueger DW, ed. *Rehabilitation Psychology*. Rockville, MD: Aspen; 1984:257–266.

van Bennekom C, Jelles F, Lankhorst G, Kuik D. Value of measuring perceived problems in a stoke population. *Clin Rehab* 1996, **10**:288–294.

Vogel LC, Klaas S, Lubicky J, Anderson C. Long-term outcomes and life satisfaction of adults who had pediatric spinal cord injuries. *Arch Phys Med Rehab* 1998, **79**:1496–1503.

Willems EP. The interface of hospital environment and patient behaviour. *Arch Phys Med Rehab* 1972, **53**:115–122.

Williams GH, Wood P. Coming to terms with chronic illness: the negotiation of autonomy in rheumatoid arthritis. *Int Disabil Studies* 1988, **10**:128–133.

Woolsey R. Rehabilitation outcome following spinal cord injury. *Arch Neurol* 1985, **42**:116–119.

Yerxa EJ, Locker S. Quality of time use by adults with spinal cord injuries. *Am J Occup Ther* 1990, **44**:318–326.

Chapter 23

Specific treatment techniques

J Jackson

INTRODUCTION

A huge variety of techniques are employed by physiotherapists working in neurological rehabilitation. When examining treatment approaches from different philosophical backgrounds, it is apparent that similar techniques may be utilised within them (see Ch. 21). A technique can be defined as a 'method or skill used for a particular task' (*Collins English Dictionary*). With this definition in mind it is important to consider to what purpose different techniques are employed and that, in order to be effective, the technique must be appropriate to help meet the treatment goals.

This chapter illustrates the diversity of the techniques used by physiotherapists. It is clear that there is a wealth of research supporting the use of some techniques and a lack of a clear evidence base to justify the use of others. Many techniques continue to rely on anecdotal evidence to support their use. In this chapter a variety of techniques are reviewed and the evidence available to support their use is considered. Some of the work cited is fairly old and that reflects the need for more research in the field of specific treatment techniques. When choosing to use a specific technique it is necessary for the physiotherapist to balance the risks and benefits of alternative sources of evidence available to support its use (Bury, 1998).

The chapter is divided into sections: some techniques have mixed effects such that they could be included in more than one section; they will be found in the section which reflects their main usage. This is not intended as a recipe-type guide to treatments but rather as a brief overview of the different treatments available, their proposed effects and their indications for use. Details of how to apply the techniques can be found in the relevant literature, some of which is cited here. Examples of where the techniques may be applied, and illustrations of their use, can be seen in the chapters on specific neurological conditions in this text.

FACILITATION

Many of the techniques used in neurological rehabilitation are applied to facilitate and enhance muscle activity and thus help achieve improved control of movement. It is thought that the use of many of these techniques may be beneficial in assisting muscle activation during the practice of functional activities (Bennett & Karnes, 1998). Many of the specific techniques used for facilitation have their origins in the work of Margaret Rood. For a comprehensive examination of the Rood approach and a modern interpretation of its relevance the reader is directed to Baily Metcalfe & Lawes (1998) and Royeen

et al. (2001). Some of those most commonly used techniques are outlined below.

Brushing

In the 1950s Rood proposed that fast brushing, using a battery-operated brush, of the skin overlying a muscle could be used to facilitate a muscle contraction. Brushing has been used widely by physiotherapists, applied either using an electrically operated brush or manually using a bottle brush, but there is little indication given about the required rate or duration of the brushing, or pressure to be applied. It would make sense that the skin being brushed and the muscle being facilitated should be supplied by the same spinal segment.

There is little evidence to support the effectiveness of brushing (O'Sullivan, 1988), although Garland & Hayes (1987) observed an effect in hemiplegic subjects with foot drop. In subjects who received a combination of brushing preceded by voluntary contraction of the tibialis anterior, a significant change in electromyographic (EMG) activity was seen both immediately and 30 min after stimulation. Brushing may be a powerful method of facilitation but it is clearly not well researched in terms of its continued effects, particularly as much of the work has been carried out on subjects with no neurological impairments. It is worth noting that caution in its use has been advised (Farber, 1982) and that Royeen et al. (2001) consider it beyond the scope of entry-level practice.

Ice – brief

Ice can be used to facilitate a response from muscle. Ice uses a combination of coolness and pain sensations to produce the desired response.

In order to facilitate a motor response, an ice cube is quickly swept over the chosen muscle belly (Umphred, 1995). Following each swipe the iced area is blotted with a towel. After three swipes the patient is asked to produce an active muscle contraction. If ice is being used to facilitate lip closure and encourage feeding and sucking, an ice lolly can be placed in the mouth with pressure on the tongue (Farber, 1982).

When using ice as a stimulating technique it is important to remember that it can be a potent stimulus and results can be unpredictable. Putting ice on the face above the level of the lips and to the midline of the trunk should be avoided, as it has been reported that undesirable behavioural and autonomic responses may be provoked (Umphred, 1995).

Tapping

Tapping is the use of a light force applied manually over a tendon or muscle belly to facilitate a voluntary contraction. Tapping over a tendon would usually be used to assess reflex activity. A normal response would be a brisk muscle contraction. It is not therefore recommended that tendon tapping be used in a treatment situation, as the response is a crude muscle contraction and will be of little use to help a patient produce a graded, functional movement (Umphred, 1995).

Rood recommended 3–5 taps over the belly of the muscle being facilitated. In addition, tapping can be applied to a muscle that has been stretched by the effect of gravity. Once the muscle responds to the stretch produced by gravity the therapist taps the muscle, using the hand, facilitating further activity (O'Sullivan, 1988). For example, with a patient who is standing, weight-bearing through both legs, if one knee gives way gravity will stretch the quadriceps muscle group. The therapist can then tap the muscle, facilitating a return to full knee extension.

Sweep tapping is a light touch sweeping movement applied by the back of the therapist's fingers over the dermatomal area innervating the muscles the patient is required to contract (Umphred, 1995). Davies (2000) described the use of sweep tapping to provide an excitatory stimulus to activate the finger extensors in hemiplegia. This is applied by providing support to the affected upper limb with one hand, while the other hand sweeps firmly and briskly over the extensors of the wrist and fingers; the sweep commences just below the elbow and continues over the dorsum of the hand and fingers. In common with other tapping techniques, an active response is requested from the patient following its application.

The use of tapping, like many of the other sensory facilitatory techniques, is mainly supported by anecdotal evidence.

Passive stretching – fast

Stretching may be applied in different ways to patients with neurological dysfunction to achieve different effects. A quick stretch is applied to facilitate a muscle contraction, and a slow or sustained stretch is given to reduce spasticity or prevent or reduce contractures. It is not within the scope of this chapter to consider the anatomy and physiology of the structures involved, including muscle, tendons, joints and the stretch reflex, as there are comprehensive texts devoted entirely to such topics.

A quick stretch is facilitatory and achieves its effect via stimulation of the muscle spindle primary endings. Quick stretching of the agonist muscle will therefore result in reflex facilitation of that muscle via the mono-synaptic reflex arc. This stretch is normally applied manually by the physiotherapist. Fast stretching is one of the

core procedures employed during proprioceptive neuromuscular facilitation (PNF) techniques (see below).

Joint compression

Receptors in joints and muscles are involved with the awareness of joint position and movement. Compression of a joint stimulates these receptors and can produce both inhibitory and facilitatory effects. Joint compression (approximation) is achieved either by normal body weight (or less) being applied through the longitudinal axis of the bone (light compression) or as heavy joint compression, where the approximation is greater than that produced by body weight (Royeen et al., 2001). Heavy joint compression is thought to facilitate cocontraction at the joint undergoing compression, whereas light joint compression is reported to produce an inhibitory (relaxing) effect on spastic muscles around joints (Royeen et al., 2001).

Bone pounding or jamming is used to inhibit plantarflexion and facilitate cocontraction around the ankle. It can be applied with the patient sitting, by pounding the heel on the floor whilst supporting the knee. Alternatively, with the patient lying prone over a pillow with some degree of flexion at the hips and knees, force can be applied to the heel by the therapist using the ulnar side of a clenched fist (Umphred, 1995).

Other techniques that use joint compression include weight-bearing through a hemiplegic arm to facilitate cocontraction and activation of the muscles around the shoulder joint (Davies, 2000). Weight belts and weighted wrist or ankle cuffs have also been used to increase joint compression. Joint compression can be applied to many joints using a variety of positions or patterns of movement. For example, using four-point kneeling as a starting position, joint compression can be applied to the shoulders and/or hips. Ideally, joint compression should be applied in a functional position but if this is not possible treatment should quickly progress to using the joint in a functional manner. Joint compression is also a procedure used in PNF and is considered in this context below.

Several authors described joint compression, either in terms of normal weight approximation or by other means, but only anecdotal evidence is given to support its use (Farber, 1982; Umphred, 1995; Davies, 2000; Royeen et al., 2001).

Vibration

Therapeutic vibration is a directly applied stimulus of high frequency (100–300 Hz) and low amplitude, which stretches the muscle spindle and activates type 1a afferent fibres. Vibration is generally applied directly to the chosen muscle or its tendon. Bishop (1974) identified three motor effects achievable by vibrating a muscle: (1) a sustained contraction of the vibrated muscle (via the tonic vibration reflex); (2) the depression of the motoneurones innervating the antagonistic muscles (reciprocal inhibition or antagonist inhibition); and (3) suppression of the monosynaptic stretch reflexes of the vibrated muscle (during the period of vibration). There appears to be disagreement, however, as to whether vibration has a sustained effect on muscle contractility (Umphred, 1995) and thus any long-term benefit.

It would appear that vibration has potential clinical applications via agonist facilitation or antagonist inhibition. Bishop (1974) identified four factors that influenced the strength of the tonic vibration reflex (TVR):

1. the location of the vibrator
2. the initial length of the muscle
3. the level of excitability of the central nervous system (CNS)
4. the parameters of the vibratory stimulus.

Application of the vibrator on to the belly of a stretched muscle or over the tendon allows easy facilitation of the TVR. It appears that the tonic neck reflexes and body-righting reflexes (Rothwell, 1994; Shepherd, 1994) interact with the TVR; so, treatment in the supine position results in an improved extensor TVR, and that in the prone position results in increased flexor TVR. Finally, increasing the amplitude of the vibration increases the stretch on the muscle but, more significantly, the TVR is greater as the frequency of the vibratory stimulus increases.

Despite the apparent theoretical basis for its use, there are few reports of vibration being used in clinical practice to facilitate muscle contraction.

Another quite different investigation involving vibration was made by Lovgreen et al. (1993) who studied the effects of muscle vibration on the voluntary movements of patients with cerebellar dysmetria. Part of the study was to consider whether vibration could improve movement accuracy and reduce hypermetria. They found that antagonist vibration reduced the amplitude of patients' movements and suggested that vibration had potential for use in both hyper- and hypometria, although the feasibility of its application would require careful thought.

Vibration has the potential to be a potent treatment technique but there are various precautions that must be considered when using it. Key points to remember include: vibration will generate heat at its point of application; and there is potential to cause damage to the skin, particularly at high amplitudes (Farber, 1982). Athetoid-like movements have been reported in patients with cerebellar disease when vibration was applied over muscle and a clear explanation to the patient is always essential.

Umphred (1995) recommend that vibrators registering 100–125 Hz be used and noted that most battery-operated hand-held vibrators register only 50–90 Hz. There is a wide range of commercially available vibrators, so the available frequency range should always be checked prior to purchase.

Vestibular stimulation

Any static position or movement will have an effect on the vestibular system, so many interventions will result in vestibular stimulation in some way or other. However, specific vestibular stimulation has not been widely used in neurological physiotherapy and was, until recently, mainly described in relation to a multisensory approach to neurological rehabilitation in paediatrics. Advocates of its use are anxious to remind others that vestibular stimulation is a powerful form of stimulation that should be used with care. Umphred (1995) stated that it is important to remember that 'the rate of vestibular stimulation determines the effects. A constant, slow rocking tends to dampen the motor system, whereas a fast spin or linear movement tends to heighten both alertness and the motor response.'

The management of vestibular dysfunction has evolved from increasing research to become recognised as a specialist area within physiotherapy. Chapter 24 explains that patients with a primary problem of vestibular dysfunction require vestibular rehabilitation, which involves specific assessment and treatment techniques.

Facilitation of movement

Facilitated movements do not require the patient to activate the nervous system to produce the required movement. This lack of self-initiation of movement has been criticised for not providing a basis for the learning of movement. However, it could be argued that once movement can be initiated in patients the possibility of the production of an active response then exists with the potential for learning of functional movements (Baily Metcalfe & Lawes, 1998).

NORMALISATION OF TONE AND THE MAINTENANCE OF SOFT-TISSUE LENGTH

The Bobath approach is widely used as a treatment approach in neurological physiotherapy (Sackley & Lincoln, 1996) and the control of tone forms a major part of the Bobath concept of stroke rehabilitation (Lennon & Ashburn, 2000; also see Ch. 21). An awareness of the potential for changes in the musculoskeletal system and the subsequent loss of range of movement associated with neurological dysfunction (Chs 25 and 30) is essential for effective management of patients with neurological disorders.

Passive stretching – slow

Slow stretch is applied to a muscle or joint such that a stretch reflex is not elicited and the effect is therefore inhibitory in terms of the neural response. The effect of prolonged, slow stretching on muscle is not entirely clear, although it certainly varies depending upon the time for which the stretch is maintained. It appears to have an influence on both the neural components of muscle, via the Golgi tendon organs and muscle spindles, and the structural components in the long term, via the number and length of sarcomeres (Hale et al., 1995).

Changes in muscle length

The presence of increased tone, possibly combined with paresis and/or weakness, can ultimately lead to joint contracture and changes in muscle length (see Ch. 30). Slow, prolonged stretching is therefore applied to maintain or prevent loss of range of movement (ROM). It has been demonstrated in animal studies that if a muscle is immobilised in a shortened position, sarcomeres will be lost and, conversely, a muscle immobilised in a lengthened position will add on sarcomeres (Goldspink & Williams, 1990). A shortened immobilised muscle will also show an increase in stiffness related to an increase in connective tissue within the muscle (Williams et al., 1988). However, it has been demonstrated in mice that a stretch of 30 min daily will prevent the loss of sarcomeres and changes in the connective tissue of an immobilised muscle (Williams, 1990). The timescale relating to changes in the mouse may not be relevant to humans.

Manual stretching

A prolonged muscle stretch can be applied manually, using the effect of gravity and body weight, or mechanically (by machine or splint). When applied, the stretch should provide sufficient force to overcome the hypertonicity and passively lengthen the muscle. When contractures are already present, it is doubtful whether the use of manual stretching alone will be sufficient to provide a sustained improvement in the ROM, if any was achieved.

Splinting

The clinical practice guidelines on splinting adults with neurological dysfunction (Association of Chartered Physiotherapists Interested in Neurology (ACPIN), 1998) identify a paucity of research in the area, making it almost impossible to adopt an evidence-based approach to the use of splints. Low-force stretching of long duration can be provided by splinting.

Recently, dynamic Lycra splints have been used as part of the management of patients with hemiplegia (Gracies et al., 2000). Lycra splints are custom-made, individually designed garments – it is claimed that Lycra splinting is effective in managing posture, and motor and sensory changes following a stroke. The study by Gracies et al. (2000) investigated acceptability and effects on swelling, resting posture, spasticity, active ROM and passive ROM of an upper-limb Lycra garment when worn for 3 h by patients with a hemiplegia. The findings from this small-scale study, using a convenience sample, indicate some support for the use of these garments in reducing spasticity and swelling. Another study, investigating the effect of a body splint made from Lycra (Blair et al., 1995), used with children with cerebral palsy, found improved postural stability and reduced involuntary movements in patients presenting with pelvic, shoulder and trunk instability.

Different types of splinting and the rationale for use are discussed in Chapter 25, with further details being provided by Edwards & Charlton (2002). Examples of splints used for peripheral nerve injuries are illustrated in photographs in Chapter 9.

Weight-bearing

Several studies report the use of weight-bearing to reduce contractures in joints of the lower limb (Richardson, 1991; Bohannon, 1993). These reports illustrate the effectiveness of using a tilt table to achieve a sustainable position in which a prolonged stretch is applied. The angle of table tilt needs to be considered when standing patients with knee joint contractures, as the supporting straps bear more of the body weight than when the knees are extended (Morgan et al., 2003). Force exerted at the supporting straps is greater the higher the degree of flexion, and is more pronounced with greater body weight but can be modified by reducing table incline, thus reducing the pressure on underlying tissues. Illustrated examples of equipment to assist standing can be seen in Chapters 8, 18 and 25.

Serial casting

Serial plaster casting is another technique used to prevent or reduce contractures, which may be most effective when the contractures result from spasticity. Serial casting methods were described and illustrated by Edwards & Charlton (2002) and a comprehensive overview of the practicalities of casting the lower limb in neurology was provided by Young & Nicklin (2000).

The use of a soft splint has been shown to be effective in the acute management of elbow hypertonicity (Wallen & Mackay, 1995). This splint has certain advantages over casting in that it is more dynamic in nature, less likely to cause unwanted pressure and provides neutral warmth (Wallen & O'Flaherty, 1991). However, it is also easily removed and thus a level of compliance is necessary!

Moseley (1997) also demonstrated the effectiveness of serial casting and stretching on regaining ROM in the ankle due to established shortening of the calf muscles. Jones (1999) undertook a series of single-system studies to examine the efficacy of lower-extremity serial casts on gait in four adults with hemiparetic gait patterns. There was an improvement in walking speed and a reduction in the level of assistance required during walking following the intervention.

When spasticity is present, physiotherapists are often reluctant to use splints or other externally applied devices for stretching as, despite the lack of supporting evidence, it is thought that splinting can lead to an increase in muscle tone. However, it has been demonstrated that inhibitory splinting can reduce contractures without causing detrimental effects to muscle tone (Mills, 1986). Indeed, the ACPIN guidelines recommend that patients suitable for splinting are those who may have, or be at risk of, contractures as a result of significant increases in muscle tone or immobility (1998).

Duration of stretch to reduce spasticity

Although it has been shown that prolonged stretching can reduce spasticity, the time needed is not clear. Hale et al. (1995) found that the most beneficial duration of stretch applied to reduce spasticity was 10 min. This study used a variety of methods to assess the level of spasticity, including both subjective and objective measures. The results illustrated the difficulties that arise when measuring spasticity (see Ch. 25), and that perhaps the concurrent problems of length-associated changes in muscle required greater consideration.

Duration of stretch to prevent contracture

Tardieu et al. (1988) investigated how long it was necessary to stretch the soleus muscle each day to prevent contracture in children with cerebral palsy and concluded that it must be stretched for 6 h a day.

Some work has been done to evaluate the effect of stretching, mainly on normal subjects. However, it is clear that further work is still required to establish the appropriate stretching techniques and the duration required to produce the desired effect in different situations.

Positioning

Positioning is used widely by physiotherapists to prevent the development of contractures and to discourage unwanted reflex activity (Carr & Kenney, 1992; Pope, 2002). A survey of current practice of positioning for stroke patients identified that one of the most common aims of physiotherapists advocating its use was to modulate muscle tone and prevent damage to affected limbs (Chatterton et al., 2001).

Specific positions are often adopted to achieve a slow maintained stretch on a particular muscle and the thinking behind this has already been explored. Bromley (1998) gave detailed guidelines for the positioning of patients following spinal cord injury and described its importance for: correct alignment of fractures; prevention of contractures; prevention of pressure sores; and inhibiting the onset of severe spasticity.

Indeed, many of the positions advocated by physiotherapists relate to the desire to avoid the development of spastic patterns of movement (Bobath, 1990). Positions are chosen to minimise the influence of the primitive reflexes. The three reflexes, which are normally under cortical control and whose release can be influenced by careful choice and use of positions, are: (1) the symmetrical tonic neck reflex; (2) the asymmetrical tonic neck reflex; and (3) the labyrinthine reflex (Carr & Kenney, 1992). These reflexes are outlined in Chapter 17.

Davies (2000) gave fairly detailed descriptions of desirable positions that should be used following stroke, urging the avoidance of supine lying as in this position the influences of the tonic neck and labyrinthine reflexes are great and this could result in an overall increase in extensor activity throughout the body.

Careful positioning to limit musculoskeletal changes is essential but it appears that there is a lack of consensus about the precise positions necessary to limit the onset of spasticity and unwanted patterns of movement, particularly after stroke (Carr & Kenney, 1992; Chatterton et al., 2001). Certainly, Bobath (1990) identified a need to be more dynamic and advocated the use of reflex-inhibiting patterns of movement, rather than static postures, to inhibit abnormal postural reactions and facilitate automatic and voluntary movements.

Positioning is sometimes adopted as a strategy to minimise shoulder pain and loss of ROM in patients following stroke. However, a recent study by Dean et al. (2000) failed to demonstrate that the inclusion of prolonged positioning of the shoulder, daily for 6 weeks, significantly altered the outcomes of patients undergoing a multidisciplinary rehabilitation programme.

These concepts are discussed in Chapter 21. Positioning is also discussed in Chapters 8, 18 and 25, where illustrations show various types of equipment used for posture and seating.

Pressure

Pressure is used by physiotherapists both to facilitate and inhibit a response in muscle, more especially in muscle tone. This pressure can be applied in a variety of ways, including the use of air-filled splints (Johnstone, 1995), tone-inhibiting casts (Zachazewski et al., 1982) or manually (Umphred, 1995). Pressure can be applied directly over a tendon (Leone & Kukulka, 1988) or over the muscle itself (Robichaud et al., 1992). The pressure can be sustained or intermittent, and variable in terms of the degree applied.

Most of the research investigating the effects of a variety of pressure conditions has measured motor neurone excitability, via change in the Hoffman reflex (H reflex). Studies have suggested that the characteristic appearance of the H reflex reflects spinal motor function and therefore it can be used to evaluate the effects of therapeutic interventions that aim to reduce motor neurone excitability (Suzuki et al., 1995). It is important to remember, however, the problems of quantifying that part of muscle tone that occurs as a direct result of reflex activity.

Leone & Kukulka (1988) investigated the effects of achilles tendon pressure on the H reflex in stroke patients. The assumption was made that any change in motoneurone excitability would be reflected in an associated alteration in tone as, again, no direct measurement of tone was made. Pressure was applied both continuously and intermittently, and under both conditions depression of the H reflex occurred. Intermittent pressure, however, was significantly more effective than continuous. Further investigation revealed that increasing the amount of pressure had no greater effect, and the effect of the pressure was sustained only during its actual application. No carryover effect was observed but it is suggested that tendon pressure could be used therapeutically, e.g. when a short-term reduction in tone would allow achievement of an improved patient position in bed.

The strongest proponent of the use of pressure during treatment was Johnstone (1995), who advocated the use of constant pressure provided by orally inflated splints and intermittent pressure produced by a machine. The uses of the splint are to: reduce the therapist's need for extra hands; provide stability to the limb; divert associated reactions; allow early weight-bearing through the affected limb; and increase sensory input (Johnstone, 1995). It was claimed that when the antigravity muscles of the upper limb are held in a position of sustained stretch using the air splints, tonic and phasic wrist flexor EMG activity is reduced (Johnstone, 1995).

Robichaud et al. (1992) supported the use of air-splint pressure to reduce motor neurone excitability of the soleus muscle when circumferential pressure was applied around the lower leg. As in the tendon pressure study, the reduction was not sustained once the pressure had been released. Conversely, an increase in motor neurone excitability following the application of muscle pressure has been reported (Kukulka et al., 1987). This may reflect the different methods employed to apply pressure, which can include tapping and massage (Umphred, 1995).

It is clear that the application of pressure has many potential effects, some of which are still not understood. Externally applied pressure over muscle or tendon must also cause a disturbance in the cutaneous mechanoreceptors. Because of the wealth of afferent activity caused by pressure, its application poses many questions yet to be answered.

Neutral warmth

When considering exteroceptive input techniques, Umphred (1995) identified an additional use for air splints – that of the provision of neutral warmth. Johnstone (1995) also advocated their use to provide sensory stimulation of soft tissues, causing inhibition of the area under which the neutral warmth is applied. Alternative techniques used for achieving neutral warmth are tepid baths, whole-body wrapping and wrapping of isolated body parts. The required range of temperatures that should be utilised for this technique is 35–37°C (Farber, 1982).

There appears to be little research to support the use of this concept of neutral warmth. Baily Metcalf & Lawes (1998) suggested that the inhibition seen is due to inhibition of tonic muscles via the stimulation of low-threshold mechanoreceptors through light touch. One study looked specifically at the effect of a wrapping technique on a passive ROM in a spastic upper extremity (Twist, 1985). Wrapping (elastic wrap bandages and gloves) was applied to spastic upper limbs for 3 h, three times a week on alternate days over a period of 2–4 weeks. Results showed statistically significant increases in passive ROM, with subjective reports of reduced pain. Although this study contained several shortcomings (small subject numbers and lack of control), it did indicate an effect.

Ice – prolonged

Prolonged use of ice reduces afferent and efferent neurotransmission. To be effective in reducing spasticity, the muscle spindles must themselves be cooled. The ice must be applied until there is no longer an excessive reflex response to stretching (Lehmann & De Lateur, 1990). It is considered that a reduction of spasticity lasting 1–2 h can be achieved, such that stretching or active exercises can be applied to greater effect.

The most common form of application of ice to reduce spasticity is local immersion; this is particularly effective for reducing flexor spasticity in the hand. A mixture of tap water and flaked ice is used, in the ratio of one-third water to two-thirds ice. Davies (2000) advocated that the hand is immersed three times for 3 s, with only a few seconds between immersions. The therapist should hold the patient's hand in the ice–water mixture. This procedure can result in a dramatic reduction in spasticity.

General immersion, where the patient sits in a bath of cold water, has been used to reduce spasticity. Patients can tolerate water temperatures of 20–22°C for 10–15 min (Lee et al., 1978). Neither local nor general cooling has been found to have any long-term effect on spasticity, so any short-term reduction achieved must be fully exploited.

When using ice it is important to remember that the patient must be receptive to its use. If ice causes the patient distress and anxiety, the inhibitory effect may be blocked (Farber, 1982). A sensory assessment of the patient should be carried out before using ice and the presence of sensory deficits is a contraindication to its use (Umphred, 1995).

Vibration

Vibration can also be used to produce inhibitory effects. In an effort to support the efficacy of its use to treat patients with disorders of muscle tone, Ageranioti & Hayes (1990) investigated the effects of vibration on hypertonia and hyperreflexia in the wrist joints of patients with spastic hemiplegia. They found that immediately after vibration, hypertonia and hyperreflexia were significantly reduced and concluded that in patients with spastic hemiplegia vibration gave short-term symptomatic relief. However, they also acknowledged that, despite using a relatively homogeneous group of subjects, there were many different patterns of hyperreflexia and this could possibly explain previous anecdotal reports where vibration was of no benefit in apparently similar cases.

Vibration has also been used at low frequencies (60–90 Hz) to normalise or reduce sensitivity in the skin (Farber, 1982; Umphred, 1995). Hochreiter et al. (1983) found that in the 'normal' hand, vibration increased the tactile threshold, with the effect lasting for at least 10 min. There appears to be a lack of clinically applied studies in this area.

Certain precautions need to be considered when applying vibration (Farber, 1982), and these are outlined above in the section on facilitation.

Massage

Massage was a core element of physiotherapy in the UK and has been described as one of the 'roots of our profession' (Murphy, 1993). How widely massage is used or should be used is the subject of much debate that will not be explored here. For an extensive overview of massage, its application and effects, the reader is directed to Holey & Cook (1997) or Cassar (1999).

Massage has two main effects – mechanical and physiological. The inhibitory effects of massage are of particular interest to the physiotherapist working in neurology when the aim is to achieve a reduction in muscle tone or muscle spasm. Slow stroking applied to patients with multiple sclerosis has been found to achieve a significant reduction in the amplitude of the H reflex (a measure of motoneurone excitability). The stroking was of light pressure and applied over the posterior primary rami (Brouwer & Sousa de Andrade, 1995).

Studies on neurologically healthy subjects have found similar results. Goldberg et al. (1992) found that deep massage produced a greater inhibitory response than light massage when applied to the leg. Sullivan et al. (1991) indicated, by their results, a specificity of the effect of massage on the muscle group being massaged. This was contrary to their expectations that the inhibitory effects of massage would extend beyond the muscle being massaged.

It is not clear whether the results of these studies could be transferred to subjects with neurological dysfunction; further studies are essential and must include measures beyond that of H-reflex amplitude as an indication of the efficacy of massage.

EXERCISE AND MOVEMENT

This section includes well-established treatments and those that are emerging in neurological rehabilitation. A major area that is not included is gait re-education, which is a vast field and the reader is referred to the chapters in this book on the different neurological conditions, as well as to Kisner & Colby (2002), Whittle (2001) and Kerrigan & Sheffler (1995).

Hydrotherapy

Immersion in water can enhance the treatment of the neurologically impaired patient and has therapeutic, psychological and social benefits. Hydrotherapy can give an individual with limited independence on dry land an ability to move freely and with confidence. It also allows a recreational activity that can be easily enjoyed by many.

It must be remembered, when hydrotherapy is incorporated into a rehabilitation programme, that the effects of gravity are altered when in water. Many of the problems associated with neurological dysfunction arise from an individual's inability to respond normally to the effect of gravity and, therefore, hydrotherapy is unlikely to be the sole method of treatment. However, water is an environment that permits a freedom of movement seldom achieved elsewhere. Water is also quite unique in being able to take over some of the physiotherapist's work (Gray, 1997), particularly in terms of supporting the patient.

Muscle stretching, reducing contractures, re-education of motor patterns, re-education of balance and equilibrium reactions, gait retraining and breathing exercises are all areas covered by Gray (1997) and Bennie (1997), along with details of examples of suitable procedures used in hydrotherapy for neurological rehabilitation. Bad Ragaz techniques, where the buoyancy of the water is used to provide support rather than resistance to the patient, is covered by Davis & Harrison (1988).

As with any technique, careful assessment of the patient before and after treatment will allow the physiotherapist to monitor the effect of hydrotherapy. There are anecdotal reports of increased tone following exercise in hot water but there is little evidence to substantiate this claim. The anxiety experienced by a patient being treated in water should be minimised by the reassurance provided by careful teaching skills (Reid Campion, 1997).

Swimming can form an integral part of hydrotherapy. The Halliwick method of swimming for the disabled (Martin, 1981; Reid Campion, 1997) is suitable for nearly any degree of disability at any age.

For further details of the principles, applications and techniques of hydrotherapy, the reader is directed to Skinner & Thomson (1983), Davis & Harrison (1988) and Reid Campion (1997).

Gymnastic balls

Gymnastic balls were originally used in orthopaedics but are now used widely by physiotherapists working in neurology. These balls are light-weight, being inflated with air to a high pressure. The ball is used to provide some support to the patient; this could range from a patient lying supine with feet resting on the ball to a patient sitting on the ball with the feet on the ground. When using the gymnastic ball, the principle

of action–reaction is followed. The patient is asked to achieve a specific action of the ball that will result in the desired reaction of body movement. With the patient sitting on the ball, feet on the floor, the action required is to roll the ball gently forwards and backwards. The reaction is flexion and extension of the lumbar spine, with associated pelvic tilt.

When using a ball it is important to remember several key points such that its potential is fully exploited.

- A ball provides an unstable surface; if it is fixed and unable to roll, its effects are significantly altered.
- The stability of a ball is influenced by the horizontal location of the centre of gravity relative to the base of support.
- The ball can be used with the patient lying, sitting or standing.
- Its uses are so extensive that it can be used with patients who have a limited ability to move independently or those who are completely independent. For example, when sitting a patient on a ball, the ball supports the weight of much of the body.
- Achieving and maintaining a correct sitting position will require continual co-ordinated activity in the muscles of the trunk and limbs to prevent the ball from rolling. This would be more demanding than having the patient sit on a stable surface, yet easier than standing.
- The patient who is functioning at a higher level can use the ball in a more dynamic manner in which controlled movement of the ball is required.

A comprehensive description of the use of the gymnastic ball can be found in Carriere (1998, 1999) and Davies (1990), and an example of use is illustrated in Chapter 8 (Fig. 8.9).

Gymnastic balls are available in a variety of different sizes and are now produced by various manufacturers. They should be made of a resilient plastic and inflated to sufficient pressure to withstand adult body weight such that little deformation of the ball occurs. The gymnastic ball is a highly portable, versatile piece of equipment and is available in many neurological physiotherapy departments, yet there is no evidence of its effectiveness and research is required to support its continued use.

Proprioceptive neuromuscular facilitation (PNF)

PNF was developed as a therapeutic approach over 40 years ago. It is a very labour-intensive method of treatment, in which the physiotherapist facilitates the achievement of specific movement patterns by the patient with particular use of the therapist's hands. The philosophy and conceptual framework of this approach have been discussed in Chapter 21. Some of the basic procedures and techniques which are utilised will be considered here in relation to their use in neurological rehabilitation. For a complete overview of PNF the reader is referred to Voss et al. (1985) and Adler et al. (1993); combined, these texts give an extensive theoretical and practical review of the thoughts of some of the proponents of PNF.

Ten basic procedures for facilitation have been identified by Adler et al. (1993):

1. resistance
2. irradiation and reinforcement
3. manual contact
4. body position and body mechanics
5. verbal commands
6. vision
7. traction and approximation
8. stretch
9. timing.
10. patterns of movement.

The application of manual resistance has been one of the core features of PNF. There has been a shift away from the use of maximal resistance to the use of resistance appropriate to the needs of the patient. How the resistance is applied will reflect the type of muscle contraction being resisted. Concentric and eccentric muscle work should be resisted so the movement is smooth and co-ordinated. Resistance to an isometric contraction should be varied, with a gradual increase and decrease such that no movement occurs. By the correct application of resistance, irradiation or reinforcement will result. An example of this could be the use of resisted hip flexion, adduction and external rotation to facilitate weak dorsiflexion.

These two procedures of resistance and the resulting irradiation and reinforcement are possibly two of the reasons why PNF is no longer used extensively for neurological rehabilitation in the UK. The use of resistance does not fit comfortably with the other neurophysiological approaches, such as the Bobath approach. This, combined with the diagonal and spiral patterns of movement in the three anatomical planes, makes its relevance to normal movement difficult to comprehend. It is interesting to note, however, that Adler et al. (1993) felt that the patterns are not essential for the application of PNF and it is possible to use only the philosophy and appropriate procedures.

The other basic procedures appear to involve the use of techniques widely employed by physiotherapists using other approaches. The use of accurate handling is stressed in PNF; the lumbrical grip is advocated to give the appropriate stimulus to the patient. The therapist's manual contact should give information to the patient,

facilitating movement in a specific direction. The position of the therapist relative to the patient allows the therapist to stay in line with the desired motion or force and to use body weight to give resistance. The use of visual feedback is promoted, with the patient following the movement to facilitate a stronger contraction. Traction and approximation may be applied to the trunk or extremities, eliciting a response via stimulation of the joint receptors.

The remaining three procedures – timing, stretch and the use of verbal commands – are extensively used in physiotherapy. Combining these in a variety of ways gives rise to the specific techniques of PNF.

Adler et al. (1993) grouped the techniques so that those with similar functions or actions were together. They gave detailed descriptions and examples of the techniques and indications for their use.

Although the core PNF texts previously cited gave examples of its use with neurological dysfunction, PNF is certainly not in common use in neurology gymnasia in the UK. One study investigated its effect on the gait of patients with hemiplegia of long and short duration and found its cumulative effects were more beneficial than the immediate effects (Wang, 1994). However, as no control groups were used, the possible inferences from this study are limited. An earlier study by Dickstein et al. (1986) compared three exercise therapy approaches including PNF and found that no substantial advantages could be attributed to any of the three therapeutic approaches used.

It has been identified that some of the underlying assumptions of the procedures and techniques used in PNF are now out of date (Morris & Sharpe, 1993) but there still appears to be a vast potential for research involving its use. An attempt has been made to explore the rationale behind the PNF relaxation techniques by studying postcontraction depression of the H reflex (Moore & Kukulka, 1991). The techniques did produce a strong but brief neuromuscular inhibition, but the results of this study, performed on subjects with no neurological dysfunction, cannot be directly applied to patients.

Cardiovascular exercise and strength training

The use of exercise to increase muscle strength in neurological rehabilitation is controversial and many physiotherapists have believed that muscle strength is not appropriate for treatment or measurement. However, there is increasing evidence that use of exercise and strength training, including the use of treadmills and static bikes, is beneficial in the management of patients with neurological dysfunction. Chapter 29 reviews the emerging literature, which reveals the benefits of exercise without the adverse effects traditionally feared by physiotherapists, such as increasing muscle tone in patients with spasticity.

Pilates–based rehabilitation

Pilates exercise has evolved from its use with elite dancers into different areas of rehabilitation (Anderson & Spector, 2000). Pilates-based rehabilitation was introduced from the USA in the 1990s and interest amongst physiotherapists is growing.

As acknowledged in the above review, research is needed to provide evidence of its effectiveness. Pilates classes in sports gyms are also very popular but people with neurological conditions would be advised to seek specialist supervision from a physiotherapist trained in Pilates, at least initially.

ELECTRICAL STIMULATION TECHNIQUES

The uses of electrical stimulation (ES) include pain relief, muscle strengthening and improving endurance, and producing functional movement. Different terms are used for the different applications (see below).

Transcutaneous electrical nerve stimulation (TENS)

TENS is a term used to describe nerve-stimulating pulses of low intensity, often used to control pain but also to reduce spasticity.

Pain relief

The management of pain in neurological rehabilitation would possibly not be identified as a key area for the physiotherapist working in neurology. However, the physiotherpist may have a significant role in the management of a patient's pain. Chapter 26 reviews the specific management of pain in neurological rehabilitation.

TENS has been used specifically in the management of hemiplegic shoulder pain. High-intensity TENS has been shown to be a valuable technique in the treatment of such shoulder pain, whereas the more traditional low-intensity TENS was not (Leandri et al., 1990). In this study a reduction in pain was achieved and increased passive ROM obtained; both of these effects were sustained to some extent for the month following cessation of treatment.

Details about TENS and its application in pain relief can be found in Kitchen (2002), which also provides a comprehensive overview of electrotherapy and its principles and practice.

Management of spasticity using TENS

An alternative use of TENS has been in the treatment of spasticity. Studies investigating its effects on spasticity have had mixed results. Goulet et al. (1994)

postulated that TENS would have an inhibitory effect on the amplitude of the soleus H reflex. They failed to demonstrate any consistent effects and no significant treatment effects were found following stimulation (at 50 or 99 Hz) on a mixed or sensory nerve. These results could reflect the difficulties of obtaining consistent H-reflex amplitudes in normal subjects and in those with neurological dysfunction.

Seib et al. (1994) used the spasticity measurement scale, in which neurophysiological and biomechanical responses are evaluated, to investigate the effect of cutaneous ES (over the tibialis anterior muscle) on spasticity of the gastrocnemius–soleus–achilles tendon unit. Using two groups of subjects, one with traumatic brain injuries and the other with spinal cord injuries, a significant reduction in spasticity was found which lasted for 6 h or more following the stimulation. Based on these results the authors proposed that TENS could be of use for decreasing spasticity prior to other physiotherapeutic interventions such as stretching.

Electrical stimulation of muscle

Surface ES to produce a muscle contraction via the motor nerves has been widely used in physiotherapy. Muscle ES has five major uses in physiotherapy in general:

1. strengthening and/or maintaining muscle bulk
2. facilitating voluntary muscle contraction
3. gaining or maintaining ROM
4. reducing spasticity
5. as an orthotic substitute to produce functional movement.

The latter three uses are those most commonly seen in neurological rehabilitation. All types of ES that produce contraction tend to be termed functional electrical stimulation (FES) but this is inaccurate (see below).

Maintaining ROM is often an important goal in neurological dysfunction. If patients are unable to maintain range by moving a joint themselves, or having it moved passively, neuromuscular ES may be used to provide assistance or as a substitute. It can provide a consistent controlled treatment that the patient can apply and use at home (Baker, 1991).

The effects of ES on shoulder subluxation, functional recovery of the upper limb and shoulder pain in stroke patients have been studied (Faghri et al., 1994). Using radiographs to assess the degree of subluxation, a significant reduction in the amount of displacement was achieved in the experimental group who received ES to supraspinatus and posterior deltoid muscles. A larger study by Chantraine et al. (1999) also supported the early use of ES in order to reduce the degree of shoulder subluxation poststroke.

Functional electrical stimulation

FES is the term used when the aim of treatment is to enhance or produce a functional movement (McDonough & Kitchen, 2002).

When used as an orthotic substitute, ES can pos-sibly be considered to be truly functional. However, opinions vary as to the efficacy of its use in this area. Petrofsky (1988) identified that FES can be used, often in conjunction with light-weight braces, to provide a method of independent ambulation, but that walking in this way is only part of a comprehensive physical training programme. Melis et al. (1995) concluded that the use of ambulatory assistive devices and FES could help patients with spinal cord injuries to regain independent locomotion and improve their quality of life. Much of the literature available about FES of the lower limbs focuses on its use in spinal cord injury. Whalley Hammell (1995) considered the financial implications of FES which, despite two decades of research, still cannot produce a functional level of walking. Another use of FES in this patient group is in the upper limb to improve hand function, but it appears that the fine control required here is as difficult to reproduce as the combination of balance and movement required in walking (Baker, 1991).

The use of FES as part of a rehabilitation programme must be accompanied by an accurate explanation to the patient, including setting achievable goals so that the patient's expectations are realistic. It should be noted that the *National Clinical Guidelines for Stroke* (Intercollegiate Working Party for Stroke, 2002) do not recommend the use of FES after stroke. This recommendation is based on the work of Glanz et al. (1995), although some studies have identified positive benefits in its use (Powell et al., 1999; Wright & Granat, 2000).

ES for reducing spasticity

Establishing the effect of ES on spasticity has been hindered by the difficulties of quantifying spasticity. Vang et al. (1995) used a single-case-study design to investigate the effect of ES on a patient experiencing problems with upper-limb function due to spasticity, secondary to cerebral palsy. Using a test of hand function to evaluate the level of spasticity, ES resulted in a measurable reduction in spasticity. However, a systematic review of the literature relating to the use of ES for preventing and treating poststroke shoulder pain concluded that there was no significant effect on upper-limb spasticity (Price & Pandyan, 2002).

Considerations when using ES

It is important to be aware of the safety aspects of using ES and the adverse effects it may have on abnormal neuromuscular systems, as much of the research has so far been conducted on normal muscle. Stokes & Cooper (1989) considered the problems of fatigue when stimulating muscles, the physiological effects of ES and the potential dangers when ES is used indiscriminately for therapeutic stimulation. Indeed, initial studies using stimulation to allow paraplegic and quadriplegic subjects to stand and walk short distances found that fatigue limited the distance walked and excessive stress was placed on the cardiorespiratory system and the legs (Petrofsky, 1988). These problems have been partly overcome by the combined use of bracing and FES, and preparation of the muscle for FES by low-frequency conditioning stimulation to improve endurance.

Increased resistance to fatigue in response to conditioning stimulation is achieved by biochemical and physiological adaptations in the muscle (Pette, 1986). Furthermore, the frequency patterns used during conditioning stimulation are important, as a single low frequency can cause muscle weakness but intermittent bursts of high frequency can maintain strength and still improve endurance (Rutherford & Jones, 1988). When ES is used to strengthen muscle, a stimulation pattern similar to the normal motor unit firing pattern has been shown to be more effective than uniform frequency or random frequencies (Oldham et al., 1995; also see Ch. 5, p. 70). This finding was in patients with rheumatoid arthritis and hand muscle weakness. Stimulation patterns have also been studied in the quadriceps in patients with patellofemoral pain (Callaghan et al., 2001). Whilst this approach appears promising, these studies involved conditions in which muscles and nerves were not diseased, so further research is required in patients with muscular and neurological disorders.

It also appears that further studies are necessary to monitor the effects of ES in specific neuromuscular disorders. Studies such as those which examined the effects of ES on patients with progressive muscular dystrophy (Zupan & Gregoric, 1995) and other neurological disorders (Scott et al., 1986) may allow physiotherapists to make informed decisions about the usefulness of ES as part of a therapeutic programme. Research is also needed to establish appropriate stimulation parameters for the different applications of ES. The reader is directed to McDonough & Kitchen (2002) for specific guidance to the use of ES.

OTHER TECHNIQUES

In this section, various unrelated techniques are discussed. Two treatments that were mainly used in orthopaedics before being applied to neurology are acupuncture and neurodynamics (for neurodynamics, see Ch. 31). Another orthopaedic treatment not discussed here is the correction of muscle imbalance (see Ch. 30).

Biofeedback

Biofeedback has been used widely in physiotherapy; a detailed description of its use in neurology can be found in McCulloch & Nelson (1995) and Low & Reed (2000). It has been defined as 'procedures whereby information about an aspect of bodily functioning is fed back by some visual or auditory signal' (Caudrey & Seeger, 1981). Biofeedback therapy seeks to allow subjects to gain conscious control over a voluntary but latent activity (Glanz et al., 1995).

The most commonly used form of biofeedback in neurological rehabilitation is EMG using surface electrodes. Most EMG feedback equipment will provide both auditory and visual feedback to the patient and therapist. For the purposes of providing feedback, changes in the EMG signal can be taken to indicate changes in muscle activity. This does not provide a measure of changes in force, since EMG and force are known to dissociate when muscle fatigues, as shown by the classic experiment of Edwards & Lippold in 1956. EMG biofeedback therefore reflects muscular effort and not force.

Force can be reflected more accurately by recording the mechanical activity of muscle, using the technique of mechanomyography or MMG (Orizio, 1993; Stokes & Blythe, 2001). A small recording device is placed on the skin to record the vibrations (often referred to as muscle sounds) produced when a muscle contracts. This technique is currently used in research to examine the contractile properties of muscle and has been used clinically, including for biofeedback. MMG can be used to record from muscles in which force cannot be measured directly, e.g. paraspinal muscles. The potential for MMG as a clinical tool is therefore very promising but some technical limitations need to be overcome before it can be used in routine clinical practice.

Reviews of EMG biofeedback therapy assessed its efficacy in rehabilitation following stroke (Glanz et al., 1995) and compared it with conventional physical therapy for upper-extremity function also following stroke (Moreland & Thomson, 1994). A study of acute stroke patients used EMG biofeedback for gait training but demonstrated no significant differences between the intervention and control groups (Bradley et al., 1998).

Glanz et al. (1995) carried out a retrospective study to determine whether biofeedback could increase the ROM of paretic limb joints after stroke. They reviewed eight published randomised controlled trials and concluded that the efficacy of biofeedback therapy in the rehabilitation of cerebrovascular disease had not been established. A particular problem identified by this meta-analysis was the number of studies with very small sample sizes. A similar conclusion was reached by Moreland & Thomson (1994). More recently, a meta-analysis by Hiraoka (2001) concluded that EMG biofeedback had a large effect on improving function of the upper limb poststroke. A subsequent meta-analysis by Moreland et al. (1998) concluded that the use of EMG biofeedback is superior to conventional therapy alone for improving ankle dorsiflexion muscle strength.

These reviews indicate that further research is required to support the use of biofeedback in physiotherapy. The doubts over its efficacy may explain why De Weerdt & Harrison (1985) found that the use of biofeedback was limited in physiotherapy departments in the UK.

Caudrey & Seeger (1981) provided a clear review of biofeedback devices other than EMG, which could be used as adjuncts to conventional physiotherapy. These include posture control equipment and the head position trainer, the limb load monitor and devices for improving orofacial control.

Another technique that is becoming a useful biofeedback tool in physiotherapy is real-time ultrasound imaging of muscle (see Stokes et al., 1997, for a review). For example, re-education of the lumbar multifidus muscle, which can be difficult to teach, was shown to be enhanced using ultrasound imaging as visual feedback (Hides et al., 1998). It is stressed that adoption of the ultrasound technique by physiotherapists requires training and knowledge of its technical aspects, and adherence to safety guidelines (see www.bmus.org).

Most biofeedback equipment provides immediate, precise feedback to the patient about some aspect of activity. It is important to remember that most physiotherapists utilise verbal feedback when treating patients, whether to provide praise, correction or instruction.

Neurodynamics

With any form of neurological dysfunction, the normal adaptive lengthening or shortening which occurs within the nervous system may be interrupted. Maintaining and restoring a mobile, extensible nervous system and a knowledge of normal neurodynamics is therefore an essential part of the management of the neurological patient and this topic is discussed in detail in Chapter 31.

Orthoses

An orthosis is a device that, when correctly applied to the appropriate external surface of the body, will achieve one or more of the following (Leonard et al., 1989):

- relief of pain
- immobilisation of musculoskeletal segments

- reduced axial loading
- prevention or correction of deformity
- improved function

In neurological rehabilitation, orthoses are most frequently used to improve function and occasionally to prevent or correct deformity. Using anatomical and physiological knowledge, functional and biomechanical abnormalities are identified and, as far as is possible, corrected.

A variety of materials and designs can be used in the construction of an orthosis. The word 'splint' suggests an orthotic device designed for temporary use; examples of some splints were considered above in the section on inhibitory stretching. Ideally, most orthoses are designed, made and fitted by an orthotist.

Orthoses tend to be named in relation to the joints they surround. Foot orthoses (FOs) are applied to the foot, either inside or outside the shoe (arch supports, heel lifts). Ankle–foot orthoses (AFOs) encompass the foot and ankle, generally extending to just below the knee (see Ch. 13, Fig. 13.1). Knee–ankle–foot orthoses (KAFOs) extend from foot to thigh; those extending above the hip are hip–knee–ankle–foot orthoses (HKAFOs; Edwards & Charlton, 2002). A hip guidance orthosis (HGO) is illustrated in Chapter 19 (Fig. 19.5) and Table 19.2 lists some uses for these orthoses in children with different levels of paralysis.

Orthoses should help the patient meet identified functional objectives; in the case of those applied to the lower limbs, this frequently relates to walking. In order to use orthoses effectively to improve walking, it is essential to consider the normal biomechanics of walking. When using an orthosis, forces are applied to the lower limb as a series of three-point force systems (Leonard et al., 1989). It is essential that these forces are correctly applied so that the desired effect is achieved.

Of particular biomechanical interest is an ability to visualise the ground reaction forces during activities of the lower limb. In a laboratory situation it is possible, using a force plate and video vector generator, to evaluate the effects of an orthosis, using a real-time ground reaction vector. Abnormal moments or turning effects on joints can be noted; energy demand is reduced by minimising the moments that must be resisted during walking, and this can be achieved by altering the forces applied by the orthosis. Butler & Nene (1991) illustrated this clearly in relation to the application of fixed AFOs used in the management of children with cerebral palsy.

Upper-limb orthoses used in neurological dysfunction are often employed to provide a dynamic force on a joint to reduce contractures (Leonard et al., 1989), a use already outlined above. Orthoses to enhance upper-limb function are illustrated in Chapter 9. Perhaps the most common orthotic device used by physiotherapists working in neurology is some form of shoulder support for patients with subluxation following stroke. Various types of shoulder support have been used; one of the most commonly used supports in the UK is based upon a method outlined by Bertha Bobath (Leddy, 1981). One study compared four different supports used to correct shoulder subluxation (Zorowitz et al., 1995). There was no evidence to show that the use of supports prevented or reduced long-term subluxation; indeed, two of the supports investigated appeared to cause lateral displacement of the humeral head. It is essential that the effects of shoulder supports are carefully evaluated and it may well be that, until evidence is provided to the contrary, there is little justification for their use.

Acupuncture

Acupuncture was recognised in 1979 by the World Health Organization (WHO) as a clinical procedure of value that should be taken seriously. Although increasingly used in the musculoskeletal field, acupuncture has not been used extensively by physiotherapists working in neurology. The exception to this is in East Asia where various papers report its use (Johansson, 1993).

In an overview of acupuncture from a medical viewpoint, Gibb (1981) identified its use in chronic pain, analgesia, chronic arthritis, autonomic dysfunction, dysmenorrhoea, insomnia and malignant pain. A randomised controlled study investigating whether acupuncture can improve the functional outcome in stroke patients, in which subjects were assigned to one of three groups, was undertaken by Gosman-Hedstrom et al. (1998). All subjects were receiving conventional physiotherapy (details not given). Subjects in two of the groups were also to receive acupuncture, either with deep needles plus ES on the affected side or with superficially situated needles. The results of this study did not support the use of acupuncture in improving function, quality of life or reducing the use of health care and social services.

String wrapping

Flowers (1988) advocated the use of string wrapping, also referred to as compressive centripetal wrapping, to help control oedema. This is an easily applied method for reducing oedema, particularly in the swollen paralysed hand. Each digit, the thumb and hand are wrapped, from distal to proximal, using string of 1–2 mm diameter. A loop is made as the wrapping commences and the wrapping is applied firmly and continuously. Once applied, the wrapping is immediately removed by pulling on the free end of the loop (Davies, 2000). The reduction of swelling allows greater facilitation of active movement. This is a treatment that can easily be applied by carers prior to, and in between, episodes of physiotherapy. It has very specific, local effects and may prove very useful when swelling is restricting functional improvement in the hand.

CONSTRAINT-INDUCED (FORCED-USE) THERAPY

It has been suggested that following the onset of certain neurological disorders some of the resulting dysfunction is as a result of learned non-use. The faster recovery seen in the lower limb following stroke is as a result of the continued lower-limb use in transferring and walking; this can be thought of as naturally occurring forced use (Fisher & Woll, 1995). The occurrence of this natural forced use is often reduced when compensation is allowed to occur. For example, patients may be able to accept and support their body weight but there is a natural tendency for patients to adopt compensatory strategies that eliminate the need for them to do so (Fisher & Woll, 1995). Encouraging a patient poststroke to take weight through the affected lower limb by stepping on to a block with the unaffected lower limb is an example of forced use. The principle of forced use is the basis for the increasing use of constraint therapy (Morris & Taub, 2001), seen particularly in relation to the upper limb (van-der-Lee et al., 1999; Charles et al., 2001), and is discussed in Chapter 29.

CONCLUSION

A variety of techniques used by physiotherapists working in neurology have been discussed. It is not possible to give detailed descriptions of their exact application but brief outlines have been given and references provided for further information. Many of the techniques used require further research either to validate their use and/or to establish appropriate guidelines for their application.

CASE HISTORIES

CASE 1 – STROKE

History and problem
Mrs S is a 62-year-old woman attending for outpatient physiotherapy following a left cardiovascular accident (CVA). At the moment she is wheelchair-dependent and has little active movement in her right upper and lower limbs. Passive ROM on the right is within normal limits and there is no resistance felt to passive movement.

Treatment
Techniques of facilitation can be combined with the use of functional positions to try and facilitate a motor response on the right. Possible techniques include approximation and tapping.

To apply approximation, Mrs S must be placed in a position that results in joint approximation. Sitting Mrs S on a low plinth, the right upper limb is placed with the shoulder laterally rotated and abducted, with the elbow extended and the hand resting on the plinth. The physiotherapist may need to give manual support to the elbow and shoulder to maintain the position while weight is taken through the hand, and joint approximation occurs.

Alternatively, Mrs S could be weight-bearing through her upper limb using a plinth in front of her while she stands and also takes weight through the lower limbs.

Tapping over the right knee extensors can be used to facilitate their action during standing. Continuing in standing, a ball could be placed on the plinth so that Mrs S can achieve some dynamic upper-limb weight-bearing, combined with continued weight-bearing through the lower limbs.

CASE 2 – HEAD INJURY

History and problem
Mr P is a 70-year-old man who has been an inpatient for some time following a head injury. He is currently working to improve his walking ability, which is severely hindered by a loss of extensibility in his right calf muscles.

Treatment
Before he starts his physiotherapy session, Mr P comes down to the gym to stand on a tilt table in order to give his calf muscles a prolonged stretch. To make this even more effective, his left leg is placed on a stool to ensure that the right limb is fully loaded. When he starts his walking practise he has EMG biofeedback applied to his right ankle dorsiflexors to help him activate these muscles during the swing phase of gait. His physiotherapist has also been using ice on his dorsiflexors to facilitate movement. This is applied by sweeping an ice cube over the muscle belly and then asking Mr P to try and dorsiflex his ankle.

References

Adler SJ, Beckers D, Buck M. *PNF in Practice*. Berlin: Springer Verlag; 1993.

Ageranioti S, Hayes K. Effects of vibration in hypertonia and hyperreflexia in the wrist joint of patients with spastic hemiparesis. *Physiother Can* 1990, **42**:24–33.

Anderson BD, Spector A. Introduction to Pilates-based rehabilitation. *Orthop Phys Ther North Am* 2000, **9**:395–410.

Association of Chartered Physiotherapists Interested in Neurology (ACPIN). *Clinical Practice Guidelines on Splinting Adults with Neurological Dysfunction*. London: Chartered Society of Physiotherapy; 1998.

Baily Metcalf A, Lawes N. A modern approach of the Rood approach. *Phys Ther Rev* 1998, **3**:195–212.

Baker L. Clinical uses of neuromuscular electrical stimulation. In: Nelson R, Currier D, eds. *Clinical Electrotherapy*, Connecticut: Appleton and Lange; 1991:143–170.

Bennettt SE, Karnes JL. *Neurological Disabilities: Assessment and Treatment*. Philadelphia: Lippincott; 1998.

Bennie A. Spinal cord injuries. In: Reid Campion M, ed. *Hydrotherapy: Principles and Practice*. Oxford: Butterworth-Heinemann; 1997:242–251.

Bishop B. Neurophysiology of motor responses evoked by vibratory stimulation. *Phys Ther* 1974, **54**:1273–1282.

Blair E, Ballantyne J, Horsman S et al. A study of a dynamic proximal stability splint in the management of children with cerebral palsy. *Dev Med Child Neurol* 1995, **37**:544–554.

Bobath B. *Adult Hemiplegia: Evaluation and Treatment*. Oxford: Heinemann; 1990.

Bohannon RW. Tilt table standing for reducing spasticity after spinal cord injury. *Arch Phys Med Rehab* 1993, **74**:1121–1122.

Bradley L, Hart BB, Mandana S et al. Electromyographic biofeedback for gait training after stroke. *Clin Rehab* 1998, **12**:11–22.

Bromley I. *Tetraplegia and Paraplegia. A Guide for Physiotherapists*. Edinburgh: Churchill Livingstone; 1998.

Brouwer B, Sousa de Andrade V. The effects of slow stroking on spasticity in patients with multiple sclerosis: a pilot study. *Physiother Theory Pract* 1995, **11**:13–21.

Bury T. Evidence-based healthcare explained. In: Bury T, Mead J, eds. *Evidence Based Healthcare*. Oxford: Butterworth Heinemann; 1998.

Butler P, Nene A. The biomechanics of fixed ankle foot orthoses and their potential in the management of cerebral palsied children. *Physiotherapy* 1991, **77**:81–88.

Callaghan MJ, Oldham JA, Winstanley J. A comparison of two types of electrical stimulation of the quadriceps in the treatment of patellofemoral pain syndrome. A pilot study. *Clin Rehab* 2001, **5**:637–646.

Carr EK, Kenney FD. Positioning of the stroke patient: a review of the literature. *Int J Nurs Stud* 1992, **29**:355–356.

Carriere B. *The Swiss Ball: Theory, Basic Exercises and Clinical Applications*. Berlin: Springer Verlag; 1998.

Carriere B. The 'Swiss ball'. *Physiotherapy* 1999, **85**:552–561.

Cassar MP. *Handbook of Massage Therapy*. Oxford: Butterworth-Heinemann; 1999.

Caudrey D, Seeger B. Biofeedback devices as an adjunct to physiotherapy. *Physiother* 1981, **67**:371–376.

Chantraine A, Baribeault A, Uebelhart D et al. Shoulder pain and dysfunction in hemiplegia. *Arch Phys Med Rehab* 1999, **80**:328–331.

Charles J, Laviner G, Gordan AM. Effects of constraint-induced therapy on hand function in children with hemiplegic cerebral palsy. *Pediatr Phys Ther* 2001, **13**:68–76.

Chatterton HJ, Pomeroy VM, Gratton J. Positioning for stroke patients: a survey of physiotherapists' aims and practices. *Disabil Rehab* 2001, **23**:413–421.

Davies PM. *Right in the Middle. Selective Trunk Activity in the Treatment of Adult Hemiplegia*. Berlin: Springer-Verlag; 1990.

Davies PM. *Steps to Follow: The Comprehensive Treatment of Patients with Hemiplegia*. Berlin: Springer-Verlag; 2000.

Davis BC, Harrison RA. *Hydrotherapy in Practice*. Edinburgh: Churchill Livingstone; 1988.

Dean CM, Mackey FH, Katrak P. Examination of shoulder positioning after stroke: a randomized controlled pilot trial. *Aust J Physiother* 2000, **46**:35–40.

De Weerdt W, Harrison M. The use of biofeedback in physiotherapy. *Physiotherapy* 1985, **71**:9–12.

Dickstein R, Hocherman S, Pillar T et al. Stroke rehabilitation three exercise therapy approaches. *Phys Ther* 1986, **66**:1233–1237.

Edwards S, Charlton P. Splinting and the use of orthoses in the management of patients with neurological disorders. In: Edwards S, ed. *Neurological Physiotherapy: A Problem-solving Approach*. Edinburgh: Churchill Livingstone; 2002:219–253.

Edwards RG, Lippold OCJ. The relation between force and integrated electrical activity in fatigued muscle. *J Physiol* 1956, **312**:677–681.

Faghri PD, Rodgers MM, Glaser RM et al. The effects of functional electrical stimulation on shoulder subluxation, arm function recovery and shoulder pain in hemiplegic stroke patients. *Arch Phys Med Rehab* 1994, **75**:73–79.

Farber S. A multisensory approach to neurorehabilitation. In: Farber S, ed. *Neurorehabilitation: A Multisensory Approach*. Philadelphia: WB Saunders; 1982:115–177.

Fisher B, Woll S. Considerations in the restoration of motor control. In: Montgomery J, ed. *Physical Therapy for Traumatic Brain Injury*. New York: Churchill Livingstone; 1995:55–78.

Flowers K. String wrapping versus massage for reducing digital volume. *Phys Ther* 1988, **68**:57–59.

Garland SJ, Hayes KC. Effects of brushing on electromyographic activity and ankle dorsiflexion in hemiplegic subjects with foot drop. *Physiother Can* 1987, **39**:239–247.

Gibb G. Acupuncture: a medical viewpoint. *NZ J Physiother* 1981, **9**:11–14.

Glanz M, Klawansky S, Stason W et al. Biofeedback therapy in poststroke rehabilitation: a meta-analysis of the randomised controlled trials. *Arch Phys Med Rehab* 1995, **76**:508–515.

Goldberg J, Sullivan SJ, Seaborne DE. The effect of two intensities of massage on H-reflex amplitude. *Phys Ther* 1992, **72**:449–457.

Goldspink G, Williams PE. Muscle fibre and connective tissue changes associated with use and disuse. In: Ada L, Canning C, eds. *Key Issues in Neurological Physiotherapy*. Oxford: Butterworth-Heinemann; 1990:197–218.

Gosman-Hedstrom G, Claesson L, Klingenstierna U et al. Effects of acupuncture treatment on daily life activities and quality of life: a controlled prospective and randomised study of acute stroke patients. *Stroke* 1998, **29**:2100–2108.

Goulet C, Arsenault AB, Levin MF et al. Absence of consistent effects of repetitive transcutaneous electrical stimulation on soleus H-reflex in normal subjects. *Arch Phys Med Rehab* 1994, **75**:1132–1136.

Gracies JM, Marosszeky E, Renton R et al. Short-term effects of dynamic lycra splints on upper limb in hemiplegic patients. *Arch Phys Med Rehab* 2000, **81**:1547–1555.

Gray S. Neurological rehabilitation. In: Reid Campion M, ed. *Hydrotherapy: Principles and Practice*. Oxford: Butterworth-Heinemann; 1997:204–224.

Hale LA, Fritz VU, Goodman M. Prolonged static muscle stretch reduces spasticity – but for how long should it be held? *SA J Physio* 1995, **51**:3–6.

Hides JA, Richardson CA, Jull GA. Use of real-time ultrasound imaging for feedback in rehabilitation. *Manual Ther* 1998, **3**:125–131.

Hiraoka K. Rehabilitation effort to improve upper extremity function in post-stroke patients: a meta-analysis. *J Phys Ther Sci* 2001, **13**:5–9.

Hochreiter NW, Jewell M, Barber L et al. Effect of vibration on tactile sensitivity. *Phys Ther* 1983, **6**:934–937.

Holey E, Cook E. *Therapeutic Massage*. London: WB Saunders; 1999.

Intercollegiate Working Party for Stroke. *National Clinical Guidelines for Stroke*, 2nd edn. London: Royal College of Physicians; 2002. Available online at: http://www.rcplondon.ac.uk/pubs/books/stroke/index.htm.

Johansson B. Has sensory stimulation a role in stroke rehabilitation? *Scand J Rehab Med* 1993, **29**:87–96.

Johnstone M. *Restoration of Normal Movement after Stroke*. Edinburgh: Churchill Livingstone; 1995.

Jones CA. Case in point. Effect of lower extremity serial casts on hemiparetic gait patterns in adults. *Phys Ther Case Rep* 1999, **2**:221–231.

Kerrigan DC, Sheffler LR. Spastic paretic gait: an approach to evaluation and treatment. *Crit Rev Rehab Med* 1995, **7**: 253–268.

Kisner C, Colby LA. *Therapeutic Exercise: Foundations and Techniques*. Philadelphia: FA Davis; 2002.

Kitchen S (ed.) *Electrotherapy Evidence Based Practice*. Edinburgh: Churchill Livingstone; 2002.

Kukulka C, Haberichter PA, Mueksch AE et al. Muscle pressure effects on motoneuron excitability: a special communication. *Phys Ther* 1987, **67**:1720–1722.

Leandri M, Parodi CI, Corrieri N et al. Comparison of TENS treatments in hemiplegic shoulder pain. *Scand J Rehab Med* 1990, **22**:69–72.

Leddy M. Sling for hemiplegic patients. *Br J Occup Ther* 1981, **44**:158–160.

Lee JM, Warren MP, Mason AM. Effects of ice on nerve conduction velocity. *Physiotherapy* 1978, **64**:2–6.

Lehmann J, De Lateur B. Application of heat and cold in the clinical setting. In: Lehmann J, ed. *Therapeutic Heat and Cold*. Baltimore: Williams & Wilkins; 1990: 633–644.

Lennon S, Ashburn A. The Bobath concept in stroke rehabilitation: a focus group study of the experienced physiotherapists' perspective. *Disabil Rehab* 2000, **22**: 665–674.

Leonard JA, Hicks JE, Nelson VS et al. Prosthetics, orthotics, and assistive devices. 1. General concepts. *Arch Phys Med Rehab* 1989, **70**:S195–S201.

Leone J, Kukulka C. Effects of tendon pressure on alpha motoneuron excitability in patients with stroke. *Phys Ther* 1988, **68**:475–480.

Lovgreen B, Cody FWJ, Schady W. Muscle vibration alters the trajectories of voluntary movements in cerebellar disorders – a method of counteracting impaired movement accuracy? *Clin Rehab* 1993, **7**:327–336.

Low J, Reed A. *Electrotherapy Explained*. Edinburgh: Butterworth-Heinemann; 2000.

Martin J. The Halliwick method. *Physiotherapy* 1981, **67**: 288–291.

McCulloch KL, Nelson CM. Electrical stimulation and electromyographic biofeedback. In: Umphred DA, ed. *Neurological Rehabilitation*. St Louis: Mosby; 1995:852–871.

McDonough S, Kitchen S. Neuromuscular and muscular electrical stimulation. In: Kitchen S, ed. *Electrotherapy Evidence Based Practice*. Edinburgh: Churchill Livingstone; 2002:241–258.

Melis EH, Torres-Moreno R, Chilco L et al. Application of ambulatory assistive devices and functional electrical stimulation to facilitate the locomotion of spinal cord injured subjects. In: *Proceedings of 12th International Congress of World Confederation for Physical Therapy*. Washington, DC: 1995:772.

Mills V. Electromyographic results of inhibitory splinting. *Phys Ther* 1986, **64**:190–193.

Moore M, Kukulka C. Depression of Hoffmann reflexes following voluntary contraction and implications for proprioceptive neuromuscular facilitation therapy. *Phys Ther* 1991, **71**:321–333.

Moreland J, Thomson MA. Efficacy of electromyographic biofeedback compared with conventional physical therapy for upper-extremity function in patients following stroke: a research overview and meta-analysis. *Phys Ther* 1994, **74**:534–545.

Moreland JD, Thomson MA, Fuoco AR. Electromyographic biofeedback to improve lower extremity function after stroke: a meta-analysis. *Arch Phys Med Rehab* 1998, **79**:134–140.

Morgan CL, Cullen GP, Stokes M et al. Effects of knee joint angle and tilt table incline on force distribution at the feet and supporting straps. *Clin Rehab* 2003, **17**:871–878.

Morris SL, Sharpe M. PNF revisited. *Physio Theory Pract* 1993, **9**:43–51.

Morris DM, Taub E. Constraint-induced therapy approach to restoring function after neurological injury. *Top Stroke Rehab* 2001, **8**:16–30.

Moseley AM. The effect of casting combined with stretching on passive ankle dorsiflexion in adults with traumatic head injury. *Phys Ther* 1997, **77**:240–247.

Murphy C. Massage – the roots of the profession. *Physio* 1993, **79**:546.

Oldham JA, Howe TE, Peterson T et al. Electrotherapeutic rehabilitation of the quadriceps in elderly osteoarthritic patients: a double blind assessment of patterned neuromuscular stimulation. *Clin Rehab* 1995, **9**:10–20.

Orizio C. Muscle sound: bases for the introduction of a mechanomyographic signal in muscle studies. *Crit Rev Biomed Eng* 1993, **21**:201–243.

O'Sullivan SB. Strategies to improve motor control. In: O'Sullivan S, Schmitz T, eds. *Physical Rehabilitation Assessment and Treatment*. Philadelphia: FA Davis; 1988.

Petrofsky J. Functional electrical stimulation and its application in the rehabilitation of neurologically injured adults. In: Finger S et al., eds. *Brain Injury and Recovery: Theoretical and Controversial Issues*. New York: Plenum Press; 1988.

Pette D. Skeletal muscle adaptation in response to chronic stimulation. In: Nix WA, Vrbová G, eds. *Electrical Stimulation and Neuromuscular Disorders*. Berlin: Springer-Verlag; 1986:12–20.

Pope PM. Postural management and special seating. In: Edwards S, ed. *Neurological Physiotherapy: A Problem-solving Approach*. Edinburgh: Churchill Livingstone; 2002:189–253.

Powell J, Pandyan AD, Granat M et al. Electrical stimulation of wrist extensors in post-stroke hemiplegia. *Stroke* 1999, **30**:1384–1389.

Price CIM, Pandyan AD. Electrical stimulation for preventing and treating post-stroke shoulder pain (Cochrane Review). In: *The Cochrane Library*, 2002, issue 2. Oxford: Update Software.

Reid Campion M. *Hydrotherapy Principles and Practice*. Oxford: Butterworth-Heinemann; 1997.

Richardson DLA. The use of the tilt table to effect passive tendo-Achilles stretch in a patient with head injury. *Physio Theory Pract* 1991, **7**:45–50.

Robichaud J, Agostinucci J, Vander Linden D. Affect of air-splint application on soleus muscle motoneuron reflex excitabilty in nondisabled subjects and subjects with cerebrovascular accidents. *Phys Ther* 1992, **72**:176–185.

Rothwell J. *Control of Human Voluntary Movement*. London: Chapman & Hall; 1994.

Royeen CB, Duncan M, McCormack GL. The Rood approach: a reconstruction. In: Pedretti LW, Early MB, eds. *Occupational Therapy: Practice Skills for Physical Dysfunction*. St Louis: Mosby; 2001:576–587.

Rutherford OM, Jones DA. Contractile properties and fatiguability of the human adductor pollicis and first dorsal interosseus: a comparison of the effect of two chronic stimulation patterns. *J Neurol Sci* 1988, **85**:319–331.

Sackley CM, Lincoln NB. Physiotherapy treatment for stroke patients: a survey of current practice. *Physiother Theory Pract* 1996, **12**:87–96.

Scott OM, Vrbová G, Hyde SA et al. Effects of electrical stimulation on normal and diseased human muscle. In: Nix WA, Vrbová G, eds. *Electrical Stimulation and Neuromuscular Disorders*. Berlin: Springer-Verlag; 1986:125–131.

Seib T, Price R, Reyes MR et al. The quantitative measurement of spasticity: effect of cutaneous electrical stimulation. *Arch Phys Med Rehab* 1994, **75**:746–750.

Shepherd GM. *Neurobiology*. New York: Oxford University Press; 1994.

Skinner AT, Thomson AM. *Duffield's Exercise in Water*. London: Baillière Tindall; 1983.

Stokes MJ & Blythe GM. *Muscle Sounds – in Physiology, Sports Science and Clinical Investigation: Applications and History of Mechanomyography*. Oxford: Medintel Publications; 2001. www.oxmedic.com.

Stokes M, Cooper R. Muscle fatigue as a limiting factor in functional electrical stimulation; a review. *Physiother Pract* 1989, **5**:93–90.

Stokes MJ, Hides JA, Nassiri D. Musculoskeletal ultrasound imaging: diagnostic and treatment aid in rehabilitation. *Phys Ther Rev* 1997, **2**:73–92.

Sullivan SJ, Williams LRT, Seaborne DE et al. Effects of massage on alpha motorneurone excitability. *Phys Ther* 1991, **71**:555–560.

Suzuki T, Fujiwara T, Yase Y et al. Electrophysiological study of spinal motor neurone function in patients with cerebrovascular diseases – characteristic appearances of the H-reflex and F-wave. In: *Proceedings of 12th International Congress of World Confederation for Physical Therapy*. Washington, DC: 1995:798.

Tardieu C, Lespargot A, Tabary C et al. For how long must the soleus muscle be stretched each day to prevent contracture? *Dev Med Child Neurol* 1988, **30**:3–10.

Twist D. Effects of a wrapping technique on passive range of motion in a spastic upper extremity. *Phys Ther* 1985, **65**:299–304.

Umphred DA. Classification of common facilitatory and inhibitory techniques. In: Umphred DA, ed. *Neurological Rehabilitation*. St Louis: Mosby; 1995:118–178.

van-der-Lee JH, Wagenaar RC, Lankhorst GJ et al. Forced use of the upper extremity in chronic stroke patients: results from a single-blind randomized clinical trial. *Stroke* 1999, **30**:2369–2375.

Vang MM, Coleman KA, Gardner MP et al. Effects of functional electrical stimulation on spasticity. In: *Proceedings of 12th International Congress of World Confederation for Physical Therapy*. Washington DC: 1995:574.

Voss DE, Ionta M, Meyers B. *Proprioceptive Neuromuscular Facilitation: Patterns and Techniques*. New York: Harper & Row; 1985.

Wallen M, O'Flaherty S. The use of the soft splint in the management of spasticity of the upper limb. *Aust Occup Ther J* 1991, **38**:227–231.

Wallen M, Mackay S. An evaluation of the soft splint in the acute management of elbow hypertonicity. *Occup Ther J Res* 1995, **15**:3–16.

Wang R. Effect of proprioceptive neuromuscular facilitation on the gait of patients with hemiplegia of long and short duration. *Phys Ther* 1994, **74**: 1108–1115.

Whalley Hammell K. *Spinal Cord Injury Rehabilitation*. London: Chapman & Hall; 1995.

Whittle MW. *Gait Analysis: An Introduction*. Edinburgh: Butterworth-Heinemann; 2001.

Williams PE. Use of intermittent stretch in the prevention of serial sarcomere loss in immobilised muscle. *Ann Rheum Dis* 1990, **49**:316–317.

Williams PE, Catanese T, Lucey EG et al. The importance of stretch and contractile activity in the prevention of connective tissue accumulation in muscle. *J Anat* 1988, **158**:109–114.

Wright PA. & Granat MH. Therapeutic effects of functional electrical stimulation of the upper limb of eight children with cerebral palsy. *Dev Med Child Neurol* 2000, **42**:724–727.

Young T, Nicklin C. Lower limb casting in neurology practical guidelines. London: Royal Hospital for Neuro-disability; 2000.

Zachazewski JE, Eberle ED, Jefferies M. Effect of tone-inhibiting casts and orthoses on gait: a case report. *Phys Ther* 1982, **62**:453–455.

Zorowitz RD, Idank D, Ikai T et al. Shoulder subluxation after stroke: a comparison of four supports. *Arch Phys Med Rehab* 1995, **76**:763–771.

Zupan A, Gregoric M. Long-lasting effects of electrical stimulation upon muscles of patients suffering from progressive muscular dystrophy. *Clin Rehab* 1995, **9**:102–109.

Vestibular and balance rehabilitation

D Meldrum   R McConn Walsh

The overwhelming vertigo, the awful sickness and the turbulent eye movements – all enhanced by the slightest movement of the head, combine to form a picture of helpless misery that has few parallels in the whole field of injury and disease (Cawthorne, 1945).

INTRODUCTION

Normal postural control or 'balance', as it is commonly known, is fundamental to activities of daily living. Visual, vestibular and somatosensory systems all have important and integrated roles in the maintenance of balance and the neurological patient can present with problems in any or all of these components.

This chapter will focus on the assessment and treatment of patients who have a primary problem in the vestibular system. Vestibular dysfunction is characterised by a number of signs and symptoms, including vertigo, gait and balance impairment, nausea and nystagmus (Table 24.1).

Patients with such dysfunction present the physiotherapist with specific problems and require specialised assessment and treatment techniques, collectively referred to as vestibular rehabilitation. Vestibular rehabilitation has its roots in the empirical work of Cawthorne and Cooksey who, in the 1940s, first documented the important role of exercise in recovery after a vestibular injury (Cooksey, 1945).

The evidence base has increased in the recent past for the effective role of physiotherapy in the management of patients with vestibular disorders and vestibular rehabilitation is now recognised as a specialist area within physiotherapy.

Table 24.1 Signs and symptoms of vestibular disorders

Primary symptoms and signs	Associated problems
Vertigo	Neck and back pain
Dizziness/light-headedness	Physical deconditioning
Nausea and vomiting	Agoraphobia
Oscillopsia	Hyperventilation
Nystagmus	Falls
Disequilibrium/impaired balance	Hearing loss/tinnitus
Panic/anxiety	
Gait abnormality	
Fatigue	

Key point

Vertigo is defined as the sensation of motion when no motion is occurring relative to the Earth's gravity (Monsell et al., 1998). The sensation can be of the patient moving in relation to the environment or the environment moving in relation to the patient. It is generally accepted that true vertigo involves a spinning sensation and usually indicates inner-ear pathology (Blakley & Goebel, 2001). The word 'dizziness' is used to describe non-rotatory vertigo

INCIDENCE AND PREVALENCE OF DIZZINESS AND BALANCE DISORDERS

The prevalence of dizziness has been estimated to be one in five in the 18–64 age group with 50% of these reporting postural unsteadiness (Yardley et al., 1998a). Prevalence rises to one in three in the over-65s (Colledge et al., 1994) and dizziness is the most common complaint of patients presenting to primary care in those aged over 75 (Sloane, 1989). However approximately 40% of patients with a complaint of dizziness do not consult their general practitioner, demonstrating a probable underestimation of the problem (Yardley et al., 1998a). There is a very low prevalence of dizziness in the under-25s and women are more likely to experience dizziness. Dizziness rarely results in hospitalisation and the majority of patients are managed at primary care level with medication (Sloane, 1989).

NORMAL ANATOMY AND PHYSIOLOGY

The anatomy and physiology of the vestibular system are extremely complex and the reader is referred to Cohen (1999) for a detailed description. A brief organisational overview is shown in Figure 24.1. The vestibular system has both sensory and motor functions and is generally divided into peripheral and central components. The peripheral system consists of the vestibular end organ and the vestibular nerve up to and including the dorsal root entry zone. The central system includes the vestibular nuclei in the brainstem and their central connections.

The vestibular end organ includes the semicircular canals (SCC) and the otoliths (utricle and saccule). There are three SCCs on each side (horizontal, anterior and posterior) and they are oriented at 90° angles to each other (Fig. 24.1). Each canal is coupled functionally with a canal in the opposite end organ, i.e. both horizontal canals are coupled, as are the left anterior and right posterior and the right posterior and left anterior canals. Specialised sensors known as hair cells are located in the semicircular canals in a region known as the cupula (Fig. 24.1) and respond to angular velocity of head movement in different planes. Each canal responds best to movement in its own plane. For example, if the head turns to the right, the hair cells in the right horizontal SCC increase their firing rate and those in the left horizontal SCC decrease their firing rate (Fig. 24.2). Thus the central nervous system (CNS) gains information relating to the velocity and direction of head movement.

The otoliths have different hair cells in a region known as the macula, and these are covered by a layer of calcium carbonate crystals called otoconia. They respond to the force of gravity and thus can provide the CNS with information on head tilt and linear acceleration (i.e. going up and down in a lift or going forwards or backwards in a car).

The peripheral system is a tonically active system, i.e. it always has a certain firing level, which will increase or decrease with head movement. The CNS interprets any asymmetry in the firing rate as movement. This fact is of utmost importance when considering a patient who has loss of vestibular function on one side (i.e. decrease or absence of firing) since there will be a relative increase of firing on the intact side even when the head is not moving (Fig. 24.2). This asymmetry and the resultant disturbance in cortical spatial orientation are thought to form the basis of vertigo (Brandt, 2000).

The vestibular nerve sends fibres to two main areas: the vestibular nuclei and the cerebellum (Fig. 24.1). The vestibular nuclei are responsible for integrating information received from the end organ with that received from other sensory systems and the cerebellum. Vestibular nuclei send fibres to the oculomotor nuclei, vestibulospinal tracts, contralateral vestibular nuclei, reticular formation, cerebellum, autonomic nervous system and the cortex. The symptoms of nausea, vomiting and

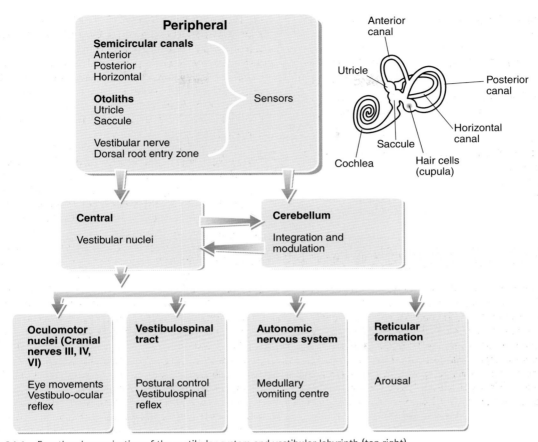

Peripheral

Semicircular canals
Anterior
Posterior
Horizontal

Otoliths
Utricle
Saccule

Vestibular nerve
Dorsal root entry zone

Sensors

Anterior canal

Utricle

Posterior canal

Horizontal canal

Saccule

Cochlea

Hair cells (cupula)

Central

Vestibular nuclei

Cerebellum

Integration and modulation

Oculomotor nuclei (Cranial nerves III, IV, VI)

Eye movements
Vestibulo-ocular reflex

Vestibulospinal tract

Postural control
Vestibulospinal reflex

Autonomic nervous system

Medullary vomiting centre

Reticular formation

Arousal

Figure 24.1 Functional organisation of the vestibular system and vestibular labyrinth (top right).

anxiety associated with vestibular disorders are thought to be a result of abnormal activation of the autonomic and reticular pathways respectively (Fig. 24.1).

Vestibulo–ocular reflex and vestibulospinal reflex

The motor functions of the vestibular system include the vestibulo-ocular reflex (VOR) and the vestibulospinal reflex (VSR). The function of the VOR is to maintain stable vision when the head is moving. A good example of this is being able to focus on an object when walking. If the eyes moved with the head as it goes up and down when walking it would be impossible to see clearly. The VOR enables the eyes (through activation of the appropriate ocular muscles) to move in the opposite direction and at an equal velocity to the head. The image of the object thus remains stable on the retina. For the VOR to function normally, the velocity of eye movement must be equal to and in the opposite direction from the head movement. This is known as the 'gain' of the VOR. Patients who have problems with the vestibular system

have impairment of the gain of the VOR and therefore demonstrate problems with gaze stability. They often describe that during self-motion stationary objects seem as if they are moving. The function of the VSR is primarily to maintain and regain postural control and this is achieved through activation of monosynaptic and polysynaptic vestibulospinal pathways.

CLASSIFICATION AND CAUSES OF VESTIBULAR DISORDERS

Vestibular disorders are classified anatomically into peripheral or central, depending on which area the pathology affects. Common peripheral and central vestibular disorders are shown in Table 24.2. It is important to note that dizziness is not always caused by pathology affecting the vestibular system; there may be many other causes, including postural hypotension, cardiac disorders, migraine, psychiatric disorders and hyperventilation, and these should be evaluated prior

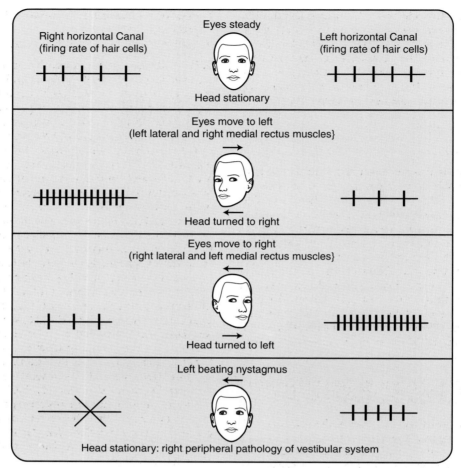

Figure 24.2 Function of the horizontal canals in generating a vestibulo-ocular reflex (VOR) during turning of the head and effect of loss of hair cell function. With loss of tonic firing on the right there is a relative increase in firing on the left; the brain interprets this as movement to the left (patient feels dizzy) and generates a VOR so that the eyes move to the right. The central nervous system corrects the eye movement with a saccadic movement to left, and a left-beating nystagmus is seen. (Firing rate for illustrative purposes only.)

Table 24.2 Peripheral and central vestibular disorders

Peripheral	Central
Viral – vestibular neuritis/labyrinthitis	Ischaemia, e.g lateral medullary syndrome
Benign paroxysmal positional vertigo (BPPV)	(Wallenberg's syndrome)
Perilymph fistula	Vertebrobasilar insufficiency
Ménière's disease	Infection
Vascular occlusion	Head injury
Iatrogenic (ototoxic drugs, surgery)	Degenerative disease, e.g. multiple sclerosis
Head injury	Friedreich's ataxia
Acoustic neuromas (may have a central component)	Base-of-skull abnormalities, e.g. Arnold–Chiari malformation
	Tumours of the cerebellopontine angle
	Drugs
	Epilepsy
	Migraine

to referral to physiotherapy. The exact cause of dizziness frequently remains uncertain and a trial of vestibular rehabilitation may be suggested in the absence of a specific diagnosis. The pathologies of disorders that can affect the central vestibular system (particularly cerebrovascular accidents, traumatic brain injury and multiple sclerosis) are considered in other chapters.

Peripheral disorders

Vestibular neuritis

This condition is also called neuronitis and is a common peripheral vestibular problem thought to be caused by a virus. It results in hair cell loss and unilateral vestibular paresis (or hypofunction). Patients present with an acute onset of vertigo, nausea and vomiting that are severely incapacitating and worsened by head and eye movements. On examination a spontaneous horizontal nystagmus can be seen, the fast phase of which beats away from the involved side. This is due to the asymmetrical tonic firing of the vestibular nerves (Fig. 24.2). Balance and gait abnormalities are also evident. Hearing is not generally affected; if it is, the condition is called labyrinthitis. These symptoms generally resolve over a period of 2–6 weeks.

> **Key point**
>
> **Nystagmus** is oscillation of the eyes. There is a slow movement or phase in one direction and a fast corrective movement in the opposite direction. By convention, nystagmus is named by the direction of the fast phase. For example, left-beating horizontal nystagmus is one in which the slow phase of the nystagmus is horizontal movement of the eyes towards the right and the fast phase of the nystagmus is horizontal eye movement towards the left. There are many causes of nystagmus. In the patient with a peripheral vestibular disorder, a spontaneous nystagmus is often seen with the fast phase beating away from the side of the lesion

Benign paroxysmal positional vertigo (BPPV)

BPPV is the commonest cause of vertigo in peripheral vestibular disorders. Its aetiology is unknown in many cases but it can occur as a result of an earlier vestibular neuritis or head trauma. The name encompasses the associated features:

- benign – the prognosis for recovery is favourable
- paroxysmal – the associated vertigo is short-lived, generally less than 1 min

- positional – the vertigo is provoked by certain head positions
- vertigo – a spinning sensation is experienced.

BPPV is thought to be caused by detached utricular otoconia entering one of the SCCs and either floating free in the canal (canalithiasis) or adhering to the cupula (apex of the cochlea; cupulolithiasis; Epley, 1980). This has the effect of making the SCCs responsive to gravity when normally they are not. The SCCs usually respond to head movement in their respective planes and increase or decrease their firing rate during head movement, returning to normal tonic firing level when the head has stopped moving. However, the displaced otoconia are heavier, continue to move in the canal and stimulate the hair cells in the canal to continue firing. The central vestibular system interprets this as further movement and generates a VOR for that canal, and the patient develops nystagmus and vertigo.

This nystagmus, following movement into the provoking position, has a latency of 1–50 s, is generally transient in nature (it stops when the otoconia come to a resting position) and is torsional towards the affected ear. If the patient repeatedly moves into the provoking position the vertigo and nystagmus will decrease due to habituation of the response (Baloh et al., 1987).

The diagnosis of BPPV is generally made using the Hallpike–Dix manoeuvre (Fig. 24.3, Table 24.3) in which the head is moved into a provocative position. BPPV is most commonly caused by canalithiasis affecting the posterior SCC but can also affect the anterior and, very rarely, the horizontal canal (Baloh et al., 1993; De la Meilleure et al., 1996).

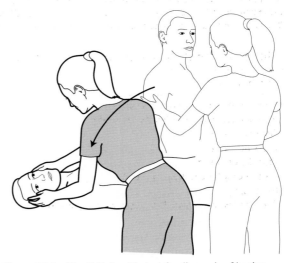

Figure 24.3 The Hallpike–Dix test for diagnosis of benign paroxysmal positional vertigo (BPPV).

Table 24.3 Oculomotor and positional tests of the vestibular patient

Oculomotor examination	Details

Spontaneous nystagmus
    Room light (visual fixation)
    Frenzel lenses (no visual fixation)
	Patient looks straight ahead. The eyes are observed for nystagmus and the direction is noted. Frenzel lenses both remove visual fixation and magnify the eyes (Fig. 24.4). Nystagmus due to a peripheral vestibular disorder can be suppressed by visual fixation

Gaze-evoked nystagmus[a]	Ability to hold eyes steady on a stationary object. If abnormal, the eyes will make jerky movements in an effort to remain on the object
Smooth pursuit[a]	Ability to track a moving object with the eyes when the head is stationary. In normal subjects the eyes make smooth movements; abnormalities include jerky movements of the eyes
Saccades[a]	Ability to move the eyes from one stationary target to another when the head is stationary. In an abnormal case the eyes may over- or undershoot the target
Vestibulo-ocular reflex cancellation[a]	Ability to suppress the vestibulo-ocular reflex and move the eyes in phase with the head. Patient is asked to follow a moving target as the examiner moves the head in the same direction

Vestibulo-ocular reflex
    Gaze stabilisation with head movement
    Slow head movement
    Fast head movement
	A normal vestibulo-ocular reflex is when the eyes can make a compensatory movement to stay on a stationary target when the head moves. Patient is asked to keep eyes steady on a target whilst the examiner moves patient's head in a small range of movement from side to side and then up and down slowly. This is repeated with faster movements of the head. Abnormalities would involve a saccadic movement of the eyes to stay on the target

Positional tests	
Hallpike–Dix test (see Fig. 24.3)	The patient is long-sitting on plinth with eyes open. The head is turned 45° to the side that is being tested. The patient is brought quickly into a lying position with the head in 30° extension by the examiner. This position is maintained for 50s and the presence, duration and direction of nystagmus are noted. Symptoms are also noted. This test is diagnostic for BPPV

[a] If this test is abnormal it is indicative of central nervous system pathology.
BPPV, benign paroxysmal positional vertigo.

Patients with BPPV complain of vertigo associated with certain head movements, i.e. rolling over in bed, looking up, bending down, and will usually avoid these movements. BPPV is more common in older patients.

Ménière's disease

The cause of Ménière's disease is an increase in volume and a problem with absorption of the endolymph (one of the fluids in the inner ear). This results in dilation of the endolymphatic spaces (endolymphatic hydrops). This happens episodically and an attack is characterised by a complaint of a fullness in the ear, reduction of hearing and tinnitus (a ringing sound in the ear). This is followed by vertigo, vomiting and postural imbalance and nystagmus is observed. The episodes may last from 30 min to 72 h and then the patient gradually improves. Episodes are generally managed with medication, diet and rest but in severe cases surgery may be indicated (see below). Vestibular rehabilitation is generally not indicated in patients with Ménière's as the attacks remit spontaneously.

Bilateral vestibular hypofunction

This condition can be caused by infections, e.g. meningitis, tumours (e.g. bilateral acoustic neuromas in neurofibromatosis), Ménière's disease, autoimmune diseases and ototoxic drugs (e.g. aminoglycoside antibiotics). In some cases the cause is unknown. Patients with bilateral vestibular hypofunction do not usually complain of vertigo when vestibular loss is symmetrical. Their main problems include balance and gait impairments. They also have decreased gaze stability due to loss of VOR function and complain that they cannot see clearly during head movements and describe their surroundings as bouncing or jumping. This is termed oscillopsia.

RECOVERY FROM VESTIBULAR PATHOLOGY: VESTIBULAR COMPENSATION

In most cases, the symptoms of patients with a unilateral vestibular loss spontaneously ameliorate over a period of weeks. The process by which the patient recovers is called vestibular compensation. The spontaneous nystagmus disappears by 2–3 days (static compensation) and the symptoms associated with movement (vertigo, visual blurring and postural unsteadiness) by 6 weeks (dynamic compensation). Hair cells have not been shown to regenerate in humans, therefore the patient must recover by other means.

Research has shown that plastic changes occur in the CNS in response to peripheral vestibular pathology and these changes are responsible for vestibular compensation (Curthoys, 2000; Zee, 2000). Three processes are thought to contribute:

1. Initially, the cerebellum inhibits firing of the vestibular nuclei of the unaffected side, probably to reduce the asymmetry produced by the lesion. The vestibular nucleus of the affected side begins spontaneously to fire tonically again, probably due to neurochemical changes produced by the loss of input (denervation supersensitivity; Curthoys, 2000).

2. The second process is known as sensory substitution. In this process the CNS reorganises to substitute or utilise inputs more efficiently from intact systems, including vision and somatosensory and cervical proprioceptive systems. The intact vestibular end organ is able to compensate for loss on the other side, as both sides respond to head movement in any direction. It is important to note also that if there is some remaining vestibular function on the pathological side, the CNS will utilise it.

3. Lastly, the process of habituation is thought to play a role in vestibular compensation. Habituation is generally defined as a reduction in response over time with repeated exposure to a specific stimulus. This is the process thought to underpin improvement with the Cawthorne Cooksey exercises (see below), in which the patient repeatedly performs head and/or eye movements that provoke symptoms of vertigo.

The reasons why some patients fail to compensate are not always clear but may be a result of abnormality in the CNS, visual, somatosensory or musculoskeletal systems. Animal studies have shown that compensation is delayed by immobilisation, reduced or absent visual inputs and is promoted by exercise (Courjon et al., 1977; Lacour & Xerri, 1981). It is thought that the CNS needs to experience the error signals in order for vestibular compensation to occur. Certain medications, including those used in the treatment of vestibular problems, can delay compensation (Zee, 1985). An intact CNS is vitally important for the process of vestibular compensation and thus patients with central vestibular problems will have a slower and more incomplete recovery (Rudge & Chambers, 1982). In bilateral vestibular loss, there may be no remaining VOR function with which to compensate, so the process of sensory substitution plays a major role in the recovery of these patients. Recovery will always be incomplete.

> **Key point**
>
> Most patients with unilateral peripheral vestibular pathology spontaneously recover over a period of a few weeks through a process known as vestibular compensation. Patients who do not spontaneously recover present for treatment and may benefit from vestibular rehabilitation

Multidisciplinary team

Patients with vestibular problems can be seen by a variety of members of the multidisciplinary team, including the physiotherapist, and communication between them facilitates optimum management. Diagnosis can be made at the level of primary care and it must be emphasised that the majority of patients are managed at this level as vestibular problems are generally associated with a favourable prognosis and spontaneous resolution. Patients who continue to experience problems are generally referred to ear, nose and throat specialists (also known as otologists or neurotologists), neurologists or neurosurgeons. Audiologists and audiological scientists carry out vestibular function testing and are involved in vestibular rehabilitation in some centres. Psychiatrists and psychologists are involved in the management of psychological problems associated with vestibular problems.

Medical and surgical management

Diagnosis/investigations

● Hearing tests (pure tone audiogram/speech discrimination): certain conditions that cause dizziness may also result in hearing loss. These include Ménière's disease, ototoxic medications, head trauma, acoustic neuromas and previous middle-ear surgery. A hearing test will provide valuable information on the inner ear (cochlea) and middle-ear function of these patients.

- Caloric/oculomotor testing: the caloric test is the most commonly used test of peripheral vestibular function and provides a separate, quantitative measure of lateral SCC function in each inner ear (Savundra & Luxon, 1997). This is performed by measuring the response of the VOR (nystagmus) to the instillation of cold and warm water down the external canal. As well as assessing peripheral vestibular function, oculomotor testing can also detect oculomotor disturbance (abnormal saccades, smooth pursuit) suggestive of a central disorder.

- Magnetic resonance imaging (MRI): any patient who presents with dizziness that is persistent or progressive should have an MRI scan (preferably with gadolinium enhancement) of the brain and cerebellopontine angle to exclude lesions such as a brain tumour, acoustic neuroma, multiple sclerosis or embolic/haemorrhagic events.

- Posturography: this provides a quantitative measure of certain functional aspects of dynamic equilibrium (Savundra & Luxon, 1997). It therefore has a role to play in the assessment of the disabled dizzy patient and can also be used in monitoring rehabilitation. To date, however, it has mainly been used as a research tool.

Medications

The acute rotatory vertigo suffered during an acute peripheral vestibular upset is due to sudden asymmetry in vestibular input to the CNS. Vestibular sedatives are a group of drugs that have a well-established record of controlling such attacks. These drugs have variable anticholinergic, antiemetic and sedative properties. They include phenothiazines (e.g. prochlorperazine, perphenazine), antihistamines (e.g. cinnarizine, dimenhydrinate, promethazine, meclizine) and benzodiazepines (e.g. diazepam, lorazepam; Moffat & Ballagh, 1997). These drugs are of particular value in the management of acute vertigo and they can be administered by intramuscular or intravenous injection, suppository, buccal absorption or orally, depending on the individual drug. However, they should be avoided in the management of chronic peripheral labyrinthine disorders as they may suppress central vestibular activity and thereby delay compensation and symptomatic recovery.

Betahistine and thiazide diuretics have been advocated in the management of Ménière's disease. Betahistine is a vasodilator that works directly on the inner ear and is thought to improve its microcirculation. Thiazide diuretics are thought to work in Ménière's disease by reducing the endolymphatic pressure by means of a systemic diuretic effect. However, much of the data reported regarding the efficacy of these drugs in Ménière's disease is conflicting.

Surgical management

Ménière's disease In those patients with unilateral Ménière's disease that is symptomatic for 6 months to 1 year despite conservative management (betahistine, thiazide diuretic, salt/caffeine restriction), then surgery should be considered (Moffat & Ballagh, 1997). The type of surgery is dependent on the level of hearing in the affected ear.

If the hearing is not serviceable or useful (<50% speech discrimination score, >50% speech reception threshold), then a labyrinthectomy is the preferred choice. This entails a mastoidectomy and drilling out the three SCCs under general anaesthesia. This is very effective at treating the vertiginous episodes by destroying all peripheral vestibular function, although all residual hearing is destroyed.

If the hearing is useful, then the surgery should attempt to preserve the remaining hearing. This can be done by means of topical gentamicin ablation therapy, endolymphatic sac decompression or by vestibular neurectomy. Topical gentamicin therapy involves the transtympanic instillation of gentamicin solution into the middle ear (Nedzelski et al., 1992). The gentamicin then diffuses into the inner ear across the round window membrane where it selectively destroys vestibular and not cochlear hair cells. Success rates of over 80% have been reported. The main disadvantage is that there is a risk of sensorineural hearing loss.

Endolymphatic sac decompression entails a mastoidectomy with removal of all bone over the endolymphatic sac/duct and possibly inserting a drain into it (Moffat, 1994). The sac is the proposed site of obstruction of endolymphatic reabsorption in Ménière's disease and this procedure enables the sac to expand during the active disease process. Vestibular neurectomy entails transecting the vestibular nerves in the posterior cranial fossa. The main disadvantages are damage to the facial and cochlear nerves together with intracranial complications. Vestibular rehabilitation is important following these procedures.

Persistent benign paroxysmal positional vertigo Cases of intractable (>1 year) and incapacitating BPPV can be treated by occlusion of the posterior semicircular canal (PSCC) (Parnes & McClure, 1990). This involves a mastoidectomy with isolation, and then occlusion of the PSCC. This is a safe and effective operation with success rates of over 90–95% (Walsh et al., 1999). Prior to this operation, singular neurectomy was advocated but this is a technically more demanding operation with a risk of sensorineural hearing loss.

Acoustic neuromas There are currently three methods of managing acoustic neuromas. These include conservative management, surgery (combined ear, nose and throat and neurosurgery) and stereotactic radiosurgery. Conservative management is reserved for small tumours that are not growing or for patients who are unfit or express a desire not to have surgery (Walsh et al., 2000). In those tumours that are growing, causing symptoms, and those tumours greater than 1–2 cm in diameter, then surgery should be considered. The aim of surgery is to remove the tumour without traumatising the facial nerve, and when indicated to preserve hearing. Three surgical approaches are possible (translabyrinthine, retrosigmoid and middle cranial fossa) and the type depends on the level of remaining hearing. If the hearing is not serviceable or useful then a translabyrinthine approach is performed (House & Hitselberger, 1985). The main advantage of this technique is that there is minimal brain retraction and the access is excellent, although all remaining hearing is sacrificed.

If the hearing is useful, then the tumour is approached either via a retrosigmoid or a middle cranial fossa approach in an attempt to preserve the hearing (Sekhar et al., 1996). The main disadvantage of the former is that there is cerebellar retraction while the latter is technically demanding.

Stereotactic radiosurgery entails the accurate application of radiotherapy from an external source to the site of the acoustic neuroma with minimal surrounding tissue damage (Kondziolka et al., 1998). This is a relatively new technique that is currently undergoing rigorous evaluation.

Physical management

Physiotherapy assessment of the vestibular patient

The assessment of the vestibular patient is a crucial prerequisite to any treatment. Although many aspects of the examination are similar to that of any physiotherapy assessment, there are specific tests that should be performed. The patient should be made aware that aspects of the examination often provoke symptoms and leave the patient feeling unwell. A history is taken of the present complaint, the nature, severity, duration and irritability of the problem, aggravating and alleviating factors. True vertigo should be differentiated from dizziness, light-headedness, giddiness and disequilibrium.

A history should also be taken of any other associated symptoms (Table 24.1). It should be ascertained how long the patient has had the symptoms, and what was the initial presentation. Any previous episodes and their outcomes should be explored. Pertinent past medical history includes problems with vision, other neurological or musculoskeletal problems and any previous vestibular surgery.

The effects of the problem on the patient's occupational and leisure activities should also be noted. Medications, type, dosage and effect and plans for cessation should also be discussed. Results of any investigations should be noted.

Physical examination The examination of the vestibular patient includes assessment of posture, tone, power, sensation, proprioception, co-ordination and reflexes. Specific oculomotor and positional tests are also carried out (Table 24.3 and Fig. 24.4). The cervical spine is always assessed prior to the oculomotor examination and a musculoskeletal examination is carried out on the lumbar spine and extremities if indicated. Gait and balance are then assessed (Table 24.4).

Outcome measures Outcome measures can include measures of balance and gait (Table 24.4). Questionnaires which allow patients to rate their symptoms and the resultant effect on daily life such as the Vertigo Handicap Questionnaire and Vertigo Symptom Scale (Yardley et al., 1992) or the Dizziness Handicap Inventory (Jacobson & Newman, 1990) are also very useful.

Physiotherapy management of vestibular disorders

Vestibular rehabilitation aims to:

- educate the patient
- maximise vestibular compensation, thus reducing vertigo, dizziness and nausea
- improve balance and gait
- reduce or alleviate secondary problems such as physical deconditioning and neck or back pain.

Patient groups that benefit most from vestibular rehabilitation are shown in Table 24.5 and there are now many texts on this subject alone (Shepard & Telian, 1996; Luxon & Davies, 1997; Herdman, 2000).

A vestibular rehabilitation programme can involve treating many impairments and possible components of a programme are summarised in Table 24.6. Patients

Table 24.4 Balance assessment and outcome measures

Balance and gait outcome measures	Balance tests are timed for a period of up to 30 s and the best of three attempts is recorded for assessment of change over time
Romberg (Black et al., 1982)	Patient stands with feet close together and eyes closed. This test can also be performed with eyes open in very severely impaired patients

Tandem Romberg
    Eyes open
    Eyes closed
	Patient stands heel to toe with preferred foot in front

One-leg stance (Bohannon et al., 1984)
    Eyes open
    Eyes closed
	Patient is asked to stand on one leg with eyes open and then closed

Tandem walking	Patient is asked to walk heel to toe on a line for a distance of 1 m and the number of steps off the line are counted
Functional reach test (Duncan et al., 1990; Mann et al., 1996)	This is the furthest distance that the patient can reach without moving the feet
Berg Balance Scale (Berg et al., 1989)	A 14-item functional balance assessment (see Box 3.6, p. 35)
Tinetti's Balance Performance Assessment (Tinetti, 1986)	A 13-item functional balance assessment and a nine-item gait assessment
Clinical assessment of postural integration of balance (CTSIB) (Shumway-Cook & Horak, 1986; Cohen et al., 1993) 1. Stand with feet together, eyes open 2. Stand with feet together, eyes closed 3. Stand with feet together and visual conflict dome 4. Stand on foam, eyes open 5. Stand on foam, eyes closed 6. Stand on foam with visual conflict dome	A six-item test of balance involving manipulation of visual, vestibular and somatosensory systems. The visual conflict dome is a modified Japanese lantern placed over the patient's head which gives erroneous information about the vertical and thus reduces the ability of the patient to use visual cues for balance. This test has been modified to contain items 1, 2, 4 and 5
Posturography	Computerised system using a specialised forceplate and visual surround which measures postural sway in conditions similar to the CTSIB

CTSIB, Clinical Test of Sensory Interaction and Balance.

often report that they think their symptoms are too severe to have a benign cause and fear a more sinister pathology (most commonly a brain tumour), despite the latter being excluded by the medical team. The first encounter with the patient thus usually requires education and reassurance about the problem.

It is essential that the patient receives an explanation about the principles of vestibular compensation and the importance of movement for this process as patients have usually been avoiding symptom-provoking movements and postures.

Shepard & Telian (1995) found that patients who received an individualised vestibular rehabilitation programme specific to their particular signs and symptoms achieved a better outcome than those who received a more generic-type programme.

Vestibular paresis/hypofunction The patient with unilateral vestibular hypofunction who has failed to compensate usually has three main problems:

1. decreased gain of the VOR, leading to decreased gaze stability during head movement
2. vertigo or associated symptoms at rest or during head/self movement (often termed motion sensitivity)
3. impaired balance and gait.

Each of these require separate treatment approaches. Gaze stability is promoted with eye–head co-ordination exercises (Szturm et al., 1994; Herdman et al., 1995). For example, the patient is asked to look at a stationary object (this could be a letter pinned to a wall) and move the head from side to side and then up and down, keeping the object in focus. The patient is

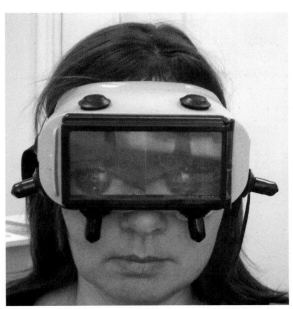

Figure 24.4 Frenzel lenses, used to remove visual fixation and magnify the eyes for ease of observation (see Table 24.3).

Table 24.5 Patient groups that benefit from vestibular rehabilitation (Shepard & Telian, 1995)

Patients with non-compensated peripheral vestibular disorders

Benign paroxysmal positional vertigo (BPPV)

Stable central vestibular lesions or mixed central and peripheral lesions (e.g. head injury)

Multifactorial balance abnormalities (e.g. elderly)

Postablative surgery (e.g. acoustic neuroma resection, labyrinthectomy)

Table 24.6 Components of a vestibular rehabilitation programme

Assessment
Education
Habituation exercises
Adaptation exercises
Balance and gait re-education
Particle-repositioning manoeuvres (e.g. Epley's; see Fig. 24.6)
Physical conditioning
Relaxation
Breathing exercises
Treatment of neck and back pain
Correction of postural abnormalities

instructed to do the exercise for a minute. The speed and duration of the exercise are increased as tolerated and the exercise can be made more difficult by having the object move out of phase with the head. The patient moves an object he or she is holding to the left and the head to the right, keeping the eyes on the object at all times, and then performs the opposite movement.

Motion sensitivity is decreased by exercises that aim to habituate the patient to movement (Norre & De Weerdt, 1980; Norre & Beckers, 1989; Johansson et al., 2001). The Cawthorne Cooksey exercises or modifications of them (Luxon & Davies, 1997) can be taught (an example of a Cawthorne Cooksey exercise programme is shown in Fig. 24.5). It is first determined what head, eye or body movements bring on the patient's symptoms. Patients are then instructed to carry out these movements three to four times a day. Each movement or exercise is repeated just to the point where symptoms begin to come on. Gradually over time the patient habituates to the movement and either the duration or the complexity of the exercise can be increased. It is very important that patients are warned that they should not feel excessively symptomatic after performing the exercises, as this may decrease compliance. Exercises should be graded gently and performed only as tolerated. In the early stages, patients may only be able to perform one exercise at a time.

Balance and gait re-education Balance exercises are customised to the patient, depending on the findings of the balance assessment, and are included in the home exercise programme. For example, if a patient has a particular dependence on vision and it is known that there is some remaining vestibular function, the therapist might choose to include exercises that minimise visual inputs in order for the patient to utilise and strengthen remaining vestibular function. Exercises with eyes closed and/or on an unstable surface (such as a foam cushion) would be included in such a programme.

Balance exercises can be graded by progressively decreasing the area of the base of support, increasing the height of the centre of gravity from the supporting surface or manipulation of the environment by the removal or alteration of visual (for example, eyes closed or head moving) or somatosensory (for example, on foam or on an uneven surface) cues. The complexity of balance tasks is progressively increased over time as the patient improves. For example, when a patient is able to walk on the flat with good postural control, he or she can be asked to walk at a faster pace, walk on an incline or walk while talking or moving the head up and down or from side to side. Care should be taken in the initial stages to avoid falls. This is best achieved by having a

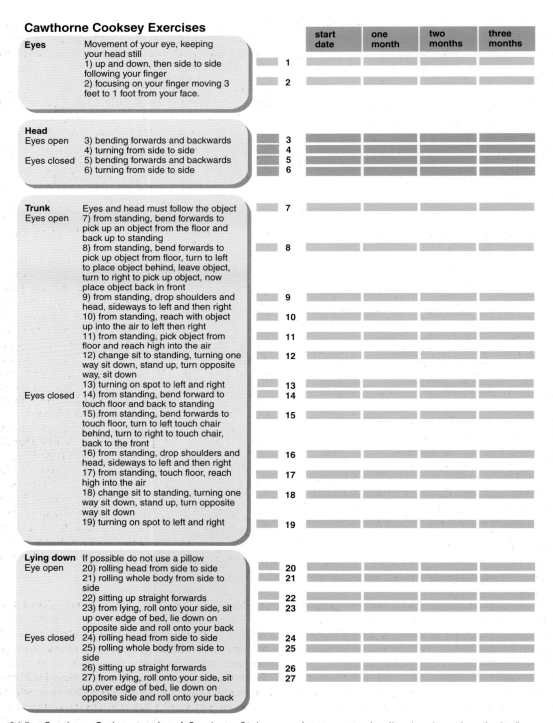

Cawthorne Cooksey Exercises

		start date	one month	two months	three months

Eyes
Movement of your eye, keeping your head still
1) up and down, then side to side following your finger
2) focusing on your finger moving 3 feet to 1 foot from your face.

Head
Eyes open   3) bending forwards and backwards
4) turning from side to side
Eyes closed   5) bending forwards and backwards
6) turning from side to side

Trunk
Eyes open   Eyes and head must follow the object
7) from standing, bend forwards to pick up an object from the floor and back up to standing
8) from standing, bend forwards to pick up object from floor, turn to left to place object behind, leave object, turn to right to pick up object, now place object back in front
9) from standing, drop shoulders and head, sideways to left and then right
10) from standing, reach with object up into the air to left then right
11) from standing, pick object from floor and reach high into the air
12) change sit to standing, turning one way sit down, stand up, turn opposite way, sit down
13) turning on spot to left and right
Eyes closed   14) from standing, bend forward to touch floor and back to standing
15) from standing, bend forwards to touch floor, turn to left touch chair behind, turn to right to touch chair, back to the front
16) from standing, drop shoulders and head, sideways to left and then right
17) from standing, touch floor, reach high into the air
18) change sit to standing, turning one way sit down, stand up, turn opposite way sit down
19) turning on spot to left and right

Lying down   If possible do not use a pillow
Eye open   20) rolling head from side to side
21) rolling whole body from side to side
22) sitting up straight forwards
23) from lying, roll onto your side, sit up over edge of bed, lie down on opposite side and roll onto your back
Eyes closed   24) rolling head from side to side
25) rolling whole body from side to side
26) sitting up straight forwards
27) from lying, roll onto your side, sit up over edge of bed, lie down on opposite side and roll onto your back

Figure 24.5.   Cawthorne Cooksey exercises. A Cawthorne Cooksey exercise programme is tailored to the patient. At the first assessment the patient is asked to perform each exercise five times and rate symptoms on a scale (0 = no symptoms, 1 = mild symptoms, 2 = moderate symptoms, 3 = severe symptoms). The patient is then given a home exercise programme doing only the exercises that cause mild to moderate symptoms. The exercises are then progressed as tolerated over time (see text for more details). (Reproduced from Luxon & Davies (1997), with kind permission of Whurr Publishers.)

relative or friend supervise or by having a supportive surface such as a wall or chair nearby.

Balance has been shown to improve with exercise in several randomised, controlled studies (Horak et al., 1992; Mruzek et al., 1995; Strupp et al., 1998; Yardley et al., 1998b).

Gait and postural re-education is also important. Patients commonly adopt abnormal postures whilst moving, and decrease the amplitude of head movement. They will turn en bloc rather than dissociating their head from their trunk. Retraining can include use of verbal and visual feedback. Gait aids may be necessary in the acute stages.

The patient with a central vestibular loss requires a similar therapeutic approach but recovery will be slower and more incomplete (Shepard & Telian, 1995; Furman & Whitney, 2000).

The mainstay of treatment of the patient with bilateral vestibular loss is to encourage substitution of visual and proprioceptive systems for vestibular function (Krebs et al., 1993). It is thought that these patients may be able to substitute pursuit and saccadic eye movements (generated by the CNS) and the cervico-ocular reflex to maintain gaze stability (Bronstein & Hood, 1986). Thus, balance exercises and functional activities incorporating saccadic and pursuit eye movements are included in programmes for these patients (Herdman, 2000).

Management of BPPV The management of the patient with BPPV is based on manoeuvres or exercises which remove the otoconia responsible for the vertiginous episodes from the involved canal back into the utricle (Harvey et al., 1994; Steenerson & Cronin, 1996; Benyon, 1997; Herdman et al., 2000). For canalithiasis (the otoconia are free-floating), Epley's manoeuvre or a modified version is commonly used (Fig. 24.6). The head is moved through different positions so that the otoconia move out of the involved SCC.

After Epley's has been performed, patients are instructed to avoid quick head movements and the supine position for 48 h. In 90% of cases one manoeuvre will alleviate symptoms, but a small number of patients will require it twice or three times. Recurrence of symptoms can occur with reports of anywhere between 3 and 21% of patients (Benyon, 1997). Patients can be taught to self-perform the manoeuvre.

If treatment is not successful or cupulolithiasis (i.e the otoconia are adherent to the cupula) is thought to be the problem, the Brandt & Daroff (1980) exercises can be performed (Fig. 24.7). These exercises aim to free crystals from the cupula and disperse particles back into the otolith. They are repeated every three waking hours until the vertigo subsides and terminated after two consecutive vertigo-free days. Recently it has been found that patients with BPPV can also have balance impairment (Blatt et al., 2000), therefore balance re-education should also form a part of rehabilitation for BBPV.

Secondary problems Patients will often complain of neck pain and, less commonly, back pain associated with vertigo. Stiffness of the cervical spine caused by avoidance of head movements is frequently observed and these patients often benefit from joint mobilisations, electrotherapy and heat therapy. Cervical spine symptoms may be severe enough to interfere with habituation exercises and therefore should be treated. Habituation exercises that avoid cervical spine movement, such as eye movements or whole-body movements, may be performed until cervical spine symptoms improve.

Physical deconditioning can also occur as patients understandably limit any activity that causes an increase in their symptoms. Promoting exercise through a graduated walking programme is usually the easiest and most acceptable way for patients to increase their exercise tolerance again. Walking is also a functional and relevant context for the patient (as opposed to a static exercise bike, for example) and head movements and visual stimulation during walking probably assist the process of vestibular compensation. As patients improve they should be encouraged to resume their normal sporting or leisure activities as tolerated.

The physiotherapist can also intervene in the symptoms of anxiety and hyperventilation. Simple education on breathing, control of breathing (breathing exercises), the adverse effects of hyperventilation on cerebral blood flow and recognition of hyperventilation can help the patient recognise and control the problem. Relaxation classes or tapes can be used to teach the patient control of anxiety and associated muscular tension. Where significant anxiety exists or the patient complains of agoraphobia, psychological evaluation and treatment are indicated.

SPECIALIST CENTRES AND SUPPORT GROUPS

There are now many centres worldwide that specialise in vestibular rehabilitation and recently a physiotherapy clinical interest group, the Association of Physiotherapists with an Interest in Vestibular Rehabilitation (ACPIVR), has been set up in the UK (contact the Chartered Society of Physiotherapy (www.csp.org.uk) for details). This interest group has a database of physiotherapists who have specialised in vestibular rehabilitation. The Royal National Institute for Deaf People (www.rnid.org.uk) and British Brain and Spine Foundation (www.bbsf.or.uk) both produce patient

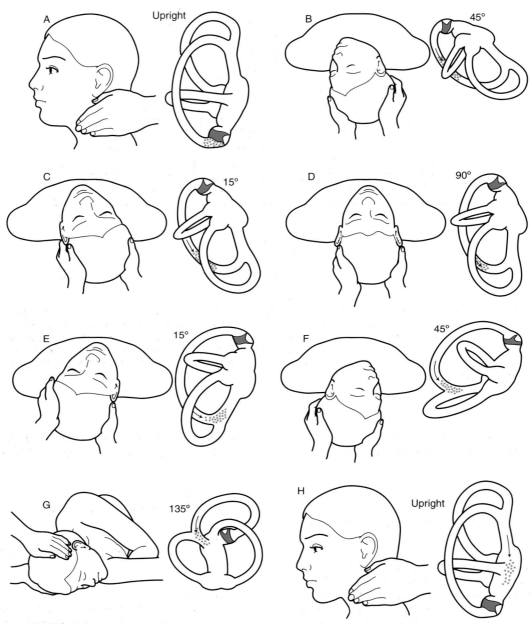

Figure 24.6 Modified Epley's manoeuvre for left-sided benign paroxysmal positional vertigo (BPPV). The patient is brought into the left Hallpike position (A, B). The head is then slowly rotated in a stepwise position to the opposite side (C–F). As this is happening, the patient turns on to the right side so that the head has turned a total of 135° (G). The head is maintained in 30° extension throughout the manoeuvre. The patient is then brought up into sitting (H). (Reproduced from Harvey et al. (1994), with permission.)

information leaflets on different aspects of vestibular and hearing problems. The Ménière's Society also provides support. See the Appendix for contact details of these organisations.

CONCLUSION

Vestibular rehabilitation is a developing area in physiotherapy. It is important that patients with

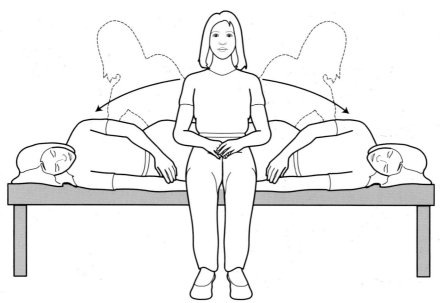

Figure 24.7 Brandt–Daroff exercises for benign paroxysmal positional vertigo (BPPV). The patient is instructed to sit in the middle of the bed with the eyes closed and turn the head 30° away from the affected side. This places the posterior semicircular canal in the coronal plane. The patient is then instructed to lie down quickly on to the affected side, keeping the head in the same position, and wait until vertigo develops and settles (movement of the otoconia crystals in the canal), usually after 30 s. The patient is then instructed to sit up and, after any further vertigo settles, lies down in the mirror-image head position. (Reproduced, with permission, from the American Medical Association (copyrighted 1980).)

vestibular problems are given access to this valuable and increasingly evidence-based treatment.

CASE HISTORIES

CASE 1: PERIPHERAL VESTIBULAR NEURITIS

History

Mr V, a 68-year-old, presented with a 6-month history of vertigo that was aggravated by walking, bending down, looking up and turning around. He described that his head constantly felt 'all mixed up and muzzy'. His symptoms began with a sudden onset of severe vertigo, vomiting and unsteadiness. He was then unable to walk unaided and was confined to bed for 4 days. Over the following few weeks his symptoms gradually decreased in severity but remained problematic.

Investigations

An MRI was normal. Hearing was normal. Electro-nystagmography (ENG) showed no positional nystagmus and all tests of smooth pursuit and saccades were normal. Caloric testing demonstrated a 100% right

canal paresis with an 88% directional preponderance to the left. A diagnosis of a right peripheral vestibular neuritis was made.

Medications

Betahistine (Serc) and prochlorperazine (Stemetil) b.i.d.

Past medical history

Prostate surgery 2 years ago. No previous history of vertigo.

Social history

Mr V was a retired accountant and was unable to pursue his usual hobbies of gardening and walking since the onset of his symptoms.

Physiotherapy assessment

Findings were normal on examination of tone, power, sensation, proprioception, reflexes and co-ordination. There were no cervical spine symptoms and the range of movement of the cervical spine was pain-free and within normal limits. On oculomotor examination there was no spontaneous nystagmus (in room light or with Frenzel lenses on). Smooth pursuit and saccadic eye movements were normal. The VOR cancellation test was normal. VOR testing revealed a catch-up saccadic movement of the eyes to the left when the head was rapidly moved to the right. Positional tests (Hallpike–Dix test) were negative bilaterally. A normal gait pattern was observed. The Romberg test was normal. Mr V was unable to maintain tandem Romberg with his eyes closed. One-leg stance (OLS) test times were normal with eyes open but were decreased with eyes closed (left OLS: 3 s/right OLS: 2 s). He could tandem walk a 1-m line but took four steps off the line. Mr V had difficulty with item 5 (he was only able to maintain the position for 5 s) of the Clinical Assessment of Postural Integration and Balance.

Assessment of motion sensitivity

When Mr V performed repeated tracking movements with his eyes he reported moderate vertigo. He also reported severe vertigo with repeated head movements in all planes with eyes open and closed, bending down to touch the floor and turning on the spot.

Physiotherapy treatment

Mr V was firstly given an explanation of why he was experiencing his symptoms and the process of vestibular compensation. He agreed that his main problems were motion sensitivity (i.e. vertigo provoked by movement) and balance impairment. His treatment programme aimed to increase the gain of the VOR through adaptation exercises and to decrease motion sensitivity.

Mr V carried out an exercise programme four times daily. Initially exercises consisted of focusing on a business card in his hand whilst moving his head from side to side and then up and down at a speed that kept the letters in focus. He also carried out habituation exercises. These included visually tracking his own thumb as he moved it from side to side and then up and down while keeping his head steady. Other exercises included head and cervical spine movements (rotation and flexion and extension), which were performed with his eyes open and closed. Each exercise was only performed until vertigo began to develop. Over 4 months the speed, complexity and duration of exercises were gradually increased as symptoms lessened. Mr V was also provided with a balance exercise programme that he performed daily. He was encouraged to discuss cessation of betahistine and prochlorperazine with his doctor and decrease use over time. He had discontinued all use of vestibular medications 2 months later.

Mr V steadily improved and had five sessions of treatment over 6 months. Two months into treatment he developed a common cold and reported that his symptoms temporarily worsened. At his final visit he reported he felt '85% of normal'. His vertigo symptom scale and vertigo handicap questionnaire scores demonstrated a significant improvement. His balance had improved, demonstrated by an increase in time on balance tests. He had resumed his hobbies.

CASE 2: BENIGN PAROXYSMAL POSITIONAL VERTIGO

History

Ms R, a 36-year-old, presented with a 2-week history of episodic vertigo which came on one morning after getting up. She described the vertigo as a severe spinning sensation associated with severe nausea. Due to the intensity of the symptoms she had been admitted to hospital for 2 days. Since the initial onset she reported several episodes of vertigo, which typically lasted 3–4 s and were associated with head movement, particularly rolling over in bed from right to left or bending down. She also described feeling unsteady and tired. Her symptoms were worse in the morning.

Investigations

A computed tomographic scan was normal. No vestibular function tests had been performed.

Medications

Prochlorperazine (Stemetil) prescribed on admission to hospital but discontinued after a week.

Social history

Ms R was a secretary and had a sedentary lifestyle.

Past medical history

Appendectomy, tonsillectomy.

Physiotherapy assessment

Findings were normal on examination of tone, power, sensation, proprioception, reflexes and co-ordination. There were no cervical spine symptoms. Oculomotor examination was unremarkable except for the left Hallpike–Dix test. This reproduced the spinning sensation and was accompanied by a rotary nystagmus (beating up and towards the left ear) which came on with a latency of 10 s and lasted for 15 s. Gait was normal. On balance testing, there was impairment of the left and right OLS tests performed with eyes closed. All other balance tests were normal. Symptoms were consistent with a diagnosis of left posterior SCC BPPV.

Physiotherapy treatment

Following explanation of the likely cause of the symptoms and treatment, a modified Epley's manoeuvre was performed for the left posterior SCC (Fig. 24.6). The patient was instructed to try and maintain the head upright for 3 days (i.e. avoid bending) and to avoid sleeping flat. Balance exercises were prescribed to perform at home.

A week later Ms R reported she had been completely symptom-free since the first visit. The left Hallpike–Dix test was normal (no nystagmus or vertigo). Ms R was advised to continue with her balance exercises and to contact the department if there were any recurrences of vertigo.

ACKNOWLEDGEMENTS

Dara Meldrum would like to acknowledge the expert teaching of Dr Susan Herdman and Dr Ronald Tusa (Emory University, Atlanta, Georgia, USA).

References

American Medical Association. Physical therapy for benign paroxysmal positional vertigo. *Arch Otolaryngol* 1980, **106**:185.

Baloh RW, Honrubia V, Jacobson K. Benign positional vertigo: clinical and oculographic features in 240 cases. *Neurology* 1987, **37**:371–378.

Baloh R, Jacobson K, Honrubia V. Horizontal semicircular canal variant of benign positional vertigo. *Neurology* 1993, **43**:2542–2549.

Black FO, Wall C, Rockette H et al. Normal subject postural sway during the Romberg test. *Am J Otolaryngol* 1982, **3**:309–318.

Blakley BW, Goebel J. The meaning of the word "vertigo". *Otolaryngol Head Neck Surg* 2001, **125**:147–150.

Blatt PJ, Georgakakis GA, Herdman SJ et al. Effect of canalith repositioning maneuver on resolving postural instability in patients with BPPV. *Am J Otolol* 2000, **21**:356–363.

Benyon GJ. A review of management of benign paroxysmal positional vertigo by exercise therapy and by repositioning manoeuvres. *Br J Audiol* 1997, **31**:11–26.

Berg K, Wood-Dauphinee S, Williams JI, Gayton D. Measuring balance in the elderly: preliminary development of an instrument. *Physiother Can* 1989, **41**:304–311.

Bohannon R, Larkin P, Cook A et al. Decreased in timed balance test scores with aging. *Phys Ther* 1984, **64**:1067–1070.

Brandt T. Management of vestibular disorders. *J Neurol* 2000, **247**:491–499.

Brandt T, Daroff RB. Physical therapy for benign paroxysmal positional vertigo. *Arch Otolaryngol* 1980, **106**:484–485.

Bronstein A, Hood J. The cervico-ocular reflex in normal subjects and patients with absent vestibular function. *Brain Res* 1986, **373**:399–408.

Cawthorne T. Vestibular injuries. *Proc R Soc Med* 1945, **39**:270–273.

Cohen H. Special senses 2: The vestibular system. In: Cohen H, ed. *Neuroscience for Rehabilitation*, 2nd edn. Philadelphia: Lippincott Williams & Wilkins; 1999: 149–167.

Cohen H, Blatchly CA, Gombash LL. A study of the clinical test of sensory interaction and balance. *Phys Ther* 1993, **73**:346–353.

Colledge NR, Wilson JA, Macintyre CC et al. The prevalence and characteristics of dizziness in an elderly community. *Age Ageing* 1994, **23**:117–120.

Cooksey F. Rehabilitation in vestibular injuries. *Proc R Soc Med* 1945, **39**:273–278.

Courjon JH, Jeannerod M, Ossuzio I et al. The role of vision in compensation of vestibulo-ocular reflex after hemi-labryrinthectomy in the cat. *Exp Brain Res* 1977, **28**:235–248.

Curthoys IS. Vestibular compensation and substitution. *Curr Opin Neurol* 2000, **13**:27–30.

De la Meilleure G, Dehaene I, Depondt M et al. Benign paroxysmal vertigo of the horizontal canal. *J Neurol Neurosurg Psychiatry* 1996, **60**:68–71.

Duncan PW, Weiner DK, Chandler J et al. Functional reach: a new clinical measure of balance. *J Gerontol* 1990, **45**:M192–M197.

Epley JM. New dimensions of benign paroxysmal positional vertigo. *Otolaryngol Head Neck Surg* 1980, **88**:599–605.

Furman JM, Whitney SL. Central causes of dizziness. *Phys Ther* 2000, **2**:179–187.

Harvey SA, Hain TC, Adamiec MS. Modified liberatory manoeuvre: effective treatment for benign paroxysmal positional vertigo. *Laryngoscope* 1994, **104**:1206–1212.

Herdman SJ. *Vestibular Rehabilitation*, 2nd edn. *Contemporary Perspectives in Rehabilitation*. Philadelphia: FA Davis; 2000.

Herdman SJ, Clendaniel RA, Mattox DE et al. Vestibular adaptation exercises and recovery: acute stage after acoustic neuroma resection. *Otolaryngol Head Neck Surg* 1995, **133**:77–87.

Herdman SJ, Blatt PJ, Schubert MC. Vestibular rehabilitation of patients with vestibular hypofunction or with benign paroxysmal positional vertigo. *Curr Opin Neurol* 2000, **13**:39–43.

Horak FB, Jones-Rycewicz C, Black O et al. Effects of vestibular rehabilitation on dizziness and imbalance. *Otolaryngol Head Neck Surg* 1992, **106**:175–180.

House WF, Hitselberger WF. The neurotologist view of the surgical management of acoustic neuromas. *Clin Neurosurg* 1985, **32**:214–222.

Jacobson GP, Newman CW. The development of the dizziness handicap inventory. *Arch Orolaryngol Head Neck Surg* 1990, **116**:424–427.

Johansson M, Akerlund D, Larsen HC et al. Randomised controlled trial of vestibular rehabilitation combined with cognitive behavioural therapy for dizziness in older people. *Otolaryngol Head Neck Surg* 2001, **125**:151–156.

Kondziolka D, Lunsford LD, McLaughlin MR et al. Long-term outcomes after radiosurgery for acoustic neuromas. *N Engl J Med* 1998, **339**:1426–1433.

Krebs D, Gill-Body K, Riley P et al. 1993 Double-blind, placebo controlled trial of rehabilitation for bilateral vestibular hypofunction; preliminary report. *Otolaryngol Head Neck Surg* 1993, **109**:735–741.

Lacour M, Xerri C. Vestibular compensation: new perspectives. In: Flohr H, Precht W, eds. *Lesion Induced Neuronal Plasticity in Sensorimotor Systems*. Berlin: Springer; 1981:240–253.

Luxon L, Davies RA. *Handbook of Vestibular Rehabilitation*. London: Whurr Publishers; 1997.

Mann GC, Whitney SL, Redfern MS et al. Functional reach and single leg stance in patients with peripheral vestibular disorders. *J Vestib Res* 1996, **6**:342–353.

Moffat DA. Endolymphatic sac surgery: analysis of 100 operations. *Clin Otol* 1994, **19**:261–266.

Moffat D, Ballagh RH. Meniere's disease. In: Booth JB, ed. *Scott Brown's Otolaryngology*, vol. 3, *Otology*. Oxford: Butterworth-Heinemann; 1997:1–50.

Monsell EM, Balkany TA, Gates GA et al. Committee on hearing and equilibrium guidelines for the diagnosis and evaluation of therapy in Meniere's disease. *Otolaryngol Head Neck Surg* 1998, **113**:181–185.

Mruzek M, Barin K, Nichols DS et al. Effects of vestibular rehabilitation and social reinforcement on recovery following ablative vestibular surgery. *Laryngoscope* 1995, **105**:686–692.

Nedzelski JM, Schessel DA, Bryce GE et al. Chemical labyrinthectomy: local application of gentamicin for the treatment of unilateral Meniere's disease. *Am J Otol* 1992, **13**:18–22.

Norre ME, Beckers A. Vestibular habituation training; exercise treatment for vertigo based upon the habituation effect. *Otolaryngol Head Neck Surg* 1989, **101**:14–19.

Norre ME, De Weerdt W. Treatment of vertigo based on habituation. *J Laryngol Otol* 1980, **94**:971–977.

Parnes LS, McClure JA. Posterior semicircular canal occlusion for intractable benign paroxysmal positional vertigo. *Ann Otol Rhinol Laryngol* 1990, **99**:330–334.

Rudge P, Chambers BR. Physiological basis for enduring vestibular symptoms. *J Neurol Neurosurg Psychiatry* 1982, **45**:126–130.

Savundra P, Luxon LM. The physiology of equilibrium and its application to the dizzy patient. In: Gleeson M, ed. *Scott Brown's Otolaryngology*, vol. 1: *Basic Sciences*. Oxford: Butterworth-Heinemann; 1997:1–65.

Sekhar LN, Gormley WB, Wright DC. The best treatment for vestibular schwannoma (acoustic neuroma): microsurgery or radiosurgery? *Am J Otol* 1996, **17**:676–689.

Shepard NT, Telian SA. Programmatic vestibular rehabilitation. *Otolaryngol Head Neck Surg* 1995, **112**:173–181.

Shepard NT, Telian SA. *Practical Management of the Balance Disorder Patient*. San Diego, CA: Singular; 1996.

Shumway-Cook A, Horak F. Assessing the influence of sensory interaction on balance. *Phys Ther* 1986, **66**:1540–1548.

Sloane PD. Dizziness in primary care. Results from the National Ambulatory Medical Care Survey. *J Fam Pract* 1989;**29**:33–38.

Steenerson RL, Cronin GW. Comparison of the canalith repositioning procedure and vestibular habituation training in forty patients with benign paroxysmal positional vertigo. *Otolaryngol Head Neck Surg* 1996, **114**:61–64.

Strupp M, Arbusow V, Maag KP et al. Vestibular exercises improve central vestibulospinal compensation after vestibular neuritis. *Neurology* 1998, **51**:838–844.

Szturm T, Ireland DJ, Lessing-Turner M. Comparison of different exercise programs in the rehabilitation of patients with chronic peripheral vestibular dysfunction. *J Vestib Res* 1994, **4**:461–479.

Tinetti ME. Performance-oriented assessment of mobility problems in elderly patients. *J Am Geriatr Soc* 1986, **34**:119–126.

Walsh RM, Bath AP, Cullen JR et al. Long-term results of posterior semicircular canal occlusion for intractable benign paroxysmal positional vertigo. *Clin Otol* 1999, **24**:316–323.

Walsh RM, Bath AP, Bance ML et al. The role of conservative management of vestibular schwannomas. *Clin Otol* 2000, **25**:28–39.

Yardley L, Masson E, Verschuur C et al. Symptoms, anxiety and handicap in dizzy patients: development of the vertigo symptom scale. *J Pyschosom Res* 1992, **36**: 731–741.

Yardley L, Owen N, Nazareth I et al. Prevalence and presentation of dizziness in a general practice community sample of working age people. *Br J Gen Pract* 1998a, **48**:1131–1135.

Yardley L, Beech S, Zander L et al. A randomized controlled trial of exercise therapy for dizziness and vertigo in primary care. *Br J Gen Pract* 1998b, **48**:1136–1140.

Zee DS. Perspectives on the pharmacotherapy of vertigo. *Arch Otolaryngol* 1985, **111**:609–612.

Zee DS. Vestibular adaptation In: Herdman SJ, ed. *Vestibular Rehabilitation*, 2nd edn. *Contemporary Perspectives in Rehabilitation*. Philadelphia: FA Davis; 2000:77–87.

Chapter 25

Physical management of abnormal tone and movement

H Thornton   C Kilbride

INTRODUCTION

Muscle tone is an integral part of movement and posture, and may be abnormally increased (hypertonic) or decreased (hypotonic). The importance of tone abnormalities has been a subject of debate, at both a physiological level and within the wider discussion of its relevance to physiotherapists treating neurological patients. Hypertonia is widely referred to as spasticity and described as a motor disorder characterised by a velocity-dependent increase in tonic stretch reflexes (Intercollegiate Working Party for Stroke, 2002).

More recently, the resistive tonal change seen in hemiplegia following stroke has been described as 'spastic dystonia', being attributed to a presence of continuous activity in the absence of movement via an efferent drive (Edwards, 2002, p. 90). As the evidence base continues to expand, it has shown that there are both peripheral and central components to this phenomenon, therefore both should be considered within the physical management and treatment of patients.

In considering the peripheral components, it is established that length-associated changes occur in the shortened (and lengthened) muscle with a loss of compliance and remodelling of connective tissue within and around muscle (see Ch. 30). Contracture, caused by muscle shortening, has been shown to be associated with loss of sarcomeres (reduction of muscle fibre length; Goldspink & Williams, 1990) but can also occur without such loss. It has been suggested that it could be due to fibre atrophy (loss of width; Shortland et al., 2002). The implications of these different mechanisms are discussed below ('Muscle strengthening') and in Chapter 29.

Changes in the muscle itself include thixotrophy (Vattanaslip et al., 2000) and even where there is no neurological damage, the normal resistance to movement is the result of such things as muscle, tendon and connective tissue inherent stiffness. To what extent these peripheral components relate to spasticity is uncertain, and O'Dwyer et al. (1996) found no relationship between spasticity and contracture. Hence, the exact causal relationship between contracture and altered tone remains unclear.

Irrespective of the underlying cause, 'spasticity' is still a recognised term and for this reason will be used throughout this chapter.

Despite the causal uncertainty, physiotherapists manage the effects of tone abnormalities using their skills of clinical reasoning to judge whether increased tone enables or inhibits an individual's function. For example, patients may use extensor spasticity to stand and transfer (Barnes, 2001); conversely, muscle spasms may be so disabling that they hinder comfortable seating. Movement disorders that include dysfunction of muscle tone are complex and challenge the interpretation and identification of which component primarily contributes to the abnormal movement.

Appropriate management of movement dysfunction, irrespective of underlying cause, requires a broad knowledge of different areas, which include:

- motor control
- biomechanics
- kinesiology
- neuroplasticity/neurophysiology
- learning theory
- anatomy and physiology.

This chapter describes the physical management of spasticity and other abnormalities of muscle tone and movement. The pathophysiology of these problems is discussed in Chapter 4. Spasticity occurs in many neurological conditions and its association with those conditions is discussed in the relevant chapters in Sections 2 and 3 of this book.

Key points

- Muscle tone is an integral part of movement and function
- Tone may be abnormally increased or decreased
- Both peripheral and central components of spasticity need to be considered in treatment

---

PHYSICAL MANAGEMENT OF SPASTICITY

Spasticity can limit function and lead to the development of contractures and other forms of soft-tissue adaptation. Management includes manual (hands-on) interventions, specific treatment techniques and education.

Use of movement

Manual techniques are the principal means available to physiotherapists in the management of spasticity. The main aims of physical treatments are:

- maintenance of soft-tissue length and underlying structures
- modulation of tone
- re-education of movement.

The importance of afferent inputs and their effects on muscle tone and postural alignment have been described by Lynch (1991) and Shumway-Cook & Woollacott (1995). Hamdy et al. (2000) demonstrated cross-system plasticity during sensory stimulation to the pharynx, which resulted in a change to motor output.

Johansson (2000) described how neuronal connections and cortical maps are being continually remodelled by experience. Such studies provide direct evidence that altering sensory input can drive motor output, hence handling is a means of altering afferent input to the patient.

Maintenance of soft-tissue length

The need for prevention of soft-tissue adaptive changes, in addition to that of contractures, is gaining wider clinical recognition. Without full range of motion, peripheral changes cause muscle imbalance (see Ch. 30) and this compounds any central motor dysfunction (Ada & Canning, 1990; Singer et al., 2001). The physiotherapist must be able to make an informed analysis of any postural deviations from the norm and recognise non-co-operative alignment of limbs in relation to each other and also to the head and trunk. This information is then used when deciding upon the primary problems and subsequent secondary compensations. For example, shortening or malalignment of muscles may be being masked by compensatory movements (Kilbride & McDonnell, 2000). Stretching has traditionally been used as a technique within a management programme to prevent contractures and early work suggests that there may also be a role for strengthening (Shortland et al., 2002; also see below, 'Muscle strengthening').

Stretching, assisted and passive movements   When handling a patient, the therapist must perceive and adapt to any changes in muscle tone that are a direct response to the movement. Changes in the motor and sensory systems (Nelles et al., 1999) can be expected even when movement is passive. If the patient is active, movement is further enhanced by the muscular contraction (Gandevia et al., 1992). The importance of carrying out active/assisted or passive movements through their full range is paramount and attention should be paid to muscles that cross two or more joints. Movements should be performed with care, confidence and variety and the patient should be taken out of his or her preferred posture. Movement should not be vigorous, and never forced, as this could be a causative factor in heterotopic ossification (HO; Ada & Canning, 1990). However, movement can prevent the development of HO and should be encouraged even when HO is present (Knight et al., 2003).

Modulation of muscle tone   Therapeutic movement and alteration in alignment of body parts are thought to be able to influence muscle tone in other areas indirectly. For example, mobilisation of the trunk and shoulder girdle can lead to a decrease in tone throughout the arm (Davies, 1985; Bobath, 1990). The trunk, head and shoulder and pelvic girdles have been found to be particularly influential in altering muscle tone (Bobath, 1990), although this is largely based on anecdotal evidence. This alteration of muscle tone may be augmented by presynaptic inhibition from the periphery, leading to neuroplastic adaptation (Kidd et al., 1992). Wolpaw & Tennissen (2001) likewise referred to spinal plasticity, that is, activity driven from the periphery and higher centers, leading to persistent changes in the central nervous system (CNS). Additional preliminary findings around therapeutic touch, such as slow stroking on hypertonic muscles in multiple sclerosis, has indicated a reduction in alpha-motor neuron excitability (Brouwer & de Andrade, 1995). The use of rotation is also thought to be important in modulating tone and the additional components of traction and compression can likewise be used (Rosche et al., 1996). Handling that incorporates support and external rotation to the glenohumeral joint has also been shown to improve range of movement in hemiplegic shoulders (Tyson & Chissim, 2002).

Each patient should be assessed for the best response to movement and handling. Table 25.1 illustrates a few basic guidelines for dealing with patients who demonstrate spasticity or other motor dysfunction.

Table 25.1   Handling techniques used in the management of abnormal muscle tone

Disorder	Speed	Range	Repetition	Voice	Base of support	Other
↑ Tone	Slow	Large	Yes	Quiet, minimal	Large	Longitudinal traction
↓ Tone	Moderate to fast	Small	Yes	Brisk, loud	Small	Graded resistance, quick stretch, compression
Dystonia	Varied	Varied	No	Cognitive, verbal cues or automatic	Use of distal key points, i.e. hands and feet	Compression
Rigidity	Slow	Large	Yes	Quiet with verbal cues	Large	Longitudinal traction

Courtesy of Mary Lynch (adapted with permission).

Re-education of movement During treatments, therapists need to ensure they achieve the balance of reducing tone and activating movement. Reduction of tone should be only part of a treatment so as not to affect function inadvertently. Many therapists believe that a 'higher quality of movement translates directly to greater functional ability' (Davidson & Waters, 2000), but this relationship has yet to be empirically proven. Treatment can be based on one or more of the various models of motor control and some of these treatment approaches are discussed in Chapters 21 and 23.

Weight-bearing Standing is a way of maintaining length in the soft tissues, modulating tone and activating extensor activity. To be most effective it should be dynamic to allow tonal changes (Massion, 1994). It is thought to be effective in altering tone via the vestibular system, which is a major source of excitatory influence to extensor muscles, whilst reciprocally inhibiting flexor muscles (Markham, 1987; Brown, 1994). Daily standing can be effective in maintaining tone and reducing the frequency of spasms, whilst maintaining joint range (Bohannon, 1993). Standing can be carried out whilst the patient is still unconscious, if medically stable, using a tilt table. Alternatively in the more awake patient, backslabs (Davies, 1994) or electrical standing frames may be used (Fig. 25.1). With the current emphasis on risk management it is recommended that, where possible and practicable, equipment should be used to minimise the manual handling risk (Association of Chartered Physiotherapists Interested in Neurology, 2001). The use of standing hoists can allow patients to weight-bear regularly in a normal functional task and so should be encouraged (Fig. 25.2).

Weight-bearing with specific alignment can also be achieved through the upper limbs to maintain length and influence tone, but must be performed with extreme care. Normal biomechanical alignment is maintained by external rotation at the shoulder and the wrist joint should not be overstretched (Ryerson & Levit, 1991).

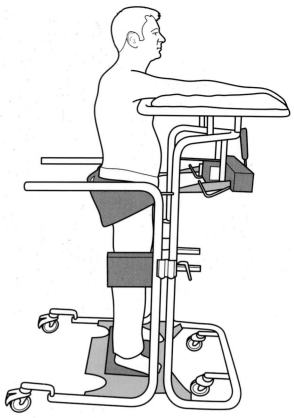

Figure 25.1 Electric standing frames can enable patients to stand for long periods, providing weight-bearing, stretching and promoting activity in the trunk.

ADJUNCTS TO MOVEMENT THERAPY

These include various approaches to management, as well as specific treatment techniques, some of which involve use of equipment:

- positioning and seating
- splinting
- muscle strengthening
- aerobic exercise
- medication

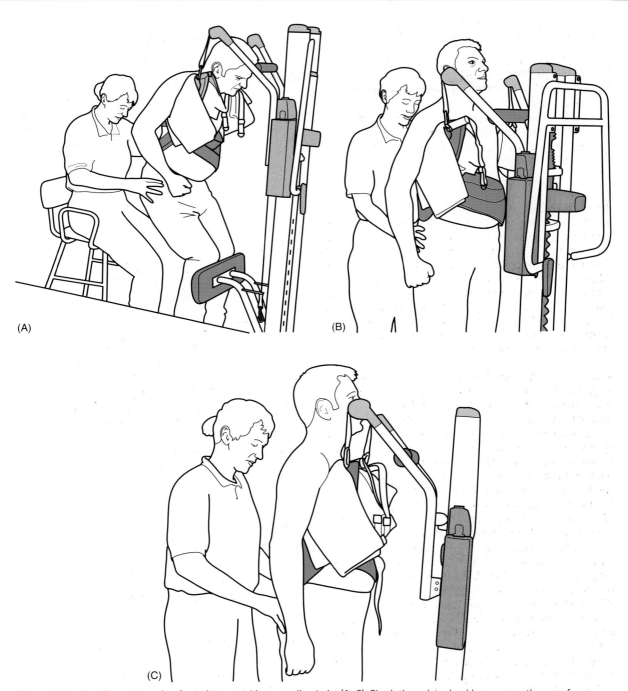

Figure 25.2 A patient progressing from sit to stand in a standing hoist (A–C). Physiotherapists should encourage the use of a standing hoist for suitable patients, as they provide weight-bearing in a functional activity.

- continuous passive motion machines
- hydrotherapy
- thermal treatments
- electrical stimulation
- biofeedback
- acupuncture.

The evidence base for these different modalities is growing and some areas are more advanced than others.

Positioning and seating

Therapeutic positioning and seating are essential to:

- maximise function
- reduce sustained postures
- prevent pressure sores
- maintain soft-tissue length
- reduce discomfort and noxious stimuli
- promote socialisation.

Sufficient support should be provided to allow the patient to cope with gravity and maintain alignment without using excessive abnormal activity, which could otherwise lead to deformity. The reader is referred to Pope (2002) for a detailed review of posture and seating. There has been limited research into its effectiveness (Rowat, 2001) but there is a consensus view in the literature advocating positioning (Goldsmith, 2000; Pope, 2002).

Liaison with occupational therapists, nurses and rehabilitation technicians is essential to ensure optimal provision of equipment. It is important to use appropriate manual handling equipment and techniques when moving patients into positions, to prevent shearing forces causing tissue breakdown (Perr, 1998). Where possible, positioning should be integrated into functional activities in a normal daily routine (Fig. 25.3).

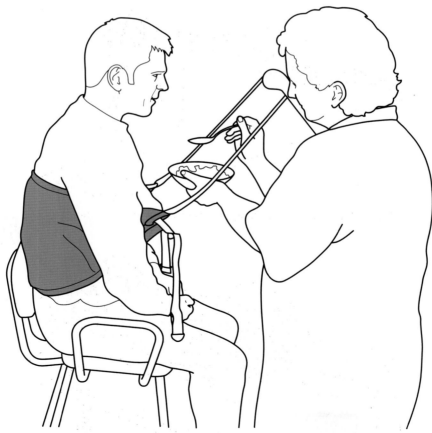

Figure 25.3 This patient uses a perching chair to sit and eat his breakfast, which encourages development of trunk stability and weight-bearing through his lower limbs, whilst carrying out a functional activity.

Positioning in bed

Lying supine is generally thought to encourage extensor spasticity (Davies, 1994). Where this position cannot be avoided, e.g. in a patient with head injury and unstable intracranial pressure (ICP), the physiotherapist must try to minimise its undesirable effects. This may be achieved by breaking up the position, using wedges to prevent mass extension and by increasing the regularity of stretches and limb movement.

The prone position can be helpful for the patient with head injury and mass extension. It can be achieved on a bed but commercially produced beanbags can be useful for gaining good shoulder protraction and for work on head extension (Fig. 25.4). However, patients with tracheotomies or severe contractures may be unable to achieve this position.

In general, side-lying can be used to break up the classic flexion and extension synergies and relieve pressure. Use of pillows, wedges and T-rolls can assist in providing adaptable support and allowing change of position (Fig. 25.5). Charts that illustrate these postures are useful to ensure consistency and for staff education.

Mattresses

Each patient should have a mattress that matches his or her needs. As nursing staff select mattresses, there should be collaboration between physiotherapists and nurses, so that the patient's pressure area and positioning needs are optimised. In many situations an air-filled mattress, designed to relieve pressure, may seem the most appropriate but these mattresses may encourage flexion and lead to flexion contractures, unless careful attention is paid to stretches and standing. Getting the patient out of a bed with an air-filled mattress can also be difficult unless an overhead hoist is available. It is generally preferable to select a mattress that offers adequate pressure relief whilst allowing ease

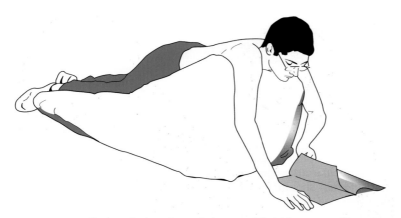

Figure 25.4 The use of a bean bag to induce a comfortable prone position.

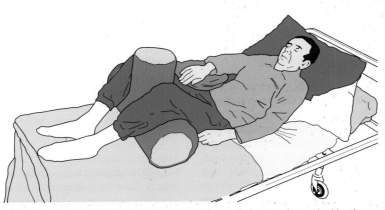

Figure 25.5 The use of a T-roll to prevent lower-limb extension and adduction.

of transfer, and to encourage regular turning and change of position.

For acute head injuries where ICP is a problem, the use of the electronic pressure beds should be considered. These constantly turn the patient, providing changing weight distribution and thereby positive effects on respiratory function. For patients with uncontrolled movements, reduced sensation, cognitive or perceptual deficits, the use of cot sides, or placing the mattress on the floor, should be considered to prevent injury from the patient falling out of bed.

Sitting

The optimal sitting position for a patient with severe disability may be achieved through the provision of a specialist wheelchair with a suitable seating system. Such an arrangement should allow a patient to move or be moved safely, promote socialisation and minimise manual handling.

For seating to be effective it must be matched to the needs of the patient (Perr, 1998; Turner, 2001). Hospitals and rehabilitation units should have a range of wheelchairs and seating systems available for short-term loan. Such an arrangement is particularly beneficial for patients in the acute stage where needs may change rapidly. For example, a patient may initially require a very supportive system, but eventually only need a basic wheelchair. Adjustable seating systems, such as the Matrix system, can be used to accommodate the patient's changing needs (Pope, 2002). Consideration for provision of head and arm supports, with particular attention for supporting hemiplegic shoulders, should be given. Support should be proximal and sufficient to allow the patient to sustain good posture, which can improve carryover of treatment (Chiu, 1995). For patients with a marked neurological deficit, regional specialist seating clinics should be used (see Pope, 2002, for a review).

Electric and patient-propelled wheelchairs

Wheelchair provision promotes independence, although there is a debate regarding self-propulsion in the early stages of rehabilitation (Blower, 1988). In hemiplegic patients, self-propelling a wheelchair is a unilateral activity involving only the sound side. Over time this can result in poor posture, asymmetry, back pain and contractures (Ashburn & Lynch, 1988), and has been shown to increase spasticity (Cornall, 1991). The debate continues as to whether early self-propulsion

should be advocated. Barrett et al. (2001) found no difference between two groups (self-propulsion encouraged or discouraged) on the chosen outcome measures.

Electric wheelchairs provide an alternative to manual chairs. Cognitive and perceptual difficulties can, however, limit a patient's ability to use an electric wheelchair, but should not automatically rule out electric wheelchair provision; each patient must be individually assessed. Other patients requiring electric wheelchairs include those with progressive neurological disorders such as multiple sclerosis and motor neurone disease. Recently the introduction of electric-powered indoor/outdoor chairs (EPIOC) provided by the EPIOC service (Frank et al., 2000) has enhanced the independence in the community of individuals with severe disability.

> **Key points**
>
> - Collaborative teamwork is essential in the management of abnormal tone
> - Effective seating and posture systems are like 'silent therapists'

Splinting

The development of contractures can have a varied timescale, depending on the underlying pathology. The best approach to contractures remains prevention, yet in some patients, despite interventions, aspects of soft-tissue adaptation may occur. O'Dwyer et al. (1996) even suggested that the presence of contractures may in itself influence the development of spasticity. Hence, it remains an important goal to prevent this potentially avoidable feature.

Unconscious immobile patients with altered tone are generally most at risk from contracture. The following factors may be useful indicators to identify other patients at risk:

- evidence of shortening with current intervention
- the patient remains medically unstable and is unable to be placed in standing
- lower-limb fractures
- low Glasgow Coma Scale (GCS) score (<9) and decerebrate rigidity.

The actual mechanism behind splinting/casting is still being investigated but both neural and musculoskeletal effects have been implicated (Stoeckmann, 2001). The length of time required to prevent contracture formation also remains an area of debate; the literature suggests intervals from 30 min to 6 h (Tardieu et al., 1988; Williams, 1990). The reader is also directed to the splinting guidelines produced by the Association of Chartered Physiotherapists Interested in Neurology (1998). Plastering may be precluded if the condition of the patient's skin or vascular system is poor, and in the aggressively behaved patient the cast may present a danger to the patient or others.

Main forms of splinting

The following section outlines the main categories of splinting (for information about application principles, see Edwards & Charlton, 2002, and for patients with severe, chronic contractures, see Young & Nicklin, 2000). Splinting carries the risk of pressure sores and tissue damage, so care should be taken. There is a place for 'off-the-shelf' splints or orthoses, especially in assessment, but often customised splints are required.

Prophylactic splinting Preventive splinting (Stoeckmann, 2001) may be necessary for patients who have a number of the risk factors identified above. If high tone is evident before plastering, a good casting position may be difficult to achieve. In collaboration with medical and nursing staff, tone can be temporarily reduced with a muscle relaxant (see Ch. 28) or a paralysing agent, to allow a better casting position to be achieved more easily, but without overstretching.

Barnard et al. (1984) reported a reduction in the overall level of spasticity after using plaster boots. Robichaud & Agostinucci (1996) speculated that this effect might be due to the reduction in input to tactile, proprioceptive and temperature receptors from wearing the cast. They suggested that the cast promotes total contact, even pressure and warmth, thus decreasing the excitability of the alpha or gamma motor neurones in the spinal cord. This hypothesis was further supported by Childers et al. (1999), who used electromyography (EMG) to look at the use of inhibitory casting to decrease spasticity in the upper limb and found that there was a reduction in the vibratory inhibition index. This correlated with a decrease in motor neurone excitability in the hypertonic upper limb. However, in the absence of activity and function, any gains in range of movement achieved may be difficult to maintain, particularly in the presence of persistent muscle tone (Hill, 1994).

As an alternative, pressure splints (Johnstone, 1995) may be used for periods during the day, and, in the presence of mildly increased tone, strapping may suffice.

Corrective splinting or serial casting Corrective splinting is used to increase range of movement in the presence of contracture. Two common methods are serial casting in the form of cylinders or drop-out casts. The advantage of the drop-out cast is that active movement can still be encouraged and function is not so compromised.

Electrical stimulation can also be applied to the appropriate muscle (Stoeckmann, 2001). Frequency of changing a corrective cast varies within clinical practice; conflicting recommendations can be found in the literature with times ranging from daily (King, 1982) to weekly (Edwards & Charlton, 2002). With lower-limb casting a platform should be built under the toes to prevent clawing and shortening of the toe flexors.

Cast braces with adjustable hinges can be useful for slowly correcting contracted joints, especially at the elbow or knee when the contracture is >90°, where serial casting is more difficult. A risk factor may be swelling, which can occur around the elbow or knee. Orthoses with a sprung hinge can assist in stretching out contractures (Farmer & James, 2001).

If a patient has established contractures, consideration should be given to surgery. A conservative approach should always be considered if handling alters tone, if movement is felt or observed or if there is a soft end-feel. A preliminary cast should be applied if there is any doubt about the approach. If casting is going to be successful, a gain in range is usually evident after the removal of the first plaster. A radiograph should be taken to exclude HO, where clinical assessment indicates this may be present.

Dynamic splinting Dynamic splinting aims to facilitate recovery and assist stability for improved function. Examples are ankle-training braces (Burdett et al., 1988), and hinged ankle–foot orthoses (AFOs; Tyson & Thornton, 2001). It is important to consider the effect on function that an orthosis may have, albeit usually a positive effect, as they can occasionally decrease function, such as in the case of a lower-limb splint and driving.

Strapping is an alternative short-term method and can be applied to virtually any joint. It can be useful for the ankle and shoulder complexes. Strapping is gaining in popularity in conjunction with greater knowledge of musculoskeletal muscle imbalance treatment approaches (see Ch. 30). Hanger et al. (2000) found that where patients had their shoulders strapped, they had a trend towards less pain and better arm and hand function on final assessment. However, the results were not statistically significant. The use of strapping for shoulder pain has now been withdrawn from the *National Clinical Guidelines for Stroke*, produced by the Royal College of Physicians (Intercollegiate Working Party for Stroke, 2002). The short-term effect of using dynamic Lycra splints on the upper limbs following hemiplegia was a reduction in finger and wrist spasticity when worn for 3 h a day (Gracies et al., 2000).

Orthotic insoles   The use of orthotic insoles should be explored with the podiatry department if available. A primary goal of foot orthoses is to aid the maintenance and redistribution of weight-bearing patterns (Edwards & Charlton, 2002). In cases where the alignment is good and there is minimal contracture, the authors have clinical experience of using orthotic insoles to 'walk out' contracture.

Muscle strengthening

Until recently, it was widely believed by physiotherapists that patients with spasticity should avoid muscle-strengthening exercises because they assumed they would further increase hypertonicity. Studies emerging in the literature for different neurological disorders are showing that this is not the case, e.g. after stroke, muscle strengthening can increase strength and improve function without adversely affecting spasticity (Bhakta, 2000; Weiss et al., 2000). As a result of this evidence and recommendations by the Intercollegiate Working Party for Stroke (2002), many clinicians are incorporating muscle-strengthening exercises into treatment programmes. Chapter 29 discusses the role of muscle strengthening in different neurological disorders and outlines the areas needed for further clinical research.

Recent research has suggested there may be a role for strengthening in the treatment of contractures. Shortland et al. (2002) found that fibre length was not reduced in the medial gastrocnemius muscles of children with spastic diplegia and plantarflexion contractures. They related this finding to results in the literature from animal studies, where fibre length was normal but diameter was reduced, and concluded that muscle shortening in bipennate muscles was due to fibre atrophy, causing shortening of the aponeurosis. Shortland et al. (2002) did not provide direct evidence of fibre atrophy but the contractures seen in the children they studied could not be explained by the accepted mechanism of sarcomere loss (see Ch. 30). Although this is only one study and was carried out in children, it may be that strengthening would prevent or reverse atrophy and thus prevent or reverse contractures; further investigation is required in adults but these initial findings are encouraging.

Aerobic exercise

Recent evidence suggests that aerobic exercise does not result in increased spasticity (see Ch. 29). Dawes et al. (2000) found that high-intensity cycling did not lead to any increase in tone. This finding was further supported by Holt et al. (2001), who studied static bicycling in chronic stroke and found beneficial effects. Aerobic treadmill training also produced a positive outcome of improved functional mobility (Silver et al., 2000).

Medication

The therapist needs a basic understanding of the pharmacological means of controlling spasticity (see Ch. 28 and chapters on specific neurological conditions). Physiotherapists' skills in assessing tone, over time, can also play a valid role in evaluating the effectiveness of drugs and when they should be administered. Medication may be appropriate where physical means are inadequate but consideration needs to be given to their use (Barnes, 2001). Pain increases spasticity and so the use of analgesia should be considered; however it needs to be recognised that not all patients are able to communicate effectively to request analgesia.

It is essential to establish if the presentation of spasticity is generalised, regional or focal. The treatment options are then clearer. For generalised spasticity, oral medication may be a first approach. For focal spasticity, injections of botulinum toxin may be a useful adjunct to therapy (Richardson & Thompson, 1999), or where more permanent paralysis is required, then phenol nerve blocks can be used. Guidelines for the use of botulinum toxin have been produced (Barnes, 2001) and emphasise the need for a multidisciplinary team approach. In some patients, intrathecal baclofen may be used (Porter, 1997), especially where spasticity is a major problem and there is virtually no function in the affected limbs.

Continuous passive movement machines

Continuous passive movement (CPM) machines are commonly used in orthopaedics. In neurological physiotherapy, CPM can be beneficial in gaining range in head-injured patients with contractures (Macfarlane & Thornton, 1997). It can also be used in the management of contractures to assist in the breakdown of abnormal cross-bridge attachments, which have been shown to contribute to the abnormal stiffness during lengthening (Carey & Burghardt, 1993). However, it is likely to require repeated use to prevent the reformation of anomalous attachments (Singer et al., 2001), unless combined with active movement.

Hydrotherapy

During hydrotherapy the water has a dual role, providing support and warmth, and has a global effect on muscle activity. Hydrotherapy can also be utilised to alter tone and joint range of movement prior to treatment on dry land. The Halliwick concept is a well-accepted intervention for children with a neurological disability (Lambeck & Stanat, 2000) and it could be extrapolated that similar benefits could be seen with adults.

The use of hydrotherapy for patients with spinal injury is widespread, although there is a diversity of provision (Mahony et al., 1993). There is some evidence that hydrotherapy may be beneficial for patients after stroke (Taylor et al., 1993). Care should be taken in using hydrotherapy for patients with multiple sclerosis as they are often adversely affected by the heat (see Ch. 10), although a recent study of exercise in water that was heated to 94°F (34°C) did not find any such effects (Peterson, 2001).

Thermal treatments

Ice can have a temporary effect in reducing tone, although it is usually applied as an adjunct and only in a specific area. It has been demonstrated to be effective in the treatment of a painful shoulder in hemiplegia (Partridge et al., 1990) and cooling has been shown to have some benefits to patients with an essential tremor (Cooper et al., 2000).

The application of heat packs can help to increase range of movement (Funk et al., 2001) by altering the properties of connective tissue that can be affected in movement dysfunction (Hardy & Woodall, 1998).

Electrical stimulation

Electrical stimulation is gaining in popularity within the field of neurological physiotherapy. The different modes of electrical stimulation are muscle stimulation via the motor nerves, which is intended to produce a muscle contraction, and transcutaneous electrical nerve stimulation (TENS), which uses lower intensity stimulation and does not produce contractions. Spasticity in specific muscles in the lower limb has been shown to be reduced by using surface spinal cord stimulation (Wang et al., 2000). A systematic Cochrane review of electrical stimulation for shoulder pain (Price & Pandyan, 2001) found that there was no significant effect on upper-limb spasticity, but some improved range of passive lateral rotation was noted. TENS was found to have no effect on spasticity or pain in the upper limb but motor function improved in the treatment group (Sonde et al., 1998). Electrical stimulation has also been used in conjunction with botulinum toxin to increase the effectiveness of the toxin (Hesse et al., 1998).

Where muscle strengthening is required, electrical stimulation may be appropriate for patients who have reduced awareness (brain-injured) or have no control over their muscles (spinal cord-injured).

Biofeedback

The effectiveness of EMG biofeedback machines in the treatment of increased tone is unproven (Moreland & Thomson, 1994) but has been found to have a positive effect on ankle strength (Moreland et al., 1998). Sackley & Lincoln (1997) used visual feedback in balance retraining and noted a more rapid recovery of balance with a reduction in disability, but there was no long-term difference from patients who had not received the visual feedback. The Royal College of Physicians has withdrawn the recommendation of using biofeedback as an adjunct to traditional therapy, stating that more research is required in this area (Intercollegiate Working Party for Stroke, 2002).

Acupuncture

Acupuncture can be utilised as an adjunct in the management of tone. Guo et al. (1997) claimed that their technique of needling deeply into the acupoints and skin needling on the inferior–spasm side was therapeutic in the short- and long-term. For patients who dislike needles, Sonde et al. (2000) stimulated acupuncture points using high-frequency TENS with a reported decrease in spasticity in the lower limb.

> **Key points**
>
> - Prevention remains the best approach for contractures
> - In established contractures, the full range of techniques and approaches should be considered before surgical intervention
> - Effective intervention will include both treatment and management
> - Adjuncts should be used to support physical means and not used in isolation
> - Increasing evidence is emerging for the use of muscle-strengthening and aerobic exercise, even in the presence of tonal changes

EDUCATION

Management of altered tone requires a 24-h approach and education is an essential component. Education needs to be tailored to the patient's abilities and desire to know. Individuals react and cope differently to changes in their abilities, so the presumption that all patients want extensive information should not be assumed. The physiotherapist must judge what information to provide and when to provide it, but it is the patient who decides when or if to use this information. It is important to empower patients in making decisions (Jones et al., 2000; also see Ch. 22); too often a paternalistic or maternalistic approach is adopted.

Patients need education so that they can identify triggers to spasms and increased tone. Nociceptive stimuli, such as those from skin, bladder and bowel (and even tight clothing and wrinkled seat cushions), can all exacerbate spasticity. In patients who have difficulty communicating or are in a comatose state, increasing spasticity can be a sign that there is another problem, such as infection or constipation.

Patients may be able to learn to exhale and breathe through spasms and so help to prevent further tensing and worsening the spasm (Livingstone, 1998). Some patients will be able to gain some further cognitive control over their spasms. Patients with clonus can be taught to push down through the long axis of the lower leg via the knee, giving a prolonged stretch to inhibit overactivity in the muscles concerned.

A home programme may be part of the overall management of tone. Even if the patient is unable to carry out all the exercises or stretches independently, he or she should be able to direct a carer and thus retain responsibility. In some cases the spouse or partner may not see this as part of his or her role and this should be respected. Patient compliance with a home programme sometimes increases if exercises are incorporated into everyday life (e.g. linking them with the washing-up).

From the outset of any education programme, the carer should be involved as appropriate, and his or her needs assessed independently. Carers may need to be taught appropriate manual handling techniques (Association of Chartered Physiotherapists Interested in Neurology, 2001) and advised on the use of equipment. Relevant information about support groups or networks (see Appendix) can also be given.

FACTORS INFLUENCING DECISION-MAKING IN MANAGEMENT OF MUSCLE TONE

Factors that influence decision-making include:

- the neurological condition
- physical and cognitive abilities of the patient
- carryover of treatment effects into everyday activities
- severity of the tonal abnormality
- current and previous function
- presence of additional pathologies.

A holistic view of the patient should be taken when making decisions about the management of tonal difficulties. Details of the patient's previous lifestyle should be considered, as well as his or her aspirations for the future. Quality of life is both personal and subjective: the individual must be consulted and goals must be set jointly (see Ch. 22). The views of family and friends should be sought if it is not possible to converse with the patient.

Diagnosis and prognosis

The approach to the management of tone will depend on the patient's diagnosis. For the patient with a rapidly deteriorating condition, such as a primary tumour of the brain or motor neurone disease, the priorities would be functionally oriented, with a stronger emphasis on monitoring and management. Importance would be placed on the provision of equipment, and timely advice to carers regarding transfers and positioning, as appropriate. It would not be prudent to carry out long impairment-focused treatments where no functional improvement was anticipated. However, it may be possible to alleviate pain from malaligned joints due to muscle spasm and thus be an appropriate goal.

Prediction of prognosis is multifactoral and individual, although there are some common factors linked to a more positive prognosis (Counsell et al., 2002). In acute head injury where the prognosis is unknown, and the patient is at particular risk of developing contractures, emphasis is often placed on respiratory problems and insufficient attention can be given to the longer-term physical problems. Where the patient does not have a diagnosis on which to base a prognostic assessment or the outcome is unclear, the physiotherapist must treat the presenting symptoms.

The ability to learn

The response to physical rehabilitation cannot be seen in isolation from cognition, motivation, premorbid ability, behavioural difficulties, and perceptual and communication dysfunction. Motor learning can be seen as a result of a complex perception–cognition–action

> ### Key point
>
> - Patients must be empowered in decision-making and so be given appropriate information and explanation

process (Shumway-Cook & Woollacott, 1995). This area is covered in more detail in Chapter 27 on psychological management.

Motivation, which is necessary to optimise learning, should similarly be assessed. Motivation is described by the World Health Organization (WHO) as a global mental function that can be both a conscious and unconscious drive that leads to an incentive to act (WHO, 2001).

Potential for physical change

When handling a patient, certain signs indicate a potentially favourable outcome for prolonged physical change. These include:

- a change in tone in response to handling or positioning
- the ability of the patient actively to engage in the movement
- the presence of any active movement
- the presence of some tone (as opposed to flaccidity).

Abnormal tone may not be constant and the wider picture should be sought by a full assessment, preferably over at least two sessions at different times of the day. The ability to make a physical alteration may then inform the clinical decision as to how to balance the management/treatment dichotomy. For instance, the patient who is unchanging with hands-on intervention will require more of a maintenance-type approach. It must be noted that preventing deterioration is a valid reason for intervention, especially in progressive conditions.

Carryover and teamwork

Carryover can be defined as the extent to which treatment gains are maintained and used functionally between treatment sessions.

Spasticity management requires a 24-h approach for maximum effectiveness and it is essential that the whole rehabilitation team works towards common goals and has the knowledge and skills necessary to provide a co-ordinated approach. Interdisciplinary working practices can help such co-ordination, but these require commitment (Davis et al., 1992). For example, the speech and language therapist could undertake treatment while the patient is in a standing frame, or a perching stool could be used to encourage a more extended posture during activities in other therapies. Similar consideration should be given to modifying physiotherapy treatments on the advice of other therapists. Regular communication between staff in the form of joint goals and treatment sessions, meetings, multidisciplinary notes and training may assist

professions to work together effectively. Team working is documented to be more effective (Langhorne & Dennis, 1998).

> **Key points**
>
> - A holistic view of the patient should be taken when making decisions about the management of tonal difficulties
> - Physiotherapy intervention needs to ensure it is not based purely on the physical presentation of the patient but also on the diagnosis and prognosis, and psychosocial factors

MEASUREMENT OF EFFECTIVENESS OF TONE MANAGEMENT

There are inherent difficulties in measuring tone in the clinical setting. Tone is dynamic and changing, according to intrinsic and extrinsic factors, such as position, mood, base of support, temperature, stress, pain or time. There is also evidence to suggest that it has a natural progression (Drolet et al., 2000). Measurement is often made clinically by assessment of resistance to passive movement of the limb, but this resistance could be multifactoral and only one component may be tone. These factors make the assessment of tone complex and suggest that repeated measures and standardisation are required for evaluation.

The subjective assessment of muscle tone is carried out routinely by physiotherapists, by passively moving the limbs.

Specific scales for tone

Commonly used scales are the Ashworth scale (Ashworth, 1964) and the modified Ashworth scale (Bohannon & Smith, 1987), having greater reliability in the upper limb (Pandyan et al., 1999). They still require standardisation when being applied, for example, the starting position and velocity of the stretch. Vattanaslip (2000) compared the measurement scales using laboratory and clinical measures, and found that there was a relationship with passive resistance, but not for reflex activity. There is yet to be developed a clinical tool with good validity and reliability that can distinguish between spasticity and contracture.

Motor scales

There are a number of scales that concentrate on the motor abilities (Wade, 1992) but these may not be sensitive to changes in tone. The Motor Assessment Scale (Carr et al., 1985) includes a measure of tone and disability items.

Functional scales

Activity (disability) scales have a limited role in the assessment of spasticity. They can assess the effects of spasticity on activity, but cannot measure spasticity directly. These include global measures such as the Barthel Index (Wade, 1992), the Functional Independence Measure (FIM) and the Functional Assessment Measure (FAM; Hall, 1992). The FIM/FAM has seven levels, and hence greater sensitivity than the Barthel.

Other measures

Other measures may be helpful at an individual patient level, although these do not assess tone directly. Walking tests, such as the timed 10-m walk (Collen et al., 1990), or a paper walkway can give useful information in the absence of a gait laboratory (i.e. stride length, step width and length). Painted footprints allow changes in weight distribution to be recorded and are a useful way of documenting the realignment of the foot complex. Similarly, periodic photographs allow comparison over time. The procedure needs to be standardised to ensure that the same perspective and distance are used each time. Video recordings are an excellent means of documenting change in posture and movement (Stillman, 1991). It is possible to use undesirable signs such as frequency of spasms (Snow et al., 1990) to assess the outcome of intervention.

Goal–setting

Goal-setting is considered good practice (Intercollegiate Working Party for Stroke, 2002) and can be meaningful to both the therapist and the patient; however, practice varies (Playford et al., 2000). Integration of the patient into all stages of the process is essential and where the patient is incapable of involvement, e.g. reduced consciousness, carers or patient advocates, such as key workers, should be substituted.

Key points

- Measurement of outcome is essential and must relate to the aims of treatment
- Measurement of tone is difficult to achieve reliably in the clinical setting

---

OTHER ABNORMALITIES OF TONE AND MOVEMENT

The clinical features and medical management of hypotonia, rigidity and dystonia are discussed in Chapter 4. Neurological disease can present in many ways and can often exhibit a mixed picture. An important role for the physiotherapist can be to provide information regarding physical impairments. Often it may be the experienced neurophysiotherapist who identifies that a patient has a tremor or specific focal abnormality. Any physical findings that are not congruent to the diagnosis of the patient should be discussed with medical staff.

Hypotonia

When dealing with persistent low tone, care must be taken to avoid damage to joints or overstretching of muscles. If muscles are elongated, this can present difficulty in recruitment due to alteration in the length–tension curve (see Ch. 30). If the patient is mobile, care must be paid to the knee joint, which may hyperextend, and orthoses may need to be considered.

The flaccid shoulder sometimes seen following damage to the CNS can lead to traction of the brachial plexus and soft tissues, causing pain. Various support devices for the arm are available that may be useful in alleviating this pain (see Ch. 23).

Rigidity

The most common presentations of rigidity occur in Parkinson's disease (see Chs 4 and 11), and decerebrate and decorticate rigidity in head injury (the latter two are better described as postures; see Ch. 4). In Parkinson's disease, the physiotherapist must understand the pharmacological management and therapy must be timed accordingly. Treatment is especially aimed at maintenance of posture through regular exercise but the effectiveness of physiotherapy intervention is not yet conclusive (Deane et al., 2001). Rigidity in the patient with head injury will rapidly result in contractures, and preventive physical measures are usually required. Some of the rarer conditions that may present with rigidity are 'stiff-man syndrome' (Barker et al., 1998), atypical spinal cord lesions and Schwartz–Jampel syndrome (Thompson, 1993).

Dystonia

Dystonia has been described as mobile rigidity or 'sustained involuntary muscle contractions' (Pentland, 1993), and has been classified in light of recent advances into four groups (Fahn et al., 1998). Focal dystonia, such as blepharospasm and cervical dystonia, is now treated using botulinum injections. Clinically, for generalised dystonia treatment should aim to increase proprioceptive input by compression or stretch. This sensory retraining should aim to prevent the patient adopting static postures; clinically, it has been noted that mobile weight-bearing through hands and feet may allow the patient to feel postural adaptation.

Ataxia

Ataxia is associated with a disturbance in the sensory or vestibular system, or a lesion in the cerebellum, and occurs in conditions such as multiple sclerosis and Friedreich's ataxia (see Ch. 10). It is important to identify, where possible, the causal factor and treat effectively. Gill-Body et al. (1997) presented two cases that illustrate the importance of individual assessment and treatment.

In cerebellar ataxia the patient generally presents with low tone and a wide-based gait. Patients may appear to have increased tone distally as they seek to gain some stability. Treatment should concentrate on creating stability around proximal joints and in the trunk, and functionally encouraging appropriate compensation strategies and using movement at one or two joints.

Where the patient uses compensatory activity, the physiotherapist needs to consider how this may best be achieved to prevent overdominance of one movement or posture. Measures available to give the patient stability include supportive seating (Fig. 25.6), weighted frames and damping devices such as the 'neater eater'. In multiple sclerosis patients, fatigue may make treatment difficult, but treatment by therapists has been shown to be effective (Jones et al., 1996) and Case history 2, below, describes a patient with ataxia.

In vestibular ataxia, habituation exercises should be used, and can lead to a decrease in symptoms (Herdman & Whitney, 2000; see also Ch. 24). In sensory ataxia the use of compensation strategies for function and advice is essential to prevent injury or skin damage.

Tremor

Tremors may occur in many neurological conditions, including Parkinson's disease, brain injury and multiple sclerosis. Drug therapy is usually effective to some extent (see Chs 4 and 28) and the provision of adaptive equipment should be considered.

Athetosis

Management and the provision of equipment are important (see Ch. 18). Clinicians may see this condition more frequently in adults in the future, as the life expectancy of people with cerebral palsy increases.

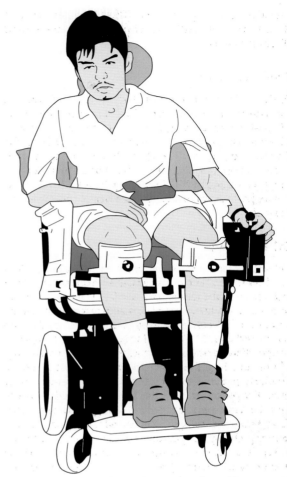

Figure 25.6 A supportive seating system allows this very ataxic young man to be able to drive a powered wheelchair.

Bradykinesia

This disorder, in which movements are slowed, is most commonly seen in conjunction with Parkinson's disease (see Ch. 11). Treatment should be concentrated at the time when drug therapy has been maximised. Exercise programmes that teach compensatory strategies may be beneficial (Kamsa et al., 1995).

Other movement disorders

There has been little evaluation of therapy in the rarer movement abnormalities. Choreiform movements are discussed in Chapter 12 on Huntington's disease. The therapist should carry out a detailed assessment and consider each individual case on the basis of the clinical presentation.

CASE HISTORIES

For each case history, a certain point in the patient's rehabilitation has been described. The aim of these presentations is to give an overview, not to provide detailed descriptions of treatment.

CASE 1 – SPASTICITY

The patient
Steve, a 24-year-old man, suffered a head injury from a climbing accident. Initially he was admitted to a neurosurgical unit where he underwent a craniotomy and removal of a haematoma from the frontoparietal region. Scanning revealed widespread contusions. He was intubated and ventilated for a week and bilateral prophylactic plaster boots were applied as he had extensor tone in both lower limbs. He developed a flexion contracture of his right arm, which could not be splinted due to a large abrasion. Four weeks after the accident he was transferred back to a general surgical ward in his local general hospital and assessed.

Problems identified
Steve was nasogastrically fed due to the risk of aspiration from dysphagia. He had marked extensor tone in the lower limbs. His left arm was functional but his right arm was flexed and contracted with no useful movement. He was unable to sit independently and had attention-seeking behaviour.

Clinical decision-making
Regular team meetings were arranged and the family were invited to therapy sessions and to a case conference where the team identified a requirement for long-term rehabilitation to maximise Steve's functional recovery; he was referred to a specialist rehabilitation centre.

Action taken
It was decided to give Steve a percutaneous endoscopic gastrostomy (PEG) in liaison with the speech and language therapist, dietician and surgeon. A joint session with the occupational therapist provided him with a temporary supportive seating package. The plaster boots were removed and, with daily standing and the use of removable night splints, range of movement was maintained. Serial drop-out casts were applied to his right arm to increase range. Staff tried to ignore inappropriate behaviour and socially reward good behaviour. The nurses and physiotherapist undertook a joint risk assessment and a standing hoist was used on the ward for transfers.

He was transferred to the rehabilitation unit after 2 months.

Evaluation of outcome
Steve's range of flexion at the elbow and ankles was measured. Baseline charts were kept to monitor periods of attention-seeking behaviour. Functional and behavioural goals were set jointly by the team, Steve and his family. He achieved the functional goals of independent sitting and dressing his upper body.

CASE 2 – ATAXIA

The patient
Jenny, a 26-year-old single mother, had been diagnosed with multiple sclerosis resulting in a partial paraplegia. She was referred for outpatient physiotherapy by a neurologist, following a relapse. Jenny had been confined to a wheelchair for 3 years and presented in low mood and with social isolation. She had fears about losing her 4-year-old daughter if she approached social services for any help. Her wheelchair was small, the canvas sagged, and she found it difficult to propel for long distances.

Problems identified
On examination, Jenny was found to have low tone in her trunk, with overactivity and moderate contractures of the hip flexors and adductors. She compensated by using her arms for support in a flexed internally rotated position. She was unable to stand and spent all day sitting. Her flexor spasms were becoming worse, and she had only flickers of activity in her lower limbs. She was very emotional on assessment and cried when asked about how she managed with daily tasks.

Decision-making
Worsening spasms concerned Jenny as they were affecting her function. Prompt action was needed to prevent this interfering with her transfers. There was also reduced range in the hips and knees. On examination she had more activity in her trunk than she was currently using. It appeared that she had developed habitual postures resulting from her relapse. She also had psychosocial needs.

Action taken
In order to give appropriate education and advice to Jenny, she kept a diary detailing when she had a spasm and why it happened. Active treatment included teaching Jenny to relax through spasms and to be much more aware of what triggered them.

Therapists made backslabs to enable her to stand with alignment of trunk on pelvis and gain activation of her trunk muscles whilst carrying out activities with her upper limbs. After a risk assessment and trial period with a standing frame, Jenny was provided with a frame for use at home and began daily standing. She was given a perching stool for use in the kitchen. She was referred for a wheelchair and an EPIOC assessment (Frank et al., 2000). Once the relationship between Jenny and her physiotherapist was established, she agreed to visit her general practitioner's counsellor and to attend the local multiple sclerosis support group.

Evaluation of outcome

The frequency of spasms was monitored and at discharge Jenny was rarely getting spasms. She was going out regularly and subjective assessment suggested that her mood had improved substantially. Following discussions with Jenny and other team members, it was organised for her daughter to attend a nursery in the morning, giving Jenny some free time to manage the household tasks. Instead of giving her a prescribed exercise programme, the emphasis was on incorporating activities such as standing into her daily life and adopting different postures that would maintain her abilities.

References

Ada L, Canning C. Anticipating and avoiding muscle shortening. In: Ada L, Canning C, eds. *Key Issues in Neurological Physiotherapy: Foundations for Practice*. Oxford: Butterworth Heinemann; 1990:219–237.

Ashburn A, Lynch M. Disadvantages of the early use of electric wheelchairs in the treatment of hemiplegia. *Clin Rehab* 1988, **2**:327–331.

Ashworth B. Preliminary trial of carisoprodal in multiple sclerosis. *Practioner* 1964, **192**:540–542.

Association of Chartered Physiotherapists Interested in Neurology (ACPIN). *Clinical Practice Guidelines on Splinting Adults with Neurological Dysfunction*. London: Chartered Society of Physiotherapy; 1998.

Association of Chartered Physiotherapists Interested in Neurology (ACPIN). *Guidance on Manual Handling in Treatment*. Norfolk: Barnwell's Print; 2001.

Barker RA, Reeves T, Thom M et al. Review of 23 patients affected by the stiff man syndrome and progressive encephalomyelitis with rigidity. *J Neurol Neurosurg Psychiatry* 1998, **65**:633–640.

Barnard P, Dill H, Eldredge P et al. Reduction of hypertonicity by early casting in a comatose head-injured individual. A case report. *Phys Ther* 1984, **64**:1540–1542.

Barnes MP. Medical management of spasticity in stroke. *Age Ageing* 2001, **30-S1**:13–16.

Barrett JA, Watkins C, Plant R et al. The COSTAR wheelchair study: a two-centre pilot study of self-propulsion in a wheelchair in early stroke rehabilitation. *Clin Rehab* 2001, **15**:32–41.

Bhakta BB. Management of spasticity in stroke. *Br Med Bull* 2000, **56**:476–485.

Blower P. The advantages of the early use of wheelchairs in the treatment of hemiplegia. *Clin Rehab* 1988, **2**:323–325.

Bobath B. *Adult Hemiplegia: Evaluation and Treatment*, 3rd edn. Oxford: Butterworth-Heinnemann; 1990.

Bohannon RW. Tilt table standing for reducing spasticity after spinal cord injury. *Arch Phys Med Rehab* 1993, **74**:1121–1122.

Bohannon RW, Smith MB. Interrater reliability of a modified Ashworth scale of muscle spasticity. *Phys Ther* 1987, **67**:206–207.

Brouwer B, de Andrade VS. The effects of slow stroking on spasticity in patients with multiple sclerosis; a pilot study. *Physiother Theory Pract* 1995, **11**:13–21.

Brown P. Pathophysiology of spasticity – editorial. *J Neurol Neurosurg Psychiatry* 1994, **57**:773–777.

Burdett RG, Borello-France D, Blatchly C et al. Gait comparison of subjects with hemiplegia walking unbraced with ankle foot orthosis and with an Air Stirrup® brace. *Phys Ther* 1988, **68**:1197–1203.

Carey JR, Burghardt TP. Movement dysfunction following central nervous system lesions: a problem of neurologic or muscular impairment? *Phys Ther* 1993, **73**:538–547.

Carr JH, Shepherd RB, Nordholm L et al. Investigation of a new motor assessment scale for stroke patients. *Phys Ther* 1985, **65**:175–176.

Childers MK, Biswass SS, Petroski G et al. Inhibitory casting decreases a vibratory inhibition index of the h reflex in the upper limb. *Arch Phys Med Rehab* 1999, **80**:714–716.

Chui ML. Wheelchair seating and positioning. In: Montgomery J, ed. *Physical Therapy for Traumatic Brain Injury*. New York: Churchill Livingstone; 1995:117–136.

Collen FM, Wade DT, Bradshaw CM. Mobility after stroke: reliability of measures of impairment and disability. *Int Disability Stud* 1990, **12**:6–9.

Cooper C, Evidente VGH, Hentz JG et al. The effect of temperature on hand function in patients with tremor. *J Hand Ther* 2000, **13**:276–288.

Cornall C. Self-propelling wheelchairs: the effects on spasticity in hemiplegic patients. *Physio Theory Pract* 1991, **7**:13–21.

Counsell C, Dennis M, McDowall M et al. Predicting outcome after acute and subacute stroke: development and validation of new prognostic models. *Stroke* 2002, **33**:1041–1047.

Davidson I , Waters K. Physiotherapists working with stroke patients: a national survey. *Physiotherapy* 2000, **86**:69–80.

Davies PM. *Steps to Follow. A Guide to the Treatment of Adult Hemiplegia*. Berlin: Springer-Verlag; 1985.

Davies PM. *Starting Again. Early Rehabilitation after Traumatic Brain Injury or other Severe Brain Lesion*. Berlin: Springer-Verlag; 1994.

Davis A, Davis S, Moss N et al. First steps towards an interdisciplinary approach to rehabilitation. *Clin Rehab* 1992, **6**:237–244.

Dawes H, Bateman A, Wade D et al. High intensity cycling exercise after stroke: a single case study. *Clin Rehab* 2000, **14**:570–573.

Deane KHO, Jones D, Playford ED et al. *Physiotherapy for Parkinson's Disease*. Oxford: Cochrane Library; 2001.

Drolet M, Noreau L, Vachon J et al. Spasticity change during and following functional rehabilitation in individuals with spinal cord injury. *J Rehab Outcomes Meas* 2000, **4**:1–14.

Edwards S. Abnormal tone and movement as a result of neurological impairment; considerations for treatment. In: Edwards S, ed. *Neurological Physiotherapy*. London: Churchill Livingstone; 2002:35–68.

Edwards S, Charlton P. Splinting and the use of orthoses in the management of patients with neurological disorder. In: Edwards S, ed. *Neurological Physiotherapy*. London: Churchill Livingstone; 2002:219–254.

Fahn S, Bressman SB, Marsden CD. Classification of dystonia. *Adv Neurol* 1998, **78**:1–10.

Farmer S, James M. Contractures in orthopaedic and neurological conditions: a review of causes and treatment. *Disabil Rehab* 2001, **23**:549–558.

Frank AO, Ward J, Orwell NJ et al. Introduction of a new NHS electric-powered indoor/outdoor chair (EPIOC) service: benefits, risks and implications for prescribers. *Clin Rehab* 2000, **14**:665–673.

Funk D, Swank AM, Adams KJ et al. Effects of moist heat pack application over static stretching on hamstring flexibility. *J Strength Condition Res* 2001, **15**:123–126.

Gandevia SC, McCloskey DI, Burke K. Kinaesthetic signals and muscle contraction. *TINS* 1992, **15**:62–65.

Gill-Body KM, Popat RA, Parker SW et al. Rehabilitation of balance in two patients with cerebellar dysfunction. *Phys Ther* 1997, **77**:534–552.

Goldsmith S. The Mansfield project: postural care at night within a community setting: a feedback study. *Physiotherapy* 2000, **86**:528–534.

Goldspink G, Williams W. Muscle fibre and connective tissue changes associated with use and disuse. In: Ada L, Canning C, eds. *Key Issues in Neurological Physiotherapy*. London: Butterworth Heinemann; 1990:25–50.

Gracies JM, Fitzpatrick R, Wilson L et al. Short term effects of dynamic Lycra splints on upper limb in hemiplegic patients. *Arch Phys Med Rehab* 2000, **81**:1547–1555.

Guo Z, Zhou M, Chen X et al. Acupuncture methods for hemiplegic muscle spasm. *J Trad Chinese Med* 1997, **17**:284–288.

Hall KM. Overview of functional assessment scales in brain injury rehabilitation. *Neuro Rehab* 1992, **2**:98–113.

Hamdy S, Rothwell JC, Aziz Q et al. Organization and reorganization of human swallowing motor cortex: implications for recovery after stroke. *Clin Sci* 2000, **99/2**:151–157.

Hanger HC, Whitewood P, Brown G et al. A randomised controlled trial of strapping to prevent post stroke shoulder pain. *Clin Rehab* 2000, **14**:370–380.

Hardy M, Woodall W. Therapeutic effects of heat, cold and stretch on connective tissue. *J Hand Ther* 1998, **11**:148–156.

Herdman SJ, Whitney SL. Assessment and management of central vestibular disorders. In: Herdman S, ed. *Vestibular Rehabilitation*, 2nd edn. Philadelphia: FA Davis; 2000.

Hesse S, Reiter F, Konrad M et al. Botulinum toxin type A and short-term electrical stimulation in the treatment of upper limb spasticity after stroke: a randomized, double-blind, placebo-controlled trial. *Clin Rehab* 1998, **12**:381–388.

Hill J. The effects of casting on upper extremity motor disorders after brain injury. *Am J Occup Ther* 1994, **48**:219–223.

Holt R, Kendrick C, McGlashan K et al. Static bicycle training for functional mobility in chronic stroke: case report. *Physiotherapy* 2001, **87**:257–260.

Intercollegiate Working Party for Stroke. *National Clinical Guidelines for Stroke*, 2nd edn. London: Royal College of Physicians; 2002. http://www.rcplondon.ac.uk/pubs/books/stroke/index.htm

Johansson BB. Brain plasticity and stroke rehabilitation: the Willis lecture. *Stroke* 2000, **31**:223–230.

Johnstone M. *Restoration of Normal Movement after Stroke*. Edinburgh: Churchill Livingstone; 1995.

Jones L, Lewis Y, Harrison J et al. The effectiveness of occupational therapy and physiotherapy in multiple sclerosis patients with ataxia of the upper limb and trunk. *Clin Rehab* 1996, **10**:277–282.

Jones F, Mandy A, Partridge C. Who's in control after a stroke? Do we disempower our patients? *Physiother Res Int* 2000, **5**:249–253.

Kamsa YPT, Browner W, Johannes PWF et al. Training of compensational strategies for impaired gross motor skills in Parkinson's disease. *Physio Theory Pract* 1995, **11**:209–229.

Kidd G, Lawes N, Musa I. *Understanding Neuromuscular Plasticity*. London: Edward Arnold; 1992:57–68.

Kilbride C, McDonnell A. Spasticity: the role of physiotherapy. *Br J Ther Rehab* 2000, **7**:61–64.

King T. Plaster splinting as a means of reducing elbow flexor spasticity: a case study. *Am J Occup Ther* 1982, **36**:671–673.

Knight LA, Thornton HA, Turner-Stokes L. Management of neurogenic heterotrophic ossification. *Physiother* 2003, **89**:471–477.

Lambeck J, Stanat FC. The Halliwick concept, part 1. *J Aquatic Phys Ther* 2000, **8**:6–11.

Langhorne P, Dennis M. *Stroke Units: An Evidence Based Approach*. London: BMJ Books; 1998.

Livingstone L. Coping with labour: what are the options? In: Sapsford R, Bullock-Saxton J, Markwell S, eds. *Women's Health. A Textbook for Physiotherapists*. London: WB Saunders; 1998.

Lynch M. The re-education of normal movement using proprioceptive information via key point control in the patients with neurological disorders. In: *Proceedings Book II World Conference of Physical Therapists*. London: 11th International Congress; 1991.

Macfarlane A, Thornton HA. Solving the problem of contractures – throw out the recipe book? *Physiother Res Int* 1997, **2**:1–6.

Mahony M, McGraw-Non K, McNamara N et al. Aquatic intervention for patients with spinal cord injury. Aquatic physical therapy. *J Aquatic Sect Am Phys Ther Assoc* 1993, **1**:10–16, 20.

Markham CH. Vestibular control of muscular tone and posture. *J Can Sci Neurol* 1987, **14**:493–496.

Massion J. Postural control system. *Curr Opin Neurobiol* 1994, **4**:877–887.

Moreland J, Thomson MA. Efficacy of electromyographic biofeedback compared with conventional physical therapy for upper-extremity function in patients following stroke: a research overview and meta-analysis. *Phys Ther* 1994, **74**:23–32.

Moreland J, Thompson MA, Fuoco AR. Electromyographic biofeedback to improve lower extremity function after stroke: a meta-analysis. *Arch Phys Med Rehab* 1998, **79**:134–140.

Nelles G, Spiekermann G, Jueptner M et al. Reorganization of sensory and motor systems in hemiplegic stroke patients. A positron emission tomography study. *Stroke* 1999, **30**:1510–1516.

O'Dwyer N, Ada L, Neilson P. Spasticity and muscle contracture following stroke. *Brain* 1996, **119**:1737–1749.

Pandyan AD, Johnson GR, Price CIM et al. A review of the properties and limitations of the Ashworth and modified Ashworth scales as measures of spasticity. *Clin Rehab* 1999, **13**:373–383.

Partridge CJ, Edwards SM, Mee R et al. Hemiplegic shoulder pain: a study of two methods of physiotherapy treatment. *Clin Rehab* 1990, **4**:43–49.

Pentland B. Parkinsonism in dystonia. In: Greenwood R, Barnes MP, McMillan TM., eds. *Neurological Rehabilitation*. Edinburgh: Churchill Livingstone; 1993:475–484.

Perr A. Elements of seating and wheeled mobility intervention. *OT Pract* 1998, **3**:16–24.

Peterson C. Exercise in 94 degree F water for a patient with multiple sclerosis. *Phys Ther* 2001, **81**:1049–1058.

Playford ED, Dawson L, Limbert V et al. Goal-setting in rehabilitation: report of a workshop to explore professionals' perceptions of goal setting. *Clin Rehab* 2000, **14**:491–496.

Pope PM. Posture management and special seating. In: Edwards S, ed. *Neurological Physiotherapy*, 2nd edn. Edinburgh: Churchill Livingstone; 2002:189–217.

Porter B. A review of intrathecal baclofen in the management of spasticity. *Br J Nurs* 1997, **6**:253–260.

Price CIM, Pandyan AD. Electrical stimulation for preventing and treating post stroke shoulder pain: a systematic Cochrane review. *Clin Rehab* 2001, **15**:5–19.

Richardson D, Thompson A. Botulinum toxin: its use in the treatment of acquired spasticity in adults. *Physiotherapy* 1999, **85**:541–551.

Robichaud JA, Agostinucci J. Air–splint pressure effect on soleus muscle alpha motoneuron reflex excitability in subjects with spinal cord injury. *Arch Phys Med Rehabil* 1996, **77**:778–782.

Rosche J, Rub B, Niemann-Delius B et al. Effects of physiotherapy on F-wave amplitudes in spasticity. *Electromyogr Clin Neurophysiol* 1996, **36**:509–511.

Rowat AM. What do nurses and therapists think about the positioning of stroke patients? *J Adv Nurs* 2001, **34**:795–803.

Ryerson S, Levit K. The shoulder in hemiplegia. In: Donatelli R, ed. *Physical Therapy of the Shoulder*, 2nd edn. New York: Churchill Livingstone; 1991:117–149.

Sackley CM, Lincoln NB. Single-blind randomised controlled trial of visual feedback after stroke: effects on stance and symmetry and function. *Disabil Rehab* 1997, **19**:536–546.

Shortland AP, Harris CA, Gough M et al. Architecture of the medial gastrocnemius in children with spastic diplegia. *Dev Med Child Neurol* 2002, **44**:158–163.

Shumway-Cook A, Woollacott M. *Motor Control. Theory and Practical Applications*. Baltimore: Williams & Wilkins; 1995.

Silver KH, Macko RF, Forrester LW et al. Effects of aerobic treadmill training on gait velocity, cadence and gait symmetry in chronic hemiparetic stroke: a preliminary report. *Neurorehab Neural Repair* 2000, **14**:65–71.

Singer B, Dunne J, Allison G. Clinical evaluation of hypertonia in the triceps surae muscles. *Phys Ther Rev* 2001, **6**:71–80.

Snow BJ, Tsui JKC, Bhatt MH et al. Treatment of spasticity with Botulinum toxin: a double blind study. *Ann Neurol* 1990, **28**:512–515.

Sonde L, Fernaeus SE, Nilsson CG et al. Stimulation with low frequency (1.7 Hz) transcutaneous electrical nerve stimulation (low-tens) increases motor function of the post-stroke paretic arm. *Scand J Rehab Med* 1998, **30**:95–99.

Sonde L, Kalimo H, Viitanen M. Stimulation with high frequency TENS – effects on lower limb spasticity after stroke. *Adv Physiother* 2000, **2**:183–187.

Stillman B. Computer-based video analysis of movement. *Aust J Physiother* 1991, **37**:219–227.

Stoeckmann T. Casting for the person with spasticity. *Topics Stroke Rehab* 2001, **8**:27–35.

Tardieu C, Lespargot A, Tabary C et al. How long must the soleus muscle be stretched each day to prevent contracture? *Dev Med Child Neurol* 1988, **30**:3–10.

Taylor EW, Morris D, Shaddeau S et al. Effects of water walking on hemiplegic gait. Aquatic physical therapy. *J Aquatic Sect Am Phys Ther Assoc* 1993, **1**:10–13.

Thompson PD. Stiff muscles. *J Neurol Neurosurg Psychiatry* 1993, **56**:121–124.

Turner C. Posture and seating for wheelchair users: an introduction. *Br J Ther Rehab* 2001, **8**:24–28.

Tyson SF, Chissim C. The immediate effect of handling technique on range of movement in the hemiplegic shoulder. *Clin Rehab* 2002, **16**:137–140.

Tyson SF, Thornton HA. The effect of a hinged ankle foot orthosis on hemiplegic gait: objective measures and users' opinions. *Clin Rehab* 2001, **15**:53–58.

Vattanaslip W, Ada L, Crosbie J. Contribution of thixotrophy, spasticity, and contracture to ankle stiffness after stroke. *J Neurol Neurosurg Psychiatry* 2000, **69**:34–39.

Wade DT. *Measurement in Neurological Rehabilitation*. New York: Oxford University; 1992.

Wang R, Chan R, Tsai M. Effects of thoraco-lumbar electric sensory stimulation on knee extensor spasticity of persons who survived cerebrovascular accident (CVA). *J Rehab Res Dev* 2000, **37**:73–79.

Weiss A, Suzuki T, Bean J et al. High intensity strength training improves strength and functional performance after stroke. *Am J Phys Med Rehab* 2000, **79**:369–376.

Williams PE. Use of intermittent stretch in the prevention of serial sarcomere loss in immobilised muscle. *Ann Rheumat Dis* 1990, **49**:3–16

Wolpaw JR, Tennissen AM. Activity dependent spinal cord plasticity in health and disease. *Annu Rev Neurosci* 2001, **24**:807–843.

World Health Organization. *International Classification of Functioning and Disability*. Geneva: WHO; 2001. Available online at http:/www.who.int/classification/icf.

Young T, Nicklin C. *Lower Limb Casting in Neurology Practical Guidelines*. London: Royal Hospital for Neuro-disability; 2000.

Chapter **26**

Pain management in neurological rehabilitation

D Langdon

CHAPTER CONTENTS

INTRODUCTION

Chronic pain syndromes pose a particular challenge to the physiotherapist in neurological practice because, whilst the psychology of a patient may be a stronger influence on outcome than is his or her physical status, instigating and maintaining change in physical activity is crucial to rehabilitation. Indeed, the role of psychology in the physiotherapy of chronic conditions has merited an editorial in a physiotherapy journal (Harding & Williams, 1995a). The same authors have argued elsewhere (1995b) that the physiotherapist working with chronic pain has the same aims as in any other specialty, i.e. to improve fitness and mobility and to educate the patient about the condition. However, the achievement of these aims for the patient in chronic pain often requires different means, based on psychological principles (Turk & Okifuji, 2002). Why should the patient's psychology affect the treatment of a physical pain syndrome?

The importance of psychological aspects to the understanding and recovery of the person with persistent pain stems from the primary experience of pain being wholly subjective. Pain cannot be observed directly. The International Association for the Study of Pain (IASP) has defined pain as 'an unpleasant and emotional experience associated with actual or potential tissue damage or described in terms of such damage'. Science has not yet made the measurement of experience a straightforward matter. Turk (1989), in a classic discussion of this dilemma, likened the investigator who was trying to measure pain to a hunter who goes into the woods to catch an animal no one has ever seen but whose damaging effects are clear to all. The only way the hunter can decide which tracks to follow is by adopting assumptions about the nature of the quarry. Similarly, clinicians and scientists attempting to investigate and treat pain know the effects of pain from their daily work, yet no precise definition for measurement exists to date.

Clinicians must rely on secondary sources from which to infer the magnitude and quality of the pain experience. Broadly, these are physiological (e.g. autonomic response), motor activity (e.g. guarding, moaning, facial expressions), self-report (e.g. visual analogue scales, numerical ratings, descriptive adjectives, questionnaires) or other indicators such as health care use and medication levels. Part of the complexity of pain phenomena is that self-reports of pain vary greatly in the extent to which they coincide with either psychophysiology or motor activity. It seems that we are interrogating at least three response systems that may correlate at times but are at best loosely coupled.

Melzack & Wall (1965) suggested that sensory, affective and cognitive factors combine to create an individual's pain experience. The sensory-discriminative dimension relates location, intensity and duration; the affective-motivational aspects are the noxious characteristics; and the cognitive-evaluative domain contributes attention, anticipation and memory (Villemure & Bushnell, 2002). Melzack (1975) designed the McGill Pain Questionnaire to assess each of these three components, by analysing the patient's selection of adjectives which best describe the pain. It is by no means certain, however, that verbal labels can accurately represent the pain experience. The complexities of the experience of pain in both the laboratory and clinic are discussed by Melzack & Wall (1984), in a text that can be helpful to both professionals and patients. The shortcomings of measurements for pain led clinicians to move towards assessing the patient, in terms of physical pathology, psychosocial and behavioural variables, rather than the pain as an isolated phenomenon (Turk & Rudy, 1987).

The role of therapists in the management of pain was detailed in a recent book by Strong et al. (2001).

NEUROPSYCHOLOGY OF PAIN

The basic anatomy and physiology of pain are outlined by Wall (1999) and Coniam & Diamond (1994). Recent advances of functional imaging techniques have increased our understanding of the central processing that affects sensation, emotion and cognition. A 'pain network' of structures that react to painful stimuli has been identified. For example, a positron emission tomography (PET) study of patients with mononeuropathies revealed activation of bilateral anterior insular, posterior parietal, lateral inferior prefrontal and posterior cingulate cortices, compared to a pain-free

state created by regional nerve blocks. In addition, both the right anterior cingulate cortex (ACC) and Brodmann area were also activated, regardless of the laterality of the neuropathy (Hsieh et al., 1995). The ACC may be important in chronic pain syndromes: it has involvement in avoidance learning, it is rich in opioid receptors and it may process the affective component of pain experience. There are two neuronal clusters in the ACC that have links with attention and motor control and motor intention; these two functions have been implicated in psychological pain management techniques that target cognition and behaviour (see 'Distraction', below). Discussion of the physiological basis of psychological pain management can sometimes be helpful in the early stages of treatment for patients who find any non-organic aspects hard to accept. Plasticity occurs with chronic pain (Ch. 5, p. 64)

PEOPLE WITH CHRONIC PAIN

Unsurprisingly, pain has a significant negative impact on the patient's quality of life (Skevington, 1998). A person with chronic pain is likely to be inactive and unable to fulfil normal social roles, such as family member, employee or leisure partner. Behavioural theory has offered a conceptual framework for understanding and treating this disability that has received considerable empirical support. It suggests that the behaviour of patients with chronic pain is influenced by social and environmental stimuli and consequences. The reinforcement schedules for well and illness behav-iour are entirely controlled by the immediate social group. Pain complaints often bear little relationship to organic pathology (Fordyce, 1976). Limping, grim-acing or verbal complaints signal pain and elicit attention and consideration from others. Some consequences of pain behaviour, such as extra care-giving by friends and relatives, or the avoidance of aversive situations such as a stressful workplace, serve to reinforce and maintain pain behaviour.

Because of his or her frequent interactions with the patient, a spouse is able to be very influential in shaping the patient's behaviour. Significant associations have been found between the responses of a spouse and the activity of the patient. Flor et al. (1987) reported that patients who viewed their spouses as highly solicitous responders to pain behaviours were more likely both to report their pain as more severe and to have low activity levels. Using a methodology that has been developed and validated to observe directly the behaviour between spouse and patient (Romano et al., 1991), Romano et al. (1995) demonstrated that solicitous responses from the spouse to the patient's pain behaviours were associated with greater pain behaviour and disability amongst patients with chronic pain. Many programmes for pain management explicitly address this issue, involving spouses and teaching them to respond positively to increased patient activity and other well behaviours and, conversely, to respond less solicitously to pain behaviours. Negative exchanges with care-givers or criticism from family members may have adverse consequences for both physical and psychological well-being that exceed the beneficial effects of positive support (Kerns et al., 1991). Prospective studies are few, but they suggest that patient hostility may precede increases in criticism by the spouse (Lane & Hobfell, 1992).

Pain and depression

Depressed patients often report pain and depression, and depressive symptoms are frequently found in patients with chronic pain. A large population survey of middle-aged people (Rajala et al., 1994) demonstrated that pain was more common amongst the depressed than the non-depressed population, and many of the depressed subjects reported pain in mul-tiple anatomical sites. Assessed according to the *International Classification of Diseases* (ICD-10; World Health Organization, 2002), the prevalence of depressive neurosis was reported to be 21% in a British pain clinic population (Tyrer et al., 1989). Depression may be a consequence of pain and the limitations it imposes on the patient's life, or it may be a sign of an underlying distress which renders a person more vulnerable to the causation and maintenance of a chronic pain syndrome. In a 10-year follow-up sample of a general population, depressive symptoms predicted future musculoskeletal pain episodes, but not vice versa (Leino & Magni, 1993).

There is evidence from correlational analyses that it is the perceived impact that the pain has on the patient's life that predicts depression, rather than the absolute level of pain experienced. A path analysis of the self-report cognitive and emotional scores of 10 chronic pain patients was conducted by Turk et al. (1995). Pain intensity significantly influenced perceptions of interference and life control, which in turn affected depression scores. However, pain intensity was not directly related to depression.

Although less well studied than depression, anger is another prominent negative emotion in chronic pain (Wade et al., 1990; Hatch et al., 1991). Fernandez & Turk (1995) have suggested a list of objects and reasons for anger (Table 26.1). If the expression of anger is inhibited, then the patient runs the risk of experiencing more pain and depression. However, unchecked expression of anger may disrupt interpersonal relations and affect treatment outcome. This analysis led Fernandez & Turk (1995) to postulate an optimal regulation of anger that represents a better adjustment by the patient to the condition.

The beliefs and expectations of patients with chronic pain have been shown to be critical facilitators of, or impediments to, their recovery. For example, DeGood & Kiernan (1996) asked outpatients with chronic pain, 'Who do you think is at fault for your pain?' The responses were grouped according to whether a patient identified his or her employer, another person or no one. Only half those patients who had experienced a work-related injury blamed their employers. The patients who faulted their employers were more likely to feel unfairly treated by the employers before and after the injury. This was despite there being no difference amongst the three groups in terms of

Table 26.1 Attributions about objects of anger and appraisals about reasons for anger amongst people with chronic pain

Agent (object of anger)	Action (reason for anger)
Causal agent of injury/illness	Chronic pain
Medical health care providers	Diagnostic ambiguity; treatment failure
Mental health professionals	Implications of psychogenicity or psychopathology
Attorneys and legal system	Adversarial dispute, scrutiny and arbitration
Insurance companies; social security system	Inadequate monetary coverage or compensation
Employer	Cessation of employment; job transfer; job retraining
Significant others	Lack of interpersonal support
God	'Predetermined' injury and consequences; ill fate
Self	Disablement, disfigurement
The whole world	Alienation

(Adapted from Fernandez & Turk (1995), with permission.)

current pain intensity or activity limitation. However, those patients who blamed their employers or another person reported greater mood and behavioural disturbance, poorer response to past treatments and lesser expectations of future benefit. It may be that the sense of suffering is increased when pain is seen as the result of others' lack of caution or concern.

Coping with chronic pain

Differences in the use of coping strategies for pain may be significant in adjusting to chronic pain. Active coping by patients with chronic pain is related to psychological well-being. In contrast, passive coping is strongly related to psychological distress and depression (Snow-Turek et al., 1996). Cross-sectional studies show that active strategies such as positive self-statements, the use of coping self-statements and increasing activities are associated with better physical and psychological functioning in patients with chronic pain. In contrast, the use of rest to cope with pain, and other passive strategies, appears to be associated with worse physical functioning. Measures of coping with pain have been developed, e.g. the Chronic Pain Coping Inventory (Jensen et al., 1995) includes positive items (such as 'imagined a calming or distracting image to help me relax') and negative items (such as 'walked with a limp to decrease the pain').

PAIN MANAGEMENT IN PRACTICE

Management of pain includes: initial assessment of the problem; planning treatment and setting goals; treatment strategies; and monitoring progress.

Assessment

Some measurement of a patient's physical function and everyday activity is an essential prerequisite to starting treatment. It provides a quantitative description of the patient's current situation, which can then be used to monitor treatment progress and maintenance. Many useful tools for measuring pain and its effects have been developed, with good reliability and validity. Provided that they are selected and used with an appreciation of their limitations, some of which were outlined in the first part of this chapter, they can be of great benefit to both the clinician and the researcher. Harding et al. (1994) have described a battery for assessing the physical functioning of patients with chronic pain, which reportedly took only 45 min to complete prior to treatment. The reliability, validity and acceptability of seven tests of speed and endurance are recorded. Some measures of pain for specific anatomical sites have been developed, which have high face validity and therefore facilitate patient

co-operation. For example, the Pain Index for the Knee (Lewis et al., 1995a) offers a clinical procedure for assessing knee pain, with some basic transportable equipment, and takes only 5–10 min for each knee. It involves 10 standardised knee movements (four active, six passive), which are then scored by the assessor, largely in terms of the subject's pain behaviour. The Curtin Back Screening Questionnaire has been demonstrated to discriminate between people with different degrees of disability resulting from occupational low-back pain (Harper et al., 1995) and has good psychometric properties. It is reportedly self-administered in 30 min and scored in 3 min, and is designed for a range of settings from primary care to the specialist clinic. A categorical scale may be as good as a visual analogue scale for a simple pain report and is quicker (Lines et al., 2001). A two-point reduction is considered clinically significant on an 11-point scale (Farrar et al., 2001).

Records

Because of the many emotional and cognitive variables that can influence a patient's understanding of his or her condition, self-report is only one facet of information-gathering. For instance, patients with pain tend to underreport their activity levels, as compared to objective measures of activity (Turk et al., 1992). Any report or rating of pain over time necessarily depends on memory for pain, which in itself is complex and problematic (Erskine et al., 1990). A structured system of record-keeping and diaries is therefore essential. For research purposes, electronic data-logging devices have been developed (Lewis et al., 1995b) and these could be adapted for clinical use.

Strategies for pain management

Medication for pain is outlined in Chapter 28 and will not be considered here, except in passing. A fairly detailed and accessible account of psychological pain management strategies can be found in Chapters 8–13 of Turk et al. (1983). It can often be a great surprise to the patient that pain levels and painful body parts are not to be the focus of treatment, but rather general fitness and activity levels, physical confidence and attitude. However, some patients with chronic pain are resigned to the persistence of their condition and may not require a great deal of persuasion, but rather welcome an approach offering constructive help and real hope, and which has only minimal risks.

Relaxation

Relaxation is often an essential part of most pain management programmes, especially in the early stages.

The classical Jacobsen exercises, involving the clenching and relaxing of various muscle groups, are not usually the technique of choice for neuropathic pain because they tend to increase muscle tension. Patients with chronic pain who receive relaxation training report greater decrease in pain, decrease in psychological distress and decrease in functional disability compared to patients on a waiting list or in attention-placebo control conditions (Turk et al., 1983). Applied relaxation training (ART) has been demonstrated to be more effective at treating upper-extremity pain associated with repetitive workplace tasks than either electromyography (EMG) biofeedback alone, or EMG biofeedback combined with ART (Spence et al., 1995). The authors suggest that, whereas ART creates feelings of control over pain by influencing muscle tension levels, any involvement of machinery reduces feelings of control and reinforces conceptions of pain as a primarily physical and mechanical phenomenon. It is certainly true that ART teaches a more flexible and portable skill, which can be employed in a variety of situations.

Distraction

Directing attention away from pain by concentrating on aspects of the environment, mental problem-solving or internally generated images is another clinical technique for increasing feelings of control over pain, which has some experimental support (Miron et al., 1989; Rode et al., 2001). Peyron et al. (1999) identified a possible physiological substrate for this phenomenon, demonstrating that insular/second somatosensory cortices responded in all experimental pain conditions, regardless of attention mode, and are therefore linked to the sensory-discriminative dimension, whereas a large network of structures was additionally recruited when attention was directed to a painful thermal stimulus (prefrontal, posterior parietal, anterior cingulate cortices and thalamus), and this was termed the attentional network. Conversely, a demanding cognitive task in addition to cold pressor pain decreased activation in somatosensory association areas, increased activation of lateral orbitofrontal regions and lowered pain ratings compared to pain experienced without a simultaneous cognitive task (Petrovic et al., 2000).

Setting goals

The setting of goals serves a number of purposes: (1) there is an explicit contract describing what is expected of the patient in terms of physical progress over the next few weeks; (2) the patient and his or her family have a clear account of a realistic rate of progress; and (3) the patient's progress can be monitored against the agreed goals, and success or failure noted.

Initially, the therapist may need to offer extensive guidance in setting goals, but it is always essential to take a careful and detailed account of the patient's preferences and current situation.

Pacing

Pacing involves the gradual increase of activity, in a structured, graded way, in line with the patient's increasing stamina and pain management skills. Most patients are surprised at how little activity they are required to perform at the outset and this can lead them to view their treatment as a step backwards; this requires careful explanation and education. The ideal baseline is far below the personal maximum level of effort. Any sign of exhaustion or pain, suggesting that a person is approaching his or her activity limit, is evidence that the baseline has been set too high. The baseline level of activity or exercise should be performed by the patient relatively easily and should be achievable on any day, not just 'good days'. Sometimes the baseline levels of activity can appear trivial to an outsider. For example, a severely disabled, bed-bound woman with chronic pain started with a baseline that amounted to little more than five slight shifts of each foot on the bed, three times a day, but that was the level at which the team could engage her and from which she could start to build her confidence.

Cognitive therapy

People with chronic pain will have a different outlook on life from that of healthy people. They will tend to fasten on negative events, predict the future negatively, denigrate themselves, experience a great deal of guilt, discount positive events and successes and catastrophise, i.e. follow trains of thoughts that lead to a disastrous potential outcome from a relatively minor setback. This skewing of their perception of themselves and their lives can be overcome and normalised by a technique known as cognitive therapy. This identifies, records and challenges mistakenly negative thoughts and attitudes; challenges them by exploring or gathering evidence related to them; and systematically and routinely counters them with replacement 'healthy' thoughts.

Self-help books

It can be extremely useful for a person with chronic pain to read about pain and its management. There are pitfalls though: the book may offend or anger the patient by being irrelevant to, or inaccurate about, his or her condition; the patient may become obsessed with the details of the condition and never move beyond diagnosis and terminology; or the patient may think that he or she could have written a more expert and insightful book, either before or after reading the one that you recommend. However, judicious timing and matching of patients to books can bring dividends. These books can extend the time each week a person thinks constructively about his or her pain; they can serve as a memo, to remind the patient and extend the contents of treatment sessions; they can introduce new topics, such as the role of the family, in a less threatening way than a face-to-face discussion might be able to do; and family members, who may not be able to attend sessions, can become acquainted with some basic principles of pain management. For physiology and anatomy, Coniam & Diamond (1994) is good. Three self-help books which have proved useful in clinical work are Shone (1987), Sternbach (1990) and White (1992).

Overview of pain strategies

It is not known which individual components or combinations of strategies are the most effective, or even necessary, within a pain management programme. No two programmes are alike, even within the same hospital and when run by the same staff, because the patients' individual personalities and experiences on the programme affect the content and emphasis. It may be that different aspects are helpful to particular patient profiles, or at particular stages of rehabilitation and maintenance. It is sometimes argued that strategies in themselves do not represent the core process in pain management and rehabilitation, but rather serve as agents that contribute to the primary process, which is one of establishing feelings of control.

There is an experimental study which provides evidence for the importance of control in the experience of pain (Holroyd et al., 1984). College students suffering from recurrent tension headache were recruited and assigned to one of four EMG biofeedback training groups. All were told that they were learning to decrease frontal EMG. All subjects were shown two graphs on a VDU, one graph showing dramatic improvement, the other showing modest improvement. Half of the subjects were told that the dramatically improving line represented their progress and the modestly improving line was an average performance (the 'high-success group'). The other half of the subjects were told that the dramatically improving line was the average performance and the modestly improving line was their own performance (the 'low-success group'). Although all subjects were led to believe that they were learning to decrease EMG activity, the high- and low-success groups were further split into two separate feedback schedules, with half the subjects in each group receiving feedback for decreasing EMG activity, but the other half receiving feedback for increasing EMG activity. Regardless of whether their experimental feedback led them to increase or decrease their actual EMG activity, the high-success group reported greater reduction in tension headache (53%) than the low-success group (26%).

Performance feedback was also related to cognitive changes, including feelings of control over pain and beliefs about being able to perform everyday activities despite pain. The authors concluded that the effectiveness of EMG training in tension headache may be mediated by cognitive changes induced by performance feedback and not primarily by reductions in EMG activity.

Clinical aspects of neuropathic pain

It is likely to be the case that your first contact with a person with chronic pain will be an uncomfortable experience. The patient may be firmly entrenched in the view that nothing can help the pain. Patients with chronic pain are often extremely bitter and distrustful of health care professionals. They may produce lengthy and colourful accounts of their pain and previous operations and treatments. They may have had, or report, previous unsuccessful or painful experiences of physiotherapy. The task of the physiotherapist in the first session is to engage them. You must somehow convince them that it is worth coming back for the next session, that changes are possible, that their lives can get better. The prolonged impact of low-back pain, at least, can be reduced be helping patients to perceive pain as a problem that can be overcome and using strategies to promote activity (Shaw et al., 2001). Strategies to effect this include: emphasising your expertise; not reinforcing exclamations of pain and other pain behaviour, whilst remaining respectful and interested; examining range of movement (as far as is possible); and offering some immediate education about joint care, sitting posture or environmental aids.

It is a great privilege if a person with chronic pain agrees to enter a treatment programme with you; the patient will almost certainly have suffered many therapeutic disappointments previously and will be risking another by daring to start hoping again. A good way of encouraging people with chronic pain to continue with pain management programmes is to induce positive change early. Relaxation will often do this, offering some modulation of pain experience and therefore evidence that the problem is not completely intractable, as the patient may have professed or believed at initial assessment.

The intractability and persistence of some neuropathic pain syndromes should not be underestimated. People experiencing neuropathic pain can be driven to extreme and even bizarre behaviours. The clinician must be aware of all possibilities and alert to them. For example, Mailis (1996) reported four cases of self-injurious behaviour in people with painful dysaesthesiae. Whilst these are the exception rather than the rule, they serve as a reminder of the range of behavioural disturbances that pain can induce.

The pain management team

A team approach to chronic pain goes some way to addressing the many interrelated factors that serve to influence and maintain a chronic pain syndrome. It should also ensure a continuity of approach. It allows a greater number of patients to receive the attention of several specialists within a short period of time, leading to savings in time and costs. However, teams are not a panacea. The individual characteristics of team members exert great influence over the team's character and effectiveness. Time must be allocated for meetings and other team functions. 'Participatory democracy tends to be a cumbersome and slow-moving process' (Segraves, 1989).

The role of the various professionals in the team is in line with each particular discipline's skills and expertise. The neurologist will be involved in the initial examination and investigations of the patient and the diagnosis. A neurosurgical opinion may be sought. Medication may be prescribed. Most pain clinics involve a pain anaesthetist, who will examine the patient, may request further investigations and may perform some procedures and adjust medication. A psychiatrist may be involved if there are reasons to consider psychotropic medication, although as a general rule most pain management programmes seek to reduce medication. A psychologist will usually be involved once pain management, as opposed to more active treatments, is under consideration. The psychologist will be involved in the psychosocial assessment of the patient and planning the cognitive aspects of treatment.

The physiotherapist will be involved in the assessment and planning of physical treatment (the role of the physiotherapist in the pain management team is discussed in detail by Harding & Williams, 1995b). In some centres, a nurse may oversee the reduction of medication and an occupational therapist may assist patients with household and work activities. Once a pain management programme is instigated, all staff must be able

to discuss and reinforce the basic principles of increasing activity and well behaviour, pacing, using relaxation strategies, maintaining the exercise programme, at least rudimentary cognitive therapy and goal-setting.

The organisation of teams has been described in sports terms by Segraves (1989), not entirely for reasons of humour. Three models are identified:

1. baseball teams, in which individuals function and are evaluated independently, hardly interacting; the team manager's concern is 'batting order'
2. football teams, which require more interaction but are basically a co-ordinated hierarchical service; this is best suited to large organisations, or many independent units
3. basketball teams, which require continuous team member awareness, co-operation, adjustment and spontaneous reaction; the coach is an enabler rather than a director; this flexible and dynamic system tends to work where numbers are small.

Outcomes

There is a growing body of evidence that psychological pain management programmes, delivered by a multidisciplinary team, result in significant benefit for a substantial proportion of recruited patients and that this improvement is generally maintained over a number of years. Changes in beliefs about pain have been associated with better outcomes; specifically, reductions in reported 'organic' pain beliefs have led to reduced disability (Walsh & Radcliffe, 2002). In a large study, Maruta et al. (1990) reported a 70% success rate at discharge from an inpatient pain management programme, which was maintained by very nearly half of those successfully treated at 3-year follow-up. These figures are similar to those reported in a previous study from the same institution. These outcomes are particularly encouraging when one considers the severe disability, emotional distress and excessive medication use typical of the patients who are admitted to these programmes. A meta-analysis of 25 trials found that cognitive-behavioural programmes were comprehensively better than wait-list control conditions, and produced greater changes in pain experience, cognitive coping and appraisal and reduced pain behaviours than alternative active treatments (Morley et al., 1999).

References

Coniam SW, Diamond AW. *Practical Pain Management*. Oxford: Oxford University Press; 1994.

DeGood DE, Kiernan B. Perception of fault in patients with chronic pain. *Pain* 1996, **64**:153–160.

Erskine A, Morley S, Pearce S. Memory for pain: a review. *Pain* 1990, **41**:255–266.

Farrar JT, Young JP, LaMoreaux L. Clinical importance of changes in chronic pain intensity measured on an

11-point numerical pain rating scale. *Pain* 2001, **94**:149–158.

Fernandez E, Turk DC. The scope and significance of anger in the experience of chronic pain. *Pain* 1995, **61**:165–175.

Flor H, Kerns RD, Turk DC. The role of spouse reinforcement, perceived pain, and activity levels of chronic pain patients. *J Psychosom Res* 1987, **31**:251–259.

Fordyce WE. *Behavioural Methods for Chronic Pain and Illness*. St Louis: Mosby; 1976.

Harding V, Williams A CdeC, Richardson PH et al. The development of a battery of measures for assessing physical functioning of chronic pain patients. *Pain* 1994, **58**:367–375.

Harding V, Williams ACdeC. Applying psychology to enhance physiotherapy outcomes. *Physiother Theory Pract* 1995a, **11**:129–132.

Harding V, Williams ACdeC. Extending physiotherapy skills using a psychological approach: cognitive-behavioural management of chronic pain. *Physiotherapy* 1995b, **81**:681–688.

Harper AC, Harper DA, Lambert LJ et al. Development and validation of the Curtin Back Screening Questionnaire (CBSQ) – a discriminative disability measure. *Pain* 1995, **60**:73–81.

Hatch JP, Schoenfeld LS, Boutros NN et al. Anger and hostility in tension-type headache. *Headache* 1991, **31**:302–304.

Holroyd KA, Penzien DB, Hursey KG et al. Change mechanisms in EMG biofeedback training: cognitive changes underlying improvement in tension headache. *J Con Clin Psychol* 1984, **52**:1039–1053.

Hsieh JC, Belfrage M, Stone-Elander S et al. Central representation of chronic ongoing neuropathic pain studied by positron emission tomography. *Pain* 1995, **63**:225–236.

Jensen MP, Turner JA, Romano JM et al. The chronic pain coping inventory: development and preliminary validation. *Pain* 1995, **60**:203–216.

Kerns RD, Southwick S, Giller EL et al. The relationship between reports of pain related social interactions and expressions of pain and affective distress. *Behav Ther* 1991, **22**:101–111.

Lane C, Hobfell SE. How loss affects anger and alienates potential supporters. *J Con Clin Psychol* 1992, **60**:935–942.

Leino P, Magni G. Depressive and distress symptoms as predictors of low back pain, neck-shoulder pain, and other musculoskeletal morbidity: a 10-year follow-up of metal industry employees. *Pain* 1993, **53**:89–94.

Lewis B, Bellamo R, Lewis D et al. A clinical procedure for assessment of severity of knee pain. *Pain* 1995a, **63**:361–364.

Lewis B, Lewis D, Cumming G. Frequent measurement of chronic pain: an electronic diary and empirical findings. *Pain* 1995b, **60**:341–347.

Lines CR, Vandormael K, Malbecq W. A comparison of visual analog scale and categorical ratings of headache pain in a randomized controlled trial with migraine patients. *Pain* 2001, **93**:185–190.

Mailis A. Compulsive targeted self-injurious behaviour in humans with neuropathic pain: a counterpart of animal

autonomy? Four case reports and a review of the literature. *Pain* 1996, **64**:569–578.

Maruta T, Swanson DW, McHardy MJ et al. Three year follow-up of patients with chronic pain who were treated in a multidisciplinary pain management centre. *Pain* 1990, **41**:47–53.

Melzack R. The McGill pain questionnaire: major properties and scoring methods. *Pain* 1975, **1**:277–299.

Melzack R, Wall PD. Pain mechanisms: a new theory. *Science* 1965, **150**:971–979.

Melzack R, Wall PD. *The Challenge of Pain*. London: Penguin; 1984.

Miron D, Duncan GH, Bushnell MC. Effects of attention on the intensity and unpleasantness of thermal pain. *Pain* 1989, **39**:345–352.

Morley S, Eccleston C, Williams A. Systematic review and meta-analysis of randomized controlled trials of cognitive behaviour therapy for chronic pain in adults, excluding headache. *Pain* 1999, **80**:1–13.

Petrovic P, Petersson KM, Ghatan PH et al. Pain-related cerebral activity is altered by a distracting cognitive task. *Brain* 2000, **85**:19–30.

Peyron R, Garcia-Larrea L, Gregoire MC et al. Haemodynamic brain responses to acute pain in humans. Sensory and attentional networks. *Brain* 1999, **122**:1765–1779.

Rajala U, Uusimaki A, Keinanen-Kiukaanniemi S et al. Prevalance of depression in a 55 year old Finnish population. *Soc Psychiatry Psychiat Epidemiol* 1994, **29**:126–130.

Rode S, Salkovkis PM, Jack T. An experimental study of attention, labelling and memory in people suffering from chronic pain. *Pain* 2001, **94**:193–203.

Romano JM, Turner JA, Friedman LS et al. Observational assessment of chronic pain patient–spouse behavioural interactions. *Behav Ther* 1991, **22**:549–567.

Romano JM, Turner JA, Jensen MP et al. Chronic pain patient–spouse behavioral interactions predict patient disability. *Pain* 1995, **63**:353–360.

Segraves KB. Bringing it all together: developing the clinical team. In: Camic PM, Brown FD, eds. *Assessing Chronic Pain: A Multidisciplinary Handbook*. New York: Springer-Verlag; 1989:229–248.

Shaw WS, Feuerstein M, Haufler AJ et al. Working with low back pain: problem-solving orientation and function. *Pain* 2001, **93**:129–137.

Shone N. *Coping Successfully with Pain*. London: Sheldon Press; 1992.

Skevington SM. Investigating the relationship between pain and discomfort and the quality of life, using the WHOQOL. *Pain* 1998, **76**:395–406.

Snow-Turek AL, Norris MP, Tan G. Active and passive coping strategies in chronic pain patients. *Pain* 1996, **64**:455–462.

Spence SH, Sharpe L, Newton-John T et al. Effect of EMG biofeedback compared to applied relaxation training with chronic, upper extremity cumulative trauma disorders. *Pain* 1995, **63**:199–206.

Sternbach R. *Mastering Pain*. London: Arlington Press; 1987.

Strong J, Unruh AM, Wright A et al. *Pain: A Textbook for Therapists*. London: Churchill Livingstone; 2001.

Turk DC. Assessment of pain: the elusiveness of a latent construct. In: Chapman CR, Loeser J, eds. *Advances in Pain Research and Therapy*, vol. 12: *Issues in Pain Measurement*. New York: Raven; 1989:267–280.

Turk DC, Okifuji A. Psychological factors in chronic pain: evolution and revolution. *J Con Clin Psychol* 2002, **70**:678–690.

Turk DC, Rudy TE. Assessment of chronic pain patients. *Behav Res Ther* 1987, **25**:237–249.

Turk DC, Meichenbaum D, Genest M. *Pain and Behavioural Medicine: A Cognitive Behavioral Approach*. New York: Guilford Press; 1983.

Turk DC, Kerns RD, Rosenberg R. Effects of marital interaction on chronic pain and disability: examining the down side of social support. *Rehabil Psychol* 1992, **37**:259–274.

Turk DC, Okifuji A, Scharff L. Chronic pain and depression: role of perceived impact and perceived control in different age cohorts. *Pain* 1995, **61**:93–101.

Tyrer SP, Capon M, Peterson DM et al. The detection of psychiatric illness and psychological handicaps in a British pain clinic population. *Pain* 1989, **36**:63–74.

Villemure C, Bushnell MC. Cognitive modulation of pain: how do attention and emotion influence pain processing? *Pain* 2002, **95**:195–199.

Wade JB, Price DD, Hamer RM et al. An emotional component analysis of chronic pain. *Pain* 1990, **40**:303–310.

Wall P. *Pain: The Science of Suffering*. London: Weidenfeld and Nicolson, 1999.

Walsh DA, Radcliffe JC. Pain beliefs and perceived physical disability of patients with chronic low back pain. *Pain* 2002, **97**:23–31.

White AA. *Your Aching Back*. New York: Simon and Schuster; 1990.

World Health Organization. *Mental disorders, glossary and guide to their Classification in Accordance with the 10th Revision of the International Classification of Diseases (ICD) and Related Health Problems*. ICD-10, Chapter V, Geneva: WHO; 2002. Available online at: www.who.int/msa/mnh/ems/icd10/icd10.htm.

Recommended Reading

Strong J, Unruh AM, Wright A et al. *Pain: A Textbook for Therapists*. London: Churchill Livingstone; 2001.

Chapter **27**

Clinical neuropsychology in rehabilitation

JG Beaumont

INTRODUCTION

The field of clinical psychology that is concerned with neurological disorders has now become known as clinical neuropsychology. Although in the UK there is no formal definition of a clinical neuropsychologist, developments are currently under way which will result in the establishment of professional qualifications in neuropsychology. In practice, clinical neuropsychologists are chartered clinical psychologists with specialist experience and expertise in the field of neuropsychology, and often title themselves 'neuropsychologist'.

Whilst clinical neuropsychology is only now emerging as an independent area of professional psychology, it has a history as long as the history of modern scientific psychology. From the end of the last century, psychologists have investigated the behavioural effects of lesions to the brain, not only for the light this study could shed on the operation of normal brain processes but also from a genuine concern to alleviate the distress and disability resulting from neurological injury and disease.

Clinical neuropsychology was given an inevitable stimulus by the two World Wars of the twentieth century, the study of missile wounds proving a fertile ground for the association of specific psychological deficits with defined regions of the brain. This research carried significant implications for a debate, inherited from nineteenth-century neurology and which occupied at least the first half of the twentieth century, about the nature of the representation of psychological functions in the brain. Put rather crudely, the opposite poles of the debate argued either for the highly localised and specific representation of functions or for a mass action view whereby psychological functions are distributed across the entire cerebral cortex. This debate has never been finally resolved, but the position that most clinical neuropsychologists now adopt is one of relative localisation: that many functions are localised to regions of the cortex but cannot be more finely localised. This is often qualified by a tertiary model of cortical function in that the primary cortex, subserving sensation and discrete motor control, is quite highly localised; the secondary cortex, subserving perception and the control of movements, is rather less localised; and the tertiary or association cortex, supporting all higher-level functions, is much less clearly localised. Current developments in connectionist theory, which suggest radical models for neuropsychological processes are, however, starting to modify these views. For a fuller discussion, see Beaumont (1996) and for illustrations see Code et al. (1996, 2001).

Only within the last two decades has rehabilitation become an active focus of interest for clinical neuropsychology. Before that time clinicians saw their role as primarily one of assessment, in the context of either diagnosis or of vocational adjustment. The widespread introduction of modern neuroimaging greatly diminished the contribution of neuropsychology to diagnosis and as a result the embarrassing period of neglect of rehabilitation, both in terms of research and of practical interventions, came to an end. Rehabilitation is now the central focus of neuropsychology and assessment is understood, quite properly, as only a significant stage in the planning of rehabilitation and management.

APPROACHES IN CLINICAL NEUROPSYCHOLOGY

Clinical psychological management involves detailed assessment, which is discussed prior to reviewing interventions.

Neuropsychological assessment

Neuropsychological assessment should be understood as the essential precursor to the planning and implementation of rehabilitation. It is not an end in itself, but is designed to provide a description in psychological terms of the client's current state with respect to the clinical problems being addressed. Such a description should provide an insight into the processes which are no longer functioning normally in that individual, and so provide the rationale upon which the intervention is based. Subsequent reassessments allow progress to be monitored and interventions to be adjusted, according to the client's current state. Rehabilitation should never proceed without an adequate assessment having been undertaken.

The three traditions

There are historically three traditions in clinical neuropsychology. The first, most eloquently expressed in the work of Luria (Christensen, 1974), is based upon behavioural neurology, although it is a much more sophisticated extension of it. The approach is based upon the presentation of simple tasks, selected in a coherent way from a wide variety of tests available, which any normal individual can be expected to complete successfully without difficulty. Any failure on the task is a pathological sign and the pattern of these signs, in skilled hands, allows a psychological description to be built up.

The second tradition, associated with work in North America, is a psychometric battery-based approach, most notably expressed in the Halstead–Reitan and Luria Nebraska Neuropsychological Test Batteries (any apparent theoretical link with the approach of Luria is quite illusory). In this approach a standard, and often large, battery of tests is administered to all clients and the resulting descriptions arise out of a psychometric analysis of the pattern of test scores.

The third approach, the normative individual-centred approach, has been dominant in Europe, particularly in the UK, but is now the leading international methodology. It relies upon the use of specific tests, associated wherever possible with adequate normative standardisation, which are selected to investigate hypotheses about the client's deficits; testing these hypotheses permits the psychological description to be built up. Whilst requiring a high level of expertise, this neuropsychological detective work can be more efficient and provide a finer degree of analysis, when applied intelligently. In practice, many neuropsychologists employ a mixture of these approaches, although the normative individual-centred approach is generally becoming more dominant.

Cognitive functions

The greater part of neuropsychological assessment concentrates upon cognitive functions: perception, learning, memory, language, thinking and reasoning. This is a reflection of the principal interests of contemporary psychology. There is a bewildering variety of test procedures available to the clinical neuropsychologist, but most involve the presentation of standardised test materials in a controlled way; this can yield reliable scores which are then interpreted with respect to appropriate normative data. These norms may be more or less adequate for the clinical population under consideration, and there are certainly some excellent, some very good, and some rather inadequate tests.

Even a partial description of the most popular tests is outside the scope of this chapter, but a good introduction may be found in Harding & Beech (1996), and a more thorough account in Crawford et al. (1992), Lezak (1995) and Spreen & Strauss (1998).

Behavioural assessment

Assessment of behaviour (as distinct from specifically cognitive performance), usually in relation to undesirable behaviours or defective interpersonal or social skills, relies more directly upon observational recording. Here the object is to identify the antecedents of the behaviour under investigation, and then to analyse the consequences of the behaviour for the individual. In this way an understanding can be gained of what causes the behaviour, and what maintains the behaviour in the individual's repertoire. This information can be used to construct a programme designed to modify the behaviour (see below) or simply be used to provide feedback to the client to assist him or her to gain the insight to modify his or her own behaviour.

Behavioural sampling – the regular observation and recording of relevant aspects of behaviour for fixed samples of time – is frequently employed, and carers may also be requested to maintain records or diaries of specific events. Video recording, sometimes with detailed analysis, may also be employed.

Affective states

Clinical neuropsychologists are also commonly asked to evaluate other aspects of behaviour: affective states, motivation, insight, adjustment to disability, pain and, often most difficult of all, the possible psychological basis of apparently organic neurological states. It is for this reason, amongst others, that a thorough training in clinical psychology is considered essential for neuropsychological practice. A certain number of standard questionnaires and rating scales are available to assist in this assessment, but the neuropsychologist must commonly rely upon clinical experience and expertise in forming a judgement.

Outcome measures and the quality of life

The political climate of health service changes in the UK has forced health care providers to consider the outcome of their interventions, and this can only be to the advantage of clients. Psychologists, because of their expertise in the measurement of behaviour, have been prominent in the development of outcome measures. Within neuropsychological rehabilitation there is a variety of measures, of which the Barthel Index (Wade, 1992) is widely used, and the Functional Independence Measure–Functional Assessment Measure (FIM–FAM: Ditunno, 1992; Cook et al., 1994) is growing in popularity as it can be linked to problem-oriented and client-centred rehabilitation planning. However, none of the available scales is adequate to assess the status of severely disabled clients (see Ch. 3), and there is also a lack of good measures of the specific outcome of psychological interventions. Research is actively being undertaken to fill these gaps, and a discussion is to be found in Fleminger & Powell (1999).

Allied to the need to assess outcomes has been a growing interest in quality of life (QoL), recognising that not only functional and physical status should be considered but also the individual's personal feelings and life experience. A central problem is that QoL is not a unitary concept and encompasses a range of ideas, from the spiritual and metaphysical to cognitions about health and happiness. What is clear is that QoL relates not in a direct, but in a very complex, way to health status, physical disability and handicap, and that the precise nature of this relationship has yet to be clarified.

Cognitive neuropsychology

Cognitive neuropsychology should be understood as a distinct, and currently very fashionable approach within neuropsychology. Of growing importance over the past decade, cognitive neuropsychology concentrates upon the single case and seeks to explain psychological deficits in terms of the components of cognitive information-processing models. Such models, which are now quite detailed in respect of functions such as reading, spelling and face recognition, are based upon experimental data derived from normal individuals and from clinical investigations. These models are modular, and dysfunction can be understood in terms of the faulty performance of either the modules or the connections between them.

Cognitive neuropsychological analysis has been of enormous importance in developing our understanding of both normal and abnormal cognitive psychological functions within the brain but, partly because of the resources required to analyse a problem fully using this approach in the individual case, it has not made such a great impact upon the clinical practice of neuropsychologists.

Neuropsychological interventions

Management strategies include cognitive and behavioural interventions as well as psychotherapy.

Cognitive interventions

Cognitive interventions aim to reduce the impact of deficits in the areas of memory, learning, perception, language, and thinking and reasoning. How this is achieved depends in part upon the model of recovery that is adopted but, in general, requires either new learning or the development of strategies which bypass the abnormal components in the system. There are often a variety of routes by which an end result may be achieved. Perhaps trivially, consider how many ways 9 may be multiplied by 9 to achieve 81. There are in fact at least nine ways. If you learnt the solution by rote learning, you may well find that your children have been taught a different method: $9 \times 10 - 9$, or the fact that the first digit of the solution is $9 - 1$ and that the two digits of the answer sum to 9. These are different strategies of finding the solution. If the previously available strategy has been lost, it may be more successful to teach a new strategy that relies upon different brain mechanisms.

Besides the explicit teaching of new strategies, appropriately structured training may be employed; this is often based upon error-free learning, which has been shown to be most effective following head injury. Aids to performance, which may be either external (such as diaries to aid memory) or internal (mnemonics), may also be successfully employed. These interventions are more fully developed in some areas than others, and have been used most extensively in the rehabilitation of memory (Wilson & Moffat, 1992; Kapur, 1994), but the basic principles can be applied in any area of cognitive function (see also Riddoch & Humphreys, 1994; Prigatano, 1999).

Behavioural interventions

Behavioural interventions are less widely employed but may be appropriate to address the remediation of undesirable behaviours and in situations where the residual cognitive function of the individual is severely limited. These interventions are based upon psychological learning theory which, put rather simply, states that behaviour is determined by its consequences. Behaviour which leads to a 'good' outcome for the individual will increase in frequency; that which has an undesirable outcome for the individual will decrease in frequency. Behaviours that are desirable (from the perspective of the rehabilitation goals) can therefore be increased by ensuring that they are positively re-inforced (given a good outcome for the individual), whilst undesirable behaviours do not receive such reinforcement. In laboratory situations, negative re-inforcement (punishment) might be used to reduce

the frequency of a behaviour, but in a clinical situation its use would be extremely exceptional (perhaps only in relation to a significant life-threatening behaviour and then only with informed consent); in practice, the lack of positive reinforcement is sufficient for the undesired behaviour to reduce in frequency.

The range of behavioural techniques is both wider and more sophisticated than this brief account might suggest, and in certain selected contexts these approaches may be highly effective (Wood, 1990). However, the demands on resources and staff skills are high, given that a behavioural programme must be applied consistently, contingently and continuously, often over a very protracted period. For this reason, behavioural approaches are less commonly employed outside specialist facilities, although they are perhaps unreasonably neglected within other rehabilitation contexts.

Psychotherapy; staff, team and organisational support; research

Psychologists in neuropsychological practice are also involved in a variety of more general clinical psychological issues. Amongst these is the provision of psychotherapy or counselling, which may follow one of a large variety of models and is often eclectic in nature, addressing issues of personal loss, life changes and adjustment to disability. Psychotherapeutic techniques appropriate to neuropsychological disability are relatively underdeveloped, and are associated with a number of specific problems such as cognitive limitations and impairment of memory.

Because of their specialist knowledge of human and social relations, and of organisational processes, psychologists will advise and provide practical support to the construction and functioning of clinical teams, besides giving staff support at an individual level. Staff stress is often high in neurological care settings, and the health and welfare of staff are important not only as ends in themselves, but also because they have consequences for the care of patients.

Psychologists, who have been trained in methods of research design and analysis, are also commonly active in research relating to neuro-disability and in supporting the research of others, and regard it as an important aspect of their role.

NEUROPSYCHOLOGICAL CONSEQUENCES OF NEUROLOGICAL DISORDERS

The consequences and management of neuropsychological problems cannot be discussed in any detail in this chapter but several useful texts exist (Riddoch & Humphreys, 1994; Beaumont et al., 1996; Kolb & Whishaw, 1996).

General considerations

The neuropsychological consequences of neurological disease depend upon a number of factors, not all of which are determined by the neurological aetiology.

Focal versus diffuse

Focal, relatively localised lesions result in quite different effects from lesions which diffusely affect the cerebral cortex. Most specific neuropsychological deficits of cognitive function are associated with relatively focal lesions (following trauma, tumours or surgical intervention), and these have generally been the area of study of neuropsychologists. By contrast, diffuse lesions (following infections, generalised degeneration or widespread closed head injury) tend to affect level of consciousness, attention, motivation and initiation and affect, rather than specific psychological functions.

Acute versus chronic

Acute lesions have greater effects than chronic lesions. In the acute period following the acquisition of a lesion there may be widespread disruption of psychological functions, together with changes in the level of consciousness, confusion and loss of orientation. Amnesia is common in the acute period, and the duration of posttraumatic amnesia, before continuous memory and full orientation return, is the best indicator of the severity of the lesion (see Ch. 7, p. 106). Neuropsychological consequences diminish over time, most of the recovery occurring within the first 6–12 months, but with further improvements occurring over the next year or a little longer.

Progressive versus static; speed of development

Lesions that continue to develop, such as tumours and degenerative conditions, have a greater impact than lesions that are essentially static after the initial acute period, such as trauma, cerebrovascular accidents and surgical interventions. The assumption is that the brain accommodates more readily the presence of a static lesion, but must continue to adapt to a developing lesion.

Within progressive lesions, those that develop more rapidly will cause greater psychological disruption than those which develop more slowly. This effect is seen most clearly in the case of tumours, where slow-growing tumours such as meningiomas have much less effect than more rapidly growing tumours such as gliomas. Indeed, meningiomas may grow to a very considerable size before they cause sufficient interference with psychological function to come to medical attention; this is most unlikely to happen in the case of the more aggressive tumours, where a much smaller lesion will have dramatic behavioural consequences.

Site and lateralisation

The site is obviously of relevance in the case of a focal lesion, and will determine the neuropsychological consequences within the principle of relative localisation (see above). Lateralisation, whether the lesion is primarily located in the left or right hemisphere of the cerebral cortex, is also of relevance as the psychological functions assumed by the two hemispheres are known to differ. There is an enormous literature on cerebral lateralisation, which was the most prominent research topic of neuropsychology for the two decades from about 1960, and most functions show some degree of differential lateralisation. The clearest case is speech, which is exclusively located in the left hemisphere of about 95% of right-handed individuals (Beaumont et al., 1996; Kolb & Whishaw, 1996).

Age of acquisition

The age at which a lesion is acquired may also be of relevance, as the effects are less in the younger patient and throughout the childhood years (the Kennard principle). This was previously attributed to an increased plasticity of the developing brain, in that alternative regions could subsume the functions previously destined to be located in the area containing the lesion. However, there is now some doubt over this hypothesis, partly due to accumulating evidence for the continuing neural adaptability of the brain in adult life (see Ch. 5). The explanation may lie at least as much in the cognitive flexibility of the developing psychological systems and the greater opportunities for alternative forms of learning in the preadult period.

Specific aetiologies

As stated above, it is not possible to describe the management of neuropsychological problems in the conditions mentioned in this section. As well as the psychology texts cited in this chapter, the reader is referred to a book on neurological rehabilitation which devotes sections to cognitive and behavioural problems (Greenwood et al., 1993).

Head injury

Head injury is the most common cause of neuro-disability for which rehabilitation is undertaken (see Ch. 7). It affects young males more than any other group and effective intervention can result in a very favourable outcome. Head injuries range from very mild to very severe and profound, with dramatic differences in the behavioural consequences up to and including prolonged coma and vegetative states. The lesions associated with head injury are generally focal or multifocal, and static, although acceleration–deceleration closed head injuries may result in widespread and diffuse lesions across the cortex. An important consideration is that even apparently very mild head injuries associated with a brief period of concussion may sometimes have significant behavioural consequences in terms of anxiety, depression, changes in personality and subtle disorders of memory, with consequent effects upon occupational performance, social activity and personal relationships.

Stroke

Stroke, perhaps because it tends to occur in the more elderly, has received less attention than head injury. The effects of strokes and other cerebrovascular accidents will depend upon the area and proportion of the arterial distribution which is lost, ranging from the whole territory of one of the main cerebral arteries, which is a substantial proportion of the cortex, down to relatively discrete focal lesions associated with a distal portion of one of these arteries (see Ch. 6). Although the neuropsychological consequences depend primarily on the area of cortex affected, the picture is often complicated by the occurrence of further, perhaps minor strokes that prevent the psychological condition being stable, and by associated arterial disease, which may result in more general and perhaps fluctuating insufficiency of the blood supply to the entire cortex.

Degenerative conditions

Interest in the degenerative conditions from a neuropsychological perspective has grown in recent years. Other than the dementias of later life, principally dementia of the Alzheimer type, which are clearly associated with deficits of cognitive function of a progressive nature, there are a number of other degenerative conditions which occur in adult life, but of which the neuropsychological consequences are only beginning to be understood. Multiple sclerosis, the most common neurological disease of the population, Parkinson's disease, Huntington's disease and motor neurone disease, sometimes referred to collectively as the subcortical dementias, are all associated with cognitive, affective and behavioural deficits in a significant proportion of those with the disease, and almost all those whose disease progresses to an advanced stage suffer psychological sequelae (see Chs 10–13). Disorders of memory, attention and affect are common as primary consequences of the disease in this group, and there are naturally significant psychological disturbances associated with being a sufferer from one of these diseases.

Spinal injuries

Spinal cord injury clearly differs from other neurological conditions in that the patient has suffered a disabling condition, but all neural systems supporting psychological functions are intact (see Ch. 8). The main issue is therefore one of adjustment to the disability, both in terms of the primary impairment dependent upon the spinal cord lesion and the secondary consequences of handicap that follow from the disability. Amongst the primary disabilities are loss of mobility and other functional capacities (especially if the upper limbs are affected), together with loss of bladder and bowel control and, most importantly for psychological health, sexual function may also be affected. Depression is very common following spinal injury, and the facilitation of insight and adjustment to the disability is a primary task for the neuropsychologist.

Neuropsychological disorders of movement

Apraxia

Apraxia refers to disorders of voluntary movement in the absence of sensory loss, paresis or motor weakness (Heilman & Valenstein, 1993; Jeannerod, 1997; Rothi & Heilman, 1997). It is normally demonstrated when the patient is asked to respond to a command, or to produce an action outside its normal context. It is therefore probably the intentional aspects of the task which are the root of the problem. A distinction is often drawn between ideomotor and ideational apraxia. Ideomotor apraxia is a disorder of simple gestures to be produced either on command or by imitation, while the ability to perform more complex tasks may be largely intact; that 'the patient knows what to do but not how to do it' is a helpful dictum. By contrast, ideational apraxia refers to the inability to perform actions requiring a well-ordered sequence of elements. However, while this is an important distinction in the literature, there is still considerable debate about the dissociability of these two conditions. Both conditions are associated with lesions in the posterior cortical regions, especially the parietal lobe, and in the dominant hemisphere. An interesting feature of both conditions is that the relevant behaviours may be performed without difficulty in everyday life; the problem only appears when conscious attention is directed to the task. Dressing apraxia has been regarded as an independent form of apraxia, but there is some reason to believe that it is only the difficulty of this particular task which involves the integration of body elements with external space, and complex personal movements in relation to highly plastic objects, that makes it appear a distinct entity. Constructional apraxia is, however, a distinct type of apraxia and involves a defect in the spatial aspects of a task in relationship to individual motor movements. The problem appears to lie in the integration of visuo-spatial information and voluntary motor acts, and may be apparent in drawing, or in the construction of three-dimensional models. The disorder is also associated with lesions of parietal cortex and some believe that it has a different flavour when the right hemisphere is involved affecting visuospatial perception, or the left hemisphere affecting motor execution.

Neglect

Unilateral neglect, or unilateral hemi-inattention, has attracted considerable research interest in recent years (Robertson & Marshall, 1993). Patients with this disorder act as if one side of space, more commonly the left side of space following right parietal lesion, did not exist. This is in the absence of any visual field defect. In extreme cases patients may only eat food on the right half of their plate, dress the right side of their body and attend to visual events to their right. It can occur in relation to imagined scenes as well as to real stimuli. There is still considerable debate about whether the problem is one of disordered internal representations, or one of attentional deficit. It seems clear, however, that patients have some semantic access to the information appearing in the neglected space, but this information does not enter consciousness, or direct behaviour. Voluntary limb activation, out of sight and on the neglected side, has proved the most effective treatment approach to date (Halligan et al., 1991; Robertson & Marshall, 1993; Antonucci et al., 1995).

Motor memory

Memory for motor acts, and in particular motor skills, has been shown to be distinct from memory for semantic or episodic information. It is noteworthy that even patients with a dense global amnesia, as in the amnesic syndrome, may retain the ability to perform previously learned motor skills. Their ability to acquire new motor skills may be less impaired than their ability to learn new semantic information or recall recent events. While disorders of motor memory are much less well researched than other aspects of memory, it is worth noting that even a serious impairment of memory will not necessarily prevent the learning of new motor tasks. We can conversely assume that there are specific disorders of motor memory in the absence of other memory problems, but these are little studied.

CONCLUSIONS

Factors that influence psychological management and that need to be considered include the cognitive ability and psychological adjustment of the patient, and a collaborative team approach.

Cognitive ability

An important determinant of the psychological effects of neurological injury or disease is the cognitive status of the individual. Besides specific cognitive deficits, which may limit both psychological and functional adjustment to the disease, more general factors such as attentional capacity, motivation and the capacity for learning and the acquisition of skills will all contribute to the eventual outcome.

Premorbid intellectual capacity will also be a factor; it is known that the best protective factor against dementia in advanced age is to be more intelligent as an adult, and the same principle applies to all neuropsychological deficits. The more you have, the less you will be affected by a given loss, and the more you have left with which to compensate. Nevertheless, those who functioned at a high intellectual level with a mentally demanding occupation before illness may also be more acutely aware of relatively subtle deficits in their ability and this may have a disproportionate effect upon their capacity to pursue a previous occupation.

Relatively intact cognitive abilities may contribute to the ability to benefit from rehabilitation interventions, and to gain insight and consequent adjustment to the disability, although in some severely affected individuals the lack of insight and memory for what has been lost may result in an unawareness which is in some respects protective, even if it cannot be regarded as psychologically healthy.

Psychological adjustment

Good psychological adjustment depends upon: satisfactory insight into the events and psychological changes that have occurred and a personal accept-ance of these changes; an appropriate adjustment of the perception of self; a modification of beliefs and personal goals; and the acquisition of appropriate strategies to compensate as far as is possible for any residual handicap. It implies not only psychological adjustment, but also the re-establishment of per-sonal, family and social relationships, both intimate and more distant. It may also involve occupational adjustment and redefinition of personal roles in all these contexts. This the psychologist must understand and have the skills to facilitate.

It should also be recognised that not all those who acquire neurological diseases had perfect psycholog-ical adjustment before the problem occurred; occa-sionally, the personality of a patient, as perceived by those close to him or her, has actually been improved by the condition. Not everyone who is neurologically intact is in good psychological health, and the goal of returning the client to this state may be confounded by circumstances quite unrelated to the neurological problem.

The process of care

Neuropsychologists generally work within a team, particularly in rehabilitation settings. They must con-tribute to the team not only by their support, but also by effectively playing the appropriate multidiscipli-nary role within the team. A psychologist who is priv-ileged to work within an expert and committed team will respect the particular contributions made by other team members. They will come to realise that it is only by the collaborative efforts of the disciplines within the team that the optimal outcome will be achieved for the patient, and that the patient will have the best chance of a good psychological adjustment to his or her condition and obtain the best quality of life that is possible.

References

Antonucci G, Gauriglia C, Judicia A et al. Effectiveness of neglect rehabilitation in a randomised group study. *J Clin Exp Neuropsychol* 1995, **17**:383–389.

Beaumont JG. Neuropsychology. In: Beaumont JG, Kenealy PM, Rogers MJC, eds. *Blackwell Dictionary of Neuropsychology*. Oxford: Blackwell Publishers; 1996;523–531.

Beaumont JG, Kenealy PM, Rogers MJC (eds). *Blackwell Dictionary of Neuropsychology*. Oxford: Blackwell Publishers; 1996.

Christensen A-L. *Luria's Neuropsychological Investigation*. Copenhagen: Munksgaard; 1974.

Code C, Wallesch C-W, Lecours AR, Joanette Y. *Classic Cases in Neuropsychology*. Hove: Psychology Press; 1996.

Code C, Wallesch C-W, Joanette Y, Lecours AR. *Classic Cases in Neuropsychology*, vol. II. Hove: Psychology Press; 2001.

Cook L, Smith DS, Truman G. Using Functional Independence Measure profiles as an index of outcome in the rehabilitation of brain-injured patients. *Arch Phys Med Rehab* 1994, **75**:390–393.

Crawford JR, Parker DM, McKinlay WW. *A Handbook of Neuropsychological Assessment*. Hove: Lawrence Erlbaum; 1992.

Ditunno JF Jr. Functional assessment measures in CNS trauma. *J Neurotrauma* 1992, **9**(Suppl. 1):S301–S305.

Fleminger S, Powell J (eds). *Evaluation of Outcomes in Brain Injury Rehabilitation*. Hove: Psychology Press; 1999.

Greenwood R, Barnes MP, McMillan TM et al. *Neurological Rehabilitation*. London: Churchill Livingstone; 1993.

Halligan PW, Manning L, Marshall JC. Hemispheric activation vs. spatio-motor cueing in visual neglect: a case study. *Neuropsychologia* 1991, **29**:165–176.

Harding L, Beech JR. *Assessment in Neuropsychology*. London: Routledge; 1996.

Heilman KM, Valenstein E (eds). *Clinical Neuropsychology*, 3rd edn. New York: Oxford University Press; 1993.

Jeannerod M. *The Cognitive Neuroscience of Action*. Oxford: Blackwell; 1997.

Kapur N. *Memory Disorders in Clinical Practice*. Hove: Lawrence Erlbaum; 1994.

Kolb B, Whishaw IQ. *Fundamentals of Human Neuropsychology*, 4th edn. New York: WH Freeman; 1996.

Lezak M. *Neuropsychological Assessment*, 3rd edn. New York: Oxford University Press; 1995.

Prigatano G. *Principles of Neuropsychological Rehabilitation*. Oxford: Oxford University Press; 1999.

Riddoch MJ, Humphreys GW. *Cognitive Neuropsychology and Cognitive Rehabilitation*. Hove: Lawrence Erlbaum; 1994.

Robertson IH, Marshall JC (eds). *Unilateral Neglect: Clinical and Experimental Studies*. Hove: Lawrence Erlbaum; 1993.

Rothi LJG, Heilman KM (eds). *Apraxia: The Neuropsychology of Action*. Hove: Psychology Press; 1997.

Spreen O, Strauss E (eds). *A Compendium of Neuropsychological Tests*, 2nd edn. New York: Oxford University Press; 1998.

Wade DT. The Barthel ADL index: guidelines. In: Wade DT, ed. *Measurement in Neurological Rehabilitation*. Oxford: Oxford University Press; 1992:177–178.

Wilson BA, Moffat N. *Clinical Management of Memory Problems*, 2nd edn. London: Chapman & Hall; 1992.

Wood RL. *Neurobehavioural Sequelae of Traumatic Brain Injury*. London: Taylor & Francis; 1990.

Chapter 28

Drug treatments in neurological rehabilitation

M Khanderia

Drug therapy in patients with neurological disorders is aimed mainly at treating and controlling symptoms of conditions for which there is usually no cure. The majority of these disorders are chronic and require multiple drug therapy. Patients vary in their response to drugs. Actions and side-effects of many drugs are dose-dependent and often exaggerate the underlying neurological condition. Therefore in planning, administering and assessing care of a patient with a neurological disorder, the combined effects of all drugs prescribed should be taken into account. Pharmacists are a valuable resource for advice on issues relating to multiple drug therapy.

This chapter, in the form of a glossary of drugs used in neurological disorders, focuses on uses and side-effects that are considered of interest to a physiotherapist. This glossary does not provide an exhaustive guide to drugs or discuss their uses in the context of pathology. The reader should refer to the relevant chapters in this book for the latter. The information about drugs included in this chapter is drawn from the *British National Formulary* (2003), *UK Medicines Compendium* (2003) and *Martindale* (2003). The reader requiring comprehensive information about a particular drug is referred to these texts.

Recommended international non-proprietary names (rINN), or generic names, have been used in this text. Where a British approved name (BAN) differs from rINN, the BAN is included in brackets after the rINN. Proprietary names used in the text (in italics following the generic name) are those used in the UK; those used outside the UK may be found in *Martindale* (2002) and/or in the respective national formulary. Table 28.1 at the end of the glossary lists a cross-reference between generic names (rINN), proprietary names (marked with asterisks) and the indication for use of these drugs in neurological conditions. Unlicensed use of drugs for clinical or research purposes is not included in this text.

1. EPILEPSY

Carbamazepine (Tegretol)

Use All forms of simple and complex partial seizures and tonic–clonic seizures. Also used in the treatment of trigeminal neuralgia and in the prophylaxis of bipolar disorder unresponsive to lithium. Has little or no use in absent seizures. May be used alone or with other anticonvulsants.

Side-effects Ataxia, diplopia, drowsiness, dizziness, vertigo, tremor, headache, nausea, diarrhoea, dry mouth, itching, behavioural disturbance and agitation.

Clonazepam (Rivotril)

Use Status epilepticus, myoclonus and all forms of epilepsy.

Side-effects Drowsiness, fatigue, dizziness, muscle hypotonia, co-ordination disturbances, paradoxical aggression, irritability and mental changes.

Ethosuximide (Zarontin)

Use Absent seizures (periods of lack of awareness or response but without convulsions).

Side-effects Drowsiness, dizziness, ataxia, dyskinesia, headache, extrapyramidal side-effects, lethargy and fatigue, gastrointestinal disturbances, weight loss, psychotic states, irritability, hyperactivity, sleep disturbances, night terrors, inability to concentrate and aggressiveness.

Gabapentin (Neurontin)

Use As an adjunct in the treatment of partial seizures with or without secondary generalisation that are not satisfactorily controlled with other antiepileptics, and for treatment of neuropathic pain.

Side-effects Drowsiness, dizziness, ataxia, fatigue, nystagmus, nervousness, headache, tremor, diplopia, nausea and vomiting, and dysarthria.

Lamotrigine (Lamictal)

Use May be used alone or as an adjunct in partial seizures, primary and secondary generalised tonic–clonic seizures.

Side-effects Drowsiness, diplopia, blurred vision, dizziness, insomnia, headache, ataxia, tiredness, gastrointestinal disturbances, aggression, tremor, agitation and confusion.

Levetiracetam (Keppra)

Use As an adjunct in treatment of partial seizures with or without secondary generalisation.

Side-effects Drowsiness, asthenia, dizziness, nausea, amnesia, ataxia, aggression, nervousness, tremor, vertigo, headache and diplopia.

Oxcarbazepine (Trileptal)

Use Treatment of partial seizures with or without secondary generalised tonic–clonic seizures.

Side-effects Ataxia, drowsiness, nausea, vomiting, abdominal pain, dizziness, headache, agitation, amnesia, asthenia, ataxia, confusion, impaired concentration, depression, tremor, vertigo, nystagmus, diplopia and angioedema.

Phenobarbital

Use Status epilepticus and all forms of epilepsy except absent seizures.

Side-effects Drowsiness, lethargy, depression, ataxia, paradoxical excitement, restlessness and confusion in elderly.

Phenytoin (Epanutin)

Use Effective in tonic–clonic and partial seizures. Has a narrow therapeutic index and the relationship between dose and plasma concentrations is not linear, thus a small increase in dosage may lead to a large rise in plasma concentration with acute toxic side-effects.

Side-effects Nystagmus, blurred vision, ataxia, slurred speech, decreased co-ordination, mental confusion, paraesthesia, drowsiness, vertigo, dizziness, insomnia, motor twitching, headache, nausea, vomiting, constipation, tremor, rarely dyskinesias, peripheral neuropathy and lymphadenopathy.

Primidone (Mysoline)

Use Essential tremor and all forms of epilepsy except absent seizures.

Side-effects Drowsiness, ataxia, headache, dizziness, nausea and vomiting, and visual disturbances.

Sodium valproate (Epilim)

Use All forms of epilepsy.

Side-effects Ataxia, tremor, sedation, gastric irritation, nausea, oedema, hyperactivity and behavioural disturbances.

Tiagabine (Gabitril)

Use As an adjunct for treatment of partial seizures with or without secondary generalisation.

Side-effects Dizziness, tiredness, nervousness, tremor, concentration difficulties, emotional lability, speech impairment, diarrhoea, drowsiness and psychosis.

Topiramate (Topamax)

Use As an adjunct in the treatment of partial seizures with or without secondary generalisation, not satisfactorily controlled with other antiepileptics.

Side-effects Ataxia, confusion, dizziness, fatigue, paraesthesia, emotional lability, aphasia, diplopia, nausea, nystagmus and speech disorder.

Vigabatrin (Sabril)

Use Chronic epilepsy not satisfactorily controlled by other antiepileptics.

Side-effects Drowsiness, fatigue, dizziness, nervousness, irritability, headache, aggression, psychosis, excitation and agitation, occasional increase in seizure frequency, diplopia and gastrointestinal disturbances.

2. SPASTICITY

The effectiveness of drugs in reducing spasticity varies with the mode of application and the condition of the patient. For example, baclofen given intrathecally may be more effective than when given orally in some patients.

Baclofen (Lioresal)

Use Chronic and severe spasticity resulting from multiple sclerosis, spinal cord lesions, cerebral palsy and brain injury.

Side-effects Sedation, light-headedness, dizziness, ataxia, headache, tremor, nystagmus, paraesthesiae, convulsions, muscular pain and weakness, gastrointestinal and urinary disturbances, increased sweating and paradoxical increase in spasticity.

Botulinum A toxin (Botox, Dysport)

Use Under investigation for treatment of chronic and severe spasticity in multiple sclerosis and brain injury; injected into muscle, e.g. to relieve hip adductor or elbow flexor spasticity.

Side-effects Muscle weakness.

Dantrolene (Dantrium)

Use Chronic severe spasticity.

Side-effects Drowsiness, dizziness, weakness, malaise, fatigue, nervousness, diarrhoea, nausea, headache, less frequently constipation, dysphagia, speech and visual disturbances, seizures, dyspnoea and urinary incontinence or retention.

Diazepam (Valium), Methocarbamol (Robaxin), Orphenadrine (Disipal)

Use For short-term symptomatic relief of muscle spasms of varied aetiology with the exception of muscle spasm resulting from coma, pre-coma, brain damage, epilepsy or myasthenia gravis.

Side-effects Light-headedness, fatigue, dizziness, drowsiness, nausea and paradoxical restlessness.

Phenol

Use Intrathecal block to reduce lower-limb spasticity and help control pain.

Side-effects Non-specific damage to other neural structures.

Tizanidine (Zanaflex)

Use Spasticity associated with multiple sclerosis or spinal cord injury or disease.

Side-effects Drowsiness, fatigue, dizziness, nausea, gastrointestinal disturbances and hypotension.

3. PARKINSON'S DISEASE

There are two groups of antiparkinsonian drugs, the dopaminergic and the antimuscarinic drugs.

Dopaminergic antiparkinsonian drugs

Amantadine (Symmetrel)

Use Parkinson's disease, with the exception of drug-induced extrapyramidal symptoms.

Side-effects Nervousness, dizziness, convulsions, blurred vision, gastrointestinal disturbances and peripheral oedema.

Apomorphine (Britaject)

Use Patients with frequent 'on–off' fluctuations in motor performance which are inadequately controlled by conventional antiparkinsonian medication.

Side-effects Dyskinesia during the 'on' periods, postural instability and falls, increase in cognitive impairment, nausea, vomiting, sedation, postural hypotension, euphoria, light-headedness, restlessness and tremors.

Bromocriptine (Parlodel)

Use Idiopathic Parkinson's disease, both alone and in combination with levodopa.

Side-effects Nausea, vomiting, headache, dizziness, postural hypotension, drowsiness, vasospasm of the fingers and toes, particularly in patients with poor peripheral circulation, confusion, psychomotor excitation, dyskinesia and leg cramps.

Cabergoline (Cabaser)

Use As an adjunct to levodopa (with dopa-decarboxylase inhibitor) in Parkinson's disease.

Side-effects Epigastric and abdominal pain, breast pain, angina, epistaxis, peripheral oedema, nausea, dizziness, postural hypotension, dyskinesia, hyperkinesias, peripheral oedema, somnolence.

Entacapone (Comtess)

Use As an adjunct to levodopa with dopa-decarboxylase inhibitor in Parkinson's disease and 'end-of-dose' motor fluctuations.

Side-effects Nausea, vomiting, abdominal pain, dry mouth, dyskinesias, dystonia, hyperkinesias and dizziness.

Levodopa (Brocadopa, Larodopa) *used with a dopa-decarboxylase inhibitor, e.g. benserazide (co-beneldopa, Madopar) or carbidopa (co-careldopa, Sinemet)*

Use Idiopathic parkinsonism, with the exception of drug-induced extrapyramidal symptoms.

Side-effects Ataxia, gait abnormalities, numbness, abnormal involuntary movements, agitation, postural hypotension, dizziness, psychiatric symptoms which include hypomania and psychosis, drowsiness, headache, flushing, sweating, nausea, vomiting, dysphagia, peripheral neuropathy, diplopia, blurred vision, urinary retention and incontinence and fatigue.

Lisuride maleate (Revanil)

Use Treatment of Parkinson's disease, as monotherapy or in combination with levodopa.

Side-effects Nausea, vomiting, sudden severe fall in blood pressure in early stages of treatment, dizziness, headache, lethargy, malaise and drowsiness.

Pergolide (Celance)

Use Treatment of Parkinson's disease, as monotherapy or in combination with levodopa.

Side-effects Body pain, abdominal pain, nausea, dyspepsia, dyskinesia, somnolence, diplopia, dyspnoea, dizziness, drowsiness and hypotension.

Pramipexole (Mirapexin)

Use Treatment of Parkinson's disease, as monotherapy or in combination with levodopa.

Side-effects Nausea, drowsiness (including sudden onset of sleep), dizziness and dyskinesia during initial dose titration, peripheral oedema.

Ropinirole (Requip)

Use Parkinson's disease, more useful as an adjunct to levodopa.

Side-effects Nausea, abdominal pain, vomiting, oedema, somnolence, dyskinesia, confusion and occasionally severe hypotension.

Selegiline (Eldepryl)

Use Idiopathic parkinsonism, with the exception of drug-induced extrapyramidal symptoms, alone or in combination with levodopa.

Side-effects Hypotension, nausea and vomiting, headache, tremor, dizziness, vertigo, back pain, muscle cramps, joint pain and agitation.

Antimuscarinic antiparkinsonian drugs

Benzatropine mesilate (Cogentin), *biperiden* (Akineton), *orphenadrine hydrochloride*, (Disipal), *procyclidine hydrochloride*, (Kemadrin), *trihexyphenidyl hydrochloride (benzhexol hydrochloride)* (Broflex)

Use Parkinson's disease and drug-induced extrapyramidal symptoms.

Side-effects Dry mouth, gastrointestinal disturbances, dizziness, blurred vision, urinary retention, nervousness, and in high doses in susceptible patients, mental confusion, excitement and sedation (with benztropine and biperiden).

4. MOVEMENT ABNORMALITIES

Movement disorders covered here include essential tremor, chorea (e.g. in Huntington's disease), tics and related disorders.

Botulinum A toxin (Botox, Dysport) *and botulinum* B toxin (NeuroBloc)

Use Blepharospasm, hemifacial spasm and spasmodic torticollis.

Side-effects Ptosis, lacrimation, eye irritation, diplopia, increased electrophysiological jitter in some distant muscles, bruising, weakness of neck muscles, dysphagia and dryness of mouth. Excessive doses may produce distant and profound neuromuscular paralysis, reversed with time.

Chlorpromazine (Largactil), *haloperidol* (Serenace, Haldol), *pimozide* (Orap), *clonidine* (Dixarit), *sulpiride* (Dolmatil)

Use Motor tics, adjunctive treatment in choreas and Gilles de la Tourette syndrome.

Side-effects Extrapyramidal symptoms such as dystonic reactions and akathisia, parkinsonism, tremor, tardive dyskinesia, drowsiness; in more rare instances, agitation, convulsions, antimuscarinic symptoms such as dry mouth, nasal congestion, constipation, difficulty in micturition and blurred vision.

Piracetam (Nootropil)

Use Myoclonus of cortical origin.

Side-effects Hyperkinesia, drowsiness and nervousness.

Primidone (Mysoline)

Use Benign essential tremor.

Side-effects Drowsiness, nystagmus, ataxia, nausea, vomiting, headache and dizziness.

Propranolol (Inderal)

Use Treatment of essential tremor or tremor associated with anxiety or thyroytoxicosis.

Side-effects Postural hypotension, peripheral vasoconstriction, paraesthesia, dizziness, mood changes, psychoses, gastrointestinal disturbances and fatigue.

Tetrabenazine (Nitoman)

Use Movement disorders due to Huntington's chorea, senile chorea and related neurological conditions.

Side-effects Drowsiness, gastrointestinal disturbances, extrapyramidal dysfunction and hypotension.

Trihexyphenidyl hydrochloride (benzhexol hydrochloride) (Broflex)

Use In some movement disorders at high doses.

Side-effects Previously described in section on antiparkinsonian drugs.

5. MULTIPLE SCLEROSIS (MS)

Corticosteroids: methylprednisolone (Depo-Medrone)

Use   To hasten recovery following a relapse.

Side–effects   Cushing's syndrome, hypotension, mental disturbances and muscle wasting.

Amantadine (Symmetrel)

Use   To treat fatigue associated with MS.

Side–effects   Nervousness, restlessness, tremor, dizziness, convulsions, headache, blurred vision, gastrointestinal disturbances, peripheral oedema, dry mouth, sweating, tics and Gilles de la Tourette's syndrome.

Beta-1a-interferon (Avonex, Rebif), *beta-1b-interferon* (Betaferon)

Use   To reduce the frequency and severity of relapses in patients with relapsing remitting MS.

Side–effects   Injection site reactions, anxiety, convulsions and confusion.

Glatiramer acetate (Copaxone)

Use   To reduce frequency of relapses in ambulatory patients with relapsing remitting MS.

Side–effects   Flushing, chest pain, palpitations, tachycardia and dyspnoea may occur within minutes of injection; injection site reactions; nausea, peripheral and facial oedema, syncope, asthenia, headache, tremor, sweating, lymphadenopathy, hypertonia, arthralgia and convulsions.

Isoniazid/pyridoxine

Use   To treat tremor associated with MS. Does not affect progression or remission of disease.

Side–effects   Nausea, vomiting, peripheral neuritis, convulsions and psychotic episodes.

Cannabis

Use   Under investigation for the treatment of tremor, spasticity, ataxia and muscle pain associated with MS; currently classed as Schedule I Controlled Drug and a licence from the Home Office is needed for investigational use.

Side–effects   Weakness, dry mouth, dizziness, impairment of posture and balance.

6. STROKE

Sequelae seen in stroke can vary depending on the site of lesion and the type of haemorrhage, thrombosis or embolism (see Ch. 6). Drug treatment is aimed at controlling the symptoms and treating the predisposing risk factors such as hypertension, diabetes, hyperlipidaemia, obesity, smoking and alcohol excess. In addition, the following may be prescribed depending upon need: anticonvulsants, antiplatelet drugs such as aspirin, antispasticity drugs such as baclofen, anticoagulant drugs such as warfarin (contraindicated following cerebral haemorrhage) and nimodipine, a calcium channel blocker to prevent vascular spasm following subarachnoid haemorrhage (SAH).

7. HEAD AND SPINAL CORD INJURY

A prolonged or incomplete recovery may follow injury, and drug treatment is aimed at treating the sequelae such as posttraumatic epilepsy (1), spasticity (2), pain (9), depression (12) and loss of autonomic functions such as bladder and bowel control (16–18). Excessive bronchial and salivary secretions are treated with oral or transdermal administration of hyoscine.

8. INFLAMMATION

Steroidal anti–inflammatory drugs

Dexamethasone (Decadron), *hydrocortisone* (Hydrocortistab), *methylprednisolone* (Depo-Medrone), *prednisolone* (Deltastab), *triamcinolone* (Adcortyl, Kenalog, Lederspan)

Use   Injected locally into soft tissue or joints for anti-inflammatory effect to relieve pain, increase mobility and reduce deformity.

Side–effects   Occasionally, reaction at the site of injection.

Non–steroidal anti–inflammatory drugs

Aspirin, *azapropazone* (Rheumox), *diclofenac* (Voltarol), *diflunisal* (Dolobid), *ibuprofen* (Brufen), *indometacin* (Indocid), *ketoprofen* (Orudis, Oruvail), *mefenamic acid* (Ponstan), *naproxen* (Naprosyn, Synflex), *phenylbutazone* (Butacote), *piroxicam* (Feldene) *and the selective cyclo-oxygenase 2 (COX2) inhibitors celecoxib* (Celebrex), *etodolac* (Lodine SR), *etoricoxib* (Arcoxia), *meloxicam* (Mobic), *rofecoxib* (Vioxx)

Use   To treat pain and inflammation.

Side-effects   Headache, dizziness, fatigue, vertigo, drowsiness, convulsions, peripheral neuropathy, muscle weakness, involuntary muscle movements, aggravation of epilepsy and parkinsonism, gastrointestinal side-effects such as nausea, dyspepsia, abdominal pain, oedema, hypotension and diplopia. There is a lower risk of upper gastrointestinal side-effects with the COX2 inhibitors.

9. PAIN

Non-opioid analgesics

Nefopam (Acupan)

Use   Moderate pain.

Side-effects   Nausea, vomiting, dry mouth, nervousness, light-headedness, drowsiness, confusion, urinary retention, blurred vision and sweating.

Paracetamol (Panadol)

Use   Mild to moderate pain, pyrexia.

Side-effects   Rash.

Non-steroidal anti-inflammatory drugs to control pain

Use   Previously described under inflammation (8).

Side-effects   Listed above (8).

Opioid analgesics

Buprenorphine (Temgesic), *codeine, dextropropoxyphene in combination with paracetamol as co-proxamol, diamorphine, dihydrocodeine* (DF 118), *dipipanone* (Diconal), *fentanyl* (Durogesic), *meptazinol* (Meptid), *morphine* (Oramorph, MST Continus), *pethidine, tramadol* (Zydol)

Use   Moderate to severe pain.

Side-effects   Nausea, vomiting, constipation, drowsiness, hypotension, difficulty with micturition, dry mouth, sweating, headache, facial flushing and vertigo.

10. TRIGEMINAL NEURALGIA

Carbamazepine (Tegretol), *oxcarbazepine* (Trileptal).

Use   In acute stage.

Side-effects   Listed under section on epilepsy (1).

Phenytoin (Epanutin)

Use   In crisis.

Side-effects   Listed under section on epilepsy (1).

Gabapentin (Neurontin), *lamotrigine* (Lamictal)

Use   In acute stage.

Side-effects   Listed under section on epilepsy (1).

11. MIGRAINE

Clonidine (Dixarit)

Use   Prophylaxis of recurrent migraine.

Side-effects   Dry mouth, sedation, dizziness and nausea.

Methysergide (Deseril)

Use   Prevention of recurrent migraine and cluster headache.

Side-effects   Nausea, vomiting, heartburn, drowsiness, dizziness, postural hypotension, mental and behavioural disturbances, oedema, rashes, leg cramps and paraesthesiae of extremities.

Pizotifen (Sanomigran)

Use   Prophylaxis of vascular headache, cluster headache and migraine.

Side-effects   Dry mouth, nausea, constipation, drowsiness and dizziness.

Propranolol (Inderal)

Use Migraine prophylaxis.

Side-effects See section on movement abnormalities (4).

Ergotamine (Cafergot, Migril)

Use Treatment of migraine.

Side-effects Nausea, vomiting, abdominal pain, paraesthesiae, peripheral vasoconstriction, pain and weakness in the extremities, numbness, muscle cramps and occasionally increased headache.

Paracetamol with an antiemetic such as metoclopramide (Paramax)

Use Treatment of migraine.

Side-effects Metoclopramide can cause extrapyramidal symptoms of dystonic type, tardive dyskinesia, neuroleptic syndrome, drowsiness, restlessness and diarrhoea.

Sumatriptan (Imigran) *and other 5HT1 agonists*

Use Treatment of migraine.

Side-effects Chest pain and tightness, sensations of tingling, heat, heaviness, pressure or tightness in any part of the body, flushing, dizziness, weakness, paraesthesiae, seizures, hypotension, nausea, vomiting, fatigue and drowsiness.

12. DEPRESSION

Tricyclic antidepressants

Amitriptyline, clomipramine (Anafranil), *dosulepin* (Prothiaden), *imipramine* (Tofranil), *lofepramine* (Gamanil), *trimipramine* (Surmontil)

Use Treatment of moderate to severe endogenous depression.

Side-effects Dry mouth, nausea, constipation, sedation, blurred vision, difficulty with micturition, syncope, postural hypotension, sweating, tremor, behavioural disturbances, movement disorders and dyskinesias, convulsions, numbness, paraesthesia of extremities, peripheral neuropathy, inco-ordination, extrapyramidal symptoms, dizziness, weakness, fatigue and headache.

Other antidepressants related to the tricyclics

Maprotiline (Ludiomil), *mianserin, trazodone* (Molipaxin)

Use Treatment of moderate to severe endogenous depression.

Side-effects As for the tricyclic antidepressants but with milder antimuscarinic side-effects.

Monoamine oxidase inhibitors

Phenelzine (Nardil), *isocarboxazid, tranylcypromine* (Parnate)

Use In patients refractory to treatment with other antidepressants.

Side-effects Postural hypotension, dizziness, drowsiness, headache, weakness, fatigue, dry mouth, constipation, other gastrointestinal disturbances, oedema, agitation, tremors, nervousness, blurred vision, difficulty in micturition, sweating, convulsions and psychotic episodes with hypomanic behaviour.

Reversible monoamine oxidase inhibitors

Moclobemide (Manerix)

Use Major depression and social phobia.

Side-effects Dizziness, nausea, headache, restlessness and agitation.

Selective serotonin reuptake inhibitors (SSRIs)

Citalopram (Cipramil), *fluoxetine* (Prozac), *fluvoxamine* (Faverin), *paroxetine* (Seroxat), *sertraline* (Lustral)

Use In patients intolerant to the side-effects of the tricyclic antidepressants.

Side-effects Nausea, vomiting, diarrhoea, dry mouth, dyspepsia, headache, agitation, drowsiness, tremor, dizziness, fatigue, seizures, dyskinesia, movement disorders and sweating.

Serotonin and noradrenaline (norepinephrine) reuptake inhibitors

Venlafaxine (Efexor)

Use Treatment of depression accompanied by anxiety.

Side-effects Nausea, constipation, dry mouth, headache, drowsiness, dizziness (and occasionally hypotension), asthenia, nervousness, sweating, weight changes, dyspnoea, paraesthesia, tremor, hypertonia, psychiatric disturbances (including agitation, anxiety, abnormal dreams), arthralgia, myalgia, visual disturbances and movement disorders.

13. PSYCHOSES

Psychoses resulting from schizophrenia, brain damage, mania, toxic delirium or agitated depression.

Phenothiazines and similar antipsychotic drugs

Chlorpromazine (Largactil), *flupentixol* (Depixol), *fluphenazine hydrochloride* (Modecate), *haloperidol* (Haldol, Serenace), *sulpiride* (Dolmatil), *thioridazine* (Melleril), *trifluoperazine* (Stelazine), *zuclopenthixol* (Clopixol)

Use Schizophrenia and other psychoses with agitated, aggressive or hostile behaviour.

Side–effects Parkinsonian symptoms (including tremor), dystonia, dyskinesia, akathisia, tardive dyskinesia, hypotension, tachycardia, electrocardiogram (ECG) changes, sweating, drowsiness, agitation, convulsions, dizziness, headache, confusion, gastrointestinal disturbances; nasal congestion; antimuscarinic symptoms (such as dry mouth, constipation, difficulty with micturition and blurred vision).

Atypical antipsychotics

Amisulpride (Solian), *clozapine* (Clozaril), *olanzapine* (Zyprexa), *quetiapine* (Seroquel), *risperidone* (Risperdal), *zotepine* (Zoleptil)

Use Schizophrenia in patients unresponsive to, or intolerant of, conventional antipsychotics.

Side–effects Dizziness, postural hypotension, extrapyramidal symptoms, tardive dyskinesia, agitation, drowsiness, gastrointestinal disorders such as constipation, nausea, vomiting, fatigue, blurred vision, dry mouth, dysphagia, headache, dizziness, hypersalivation, urinary incontinence and retention, arrhythmias, tachycardia, convulsions, oedema, electroencephalogram changes (QT interval prolongation) and oedema.

Antimanic drugs

Carbamazepine (Tegretol)

Use Prophylaxis of manic-depressive disorder.

Side–effects Listed under section on epilepsy (1).

Valproic acid (Depakote)

Use Treatment of manic episodes associated with bipolar disorder.

Side–effects Listed under section on epilepsy (1).

Lithium (Priadel)

Use Prophylaxis and treatment of mania, bipolar disorder and in the prophylaxis of recurrent disorder.

Side–effects Gastrointestinal disturbances, fine tremor, oedema, mild drowsiness and sluggishness.

14. VESTIBULAR AND BALANCE DISORDERS

Antihistaminics

Cinnarizine (Stugeron), *promethazine* (Avomine, Phenergan), *meclozine* (Sea-legs)

Use Vertigo, tinnitus, nausea, and vomiting in Ménière's disease and motion sickness.

Side–effects Drowsiness, occasional dry mouth and blurred vision, fatigue, extrapyramidal symptoms (rarely).

Phenothiazines

Chlorpromazine (Largactil), *prochlorperazine* (Stemetil), *perphenazine*, *trifluoperazine* (Stelazine)

Use Severe nausea, vomiting, vertigo and labyrinthine disorders.

Side–effects Listed under section on psychoses (13).

Metoclopramide (Maxolon)

Use Nausea and vomiting in adults.

Side–effects Extrapyramidal effects, drowsiness, restlessness, diarrhoea, depression, oedema and occasionally tardive dyskinesia on prolonged administration.

Domperidone (Motilium)

Use Nausea and vomiting.

Side–effects Acute dystonic reactions.

Betahistine (Serc)

Use Vertigo, tinnitus and hearing loss associated with Ménière's disease.

Side-effects Gastrointestinal disturbances; headache, rashes and pruritus.

15. ATTENTION DEFICIT DISORDER

Dexamfetamine sulphate (Dexedrine)

Use As an adjunct in the management of attention deficit-hyperactivity disorder.

Side-effects Restlessness, irritability, excitability, nervousness, tremor, dizziness, convulsions, sweating, tachycardia, palpitations and visual disturbances.

Methylphenidate hydrochloride (Ritalin)

Use Treatment of attention deficit-hyperactivity disorder.

Side-effects As for dexamfetamine sulphate; also skin reactions, fever and arthralgia.

16. BOWEL DISORDERS

Bulk-forming laxatives

Bran (Trifyba), *ispaghula husk* (Fybogel, Isogel, Regulan), *methylcellulose* (Celevac), *sterculia* (Normacol)

Side-effects Flatulence, abdominal distension and gastrointestinal obstruction or impaction.

Faecal softeners

Arachis oil (rectally), docusate (orally)

Side-effects Abdominal cramps.

Osmotic laxatives

Lactitol, lactulose, magnesium salts (Epsom salts), *phosphates* (Fletchers' Phosphate Enemas), *sodium citrate* (Microlette)

Side-effects Flatulence, cramps and abdominal discomfort.

Stimulant laxatives

Bisacodyl (Dulcolax), *Dantron* (Co-danthramer, Co-danthrusate), *docusate sodium* (Dioctyl),

glycerol, senna (Senokot), *sodium picosulfate* (Picolax)

Side-effects Increased intestinal motility and abdominal cramps; prolonged use can precipitate atonic colon and hypokalaemia.

17. DIARRHOEA/FAECAL INCONTINENCE

Codeine phosphate

Side-effects Nausea, vomiting, difficulty with micturition and dry mouth.

Loperamide (Imodium)

Side-effects Abdominal cramps and abdominal bloating.

Diphenoxylate/atropine combination (Lomotil)

Side-effects As for codeine.

18. BLADDER DISORDERS

Urinary retention

Alpha-blockers: alfuzosin (Xatral), *doxazosin* (Cardura), *indoramin* (Doralese), *prazosin* (Hypovase), *terazosin* (Hytrin)

Side-effects Sedation, dizziness, postural hypotension, weakness, lack of energy, headache, dry mouth, nausea, urinary frequency and incontinence.

Parasympathomimetic agents: bethanechol (Myotonine), *distigmine* (Ubretid)

Side-effects Nausea, vomiting, sweating and blurred vision.

Urinary frequency, enuresis, incontinence

Flavoxate (Urispas), *oxybutynin* (Cystrin, Ditropan), *propantheline* (Pro-Banthine), *tolterodine tartrate* (Detrusitol)

Side-effects Dry mouth, constipation, diarrhoea, blurred vision, nausea, abdominal discomfort, facial flushing, difficulty in micturition, headache, dizziness and drowsiness.

Table 28.1 Cross-reference of generic and proprietary drug names and their use in neurological disorders

Drug name	Drug name	Drug use (cross-reference to sections in this chapter)
Acupan*	Nefopam	Pain (9)
Adcortyl*	Triamcinolone	Inflammation (8)
Akineton	Biperiden*	Parkinson's (3)
Alfuzosin	Xatral*	Urinary retention (18)
Alrheumet*	Ketoprofen	Inflammation, pain (8, 9)
Amantadine	Symmetrel*	Parkinson's (3), fatigue in MS (5)
Amisulpride	Solian*	Psychoses (13)
Amitriptyline		Trigeminal neuralgia (10), depression (12)
Anafranil*	Clomipramine	Trigeminal neuralgia (10), depression (12)
Apomorphine	Britaject*	Parkinson's (3)
Arachis oil		Laxative (16)
Arcoxia*	Etoricoxib	Inflammation, pain (8, 9)
Aspirin		Inflammation, pain (8, 9)
Avomine*	Promethazine	Vestibular disorders (14)
Avonex*	Beta-1a-interferon	MS (5)
Azapropazone	Rheumox*	Inflammation, pain (8, 9)
Baclofen	Lioresal*	Spasticity (2)
Benzatropine	Cogentin*	Parkinson's (3)
Beta-1a-interferon	Avonex*, Rebif*	MS (5)
Beta-1b-interferon	Betaferon*	MS (5)
Betaferon*	Beta-1b-Interferon	MS (5)
Betahistine	Serc*	Vestibular disorders (14)
Bethanechol	Myotonine*	Urinary retention (18)
Biperiden	Akineton*	Parkinson's (3)
Bisacodyl	Dulcolax*	Laxative (16)
Botox*	Botulinum A toxin	Torticollis, blepharospasm (4), spasticity (2)
Botulinum A toxin	Botox*, Dysport*	Torticollis, blepharospasm (4), spasticity (2)
Botulinum B toxin	NeuroBloc*	Torticollis (4)
Britaject*	Apomorphine	Parkinson's (3)
Brocadopa*	Levodopa	Parkinson's (3)
Broflex*	Trihexyphenidyl (Benzhexol)	Parkinson's (3), tremor (4), chorea (4), tics (4)
Bromocriptine	Parlodel*	Parkinson's (3)
Brufen*	Ibuprofen	Inflammation, pain (8, 9)
Buprenorphine	Temgesic*	Pain (9)
Butacote*	Phenylbutazone	Inflammation, pain (8, 9)
Cabaser*	Cabergoline	Parkinson's (3)
Cabergoline	Cabaser*	Parkinson's (3)
Cafergot*	Ergotamine	Migraine (11)
Cannabis		MS (5)
Carbamazepine	Tegretol*	Epilepsy (1), trigeminal neuralgia (10), psychoses (13)
Cardura*	Doxazosin	Urinary retention (18)
Celance*	Pergolide	Parkinson's (3)
Celebrex*	Celecoxib	Inflammation, pain (8, 9)
Celecoxib	Celebrex*	Inflammation, pain (8, 9)
Chlorpromazine	Largactil*	Motor tics, chorea (4), psychoses (13), vestibular disorders (14)
Cinnarizine	Stugeron*	Vestibular disorders (14)

Continued

Table 28.1 (*Continued*)

Drug name	Drug name	Drug use (cross-reference to sections in this chapter)
Cipramil*	Citalopram	Depression (12)
Citalopram	Cipramil*	Depression (12)
Clomipramine	Anafranil*	Trigeminal neuralgia (10), depression (12)
Clonazepam	Rivotril*	Epilepsy (1)
Clonidine	Dixarit*	Motor tics, chorea (4), migraine (11)
Clopixol*	Zuclopenthixol	Psychoses (13)
Clozapine	Clozaril*	Psychoses (13)
Clozaril*	Clozapine	Psychoses (13)
Co-beneldopa	Madopar*	Parkinson's (3)
Co-careldopa	Sinemet*	Parkinson's (3)
Co-proxamol	Dextropropoxyphene/ paracetamol	Pain (9)
Codeine		Pain (9), diarrhoea (17)
Cogentin*	Benzatropine	Parkinson's (3)
Comtess*	Entacapone	Parkinson's (3)
Copaxone*	Glatiramer acetate	MS (5)
Cystrin*	Oxybutynin	Urinary frequency (18)
Dantrium*	Dantrolene	Spasticity (2)
Dantrolene	Dantrium*	Spasticity (2)
Decadron*	Dexamethasone	Inflammation (8)
Deltastab*	Prednisolone	Inflammation (8)
Depakote*	Valproic acid	Psychoses (13)
Depixol*	Flupentixol	Psychoses (13)
Depo-Medrone*	Methylprednisolone	Inflammation (8)
Deseril*	Methysergide	Migraine (11)
Detrusitol*	Tolterodine	Urinary frequency (18)
Dexamethasone	Decadron*	Inflammation (8)
Dextropropoxyphene/ paracetamol	Co-proxamol	Pain (9)
Dexamfetamine sulphate	Dexedrine*	Attention deficit syndrome (15)
Dexedrine*	Dexamfetamine sulphate	Attention deficit syndrome (15)
DF 118*	Dihydrocodeine	Pain (9)
Diamorphine		Pain (9)
Diazepam	Valium*	Status epilepticus (1), spasticity (2)
Diclofenac*	Voltarol*	Inflammation, pain (8, 9)
Diconal*	Dipipanone	Pain (9)
Diflunisal	Dolobid*	Inflammation, pain (8, 9)
Dihydrocodeine	DF 118*	Pain (9)
Dimenhydrinate	Dramamine*	Vestibular disorders (14)
Dioctyl*	Docusate sodium	Laxative (16)
Diphenoxylate/atropine	Lomotil*	Diarrhoea (17)
Dipipanone	Diconal*	Pain (9)
Disipal*	Orphenadrine	Parkinson's (3), spasticity (2)
Distigmine	Ubretid*	Urinary retention (18)
Ditropan*	Oxybutynin	Urinary frequency (18)
Dixarit*	Clonidine	Motor tics, chorea (4), migraine (11)
Docusate sodium	Dioctyl*	Laxative (15)
Dolmatil*	Sulpiride	Motor tics, chorea (4), psychoses (13)
Dolobid*	Diflunisal	Inflammation, pain (8, 9)

Continued

Table 28.1 (*Continued*)

Drug name	Drug name	Drug use (cross-reference to sections in this chapter)
Domperidone	Motilium*	Vestibular disorders (14)
Doralese*	Indoramin	Urinary retention (18)
Dosulepin	Prothiaden*	Trigeminal neuralgia (10), depression (12)
Doxazosin	Cardura*	Urinary retention (18)
Dramamine*	Dimenhydrinate	Vestibular disorders (14)
Dulcolax*	Bisacodyl	Laxative (16)
Durogesic*	Fentanyl	Pain (9)
Dysport*	Botulinum A toxin	Torticollis, blepharospasm (4), spasticity (2)
Efexor*	Venlafaxine	Depression (12)
Eldepryl*	Selegiline	Parkinson's (3)
Entacapone	Comtess*	Parkinson's (3)
Epanutin*	Phenytoin	Epilepsy, status epilepticus (1)
Epilim*	Sodium valproate	Epilepsy (1)
Epsom salts*	Magnesium sulphate	Laxative (16)
Ergotamine	Cafergot*, Migril*	Migraine (11)
Ethosuximide	Zarontin*	Epilepsy (1)
Etodolac	Lodine SR*	Inflammation, pain (8,. 9)
Etoricoxib	Arcoxia*	Inflammation, pain (8, 9)
Faverin*	Fluvoxamine	Depression (12)
Feldene*	Piroxicam	Inflammation, pain (8, 9)
Fentanyl	Durogesic*	Pain (9)
Fibre	Isogel*, Fybogel*, Normacol*, Trifyba*, Regulan*	Laxative (16)
Flavoxate	Urispas*	Urinary frequency (18)
Fletcher's Phosphate Enemas*	Phosphate enemas	Laxative (16)
Fluoxetine	Prozac*	Depression (12)
Flupentixol	Depixol*	Psychoses (13)
Fluphenazine	Modecate*	Psychoses (13)
Fluvoxamine	Faverin*	Depression (12)
Gabapentin	Neurontin*	Epilepsy (1), trigeminal neuralgia (10)
Gabitril*	Tigabine	Epilepsy (1)
Gamanil*	Lofepramine	Trigeminal neuralgia (10), depression (12)
Glatiramer acetate	Copaxone*	MS (5)
Glycerol		Laxative (16)
Haldol*	Haloperidol	Motor tics, chorea (4), psychoses (13)
Haloperidol	Haldol*, Serenace*	Motor tics, chorea (4), psychoses (13)
Hydrocortisone	Hydrocortistab*	Inflammation (8)
Hydrocortistab*	Hydrocortisone	Inflammation (8)
Hyoscine	Kwells*, Scopaderm*	Reduce secretions (7)
Hypovase*	Prazosin	Urinary retention (18)
Hytrin*	Terazosin	Urinary retention (18)
Ibuprofen	Brufen*	Inflammation, pain (8, 9)
Imigran*	Sumatriptan	Migraine (11)
Imipramine	Tofranil*	Trigeminal neuralgia (10), depression (12)
Imodium*	Loperamide	Diarrhoea (17)
Inderal*	Propranolol	Essential tremor (4), migraine (11)
Indocid*	Indometacin	Inflammation, pain (8, 9)
Indometacin	Indocid*	Inflammation, pain (8, 9)

Continued

Table 28.1 (*Continued*)

Drug name	Drug name	Drug use (cross–reference to sections in this chapter)
Indoramin	Doralese*	Urinary retention (18)
Isocarboxazid		Depression (12)
Isogel*, Fybogel*, Normacol*, Trifyba*, Regulan*	Fibre	Laxative (16)
Isoniazid/pyridoxine		MS (5)
Kemadrin*	Procyclidine	Parkinson's (3)
Kenalog*	Triamcinolone	Inflammation (8)
Keppra*	Levetiracetam	Epilepsy (1)
Ketoprofen	Alrheumet*, Orudis*, Oruvail*	Inflammation, pain (8, 9)
Kwells*	Hyoscine	Reduce secretions (7)
Lactitol		Laxative (16)
Lactulose		Laxative (16)
Lamictal*	Lamotrigine	Epilepsy (1)
Lamotrigine	Lamictal*	Epilepsy (1)
Largactil*	Chlorpromazine	Motor tics, chorea (4), psychoses (13), vestibular disorders (14)
Larodopa*	Levodopa	Parkinson's (3)
Lederspan*	Triamcinolone	Inflammation (8)
Levetiracetam	Keppra*	Epilepsy (1)
Levodopa	Brocadopa*, Larodopa*	Parkinson's (3)
Lioresal*	Baclofen	Spasticity (2)
Lisuride	Revanil*	Parkinson's (3)
Lithium	Priadel*	Psychoses (13)
Lodine SR*	Etodolac	Inflammation, pain (8, 9)
Lofepramine	Gamanil*	Trigeminal neuralgia (10), depression (12)
Lomotil*	Diphenoxylate/atropine	Diarrhoea (17)
Loperamide	Imodium*	Diarrhoea (17)
Ludiomil*	Maprotiline	Depression (12)
Lustral*	Sertraline	Depression (12)
Lisuride	Revanil*	Parkinson's disease (3)
Madopar*	Co-beneldopa	Parkinson's disease (3)
Magnesium sulphate	Epsom salts*	Laxative (16)
Manerix*	Moclobemide	Depression (12)
Maprotiline	Ludiomil*	Depression (12)
Maxolon*	Metoclopramide	Vestibular disorders (14)
Meclozine	Sea-legs*	Vestibular disorders (14)
Mefenamic acid	Ponstan*	Inflammation, pain (8, 9)
Melleril*	Thioridazine	Psychoses (13)
Meloxicam	Mobic*	Inflammation, pain (8, 9)
Meptazinol	Meptid*	Pain (9)
Meptid*	Meptazinol	Pain (9)
Methocarbamol	Robaxin*	Spasticity (2)
Methylprednisolone	Depo-Medrone*	Inflammation (8)
Methylphenidate hydrochloride	Ritalin*	Attention deficit syndrome (15)
Methysergide	Deseril*	Migraine (11)
Metoclopramide	Maxolon*	Vestibular disorders (14)
Mianserin		Depression (12)
Microlette*	Sodium citrate solution	Laxative (16)
Migril*	Ergotamine	Migraine (11)

Continued

Table 28.1 (*Continued*)

Drug name	Drug name	Drug use (cross-reference to sections in this chapter)
Mirapexin*	Pramipexole	Parkinson's disease (3)
Mobic*	Meloxicam	Inflammation, pain (8, 9)
Moclobemide	Manerix*	Depression (12)
Modecate*	Fluphenazine	Psychoses (13)
Molipaxin*	Trazodone	Depression (12)
Motilium*	Domperidone	Vestibular disorders (14)
Morphine	MST Continus*, Oramorph*	Pain (9)
MST Continus*	Morphine	Pain (9)
Myotonine*	Bethanechol	Urinary retention (18)
Mysoline*	Primidone	Essential tremor (4), epilepsy (1)
Naprosyn*	Naproxen	Inflammation, pain (8, 9)
Naproxen	Naprosyn*, Synflex*	Inflammation, pain (8, 9)
Nardil*	Phenelzine	Depression (12)
Nefopam	Acupan*	Pain (9)
NeuroBloc*	Botulinum B toxin	Torticollis (4)
Neurontin*	Gabapentin	Epilepsy (1), trigeminal neuralgia (10)
Nimodipine	Nimotop*	Subarachnoid haemorrhage (6)
Nimotop*	Nimodipine	Subarachnoid haemorrhage (6)
Nitoman*	Tetrabenazine	Chorea (4)
Nootropil*	Piracetam	Myoclonus (4)
Olanzapine	Zyprexa*	Psychoses (13)
Oramorph*	Morphine	Pain (9)
Orap*	Pimozide	Motor tics, chorea (4)
Orphenadrine	Disipal*	Parkinson's (3), spasticity (2)
Orudis*	Ketoprofen	Inflammation, pain (8, 9)
Oruvail*	Ketoprofen	Inflammation, pain (8, 9)
Oxcarbazepine	Trileptal*	Epilepsy (1), trigeminal neuralgia (10)
Oxybutynin	Cystrin*, Ditropan*	Urinary frequency (17)
Panadol*	Paracetamol	Pain (9)
Paracetamol	Panadol*	Pain (9)
Paracetamol/metoclopramide	Paramax*	Migraine (11)
Paramax*	Paracetamol/metoclopramide	Migraine (11)
Parlodel*	Bromocriptine	Parkinson's (3)
Parnate*	Tranylcypromine	Depression (12)
Paroxetine	Seroxat*	Depression (12)
Pergolide	Celance*	Parkinson's (3)
Perphenazine		Vestibular disorders (14)
Pethidine		Pain (9)
Phenelzine	Nardil*	Depression (12)
Phenergan*	Promethazine	Vestibular disorders (14)
Phenobarbital		Epilepsy (1)
Phenol		Spasticity (2)
Phenylbutazone	Butacote*	Inflammation, pain (8, 9)
Phenytoin	Epanutin*	Status epilepticus (1), epilepsy (1)
Phosphate enemas	Fletchers' Phosphate Enemas*	Laxative (16)
Picolax*	Sodium picosulfate	Laxative (16)
Pimozide	Orap*	Motor tics, chorea (4)
Piracetam	Nootropil*	Myoclonus (4)
Piroxicam	Feldene*	Inflammation, pain (8, 9)

Continued

Table 28.1 (*Continued*)

Drug name	Drug name	Drug use (cross-reference to sections in this chapter)
Pizotifen	Sanomigran*	Migraine (11)
Ponstan*	Mefenamic acid	Inflammation, pain (8, 9)
Prazosin	Hypovase*	Urinary retention (18)
Prednisolone	Deltastab*	Inflammation (8)
Pramipexole	Mirapexin*	Parkinson's (3)
Priadel*	Lithium	Psychoses (13)
Primidone	Mysoline*	Essential tremor (4), epilepsy (1)
Probanthine*	Propantheline	Urinary frequency (18)
Prochlorperazine	Stemetil*	Vestibular disorders (14)
Procyclidine	Kemadrin*	Parkinson's (3)
Promethazine	Avomine*, Phenergan*	Vestibular disorders (14)
Propantheline	Pro-Banthine*	Urinary frequency (18)
Propranolol	Inderal*	Essential tremor (4), migraine (11)
Prothiaden*	Dosulepin	Trigeminal neuralgia (10), depression (12)
Prozac*	Fluoxetine	Depression (12)
Quetiapine	Seroquel*	Psychoses (13)
Rebif*	Beta-1a-interferon	MS (5)
Requip*	Ropinirole	Parkinson's (3)
Revanil*	Lisuride	Parkinson's (3)
Rheumox*	Azapropazone	Inflammation, pain (8, 9)
Risperdal*	Risperidone	Psychoses (13)
Risperidone	Risperdal*	Psychoses (13)
Ritalin*	Methylphenidate hydrochloride	Attention deficit syndrome (15)
Rivotril*	Clonazepam	Epilepsy (1)
Robaxin*	Methocarbamol	Spasticity (2)
Rofecoxib	Vioxx*	Inflammation, pain (8, 9)
Ropinirole	Requip*	Parkinson's (3)
Sabril*	Vigabatrin	Epilepsy (1)
Sanomigran*	Pizotifen	Migraine (11)
Scopaderm*	Hyoscine	Reduce secretions (7)
Sea-legs*	Meclozine	Vestibular disorders (14)
Selegiline	Eldepryl*	Parkinson's (3)
Senna	Senokot*	Laxative (16)
Senokot*	Senna	Laxative (16)
Serc*	Betahistine	Vestibular disorders (14)
Serenace*	Haloperidol	Motor tics, chorea (4), psychoses (13)
Seroquel*	Quetiapine	Psychoses (13)
Seroxat*	Paroxetine	Depression (12)
Sertraline	Lustral*	Depression (12)
Sinemet*	Co-careldopa	Parkinson's (3)
Sodium citrate solution	Microlette*	Laxative (16)
Sodium picosulfate	Picolax*	Laxative (16)
Sodium valproate	Epilim*	Epilepsy (1)
Solian*	Amisulpride	Psychoses (13)
Stelazine*	Trifluoperazine	Psychoses (13), vestibular disorders (14)
Stemetil*	Prochlorperazine	Vestibular disorders (14)
Stugeron*	Cinnarizine	Vestibular disorders (14)
Sulpiride	Dolmatil*	Motor tics, chorea (4), psychoses (13)
Sumatriptan	Imigran*	Migraine (11)

Continued

Table 28.1 (*Continued*)

Drug name	Drug name	Drug use (cross-reference to sections in this chapter)
Surmontil*	Trimipramine	Trigeminal neuralgia (10), depression (12)
Symmetrel*	Amantadine	Parkinson's (3), fatigue in MS (5)
Synflex*	Naproxen	Inflammation, pain (8, 9)
Tegretol*	Carbamazepine	Epilepsy (1), trigeminal neuralgia (10), psychoses (13)
Temgesic*	Buprenorphine	Pain (9)
Terazosin	Hytrin*	Urinary retention (18)
Tetrabenazine	Nitoman*	Chorea (4)
Thioridazine	Melleril*	Psychoses (13)
Tiagabine	Gabitril*	Epilepsy (1)
Tizanidine	Zanaflex*	Spasticity (2)
Tofranil*	Imipramine	Trigeminal neuralgia (10), depression (12)
Tolterodine	Detrusitol*	Urinary frequency (18)
Topamax*	Topiramate	Epilepsy (1)
Topiramate	Topamax*	Epilepsy (1)
Tramadol	Zydol*	Pain (9)
Tranylcypromine	Parnate*	Depression (12)
Trazodone	Molipaxin*	Depression (12)
Triamcinolone	Adcortyl*, Kenalog*, Lederspan	Inflammation (8)
Trifluoperazine	Stelazine*	Psychoses (13), vestibular disorders (14)
Trihexyphenidyl (benzhexol)	Broflex*	Parkinson's (3), tremor (4), chorea (4), tics (4)
Trimipramine	Surmontil*	Trigeminal neuralgia (10), depression (12)
Trileptal*	Oxcarbazepine	Epilepsy (1), trigeminal neuralgia (10)
Ubretid*	Distigmine	Urinary retention (18)
Urispas*	Flavoxate	Urinary retention (18)
Valium*	Diazepam	Status epilepticus (1), spasticity (2)
Valproic acid	Depakote*	Psychoses (13)
Venlafaxine	Efexor*	Depression (12)
Vigabatrin	Sabril*	Epilepsy (1)
Vioxx	Rofecoxib	Inflammation, pain (8, 9)
Voltarol*	Diclofenac*	Inflammation, pain (8, 9)
Xatral*	Alfuzosin	Urinary retention (17)
Zanaflex*	Tizanidine	Spasticity (2)
Zarontin*	Ethosuximide	Epilepsy (1)
Zoleptil*	Zotepine	Psychoses (13)
Zotepine	Zoleptil*	Psychoses (13)
Zuclopenthixol	Clopixol*	Psychoses (13)
Zydol*	Tramadol	Pain (9)
Zyprexa*	Olanzapine	Psychoses (13)

* Proprietary drug name.
MS, multiple sclerosis.

References

British National Formulary, no. 46. London: British Medical Association & Royal Pharmaceutical Society of Great Britain; 2003.

Martindale: The Complete Drug Reference, 34th edn. London: Pharmaceutical Press; 2003.

UK Medicines Compendium. London: Datapharm Communications; 2003.

Skill acquisition and neurological adaptations

Chapter 29

Physical activity and exercise in neurological rehabilitation

BM Haas   F Jones

INTRODUCTION

Individuals with neurological conditions can show signs of muscle weakness and cardiovascular deconditioning similar to the general population. This chapter will outline the importance of exercise and task-specificity of practice, with particular reference to constraint-induced movement therapy (CIMT) and treadmill training. The effects of muscle-strengthening programmes and aerobic exercises in this patient group will also be reviewed.

TERMINOLOGY

- *External restraints* to a movement are restrictions imposed by the environment or the task itself; *internal constraints* are the individual's biomechanical, physiological and psychological characteristics (Wu et al., 2001).

- A *skill* is the competence to achieve a goal with consistency and economy under a wide variety of conditions (Higgins, 1991).

- *Motor learning* is a relatively permanent change in motor behaviour emerging from processes including cognition, perception and action (Shumway-Cook & Woollacott, 2001).

- *Physical activity* can be defined as the movements of the body brought about by muscle power and the expenditure of energy (Pfaffenbarger et al., 1988).

- *Exercise* is physical activity which is planned, structured, purposeful and repetitive (McArdle et al., 1996).

- *Strength* is the capacity of a muscle or a group of muscles to produce the force necessary for initiating, maintaining and controlling movement (Ng & Shepherd, 2000).

TASK-SPECIFIC ACTIVITY

The natural problem-solving responses of an individual with a damaged nervous system, whether by single incident such as a stroke, or a degenerative condition, such as multiple sclerosis or Parkinson's disease, consist of an interaction between their problems, individual resources/characteristics and the environment (Higgins, 1991). Successful motor behaviour is the product of an interaction between the individual and the desired task.

Neurological impairment limits the ability to perform some actions which may have previously been performed with ease. External and internal constraints together will impact on the potential for successful completion of a task. Individuals may become more skilled when they achieve the ability to interact between internal and external constraints and use their own resources. The ongoing challenge of maintaining independent function in their daily life will also provide an opportunity to develop a degree of competence (Higgins, 1991).

Goals will vary between individuals and can be reached if an individual manages to achieve an action through independent movement. Motor learning is achieved when there is a relatively permanent change in motor behaviour. In general, treatment programmes that aim to facilitate motor learning have to work within the limits imposed by many other factors, such as age, genetics, the severity of damage and quality of the environmental stimulus (Neistadt, 1993).

Physiotherapy programmes which incorporate existing knowledge about human movement and encompass theories of learning and motor control are becoming more widely accepted, especially as studies that have examined other neurofacilitatory methods (e.g. Bobath, proprioceptive neuromuscular facilitation and Brunström) have not produced optimal results (Woods Duncan, 1997). The *National Clinical Guidelines for Stroke* (Intercollegiate Working Party for Stroke, 2002a) also suggest that a task-specific training or practice approach is showing enhanced evidence over impairment-focused approaches. They recommend giving the patient the opportunity to practise tasks. Programmes which focus on practice of specific skill acquisition may also help to modify some of the external constraints. Modifications could include enrichment of the environment, consideration of the motivational aspect of the programme including personal preferences for the chosen task, and level of demand and intensity required to produce a particular task.

Studies involving task-specific training, despite some methodological inconsistencies, have produced some encouraging results (Dean & Shepherd, 1997; Wu et al., 2001). Woods Duncan (1997) supports the view that programmes must be intensive and provide individuals with many practice opportunities if motor control is going to improve. However, physical fatigue can be a problem and limit active participation.

Harrison & Jackson (1994) suggested that mental practice may offer an alternative and could intersperse physical practice. An essential part of mental practice is the ability to create a clear powerful image of the required task on demand. Therefore the choice of tasks is important. The practice must have functional relevance and meaning to the individual to enable more successful visualisation. The evidence to support these methods is currently scarce, but with the advancement in neuroimaging techniques, a fuller exploration of mental rehearsal may be forthcoming. Nevertheless an implicit component of the technique is the emphasis on individuals to be responsible for their own practice. This may offer the potential to improve motivation in individuals who cannot sustain physical practice for long periods of time.

Constraint–induced movement therapy (CIMT)

Programmes that incorporate an intensive therapy programme described as forced-use or CIMT have shown some of the most promising evidence thus far that motor recovery can be facilitated over and above the natural period of recovery after a stroke (Liepert et al., 2000). Following any severe and sudden neurological insult there may be a period of shock or diaschesis; the threshold necessary for motor output then becomes elevated. It has been suggested that if successful motor output is not achieved, a conditioned suppression of activity may be the result (Taub et al., 1998). Failure or difficulty in the attempt to move may then further suppress limb use. In humans poststroke, actual use of the affected limb can be inferior to potential use (Andrews & Stewart, 1979). Constraining the stronger limb will encourage the use of the weaker limb. The motivation for motor output changes and subsequent accomplishment of a task then serves as a positive reinforcement for future attempts.

After brain damage, such as that resulting from stroke, a complex pattern of neurological reorganisation occurs (see Chs 1 and 5) – not only a reduction in motor cortex excitability, but also a reduction in the cortical representation of the paralysed muscles (Liepert et al., 2000). This has also been supported by studies which have examined use-dependent cortical reorganisation. Programmes using CIMT focus attention towards the weaker limb and use repeated and extensive practice for up to 6 h per day. The stronger arm is constrained in a sling and/or padded mitt. Many of the studies that have evaluated CIMT have included chronic stroke patients and findings have been encouraging, showing significant and large treatment effects even in individuals as much as 17 years poststroke (Miltner et al., 1999).

Some researchers and clinicians have questioned the suitability of all patients for CIMT. Inclusion criteria used in a number of studies were stringent and excluded a large proportion of stroke patients with significant impairments. Despite more relaxed criteria suggested by Taub et al. (1998), approximately 50% of patients may still be excluded from CIMT programmes.

Concerns over safety for patients with significant balance problems have also been raised. For such people, some researchers have opted to use a padded mitt in place of a sling (Dromerick et al., 2000). In this way the arm is restrained from activities using dexterity but patients can still use their arm for balance if required. Therapists and patients have raised some concerns about the practicalities of administering such an intensive programme, questioning patients' ability to engage actively during the proposed hours of practice (Page et al., 2002). Modification of some of the stringent aspects of the programmes may be necessary to broaden the appeal of CIMT.

However, the relative contributions of the individual aspects of CIMT (frequency and intensity of treatment, constraint of stronger limb and positive encouragement during practice of functional tasks) have not been fully evaluated.

Treadmill training

The incentive to provide a challenging environment, in which there is an opportunity to practise repetitively missing components of gait, has underpinned another task-specific activity. This involves using a treadmill for gait training. A harness can be used for individuals with significant functional limitations, and this also offers the opportunity to grade the amount of body weight support provided. Therapists help to facilitate alternating stepping and weight-bearing, and as many as three therapists may be required to assist with the complete gait cycle.

Shepherd & Carr (1999) argued that there are three reasons why treadmill training can support gait re-education:

- allows a complete practice of the gait cycle
- provides opportunity for gaining improvements in speed and endurance
- optimises aerobic fitness.

The original work on the effects of treadmill training involved animal studies (Barbeau et al., 1999). Animals with transected spinal cords were able to generate activity in lower-limb muscles and produce a stepping

motion. Research carried out on humans with incomplete spinal cord injury also showed it was possible to elicit similar activity when the individual was suspended in a harness and stepping was facilitated on a treadmill (Dobkin, 1999). This served to support the theory that humans may possess specific neural circuitry in the lumbar spinal cord that may have the ability for motor learning. The mechanism for motor learning appears as a consequence of repeated sensory inputs into lumbosacral motoneurones and interneurones, which leads to long-term potentiation. Repeated practice of the gait cycle, involving alternating loading and unloading of the lower-limbs and hip extension, seems to be the main sensory drive to promote the motor activity (Hesse, 1999). Task-specific training on a treadmill is likely to induce expansion of subcortical and cortical locomotion areas in individuals following stroke and spinal cord injury (Dobkin, 1999; Hesse, 1999).

Key points

Treadmill training:
- can be used safely
- with added harness systems provides security
- offers task-specific practice of ambulation
- improves gait parameters
- has not been found to increase spasticity

Treadmill training following stroke

Gait rehabilitation using treadmill training with partial body weight support offers the possibility for active and task-specific gait training following stroke, even with individuals with low levels of functional ability (Hesse et al., 1999). Hesse et al. (1995a, b) investigated the use of treadmill training and partial body weight support with individuals following chronic stroke. These early studies showed some encouraging results with changes in gait parameters such as stride length, cadence and velocity following the intervention. Outcome measures which showed change were those that reflected the specificity of the training, such as the Functional Ambulation Classification test (Holden et al., 1986). All the subjects in these studies had been previously treated with a neurodevelopmental approach and had not regained walking despite lengthy rehabilitation. After the treadmill training all subjects improved their walking ability, although some still needed standby supervision.

Smith et al. (1998) found normalisation of reflexive activity in some individuals by the end of their programme, implying that reductions in spasticity could

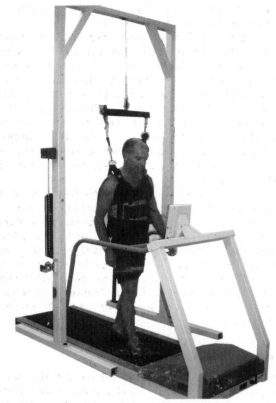

Figure 29.1 A man with incomplete spinal cord injury at C5–C6 using a treadmill with harness body weight support system.

also accompany the strength gains seen in treadmill training. This indicates that there is no evidence to support the fear that treadmill training increases mass synergistic activity in the weaker side (Hassid et al., 1997; Hesse, 1999; Smith et al., 1999). However, it is important to note that actual spasticity levels in these studies were not described clearly.

Treadmill training following spinal cord injury

The role of treadmill training in the rehabilitation of individuals with spinal cord injury is gaining support in a similar way to stroke. Evidence suggests that individuals with incomplete spinal cord injury benefit more from this approach (Nymark et al., 1998). Figure 29.1 shows a man with incomplete spinal cord injury at C5–C6 using a treadmill with harness support system.

Both acute and chronic patients have seen improvements in their independent walking ability, even in cases several years after the initial injury (Gardner et al., 1998; Wernig, 1999). Behrman & Harkema (2000) described the range of sensory cues needed to induce a normal reciprocal gait pattern when using treadmill training following spinal cord injury. Listed below, they could just as easily be adopted as aims for any treadmill training programme attempting to normalise gait:

- generation of speeds which induce normal stepping responses
- applying a maximal sustainable load on the supporting limb during stance phase
- maintaining upright trunk and head posture
- obtaining near-normal ankle, knee and hip kinematics throughout gait cycle
- synchronising the timing of extension and loading of supporting limb, with simultaneous unloading of the contralateral limb
- decreasing weight-bearing through handrails by encouraging arm swing.

Body weight support and mechanised gait training

The optimum level of body weight support seems to be that which allows maximum loading of the limb during the stance phase, whilst providing support for those individuals who are unable to maintain an upright posture independently. There is also agreement that as soon as an individual is progressing towards being able to balance independently whilst taking a step, the inclusion of practice of overground walking should be given more priority (Wernig, 1999; Behrman & Harkema, 2000).

Hesse et al. (1997) suggested using a limit of 30% body weight support; above this level heel strike and limb loading are compromised. Body weight support has been shown to reduce double support time, and therefore may offer more scope to compensate for balance deficits, whilst maintaining an upright posture and producing a stepping motion (Barbeau et al., 1999).

The effort required by physiotherapists to assist with the gait cycle may be reduced with body weight support systems, but still needs careful consideration. Training programmes often describe the involvement of three therapists for individuals with a spinal cord injury and two for stroke. One therapist stands astride the treadmill and behind the patient, facilitating lateral pelvic tilt and weight shift. The other one or two therapists crouch alongside the treadmill to lift and position the patient's lower-limb(s).

Understandable concerns about the effort required by therapists during the treatment has led researchers to look at developing other assistive devices such as a mechanised gait trainer developed by Hesse et al. (1999, 2000). The work involved by the therapist lifting an individual's leg for the swing phase is replaced by a mechanised footplate, which induces a step and stance phase. Step and stance phase are on the same arc of movement using reversed actions, and the activity in hip flexors and anterior tibialis is subsequently reduced. However, the activity in lower-limb extensor muscles during stance is comparable to ordinary body weight support treadmill training.

A few studies have examined the effect of treadmill training with other patient groups, such as individuals with Parkinson's disease, cerebral palsy and multi-infarct dementia (Liston et al., 2000; Miyai et al., 2000; Schindl et al., 2000). Evidence is inconclusive at present; none the less, treadmill training has been well tolerated, and the study carried out on children with cerebral palsy demonstrated results comparable to those found in individuals following spinal cord injury.

It has been argued that treadmill training is unsuitable for gait re-education, because it does not allow for the complexities and the unpredictable nature of overground walking. The notion that each step on a treadmill is active and not reactive because of the direction of the treadmill belt, that body weight support may induce unfamiliar sensory input, and the harness may hamper active balance reactions are some of the points raised by Davies (1999). However, the weight of evidence to support treadmill training in neurorehabilitation is becoming impossible for physiotherapists to ignore. It would therefore be prudent to consider structured training protocols for both patients and physiotherapists before embarking on the purchase of body weight support treadmill systems. Treadmill training will not replace overground walking practice within neurorehabilitation but provides an exciting addition to the repertoire of task-specific training programmes that have gained credibility in recent years.

MUSCLE STRENGTH AND AEROBIC FITNESS

The general population has the potential to gain health benefits from regular exercise. These benefits could include improved fitness and muscle strength, improved mood and sense of well-being, weight control, improved bone density and improved co-ordination. Physical activity and regular exercise can also have positive effects on a number of disease states which include atherosclerosis, diabetes, heart disease, stroke, hypertension, obesity, osteoporosis, chronic airway obstruction and depression (Pfaffenbarger et al., 1988). However, participation in regular exercise sufficient to produce these health gains is low. Sixty per cent of North Americans and 70% of the English population do not participate in regular exercise (Hillsdon & Thorogood,

1996; McArdle et al., 1996). The reasons for non-participation in exercise are complex.

Oman & King (2000) focused their attention on life events with a negative effect on exercise behaviour. These life events include major changes in health, injury and illness. This could imply that the adoption of exercise behaviour for individuals with a neurological impairment would present a number of challenges. However, it would seem critical to promote exercise for individuals who may be at a higher risk of cardiovascular deconditioning or whose activity limitations and participation restrictions force them to lead a sedentary lifestyle.

Individuals with physical impairments will need a great deal of encouragement to engage in regular intensive exercise. This encouragement may not always be forthcoming from therapists who have been led to believe that effortful activity is harmful to their patients and must be avoided. However, recent evidence shows that this is not the case and that exercise should be an integral part of an overall rehabilitation programme (Miller & Light, 1997; Sharp & Brouwer, 1997; Fowler et al., 2001).

Muscle strength

A minimum level of muscle strength is required to carry out physical activities and weakness may lead to substantial activity limitations. Brill et al. (2000) found evidence for this in the healthy population and studies of muscle strength of individuals with neurological problems have reached similar conclusions. There is now a consensus that muscle weakness is a feature in many neurological pathologies. The notion that increased coactivation of antagonistic muscles rather than muscular weakness is responsible for motor control problems has not been confirmed by scientific evidence.

Investigations into muscle weakness following stroke have concluded that there is reduced muscle strength in the limbs contralateral to the side of the brain lesion (Bohannon & Walsh, 1992; Bohannon, 1997b; Sunnerhagen et al., 1999; Andrews & Bohannon, 2000). It must also be remembered that the limbs ipsilateral to the brain lesion are not 'normal' but also show signs of muscular weakness (Andrews & Bohannon, 2000; Harris et al., 2001). The trunk muscles, both contralateral and ipsilateral to the brain lesion, are weakened, with all trunk movements being affected by the weakness (Bohannon, 1995; Bohannon et al., 1995; Tanaka et al., 1997, 1998). The muscle weakness found in stroke contributes to reduced dexterity, hand grip and hand function (Ada et al., 2000; Ng & Shepherd, 2000). Contrary to common beliefs, flexor muscles in the upper limb are weaker than the extensor muscles (Andrews & Bohannon, 2000).

Disuse atrophy can be found in many muscle groups on both the weaker and the stronger side, even in individuals with a good rehabilitation outcome and who are physically active (Hachisuka et al., 1997). However, disuse atrophy is not the only underlying cause of the muscle weakness because weakness is evident early after stroke. Therefore, the lesion itself may actually be the primary cause of the weakness (Newham & Hsiao, 2001). Muscle weakness in the lower-limb is associated with reduced gait speed (Bohannon & Walsh, 1992) and reduced levels of activity (Hachisuka et al., 1997) in individuals following stroke. There is also slowness to produce muscular force.

Strength measurements are not frequently used in stroke rehabilitation. However, Bohannon (1997a) and Bohannon & Walsh (1992) have established that, despite their limitations, strength measurements can give useful information and can be reliable, provided that standardised procedures are followed.

Muscle weakness has also been demonstrated in individuals with cerebral palsy (Maruishi et al., 2001), Parkinson's disease (Nogaki et al., 1999) and multiple sclerosis (Ponichtera-Mulcare, 1993).

Muscle strengthening in neurological rehabilitation

The use of resisted strengthening exercises in neurological rehabilitation has previously been avoided because it was believed that effort in the presence of spasticity would increase cocontraction, produce associated reactions and worsen motor function (Bobath, 1990). However, this belief has not been confirmed by scientific evidence. On the contrary, several researchers have found that spasticity does not worsen following a short burst of resisted muscle work and that cocontraction of agonists and antagonists may actually improve (Miller & Light, 1997; Fowler et al., 2001). Both of these studies included individuals with mild to moderate spasticity and Fowler et al. (2001) also included some with severe spasticity (grade 4 on the Ashworth scale).

Longer periods of incremental resisted muscle-strengthening programmes have also failed to produce adverse effects on spasticity (Sharp & Brouwer, 1997; Teixeira-Salmela et al., 1999). However, it is important to note that neither of these studies reported the actual spasticity grading of their participants, who were independently mobile and had no contractures.

Muscle strengthening can be safely and usefully incorporated into the overall rehabilitation of individuals with a variety of neurological conditions. Resisted muscle-strengthening programmes led to an increase in muscle strength as well as improvements in the activity levels of the individual.

> **Key points**
>
> Muscle-strengthening programmes:
> - can be used safely
> - increase muscle strength
> - improve a patient's activity level
> - have not been found to increase spasticity

Stroke

The *National Clinical Guidelines for Stroke* (Intercollegiate Working Party for Stroke, 2002b) recently included a new section on resisted exercises because the evidence for this type of intervention is now growing. Their recommendation is to consider resisted exercises in targeted muscles. It has also been found that, following stroke, lower-limb muscle strength can be increased and function improved without adversely affecting spasticity (Bhakta, 2000; Weiss et al., 2000). Eccentric training was found to be slightly superior to concentric training (Enghardt et al., 1995). Gait parameters can change following strength training, with improved gait speed reported by a number of researchers (Sharp & Brouwer, 1997; Teixeira-Salmela et al., 1999, 2001).

Multiple sclerosis

Limited research in multiple sclerosis has indicated that strengthening exercises in this patient group can produce increases in muscle strength. The effects on activity and participation have not been sufficiently tested. The literature cautions against overload and advises careful exercise prescription in individuals who suffer from heat-sensitivity (see Ch. 10, p. 182, 191). Exercising should be safe in these individuals as long as their body core temperature does not rise significantly, so appropriate steps should be taken to avoid overheating (Costello et al., 1996). The effects noted on p. 191 could have been due to heat sensitivity. Useful strategies could include exercising with equipment with built-in fans or in air-conditioned rooms, and some have used cooling suits during the exercise. Exercising in the early part of the day may also be better as the circadian rhythm of lower body temperature in the morning could be more conducive to the individual. These recommendations relate to individuals in stable phases of the disease, as no research on exercise during acute exacerbations has been conducted.

Parkinson's disease

Glendinning (1997) provided a rationale for strength training in Parkinson's disease and suggested that it has the potential to combat weakness, increase agonist activation and influence well-being. A limited number of small studies have provided some evidence to support these suggestions and indicate that a combined strengthening and balance exercise programme can improve balance and muscle strength (Toole et al., 2000) and that gait improvements can be achieved (Scandalis et al., 2001).

Cerebral palsy

Darrah et al. (1997) conducted a consensus on muscle strengthening in cerebral palsy. They felt that evidence was limited to support the use of strengthening in this patient group. Conversely, there was no evidence to suggest that strengthening exercises may be harmful to children or adults with cerebral palsy. Since then, further small-scale evidence has been added and this continues to show that specific muscle strengthening in this patient group can produce beneficial results. The benefits include improved gait parameters (Johnson et al., 1998) and increased gross motor function measures (Damiano & Abel, 1998).

Possible effect of strength training on muscle length

It has been suggested that loss of muscle fibre diameter may cause contracture in pennate muscles, through shortening of the aponeuroses. A recent study, using ultrasound imaging to examine the architecture of medial gastrocnemius, found no difference in fibre length between normal children and those with spastic diplegia and plantarflexion contractures (Shortland et al., 2002). On relating the findings to those in the literature from animal studies, where fibre length was normal but diameter was reduced, the investigators concluded that muscle shortening was due to fibre atrophy.

Although the study by Shortland et al. (2002) did not provide direct evidence of fibre atrophy, contractures seen in the children with spastic diplegia could not be explained by the commonly accepted mechanism of sarcomere loss (see Ch. 30, p. 505), since they did not find any loss of fibre length.

An important clinical implication of this conclusion is that strengthening may have a role to play in preventing and reversing contractures, but this requires investigation.

Guidelines for strength training in neurological conditions

Further research is urgently needed to establish suitable muscle-strengthening protocols for individuals with neurological conditions. In the absence of any tested protocols for patient groups, researchers and clinicians have successfully utilised protocols from the weight-training literature. It is unclear at this stage how much these protocols need to be modified for patients with neurological conditions. However, a useful starting point may be adoption of the guidelines published by the American College of Sports Medicine (1995) for anyone prescribing resistance exercises to individuals with neurological conditions:

- The strengthening programme should involve 8–10 separate exercises for major muscle groups.
- Eight to 12 repetitions of each exercise should be performed. Indications are that weak patients benefit from reducing the weights so that they can perform 15 repetitions.
- The programme should be carried out at least twice per week.
- Work muscle groups concentrically as well as eccentrically.
- Normal breathing should be maintained during the exercises.
- Most patients will need supervision.
- Exercises should be performed through a full as possible range of motion.

In addition, researchers have tended to apply loads of about 60–65% of the muscle's force-generating capacity, which was measured at the beginning of the strengthening programme and then regularly throughout. Therefore, it is important to remember that strength training should be individualised and be specific to the muscle groups that require strengthening. Free weights, resistance apparatus and isokinetic machines, as well as resistance arm and leg ergometers, can be used for strengthening exercise programmes.

It has been suggested that the respiratory muscles may also be weakened in certain neurological conditions, such as Parkinson's disease (deBruin et al., 1993; Haas et al., 2001). Hand-held respiratory muscle trainers, designed for strengthening the inspiratory muscles, are being used in the training of athletes and are now widely available. Their use and effectiveness in patients with neurological conditions have not been systematically evaluated and therefore it is not possible to make recommendations about their use.

Aerobic fitness in neurological rehabilitation

Aerobic fitness may not seem a rehabilitation priority. One reason for this may be that a person with significant activity limitations may never be active enough to notice any loss in aerobic fitness. Once the individual has been discharged from early rehabilitation, the support and encouragement for starting and maintaining a fitness programme may not be forthcoming.

The link between fitness and activity and participation is also not fully clear. Individuals with Parkinson's have demonstrated reduced fitness, which correlated with reduced quality of life; however, this was not a cause-and-effect relationship (Haas et al., 2001). Improved fitness does not necessarily lead to increased participation, as Petajan et al. (1996) showed in their study involving individuals with multiple sclerosis. However, Potempa et al. (1996) suggested that they may be able to carry out activities of daily living at a lower percentage of their maximum oxygen uptake.

Individuals with neurological conditions have reduced exercise capacity, which is demonstrated as reduced maximal and peak oxygen uptake, reduced workload and heart rate. This has been shown in post-polio syndrome (Willen et al., 1999), Parkinson's disease (Canning et al., 1997; Reuter et al., 1999; Haas et al., 2001), and stroke (Potempa et al., 1996). Hemiparesis due to stroke limits the number of recruitable motor units and therefore endurance. This has undoubted implications for fatiguability and overwork in these individuals (Potempa et al., 1996).

Intervention studies using aerobic exercises, or in some instances a combination of aerobic and strengthening exercises, demonstrated improvements in these individuals poststroke. No study to date has shown an increase in spasticity or worsening of any other neurological signs with the effort of aerobic exercise. In Parkinson's disease, normal exercise capacity can be maintained with regular exercise, despite respiratory and/or gait abnormalities (Canning et al., 1997). Both upper-limb and lower-limb exercises can be used safely and effectively in this patient group (Protas et al., 1996). Cycle ergometer training has improved the workload capacity in individuals following traumatic brain injury (Wolman et al., 1994). While it is not known how this affected their levels of activity or participation, the enhanced endurance may have contributed to the overall success of rehabilitation.

The appropriate timing for introducing aerobic exercises is currently difficult to assess. Indications are that persons who have certain chronic conditions, such as multiple sclerosis or Parkinson's disease, should start as early as possible. In multiple sclerosis this may be exactly the time when exercise is most beneficial (Ponichtera-Mulcare, 1993; Costello et al., 1996). The optimal timing for stroke patients is unknown.

Guidelines for aerobic training

Patients will need careful initial screening and monitoring prior to starting fitness programmes and during the exercises. The procedures recommended by the American College of Sports Medicine (1995) should be followed. Some of the key issues have been summarised but anyone considering setting up aerobic exercise programmes for individuals with neurological conditions must ensure that appropriate health and safety procedures are in place. An exercise test or exercise intervention must be terminated when any of the following occurs:

- onset of angina or angina-like symptoms
- signs of poor perfusion (light-headedness, confusion, ataxia, pallor, cyanosis, nausea, cold and clammy skin)
- failure of heart rate to increase with increased exercise intensity
- noticeable change in heart rhythm
- blood pressure rises to above 240/120 mmHg
- physical or verbal manifestation of severe fatigue
- failure of the testing or monitoring equipment
- patient requests to stop.

No research has investigated maximal exercises in individuals with neurological conditions and therefore only submaximal interventions can be recommended at this stage. Very few clear indications about the optimum intensity and frequency of exercising have emerged from the literature. General guidelines for healthy populations may be somewhat advanced for individuals with motor problems and muscles insufficiently innervated.

Measurements and monitoring of heart rate during the exercises has been used widely in research and calculation of the heart rate reserve (also known as the Karvonnen formula, which involves subtracting the resting heart rate from the estimated maximal heart rate) has been used to determine exercise intensity (American College of Sports Medicine, 1995). Forty to 50% of a person's heart rate reserve appears to be a useful intensity starting point, with a frequency of three to five sessions of up to 30 min. Individuals commencing an exercise programme may not be able to maintain this intensity for the full 30 min. An initial aim of the exercise programme should be a steady increase in the exercise duration from about 10 min towards the full 30 min.

Mode of aerobic exercise

The mode of exercise could be any activity that uses large muscle groups and which can be maintained continuously and is rhythmical and aerobic in nature (Pollock et al., 1998). Many different types of equipment, such as arm and leg cycle ergometers, have been utilised. However, a firm favourite activity that emerges from the literature is walking. Hillsdon & Thorogood (1996) see brisk walking as the exercise with the greatest potential for increasing the overall activity levels of a sedentary population and walking was seen as the type of exercise most likely to be adopted by a wide range of ages, socioeconomic and ethnic groups. Although their work refers to healthy populations, walking may also provide a useful exercise for those individuals with neurological conditions who are sufficiently mobile. The treadmill may be a useful piece of equipment for initiating a walking programme but this has not been fully explored. Macko et al. (1997) investigated the effect of a 6-month low-intensity aerobic training programme consisting of graded treadmill walking at 50–60% of heart rate reserve. They found that the programme was well tolerated and a feasible method of cardiovascular conditioning using submaximal training methods.

CONCLUSIONS

The evidence supports the need for therapists to create opportunities in which an individual is encouraged to persevere with tasks which are meaningful and at a level sufficient to induce changes in strength and fitness. Therapists require knowledge about how to help facilitate a change in exercise behaviour, so that activity is maintained long-term in order to prevent secondary deconditioning.

Therapists may need to think beyond the restraints of the neurogym, and consider more active collaboration with agencies providing leisure and social pursuits.

References

Ada L, Canning CG, Dwyer T. Effect of muscle length on strength and dexterity after stroke. *Clin Rehab* 2000, **14**:55–61.

American College of Sports Medicine. *ACSM's Guidelines for Exercise Testing and Prescription*. Baltimore: Williams & Wilkins; 1995.

Andrews AW, Bohannon RW. Distribution of muscle strength impairments following stroke. *Clin Rehab* 2000, **14**:79–87.

Andrews K, Stewart J. Stroke recovery: he can but does he? *Rheumatol Rehab* 1979, **18**:43–48.

Barbeau H, Fung J, Visintin M. New approach to retrain gait in stroke and spinal cord injured subjects. *Neurorehab Neural Repair* 1999, **13**:177–178.

Behrman AL, Harkema SJ. Locomotor training after human spinal cord injury: a series of case studies. *Phys Ther* 2000, **80**:688–700.

Bhakta BB. Management of spasticity in stroke. *Br Med Bull* 2000, **56**:476–485.

Bobath B. *Adult Hemiplegia – Evaluation and Treatment*. Oxford: Heinemann; 1990.

Bohannon RW. Recovery and correlates of trunk muscle strength after stroke. *Int J Rehab Res* 1995, **18**:162–167.

Bohannon RW. Reference values for extremity muscle strength obtained by hand-held dynamometry from adults aged 20–79 years. *Arch Phys Med Rehab* 1997a, **78**:26–32.

Bohannon RW. Measurement and nature of muscle strength in patients with stroke. *J Neurol Rehab* 1997b, **11**:115–125.

Bohannon R, Walsh S. Nature, reliability and predictive value of muscle performance measures in patients with hemiparesis following stroke. *Arch Phys Med Rehab* 1992, **73**:721–725.

Bohannon RW, Cassidy D, Walsh S. Trunk muscle strength is impaired multidirectionally after stroke. *Clin Rehab* 1995, **9**:47–51.

Brill PA, Macera CA, Davis DR et al. Muscular strength and physical function. *Med Sci Sports Exerc* 2000, **32**:412–416.

Canning CG, Alison JA, Allen NE et al. Parkinson's disease: an investigation of exercise capacity, respiratory function and gait. *Arch Phys Med Rehab* 1997, **78**:199–207.

Costello E, Curtis CL, Sandel IB et al. Exercise prescription for individuals with multiple sclerosis. *Neurol Rep* 1996, **20**:24–30.

Damiano DL, Abel MF. Functional outcomes of strength training in spastic cerebral palsy. *Arch Phys Med Rehab* 1998, **79**:119–125.

Darrah J, Fan JSW, Chen LC et al. Review of the effects of progressive resisted muscle strengthening in children with cerebral palsy: a clinical consensus exercise. *Pediatr Phys Ther* 1997, **9**:12–17.

Davies PM. Weight-supported treadmill training. *Neurorehab Neural Repair* 1999, **13**:167–169.

Dean CM, Shepherd RB. Task-related training improves performance of seated reaching tasks after stroke. *Stroke* 1997, **28**:722–728.

deBruin PFC, deBruin VMS, Lees AJ et al. Effects of treatment on airway dynamics and respiratory muscle strength in Parkinson's disease. *Am Rev Resp Dis* 1993, **148**:1576–1580.

Dobkin BH. An overview of treadmill locomotor training with partial body weight support: a neurologically sound approach whose time has come for randomized clinical trials. *Neurorehab Neural Repair* 1999, **13**:157–165.

Dromerick A, Edwards D, Hahn M. Does the application of constraint-induced movement therapy during acute rehabilitation reduce arm impairment after ischemic stroke? *Stroke* 2000, **31**:2984–2988.

Enghardt M, Knutson E, Jonsson M et al. Dynamic muscle strength training in stroke patients: effects on knee extension torque, electromyographic activity and motor function. *Arch Phys Med Rehab* 1995, **76**:419–425.

Fowler EG, Ho TW, Nwigwe AI et al. The effects of quadriceps femoris muscle strengthening exercises on spasticity in children with cerebral palsy. *Phys Ther* 2001, **81**:1215–1223.

Gardner MB, Holden MK, Leikauskas JM et al. Partial body weight support with treadmill locomotion to improve gait after incomplete spinal cord injury: a single-subject experimental design. *Phys Ther* 1998, **78**:361–374.

Glendinning DA. Rationale for strength training in patients with Parkinson's disease. *Neurol Rep* 1997, **21**:132–135.

Haas BM, Trew M, Castle PC et al. *Respiratory Muscle Strength, Quality of Life, ADL Function and Mobility in Individuals with Parkinson's disease – Preliminary Results. Multidisciplinary Care in Parkinson's Disease and Parkinsonism – From Science to Practice*. London: Royal Collage of Physicians; 2001.

Hachisuka K, Umezu Y, Ogata H. Disuse muscle atrophy of lower-limbs in hemiplegic patients. *Arch Phys Med Rehab* 1997, **78**:13–18.

Harris ML, Polkey MI, Bath PMW et al. Quadriceps muscle weakness following acute hemiplegic stroke. *Clin Rehab* 2001, **15**:274–281.

Harrison K, Jackson J. Relationship between mental practice and motor performance. *Br J Ther Rehab* 1994, **1**:14–18.

Hassid E, Rose D, Commisarow J et al. Improved gait symmetry in hemiparetic stroke patients induced during body weight-supported treadmill stepping. *J Neurol Rehab* 1997, **11**:21–26.

Hesse S. Treadmill training with partial body weight support in hemiparetic patients – further research needed. *Neurorehab Neural Repair* 1999, **13**:179–181.

Hesse S, Bertelt C, Jahnke M et al. Treadmill training with partial body weight support compared with physio-therapy in nonambulatory hemiparetic patients. *Stroke* 1995a, **26**:976–981.

Hesse S, Malezic M, Schaffrin A et al. Restoration of gait by combined treadmill training and multichannel electrical stimulation in non-ambulatory hemiparetic patients. *Scand J Rehab Med* 1995b, **27**:199–204.

Hesse S, Helm B, Krajnick J. Treadmill training with partial body weight support: influence of body weight release on the gait of hemiparetic patients. *J Neurol Rehab* 1997, **11**:15–20.

Hesse S, Uhlenbrock D, Sarkodie-Gyan T. Gait pattern of severely disabled hemiparetic subjects on a new controlled gait trainer as compared to assisted treadmill walking with partial body weight support. *Clin Rehab* 1999, **13**:401–410.

Hesse S, Uhlenbrock D, Werner C et al. A mechanized gait trainer for restoring gait in nonambulatory subjects. *Arch Phys Med Rehab* 2000, **81**:1158–1161.

Higgins S. Motor skill acquisition. *Phys Ther* 1991, **71**:123–139.

Hillsdon M, Thorogood M. A systematic review of physical activity promotion strategies. *Br J Sports Med* 1996, **30**:84–89.

Holden MK, Gill KM, Magliozzi MR. Gait assessment for neurologically impaired patients – standards for outcome assessments. *Phys Ther* 1986, **66**:1530–1539.

Intercollegiate Working Party for Stroke. *National Clinical Guidelines for Stroke Section 4: Approaches to Therapy – Update*. London: Royal College of Physicians, 2002a. Available online at www.rcplondon.ac.uk/pubs/books/stroke/.

Intercollegiate Working Party for Stroke. *National Clinical Guidelines for Stroke Section 9.3.6. Strength Training – New Section*. London: Royal College of Physicians; 2002b. www.rcplondon.ac.uk/pubs/books/stroke/.

Johnson LM, Nelson MJ, McCormack CM et al. The effects of plantarflexor muscle strengthening on the gait and range of motion at the ankle in ambulant children with cerebral palsy. *NZ J Physiother* 1998, **26**:8–14.

Liepert J, Bauder H, Miltner W et al. Treatment-induced cortical reorganisation after stroke in humans. *Stroke* 2000, **31**:1210–1216.

Liston RAL, Mickelborough J, Harris B et al. Conventional physiotherapy and treadmill re-training for higher-level gait disorders in cerebrovascular disease. *Age Ageing* 2000, **29**:311–318.

Macko RF, DeSouza CA, Tretter LD et al. Treadmill aerobic exercise training reduces the energy expenditure and cardiovascular demands of hemiparetic gait in chronic stroke patients. *Stroke* 1997, **28**:326–330.

Maruishi M, Mano Y, Sasaki T et al. Cerebral palsy in adults: independent effects of muscle strength and muscle tone. *Arch Phys Med Rehab* 2001, **82**:637–641.

McArdle WD, Katch FI, Katch VL. *Exercise Physiology*. Baltimore: Williams & Wilkins; 1996.

Miller GJT, Light KE. Strength training in spastic hemiparesis: should it be avoided? *NeuroRehabilitation* 1997, **9**:17–28.

Miltner WHR, Bauder H, Sommer M et al. Effects of constraint-induced movement therapy on patients with chronic motor deficits after stroke. *Stroke* 1999, **30**:586–592.

Miyai I, Fujimoato Y, Ueda Y et al. Treadmill training with body weight support: its effect on Parkinson's disease. *Arch Phys Med Rehab* 2000, **81**:849–852.

Neistadt ME. The neurobiology of learning: implications for treatment of adults with brain injury. *Am J Occup Ther* 1993, **48**:421–430.

Newham DJ, Hsiao S-F. Knee muscle isometric strength, voluntary activation and antagonist co-contraction in the first six months after stroke. *Disabil Rehab* 2001, **23**:379–386.

Ng SSM, Shepherd RB. Weakness in patients with stroke: implications for strength training in neurorehabilitation. *Phys Ther Rev* 2000, **5**:227–238.

Nogaki H, Kakinuma S, Morimatsu M. Movement velocity dependent muscle strength in Parkinson's disease. *Acta Neurol Scand* 1999, **99**:152–157.

Nymark J, DeForge D, Barbau H et al. Body weight support treadmill gait training in the subacute recovery phase of incomplete spinal cord injury. *J Neurol Rehab* 1998, **12**:119–138.

Oman RF, King AC. The effect of life events and exercise program format on the adoption and maintenance of exercise behaviour. *Health Psychol* 2000, **19**:605–612.

Page S, Levine P, Sisto S et al. Stroke patients' and therapists' opinions of constraint-induced movement therapy. *Clin Rehab* 2002, **16**:55–60.

Petajan JH, Gappmaier E, White AT et al. Impact of aerobic training on fitness and quality of life in multiple sclerosis. *Ann Neurol* 1996, **39**:432–441.

Pfaffenbarger RS, Hyde RT, Wing AL. Physical activity and physical fitness as determinants of health and longevity. In: Bouchard C, Shephard RJ, Stephens T et al., eds. *Exercise, Fitness and Health*. Champaign, Illinois: Human Kinetics; 1988:33–48.

Pollock ML, Gaesser GA, Butcher JD et al. The recommended quantity and quality of exercise for developing and maintaining cardiorespiratory and muscular fitness and flexibility in healthy adults. American College of Sports Medicine position stand. *Med Sci Sports Exerc* 1998, **30**:975–991.

Ponichtera-Mulcare JA. Exercise and multiple sclerosis. *Med Sci Sports Exerc* 1993, **4**:451–465.

Potempa K, Brown LT, Tinknell T et al. Benefits of aerobic exercise after stroke. *Sports Med* 1996, **21**:337–346.

Protas EJ, Stanley RK, Jankovic J et al. Cardiovascular and metabolic responses to upper and lower extremity exercises in men with idiopathic parkinson's disease. *Phys Ther* 1996, **76**:34–40.

Reuter I, Engelhardt M, Stecker K et al. Therapeutic value of exercise training in Parkinson's disease. *Med Sci Sports Exerc* 1999, **31**:1544–1549.

Scandalis TA, Bosak A, Berliner JC et al. Resistance training and gait function in patients with Parkinson's disease. *Am J Phys Med Rehab* 2001, **80**:38–43.

Schindl MR, Forstner C, Kern H et al. Treadmill training with partial body weight support in nonambulatory patients with cerebral palsy. *Arch Phys Med Rehab* 2000, **81**:301–306.

Sharp SA, Brouwer BJ. Isokinetic strength training of the hemiparetic knee: effects on function and spasticity. *Arch Phys Med Rehab* 1997, **78**:1231–1236.

Shepherd RB, Carr JH. Treadmill walking in neuro-rehabilitation. *Neurorehab Neural Repair* 1999, **13**: 171–173.

Shortland AP, Harris CA, Gough M et al. Architecture of the medial gastrocnemius in children with spastic diplegia. *Dev Med Child Neurol* 2002, **44**:158–163.

Shumway-Cook A, Woollacott M. *Motor Control*. Baltimore: Williams and Wilkins; 2001.

Smith GV, Macko RF, Silver KHC et al. Treadmill aerobic exercise improves quadriceps strength in patients with chronic hemiparesis following stroke: a preliminary report. *J Neurol Rehab* 1998, **12**:111–117.

Smith GV, Silver KHC, Goldberg AP et al. 'Task-orientated' exercise improves hamstring strength and spastic reflexes in chronic stroke patients. *Stroke* 1999, **30**:2112–2118.

Sunnerhagen KS, Svantesson U, Lonn L et al. Upper motor neurone lesion: their effects on mucle performance and appearance in stroke patients with minor motor impairment. *Arch Phys Med Rehab* 1999, **80**:155–161.

Tanaka S, Hachisuka K, Ogata H. Trunk rotatory muscle performance in post-stroke hemiplegic patients. *Am J Phys Med Rehab* 1997, **76**:366–369.

Tanaka S, Hashisuka K, Ogata H. Muscle strength of trunk flexion-extension in post-stroke hemiplegic patients. *Am J Phys Med Rehab* 1998, **77**:288–290.

Taub E, Crago J, Uswatte G. Constraint-induced movement therapy: a new approach to treatment in physical rehabilitation. *Rehab Psychol* 1998, **43**:152–170.

Teixeira-Salmela LF, Olney SJ, Nadeau S et al. Muscle strengthening and physical conditioning to reduce impairment and disability in chronic stroke survivors. *Arch Phys Med Rehab* 1999, **80**:1211–1218.

Teixeira-Salmela LF, Nadeau S, McBride ID et al. Effects of muscle strengthening and physical conditioning training on temporal, kinematic and kinetic variables during gait in chronic stroke survivors. *J Rehab Med* 2001, **33**:53–60.

Toole T, Hirsch MA, Forkink A et al. The effects of a balance and strength training program on equilibrium in Parkinson's disease: a preliminary study. *NeuroRehabilitation* 2000, **14**:165–174.

Weiss A, Suzuki T, Bean J et al. High intensity strength training improves strength and functional performance after stroke. *Am J Phys Med Rehab* 2000, **79**:369–376.

Wernig A. Laufband (treadmill) therapy in SCI persons. *Neurorehab Neural Repair* 1999, **13**:175–176.

Willen C, Cider A, Sunnerhagen KS. Physical performance in individuals with late effect of polio. *Scand J Rehab Med* 1999, **31**:244–249.

Wolman RL, Cornell C, Fulcher K et al. Aerobic training in brain injured patients. *Clin Rehab* 1994, **8**:253–257.

Woods Duncan P. Synthesis of intervention trails to improve motor recovery following stroke. *Top Stroke Rehab* 1997, **3**:1–20.

Wu C, Wong M, Lin K et al. Effects of task goal and personal preference on seated reaching kinematics after stroke. *Stroke* 2001, **32**:70–76.

Muscle imbalance in neurological conditions

D Fitzgerald   M Stokes

INTRODUCTION

Muscle imbalance is said to occur when relative changes in muscle length and recruitment patterns take place between agonist/antagonist and synergist muscle groups. The ratio of muscle strength and flexibility alters, and functional consequences include abnormal movement patterns, pain and instability.

The concept of muscle imbalance has emerged from several different sources over the latter half of the twentieth century. The most noted contributors were Kendall & Kendall (1938), Lewitt (1991), Janda (1978), Klein Vogelback (1990), Bobath (1990), Carr & Shepherd (1999) and, more recently, Sahrmann (2002) and Richardson et al. (1999). The common ideology amongst these systems of approach is an attempt to quantify the efficiency of muscle activity during functional movement. All systems are largely derived from clinical practice and hypothesise regarding the efficiency of movement but also draw on an increasing body of substantive scientific data.

Whilst it is acknowledged that the detail of our understanding of muscle control in functional movement is in its infancy, there is an accumulating evidence derived from biomechanics, neurophysiology, motor control and skill acquisition, together with basic sciences of muscle physiology, anatomy and human movement. Much of the analysis centres around evaluating the interaction between agonist, antagonist and synergist muscle activity.

The clinical application of this approach is to optimise stress within the musculoskeletal system and prevent or treat regions where dysfunctional movement has produced tissue overload. These concepts are also used in an attempt to optimise movement patterns and hence functional efficiency.

Table 30.1 Examples of muscles with a mainly postural or dynamic function

Mainly postural function	Dynamic function (phasic)
Stenocleidomastoid	Scaleni
Pectoralis major	Pectoralis major
Trapezius	Subscapularis
Levator scapulae	Extensors of the upper extremity
Flexors of the upper extremity	Trapezius
Quadratus lumborum	Rhomboids
Back extensors	Serratus anterior
Hip flexors	Rectus abdominis
Lateral hip rotators	Obliquus abdominis externus
Medial hip rotators	Obliquus abdominis internus
Hamstrings	Gluteus minimus, medius and maximus
Plantarflexors	Vastus medialis and lateralis
	Tibalis anterior
	Peronei

THEORETICAL BASIS OF MUSCLE IMBALANCE

Kinetic data (forces and movement causing motion) and kinematic data (analysis of body segment motion) are the scientific methods used to measure human function (Durward et al., 1999). Notwithstanding the impressive developments in this area, there are significant technical limitations in the ability to determine the precise interaction between multiple muscles involved in a movement and the distribution of stress within the system. Consequently, clinicians developed a battery of tests involving components of:

- functional movement patterns
- isolated muscle strength tests
- isolated muscle flexibility tests.

These three components are the essential elements of applying muscle imbalance concepts in clinical practice. Initial clinical observations (Janda, 1983; Lewitt, 1991) suggested characteristic alterations in muscle function associated with variation in postural alignment. Essentially some muscles show a tendency to *shorten* and become *hyperactive*, and some muscles show a tendency to *lengthen* and become *inhibited*. Examples of these muscles are outlined in Table 30.1.

These observations were initially made in patients who had lesions of the central nervous system (CNS), who developed characteristic postural deformities associated with changes in muscle tone (both hyper- and hypotonicity). This clinical subgroup constitutes the most extreme end of the muscle imbalance spectrum, whilst non-CNS lesion cases represent the other end of the clinical spectrum, displaying similarities in movement pattern disturbance without gross neurological disruption. Attempts to determine the underlying mechanism have speculated a relationship to muscle fibre-type characteristics, muscle morphology, phylogenetic characteristics and muscle architecture, but without consensus. At present, it seems unlikely that any of these hypotheses offers a complete explanation of clinical observations.

Key points

Possible underlying mechanism of muscle imbalance:
- Muscle fibre-type characteristics
- Muscle morphology
- Phylogenetic characteristics
- Muscle architecture

No consensus has yet been reached

The assessment of muscle in relation to movement dysfunction takes into account the anatomical, biomechanical, physiological and biochemical properties of the muscles, and the motor control patterns in which they operate. Precise classification of muscle into postural or phasic characteristics is not always possible and leads to confusion reviewing literature, which classifies muscle according to putative function. Problems with terminology arise if the terms 'postural' and 'phasic muscles' are used, as the two systems no longer appear to concur, due to Janda's altered meaning of the words.

Some conflicts include tensor fascia lata, hamstrings and gastrocnemius, which are movement synergists in one classification (Richardson, 1992) and postural muscles in the other (Jull & Janda, 1987). Inconsistencies are less apparent if muscle length (short/hyperactive, lengthened/inhibited) concepts are applied and it may help to bear this in mind when reading any literature by Janda or any reviews which mention this classification (Norris, 1995a).

Global and local muscle systems

It is known that the neuromuscular system employs complex and varying strategies of cocontraction to provide stiffness and stability during functional movement (Pope et al., 1986; Roy et al., 1989; Lavender et al., 1993a, b; Thelen et al., 1995; O'Sullivan & Taylor, 2000). Stability is required to produce movement about a controlled axis and to equilibrate moments created at other joints as a consequence of motion. This has led to

Table 30.2 Features of the upper motor neurone (corticofugal) syndrome

NEGATIVE	
Acute hypotonia (shock)	
Weakness due to inadequate muscle activation	
Loss of dexterity	
Loss of cutaneous reflexes	
Fatiguability	
POSITIVE	
At rest, in response to peripheral stimulation	
Proprioceptive	Nociceptive
Increased tendon reflexes	Positive Babinsky
with radiation	Extensor spasms
Clonus	Flexor spasms
Spasticity	Mass reflex
During movement (spastic dystonias)	
Dyssynergic patterns of co-contraction	
Associated reactions	
Flexor withdrawal reflexes	
Positive support reaction	
Extensor thrust	
'Pushing' reactions	

Adapted from Greenwood (1998), with permission.

the concept of *global* and *local* muscle systems (Bergmark, 1989). The global muscle system consists of large torque-producing muscles that act upon the region they cross, without having direct anatomical attachments to the area. The local muscle system consists of deep, local muscles positioned close to the joint axis, inserted into adjacent segments and producing significant compressive force components, as opposed to torque.

This concept has provided a framework for much of the contemporary research into muscle imbalance, particularly with regard to the spine and pelvis (Richardson et al., 1999). There is some experimental evidence to support the stability/mobility concept in normally functioning muscles, in that rapid movements which mainly involve type II muscle fibres have been shown selectively to recruit mobility muscles and conversely inhibit synergic stabilising musculature. Examples include: rapid knee extension involving greater rectus femoris activity than vastii activity (Richardson & Bullock, 1986); rapid ankle plantarflexion producing greater activity and a training effect in gastrocnemius rather than soleus (Ng & Richardson, 1990); rapid trunk flexion involving greater activity of rectus abdominis than the oblique abdominal muscles (Thorstensson et al., 1985; Wohlfahrt et al., 1993); and, in cyclists, lengthening and reduced activity of gluteus

maximus (Richardson & Sims, 1991). Richardson (1992) suggested that the movement synergists take over a stability role, as the stability synergists are activated less than the movement synergists.

Since the stability synergists are thought to be used less in muscle imbalance syndromes displaying a tendency to lengthen, presumably by reduced tonic activity and increased phasic activity reducing endurance, the movement synergists become more active and increase their tonic activity to take over the stabilising role of the joints.

In the neurologically impaired patient the application of these concepts is confounded by pathology which affects the spinal or upper motor neurone pools. This pathophysiology results in alterations in muscle tone (either increases or decreases) and consequent disturbances in movement, as outlined in Table 30.2 (Greenwood, 1998).

Evidence for specific postural muscle function

Much of the scientific investigation has been directed towards the lumbopelvic region (Richardson et al., 1999) but there are also data accumulating for the cervical spine, shoulder girdle, knee and ankle, as discussed below.

Cresswell et al. (1992) initially observed continual activation of transversus abdominis, regardless of the direction of trunk motion. Other trunk musculature showed variations in activity, predictable from the direction of displacement. Multifidus, lumbar longissimus and illiocostalis showed sustained activation in upright postures such as standing and walking (Richardson et al., 1999, Ch. 3). Whilst muscles such as lumbar multifidus can provide up to two-thirds of the control of intersegmental motion in certain directions (sagittal plane), it is limited in its ability to control rotation (Wilke et al., 1995). Therefore co-ordinated patterns of muscle recruitment are essential between the global and local muscle systems of the trunk in order to compensate for changing demands of daily life and to ensure that the dynamic stability of the spine is preserved (Gardner Morse et al., 1995; Cholewicki et al., 1996).

Co-contraction between transverse abdominis and lumbar multifidus has been observed in static postures and dynamic movements of the spine (Cresswell et al., 1992, 1994). Increasing levels of postural load are associated with an increase in co-activation of both global and local muscle systems to meet the increasing demands (McGill, 1992). Increasing the speed of dynamic load has been shown to increase the recruitment of postural stabilising muscles and influence their level of activity (Cresswell et al., 1994; Hodges, 1999).

The evidence for neuromuscular dysfunction has come from investigating patients with low-back pain. These observations primarily relate to disturbances in the pattern of muscle recruitment and the co-contraction between different muscle synergies. The types of changes observed relate to delayed/absence of firing, inappropriate increase in muscle co-contraction enhancing stiffness and impaired anticipatory/ feedforward motor relegation (Hodges, 1999; O'Sullivan & Taylor, 2000).

Deficits in control of the neuromuscular system have also been noted in subjects with functional shoulder instability (Lephart et al., 1993; Sainburg et al., 1993) and shoulder impingement syndromes (Pink, 2000). Knee patients with anterior cruciate ligament deficiencies show disturbed firing patterns between quadriceps and hamstrings in specific ranges of the gait cycle and different patterns of activation under functional load (Andriacchi, 1990; Noyes et al., 1992).

Subjects with chronic ankle instability also display impaired joint stability (Gottlieb et al., 1996), impaired proprioceptive function (Jerosch & Bischof, 1996) and alterations in contraction timing (Lynch et al., 1996).

From the above overview it is evident that the debate has moved beyond issues of strength and flexibility, which have historically been the focus of rehabilitation research. The focus of critical research now includes issues regarding:

- the recruitment, co-ordination and regulation of muscle activity
- together with feedforward/feedback control mechanisms during functional tasks.

We also require greater understanding of:

- the observed alterations in muscle control outlined above, particularly the cause-and-effect relationship in the pathological process
- the variability in motor control of movement patterns in order to determine the clinical significance of these variations and whether they represent legitimate targets for rehabilitation.

Key points

- The debate has moved beyond strength and flexibility
- Motor control mechanisms during functional tasks are now the focus of research in rehabilitation
- Need to determine the clinical significance of variability of motor control in movement patterns

CAUSES OF MUSCLE IMBALANCE

Several factors have been suggested as causes of muscle imbalance, based on clinical observation (reviewed by Norris, 1995a):

- habitual poor posture and alignment problems (Sahrmann, 2002)
- pain may lead to postures that reduce pain but cause imbalance and abnormal alignment
- joint pathology can cause reflex inhibition of muscle activity, which tends to inhibit selectively certain muscles associated with a joint (Stokes & Young, 1984) and may therefore lead to imbalance
- muscle imbalance has been suggested as a cause of injury (Grace, 1985)
- modern lifestyle activities at work and in sport may lead to muscles changing their activation pattern and thus functional role, therefore leading to imbalance (Richardson, 1992).

Clearly, any of these causal factors can become involved in a vicious cycle in which it may not be possible to state which came first, i.e. imbalance, altered length, strength or recruitment, or injury.

PHYSIOLOGICAL CONSEQUENCES OF ALTERED MUSCLE FUNCTION

The strength and excitability of a muscle alter with changes in length (Sahrmann, 1987, 2002). The effects of variation in resting muscle length can be considered in biomechanical, neurophysiological and biochemical terms.

Mechanical consequences of altered muscle function

The most obvious implications of changing muscle length relate to musculotendinous shortening with reduced elasticity, resulting in compromised available range of motion or increased tensile load induced by changes in the associated joint kinematics. A typical example of this relates to hip flexor tightness associated with increased lumbar lordosis and anterior pelvic tilt. The mechanical consequences of hip flexor tightness are to interfere with the normal mechanics of hip extension.

Moderate tightness may not produce an overt restriction in hip extension range but manifest itself as anterior hip pain as a consequence of increased tissue load. Soft-tissue adaptations initiate progressive loss of elasticity in association with impairment of joint motion. These adaptive changes relating to changes in muscle fibre length are well recognised from studies assessing the effect of immobilisation/postsurgical interventions (Thompson, 2002), and from muscle length-testing protocols (Janda, 1983; Kendall et al., 1993). The more recent concept of muscle fibre atrophy causing shortening (Shortland et al., 2002; discussed below) has yet to be explored in rehabilitation research.

Changes in muscle tissue

The length/tension relationship for muscle defines the ability of a muscle to generate force as a consequence of its length. The length/tension relationships have been shown to alter due to changes in muscle length (Williams & Goldspink, 1978; Goldspink & Williams, 1990).

Changes in fibre length It has been demonstrated that lengthened muscles gain sarcomeres and shortened muscles lose sarcomeres, with normal sarcomere numbers being restored when immobilisation is discontinued (Williams & Goldspink, 1978; Goldspink & Williams, 1990; Thompson et al., 1998; Thompson, 2002).

Changes in fibre diameter Muscle shortening can also occur without loss of sarcomeres. Fibre length was not reduced in the gastrocnemius muscles of children with spastic diplegia and plantarflexion contractures (Shortland et al., 2002). Extrapolating from the findings of animal studies, where fibre length was normal but diameter was reduced, the investigators concluded that muscle shortening was due to fibre atrophy; the proposed mechanism is loss of muscle fibre diameter in pennate muscles causing shortening of the aponeuroses, thus shortening the muscle and leading to contracture.

Although only indirect evidence was provided for atrophy producing shortening, the contractures seen in the children studied could not be explained by sarcomere loss. This phenomenon needs to be studied in other disorders. It may transpire that, in certain conditions, loss of both fibre diameter and length coexist.

The clinical implications of this observation, regarding muscle strengthening as a means of treating and preventing contractures, are discussed in Chapters 25 and 29.

Effects on function The effect of these adaptations to muscle length on physiological function is to cause a shift in the length/tension relationship (Fig. 30.1). In lengthened muscles, the curve is shifted to the right so that peak tension occurs at a longer length than normal (in the position in which it has been immobilised). Also, because the muscle is longer and has a greater mechanical advantage, its absolute peak tension is greater that that of a muscle of normal length. In the shortened muscle, the curve is shifted to the left of

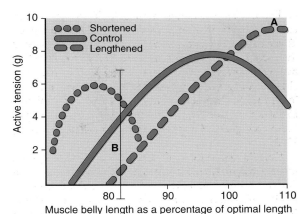

Figure 30.1 Changes in the length/tension curve for muscles immobilised in lengthened and shortened positions. (Redrawn from Norris (1995a), adapted from Gossman et al. (1982), with permission.)

normal, giving a lower peak tension. Therefore, the normal length/tension relationship for individual muscles applies to situations where sarcomere number remains constant and sarcomere number corresponds to anatomical muscle length parameters.

The spontaneous return to normal sarcomere number following the removal of external constraints suggests a physiological mechanism to restore homeostasis and optimal muscle mechanics.

From Figure 30.1 it can be seen that lengthened muscles are stronger that normal and shorter muscles are weaker than normal when tested at their optimal length; this can be achieved under laboratory conditions. The optimal length of a lengthened muscle (point A in Fig. 30.1) can produce a peak tension which is up to 35% greater than that of a muscle of normal length (Williams & Goldspink, 1978). However, consider a muscle tested in inner range, which is approximately just over 80% of the optimal length for a muscle of normal length (point B in Fig. 30.1). At this point of the range, optimal length is not achieved for any length of muscle and favours greatest tension in the shortened muscles. This is because in inner range, the myofilaments of the lengthened muscle would overlap excessively, with redundant cross-bridge formation and a consequent reduction in power output.

Under clinical conditions, therefore, lengthened muscles appear weaker than short muscles (length/tension adaptive changes), particularly if tested in neutral anatomical positions (mid or inner range). It is therefore imperative in clinical testing that muscle strength should be assessed throughout its operational range and not just in one anatomical position.

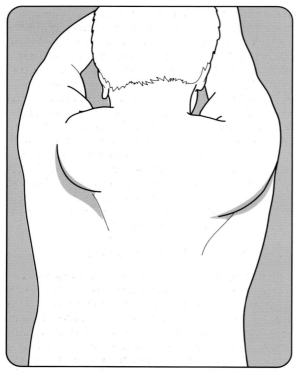

Figure 30.2 Superior scapular migration (left) indicative of alteration in synergic control of scapular position on thorax. There is dominance of the scapular suspensory muscles.

Key point

Clinical testing
Strength should be assessed throughout the operational range of a muscle and not just one anatomical position

---

If muscles are incapable of generating force throughout their operational range, then either range of motion will be impaired or compensatory movement strategies will be employed to achieve functional range.

This compensatory movement strategy is considered to be a typical finding in muscle imbalance syndromes and an example in the shoulder may serve to illustrate. Assessing the pattern of scapular motion during arm elevation can yield useful information regarding the synergic function of scapular muscles (Janda, 1983; Lewitt, 1991; Culham & Peat, 1993). When evaluating arm elevation, the therapist monitors the contour of the upper trapezius and the tendency for superior scapular migration (Fig. 30.2).

Biomechanically, the function of the scapula is to rotate the glenoid upwards during arm elevation and this is primarily accomplished by scapular protraction and upward rotation, producing movement of the inferior angle around the chest wall. The force couple is generated by upper and lower fibres of trapezius and serratus anterior, while middle trapezius and rhomboids act to stabilise the scapula on the thorax. A tendency for superior scapular migration during this movement pattern implies that the upper trapezius is more dominant in the synergy. Whether the cause is primary trapezius hyperactivity or weakness or inhibition of lower trapezius and serratus anterior, the therapeutic goal is to reduce or diminish the tendency for superior scapular migration. This can be achieved by the therapist either applying a downward force on the scapula as the motion occurs in order to give feedback or by prescribing specific scapular stabilisation exercises (Bryden & Fitzgerald, 2001), if adaptive changes have occurred in the upper limb, i.e. biceps.

In summary, the physiological consequences of alterations in muscle length produce increasing discrepancy between the joint angle, giving rise to optimal muscle torque and the normal joint mechanics. In practical terms this means that, for example, the lengthening produced in middle and lower trapezius as a consequence of upper-limb spasticity effectively changes a neutral scapular alignment to an inner range of motion for these muscles. Similar analogies apply to a lengthened gluteus maximus associated with tight hip flexors, or a lengthened anterolateral abdominal wall associated with a sway-back posture.

Connective tissue changes

The physical changes in muscle length are associated with connective tissue adaptation. As described above, Williams & Goldspink (1973) demonstrated the addition and subtraction of sarcomeres to muscle fibres, depending on the position of immobilisation. There is a proliferation of extracellular connective tissue, with resultant increase in passive stiffness and muscle shortening (Lieber, 1992, Ch. 5). The remodelling of dense connective tissue can be considered in two phases – the initial gross disorganisation of unstressed collagen bundles (with associated weakness) evident within a few days of immobilisation (Enwemeka, 1990), and the second stage of remodelling producing consolidation of the randomly aligned collagen to form contracture (Cummings & Tillman, 1992). Ten weeks of connective tissue proliferation with resultant shortening has been shown to be fully reversible (Lieber, 1992) and clinical experience would suggest that it extends well beyond this point. However, determining the point at which contracture is irreversible is largely based on response to appropriate treatment techniques and may ultimately require surgical intervention.

Neurophysiological aspects of altered muscle function

Preferential recruitment theory

The suggestion made in this theory, that shortened muscles are recruited first in a movement pattern, was based on the clinical observations of Sahrmann (1987, 2002). The hypothesis suggests that the neural drive or gain is enhanced in physiologically shortened muscles, thus lowering the recruitment threshold and making them more dominant in a movement synergy. There is some evidence to substantiate this. Hodges & Richardson (1997a, b) have demonstrated a delay in recruitment of the transverse abdominis muscles in patients with low-back pain. Babyar (1996) demonstrated that patients with shoulder pain have excessive scapular elevation which persists in the absence of pain. Mueller et al. (1994) have shown that diabetic patients with impaired ankle dorsiflexion use a hip-dominant strategy for walking.

Co-activation

The co-activation of abdominal and hamstring muscles has been investigated, demonstrating that a decrease in activity of one muscle in a force couple is accompanied by an increase in activity of another (Mayhew et al., 1983). Richardson & Sims (1991) have shown reduced activation of the lengthened gluteus maximus in cyclists. This type of subtle alteration in the reciprocal participation of muscle synergies is thought to contribute to muscle imbalances by reinforcing the demands of a stronger muscle and minimising the demands of the weaker muscles (Sahrmann, 2002).

Proprioception

Alterations in neuronal control profoundly influence the sensory input and motor control required for purposeful movement (Lephart & Fu, 2001). Historically, these issues have been considered as proprioception (Sherrington, 1906). In physiological terms, this requires many afferent receptors to convert mechanical stimuli into neural signals for CNS processing to produce controlled motor output. The current challenge is to understand the integration of these systems to provide the optimal treatment protocols.

In neurologically impaired patients, a major clinical challenge is to achieve adequate limb alignment in order to approximate normal afferent input. This is an important distinction between rehabilitation which is purely focused on achieving functional objectives regardless of the muscle recruitment strategy (motor relearning theory), as opposed to 'normal' movement advocates (Bobath, 1990), who focus on optimising limb alignment and muscle tone as a prerequisite to rehabilitation of functional goals. The clinician has several therapeutic options to enhance proprioceptive function, such as using unstable surfaces, cutaneous stimulation around the muscle, verbal, visual or auditory feedback using mirrors or video, electromyogram (EMG) biofeedback or palpatory facilitation of the target muscles. In terms of motor control theory, there is a putative hierarchy of progression from cognitive activation to associative motor learning to autonomous (Shumway-Cook & Woollacott, 1995).

Pain associated with tightened muscles

Painful trigger points, which are areas of hypersensitive tissue, can occur in shortened hyperactive muscles observed in myofascial pain syndromes (Travell & Simons, 1983). There is deep tenderness and increased tone (the so-called twitch response), which is palpable and easily demonstrated clinically. Each muscle has a characteristic pain referral pattern and can also mimic autonomic dysfunction or peripheral neuropathic pain. There is much debate regarding the pathophysiology of trigger points (Wall, 1993) but they are frequently demonstrable in high-tone patients and are amenable to a variety of treatment techniques, such as sustained pressure, stretching, coolant spray, soft-tissue massage or modalities such as laser or acupuncture.

Biochemical consequences of altered muscle function

Skeletal muscle adaptation through inactivity, therapeutic exercise, training and overload has been well investigated and reviewed (Lieber, 1992; Baechle & Earle, 2000). Adult skeletal muscle contains at least three distinct fibre types, classified because of their functional and metabolic properties as fast glycolytic (type IIa), fast oxidative glycolytic (type IIb) and slow oxidative (type I).

Fast glycolytic and fast oxidative glycolytic fibre types are fast-twitch fibres, characterised by fast myofibrillar adenosine triphosphatase (ATPase) and sarcoplasmic reticulum calcium (Ca)-ATPase activities, and correspondingly short isometric twitch durations and fast maximal shortening velocities.

In contrast, the slow oxidative fibre possesses slow sarcoplasmic reticulum Ca-ATPase and myofibrillar ATPase activities, prolonged twitch duration and slow maximal shortening velocities compared with those of the fast-twitch fibre types (Thompson, 2002).

Classically, skeletal muscle fibres are identified because of their histochemically determined myosin ATPase activity as type I, IIa or IIb. Slow-fibre-dominant musculature, such as soleus, transversus abdominis and lumbar multifidus, contain primarily type I fibres, whereas extensor digitorum longus, gastrocnemius and vastus lateralis contain primarily a mixture of fast type IIa or type IIb fibres.

Information regarding skeletal muscle adaptation to decreased loading/inactivity is derived from varied sources of investigation such as complete limb immobilisation models, limb unloading animal models and space flight. In both animals and humans muscle wasting is associated with selective loss and atrophy of specific muscles and of specific fibre-types (Oganov et al., 1980; Ohira et al., 1992; Edgerton et al., 1995; Alley & Thompson, 1997; Sandmann et al., 1998; Thompson et al., 1998; Widrick et al., 1999).

Antigravity, predominantly slow-twitch type 1 fibre muscle, such as soleus, atrophies more than primarily fast-twitch type II muscles and extensors are more affected than flexors. This atrophic response occurs rapidly, with a reduction in soleus mass of up to 37% after 4–7 days of inactivity (Desplanches et al., 1990; Jiang et al., 1993; Caiozzo et al., 1994; Alley & Thompson, 1997; Sandmann et al., 1998; Thompson et al., 1998). Inactivity also induces a fibre-type transformation within specific muscles. Within a relatively short period of inactivity, the number of type 1 fibres in the antigravity muscles decreases, whereas the number of fibres containing fast-type myosin increases. After 7 days of inactivity the soleus and adductor longus muscles have an increased percentage of dark ATPase (fast) fibres – 11 and 26% respectively (Martin et al., 1989). In contrast, 7 days of inactivity has no effect on the percentage fibre-type distribution in the fast plantaris and superficial region of the medial gastrocnemius (extensor muscles), or the fast extensor digitorum longus.

Importantly, these changes in muscle fibre-type composition impact upon the contractile functions of the muscles and the underlying mechanism responsible for the change in fibre-type composition is probably due to removal of the weight-bearing stimulus.

Myofibril degradation in the early stages of atrophy can be attributed almost entirely to the reduced synthesis of protein. After the initial few days of inactivity the synthesis rate remains steady, whereas the degradation rates show a large increase, thus the majority of the protein loss after 3 days of inactivity can be attributed to the increased degradation rate (Baldwin et al., 1990). These findings suggest that both protein synthesis and degradation rates are altered with inactivity and play a role in skeletal muscle atrophy. The consistent feature of inactivity is limb muscle atrophy and the loss of peak force and power. Differences exist in the rate and mechanisms of muscle wasting and in the susceptibility of a given fibre-type to atrophy. Whilst these data are derived from both experimental animal and human studies undergoing space flight or bed rest, it is reasonable to argue that they may not fully replicate the situation in patients with neurological disease. However, given that the majority of these patients may have been on bed rest and have impaired ability to resist gravity, reduced exercise tolerance and certain conditions that constitute a relatively older age profile, it is likely that this information bears some relevance. In the clinical situation one rarely has the luxury of biochemical or histological profiles regarding muscle characteristics and clinical decisions regarding muscle loading and movement capacity must be judged on an empirical basis in the knowledge of pathophysiological processes.

ASSESSMENT OF MUSCLE IMBALANCE

Muscle imbalance assessment is concerned with evaluating the capacity of the musculoskeletal system to execute the motor commands of the CNS.

Aspects of function should include assessment of:

- postural alignment
- muscle length
- muscle strength
- muscle endurance
- movement patterns.

Postural alignment

Evaluation of postural alignment allows the clinician to generate hypotheses regarding resting muscle length and the likely implications upon movement patterns. It must be emphasised that at this point they are simply clinical hypotheses which must be confirmed or refuted by the appropriate clinical tests.

Classic postural alignment has been described by Kendall et al. (1993), and variants of this alignment have also been described largely in relation to orthopaedic dysfunction. These variants are outlined in Figure 30.3.

In patients with neurological damage, the spectrum of presentation is so variable that assessing posture in an upright stance position relative to a plumbline is often not practical. In these situations, a seated assessment may be necessary and localised assessment of posture, e.g. head/neck alignment or scapulothoracic alignment, may be an appropriate objective.

Figure 30.4 outlines a classic postural alignment in a hemiparietic patient. Evidence of trunk or lower limb malalignment can also be obtained in supine lying, from which the therapist can determine the primary

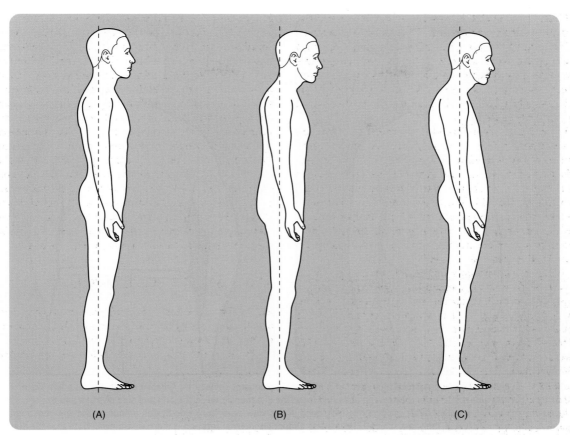

Figure 30.3   Optimal postural alignment in orthopaedic evaluation indicative of minimal muscle activity and joint stress. (A) Kypholordotic pressure; (A) flat-back posture; (C) sway-back posture. (Adapted from Bryden & Fitzgerald (2001), with permission.)

areas of malalignment and the intervention necessary to address these discrepancies.

Muscle length

A preliminary evaluation of muscle length can be determined by attempting passively to realign the deviant segments. This may involve attempting to realign a scapula that has become protracted and elevated (Fig. 30.5), or facilitating trunk extension in a patient who has adopted a flexed posture. If the therapist can facilitate a more efficient alignment by these relatively simple measures, then the direction of therapy must be to try to facilitate activity in the muscles which will provide the necessary mechanical realignment. If the therapist is unable to achieve efficient alignment through facilitation, then mechanical/hypertonicity issues potentially restricting movement must be explored.

Specific muscle length tests can be performed based on a knowledge of functional anatomy and well-described muscle length tests (Janda, 1978; Kendall et al., 1993).

In the hypertonic patient, one of the greatest clinical challenges is to determine whether muscle length changes are a consequence of mechanical adaptations within the connective tissue or of increased activity in the relevant muscle. Very often these are coexisting phenomena and the therapist may need to employ inhibitory techniques or positions prior to assessing muscle length with more formal tests. Therapists must also consider the possibility of articular restriction as a feature limiting movement, which must be evaluated and treated. The procedures for evaluating joint restriction are beyond the scope of this text but have been outlined in other sources (Maitland, 1986; Fitzgerald, 1992).

Muscle strength

As previously discussed, absolute strength is of limited relevance in relation to functional tasks and activities of daily living. It is therefore more appropriate to

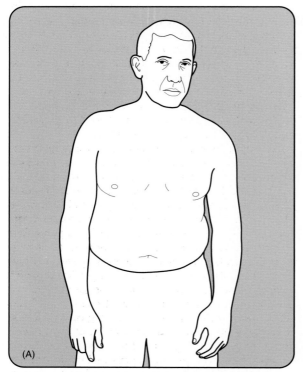
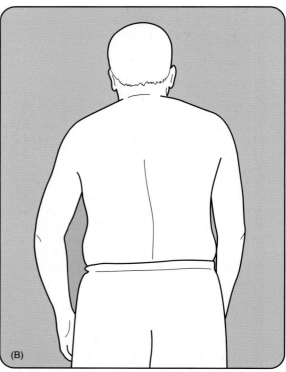

Figure 30.4 Typical hemiparetic postural alignment of a high-level, ambulant subject. (A) Anterior perspective of a left-sided hemiparesis. The left arm is internally rotated and abducted (note the distance between the arm and side of trunk and the orientation of the cubital fossa). The shoulder girdle appears relatively good in this view, with trunk side flexion producing the apparent alignment difference. (B) Posterior view of the same subject. The left arm abduction/internal rotation is more visible here. Note that the point of the left shoulder is lower (due to trunk side flexion) but the contour of the shoulder appears elevated and protracted. This illustrates the importance of determining the position of bony landmarks in order to evaluate the dominant muscle synergies.

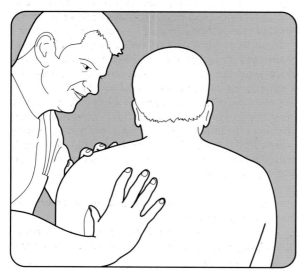

Figure 30.5 Preliminary realignment of scapula with therapist facilitation.

determine the force required to move limbs and trunk rather than that required to move external resistance, as indicated in the DeLorme philosophies and general muscle hypertrophy training programmes.

The level of loading applied is determined by the anatomical location. Lower-limb musculature needs to have adequate strength to tolerate body weight in varying combinations of trunk and leg position. Trunk musculature must be sufficient to maintain trunk stability, whilst allowing independent limb movement. The commonly observed clinical phenomenon in neurologically impaired patients is the inability to move limb and body segments independently because of lack of specific muscle control or more generalised muscle hyperactivity to maintain functional stability.

A wide combination of strengthening techniques is available when using a functional approach and has been well reviewed by Davies (1994), Edwards (2002) and in Chapter 29. A key aspect of strength training is to provide adequate training stimulus, which will produce physiological adaptation towards achieving a functional goal and minimise the risk of overload, which may stimulate altered patterns of muscle synergy.

Holding capacity (endurance)

The ability of antigravity muscles (postural muscles in the traditional sense and stability synergists) to maintain low-force isometric contractions is vital to their functional requirements. This ability can be tested in the usual muscle-testing positions in the middle or inner range, by asking the subject to hold the contraction. It is not the total time of static hold that is of interest, but the length of time the contraction is held without jerky (phasic) movements occurring (Richardson, 1992). For example, the trunk-stabilising muscles need to provide sustained contraction to stabilise the torso allowing limb motion. This can be assessed by asking a seated patient to lift a leg into flexion, thereby creating forces tending to displace the body. If this can be counteracted using muscle control, then the therapist can grade the stability endurance.

Movement patterns

Muscle imbalance leads to abnormal movement patterns in which a functional activity may be achieved and be apparently normal but compensatory strategies and 'trick movements' may have been used (Jull & Janda, 1987; Kendall et al., 1993). Analysis of functional movement patterns is necessary to detect these abnormalities so that treatment can be planned for their correction. For example, a patient may use excessive spinal extension to achieve a functional goal of elevating the arm overhead. This is commonly seen as a substitution when there is an impairment of upper-limb function. Similarly, a patient with limited trunk control may use mass muscle activation in order to achieve a sense of stability. This often leads to compromised upper-limb function (as it is being used to provide fixation as opposed to prehensile tasks) or gross gait disturbance as dissociated trunk and limb motion is compromised.

CORRECTION OF MUSCLE IMBALANCE

The essential criterion in attempting to correct movement impairment in the musculoskeletal system is to identify the underlying cause. Movement patterns may be altered as a consequence of mechanical restriction in one or more elements involved with the movement pattern. Careful testing can elucidate if these mechanical restrictions reside in the joints or the periarticular tissues and help to select the appropriate treatment techniques.

Movement patterns that are deviant from optimal but are not associated with specific mechanical restrictions can be considered as a consequence of alteration in specific muscle co-ordination. This may be due to a lack of appropriate strength for the functional task (e.g. the ability of the lower-limb muscles to control body weight), overrecruitment of dominant/hyperactive muscles in the movement synergy or inadequate activation on the relevant synergic stabilising musculature. These are important aspects of movement impairment for the clinician to quantify because they directly dictate the direction of therapeutic intervention.

The conventional hierarchy of exercise progression is to achieve isolated contraction in low-load situations of individual target muscles (Shumway-Cook & Woolacott, 1995). Following the acquisition of this level of skill, the therapeutic progressions are to increase the level of load and the complexity of the movement pattern to involve greater combinations of synergic stability and mobility demands. The majority of research regarding treatment protocols has been specific to musculoskeletal disorders in non-neurologically impaired patients. Whilst this body of data has shown validity in these aspects of rehabilitation, it has not yet been determined to be efficacious in neurological conditions. However, it must be acknowledged that it has been used routinely in many clinical centres worldwide but has yet to be exposed to the rigours of scientific scrutiny.

Sahrmann (1987) gave an example of muscle imbalance syndrome in hemiplegia involving tightness of the iliotibial band. The typical hemiplegic limb position of abduction and medial rotation with knee extension reciprocates shortening of the iliotibial band. Adaptive changes within the upper limb have already been described earlier in this chapter and some graphic illustrations will follow in the case history below. The use of cycle ergometry and EMG biofeedback was proposed for correction of muscle imbalance in the stroke patients (Brown & DeBacher, 1987). Treatment involved retraining the activation of antagonistic muscle groups of the hemiplegic limb, as well as reciprocal exercise with some symmetry between the two limbs.

Unloaded treadmill walking has also been utilised therapeutically in a variety of neurological conditions, such as partial and complete spinal cord injury, as well as stroke (Dietz et al., 1997; Liston et al., 2000; Kendrick et al., 2001). A number of conclusions can be drawn from these studies:

1. Spinal locomotor centres can be activated in paraplegic patients.
2. Increased leg extensor EMG is related to greater weight-bearing function and the ability to tolerate increasing load.
3. Successive reloading of the body is seen as a stimulus for extensor load receptors.

4. The speed requires adjustment to the optimal rhythm in order to facilitate minimal assistance during the movement pattern.
5. The pelvis may need to be fixed to avoid deviation (lateral/posterior) so that limb loading occurs in a physiological manner.
6. In stroke there is a decrease in premature activity in plantarflexion caused by calf activation in terminal swing.
7. Following training, timing and structure of patterns of leg activity were similar to those seen in healthy subjects (Mulholland, 2002).

Retraining muscle activation

Muscle activation patterns could be altered by increasing tonic input to the stability synergists or by reducing tonic input to the movement synergists. Richardson (1992) explained that the former method was thought to be more effective clinically and described strategies for retraining tonic activity. The first step is to isolate the stability synergist so that the movement synergist is not contracting.

Tonic activity to re-educate slow-twitch muscle fibre function can be achieved by voluntary exercise or electrical stimulation. Richardson (1992) suggested voluntary activity involving low-force (20–30% of maximum voluntary contraction), sustained contractions of about 10 s each. Presumably rest periods, numbers of repetitions and frequency of exercise have yet to be researched but would also depend on the individual. Low-frequency electrical stimulation can be used to change the muscle fibre properties but care must be taken as this can weaken muscle, and further research is required to establish appropriate frequency patterns (see Ch. 23).

Restoration of muscle length

Techniques for restoring muscle length were described by Kendall et al. (1993). Briefly, shortened muscles can be lengthened using standard manual stretching or proprioceptive neuromuscular facilitation (PNF) techniques (see Ch. 23). A recent study has challenged this accepted approach to managing contractures using stretching (Shortland et al., 2002; see also Ch. 29). The investigators concluded that contracture of pennate muscles was due to loss of muscle fibre diameter, causing shortening of the aponeuroses. They therefore suggested that strengthening exercises would prevent or restore muscle length, but evidence to support this suggestion is required.

Lengthened muscles can be shortened by exercising them using low-load contractions held for about 10 s in the shortened, inner range or by splinting them in this position (Kendall et al., 1993).

Norris (1995a) discussed the problems of muscle imbalance around the lumbar spine and techniques for correcting length changes in specific muscle groups.

Restoring stability

The functional interaction between synergists is restored by gradually increasing loads and speed (Richardson, 1992). Exercise programmes have been developed to improve the stability of the lumbar spine (Jull & Richardson, 1994; Norris, 1995b; Sahrmann, 2002). The principles of restoring stability fall into four stages, which were summarised by Norris (1995b) and involve: re-education of stabilising muscles; exercise progressions for static stabilisation; exercise progressions for dynamic stabilisation; and occupational or activity-specific stabilisation. Jull & Richardson (1994) described the use of feedback devices to aid in the isolation of specific muscles for assessment and retraining purposes.

CONCLUSIONS

The potential impact of the muscle imbalance concept for improving the effectiveness of physiotherapy appears to be substantial but its future depends on research to establish its place in clinical practice. Collaborative research between physiotherapists, physiologists and biomechanical engineers should prove fruitful in elucidating the theory, producing guidelines for assessment and treatment and providing evidence of the effectiveness of corrective techniques. Neurological physiotherapists need to take part in research in this area so that application of the concept to neurological patients is applied and evaluated appropriately.

CASE HISTORY

MQ was a 58-year-old man who suffered a left hemiparesis 1 year ago following surgery for removal of a brain tumour. His main difficulties were as follows:

1. severely painful left shoulder
2. gross limitation of left shoulder movement
3. impaired functional use of the left arm, as a consequence of shoulder girdle dysfunction, despite good disassociated motion in wrist, forehand and fingers
4. instability in standing due to poor alignment of the left lower limb, as a consequence of extensor spasticity

5. compromised gait pattern due to extensor spasticity in the stance phase using knee hyperextension, internal rotation and abduction under load
6. no active ankle motion, with extensor spasticity dominant in weight-bearing.

The treatment approach for the left shoulder involved a combination of graded joint mobilisations, initially in neutral positions and then progressing through various degrees of flexion and abduction (Figs 30.6 and 30.7). These were small-amplitude movements short of pain and ensuring not to produce hypertonicity. Joint mobilisation was supplemented with soft-tissue mobilisation and massage to increase compliance of the congested connective tissue.

With improvement in pain-free motion, initially in flexion and subsequently abduction, the progression was to achieve some degree of active control within the available range. The strategies used were first to facilitate active scapular positioning on the thoracic wall and then to progress to maintaining scapular

control with the addition of arm motion. This needed to be facilitated by the therapist until adequate strength and control were achieved (Fig. 30.8).

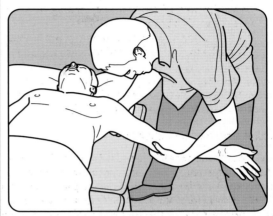

Figure 30.7   Inferior humeral glide in abduction (within patient tolerance) to facilitate arthrokinematics of shoulder abduction and counterimpingement.

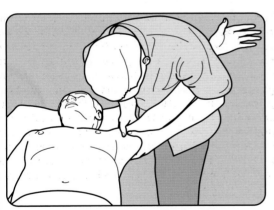

Figure 30.6   Inferior humeral glide in flexion (within patient tolerance) to facilitate arthrokinematics of shoulder flexion. The humeral head should translate inferiorly during arm elevation to prevent impingement. This requires a prerequisite degree of capsular compliance.

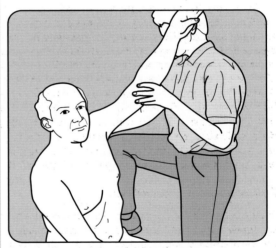

Figure 30.8   Therapist facilitation of active flexion, preventing superior scapular migration, supporting the weight of the limb and stimulating proprioceptive input.

References

Alley KA, Thompson LV. Influence of simulated bed rest and intermittent weight bearing exercise on single skeletal fibre function in aged rats. *Arch Phys Med Rehab* 1997, **78**:19–25.

Andriacchi TP. Dynamics of pathological motion applied to the anterior cruciate deficient knee. *J Biomechanics* 1990, **23** (Suppl.):99–105.

Babyar SR. Excessive scapular motion in individuals recovering from painful and stiff shoulders: causes and treatment strategies. *Phys Ther* 1996, **76**:226–232.

Baechle TR, Earle RW. *Essentials of Strength Training and Conditioning*. Champaign, Illinois: Human Kinetics; 2000.

Baldwin KM, Herrick RE, Ilyina-Kakueva E, Oganov VS. Effect of zero gravity on myofibril content and isomyosin distribution in rodent skeletal muscle. *FASEB J* 1990, **4**:79–83.

Bergmark A. Stability of the lumbar spine. A study in mechanical engineering. *Acta Orthop Scand* 1989, **230** (Suppl.):1–54.

Bobath B. *Adult Hemiplegia: Evaluation and Treatment*. Oxford: Heinemann Medical Books; 1990.

Brown DA, DeBacher GA. Bicycle ergometer and electromyographic feedback for treatment of muscle imbalance in patients with spastic hemiparesis. *Phys Ther* 1987, **67**:1715–1719.

Bryden L, Fitzgerald D. The influence of posture and alteration of function upon the craniocervical and craniofacial region. In: Von Piekartz H, Bryden L, eds. *Craniofacial Dysfunction and Pain*. Oxford: Butterworth Heinemann; 2001:163–188.

Caiozzo VJ, Baker MJ, Herrick RE, Tao M, Baldwin KM. Effect of spaceflight on skeletal muscle: mechanical properties and myosin isoform content of a slow muscle. *J Appl Physiol* 1994, **76**:1764–1773.

Carr J, Shepherd R. *Neurological Rehabilitation: Optimising Motor Performance*. Oxford: Butterworth-Heinemann; 1999.

Cholewicki J, McGill SM. Mechanical stability of the in vivo lumbar spine: implications for injury and low back pain. *Clin Biomech* 1996, **11**:1–15.

Cholewicki J, Panjabi MM, Kachatryan A. Stabilising function of trunk flexor–extensor muscles around a neutral spine posture. *Spine* 1997, **22**:2207–2212.

Cresswell AG, Grundstrom H, Thorstensson A. Observations on intra-abdominal pressure and patterns of abdominal intra muscular activity in man. *Acta Physiol Scand* 1992, **144**:409–418.

Cresswell AG, Oddsson L, Thorstensson A. The influence of sudden perturbations on trunk muscle activity and intra-abdominal pressure while standing. *Exp Brain Res* 1994, **98**:336–341.

Culham E, Peat M. Functional anatomy of the shoulder complex. *J Orthop Sports Phys Ther* 1993, **18**:342–350.

Cummings G, Tillman L. Remodelling of dense connective tissue in normal abdominal tissues. In: Currier DP, Nelson RM, eds. *Dynamics of Human Biologic Tissues*. Philadelphia: FA Davis; 1992:45–74.

Davies PM. *Starting Again*. Berlin: Springer-Verlag; 1994.

Desplanches D, Mayet MH, Ilynia-Kakueva EI, Sempore B, Flandrois R. Skeletal muscle adaptation in rats flown on Cosmos 1667. *J Appl Physiol* 1990, **68**:48–52.

Dietz V, Wirtz M, Jensen L. Locomotion in patients with spinal cord injuries. *Phys Ther* 1997, **77**:508–516.

Durward BR, Baer GD, Rowe PJ. Measurement issues in functional human movement. In: Durward BR, Baer GD, Rowe PJ, eds. *Functional Human Movement*. Oxford: Butterworth-Heinemann; 1999:2–12.

Edgerton VR, Zhou M-Y, Ohira Y et al. Human fibre size and enzymatic properties after 5 and 11 days of spaceflight. *J Appl Physiol* 1995, **78**:1733–1739.

Edwards S. *Neurological Physiotherapy*. Edinburgh: Churchill Livingstone; 2002.

Enwemeka CS. Ultrastructural changes induced by cast immobilisation in the soleus tendon. In:

Proceedings of the 65th Annual Conference of the American Physical Therapy Association. Anaheim, CA: 1990:58–65.

Fitzgerald D. *Muscle Imbalance in Neurological Disorders. Instructional Course Notes*. Dublin: Dublin Physiotherapy Clinic; 1992.

Gardner-Morse M, Stokes IAF, Laible JP. Role of muscles in lumbar spine stability in maximum extension efforts. *J Orthop Res* 1995, **13**:802–808.

Goldspink G, Williams PE. Muscle fibre and connective tissue changes associated with use and disuse. In: Ada L, Canning C, eds. *Key Issues in Neurological Physiotherapy*. Oxford: Butterworth-Heinemann; 1990:197–218.

Gossman MR, Sahrmann SA, Rose SJ. Review of length-associated changes in muscle: experimental evidence and clinical implication. *Phys Ther* 1982, **62**:1799–1808.

Gottlieb DJ, Huber BM, Roos EM, et al. *Stability in Unilateral, Chronic Ankle Instability*. ORS: 1996.

Grace TG. Muscle imbalance and extremity injury: a perplexing relationship. *Sport Med* 1985, **2**:77–82.

Greenwood R. Spasticity and upper motor neurone syndrome in spasticity rehabilitation. In: Sheean G, ed. *Spasticity Rehabilitation*. London: Churchill Communication: 1998:1–5.

Hodges P. Is there a role for transversus abdominis in lumbo pelvic stability? *Manual Ther* 1999, **4**:74–86.

Hodges PW, Richardson CA. Contraction of the abdominal muscles associated with movement of the lower limb. *Phys Ther* 1997a, **77**:132–144.

Hodges PW, Richardson CA. Feedforward contraction of transversus abdominis is not influenced by the direction of arm movement. *Exp Brain Res* 1997b, **114**:62–370.

Janda V. *Muscle Testing and Function*. London: Butterworth-Heinemann; 1978.

Jerosch J, Bischof M. Proprioceptive capabilities of the ankle in stable and unstable joints. *Sports Exerc Inj* 1996, **2**:100–109.

Jiang B, Roy RR, Navarro C et al. Absence of a growth hormone on rat soleus atrophy during a 4-day spaceflight. *J Appl Physiol* 1993, **74**:527–531.

Jull GA, Janda V. Muscles and motor control in low back pain: assessment and management. In: Twomey L, Taylor JR, eds. *Physical Therapy of the Low Back*, 1st edn. Edinburgh: Churchill Livingstone; 1987:253–278.

Jull GA, Richardson CA. Rehabilitation of active stabilisation of the lumbar spine. In: Twomey L, Taylor JR, eds. *Physical Therapy of the Low Back*, 2nd edn. Edinburgh: Churchill Livingstone; 1994:251–273.

Kendall HO, Kendall FP. Care during the recovery period in paralytic poliomyelitis. *Pub Health Bull* 1938, **242**:1–9.

Kendall FP, Kendall HO, McCreary E. *Muscles, Testing and Function*, 4th edn. Baltimore: Williams & Wilkins; 1993.

Kendrick C, Holt R, McGlashan K, Jenner J, Kirker S. Exercising on a treadmill to improve functional mobility in chronic stroke. *Physiotherapy* 2001, **87**:261–265.

Klein Vogelback S. *Functional Kinetics*. Berlin: Springer-Verlag; 1990.

Lavender S, Marras W, Miller R. The development of response strategies in preparation for sudden loading to the torso. *Spine* 1993a, **18**:2097–3002.

Lavender S, Tsuang Y, Andersson G. Trunk muscle activation and co-contraction while resisting applied moments in a twisted posture. *Ergonomics* 1993b, **36**:1145–1150.

Lephart SM, Fu FH. Proprioception and neuromuscular control in joint stability. USA: Human Kinetics; 2001: xv–xxiv.

Lephart SM, Warner JP, Borsa PA et al. Proprioception in athletic individuals with unilateral shoulder instability. In: *Proceedings of the American Shoulder and Elbow Surgeons Annual Meeting*. Williamsburg, VA: 1993:98–107.

Lewitt K. *Manipulative Therapy in Rehabilitation of the Locomotor System*, 2nd edn. Oxford: Butterworth-Heinemann; 1991.

Lieber R. *Skeletal Muscle Structure and Function*. Baltimore: Williams & Wilkins; 1992.

Liston R, Mickleborough J, Harris B, Hann A, Tallis R. Conventional physiotherapy and treadmill re-training for higher level gait disorders in cerebrovascular disease. *Age Ageing* 2000, **29**:311–318.

Lynch SA, Eklund U, Gottlieb D, Renstrom PA, Beynnon B. Electromyographic latency changes in the ankle musculature during inversion moments. *Am J Sports Med* 1996, **24**:362–369.

Maitland GD. *Peripheral Manipulation*. London: Butterworths; 1986.

Martin TP, Edgerton VR, Grindeland RE. Influence of spaceflight on rat skeletal muscle. *J Appl Physiol* 1989, **65**:2318–2325.

Mayhew T, Norton BJ, Sahrmann SA. Electromyographic study of the relationship between hamstring and abdominal muscles during a unilateral straight-leg raise. *Phys Ther* 1983, **63**:1769–1775.

McGill S. A myoelectrically based dynamic three-dimensional model to predict loads on lumber spine tissues during lateral bending. *J Biomech* 1992, **25**:395–414.

Mueller MJ, Minor SD, Sahrmann SA et al. Differences in the gait characteristics of patients with diabetes and peripheral neuropathy compared with age-matched controls. *Phys Ther* 1994, **74**:299–308.

Mulholland P. *Neurophysiology and Clinical Practice: Instructional Course Notes*. Lancashire, UK: Preston Royal Infirmary; 2002.

Ng G, Richardson CA. The effects of training triceps surae using progressive speed loading. *Physiother Pract* 1990, **6**:77–84.

Norris CM. Spinal stabilisation: 4. Muscle imbalance and the low back. *Physiotherapy* 1995a, **81**:127–138.

Norris CM. Spinal stabilisation: 5. An exercise programme to enhance lumbar stabilisation. *Physiotherapy* 1995b, **81**:138–145.

Noyes FR, Schipplein OD, Andriacchi TP et al. The anterior cruciate ligament-deficient knee with varus alignment: an analysis of gait adaptations and dynamic joint loadings. *Am J Sport Med* 1992, **20**:707–716.

Oganov VS, Skuratova SA, Potapov AN et al. Physiological mechanisms of adaptation of rat skeletal muscles to the weightlessness and similar functional requirements. *Physiologist* 1980, **23**:S16–S21.

Ohira Y, Jiang B, Roy RR et al. Rat soleus muscle fibre responses to 14 days of spaceflight and hind limb suspension. *J Appl Physiol* 1992, **73**:51S–57S.

O'Sullivan P, Taylor RJ. Lumbar segmental instability: pathology, diagnosis and conservative management. In: Twomey LT, Taylor JR, eds. *Physical Therapy of the Low Back*. New York: Churchill Livingstone; 2000:201–248.

O'Sullivan PB, Twomey LT, Allison GT. Evaluation of specific stabilizing exercise in the treatment of chronic low back pain with radiologic diagnosis of spondylolysis or spondylolisthesis. *Spine* 1997, **22**:2959–2967.

Pink M. Scapulohumeral rhythm. In: Singer KP, ed. *Proceedings of the 7th Scientific Conference of the IFOMT; Manipulative Physiotherapy Association of Australia*. 2000:381–386.

Pope M, Anderson G, Broman H et al. Electromyographic studies of the lumbar trunk musculature during development of axial torques. *J Orthop Res* 1986, **4**:288–293.

Richardson CA. Muscle imbalance: principles of treatment and assessment. In: *Proceedings of the New Zealand Society for Physiotherapists Challenges Conference*. Christchurch, New Zealand: New Zealand Physiotherapy Association; 1992:127–138.

Richardson CA, Bullock MI. Changes in muscle activity during fast, alternating flexion–extension movements of the knee. *J Rehab Med* 1986, **18**:51–58.

Richardson CA, Sims K. An inner range holding contraction. An objective measure of stabilising function of an antigravity muscle. In: *Proceedings of the World Confederation for Physical Therapy, 11th International Congress*. London: 1991:829–831.

Richardson CA, Jull GA, Hodges PW et al. *Therapeutic Exercise for Spinal Segmental Stabilisation in Low Back Pain: Scientific Basis and Clinical Approach*. Edinburgh: Churchill Livingstone; 1999.

Roy S, Deluca C, Casavant D. Lumbar muscle fatigue and chronic low back pain. *Spine* 1989, **14**:992–998.

Sahrmann SA. Muscle imbalances in orthopaedic and neurological patient. In: *Proceedings of Tenth International Congress of the World Confederation for Physical Therapy*. Sydney, Australia: 1987:836–841.

Sahrmann S. *Movement Impairment Syndromes*. St Louis: Mosby; 2002.

Sainburg RL, Poizner H, Ghez C. Loss of proprioception deficits in interjoint coordination. *J Neurophysical* 1993, **70**:2136–2147.

Sandmann ME, Shoeman JA, Thompson LV. The fibre-type-specific effect of inactivity and intermittent weight-bearing on the gastrocnemius muscle of 30-month-old rats. *Arch Phys Med Rehab* 1998, **79**:658–662.

Sherrington CS. *The Integrative Action of the Nervous System*. New Haven, CT: Yale University Press; 1906.

Shortland AP, Harris CA, Gough M et al. Architecture of the medial gastrocnemius in children with spastic diplegia. *Dev Med Child Neurol* 2002, **44**:158–163.

Shumway-Cook A, Woolacott M. *Motor Control – Theory and Practical Applications*. Baltimore: Williams & Wilkins; 1995.

Stokes M, Young A. The contribution of reflex inhibition to arthrogenous muscle weakness. *Clin Sci* 1984, **67**:1–14.

Thelen D, Schultz A, Ashton-Miller J. Co-contraction of lumbar muscles during development of tome-varying triaxial moments. *J Orthop Res* 1995, **13**:390–396.

Thompson LV. Skeletal muscle adaptations with age, inactivity and therapeutic exercise. *J Orthop Sports Phys Ther* 2002, **32**:44–57.

Thompson LV, Johnson SA, Shoeman JA. Single soleus muscle fibre function after hindlimb unweighting in adult and aged rats. *J Appl Physiol* 1998, **84**:1937–1942.

Thorstensson A, Oddsson L, Carlson HJ. Motor control of voluntary trunk movements in standing. *Acta Physiol Scand* 1985, **125**:309–321.

Travell JG, Simons DG. *Myofascial Pain and Dysfunction*. Baltimore: Williams & Wilkins; 1983.

Wall P. The mechanisms of fibromyalgia. In: Vaeroy H, Merskey H, eds. *Progress in Fibromyalgia and Myofascial Pain*. Amsterdam: Elsevier, 1993:53–60.

Widrick JJ, Knuth St, Norenberg KM et al. Effect of a 17 day spaceflight on contractile properties of human soleus muscle fibres. *J Physiol* 1999, **516**:915–930.

Wilke HJ, Wolf S, Claes LE, Arand M, Wiesend A. Stability increase of the lumbar spine with different muscle groups: a biomechanical in vitro study. *Spine* 1995, **20**:192–198.

Williams P, Goldspink G. The effect of immobilization on the longitudinal growth of striated muscle fibres. *J Anat* 1973, **116**:45–52.

Williams P, Goldspink G. Changes in sarcomere length and physiologic properties in immobilized muscle. *J Anat* 1978, **127**:459–468.

Wohlfahrt DA, Jull GA, Richardson CA. The relationship between the dynamic and static function of the abdominal muscles. *Aust J Physiother* 1993, **39**:9–15.

Chapter 31

Neurodynamics

E Panturin

INTRODUCTION

The purpose of physiotherapy treatment in general, and of physiotherapy of neurological conditions in particular, is to help the individual to return to full function of as near to normal quality as is achievable, depending, obviously, on the severity of the condition. Neurodynamics addresses impairment-based problems and it is important to consider their impact on different aspects of a patient's life, as described in the World Health Organization's (WHO) *International Classification of Functioning, Disability and Health* (WHO, 2001).

There are many causes that may prevent normal function in people, e.g. limited joint movements, muscle weakness, shortening of soft tissues, increased and/or decreased muscle tone, impaired sensation, cognitive and perceptual restrictions. Over recent years, orthopaedically oriented physiotherapists such as Elvey (1986), Maitland (1986) and Butler & Gifford (1989) have all mentioned another cause for restricted function – restricted movement of the nervous system, then termed adverse mechanical, or neural, tension (AMT or ANT). That is to say, impairment of movement and/or elasticity of the nervous system may cause symptoms from within its own tissues, such as pain and restriction of movements in different parts of the body.

Recently, Shacklock (1995a, b) emphasised not only the mechanics of the nervous system, but also the link between the pathomechanics and pathophysiology of the nervous system. Shacklock suggested using the term 'neurodynamics' when discussing interaction between nervous system mechanics and physiology.

Can we presume that the difficulty displayed by the hemiplegic or severely head-injured person in straightening his or her knee on gentle heel landing when walking is always due to a restriction in the knee joint itself? Perhaps it may be caused by increased tone, shortening of the gastrocnemius muscle or hamstrings or, possibly, by an abnormality in the movement of, or physical changes in, the nervous system. Following this theme, why may a person suffering central nervous system (CNS) damage have difficulty in extending his or her hip in the stance phase? Or, are we aware of all the causes of pain and restriction of movement in the shoulder of the person with hemiplegia or incomplete spinal cord injury? Do we know why the person is unable to stretch out his or her arm to pick up an object or grasp a glass in a normal manner? Why does the hemiplegic or head-injured person display a certain posture (Rolf, 1999)? How can the loss of selective movements and/or the complex regional pain syndrome (CRPS) be explained? (CRPS was previously known as reflex sympathetic dystrophy, which was inaccurate because symptoms of this syndrome are not only of sympathetic origin). We must add here another tissue to this long list of known causes – the restriction of movement in the nervous system.

In central neurological, as in orthopaedic, conditions one must always look for further causes of restricted function:

- by examining the ability of movement, or elasticity, of the nervous system
- by understanding the effect of the physiological changes of the nervous system caused as a direct result of the injury itself
- by understanding the origins of pain in general and particularly central pain and central sensitisation (Wright, 1999; Butler, 2000). Central sensitisation describes changes occurring at a cellular level to support the process of neural plasticity that occurs in nociceptive system neurones in the spinal cord and supraspinal centres, as a result of activation of the nociceptive system (Wright, 1999). There are three ways in which central sensitisation is manifested in the CNS:
  - the threshold of firing will be reduced
  - neurone responsiveness increases
  - the receptive field of the neurone increases (Butler, 2000).

According to Butler (1991a), the nervous system should be considered as another organ of the body, where a change occurring in part of the system may cause repercussions in the system as a whole. This is an inevitable phenomenon in a continuous tract; and, as the peripheral, central and autonomic nervous systems form continuous tracts they can be considered as a body organ system.

This relatively new concept of neurodynamics is beginning to be applied in neurological practice; a brief overview of its proposed mechanisms and applications is given here, and the reader is referred to the growing literature on this subject. There are, as yet, no randomised controlled trials providing evidence for the use of neurodynamics in clinical practice (see 'Proposed explanation of the neurodynamic phenomenon', below, for a discussion on research required).

MOVEMENT OF NEURAL TISSUE

As explained above, the nervous system is a continuum and can be likened to the letter H in that it joins together all the parts of the body (Butler, 1991a). We can therefore understand how movement in one part of the body can produce either an enhancing or restricting effect in other parts of the body.

A study in the monkey showed that the addition of dorsiflexion on straight-leg raising (SLR) may either stretch and/or move the nervous system up as far as the cerebellum (Smith, 1956). The spinal cord is moved, and the meninges stretched as far as the sciatic nerve, by passively flexing the neck (Breig, 1978). Breig & Troup (1979) demonstrated the influence of dorsiflexion on lumbosacral nerve roots, and even reaching as far as the brain, thus illustrating the continuous nature of the nervous system. Butler (2000) mentioned in vivo studies which demonstrated that cervical flexion has a mechanical influence on the neural tissue of the lumbar spine. Movement of the wrist has been shown to produce a direct mechanical effect on the nervous system in the upper arm (McLellan & Swash, 1976; Coppieters et al., 2001).

In 1980, Maitland demonstrated that the position of the head whilst performing the slump test (slump sitting, neck in flexion, straightening the knee and dorsiflexing the foot) altered the amount of dorsiflexion achieved and affected the ability to extend the knee. Davidson (1987) demonstrated that, while extending the hip in side-lying with knee flexed (slump-prone knee-bending – SPKB), the position of the head changes the amount of hip extension achieved.

A direct connection has been shown between movement of the nervous system and the symptoms displayed by patients with orthopaedic problems. One of the first to demonstrate the clinical effect was Maitland (1979) while performing the slump test in sitting. Elvey (1986) showed that symptoms in an arm were altered by movement of the contralateral arm or by SLR.

Lewis et al. (1998), in a study on five cadavers, found a significant increase in tension in the median nerve when ipsilateral movements of elbow and wrist extension were applied. Contralateral cervical side flexion and ipsilateral SLR also increased tension significantly, but not when the same movements were made on the contralateral side. Many further examples can be seen in the growing literature on this topic. Clinical experience has found that SLR, performed either ipsi- or contralaterally to the treated upper extremity, may either decrease or increase tension.

TREATMENT IN ORTHOPAEDIC PRACTICE

The development of the concept of neurodynamic treatment is based on earlier observations (Elvey, 1986; Butler & Gifford, 1989; Butler, 1991a). Various techniques for examining, moving and treating the nervous system have been devised. All the techniques (movements) are based on the anatomical pathways of different nerves: passive neck flexion – spinal cord (Troup, 1981); SLR – sciatic nerve (Maitland, 1979); prone knee bending (PKB) and SPKB – femoral nerve (Davidson, 1987); and the upper-limb tension tests (ULTT: Elvey, 1986; Butler, 1991a). As the concept is now known as neurodynamics and as the emphasis is now on movement rather than tension, the ULTT is now known as upper-limb neurodynamic test – ULNT (Butler, 2000).

Names of the commonly used movement tests of the upper extremity are:

- ULNT1 – median nerve (Butler, 2000)
- modification of the ULTT1 (Yaxley & Jull, 1991)
- ULNT2a – median nerve
- ULNT2b – radial nerve
- ULNT3 – ulnar nerve (Butler & Gifford, 1989; Butler, 1991a).

The great variety of responses witnessed (e.g. median nerve movement may cause ulnar nerve symptoms) when using these techniques may be explained by the following:

- To date, 38 variations of the structure of the brachial plexus have been described (Tountas & Bergman, 1993), e.g. a connection between the ulnar and median nerves in the forearm was found in 20% of the population (Lebovic & Hastings, 1992). Therefore it will be necessary to change treatment techniques accordingly, in order to reproduce the patient's symptoms.
- The starting body position may affect the results (Butler, 1991a). For example, symptoms of sciatic pain while performing SLR may differ between supine and side-lying positions.
- Passive and/or active movements may produce different results (Butler, 1991a).

- Physiological changes of the nerve, such as those occurring in diabetic patients rendering the nerve more vulnerable, may also affect results (Shacklock, 1995b).
- Central sensitivity (Wright, 1999; Butler, 2000). This concept proposes that the CNS's sensitivity or activation threshold is reduced, thus enabling stimulation that would not normally be able to access central neurones to have an effect (Butler, 2000).

Clinically it was found that the sequence of application of the techniques (which joint or part of the nerve is moved first) influences the response. If the nervous system in the examined limb is relaxed, it can be presumed that the first component of the test chosen will effectually evaluate the movement of the nerve in relation to its surroundings. As Butler (2000) said: 'First load the area you want to challenge most', or, 'The first movement tested "borrows" the neural tissue first and thus allows a better examination'. Following this it is necessary to sensitise the test, which means adding body movement likely to place more mechanical force (loading) upon the nervous system. Butler et al. (1994) introduced the slider/tension principle: tension – placing a load on the nervous system from 'both ends' simultaneously and slider – placing load on the nervous system at alternate ends. Slider allows better movement of the nerve with less tension.

In orthopaedics, neurodynamics is used for treating various pathologies: in sport, ankle sprains, hamstring strains, tennis elbow and thoracic outlet syndrome (Gallant, 1998); mechanical allodynia following hand injury (Sweeney & Harnos, 1996); problems of the foot and fitting of orthoses (Chapman, 2001). Needless to say, the sympathetic nervous system must be taken into consideration during treatment (Manning, 2000). Because the sympathetic system is part of the CNS, every peripheral nerve possesses a sympathetic component, e.g. SLR moves the sympathetic ganglion chain (Breig, 1978).

A relationship has been observed between the appearance of symptoms in the ULNT and those of Colles fracture (Young & Bell, 1991), tennis elbow (Yaxley & Jull, 1993), whiplash injury (Quinter, 1989; Yeung et al., 1997) and overuse syndrome in keyboard workers (Byng, 1997). Turl & George (1998) found a connection between SLR symptoms and repetitive hamstring strain and Pahor & Toppenberg (1996) found altered neurodynamic function following ankle inversion sprain. Positive signs of neural tension have also been observed in asymptomatic athletes, e.g. swimmers (Heighway & Monteith, 1991) and in keyboard workers (Byng, 1997).

Neurodynamic techniques do not stand on their own. They are components of a complete treatment, aiming to improve meaningful and purposeful activity. Treatment is combined: with direct mobilisation of a nerve (Rolf, 1999; Butler, 2000); with treatment of anatomical structures such as joints (Tal-Akabi & Rushton, 2000), muscles and connective tissues (Hall & Elvey, 1999). The treatment of acute conditions is mainly passive, but, as the condition improves, and in more chronic conditions, the treatment is active (Butler, 2000). Treatment should take into consideration self-mobilisation, improving posture, ergonomics and function.

PROPOSED EXPLANATION OF THE NEURODYNAMIC PHENOMENON

In an attempt to explain the neurodynamic phenomenon a gap exists between practice and research. Clear diagnostic validity for most of the tests is still lacking, but there are neuroanatomical and neuropathological bases for them (Matheson, 2000).

To date, diagnostic validity exists only for ULNT1 (Kleinrensink et al., 2000; Coppieters et al., 2001) and ULNT3 (Shacklock, 1996). Kleinrensink et al. (2000) examined ULNT of the median, ulnar and radial nerves. This study demonstrated that only ULNT1 had both high sensitivity and specificity. Although the radial and ulnar ULNT increased tension in their corresponding nerves, it was not significantly greater or specific in the nerve named in the test. One of the problems is that when performing the movements, not only are nerves moved but other tissues also. For example, when examining the median nerve with cervical side flexion to the opposite side, segments of the subclavian artery (Wilson et al., 1994) and the posterior longitudinal ligament (Moses & Carmass, 1996) are also moved.

Existence of movement of the nervous system has been seen in peripheral nerves and demonstrated by Gelberman et al. (1998) on magnetic resonance imaging (MRI) examination of the spinal cord. Shortening of the ulnar nerve and elongation of the radial and median nerves occur on flexing the elbow. The bed of the median nerve is 20% longer when the elbow and wrist are extended than when they are flexed (Millesi, 1986). The spinal canal is 5–9 cm longer in flexion than in extension of the spine (Breig, 1978; Louis, 1981).

The nervous system possesses an adaptive mechanism of movement and, according to Butler (1991a), this is achieved by:

- the presence of excess length in the nervous system (Breig, 1978; Millesi, 1986)

- the nerve moving in relation to the tissue surrounding it (e.g. the posterior interosseous branch of the radial nerve moves within the supinator muscle), or

movement within the nerve itself, when the fascicles move against the external epineurium and each fascicle moves against its neighbour (McKibbin, 1995).

As already stated, the connection between movement of the nervous system and symptoms demonstrated by orthopaedic patients can be explained by the fact that the nervous system may be damaged by physical injury, endangering the neural and connective tissues. The pathology caused may be extra- and/or intraneural. Normally the nerve is situated in contact with various tissues, named by Butler (1989) as mechanical interfaces and, more recently by Shacklock (1995a, b) as neural containers. Mechanical interfaces are defined as 'that tissue or material adjacent to the nervous system that can move independently to the system'. They may be pathological features, such as haemorrhage, oedema or scar tissue, or plaster casts, and perhaps hypertonic and rigid muscles.

The injury may be to the blood supply of the nerve, to the nerve itself or to the axoplasmic flow. The nervous system consumes 20% of the oxygen in the arterial circulation, which is required for impulse conduction (Dommisse, 1994). An increase of 8% of the normal length of a nerve decreases the blood flow, and an increase of 15% in nerve length will cause complete occlusion of the blood supply (Ogata & Naito, 1986). The blood vessels in the spinal cord and of the peripheral nerves possess extra length and anatomical organisation, affording both movement and normal blood flow (Breig, 1978).

The axoplasmic flow described by Delcomyn (1998) includes anti- and retrograde movements (flow) of substances. The importance of this flow is described by Butler (1991b), and the importance of axonal transport can be learned from researches connected with the function of the CNS. For example, axonal transport is used as a strategy for tracing long axonal pathways in the CNS (Chamberlin et al., 1998); direct and indirect pathways of the flow of cortical information through the basal ganglia (Smith et al., 1998) and also, in the understanding of the pathology of illnesses, such as Huntington's disease (Sapp et al., 1999) and amyotrophic lateral sclerosis (Susaki & Twata, 1999). Changes in the flow are expressed by trophic changes in the target tissue, damage to the neurone and its axon, and in the action potential of the nerve. It was found, in rabbits, that the axoplasmic flow was affected by very low pressure (Shacklock, 1995a, b). Miura et al. (1997) found that inhibition of distal sprouting in rabbits was probably caused by a local disturbance of axonal transport resulting from proximal constriction.

According to Butler (2000), damage to the function of the nerve begins at pressures of 30–40 mm of mercury (mmHg). In a healthy person, the pressure in the carpel tunnel, with the wrist joint in a neutral position, is 3 mmHg. With injury, the pressure with the wrist in neutral position reaches 30 mmHg and with the wrist in flexion the pressure can reach as high as 100 mmHg. If this is so, it can be presumed that flexor spasticity seen around the wrist joint in a hemiplegic person causes abnormal pressure on the median nerve. Therefore, the symptoms frequently seen in the hemiplegic hand may arise from, among other causes, damage to the axonal transport. Thus, it is possible that some of the physiological changes seen in the hemiplegic person are caused by spasticity (mechanical interface) influencing the axonal flow. The axoplasma has thixotrophic properties, meaning that it flows better when kept moving (Baker et al., 1977).

As the nervous system is a continuum, symptoms may develop in areas distant from the area of injury (Butler, 1991a). This concept was first described by Upton & McComas (1973), and described in many sources as the 'double crush' phenomenon (appearance of symptoms in a part of the body, or nervous system, distant from the original injury). The concept was developed further by Butler (1991a), who described the 'multicrush syndrome' and its many causes. This idea was challenged by Morgan & Wilbourn (1998), who claimed that not all symptoms develop in areas distant to the injury. Therefore, when evaluating a patient with two symptomatic areas, it is important to find out if they are connected by one or more causes.

In a literature review, Matheson (2000) did not find many studies demonstrating the value of using neurodynamics. Only some of the studies claimed significant improvement when using neurodynamics in treatment. In neurological treatment, the use of neurodynamics is gaining good clinical but not, as yet, scientific evidence required to endorse practice. It is essential that research is undertaken to verify the use of neurodynamics in the different clinical areas in which it is being applied.

NEURODYNAMICS IN NEUROLOGICAL DISORDERS

According to Davies (1994, 2000), Rolf (1999) and Simionato et al. (1988), who described neural tension signs in Guillain–Barré syndrome, and the author's clinical experience; it appears that the effect of movement of the nervous system may also be applied to injuries of the CNS. When examining patients with hemiplegia, spinal cord injuries or cerebral palsy, it can frequently be observed that the range of motion in one part of the body is altered by passive movement of another part distant from the original movement

(Davies, 1994). According to Davies (2000), clinical experience shows that there is loss of movement of the neuraxis and peripheral nerves following head injury. This loss gives rise to pathological postures (which are difficult to correct voluntarily), great resistance to movement and loss of selective movements of the trunk and extremities, for example, straightening of the elbow when the glenohumeral joint (GHJ) is in abduction, or extension of the knee when the hip is flexed, or flexion of the knee when the hip is extended. The kyphotic sitting position seen in hemiplegic and Parkinson patients causes overstretching of the sympathetic nervous system.

Clinical experience shows that flexing the neck of a person with cerebral palsy may increase the range of movement in SLR. With hemiplegic patients, movement of the head affects range of movement of the shoulder or elbow and performing ULNT1 on the unaffected arm or SLR on one (ipsi- or contralateral) or both legs can affect movement and/or pain in the plegic arm. It has also been observed clinically (by the author) that hip flexion in SLR is affected by hip extension in SPKB and vice versa. The slump test technique reduces tension in the involved upper extremity and may cause retraction of the scapula in the patient with hemiparesis (Davies, 1994). Davies also suggests using abduction of the hip in the slump technique in cases of adductor spasticity.

Davies (1994) recommended including the neurodynamic techniques within holistic treatment, giving an example of the positive effects of treatment in head-injured persons even 10 years after injury. As stated earlier, and as will be described in a case history later, the physiotherapist must remember that treatment by movements means not only moving joints and muscles or influencing tone, but also moving the nervous system. It is therefore suggested that the physiotherapist include: (1) movement of parts distal to all movements performed during treatment; (2) mobilisation of the nerve itself; (3) movement of the trunk, enhancing movement of the nervous system and affecting the sympathetic chain (Breig, 1978; Butler, 1991a; Davies, 1994, 2000).

Where does treatment begin? Physiotherapists treat symptoms and, therefore, carefully selected movements of different parts of the body and their effect on the functional ability of the patient must be considered. The variety of available movements is very large, and the effect is varied and individual to each patient. For example, while performing ULNT1 on a plegic arm, a similar movement of the other arm may improve movement of the affected arm in some hemiplegics, whilst in others it may increase pain and restrict movement (Davies, 1994).

When does treatment begin? In order to maintain free mobility of joints, muscles and the nervous system, treatment should start early (Davies, 1994). Furthermore, movement preserves the viscosity of exoplasm (thixotrophic characteristics) required for normal axonal transport.

Treatment of the patient with a neurological condition should not be solely passive and local. The integration of neurodynamics into general treatment and active function is desirable. If no active ability exists, passive techniques contribute greatly to the patient's well-being and help to prevent contractures.

Each improvement in range gained passively needs to be integrated immediately into the patient's active control and function, depending on the degree of damage (Davies, 1994). The patient should be encouraged to perform self-mobilisation at home.

CASE HISTORY

HG, an active 64-year-old man with right hemiparesis following a cerebrovascular accident, complained of

difficulty in grasping objects with his paretic hand or with both hands. He also did not extend his right hip sufficiently when standing or walking. The aim of treatment was to improve his ability to drink from a cup, held in both hands, whilst sitting and standing.

As part of HG's holistic care, some therapeutic components of neurodynamics were included. Treatment possibilities are many and it is often worthwhile starting with cervical movements which, from the neurodynamic point of view, enable the nerves in the trunk and extremities to move without moving the container. This was followed by movements of the trunk and scapula (rotatory movements of the trunk affect the sympathetic nervous system). Then ULNT1 was performed in lying (Fig. 31.1).

The sequence of ULNT1 is:

- abduction of the arm to between 90° and 100°
- wrist and finger extension
- supination
- external rotation of the arm
- careful extension of the elbow

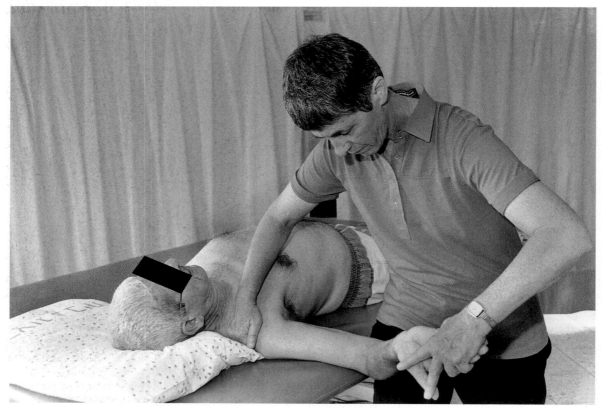

Figure 31.1   Upper–limb neurodynamic test (ULNT1). Abduction of glenohumeral joint to 90–100°, extension of wrist and fingers, supination of forearm, lateral rotation of glenohumeral joint and elbow extension. Restriction of fingers, wrist and elbow extension is demonstrated. The therapist's right hand feels the movement while preventing anterior subluxation of the head of the humerus.

- and, if achievable, lateral flexion of the neck towards the contralateral side (Butler, 1991a). This movement produced tension, causing restriction of wrist, fingers and elbow extension, and HG complained of slight pain.

Other movements of the body which might alter these restrictions and pain were then sought. Of the many possibilities, ULNT1 of the opposite limb was chosen and found to reduce the restriction and pain in the plegic arm. If symptoms had been increased by this manoeuvre, it would not have been repeated. Attempts were also made to find movements in other limbs (such as SLR) which might relieve the symptoms. If symptoms are worsened by neurodynamic tests already performed, there are other possibilities for continuing treatment: (1) to perform slider movements (movement of the nerve without tension); (2) to change the order of the components of the test.

Since the ULNT1 on the contralateral arm improved HG's symptoms, this was followed by straightening the elbow and/or wrist of the paretic arm. Passive movements of the wrist were performed whilst the elbow was flexed, as well as passive movements of the elbow while the wrist was released from tension (slide). This was combined with mobilisation of the muscles and the median nerve in the anterior forearm. Active movements followed immediately after the passive movements, e.g. flexion and extension of the elbow while maintaining wrist extension.

Another treatment possibility is performing ULNT3 and this was used on HG. According to Butler (2000), the sequence of this test is:

- extension of wrist and fingers
- pronation and flexion of the elbow
- external rotation of the arm
- depression of the shoulder girdle
- abduction of the arm
- and, if attainable, lateral flexion of the neck towards the contralateral side.

This can be followed with slider movements, changing the order of the components of the test, soft-tissue and ulnar nerve mobilisation. This should be followed immediately by active movements. All the upper-limb movements were performed while paying attention to the position of the neck, trunk and lower extremities.

Attention was then paid to the restricted extension of the hip joint. Here, also, many possibilities of treatment were available, preferably beginning with movements of the trunk. Extending the affected hip in side-lying (SPKB), with both knees flexed, was chosen.

The passive movements, here also, were followed immediately with active extension of the hip and slider movements. Still in side-lying, the patient rotated his upper trunk towards the bed, enabling increased hip extension, extended his arm diagonally downwards, while the therapist added supination and extension of the wrist and fingers and performed various assisted active movements (Fig. 31.2). This combination of movements can also be used as slider movements. Here too soft-tissue and nerve mobilisation can be added. It should be remembered that SLR may also influence extension of the hip.

Following treatment in lying, HG stood in step position, affording hip extension, while repeating, passively and actively, neurodynamic movements of the upper limb. Treatment ended with a re-evaluation of the function. HG was able to grasp and hold the cup with better control while standing, and was encouraged to repeat some of the treatment movements at home.

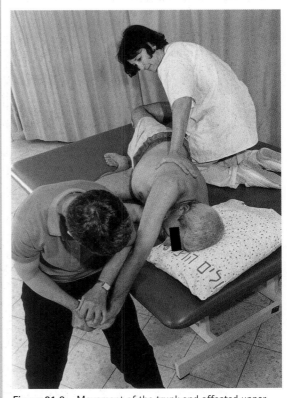

Figure 31.2 Movement of the trunk and affected upper extremity. Supination and extension of the wrist and fingers whilst maintaining slump-prone knee-bending (SPKB). This can be performed as tension or slide. SPKB involves side-lying with lower hip and knee fully flexed, upper hip extended and upper knee flexed.

Since mobilisation of the muscles and other soft tissues was included in the treatment, it is not possible to conclude that the treatment effects were solely due to neurodynamic changes.

PRECAUTIONS WITH NEURODYNAMIC TREATMENT

1. Some neurological patients will have a history of back pain and symptoms may still be present; the therapist must therefore always perform neurological examinations and treatments with the greatest caution and care (Butler & Gifford, 1989).
2. As the nervous system is delicate and superficial in certain areas, all movement and treatment progress must be performed slowly (Butler & Gifford, 1989).
3. Joints must be kept in normal alignment during each movement.
4. Attention must be given to the effect of every movement on the body as a whole.
5. Special care should be taken when treating unconscious patients or those without sensation (Davies, 1994).
6. Pain of neural origin can appear some hours after the nerve has been irritated.
7. Pain may have many causes, one possibly being sensitisation of the nervous system.
8. Clinical experience shows that, despite the resistance to movement that may be felt by the therapist, the patient may not feel any discomfort or limitation. In this instance, the therapist must treat according to the symptoms he or she feels (Butler & Gifford, 1989; Davies, 1994).
9. It has been demonstrated that frequent repetition of SLR, even in a healthy person, can give rise to symptoms such as headache, nausea and 'floating'. A possible explanation may be that SLR moves the sympathetic chain (Breig, 1978).
10. The pathomechanical and pathophysiological aspects of both symptoms and treatment must be considered (Shacklock, 1995a, b; Rolf, 1999).

Always remember that neurodynamic treatment may aggravate symptoms if not performed appropriately. Therefore, every component in the chain of movements should be added with great care. It is better to start with a few movements without full extension (remembering that it is possible to start with slide). Acute symptoms should be treated passively.

CONCLUSIONS

As yet, there is no scientific research or direct proof of the effect of using neurodynamic movements in neurological treatment. There is still insufficient knowledge available to explain the physiological effect of the treatment. Clinical experience in this field is growing, and research is required to underpin its use and develop it further.

The therapist must remember that treatment of the neurological patient is holistic and that the use of neurodynamic movements is only one part of the integral treatment. In the opinion of the author:

- Neurodynamics should be used not only as tests, but also as movement or techniques.
- Neurodynamic movements can be successfully integrated within other treatment concepts such as proprioceptive neuromuscular facilitation (PNF), Bobath (neurodevelopmental therapy or NDT) and motor relearning programmes.

References

Baker P, Ladds M, Rubinson K. Measurement of the flow properties of isolated axoplasm in a defined chemical environment. *J Physiol* 1977, **269**:10–11.

Breig A. *Adverse Mechanical Tension in the Central Nervous System*. Stockholm, Sweden: Almquist & Wiksell; 1978.

Breig A, Troup JDC. Biomechanical considerations in the SLR test. *Spine* 1979, **4**:242–250.

Butler D. Adverse mechanical tension in the nervous system: a model for assessment and treatment. *Aust J Physiother* 1989, **35**:227–238.

Butler D. *Mobilisation of the Nervous System*. Melbourne, Australia: Churchill Livingstone; 1991a.

Butler D. Axoplasmic flow and manipulative physiotherapy. In: *Proceedings of 7th Biennial Conference of Manipulative Physiotherapists Association*. New South Wales, Australia: Australian Association of Manual Therapists; 1991b:206–213.

Butler DS. *The Sensitive Nervous System*. Adelaide, Australia: Noigroup Publications; 2000.

Butler D, Gifford L. The concept of adverse mechanical tension in the nervous system. *Physiotherapy* 1989, **75**:622–636.

Butler DS, Shacklock MO, Slater H. Treatment of altered nervous system mechanics. In: Boyling JD, Palastanga N, eds. *Grieve's Modern Manual Therapy*, 2nd edn. Edinburgh: Churchill Livingstone; 1994:693–704.

Byng J. Over use syndromes of the upper limb and the upper limb tension test: a comparison between patients, asymptomatic keyboard workers and asymptomatic non keyboard workers. *Man Ther* 1997, **3**:157–164.

Chamberlin NL, Du B, de-Lacalle S, Saper CB. Recombinant adeno-associated virus vector: use for trangene expression and anterograde tract in the central nervous system. *Brain Res* 1998, **793**:169–175.

Chapman C. Neurodynamic testing as an approach to diagnosis in podiatry. *Br J Podiatr* 2001, **3**:101–109.

Coppieters MW, Stappaerts KH, Everaert DG, Staes FF. Addition of test components during neurodynamic testing: effect on range of motion and sensory responses. *J Orthop Sport Phys Ther* 2001, **5**:226–237.

Davidson S. Prone knee bend: an investigation into the effect of cervical flexion and extension. In: Dalziell RA, Snowcill JC, eds. *Proceedings of the Manipulative Therapists Association of Australia. 5th Biennial Conference.* Melbourne, Australia: Australian Association of Manual Therapists; 1987:235–246.

Davies PM. *Starting Again.* London: Springer Verlag; 1994:121–179.

Davies PM. *Steps to Follow,* 2nd edn. London: Springer Verlag; 2000:429–469.

Delcomyn F. *Foundation of Neurobiology.* New York: WH Freeman; 1998.

Dommisse GF. The blood supply of the spinal cord. In: Boyling JD, Palastanga N, eds. *Grieve's Modern Manual Therapy – The Vertebral Column,* 2nd edn. London: Churchill Livingstone; 1994:3–20.

Elvey RL. Treatment of arm pain associated with abnormal brachial plexus tension. *Aust J Physiother* 1986, **32**:225–230.

Gallant S. Clinical perspectives. Assessing adverse neural tension in athletes. *J Sport Rehab* 1998, **2**:128–129.

Gelberman RH, Yamaguchi K, Hallstein SB. Changes in interstitial pressure and cross-section area of the cubital tunnel and the ulner nerve with flexion of the elbow. *J Bone Joint Surg* 1998, **80A**:492–501.

Hall TM, Elvey RL. Nerve trunk pain: physical diagnosis and treatment. *Man Ther* 1999, **4**:63–73.

Heighway S, Monteith G. Swimmer's shoulder: incidence of upper limb neural tension signs in swimmers. *Aust J Physiother* 1991, **37**:52.

Kleinrensink GJ, Stoeckart R, Mulder PGH. Upper limb tension tests as tools in the diagnosis of nerve and plexus lesions. *Clin Biomech* 2000, **15**:9–14.

Lebovic CJ, Hastings H. Martin Gruber revisited. *J Hand Surg* 1992, **17A**:47–53.

Lewis J, Ramot R, Green A. Change in mechanical tension in the median nerve: possible complications for the upper limb tension test. *Physiotherapy* 1998, **6**:254–261.

Louis R. Vertebroradicular and vertebromedullar dynamics. *Anat Clin* 1981, **3**:1–11.

Maitland GD. Negative disc exploration: practical canal signs. *Aust J Physiother* 1979, **25**:129–134.

Maitland GD. Movement of pain sensitive structures in the vertebral canal in a group of physiotherapy students. *South Afr J Physiother* 1980, **36**:4–12.

Maitland GD. *Vertebral Manipulation,* 5th edn. London: Butterworths; 1986.

Manning DC. Reflex sympathetic dystrophy, sympathetically maintained pain, and complex regional pain syndrome. *J Hand Ther* 2000, **4**:260–268.

Matheson JW. Research and neurodynamics. In: Butler DS, ed. *The Sensitive Nervous System.* Adelaide, Australia: Noigroup Publications; 2000: 343–365.

McKibbin H. Neurodynamics related to the treatment of patients following a cerebrovascular accident. In: Harrison MA, ed. *Physiotherapy in Stroke Management.* Edinburgh: Churchill Livingstone; 1995.

McLellan DL, Swash M. Longitudinal sliding of the median nerve during movements of the upper limb. *J Neurol Neurosurg Psychiatry* 1976, **39**:556–570.

Millesi H. The nerve gap: theory and clinical practice. *Hand Clin* 1986, **4**:651–663.

Miura H, Baba M, Matsuniga M, Oda K. Changes in motor nerve terminals following proximal constriction by a ligature. *J Peripher Nerve Syst* 1997, **1**:170–176.

Morgan G, Wilbourn AJ. Cervical radiculopathy and coexisting distal entrapment neuropathies: double-crush syndromes? *Neurology* 1998, **1**:78–83.

Moses AS, Carmass JB. Anatomy of the cervical spine: implications for the ALTT. *Aust J Physiother* 1996, **42**:31–35.

Ogata K, Naito M. Blood flow of peripheral nerve effects of dissection, stretching and compression. *J Hand Surg* 1986, **11**:10–14.

Pahor S, Toppenberg R. An investigation of neural tissue involvement in ankle inversion sprains. *Man Ther* 1996, **1**:192–197.

Quinter TI. A study of upper limb pain and paraesthesia following neck injury in motor vehicle accidents: assessment of the brachial plexus tension nest of Elvey. *Br J Rheumatol* 1989, **28**:528–533.

Rolf G. *Patho-neurodynamics Following Lesions of the Central Nervous System.* Unpublished lecture. IBITA course for instructors and candidates. Burgau, Germany: 1999.

Sapp E, Penney J, Young A, Aronin N, Vonsattel JP, DiFiglio M. Axonal transport of N-terminal huntingtin suggests early pathology of corticastriated projections in huntington disease. *Neuropathol Exp Neurol* 1999, **2**: 165–173.

Shacklock M. Neurodynamics. *Physiotherapy* 1995a, **81**:9–16.

Shacklock M. Clinical application of neurodynamics. In: Shacklock M, ed. *Moving in on Pain.* Chatswood, Australia: Butterworth-Heinemann; 1995b.

Shacklock MO. Positive upper limb tension test in a case of surgically proven neuropathy. *Man Ther* 1996, **1**:154–161.

Simionato R, Stiller K, Butler D. Neural tension signs in Guillain–Barré syndrome: two case reports. *Aust J Physiother* 1988, **34**:257–259.

Smith CG. Changes in length and posture of the segments of the spinal cord in posture in the monkey. *Radiology* 1956, **66**:259–265.

Smith Y, Bevan MD, Shink E, Bolam JP. Microcircuitry of the direct and indirect pathways of the basal ganglia. *Neuroscience* 1998, **2**:358–387.

Susaki S, Twata M. Immunoreactivity of beta-amyloid precursor protein in amyotrophic lateral sclerosis. *Acta Neuropathol* 1999, **5**:463–468.

Sweeney J, Harnos A. Persistent mechanical allodynia following injury of the hand: treatment through mobilisation of the nervous system. *J Hand Ther* 1996, **4**:328–338.

Tal-Akabi A, Rushton A. An investigation to compare the effectiveness of a carpal bone mobilisation and neurodynamic mobilisation as methods of treatment for carpal tunnel syndrome. *Man Ther* 2000, **4**:214–222.

Tountas CP, Bergman RA. *Anatomic Variations of the Upper Extremity*. New York: Churchill Livingstone; 1993.

Troup JDG. Straight leg raising (SLR) and the qualifying tests for increased root tension. *Spine* 1981, **6**:526–527.

Turl SE, George KP. Adverse neural tension: a factor in repetitive hamstring strain. *J Ortho Sport Phys Ther* 1998, **1**:16–21.

Upton ARM, McComas AJ. The double crush in nerve entrapment syndromes. *Lancet* 1973, **2**:359–362.

Wilson S, Selvaratnam PJ, Briggs C. Strain at the subclavian artery during the upper limb tension test. *Aust J Physiother* 1994, **40**:243–248.

WHO. *International Classification of Functioning, Disability and Health* (ICF). Geneva: World Health Organization; 2001.

Available online at: http://www.who.int/classification/icf.

Wright A. Recent concepts in neurophysiology of pain. *Man Ther* 1999, **4**:196–202.

Yaxley GA, Jull GA. A modified upper limb tension test: an investigation of responses in normal subjects. *Aust J Physiother* 1991, **37**:143–152.

Yaxley GA, Jull GA. Adverse tension in the neural system, a preliminary study of tennis elbow. *Aust J Physiother* 1993, **39**:15–22.

Yeung E, Jones M, Hall B. The response to the slump test in a group of female whiplash patients. *Aust J Physiother* 1997, **4**:245–252.

Young L, Bell A. The upper limb tension test response in a group of post Colles fracture patients. In: *Proceedings of 7th Biennial Conference of Manipulative Therapists Association*. New South Wales, Australia: Australian Association of Manual Therapists; 1991: 226–231.

Appendix

Associations and Support Groups

This appendix lists some national charities which provide support to those with neurological disabilities and their carers. The list is not exhaustive, as other groups exist locally and there may also be national groups for rarer disorders. National offices will have contact details for different parts of the UK and internationally, where they exist. Some of these charities also fund medical research.

ATAXIA

Ataxia

(formally known as Friedreich's Ataxia Group)
Rooms 10–10A Winchester House
Kennington Park
Cranmer Road
London SW9 6EJ
Tel: 020 7582 1444
e-mail: office@ataxia.org.uk
www.ataxia.org.uk

BALANCE DISORDERS

British Brain and Spine Foundation

See 'Brain injury', below.

Ménière's Society

98 Maybury Road
Woking
Surrey GU21 5HX
Tel: 01483 740597
e-mail: info@menieres.co.uk
www.menieres.co.uk

Royal National Institute for Deaf People

See 'Communication', below.

BRAIN INJURY

Basic

The Neurocentre
554 Eccles New Road
Salford M5 1AL
Tel: 0161 707 6441
Helpline: 0870 750 0000
e-mail: basic_charity@compuserve.com
www.basiccharity.org.uk

Brain & Spine Foundation

7 Winchester House
Kennington Park
Cranmer Road
London SW9 6EJ
Tel: 020 7793 5900
e-mail: info@bbsf.org.uk
www.bbsf.org.uk

British Epilepsy Association

New Anstey House
Gate Way Drive
Yeadon
Leeds LS19 7XY
Tel: 0113 210 8800
www.epilepsy.org.uk

Children's Brain Injury Trust (CBIT)

The Radcliffe Infirmary
Woodstock Road

Oxford OX2 6HE
Tel: 01865 522467
Helpline: 0845 601 4939
www.cbituk.org

Encephalitis Support Group

44a Market Place
Malton
North Yorkshire YO17 7LW
Tel: 01653 699599
www.esg.org.uk

Headway

National Head Injuries Association
7 King Edward Court
King Edward Street
Nottingham NG1 1EW
Tel: 0115 924 0800
Fax: 0115 924 0432
e-mail: enquiries@headway.org.uk
www.headway.org.uk

National Meningitis Trust

Fern House
Bath Road
Stroud
Gloucester GL5 3TJ
Tel: 01453 768000
24-hour helpline UK: 0845 6000 800 (LoCall)
24-hour helpline Republic of Ireland: 1800 523196
(freephone)
24-hour helpline International: +44 870124 7000
Fax: 01453 768001
e-mail: info@meningitis-trust.org
www.meningitis-trust.org.uk

UKABIF (United Kingdom Acquired Brain Injury Foundation)

c/o Royal Hospital for Neuro-disability
West Hill
Putney
London SW15 3SW
Tel: 020 7878 4569
www.ukabif.org.uk

CARE AND RESPITE

Crossroads – Caring for Carers

Association Office
10 Regent Place
Rugby

Warks CV21 2PN
Tel: 01788 573653
Fax: 01788 565498
e-mail: association.office@crossroads.org.uk
www.crossroads.org.uk

Leonard Cheshire Foundation

National Information Officer
30 Millbank
London SW1P 4QD
Tel: 020 7802 8200
Fax: 020 7802 8250
e-mail: info@london.leonard-cheshire.org.uk
www.leonard-cheshire.org.uk

CEREBRAL PALSY

Hare Association

c/o Chartered Society of Physiotherapy (CSP)
14 Bedford Row
London WC1R 4ED

SCOPE

PO Box 833
Milton Keynes MK12 5NY
Tel: CPHelpline: 08088 003333
e-mail: cphelpline@scope.org.uk
www.scope.org.uk

COMMUNICATION (ASSISTIVE DEVICES AND COMMUNICATIONS AIDS)

Ability Net

PO Box 94
Warwick CV34 5WS
Tel: 0800 269545
www.abilitynet.org.uk

ACE Centre Advisory Trust

92 Windmill Road
Headington
Oxford OX3 7DR
Tel: 01865 759800
Fax: 01865 759810
e-mail: info@ace-centre.org.uk
www.ace-centre.org.uk

Royal National Institute for Deaf People

19–23 Featherstone Street
London EC1 Y8SL

Tel: 0808 808 0123 (freephone)
Textphone: 0808 808 9000 (freephone)
Fax: 020 7296 8199
e-mail: infomationline@rnid.org.uk
www.rnid.org.uk

Typetalk

RNID Typetalk
PO Box 284
Liverpool L69 3UZ
Tel: 0151 709 9494
e-mail: helpline@rnid-typetalk.org.uk
www.typetalk.org.uk

GENERAL SUPPORT SERVICES

Association of Medical Research Charities (AMRC)

61 Gray's Inn Road
London WC1X 8TL
Tel: 020 7269 8820
Fax: 020 7242 2484
e-mail: info@amrc.org.uk
www.amrc.org.uk

Capability Scotland
ASCS (Advice Service Capability Scotland)

11 Ellersly Road
Edinburgh
Scotland EH12 6HY
Tel: 0131 313 5510
Textphone: 0131 346 2529
Fax: 0131 346 1681
e-mail: ascs@capability-scotland.org.uk
www.capability-scotland.org.uk

Disability Action – Northern Ireland

2 Annadale Avenue
Belfast BT7 3JH
Tel: 028 9029 7880
Fax: 028 9029 7881
e-mail: hq@disabilityaction.org
www.disabilityaction.org

Disabled Living Foundation (DLF)

380/384 Harrow Road
London W9 2HU
Tel: 020 7289 6111
Fax: 020 7266 2922
e-mail: dlf@dlf.org.uk
www.dlf.org.uk

Physically Handicapped and Able Bodied (PHAB)

Summit House
Wandle Road
Croydon
London CR0 1DF
Tel: 020 8667 9443
Fax: 020 8681 1399
e-mail: info@phabengland.org.uk
www.phabengland.org.uk

Royal Association for Disability and Rehabilitation (RADAR)

12 City Forum
250 City Road
London EC1V 8AF
Tel: 020 7250 3222
Fax: 020 7250 0212
e-mail: radar@radar.org.uk
www.radar.org.uk

HUNTINGTON'S DISEASE

Huntington's Disease Association

108 Battersea High Street
Battersea
London SW11 3HP
Tel: 020 7223 7000
Fax: 020 7223 9489
e-mail: info@hda.org.uk
www.hda.org.uk

MOTOR NEURONE DISEASE (MND)

Motor Neurone Disease Association

PO Box 246
Northampton NN1 2PR
Tel: 01604 250505
Fax: 01604 24726
Helpline: 08457 62 62 62
e-mail: enquiries@mndassociation.org
www.mndassociation.org.uk

Motor Neurone Disease Care and Research Centres

Contact the MND helpline (see above) if you have difficulty contacting any of the centres:

- King's College Hospital, London
  Tel: 020 7848 5172
  www.mndcentre.org.uk

- Queen Elizabeth II Hospital, Birmingham
  Tel: 0121 472 1311 ext. 8626
- Queens Medical Centre University Hospital, Nottingham
  Tel: 0115 924 9924 ext. 43179
- Radcliffe Infirmary, Oxford
  Tel: 01865 224310
- Rookwood Hospital, Cardiff
  Tel: 029 2056 6281 ext. 3749
- Royal Hallamshire Hospital, Sheffield
  Tel: 0114 271 3431
- Royal Victoria Infirmary, Newcastle
  Tel: 0191 227 5267
- The Walton Centre, Liverpool
  Tel: 0151 529 5070

Regional care advisers (RCAs) for MND

Listed on the MND website
e-mail: care@mndassociation.org

MULTIPLE SCLEROSIS

Multiple Sclerosis Society of Great Britain

MS National Centre
372 Edgware Road
London NW2 6ND
Tel: 020 8438 0700
Fax: 020 8438 0701
e-mail: info@mssociety.org.uk
www.mssociety.org.uk

Multiple Sclerosis Society in Scotland

National Office
Ratho Park
88 Glasgow Road
Ratho Station
Edinburgh
Scotland EH28 8PP
Tel: 0131 335 4050
Fax: 0131 335 4051
e-mail: through the website
www.mssocietyscotland.org.uk

NERVE INJURIES

Obstetric brachial plexus palsy (OBPP)

Several groups exist locally – a national contact address is not available.

NEUROCUTANEOUS DISORDERS

Dystrophic Epidermolysis Bullosa Research Association (DEBRA)

DEBRA House
13 Wellington Business Park
Dukes Ride
Crowthorne
Berks RG45 6LS
Tel: 01344 771961
Fax: 01344 762661
e-mail: debra.uk@btinternet.com
www.debra.org.uk

The Neurofibromatosis Association

82 London Road
Kingston upon Thames
Surrey KT2 6PX
Tel: 020 8547 1636
Fax: 020 8947 5601
e-mail: nfa@zetnet.co.uk
www.nfa.zetnet.co.uk

NEUROMUSCULAR DISORDERS

Muscular Dystrophy Campaign

7–11 Prescott Place
London SW4 6BS
Tel: 020 7720 8055
Fax: 020 7498 0670
e-mail: info@muscular-dystrophy.org
www.muscular-dystrophy.org

Myasthenia Gravis Association

Central Office
Keynes House
Chester Park
Alfreton Road
Derby DE21 4AS
Tel: 01332 290219
Fax: 01332 293641
e-mail: mg@mgauk.org.uk
www.mgauk.org

PARKINSON'S DISEASE

Parkinson's Disease Society of the UK

215 Vauxhall Bridge Road
London SW1V 1EJ
Tel: 020 7932 1346
Helpline: 0808 8000 303 (freephone)

Fax: 020 7233 9908
e-mail: enquiries@parkinsons.org.uk
www.parkinsons.org.uk

POLYNEUROPATHIES

Charot–Marie–Tooth (CMT)

CMT United Kingdom
36E Melbourne Road
Christchurch
Dorset BH23 2HZ
Tel: 01202 480285
e-mail: membership@cmt.org.uk
www.cmt.org.uk

Guillain–Barré Syndrome (GBS) Support Group

GBS Support Group of the UK
Lincolnshire County Council Offices
Eastgate
Sleaford
Lincolnshire NG34 7EB
Tel/fax: 01529 304615
Freephone helpline UK: 0800 374803
Freephone helpline Republic of Ireland: 00 44
1529 415278
e-mail: admin@gbs.org.uk
www.gbs.org.uk

SEXUAL COUNSELLING

SPOD

Association to Aid Sexual and Personal
Relationships of People with a Disability
286 Camden Road
London N7 0BJ
Tel: 020 7607 8851
e-mail: spod.uk@aol.com
www.spod-uk.org

SPINA BIFIDA

Association for Spina Bifida and Hydrocephalus (ASBAH)

ASBAH House
42 Park Road
Peterborough
Cambridgeshire PE1 2UQ
Tel: 01733 555 988
Fax: 01733 555 985
e-mail: postmaster@asbah.org
www.asbah.org

Scottish Spina Bifida Association

190 Queensferry Road
Edinburgh
Scotland EH4 2BW
Tel: 0131 332 0743
Fax: 0131 343 3651
e-mail: mail@ssba.org.uk
www.ssba.org.uk

SPINAL CORD INJURY

Association of Spinal Injury Research, Rehabilitation and Reintegration (ASPIRE)

Wood Lane
Stanmore, Middlesex
London HA7 4AP
Tel: 020 8954 5759
e-mail: info@aspire.org.uk
www.aspire.org.uk

Back Up Trust

Room 102, The Business Village
Broomhill Road
London SW18 4JQ
Tel: 020 8875 1805
Fax: 020 8870 3619
e-mail: admin@backuptrust.org.uk
www.backuptrust.org.uk

Spinal Injuries Association

Newpoint House
76 St James' Lane
London N10 3DF
Tel: 020 8444 2121
Fax: 020 8444 3761
e-mail: sia@spinal.co.uk
www.spinal.co.uk

SPORT

British Wheelchair Sports Foundation

Guttman Road
Stoke Mandeville
Aylesbury
Bucks HP21 9PP
Tel: 01296 395995
Fax: 01296 424171
e-mail: enquiries@britishwheelchairsports.org
www.britishwheelchairsports.org

Pashby Sports Fund Concussion Site

Online. Available: http://www.concussionsafety.com

Riding for the Disabled Association (RDA), incorporating carriage driving

Lavinia Norfolk House
Avenue R, National Agricultural Centre
Kenilworth
Warwickshire CV8 2LY
Tel: 01203 696510
Fax: 01203 696532
www.charitiesdirect.com

STROKE

Chest, Heart and Stroke Association (Scotland)

65 North Castle Street
Edinburgh EH2 3LT
Tel: 0131 225 6963
Fax: 0131 220 6313
e-mail: info@chss.org.uk
www.chss.org.uk

Northern Ireland Chest, Heart and Stroke Association

21 Dublin Road
Belfast BT2 7HB
Tel: 028 9032 0184
Helpline: 08457 697 299
Fax: 028 9033 3487
e-mail: mail@nichsa.com
www.nichsa.com

The Stroke Association

CHSA House
Whitecross Street
London EC1Y 8JJ
Tel: 020 7566 0300
Fax: 020 7490 2686
e-mail: stroke@stroke.org.uk
www.stroke.org

OTHER LOCAL SERVICES

Crossroads (Care Attendants Scheme Ltd)
Dial-a-ride
Meals on wheels
Stroke clubs

PROFESSIONAL GROUPS FOR PHYSIOTHERAPISTS

These groups are relevant to neurological rehabilitation and are contactable via:

The Chartered Society of Physiotherapy

14 Bedford Row
London WC1R 4ED
Tel: 020 7306 6666
Fax: 020 7306 6611
e-mail: through the website
www.csp.org.uk

AGILE – Chartered Physiotherapists Working with Older People
Association of Chartered Physiotherapists Interested in Neurology (ACPIN)
Association of Chartered Physiotherapists in Oncology and Palliative Care (ACPOPC)
Association of Community Physiotherapists
Association of Paediatric Chartered Physiotherapists for People with Learning Disabilities
Association of Chartered Physiotherapists in Mental Health Care
Association of Chartered Physiotherapists in Riding for the Disabled
Association of Chartered Physiotherapists in Women's Health
Association of Chartered Therapists Interested in Electrotherapy
Association of Chartered Physiotherapists Interested in Vestibular Rehabilitation (ACPIVR)
British Association of Bobath Trained Therapists
British Association of Hand Therapists
Hydrotherapy Association of Chartered Physiotherapists
Physiotherapists interested/specialising in balance and vestibular disorders – list of names available

CONFERENCES FOR PROFESSIONALS

Organisations holding conferences/seminars relevant to neurological rehabilitation include:

Association of Chartered Physiotherapists Interested in Neurology (ACPIN)
c/o Chartered Society of Physiotherapy
www.csp.org.uk

British Society of Rehabilitation Medicine (BSRM)
www.bsrm.co.uk

Society for Research in Rehabilitation (SRR)
www.srr.org.uk

Other organisations can be found in various physiotherapy and rehabilitation journals, in sections listing conferences.

Index

Note: page numbers in *italics* refer to figures and/or tables
for specific drugs *see* Table 28.1, pp 479–485
for associations and support group *see* Appendix, pp 527–532.

Strategic Management

text and cases

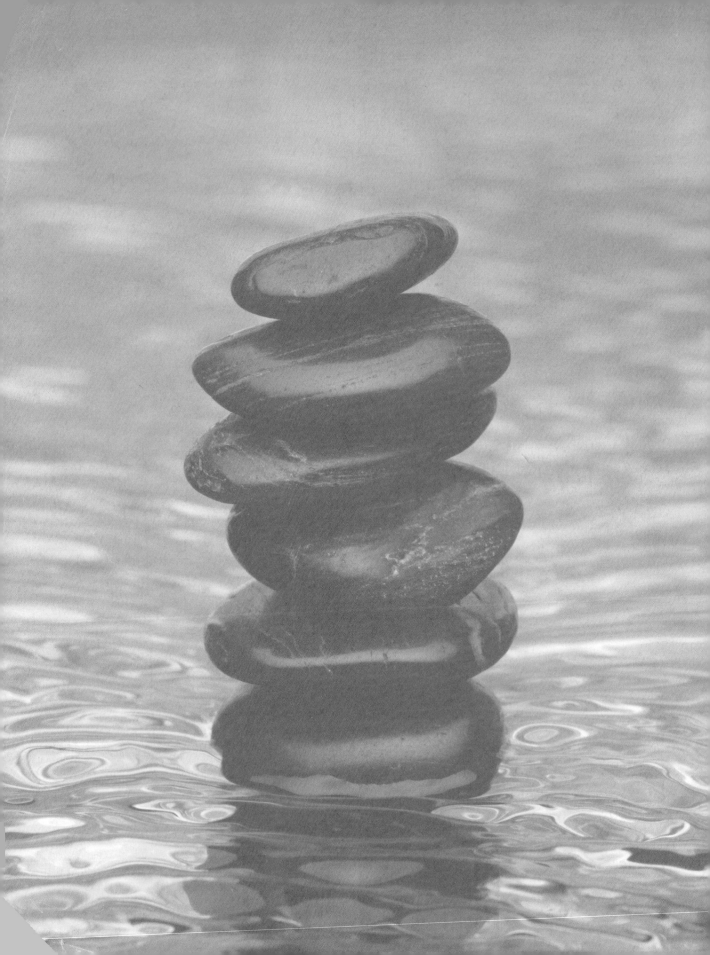

Gregory G. Dess
University of Texas at
Dallas

G. T. Lumpkin
Syracuse University

Alan B. Eisner
Pace University

Gerry McNamara
Michigan State
University

Bongjin Kim
Ewha Womans University

Strategic
Management

text and cases

sixth edition

GLOBAL EDITION

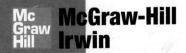

Mc
Graw **McGraw-Hill**
Hill **Irwin**

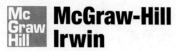

The *McGraw-Hill* Companies

McGraw-Hill
Irwin

Dedication

To my family, Margie and Taylor;
my parents, Bill and Mary Dess;
and Glenn F. Kirk
–Greg

To my lovely wife, Vicki,
and my students and colleagues
–Tom

To my family, Helaine, Rachel, and Jacob
–Alan

To my wonderful wife, Gaelen;
my children, Megan and AJ;
and my parents, Gene and Jane
–Gerry

To my wife, Youngae;
my children, Terry and David;
and my parents, Moonkyung and Sunhee
–Bongjin

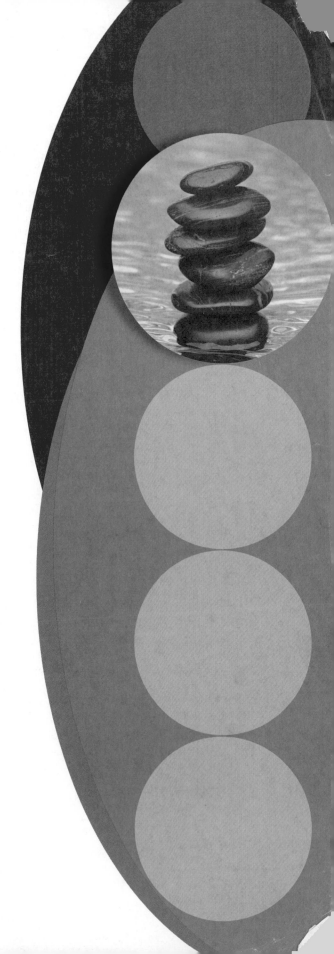

About the Authors

Gregory G. Dess is the Andrew R. Cecil Endowed Chair in Management at the University of Texas at Dallas. His primary research interests are in strategic management, organization–environment relationships, and knowledge management. He has published numerous articles on these subjects in both academic and practitioner-oriented journals. He also serves on the editorial boards of a wide range of practitioner-oriented and academic journals. In August 2000, he was inducted into the *Academy of Management Journal*'s Hall of Fame as one of its charter members. Professor Dess has conducted executive programs in the United States, Europe, Africa, Hong Kong, and Australia. During 1994 he was a Fulbright Scholar in Oporto, Portugal. In 2009, he received an honorary doctorate from the University of Bern (Switzerland). He received his PhD in Business Administration from the University of Washington (Seattle) and a BIE degree from Georgia Tech.

G. T. (Tom) Lumpkin is the Chris J. Witting Chair and Professor of Entrepreneurship at Syracuse University in New York. Prior to joining the faculty at Syracuse, Tom was the Kent Hance Regents Endowed Chair and Professor of Entrepreneurship at Texas Tech University. His research interests include entrepreneurial orientation, opportunity recognition, strategy-making processes, social entrepreneurship, and innovative forms of organizing work. He has published numerous research articles in journals such as *Strategic Management Journal, Academy of Management Journal, Academy of Management Review, Journal of Business Venturing,* and *Entrepreneurship: Theory and Practice.* He is a member of the editorial review boards of *Strategic Entrepreneurship Journal, Entrepreneurship Theory & Practice,* and the *Journal of Business Venturing.* He received his PhD in management from the University of Texas at Arlington and MBA from the University of Southern California.

Alan B. Eisner is Professor of Management and Department Chair, Management and Management Science Department, at the Lubin School of Business, Pace University. He received his PhD in management from the Stern School of Business, New York University. His primary research interests are in strategic management, technology management, organizational learning, and managerial decision making. He has published research articles and cases in journals such as *Advances in Strategic Management, International Journal of Electronic Commerce, International Journal of Technology Management, American Business Review, Journal of Behavioral and Applied Management,* and *Journal of the International Academy for Case Studies.* He is the former Associate Editor of the Case Association's peer reviewed journal, *The CASE Journal.*

Gerry McNamara is Professor of Management at Michigan State University. He received his PhD from the Carlson School of Management at the University of Minnesota. His research focuses on strategic decision making, organizational risk taking, and mergers and acquisitions. His research has been published in numerous journals, including the *Academy of Management Journal, Strategic Management Journal, Organization Science, Organizational Behavior and Human Decision Processes, Journal of Management,* and *Journal of International Business Studies.* His research on mergers and acquisitions has been abstracted in the *New York Times, Bloomberg Businessweek, The Economist,* and *Financial Week.* He is currently an Associate Editor for the *Academy of Management Journal.*

Bongjin Kim is Associate Professor of Strategic Management and Associate Dean at the Ewha School of Business, Ewha Womans University in Korea. Prior to joining the faculty at Ewha, Bongjin was on the faculty at the University of Texas at San Antonio, California State University, Northridge, and Tilburg University in the Netherlands. He received his PhD in management from the Joseph M. Katz Graduate School of Business at the University of Pittsburgh, MS in management from the University of Wisconsin-Madison, and MBA from Syracuse University. His research focuses on strategic decision making, corporate governance, strategic change, and international management. He has published research articles in journals such as *Academy of Management Review, Journal of Business Research, Corporate Governance: An International Review,* and *Journal of International Management.*

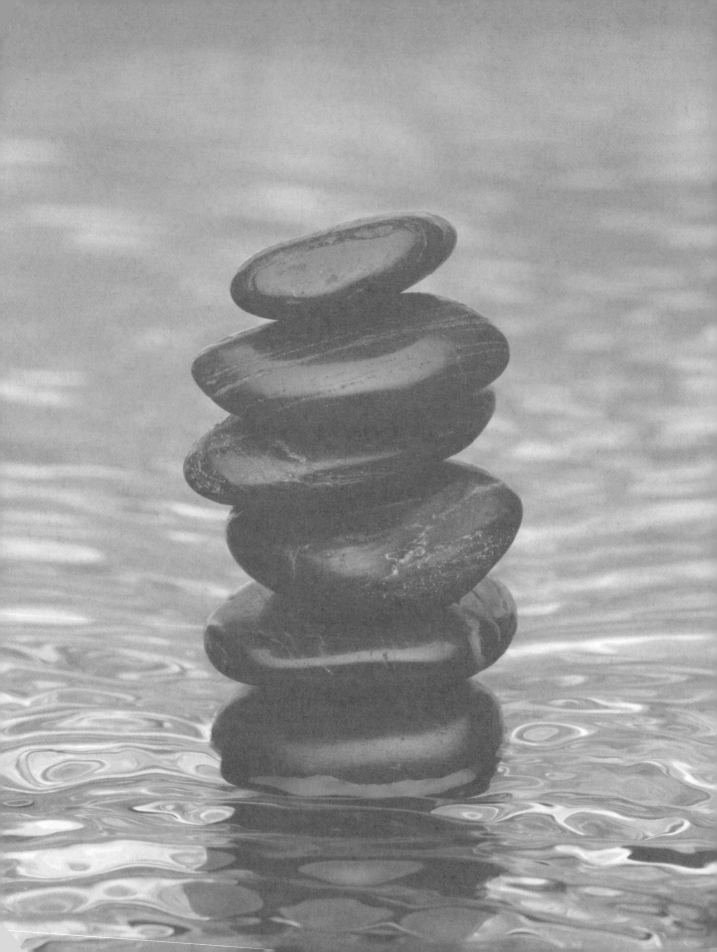

Preface

Welcome to the Global Edition of *Strategic Management: Text and Cases*. As economic turbulence continues to have a significant impact on organizations around the world, decision makers at all levels face strategic, organizational, and environmental factors that challenge the overall success of their respective firms. Despite the unsettled business environment, students must gain a worldwide perspective in understanding the key factors that can make or break a company's ability to maintain or improve its position in the global marketplace.

Strategic Management Courses Outside the United States

In countries such as Korea and the Netherlands, contrary to our expectations, students do not know much about U.S. corporations, except for the very famous ones. At Ewha Womans University, where Professor Kim currently teaches, there are many European exchange students. Surprisingly, he has discovered that they don't know much about U.S. corporations either. Consequently, the examples of non–U.S. corporations we discuss in the Global Edition—in new Strategy Spotlights, in new in-text examples, and in revised chapter exhibits—will help global students understand the topics and issues discussed in each chapter.

In his international teaching experience, Professor Kim has also learned that students in Asia and Europe are not exposed routinely to debate and discussion of teaching cases as part of the strategic management curriculum. The Global Edition of *Strategic Management: Text and Cases* provides instructors in other countries with the opportunity to use the case method as an integral part of teaching and student learning.

Chapter Features

The Global Edition draws on the comprehensive content and conceptual approach used in the U.S. edition of *Strategic Management* by Dess, Lumpkin, Eisner, and McNamara and includes new examples and cases that provide a worldly view of business strategies while maintaining the central themes of technology, ethics, sustainability, and entrepreneurship.

Chapters are divided logically into the traditional sequence of strategy analysis, strategy formulation, and strategy implementation. Unlike other strategy texts, three chapters discuss relevant topics such as intellectual capital/knowledge management; entrepreneurial strategy and competitive dynamics; and fostering corporate entrepreneurship and new ventures.

"Learning from Mistakes" vignettes lead off each chapter and serve as a springboard for classroom discussion.

"Strategy Spotlights" focus on key concepts in a concise, readable presentation. The Global Edition includes new Spotlights that provide a worldwide focus. Examples include why Japan's Bridgestone Company refined its environmental mission statement

(Chapter 1); how scenario planning at Nissan Motors in Great Britain helped expand the company's European business (Chapter 2); what happened when senior executives at an Indian firm were mentored by their subordinates (Chapter 4); how a fruitful combination of low-cost and differentiation advantages has provided AirAsia with sustainable competitive advantages (Chapter 5); how a multinational firm such as BP has dealt with serious risks of bribery and corruption in the course of its businesses (Chapter 7); how plastic manufacturers in Europe committed themselves to enhancing efficiency and quality by actively focusing on recycling (Chapter 8); how Norway's DnB NOR has created potential synergies by adopting a functional organizational structure (Chapter 10); how a simple twist on innovation gave Dyson a new product that has gained worldwide attention (Chapter 12); and how The Body Shop, a global retailer, continues to be committed to its founder's sense of social responsibility more than 35 years after its start (Chapter 12).

Many new in-text examples have been added to provide a global perspective to key text discussions. Highlighted companies and featured topics include Baidu's CEO in China (Chapter 1); London's 2012 Olympic committee and how it abandoned its low-carbon energy promise (Chapter 2); Royal Dutch Shell's decentralized management structure (Chapter 3); Taiwan's emerging knowledge economy (Chapter 4); BASF's online social platform for employees (Chapter 4); Singapore Airlines and its strong interconnected elements (Chapter 5); Internet coupon company, Groupon, and its many imitators (Chapter 5); Shire Limited's acquisition of German pharmaceutical company Jerini AG (Chapter 6); Hyundai Motor Group's vertical integration into the steel industry (Chapter 6); business financing in the European Union and the UK (Chapter 8); successful foundation of UK's Last.fm, an European version of Pandora (Chapter 8); Nokia's failures in the smartphone business (Chapter 9); Parmalat's fraud scandal in Italy (Chapter 9); Lego and its unsuccessful outsourcing experience (Chapter 10); Xerox's decision to benchmark Canon's practices, which led to its remarkable turnaround in the United States (Chapter 11); Denmark and its green energy efforts to curb global warming (Chapter 11); Dutch retailer HEMA and its code of conduct for employees and vendors (Chapter 11); and Teijin of Japan's environmentally sensitive products (Chapter 12).

Cases in the Global Edition

As mentioned previously, the case teaching method is not routinely used in strategy courses taught outside of the United States. Thus, the inclusion of cases in this Global Edition provides students with the opportunity to place themselves in the role of strategic decision makers at well-known companies from around the world. The cases help students analyze, interpret, and apply strategic management concepts in a real-world setting. The cases vary in length and discuss a wide range of businesses. We took great care in selecting cases that would provide a broad mix of global companies in a variety of business sectors. Companies featured in the cases include Google, Apple, Samsung, Gazprom, Tata Group, HTC, DeBeers, Porsche, Ryanair, Novartis, and ePlanet Ventures. Business sectors discussed include aviation, automotive, energy, food service, consumer electronics, Internet, entertainment, pharmaceutical, and not-for-profit.

Approximately half of the cases are written by text author Alan Eisner and other case specialists; several others are "classics" and favorites from Harvard Business School; and others are new to this Global Edition. This approach promotes a strong link between case and chapter content and ensures that students learn to apply key strategic management concepts effectively. The following summaries highlight the new cases in the Global Edition.

Case 7—Gazprom

The case documents the growth strategies of Gazprom, which started in its early days as an experiment in privatization of oil and gas, and follows the company's progress after the rapid breakup of the Soviet Union. The case offers a rich mix of insights into the contextual forces at work in shaping the destiny of Gazprom, the political pressures it faces as Russia's largest company, and its stutter-step approach to globalization.

Case 8—Ryanair

The case discusses Ryanair's operations and its strategies to maintain high efficiency at lower costs and offers ideas on how the company's success could be sustained in the European airline industry. The leading low-cost airline in Europe, Ryanair began its operations in 1985 in Ireland. The company was able to establish itself in the UK and then extended its wings to other parts of Europe. With successful pricing and cost-cutting strategies, Ryanair maintained a cost gap of 64% compared to other scheduled airlines.

Case 9—DeBeers

The synthetic diamond industry has become a potentially disruptive technology for South Africa's diamond giant, DeBeers. The question facing the firm is how it should respond to the threat. The case's objective is to explore issues of strategy that arise in markets for status goods and to appreciate how a major player's strategic moves can transform a market. The case also provides the opportunity to discuss the source of diamonds' value to consumers, and how that value can be shaped through DeBeers' strategic choices.

Case 11—What's Driving Porsche?

In 2008, German sports car maker Porsche announced its intention to acquire a majority stake in Volkswagen. At a time when Porsche was entering into new car markets with its SUV and luxury sedans observers voiced concerns as to whether Porsche would be able to retain its legendary reputation as an engineering powerhouse as it folds Volkswagen into its corporate mix. The case highlights the challenges of managing human capital and corporate strategy amidst a merger of two very different companies.

Case 13—HTC

This case describes how HTC, a pioneer of mobile computing from Taiwan, evolved from a local subcontractor for PDA (personal data assistant) devices to a global contender in the smartphone industry. The key issue in this case is the introduction of the HTC brand carried by products delivered to network operators worldwide, such as AT&T, British Telecom, NTT DoCoMo, Rogers, Verizon, and Vodafone. This case identifies the structural issues between a subcontractor and a client that can potentially dictate the branding status of the final product sold to end-users, namely, when a subcontractor should remain anonymous to end-users and when it should appeal to end-users by branding its own product.

Case 16—Tata Inc.

The Tata Group is an Indian conglomerate founded by noted industrialist JRD Tata. The company has a significant presence on the global business scene. In 2008, Tata ranked sixth in the list of Boston Consulting Group's most innovative companies across the world. The case delves into the challenges faced by a global conglomerate adopting an innovation strategy. The pedagogical objectives are to: (1) understand Tata Group's various innovative moves; (2) study the challenges faced by the company when it made these innovative moves; and (3) comprehend if innovation can be used as a brand-building strategy.

Case 18—Google in China

The case describes the circumstances surrounding Google's reconsideration of its China Internet strategy. Google officially announced in January 2010 that its Chinese website, Google.cn, experienced cyber attacks from within China. Google then announced that, as a result, it had decided to reconsider its approach to China, including the option of a complete exit from the Chinese market. The case presents Google's performance in China, the details of the cyber attack, and the heated public discussion that followed Google's announcement. The case offers an opportunity to consider actions that Google should take and the corresponding, underlying rationale for these actions.

Case 19—ePlanet Ventures and Pakistan

Asad Jamal, a Pakistani born entrepreneur and founder of ePlanet Ventures, a technology-based fund, is considering whether he wants his firm to be one of the first entrants into the largely untapped market of Pakistan. The case describes the opportunities and risks of doing so, leaving readers to decide what makes the most sense for ePlanet. This case highlights Pakistan's explosive growth during the tenure of General Pervez Musharraf from 1999 to 2007, and the power of a diaspora in facilitating entrepreneurship.

Case 21—Building a New Company

After Bosco Pharmaceutical's acquisition of Zeta AG, Bosco's chairman is unsure whether to merge the two firms using only internal resources or accept the help of Deloitte Consulting. Deloitte advocates an overhaul of Bosco's organizational structure to accommodate Zeta, a company one-fifth Bosco's size. The chairman is uncertain whether to adopt Zeta's worldwide product structure or whether Zeta should be required to conform to Bosco's more geographic management and operating structure. This merger would be the biggest in Bosco's 110-year history, and it is imperative for the company to extract benefits from the merger—primarily by meshing corporate cultures and achieving ambitious cost savings.

Case 23—The Novartis Foundation

In 1998, Klaus Leisinger and Karin Schmitt of the Novartis Foundation for Sustainable Development in Basel, Switzerland, were approached by a sociologist who wanted help in launching a pilot program in Tanzania to deal with the crisis of the more than 8 million HIV/AIDS-orphaned children in sub-Saharan Africa. The proposed program was unusual in that it addressed the psychological and social traumas these children experienced. The other unusual aspect of this request was that Novartis, at that time the second-largest pharmaceutical company in the world, did not make, sell, or distribute any products related to HIV/AIDS. Novartis and its philanthropic foundation were committed to helping the neediest persons in developing countries. However, Leisinger and Schmitt did not believe that "throwing money" at problems resulted in solutions; rather, they looked for innovative ways to address problems and crises.

Student Support Materials

Online Learning Center (OLC)

The following resources are available to students via the publisher's OLC at www.mhhe
.com/dess6e:

- Chapter quizzes students can take to gauge their understanding of material covered in each chapter.
- A selection of PowerPoint slides for each chapter.
- Links to strategy simulations the Business Strategy Game & GLO-BUS. Both provide a powerful and constructive way of connecting students to the subject matter of the course with a competition among classmates on campus and around the world.

Instructor Support Materials

Instructor's Manual (IM)

Prepared by the textbook authors, the accompanying IM contains summary/objectives, lecture/discussion outlines, discussion questions, extra examples not included in the text, teaching tips, reflecting on career implications, experiential exercises, and more.

Test Bank

Prepared by the authors, the test bank contains more than 1,000 true/false, multiple-choice, and essay questions. It has now been tagged with learning objectives as well as Bloom's Taxonomy and AACSB criteria.

- **Assurance of Learning Ready.** Assurance of Learning is an important element of many accreditation standards. Dess 6e is designed specifically to support your Assurance of Learning initiatives. Each chapter in the book begins with a list of numbered learning objectives that appear throughout the chapter, as well as in the end-of-chapter questions and exercises. Every test bank question is also linked to one of these objectives, in addition to level of difficulty, topic area, Bloom's Taxonomy level, and AACSB skill area. *EZ Test,* McGraw-Hill's easy-to-use test bank software, can search the test bank by these and other categories, providing an engine for targeted Assurance of Learning analysis and assessment.
- **AACSB Statement.** The McGraw-Hill Companies is a proud corporate member of AACSB International. Understanding the importance and value of AACSB accreditation, Dess 6e has sought to recognize the curricula guidelines detailed in the AACSB standards for business accreditation by connecting selected questions in Dess 6e and the test bank to the general knowledge and skill guidelines found in the AACSB standards. The statements contained in Dess 6e are provided only as a guide for the users of this text. The AACSB leaves content coverage and assessment within the purview of individual schools, the mission of the school, and the faculty. While Dess 6e and the teaching package make no claim of any specific AACSB qualification or evaluation, we have labeled selected questions within Dess 6e according to the six general knowledge and skills areas.

- **Computerized Test Bank Online.** A comprehensive bank of test questions is provided within a computerized test bank powered by McGraw-Hill's flexible electronic testing program, *EZ Test Online* (www.eztestonline.com). *EZ Test Online* allows you to create paper and online tests or quizzes in this easy-to-use program! Imagine being able to create and access your test or quiz anywhere, at any time without installing the testing software. Now, with *EZ Test Online,* instructors can select questions from multiple McGraw-Hill test banks or author their own, and then either print the test for paper distribution or give it online.
- **Test Creation.**
  - Author/edit questions online using the 14 different question type templates.
  - Create printed tests or deliver online to get instant scoring and feedback.
  - Create questions pools to offer multiple versions online – great for practice.
  - Export your tests for use in *WebCT, Blackboard, PageOut,* and Apple's *iQuiz.*
  - Compatible with *EZ Test Desktop* tests you've already created.
  - Sharing tests with colleagues, adjuncts, TAs is easy.
- **Online Test Management.**
  - Set availability dates and time limits for your quiz or test.
  - Control how your test will be presented.
  - Assign points by question or question type with drop-down menu.
  - Provide immediate feedback to students or delay until all finish the test.
  - Create practice tests online to enable student mastery.
  - Your roster can be uploaded to enable student self-registration.
- **Online Scoring and Reporting.**
  - Automated scoring for most of *EZ Test*'s numerous question types.
  - Allows manual scoring for essay and other open response questions.
  - Manual rescoring and feedback is also available.
  - *EZ Test*'s grade book is designed to easily export to your grade book.
  - View basic statistical reports.
- **Support and Help.**
  - User's guide and built-in page-specific help.
  - Flash tutorials for getting started on the support site.
  - Support website: *www.mhhe.com/eztest.*
  - Product specialist available at 1-800-331-5094.
  - Online Training: *http://auth.mhhe.com/mpss/workshops/.*

PowerPoint Presentation

Prepared by Brad Cox of Midlands Tech, it consists of more than 400 slides incorporating an outline for the chapters tied to learning objectives. Also included are multiple-choice questions that can be used as Classroom Performance System (CPS) questions as well as additional examples outside of the text to promote class discussion.

Instructor's Resource CD-ROM

All instructor supplements are available in this one-stop multimedia resource, which includes the Instructor's Manual, Test Bank, PowerPoint Presentations, and Case Study Teaching Notes.

Online Learning Center (OLC)

The instructor section of *www.mhhe.com/dess6e* also includes the Instructor's Manual, PowerPoint Presentations, Case Grid, and Case Study Teaching Notes as well as additional resources.

The Business Strategy Game and GLO-BUS Online Simulations

Both allow teams of students to manage companies in a head-to-head contest for global market leadership. These simulations give students the immediate opportunity to experiment with various strategy options and to gain proficiency in applying the concepts and tools they have been reading about in the chapters. To find out more or to register, please visit *www.mmhe.com/thompsonsims*.

Additional Resources

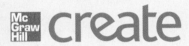

Create

Craft your teaching resources to match the way you teach! With McGraw-Hill *Create, www.mcgrawhillcreate.com* you can easily rearrange chapters, combine material from other content sources, and quickly upload content you have written, like your course syllabus or teaching notes. Find the content you need in *Create* by searching through thousands of leading McGraw-Hill textbooks. Arrange your book to fit your teaching style. *Create* even allows you to personalize your book's appearance by selecting the cover and adding your name, school, and course information. Order a *Create* book and you'll receive a complimentary print review copy in 3–5 business days or a complimentary electronic review copy (eComp) via e-mail in about one hour. Go to *www.mcgrawhillcreate.com* today and register. Experience how McGraw-Hill *Create* empowers you to teach *your* students *your* way.

McGraw-Hill Higher Education and Blackboard

McGraw-Hill Higher Education and Blackboard have teamed up. What does this mean for you?

1. **Your life, simplified.** Now you and your students can access McGraw-Hill's *Create* right from within your Blackboard course—all with one single sign-on. Say goodbye to the days of logging in to multiple applications.
2. **Deep integration of content and tools.** Not only do you get single sign-on with *Create,* you also get deep integration of McGraw-Hill content and content engines right in Blackboard. Whether you're choosing a book for your course or building assignments, all the tools you need are right where you want them—inside of Blackboard.
3. **Seamless gradebooks.** Are you tired of keeping multiple gradebooks and manually synchronizing grades into Blackboard? We thought so. When a student completes an integrated assignment, the grade for that assignment automatically (and instantly) feeds your Blackboard grade center.
4. **A solution for everyone.** Whether your institution is already using Blackboard or you just want to try Blackboard on your own, we have a solution for you.

McGraw-Hill and Blackboard can now offer you easy access to industry-leading technology and content, whether your campus hosts it or we do. Be sure to ask your local McGraw-Hill representative for details.

McGraw-Hill Customer Care Contact Information

At McGraw-Hill, we understand that getting the most from new technology can be challenging. That's why our services don't stop after you purchase our products. You can e-mail our product specialists 24 hours a day to get product training online. Or you can search our knowledge bank of Frequently Asked Questions on our support website. For customer support, call 800-331-5094, e-mail *hmsupport@mcgraw-hill.com*, or visit *www.mhhe.com/support*. One of our technical support analysts will be able to assist you in a timely fashion.

The Best of Both Worlds

Mc Graw Hill

Bb
Blackboard

Do More

Acknowledgments

Strategic Management represents far more than just the joint efforts of the five co-authors. Rather, it is the product of the collaborative input of many people. Some of these individuals are academic colleagues, others are the outstanding team of professionals at McGraw-Hill/Irwin, and still others are those who are closest to us—our families. It is time to express our sincere gratitude.

First, we'd like to acknowledge the dedicated instructors who have graciously provided their insights since the inception of the U.S. version of the text. Their input has been very helpful in both pointing out errors in the manuscript and suggesting areas that needed further development as additional topics. We sincerely believe that the incorporation of their ideas has been critical to improving the final product. These professionals and their affiliations are:

The Reviewer Hall of Fame

Moses Acquaah, *University of North Carolina–Greensboro*

Todd Alessandri, *Northeastern University*

Larry Alexander, *Virginia Polytechnic Institute*

Brent B. Allred, *College of William & Mary*

Allen C. Amason, *University of Georgia*

Kathy Anders, *Arizona State University*

Peter H. Antoniou, *California State University, San Marcos*

Dave Arnott, *Dallas Baptist University*

Marne L. Arthaud-Day, *Kansas State University*

Jay Azriel, *York University of Pennsylvania*

Jeffrey J. Bailey, *University of Idaho*

Dennis R. Balch, *University of North Alabama*

Bruce Barringer, *University of Central Florida*

Barbara R. Bartkus, *Old Dominion University*

Barry Bayon, *Bryant University*

Brent D. Beal, *Louisiana State University*

Joyce Beggs, *University of North Carolina–Charlotte*

Michael Behnam, *Suffolk University*

Kristen Bell DeTienne, *Brigham Young University*

Eldon Bernstein, *Lynn University*

Daniela Blettner, *Tilburg University*

Dusty Bodie, *Boise State University*

William Bogner, *Georgia State University*

Jon Bryan, *Bridgewater State College*

Charles M. Byles, *Virginia Commonwealth University*

Mikelle A. Calhoun, *Valparaiso University*

Thomas J. Callahan, *University of Michigan, Dearborn*

Samuel D. Cappel, *Southeastern Louisiana State University*

Gary Carini, *Baylor University*

Shawn M. Carraher, *Texas A&M University, Commerce*

Tim Carroll, *University of South Carolina*

Don Caruth, *Amberton University*

Maureen Casile, *Bowling Green State University*

Gary J. Castrogiovanni, *Florida Atlantic University*

Radha Chaganti, *Rider University*

Erick PC Chang, *Arkansas State University*

Theresa Cho, *Rutgers University*

Bruce Clemens, *Western New England College*

Betty S. Coffey, *Appalachian State University*

Wade Coggins, *Webster University, Fort Smith Metro Campus*

Susan Cohen, *University of Pittsburgh*

George S. Cole, *Shippensburg University*

Joseph Coombs, *Texas A & M University*

Christine Cope Pence, *University of California, Riverside*

James J. Cordeiro, *SUNY Brockport*

Jeffrey Covin, *Indiana University*

Keith Credo, *Auburn University*

Deepak Datta, *University of Texas at Arlington*

James Davis, *University of Notre Dame*

David Dawley, *West Virginia University*

Helen Deresky, *State University of New York, Plattsburgh*

Rocki-Lee DeWitt, *University of Vermont*

Jay Dial, *Ohio State University*

Michael E. Dobbs, *Arkansas State University*

Jonathan Doh, *Villanova University*

Tom Douglas, *Clemson University*

Jon Down, *Oregon State University*

Alan E. Ellstrand, *University of Arkansas*

Dean S. Elmuti, *Eastern Illinois University*

Clare Engle, *Concordia University*

Tracy Ethridge, *Tri-County Technical College*

William A. Evans, *Troy State University, Dothan*

Frances H. Fabian, *University of Memphis*

Angelo Fanelli, *Warrington College of Business*

Michael Fathi, *Georgia Southwestern University*

Carolyn J. Fausnaugh, *Florida Institute of Technology*

Tamela D. Ferguson, *University of Louisiana at Lafayette*

David Flanagan, *Western Michigan University*

Dave Foster, *Montana State University*

Isaac Fox, *University of Minnesota*

Deborah Francis, *Brevard College*

Steven A. Frankforter, *Winthrop University*

Vance Fried, *Oklahoma State University*

Naomi A. Gardberg, *CNNY Baruch College*

Mehmet Erdem Genc, *Baruch College, CUNY*

J. Michael Geringer, *California Polytechnic State University*

Diana L. Gilbertson, *California State University, Fresno*

Matt Gilley, *St. Mary's University*

Debbie Gilliard, *Metropolitan State College–Denver*

Yezdi H. Godiwalla, *University of Wisconsin–Whitewater*

Sanjay Goel, *University of Minnesota, Duluth*

Sandy Gough, *Boise State University*

Allen Harmon, *University of Minnesota, Duluth*

Niran Harrison, *University of Oregon*

Paula Harveston, *Berry College*

Ahmad Hassan, *Morehead State University*

Donald Hatfield, *Virginia Polytechnic Institute*

Kim Hester, *Arkansas State University*

John Hironaka, *California State University, Sacramento*

Alan Hoffman, *Bentley College*

Gordon Holbein, *University of Kentucky*

Stephen V. Horner, *Arkansas State University*

Jill Hough, *University of Tulsa*

John Humphreys, *Eastern New Mexico University*

James G. Ibe, *Morris College*

Jay J. Janney, *University of Dayton*

Lawrence Jauch, *University of Louisiana–Monroe*

Dana M. Johnson, *Michigan Technical University*

Homer Johnson, *Loyola University, Chicago*

James Katzenstein, *California State University, Dominguez Hills*

Joseph Kavanaugh, *Sam Houston State University*

Franz Kellermanns, *University of Tennessee*

Craig Kelley, *California State University, Sacramento*

Donna Kelley, *Babson College*

Dave Ketchen, *Auburn University*

John A. Kilpatrick, *Idaho State University*

Helaine J. Korn, *Baruch College, CUNY*

Stan Kowalczyk, *San Francisco State University*

Daniel Kraska, *North Central State College*

Donald E. Kreps, *Kutztown University*

Jim Kroeger, *Cleveland State University*

Subdoh P. Kulkarni, *Howard University*

Ron Lambert, *Faulkner University*

Theresa Lant, *New York University*

Ted Legatski, *Texas Christian University*

David J. Lemak, *Washington State University–Tri-Cities*

Cynthia Lengnick-Hall, *University of Texas at San Antonio*

Donald L. Lester, *Arkansas State University*

Wanda Lester, *North Carolina A&T State University*

Benyamin Lichtenstein, *University of Massachusetts at Boston*

Jun Lin, *SUNY at New Paltz*

Zhiang (John) Lin, *University of Texas at Dallas*

Dan Lockhart, *University of Kentucky*

John Logan, *University of South Carolina*

Kevin Lowe, *University of North Carolina, Greensboro*

Doug Lyon, *Fort Lewis College*

Hao Ma, *Bryant College*

Rickey Madden, *Ph.D., Presbyterian College*

James Maddox, *Friends University*

Ravi Madhavan, *University of Pittsburgh*

Paul Mallette, *Colorado State University*

Santo D. Marabella, *Moravian College*

Catherine Maritan, *Syracuse University*

Daniel Marrone, *Farmingdale State College, SUNY*

Sarah Marsh, *Northern Illinois University*

John R. Massaua, *University of Southern Maine*

Larry McDaniel, *Alabama A&M University*

Abagail McWilliams, *University of Illinois, Chicago*

John E. Merchant, *California State University, Sacramento*

John M. Mezias, *University of Miami*

Michael Michalisin, *Southern Illinois University at Carbondale*

Doug Moesel, *University of Missouri–Columbia*

Fatma Mohamed, *Morehead State University*

Mike Montalbano, *Bentley University*

Debra Moody, *University of North Carolina, Charlotte*

Gregory A. Moore, *Middle Tennessee State University*

James R. Morgan, *Dominican University and UC Berkeley Extension*

Sara A. Morris, *Old Dominion University*

Carolyn Mu, *Baylor University*

Stephen Mueller, *Northern Kentucky University*

John Mullane, *Middle Tennessee State University*

Gerry Nkombo Muuka, *Murray State University*

Chandran Mylvaganam, *Northwood University*

Anil Nair, *Old Dominion University*

V.K. Narayanan, *Drexel University*

Maria L. Nathan, *Lynchburg College*

Louise Nemanich, *Arizona State University*

Charles Newman, *University of Maryland, University College*

Stephanie Newport, *Austin Peay State University*

Bill Norton, *University of Louisville*

Yusuf A. Nur, *SUNY Brockport*

Jeffrey R. Nystrom, *University of Colorado*

d.t. ogilvie, *Rutgers University*

William Ross O'Brien, *Dallas Baptist University*

Floyd Ormsbee, *Clarkson University*

Karen L. Page, *University of Wyoming*

Jacquelyn W. Palmer, *University of Cincinnati*

Julie Palmer, *University of Missouri, Columbia*

Daewoo Park, *Xavier University*

Gerald Parker, *Saint Louis University*

Ralph Parrish, *University of Central Oklahoma*

Douglas K. Peterson, *Indiana State University*

Edward Petkus, *Mary Baldwin College*

Michael C. Pickett, *National University*

Peter Ping Li, *California State University, Stanislaus*

Michael W. Pitts, *Virginia Commonwealth University*

Laura Poppo, *Virginia Tech*

Steve Porth, *Saint Joseph's University*

Jodi A. Potter, *Robert Morris University*

Scott A. Quatro, *Grand Canyon University*

Nandini Rajagopalan, *University of Southern California*

Annette L. Ranft, *Florida State University*

Abdul Rasheed, *University of Texas at Arlington*

Devaki Rau, *Northern Illinois University*

George Redmond, *Franklin University*

Kira Reed, *Syracuse University*

Clint Relyea, *Arkansas State University*

Barbara Ribbens, *Western Illinois University*

Maurice Rice, *University of Washington*

Violina P. Rindova, *University of Maryland, College Park*

Ron Rivas, *Canisius College*

David Robinson, *Indiana State University–Terre Haute*

Kenneth Robinson, *Kennesaw State University*

Simon Rodan, *San Jose State University*

Patrick R. Rogers, *North Carolina A&T State University*

John K. Ross III, *Texas State University, San Marcos*

Robert Rottman, *Kentucky State University*

Matthew R. Rutherford, *Gonzaga University*

Carol M. Sanchez, *Grand Valley State University*

William W. Sannwald, *San Diego State University*

Yolanda Sarason, *Colorado State University*

Marguerite Schneider, *New Jersey Institute of Technology*

Roger R. Schnorbus, *University of Richmond*

Terry Sebora, *University of Nebraska–Lincoln*

John Seeger, *Bentley College*

Jamal Shamsie, *Michigan State University*

Mark Shanley, *University of Illinois at Chicago*

Lois Shelton, *California State University, Northridge*

Herbert Sherman, *Long Island University*

Weilei Shi, *Baruch College–CUNY*

Chris Shook, *Auburn University*

Jeremy Short, *Texas Tech University*

Mark Simon, *Oakland University, Michigan*

Rob Singh, *Morgan State University*

Bruce Skaggs, *University of Kentucky*

Wayne Smeltz, *Rider University*

Anne Smith, *University of Tennessee*

Andrew Spicer, *University of South Carolina*

James D. Spina, *University of Maryland*

John Stanbury, *George Mason University & Inter-University Institute of Macau, SAR China*

Timothy Stearns, *California State University, Fresno*

Elton Stephen, *Austin State University*

Alice Stewart, *Ohio State University*

Ram Subramanian, *Grand Valley State University*

Roy Suddaby, *University of Iowa*

Michael Sullivan, *UC Berkeley Extension*

Marta Szabo White, *Georgia State University*

Justin Tan, *York University, Canada*

Qingju Tao, *Lehigh University*

Linda Teagarden, *Virginia Tech*

Bing-Sheng Teng, *George Washington University*

Alan Theriault, *University of California– Riverside*

Tracy Thompson, *University of Washington, Tacoma*

Karen Torres, *Angelo State University*

Robert Trumble, *Virginia Commonwealth University*

K.J. Tullis, *University of Central Oklahoma*

Craig A. Turner, *Ph.D., East Tennessee State University*

Beverly Tyler, *North Carolina State University*

Rajaram Veliyath, *Kennesaw State University*

S. Stephen Vitucci, *Tarleton State University–Central Texas*

Jay A. Vora, *St. Cloud State University*

Jorge Walter, *Portland State University*

Bruce Walters, *Louisiana Tech University*

Edward Ward, *St. Cloud State University*

N. Wasilewski, *Pepperdine University*

Andrew Watson, *Northeastern University*

Larry Watts, *Stephen F. Austin University*

Paula S. Weber, *St. Cloud State University*

Kenneth E. A. Wendeln, *Indiana University*

Robert R. Wharton, *Western Kentucky University*

Laura Whitcomb, *California State University–Los Angeles*

Scott Williams, *Wright State University*

Diana Wong, *Bowling Green State University*

Beth Woodard, *Belmont University*

John E. Wroblewski, *State University of New York–Fredonia*

Anne York, *University of Nebraska, Omaha*

Michael Zhang, *Sacred Heart University*

Monica Zimmerman, *Temple University*

Second, the authors would like to thank several faculty colleagues who were particularly helpful in the review, critique, and development of the book and supplementary materials. Greg's colleagues at the University of Texas at Dallas also have been helpful and supportive. These individuals include Mike Peng, Joe Picken, Kumar Nair, John Lin, Roberto Ragozzino, Seung-Hyun Lee, Tev Dalgic, and Jane Salk. His administrative assistant, Mary Vice, has been extremely helpful. Two doctoral students, Brian Pinkham and

Ciprian Stan, have provided many useful inputs and ideas, along with a research associate, Yolanda Tsang. He also appreciates the support of his dean and associate dean, Hasan Pirkul and Varghese Jacob, respectively. Tom would like to thank Gerry Hills, Abagail McWilliams, Rod Shrader, Mike Miller, James Gillespie, Ron Mitchell, Kim Boal, Keith Brigham, Jeremy Short, Tyge Payne, Bill Wan, Andy Yu, Abby Wang, Johan Wiklund, Mike Haynie, Alex McKelvie, Cathy Maritan, Ravi Dharwadkar, and Pam Brandes. Special thanks also to Jeff Stambaugh for his vital contribution to new materials. Tom also extends a special thanks to Benyamin Lichtenstein for his support and encouragement. Both Greg and Tom wish to thank a special colleague, Abdul Rasheed at the University of Texas at Arlington, who certainly has been a valued source of friendship and ideas for us for many years. He provided many valuable contributions to all editions. Alan thanks his colleagues at Pace University and the Case Association for their support in developing these fine case selections. Special thanks go to Jamal Shamsie at Michigan State University for his support in developing the case selections for this edition. He is also very grateful to Pauline Assenza at Berkeley College for her superb work as case teaching notes and powerpoints editor. And we appreciate Doug Sanford, at University of Towson for his expertise with one of our key pedagogical features—the key terms in each chapter. Gerry thanks all of his colleagues at Michigan State University for their help and support over the years. He also thanks his co-authors, including Phil Bromiley, Paul Vaaler, Cindy Devers, Federico Aime, Mike Mannor, John Haleblian, Kalin Kolev, Seungho Choi, Don Conlon, Bob Wiseman, Rebecca Luce, Kathie Sutcliffe, Jody Tompson, David Deephouse, Bernadine Dykes, Mathias Arrfelt, Mason Carpenter, Rob Davison, and Dustin Sleesman, for their role in helping him grow as a scholar.

Third, we would like to thank the team at McGraw-Hill/Irwin for their outstanding support throughout the process. This begins with John Biernat, formerly Publisher, who signed us to our original contract. John was always available to provide support and valued input during the entire process. In editorial, Paul Ducham, editorial director, executive editor Mike Ablassmeir, development editor Laura Griffin, and editorial coordinator Andrea Heirendt, kept things on track, responded quickly to our never-ending needs and requests, and offered insights and encouragement. Once the manuscript was completed and revised, lead project manager Harvey Yep expertly guided us through the production process. Rachel Townsend, media project manager, did an outstanding job in helping us with the digital materials. Jeremy Cheshareck, senior photo research coordinator, and freelance designer Pam Verros provided excellent design, photo, and art work. We also appreciate executive marketing manager Anke Weekes and marketing specialist Liz Steiner for their energetic, competent, and thorough marketing efforts. Last, but certainly not least, we thank MHI's 70 plus outstanding book reps—who serve on the "front lines"—as well as many in-house sales professionals based in Dubuque, Iowa. Clearly, they deserve a lot of credit for our success.

Finally, we would like to thank our families. For Greg this includes his parents, William and Mary Dess, who have always been there for him. His wife, Margie, and daughter, Taylor, have been a constant source of love and companionship. Greg would also like to recognize Glenn F. Kirk. He was one of Greg's first managers in industry (Western Electric Company), and he certainly led by example. Glenn was also very patient (and forgiving) with Greg's limited engineering and "collaboration" skills(!). Tom thanks his wife Vicki for her constant love and companionship. Tom also thanks Lee Hetherington and Thelma Lumpkin for their inspiration, as well as his mom Katy, and his sister Kitty, for a lifetime of support. Alan thanks his family—his wife Helaine and his children Rachel

22

and Jacob—for their love and support. He also thanks his parents, Gail Eisner and the late Marvin Eisner, for their support and encouragement. Gerry thanks his wife, Gaelen, for her love, support, and friendship and his children, Megan and AJ, for their love and the joy they bring to his life. He also thanks his parents, Gene and Jane, for their encouragement and support in all phases of his life. Gerry thanks Phil Bromiley, his academic mentor, for helping him grow as a scholar. Bongjin thanks his family—his wife Youngae and his children Terry and David—for their love and support. He also thanks his parents, Moonkyung and Sunhee.

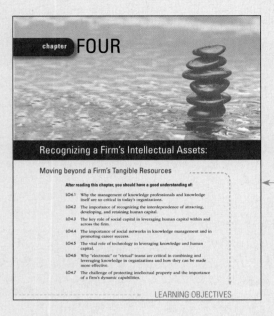

Learning Objectives

Learning Objectives numbered LO4.1, LO4.2, LO4.3, etc. with corresponding icons in the margins to indicate where learning objectives are covered in the text.

Learning from Mistakes

Learning from Mistakes are examples of where things went wrong. Failures are not only interesting but also sometimes easier to learn from. And students realize strategy is not just about "right or wrong" answers, but requires critical thinking.

Learning from Mistakes

Toyota Motor Company had developed an industry-leading strategy that focused on value innovation and cost reduction.[1] For many years it was a solid strategy for both the company and its customers. Over the years, Toyota built a reputation for engineering excellence and cost cutting. Its engineers collaborated with suppliers to extract cost-savings without compromising quality. Yet, by the middle of the last decade, Toyota's virtue had become a vice and eventually led to recalled vehicles, lawsuits, and a damaged reputation. What went wrong?

Toyota's problems stemmed from an overwhelming desire to cut costs. This, in turn, led to a product that did not meet the same high quality that its customers had come to expect. When a North American parts supplier interested in working with the automaker did a teardown of a 2007 Camry, its engineers were surprised by how much the traditional Toyota craftsmanship had been watered down by years of nips and tucks. One example of this came to light in 2006, when a redesigned Camry revealed an embarrassing flaw in its headliner (the lining that covers the inside of the roof). Under pressure to cut costs, a Toyota affiliate chose a carbon fiber material that had not yet been approved by Toyota engineers. Unfortunately, the new carbon fiber material required so much heat to mold during production that it would catch fire. Thus, as many as 30 percent of the parts were scrapped—compared to a normal scrap rate for headliners of about 5 percent.

Strategy Spotlight

These boxes weave themes of ethics, globalization, and technology into every chapter of the text, providing students with a thorough grounding necessary for understanding strategic management. Select boxes incorporating crowdsourcing, environmental sustainability, and ethical themes include the following icons:

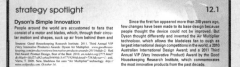

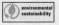

Key Terms

Key Terms defined in the margins have been added to improve students' understanding of core strategy concepts.

human capital the individual capabilities, knowledge, skills, and experience of a company's employees and managers.

Reflecting on Career Implications

This new section before the summary of every chapter consists of examples on how understanding of key concepts helps business students early in their careers.

Reflecting on Career Implications . . .

- *Creating the Environmentally Aware Organization:* In your career, what are some ways in which you can engage in scanning, monitoring, and intelligence gathering for future job opportunities? Consider, for example, subscribing to your field's professional publications and becoming actively involved in relevant professional organizations.
- *SWOT Analysis:* From a career standpoint, periodically evaluate your strengths and weaknesses as well as potential opportunities and threats to your career. In addition, strive to seek input from trusted peers and superiors.
- *General Environment:* Carefully evaluate the elements of the general environment facing your firm. Identify factors (e.g., rapid technological change) that can provide promising career opportunities as well as possibilities for you to add value for your organization. In doing this, don't focus solely on "internal factors" of your organization.
- *Five-Forces Analysis:* Consider the five forces affecting the industry within which your organization competes. If the "forces" are unfavorable, the long-term profit potential of the industry may be unattractive. And, there will likely be fewer resources available and—all other things being equal—fewer career opportunities.

Exhibits

Both new and improved exhibits in every chapter provide visual presentations of the most complex concepts covered to support student comprehension.

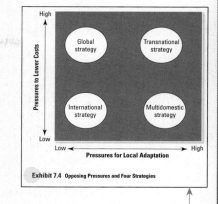

Exhibit 7.4 Opposing Pressures and Four Strategies

Cases

Case lineup for the Global Edition provides 10 new cases. Companies featured in the new cases include Porsche, HTC, Gazprom, DeBeers, Ryanair, Tata Group, and Google.

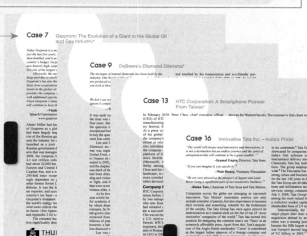

support materials

Online Learning Center (OLC)

The website *www.mhhe.com/dess6e* follows the text chapter-by-chapter. OLC content is ancillary and supplementary germane to the textbook. As students read the book, they can go online to take self-grading quizzes, review material, or work through interactive exercises. It includes chapter quizzes, student PowerPoint slides, and links to strategy simulations The *Business Strategy Game* and GLO-BUS.

The instructor section also includes the Instructor's Manual, PowerPoint Presentations, Case Study Teaching Notes, Case Grid, and Video Guide as well as all student resources.

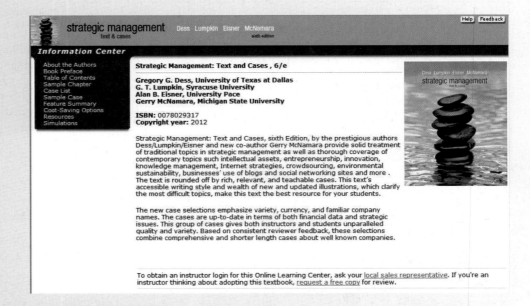

Brief Contents

Contents

Chapter 3
Assessing the Internal Environment of the Firm. 118

Chapter 4
Recognizing a Firm's Intellectual Assets: Moving Beyond a Firm's Tangible Resources 162

part 2   Strategic Formulation

Chapter 5

Business-Level Strategy: Creating and Sustaining Competitive Advantages 200

Chapter 6

Corporate-Level Strategy: Creating Value through Diversification 242

part 4 Case Analysis

Cases

The Strategic Management Process

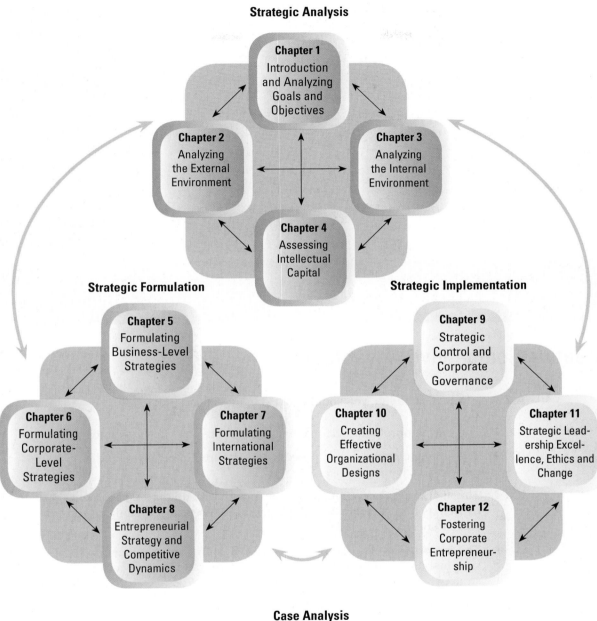

Strategic Analysis

Chapter 1
Introduction and Analyzing Goals and Objectives

Chapter 2
Analyzing the External Environment

Chapter 3
Analyzing the Internal Environment

Chapter 4
Assessing Intellectual Capital

Strategic Formulation

Chapter 5
Formulating Business-Level Strategies

Chapter 6
Formulating Corporate-Level Strategies

Chapter 7
Formulating International Strategies

Chapter 8
Entrepreneurial Strategy and Competitive Dynamics

Strategic Implementation

Chapter 9
Strategic Control and Corporate Governance

Chapter 10
Creating Effective Organizational Designs

Chapter 11
Strategic Leadership Excellence, Ethics and Change

Chapter 12
Fostering Corporate Entrepreneurship

Case Analysis

Chapter 13
Case Analysis

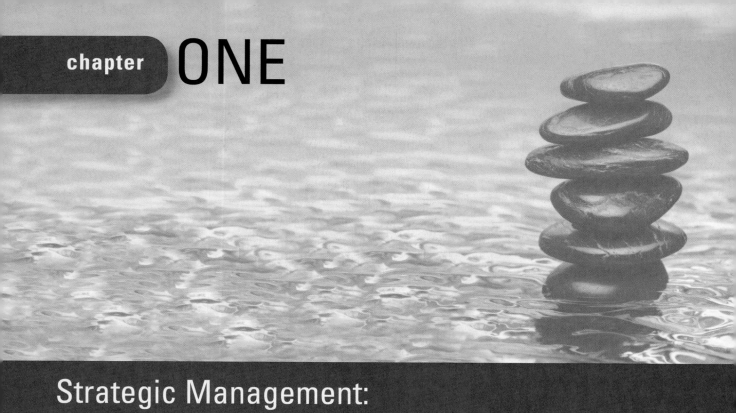

chapter ONE

Strategic Management:

Creating Competitive Advantages

After reading this chapter, you should have a good understanding of:

LO1.1 The definition of strategic management and its four key attributes.

LO1.2 The strategic management process and its three interrelated and principal activities.

LO1.3 The vital role of corporate governance and stakeholder management as well as how "symbiosis" can be achieved among an organization's stakeholders.

LO1.4 The importance of social responsibility, including environmental sustainability, and how it can enhance a corporation's innovation strategy.

LO1.5 The need for greater empowerment throughout the organization.

LO1.6 How an awareness of a hierarchy of strategic goals can help an organization achieve coherence in its strategic direction.

LEARNING OBJECTIVES

We define strategic management as *consisting of the analyses, decisions, and actions an organization undertakes in order to create and sustain competitive advantages.* At the heart of strategic management is the question: How and why do some firms outperform others? Thus, the challenge to managers is to decide on strategies that provide advantages that can be sustained over time. There are four key attributes of strategic management. It is directed at overall organizational goals, includes multiple stakeholders, incorporates short-term as well as long-term perspectives, and recognizes trade-offs between effectiveness and efficiency. We discuss the above definition and the four key attributes in the first section.

The second section addresses the strategic management process. The three major processes are strategy analysis, strategy formulation, and strategy implementation. These three components parallel the analyses, decisions, and actions in the above definition. We discuss how each of the 12 chapters addresses these three processes and provide examples from each chapter.

The third section discusses two important and interrelated concepts: corporate governance and stakeholder management. Corporate governance addresses the issue of who "governs" the corporation and determines its direction. It consists of three primary participants: stockholders (owners), management (led by the chief executive officer), and the board of directors (elected to monitor management). Stakeholder management recognizes that the interests of various stakeholders, such as owners, customers, and employees, can often conflict and create challenging decision-making dilemmas for managers. However, we discuss how some firms have been able to achieve "symbiosis" among stakeholders wherein their interests are considered interdependent and can be achieved simultaneously. We also discuss the important role of social responsibility and explain the concept of "shared value." Further, we emphasize the need for corporations to incorporate environmental sustainability in their strategic actions.

The fourth section addresses factors in the business environment that have increased the level of unpredictable change for today's leaders. Such factors have also created the need for a greater strategic management perspective and reinforced the role of empowerment throughout the organization.

The final section focuses on the need for organizations to ensure consistency in their vision, mission, and strategic objectives, which, collectively, form a hierarchy of goals. While visions may lack specificity, they must evoke powerful and compelling mental images. Strategic objectives are much more specific and are essential for driving toward overall goals.

⬛ Learning from Mistakes

What makes the study of strategic management so interesting? For one, struggling firms can become stars, while high flyers can become earthbound very rapidly. As colorfully noted by Arthur Martinez, Sears' former chairman: "Today's peacock is tomorrow's feather duster." Consider, for example, the change in membership on the prestigious *Fortune 500* list of the largest U.S. firms:[1]

- Of the 500 companies that appeared on the first list in 1955, only 62, ranked by revenue, have appeared on the list every year since.
- Some of the most powerful companies on today's list—businesses like Intel, Apple, and Google—grew from nothing to great on the strength of new technologies, bumping venerable old companies off the list.

Let's take a look at another fallen star, Nokia, the Finnish phone manufacturer. Nokia captured the emerging market for mobile phones and built the industry's most powerful brand in the 1990s.[2] Its handsets virtually defined the industry from the time it launched the first GSM phone in 1992. Then from 1996 to 2001, its revenues increased almost fivefold, and in 1998 it was the world's largest mobile manufacturer. In 2005 it sold its billionth handset, an 1100 model, to a customer in Nigeria. Unfortunately, Nokia's market dominance was short-lived. What happened?

While Nokia focused on emerging markets, it took its eye off the ball in developed economies, where the smartphone revolution was on its way. Nokia's focus on mobile phones for voice communication turned out to be their most disastrous call in the past 10 years. In addition to voice communications, customers also demanded interactive applications, web browsing, and global positioning systems—as provided by Apple's iPhone and RIM's BlackBerry. As noted in *The Economist:* "Apple's iPhone and Google's Android range compete on 'cool.' BlackBerry is synonymous with business. But what does Nokia stand for?"

Nokia's inability to meet customer needs in both established and emerging markets resulted in a significant drop in its market share. It dropped from almost 51 percent in the fourth quarter of 2007 to less than 41 percent in the fourth quarter of 2008.

Since Apple introduced its first iPhone on January 9, 2007, Nokia's stock dropped 45 percent over the next three years—wiping out about $77 billion in the firm's market capitalization. Over the same period, Apple's shares soared 234 percent! Further, the 2010 global brands ranking by Millward Brown Optimor, placed Nokia in 43rd place, i.e., 30 places down compared to its position in 2009. Its profit margins had also been shrinking, along with its market share and the average price of its phones. Finally, at its peak, Nokia accounted for 4 percent of Finland's gross national product—by 2009, that share was down to only 1.6 percent, according to Helsinki-based economic research institute ETLA.

Nokia also suffered from its location. Building a mobile telephone giant in Finland was a great achievement. However, Nokia wasn't surrounded by Internet companies or consumer electronics manufacturers. It wasn't exposed to a culture of innovation, which would have forced it to question its assumptions and business decisions. Maybe, in short, Nokia needed to be where the action was, that is, in the middle of the computer industry as well as the film, music, and Internet businesses. As suggested by *Bloomberg Businessweek:*

> Nokia should have relocated to California a decade ago. It would have caused an outcry in Finland, and probably Brussels as well. And it would have been worth it. Nokia needed to pitch itself into the cauldron of technological change. Maybe that way it could have held onto its brand leadership, rather than surrender it to a computer manufacturer that looked dead on its feet a decade ago.
>
> The cruel truth—for all its residual market share—is that Nokia misread the way the mobile phone industry was merging with the computer industry and social networking. And now, maybe it's too late to turn that around.

Today's leaders, such as those at Nokia, face a large number of complex challenges in the global marketplace. In considering how much credit (or blame) they deserve, two perspectives of leadership come immediately to mind: the "romantic" and "external control" perspectives.[3] First, let's look at the **romantic view of leadership.** Here, the implicit assumption is that the leader is the key force in determining an organization's success—or lack thereof.[4] This view dominates the popular press in business magazines such as *Fortune, BusinessWeek,* and *Forbes,* wherein the CEO is either lauded for his or her firm's success or chided for the organization's demise.[5] Consider, for example, the credit that has been bestowed on leaders such as Akio Toyota, Richard Branson, and Lee Kun-Hee for the tremendous accomplishments of their firms, Toyota Motors, Virgin Group, and Samsung, respectively.

romantic view of leadership situations in which the leader is the key force determining the organization's success—or lack thereof.

Similarly, Apple's success in the last decade has been attributed almost entirely to Steve Jobs, its late founder and CEO, who passed away in October of 2011.[6] Apple's hit products, such as iPads, iPods, and iPhones (not to mention iMac computers) are a lasting testament to his genius for developing innovative, user-friendly, and aesthetically pleasing products. In addition to being a perfectionist in product design, Jobs was also a master showman with a cult following. When he announced in January 2009 that he was taking medical leave through June of that year, Apple's stock immediately dropped 10 percent. And almost two years later, in January 2011, he announced he was taking another medical leave—Apple shares went down 6 percent, reflecting a drop of around $20 billion in the firm's market value. Two days after Jobs' passing, Apple introduced its new iPhone 4S, which topped 4 million orders in the first three days after its release.[7]

Finally, consider how George Buckley reinvigorated 3M's focus on innovation. 3M, with $23 billion in 2010 revenues, produces an astonishing 55,000 different products. Its goal has always been to generate 30 percent of its sales from products introduced in the past five years. However, when the board asked Buckley in 2005 to assume the CEO position, this benchmark had dropped to only 21 percent. Strategy Spotlight 1.1 describes Buckley's strong initiatives to accelerate 3M's rate of innovation.

On the other hand, when things don't go well, much of the failure of an organization can also, rightfully, be attributed to the leader.[8] Nokia's leadership failed to see the changes taking place in the mobile phone industry. In contrast, Apple fully capitalized on the emerging trend toward sophisticated smartphones.

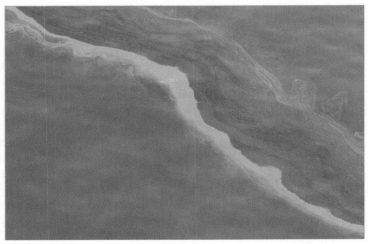

● The BP oil spill in April 2010, severely affected many industries along the U.S. Gulf Coast.

How CEO George Buckley Turned Around 3M

Why is innovation important to 3M? As their older products become outmoded or become commodities, they must be replaced. According to Larry Wendling, head of 3M's corporate research, "Our business model is literally new-product innovation." However, when James McNerney left the company to become Boeing's CEO, the percentage had slid to 21 percent. And, what's worse, much of the new product revenue came from a single category: optical films.

The board went outside the firm for its new CEO and appointed George Buckley, who had previously served as CEO of Brunswick, an Illinois company known for bowling gear and boats. What is perhaps most important to know about Buckley, however, is that he has a PhD in electrical engineering and is a scientist at heart, with several patents to his name. He states: "This is to me an engineer's and scientist's Toys'R'Us," and "There is no company like it in America. There is no company like it in the world."

When Buckley took over 3M, he quickly set some clear business goals for the company. He wanted his managers to protect and strengthen 3M's core businesses, which included abrasives, optical film, and industrial tapes. He also wanted 3M to develop lower-cost products to compete in emerging markets, as well as for the firm to play a key role in future growth markets such as renewable energy, water infrastructure, and mobile digital media.

Perhaps most important, Buckley has been an outspoken champion for 3M's labs. In 2009, despite the deep recession, he kept R&D spending at more than $1 billion and asserted that "even in the worst economic times in memory, we released over 1,000 new products." He also removed the stringent focus on efficiency, particularly in basic research. This had a huge psychic payoff for staff at the science-centric company. Ram Charan, a world-famous consultant who advises the firm claims "George has accelerated the innovation machine by devoting his personal time, his energy, his focus, to empowering the researchers, opening up their minds and urging them to restore the luster of 3M." Buckley's results are impressive: The percentage of 3M's revenue from products introduced in the past five years is back to 30 percent and is expected to reach the mid-30s by 2012.

In closing, Marc Gunther, a contributing editor at *Fortune* magazine, provides some interesting personal insights: "Buckley is a charming and, above all, enthusiastic guy . . . who, in his spare time, likes taking apart and putting together old motorcycles or restoring Victorian furniture . . . While he surely needs traditional management skills to oversee a global company of 75,000 people, my sense is that his scientific curiosity about how the world works and boyish delight in how things get invented make him a perfect fit for 3M."

Sources: Gunther, M. 2010. 3M's innovation revival. *Fortune*. September 27: 73–76; Hindo, B. 2007. 3M chief plants a money tree. *www.businessweek.com*. June 11: np; and, Gunther, M. Why 3M is unique. *theenergycollective.com*. December 10: np.

The contrasting fortunes of Hewlett-Packard under two different CEOs also demonstrate the influence leadership has on firm performance.[9] When Carly Fiorina was fired as CEO of the firm, HP enjoyed an immediate increase in its stock price of 7 percent—hardly a strong endorsement of her leadership! Her successor, Mark Hurd, led the firm to five years of outstanding financial results. Interestingly, when he abruptly resigned on August 6, 2010, the firm's stock dropped 12 percent almost instantly! (To provide some perspective, this represents a decrease in HP's market value of about $12 billion.)

However, this reflects only part of the picture. Consider another perspective called the **external control view of leadership.** Here, rather than making the implicit assumption that the leader is the most important factor in determining organizational outcomes, the focus is on external factors that may positively (or negatively) affect a firm's success. We don't have to look far to support this perspective. Developments in the general environment, such as economic downturns, governmental legislation, or an outbreak of major internal conflict or war, can greatly restrict the choices that are available to a firm's

external control view of leadership situations in which external forces—where the leader has limited influence—determine the organization's success.

executives. In addition, major unanticipated developments can often have very negative consequences for businesses regardless of how well formulated their strategies are.

Let's look at a few recent examples:[10]

- The financial meltdown of 2008 and the resultant deep recession during the following three years forced once proud corporations like Fortis Bank in Belgium and Munich's Hypo Real Estate in Germany to ask for government bailouts. Others, such as Merrill Lynch in the United States, had to be acquired by other firms.
- In the aftermath of BP's disastrous oil well explosion on April 20, 2010, along the U.S. Gulf Coast, the fishing and tourism industries in the region suffered significant downturns. BP itself was forced to pay a $20 billion fine to the U.S. government.
- In April 2010, a volcanic eruption in Iceland disrupted air traffic all over Europe for well over a week. It is estimated that major airlines lost approximately $1.7 billion.
- On March 11, 2011, a 9.0 earthquake and tsunami devastated Japan and resulted in the loss of more than 20,000 lives. During the next two trading days, the country's stock exchange (Nikkei) suffered its biggest loss in 40 years. The disaster hit nearly every industry hard—especially energy companies. For example, Tokyo Electric Power Co., which operates a nuclear power plant that was severely damaged, fell 24.7 percent, and Toshiba Corp., a maker of nuclear power plants, slid 19.5 percent. Firms as diverse as Toyota, Honda, and Sony were forced to halt production because extensive damage to roads and distribution systems made it nearly impossible to move products.

Before moving on, it is important to point out that successful executives are often able to navigate around the difficult circumstances that they face. At times it can be refreshing to see the optimistic position they take when they encounter seemingly insurmountable odds. Of course, that's not to say that one should be naïve or Pollyannaish. Consider, for example, how one CEO is handling trying times:[11]

Name a general economic woe, and the chances are that Charles Needham is dealing with it.

- Market turmoil has knocked 80 percent off the shares of South Africa's Metorex, the mining company that he heads.
- The plunge in global commodities is slamming prices for the copper, cobalt, and other minerals Metorex unearths across Africa. The credit crisis makes it harder to raise money.
- And fighting has again broken out in the Democratic Republic of Congo, where Metorex has a mine and several projects in development.

Such problems might send many executives to the window ledge. Yet Needham appears unruffled as he sits down at a conference table in the company's modest offices in a Johannesburg suburb. The combat in northeast Congo, he notes, is far from Metorex's mine. Commodity prices are still high, in historical terms. And Needham is confident he can raise enough capital, drawing on relationships with South African banks. "These are the kinds of things you deal with, doing business in Africa," he says.

What Is Strategic Management?

Given the many challenges and opportunities in the global marketplace, today's managers must do more than set long-term strategies and hope for the best.[12] They must go beyond what some have called "incremental management," whereby they view their job as making a series of small, minor changes to improve the efficiency of their firm's operations.[13]

strategic management the analyses, decisions, and actions an organization undertakes in order to create and sustain competitive advantages.

That is fine if your firm is competing in a very stable, simple, and unchanging industry. But there aren't many of those left. The pace of change is accelerating, and the pressure on managers to make both major and minor changes in a firm's strategic direction is increasing.

Rather than seeing their role as merely custodians of the status quo, today's leaders must be proactive, anticipate change, and continually refine and, when necessary, make dramatic changes to their strategies. The strategic management of the organization must become both a process and a way of thinking throughout the organization.

Defining Strategic Management

>LO1.1

The definition of strategic management and its four key attributes.

Strategic management consists of the analyses, decisions, and actions an organization undertakes in order to create and sustain competitive advantages. This definition captures two main elements that go to the heart of the field of strategic management.

First, the strategic management of an organization entails three ongoing processes: *analyses, decisions,* and *actions.* Strategic management is concerned with the *analysis* of strategic goals (vision, mission, and strategic objectives) along with the analysis of the internal and external environment of the organization. Next, leaders must make strategic *decisions.* These *decisions,* broadly speaking, address two basic questions: What industries should we compete in? How should we compete in those industries? These questions also often involve an organization's domestic and international operations. And last are the *actions* that must be taken. Decisions are of little use, of course, unless they are acted on. Firms must take the necessary actions to implement their **strategies.** This requires leaders to allocate the necessary resources and to design the organization to bring the intended strategies to reality.

strategy the analyses, decisions, and actions that enable a firm to succeed.

Second, the essence of strategic management is the study of why some firms outperform others.[14] Thus, managers need to determine how a firm is to compete so that it can obtain advantages that are sustainable over a lengthy period of time. That means focusing on two fundamental questions:

competitive advantage a firm's resources and capabilities that enable it to overcome the competitive forces in its industry(ies).

- *How should we compete in order to create **competitive advantages** in the marketplace?* Managers need to determine if the firm should position itself as the low-cost producer or develop products and services that are unique and will enable the firm to charge premium prices. Or should they do some combination of both?
- *How can we create competitive advantages in the marketplace that are unique, valuable, and difficult for rivals to copy or substitute?* That is, managers need to make such advantages sustainable, instead of temporary.

Rivals almost always copy ideas that work. In the 1980s, American Airlines tried to establish a competitive advantage by introducing the frequent flyer program. Within weeks, all the airlines did the same thing. Overnight, frequent flyer programs became a necessary tool for competitive parity instead of a competitive advantage. The challenge, therefore, is to create competitive advantages that are sustainable.

Sustainable competitive advantage cannot be achieved through operational effectiveness alone.[15] The popular management innovations of the last two decades—total quality, just-in-time, benchmarking, business process reengineering, outsourcing—are all about operational effectiveness. **Operational effectiveness** means performing similar activities better than rivals. Each of these is important, but none lead to sustainable competitive advantage because everyone is doing them. Strategy is all about being different. Sustainable competitive advantage is possible only by performing different activities from rivals or performing similar activities in different ways. Companies such as British Airways, Walmart, and IKEA have developed unique, internally consistent, and difficult-to-imitate activity systems that have provided them with sustained competitive advantages. A company with

operational effectiveness performing similar activities better than rivals.

a good strategy must make clear choices about what it wants to accomplish. Trying to do everything that your rivals do eventually leads to mutually destructive price competition, not long-term advantage.

The Four Key Attributes of Strategic Management

Before discussing the strategic management process, let's briefly talk about four attributes of strategic management.[16] It should become clear how this course differs from other courses that you have had in functional areas, such as accounting, marketing, operations, and finance. Exhibit 1.1 provides a definition and the four attributes of strategic management.

First, strategic management is *directed toward overall organizational goals and objectives.* That is, effort must be directed at what is best for the total organization, not just a single functional area. Some authors have referred to this perspective as "organizational versus individual rationality."[17] That is, what might look "rational" or ideal for one functional area, such as operations, may not be in the best interest of the overall firm. For example, operations may decide to schedule long production runs of similar products to lower unit costs. However, the standardized output may be counter to what the marketing department needs to appeal to a demanding target market. Similarly, research and development may "overengineer" the product to develop a far superior offering, but the design may make the product so expensive that market demand is minimal. Therefore, in this course you will look at cases and strategic issues from the perspective of the organization rather than that of the functional area(s) in which you have the strongest background.

Second, strategic management *includes multiple stakeholders in decision making.*[18] **Stakeholders** are those individuals, groups, and organizations who have a "stake" in the success of the organization, including owners (shareholders in a publicly held corporation), employees, customers, suppliers, the community at large, and so on. (We'll discuss this in more detail later in this chapter.) Managers will not be successful if they focus on a single stakeholder. For example, if the overwhelming emphasis is on generating profits for the owners, employees may become alienated, customer service may suffer, and the suppliers may resent demands for pricing concessions. However, many organizations can satisfy multiple stakeholder needs simultaneously. For example, financial performance may increase because employees who are satisfied with their jobs work harder to enhance customer satisfaction—leading to higher profits.

Third, strategic management *requires incorporating both short-term and long-term perspectives.*[19] Peter Senge, a leading strategic management author, has referred to this need as a "creative tension."[20] That is, managers must maintain both a vision for the future of the organization as well as a focus on its present operating needs. However, financial markets can exert significant pressures on executives to meet short-term performance

stakeholders individuals, groups, and organizations who have a stake in the success of the organization, including owners (shareholders in a publicly held corporation), employees, customers, suppliers, and the community at large.

Definition: Strategic management consists of the analyses, decisions, and actions an organization undertakes in order to create and sustain competitive advantages.

Key Attributes of Strategic Management

- Directs the organization toward overall goals and objectives.
- Includes multiple stakeholders in decision making.
- Needs to incorporate short-term and long-term perspectives.
- Recognizes trade-offs between efficiency and effectiveness.

Exhibit 1.1
Strategic Management Concepts

targets. Studies have shown that corporate leaders often take a short-term approach to the detriment of creating long-term shareholder value. Consider the following:

> According to recent studies, only 59 percent of financial executives say they would pursue a positive net present value project if it meant missing the quarter's consensus earnings per-share estimate. Worse, 78 percent say they would sacrifice value—often a great deal of value—to smooth earnings. Similarly, managers are more likely to cut R&D to reverse an earning slide if a significant amount of the company's equity is owned by institutions with high portfolio turnover. Many companies have the same philosophy about long-term investments such as infrastructure and employee training.[21]

Fourth, strategic management *involves the recognition of trade-offs between effectiveness and efficiency.* Some authors have referred to this as the difference between "doing the right thing" (**effectiveness**) and "doing things right" (**efficiency**).[22] While managers must allocate and use resources wisely, they must still direct their efforts toward the attainment of overall organizational objectives. Managers who only focus on meeting short-term budgets and targets may fail to attain the broader goals. Consider the following amusing story told by Norman Augustine, former CEO of defense giant Martin Marietta (now Lockheed Martin):

> I am reminded of an article I once read in a British newspaper which described a problem with the local bus service between the towns of Bagnall and Greenfields. It seemed that, to the great annoyance of customers, drivers had been passing long queues of would-be passengers with a smile and a wave of the hand. This practice was, however, clarified by a bus company official who explained, "It is impossible for the drivers to keep their timetables if they must stop for passengers."[23]

Clearly, the drivers who were trying to stay on schedule had ignored the overall mission. As Augustine noted, "Impeccable logic but something seems to be missing!"

Successful managers must make many trade-offs. It is central to the practice of strategic management. At times, managers must focus on the short term and efficiency; at other times the emphasis is on the long term and expanding a firm's product-market scope in order to anticipate opportunities in the competitive environment. For example, consider Robin Li's approach. Li is CEO and chairman of Baidu, China's leading Internet search engine.

> He leads the company with trust and efficiency. He quickly built up the search engine, network communities, MP3 search engine, and consumer-to-consumer (C2C) site and sponsored numerous cultural seminars to spread the use of Baidu across the vast areas of China. In this process, Li emphasized the importance of speed. At the same time, he is a man of great patience, who took his time to select talented people who would be with the company for the long term. In addition, he innovates through constantly evolving the company's information technology (IT) business model and understands global market needs and the importance of change.[24]

Some authors have developed the concept of **"ambidexterity"** which refers to a manager's challenge to both align resources to take advantage of existing product markets as well as proactively explore new opportunities.[25] Strategy Spotlight 1.2 discusses ambidextrous behaviors that are required for success in today's challenging marketplace.

The Strategic Management Process

We've identified three ongoing processes—analyses, decisions, and actions—that are central to strategic management. In practice, these three processes—often referred to as strategy analysis, strategy formulation, and strategy implementation—are highly interdependent and do not take place one after the other in a sequential fashion in most companies.

effectiveness
tailoring actions to the needs of an organization rather than wasting effort, or "doing the right thing."

efficiency
performing actions at a low cost relative to a benchmark, or "doing things right."

ambidexterity the challenge managers face of both aligning resources to take advantage of existing product markets as well as proactively exploring new opportunities.

strategic management process strategy analysis, strategy formulation, and strategy implementation

>LO1.2
The strategic management process and its three interrelated and principal activities.

Ambidextrous Behaviors: Combining Alignment and Adaptability

A recent study involving 41 business units in 10 multinational companies identified four ambidextrous behaviors in individuals. Such behaviors are the essence of ambidexterity, and they illustrate how a dual capacity for alignment and adaptability can be woven into the fabric of an organization at the individual level.

They take time and are alert to opportunities beyond the confines of their own jobs. A large computer company's sales manager became aware of a need for a new software module that nobody currently offered. Instead of selling the customer something else, he worked up a business case for the new module. With management's approval, he began working full time on its development.

They are cooperative and seek out opportunities to combine their efforts with others. A marketing manager for Italy was responsible for supporting a newly acquired subsidiary. When frustrated about the limited amount of contact she had with her peers in other countries, she began discussions with them. This led to the creation of a European marketing forum which meets quarterly to discuss issues, share best practices, and collaborate on marketing plans.

They are brokers, always looking to build internal networks. When visiting the head office in St. Louis, a Canadian plant manager heard about plans for a $10 million investment for a new tape manufacturing plant. After inquiring further about the plans and returning to

Canada, he contacted a regional manager in Manitoba, who he knew was looking for ways to build his business. With some generous support from the Manitoba government, the regional manager bid for, and ultimately won, the $10 million investment.

They are multitaskers who are comfortable wearing more than one hat. Although an operations manager for a major coffee and tea distributor was charged with running his plant as efficiently as possible, he took it upon himself to identify value-added services for his clients. By developing a dual role, he was able to manage operations and develop a promising electronic module that automatically reported impending problems inside a coffee vending machine. With corporate funding, he found a subcontractor to develop the software, and he then piloted the module in his own operations. It was so successful that it was eventually adopted by operations managers in several other countries.

A recent *Harvard Business Review* article provides some useful insights on how one can become a more ambidextrous leader. Consider the following questions:

- **Do you meet your numbers?**
- **Do you help others?**
- **What do you do for your peers?** Are you just their in-house competitor?
- **When you manage up, do you bring problems—or problems with possible solutions?**
- **Are you transparent?** Managers who get a reputation for spinning events gradually lose the trust of peers and superiors.
- **Are you developing a group of senior managers who know you and are willing to back your original ideas with resources?**

Source: Birkinshaw, J. & Gibson, C. 2004. Building ambidexterity into an organization. *MIT Sloan Management Review,* 45(4): 47–55; and, Bower, J. L. 2007. Solve the succession crisis by growing inside-out leaders. *Harvard Business Review,* 85(11): 90–99.

Intended versus Realized Strategies

Henry Mintzberg, a management scholar at McGill University in Canada, argues that viewing the strategic management process as one in which analysis is followed by optimal decisions and their subsequent meticulous implementation neither describes the strategic management process accurately nor prescribes ideal practice.[26] He sees the business environment as far from predictable, thus limiting our ability for analysis. Further, decisions are seldom based on optimal rationality alone, given the political processes that occur in all organizations.[27]

Taking into consideration the limitations discussed above, Mintzberg proposed an alternative model. As depicted in Exhibit 1.2, decisions following from analysis, in this model, constitute the ***intended*** **strategy** of the firm. For a variety of reasons, the intended

intended strategy
strategy in which organizational decisions are determined only by analysis.

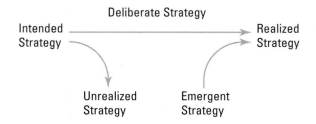

Exhibit 1.2 **Realized Strategy and Intended Strategy: Usually Not the Same**

Source: From Mintzberg, H. & Waters, J. A., "Of Strategies: Deliberate and Emergent," *Strategic Management Journal,* Vol. 6, 1985, pp. 257–272. Copyright © John Wiley & Sons Limited. Reproduced with permission.

strategy rarely survives in its original form. Unforeseen environmental developments, unanticipated resource constraints, or changes in managerial preferences may result in at least some parts of the intended strategy remaining *unrealized.* On the other hand, good managers will want to take advantage of a new opportunity presented by the environment, even if it was not part of the original set of intentions. For example, consider the carbon energy industry.

> In September 2011, the European Union approved funds for low carbon energy. Specifically in the UK, organizers of the London 2012 Olympic Games dropped a plan to cut carbon emissions during the sporting showcase, abandoning a pledge made when London defeated eight other global cities to host the event. Games administrators will "no longer pursue formal offsetting procedures" to mitigate Olympics-related emissions, documents posted on the London Olympics website said.
>
> David Stubbs, head of sustainability at the London Organising Committee for both the Olympic and Paralympics Games (LOCOG), said in an interview that going ahead with the plan would have shifted the focus away from Britain. Scrapping the plan, which would have involved offsetting the emissions generated by the games by investing in clean-energy projects in poor countries, underlines how carbon-saving measures are being overlooked to save money as the UK cuts spending and increases taxes amid an economic slowdown. By ditching the program, LOCOG may avoid spending as much as 2.7 million pounds ($4.4 million USD), according to prices quoted by broker MF Global. "Officially, if you want to [be certified as carbon-offsetting,] all projects have to be overseas, so if we plant a lot of trees in Essex that just doesn't count," Stubbs said, referring to the English county. "Because the games are in the UK, we wanted to maximize the games locally. Doing formal offsetting would be diverting things." [28]

realized strategy
strategy in which organizational decisions are determined by both analysis and unforeseen environmental developments, unanticipated resource constraints, and/or changes in managerial preferences.

Thus, the final **realized strategy** of any firm is a combination of deliberate and emergent strategies.

Next, we will address each of the three key strategic management processes: strategy analysis, strategy formulation, and strategy implementation and provide a brief overview of the chapters.

Exhibit 1.3 depicts the strategic management process and indicates how it ties into the chapters in the book. Consistent with our discussion above, we use two-way arrows to convey the interactive nature of the processes.

Strategy Analysis

strategy analysis
study of firms' external and internal environments, and their fit with organizational vision and goals.

Strategy analysis may be looked upon as the starting point of the strategic management process. It consists of the "advance work" that must be done in order to effectively formulate and implement strategies. Many strategies fail because managers may want to

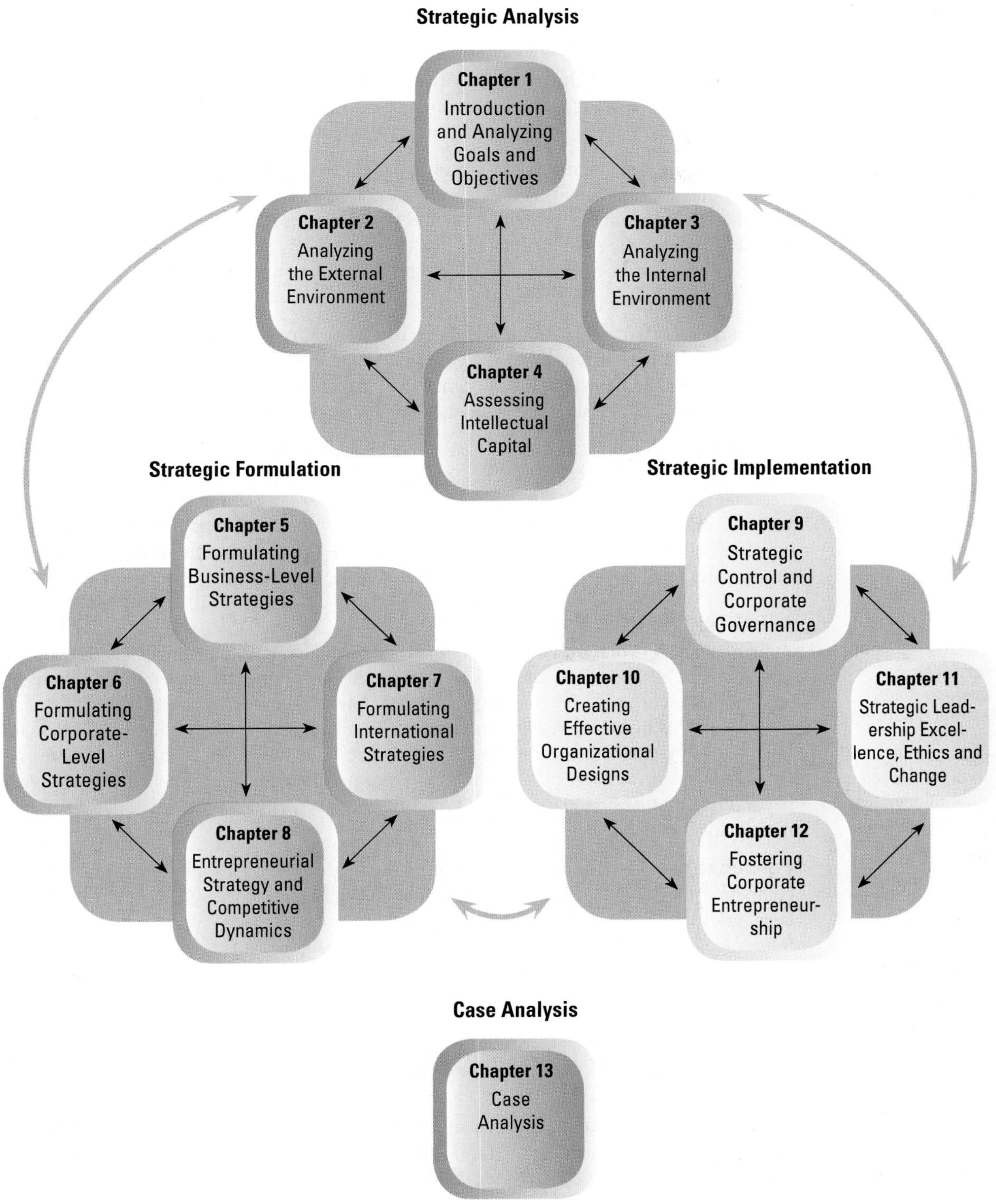

Strategic Analysis

Chapter 1
Introduction and Analyzing Goals and Objectives

Chapter 2
Analyzing the External Environment

Chapter 3
Analyzing the Internal Environment

Chapter 4
Assessing Intellectual Capital

Strategic Formulation

Chapter 5
Formulating Business-Level Strategies

Chapter 6
Formulating Corporate-Level Strategies

Chapter 7
Formulating International Strategies

Chapter 8
Entrepreneurial Strategy and Competitive Dynamics

Strategic Implementation

Chapter 9
Strategic Control and Corporate Governance

Chapter 10
Creating Effective Organizational Designs

Chapter 11
Strategic Leadership Excellence, Ethics and Change

Chapter 12
Fostering Corporate Entrepreneurship

Case Analysis

Chapter 13
Case Analysis

Exhibit 1.3 The Strategic Management Process

formulate and implement strategies without a careful analysis of the overarching goals of the organization and without a thorough analysis of its external and internal environment.

Analyzing Organizational Goals and Objectives (Chapter 1)   A firm's vision, mission, and strategic objectives form a hierarchy of goals that range from broad statements of intent and bases for competitive advantage to specific, measurable strategic objectives.

Analyzing the External Environment of the Firm (Chapter 2)   Managers must monitor and scan the environment as well as analyze competitors. Two frameworks of the external environment are provided: (1) the general environment consists of several elements, such as demographic, technological, and economic segments, and (2) the industry environment consists of competitors and other organizations that may threaten the success of a firm's products and services.

Assessing the Internal Environment of the Firm (Chapter 3)   Analyzing the strengths and relationships among the activities that constitute a firm's value chain (e.g., operations, marketing and sales, and human resource management) can be a means of uncovering potential sources of competitive advantage for the firm.[29]

Assessing a Firm's Intellectual Assets (Chapter 4)   The knowledge worker and a firm's other intellectual assets (e.g., patents, trademarks) are becoming increasingly important as the drivers of competitive advantages and wealth creation. We also assess how well the organization creates networks and relationships as well as how technology can enhance collaboration among employees and provide a means of accumulating and storing knowledge.[30]

Strategy Formulation

strategy formulation
decisions made by firms regarding investments, commitments, and other aspects of operations that create and sustain competitive advantage.

A firm's **strategy formulation** is developed at several levels. First, business-level strategy addresses the issue of how to compete in a given business to attain competitive advantage. Second, corporate-level strategy focuses on two issues: (a) what businesses to compete in and (b) how businesses can be managed to achieve synergy; that is, they create more value by working together than if they operate as stand-alone businesses. Third, a firm must determine the best method to develop international strategies as it ventures beyond its national boundaries. Fourth, managers must formulate effective entrepreneurial initiatives.

Formulating Business-Level Strategy (Chapter 5)   The question of how firms compete and outperform their rivals and how they achieve and sustain competitive advantages goes to the heart of strategic management. Successful firms strive to develop bases for competitive advantage, which can be achieved through cost leadership and/or differentiation as well as by focusing on a narrow or industrywide market segment.[31]

Formulating Corporate-Level Strategy (Chapter 6)   Corporate-level strategy addresses a firm's portfolio (or group) of businesses. It asks (1) What business (or businesses) should we compete in? and (2) How can we manage this portfolio of businesses to create synergies among the businesses?

Formulating International Strategy (Chapter 7)   When firms enter foreign markets, they face both opportunities and pitfalls.[32] Managers must decide not only on the most appropriate entry strategy but also how they will go about attaining competitive advantages in international markets.[33]

Entrepreneurial Strategy and Competitive Dynamics (Chapter 8)   Entrepreneurial activity aimed at new value creation is a major engine for economic growth. For entrepreneurial initiatives to succeed, viable opportunities must be recognized and effective strategies must be formulated.

Strategy Implementation

Clearly, sound strategies are of no value if they are not properly implemented.[34] **Strategy implementation** involves ensuring proper strategic controls and organizational designs, which includes establishing effective means to coordinate and integrate activities within the firm as well as with its suppliers, customers, and alliance partners.[35] Leadership plays a central role, including ensuring that the organization is committed to excellence and ethical behavior. It also promotes learning and continuous improvement and acts entrepreneurially in creating and taking advantage of new opportunities.

Strategic Control and Corporate Governance (Chapter 9)   Firms must exercise two types of strategic control. First, informational control requires that organizations continually monitor and scan the environment and respond to threats and opportunities. Second, behavioral control involves the proper balance of rewards and incentives as well as cultures and boundaries (or constraints). Further, successful firms (those that are incorporated) practice effective corporate governance.

Creating Effective Organizational Designs (Chapter 10)   To succeed, firms must have organizational structures and designs that are consistent with their strategy. And, in today's rapidly changing competitive environments, firms must ensure that their organizational boundaries—those internal to the firm and external—are more flexible and permeable.[36] Often, organizations develop strategic alliances to capitalize on the capabilities of other organizations.

Creating a Learning Organization and an Ethical Organization (Chapter 11)   Effective leaders set a direction, design the organization, and develop an organization that is committed to excellence and ethical behavior. In addition, given rapid and unpredictable change, leaders must create a "learning organization" to ensure that the entire organization can benefit from individual and collective talents.

Fostering Corporate Entrepreneurship (Chapter 12)   With rapid and unpredictable change in the global marketplace, firms must continually improve and grow as well as find new ways to renew their organizations. Corporate entrepreneurship and innovation provide firms with new opportunities, and strategies should be formulated that enhance a firm's innovative capacity.

Analyzing Strategic Management Cases (Chapter 13)   Provides guidelines and suggestions on how to evaluate cases in this course. Thus, the concepts and techniques discussed in these 12 chapters can be applied to real-world organizations.

Let's now address two concepts—corporate governance and stakeholder management—that are critical to the strategic management process.

The Role of Corporate Governance and Stakeholder Management

Most business enterprises that employ more than a few dozen people are organized as corporations. As you recall from your finance classes, the overall purpose of a corporation is to maximize the long-term return to the owners (shareholders). Thus, we may ask: Who is really responsible for fulfilling this purpose? Robert Monks and Neil Minow provide a useful definition of **corporate governance** as "the relationship among various participants in determining the direction and performance of corporations. The primary participants are (1) the shareholders, (2) the management (led by the chief executive officer), and (3) the board of directors."[37] This relationship is illustrated in Exhibit 1.4.

The board of directors (BOD) are the elected representatives of the shareholders charged with ensuring that the interests and motives of management are aligned with those

strategy implementation actions made by firms that carry out the formulated strategy, including strategic controls, organizational design, and leadership.

corporate governance the relationship among various participants in determining the direction and performance of corporations. The primary participants are (1) the shareholders, (2) the management (led by the chief executive officer), and (3) the board of directors.

>LO1.3
The vital role of corporate governance and stakeholder management as well as how "symbiosis" can be achieved among an organization's stakeholders.

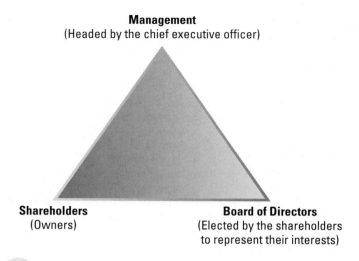

Management
(Headed by the chief executive officer)

Shareholders
(Owners)

Board of Directors
(Elected by the shareholders
to represent their interests)

Exhibit 1.4 The Key Elements of Corporate Governance

of the owners (i.e., shareholders). In many cases, the BOD is diligent in fulfilling its purpose. For example, Intel Corporation, the giant $43 billion maker of microprocessor chips, is widely recognized as an excellent example of sound governance practices. Its BOD follows guidelines to ensure that its members are independent (i.e., not members of the executive management team and do not have close personal ties to top executives) so that they can provide proper oversight, it has explicit guidelines on the selection of director candidates (to avoid "cronyism"), and it provides detailed procedures for formal evaluations of directors and the firm's top officers.[38] Such guidelines serve to ensure that management is acting in the best interests of shareholders.[39]

Recently, there has been much criticism as well as cynicism by both citizens and the business press about the poor job that management and the BODs of large corporations are doing. We only have to look at the scandals at firms such as Satyam in India and Arthur Andersen and Enron in the United States.[40] Such malfeasance has led to an erosion of the public's trust in the governance of corporations. For example, a recent Gallup poll found that 90 percent of Americans felt that people leading corporations could not be trusted to look after the interests of their employees, and only 18 percent thought that corporations looked after their shareholders. Forty-three percent, in fact, believed that senior executives were in it only for themselves. In Britain, that figure, according to another poll, was an astonishing 95 percent.[41] Perhaps worst of all, in another study, 60 percent of directors (the very people who decide how much executives should earn) felt that executives were "dramatically overpaid"![42]

It is now clear that much of the bonus pay awarded to global executives in the past few years was richly undeserved.[43] Let's take a closer look at a few of these payouts (the amounts below represent bonus pay, severance, and gains from stock sales from 2005 to 2011):

- Richard Fuld, Lehman Brothers, in the U.S. ($172 million)
- Kenneth Thompson, Wachovia Corporation, in the U.S. ($14 million)
- Edward Sampson, Niko Resources Ltd., in Canada ($11 million)
- Paul Walsh, Diageo PLC, in England ($10 million)

Clearly, there is a strong need for improved corporate governance, and we will address this topic in Chapter 9.[44] We focus on three important mechanisms to ensure effective corporate governance: an effective and engaged board of directors, shareholder activism, and proper managerial rewards and incentives.[45] In addition to these internal controls, a key role is played by various external control mechanisms.[46] These include the auditors, banks, analysts, an active financial press, and the threat of hostile takeovers.

Alternative Perspectives of Stakeholder Management

Generating long-term returns for the shareholders is the primary goal of a publicly held corporation.[47] As noted by former Chrysler vice chairman Robert Lutz, "We are here to serve the shareholder and create shareholder value. I insist that the only person who owns the company is the person who paid good money for it."[48]

Despite the primacy of generating shareholder value, managers who focus solely on the interests of the owners of the business will often make poor decisions that lead to negative, unanticipated outcomes.[49] For example, decisions such as mass layoffs to increase profits, ignoring issues related to conservation of the natural environment to save money, and exerting excessive pressure on suppliers to lower prices can certainly harm the firm in the long run. Such actions would likely lead to negative outcomes such as alienated employees, increased governmental oversight and fines, and disloyal suppliers.

Clearly, in addition to *shareholders,* there are other *stakeholders* (e.g., suppliers, customers) who must be explicitly taken into account in the strategic management process.[50] A stakeholder can be defined as an individual or group, inside or outside the company, that has a stake in and can influence an organization's performance. Each stakeholder group makes various claims on the company.[51] Exhibit 1.5 provides a list of major stakeholder groups and the nature of their claims on the company.

Zero Sum or Symbiosis?   There are two opposing ways of looking at the role of **stakeholder management** in the strategic management process.[52] The first one can be termed "zero sum." In this view, the role of management is to look upon the various stakeholders as competing for the organization's resources. In essence, the gain of one individual or group is the loss of another individual or group. For example, employees want higher wages (which drive down profits), suppliers want higher prices for their inputs and slower, more flexible delivery times (which drive up costs), customers want fast deliveries and higher quality (which drive up costs), the community at large wants charitable contributions (which take money from company goals), and so on. This zero-sum thinking is rooted, in part, in the traditional conflict between workers and management, leading to the formation of unions and sometimes ending in adversarial union–management negotiations and long, bitter strikes.

stakeholder management a firm's strategy for recognizing and responding to the interests of all its salient stakeholders.

Stakeholder Group	Nature of Claim
Stockholders	Dividends, capital appreciation
Employees	Wages, benefits, safe working environment, job security
Suppliers	Payment on time, assurance of continued relationship
Creditors	Payment of interest, repayment of principal
Customers	Value, warranties
Government	Taxes, compliance with regulations
Communities	Good citizenship behavior such as charities, employment, not polluting the environment

Exhibit 1.5
An Organization's Key Stakeholders and the Nature of Their Claims

Consider, for example, the many stakeholder challenges facing Walmart, the world's largest retailer.

> Walmart strives to ramp up growth while many stakeholders are watching nervously: employees and trade unions; shareholders, investors, and creditors; suppliers and joint venture partners; the governments of the U.S. and other nations where the retailer operates; and customers. In addition many non-governmental organizations (NGOs), particularly in countries where the retailer buys its products, are closely monitoring Walmart. Walmart's stakeholders have different interests, and not all of them share the firm's goals. Each group has the ability, in various degrees, to influence the firm's choices and results. Clearly, this wasn't the case when Sam Walton built his first store in Rogers, Arkansas, in 1962![53]

There will always be conflicting demands on organizations. However, organizations can achieve mutual benefit through stakeholder symbiosis, which recognizes that stakeholders are dependent upon each other for their success and well-being.[54] Consider Procter & Gamble's "laundry detergent compaction," a technique for compressing even more cleaning power into ever smaller concentrations.

In the early 2000s, P&G perfected a technique that could compact two or three times as much cleaning powder into a liquid concentration. This remarkable breakthrough has led to a change not only in consumer shopping habits, but also a revolution in industry supply-chain economics. Let's look at how several key stakeholders are affected along the supply chain:[55]

> *Consumers* love concentrated liquids because they are easier to carry, pour, and store. *Retailers,* meanwhile, prefer them because they take up less floor and shelf space, which leads to higher sales-per-square-foot—a big deal for Walmart, Target, and other big retailers. *Shipping and wholesalers,* meanwhile, prefer reduced-sized products because smaller bottles translate into reduced fuel consumption and improved warehouse space utilization. And, finally, *environmentalists* favor such products because they use less packaging and produce less waste than conventional products.

Strategy Spotlight 1.3 discusses the role of NGOs and their potential influence on companies' operations. While some organizations have been confronted for their controversial impact on the environment, others have made environmental concerns part of their business strategies and have been praised by watchdog groups for being proactive.

Crowdsourcing: Stakeholders Can Fulfill Multiple Roles   To show how stakeholder roles are becoming more fluid, we'd like to introduce a concept that will be a theme through the text: **crowdsourcing.**[56] When and where did the term originate? In January 2006, open sourcing was, for most businesspeople, little more than an online curiosity. At that time, Jeff Howe of *Wired* magazine started to write an article about the phenomenon. However, he soon discovered a far more important story to be told: Large—as well as small—companies in a wide variety of industries had begun farming out serious tasks to individuals and groups on the Internet. Together with his editor, Mark Robinson, they coined a new term to describe the phenomenon. In June 2006, the article appeared in which *crowdsourcing* was defined as the tapping of the "latent talent of the (online) crowd." It has become the term of choice for a process that is infiltrating many aspects of business life.

Clearly, *crowdsourcing* has claimed some well-known successes, particularly on the product development front. Consider:

- The Linux operating system, created as an open-source alternative to Windows and UNIX, can be downloaded free and altered to suit any user's needs. And, with all the firepower brought to bear by the online open-source community, bugs in the system get fixed in a matter of hours.
- One of Amazon's smartest moves was to invite their customers to write online reviews. The customers are neither paid nor controlled by the company, but the content that they create adds enormous value to other customers and, therefore, to Amazon.

crowdsourcing
practice wherein the Internet is used to tap a broad range of individuals and groups to generate ideas and solve problems.

NGOs: A Key Stakeholder Group

Although the number of NGOs worldwide is hard to determine, according to a recent study there are at least 40,000 multinational NGOs. In addition, there are also hundreds of thousands based in individual countries. The focus of most of these is, at least partially, on the welfare of the environment.

What are NGOs? NGOs describe a wide array of groups and organizations—from activist groups "reclaiming the streets" to development organizations delivering aid and providing essential public services. Other NGOs are research-driven policy organizations, looking to engage with decision makers. Still others see themselves as watchdogs, casting a critical eye over current events.

The largest NGOs are multinational operations with enormous reach and influence. They include well-established organizations such as Greenpeace, Sierra Club, World Wildlife Fund, Nature Conservancy, Environmental Defense, Natural Resources Defense Council, Conservation International, Friends of the Earth, and National Wildlife Federation. Many of these established groups have been around for more than 30 years and can still have a major public influence. In fact, according to a recent study that polled opinion leaders, 55 percent trust NGOs, versus only 6 percent that trust businesses.

Some of these organizations are confrontational, taking a range of actions to reach their goals, from making waves in courts (National Resources Defense Council), to boarding oil rigs (Greenpeace), to illegal activities, exemplified by arsonists' actions in the Colorado mountain resort of Vail. It is impossible for firms to predict all potential actions, especially irrational ones. However, they can reduce the odds of being attacked. In contrast to Vail, other ski resorts, such as Aspen, have confronted environmental issues and made them a central focus of their business strategies. For example, Aspen ski company decided to rely solely on wind power to power all of its operations. As a result, the company was rated as the number one ski resort in the West in addressing environmental issues by respected watchdog groups. Vail, on the other hand, is still trying to catch up.

As another example of a firm's environmentally sensitive behavior, Nike recently announced that it would not source any leather from the Amazon until deforestation for cattle expansion is halted. Their announcement, coupled with a similar one by Timberland, followed the release of a Greenpeace report entitled "Slaughtering the Amazon." It documented a three-year investigation that tracked beef, leather, and other cattle products from ranches involved in deforestation at the heart of the Amazon rainforest.

Sources: Esty, D. C. & Winston, A. S. 2009. *Green to Gold.* Hoboken, NJ: Wiley: 69–70; Anonymous. 2009. Timberland Steps It Up a Notch, Commit to Amazon Protections. *www.greenpeace.org.* July 29: np; and, Anonymous. Undated. The Rise and Role of NGOs in Sustainable Development. *www.iisd.org.* np.

ethics

- Roughly five million users per month swear by Wikipedia, the free online encyclopedia created and updated by Internet volunteers to the tune of roughly two million articles and counting.

Throughout the book, we will introduce examples of *crowdsourcing* to show its relevance to key strategy concepts.

Strategy Spotlight 1.4 describes how Goldcorp, a Toronto-based mining company, crowdsourced the expertise required to identify the best location to mine gold on the firm's property. Goldcorp invited geologists around the world to compete for $575,000 in prize money for analyzing its geological data. It was a remarkable success!

Social Responsibility and Environmental Sustainability: Moving beyond the Immediate Stakeholders

Organizations cannot ignore the interests and demands of stakeholders such as citizens and society in general that are beyond its immediate constituencies—customers, owners,

How Toronto-Based Goldcorp Used Crowdsourcing to Strike It Rich

A little over a decade ago, Toronto-based gold mining company Goldcorp was in big trouble. Besieged by strikes, lingering debts, and an exceedingly high cost of production, the firm had terminated mining operations. Conditions in the marketplace were quite poor and the gold market was contracting. Most analysts assumed that the company's 50-year-old mine in Red Lake, Ontario, was nearly dead. Without solid evidence of substantial new gold deposits, Goldcorp was likely to fold.

Clearly, CEO Robert McEwen needed a miracle. He was frustrated with his in-house geologists' reliability in estimating the value and location of gold on his property. He did something that was unprecedented in the industry: He published his geological data on the Web for all to see and he challenged the world to do the prospecting. The "Goldcorp Challenge" posted a total of $575,000 in prize money to be awarded to the participants who submitted the best methods and estimates.

His reasoning: If he could attract the attention of world-class talent to the problem of finding more gold in Red Lake, just as Linux managed to attract world-class programmers to the cause of better software, he could tap into thousands of minds that he wouldn't otherwise

have access to. He could also speed up exploration and improve his odds of discovery.

Although his geologists were appalled at the idea of exposing their super-secret data to the world, the response was immediate. More than 1,400 scientists, engineers, and geologists from 50 countries downloaded the company's data and started their viral exploration. Says McEwen: "We had math, advanced physics, intelligent systems, computer graphics, and organic solutions to inorganic problems. There were capabilities I had never seen before in the industry. When I saw the computer graphics, I almost fell out of my chair."

The panel of five judges was astonished by the creativity of the submissions. The top winner, which won $105,000, was a collaboration by two groups in Australia: Fractal Graphics, of West Perth, and Taylor Wall & Associates, in Queensland, which together had developed a powerful 3-D graphical depiction of the mine. One of the team members humorously stated: "I've never been to a mine. I'd never even been to Canada." Overall, the contestants identified 110 targets on the Red Lake property, more than 80 percent of which yielded substantial quantities of gold. In fact, since the challenge was initiated, an astounding 8 million ounces of gold have been found—worth well over $3 billion (given gold's fluctuating market value). Not a bad return on a half million dollar investment.

As of early 2011, Goldcorp had annual revenues of $3 billion and a market value of $33 billion! Not bad for a once failing firm . . .

Sources: de Castella, T. 2010. Should We Trust the Wisdom of Crowds? *news .bbc.co.uk.* July 5: np; Libert, B. & Spector, J. 2008. *We Are Smarter Than Me.* Philadelphia, PA: Wharton School Publishing; Tapscott, D. & Williams, A. D. 2007. Innovation in the Age of Mass Collaboration. *www.businessweek.com.* February 1: np; and, Tischler, L. 2002. He Struck Gold on the Net (Really). *fastcompany.com.* May 2: np.

crowdsourcing

suppliers, and employees. The realization that firms have multiple stakeholders and that evaluating their performance must go beyond analyzing their financial results has led to a new way of thinking about businesses and their relationship to society. We address this important issue in the following three sections.

First, *social responsibility* recognizes that businesses must respond to society's expectations regarding their obligations to society. Second, an emerging perspective, *shared value,* views social responsibility not just as an added cost to businesses. Instead, it views businesses as creators of value that they then share with society in a mutually beneficial relationship. Finally, we discuss the *triple bottom line approach* to evaluating a firm's performance. This perspective takes into account financial, social, and environmental performance.

Social Responsibility   **Social responsibility** is the expectation that businesses or individuals will strive to improve the overall welfare of society.[57] From the perspective of a business, this means that managers must take active steps to make society better by virtue

social responsibility
the expectation that businesses or individuals will strive to improve the overall welfare of society.

of the business being in existence.[58] Similar to norms and values, actions that constitute socially responsible behavior tend to change over time. In the 1970s affirmative action was a high priority, and during the 1990s and up to the present time, the public has been concerned about environmental quality. Many firms have responded to this by engaging in recycling and reducing waste. And in the wake of terrorist attacks on New York City and the Pentagon, as well as the continuing threat from terrorists worldwide, a new kind of priority has arisen: the need to be vigilant concerning public safety.

>LO1.4
The importance of social responsibility, including environmental sustainability, and how it can enhance a corporation's innovation strategy.

Today, demands for greater corporate responsibility have accelerated.[59] These include corporate critics, social investors, activists, and, increasingly, customers who claim to assess corporate responsibility when making purchasing decisions. Such demands go well beyond product and service quality.[60] They include a focus on issues such as labor standards, environmental sustainability, financial and accounting reporting, procurement, and environmental practices.[61] At times, a firm's reputation can be tarnished by exceedingly poor judgment on the part of one of its managers. For example, BP CEO Tony Hayward's decision to withhold information from the public about the magnitude of the oil spill in the Gulf of Mexico further damaged the firm's reputation.

A key stakeholder group that appears to be particularly susceptible to corporate social responsibility (CSR) initiatives is customers.[62] Surveys indicate a strong positive relationship between CSR behaviors and consumers' reactions to a firm's products and services.[63] For example:

- A study by GlobalScan, which included interviews with more than 30,000 people across 34 countries, found that more than 80 percent of Chinese consumers felt companies communicated "honestly and truthfully" about their social and environmental performances.[64]
- An Ipsos Reid/Canadian Business for Social Responsibility poll of Canadian businesses and consumers found that 68 percent pay close attention to issues related to corporate social responsibility.[65]

Such findings are consistent with a large body of research that confirms the positive influence of CSR on consumers' company evaluations and product purchase intentions across a broad range of product categories.

The Concept of "Shared Value"   Capitalism is typically viewed as an unparalleled vehicle for meeting human needs, improving efficiency, creating jobs, and building wealth.[66] However, a narrow conceptualization of capitalism has prevented business from harnessing its full potential to meet society's broader challenges. The opportunities have always been there but have been overlooked. It is increasingly acknowledged that businesses acting as businesses, not as charitable donors, are the most powerful force for addressing the pressing issues that we face. This new conception of capitalism redefines the purpose of the corporation as creating shared value, not just profit per se. This will drive the next wave of innovation and productivity growth in the global economy.

Shared value can be defined as policies and operating practices that enhance the competitiveness of a company while simultaneously advancing the economic and social conditions in which it operates. Shared value creation focuses on identifying and expanding the connections between societal and economic progress.[67]

Shared value is not about personal values. Nor is it about "sharing" the value created by firms—a redistribution approach. Instead, it is about expanding the total pool of economic and social value. A good example of this difference is the fair trade movement:

> Fair trade aims to increase the proportion of revenue that goes to poor farmers by paying them higher prices for the same crops. Though this may be a noble sentiment, fair trade is mostly about redistribution rather than expanding the overall amount of value created.

shared value policies and operating practices that enhance the competitiveness of a company while simultaneously advancing the economic and social conditions in which it operates.

A shared value perspective, however, focuses on improving growing techniques and strengthening the local cluster of supporting suppliers and other institutions in order to increase farmers' efficiency, yields, product quality, and sustainability. This leads to a bigger pie of revenue and profits that benefits both farmers and the companies that buy from them. Early studies of cocoa farmers in the Ivory Coast, for example, suggest that while fair trade can increase farmers' incomes by 10 to 20 percent, shared value investments can raise their incomes by more than 300 percent! Initial investment and time may be required to implement new procurement practices and develop the cluster. However, the return will be greater economic value and broader strategic benefits for all participants.

A firm's value chain inevitably affects—and is affected by—numerous societal issues. Opportunities to create shared value arise because societal problems can create economic costs in the firm's value chain. Such external factors inflict internal costs to the firm, even in the absence of regulation or resource taxes. For example, excess product packaging and greenhouse gases are not just costly to the environment but also costly to businesses.

The shared value perspective acknowledges that the congruence between societal progress and value chain productivity is far greater than traditionally believed. The synergy increases when firms consider societal issues from a shared value perspective and invent new ways of operating to address them. So far, however, relatively few firms have reaped the full productivity benefits.

Let's look at what a few companies are doing to reap "win-win" benefits by addressing societal challenges and, in so doing, enjoying higher productivity and profitability:

- Hindustan Unilever is creating a new direct-to-home distribution system. It is operated by underprivileged female entrepreneurs in Indian villages of fewer than 2,000 people. The firm provides microcredit and training and has more than 45,000 entrepreneurs covering about 100,000 villages across 15 Indian states. Project Shakti, the name of the distribution system, provides benefits to communities not only by giving women skills that often double their household income but also by reducing the spread of communicable diseases through increased access to hygiene products. Thus, the unique ability of business to market to hard-to-reach consumers can benefit society by getting life-altering products into the hands of people that need them. Project Shakti now accounts for 5 percent of Unilever's total revenues in India. It has also extended the company's reach into rural areas and built its brand in media-dark regions, creating major economic value for the company.

- Leading companies have learned that because of lost workdays and diminished employee productivity, poor health costs them far more than health benefits do. For example, Johnson & Johnson has helped employees stop smoking (a two-thirds reduction in the past 15 years) and has implemented many other new wellness programs at its divisions around the globe. Such initiatives have saved the company $250 million on health care costs, a return of $2.71 for every dollar spent on wellness from 2002 to 2008. Further, Johnson & Johnson has benefited from a more present and productive workforce.

- Olam International, a leading cashew producer, traditionally shipped its nuts from Africa to Asia for processing. By opening local processing plants and training workers in Tanzania, Mozambique, Nigeria, and the Ivory Coast, Olam cut its processing and shipping costs by as much as 25 percent and greatly reduced carbon emissions! Further, Olam built preferred relationships with local farmers. It has provided direct employment to 17,000 people—95 percent of whom are women—and indirect employment to an equal number of people, in rural areas where jobs otherwise were not available.

The Triple Bottom Line: Incorporating Financial as Well as Environmental and Social Costs

Many companies are now measuring what has been called a **"triple bottom line."** This involves assessing financial, social, and environmental performance. Shell, NEC, Procter & Gamble, and others have recognized that failing to account for the environmental and social costs of doing business poses risks to the company and its community.[68]

The environmental revolution has been almost four decades in the making.[69] In the 1960s and 1970s, companies were in a state of denial regarding their firms' impact on the natural environment. However, a series of visible ecological problems created a groundswell for strict governmental regulation. In the U.S., Lake Erie was "dead," and in Japan, people died of mercury poisoning. Clearly, the effects of global warming are being felt throughout the world. Some other examples include the following:

> **triple bottom line**
> assessment of a firm's financial, social, and environmental performance.

- Ice roads are melting, so Canadian diamond miners must airlift equipment at great cost instead of trucking it in.
- More severe storms and rising seas mean oil companies must build stronger rigs, and cities must build higher seawalls.
- The loss of permafrost and protective sea ice may force villages like Alaska's Shismaref to relocate.
- Yukon River salmon and fisheries are threatened by a surge of parasites associated with a jump in water temperature.
- Later winters have let beetles spread in British Columbia, killing 22 million acres of pine forests, an area the size of Maine.
- In Mali, Africa, crops are threatened. The rainy season is now too short for rice, and the dry season is too hot for potatoes.[70]

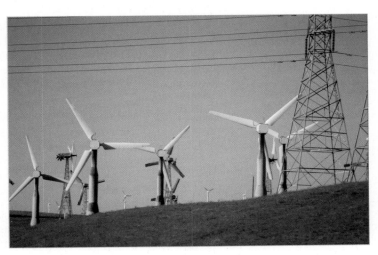

● Windpower is a more sustainable, environmentally friendly option than nuclear power plants or coal- or oil-fired power plants.

Stuart Hart, writing in the *Harvard Business Review,* addresses the magnitude of problems and challenges associated with the natural environment:

> The challenge is to develop a *sustainable global economy:* an economy that the planet is capable of supporting indefinitely. Although we may be approaching ecological recovery in the developed world, the planet as a whole remains on an unsustainable course. Increasingly, the scourges of the late twentieth century—depleted farmland, fisheries, and forests; choking urban pollution; poverty; infectious disease; and migration—are spilling over geopolitical borders. The simple fact is this: in meeting our needs, we are destroying the ability of future generations to meet theirs . . . corporations are the only organizations with the resources, the technology, the global reach, and, ultimately, the motivation to achieve sustainability.[71]

Environmental sustainability is now a value embraced by the most competitive and successful multinational companies.[72] McKinsey & Company's survey of more than 400 senior executives of companies around the world found that 92 percent agreed with former Sony President Akio Morita's contention that the environmental challenge will be one of the central issues in the 21st century.[73] Virtually all executives acknowledged their firm's responsibility to control pollution, and 83 percent agreed that corporations have an environmental responsibility for their products even after they are sold.

For many successful firms, environmental values are now becoming a central part of their cultures and management processes.[74] And, as noted earlier, environmental impacts are being audited and accounted for as the "third bottom line." According to one 2004 corporate report, "If we aren't good corporate citizens as reflected in a Triple Bottom Line that takes into account social and environmental responsibilities along with financial ones—eventually our stock price, our profits, and our entire business could suffer."[75]

Let's take a look at how Dell is making money and helping their customers at the end of their product's technology life cycle:[76]

Since computers generally have a rather short life cycle, companies are faced with real challenges over environmental and data liabilities when they need to dispose of obsolete equipment. Dell's Asset Recovery System helps customers deal with both the software and environmental cleanup they need.

For about $25 for a piece of equipment, Dell comes to your office and takes your computer away. They first perform a "destructive data overwrite" to eliminate all digital information on the computer, and then they dismantle the machine. Dell refurbishes and reuses some of the parts, and recycles the plastic. In the end, only 1 percent of the old computer's volume goes to a landfill.

This environmentally sustainable service enhances customer relationships and helps to drive sales. Dell discovered that the take-back role comes, conveniently, when Dell is delivering the next generation of equipment. Dell's executives would be happy if this service was just breaking even—but they are turning a profit on it. As noted by Daniel Esty and Andrew Winston in their book *Green to Gold,* "They seem a bit sheepish about doing so. We see no need to apologize."

Clearly, there are many other examples of how firms have profited by investing in socially responsible behavior, including those activities that enhance environmental sustainability. However, how do such "socially responsible" companies fare in terms of shareholder returns compared to benchmarks such as the Standard & Poor's 500 index? Strategy Spotlight 1.5 focuses on this issue.

>LO1.5
The need for greater empowerment throughout the organization.

The Strategic Management Perspective: An Imperative throughout the Organization

Strategic management requires managers to take an integrative view of the organization and assess how all of the functional areas and activities fit together to help an organization achieve its goals and objectives. This cannot be accomplished if only the top managers in the organization take an integrative, strategic perspective of issues facing the firm and everyone else "fends for themselves" in their independent, isolated functional areas. Instead, people throughout the organization must strive toward overall goals.

The need for such a perspective is accelerating in today's increasingly complex, interconnected, ever-changing, global economy. As noted by Peter Senge of MIT, the days when Henry Ford, Alfred Sloan, and Tom Watson (top executives at Ford, General Motors, and IBM, respectively) "learned for the organization are gone." He goes on to say:

In an increasingly dynamic, interdependent, and unpredictable world, it is simply no longer possible for anyone to "figure it all out at the top." The old model, "the top thinks and the local acts," must now give way to integrating thinking and acting at all levels. While the challenge is great, so is the potential payoff. "The person who figures out how to harness the collective genius of the people in his or her organization," according to former Citibank CEO Walter Wriston, "is going to blow the competition away."[77]

Socially Responsible Investing (SRI): Can You Do Well by Doing Good?

SRI is a broad-based approach to investing that now encompasses an estimated $3.07 trillion out of $25.2 trillion in the U.S. investment marketplace today. SRI recognizes that corporate responsibility and societal concerns are valid parts of investment decisions. With SRI, investors have the opportunity to put their money to work to build a more sustainable world while earning competitive returns both today and over time.

And, as the saying goes, nice guys don't have to finish last. The ING SRI, which tracks the stocks of 50 companies, enjoyed a 47.4 percent return in 2009. That easily beat the 26.5 percent gain of the Standard & Poor's 500-stock index. And a review of the 145 socially responsible equity mutual and exchange-traded funds tracked by Morningstar shows that 65 percent of them outperformed the S&P 500 last year.

Many socially responsible investing funds shun alcohol, tobacco, gambling, and defense companies—while embracing tech. Thus, they clearly benefitted from the 2009 returns of popular holdings, including Cisco (+46.9%), Microsoft (+60.5%), Google (+101.5%), and Intel (+43.9%). Over the recent 10-year period, Parnassus Equity Income and New Alternatives gained nearly 7 percent a year, on average, versus a 9 percent cumulative loss for the S&P 500 over the same period.

Another indication of the competitive performance of SRI funds is the performance of SRI indices over the long term. The longest running SRI index, the FTSE KLD 400, was started in 1990. Since that time, it has continued to perform competitively. It returned an average of 9.51 percent a year from inception through December 31, 2009, compared to 8.66 percent for the S&P 500 over the same period.

Sources: Kalwarski, T. 2010. It Pays to Be Good. *Bloomberg Businessweek.* February 1 & 8: 69; Anonymous. Undated. Performance and Socially Responsible Investments. *www.socialinvest.org.* np; Anonymous. Undated. Socially Responsible Investing Facts. *www.socialinvest.* np.

ethics

To develop and mobilize people and other assets, leaders are needed throughout the organization.[78] No longer can organizations be effective if the top "does the thinking" and the rest of the organization "does the work." Everyone must be involved in the strategic management process. There is a critical need for three types of leaders:

- *Local line leaders* who have significant profit-and-loss responsibility.
- *Executive leaders* who champion and guide ideas, create a learning infrastructure, and establish a domain for taking action.
- *Internal networkers* who, although they have little positional power and formal authority, generate their power through the conviction and clarity of their ideas.[79]

Sally Helgesen, author of *The Web of Inclusion: A New Architecture for Building Great Organizations,* also expressed the need for leaders throughout the organization. She asserted that many organizations "fall prey to the heroes-and-drones syndrome, exalting the value of those in powerful positions while implicitly demeaning the contributions of those who fail to achieve top rank."[80] Culture and processes in which leaders emerge at all levels, both up and down as well as across the organization, typify today's high-performing firms.[81]

Top-level executives are key in setting the tone for the empowerment of employees. Consider Richard Branson, founder of the Virgin Group, whose core businesses include retail operations, hotels, communications, and an airline. He is well known for creating a culture and an informal structure where anybody in the organization can be involved in generating and acting upon new business ideas. In an interview, he stated,

> [S]peed is something that we are better at than most companies. We don't have formal board meetings, committees, etc. If someone has an idea, they can pick up the phone and talk to me. I can vote "done, let's do it." Or, better still, they can just go ahead and do it. They know that they are not going to get a mouthful from me if they make a mistake. Rules and regulations are not our forte. Analyzing things to death is not our kind of thing. We very rarely sit back and analyze what we do.[82]

To inculcate a strategic management perspective throughout the organization, managers must often make a major effort to effect transformational change. This involves extensive communication, incentives, training, and development. For example, under the direction of Nancy Snyder, a corporate vice president, Whirlpool, the world's largest producer of household appliances, brought about a significant shift in the firm's reputation as an innovator.[83] This five-year initiative included both financial investments in capital spending as well as a series of changes in management processes, including training innovation mentors, making innovation a significant portion of leadership development programs, enrolling all salaried employees in online courses in business innovation, and providing employees with an innovation portal that allows them access to multiple innovation tools and data.

We'd like to close with our favorite example of how inexperience can be a virtue. It further reinforces the benefits of having broad involvement throughout the organization in the strategic management process (see Strategy Spotlight 1.6).

hierarchy of goals
organizational goals ranging from, at the top, those that are less specific yet able to evoke powerful and compelling mental images to, at the bottom, those that are more specific and measurable.

>LO1.6
How an awareness of a hierarchy of strategic goals can help an organization achieve coherence in its strategic direction.

Ensuring Coherence in Strategic Direction

Employees and managers throughout the organization must strive toward common goals and objectives.[84] By specifying desired results, it becomes much easier to move forward. Otherwise, when no one knows what the firm is striving to accomplish, they have no idea of what to work toward.

Organizations express priorities best through stated goals and objectives that form a **hierarchy of goals,** which includes its vision, mission, and strategic objectives.[85] What visions may lack in specificity, they make up for in their ability to evoke powerful and compelling mental images. On the other hand, strategic objectives tend to be more specific and provide a more direct means of determining if the organization is moving toward broader, overall goals.[86] Visions, as one would expect, also have longer time horizons than either mission statements or strategic objectives. Exhibit 1.6 depicts the hierarchy of goals and its relationship to two attributes: general versus specific and time horizon.

Organizational Vision

vision
organizational goal(s) that evoke(s) powerful and compelling mental images.

A **vision** is a goal that is "massively inspiring, overarching, and long term."[87] It represents a destination that is driven by and evokes passion. A vision may or may not succeed; it depends on whether everything else happens according to a firm's strategy. As Mark Hurd, Hewlett-Packard's CEO, humorously pointed out, "Without execution, vision is just another word for hallucination."[88]

Leaders must develop and implement a vision. In a survey of executives from 20 different countries, respondents were asked what they believed were a leader's key traits.[89] Ninety-eight percent responded that "a strong sense of vision" was the most important. Similarly, when asked about the critical knowledge skills, the leaders cited "strategy formulation to achieve a vision" as the most important skill. In other words, managers need to have not only a vision but also a plan to implement it. Regretfully, 90 percent reported a lack of confidence in their own skills and ability to conceive a vision.

Strategy and the Value of Inexperience

Peter Gruber, chairman of Mandalay Entertainment, explained how his firm benefited from the creative insights of an inexperienced intern.

Sometimes life is all about solving problems. In the movie business, at least, there seems to be one around every corner. One of the most effective lessons I've learned about tackling problems is to start by asking not "How to?" but rather "What if?" I learned that lesson from a young woman who was interning on a film I was producing. She actually saved the movie from being shelved by the studio.

The movie, *Gorillas in the Mist*, had turned into a logistical nightmare. We wanted to film at an altitude of 11,000 feet, in the middle of the jungle, in Rwanda—then on the verge of a revolution—and to use more than 200 animals. Warner Brothers, the studio financing the movie, worried that we would exceed our budget. But our biggest problem was that the screenplay required the gorillas to do what we wrote—in other words, to "act." If they couldn't or wouldn't, we'd have to fall back on a formula that the studio had seen fail before: using dwarfs in gorilla suits on a soundstage.

We called an emergency meeting to solve these problems. In the middle of it, a young intern asked, "What if you let the gorillas write the story?" Everyone laughed and wondered what she was doing in the meeting with experienced filmmakers. Hours later, someone casually asked her what she had meant. She said, "What if you sent a really good cinematographer into the jungle with a ton of film to shoot the gorillas. Then you could write a story around what the gorillas did on film." It was a brilliant idea. And we did exactly what she suggested: We sent Alan Root, an Academy Award–nominated cinematographer, into the jungle for three weeks. He came back with phenomenal footage that practically wrote the story for us. We shot the film for $20 million—half of the original budget!

This woman's inexperience enabled her to see opportunities where we saw only boundaries. This experience taught me three things. First, ask high-quality questions, like "What if?" Second, find people who add new perspectives and create new conversations. As experienced filmmakers, we believed that our way was the only way—and that the intern lacked the experience to have an opinion. Third, pay attention to those with new voices. If you want unlimited options for solving a problem, engage the "what if" before you lock onto the "how to." You'll be surprised by what you discover.

Source: Gruber, P. 1998. My greatest lesson. *Fast Company*, 15: 88, 90.

One of the most famous examples of a vision is Disneyland's: "To be the happiest place on earth." Other examples are:

- "Inspire the World, Create the Future." (Samsung Electronics)
- "Our vision is to be the world's best quick-service restaurant." (McDonald's)
- "To organize the world's information and make it universally accessible and useful." (Google)

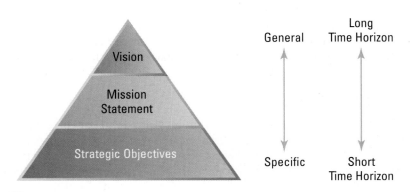

Exhibit 1.6 A Hierarchy of Goals

Although such visions cannot be accurately measured by a specific indicator of how well they are being achieved, they do provide a fundamental statement of an organization's values, aspirations, and goals. Such visions go well beyond narrow financial objectives, of course, and strive to capture both the minds and hearts of employees.

The vision statement may also contain a slogan, diagram, or picture—whatever grabs attention.[90] The aim is to capture the essence of the more formal parts of the vision in a few words that are easily remembered, yet that evoke the spirit of the entire vision statement. In its 20-year battle with Xerox, Canon's slogan, or battle cry, was "Beat Xerox." Motorola's slogan is "Total Customer Satisfaction." Panasonic's slogan is "Ideas for Life."

Clearly, vision statements are not a cure-all. Sometimes they backfire and erode a company's credibility. Visions fail for many reasons, including the following:[91]

The Walk Doesn't Match the Talk   An idealistic vision can arouse employee enthusiasm. However, that same enthusiasm can be quickly dashed if employees find that senior management's behavior is not consistent with the vision. Often, vision is a sloganeering campaign of new buzzwords and empty platitudes like "devotion to the customer," "teamwork," or "total quality" that aren't consistently backed by management's action.

Irrelevance   Visions created in a vacuum—unrelated to environmental threats or opportunities or an organization's resources and capabilities—often ignore the needs of those who are expected to buy into them. Employees reject visions that are not anchored in reality.

Not the Holy Grail   Managers often search continually for the one elusive solution that will solve their firm's problems—that is, the next "holy grail" of management. They may have tried other management fads only to find that they fell short of their expectations. However, they remain convinced that one exists. A vision simply cannot be viewed as a magic cure for an organization's illness.

Too Much Focus Leads to Missed Opportunities   The downside of too much focus is that, in directing people and resources toward a grandiose vision, losses can be devastating. Consider, Samsung's ambitious venture into automobile manufacturing:

> In 1992, Kun-Hee Lee, chairman of South Korea's Samsung Group, created a bold strategy to become one of the 10 largest car makers by 2010. Seduced by the clarity of the vision, Samsung bypassed staged entry through a joint venture or initial supply contract. Instead, Samsung borrowed heavily to build a state-of-the-art research and design facility and erect a greenfield factory, complete with cutting-edge robotics. Samsung Auto suffered operating losses and crushing interest charges from the beginning. And within a few years the business was divested for a fraction of the initial investment.[92]

An Ideal Future Irreconciled with the Present   Although visions are not designed to mirror reality, they must be anchored somehow in it. People have difficulty identifying with a vision that paints a rosy picture of the future but does not account for the often hostile environment in which the firm competes or that ignores some of the firm's weaknesses.

mission statement
a set of organizational goals that include the purpose of the organization, its scope of operations, and the basis of its competitive advantage.

Mission Statements

A company's **mission statement** differs from its vision in that it encompasses both the purpose of the company as well as the basis of competition and competitive advantage.

Exhibit 1.7 contains the vision statement and mission statement of McDonald's Corporation. Note that while the vision statement is broad based, the mission statement is more specific and focused on the means by which the firm will compete.

Exhibit 1.7
Comparing McDonald's Vision and Mission

Vision
To be the world's best quick-service restaurant experience.

Mission
Be the best employer for our people in each community around the world and deliver operational excellence to our customers in each of our restaurants.

Effective mission statements incorporate the concept of stakeholder management, suggesting that organizations must respond to multiple constituencies. Customers, employees, suppliers, and owners are the primary stakeholders, but others may also play an important role. Mission statements also have the greatest impact when they reflect an organization's enduring, overarching strategic priorities and competitive positioning. Mission statements also can vary in length and specificity. The two mission statements below illustrate these issues.

- To produce superior financial returns for our shareholders as we serve our customers with the highest quality transportation, logistics, and e-commerce. (Federal Express)
- Adidas-Salomon strives to be the global leader in the sporting goods industry, with sports brands built on a passion for sports and a sporting lifestyle. We are consumer focused. That means we continuously improve the quality, look, feel, and image of our products and our organizational structures to match and exceed consumer expectations and to provide them with the highest value. We are innovation and design leaders who seek to help athletes of all skill levels achieve peak performance with every product we bring to market. We are a global organization that is socially and environmentally responsible, creative and financially rewarding for our employees and shareholders. We are committed to continuously strengthening our brands and products to improve our competitive position and financial performance. In the medium term, we will extend our leading market position in Europe, expand our share of the U.S. footwear market and be the fastest-growing major sporting goods supplier in Asia and Latin America. The resulting top-line growth, together with strict cost control and working capital improvements, will drive over-proportionate earnings growth. (Adidas Group, global sporting goods manufacturer)[93]

Few mission statements identify profit or any other financial indicator as the sole purpose of the firm. Indeed, many do not even mention profit or shareholder return.[94] Employees of organizations or departments are usually the mission's most important audience. For them, the mission should help to build a common understanding of purpose and commitment to nurture.

A good mission statement, by addressing each principal theme, must communicate why an organization is special and different. Two studies that linked corporate values and mission statements with financial performance found that the most successful firms mentioned values other than profits. The less successful firms focused almost entirely on profitability.[95] In essence, profit is the metaphorical equivalent of oxygen, food, and water that the body requires. They are not the point of life, but without them, there is no life.

Vision statements tend to be quite enduring and seldom change. However, a firm's mission can and should change when competitive conditions dramatically change or the firm is faced with new threats or opportunities.

Strategy Spotlight 1.7 focuses on how Bridgestone Corporation refined its environmental mission statement to reflect its overall commitment to sustainability.

strategic objectives A set of organizational goals that are used to operationalize the mission statement and that are specific and cover a well-defined time frame.

Strategic Objectives

Strategic objectives are used to operationalize the mission statement.[96] That is, they help to provide guidance on how the organization can fulfill or move toward the "higher goals" in the goal hierarchy—the mission and vision. Thus, they are more specific and cover a more well-defined time frame. Setting objectives demands a yardstick to measure the fulfillment of the objectives.[97]

Exhibit 1.8 lists several firms' strategic objectives—both financial and nonfinancial. While most of them are directed toward generating greater profits and returns for the owners of the business, others are directed at customers or society at large.

For objectives to be meaningful, they need to satisfy several criteria. They must be:

- *Measurable.* There must be at least one indicator (or yardstick) that measures progress against fulfilling the objective.
- *Specific.* This provides a clear message as to what needs to be accomplished.
- *Appropriate.* It must be consistent with the organization's vision and mission.
- *Realistic.* It must be an achievable target given the organization's capabilities and opportunities in the environment. In essence, it must be challenging but doable.
- *Timely.* There must be a time frame for achieving the objective. As the economist John Maynard Keynes once said, "In the long run, we are all dead!"

When objectives satisfy the above criteria, there are many benefits. First, they help to channel all employees' efforts toward common goals. This helps the organization concentrate and conserve valuable resources and work collectively in a timely manner.

Exhibit 1.8
Strategic Objectives

Strategic Objectives (Financial)

- Increase sales growth 6 percent to 8 percent and accelerate core net earnings growth from 13 percent to 15 percent per share in each of the next 5 years. (Procter & Gamble)
- Increase the contribution of Banking Group earnings from investments, brokerage, and insurance from 16 percent to 25 percent. (Wells Fargo)
- Growth in earnings per share averaging 10 percent a year or better. (3M)

Strategic Objectives (Nonfinancial)

- We want a majority of our customers, when surveyed, to say they consider Wells Fargo the best financial institution in the community. (Wells Fargo)
- We want to operate 6,000 stores by 2010—up from 3,000 in the year 2000. (Walgreen's)
- Reduce greenhouse gases by 10 percent (from a 1990 base) by 2012. (BP Amoco)

Sources: Company documents and annual reports.

Bridgestone Refines Its Environmental Mission Statement

On behalf of its worldwide family of companies, Bridgestone Corporation released a refined global environmental mission statement in 2011. First released in 2009, the mission statement now clarifies the direction of Bridgestone's long-term environmental commitment and uses simpler language. Bridgestone updated the statement to help raise environmental awareness among its employees worldwide, "which in turn will lend strength to the company's efforts to develop and maintain a sustainable society," the company stated.

Source: Bridgestone Corporation website, *www.bridgestone.com/responsibilities/environment/index.html* and *www.bridgestone.com/corporate/news/2011052001.html*, accessed September 3, 2011.

Per the updated statement, the company is focusing on three objectives: "In order to exist *in harmony with nature,* Bridgestone will develop and utilize technologies that *value natural resources* while addressing the urgent matter of global warming through efforts to *reduce CO2 emissions."* The company clarified the direction of its long-term environmental aspirations while taking decisive action with respect to three important environmental issues: ecological conservation, resource conservation, and reduction of emissions.

The environmental mission statement continues to support Bridgestone's unchanging environmental philosophy, "to help ensure a healthy environment for current and future generations." But the statement update enables Bridgestone to enhance its commitment to a diverse range of environmental activities that go beyond its already wide-ranging areas of business.

Second, challenging objectives can help to motivate and inspire employees to higher levels of commitment and effort. Much research has supported the notion that people work harder when they are striving toward specific goals instead of being asked simply to "do their best."

Third, as we noted earlier in the chapter, there is always the potential for different parts of an organization to pursue their own goals rather than overall company goals. Although well intentioned, these may work at cross-purposes to the organization as a whole. Meaningful objectives thus help to resolve conflicts when they arise.

Finally, proper objectives provide a yardstick for rewards and incentives. They will ensure a greater sense of equity or fairness when rewards are allocated.

In summary, an organization must take care to ensure consistency throughout in how it implements strategic objectives. Consider how Textron, an $11 billion conglomerate, ensures that its corporate goals are effectively implemented:

> At Textron, each business unit identifies "improvement priorities" that it must act upon to realize the performance outlined in the firm's overall strategic plan. Each improvement priority is translated into action items with clearly defined accountabilities, timetables, and key performance indicators (KPIs) that enable executives to tell how a unit is delivering on a priority. Improvement priorities and action items cascade to every level at the firm—from the management committee (consisting of Textron's top five executives) down to the lowest levels in each of the company's 10 business units. Says Lewis Campbell, Textron's CEO, "Everyone needs to know: 'If I have only one hour to work, here's what I'm going to focus on.' Our goal deployment process makes each individual's accountabilities and priorities clear."[98]

As indicated in this example, organizations have lower-level objectives that are more specific than strategic objectives. These are often referred to as short-term objectives—essential components of a firm's "action plan" that are critical in implementing the firm's chosen strategy. We discuss these issues in detail in Chapter 9.

Reflecting on Career Implications . . .

- *Attributes of Strategic Management:* How do your activities and actions contribute to the goals of your organization? Observe the decisions you make on the job. What are the short-term and long-term implications of your decisions and actions? Have you recently made a decision that might yield short-term profits but might negatively impact the long-term goals of the organization (e.g., cutting maintenance expenses to meet a quarterly profit target)?
- *Intended versus Emergent Strategies:* Don't be too inflexible in your career strategies; strive to take advantage of new opportunities as they arise. Many promising career opportunities may "emerge" that were not part of your intended career strategy or your specific job assignment. Take initiative by pursuing opportunities to get additional training (e.g., learn a software or a statistical package), volunteering for a short-term overseas assignment, etc.
- *Ambidexterity:* Avoid defining your role in the organization too narrowly; look for opportunities to leverage your talents and your organization's resources to create value for your organization. This often involves collaborating with people in other departments or with your organization's customers and suppliers.
- *Strategic Coherence:* Focus your efforts on the "big picture" in your organization. In doing this, you should always strive to assure that your efforts are directed toward your organization's vision, mission, and strategic objectives.

Summary

We began this introductory chapter by defining strategic management and articulating some of its key attributes. Strategic management is defined as "consisting of the analyses, decisions, and actions an organization undertakes in order to create and sustain competitive advantages." The issue of how and why some firms outperform others in the marketplace is central to the study of strategic management. Strategic management has four key attributes: It is directed at overall organizational goals, includes multiple stakeholders, incorporates both short-term and long-term perspectives, and incorporates trade-offs between efficiency and effectiveness.

The second section discussed the strategic management process. Here, we paralleled the above definition of strategic management and focused on three core activities in the strategic management process—strategy analysis, strategy formulation, and strategy implementation. We noted how each of these activities is highly interrelated to and interdependent on the others. We also discussed how each of the 12 chapters in this text fits into the three core activities.

Next, we introduced two important concepts—corporate governance and stakeholder management—which must be taken into account throughout the strategic management process. Governance mechanisms can be broadly divided into two groups: internal and external. Internal governance mechanisms include shareholders (owners), management (led by the chief executive officer), and the board of directors. External control is exercised by auditors, banks, analysts, and an active business press as well as the threat of takeovers. We identified five key stakeholders in all organizations: owners, customers, suppliers, employees, and society at large. Successful firms go beyond an overriding focus on satisfying solely the interests of owners. Rather, they recognize the inherent conflicts that arise among the demands of the various stakeholders as well as the need to endeavor to attain "symbiosis"—that is, interdependence and mutual benefit—among the various stakeholder groups. The emerging practice of crowdsourcing, wherein the Internet is used to generate ideas and solve problems, is leading to an evolution in stakeholder roles. Managers must also recognize the need to act in a socially responsible manner, which, if done effectively, can enhance a firm's innovativeness. The "shared value" approach represents an innovative perspective on creating value for the firm and society at the same time. The managers also should recognize and incorporate issues related to environmental sustainability in their strategic actions.

In the fourth section, we discussed factors that have accelerated the rate of unpredictable change that managers face today. Such factors, and the combination of them, have increased the need for managers and employees throughout the organization to have a strategic management perspective and to become more empowered.

The final section addressed the need for consistency among a firm's vision, mission, and strategic objectives. Collectively, they form an organization's hierarchy of goals. Visions should evoke powerful and compelling mental images. However, they are not very specific. Strategic objectives, on the other hand, are much more specific and are vital to ensuring that the organization is striving toward fulfilling its vision and mission.

Summary Review Questions

1. How is "strategic management" defined in the text, and what are its four key attributes?

2. Briefly discuss the three key activities in the strategic management process. Why is it important for managers to recognize the interdependent nature of these activities?

3. Explain the concept of "stakeholder management." Why shouldn't managers be solely interested in stockholder management, that is, maximizing the returns for owners of the firm—its shareholders?

4. What is "corporate governance"? What are its three key elements and how can it be improved?

5. How can "symbiosis" (interdependence, mutual benefit) be achieved among a firm's stakeholders?

6. Why do firms need to have a greater strategic management perspective and empowerment in the strategic management process throughout the organization?

7. What is meant by a "hierarchy of goals"? What are the main components of it, and why must consistency be achieved among them?

Key Terms

romantic view of leadership, 45
external control view of leadership, 46
strategic management, 48
strategy, 48
competitive advantage, 48
operational effectiveness, 48
stakeholders, 49
effectiveness, 50
efficiency, 50
ambidexterity, 50
strategic management process, 50
intended strategy, 51
realized strategy, 52
strategy analysis, 52
strategy formulation, 54
strategy implementation, 55
corporate governance, 55
stakeholder management, 57
crowdsourcing, 58
social responsibility, 60
shared value, 61
triple bottom line, 63
hierarchy of goals, 66
vision, 66
mission statement, 68
strategic objectives, 70

Experiential Exercise

Using the Internet or library sources, select four organizations—two in the private sector and two in the public sector. Find their mission statements. Complete the following exhibit by identifying the stakeholders that are mentioned. Evaluate the differences between firms in the private sector and those in the public sector.

Name			
Mission Statement			
Stakeholders (✓ = mentioned)			
1. Customers			
2. Suppliers			
3. Managers/employees			
4. Community-at-large			
5. Owners			
6. Others?			
7. Others?			

Application Questions & Exercises

1. Go to the Internet and look up one of these company sites: *www.walmart.com, www.ge.com*, or *www.lgcorp.com*. What are some of the key events that would represent the "romantic" perspective of leadership? What are some of the key events that depict the "external control" perspective of leadership?

2. Select a company that competes in an industry in which you are interested. What are some of the recent demands that stakeholders have placed on this company? Can you find examples of how the company is trying to develop "symbiosis" (interdependence and mutual benefit) among its stakeholders? (Use the Internet and other resources.)

3. Provide examples of companies that are actively trying to increase the amount of empowerment in the strategic management process throughout the organization. Do these companies seem to be having positive outcomes? Why? Why not?

4. Look up the vision statements and/or mission statements for several companies from around the world. Do you feel that they are constructive and useful as a means of motivating employees and providing a strong strategic direction? Why? Why not? (*Note:* Annual reports, along with the Internet, may be good sources of information.)

Ethics Questions

1. A company focuses solely on short-term profits to provide the greatest return to the owners of the business (i.e., the shareholders in a publicly held firm). What ethical issues could this raise?

2. A firm has spent some time—with input from managers at all levels—in developing a vision statement and a mission statement. Over time, however, the behavior of some executives is contrary to these statements. Could this raise some ethical issues?

References

1. Gunther, M. 2010. Fallen angels. *Fortune,* November 1: 75–78.

2. Sidhu, I. 2010. *Doing both.* East Saddle River, NJ & London: FT Press; ben-Aaron, D. 2010. After Nokia, can angry birds propel Finland? *Bloomberg Businessweek,* December 6–December 12: 48–50; ben-Aaron, D. 2010. Nokia board faces call for change on $77 billion lost value. *www.bloomberg.com/news.* July 15: np; Anonymous. 2010. The curse of the alien boss. *The Economist.* August 7: 65; and, Lynn, M. 2010. The fallen king of Finland. *Bloomberg Businessweek,* September 26: 6–7. We thank Pratik Kapadia for his valued contribution.

3. For a discussion of the "romantic" versus "external control" perspective, refer to Meindl, J. R. 1987. The romance of leadership and the evaluation of organizational performance. *Academy of Management Journal,* 30: 92–109; and Pfeffer, J. & Salancik, G. R. 1978. *The external control of organizations: A resource dependence perspective.* New York: Harper & Row.

4. A recent perspective on the "romantic view" of leadership is provided by Mintzberg, H. 2004. Leadership and management development: An afterword. *Academy of Management Executive,* 18(3): 140–142.

5. For a discussion of the best and worst managers for 2008, read: Anonymous. 2009. The best managers. *BusinessWeek,* January 19: 40–41; and, The worst managers. On page 42 in the same issue.

6. Burrows, P. 2009. Apple without its core? *BusinessWeek,* January 26/February 2: 31.

7. For an insightful discussion of Steve Jobs's impact on Apple, read: Satariano, A. 2011. The essence of Apple. *Bloomberg Businessweek,* January 24–January 30: 6–8; Friedman, L. October 17, 2011. iPhone 4S sales top 4 million; 25 million iOS 5 upgrades. Accessed at *www.macworld.com.*

8. For a study on the effects of CEOs on firm performance, refer to: Kor, Y. Y. & Misangyi, V. F. 2008. *Strategic Management Journal,* 29(11): 1357–1368.

9. Charan, R. & Colvin, G. 2010. Directors: A harsh new reality. *money.cnn.com.* October 6: np.

10. Dobson, C. 2010. Global airlines lost $1.7 billion due to Iceland ash cloud. *www.theepochtimes.com.* May 23: np; and Pylas, P. 2011. Nikkei slides 11 percent on radiation fears. *www.finance.yahoo.com.* March 14: np.

11. Ewing, J. 2008. South Africa emerges from the shadows. *BusinessWeek,* December 15: 52–56.

12. For an interesting perspective on the need for strategists to maintain a global mind-set, refer to Begley, T. M. & Boyd, D. P. 2003. The need for a global mind-set. *MIT Sloan Management Review,* 44(2): 25–32.

13. Porter, M. E. 1996. What is strategy? *Harvard Business Review,* 74(6): 61–78.

14. See, for example, Barney, J. B. & Arikan, A. M. 2001. The resource-based view: Origins and implications. In Hitt, M. A., Freeman, R. E., & Harrison, J. S. (Eds.), *Handbook of strategic management:* 124–189. Malden, MA: Blackwell.

15. Porter, M. E. 1996. What is strategy? *Harvard Business Review,* 74(6): 61–78; and Hammonds, K. H. 2001. Michael Porter's big ideas. *Fast Company,* March: 55–56.

16. This section draws upon Dess, G. G. & Miller, A. 1993. *Strategic management.* New York: McGraw-Hill.

17. See, for example, Hrebiniak, L. G. & Joyce, W. F. 1986. The strategic

importance of managing myopia. *Sloan Management Review,* 28(1): 5–14.

18. For an insightful discussion on how to manage diverse stakeholder groups, refer to Rondinelli, D. A. & London, T. 2003. How corporations and environmental groups cooperate: Assessing cross-sector alliances and collaborations. *Academy of Management Executive,* 17(1): 61–76.

19. Some dangers of a short-term perspective are addressed in: Van Buren, M. E. & Safferstone, T. 2009. The quick wins paradox. *Harvard Business Review,* 67(1): 54–61.

20. Senge, P. 1996. Leading learning organizations: The bold, the powerful, and the invisible. In Hesselbein, F., Goldsmith, M., & Beckhard, R. (Eds.), *The leader of the future:* 41–58. San Francisco: Jossey-Bass.

21. Samuelson, J. 2006. A critical mass for the long term. *Harvard Business Review,* 84(2): 62, 64; and, Anonymous. 2007. Power play. *The Economist,* January 20: 10–12.

22. Loeb, M. 1994. Where leaders come from. *Fortune,* September 19: 241 (quoting Warren Bennis).

23. Address by Norman R. Augustine at the Crummer Business School, Rollins College, Winter Park, FL, October 20, 1989.

24. Cheng, D. S. 2009. *The Baidu World of Li Yanhong.* Shanghai: Zhongxin Publishing Group.

25. New perspectives on "management models" are addressed in: Birkinshaw, J. & Goddard, J. 2009. What is your management model? *MIT Sloan Management Review,* 50(2): 81–90.

26. Mintzberg, H. 1985. Of strategies: Deliberate and emergent. *Strategic Management Journal,* 6: 257–272.

27. Some interesting insights on decision-making processes are found in: Nutt, P. C. 2008. Investigating the success of decision making processes. *Journal of Management Studies,* 45(2): 425–455.

28. Halls, S. 2011. London Olympics Drops Carbon-Offset Plan. *www.bloomberg.com/news.* August 31.

29. A study investigating the sustainability of competitive advantage is: Newbert, S. L. 2008. Value, rareness, competitive advantages, and performance: A conceptual-level empirical investigation of the resource-based view of the firm. *Strategic Management Journal,* 29(7): 745–768.

30. Good insights on mentoring are addressed in: DeLong, T. J., Gabarro, J. J., & Lees, R. J. 2008. Why mentoring matters in a hypercompetitive world. *Harvard Business Review,* 66(1): 115–121.

31. A unique perspective on differentiation strategies is: Austin, R. D. 2008. High margins and the quest for aesthetic coherence. *Harvard Business Review,* 86(1): 18–19.

32. Some insights on partnering in the global area are discussed in: MacCormack, A. & Forbath, T. 2008. *Harvard Business Review,* 66(1): 24, 26.

33. For insights on how firms can be successful in entering new markets in emerging economies, refer to: Eyring, M. J., Johnson, M. W., & Nair, H. 2011. New business models in emerging markets. *Harvard Business Review,* 89(1/2): 88–95.

34. An interesting discussion of the challenges of strategy implementation is: Neilson, G. L., Martin, K. L., & Powers, E. 2008. The secrets of strategy execution. *Harvard Business Review,* 86(6): 61–70.

35. Interesting perspectives on strategy execution involving the link between strategy and operations are addressed in: Kaplan, R. S. & Norton, D. P. 2008. Mastering the management system. *Harvard Business Review,* 66(1): 62–77.

36. An innovative perspective on organizational design is found in: Garvin, D. A. & Levesque, L. C. 2008. The multiunit enterprise. *Harvard Business Review,* 86(6): 106–117.

37. Monks, R. & Minow, N. 2001. *Corporate governance* (2nd ed.). Malden, MA: Blackwell.

38. Intel Corp. 2007. *Intel Corporation board of directors' guidelines on significant corporate governance issues. www.intel.com.*

39. Jones, T. J., Felps, W., & Bigley, G. A. 2007. Ethical theory and stakeholder-related decisions: The role of stakeholder culture. *Academy of Management Review,* 32(1): 137–155.

40. For example, see: The best (& worst) managers of the year, 2003. *Businessweek,* January 13: 58–92; and Lavelle, M. 2003. Rogues of the year. *Time,* January 6: 33–45.

41. Handy, C. 2002. What's a business for? *Harvard Business Review,* 80(12): 49–55.

42. Anonymous, 2007. In the money. *Economist,* January 20: 3–6.

43. Hessel, E. & Woolley, S. 2008. Your money or your life. *Forbes,* October 27: 52.

44. Some interesting insights on the role of activist investors can be found in: Greenwood, R. & Schol, M. 2008. When (not) to listen to activist investors. *Harvard Business Review,* 66(1): 23–24.

45. For an interesting perspective on the changing role of boards of directors, refer to Lawler, E. & Finegold, D. 2005. Rethinking governance. *MIT Sloan Management Review,* 46(2): 67–70.

46. Benz, M. & Frey, B. S. 2007. Corporate governance: What can we learn from public governance? *Academy of Management Review,* 32(1): 92–104.

47. The salience of shareholder value is addressed in: Carrott, G. T. & Jackson, S. E. 2009. Shareholder value must top the CEO's agenda. *Harvard Business Review,* 67(1): 22–24.

48. Stakeholder symbiosis. 1998. *Fortune,* March 30: S2.

49. An excellent review of stakeholder management theory can be found in: Laplume, A. O., Sonpar, K., & Litz, R. A. 2008. Stakeholder theory: Reviewing a theory that moves us. *Journal of Management,* 34(6): 1152–1189.

50. For a definitive, recent discussion of the stakeholder concept, refer to Freeman, R. E. & McVae, J. 2001. A stakeholder approach to strategic management. In Hitt, M. A., Freeman, R. E., & Harrison, J. S. (Eds.). *Handbook of strategic management:* 189–207. Malden, MA: Blackwell.

51. Harrison, J. S., Bosse, D. A., & Phillips, R. A. 2010. Managing for stakeholders, stakeholder utility

functions, and competitive advantage. *Strategic Management Journal,* 31(1): 58–74.

52. For an insightful discussion on the role of business in society, refer to Handy, op. cit.

53. Camillus, J. 2008. Strategy as a wicked problem. *Harvard Business Review,* 86(5): 100–101.

54. Stakeholder symbiosis, op. cit., p. S3.

55. Sidhu, I. 2010. *Doing both.* FT Press: Upper Saddle River, NJ: 7–8.

56. Our discussion of crowdsourcing draws on the first two books that have addressed this concept: Libert, B. & Spector, J. 2008. *We are smarter than me.* Philadelphia: Wharton Publishing; and, Howe, J. 2008. *Crowdsourcing.* New York: Crown Business. Eric von Hippel has addressed similar ideas in his earlier book (2005. *Democratizing innovation.* Cambridge, MA: MIT Press).

57. Thomas, J. G. 2000. Macroenvironmetal forces. In Helms, M. M. (Ed.), *Encyclopedia of management.* (4th ed.): 516–520. Farmington Hills, MI: Gale Group.

58. For a strong advocacy position on the need for corporate values and social responsibility, read Hollender, J. 2004. What matters most: Corporate values and social responsibility. *California Management Review,* 46(4): 111–119.

59. Waddock, S. & Bodwell, C. 2004. Managing responsibility: What can be learned from the quality movement. *California Management Review,* 47(1): 25–37.

60. For a discussion of the role of alliances and collaboration on corporate social responsibility initiatives, refer to Pearce, J. A., II & Doh, J. P. 2005. The high impact of collaborative social initiatives. *MIT Sloan Management Review,* 46(3): 30–40.

61. Insights on ethical behavior and performance are addressed in: Trudel, R. & Cotte, J. 2009. *MIT Sloan Management Review,* 50(2): 61–68.

62. Bhattacharya, C. B. & Sen, S. 2004. Doing better at doing good: When, why, and how consumers respond to corporate social initiatives. *California Management Review,* 47(1): 9–24.

63. For some findings on the relationship between corporate social responsibility and firm performance, see: Margolis, J. D. & Elfenbein, H. A. 2008. *Harvard Business Review,* 86(1): 19–20.

64. GlobalScan Study. 2005. *www .globalscan.com.*.

65. Ipsos Reid Survey. 2006. *www.ipsosna.com.*

66. This section draws on: Porter, M. E. & Kramer, M. R. 2011. Creating shared value. *Harvard Business Review,* 89 (1/2): 62–77.

67. A similar concept is conscious capitalism. Refer, for example, to: Sheth, J. N. 2007. *Firms of endearment: How world-class companies profit from passion and purpose.* Philadelphia, PA: Wharton Publishing.

68. An insightful discussion of the risks and opportunities associated with global warming, refer to: Lash, J. & Wellington, F. 2007. Competitive advantage on a warming planet. *Harvard Business Review,* 85(3): 94–102.

69. This section draws on Hart, S. L. 1997. Beyond greening: Strategies for a sustainable world. *Harvard Business Review,* 75(1): 66–76; and, Berry, M. A. & Rondinelli, D. A. 1998. Proactive corporate environmental management: A new industrial revolution. *Academy of Management Executive,* 12(2): 38–50.

70. Carey, J. 2006. Business on a warmer planet. *BusinessWeek,* July 17: 26–29.

71. Hart, op. cit., p. 67.

72. For a creative perspective on environmental sustainability and competitive advantage as well as ethical implications, read Ehrenfeld, J. R. 2005. The roots of sustainability. *MIT Sloan Management Review,* 46(2): 23–25.

73. McKinsey & Company. 1991. *The corporate response to the environmental challenge.* Summary Report, Amsterdam: McKinsey & Company.

74. Delmas, M. A. & Montes-Sancho, M. J. 2010. Voluntary agreements to improve environmental quality: Symbolic and substantive cooperation. *Strategic Management Journal,* 31(6): 575–601.

75. Vogel, D. J. 2005. Is there a market for virtue? The business case

for corporate social responsibility. *California Management Review,* 47(4): 19–36.

76. Esty, D. C. & Winston, A. S. 2009. *Green to gold.* Hoboken, NJ: Wiley: 124–125.

77. Senge, P. M. 1990. The leader's new work: Building learning organizations. *Sloan Management Review,* 32(1): 7–23.

78. For an interesting perspective on the role of middle managers in the strategic management process, refer to Huy, Q. H. 2001. In praise of middle managers. *Harvard Business Review,* 79(8): 72–81.

79. Senge, 1996, op. cit., pp. 41–58.

80. Helgesen, S. 1996. Leading from the grass roots. In Hesselbein, F., Goldsmith, M., & Beckhard, R. (Eds.), *The leader of the future:* 19–24. San Francisco: Jossey-Bass.

81. Wetlaufer, S. 1999. Organizing for empowerment: An interview with AES's Roger Sant and Dennis Blake. *Harvard Business Review,* 77(1): 110–126.

82. Kets de Vries, M. F. R. 1998. Charisma in action: The transformational abilities of Virgin's Richard Branson and ABB's Percy Barnevik. *Organizational Dynamics,* 26(3): 7–21.

83. Hamel, G. 2006. The why, what, and how of management innovation. *Harvard Business Review,* 84(2): 72–84.

84. An interesting discussion on how to translate top management's goals into concrete actions is found in: Bungay, S. 2011. How to make the most of your company's strategy. *Harvard Business Review,* 89(1/2): 132–40.

85. An insightful discussion about the role of vision, mission, and strategic objectives can be found in: Collis, D. J. & Rukstad, M. G. 2008. Can you say what your strategy is? *Harvard Business Review,* 66(4): 82–90.

86. Our discussion draws on a variety of sources. These include Lipton, M. 1996. Demystifying the development of an organizational vision. *Sloan Management Review,* 37(4): 83–92; Bart, C. K. 2000. Lasting inspiration. *CA Magazine,* May: 49–50; and Quigley, J. V. 1994. Vision:

How leaders develop it, share it, and sustain it. *Business Horizons,* September–October: 37–40.

87. Lipton, op. cit.

88. Hardy, Q. 2007. The UnCarly. *Forbes,* March 12: 82–90.

89. Some interesting perspective on gender differences in organizational vision are discussed in: Ibarra, H. & Obodaru, O. 2009. Women and the vision thing. *Harvard Business Review,* 67(1): 62–70.

90. Quigley, op. cit.

91. Lipton, op. cit. Additional pitfalls are addressed in this article.

92. Sull, D. N. 2005. Strategy as active waiting. *Harvard Business Review,* 83(9): 120–130.

93. Adidas Group corporate website, Our Group page, accessed at *www.adidas-group.com/en/ourgroup/OurGroup_AreaStart.aspx.*

94. Lipton, op. cit.

95. Sexton, D. A. & Van Aukun, P. M. 1985. A longitudinal study of small business strategic planning. *Journal of Small Business Management,* January: 8–15, cited in Lipton, op. cit.

96. For an insightful perspective on the use of strategic objectives, refer to Chatterjee, S. 2005. Core objectives: Clarity in designing strategy. *California Management Review,* 47(2): 33–49.

97. Ibid.

98. Mankins, M. M. & Steele, R. 2005. Turning great strategy into great performance. *Harvard Business Review,* 83(5): 66–73.

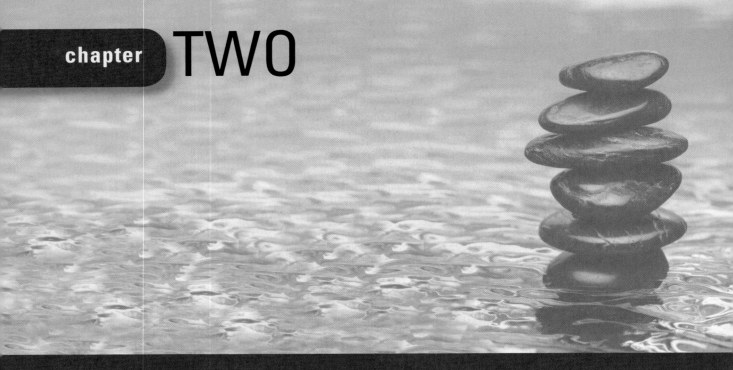

chapter TWO

Analyzing the External Environment of the Firm

Creating Competitive Advantages

After reading this chapter, you should have a good understanding of:

LO2.1 The importance of developing forecasts of the business environment.

LO2.2 Why environmental scanning, environmental monitoring, and collecting competitive intelligence are critical inputs to forecasting.

LO2.3 Why scenario planning is a useful technique for firms competing in industries characterized by unpredictability and change.

LO2.4 The impact of the general environment on a firm's strategies and performance.

LO2.5 How forces in the competitive environment can affect profitability, and how a firm can improve its competitive position by increasing its power vis-à-vis these forces.

LO2.6 How the Internet and digitally based capabilities are affecting the five competitive forces and industry profitability.

LO2.7 The concept of strategic groups and their strategy and performance implications.

LEARNING OBJECTIVES

Strategies are not and should not be developed in a vacuum. They must be responsive to the external business environment. Otherwise, your firm could become, in effect, the most efficient producer of buggy whips, leisure suits, or typewriters. To avoid such strategic mistakes, firms must become knowledgeable about the business environment. One tool for analyzing trends is forecasting. In the development of forecasts, environmental scanning and environmental monitoring are important in detecting key trends and events. Managers also must aggressively collect and disseminate competitor intelligence. The information gleaned from these three activities is invaluable in developing forecasts and scenarios to minimize present and future threats as well as to exploit opportunities. We address these issues in the first part of this chapter. We also introduce a basic tool of strategy analysis—the concept of SWOT analysis (strengths, weaknesses, opportunities, and threats).

In the second part of the chapter, we present two frameworks for analyzing the external environment—the general environment and the competitive environment. The general environment consists of six segments—demographic, sociocultural, political/legal, technological, economic, and global. Trends and events in these segments can have a dramatic impact on your firm.

The competitive environment is closer to home. It consists of five industry-related factors that can dramatically affect the average level of industry profitability. An awareness of these factors is critical in making decisions such as which industries to enter and how to improve your firm's current position within an industry. This awareness is helpful in neutralizing competitive threats and increasing power over customers and suppliers. We also address how industry and competitive practices are being affected by the capabilities provided by Internet technologies. In the final part of this section, we place firms within an industry into strategic groups based on similarities in resources and strategies. As we will see, the concept of strategic groups has important implications for the intensity of rivalry and how the effects of a given environmental trend or event differ across groups.

Learning from Mistakes

The emerging middle-class market in China has grown rapidly, and its appetite for consumerism and savings has skyrocketed.[1] Currently the upper tier of China's wealthiest account for 25 percent of Chinese household savings and will continue to control the bulk of the nation's accumulated wealth—60 percent by 2025. Their importance to banks and other financial-services firms will therefore increase. As the first foreign bank—and now the largest foreign financial institution in Hong Kong—Citibank Hong Kong was counting on over 100 years of successful, award-winning business strategies to help it grow along with China's economy and its increasing consumer financial needs. But it suffered from a misstep . . .

The company expected favorable results after launching a 15 percent customer discount program in partnership with a restaurant chain. However, Citibank found itself in the hot seat, or bowl for that matter, with many environmentally conscious customers. In a matter of days, social media campaigns had sprung up condemning the promotion. Citibank Hong Kong quickly removed the promotion after being inundated with emails and calls to action. So how did this shining example of a foreign company tarnish its reputation abroad?

Well . . . the cultural delicacy item that Citibank Hong Kong promoted (with partner Maxim's Chinese Cuisine outlets) was shark fin soup, a soup that is increasingly known for contributing to an estimated 90–100 million shark deaths per year due to definning. The prized fins are collected from live sharks by removing them and then throwing the sharks back in the ocean to die. The company tried to promote a rare, high-status item (US$150/bowl), but ignored the growing sensitivity the market had toward shark fin soup. Citibank Hong Kong lost sight of its environmentally informed market and paid the price when this issue was widely publicized.

Successful managers must recognize opportunities and threats in their firm's external environment. They must be aware of what's going on outside their company. If they focus exclusively on the efficiency of internal operations, the firm may degenerate into the world's most efficient producer of buggy whips, typewriters, or carbon paper. But if they miscalculate the market, opportunities will be lost—hardly an enviable position for their firm. As we saw from the Citibank Hong Kong example, misreading the market can lead to negative consequences—and even adversely affect a firm's reputation.

In *Competing for the Future,* Gary Hamel and C. K. Prahalad suggest that "every manager carries around in his or her head a set of biases, assumptions, and presuppositions about the structure of the relevant 'industry,' about how one makes money in the industry, about who the competition is and isn't, about who the customers are and aren't, and so on."[2] Environmental analysis requires you to continually question such assumptions. Peter Drucker labeled these interrelated sets of assumptions the "theory of the business."[3] The sudden reversal in Nokia's fortunes (discussed in chapter 1) clearly illustrates that if a company does not keep pace with changes in the external environment, sustaining competitive advantages and delivering strong financial results become difficult.

● Citibank Hong Kong paid a high price for promoting shark fin soup for a sales promotion in China.

A firm's strategy may be good at one point in time, but it may go astray when management's frame of reference gets out of touch with the realities of the actual business situation. This results when management's assumptions, premises, or beliefs are incorrect or when internal inconsistencies among them render the overall "theory of the business" invalid. As Warren Buffett, investor extraordinaire, colorfully notes, "Beware of past performance 'proofs.' If history books were the key to riches, the Forbes 400 would consist of librarians."

In the business world, many once successful firms have fallen. Consider the high-tech company Novell, which went head-to-head with Microsoft. Novell bought market-share loser WordPerfect to compete with Microsoft Word. The result? A $1.3 billion loss when Novell sold WordPerfect to Corel. And today we may wonder who will be the next Blockbuster, Circuit City, or *Encyclopaedia Britannica*.

Creating the Environmentally Aware Organization

So how do managers become environmentally aware?[4] We will now address three important processes—scanning, monitoring, and gathering competitive intelligence—used to develop forecasts.[5] Exhibit 2.1 illustrates relationships among these important activities. We also discuss the importance of scenario planning in anticipating major future changes in the external environment and the role of SWOT analysis.[6]

>LO2.1
The importance of developing forecasts of the business environment.

The Role of Scanning, Monitoring, Competitive Intelligence, and Forecasting

Environmental Scanning   **Environmental scanning** involves surveillance of a firm's external environment to predict environmental changes and detect changes already under way.[7] This alerts the organization to critical trends and events before changes develop a discernible pattern and before competitors recognize them.[8] Otherwise, the firm may be forced into a reactive mode.[9]

Experts agree that spotting key trends requires a combination of knowing your business and your customer as well as keeping an eye on what's happening around you.[10] Such a big-picture/small-picture view enables you to better identify the emerging trends that will affect your business. We suggest a few tips in Exhibit 2.2.

Leading firms in an industry can also be a key indicator of emerging trends.[11] For example, with its wide range of household goods, global giant Procter & Gamble is a barometer for consumer spending. Any sign that it can sell more of its premium products without cutting prices sharply indicates that shoppers may finally be becoming

>LO2.2
Why environmental scanning, environmental monitoring, and collecting competitive intelligence are critical inputs to forecasting.

environmental scanning surveillance of a firm's external environment to predict environmental changes and detect changes already under way.

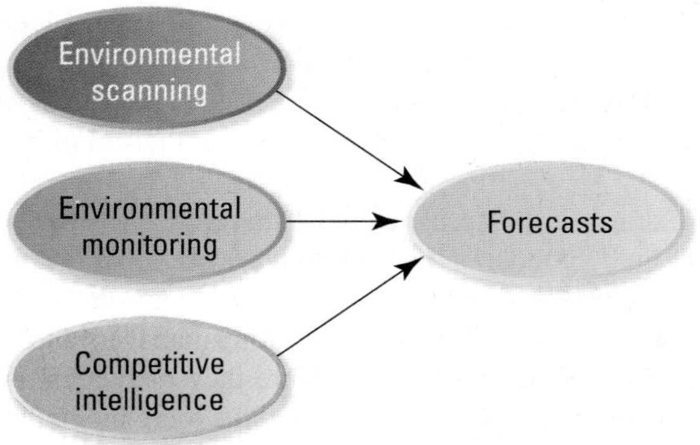

Exhibit 2.1   **Inputs to Forecasting**

Exhibit 2.2
Some Suggestions on
How to Spot Hot Trends

- **Listen.** Ask your customers questions about your products and services. Ask what they are looking for next. Find out what media they're watching and what they think of current events.
- **Pay attention.** Read trade publications related to your industry to identify key issues. Watch industries that are always on the cutting edge, such as technology, music, and fashion, in order to discover emerging trends that may affect your business.
- **Follow trends online.** Trend-hunting websites such as *trendhunter.com* and *jwtintelligence.com* offer up the trends du jour. Add them to your regular web-surfing itinerary.
- **Go old school.** Ask your customers what they think. Organize online or in-person focus groups to find out what people are thinking. You can also launch social media groups or chat rooms to gather feedback from your audience.

Source: Moran, G. 2008. Be Your Own Trendspotter. *Entrepreneur*, December: 17.

less price-sensitive with everyday purchases. In particular, investors will examine the performance of beauty products such as Bourjois cosmetics (France) and Nivea lotion products (Germany) for evidence that spending on small, discretionary pick-me-ups is improving.

Strategy Spotlight 2.1 addresses how Zara, a Spanish fashion retailer, keeps abreast of trends and promising opportunities.

Environmental Monitoring **Environmental monitoring** tracks the evolution of environmental trends, sequences of events, or streams of activities. They may be trends that the firm came across by accident or ones that were brought to its attention from outside the organization.[12] Monitoring enables firms to evaluate how dramatically environmental trends are changing the competitive landscape. Such indices are critical for managers in determining a firm's strategic direction and resource allocation.

Competitive Intelligence **Competitive intelligence** (CI) helps firms define and understand their industry and identify rivals' strengths and weaknesses.[13] This includes the intelligence gathering associated with collecting data on competitors and interpreting such data. Done properly, competitive intelligence helps a company avoid surprises by anticipating competitors' moves and decreasing response time.[14]

Examples of competitive analysis are evident in daily newspapers and periodicals throughout the world such as the *Financial Times* (with regional editions around the globe). For example, banks continually track home loan, auto loan, and certificate of deposit (CD) interest rates charged by rivals. Major airlines change hundreds of fares daily in response to competitors' tactics. Car manufacturers are keenly aware of announced cuts or increases in rivals' production volume, sales, and sales incentives (e.g., rebates and low interest rates on financing). This information is used in their marketing, pricing, and production strategies.

The Internet has dramatically accelerated the speed at which firms can find competitive intelligence. Leonard Fuld, founder of the Cambridge, Massachusetts, training and consulting firm Fuld & Co., specializes in competitive intelligence for companies around the world.[15] His firm often profiles top company and business group managers and considers these issues: What is their background? What is their style? Are they marketers? Are they cost cutters? Fuld has found that the more articles he collects and the more biographies he downloads, the better he can develop profiles.

One of Fuld & Co.'s clients asked it to determine the size, strength, and technical capabilities of a privately held company. Initially, it was difficult to get detailed information.

environmental monitoring a firm's analysis of the external environment that tracks the evolution of environmental trends, sequences of events, or streams of activities.

competitive intelligence a firm's activities of collecting and interpreting data on competitors, defining and understanding the industry, and identifying competitors' strengths and weaknesses.

strategy spotlight

How Zara, a Spanish Retailer, Spots Opportunities

After massive investments in sophisticated IT systems, many companies continue to miss market shifts that their rivals exploit. With IT investments, however, it's not how much you spend but how you spend it. To continually identify gaps in the market, firms need real-time data and the ability to share it widely throughout the organization. Those hard data must be supplemented with direct observations from the field.

Consider Spanish retailer, Zara, whose success is often attributed to its flexible supply chain. Equally impressive is Zara's ability to spot changing preferences among its fickle customers—despite spending only one-quarter of the industry average on IT. Zara's designers, marketing managers, and buyers work side by side in the company's sprawling headquarters. The open office plan fosters frequent discussions and promotes the sharing of real-time data as well as field observations and anecdotes. By co-locating employees from different functions, Zara allows them to break out of their silos and develop a holistic feel for the market, see how their work fits, and sense new opportunities as they arise.

For instance, in the summer of 2007, Zara launched a line of slim-fit clothes, including pencil skirts and tapered jeans, in response to catwalk trends and what celebrities were wearing. Marketing executives projected that the new items would fly off the racks, but the daily statistics revealed that the items were not selling. So Zara marketing managers immediately went into the field to see firsthand what was happening. They talked to managers, employees, and customers and quickly realized that women loved how the clothes looked but struggled to squeeze into their usual size in the dressing room. Zara responded by recalling the items and relabeling them one size smaller. The company then watched sales boom as customers happily fit into their usual size. The shared, real-time data supplemented with firsthand observation helped employees respond quickly and tip the balance from failure to success.

Zara has experienced tremendous growth and increasing market power. By 2007, it was the biggest fashion company in Europe, outpacing H&M as queen of cheap chic. It is committed to international expansion. In 2008, Korea, Ukraine, Montenegro, Egypt, and Honduras were conquered, and, in 2009, Zara announced a joint venture with India's Tata Group to open stores in India.

Finally, in September 2010, Zara launched its first online retail stores in France, Spain, Italy, Portugal, and the United Kingdom. Since Zara is "liked" by more than 4.5 million people who have signed up as fans on Facebook, the key to its success will now be to convert those fans to customers.

Source: Sull, D. 2010. Are you ready to rebound? *Harvard Business Review*, 88(3): 72; D'Aveni, R. A. 2010. *Beating the commodity trap*. Boston: Harvard Business Press; and, Caesar, J. 2010. Zara launches online retail store. *www.bbc.co.uk*. September 2: np.

Then one analyst used Deja News (*www.dejanews.com*), now part of Google, to tap into some online discussion groups. The analyst's research determined that the company had posted 14 job openings on one Usenet group. That posting was a road map to the competitor's development strategy.

At times, a firm's aggressive efforts to gather competitive intelligence may lead to unethical or illegal behaviors.[16] Strategy Spotlight 2.2 provides an example of a company, United Technologies, that has set clear guidelines to help prevent unethical behavior.

A word of caution: Executives must be careful to avoid spending so much time and effort tracking the actions of traditional competitors that they ignore new competitors. Further, broad environmental changes and events may have a dramatic impact on a firm's viability. Peter Drucker, considered the father of modern management, wrote:

> Increasingly, a winning strategy will require information about events and conditions outside the institution: noncustomers, technologies other than those currently used by the company and its present competitors, markets not currently served, and so on.[17]

Consider the fall of the once-mighty U.S.-based *Encyclopaedia Britannica*.[18] Its demise was not caused by a traditional competitor in the encyclopedia industry. It was caused by new technology. CD-ROMs came out of nowhere and devastated the printed encyclopedia industry. Why? A full set of the *Encyclopaedia Britannica* sells for about

strategy spotlight

2.2

Ethical Guidelines on Competitive Intelligence: United Technologies

United Technologies (UT) is a $53 billion global conglomerate composed of world-leading businesses with rich histories of technological pioneering, such as Otis Elevator, Carrier Air Conditioning, and Sikorsky (helicopters). It was founded in 1853 and has an impressive history of technological accomplishments. UT built the first working helicopter, developed the first commercially available hydrogen cells, and designed complete life support systems for space shuttles. UT believes strongly in a robust code of ethics. In the last decade, it has clearly articulated its principles governing business conduct. These include an antitrust guide, an ethics guide when contracting with the U.S. government and foreign governments, a policy on accepting gifts from suppliers, and guidelines for proper usage of e-mail. One such document is the Code of Ethics Guide on Competitive Intelligence. This encourages managers and workers to ask themselves these five questions whenever they have ethical concerns.

1. Have I done anything that coerced somebody to share this information? Have I, for example, threatened a supplier by indicating that future business opportunities will be influenced by the receipt of information with respect to a competitor?

2. Am I in a place where I should not be? If, for example, I am a field representative with privileges to move around in a customer's facility, have I gone outside the areas permitted? Have I misled anybody in order to gain access?

3. Is the contemplated technique for gathering information evasive, such as sifting through trash or setting up an electronic "snooping" device directed at a competitor's facility from across the street?

4. Have I misled somebody in a way that the person believed sharing information with me was required or would be protected by a confidentiality agreement? Have I, for example, called and misrepresented myself as a government official who was seeking some information for some official purpose?

5. Have I done something to evade or circumvent a system intended to secure or protect information?

Sources: Nelson, B. 2003. The thinker. *Forbes,* March 3: 62–64; and The Fuld war room—Survival Kit 010. Code of ethics (printed 2/26/01); and, *www.yahoo.com.*

ethics

---

environmental forecasting the development of plausible projections about the direction, scope, speed, and intensity of environmental change.

> **>LO2.3**
>
> Why scenario planning is a useful technique for firms competing in industries characterized by unpredictability and change.

$2,000, but an encyclopedia on CD-ROM, such as Microsoft *Encarta,* sells for about $50. To make matters worse, many people receive *Encarta* free with their personal computers.

Environmental Forecasting Environmental scanning, monitoring, and competitive intelligence are important inputs for analyzing the external environment. **Environmental forecasting** involves the development of plausible projections about the direction, scope, speed, and intensity of environmental change.[19] Its purpose is to predict change.[20] It asks: How long will it take a new technology to reach the marketplace? Will the present social concern about an issue result in new legislation? Are current lifestyle trends likely to continue?

Some forecasting issues are much more specific to a particular firm and the industry in which it competes. Consider how important it is for Best Western to predict future indicators, such as the number of rooms, in the budget segment of the industry. If its predictions are low, it will build too many units, creating a surplus of room capacity that would drive down room rates.

A danger of forecasting is that managers may view uncertainty as black and white and ignore important gray areas.[21] The problem is that underestimating uncertainty can lead to strategies that neither defend against threats nor take advantage of opportunities.

In 1977 one of the colossal underestimations in business history occurred when Kenneth H. Olsen, president of Digital Equipment Corp., announced, "There is no reason for individuals to have a computer in their home." The explosion in the personal computer market was not easy to detect in 1977, but it was clearly within the range of possibilities at the time. And, historically, there have been underestimates of the growth potential of new telecommunication services. The electric telegraph was derided by Ralph Waldo Emerson, and the telephone had its skeptics. More recently, an "infamous" McKinsey study in the early 1980s predicted fewer than 1 million cellular users in the United States by 2000. Actually, there were nearly 100 million.[22]

Obviously, poor predictions never go out of vogue. Consider some of the "gems" associated with the global financial crisis that began in 2008.[23]

- "Freddie Mac and Fannie Mae are fundamentally sound. . . . I think they are in good shape going forward."—Barney Frank (D-Mass.), House Financial Services Committee Chairman, July 14, 2008. (*Two months later, the government forced the mortgage giants into conservatorships.*)
- "Existing home sales to trend up in 2008"—Headline of a National Association of Realtors press release, December 9, 2007. (*On December 23, 2007, the group said November sales were down 11 percent from a year earlier in the worst housing slump since the Great Depression.*)
- "I think you'll see $150 a barrel [of oil] by the end of the year."—T. Boone Pickens, June 20, 2008. (*Oil was then around $135 a barrel. By late December it was around $40.*)
- "I expect there will be some failures. . . . I don't anticipate any serious problems of that sort among the large internationally active banks."—Ben Bernanke, Federal Reserve Chairman, February 28, 2008. (*In September, Washington Mutual became the largest financial institution in U.S. history to fail. Citigroup needed an even bigger rescue in November.*)
- "In today's regulatory environment, it's virtually impossible to violate rules." —Bernard Madoff, money manager, October 20, 2007. (*On December 11, 2008, Madoff was arrested for allegedly running a Ponzi scheme that may have lost investors $50 billion. He was sentenced to 150 years in prison on July 29, 2009.*)

Scenario Analysis **Scenario analysis** is a more in-depth approach to forecasting. It draws on a range of disciplines and interests, among them economics, psychology, sociology, and demographics. It usually begins with a discussion of participants' thoughts on ways in which societal trends, economics, politics, and technology may affect an issue.[24] For example, consider Lego. The popular Danish toy manufacturer has a strong position in the construction toys market. But what would happen if this broadly defined market should change dramatically? After all, Lego is competing not only with producers of similar products but also on a much broader canvas for a share of children's playtime. In this market, Lego has a host of competitors, many of them computer based; still others have not yet been invented. Lego may end up with an increasing share of a narrow, shrinking market (much like IBM in the declining days of the mainframe computer). To avoid such a fate, managers must consider a wider context than their narrow, traditional markets, by laying down guidelines for at least 10 years in the future to anticipate rapid change. Strategy Spotlight 2.3 provides an example of scenario planning at Nissan Motors GB.

scenario analysis an in-depth approach to environmental forecasting that involves experts' detailed assessments of societal trends, economics, politics, technology, or other dimensions of the external environment.

SWOT Analysis

To understand the business environment of a particular firm, you need to analyze both the general environment and the firm's industry and competitive environment. Generally, firms compete with other firms in the same industry. An industry is composed of a set of firms that produce similar products or services, sell to similar customers, and use similar methods of production. Gathering industry information and understanding competitive dynamics among the different companies in your industry is key to successful strategic management.

strategy spotlight

Scenario Planning at Nissan Motors GB

In the mid-1990s, Nissan Motors GB (NMGB) was a newly formed sales and marketing company wholly owned by Nissan Japan Ltd. NMGB's first main task was to evaluate the possibility of setting up and running its own dealer network. As a maker and distributor of cars and spare parts, Nissan had a vast amount of experience and expertise with that side of the business. After all, in Sunderland, UK, it had created the most efficient car manufacturing plant in Europe. But it lacked a deeper understanding of the retail side of the business—how car dealerships handled sales, servicing and repairs, and customer service. Within NMGB there was some skepticism about the full vertical integration model. There had been very few, if any, past successes where manufacturers had also run dealerships profitably. Moreover, doing so was likely to require a large investment commitment and acceptance of a significant degree of risk arising from major uncertainties in the retailing world, including the likelihood of the EU Block Exemption for car manufacturers being abolished. So, for Nissan, would ownership of retail distribution be a viable route into the future?

In order to confidently forecast viable options, the company decided to test an alternative approach—scenario planning—to understand future uncertainties and explore the range of possible outcomes. Nissan was no stranger to scenario planning, having used it in its American operations since the early 1980s. NMGB began working with SAMI Consulting on an exercise called "Future Purchasing of Personal Transportation," which led to "Scenarios for Motor Retailing in the UK." An open scenario planning methodology was used, in which the NMGB management team (as the "owners of the problem"), together with selected others from inside and outside the company and the industry, were interviewed to explore their individual strategic thinking. The inputs were synthesized to identify the range of ideas about what might be important for the future, resulting in the following three diverse views of the future:

- *Sands of Time,* in which economic growth of 3 percent reduces pressure for change in the short term but allows traffic, pollution, and safety concerns to build up inexorably. Current business trends continue: Company cars remain popular, leasing grows slowly,

the block exemption continues, dealerships concentrate slowly as the weakest "go to the wall."

- *Lean Retailing,* in which economic growth of 1 to 2 percent forces competition in the car industry, and the block exemption from trade restraint is removed. The slower growth curbs margins, limits road expansion and repair, and lengthens car life. New distributors with wider retail experience and a lean mentality drive existing distributors to concentrate faster. Greater emphasis is given to used car sales ("nearly new" market approach) and on financing used cars. Growth of imports from cheaper manufacturing sources, such as the Far East and Eastern Europe, occurs.

- *Screen and Lean,* in which there is economic growth of 1.0 to 1.5 percent and lower employment and market growth. Competition drives web-enabled operations (enabling staff reductions), car life is much longer, and public transport is neglected. Manufacturers fight back by moving into the "whole life" value chain. They invest in new showrooms and multimedia support and communication facilities. Greater use is made of web-driven sales (also in the aftermarket).

The Wider Impact

The project yielded wider and longer-term benefits too. NMGB found the scenarios process very rewarding. It brought an added dimension to the conventional strategic planning methods, making scenario planning a potent tool in the armory of the leadership team. The three scenarios made for much more confident strategic decision making and contributed substantially to the success in meeting corporate objectives over the long term. Even more significantly, once UK strategy had been established, Nissan turned its sights to beyond the Channel. Scenarios were employed to examine the future of Nissan in all of Europe. This project brought not only the adoption of similar business models and a significant increase in profitability, but also a much wider perspective of Nissan's business on the global stage. The realization that Nissan needed to strengthen its global position led to the alliance with French automotive manufacturer Renault, involving substantial cross-shareholdings and the creation of Renault-Nissan BV, a company incorporated under Dutch law, which forms the strategic management structure for the group. Prior to the outcomes of the scenarios work, such a bold, radical move would not have been contemplated.

Source: Modha, N. Sowing the Seeds of Global Strength. Vector (SAMI Consulting), February 2005, accessed at *www.samiconsulting.co.uk/4vectorpdfs.html.*

One of the most basic techniques for analyzing firm and industry conditions is **SWOT analysis.** SWOT stands for strengths, weaknesses, opportunities, and threats. It provides "raw material"—a basic listing of conditions both inside and surrounding your company.

The Strengths and Weaknesses refer to the internal conditions of the firm—where your firm excels (strengths) and where it may be lacking relative to competitors (weaknesses). Opportunities and Threats are environmental conditions external to the firm. These could be factors either in the general or competitive environment. In the general environment, one might experience developments that are beneficial for most companies, such as improving economic conditions that lower borrowing costs, or trends that benefit some companies and harm others. An example is the heightened concern with fitness, which is a threat to some companies (e.g., tobacco) and an opportunity to others (e.g., health clubs). Opportunities and threats are also present in the competitive environment among firms competing for the same customers.

The general idea of SWOT analysis is that a firm's strategy must:

- build on its strengths,
- remedy the weaknesses or work around them,
- take advantage of the opportunities presented by the environment, and,
- protect the firm from the threats.

Despite its apparent simplicity, the SWOT approach has been very popular. First, it forces managers to consider both internal and external factors simultaneously. Second, its emphasis on identifying opportunities and threats makes firms act proactively rather than reactively. Third, it raises awareness about the role of strategy in creating a match between the environmental conditions and the firm's internal strengths and weaknesses. Finally, its conceptual simplicity is achieved without sacrificing analytical rigor. (We will also address some of the limitations of SWOT analysis in Chapter 3.)

The General Environment

The **general environment** is composed of factors that can have dramatic effects on firm strategy.[25] Typically, a firm has little ability to predict trends and events in the general environment and even less ability to control them. When listening to CNBC, for example, you can hear many experts espouse different perspectives on what action the Federal Reserve Board may take on short-term interest rates—an action that can have huge effects on the valuation of entire economic sectors. Also, it's difficult to predict future political events such as the ongoing Middle East peace negotiations and tensions on the Korean peninsula. Dramatic innovations in information technology (e.g., the Internet) have helped keep inflation in check by lowering the cost of doing business in the United States at the beginning of the 21st century.[26]

We divide the general environment into six segments: **demographic, sociocultural, political/legal, technological, economic,** and **global.** Exhibit 2.3 provides examples of key trends and events in each of the six segments of the general environment.

The Demographic Segment

Demographics are the most easily understood and quantifiable elements of the general environment. They are at the root of many changes in society. Demographics include elements such as the aging population,[27] rising or declining affluence, changes in ethnic composition, geographic distribution of the population, and disparities in income level.[28]

SWOT analysis
a framework for analyzing a company's internal and external environment and that stands for strengths, weaknesses, opportunities, and threats.

general environment
factors external to an industry, and usually beyond a firm's control, that affect a firm's strategy.

>LO2.4
The impact of the general environment on a firm's strategies and performance.

demographic segment of the general environment
genetic and observable characteristics of a population, including the levels and growth of age, density, sex, race, ethnicity, education, geographic region, and income.

Exhibit 2.3
**General Environment:
Key Trends and Events**

Demographic

- Aging population
- Rising affluence
- Changes in ethnic composition
- Geographic distribution of population
- Greater disparities in income levels

Sociocultural

- More women in the workforce
- Increase in temporary workers
- Greater concern for fitness
- Greater concern for environment
- Postponement of family formation

Political/Legal

- UK Combined Code on Corporate Governance
- French Vienot Report
- Italian Preda Code
- Spanish Olivecia and Aldama Reports
- German Corporate Governance Code
- U.S. legislation on corporate governance reforms in bookkeeping, stock options, etc. (Sarbanes-Oxley Act of 2002)

Technological

- Genetic engineering
- Emergence of Internet technology
- Computer-aided design/computer-aided manufacturing (CAD/CAM) systems
- Research in synthetic and exotic materials
- Pollution/global warming
- Miniaturization of computing technologies
- Wireless communications
- Nanotechnology

Economic

- Interest rates
- Unemployment rates
- Consumer Price Index
- Trends in GDP
- Changes in stock market valuations

Global

- Increasing global trade
- Currency exchange rates
- Emergence of the Indian and Chinese economies
- Trade agreements among regional blocs (e.g., FTAA, CAFTA, APEC)
- Creation of WTO (leading to decreasing tariffs/free trade in services)
- Increased risks associated with terrorism

China's Growing Middle Class Helps Cargo Carriers Rebound from the Recession

Increasingly, wealthy Chinese consumers eat more imported fresh fish, lobster, and cheese and wear imported fashions. One implication: They are helping global air cargo revenue rebound from the decline in 2009, the worst year in five decades.

China, with its soaring demand for luxury goods and perishable foods from overseas, lead an 18.5 percent recovery in air shipments in 2010, according to the International Air Transport Association. "China has attracted more investment and luxury brands, as purchasing power has gotten much stronger," said Kelvin Lau, an equity analyst at Daiwa Institute of Research in Hong Kong. For example,

Source: Leung, W. & Ling, C. S. 2010. Chinese consumers' appetites fatten air shippers. *International Herald Tribune.* July 30: 15; Wong, F. & Lian, R. 2011. Shanghai international port posts 44 percent jump in 2010 Net. *www.reuters .com.* January 11: np; and, Park, K. 2011. Global logistic to expand in smaller China cities to tap on rental growth. *www.bloomberg.com.* January 4: np.

Cathay Pacific, the biggest carrier in Hong Kong, is flying 100 tons of lobster and 150 tons of grouper to China and Hong Kong every month from Australia and Indonesia. It also increased shipments of sashimi-grade fish to the country from Tokyo by 60 percent in the first four months of 2010.

The size of China's middle class could rise to 46 percent of all households by 2020, from 32 percent in 2010, claims the research firm Euromonitor International. The firm defines middle-class households as those with annual disposable incomes equivalent to $5,000 to $15,000.

United Parcel Service, the world's largest package-delivery firm, added two cargo planes in Hong Kong and one in Shanghai in 2010. FedEx, the world's largest air cargo carrier, is planning to buy more air freighters for its longest routes to Asia.

Shanghai International Port, China's largest port group, had a throughput of 428 million tons in 2010—up from 365 tons the previous year. And Global Logistic Properties Ltd., a logistics company whose customers include Walmart China and FedEx, expects cargo demand through the Beijing airport to increase by 15 percent a year from 2010 to 2015.

The impact of a demographic trend, like all segments of the general environment, varies across industries. Rising levels of affluence in many developed countries bode well for brokerage services as well as for upscale pets and supplies. However, this trend may adversely affect fast-food restaurants because people can afford to dine at higher-priced restaurants. Fast-food restaurants depend on minimum-wage employees to operate efficiently, but the competition for labor intensifies as more attractive employment opportunities become prevalent, thus threatening the employment base for restaurants. Let's look at the details of one of these trends.

The aging population in the United States and other developed countries has important implications. The U.S. Bureau of Statistics states that only 18 percent of American workers were 55 and older in 2008. However, by 2012 that figure will increase to 24 percent, or about one in four, of all U.S. workers. At the same time, the United States is expected to experience a significant drop in younger workers aged 25 to 44 from 68 percent to 64 percent by 2018, making it increasingly important for employers to recruit and retain older workers.

As a result of declining fertility and increasing longevity, the populations of a growing number of countries are aging rapidly. Between 2005 and 2050, half of the increase in the world population will be accounted for by a rise in the population aged 60 years or over, whereas the number of children (persons under age 15) will decline slightly. Furthermore, in the more developed regions, the population aged 60 or over is expected nearly to double (from 245 million in 2005 to 406 million in 2050), whereas the population under age 60 will likely decline (from 971 million in 2005 to 839 million in 2050). In China, for example, by 2040 more than 400 million people will be over the age of 60.[29]

Strategy Spotlight 2.4 discusses how the increasing appetite for high-end consumer goods by China's growing middle class has boosted the revenues for air cargo carriers. This comes at a time when many western economies are still reeling from a recession.

The Sociocultural Segment

Sociocultural forces influence the values, beliefs, and lifestyles of a society. Examples include a higher percentage of women in the workforce, dual-income families, increases in the number of temporary workers, greater concern for healthy diets and physical fitness, greater interest in the environment, and postponement of having children. Such forces enhance sales of products and services in many industries but depress sales in others. The increased number of women in the workforce has increased the need for business clothing merchandise but decreased the demand for baking product staples (since people would have less time to cook from scratch). This health and fitness trend has helped industries that manufacture exercise equipment and healthful foods but harmed industries that produce unhealthful foods.

Increased educational attainment by women in the workplace has led to more women in upper management positions.[30] Given such educational attainment, it is hardly surprising that companies owned by women have been one of the driving forces of the U.S. economy; these companies (now more than 9 million in number) account for 40 percent of all U.S. businesses and have generated more than $3.6 trillion in annual revenue. In addition, women have a tremendous impact on consumer spending decisions. Not surprisingly, many companies have focused their advertising and promotion efforts on female consumers. Consider, for example, video game companies' efforts to attract female players:

> Video game publishers, pushing to expand their businesses, are making games that target girls and women a new industry battleground. Video games have long been considered the domain of teenage boys and young men. Though a few publishers have developed computer games for women, the genre wasn't considered significant until the past several years. Nintendo helped fuel the change with its touch-screen DS portable device five years ago and Wii console three years ago, providing easy-to-play games that appealed to a broader audience—including women—and helped spur sales. Since then, publishers have made a serious effort to develop mass-market games beyond the usual shooter, racing, and sports titles. According to financial firm Wedbush Morgan, female game players now account for about 40 percent of the overall market, compared with research firm IDC's estimate of less than 12 percent in 2001. Wedbush calculates that a 5 percent increase in female players could translate into as much as $1 billion in new revenue every year.[31]

The Political/Legal Segment

Political processes and legislation influence environmental regulations with which industry must comply.[32,33] Government legislation can also have a significant impact on the governance of corporations. In Germany, the Government Commission appointed by the Justice Minister adopted the German Corporate Governance Code on February 26, 2002. The aim of the code is to make Germany's corporate governance rules transparent for both national and international investors, thus strengthening confidence in the management of German corporations.[34]

The U. S. Congress passed the Sarbanes-Oxley Act in 2002, which also greatly increases the accountability of auditors, executives, and corporate lawyers. This act responded to the widespread perception that existing governance mechanisms failed to protect the interests of shareholders, employees, and creditors. Clearly, the German Corporate Governance Code and the Sarbanes-Oxley law have also created a tremendous demand for professional accounting services.

Legislation can also affect firms in the high-tech sector of the economy by expanding the number of temporary visas available for highly skilled foreign professionals.[35] For example, a bill passed by the U.S. Congress in October 2000 allowed 195,000 H-1B visas for

How Microsoft "Gets Around" H-1B Visa Restrictions

In March 2008, Microsoft Chairman Bill Gates took one of his company's most problematic issues to the U.S. Senate. During his testimony, he criticized U.S. immigration policy that limits the H-1B visas issued to skilled workers from foreign countries—workers that Microsoft would urgently like to hire. Gates told the lawmakers: "It makes no sense to tell well-trained, highly skilled individuals—many of whom are educated at top universities—that the U.S. does not welcome or value them" and that the U.S. "will find it far more difficult to maintain its competitive edge over the next 50 years if it excludes those who are able and willing to help

Sources: Elliott, M. 2010. Opinion. *Fortune.* June 14: 56; MacDonald, I. 2008. Finesse the visa crisis with a worker-mobility plan. *Harvard Business Review,* 86(11): 28–29; Greene, J. 2008. Case study: Microsoft's Canadian solution. *BusinessWeek,* January 28: 51; MacDonald, I. 2008. Tech firms get creative in employing foreigners. *Dallas Morning News,* November 16: 5D; and, Anonymous. 2007. Microsoft to open Canada center in response to U.S. immigration. *www.workpermit.com.* July 10: np.

us compete." Gates also claimed that Microsoft hires four Americans in supporting roles for every high-skilled H-1B visa holder it hires. (This claim was also made in a June 2010 editorial in *Fortune* magazine.) Despite his efforts, the senators ignored his pleas and the visa policy went unchanged.

What to do? Six months later, Microsoft opened an office in Richmond, British Columbia, a suburb of Vancouver. Here, it hopes to place hundreds of workers unable to obtain U.S. visas. Placing workers in the same time zone will help them to collaborate—given that the facility is located just 130 miles north of Microsoft's Redmond, Washington, campus. And it is just a 2½ hour drive on Interstate 5 if one needs face time. It certainly doesn't hurt that Canada does not place limits on visas for skilled workers. An unusually pointed press release by Microsoft stated: "The Vancouver area is a global gateway with a diverse population, is close to Microsoft's offices in Redmond, and allows the company to recruit and retain highly skilled people affected by immigration issues in the U.S."

each of the following three years—up from a cap of 115,000. However, beginning in 2006 and continuing through 2010, the annual cap on H-1B visas shrunk to only 65,000—with an additional 20,000 visas available for foreigners with a master's or higher degree from a U.S. institution. Many of the visas are for professionals from India with computer and software expertise. As one would expect, this is a political "hot potato" for industry executives as well as U.S. labor and workers' right groups. The key arguments against increases in H-1B visas are that H-1B workers drive down wages and take jobs from Americans.

Strategy Spotlight 2.5 discusses one of the proactive steps that Microsoft has taken to address this issue.

The Technological Segment

Developments in technology lead to new products and services and improve how they are produced and delivered to the end user.[36] Innovations can create entirely new industries and alter the boundaries of existing industries.[37] Technological developments and trends include genetic engineering, Internet technology, computer-aided design/computer-aided manufacturing (CAD/CAM), research in artificial and exotic materials, and, on the downside, pollution and global warming.[38] Petroleum and primary metals industries spend significantly to reduce their pollution. Engineering and consulting firms that work with polluting industries derive financial benefits from solving such problems.

Nanotechnology is becoming a very promising area of research with many potentially useful applications.[39] Nanotechnology takes place at industry's tiniest stage: one-billionth of a meter. Remarkably, this is the size of 10 hydrogen atoms in a row. Matter at such a tiny scale behaves very differently. Familiar materials—from gold to carbon soot—display startling and useful new properties. Some transmit light or electricity. Others become harder than diamonds or turn into potent chemical catalysts. What's more,

technological segment of the general environment innovation and state of knowledge in industrial arts, engineering, applied sciences, and pure science; and their interaction with society.

researchers have found that a tiny dose of nanoparticles can transform the chemistry and nature of far bigger things.

However, transforming the power of new technologies to commercially viable products can be difficult.[40] For example, the East Japan Railway Company tried to capture tiny amounts of energy from the footsteps of the thousands of commuters who passed through their gates. Unfortunately, they found out that all the energy generated in a day at the station was miniscule: enough to light a 100-watt bulb for a few minutes!

The Economic Segment

economic segment of the general environment characteristics of the economy, including national income and monetary conditions.

The economy affects all industries, from suppliers of raw materials to manufacturers of finished goods and services, as well as all organizations in the service, wholesale, retail, government, and nonprofit sectors.[41] Key economic indicators include interest rates, unemployment rates, the Consumer Price Index, the gross domestic product, and net disposable income.[42] Interest-rate increases have a negative impact on the residential home construction industry but a negligible (or neutral) effect on industries that produce consumer necessities such as prescription drugs or common grocery items.

Other economic indicators are associated with equity markets. Perhaps the most watched is the Dow Jones Industrial Average (DJIA), which is composed of 30 large industrial firms' stock values. When stock market indexes increase, consumers' discretionary income rises and there is often an increased demand for luxury items such as jewelry and automobiles. But when stock valuations decrease, demand for these items shrinks. For example, Exhibit 2.4 shows that the sales of value-priced liquor, wine, and beer actually went up, while sales of higher priced alcoholic beverages did not fare so well during the recent global recession.

The Global Segment

global segment of the general environment influences from foreign countries, including foreign market opportunities, foreign-based competition, and expanded capital markets.

More firms are expanding their operations and market reach beyond the borders of their "home" country. Globalization provides opportunities to access both larger potential markets and a broad base of production factors such as raw materials, labor, skilled managers, and technical professionals. However, such endeavors also carry many political, social, and economic risks.[43]

Examples of key elements include currency exchange rates, increasing global trade, the economic emergence of China, trade agreements among regional blocs (e.g., North American Free Trade Agreement, European Union, and Asia-Pacific Economic Cooperation), and the General Agreement on Tariffs and Trade (GATT) (lowering of tariffs).[44] Increases in trade across national boundaries also provide benefits to air cargo and shipping industries but have a minimal impact on service industries such as bookkeeping and

Exhibit 2.4
Alcoholic Beverage Sales during the Recession: Low End versus Premium Products

	Percentage changes in sales compared to a year earlier (52 weeks ended March 6, 2010, in US$)	
Spirits	Increase in value-priced liquors	+1.4%
	Top-shelf spirits	Flat
Wine	Growth of $9–$12 bottles of table wine	+6.0%
	Decline of $20 bottles of table wine	−1.6%
Beer	Growth of cheapest beer segment	+7.3%
	Decline in sales of imported beers	−3.8%

Source: Kalwarski, T. 2010. No recession hangover for the booze business. *Bloomberg Businessweek*, April, 19: 17.

routine medical services. The emergence of China as an economic power has benefited many industries, such as construction, soft drinks, and computers. However, it has had a negative impact on the defense industry in the United States as diplomatic relations between the two nations improve.

A key factor in the global economy is the rapid rise of the middle class in emerging countries. By 2015, for the first time, the number of consumers in Asia's middle class will equal those in Europe and North America combined. An important implication of this trend is the dramatic change in hiring practices of U.S. multinationals. In 2010, for example, American companies created 1.4 million jobs overseas—but only 1 million in the United States.[45]

Also, consider the cost of terrorism. A recent survey indicates that for S&P 500 firms, the threat has caused direct and indirect costs of $107 billion a year. This figure includes extra spending (on insurance and redundant capacity, for instance) as well as lost revenues (from fearful consumers' decreased activity).[46]

Relationships among Elements of the General Environment

In our discussion of the general environment, we see many relationships among the various elements.[47] For example, a demographic trend in the United States, the aging of the population, has important implications for the economic segment (in terms of tax policies to provide benefits to increasing numbers of older citizens). Another example is the emergence of information technology as a means to increase the rate of productivity gains in the United States and other developed countries. Such use of IT results in lower inflation (an important element of the economic segment) and helps offset costs associated with higher labor rates.

The effects of a trend or event in the general environment vary across industries. Governmental legislation (political/legal) to permit the importation of prescription drugs from foreign countries is a very positive development for drugstores but a very negative event for U.S. drug manufacturers. Exhibit 2.5 provides other examples of how the impact of trends or events in the general environment can vary across industries.

Before moving on, let's consider the Internet. The Internet has been a leading and highly visible component of a broader technological phenomenon—the emergence of digital technology. These technologies are altering the way business is conducted and having an impact on nearly every business domain. Strategy Spotlight 2.6 addresses the impact of the Internet and digital technologies on the business environment.

> **industry**
> a group of firms that produce similar goods or services.

The Competitive Environment

Managers must consider the competitive environment (also sometimes referred to as the task or **industry** environment). The nature of competition in an industry, as well as the profitability of a firm, is often more directly influenced by developments in the competitive environment.

The **competitive environment** consists of many factors that are particularly relevant to a firm's strategy. These include competitors (existing or potential), customers, and suppliers. Potential competitors may include a supplier considering forward integration, such as an automobile manufacturer acquiring a rental car company, or a firm in an entirely new industry introducing a similar product that uses a more efficient technology.

Next, we will discuss key concepts and analytical techniques that managers should use to assess their competitive environments. First, we examine Michael Porter's five-forces model that illustrates how these forces can be used to explain an industry's profitability.[48] Second, we discuss how the five forces are being affected by the capabilities provided by Internet technologies. Third, we address some of the limitations, or "caveats," that managers should be familiar with when conducting industry analysis. Finally, we address the

> **>LO2.5**
> How forces in the competitive environment can affect profitability, and how a firm can improve its competitive position by increasing its power vis-à-vis these forces.

> **competitive environment**
> factors that pertain to an industry and affect a firm's strategies.

Exhibit 2.5 The Impact of General Environmental Trends on Various Industries

Segment/Trends and Events	Industry	Positive	Neutral	Negative
Demographic				
Aging population	Health care	✓		
	Baby products			✓
Rising affluence	Brokerage services	✓		
	Fast foods			✓
	Upscale pets and supplies	✓		
Sociocultural				
More women in the workforce	Clothing	✓		
	Baking products (staples)			✓
Greater concern for health and fitness	Home exercise equipment	✓		
	Meat products			✓
Political/legal				
Tort reform	Legal services			✓
	Auto manufacturing	✓		
Technological				
Genetic engineering	Pharmaceutical	✓		
	Publishing		✓	
Pollution/global warming	Engineering services	✓		
	Petroleum			✓
Economic				
Interest rate increases	Residential construction			✓
	Most common grocery products		✓	
Global				
Increasing global trade	Shipping	✓		
	Personal service		✓	
Emergence of China as an economic power	Soft drinks	✓		
	Defense			✓

concept of strategic groups, because even within an industry it is often useful to group firms on the basis of similarities of their strategies. As we will see, competition tends to be more intense among firms *within* a strategic group than between strategic groups.

Porter's Five-Forces Model of Industry Competition

The **five-forces model** developed by Michael E. Porter has been the most commonly used analytical tool for examining the competitive environment. It describes the competitive environment in terms of five basic competitive forces.[49]

1. The threat of new entrants.
2. The bargaining power of buyers.
3. The bargaining power of suppliers.

Porter's five-forces model of industry competition
a tool for examining the industry-level competitive environment, especially the ability of firms in that industry to set prices and minimize costs.

strategy spotlight

The Internet and Digital Technologies: Affecting Many Environmental Segments

The Internet has dramatically changed the way business is conducted in every corner of the globe. According to digital economy visionary Don Tapscott:

> The Net is much more than just another technology development; the Net represents something qualitatively new—an unprecedented, powerful, universal communications medium. Far surpassing radio and television, this medium is digital, infinitely richer, and interactive. . . . Mobile computing devices, broadband access, wireless networks, and computing power embedded in everything from refrigerators to automobiles are converging into a global network that will enable people to use the Net just about anywhere and anytime.

The Internet provides a platform or staging area for the application of numerous technologies, rapid advances in knowledge, and unprecedented levels of global communication and commerce. Even technologies that don't require the Internet to function, such as wireless phones and GPS, rely on the Internet for data transfer and communications.

Sources: Anonymous. 2005. SMBs believe in the Web. *www.emarketer.com*, May 16; Downes, L. & Mui, C. 1998. *Unleashing the killer app.* Boston: Harvard Business School Press: Green, H. 2003. Wi-fi means business. *BusinessWeek,* April 28: 86–92; McGann, R. 2005. Broadband: High speed, high spend. *ClickZ Network, www.clickz.com*, January 24; Tapscott, D. 2001. Rethinking strategy in a Networked World. *Strategy and Business,* Third Quarter: 34–41; and, Yang, C. 2003. Beyond wi-fi: A new wireless age. *BusinessWeek,* December 15: 84–88.

Growth in Internet usage has surged in recent years both among individual users as well as businesses. Exhibit 2.6 illustrates (2000–2010) worldwide growth trends in Internet use. Business use of the Internet has become nearly ubiquitous throughout the economy. Major corporations all have a web presence, and many companies use the Internet to interact with key stakeholders. For example, some companies have direct links with suppliers through online procurement systems that automatically reorder inventories and supplies. Companies such as Cisco Systems even interact with their own employees using the Internet to update employment records, such as health care information and benefits.

Small and medium-sized enterprises (SMEs) are also relying on the Internet more than ever. A recent study found that 87 percent of SMEs are receiving monthly revenue from their website, and 42 percent derive more than a quarter of their monthly revenue from their Internet presence. According to Joel Kocher, CEO of Interland, "We are getting to the point in most small-business categories where it will soon be safe to say that if you're not online, you're not really serious about being in business."

Despite these advances, the Internet and digital technologies still face numerous challenges. For example, international standards for digital and wireless communications are still in flux. As a result, cell phones and other devices that work in the United States are often useless in many parts of Europe and Asia. And, unlike analog systems, electronic bits of data that are zooming through space can be more easily lost, stolen, or manipulated. However, even with these problems, Internet and digital technologies will continue to be a growing global phenomenon. As Andy Grove, former chairman of Intel, stated, "The world now runs on Internet time."

Geographic Regions	Internet Users, 2000 (1000s)	Internet Users, 2010 (1000s)	Population Penetration	Usage Growth, 2000–2010
Africa	4,514	110,932	10.9%	2,357%
Asia	114,304	825,094	21.5%	622%
Europe	105,096	475,069	58.4%	352%
Middle East	3,285	63,241	29.8%	1,825%
North America	108,097	266,225	77.4%	146%
Latin America/Caribbean	18,069	204,690	34.5%	1,033%
Oceania/Australia	7,620	21,264	61.3%	179%
World Total	360,985	1,966,515	28.7%	445%

Source: *www.internetworldstats.com*

Exhibit 2.6 **Growth in Internet Activity**

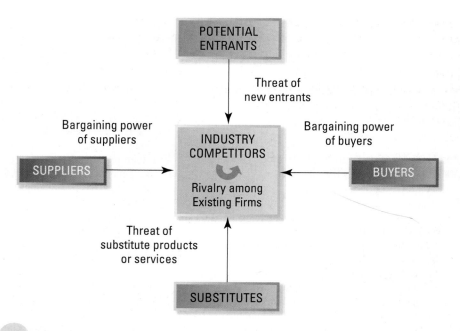

Exhibit 2.7 **Porter's Five-Forces Model of Industry Competition**

Source: Adapted and reprinted with permission of The Free Press, a division of Simon & Schuster Adult Publishing Group, from *Competitive Strategy: Techniques for Analyzing Industries and Competitors* by Michael E. Porter. Copyright © 1980, 1998 by The Free Press. All rights reserved.

4. The threat of substitute products and services.
5. The intensity of rivalry among competitors in an industry.

Each of these forces affects a firm's ability to compete in a given market. Together, they determine the profit potential for a particular industry. The model is shown in Exhibit 2.7. A manager should be familiar with the five-forces model for several reasons. It helps you decide whether your firm should remain in or exit an industry. It provides the rationale for increasing or decreasing resource commitments. The model helps you assess how to improve your firm's competitive position with regard to each of the five forces.[50] For example, you can use insights provided by the five-forces model to create higher entry barriers that discourage new rivals from competing with you.[51] Or you may develop strong relationships with your distribution channels. You may decide to find suppliers who satisfy the price/performance criteria needed to make your product or service a top performer.

The Threat of New Entrants   The **threat of new entrants** refers to the possibility that the profits of established firms in the industry may be eroded by new competitors.[52] The extent of the threat depends on existing barriers to entry and the combined reactions from existing competitors.[53] If entry barriers are high and/or the newcomer can anticipate a sharp retaliation from established competitors, the threat of entry is low. These circumstances discourage new competitors. There are six major sources of entry barriers.

Economies of Scale Economies of scale refers to spreading the costs of production over the number of units produced. The cost of a product per unit declines as the absolute volume per period increases. This deters entry by forcing the entrant to come in at a large scale and risk strong reaction from existing firms or come in at a small scale and accept a cost disadvantage. Both are undesirable options.

threat of new entrants the possibility that the profits of established firms in the industry may be eroded by new competitors.

economies of scale decreases in cost per unit as absolute output per period increases.

Product Differentiation When existing competitors have strong brand identification and customer loyalty, differentiation creates a barrier to entry by forcing entrants to spend heavily to overcome existing customer loyalties.

Capital Requirements The need to invest large financial resources to compete creates a barrier to entry, especially if the capital is required for risky or unrecoverable up-front advertising or research and development (R&D).

Switching Costs A barrier to entry is created by the existence of one-time costs that the buyer faces when switching from one supplier's product or service to another.

Access to Distribution Channels The new entrant's need to secure distribution for its product can create a barrier to entry.

Cost Disadvantages Independent of Scale Some existing competitors may have advantages that are independent of size or economies of scale. These derive from:

- Proprietary products
- Favorable access to raw materials
- Government subsidies
- Favorable government policies

In an environment where few, if any, of these entry barriers are present, the threat of new entry is high. For example, if a new firm can launch its business with a low capital investment and operate efficiently despite its small scale of operation, it is likely to be a threat. One company that failed because of low entry barriers in an industry is ProCD.[54] You probably have never heard of this company. It didn't last very long. ProCD provides an example of a firm that failed because it entered an industry with very low entry barriers.

The story begins in 1986 when Nynex (a former Baby Bell company) issued the first electronic phone book, a compact disk containing all listings for the New York City area. It charged $10,000 per copy and sold the CDs to the FBI, IRS, and other large commercial and government organizations. James Bryant, the Nynex executive in charge of the project, smelled a fantastic business opportunity. He quit Nynex and set up his own firm, ProCD, with the ambitious goal of producing an electronic directory covering the entire United States.

The telephone companies, fearing an attack on their highly profitable Yellow Pages business, refused to license digital copies of their listings. Bryant was not deterred. He hired Chinese workers at $3.50 a day to type every listing from every U.S. telephone book into a database. The result contained more than 70 million phone numbers and was used to create a master disk that enabled ProCD to make hundreds of thousands of copies. Each CD sold for hundreds of dollars and cost less than a dollar each to produce.

It was a profitable business indeed! However, success was fleeting. Competitors such as Digital Directory Assistance and American Business Information quickly launched competing products with the same information. Since customers couldn't tell one product from the next, the players were forced to compete on price alone. Prices for the CD soon plummeted to a few dollars each. A high-priced, high-margin product just months earlier, the CD phone book became little more than a cheap commodity.

The Bargaining Power of Buyers

Buyers threaten an industry by forcing down prices, bargaining for higher quality or more services, and playing competitors against each other. These actions erode industry profitability.[55] The power of each large buyer group depends on attributes of the market situation and the importance of purchases from that group compared with the industry's overall business. A buyer group is powerful when:

- ***It is concentrated or purchases large volumes relative to seller sales.*** If a large percentage of a supplier's sales are purchased by a single buyer, the importance of the buyer's business to the supplier increases. Large-volume buyers also are powerful in industries with high fixed costs (e.g., steel manufacturing).

---

product differentiation the degree that a product has strong brand loyalty or customer loyalty.

switching cost one-time costs that a buyer/supplier faces when switching from one supplier/buyer to another.

bargaining power of buyers the threat that buyers may force down prices, bargain for higher quality or more services, and play competitors against each other.

- *The products it purchases from the industry are standard or undifferentiated.* Confident they can always find alternative suppliers, buyers play one company against the other, as in commodity grain products.
- *The buyer faces few switching costs.* Switching costs lock the buyer to particular sellers. Conversely, the buyer's power is enhanced if the seller faces high switching costs.
- *It earns low profits.* Low profits create incentives to lower purchasing costs. On the other hand, highly profitable buyers are generally less price sensitive.
- *The buyers pose a credible threat of backward integration.* If buyers are either partially integrated or pose a credible threat of backward integration, they are typically able to secure bargaining concessions.
- *The industry's product is unimportant to the quality of the buyer's products or services.* When the quality of the buyer's products is not affected by the industry's product, the buyer is more price sensitive.

At times, a firm or set of firms in an industry may increase its buyer power by using the services of a third party. FreeMarkets Online is one such third party.[56] U.S.-based FreeMarkets has developed software enabling large industrial buyers to organize online auctions for qualified suppliers of semistandard parts such as fabricated components, packaging materials, metal stampings, and services. By aggregating buyers, FreeMarkets increases the buyers' bargaining power. The results are impressive. In its first 48 auctions, most participating companies saved over 15 percent; some saved as much as 50 percent.

Although a firm may be tempted to take advantage of its suppliers because of high buyer power, it must be aware of the potential long-term backlash from such actions. A recent example is the growing resentment that students have toward Britain's Oxford University because of steep increases in fees scheduled for 2012. Unfortunately, students are essentially a captive market and have relatively little bargaining power.

bargaining power of suppliers the threat that suppliers may raise prices or reduce the quality of purchased goods and services.

The Bargaining Power of Suppliers Suppliers can exert bargaining power by threatening to raise prices or reduce the quality of purchased goods and services. Powerful suppliers can squeeze the profitability of firms so far that they can't recover the costs of raw material inputs.[57] The factors that make suppliers powerful tend to mirror those that make buyers powerful. A supplier group will be powerful when:

- *The supplier group is dominated by a few companies and is more concentrated (few firms dominate the industry) than the industry it sells to.* Suppliers selling to fragmented industries influence prices, quality, and terms.
- *The supplier group is not obliged to contend with substitute products for sale to the industry.* The power of even large, powerful suppliers can be checked if they compete with substitutes.
- *The industry is not an important customer of the supplier group.* When suppliers sell to several industries and a particular industry does not represent a significant fraction of its sales, suppliers are more prone to exert power.
- *The supplier's product is an important input to the buyer's business.* When such inputs are important to the success of the buyer's manufacturing process or product quality, the bargaining power of suppliers is high.
- *The supplier group's products are differentiated or it has built up switching costs for the buyer.* Differentiation or switching costs facing the buyers cut off their options to play one supplier against another.
- *The supplier group poses a credible threat of forward integration.* This provides a check against the industry's ability to improve the terms by which it purchases.

threat of substitute products and services the threat of limiting the potential returns of an industry by placing a ceiling on the prices that firms in that industry can profitably charge without losing too many customers to substitute products.

The Threat of Substitute Products and Services All firms within an industry compete with industries producing **substitute products and services.**[58] Substitutes limit the potential returns of an industry by placing a ceiling on the prices that firms in that industry can profitably charge. The more attractive the price/performance ratio of substitute products, the tighter the lid on an industry's profits.

Identifying substitute products involves searching for other products or services that can perform the same function as the industry's offerings. This may lead a manager into businesses seemingly far removed from the industry. For example, the airline industry might not consider video cameras much of a threat. But as digital technology has improved and wireless and other forms of telecommunication have become more efficient, teleconferencing has become a viable substitute for business travel. That is, the rate of improvement in the price–performance relationship of the substitute product (or service) is high.

Teleconferencing can save both time and money, as IBM found out with its Manager Jam idea.[59] With 319,000 employees scattered around six continents, it is one of the world's largest businesses (including 32,000 managers) and can be a pretty confusing place. The shift to an increasingly mobile workplace means many managers supervise employees they rarely see face-to-face. To enhance coordination, Samuel Palmisano, IBM's new CEO, launched one of his first big initiatives: a two-year program exploring the role of the manager in the 21st century. Manager Jam, as the project was nicknamed, was a 48-hour real-time web event in which managers from 50 different countries swapped ideas and strategies for dealing with problems shared by all of them, regardless of geography. Some 8,100 managers logged on to the company's intranet to participate in the discussion forums.

Renewable energy resources are also a promising substitute product and are rapidly becoming more economically competitive with fossil fuels. Strategy Spotlight 2.7 addresses this critical issue.

The Intensity of Rivalry among Competitors in an Industry   Firms use tactics like price competition, advertising battles, product introductions, and increased customer service or warranties. Rivalry occurs when competitors sense the pressure or act on an opportunity to improve their position.[60]

Some forms of competition, such as price competition, are typically highly destabilizing and are likely to erode the average level of profitability in an industry.[61] Rivals easily match price cuts, an action that lowers profits for all firms. On the other hand, advertising battles expand overall demand or enhance the level of product differentiation for the benefit of all firms in the industry. Rivalry, of course, differs across industries. In some instances it is characterized as warlike, bitter, or cutthroat, whereas in other industries it is referred to as polite and respectful. Intense rivalry is the result of several interacting factors, including the following:

- *Numerous or equally balanced competitors.* When there are many firms in an industry, the likelihood of mavericks is great. Some firms believe they can make moves without being noticed. Even when there are relatively few firms, and they are nearly equal in size and resources, instability results from fighting among companies having the resources for sustained and vigorous retaliation.
- *Slow industry growth.* Slow industry growth turns competition into a fight for market share, since firms seek to expand their sales.
- *High fixed or storage costs.* High fixed costs create strong pressures for all firms to increase capacity. Excess capacity often leads to escalating price cutting.
- *Lack of differentiation or switching costs.* Where the product or service is perceived as a commodity or near commodity, the buyer's choice is typically based on price and service, resulting in pressures for intense price and service competition. Lack of switching costs, described earlier, has the same effect.
- *Capacity augmented in large increments.* Where economies of scale require that capacity must be added in large increments, capacity additions can be very disruptive to the industry supply/demand balance.

substitute products and services products and services outside the industry that serve the same customer needs as the industry's products and services.

intensity of rivalry among competitors in an industry the threat that customers will switch their business to competitors within the industry.

strategy spotlight

2.7

The Growing Viability of Renewable Energy

Renewable energy supplied 16 percent of global final energy consumption and almost 20 percent of electricity production in 2010, according to REN21 (Renewable Energy Policy Network for the 21st Century). At the same time, global investment in renewable energy increased more than 20 percent to US$211 billion, and renewable energy capacity accounted for about a quarter of global power-generating capacity if including hydropower. In terms of added capacity, renewable energy accounted for around half of total added power capacity in 2010. Excluding hydropower, the top five countries for renewable energy capacity were the United States, China, Germany, Spain, and India.

Solar photovoltaics (PV) more than doubled in 2010, and Germany installed more solar PV in 2010 than was installed globally in 2009. Solar PV in the United States and Japan almost doubled from 2009 levels. Over 100 countries saw solar PV capacity increase.

Wind accounted for most of the electricity capacity, although in Europe more solar was installed than wind. "Wind power continues to lead the renewable electricity sector, with more new capacity installed in 2010 than

for any other technology," said Steve Sawyer, secretary general of the Global Wind Energy Council (GWEC) and a member of REN21's steering committee. "Equally important to note is that in 2010, for the first time, more wind power was added in developing countries and emerging markets than in the industrialized world." Average wind turbine sizes are continuing to grow, and direct drive designs have now captured 18 percent of the global market, according to GWEC.

By the beginning of 2011, 119 countries had some sort of policy target or renewable energy support policy—more than half of these in the developing world. Investment in renewable energy companies and in utility-scale generation and biofuel projects reached US$143 billion, with China alone attracting a third of this amount with US$48.5 billion.

"The increased renewable energy activity in developing countries highlighted in this year's report is very encouraging, since most of the future growth in energy demand is expected to occur in developing countries," said Mohamed El-Ashry, chairman of REN21's steering committee. "More and more of the word's people are gaining access to energy services through renewables, not only to meet their basic needs, but also to enable them to develop economically."

Sources: Renewable energy produced 20% of 2010 global electricity. www .renewableenergyfocus.com. July 13, 2011.

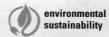 **environmental sustainability**

- ***High exit barriers.*** Exit barriers are economic, strategic, and emotional factors that keep firms competing even though they may be earning low or negative returns on their investments. Some exit barriers are specialized assets, fixed costs of exit, strategic interrelationships (e.g., relationships between the business units and others within a company in terms of image, marketing, shared facilities, and so on), emotional barriers, and government and social pressures (e.g., governmental discouragement of exit out of concern for job loss).

Rivalry between firms is often based solely on price, but it can involve other factors. Take Pfizer's market position in the impotence treatment market. Pfizer was the first pharmaceutical firm to develop Viagra, a highly successful drug that treats impotence.

In several countries, the United Kingdom among them, Pfizer faced a lawsuit by Eli Lilly & Co. and ICOS Corp. challenging its patent protection. These two pharmaceutical firms entered into a joint venture to market Cialis, a drug to compete with Viagra. The U.K. courts agreed and lifted the patent.

This opened the door for Eli Lilly and ICOS to proceed with challenging Pfizer's market position. Because Cialis has fewer side effects than Viagra, U.K. physicians switched prescriptions from Viagra to Cialis, which eroded Viagra's market share rapidly. By 2004, Cialis had 40% of the U.K. market; by 2011, it had overtaken Viagra as the global market leader.[62]

Exhibit 2.8 summarizes our discussion of industry five-forces analysis. It points out how various factors such as economies of scale and capital requirements affect each "force."

How the Internet and Digital Technologies Are Affecting the Five Competitive Forces

The **Internet** and other digital technologies are having a significant impact on nearly every industry. These technologies have fundamentally changed the ways businesses interact with each other and with consumers. In most cases, these changes have affected industry forces in ways that have created many new strategic challenges. In this section, we will evaluate Michael Porter's five-forces model in terms of the actual use of the Internet and the new technological capabilities that it makes possible.

The Threat of New Entrants   In most industries, the threat of new entrants has increased because digital and Internet-based technologies lower barriers to entry. For example, businesses that reach customers primarily through the Internet may enjoy savings on other traditional expenses such as office rent, sales-force salaries, printing, and postage. This may encourage more entrants who, because of the lower start-up expenses, see an opportunity to capture market share by offering a product or performing a service more efficiently than existing competitors. Thus, a new cyber entrant can use the savings provided by the Internet to charge lower prices and compete on price despite the incumbent's scale advantages.

Alternatively, because digital technologies often make it possible for young firms to provide services that are equivalent or superior to an incumbent, a new entrant may be able to serve a market more effectively, with more personalized services and greater attention to product details. A new firm may be able to build a reputation in its niche and charge premium prices. By so doing, it can capture part of an incumbent's business and erode profitability. Consider voice over Internet protocol (VOIP), a fast growing alternative to traditional phone service, which is expected to reach 25 million U.S. households by 2012.[63] Savings of 20 to 30 percent are common for VOIP consumers. This is driving prices down and lowering telecom industry profits. More importantly it threatens the value of the phone line infrastructure that the major carriers have invested in so heavily.

Another potential benefit of web-based business is access to distribution channels. Manufacturers or distributors that can reach potential outlets for their products more efficiently by means of the Internet may enter markets that were previously closed to them. Access is not guaranteed, however, because strong barriers to entry exist in certain industries.[64]

The Bargaining Power of Buyers   The Internet and wireless technologies may increase buyer power by providing consumers with more information to make buying decisions and by lowering switching costs. But these technologies may also suppress the power of traditional buyer channels that have concentrated buying power in the hands of a few, giving buyers new ways to access sellers. To sort out these differences, let's first distinguish between two types of buyers: end users and buyer channel intermediaries.

End users are the final customers in a distribution channel. Internet sales activity that is labeled "B2C"—that is, business-to-consumer—is concerned with end users. The Internet is likely to increase the power of these buyers for several reasons. First, the Internet

Internet a global network of linked computers that use a common transmission format, exchange information, and store data.

>LO2.6
How the Internet and digitally based capabilities are affecting the five competitive forces and industry profitability.

Threat of New Entrants Is High When:	High	Low
Economies of scale are		X
Product differentiation is		X
Capital requirements are		X
Switching costs are		X
Incumbent's control of distribution channels is		X
Incumbent's proprietary knowledge is		X
Incumbent's access to raw materials is		X
Incumbent's access to government subsidies is		X

Power of Buyers Is High When:	High	Low
Concentration of buyers relative to suppliers is	X	
Switching costs are		X
Product differentiation of suppliers is		X
Threat of backward integration by buyers is	X	
Extent of buyer's profits is		X
Importance of the supplier's input to quality of buyer's final product is		X

Power of Suppliers Is High When:	High	Low
Concentration relative to buyer industry is	X	
Availability of substitute products is		X
Importance of customer to the supplier is		X
Differentiation of the supplier's products and services is	X	
Switching costs of the buyer are	X	
Threat of forward integration by the supplier is	X	

Threat of Substitute Products Is High When:	High	Low
The differentiation of the substitute product is	X	
Rate of improvement in price–performance relationship of substitute product is	X	

Intensity of Competitive Rivalry Is High When:	High	Low
Number of competitors is	X	
Industry growth rate is		X
Fixed costs are	X	
Storage costs are	X	
Product differentiation is		X
Switching costs are		X
Exit barriers are	X	
Strategic stakes are	X	

Exhibit 2.8   **Competitive Analysis Checklist**

provides large amounts of consumer information. This gives end users the information they need to shop for quality merchandise and bargain for price concessions. The automobile industry provides an excellent example. For a small fee, agencies such as Consumers Union (publishers of *Consumer Reports*) will provide customers with detailed information about actual automobile manufacturer costs.[65] This information, available online, can be used to bid down dealers' profits. Second, an end user's switching costs are also potentially much lower because of the Internet. Switching may involve only a few clicks of the mouse to find and view a competing product or service online.

In contrast, the bargaining power of distribution channel buyers may decrease because of the Internet. *Buyer channel intermediaries* are the wholesalers, distributors, and retailers who serve as intermediaries between manufacturers and end users. In some industries, they are dominated by powerful players that control who gains access to the latest goods or the best merchandise. The Internet and wireless communications, however, make it much easier and less expensive for businesses to reach customers directly. Thus, the Internet may increase the power of incumbent firms relative to that of traditional buyer channels. Strategy Spotlight 2.8 illustrates some of the changes brought on by the Internet that have affected the industry's two types of buyers.

The Bargaining Power of Suppliers   Use of the Internet and digital technologies to speed up and streamline the process of acquiring supplies is already benefiting many sectors of the economy. But the net effect of the Internet on supplier power will depend on the nature of competition in a given industry. As with buyer power, the extent to which the Internet is a benefit or a detriment also hinges on the supplier's position along the supply chain.

The role of suppliers involves providing products or services to other businesses. The term "B2B"—that is, business-to-business—often refers to businesses that supply or sell to other businesses. The effect of the Internet on the bargaining power of suppliers is a double-edged sword. On the one hand, suppliers may find it difficult to hold onto customers because buyers can do comparative shopping and price negotiations so much faster on the Internet. This is especially damaging to supply-chain intermediaries, such as product distributors, who cannot stop suppliers from directly accessing other potential business customers. In addition, the Internet inhibits the ability of suppliers to offer highly differentiated products or unique services. Most procurement technologies can be imitated by competing suppliers, and the technologies that make it possible to design and customize new products rapidly are being used by all competitors.

On the other hand, several factors may also contribute to stronger supplier power. First, the growth of new web-based business may create more downstream outlets for suppliers to sell to. Second, suppliers may be able to create web-based purchasing arrangements that make purchasing easier and discourage their customers from switching. Online procurement systems directly link suppliers and customers, reducing transaction costs and paperwork.[66] Third, the use of proprietary software that links buyers to a supplier's website may create a rapid, low-cost ordering capability that discourages the buyer from seeking other sources of supply. *Amazon.com*, for example, created and patented One-Click purchasing technology that speeds up the ordering process for customers who enroll in the service.[67]

Finally, suppliers will have greater power to the extent that they can reach end users directly without intermediaries. Previously, suppliers often had to work through intermediaries who brought their products or services to market for a fee. But a process known as *disintermediation* is removing the organizations or business process layers responsible for intermediary steps in the value chain of many industries.[68] Just as the Internet is eliminating some business functions, it is creating an opening for new functions. These new activities are entering the value chain by a process known as *reintermediation*—the introduction of new types of intermediaries. Many of these new functions are affecting

Buyer Power in the Book Industry: The Role of the Internet

The $25 billion book publishing industry illustrates some of the changes brought on by the Internet that have affected buying power among two types of buyers—end users and buyer channel intermediaries. Prior to the Internet, book publishers worked primarily through large distributors. These intermediaries such as Tennessee-based Ingram, one of the largest and most powerful distributors, exercised strong control over the movement of books from publishers to bookstores. This power was especially strong relative to small, independent publishers who often found it difficult to get their books into bookstores and in front of potential customers.

Sources: Healy, M. 2009. Book industry trends 2009 shows publishers' net revenues rose 1.0 percent in 2007 to reach $40.3 billion. *www.bisg.org.* May 29: np; Books "most popular online buy." 2008. *newsvote.bbc.co.uk.* January 29: np. Hoynes, M. 2002. Is it the same for book sales? *www.bookweb.org.* March 20; *www.parapublishing.com;* Teague, D. 2005. U.S. book production reaches new high of 195,000 titles in 2004; Fiction soars. *www.bowker.com.* May 24; Teicher, C. M. 2007. March of the small presses. *www.publishersweekly.com,* March 26; and, The Nielsen Company. 2010. Global trends in online: A Nielsen global consumer report.

The Internet has significantly changed these relationships. Publishers can now negotiate distribution agreements directly with online retailers such as Amazon and Books-A-Million. Such online bookstores now account for about $4 billion in annual sales. And small publishers can use the Internet to sell directly to end users and publicize new titles, without depending on buyer channel intermediaries to handle their books. By using the Internet to appeal to niche markets, 63,000 small publishers with revenues of less than $50 million each, generated $14.2 billion in sales in 2005—over half of the industry's total sales.

Future trends for the intermediary industry do not look favorable. The Book Industry Study Group (BISG) released figures in May 2009 that estimated that publishers' revenues in 2008 reached $40.3 billion, up 1 percent from 2007's total. BISG expects revenues to increase to $43.5 billion by the end of 2012. There is also good news for online booksellers: According to results from a 2010 worldwide survey by Nielsen Online, 44 percent of users had bought books online—up from 34 percent just three years earlier.

traditional supply chains. For example, delivery services are enjoying a boom because of the Internet. Many more consumers are choosing to have products delivered to their door rather than going out to pick them up.

The Threat of Substitutes Along with traditional marketplaces, the Internet has created a new marketplace and a new channel. In general, therefore, the threat of substitutes is heightened because the Internet introduces new ways to accomplish the same tasks.

Consumers will generally choose to use a product or service until a substitute that meets the same need becomes available at a lower cost. The economies created by Internet technologies have led to the development of numerous substitutes for traditional ways of doing business. For example, a company called Conferenza is offering an alternative way to participate in conferences for people who don't want to spend the time and money to attend. Conferenza's website provides summaries of many conference events, quality ratings using an "event intelligence" score, and schedules of upcoming events.[69]

Another example of substitution is in the realm of electronic storage. With expanded desktop computing, the need to store information electronically has increased dramatically. Until recently, the trend has been to create increasingly larger desktop storage capabilities and techniques for compressing information that create storage efficiencies. But a viable substitute has recently emerged: storing information digitally on the Internet. Companies such as My Docs Online Inc. are providing web-based storage that firms can access simply by leasing space online. Since these storage places are virtual, they can be accessed anywhere the web can be accessed. Travelers can access important documents and files without transporting them physically from place to place. Cyberstorage is not free, but it is cheaper and more convenient than purchasing and carrying disk storage.[70]

The Intensity of Competitive Rivalry Because the Internet creates more tools and means for competing, rivalry among competitors is likely to be more intense. Only those competitors that can use digital technologies and the web to give themselves a distinct image, create unique product offerings, or provide "faster, smarter, cheaper" services are likely to capture greater profitability with the new technology. Such gains are hard to sustain, however, because in most cases the new technology can be imitated quickly. Thus, the Internet tends to increase rivalry by making it difficult for firms to differentiate themselves and by shifting customer attention to issues of price.

Rivalry is more intense when switching costs are low and product or service differentiation is minimized. Because the Internet makes it possible to shop around, it has "commoditized" products that might previously have been regarded as rare or unique. Since the Internet reduces the importance of location, products that previously had to be sought out in geographically distant outlets are now readily available online. This makes competitors in cyberspace seem more equally balanced, thus intensifying rivalry.

The problem is made worse for marketers by the presence of shopping robots ("bots") and infomediaries that search the web for the best possible prices. Consumer websites like mySimon and PriceSCAN seek out all the web locations that sell similar products and provide price comparisons.[71] Obviously, this focuses the consumer exclusively on price. Some shopping infomediaries, such as BizRate and CNET, not only search for the lowest prices on many different products but also rank the customer service quality of different sites that sell similarly priced items.[72] Such infomediary services are good for consumers because they give them the chance to compare services as well as price. For businesses, however, they increase rivalry by consolidating the marketing message that consumers use to make a purchase decision into a few key pieces of information over which the selling company has little control.

Exhibit 2.9 summarizes many of the ways the Internet is affecting industry structure. These influences will also change how companies develop and deploy strategies to generate above-average profits and sustainable competitive advantage.

Using Industry Analysis: A Few Caveats

For industry analysis to be valuable, a company must collect and evaluate a wide variety of information. As the trend toward globalization accelerates, information on foreign markets as well as on a wider variety of competitors, suppliers, customers, substitutes, and potential new entrants becomes more critical. Industry analysis helps a firm not only to evaluate the profit potential of an industry but also consider various ways to strengthen its position vis-à-vis the five forces. However, we'd like to address a few caveats.

First, *managers must not always avoid low profit industries (or low profit segments in profitable industries).*[73] Such industries can still yield high returns for some players who pursue sound strategies. As an example, consider Paychex, a payroll-processing company.[74]

> Paychex, with $2 billion in revenues, became successful by serving small businesses. Existing firms had ignored them because they assumed that such businesses could not afford the service. When Paychex's founder, Tom Golisano, failed to convince his bosses at Electronic Accounting Systems that they were missing a great opportunity, he launched the firm. It now serves nearly 600,000 clients in the United States and Germany. Paychex's after-tax-return on sales is a stunning 24 percent.

Second, five-forces analysis implicitly *assumes a zero-sum game, determining how a firm can enhance its position relative to the forces.* Yet such an approach can often be short-sighted; that is, it can overlook the many potential benefits of developing constructive win–win relationships with suppliers and customers. Establishing long-term mutually beneficial relationships with suppliers improves a firm's ability to implement just-in-time (JIT)

zero-sum game a situation in which multiple players interact, and winners win only by taking from other players.

Exhibit 2.9   How the Internet and Digital Technologies Influence Industry

	Benefits to Industry (+)	Disadvantages to Industry (−)
Threat of New Entrants		• Lower barriers to entry increase number of new entrants. • Many Internet-based capabilities can be easily imitated.
Bargaining Power of Buyers	• Reduces the power of buyer intermediaries in many distribution channels.	• Switching costs decrease. • Information availability online empowers end users.
Bargaining Power of Suppliers	• Online procurement methods can increase bargaining power over suppliers.	• The Internet gives suppliers access to more customers and makes it easier to reach end users. • Online procurement practices deter competition and reduce differentiating features.
Threat of Substitutes	• Internet-based increases in overall efficiency can expand industry sales.	• Internet-based capabilities create more opportunities for substitution.
Intensity of Rivalry		• Since location is less important, the number of competitors increases. • Differences among competitors are harder to perceive online. • Rivalry tends to focus on price and differentiating features are minimized.

Sources: Bodily, S. & Venkataraman, S. 2004. Not walls, windows: Capturing value in the digital age. *Journal of Business Strategy,* 25(3): 15–25; and, Lumpkin, G. T., Droege, S. B., & Dess, G. G. 2002. E-commerce strategies: Achieving sustainable competitive advantage and avoiding pitfalls. *Organizational Dynamics,* 30 (Spring): 1–17.

inventory systems, which let it manage inventories better and respond quickly to market demands. A recent study found that if a company exploits its powerful position against a supplier, that action may come back to haunt the company.[75] Consider, for example, General Motors' heavy-handed dealings with its suppliers:[76]

> GM has a reputation for particularly aggressive tactics. Although it is striving to crack down on the most egregious of these, it continues to rank dead last in the annual supplier satisfaction survey. "It's a brutal process," says David E. Cole, who is head of the Center for Automotive Research in Ann Arbor [Mich.]. "There are bodies lying by the side of the road."
>
> Suppliers point to one particularly nasty tactic: shopping their technology out the back door to see if rivals can make it cheaper. In one case, a GM purchasing manager showed a supplier's new brake design to Delphi Corporation. He was fired. However, in a recent survey, parts executives said they tend to bring hot new technology to other carmakers first. This is yet another reason GM finds it hard to compete in an intensely competitive industry.

Third, the five-forces analysis also has been criticized for *being essentially a static analysis.* External forces as well as strategies of individual firms are continually changing the structure of all industries. The search for a dynamic theory of strategy has led to greater use of game theory in industrial organization economics research and strategy research.

Based on game-theoretic considerations, Brandenburger and Nalebuff introduced the concept of the value net,[77] which in many ways is an extension of the five-forces analysis. It is illustrated in Exhibit 2.10. The value net represents all the players in the game and analyzes how their interactions affect a firm's ability to generate and appropriate value. The vertical dimension of the net includes suppliers and customers. The firm has direct transactions with them. On the horizontal dimension are substitutes and complements, players with whom a firm interacts but may not necessarily transact. The concept of complementors is perhaps the single most important contribution of value net analysis and is explained in more detail below.

Complements typically are products or services that have a potential impact on the value of a firm's own products or services. Those who produce complements are usually referred to as complementors.[78] Powerful hardware is of no value to a user unless there is software that runs on it. Similarly, new and better software is possible only if the hardware on which it can be run is available. This is equally true in the video game industry, where the sales of game consoles and video games complement each other. Nintendo's success in the early 1990s was a result of its ability to manage its relationship with its complementors. It built a security chip into the hardware and then licensed the right to develop games to outside firms. These firms paid a royalty to Nintendo for each copy of the game sold. The royalty revenue enabled Nintendo to sell game consoles at close to its cost, thereby increasing its market share, which, in turn, caused more games to be sold and more royalties to be generated.[79]

Despite efforts to create win–win scenarios, conflict among complementors is inevitable.[80] After all, it is naive to expect that even the closest of partners will do you the favor of abandoning their own interests. And even the most successful partnerships are seldom trouble free. Power is a factor that comes into play as we see in Strategy Spotlight 2.9 with the example of Apple's iPod—an enormously successful product.

complements
products or services that have a impact on the value of a firm's products or services.

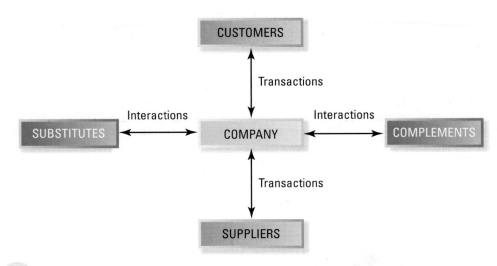

Exhibit 2.10   The Value Net

Source: Reprinted by permission of *Harvard Business Review.* Exhibit from "The Right Game: Use Game Theory to Shape Strategy," by A. Brandenburger and B. J. Nalebuff, July–August 1995. Copyright © 1995 by the Harvard Business School Publishing Corporation. All rights reserved.

We would like to close this section with some recent insights from Michael Porter, the originator of the five-forces analysis.[81] He addresses two critical issues in conducting a good industry analysis, which will yield an improved understanding of the root causes of profitability: (1) choosing the appropriate time frame and (2) a rigorous quantification of the five forces.

- *Good industry analysis looks rigorously at the structural underpinnings of profitability. A first step is to understand the time horizon.* One of the essential tasks in industry analysis is to distinguish short-term fluctuations from structural changes. A good guideline for the appropriate time horizon is the full business cycle for the particular industry. For most industries, a three- to five-year horizon is appropriate. However, for some industries with long lead times, such as mining, the appropriate horizon may be a decade or more. It is average profitability over this period, not profitability in any particular year, which should be the focus of analysis.
- *The point of industry analysis is not to declare the industry attractive or unattractive but to understand the underpinnings of competition and the root causes of profitability.* As much as possible, analysts should look at industry structure quantitatively, rather than be satisfied with lists of qualitative factors. Many elements of five forces can be quantified: the percentage of the buyer's total cost accounted for by the industry's product (to understand buyer price sensitivity); the percentage of industry sales required to fill a plant or operate a logistical network to efficient scale (to help assess barriers to entry); and the buyer's switching cost (determining the inducement an entrant or rival must offer customers).

Strategic Groups within Industries

In an industry analysis, two assumptions are unassailable: (1) No two firms are totally different, and (2) no two firms are exactly the same. The issue becomes one of identifying groups of firms that are more similar to each other than firms that are not, otherwise known as **strategic groups.**[82] This is important because rivalry tends to be greater among firms that are alike. Strategic groups are clusters of firms that share similar strategies. After all, is C&A in France more concerned about Galeries Lafayette or Carrefour? Is Mercedes more concerned about Hyundai or BMW? The answers are straightforward.[83]

> **strategic groups**
> clusters of firms that share similar strategies.

These examples are not meant to trivialize the strategic groups concept.[84] Classifying an industry into strategic groups involves judgment. If it is useful as an analytical tool, we must exercise caution in deciding what dimensions to use to map these firms. Dimensions include breadth of product and geographic scope, price/quality, degree of vertical integration, type of distribution (e.g., dealers, mass merchandisers, private label), and so on. Dimensions should also be selected to reflect the variety of strategic combinations in an industry. For example, if all firms in an industry have roughly the same level of product differentiation (or R&D intensity), this would not be a good dimension to select.

> **>LO2.7**
> The concept of strategic groups and their strategy and performance implications.

What value is the strategic groups concept as an analytical tool? *First, strategic groupings help a firm identify barriers to mobility that protect a group from attacks by other groups.*[85] Mobility barriers are factors that deter the movement of firms from one strategic position to another. For example, in the chainsaw industry, the major barriers protecting the high-quality/dealer-oriented group are technology, brand image, and an established network of servicing dealers.

The second value of strategic grouping is that it *helps a firm identify groups whose competitive position may be marginal or tenuous.* We may anticipate that these competitors may exit the industry or try to move into another group. In recent years in the retail department store industry, firms such as Super U and Champion in France have experienced

Apple's iPod: Relationships with Its Complementors

In 2002, Steve Jobs began his campaign to cajole the major music companies into selling tracks to iPod users through the iTunes Music Store, an online retail site. Most industry executives, after being burned by illegal file-sharing services like Napster and Kazaa, just wanted digital music to disappear. However, Jobs's passionate vision persuaded them to climb on board. He promised to reduce the risks that they faced by offering safeguards against piracy, as well as a hip product (iPod and iPad Touch) that would drive sales.

However, Apple had a much stronger bargaining position when its contracts with the music companies came up for renewal in April 2005. By then, iTunes had captured 80 percent of the market for legal downloads. The music companies, which were receiving between 60 and 70 cents per download, wanted more. Their reasoning: If the iTunes Music Store would only charge $1.50 or $2.00 per track, they could double or triple their revenues and profits. Since Jobs knew that he could sell more iPods if the music was cheap, he was determined to keep the price of a download at 99 cents and to maintain Apple's

margins. Given iTunes' dominant position, the music companies had little choice but to relent.

Apple's foray into music has been tremendously successful. Between 2006 and 2009, iPod sales increased from $7.7 billion to $9.4 billion—a 22 percent increase. And other music-related products and services soared from $4 billion to $5 billion over the same period. Despite tough competition, Apple still dominates the music player business.

Source: Hesseldahl, A. 2008. Now that we all have iPods. *BusinessWeek*, December 15: 36; Apple Computer Inc. 10-K, 2010; and, Yoffie, D. B. & Kwak, M. 2006. With friends like these: The art of managing complementors. *Harvard Business Review*, 84(9): 88–98.

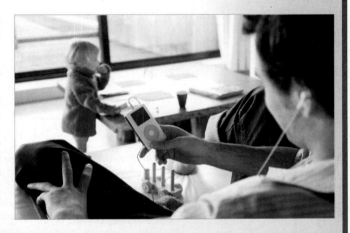

● Apple's iPod was largely responsible for the company's stellar financial performance between 2006 and 2009.

extremely difficult times because they were stuck in the middle, neither an aggressive discount player like Carrefour nor a prestigious upscale player like Au Printemps.

Third, strategic groupings *help chart the future directions of firms' strategies.* Arrows emanating from each strategic group can represent the direction in which the group (or a firm within the group) seems to be moving. If all strategic groups are moving in a similar direction, this could indicate a high degree of future volatility and intensity of competition. In the automobile industry, for example, the competition in the minivan and sport utility segments has intensified in recent years as many firms have entered those product segments.

Fourth, strategic groups are *helpful in thinking through the implications of each industry trend for the strategic group as a whole.* Is the trend decreasing the viability of a group? If so, in what direction should the strategic group move? Is the trend increasing or decreasing entry barriers? Will the trend decrease the ability of one group to separate itself from other groups? Such analysis can help in making predictions about industry evolution. A sharp increase in interest rates, for example, tends to have less impact on providers of higher-priced goods (e.g., Porsche) than on providers of lower-priced goods (e.g., Chevrolet Cobalt) whose customer base is much more price sensitive.

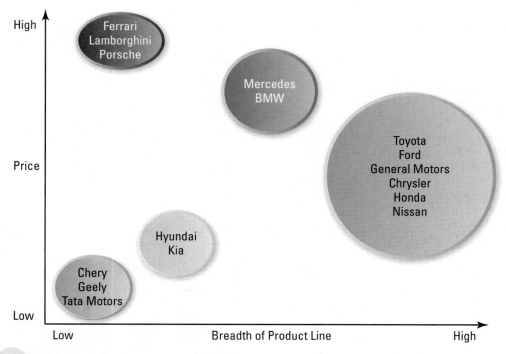

Exhibit 2.11   **The World Automobile Industry: Strategic Groups**

Note: Members of each strategic group are not inclusive, only illustrative.

Exhibit 2.11 provides a strategic grouping of the worldwide automobile industry.[86] The firms in each group are representative; not all firms are included in the mapping. We have identified five strategic groups. In the top left-hand corner are high-end luxury automakers who focus on a very narrow product market. Most of the cars produced by the members of this group cost well over $100,000. Some cost many times that amount. The 2012 Ferrari 458 Italia Spider started at $257,000, and the 2012 Lamborghini Aventador LP700-4 set you back about $387,000 (in case you were wondering how to spend your employment signing bonus). Players in this market have a very exclusive clientele and face little rivalry from other strategic groups. At the other extreme, in the lower left-hand corner is a strategic group that has low-price/low-quality attributes and targets a narrow market. These players, Chery, Geely, and Tata Motors, limit competition from other strategic groups by pricing their products very low. The third group (Mercedes and BMW) consists of firms high in product pricing/quality and average in their product-line breadth. The fourth group (at the far right) consists of firms with a broad range of products and multiple price points. These firms have entries that compete at both the lower end of the market (e.g., the Ford Focus) and the higher end (e.g., Chevrolet Corvette). The final group (near the middle), Hyundai and Kia, started off in the lower left-hand corner, now compete more with those firms to the far right (see more on this later in this section).

The auto market has been very dynamic and competition has intensified in recent years.[87] Many firms in different strategic groups compete in the same product markets, such as minivans and sport utility vehicles. In the late 1990s Mercedes entered the fray with its M series, and Porsche had an entry as well with its Cayenne, starting in 2004.

Some players are also going more upscale with their product offerings. Recently, Hyundai introduced its Genesis, starting at $33,000. This brings Hyundai into direct competition with entries from other strategic groups such as Toyota's Camry and Honda's

Accord. Hyundai is offering an extensive warranty (10 years, 100,000 miles) in an effort to offset customer perceptions of its lower quality. To further intensify competition, some key automakers are providing offerings in lower-priced segments. BMW, with its 1-series, is a well-known example. Such cars, priced in the low $30,000s, compete more directly with products from broad-line manufacturers like Ford, General Motors, and Toyota.

Such models are competing in an industry that has experienced relatively flat unit sales in the first half of the last decade. However, in recent years things have turned increasingly sour. U.S. automobile sales dropped from 13.2 million units in 2008 to only 10.4 million units in 2009 (the fewest units since 1982) and 11.3 million units in 2010. This compares to an average of 16.4 million units between 2000 and 2007. And J. D. Power predicts sales of only 13.2 million units for 2011, as the economy emerges from the recession.[88] One can certainly expect incentive-laden offerings to appear on dealer lots for some time to come.

Our discussion would not be complete, of course, without paying some attention to recent entries in the automobile industry that will likely lead to the formation of a new strategic group—placed at the bottom left corner of the grid in Exhibit 2.11. Three firms— China's Zhejiang Geely Holding Company, China's Chery Automobile Company, and India's Tata Motors—have introduced models that bring new meaning to the term "sub-compact."[89] Let's take a look at these econoboxes.

> Chery's QQ model sells for between $4,000 and $7,000 in the Chinese market and sports horsepower in the range of 51 to 74. Geely's best-selling four-door sedan, the Free Cruiser, retails from $6,300 and $6,900. The firm is planning to go more upscale with the Geely KingKong ($7,500−$10,000), a four-door 1.5- to 1.8-liter sedan, and the Vision ($9,700−$15,300), a 1.8-liter four-door sedan. But, for price-points, India's Tata Motors has everyone beat. In January 2008, it unveiled the Nano with an astonishing retail price of only $2,500. It is a four-door, five-seat hatchback that gets 54 miles per gallon. But before you order one—keep in mind that it only comes with a 30 horsepower engine.

Reflecting on Career Implications . . .

- *Creating the Environmentally Aware Organization:* In your career, what are some ways in which you can engage in scanning, monitoring, and intelligence gathering for future job opportunities? Consider, for example, subscribing to your field's professional publications and becoming actively involved in relevant professional organizations.
- *SWOT Analysis:* From a career standpoint, periodically evaluate your strengths and weaknesses as well as potential opportunities and threats to your career. In addition, strive to seek input from trusted peers and superiors.
- *General Environment:* Carefully evaluate the elements of the general environment facing your firm. Identify factors (e.g., rapid technological change) that can provide promising career opportunities as well as possibilities for you to add value for your organization. In doing this, don't focus solely on "internal factors" of your organization.
- *Five-Forces Analysis:* Consider the five forces affecting the industry within which your organization competes. If the "forces" are unfavorable, the long-term profit potential of the industry may be unattractive. And there will likely be fewer resources available and—all other things being equal—fewer career opportunities.

Summary

Managers must analyze the external environment to minimize or eliminate threats and exploit opportunities. This involves a continuous process of environmental scanning and monitoring as well as obtaining competitive intelligence on present and potential rivals. These activities provide valuable inputs for developing forecasts. In addition, many firms use scenario planning to anticipate and respond to volatile and disruptive environmental changes.

We identified two types of environments: the general environment and the competitive environment. The six segments of the general environment are demographic, sociocultural, political/legal, technological, economic, and global. Trends and events occurring in these segments, such as the aging of the population, higher percentages of women in the workplace, governmental legislation, and increasing (or decreasing) interest rates, can have a dramatic effect on a firm. A given trend or event may have a positive impact on some industries and a negative, a neutral, or no impact at all on others.

The competitive environment consists of industry-related factors and has a more direct impact than the general environment. Porter's five-forces model of industry analysis includes the threat of new entrants, buyer power, supplier power, threat of substitutes, and rivalry among competitors. The intensity of these factors determines, in large part, the average expected level of profitability in an industry. A sound awareness of such factors, both individually and in combination, is beneficial not only for deciding what industries to enter but also for assessing how a firm can improve its competitive position. We discussed how many of the changes brought about by the digital economy can be understood in the context of five-forces analysis. The limitations of five-forces analysis include its static nature and its inability to acknowledge the role of complementors. Although we addressed the general environment and competitive environment in separate sections, they are quite interdependent. A given environmental trend or event, such as changes in the ethnic composition of a population or a technological innovation, typically has a much greater impact on some industries than on others.

The concept of strategic groups is also important to the external environment of a firm. No two organizations are completely different nor are they exactly the same. The question is how to group firms in an industry on the basis of similarities in their resources and strategies. The strategic groups concept is valuable for determining mobility barriers across groups, identifying groups with marginal competitive positions, charting the future directions of firm strategies, and assessing the implications of industry trends for the strategic group as a whole.

Summary Review Questions

1. Why must managers be aware of a firm's external environment?

2. What is gathering and analyzing competitive intelligence and why is it important for firms to engage in it?

3. Discuss and describe the six elements of the external environment.

4. Select one of these elements and describe some changes relating to it in an industry that interests you.

5. Describe how the five forces can be used to determine the average expected profitability in an industry.

6. What are some of the limitations (or caveats) in using five-forces analysis?

7. Explain how the general environment and industry environment are highly related. How can such interrelationships affect the profitability of a firm or industry?

8. Explain the concept of strategic groups. What are the performance implications?

Key Terms

Experiential Exercise

Select one of the following industries: personal computers, airlines, or automobiles. For this industry, evaluate the strength of each of Porter's five forces as well as complementors.

Industry Force	High? Medium? Low?	Why?
1. Threat of new entrants		
2. Power of buyers		
3. Power of suppliers		
4. Threat of substitutes		
5. Rivalry among competitors		
6. Complementors		

Application Questions & Exercises

1. Imagine yourself as the CEO of a large firm in an industry in which you are interested. Please (1) identify major trends in the general environment, (2) analyze their impact on the firm, and (3) identify major sources of information to monitor these trends. (Use Internet and library resources.)

2. Analyze movements across the strategic groups in the UK retail industry. How do these movements within this industry change the nature of competition?

3. What are the major trends in the general environment that have impacted the German pharmaceutical industry?

4. Go to the Internet and look up *www.carrefour.com*. What are some of the five forces driving industry competition that are affecting the profitability of this firm?

Ethics Questions

1. What are some of the legal and ethical issues involved in collecting competitor intelligence in the following situations?

   a. Hotel A sends an employee posing as a potential client to Hotel B to find out who Hotel B's major corporate customers are.

   b. A firm hires an MBA student to collect information directly from a competitor while claiming the information is for a course project.

   c. A firm advertises a nonexistent position and interviews a rival's employees with the intention of obtaining competitor information.

2. What are some of the ethical implications that arise when a firm tries to exploit its power over a supplier?

References

1. Heimbuch, J. 2010. Hooray! Hawaii outlaws shark fin soup. *www.treehugger.com*. October 27: np.; Anonymous. 2006. The value of China's emerging middle class. *www.mkqpreview.com*. June: np; Wassener, B. 2010. A shark fin promotion backfires. *www.green.blogs.nytimes.com*. July 22: np; and, *www.citigroup.com*. We thank Kimberly Kentfield for her valued contributions.

2. Hamel, G. & Prahalad, C. K. 1994. *Competing for the future*. Boston: Harvard Business School Press.

3. Drucker, P. F. 1994. Theory of the business. *Harvard Business Review*, 72: 95–104.

4. For an insightful discussion on managers' assessment of the external environment, refer to Sutcliffe, K. M. & Weber, K. 2003. The high cost of accurate knowledge. *Harvard Business Review*, 81(5): 74–86.

5. For insights on recognizing and acting on environmental opportunities, refer to: Alvarez, S. A. & Barney, J. B. 2008. Opportunities, organizations, and entrepreneurship: Theory and debate. *Strategic Entrepreneurship Journal*, 2(3): entire issue.

6. Charitou, C. D. & Markides, C. C. 2003. Responses to disruptive strategic innovation. *MIT Sloan Management Review*, 44(2): 55–64.

7. Our discussion of scanning, monitoring, competitive intelligence, and forecasting concepts draws on several sources. These include Fahey, L. & Narayanan, V. K. 1983. *Macroenvironmental analysis for strategic management*. St. Paul, MN: West; Lorange, P., Scott, F. S., & Ghoshal, S.

1986. *Strategic control.* St. Paul, MN: West; Ansoff, H. I. 1984. *Implementing strategic management.* Englewood Cliffs, NJ: Prentice Hall; and, Schreyogg, G. & Stienmann, H. 1987. Strategic control: A new perspective. *Academy of Management Review,* 12: 91–103. An insightful discussion on how leaders can develop "peripheral vision" in environmental scanning is found in: Day, G. S. & Schoemaker, P. J. H. 2008. Are you a "vigilant leader"? *MIT Sloan Management Review,* 49 (3): 43–51.

8. Day & Schoemaker, op. cit.

9. Elenkov, D. S. 1997. Strategic uncertainty and environmental scanning: The case for institutional influences on scanning behavior. *Strategic Management Journal,* 18: 287–302.

10. For an interesting perspective on environmental scanning in emerging economies, see: May, R. C., Stewart, W. H., & Sweo, R. 2000. Environmental scanning behavior in a transitional economy: Evidence from Russia. *Academy of Management Journal,* 43(3): 403–27.

11. Bryon, E. 2010. For insight into P&G, check Olay numbers. *The Wall Street Journal,* October 27: C1.

12. Tang, J. 2010. How entrepreneurs discover opportunities in China: An institutional view. *Asia Pacific Journal of Management,* 27(3): 461–480.

13. Walters, B. A. & Priem, R. L. 1999. Business strategy and CEO intelligence acquisition. *Competitive Intelligence Review,* 10(2): 15–22.

14. Prior, V. 1999. The language of competitive intelligence, Part 4. *Competitive Intelligence Review,* 10(1): 84–87.

15. Zahra, S. A. & Charples, S. S. 1993. Blind spots in competitive analysis. *Academy of Management Executive,* 7(2): 7–27.

16. Wolfenson, J. 1999. The world in 1999: A battle for corporate honesty. *The Economist,* 38: 13–30.

17. Drucker, P. F. 1997. The future that has already happened. *Harvard Business Review,* 75(6): 22.

18. Evans, P. B. & Wurster, T. S. 1997. Strategy and the new economics of information. *Harvard Business Review,* 75(5): 71–82.

19. Fahey & Narayanan, op. cit., p. 41.

20. Insights on how to improve predictions can be found in: Cross, R., Thomas, R. J., & Light, D. A. 2009. The prediction lover's handbook. *MIT Sloan Management Review,* 50 (2): 32–34.

21. Courtney, H., Kirkland, J., & Viguerie, P. 1997. Strategy under uncertainty. *Harvard Business Review,* 75(6): 66–79.

22. Odlyzko, A. 2003. False hopes. *Red Herring,* March: 31.

23. Coy, P. 2009. Worst predictions about 2008. *BusinessWeek,* January 12: 15–16.

24. For an interesting perspective on how Accenture practices and has developed its approach to scenario planning, refer to Ferguson, G., Mathur, S., & Shah, B. 2005. Evolving from information to insight. *MIT Sloan Management Review,* 46(2): 51–58.

25. Dean, T. J., Brown, R. L., & Bamford, C. E. 1998. Differences in large and small firm responses to environmental context: Strategic implications from a comparative analysis of business formations. *Strategic Management Journal,* 19: 709–728.

26. Some insights on management during economic downturns are in: Colvin, G. 2009. How to manage your business in a recession. *Fortune,* January 19: 88–93.

27. Colvin, G. 1997. How to beat the boomer rush. *Fortune,* August 18: 59–63.

28. Porter, M. E. 2010. Discovering—and lowering—the real costs of health care. *Harvard Business Review,* 89 (1/2): 49–50.

29. U.S. Bureau of Labor Statistics. 2009. *Occupational handbook, 2010–2011 edition.* December 19. www.bls.gov/oco/oco203.htm, and World population prospects: The 2006 revision. *www.esa.un.org.* May 5, 2007.

30. Challenger, J. 2000. Women's corporate rise has reduced relocations. *Lexington* (KY) *Herald-Leader,* October 29: D1.

31. Kane, Y. 2009. Videogame firms make a play for women: Publishers roll out fashion-themed games for girls, workout and dance titles for older females. *The Wall Street Journal,* October 13.

32. Watkins, M. D. 2003. Government games. *MIT Sloan Management Review,* 44(2): 91–95.

33. A discussion of the political issues surrounding caloric content on meals is in: Orey, M. 2008. A food fight over calorie counts. *BusinessWeek,* February 11: 36.

34. www.corporate-governance-code.de/index-e.html. Accessed October 24, 2011.

35. Davies, A. 2000. The welcome mat is out for nerds. *BusinessWeek,* May 21: 17; Broache, A. 2007. Annual H-1B visa cap met—already. *news.cnet.com,* April 3: np; and, Anonymous. Undated. Cap count for H-1B and H-2B workers for fiscal year 2009. *www.uscis.gov:* np.

36. Hout, T. M., Ghemawat, P. 2010. China vs. the world: Whose technology is it? *Harvard Business Review,* 88(12): 94–103.

37. Anonymous. 1999. Business ready for Internet revolution. *Financial Times,* May 21: 17.

38. A discussion of an alternate energy—marine energy—is the topic of: Boyle, M. 2008. Scottish power. *Fortune,* March 17: 28.

39. Baker, S. & Aston, A. 2005. The business of nanotech. *BusinessWeek,* February 14: 64–71.

40. Morse, G. 2009. The power of unwitting workers. *Harvard Business Review,* 87(10): 26.

41. For an insightful discussion of the causes of the global financial crisis, read: Johnson, S. 2009. The global financial crisis—what really precipitated it? *MIT Sloan Management Review,* 50(2): 16–18.

42. Tyson, L. D. 2011. A better stimulus for the U.S. economy. *Harvard Business Review,* 89(1/2): 53.

43. A interesting and balanced discussion on the merits of multinationals to the U.S. economy is found in: Mandel, M. 2008. Multinationals: Are they good for America? *BusinessWeek,* March 10: 41–64.

44. Insights on risk perception across countries are addressed in: Purda, L. D. 2008. Risk perception and the financial system. *Journal of International Business Studies,* 39(7): 1178–1196.

45. Gogoi, P. 2010. Many U.S. companies are hiring . . . overseas. *www.msn.com*. December 28: np.

46. Byrnes, N. 2006. The high cost of fear. *BusinessWeek,* November 6: 16.

47. Goll, I. & Rasheed, M. A. 1997. Rational decision-making and firm performance: The moderating role of environment. *Strategic Management Journal,* 18: 583–591.

48. This discussion draws heavily on Porter, M. E. 1980. *Competitive strategy.* New York: Free Press. Chapter 1.

49. Ibid.

50. Rivalry in the airline industry is discussed in: Foust, D. 2009. Which airlines will disappear in 2009? *BusinessWeek,* January 19: 46–47.

51. Fryer, B. 2001. Leading through rough times: An interview with Novell's Eric Schmidt. *Harvard Business Review,* 78(5): 117–123.

52. For a discussion on the importance of barriers to entry within industries, read: Greenwald, B. & Kahn, J. 2005. *Competition demystified: A radically simplified approach to business strategy.* East Rutherford, NJ: Portfolio.

53. A discussion of how the medical industry has erected entry barriers that have resulted in lawsuits is found in: Whelan, D. 2008. Bad medicine. *BusinessWeek,* March 10: 86–98.

54. The ProCD example draws heavily upon Shapiro, C. & Varian, H. R. 2000. Versioning: The smart way to sell information. *Harvard Business Review,* 78(1): 106–114.

55. Wise, R. & Baumgarter, P. 1999. Go downstream: The new profit imperative in manufacturing. *Harvard Business Review,* 77(5): 133–141.

56. Salman, W. A. 2000. The new economy is stronger than you think. *Harvard Business Review,* 77(6): 99–106.

57. Mudambi, R. & Helper, S. 1998. The "close but adversarial" model of supplier relations in the U.S. auto industry. *Strategic Management Journal,* 19: 775–792.

58. Trends in the solar industry are discussed in: Carey, J. 2009. Solar: The sun will come out tomorrow. *BusinessWeek,* January 12: 51.

59. Tischler, L. 2002. IBM: Manager jam. *Fast Company,* October: 48.

60. An interesting analysis of self-regulation in an industry (chemical) is in: Barnett, M. L. & King, A. A. 2008. Good fences make good neighbors: A longitudinal analysis of an industry self-regulatory institution. *Academy of Management Journal,* 51(6): 1053–1078.

61. For an interesting perspective on the intensity of competition in the supermarket industry, refer to Anonymous. 2005. Warfare in the aisles. *The Economist,* April 2: 6–8.

62. Walker, S. 2011. Cialis overtakes Viagra as market leader. July 13. *http://www.medical-specialists.co.uk/news/2011/07/13/cialis-overtakes-viagra-as-market-leader/*; Gumbel, A. 2004. Viagra rival Cialis boasts 40% market share. March 24. *http://www.independent.co.uk/news/business/news/viagra-rival-cialis-boasts-40-market-share-6172207.html*; and Marcial, G. 2000. Giving Viagra arun for its money. BusinessWeek, October 23: 173.

63. McGann, R. 2005. VOIP poised to take flight? *ClickZ.com.* February 23.

64. For an interesting perspective on changing features of firm boundaries, refer to Afuah, A. 2003. Redefining firm boundaries in the face of Internet: Are firms really shrinking? *Academy of Management Review,* 28(1): 34–53.

65. *www.consumerreports.org.*

66. Time to rebuild. 2001. *Economist,* May 19: 55–56.

67. *www.amazon.com.*

68. For more on the role of the Internet as an electronic intermediary, refer to Carr, N. G. 2000. Hypermediation: Commerce as clickstream. *Harvard Business Review,* 78(1): 46–48.

69. Olofson, C. 2001. The next best thing to being there. *Fast Company,* April: 175; and, *www.conferenza.com.*

70. Lelii, S. R. 2001. Free online storage a thing of the past? *eWEEK,* April 22.

71. *www.mysimon.com* and *www.pricescan.com.*

72. *www.cnet.com* and *www.bizrate.com.*

73. For insights into strategies in a low-profit industry, refer to: Hopkins, M. S. 2008. The management lessons of a beleaguered industry. *MIT Sloan Management Review,* 50(1): 25–31.

74. Foust, D. 2007. The best performers. *BusinessWeek,* March 26: 58–95; Rosenblum, D., Tomlinson, D., & Scott, L. 2003. Bottom-feeding for blockbuster businesses. *Harvard Business Review,* 81(3): 52–59; *Paychex 2006 Annual Report;* and, *WellPoint Health Network 2005 Annual Report.*

75. Kumar, N. 1996. The power of trust in manufacturer–retailer relationship. *Harvard Business Review,* 74(6): 92–110.

76. Welch, D. 2006. Renault-Nissan: Say hello to Bo. *BusinessWeek,* July 31: 56–57.

77. Brandenburger, A. & Nalebuff, B. J. 1995. The right game: Use game theory to shape strategy. *Harvard Business Review,* 73(4): 57–71.

78. For a scholarly discussion of complementary assets and their relationship to competitive advantage, refer to Stieglitz, N. & Heine, K. 2007. Innovations and the role of complementarities in a strategic theory of the firm. *Strategic Management Journal,* 28(1): 1–15.

79. A useful framework for the analysis of industry evolution has been proposed by Professor Anita McGahan of Boston University. Her analysis is based on the identification of the core activities and the core assets of an industry and the threats they face. She suggests that an industry may follow one of four possible evolutionary trajectories—radical change, creative change, intermediating change, or progressive change—based on these two types of threats of obsolescence. Refer to: McGahan, A. M. 2004. How industries change. *Harvard Business Review,* 82(10): 87–94.

80. Yoffie, D. B. & Kwak, M. 2006. With friends like these: The art of managing complementors. *Harvard Business Review,* 84(9): 88–98.

81. Porter, M. I. 2008. The five competitive forces that shape strategy. *Harvard Business Review,* 86 (1): 79–93.

82. Peteraf, M. & Shanley, M. 1997. Getting to know you: A theory of strategic group identity. *Strategic Management Journal,* 18 (Special Issue): 165–186.

83. An interesting scholarly perspective on strategic groups may be found in Dranove, D., Perteraf, M., &

Shanley, M. 1998. Do strategic groups exist? An economic framework for analysis. *Strategic Management Journal,* 19(11): 1029–1044.

84. For an empirical study on strategic groups and predictors of performance, refer to Short, J. C., Ketchen, D. J., Jr., Palmer, T. B., & Hult, T. M. 2007. Firm, strategic group, and industry influences on performance. *Strategic Management Journal,* 28(2): 147–167.

85. This section draws on several sources, including Kerwin, K. R. & Haughton, K. 1997. Can Detroit make cars that baby boomers like? *BusinessWeek,* December 1: 134–148; and, Taylor, A., III. 1994. The new golden age of autos. *Fortune,* April 4: 50–66.

86. Csere, C. 2001. Supercar supermarket. *Car and Driver,* January: 118–127.

87. For a discussion of the extent of overcapacity in the worldwide automobile industry, read: Roberts, D., Matlack, C., Busyh, J., & Rowley, I. 2009. A hundred factories too many. *BusinessWeek,* January 19: 42–43.

88. Naughton, K. 2010. HIS auto trims 2010 U.S. vehicle sales forecast to 11.3 million units. *www.bloomberg.com/news.* September 27: np; and, Woodall, B. 2011. J. D. Power lowers U.S. auto sales forecast. *www.reuters.com.* August 10: np.

89. This discussion draws on: Wojdyla, B. 2008. The $2500 Tata Nano, unveiled in India. *jalopnik.com.* January 10: np; Roberts, D. 2008. China's Geely has global auto ambitions. *businessweek.com,* July 27: np; and, Fairclough, G. 2007. In China, Chery automobile drives an industry shift. *The Wall Street Journal,* December 4: A1, A17.

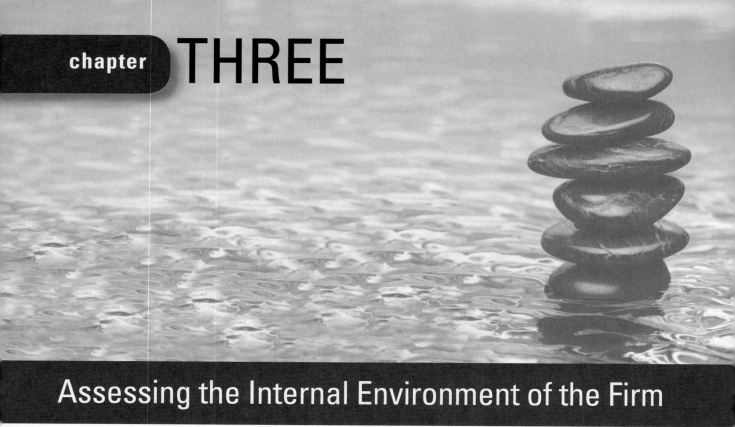

chapter THREE

Assessing the Internal Environment of the Firm

After reading this chapter, you should have a good understanding of:

LO3.1 The benefits and limitations of SWOT analysis in conducting an internal analysis of the firm.

LO3.2 The primary and support activities of a firm's value chain.

LO3.3 How value-chain analysis can help managers create value by investigating relationships among activities within the firm and between the firm and its customers and suppliers.

LO3.4 The resource-based view of the firm and the different types of tangible and intangible resources, as well as organizational capabilities.

LO3.5 The four criteria that a firm's resources must possess to maintain a sustainable advantage and how value created can be appropriated by employees and managers.

LO3.6 The usefulness of financial ratio analysis, its inherent limitations, and how to make meaningful comparisons of performance across firms.

LO3.7 The value of the "balanced scorecard" in recognizing how the interests of a variety of stakeholders can be interrelated.

LO3.8 How firms are using Internet technologies to add value and achieve unique advantages. (Appendix)

LEARNING OBJECTIVES

Two firms compete in the same industry and both have many strengths in a variety of functional areas: marketing, operations, logistics, and so on. However, one of these firms outperforms the other by a wide margin over a long period of time. How can this be so? This chapter endeavors to answer that question.

We begin with two sections that include frameworks for gaining key insights into a firm's internal environment: value-chain analysis and the resource-based view of the firm. In value-chain analysis, we divide a firm's activities into a series of value-creating steps. We then explore how individual activities within the firm add value, and also how *interrelationships* among activities within the firm, and between the firm and its suppliers and customers, create value.

In the resource-based view of the firm, we analyze the firm as a collection of tangible and intangible resources as well as organizational capabilities. Advantages that tend to be sustainable over time typically arise from creating *bundles* of resources and capabilities that satisfy four criteria: they are valuable, rare, difficult to imitate, and difficult to substitute. Not all of the value created by a firm will necessarily be kept (or appropriated) by the owners. We discuss the four key factors that determine how profits will be distributed between owners as well as employees and managers.

In the closing sections, we discuss how to evaluate a firm's performance and make comparisons across firms. We emphasize both the inclusion of financial resources and the interests of multiple stakeholders. Central to our discussion is the concept of the balanced scorecard, which recognizes that the interests of different stakeholders can be interrelated. We also consider how a firm's performance evolves over time and how it compares with industry norms and key competitors.

In an appendix to this chapter, we explore how Internet-based businesses and incumbent firms are using digital technologies to add value. We consider four activities—search, evaluation, problem solving, and transaction—as well as three types of content—customer feedback, expertise, and entertainment programming. Such technology-enhanced capabilities are providing new means with which firms can achieve competitive advantages.

Learning from Mistakes

Toyota Motor Company had developed an industry-leading strategy that focused on value innovation and cost reduction.[1] For many years it was a solid strategy for both the company and its customers. Over the years, Toyota built a reputation for engineering excellence and cost cutting. Its engineers collaborated with suppliers to extract cost savings without compromising quality. Yet, by the middle of the last decade, Toyota's virtue had become a vice and eventually led to recalled vehicles, lawsuits, and a damaged reputation. What went wrong?

Toyota's problems stemmed from an overwhelming desire to cut costs. This, in turn, led to a product that did not meet the same high quality that its customers had come to expect. When a North American parts supplier interested in working with the automaker did a teardown of a 2007 Camry, its engineers were surprised by how much the traditional Toyota craftsmanship had been watered down by years of nips and tucks. One example of this came to light in 2006, when a redesigned Camry revealed an embarrassing flaw in its headliner (the lining that covers the inside of the roof). Under pressure to cut costs, a Toyota affiliate chose a carbon fiber material that had not yet been approved by Toyota engineers. Unfortunately, the new carbon fiber material required so much heat to mold during production that it would catch fire. Thus, as many as 30 percent of the parts were scrapped—compared to a normal scrap rate for headliners of about 5 percent.

The worst of Toyota's problems came in early 2010 when the company recalled around 3.8 million vehicles. The problem with these vehicles occurred when customers complained that their car would suddenly accelerate to speeds of over 100 mph without warning. This recall included America's most popular passenger vehicle, the Camry, and the best-selling gas-electric hybrid, the Prius. Recalls came after the National Highway Traffic Safety Administration received reports of 102 incidents in which the accelerator became stuck. However, safety analysts estimated that there were approximately 2,000 cases in which owners of Toyota vehicles, including Camry, Prius, and Lexus, experienced "runaway cars."

A well-publicized incident that further tarnished Toyota's reputation was the tragic death of the Saylor family. On August 28, 2009, Mark Saylor died alongside his wife Cleofe, and their daughter Mahala, 13, and Mrs. Saylor's brother, Chris Lastrella, when the Lexus they had rented accelerated out of control on a highway in San Diego. In the emergency call, Mr. Lastrella was heard saying: "We're in a Lexus . . . and we're going north on 125 and our accelerator is stuck . . . there's no brakes . . . we're approaching the intersection . . . Hold on . . . hold on and pray . . . pray."

Clearly, Toyota got carried away chasing high-speed growth, market share, and productivity gains year in and year out. This focus slowly dulled the commitment to quality embedded in Toyota's corporate culture. In February 2010, Kiichiro Toyoda, the grandson of the company's founder, told a congressional committee: "I fear the pace at which we have grown may have been too quick . . . Priorities became confused, and we were not able to stop, think and make improvements as much as we were able to do before."

Toyota aggressively tried to cut costs at a rate its product could not keep up with. By ignoring key aspects of the value chain, such as operations and R&D, quality was sacrificed within Toyota. This led to products that were faulty as well as a recall that has cost it billions of dollars in repairs and lost revenue—plus a damaged reputation.

In this chapter we will place heavy emphasis on the value-chain concept. That is, we focus on the key value-creating activities (e.g., operations, marketing and sales, and procurement) that a firm must effectively manage and integrate in order to attain competitive advantages in the marketplace. However, firms must not only pay close attention to their own value-creating activities but must also maintain close and effective relationships with key organizations outside the firm boundaries such as suppliers, customers, and alliance partners. Clearly, Toyota's overemphasis on cost cutting—both within the firm and with its suppliers—eroded the quality of its cars as well as its reputation with customers.

Before moving to value-chain analysis, let's briefly revisit the benefits and limitations of SWOT analysis. As discussed in Chapter 2, a SWOT analysis consists of a careful listing of a firm's strengths, weaknesses, opportunities, and threats. While we believe SWOT analysis is very helpful as a starting point, it should not form the primary basis for evaluating a firm's internal strengths and weaknesses or the opportunities and threats in the environment. Strategy Spotlight 3.1 elaborates on the limitations of the traditional SWOT approach.

We will now turn to value-chain analysis. As you will see, it provides greater insights into analyzing a firm's competitive position than SWOT analysis does by itself.

>LO3.1
The benefits and limitations of SWOT analysis in conducting an internal analysis of the firm.

Value-Chain Analysis

Value-chain analysis views the organization as a sequential process of value-creating activities. The approach is useful for understanding the building blocks of competitive advantage and was described in Michael Porter's seminal book *Competitive Advantage*.[2] Value is the amount that buyers are willing to pay for what a firm provides them and is measured by total revenue, a reflection of the price a firm's product commands and the quantity it can sell. A firm is profitable when the value it receives exceeds the total costs involved in creating its product or service. Creating value for buyers that exceeds the costs of production (i.e., margin) is a key concept used in analyzing a firm's competitive position.

Porter described two different categories of activities. First, five **primary activities**—inbound logistics, operations, outbound logistics, marketing and sales, and service—contribute to the physical creation of the product or service, its sale and transfer to the buyer, and its service after the sale. Second, **support activities**—procurement, technology development, human resource management, and general administration—either add value by themselves or add value through important relationships with both primary activities and other support activities. Exhibit 3.1 illustrates Porter's value chain.

value-chain analysis a strategic analysis of an organization that uses value-creating activities.

primary activities sequential activities of the value chain that refer to the physical creation of the product or service, its sale and transfer to the buyer, and its service after sale, including inbound logistics, operations, outbound logistics, marketing and sales, and service.

support activities activities of the value chain that either add value by themselves or add value through important relationships with both primary activities and other support activities; including procurement, technology development, human resource management, and general administration.

The Value Chain

Support Activities

| General administration |
| Human resource management |
| Technology development |
| Procurement |

Margin

| Inbound logistics | Operations | Outbound logistics | Marketing and sales | Service |

Margin

Primary Activities

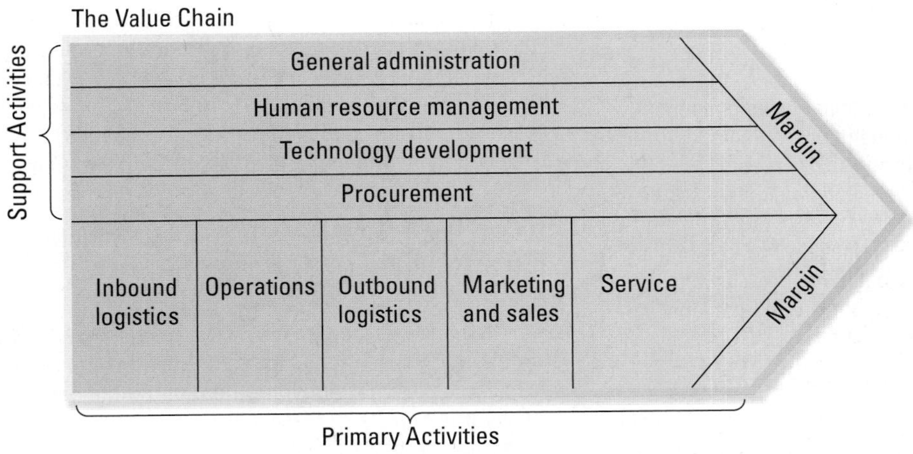

Exhibit 3.1 **The Value Chain: Primary and Support Activities**

Source: Reprinted with the permission of Free Press, a division of Simon & Schuster Inc., from *Competitive Advantage: Creating and Sustaining Superior Performance* by Michael E. Porter. Copyright © 1985, 1998 The Free Press. All rights reserved.

The Limitations of SWOT Analysis

SWOT analysis is a tried-and-true tool of strategic analysis. SWOT (strengths, weaknesses, opportunities, threats) analysis is used regularly in business to initially evaluate the opportunities and threats in the business environment as well as the strengths and weaknesses of a firm's internal environment. Top managers rely on SWOT to stimulate self-reflection and group discussions about how to improve their firm and position it for success.

But SWOT has its limitations. It is just a starting point for discussion. By listing the firm's attributes, managers have the raw material needed to perform more in-depth strategic analysis. However, SWOT cannot show them how to achieve a competitive advantage. They must not make SWOT analysis an end in itself, temporarily raising awareness about important issues but failing to lead to the kind of action steps necessary to enact strategic change.

Consider the ProCD example from Chapter 2, page 97. A brief SWOT analysis might include the following:

Strengths	Opportunities
First-mover advantage	Demand for electronic phone books
Low labor cost	Sudden growth in use of digital technology

Weaknesses	Threats
Inexperienced new company	Easily duplicated product
No proprietary information	Market power of incumbent firms

The combination of low production costs and an early-mover advantage in an environment where demand for CD-based phone books was growing rapidly seems to indicate that ProCD founder James Bryant had a golden opportunity. But the SWOT analysis did not reveal how to turn those strengths into a competitive advantage, nor did it highlight how rapidly the environment would change, allowing imitators to come into the market and erode his first-mover advantage. Let's look at some of the limitations of SWOT analysis.

Strengths May Not Lead to an Advantage

A firm's strengths and capabilities, no matter how unique or impressive, may not enable it to achieve a competitive advantage in the marketplace. It is akin to recruiting a concert pianist to join a gang of thugs—even though such

Sources: Shapiro, C. & Varian, H. R. 2000. Versioning: The Smart Way to Sell Information. *Harvard Business Review*, 78(1): 99–106; and, Picken, J. C. & Dess, G. G. 1997. *Mission Critical*. Burr Ridge, IL: Irwin Professional Publishing.

an ability is rare and valuable, it hardly helps the organization attain its goals and objectives! Similarly, the skills of a highly creative product designer would offer little competitive advantage to a firm that produces low-cost commodity products. Indeed, the additional expense of hiring such an individual could erode the firm's cost advantages. If a firm builds its strategy on a capability that cannot, by itself, create or sustain competitive advantage, it is essentially a wasted use of resources. ProCD had several key strengths, but it did not translate them into lasting advantages in the marketplace.

SWOT's Focus on the External Environment Is Too Narrow

Strategists who rely on traditional definitions of their industry and competitive environment often focus their sights too narrowly on current customers, technologies, and competitors. Hence they fail to notice important changes on the periphery of their environment that may trigger the need to redefine industry boundaries and identify a whole new set of competitive relationships. Reconsider the example from Chapter 2 of *Encyclopaedia Britannica*, whose competitive position was severely eroded by a "nontraditional" competitor—CD-based encyclopedias (e.g., Microsoft *Encarta*) that could be used on home computers.

SWOT Gives a One-Shot View of a Moving Target

A key weakness of SWOT is that it is primarily a static assessment. It focuses too much of a firm's attention on one moment in time. Essentially, this is like studying a single frame of a motion picture. You may be able to identify the principal actors and learn something about the setting, but it doesn't tell you much about the plot. Competition among organizations is played out over time. As circumstances, capabilities, and strategies change, static analysis techniques do not reveal the dynamics of the competitive environment. Clearly, ProCD was unaware that its competitiveness was being eroded so quickly.

SWOT Overemphasizes a Single Dimension of Strategy

Sometimes firms become preoccupied with a single strength or a key feature of the product or service they are offering and ignore other factors needed for competitive success. For example, Toyota, the giant automaker, paid a heavy price for its excessive emphasis on cost control. The resulting problems with quality and the negative publicity led to severe financial losses and an erosion of its reputation in many markets.

SWOT analysis has much to offer, but only as a starting point. By itself, it rarely helps a firm develop competitive advantages that it can sustain over time.

To get the most out of value-chain analysis, view the concept in its broadest context, without regard to the boundaries of your own organization. That is, place your organization within a more encompassing value chain that includes your firm's suppliers, customers, and alliance partners. Thus, in addition to thoroughly understanding how value is created within the organization, be aware of how value is created for other organizations in the overall supply chain or distribution channel.[3]

>LO3.2
The primary and support activities of a firm's value chain.

Next, we'll describe and provide examples of each of the primary and support activities. Then, we'll provide examples of how companies add value by means of relationships among activities within the organization as well as activities outside the organization, such as those activities associated with customers and suppliers.[4]

Primary Activities

Five generic categories of primary activities are involved in competing in any industry, as shown in Exhibit 3.2. Each category is divisible into a number of distinct activities that depend on the particular industry and the firm's strategy.[5]

Inbound Logistics   **Inbound logistics** is primarily associated with receiving, storing, and distributing inputs to the product. It includes material handling, warehousing, inventory control, vehicle scheduling, and returns to suppliers.

inbound logistics receiving, storing, and distributing inputs of a product.

Just-in-time (JIT) inventory systems, for example, were designed to achieve efficient inbound logistics. In essence, Toyota epitomizes JIT inventory systems, in which parts deliveries arrive at the assembly plants only hours before they are needed. JIT systems play a vital role in fulfilling Toyota's commitment to fill a buyer's new car order in just five days.[6] This standard is in sharp contrast to most competitors that require approximately 30 days' notice to build vehicles. Toyota's standard is three times faster than even Honda Motors, considered to be the industry's most efficient in order follow-through. The five

Exhibit 3.2
The Value Chain: Some Factors to Consider in Assessing a Firm's Primary Activities

Inbound Logistics

- Location of distribution facilities to minimize shipping times.
- Warehouse layout and designs to increase efficiency of operations for incoming materials.

Operations

- Efficient plant operations to minimize costs.
- Efficient plant layout and workflow design.
- Incorporation of appropriate process technology.

Outbound Logistics

- Effective shipping processes to provide quick delivery and minimize damages.
- Shipping of goods in large lot sizes to minimize transportation costs.

Marketing and Sales

- Innovative approaches to promotion and advertising.
- Proper identification of customer segments and needs.

Service

- Quick response to customer needs and emergencies.
- Quality of service personnel and ongoing training.

Source: Adapted from Porter, M.E. 1985. *Competitive Advantage: Creating and Sustaining Superior Performance.* New York: Free Press.

days represent the time from the company's receipt of an order to the time the car leaves the assembly plant. Actual delivery may take longer, depending on where a customer lives. How can Toyota achieve such fast turnaround?

- Its 360 key suppliers are linked to the company by way of computer on a virtual assembly line.
- Suppliers load parts onto trucks in the order in which they will be installed.
- Parts are stacked on trucks in the same place each time to help workers unload them quickly.
- Deliveries are required to meet a rigid schedule with as many as 12 trucks a day and no more than four hours between trucks.

operations all activities associated with transforming inputs into the final product form.

Operations Operations include all activities associated with transforming inputs into the final product form, such as machining, packaging, assembly, testing, printing, and facility operations.

Creating environmentally friendly manufacturing is one way to use operations to achieve competitive advantage. Shaw Industries (now part of Berkshire Hathaway), a world-class competitor in the floor-covering industry, is well known for its concern for the environment.[7] It has been successful in reducing the expenses associated with the disposal of dangerous chemicals and other waste products from its manufacturing operations. Its environmental endeavors have multiple payoffs. Shaw has received many awards for its recycling efforts—awards that enhance its reputation.

outbound logistics collecting, storing, and distributing the product or service to buyers.

Outbound Logistics Outbound logistics is associated with collecting, storing, and distributing the product or service to buyers. These activities include finished goods, warehousing, material handling, delivery vehicle operation, order processing, and scheduling.

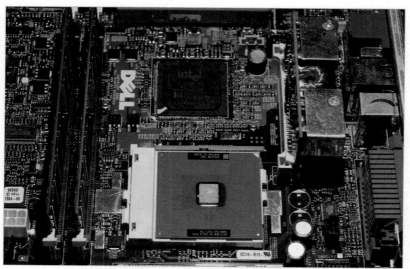

● Despite superb logistics and excellent manufacturing operations, Dell's competitive position in personal computers—including desktops and laptops—has eroded in recent years.

Yemeksepeti.com, the world's largest online food delivery portal, helps restaurants connect with potential customers all online. First launched in Turkey in 2000 and more recently expanded to Russia, the e-commerce site is now launching a joint venture in the United Arab Emirates (UAE) under the name Foodonclick.com.

The website's unique business model benefits both consumers and restaurants. Unlike with other food delivery websites, customers pay neither a premium for the service nor delivery charges. The online aspect allows the service to keep all menus up-to-date with food choices and promotions, and new outlets are listed immediately.

Users place their orders online at foodonclick.com, and the order is then transmitted in written form to the restaurant in less than a minute. Mistakes are minimized due to less margin of error than with telephone orders. All orders are delivered directly by the restaurant that receives payment. Orders can also be placed in advance.

The UAE restaurant sector is particularly diverse with numerous outlets spread across the city; Foodonclick.com was designed to bring Internet users together with restaurants that have delivery service—giving the restaurants another channel through which to increase revenue. The service requires no initial investment from outlets. The fee structure is commission-based: Participating restaurants must receive orders before the website charges them any fees.

strategy s

Security Risks in Mexico Have Led to Higher Shipping Costs

A report in January 2009 by the U.S. Joint Forces Command caught some by surprise with its warning about Mexico's political instability. It stated: "In terms of worst-case scenarios for the Joint Force and indeed the world, two large and important states bear consideration for a rapid and sudden collapse: Pakistan and Mexico." While the report stated that a collapse in Mexico was considered less likely, it went on to say, "The government, its politicians and judicial infrastructure are all under sustained assault and pressure by criminal gangs and drug cartels. How that internal conflict turns out over the next several years will have a major impact on the stability of the Mexican state."

A December 17, 2010, *Wall Street Journal* article also claimed that fights between drug cartels claimed more than 31,000 lives over the most recent four-year period—including 11,000 lives in 2010. Further, crimes such as robbery, extortion, and kidnapping increased. For some companies—especially those that don't yet have operations in Mexico—the violence has become daunting.

Sources: Casey, N. & Hagerty, J. R. 2010. Companies shun violent Mexico. *www.wsj.com.* December 17: np; Anonymous. 2009. Just how risky has Mexico become as a sourcing location? *www.scdigest.com.* February 9: np; and, Villagran, L. 2010, Companies grapple with Mexico security risks. *Dallas Morning News.* August 20: 1D, 3D.

Not surprisingly, such instability h[as] quality of life and economic developme[nt] cost of doing business. Let's take a lo[ok] costs are affected.

Ryder Systems, for example, doesn't take any chances when it comes to securing its shipping operations in Mexico. It uses GPS to track every one of its trucks moving manufactured goods in Mexico to the border. Private security agents escort every container before it heads to Texas or elsewhere. It handles about 3,000 border crossings weekly. And if a load arrives late, alarms are raised and the dogs do their inspections—not once, but three times.

Faced with the threat of smuggling attempts by criminal organizations in Mexico, foreign companies are simply forced to do more and spend more. In the process, they are charging consumers more to shore up security in a country where killings, extortions, and kidnappings have become part of daily life. While it is difficult to define the full scope of the problem, those who provide risk analysis can offer some insights.

The share of corporate operating costs dedicated to security has risen by roughly a third in the past two years, according to Julio Millan, a Mexico City–based business consultant. He estimates that security spending in 2010 accounted for 3 percent of corporate operating costs in the northern part of the country versus only 2 percent in 2009. "That's a huge jump," claimed Millan. "The public is paying the cost of security through the price of products."

"We have already seen a fantastic response from restaurants [that] want to be closer to potential customers, and we believe Foodonclick.com will see strong growth in user and restaurant numbers over the coming months," according to Shekhar Rao, regional CEO for Foodonclick.com.

That growth seems likely, if the model works as well in the UAE as the parent website Yemeksepeti.com does in Turkey. The original website has more than 500,000 users and 3,500 restaurants in Turkey, with more than 22,000 orders received per day. Approximately 45,000 people order out daily using the website, with more than 400 new users joining on a daily basis. That and the fact that Foodonclick.com has already partnered with more than 600 restaurants in the UAE, including a broad spectrum of eateries such as Wagamama, Pizza Express, Gourmet Burger Kitchen, Domino's Pizza, Labneh wa Zaatar, and Chili's. [8]

The Yemeksepeti.com example illustrates the win–win benefits of exemplary value-chain activities. Both the supplier (Foodonclick.com) and its buyers (restaurants) come out ahead, as do end users (diners).

Many U.S. companies with manufacturing plants in Mexico took advantage of low labor costs. However, they have experienced a sharp increase in their shipping costs. This is because they have been forced to spend more on security as a result of increasing drug-related violence (see Strategy Spotlight 3.2).

Marketing and Sales

Marketing and Sales Marketing and sales activities are associated with purchases of products and services by end users and the inducements used to get them to make purchases.[9] They include advertising, promotion, sales force, quoting, channel selection, channel relations, and pricing.[10,11]

It is not always enough to have a great product.[12] The key is to convince your channel partners that it is in their best interests not only to carry your product but also to market it in a way that is consistent with your strategy.[13] Consider Monsanto's efforts at educating distributors to improve the value proposition of its line of Saflex® windows.[14] The products had a superior attribute: The window design permitted laminators to form an exceptional type of glass by sandwiching a plastic sheet interlayer between two pieces of glass. This product is not only stronger and offers better ultraviolet protection than regular glass, but also when cracked, it adheres to the plastic sheet—an excellent safety feature for both cars and homes.

Despite these benefits, Monsanto had a hard time convincing laminators and window manufacturers to carry these products. According to Melissa Toledo, brand manager at Monsanto, "Saflex was priced at a 30 percent premium above traditional glass, and the various stages in the value chain (distributors and retailers) didn't think there would be a demand for such an expensive glass product." What did Monsanto do? It reintroduced Saflex as KeepSafe® and worked to coordinate the product's value propositions. By analyzing the experiences of all of the players in the supply chain, it was able to create marketing programs that helped each build a business aimed at selling its products. Said Toledo, "We want to know how they go about selling those types of products, what challenges they face, and what they think they need to sell our products. This helps us a lot when we try to provide them with these needs."[15]

At times, a firm's marketing initiatives may become overly aggressive and lead to actions that are both unethical and illegal.[16] For example:

- **Burdines.** This department store chain is under investigation for allegedly adding club memberships to its customers' credit cards without prior approval.
- **Fleet Mortgage.** This company has been accused of adding insurance fees for dental coverage and home insurance to its customers' mortgage loans without the customers' knowledge.
- **HCI Direct.** Eleven states have accused this direct-mail firm with charging for panty hose samples that customers did not order.
- **Juno Online Services.** The Federal Trade Commission brought charges against this Internet service provider for failing to provide customers with a telephone number to cancel service.

Strategy Spotlight. 3.3 discusses RYZ, a company which has almost no marketing costs. Why? It relies exclusively on social media such as Myspace and Facebook to create demand for its products.

Service

Service The primary activity of **service** includes all actions associated with providing service to enhance or maintain the value of the product, such as installation, repair, training, parts supply, and product adjustment.

Let's see how two retailers are providing exemplary customer service. At Sephora .com, a customer service representative taking a phone call from a repeat customer has instant access to what shade of lipstick she likes best. This will help the rep cross-sell by suggesting a matching shade of lip gloss. CEO Jim Wiggett expects such personalization to build loyalty and boost sales per customer. Nordstrom, the Seattle-based department store chain, goes a step further. It offers a cyber-assist: A service rep can take control of a customer's web browser and literally lead her to just the silk scarf that she is looking for. CEO Dan Nordstrom believes that such a capability will close enough additional purchases to pay for the $1 million investment in software.

Crowdsourcing: RYZ's Potential Customers Become Its Marketing and Design Staff

What happens when a company lets consumers design and vote on their own products? Quite often, the firm's overhead goes down and profits go up. This business model is an example of using crowdsourcing as a means of community-based design.

One of these companies is RYZ, founded in 2008, with over $1 million in revenues. It doesn't need a large marketing or design staff. Rather, it relies on potential customers for that. Would-be designers use a template from the company's website to create a pair of high-rise sneakers. The designs are posted online, and viewers vote on which ones they like. Winning designs are produced, and designers get $1,000 plus 1 percent of royalties for their efforts.

Sources: Britten, F. 2010. The Youdesign Movement. *www.nyt.com*. February 25: np; Kaufman, W. 2009. Crowdsourcing Turns Business on Its Head. *www.npr.org*. August 20: np; and *www.ryz.com*.

RYZ runs a weekly contest to cherry pick the best submitted sneaker design, which is then manufactured in a limited edition and sold for $54.99 to $99. And encouraging winners to promote their work makes sense: After all, you are more likely to try to make your design a success when you've invested time and effort. As an additional inducement, the winners get their picture on the company's website—along with a statement touting their work.

Not surprisingly, marketing costs are virtually nil, and relying on customers for design and market research enables the firm to move much more quickly, claims Rob Langstaff, the firm's founder and CEO. Previously head of Adidas North America, he says that it would take about 12 months and a substantial investment to get a design to market in the traditional, large shoe companies. In contrast, he asserts that RYZ can go from design to final product in only about six weeks.

crowdsourcing

Support Activities

Support activities in the value chain can be divided into four generic categories, as shown in Exhibit 3.3. Each category of the support activity is divisible into a number of distinct value activities that are specific to a particular industry. For example, technology development's discrete activities may include component design, feature design, field testing, process engineering, and technology selection. Similarly, procurement may include activities such as qualifying new suppliers, purchasing different groups of inputs, and monitoring supplier performance.

Procurement   **Procurement** refers to the function of purchasing inputs used in the firm's value chain, not to the purchased inputs themselves.[17] Purchased inputs include raw materials, supplies, and other consumable items as well as assets such as machinery, laboratory equipment, office equipment, and buildings.[18,19]

Microsoft has improved its procurement process (and the quality of its suppliers) by providing formal reviews of its suppliers. One of Microsoft's divisions has extended the review process used for employees to its outside suppliers.[20] The employee services group, which is responsible for everything from travel to 401(k) programs to the on-site library, outsources more than 60 percent of the services it provides. Unfortunately, the employee services group was not providing suppliers with enough feedback. This was feedback that the suppliers wanted to get and that Microsoft wanted to give.

The evaluation system that Microsoft developed helped clarify its expectations to suppliers. An executive noted: "We had one supplier—this was before the new system—that would have scored a 1.2 out of 5. After we started giving this feedback, and the supplier understood our expectations, its performance improved dramatically. Within six months, it scored a 4. If you'd asked me before we began the feedback system, I would have said that was impossible."

> **procurement** the function of purchasing inputs used in the firm's value chain, including raw materials, supplies, and other consumable items as well as assets such as machinery, laboratory equipment, office equipment, and buildings.

Exhibit 3.3 **The Value Chain: Some Factors to Consider in Assessing a Firm's Support Activities**

General Administration

- Effective planning systems to attain overall goals and objectives.
- Excellent relationships with diverse stakeholder groups.
- Effective information technology to integrate value-creating activities.

Human Resource Management

- Effective recruiting, development, and retention mechanisms for employees.
- Quality relations with trade unions.
- Reward and incentive programs to motivate all employees.

Technology Development

- Effective R&D activities for process and product initiatives.
- Positive collaborative relationships between R&D and other departments.
- Excellent professional qualifications of personnel.

Procurement

- Procurement of raw material inputs to optimize quality and speed and to minimize the associated costs.
- Development of collaborative win–win relationships with suppliers.
- Analysis and selection of alternative sources of inputs to minimize dependence on one supplier.

Source: Adapted from Porter, M.E. 1985. *Competitive Advantage: Creating and Sustaining Superior Performance.* New York: Free Press.

Technology Development   Every value activity embodies technology.[21] The array of technologies employed in most firms is very broad, ranging from technologies used to prepare documents and transport goods to those embodied in processes and equipment or the product itself.[22] **Technology development** related to the product and its features supports the entire value chain, while other technology development is associated with particular primary or support activities.

In 1984, General Motors (GM) and Daewoo formed a 50/50 joint venture called Daewoo Motor Company. As a win–win strategy, GM wanted to tackle the small-car market in North America and eventually expand into Asia while Daewoo was hoping to gain access to superior technology. In 1992, GM and Daewoo divorced. After the 1997 Asian economic crisis, GM and Daewoo joined hands again, eventually forming a new joint venture called GM Daewoo Auto and Technology Company in 2001. This time, GM fully integrated GM Daewoo into its global strategy.

GM Daewoo makes cars in South Korea and Vietnam and exports them to more than 140 countries. One of the most decisive moves it made was to phase out the Daewoo brand tarnished by quality problems and financial turbulence, except in South Korea and Vietnam. GM labeled a vast majority of cars built by GM Daewoo as Chevrolet, a brand that GM usually pitched as more American than the Stars and Stripes. In the United States, Latin America, and Eastern Europe, the GM Daewoo–built Chevrolet Aveo became one of the best-selling compact cars, beating the Toyota Echo and the Hyundai Excel. In addition to finished cars, GM Daewoo also made kits to be assembled by local factories in China, Colombia, India, Thailand, and Venezuela. In three years, GM Daewoo's worldwide sales

technology development
activities associated with the development of new knowledge that is applied to the firm's operations.

Removing Individual Metrics in Performance Evaluations

ITT China President William Taylor wanted to know why employee turnover was so high in the Shanghai sales office. The local manager knew the answer: If the sales manager gave workers an average "3" on the 1–5 performance scale, they'd stop talking to him and, in some cases, quit shortly thereafter. The manager lamented: "They're losing face in the organization. It would be great if we could do something about the scores."

Comments like that popped up around the world. For example, in southern Europe, the focus on individual performance didn't sit well with the region's more "collective

Source: McGregor, J. 2008. Case study: To adapt, ITT lets go of unpopular ratings. *BusinessWeek*, January 28: 46.

ethos," claimed James Duncan, director of ITT's talent development. And in Scandinavia, where there's more of "a sense of equality between bosses and workers," said Duncan, some workers asked, "What gives you the right to rate me a 3?" That led ITT to make the radical decision to ditch performance ratings altogether.

Most employees, who still require a detailed evaluation, cheered the changes. In one of the ITT plants in Shenyang, China, the new system has helped to cut the plant's attrition rate in half. The change isn't as popular in the U.S., where some metrics-loving engineers in the defense business remain attached to the old rankings. Still, most people have come around. Said Duncan, "It's not just Asia and Europe." No matter what culture you are from, everyone "likes the fact that they're treated like an adult in this discussion."

---

of cars and kits reached 1 million, up from 400,000 when GM took over. That made GM Daewoo one of the best-performing units of GM.[23]

Human Resource Management   **Human resource management** consists of activities involved in the recruiting, hiring, training, development, and compensation of all types of personnel.[24] It supports both individual primary and support activities (e.g., hiring of engineers and scientists) and the entire value chain (e.g., negotiations with labor unions).[25]

> Like all great service companies, JetBlue Airways Corporation is obsessed with hiring superior employees.[26] But it found it difficult to attract college graduates to commit to careers as flight attendants. JetBlue developed a highly innovative recruitment program for flight attendants—a one-year contract that gives them a chance to travel, meet lots of people, and then decide what else they might like to do. It also introduced the idea of training a friend and employee together so that they could share a job. With such employee-friendly initiatives, JetBlue has been very successful in attracting talent.

Jeffrey Immelt, GE's chairman, addresses the importance of effective human resource management:[27]

> Human resources has to be more than a department. GE recognized early on—50 or 60 years ago—that in a multibusiness company, the common denominators are people and culture. From an employee's first day at GE, she discovers that she's in the people-development business as much as anything else. You'll find that most good companies have the same basic HR processes that we have, but they're discrete. HR at GE is not an agenda item; it is the agenda.

Strategy Spotlight 3.4 discusses a rather unique approach to individual performance evaluations: Eliminate the metrics!

General Administration   **General administration** consists of a number of activities, including general management, planning, finance, accounting, legal and government affairs, quality management, and information systems. Administration (unlike the other support activities) typically supports the entire value chain and not individual activities.[28]

human resource management activities involved in the recruiting, hiring, training, development, and compensation of all types of personnel.

general administration general management, planning, finance, accounting, legal and government affairs, quality management, and information systems; activities that support the entire value chain and not individual activities.

Although general administration is sometimes viewed only as overhead, it can be a powerful source of competitive advantage. In a telephone operating company, for example, negotiating and maintaining ongoing relations with regulatory bodies can be among the most important activities for competitive advantage. Also, in some industries top management plays a vital role in dealing with important buyers.[29]

The strong and effective leadership of top executives can also make a significant contribution to an organization's success. As we discussed in Chapter 1, chief executive officers (CEOs) such as Lee Kun-Hee, Akio Toyoda, Andrew Grove, and Jack Welch have been credited with playing critical roles in the success of Samsung, Toyota Motor, Intel, and General Electric, respectively.

Information systems can also play a key role in increasing operating efficiencies and enhancing a firm's performance.[30] Consider UK pharmacy chain Boots' introduction of the Boots' Free Repeat Prescriptions Service and Walgreen Co.'s introduction of Intercom Plus, a computer-based prescription management system. Linked by computer to both doctors' offices and third-party payment plans, the Walgreen's system automates telephone refills, store-to-store prescription transfers, and drug reordering. It also provides information on drug interactions and, coupled with revised workflows, frees up pharmacists from administrative tasks to devote more time to patient counseling.[31]

Interrelationships among Value-Chain Activities within and across Organizations

We have defined each of the value-chain activities separately for clarity of presentation. Managers must not ignore, however, the importance of relationships among value-chain activities.[32] There are two levels: (1) **interrelationships** among activities within the firm and (2) relationships among activities within the firm and with other stakeholders (e.g., customers and suppliers) that are part of the firm's expanded value chain.[33]

With regard to the first level, consider AT&T's innovative Resource Link program. Here, employees who have reached their plateau may apply for temporary positions in other parts of the organization. Clearly, this program has the potential to benefit all activities within the firm's value chain because it creates opportunities for top employees to lend their expertise to all of the organization's value-creating activities.

With regard to the second level, Campbell Soup's use of electronic networks enabled it to improve the efficiency of outbound logistics.[34] However, it also helped Campbell manage the ordering of raw materials more effectively, improve its production scheduling, and help its customers better manage their inbound logistics operations.

Strategy Spotlight 3.5 discusses an innovative initiative by Timberland, a leading shoe manufacturer, to eliminate toxic adhesives from its shoes. This effort has the potential for long-term cost savings for its suppliers as well as increased market share for its product line.

The "Prosumer" Concept: Integrating Customers into the Value Chain

When addressing the value-chain concept, it is important to focus on the interrelationship between the organization and its most important stakeholder—its customers.[35] A key to success for some leading-edge firms is to team up with their customers to satisfy their particular need(s). As stated in a recent IBM Global CEO Study:

> In the future, we will be talking more and more about the "prosumer"—a customer/producer who is even more extensively integrated into the value chain. As a consequence, production processes will be customized more precisely and individually.[36]

Including customers in the actual production process can create greater satisfaction among them. It also has the potential to result in significant cost savings and to generate

Timberland's Detoxification Initiative

Making shoes is a surprisingly toxic business. Both the materials and the adhesives that connect them are made of chemicals that are known dangers to the cardiac, respiratory, and nervous systems. One pair of running shoes will hardly harm you. However, workers in the industry face real risks.

Timberland, the second largest company in the outdoor industry, with $1.3 billion in revenues, realized that it needed to rethink the industry's traditional reliance on toxic chemicals. It became the first footwear company to test new water-based adhesives on nonathletic shoes. (Nike and others had already taken the initiatives in the "white shoe," or athletic, part of the industry.) Making such a change required the firm to work closely with Asian suppliers. According to Timberland's website, the company released its long-term strategy in 2008, which included its goal to create products at lower cost and with less harm to the environment. The strategy included eliminating polyvinylchloride (PVC) from its product line and increasing the use of water-based adhesives in its footwear in order to reduce the use of solvents.

Common sense would suggest that Timberland's detoxification efforts would be very costly for its suppliers. And during the test phase it *was* quite expensive. The new adhesives cost more because economies of scale hadn't yet been achieved. However, over time, Timberland fully expects the process to be at least cost neutral for its business and a moneymaker for the full value chain.

Sources: Esty, D. C. & Winston, A. S. *Green to Gold.* Hoboken, NJ: Wiley, p: 112–113; *www.community.timberland.com*; and *finance.yahoo.com*.

Why? Water-based adhesives eliminate almost entirely the supplier's expense for handling hazardous materials, including waste disposal, insurance, and training. Manufacturing expenses had already declined during the testing phase, because water-based adhesives go on with one coat instead of two, and the application equipment requires less cleaning. Thus, suppliers can run

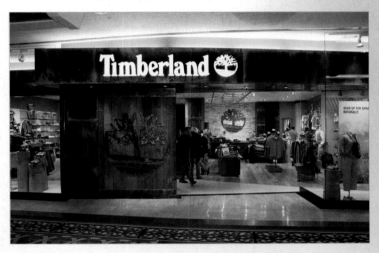

● Timberland is well known for its environmental sustainability initiatives.

longer without interruption. The change also improves worker safety as well as reduces both labor costs and time.

Sounds good. But will Timberland be able to capture these supplier savings down the road? Probably not, but over time this strategy should help the firm win market share and drive revenues.

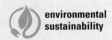

environmental sustainability

innovative ideas for the firm, which can be transferred to the customer in terms of lower prices and higher quality products and services.

In terms of how a firm views its customers, the move to create the prosumer stands in rather stark contrast to the conventional marketing approach in which the customer merely consumes the products produced by the company. Another area where this approach differs from conventional thinking concerns the notion of tying the customer into the company through, for example, loyalty programs and individualized relationship marketing.

How Procter & Gamble Embraced the Prosumer Concept In the early 2000s P&G's people were not clearly oriented toward any common purpose. The corporate mission "To meaningfully improve the everyday lives of the customers" had not been explicitly or inspirationally rolled out to the employees. To more clearly focus everyone's efforts, P&G expanded the mission to include the idea that "the consumer is the boss." This philosophy became one in which people who buy and use P&G products are valued not just for their money but also as *a rich source of information and direction.* "The consumer is the boss" became far more than a slogan in P&G. It became a clear, simple, and inclusive cultural priority for both employees and the external stakeholders such as suppliers.

The P&G efforts in the fragrance areas are one example. P&G transformed this small underperforming business area into a global leader and the world's largest fine fragrance company. It accomplished this by clearly and precisely defining the target consumer for each fragrance brand and by identifying subgroups of consumers for some brands. P&G still kept the partnerships with established fashion houses such as Dolce & Gabbana, Gucci, and Lacoste. However, the main point was to make the consumer the boss, focusing on innovations that were meaningful to consumers, including, for instance, fresh new scents, distinctive packaging, and proactive marketing. In addition, P&G streamlined the supply chain to reduce complexity and lower its cost structure.

"The consumer is the boss" idea goes even further. It also means that P&G tries to build social connections through digital media and other forms of interactions (thus incorporating the crowdsourcing concept that we introduced in Chapter 1). Baby diapers are one example. P&G used to use handmade diapers for its product tests. Today, however, this product is shown digitally and created in alternatives in an on-screen virtual world. Changes can be made immediately as new ideas emerge, and it can be redesigned on screen. Thus, P&G is creating a social system with the consumers (and potential consumers) that enable the firm to co-design and co-engineer new innovations with buyers. At P&G the philosophy of "the consumer is the boss" set a new standard.

Applying the Value Chain to Service Organizations

The concepts of inbound logistics, operations, and outbound logistics suggest managing the raw materials that might be manufactured into finished products and delivered to customers. However, these three steps do not apply only to manufacturing. They correspond to any transformation process in which inputs are converted through a work process into outputs that add value. For example, accounting is a sort of transformation process that converts daily records of individual transactions into monthly financial reports. In this example, the transaction records are the inputs, accounting is the operation that adds value, and financial statements are the outputs.

What are the "operations," or transformation processes, of service organizations? At times, the difference between manufacturing and service is in providing a customized solution rather than mass production as is common in manufacturing. For example, a travel agent adds value by creating an itinerary that includes transportation, accommodations, and activities that are customized to your budget and travel dates. A law firm renders services that are specific to a client's needs and circumstances. In both cases, the work process (operation) involves the application of specialized knowledge based on the specifics of a situation (inputs) and the outcome that the client desires (outputs).

The application of the value chain to service organizations suggests that the value-adding process may be configured differently depending on the type of business a firm is engaged in. As the preceding discussion on support activities suggests, activities such as procurement and legal services are critical for adding value. Indeed, the activities that may only provide support to one company may be critical to the primary value-adding activity of another firm.

Exhibit 3.4 provides two models of how the value chain might look in service industries. In the retail industry, there are no manufacturing operations. A firm, such as Dixons in the UK, adds value by developing expertise in the procurement of finished goods and by displaying them in their stores in a way that enhances sales. Thus, the value chain

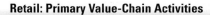

Retail: Primary Value-Chain Activities

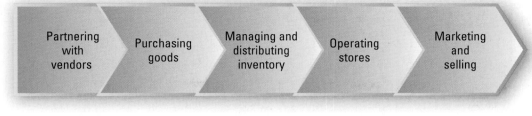

Engineering Services: Primary Value-Chain Activities

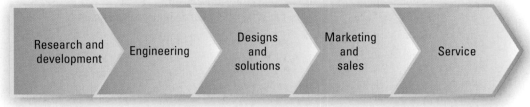

Exhibit 3.4 **Some Examples of Value Chains in Service Industries**

makes procurement activities (i.e., partnering with vendors and purchasing goods) a primary rather than a support activity. Operations refer to the task of operating Dixons' stores.

For an engineering services firm, research and development provides inputs, the transformation process is the engineering itself, and innovative designs and practical solutions are the outputs. Arthur D. Little, for example, is a large consulting firm with offices in 20 countries. In its technology and innovation management practice, A. D. Little strives to make the best use of the science, technology, and knowledge resources available to create value for a wide range of industries and client sectors. This involves activities associated with research and development, engineering, and creating solutions as well as downstream activities such as marketing, sales, and service. How the primary and support activities of a given firm are configured and deployed will often depend on industry conditions and whether the company is service and/or manufacturing oriented.

Resource-Based View of the Firm

The **resource-based view (RBV) of the firm** combines two perspectives: (1) the internal analysis of phenomena within a company and (2) an external analysis of the industry and its competitive environment.[37] It goes beyond the traditional SWOT (strengths, weaknesses, opportunities, threats) analysis by integrating internal and external perspectives. The ability of a firm's resources to confer competitive advantage(s) cannot be determined without taking into consideration the broader competitive context. A firm's resources must be evaluated in terms of how valuable, rare, and hard they are for competitors to duplicate. Otherwise, the firm attains only competitive parity.

As noted earlier (in Strategy Spotlight 3.1), a firm's strengths and capabilities—no matter how unique or impressive—do not necessarily lead to competitive advantages in the marketplace. The criteria for whether advantages are created and whether or not they can be sustained over time will be addressed later in this section. Thus, the RBV is a very useful framework for gaining insights as to why some competitors are more profitable than others. As we will see later in the book, the RBV is also helpful in developing strategies for

resource-based view (RBV) of the firm perspective that firms' competitive advantages are due to their endowment of strategic resources that are valuable, rare, costly to imitate, and costly to substitute.

>LO3.4
The resource-based view of the firm and the different types of tangible and intangible resources, as well as organizational capabilities.

Tangible Resources	
Financial	• Firm's cash account and cash equivalents
	• Firm's capacity to raise equity
	• Firm's borrowing capacity
Physical	• Modern plant and facilities
	• Favorable manufacturing locations
	• State-of-the-art machinery and equipment
Technological	• Trade secrets
	• Innovative production processes
	• Patents, copyrights, trademarks
Organizational	• Effective strategic planning processes
	• Excellent evaluation and control systems

Intangible Resources	
Human	• Experience and capabilities of employees
	• Trust
	• Managerial skills
	• Firm-specific practices and procedures
Innovation and creativity	• Technical and scientific skills
	• Innovation capacities
Reputation	• Brand name
	• Reputation with customers for quality and reliability
	• Reputation with suppliers for fairness, non–zero-sum relationships

Organizational Capabilities

• Firm competencies or skills the firm employs to transfer inputs to outputs
• Capacity to combine tangible and intangible resources, using organizational processes to attain desired end

EXAMPLES:

• Outstanding customer service
• Excellent product development capabilities
• Innovativeness of products and services
• Ability to hire, motivate, and retain human capital

Source: Adapted from Barney, J. B. 1991. Firm Resources and Sustained Competitive Advantage. *Journal of Management,* 17: 101; Grant, R. M. 1991. *Contemporary Strategy Analysis.* Cambridge England: Blackwell Business , pp. 100–102; and, Hitt, M. A., Ireland, R. D., & Hoskisson, R. E. 2001. *Strategic Management: Competitiveness and Globalization* (4th ed.). Cincinnati: South-Western College Publishing.

individual businesses and diversified firms by revealing how core competencies embedded in a firm can help it exploit new product and market opportunities.

In the two sections that follow, we will discuss the three key types of resources that firms possess (summarized in Exhibit 3.5): tangible resources, intangible resources, and organizational capabilities. Then we will address the conditions under which such assets and capabilities can enable a firm to attain a sustainable competitive advantage.[38]

It is important to note that resources by themselves typically do not yield a competitive advantage. Even if a basketball team recruited an all-star center, there would be little chance of victory if the other members of the team were continually outplayed by their opponents or if the coach's attitude was so negative that everyone, including the center, became unwilling to put forth their best efforts.

In a business context, a firm's excellent value-creating activities (e.g., logistics) would not be a source of competitive advantage if those activities were not integrated with other important value-creating activities such as marketing and sales. Thus, a central theme of the resource-based view of the firm is that competitive advantages are created (and sustained) through the bundling of several resources in unique combinations.[39]

Types of Firm Resources

Firm resources are all assets, capabilities, organizational processes, information, knowledge and so forth controlled by a firm that enable it to develop and implement value-creating strategies.

Tangible Resources These are assets that are relatively easy to identify. **Tangible resources** include the physical and financial assets that an organization uses to create value for its customers. Among them are financial resources (e.g., a firm's cash, accounts receivables, and its ability to borrow funds); physical resources (e.g., the company's plant, equipment, and machinery as well as its proximity to customers and suppliers); organizational resources (e.g., the company's strategic planning process and its employee development, evaluation, and reward systems); and technological resources (e.g., trade secrets, patents, and copyrights).

Many firms are finding that high-tech, computerized training has dual benefits: It develops more effective employees and reduces costs at the same time. Employees at FedEx take computer-based job competency tests every 6 to 12 months.[40] The 90-minute computer-based tests identify areas of individual weakness and provide input to a computer database of employee skills—information the firm uses in promotion decisions.

tangible resources organizational assets that are relatively easy to identify, including physical assets, financial resources, organizational resources, and technological resources.

Intangible Resources Much more difficult for competitors (and, for that matter, a firm's own managers) to account for or imitate are **intangible resources**, which are typically embedded in unique routines and practices that have evolved and accumulated over time. These include human resources (e.g., experience and capability of employees, trust, effectiveness of work teams, managerial skills), innovation resources (e.g., technical and scientific expertise, ideas), and reputation resources (e.g., brand name, reputation with suppliers for fairness and with customers for reliability and product quality).[41] A firm's culture may also be a resource that provides competitive advantage.[42]

For example, you might not think that motorcycles, clothes, toys, and restaurants have much in common. Yet Harley-Davidson has entered all of these product and service markets by capitalizing on its strong brand image—a valuable intangible resource.[43] It has used that image to sell accessories, clothing, and toys, and it has licensed the Harley-Davidson Café in New York City to provide further exposure for its brand name and products.

Strategy Spotlight 3.6 discusses how various social networking sites have the potential to play havoc with a firm's reputation.

intangible resources organizational assets that are difficult to identify and account for and are typically embedded in unique routines and practices, including human resources, innovation resources, and reputation resources.

Organizational Capabilities **Organizational capabilities** are not specific tangible or intangible assets, but rather the competencies or skills that a firm employs to transform inputs into outputs.[44] In short, they refer to an organization's capacity to deploy tangible and intangible resources over time and generally in combination, and to leverage those capabilities to bring about a desired end.[45] Examples of organizational capabilities are outstanding customer service, excellent product development capabilities, superb innovation processes, and flexibility in manufacturing processes.[46]

organizational capabilities the competencies and skills that a firm employs to transform inputs into outputs.

strategy spotlight

Blogs, Social Networking Sites, and Corporate Reputations: A Lethal Combination?

Customers are now connecting with and drawing power from one another. The mechanism: online social technologies such as blogs, social networking sites like Facebook and Twitter, user-generated content sites like YouTube, and countless communities across the web. They are defining their own perspective on companies and brands—a perspective that is often at odds with the image a company wants to project. This groundswell of people using technologies to get the things they need from one another, rather than from the companies, has tilted the balance of power from company to customer.

Let's look at an example: Brian Finkelstein, a law student, had trouble with the cable modem in his home. A Comcast Cable repairman arrived to fix the problem. However, when the technician had to call the home office for a key piece of information, he was put on hold for so long that he fell asleep on Finkelstein's couch. Outraged, Finkelstein made a video of the sleeping technician and posted it on YouTube. The clip became a hit—with more than a million viewings. And, to this day, it continues to undermine Comcast's efforts to improve its reputation for customer service.

Source: Bernoff, J. & Li, C. 2008. Harnessing the power of the oh-so-social web. *MIT Sloan Management Review*, 49(3): 36–42; and, Stelter, B. 2008. Griping online? Comcast hears and talks back. *nytimes.com*. July 25: np.

But Comcast is working hard to improve its reputation. It has a lot of work to do—after all, the company was ranked at the bottom of a recent American Customer Satisfaction Index, which tracks consumer opinions of more than 200 companies. And hundreds of customers have filed grievances on a site called Comcastmustdie.com.

One of Comcast's initiatives to try to turn things around is headed by Frank Eliason, its digital care manager. He uses readily available online tools to monitor public comments on blogs, message boards, and social networks for any mention of Comcast. When Eliason sees a complaint, he contacts the source and tries to defuse the problem. "When you're having a two-way conversation, you really get to clear the air," said Eliason.

Comcast said the online outreach is part of a larger effort to revamp its customer service. In just five months, Eliason, whose job redefines customer service, has reached out to well over 1,000 customers online.

Comcast is not the only company trying to reach out to customers online. Using the social messaging service Twitter, Southwest Airlines answers customer questions about ticket prices and flight delays, Whole Foods Market posts details about discounts, and the chief executive of the online shoe store Zappos shares details of his life with 7,200 "followers." Many other companies also monitor online discussion groups. But given its track record, Comcast felt it needed to take the extra step: contacting customers who are discussing the company online.

In the case of Apple, the majority of components used in its products can be characterized as proven technology, such as touch screen and MP3 player functionality.[47] However, Apple combines and packages these in new and innovative ways while also seeking to integrate the value chain. This is the case with iTunes, for example, where suppliers of downloadable music are a vital component of the success Apple has enjoyed with its iPod series of MP3 players. Thus, Apple draws on proven technologies and its ability to offer innovative combinations of these.

Firm Resources and Sustainable Competitive Advantages

As we have mentioned, resources alone are not a basis for competitive advantages, nor are advantages sustainable over time.[48] In some cases, a resource or capability helps a firm to increase its revenues or to lower costs but the firm derives only a temporary advantage because competitors quickly imitate or substitute for it.[49] Many e-commerce businesses in the early 2000s saw their profits seriously eroded because new (or existing) competitors easily duplicated their business model. For example, Priceline.com expanded its offerings from enabling customers to place bids online for airline tickets to a wide variety of

> **>LO3.5**
> The four criteria that a firm's resources must possess to maintain a sustainable advantage and how value created can be appropriated by employees and managers.

Is the resource or capability . . .	Implications
Valuable?	• Neutralize threats and exploit opportunities
Rare?	• Not many firms possess
Difficult to imitate?	• Physically unique
	• Path dependency (how accumulated over time)
	• Causal ambiguity (difficult to disentangle what it is or how it could be re-created)
	• Social complexity (trust, interpersonal relationships, culture, reputation)
Difficult to substitute?	• No equivalent strategic resources or capabilities

Exhibit 3.6
Four Criteria for Assessing Sustainability of Resources and Capabilities

other products. However, it was easy for competitors (e.g., a consortium of major airlines) to duplicate Priceline's products and services. Ultimately, its market capitalization plummeted roughly 98 percent from its all-time high.

For a resource to provide a firm with the potential for a sustainable competitive advantage, it must have four attributes.[50] First, the **strategic resource** must be valuable in the sense that it exploits opportunities and/or neutralizes threats in the firm's environment. Second, it must be rare among the firm's current and potential competitors. Third, the resource must be difficult for competitors to imitate. Fourth, the resource must have no strategically equivalent substitutes. These criteria are summarized in Exhibit 3.6. We will now discuss each of these criteria. Then, we will examine how Dell's competitive advantage, which seemed secure as late as 2006, has eroded.

strategic resources (also **firm resources** or **organizational resources**) firms' capabilities that are valuable, rare, costly to imitate, and costly to substitute.

Is the Resource Valuable?   Organizational resources can be a source of competitive advantage only when they are valuable. Resources are valuable when they enable a firm to formulate and implement strategies that improve its efficiency or effectiveness. The SWOT framework suggests that firms improve their performance only when they exploit opportunities or neutralize (or minimize) threats.

The fact that firm attributes must be valuable in order to be considered resources (as well as potential sources of competitive advantage) reveals an important complementary relationship among environmental models (e.g., SWOT and five-forces analyses) and the resource-based model. Environmental models isolate those firm attributes that exploit opportunities and/or neutralize threats. Thus, they specify what firm attributes may be considered as resources. The resource-based model then suggests what additional characteristics these resources must possess if they are to develop a sustained competitive advantage.

Is the Resource Rare?   If competitors or potential competitors also possess the same valuable resource, it is not a source of a competitive advantage because all of these firms have the capability to exploit that resource in the same way. Common strategies based on such a resource would give no one firm an advantage. For a resource to provide competitive advantages, it must be uncommon, that is, rare relative to other competitors.

This argument can apply to bundles of valuable firm resources that are used to formulate and develop strategies. Some strategies require a mix of multiple types of resources—tangible assets, intangible assets, and organizational capabilities. If a particular bundle of firm resources is not rare, then relatively large numbers of firms will be able to conceive of and implement the strategies in question. Thus, such strategies will not be a source of competitive advantage, even if the resource in question is valuable.

Can the Resource Be Imitated Easily?   Inimitability (difficulty in imitating) is a key to value creation because it constrains competition.[51] If a resource is inimitable, then any profits generated are more likely to be sustainable.[52] Having a resource that competitors can easily copy generates only temporary value.[53] This has important implications. Since managers often fail to apply this test, they tend to base long-term strategies on resources that are imitable. IBP (Iowa Beef Processors) became the first meatpacking company in the United States to modernize by building a set of assets (automated plants located in cattle-producing states) and capabilities (low-cost "disassembly" of carcasses) that earned returns on assets of 1.3 percent in the 1970s. By the late 1980s, however, ConAgra and Cargill had imitated these resources, and IBP's profitability fell by nearly 70 percent, to 0.4 percent.

Monster.com entered the executive recruiting market by providing, in essence, a substitute for traditional bricks-and-mortar headhunting firms. Although Monster.com's resources are rare and valuable, they are subject to imitation by new rivals—other dot-com firms. Why? There are very low entry barriers for firms wanting to try their hand at recruitment. For example, many job search dot-coms around the world have emerged in recent years, including allarabia.com (in the Middle East); redgoldfish.co.uk (in the UK); and jobkorea.co.kr (in South Korea). In all, there are more than 40,000 online job boards available to job seekers. It would be most difficult for a firm to attain a sustainable advantage in this industry.

Clearly, an advantage based on inimitability won't last forever. Competitors will eventually discover a way to copy most valuable resources. However, managers can forestall them and sustain profits for a while by developing strategies around resources that have at least one of the following four characteristics.[54]

Physical Uniqueness The first source of inimitability is physical uniqueness, which by definition is inherently difficult to copy. A beautiful resort location, mineral rights, or Pfizer's pharmaceutical patents simply cannot be imitated. Many managers believe that several of their resources may fall into this category, but on close inspection, few do.

path dependency
a characteristic of resources that is developed and/or accumulated through a unique series of events.

Path Dependency A greater number of resources cannot be imitated because of what economists refer to as **path dependency.** This simply means that resources are unique and therefore scarce because of all that has happened along the path followed in their development and/or accumulation. Competitors cannot go out and buy these resources quickly and easily; they must be built up over time in ways that are difficult to accelerate.

Royal Dutch/Shell Group is known for its decentralized, international management capabilities, in particular its adaptability to a wide variety of national environments. Shell was established to sell Russian oil in China and the Far East, while Royal Dutch was established to exploit Indonesian oil reserves. With head offices thousands of miles away in Europe, it is little wonder that the group developed a decentralized, adaptable management style.

causal ambiguity
a characteristic of a firm's resources that is costly to imitate because a competitor cannot determine what the resource is and/or how it can be re-created.

Causal Ambiguity The third source of inimitability is termed **causal ambiguity.** This means that would-be competitors may be thwarted because it is impossible to disentangle the causes (or possible explanations) of either what the valuable resource is or how it can be re-created. What is the root of 3M's innovation process? You can study it and draw up a list of possible factors. But it is a complex, unfolding (or folding) process that is hard to understand and would be hard to imitate.

Often, causally ambiguous resources are organizational capabilities, involving a complex web of social interactions that may even depend on particular individuals. When Continental and United tried to mimic the successful low-cost strategy of Southwest Airlines, the planes, routes, and fast gate turnarounds were not the most difficult aspects for them to copy. Those were all rather easy to observe and, at least in principle, easy to duplicate. However, they could not replicate Southwest's culture of fun, family, frugality, and focus since no one can clearly specify exactly what that culture is or how it came to be.

strategy spotlight

Amazon Prime: Very Difficult for Rivals to Copy

Amazon Prime is a free shipping service that guarantees delivery of products within two days for an annual fee of $79. According to *Bloomberg Businessweek,* it may be the most ingenious and effective customer loyalty program in all of e-commerce, if not retail in general. It converts casual shoppers, who gorge on the gratification of having purchases reliably appear two days after they order, into Amazon addicts. Analysts describe Prime as one of the main factors driving Amazon's stock price—up nearly 300 percent from 2008 to 2010. Also, it is one of the main reasons why Amazon's sales grew 30 percent during the recession while other retailers suffered.

Analysts estimate that Amazon Prime has more than 4 million members in the United States, a small slice of Amazon's 121 million active buyers worldwide. However, analysts claim that Prime members increase their purchases on the site by about 150 percent after they join and may be responsible for as much as 20 percent of Amazon's overall sales in the United States. Such shoppers are considered the "whales" of the $140 billion U.S. e-commerce market, one of the fastest-growing parts of U.S. retail. And, according to Hudson Square Research, Amazon, with a hefty 8 percent of the U.S. e-commerce market, is the single biggest online retailer in the United States.

Source: Stone, B. 2010. What's in the box? Instant gratification. *Bloomberg Businessweek.* November 29–December 5: 39–40; Klein, E. 2010. The genius of Amazon Prime. *www.voices.washingtonpost.com.* November 29: np; and, Fowler, G. A. 2010. Retailers team up against Amazon. *www.wsj.com.* October 6: np.

Prime was introduced in 2004. It was the result of a years-long search for the right loyalty program. An Amazon software engineer named Charlie Ward first suggested the idea of a free shipping service via a suggestion box feature on Amazon's internal website. Bing Gordon, an Amazon board member and venture capitalist, came up with the "Prime" name. Other executives, including Chief Executive Jeffrey Bezos, devised the two-day shipping offer—which exploited Amazon's ability to accelerate the handling of individual items in its distribution centers.

Amazon Prime has proven to be extremely hard for rivals to copy. Why? It enables Amazon to exploit its wide selection, low prices, network of third-party merchants, and finely tuned distribution system. All that while also keying off that faintly irrational human need to maximize the benefits of a club that you have already paid to join.

Now, several years after the program's creation, rivals—both online and off—have realized the increasing threat posed by Prime and are rushing to try to respond. For example, in October 2010, a consortium of more than 20 retailers, including Barnes & Noble, Sports Authority, and Toys 'R' Us, banded together to offer their own copycat $79, two-day shipping program, ShopRunner, which applies to products across their websites. However, as noted by Fiona Dias, the executive who administers the program, "As Amazon added more merchandising categories to Prime, retailers started feeling the pain. They have finally come to understand that Amazon is an existential threat and that Prime is the fuel of the engine."

Strategy Spotlight 3.7 describes Amazon's continued success as the world's largest online marketplace. Competitors recently tried to imitate Amazon's free shipping strategy, but with limited success. The reason is that Amazon has developed an array of interrelated elements of strategy which its rivals find too difficult to imitate.

Social Complexity A firm's resources may be imperfectly inimitable because they reflect a high level of **social complexity**. Such phenomena are typically beyond the ability of firms to systematically manage or influence. When competitive advantages are based on social complexity, it is difficult for other firms to imitate them.

A wide variety of firm resources may be considered socially complex. Examples include interpersonal relations among the managers in a firm, its culture, and its reputation with its suppliers and customers. In many of these cases, it is easy to specify how these socially complex resources add value to a firm. Hence, there is little or no causal ambiguity surrounding the link between them and competitive advantage. But an understanding that certain firm attributes, such as quality relations among managers, can improve a firm's efficiency does not necessarily lead to systematic efforts to imitate them. Such social engineering efforts are beyond the capabilities of most firms.

social complexity
a characteristic of a firm's resources that is costly to imitate because the social engineering required is beyond the capability of competitors, including interpersonal relations among managers, organizational culture, and reputation with suppliers and customers.

How a Chinese Beverage Company Succeeded by Creating Close Partnerships with Its Distributors

In 1998, when Hangzhou Wahaha Co. Ltd. (Wahaha), the largest Chinese beverage producer, decided to take on Coca-Cola and PepsiCo, it began its attack in the rural areas of China. Why? It believed that it possessed a competitive advantage over the international giants because of the partnerships that it had built with the distributors across the more remote locations in China. ("Wa ha ha," which sounds like a child laughing, comes from a children's folk song.)

Four years prior to the launch of the "Wahaha Future Cola," the firm developed a policy for how to tie in "channel members" over the long term as a response to the increasing problem of accounts receivable and bad debt. This policy provided incentives for the channel members to pay an annual deposit in advance to cover any potential future bad debt and to operate according to Wahaha's payment policy.

Sounds OK, but what did the distributors get in return? They received an interest rate from Wahaha that was superior to the bank rate. In addition, further discounts were offered for early payment, and annual bonuses were awarded to distributors that met the criterion for prompt payment.

Wahaha implemented this model over a two-year period. It effectively struck financial partnerships with existing distributors that led to higher commitment from distributors. This creative strategy became instrumental to Wahaha's success and its ability to deliver products to the rural areas of China. Here, logistics often create unique challenges.

Wahaha's distribution network now consists of about 4,000 first-tier domestic wholesalers and a large number of second- and third-tier wholesalers and outlets to ensure that Wahaha's products reach millions of retailers nationwide within one week of leaving the factory—no small feat with China's vast rural areas and provinces as far out as Xinjiang and Tibet. As CEO Zong Qinghou colorfully pointed out: "Our rapid and sound network serves as human blood vessels which circulate the bloodstream to every part of the body once the products are ready."

In contrast, domestic and multinational companies established their own distribution networks—not partnerships with local distributors as Wahaha had done. Not surprisingly, Wahaha has managed to capture impressive market share increases in markets traditionally dominated by Coca-Cola and PepsiCo. And its financial results have been stunning. From 2003 to 2009, its revenues have increased from $1.24 billion to $5.2 billion, and its profits have increased from $165 million to $1.5 billion. These figures represent annual compound rate increases of 27 and 45 percent, respectively!

Source: Anonymous. 2010. Wahaha . . . China's leading beverage producer. *www.chinabevnews.com*. April 11: np; Andersen, M. M., Froholdt, M., & Poulfelt, F. 2010. *Return on Strategy*. New York: Routledge; and, Miller, P. M. 2004. The Chinese beverage company's expansion is no laughing matter. *www.chinabuisnessreview*. September–October: np.

Although complex physical technology is not included in this category of sources of imperfect inimitability, the exploitation of physical technology in a firm typically involves the use of socially complex resources. That is, several firms may possess the same physical technology, but only one of them may have the social relations, culture, group norms, and so on to fully exploit the technology in implementing its strategies. If such complex social resources are not subject to imitation (and assuming they are valuable and rare and no substitutes exist), this firm may obtain a sustained competitive advantage from exploiting its physical technology more effectively than other firms.

Strategy Spotlight 3.8 describes how a Chinese beverage firm captured a significant market share in rural China by establishing close relationships with its distributors.

Are Substitutes Readily Available?   The fourth requirement for a firm resource to be a source of sustainable competitive advantage is that there must be no strategically equivalent valuable resources that are themselves not rare or inimitable. Two valuable firm resources (or two bundles of resources) are strategically equivalent when each one can be exploited separately to implement the same strategies.

Substitutability may take at least two forms. First, though it may be impossible for a firm to imitate exactly another firm's resource, it may be able to substitute a similar resource that enables it to develop and implement the same strategy. Clearly, a firm seeking to imitate another firm's high-quality top management team would be unable to copy the team exactly. However, it might be able to develop its own unique management team. Though these two teams would have different ages, functional backgrounds, experience, and so on, they could be strategically equivalent and thus substitutes for one another.

Second, very different firm resources can become strategic substitutes. For example, Internet booksellers such as Amazon.com compete as substitutes for bricks-and-mortar booksellers such as Barnes & Noble. The result is that resources such as premier retail locations become less valuable. In a similar vein, several pharmaceutical firms have seen the value of patent protection erode in the face of new drugs that are based on different production processes and act in different ways, but can be used in similar treatment regimes. The coming years will likely see even more radical change in the pharmaceutical industry as the substitution of genetic therapies eliminates certain uses of chemotherapy.[55]

To recap this section, recall that resources and capabilities must be rare and valuable as well as difficult to imitate or substitute in order for a firm to attain competitive advantages that are sustainable over time.[56] Exhibit 3.7 illustrates the relationship among the four criteria of sustainability and shows the competitive implications.

In firms represented by the first row of Exhibit 3.7, managers are in a difficult situation. When their resources and capabilities do not meet any of the four criteria, it would be difficult to develop any type of competitive advantage, in the short or long term. The resources and capabilities they possess enable the firm neither to exploit environmental opportunities nor neutralize environmental threats. In the second and third rows, firms have resources and capabilities that are valuable as well as rare, respectively. However, in both cases the resources and capabilities are not difficult for competitors to imitate or substitute. Here, the firms could attain some level of competitive parity. They could perform on par with equally endowed rivals or attain a temporary competitive advantage. But their advantages would be easy for competitors to match. It is only in the fourth row, where all four criteria are satisfied, that competitive advantages can be sustained over time. Next, let's look at Dell and see how its competitive advantage, which seemed to be sustainable for a rather long period of time, has eroded.

Dell's Eroding (Sustainable?) Competitive Advantage   In 1984, Michael Dell started Dell Inc. in a University of Texas dorm room with an investment of $1,000.[57] By 2006, Dell had attained annual revenues of $56 billion and a net income of $3.6 billion—making Michael Dell one of the richest people in the world. Dell achieved this meteoric growth by differentiating itself through the direct sales approach that it pioneered.

Exhibit 3.7
Criteria for Sustainable Competitive Advantage and Strategic Implications

Is a resource or capability . . .				
Valuable?	Rare?	Difficult to Imitate?	Without Substitutes?	Implications for Competitiveness
No	No	No	No	Competitive disadvantage
Yes	No	No	No	Competitive parity
Yes	Yes	No	No	Temporary competitive advantage
Yes	Yes	Yes	Yes	Sustainable competitive advantage

Source: Adapted from Barney, J. B. 1991. Firm Resources and Sustained Competitive Advantage. *Journal of Management,* 17: 99–120.

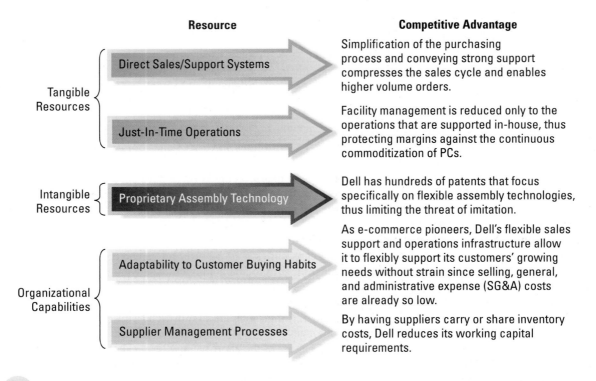

Resource	Competitive Advantage
Direct Sales/Support Systems	Simplification of the purchasing process and conveying strong support compresses the sales cycle and enables higher volume orders.
Just-In-Time Operations	Facility management is reduced only to the operations that are supported in-house, thus protecting margins against the continuous commoditization of PCs.
Proprietary Assembly Technology	Dell has hundreds of patents that focus specifically on flexible assembly technologies, thus limiting the threat of imitation.
Adaptability to Customer Buying Habits	As e-commerce pioneers, Dell's flexible sales support and operations infrastructure allow it to flexibly support its customers' growing needs without strain since selling, general, and administrative expense (SG&A) costs are already so low.
Supplier Management Processes	By having suppliers carry or share inventory costs, Dell reduces its working capital requirements.

Exhibit 3.8 Dell's Tangible Resources, Intangible Resources, and Organizational Capabilities

Its user-configurable products met the diverse needs of its corporate and institutional customer base. Exhibit 3.8 summarizes how Dell achieved its remarkable success by integrating its tangible resources, intangible resources, and organizational capabilities.

Dell continued to maintain this competitive advantage by strengthening its value-chain activities and interrelationships that are critical to satisfying the largest market opportunities. It achieved this by (1) implementing e-commerce direct sales and support processes that accounted for the sophisticated buying habits of the largest markets and (2) matching its inventory management to its extensive supplier network. Dell also sustained these advantages by investing in intangible resources, such as proprietary assembly methods and packaging configurations, that helped to protect against the threat of imitation.

Dell recognized that the PC is a complex product with components sourced from several different technologies and manufacturers. Thus, in working backward from the customer's purchasing habits, Dell saw that the company could build valuable solutions by organizing its resources and capabilities around build-to-specification tastes, making both the sales and integration processes flexible, and passing on overhead expenses to its suppliers. Even as the PC industry became further commoditized, Dell was one of the few competitors that was able to retain solid margins. It accomplished this by adapting its manufacturing and assembly capabilities to match the PC market's trend toward user compatibility.

For many years, it looked as if Dell's competitive advantage over its rivals would be sustainable for a very long period of time. However, by early 2007, Dell began falling behind its rivals in market share. This led to a significant decline in its stock price—followed by a complete shake-up of the top management team. But what led to Dell's competitive decline in the first place?[58]

- Dell had become so focused on cost that it failed to pay attention to the design of the brand. Customers increasingly began to see the product as a commodity.

- Much of the growth in the PC industry today is in laptops. Customers demand a sleeker, better-designed machine instead of just the cheapest laptop. Also, they often want to see the laptop before they buy it.
- When Dell outsourced its customer service function to foreign locations, it led to a decline in customer support. This eroded Dell's brand value.
- Dell's efforts to replicate its made-to-order, no-middleman strategy to other products such as printers and storage devices proved to be a failure. This is because customers saw little need for customization of these products.
- Rivals such as HP have been improving their product design and reducing their costs.[59] Thus, they gained cost parity with Dell, while enjoying a better brand image and the support of an extensive dealer network.

Not surprisingly, Dell's performance has suffered. Between 2006 and 2010, its revenues and net income have slumped from $56 billion to $53 billion and $3.6 billion and $1.4 billion, respectively. Inder Sidhu, the author of *Doing Both* (2010), provides a succinct summary of the central lesson in the Dell story:[60]

> Dell illustrates what can happen when a company emphasizes optimization to the exclusion of reinvention. Dell's obsession with operational excellence prevented it from delivering innovations that the market wanted, costing it a great deal of goodwill and prestige. When *Fortune* announced its annual list of "Most Admired Companies" in 2009, Dell, the leader from just four years prior, wasn't even mentioned in the top 50.

The Generation and Distribution of a Firm's Profits: Extending the Resource-Based View of the Firm

The resource-based view of the firm has been useful in determining when firms will create competitive advantages and enjoy high levels of profitability. However, it has not been developed to address how a firm's profits (often referred to as "rents" by economists) will be distributed to a firm's management and employees or other stakeholders such as customers, suppliers, or governments.[61] This becomes an important issue because firms may be successful in creating competitive advantages that can be sustainable for a period of time. However, much of the profits can be retained (or "appropriated") by its employees and managers or other stakeholders instead of flowing to the owners of the firm (i.e., the stockholders).[*]

Consider Viewpoint DataLabs International, a U.S.-based company in Salt Lake City that makes sophisticated three-dimensional models and textures for film production houses, video games, and car manufacturers. This example will help to show how employees are often able to obtain (or "appropriate") a high proportion of a firm's profits:

> Walter Noot, head of production, was having trouble keeping his highly skilled Generation X employees happy with their compensation. Each time one of them was lured away for more money, everyone would want a raise. "We were having to give out raises every six months—30 to 40 percent—then six months later they'd expect the same. It was a big struggle to keep people happy."[62]

At Viewpoint DataLabs, much of the profits are being generated by the highly skilled professionals working together. They are able to exercise their power by successfully demanding more financial compensation. In part, management has responded favorably because they are united in their demands, and their work involves a certain amount of social complexity and causal ambiguity—given the complex, coordinated efforts that their work entails.

Four factors help explain the extent to which employees and managers will be able to obtain a proportionately high level of the profits that they generate:[63]

---

[*] Economists define rents as profits (or prices) in excess of what is required to provide a normal return.

- **Employee Bargaining Power.** If employees are vital to forming a firm's unique capability, they will earn disproportionately high wages. For example, marketing professionals may have access to valuable information that helps them to understand the intricacies of customer demands and expectations, or engineers may understand unique technical aspects of the products or services. Additionally, in some industries such as consulting, advertising, and tax preparation, clients tend to be very loyal to individual professionals employed by the firm, instead of to the firm itself. This enables them to "take the clients with them" if they leave. This enhances their bargaining power.
- **Employee Replacement Cost.** If employees' skills are idiosyncratic and rare (a source of resource-based advantages), they should have high bargaining power based on the high cost required by the firm to replace them. For example, Raymond Ozzie, the software designer who was critical in the development of Lotus Notes, was able to dictate the terms under which IBM acquired Lotus.
- **Employee Exit Costs.** This factor may tend to reduce an employee's bargaining power. An individual may face high personal costs when leaving the organization. Thus, that individual's threat of leaving may not be credible. In addition, an employee's expertise may be firm-specific and of limited value to other firms. Causal ambiguity may make it difficult for the employee to explain his or her specific contribution to a given project. Thus, a rival firm might be less likely to pay a high wage premium since it would be unsure of the employee's unique contribution.
- **Manager Bargaining Power.** Managers' power is based on how well they create resource-based advantages. They are generally charged with creating value through the process of organizing, coordinating, and leveraging employees as well as other forms of capital such as plant, equipment, and financial capital (addressed further in Chapter 4). Such activities provide managers with sources of information that may not be readily available to others. Thus, although managers may not know as much about the specific nature of customers and technologies, they are in a position to have a more thorough, integrated understanding of the total operation.

Chapter 9 addresses the conditions under which top-level managers (such as CEOs) of large corporations have been, at times, able to obtain levels of total compensation that would appear to be significantly disproportionate to their contributions to wealth generation as well as to top executives in peer organizations. Here, corporate governance becomes a critical control mechanism. For example, William Esrey and Ronald T. LeMay (the former two top executives at Sprint Corporation) earned more than $130 million in stock options because of "cozy" relationships with members of their board of directors, who tended to approve with little debate huge compensation packages.[64]

Such diversion of profits from the owners of the business to top management is far less likely when the board members are truly independent outsiders (i.e., they do not have close ties to management). In general, given the external market for top talent, the level of compensation that executives receive is based on factors similar to the ones just discussed that determine the level of their bargaining power.[65]

In addition to employees and managers, other stakeholder groups can also appropriate a portion of the rents generated by a firm. If, for example, a critical input is controlled by a monopoly supplier or if a single buyer accounts for most of a firm's sales, their bargaining power can greatly erode the potential profits of a firm. Similarly, excessive taxation by governments can also reduce what is available to a firm's stockholders.

financial ratio analysis a technique for measuring the performance of a firm according to its balance sheet, income statement, and market valuation.

Evaluating Firm Performance: Two Approaches

This section addresses two approaches to use when evaluating a firm's performance. The first is **financial ratio analysis,** which, generally speaking, identifies how a firm is performing according to its balance sheet, income statement, and market valuation. As we will discuss, when performing a financial ratio analysis, you must take into account the firm's performance from a historical perspective (not just at one point in time) as well as how it compares with both industry norms and key competitors.[66]

The second perspective takes a broader stakeholder view. Firms must satisfy a broad range of stakeholders, including employees, customers, and owners, to ensure their long-term viability. Central to our discussion will be a well-known approach—the balanced scorecard—that has been popularized by Robert Kaplan and David Norton.[67]

Financial Ratio Analysis

The beginning point in analyzing the financial position of a firm is to compute and analyze five different types of financial ratios:

- Short-term solvency or liquidity
- Long-term solvency measures
- Asset management (or turnover)
- Profitability
- Market value

Exhibit 3.9 summarizes each of these five ratios.

I. Short-term solvency, or liquidity, ratios

$$\text{Current ratio} = \frac{\text{Current assets}}{\text{Current liabilities}}$$

$$\text{Quick ratio} = \frac{\text{Current assets} - \text{Inventory}}{\text{Current liabilities}}$$

$$\text{Cash ratio} = \frac{\text{Cash}}{\text{Current liabilities}}$$

II. Long-term solvency, or financial leverage, ratios

$$\text{Total debt ratio} = \frac{\text{Total assets} - \text{Total equity}}{\text{Total assets}}$$

$$\text{Debt-equity ratio} = \text{Total debt/Total equity}$$

$$\text{Equity multiplier} = \text{Total assets/Total equity}$$

$$\text{Times interest earned ratio} = \frac{\text{EBIT}}{\text{Interest}}$$

$$\text{Cash coverage ratio} = \frac{\text{EBIT} + \text{Depreciation}}{\text{Interest}}$$

III. Asset utilization, or turnover, ratios

$$\text{Inventory turnover} = \frac{\text{Cost of goods sold}}{\text{Inventory}}$$

$$\text{Days' sales in inventory} = \frac{365 \text{ days}}{\text{Inventory turnover}}$$

$$\text{Receivables turnover} = \frac{\text{Sales}}{\text{Accounts receivable}}$$

$$\text{Days' sales in receivables} = \frac{365 \text{ days}}{\text{Receivables turnover}}$$

$$\text{Total asset turnover} = \frac{\text{Sales}}{\text{Total assets}}$$

$$\text{Capital intensity} = \frac{\text{Total assets}}{\text{Sales}}$$

IV. Profitability ratios

$$\text{Profit margin} = \frac{\text{Net income}}{\text{Sales}}$$

$$\text{Return on assets (ROA)} = \frac{\text{Net income}}{\text{Total assets}}$$

$$\text{Return on equity (ROE)} = \frac{\text{Net income}}{\text{Total equity}}$$

$$\text{ROE} = \frac{\text{Net income}}{\text{Sales}} \times \frac{\text{Sales}}{\text{Assets}} \times \frac{\text{Assets}}{\text{Equity}}$$

V. Market value ratios

$$\text{Price-earnings ratio} = \frac{\text{Price per share}}{\text{Earnings per share}}$$

$$\text{Market-to-book ratio} = \frac{\text{Market value per share}}{\text{Book value per share}}$$

Exhibit 3.9 A Summary of Five Types of Financial Ratios

Appendix 1 to Chapter 13 (the Case Analysis chapter) provides detailed definitions for and discussions of each of these types of ratios as well as examples of how
each is calculated. Refer to pages 533 to 542.

>LO3.6

The usefulness
of financial
ratio analysis,
its inherent
limitations, and
how to make
meaningful
comparisons
of performance
across firms.

A meaningful ratio analysis must go beyond the calculation and interpretation of
financial ratios.[68] It must include how ratios change over time as well as how they are
interrelated. For example, a firm that takes on too much long-term debt to finance operations will see an immediate impact on its indicators of long-term financial leverage. The
additional debt will negatively affect the firm's short-term liquidity ratio (i.e., current and
quick ratios) since the firm must pay interest and principal on the additional debt each year
until it is retired. Additionally, the interest expenses deducted from revenues reduce the
firm's profitability.

A firm's financial position should not be analyzed in isolation. Important reference
points are needed. We will address some issues that must be taken into account to make
financial analysis more meaningful: historical comparisons, comparisons with industry
norms, and comparisons with key competitors.

Historical Comparisons   When you evaluate a firm's financial performance, it is
very useful to compare its financial position over time. This provides a means of evaluating trends. For example, Apple Inc. reported revenues of $65 billion and net income of $14
billion in 2010. Virtually all firms would be very happy with such financial success. These
figures represent a stunning annual growth in revenue and net income of 100 percent and
190 percent, respectively, for the 2008 to 2010 time period. Had Apple's revenues and
net income in 2010 been $40 billion and $6 billion, respectively, it would still be a very
large and highly profitable enterprise. However, such performance would have significantly damaged Apple's market valuation and reputation as well as the careers of many
of its executives.

Exhibit 3.10 illustrates a 10-year period of return on sales (ROS) for a hypothetical
company. As indicated by the dotted trend lines, the rate of growth (or decline) differs substantially over time periods.

Comparisons with Industry Norms   When you are evaluating a firm's financial
performance, remember also to compare it with industry norms. A firm's current ratio or
profitability may appear impressive at first glance. However, it may pale when compared
with industry standards or norms.

Exhibit 3.10
**Historical Trends: Return
on Sales (ROS) for a
Hypothetical Company**

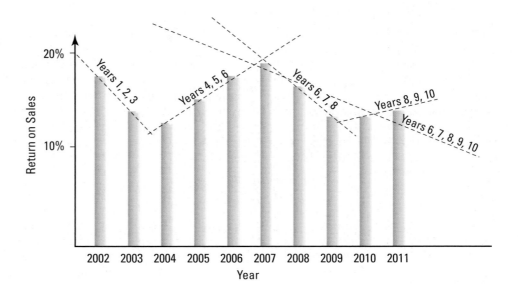

Exhibit 3.11
How Financial Ratios
Differ across Industries

Financial Ratio	Semiconductors	Grocery Stores	Skilled-Nursing Facilities
Quick ratio (times)	1.9	0.6	1.2
Current ratio (times)	3.9	1.9	1.6
Total liabilities to net worth (%)	30.2	71.4	156.9
Collection period (days)	49.0	2.6	30.3
Assets to sales (%)	147.3	19.5	113.9
Return on sales (%)	24	1.1	2.4

Source: Dun & Bradstreet. *Industry Norms and Key Business Ratios, 2007–2008*. One Year Edition, SIC #3600–3699 (Semiconductors); SIC #5400–5499 (Grocery Stores); SIC #8000–8099 (Skilled-Nursing Facilities). New York: Dun & Bradstreet Credit Services.

Comparing your firm with all other firms in your industry assesses relative performance. Banks often use such comparisons when evaluating a firm's creditworthiness. Exhibit 3.11 includes a variety of financial ratios for three industries: semiconductors, grocery stores, and skilled-nursing facilities. Why is there such variation among the financial ratios for these three industries? There are several reasons. With regard to the collection period, grocery stores operate mostly on a cash basis, hence a very short collection period. Semiconductor manufacturers sell their output to other manufacturers (e.g., computer makers) on terms such as 2/15 net 45, which means they give a 2 percent discount on bills paid within 15 days and start charging interest after 45 days. Skilled-nursing facilities also have a longer collection period than grocery stores because they typically rely on payments from insurance companies.

The industry norms for return on sales also highlight differences among these industries. Grocers, with very slim margins, have a lower return on sales than either skilled-nursing facilities or semiconductor manufacturers. But how might we explain the differences between skilled-nursing facilities and semiconductor manufacturers? Health care facilities, in general, are limited in their pricing structures by Medicare/Medicaid regulations and by insurance reimbursement limits, but semiconductor producers have pricing structures determined by the market. If their products have superior performance, semiconductor manufacturers can charge premium prices.

Comparisons with Key Competitors   Recall from Chapter 2 that firms with similar strategies are members of a strategic group in an industry. Furthermore, competition is more intense among competitors within groups than across groups. Thus, you can gain valuable insights into a firm's financial and competitive position if you make comparisons between a firm and its most direct rivals. Consider a firm trying to diversify into the highly profitable pharmaceutical industry. Even if it was willing to invest several hundred million dollars, it would be virtually impossible to compete effectively against industry giants such as Pfizer and Merck. These two firms have 2010 revenues of $68 billion and $46 billion, respectively, and R&D budgets of $9 billion and $11 billion, respectively.[69]

Integrating Financial Analysis and Stakeholder Perspectives: The Balanced Scorecard

It is useful to see how a firm is performing over time in terms of several ratios. However, such traditional approaches to performance assessments can be a double-edged sword.[70] Many important transactions that managers make—investments in research and development, employee training and development, and advertising and promotion of key

>LO3.7
The value of the "balanced scorecard" in recognizing how the interests of a variety of stakeholders can be interrelated.

Exhibit 3.12
**The Balanced
Scorecard's Four
Perspectives**

- How do customers see us? (customer perspective)
- What must we excel at? (internal business perspective)
- Can we continue to improve and create value? (innovation and learning perspective)
- How do we look to shareholders? (financial perspective)

brands—may greatly expand a firm's market potential and create significant long-term shareholder value. But such critical investments are not reflected positively in short-term financial reports. Financial reports typically measure expenses, not the value created. Thus, managers may be penalized for spending money in the short term to improve their firm's long-term competitive viability!

Now consider the other side of the coin. A manager may destroy the firm's future value by dissatisfying customers, depleting the firm's stock of good products coming out of R&D, or damaging the morale of valued employees. Such budget cuts, however, may lead to very good short-term financials. The manager may look good in the short run and even receive credit for improving the firm's performance. In essence, such a manager has mastered "denominator management," whereby decreasing investments makes the return on investment (ROI) ratio larger, even though the actual return remains constant or shrinks.

The Balanced Scorecard: Description and Benefits   To provide a meaningful integration of the many issues that come into evaluating a firm's performance, Kaplan and Norton developed a **"balanced scorecard."**[71] This provides top managers with a fast but comprehensive view of the business. In a nutshell, it includes financial measures that reflect the results of actions already taken, but it complements these indicators with measures of customer satisfaction, internal processes, and the organization's innovation and improvement activities—operational measures that drive future financial performance.

The balanced scorecard enables managers to consider their business from four key perspectives: customer, internal business, innovation and learning, and financial. These are briefly described in Exhibit 3.12.

Customer Perspective Clearly, how a company is performing from its **customers' perspective** is a top priority for management. The balanced scorecard requires that managers translate their general mission statements on customer service into specific measures that reflect the factors that really matter to customers. For the balanced scorecard to work, managers must articulate goals for four key categories of customer concerns: time, quality, performance and service, and cost. For example, lead time may be measured as the time from the company's receipt of an order to the time it actually delivers the product or service to the customer.

Internal Business Perspective Customer-based measures are important. However, they must be translated into indicators of what the firm must do internally to meet customers' expectations. Excellent customer performance results from processes, decisions, and actions that occur throughout organizations in a coordinated fashion, and, using the **internal business perspective,** managers must focus on those critical internal operations that enable them to satisfy customer needs. The internal measures should reflect business processes that have the greatest impact on customer satisfaction. These include factors that affect cycle time, quality, employee skills, and productivity. Firms also must identify and measure the key resources and capabilities they need for continued success.

Innovation and Learning Perspective Given the rapid rate of markets, technologies, and global competition, the criteria for success are constantly changing. To survive and prosper, managers must make frequent changes to existing products and services as

balanced scorecard
a method of evaluating a firm's performance using performance measures from the customers', internal, innovation and learning, and financial perspectives.

customer perspective
measures of firm performance that indicate how well firms are satisfying customers' expectations.

internal business perspective
measures of firm performance that indicate how well firms' internal processes, decisions and actions are contributing to customer satisfaction.

well as introduce entirely new products with expanded capabilities. A firm's ability to improve, innovate, and learn is tied directly to its value. Simply put, only by developing new products and services, creating greater value for customers, and increasing operating efficiencies can a company penetrate new markets, increase revenues and margins, and enhance shareholder value. A firm's ability to do well from an **innovation and learning perspective** is more dependent on its intangible than tangible assets. Three categories of intangible assets are critically important: human capital (skills, talent, and knowledge), information capital (information systems, networks), and organization capital (culture, leadership).

Financial Perspective Measures of financial performance indicate whether the company's strategy, implementation, and execution are indeed contributing to bottom-line improvement. Typical financial goals include profitability, growth, and shareholder value. Periodic financial statements remind managers that improved quality, response time, productivity, and innovative products benefit the firm only when they result in improved sales, increased market share, reduced operating expenses, or higher asset turnover.[72]

Consider how Sears, the huge retailer, found a strong causal relationship between employee attitudes, customer attitudes, and financial outcomes.[73] Through an ongoing study, Sears developed (and continues to refine) what it calls its total performance indicators, or TPI—a set of indicators for assessing their performance with customers, employees, and investors. Sears's quantitative model has shown that a 5.0 percent improvement in employee attitudes leads to a 1.3 percent improvement in customer satisfaction, which in turn drives a 0.5 percent improvement in revenue. Thus, if a single store improved its employee attitude by 5.0 percent, Sears could predict with confidence that if the revenue growth in the district as a whole were 5.0 percent, the revenue growth in this particular store would be 5.5 percent. Interestingly, Sears's managers consider such numbers as rigorous as any others that they work with every year. The company's accounting firm audits management as closely as it audits the financial statements.

A key implication is that managers do not need to look at their job as balancing stakeholder demands. They must avoid the following mind-set: "How many units in employee satisfaction do I have to give up to get some additional units of customer satisfaction or profits?" Instead, the balanced scorecard provides a win–win approach—increasing satisfaction among a wide variety of organizational stakeholders, including employees (at all levels), customers, and stockholders.

Limitations and Potential Downsides of the Balanced Scorecard There is general agreement that there is nothing inherently wrong with the concept of the balanced scorecard.[74] The key limitation is that some executives may view it as a "quick fix" that can be easily installed. However, implementing a balanced metrics system is an evolutionary process. It is not a one-time task that can be quickly checked off as "completed." If managers do not recognize this from the beginning and fail to commit to it long term, the organization will be disappointed. Poor execution becomes the cause of such performance outcomes. And organizational scorecards must be aligned with individuals' scorecards to turn the balanced scorecards into a powerful tool for sustained performance.[*]

In a recent study of 50 Canadian medium-size and large organizations, the number of users expressing skepticism about scorecard performance was much greater than the

---

innovation and learning perspective measures of firm performance that indicate how well firms are changing their product and service offerings to adapt to changes in the internal and external environments.

financial perspective measures of firms' financial performance that indicate how well strategy, implementation and execution are contributing to bottom-line improvement.

---

[*] Building on the concepts that are the foundation of the balanced scorecard approach, Kaplan and Norton have recently developed a useful tool called the strategy map. Strategy maps show the cause and effect links by which specific improvements in different areas lead to a desired outcome. Strategy maps also help employees see how their jobs are related to the overall objectives of the organization. They also help us understand how an organization can convert its assets—both tangible and intangible—into tangible outcomes. Refer to Kaplan, R. S. & Norton, D. P. 2000. Having trouble with your strategy? Then map it. *Harvard Business Review,* 78(10): 167–176.

number claiming positive results. However, the overwhelming perspective was that balanced scorecards can be worthwhile in clarifying an organization's strategy, and if this can be accomplished, better results will follow. A few companies stated categorically that scorecards have improved their firm's financial results. For example, one respondent claimed that "We did not meet our financial goals previously, but since implementing our balanced scorecard, we have now met our goals three years running."

On the other hand, a greater number of respondents agreed with the statement "Balanced scorecards don't really work." Some representative comments included: "It became just a number-crunching exercise by accountants after the first year," "It is just the latest management fad and is already dropping lower on management's list of priorities as all fads eventually do," and "If scorecards are supposed to be a measurement tool, why is it so hard to measure their results?" There is much work to do before scorecards can become a viable framework to measure sustained strategic performance.

Problems often occur in the balanced scorecard implementation efforts when there is an insufficient commitment to learning and the inclusion of employees' personal ambitions. Without a set of rules for employees that address continuous process improvement and the personal improvement of individual employees, there will be limited employee buy-in and insufficient cultural change. Thus, many improvements may be temporary and superficial. Often, scorecards that failed to attain alignment and improvements dissipated very quickly. And, in many cases, management's efforts to improve performance were seen as divisive and were viewed by employees as aimed at benefiting senior management compensation. This fostered a "What's in it for me?" attitude. Exhibit 3.13 summarizes some of the potential downsides of the balanced scorecard.

Exhibit 3.13
Potential Limitations of the Balanced Scorecard

Most agree that the balanced scorecard concept is a useful and an appropriate management tool. However, there are many design and implementation issues that may short-circuit its value, including the following:

- *Lack of a Clear Strategy.* A scorecard can be developed without the aid of a strategy. However, it then becomes a key performance indicator or stakeholder system, lacking in many of the attributes offered from a true balanced scorecard.
- *Limited or Ineffective Executive Sponsorship.* Although training and education are important, without tenacious leadership and support of a scorecard project, the effort is most likely doomed.
- *Too Much Emphasis on Financial Measures Rather Than Nonfinancial Measures.* This leads to measures that do not connect to the drivers of the business and are not relevant to performance improvement.
- *Poor Data on Actual Performance.* This can negate most of the effort invested in defining performance measures because a company can't monitor actual changes in results from changes in behavior.
- *Inappropriate Links of Scorecard Measures to Compensation.* Although this can focus managerial and employee attention, exercising it too soon can produce many unintended side effects such as dysfunctional decision making by managers looking to cash in.
- *Inconsistent or Inappropriate Terminology.* Everyone must speak the same language if measurement is to be used to guide change within an organization. Translating strategy into measures becomes even more difficult if everyone cannot agree on (or understand) the same language and terminology.

Sources: Angel, R. & Rampersad, H. 2005. Do scorecards add up? *Camagazine.com.* May: np; and, Niven, P. 2002. *Balanced Scorecard Step by Step: Maximizing Performance and Maintaining Results.* New York: John Wiley & Sons.

Reflecting on Career Implications . . .

- **The Value Chain:** Carefully analyze where you can add value in your firm's value chain. How might your firm's support activities (e.g., information technology, human resource practices) help you accomplish your assigned tasks more effectively?
- **The Value Chain:** Consider important relationships among activities both within your firm as well as between your firm and its suppliers, customers, and alliance partners.
- **Resource-Based View of the Firm:** Are your skills and talents rare, valuable, difficult to imitate, and difficult to substitute? If so, you are in a better position to add value for your firm—and earn rewards and incentives. How can your skills and talents be enhanced to help satisfy these criteria to a greater extent? More training? Changing positions within the firm? Considering career options at other organizations?
- **Balanced Scorecard:** In your decision making, strive to "balance" the four perspectives: customer, internal business, innovation and learning, and financial. Do not focus too much on short-term profits. Do your personal career goals provide opportunities to develop your skills in all four directions?

Summary

In the traditional approaches to assessing a firm's internal environment, the primary goal of managers would be to determine their firm's relative strengths and weaknesses. Such is the role of SWOT analysis, wherein managers analyze their firm's strengths and weaknesses as well as the opportunities and threats in the external environment. In this chapter, we discussed why this may be a good starting point but hardly the best approach to take in performing a sound analysis. There are many limitations to SWOT analysis, including its static perspective, its potential to overemphasize a single dimension of a firm's strategy, and the likelihood that a firm's strengths do not necessarily help the firm create value or competitive advantages.

We identified two frameworks that serve to complement SWOT analysis in assessing a firm's internal environment: value-chain analysis and the resource-based view of the firm. In conducting a value-chain analysis, first divide the firm into a series of value-creating activities. These include primary activities such as inbound logistics, operations, and service as well as support activities such as procurement and human resources management. Then analyze how each activity adds value as well as how *interrelationships* among value activities in the firm and among the firm and its customers and suppliers add value. Thus, instead of merely determining a firm's strengths and weaknesses per se, you analyze them in the overall context of the firm and its relationships with customers and suppliers—the value system.

The resource-based view of the firm considers the firm as a bundle of resources: tangible resources, intangible resources, and organizational capabilities. Competitive advantages that are sustainable over time generally arise from the creation of bundles of resources and capabilities. For advantages to be sustainable, four criteria must be satisfied: value, rarity, difficulty in imitation, and difficulty in substitution. Such an evaluation requires a sound knowledge of the competitive context in which the firm exists. The owners of a business may not capture all of the value created by the firm. The appropriation of value created by a firm between the owners and employees is determined by four factors: employee bargaining power, replacement cost, employee exit costs, and manager bargaining power.

An internal analysis of the firm would not be complete unless you evaluate its performance and make the appropriate comparisons. Determining a firm's performance requires an analysis of its financial situation as well as a review of how well it is satisfying a broad range of stakeholders, including customers, employees, and stockholders. We discussed the concept of the balanced scorecard, in which four perspectives must be addressed: customer, internal business, innovation and learning, and financial. Central to this concept is the idea that the interests of various stakeholders can be interrelated. We provide examples of how indicators of employee satisfaction lead to higher levels of customer satisfaction, which in turn lead to higher levels of financial performance.

Thus, improving a firm's performance does not need to involve making trade-offs among different stakeholders. Assessing the firm's performance is also more useful if it is evaluated in terms of how it changes over time, compares with industry norms, and compares with key competitors.

In the Appendix to Chapter 3, we discuss how Internet and digital technologies have created new opportunities for firms to add value. Four value-adding activities that have been enhanced by Internet capabilities are search, evaluation, problem solving, and transaction. These four activities are supported by three different types of content that Internet businesses often use—customer feedback, expertise, and entertainment programming. Seven business models have been identified that are proving successful for use by Internet firms. These include commission-, advertising-, markup-, production-, referral-, subscription-, and fee-for-service–based models. Firms also are finding that combinations of these business models can contribute to greater success.

Summary Review Questions

1. SWOT analysis is a technique to analyze the internal and external environment of a firm. What are its advantages and disadvantages?

2. Briefly describe the primary and support activities in a firm's value chain.

3. How can managers create value by establishing important relationships among the value-chain activities both within their firm and between the firm and its customers and suppliers?

4. Briefly explain the four criteria for sustainability of competitive advantages.

5. Under what conditions are employees and managers able to appropriate some of the value created by their firm?

6. What are the advantages and disadvantages of conducting a financial ratio analysis of a firm?

7. Summarize the concept of the balanced scorecard. What are its main advantages?

Key Terms

value-chain analysis, 121
primary activities, 121
support activities, 121
inbound logistics, 123
operations, 124
outbound logistics, 124
marketing and sales, 126
service, 126
procurement, 127
technology
    development, 128
human resource
    management, 129
general
    administration, 129
interrelationships, 130
resource-based view
    (RBV) of the
    firm, 133
tangible resources, 135
intangible resources, 135
organizational
    capabilities, 135
strategic resources
    (*also* firm resources
    or organizational
    resources), 137
path dependency, 138
causal ambiguity, 138
social complexity, 139
financial ratio
    analysis, 144
balanced scorecard, 148
customer perspective, 148
internal business
    perspective, 148
innovation and learning
    perspective, 149
financial perspective, 149
search activities, 157
evaluation activities, 157
problem-solving
    activities, 158
transaction
    activities, 158
business model, 159

Experiential Exercise

Dell Computer is a leading firm in the personal computer industry, with annual revenues of $53 billion during its 2010 fiscal year. Dell had created a very strong competitive position via its "direct model," whereby it manufactures its personal computers to detailed customer specifications. However, its advantage has been eroded recently by strong rivals such as HP.

Below we address several questions that focus on Dell's value-chain activities and interrelationships among them as well as whether it is able to attain sustainable competitive advantage(s). (We discuss Dell in this chapter on pages 141–143.)

1. Where in its value chain is Dell creating value for its customer?

Value-Chain Activity	Yes/No	How Does Dell Create Value for the Customer?
Primary:		
Inbound logistics		
Operations		
Outbound logistics		
Marketing and sales		
Service		
Support:		
Procurement		
Technology development		
Human resource management		
General administration		

2. What are the important relationships among Dell's value-chain activities? What are the important interdependencies? For each activity, identify the relationships and interdependencies.

	Inbound logistics	Operations	Outbound logistics	Marketing and sales	Service	Procurement	Technology development	Human resource management	General administration
Inbound logistics									
Operations									
Outbound logistics									
Marketing and sales									
Service									
Procurement									
Technology development									
Human resource management									
General administration									

3. What resources, activities, and relationships enable Dell to achieve a sustainable competitive advantage?

Resource/Activity	Is It Valuable?	Is It Rare?	Are There Few Substitutes?	Is It Difficult to Make?
Inbound logistics				
Operations				
Outbound logistics				
Marketing and sales				
Service				
Procurement				
Technology development				
Human resource management				
General administration				

Application Questions & Exercises

1. Using published reports, select two CEOs who have recently made public statements regarding a major change in their firm's strategy. Discuss how the successful implementation of such strategies requires changes in the firm's primary and support activities.

2. Select a firm that competes in an industry in which you are interested. Drawing upon published financial reports, complete a financial ratio analysis. Evaluate the firm's strengths and weaknesses in terms of its financial position, based on changes over time and a comparison with industry norms.

3. How might exemplary human resource practices enhance and strengthen a firm's value-chain activities?

4. Using the Internet, look up your university or college. What are some of its key value-creating activities that provide competitive advantages? Why?

Ethics Questions

1. What are some of the ethical issues that arise when a firm becomes overly zealous in advertising its products?

2. What are some of the ethical issues that may arise from a firm's procurement activities? Are you aware of any of these issues from your personal experience or businesses you are familiar with?

References

1. Anonymous. 2010. 'There's no brakes . . . hold on and pray': Last words of man before he and his family died in Toyota Lexus crash. *www.dailymail .co.uk*. February 3: np; Ohnsman, A. 2010. The Humbling of Toyota. *Bloomberg Businessweek,* March 22: 32–36;

Anonymous. 2009. Toyota recalls 3.8 million vehicles. *www.msnbc.com*. September 29: np; Ross, B. 2009. Owners of Toyota cars in rebellion over series of accidents caused by sudden acceleration, part one. *www.abcnews .go.com*. November 3: np; and,

Ohnsman, A. 2009. Toyota recall crisis said to lie in cost cuts, growth ambitions, *www.bloomberg.com*. February 26: np. We thank Jason Hirsch for his valued contributions.

2. Our discussion of the value chain will draw on Porter, M. E. 1985.

Competitive advantage: chapter. 2. New York: Free Press.

3. Dyer, J. H. 1996. Specialized supplier networks as a source of competitive advantage: Evidence from the auto industry. *Strategic Management Journal,* 17: 271–291.

4. For an insightful perspective on value-chain analysis, refer to: Stabell, C. B. & Fjeldstad, O. D. 1998. Configuring value for competitive advantage: On chains, shops, and networks. *Strategic Management Journal,* 19: 413–437. The authors develop concepts of value chains, value shops, and value networks to extend the value-creation logic across a broad range of industries. Their work builds on the seminal contributions of Porter, 1985, op. cit., and others who have addressed how firms create value through key interrelationships among value-creating activities.

5. Ibid.

6. Maynard, M. 1999. Toyota promises custom order in 5 days. *USA Today,* August 6: B1.

7. Shaw Industries. 1999. Annual report: 14–15.

8. Odiabat, H. 2010. Foodonclick.com launches in United Arab Emirates. *www.ameinfo.com/236286.html.* June 27.

9. Jackson. M. 2001. Bringing a dying brand back to life. *Harvard Business Review,* 79(5): 53–61.

10. Anderson, J. C. & Nmarus, J. A. 2003. Selectively pursuing more of your customer's business. *MIT Sloan Management Review,* 44(3): 42–50.

11. Insights on advertising are addressed in: Rayport, J. F. 2008. Where is advertising? Into 'stitials. *Harvard Business Review,* 66(5): 18–20.

12. An insightful discussion of the role of identity marketing—that is, the myriad labels that people use to express who they are—in successful marketing activities is found in: Reed, A., II & Bolton, L. E. 2005. The complexity of identity. *MIT Sloan Management Review,* 46(3): 18–22.

13. Insights on the usefulness of off-line ads are the focus of: Abraham, M. 2008. The off-line impact of online ads. *Harvard Business Review,* 66(4): 28.

14. Berggren, E. & Nacher, T. 2000. Why good ideas go bust. *Management Review,* February: 32–36.

15. For an insightful perspective on creating effective brand portfolios, refer to: Hill, S., Ettenson, R., & Tyson, D. 2005. Achieving the ideal brand portfolio. *MIT Sloan Management Review,* 46(2): 85–90.

16. Haddad, C. & Grow, B. 2001. Wait a second—I didn't order that! *BusinessWeek,* July 16: 45.

17. For a scholarly discussion on the procurement of technology components, read: Hoetker, G. 2005. How much you know versus how well I know you: Selecting a supplier for a technically innovative component. *Strategic Management Journal,* 26(1): 75–96.

18. For a discussion on criteria to use when screening suppliers for back-office functions, read: Feeny, D., Lacity, M., & Willcocks, L. P. 2005. Taking the measure of outsourcing providers. *MIT Sloan Management Review,* 46(3): 41–48.

19. For a study investigating sourcing practices, refer to: Safizadeh, M. H., Field, J. M., & Ritzman, L. P. 2008. Sourcing practices and boundaries of the firm in the financial services industry. *Strategic Management Journal,* 29(1): 79–92.

20. Imperato, G. 1998. How to give good feedback. *Fast Company,* September: 144–156.

21. Bensaou, B. M. & Earl, M. 1998. The right mindset for managing information technology. *Harvard Business Review,* 96(5): 118–128.

22. A discussion of R&D in the pharmaceutical industry is in: Garnier, J-P. 2008. Rebuilding the R&D engine in big pharma. *Harvard Business Review,* 66(5): 68–76.

23. Anonymous. 2005. Made in Korea, assembled in China. *Bloomberg Businessweek,* August 1, p. 48; Anonymous. 2004. Daewoo: GM's hot new engine. *Bloomberg Businessweek,* November 29, pp. 52–53; and, Wikipedia. 2007. GM Daewoo. *http://en.wikipedia.org.*

24. Ulrich, D. 1998. A new mandate for human resources. *Harvard Business Review,* 96(1): 124–134.

25. A study of human resource management in China is: Li, J., Lam, K., Sun, J. J. M., & Liu, S. X. Y. 2008. Strategic resource management, institutionalization, and employment modes: An empirical study in China. *Strategic Management Journal,* 29(3): 337–342.

26. Wood, J. 2003. Sharing jobs and working from home: The new face of the airline industry. AviationCareer.net. February 21.

27. Green, S., Hasan, F., Immelt, J., Marks, M., & Meiland, D. 2003. In search of global leaders. *Harvard Business Review,* 81(8): 38–45.

28. For insights on the role of information systems integration in fostering innovation refer to: Cash, J. I., Jr., Earl, M. J., & Morison, R. 2008. Teaming up to crack innovation and enterprise integration. *Harvard Business Review,* 66(11): 90–100.

29. For a cautionary note on the use of IT, refer to McAfee, A. 2003. When too much IT knowledge is a dangerous thing. *MIT Sloan Management Review,* 44(2): 83–90.

30. The important role in IT for a Japanese bank is addressed in: Upton, D. M. & Staats, B. R. 2008. Radically simple IT. *Harvard Business Review,* 66(3): 118–124.

31. Walgreen Co. 1996. *Information technology and Walgreens: Opportunities for employment.* January; *www.boots-uk.com;* and, Dess, G. G. & Picken, J. C. 1997. *Beyond productivity.* New York: AMACOM.

32. For an interesting perspective on some of the potential downsides of close customer and supplier relationships, refer to: Anderson, E. & Jap, S. D. 2005. The dark side of close relationships. *MIT Sloan Management Review,* 46(3): 75–82.

33. Day, G. S. 2003. Creating a superior customer-relating capability. *MIT Sloan Management Review,* 44(3): 77–82.

34. To gain insights on the role of electronic technologies in enhancing a firm's connections to outside suppliers and customers, refer to: Lawrence, T. B., Morse, E. A., & Fowler, S. W. 2005. Managing your portfolio of connections. *MIT Sloan Management Review,* 46(2): 59–66.

35. This section draws on: Andersen, M. M., Froholdt, M., & Poulfelt, F. 2010. *Return on strategy*, 96–100. New York: Routledge.

36. Quote from Hartmut Jenner, CEO, Alfred Karcher GmbH, IBM Global CEO Study, p. 27.

37. Collis, D. J. & Montgomery, C. A. 1995. Competing on resources: Strategy in the 1990s. *Harvard Business Review,* 73(4): 119–128; and, Barney, J. 1991. Firm resources and sustained competitive advantage. *Journal of Management,* 17(1): 99–120.

38. For recent critiques of the resource-based view of the firm, refer to: Sirmon, D. G., Hitt, M. A., & Ireland, R. D. 2007. Managing firm resources in dynamic environments to create value: Looking inside the black box. *Academy of Management Review,* 32(1): 273–292; and, Newbert, S. L. Empirical research on the resource-based view of the firm: An assessment and suggestions for future research. *Strategic Management Journal,* 28(2): 121–146.

39. For insights into research findings on the linkage between resources and performance, refer to: Crook, T. R., Ketchen, D. J., Jr., Combs, J. G., & Todd, S. Y. 2008. Strategic resources and performance: A meta-analysis. *Strategic Management Journal,* 29(11): 1141–1154.

40. Henkoff, R. 1993. Companies that train the best. *Fortune,* March 22: 83; and, Dess & Picken, *op. cit.,* p. 98.

41. Gaines-Ross, L. 2010. Reputation warfare. *Harvard Business Review,* 88(12): 70–76.

42. Barney, J. B. 1986. Types of competition and the theory of strategy: Towards an integrative framework. *Academy of Management Review,* 11(4): 791–800.

43. Harley-Davidson. 1993. Annual report.

44. For a rigorous, academic treatment of the origin of capabilities, refer to: Ethiraj, S. K., Kale, P., Krishnan, M. S., & Singh, J. V. 2005. Where do capabilities come from and how do they matter? A study of the software services industry. *Strategic Management Journal,* 26(1): 25–46.

45. For an academic discussion on methods associated with organizational capabilities, refer to: Dutta, S., Narasimhan, O., & Rajiv, S. 2005. Conceptualizing and measuring capabilities: Methodology and empirical application. *Strategic Management Journal,* 26(3): 277–286.

46. Lorenzoni, G. & Lipparini, A. 1999. The leveraging of interfirm relationships as a distinctive organizational capability: A longitudinal study. *Strategic Management Journal,* 20: 317–338.

47. Andersen, M. M. op. cit. 209.

48. A study investigating the sustainability of competitive advantage is: Newbert, S. L. 2008. Value, rareness, competitive advantages, and performance: A conceptual-level empirical investigation of the resource-based view of the firm. *Strategic Management Journal,* 29(7): 745–768.

49. Arikan, A. M. & McGahan, A. M. 2010. The development of capabilities in new firms. *Strategic Management Journal,* 31(1): 1–18.

50. Barney, J. 1991. Firm resources and sustained competitive advantage. *Journal of Management,* 17(1): 99–120.

51. Barney, 1986, op. cit. Our discussion of inimitability and substitution draws upon this source.

52. A study that investigates the performance implications of imitation is: Ethiraj, S. K. & Zhu, D. H. 2008. Performance effects of imitative entry. *Strategic Management Journal,* 29(8): 797–818.

53. Sirmon, D. G., Hitt, M. A., Arregale, J.-L., & Campbell, J. T. 2010. The dynamic interplay of capability strengths and weaknesses: Investigating the bases of temporary competitive advantage. *Strategic Management Journal,* 31(13): 1386–1409.

54. Deephouse, D. L. 1999. To be different, or to be the same? It's a question (and theory) of strategic balance. *Strategic Management Journal,* 20: 147–166.

55. Yeoh, P. L. & Roth, K. 1999. An empirical analysis of sustained advantage in the U.S. pharmaceutical industry: Impact of firm resources and capabilities. *Strategic Management Journal,* 20: 637–653.

56. Robins, J. A. & Wiersema, M. F. 2000. Strategies for unstructured competitive environments: Using scarce resources to create new markets. In Bresser, R. F., et al., (Eds.). *Winning strategies in a deconstructing world:* 201–220. New York: John Wiley.

57. For an insightful case on how Dell was able to build its seemingly sustainable competitive advantage in the marketplace, refer to: Rivkin, J. W. & Porter, M. E. 1999. Matching Dell. Harvard Business School Case 9-799-158 June 6.

58. Byrnes, N. & Burrows, P. 2007. Where Dell went wrong. *BusinessWeek,* February 18: 62–63; and, Smith, A. D. 2007. Dell's moves create buzz. *Dallas Morning News.* February 21: D1.

59. For an insightful perspective on how HP has increased its market share and profitability in the personal computer market, refer to: Edwards, C. 2008. How HP got the wow! back. *BusinessWeek,* December 22: 60–61. HP surpassed Dell in Fall 2006 to become the world's largest PC manufacturer, and it increased its market share from 14.5 percent to 18.8 percent between June 2005 and September 2008.

60. Sidhu, I. 2010. *Doing both:* 61. Upper Saddle River, NJ: FT Press.

61. Amit, R. & Schoemaker, J. H. 1993. Strategic assets and organizational rent. *Strategic Management Journal,* 14(1): 33–46; Collis, D. J. & Montgomery, C. A. 1995. Competing on resources: Strategy in the 1990s. *Harvard Business Review,* 73(4): 118–128; Coff, R. W. 1999. When competitive advantage doesn't lead to performance: The resource-based view and stakeholder bargaining power. *Organization Science,* 10(2): 119–133; and, Blyler, M. & Coff, R. W. 2003. Dynamic capabilities, social capital, and rent appropriation: Ties that split pies. *Strategic Management Journal,* 24: 677–686.

62. Munk, N. 1998. The new organization man. *Fortune,* March 16: 62–74.

63. Coff, 1999, op. cit.

64. Lavelle, L. 2003. Sprint's board needs a good sweeping, too. *BusinessWeek,* February 24: 40; Anonymous. 2003. Another nail in the

coffin. *The Economist,* February 15: 69–70; and, Byrnes, N., Dwyer, P., & McNamee, M. 2003. Hacking away at tax shelters, *BusinessWeek,* February 24: 41.

65. We have focused our discussion on how internal stakeholders (e.g., employees, managers, and top executives) may appropriate a firm's profits (or rents). For an interesting discussion of how a firm's innovations may be appropriated by external stakeholders (e.g., customers, suppliers) as well as competitors, refer to: Grant, R. M. 2002. *Contemporary strategy analysis* (4th ed.): 335–340. Malden, MA: Blackwell.

66. Luehrman, T. A. 1997. What's it worth? A general manager's guide to valuation. *Harvard Business Review,* 45(3): 132–142.

67. See, for example, Kaplan, R. S. & Norton, D. P. 1992. The balanced scorecard: Measures that drive performance. *Harvard Business Review,* 69(1): 71–79.

68. Hitt, M. A., Ireland, R. D., & Stadter, G. 1982. Functional importance of company performance: Moderating effects of grand strategy and industry type. *Strategic Management Journal,* 3: 315–330.

69. finance.yahoo.com.

70. Kaplan & Norton, op. cit.

71. Ibid.

72. For a discussion of the relative value of growth versus increasing margins, read: Mass, N. J. 2005. The relative value of growth. *Harvard Business Review,* 83(4): 102–112.

73. Rucci, A. J., Kirn, S. P., & Quinn, R. T. 1998. The employee-customer-profit chain at Sears. *Harvard Business Review,* 76(1): 82–97.

74. Our discussion draws upon: Angel, R. & Rampersad, H. 2005. Do scorecards add up? camagazine.com. May: np.; and, Niven, P. 2002. *Balanced scorecard step by step: Maximizing performance and maintaining results.* New York: John Wiley & Sons.

APPENDIX TO CHAPTER 3

How the Internet and Digital Technologies Add Value

> **>LO3.8**
> How firms are using Internet technologies to add value and achieve unique advantages. (Appendix)

The Internet has changed the way business is conducted. By providing new ways to interact with customers and using digital technologies to streamline operations, the Internet is helping companies create new value propositions. Let's take a look at several ways these changes have added new value. Exhibit 3A.1 illustrates four related activities that are being revolutionized by the Internet—search, evaluation, problem solving, and transactions.[1]

Search Activities

Search refers to the process of gathering information and identifying purchase options. Through **search activities,** the Internet has enhanced both the speed of information gathering and the breadth of information that can be accessed. This enhanced search capability is one of the key reasons the Internet has lowered switching costs—by decreasing the cost of search. These efficiency gains have greatly benefited buyers. Suppliers also have benefited. Small suppliers that had difficulty getting noticed can be found more easily, and large suppliers can publish thousands of pages of information for a fraction of the cost that hard-copy catalogs once required. Additionally, online search engines such as Google, Yahoo, and Bing have accelerated the search process to incredible speeds.

search activities a way that digital technologies and the Internet have added value to firms' operations by enhancing the gathering of information and identifying purchase options.

Evaluation Activities

Evaluation refers to the process of considering alternatives and comparing the costs and benefits of various options. Online services that facilitate comparative shopping, provide product reviews, and catalog customer evaluations of performance have made the Internet's **evaluation activities** a valuable resource.[2] For example, BizRate.com offers extensive product ratings that can help evaluate products. Sites such as CNET that provide comparative pricing have helped lower prices even for quality products that have traditionally maintained premium prices. Opinion-based sites such as ePinions.com and PlanetFeedback.com provide reports of consumer experiences with various vendors.

evaluation activities a way that digital technologies and the Internet have added value to firms' operations by facilitating the comparison of the costs and benefits of various options.

---

[1] The ideas in this section draw on several sources, including : Zeng, M. & Reinartz, W. 2003. Beyond online search: The road to profitability. *California Management Review,* Winter: 107–130; and, Stabell, C. B. & Fjeldstad, O. D. 1998. Configuring value for competitive advantage: On chains, shops, and networks. *Strategic Management Journal,* 19: 413–437.

[2] For an interesting discussion of how successful Internet-based companies are using evaluation to add value see Weiss, L. M., Capozzi, M. M., & Prusak, L. 2004. Learning from the Internet giants. *Sloan Management Review,* 45(4): 79–84.

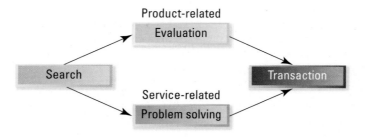

Exhibit 3A.1 Internet Activities that Add Value

Sources: Adapted from Zeng, M. & Reinartz, W. 2003. Beyond online search: The road to profitability. *California Management Review.* Winter: 107–130; and, Stabell, C. B. & Fjeldstad, O. D. 1998. Configuring value for competitive advantage: On chains, shops, and networks. *Strategic Management Journal,* 19: 413–437.

Many Internet businesses, according to digital business experts Ming Zeng and Werner Reinartz, could improve their performance by making a stronger effort to help buyers evaluate purchases.[3] Even so, only certain types of products can be evaluated online. Products such as CDs that appeal primarily to the sense of sound sell well on the Internet. But products that appeal to multiple senses are harder to evaluate online. This explains why products such as furniture and fashion have never been strong online sellers. It's one thing to look at a leather sofa, but to be able to sit on it, touch, and smell the leather online are impossible.

Problem-Solving Activities

Problem solving refers to the process of identifying problems or needs and generating ideas and action plans to address those needs. Whereas evaluation activities are primarily product-related, **problem solving activities** are typically used in the context of services. Customers usually have unique problems that are handled one at a time. For example, online travel services such as Travelocity help customers select from many options to form a unique travel package. Furthermore, problem solving often involves providing answers immediately (compared to the creation of a new product). Firms in industries such as medicine, law, and engineering are using the Internet and digital technologies to deliver many new solutions.

Many products involve both a service and a product component; therefore, both problem solving and evaluation may be needed. Dell Computer's website is an example of a site that has combined the benefits of both. By creating a website that allows for customization of individual computers, it addresses the unique concerns of customers "one computer at a time." But the site also features a strong evaluative component because it allows users to compare the costs and features of various options. Shoppers can even compare their customized selection to refurbished Dell computers that are available at a substantially lower cost.

> **problem-solving activities** a way that digital technologies and the Internet have added value to firms' operations by identifying problems or needs and generating ideas and action plans to address those needs.

Transaction Activities

Transaction refers to the process of completing the sale, including negotiating and agreeing contractually, making payments, and taking delivery. Numerous types of Internet-enabled **transaction activities** have contributed to lowering this aspect of overall transaction costs. Auctions of various sorts, from raw materials used in manufacturing to collectibles sold on eBay, facilitate the process of arriving at mutually agreed-on prices. Services such as PayPal provide a third-party intermediary that facilitates transactions between parties who never have (and probably never will) meet. Amazon.com's One-Click technology allows for very rapid purchases, and Amazon's overall superiority in managing order fulfillment has made its transactions process rapid and reliable. Amazon's success today can be attributed to a large extent to its having sold this transaction capability to other companies such as Target and Toys "R" Us.[4]

> **transaction activities** a way that digital technologies and the Internet have added value to firms' operations by completing sales efficiently, including negotiating and agreeing contractually, making payments, and taking delivery.

[3] Zeng & Reinartz, op. cit.

[4] Bayers, C. 2002. The last laugh. *Business 2.0,* September: 86–93.

Other Sources of Competitive Advantage

There are other factors that can be important sources of competitive advantage. One of the most important of these is content. The Internet makes it possible to capture vast amounts of content at a very low cost. Three types of content can improve the value proposition of a website—customer feedback, expertise, and entertainment programming.

- *Customer Feedback.* Buyers often trust what other buyers say more than a company's promises. One type of content that can enhance a website is customer testimonials. Remember the leather sofa online? The testimonials of other buyers can build confidence and add to the chances that the purchaser will buy online sight unseen. This is one way that content can be a source of competitive advantage. Being able to interact with like-minded customers by reading their experiences or hearing how they have responded to a new product offering builds a sense of belonging that is otherwise hard to create.

- *Expertise.* The Internet has emerged as a tremendously important learning tool. Fifty-one percent of users compare the Internet to a library.[5] The prime reason many users go to the web is to gain expertise. Websites that provide new knowledge or unbiased information are highly valuable. Additionally the problem-solving function often involves educating consumers regarding options and implications of various choices. For example, LendingTree.com, the online loan company, provides a help center that includes extensive information and resources about obtaining loans, maintaining good credit, and so forth. Further, the expertise function is not limited to consumer sites. In the case of B2B businesses, websites that facilitate sharing expert knowledge help build a sense of community in industry or professional groups.

- *Entertainment Programming.* The Internet is being used by more and more people as an entertainment medium. With technologies such as streaming media, which allows the Internet to send televisionlike images and sound, computers can provide everything from breaking news to video games to online movies. A study by the Pew Internet and American Life Project indicates that among people using high-speed broadband service, TV viewing is down and online activity has increased. One reason is that the technology is interactive, which means that viewers don't just passively watch, but they use the web to create art or play online games. Businesses have noticed this trend, of course, and are creating web content that is not just informative but entertaining.

These three types of content—customer feedback, expertise, and entertainment programming—are potential sources of competitive advantage. That is, they create advantages by making the value creation process even stronger. Or, if they are handled poorly, they diminish performance.

Business Models

The Internet provides a unique platform or staging area for business activity, which has become, in some ways, like a new marketplace. How do firms conduct business in this new arena? One way of addressing this question is by describing various Internet business models. A **business model** is a method and a set of assumptions that explain how a business creates value and earns profits in a competitive environment. Some of these models are quite simple and traditional even when applied in an Internet context. Others have features that are unique to the digitally networked, online environment. In this section, we discuss seven Internet business models that account for the vast majority of business conducted online.[6]

> **business model** a method and a set of assumptions that explain how a business creates value and earns profits in a competitive environment.

- *Commission-Based Models* are used by businesses that provide services for a fee. The business is usually a third-party intermediary, and the commission charged is often based on the size of the transaction. The most common type is a brokerage service, such as a stockbroker (e.g., Schwab.com), real estate broker (e.g., Remax.com), or transaction broker (e.g., PayPal .com). This category also includes auction companies such as eBay. In exchange for putting buyers and sellers together, eBay earns a commission.

- *Advertising-Based Models* are used by companies that provide content and/or services to visitors and sell advertising to businesses that want to reach those visitors. It is similar to the

[5] Greenspan, R. 2003. Internet not for everyone. *www.cyberatlas.com.* April 16.
[6] Afuah, A. & Tucci, C.L. 2003. *Internet Business Models and Strategies* (2nd ed). New York: McGraw-Hill; and, Timmers, P. 1999. *Electronic Commerce.* New York: Wiley.

broadcast television model, in which viewers watch shows produced with advertising dollars. A key difference is that online visitors can interact with both the ads and the content. Large portals such as Yahoo.com are in this category as well as specialty portals such as iNest.com, which provides services for buyers of newly constructed homes. Epinions.com, a recommender system, is just one example of the many types of content that are often available.

- *Markup-Based Models* are used by businesses that add value in marketing and sales (rather than production) by acquiring products, marking up the price, and reselling them at a profit. Also known as the merchant model, it applies to both wholesalers and retailers. Amazon.com is the best-known example in this category. It also includes bricks-and-mortar companies such as Walmart, which has a very successful online operation, and vendors whose products are purely digital such as Fonts.com, which sells downloadable fonts and photographs.

- *Production-Based Models* are used by companies that add value in the production process by converting raw materials into value-added products. Thus, it is also referred to as the manufacturing model. The Internet adds value to this model in two key ways. First, it lowers marketing costs by enabling direct contact with end users. Second, such direct contact facilitates customization and problem solving. Dell's online ordering system is supported by a state-of-the-art customized manufacturing process. Travelocity uses its rich database of travel options and customer profiles to identify, produce, and deliver unique solutions.

- *Referral-Based Models* are used by firms that steer customers to another company for a fee. One type is the affiliate model, in which a vendor pays an affiliate a fee each time a visitor clicks through the affiliate's website and makes a purchase from the vendor. Many name-brand companies use affiliate programs. For example, WeddingChannel.com, which provides a bridal registry where wedding guests can buy gifts from companies such as Tiffany's, Macy's, or Crate & Barrel, receives a fee each time a sale is made through its website. Another referral-based example is Yesmail.com, which generates leads using e-mail marketing.

- *Subscription-Based Models* are used by businesses that charge a flat fee for providing either a service or proprietary content. Internet service providers are one example of this model. Companies such as America Online and Earthlink supply Internet connections for fees that are charged whether buyers use the service or not. Subscription-based models are also used by content creators such as *The Economist* or *The New York Times*. Although these recognizable brands often provide free content, only a small portion is available free. *The Economist,* for example, advertises that 70 percent of its content is available only to subscribers.

- *Fee-for-Service–Based Models* are used by companies that provide ongoing services similar to a utility company. Unlike the commission-based model, the fee-for-service model involves a pay-as-you-go system. That is, activities are metered and companies pay only for the amount of service used. Application service providers fall in this category. For example, eProject.com provides virtual work space where people in different physical locations can collaborate online. Users essentially rent Internet space, and a host of tools that make it easy to interact, for a fee based on their usage.

Exhibit 3A.2 summarizes the key feature of each Internet business model, suggests what role content may play in the model, and addresses how the four value-adding activities—search, evaluation, problem solving, and transaction—can be sources of competitive advantage.

Type	Features and Content	Sources of Competitive Advantage
Commission-Based	Charges commissions for brokerage or intermediary services. Adds value by providing expertise and/or access to a wide network of alternatives.	Search Evaluation Problem solving Transaction
Advertising-Based	Web content paid for by advertisers. Adds value by providing free or low-cost content—including customer feedback, expertise, and entertainment programming—to audiences that range from very broad (general content) to highly targeted (specialized content).	Search Evaluation
Markup-Based	Resells marked-up merchandise. Adds value through selection, through distribution efficiencies, and by leveraging brand image and reputation. May use entertainment programming to enhance sales.	Search Transaction
Production-Based	Sells manufactured goods and custom services. Adds value by increasing production efficiencies, capturing customer preferences, and improving customer service.	Search Problem solving
Referral-Based	Charges fees for referring customers. Adds value by enhancing a company's product or service offering, tracking referrals electronically, and generating demographic data. Expertise and customer feedback often included with referral information.	Search Problem solving Transaction
Subscription-Based	Charges fees for unlimited use of service or content. Adds value by leveraging strong brand name, providing high-quality information to specialized markets, or providing access to essential services. May consist entirely of entertainment programming.	Evaluation Problem solving
Fee-for-Service–Based	Charges fees for metered services. Adds value by providing service efficiencies, expertise, and practical outsourcing solutions.	Problem solving Transaction

Sources: Afuah, A. & Tucci, C. L. 2003. *Internet Business Models and Strategies* (2nd ed). New York: McGraw-Hill; Rappa, M. 2005. Business Models on the Web. *digitalenterprise.org/models/models.html*; and, Timmers, P. 1999. *Electronic Commerce*. New York: Wiley.

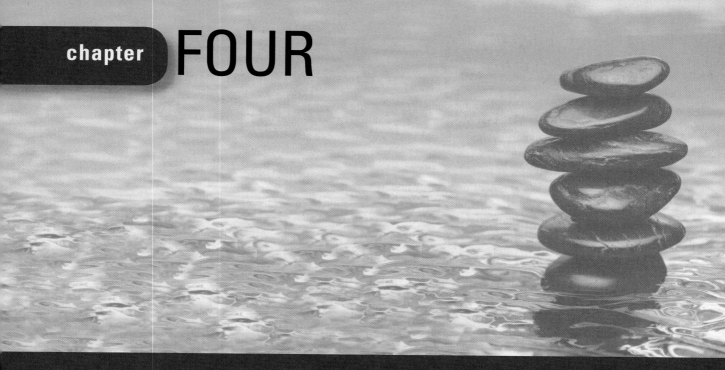

chapter FOUR

Recognizing a Firm's Intellectual Assets:

Moving Beyond a Firm's Tangible Resources

After reading this chapter, you should have a good understanding of:

LO4.1   Why the management of knowledge professionals and knowledge itself are so critical in today's organizations.

LO4.2   The importance of recognizing the interdependence of attracting, developing, and retaining human capital.

LO4.3   The key role of social capital in leveraging human capital within and across the firm.

LO4.4   The importance of social networks in knowledge management and in promoting career success.

LO4.5   The vital role of technology in leveraging knowledge and human capital.

LO4.6   Why "electronic" or "virtual" teams are critical in combining and leveraging knowledge in organizations and how they can be made more effective.

LO4.7   The challenge of protecting intellectual property and the importance of a firm's dynamic capabilities.

LEARNING OBJECTIVES

One of the most important trends that managers must consider is the significance of the knowledge worker in today's economy. Managers must both recognize the importance of top talent and provide mechanisms to leverage human capital to innovate and, in the end, develop products and services that create value.

The first section addresses the increasing role of knowledge as the primary means of wealth generation in today's economy. A company's value is not derived solely from its physical assets, such as plant, equipment, and machinery. Rather, it is based on knowledge, know-how, and intellectual assets—all embedded in people.

The second section discusses the key resource itself, human capital, which is the foundation of intellectual capital. We explore ways in which the organization can attract, develop, and retain top talent—three important, interdependent activities. With regard to attracting human capital, we address issues such as "hiring for attitude, training for skill." One of the issues regarding developing human capital is encouraging widespread involvement throughout the organization. Our discussion on retaining human capital addresses issues such as the importance of having employees identify with an organization's mission and values. We also address the value of a diverse workforce.

The attraction, development, and retention of human capital are necessary but not sufficient conditions for organizational success. In the third section we address social capital—networks of relationships among a firm's members. This is especially important where collaboration and sharing information are critical. We address why social capital can be particularly important in attracting human capital and making teams effective. We also address the vital role of social networks—both in improving knowledge management and in promoting career success.

The fourth section addresses the role of technology in leveraging human capital. Examples range from e-mail and the use of networks to facilitate collaboration among individuals to more complex forms of technologies, such as sophisticated knowledge management systems. We discuss how electronic teams can be effectively managed. We also address how technology can help to retain knowledge.

The last section discusses the differences between protection of physical property and intellectual property. We suggest that the development of dynamic capabilities may be one of the best ways that a firm can protect its intellectual property.

Learning from Mistakes

Hitachi Ltd., a Japanese multinational corporation, is the world's third largest tech firm.[1] Its first president, Namihei Odaira, believed that "inventions are an engineer's lifeblood," and, not surprisingly, he focused on the company's inventions from the very beginning. He demanded that his tech people apply their engineering skills toward generating inventions and patents. This, he felt, could be the key to value creation and competitive advantage. Sounds good . . . but what problems arose?

In 1970 alone, Hitachi filed 20,000 patent applications. Unfortunately, the emphasis was on the sheer number rather than the quality of each patent. At that time, the company earned a mere $5 million in licensing income but paid out $95 million in licensing fees.

In 1979, Hitachi faced major patent litigation. Westinghouse charged Hitachi, a Hitachi-GE joint venture, and a few other companies with patent infringement and petitioned the U.S. International Trade Commission to block the import of circuit breakers from Japan. By then, Hitachi already had several dozen U.S. patents for electrical power transmission equipment. However, it found that they were all patents for features distinctive to Hitachi products and were not the type that other companies could use. Thus, there were no grounds for countersuing Westinghouse for patent infringement.

Hitachi's second big patent problem occurred in 1986. Texas Instruments sued a total of nine Japanese and Korean semiconductor manufacturers in the U.S. International Trade Commission and Texas courts, arguing that its licensing fee was too low and that it could not renew Hitachi's contract at the terms proposed. It demanded to set the licensing fee for DRAM manufacturing technology at 10 percent of sales.

These were bitter lessons for Hitachi. It initiated four campaigns to double its number of "strategic patents" in 1981, 1985, 1990, and 1995, respectively. The goal was to focus its resources on patents that would create the most value for the firm as well as to gain global patent coverage for the company's world-class products and technologies.

Patents can be very valuable. However, a company must effectively use them to create value. Hitachi realized that there was no point in obtaining a mountain of patents if they were not going to help the company compete in the competitive marketplace.

Managers are always looking for stellar professionals who can take their organizations to the next level. However, attracting talent is a necessary but *not* sufficient condition for success. In today's knowledge economy, it does not matter how big your stock of resources is—whether it be top talent, physical resources, or financial capital. Rather, the question becomes: How good is the organization at attracting top talent and leveraging that talent to produce a stream of products and services valued by the marketplace?

We also address issues associated with intellectual property (IP) and its potential to create value for the firm. The Hitachi example shows how heavy investment in IP alone is insufficient for value creation in the competitive marketplace.

>LO4.1

Why the management of knowledge professionals and knowledge itself are so critical in today's organizations.

The Central Role of Knowledge in Today's Economy

Central to our discussion is an enormous change that has accelerated over the past few decades and its implications for the strategic management of organizations.[2] For most of the 20th century, managers focused on tangible resources such as land, equipment, and money as well as intangibles such as brands, image, and customer loyalty. Efforts were directed more toward the efficient allocation of labor and capital—the two traditional factors of production.

How times have changed. Today, more than 50 percent of the gross domestic product (GDP) in developed economies is knowledge-based; it is based on intellectual assets and intangible people skills.[3] In the U.S., intellectual and information processes create most of the value for firms in large service industries (e.g., software, medical care, communications, and education), which make up 77 percent of the U.S. GDP. In the manufacturing sector, intellectual activities like R&D, process design, product design, logistics, marketing, and technological innovation produce the preponderance of value added.[4]

Taiwan is a good example of an emerging knowledge economy. According to the Global Competitiveness Report 2011–2012 of the World Economic Forum, Taiwan ranks thirteenth (out of 142 economies) on the Growth Competitiveness Index (GCI). The country ranks ninth in the world in innovation. Interestingly enough, according to the report, Taiwan holds more U.S. patents per capita than the United States. Taiwan's capacity for innovation is further supported by its excellent educational system, with the country ranking tenth in higher education and training. These statistics illustrate how promoting education and technological development have successfully fostered innovation and established a knowledge-oriented nation.[5]

To drive home the point, Gary Hamel and the late C. K. Prahalad, two leading writers in strategic management, state:

> The machine age was a physical world. It consisted of things. Companies made and distributed things (physical products). Management allocated things (capital budgets); management invested in things (plant and equipment).
>
> In the machine age, people were ancillary, and things were central. In the information age, things are ancillary, knowledge is central. A company's value derives not from things, but from knowledge, know-how, intellectual assets, competencies—all embedded in people.[6]

In the **knowledge economy,** wealth is increasingly created by effective management of knowledge workers instead of by the efficient control of physical and financial assets. The growing importance of knowledge, coupled with the move by labor markets to reward knowledge work, tells us that investing in a company is, in essence, buying a set of talents, capabilities, skills, and ideas—intellectual capital—not physical and financial resources.[7]

Let's provide a few examples. People don't buy Microsoft's stock because of its software factories; it doesn't own any. Rather, the value of Microsoft is bid up because it sets standards for personal-computing software, exploits the value of its name, and forges alliances with other companies. Similarly, Merck didn't become the "Most Admired" company, for seven consecutive years in *Fortune*'s annual survey, because it can manufacture pills, but because its scientists can discover medicines. P. Roy Vagelos, who was CEO of Merck, the $44 billion pharmaceutical giant, during its long run atop the "Most Admired" survey, said, "A low-value product can be made by anyone anywhere. When you have knowledge no one else has access to—that's dynamite. We guard our research even more carefully than our financial assets."[8]

To apply some numbers to our arguments, let's ask, What's a company worth?[9] Start with the "big three" financial statements: income statement, balance sheet, and statement of cash flow. If these statements tell a story that investors find useful, then a company's market value* should roughly (but not precisely, because the market looks forward and the books look backward) be the same as the value that accountants ascribe to it—the book value of the firm. However, this is not the case. A study compared the market value with

knowledge economy an economy where wealth is created through the effective management of knowledge workers instead of by the efficient control of physical and financial assets.

---

*The market value of a firm is equal to the value of a share of its common stock times the number of shares outstanding. The book value of a firm is primarily a measure of the value of its tangible assets. It can be calculated by the formula: Total assets − Total liabilities.

the book value of 3,500 U.S. companies over a period of two decades. In 1978 the two were similar: Book value was 95 percent of market value. However, market values and book values have diverged significantly. Within 20 years, the S&P industrials were—on average—trading at 2.2 times book value.[10] Robert A. Howell, an expert on the changing role of finance and accounting, muses that "The big three financial statements . . . are about as useful as an 80-year-old Los Angeles road map."

The gap between a firm's market value and book value is far greater for knowledge-intensive corporations than for firms with strategies based primarily on tangible assets.[11] Exhibit 4.1 shows the ratio of market-to-book value for some well-known companies. In firms where knowledge and the management of knowledge workers are relatively important contributors to developing products and services—and physical resources are less critical—the ratio of market-to-book value tends to be much higher.

As shown in Exhibit 4.1, firms such as Apple, Google, Microsoft, and Oracle have very high market value to book value ratios because of their high investment in knowledge resources and technological expertise. In contrast, firms in more traditional industry sectors such as Bayer, Toyota, and BMW have relatively low market-to-book ratios. This reflects their greater investments in physical resources and lower investment in knowledge resources. A firm like Intel has a market-to-book value ratio that falls between the above two groups of firms. This is because its high level of investment in knowledge resources is matched by a correspondingly huge investment in plant and equipment. For example, in 2007, Intel invested $3 billion to build a fabrication facility in Chandler, Arizona.[12]

Many writers have defined **intellectual capital** as the difference between a firm's market value and book value—that is, a measure of the value of a firm's intangible assets.[13] This broad definition includes assets such as reputation, employee loyalty and commitment, customer relationships, company values, brand names, and the experience and skills of employees.[14] Thus, simplifying, we have:

Intellectual capital = Market value of firm − Book value of the firm

How do companies create value in the knowledge-intensive economy? The general answer is to attract and leverage human capital effectively through mechanisms that create products and services of value over time.

intellectual capital the difference between the market value of the firm and the book value of the firm, including assets such as reputation, employee loyalty and commitment, customer relationships, company values, brand names, and the experience and skills of employees.

Exhibit 4.1 Ratio of Market Value to Book Value for Selected Companies

Company	Annual Sales ($ billions)	Market Value ($ billions)	Book Value ($ billions)	Ratio of Market-to-Book Value
Apple	65.2	314.6	47.8	6.6
Google	20.9	196.4	36.0	5.4
Microsoft	65.8	241.3	46.2	5.2
Oracle	32.0	157.0	30.8	5.1
Intel	42.7	116.1	41.7	2.8
LVMH	10.9	56.0	19.8	2.8
Bayer	18.0	45.3	26.0	1.7
Toyota Motor	28.7	222.0	133.7	1.6
BMW	7.9	37.2	25.5	1.4

Note: The data on market valuations are as of January 11, 2011. All other financial data are based on the most recently available balance sheets and income statements.

Source: *www.finance.yahoo.com*.

First, **human capital** is the "*individual* capabilities, knowledge, skills, and experience of the company's employees and managers."[15] This knowledge is relevant to the task at hand, as well as the capacity to add to this reservoir of knowledge, skills, and experience through learning.[16]

Second, **social capital** is "the network of relationships that individuals have throughout the organization." Relationships are critical in sharing and leveraging knowledge and in acquiring resources.[17] Social capital can extend beyond the organizational boundaries to include relationships between the firm and its suppliers, customers, and alliance partners.[18]

Third is the concept of "knowledge," which comes in two different forms. First, there is **explicit knowledge** that is codified, documented, easily reproduced, and widely distributed, such as engineering drawings, software code, and patents.[19] The other type of knowledge is **tacit knowledge.** That is in the minds of employees and is based on their experiences and backgrounds.[20] Tacit knowledge is shared only with the consent and participation of the indivivdual.

New knowledge is constantly created through the continual interaction of explicit and tacit knowledge. Consider two software engineers working together on a computer code. The computer code is the explicit knowledge. By sharing ideas based on each individual's experience—that is, their tacit knowledge—they create new knowledge when they modify the code. Another important issue is the role of "socially complex processes," which include leadership, culture, and trust.[21] These processes play a central role in the creation of knowledge.[22] They represent the "glue" that holds the organization together and helps to create a working environment where individuals are more willing to share their ideas, work in teams, and, in the end, create products and services of value.[23]

Numerous books have been written on the subject of knowledge management and the central role that it has played in creating wealth in organizations and countries throughout the developed world.[24] Here, we focus on some of the key issues that organizations must address to compete through knowledge.

We will now turn our discussion to the central resource itself—human capital—and some guidelines on how it can be attracted/selected, developed, and retained.[25] Tom Stewart, editor of the *Harvard Business Review,* noted that organizations must also undergo significant efforts to protect their human capital. A firm may "diversify the ownership of vital knowledge by emphasizing teamwork, guard against obsolescence by developing learning programs, and shackle key people with golden handcuffs."[26] In addition, people are less likely to leave an organization if there are effective structures to promote teamwork and information sharing, strong leadership that encourages innovation, and cultures that demand excellence and ethical behavior. Such issues are central to this chapter. Although we touch on these issues throughout this chapter, we provide more detail in later chapters. We discuss organizational controls (culture, rewards, and boundaries) in Chapter 9, organization structure and design in Chapter 10, and a variety of leadership and entrepreneurship topics in Chapters 11 and 12.

human capital
the individual capabilities, knowledge, skills, and experience of a company's employees and managers.

social capital
the network of friendships and working relationships between talented people both inside and outside the organization.

explicit knowledge
knowledge that is codified, documented, easily reproduced, and widely distributed.

tacit knowledge
knowledge that is in the minds of employees and is based on their experiences and backgrounds.

Human Capital: The Foundation of Intellectual Capital

Organizations must recruit talented people—employees at all levels with the proper sets of skills and capabilities coupled with the right values and attitudes. Such skills and attitudes must be continually developed, strengthened, and reinforced, and each employee must be motivated and her efforts focused on the organization's goals and objectives.[27]

The rise to prominence of knowledge workers as a vital source of competitive advantage is changing the balance of power in today's organization.[28] Knowledge workers place professional development and personal enrichment (financial and otherwise) above company loyalty. Attracting, recruiting, and hiring the "best and the brightest" is a critical first

>LO4.2

The importance of recognizing the interdependence of attracting, developing, and retaining human capital.

step in the process of building intellectual capital. At a symposium for CEOs, Bill Gates said, "The thing that is holding Microsoft back . . . is simply how [hard] we find it to go out and recruit the kind of people we want to grow our research team."[29]

Hiring is only the first of three processes in which all successful organizations must engage to build and leverage their human capital. Firms must also *develop* employees to fulfill their full potential to maximize their joint contributions.[30] Finally, the first two processes are for naught if firms can't provide the working environment and intrinsic and extrinsic rewards to *retain* their best and brightest.[31]

These activities are highly interrelated. We would like to suggest the imagery of a three-legged stool (see Exhibit 4.2).[32] If one leg is weak or broken, the stool collapses.

To illustrate such interdependence, poor hiring impedes the effectiveness of development and retention processes. In a similar vein, ineffective retention efforts place additional burdens on hiring and development. Consider the following anecdote, provided by Jeffrey Pfeffer of the Stanford University Business School:

> Not long ago, I went to a large, fancy San Francisco law firm—where they treat their associates like dog doo and where the turnover is very high. I asked the managing partner about the turnover rate. He said, "A few years ago, it was 25 percent, and now we're up to 30 percent." I asked him how the firm had responded to that trend. He said, "We increased our recruiting." So I asked him, "What kind of doctor would you be if your patient was bleeding faster and faster, and your only response was to increase the speed of the transfusion?"[33]

Clearly, stepped-up recruiting is a poor substitute for weak retention.[34] Although there are no simple, easy-to-apply answers, we can learn from what leading-edge firms are doing to attract, develop, and retain human capital in today's highly competitive marketplace.[35] Before moving on, Strategy Spotlight 4.1 addresses the importance of a firm's "green" or environmental sustainability strategy in attracting young talent.

Attracting Human Capital

All we can do is bet on the people we pick. So my whole job is picking the right people.

Jack Welch, former chairman, General Electric Company[36]

The first step in the process of building superior human capital is input control: attracting and selecting the right person.[37] Human resource professionals often approach employee

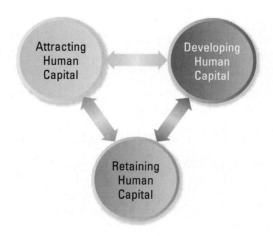

Exhibit 4.2 Human Capital: Three Interdependent Activities

Going "Green" Helps Attract Talent

When companies go "green," they often find that the benefits extend beyond the environment. Eco-friendly strategies can also help attract young talent and reduce costs. According to Lindsey Pollack, author of *Getting from College to Career:*

> Students are looking to work for companies that care about the environment. They are almost expecting greenness like they expect work–life balance, ethnic diversity, and globalization.

A recent poll on green employment by MonsterTRAK. com, a job website geared toward students and entry-level hires, found that 80 percent of young professionals are interested in securing a job that has a positive impact on the environment, and 92 percent would be more inclined to work for a company that is environmentally friendly. And, in another survey, 68 percent of Millennials said they would refuse to work for an employer that is not socially responsible.

In response, paper maker NewPage Corp. distributes a brochure that highlights the firm's commitment to environmental responsibility when it recruits on campuses. It showcases the company's new corporate headquarters, in Miamisburg, Ohio, that uses 28 percent to 39 percent less energy than a standard office building and is furnished with environmentally friendly materials. Said NewPage CEO Mark Sunwyn, "At the end of the day, we are competing with everyone else for the best talent, and this is a generation that is very concerned with the environment."

To meet the growing demand for students interested in working for green companies, MonsterTRAK, a unit of the giant employment firm Monster.com, launched GreenCareers. It was the first online recruitment service that focuses on green employment. EcoAmerica and the Environmental Defense Fund, two environmental non-profits, are adding their expertise in partnership with MonsterTRAK. "EcoAmerica approached MonsterTRAK to create GreenCareers because there is an urgent need to reach and educate environmentally 'agnostic' audiences, in this case college students, about the ways they can address climate change and other serious environmental problems," claimed Mark Charnock, vice president and general manager at MonsterTRAK.

Sources: Luhby, T. 2008. How to lure Gen Y workers? *CNNMoney.com.* August 17: np; Mattioli. 2007. How going green draws talent, cut costs. *The Wall Street Journal,* November 13: B10; and, Odell, A. M. 2007. Working for the Earth: Green companies and green jobs attract employees. *www .socialfunds.com,* October 9: np.

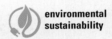 **environmental sustainability**

---

selection from a "lock and key" mentality—that is, fit a key (a job candidate) into a lock (the job). Such an approach involves a thorough analysis of the person and the job. Only then can the right decision be made as to how well the two will fit together. How can you fail, the theory goes, if you get a precise match of knowledge, ability, and skill profiles? Frequently, however, the precise matching approach places its emphasis on task-specific skills (e.g., motor skills, specific information processing capabilities, and communication skills) and puts less emphasis on the broad general knowledge and experience, social skills, values, beliefs, and attitudes of employees.[38]

Many have questioned the precise matching approach. They argue that firms can identify top performers by focusing on key employee mind-sets, attitudes, social skills, and general orientations. If they get these elements right, the task-specific skills can be learned quickly. (This does not imply, however, that task-specific skills are unimportant; rather, it suggests that the requisite skill sets must be viewed as a necessary but not sufficient condition.) This leads us to a popular phrase today that serves as the title of the next section.

"Hire for Attitude, Train for Skill" Organizations are increasingly emphasizing general knowledge and experience, social skills, values, beliefs, and attitudes of employees.[39] Consider Finland's Nokia Corp., which transformed itself into the world's largest supplier of high-tech mobile phones well into the last decade, creating along the way an innovative and entrepreneurial culture in the telecommunications sector. To retain an entrepreneurial spirit, Nokia established a set of values and behaviors across all units and embedded them directly into its screening and selection processes. A key component of its hiring strategies was a focus on not only technical skills but also attitudes and behaviors critical to the creative spirit of the company. In other words, when hiring researchers and engineers, Nokia was almost as interested in temperament as it was technical credentials. Its motto: You can teach technology in the company much easier than you can teach interpersonal skills, if at all.[40]

Alan Cooper, president of Cooper Software, Inc., in Palo Alto, California, goes further. He cleverly *uses technology* to hone in on the problem-solving ability of his applicants and their attitudes before an interview even takes place. He has devised a "Bozo Filter," an online test that can be applied to any industry. Before you spend time on whether job candidates will work out satisfactorily, find out how their minds work. Cooper advised, "Hiring was a black hole. I don't talk to bozos anymore, because 90 percent of them turn away when they see our test. It's a self-administering bozo filter."[41] How does it work?

> The online test asks questions designed to see how prospective employees approach problem-solving tasks. For example, one key question asks software engineer applicants to design a table-creation software program for Microsoft Word. Candidates provide pencil sketches and a description of the new user interface. Another question used for design communicators asks them to develop a marketing strategy for a new touch-tone phone—directed at consumers in the year 1850. Candidates e-mail their answers back to the company, and the answers are circulated around the firm to solicit feedback. Only candidates with the highest marks get interviews.

Sound Recruiting Approaches and Networking Companies that take hiring seriously must also take recruiting seriously. The number of jobs that successful knowledge-intensive companies must fill is astonishing. Ironically, many companies still have no shortage of applicants. For example, ICICI Bank, one of India's largest private lenders, ranked ninth in *Business Today's* "2010 Best Companies to Work For," is planning to hire thousands of employees—even though its hiring rate has slowed.[42] The challenge becomes having the right job candidates, not the greatest number of them.

GE Medical Systems, which builds CT scanners and magnetic resonance imaging (MRI) systems, relies extensively on networking. It has found that current employees are the best source for new ones. Recently, Steven Patscot, head of staffing and leadership development, made a few simple changes to double the number of referrals. First, he simplified the process—no complex forms, no bureaucracy, and so on. Second, he increased incentives. Everyone referring a qualified candidate received a gift certificate from Sears. For referrals who were hired, the "bounty" increases to $2,000. Although this may sound like a lot of money, it is "peanuts" compared to the $15,000 to $20,000 fees that GE typically pays to headhunters for each person hired.[43] Also, when someone refers a former colleague or friend for a job, his or her credibility is on the line. Thus, employees will be careful in recommending people for employment unless they are reasonably confident that these people are good candidates. This provides a good "screen" for the firm in deciding whom to hire. Hiring the right people makes things a lot easier: fewer rules and regulations, less need for monitoring and hierarchy, and greater internalization of organizational norms and objectives.

Consider some of the approaches that companies are currently using to recruit and retain young talent. As baby boomers retire, people in this demographic group are becoming more and more important in today's workforce. We also provide some tips on how to get hired. We address these issues in Exhibit 4.3.

Exhibit 4.3
**What Companies Are
Doing to Attract and
Retain Young Talent . . .
and What You Should Do
to Get Hired**

Here are some "best practices" that companies are using to help recruit and retain today's high-maintenance Millennials. This generation has also been termed Generation Y or Echo Boom and includes people born after 1982:

- ***Don't fudge the sales pitch.*** High-tech presentations and one-on-one attention may be attractive to undergrads, but the pitch had better match the experience. Today's ultraconnected students can get the lowdown on a company by spending five minutes on a social networking site.

- ***Let them have a life.*** Wary of their parents' 80-hour workweeks, Millennials strive for more balance, so liberal vacations are a must. They also want assurances they'll be able to use it. At KPMG, 80 percent of employees used 40 hours of paid time off in the six months through May 2006.

- ***No time clocks, please.*** Recent grads don't mind long hours if they can work them on their own time. Lockheed Martin allows employees to work nine-hour days and take every other Friday off.

- ***Give them responsibility.*** A chance to work on fulfilling projects and develop ones of their own is important to Millennials. Google urges entry-level employees to spend 20 percent of their time developing new ideas. PepsiCo allows promising young employees to manage small teams in six months.

- ***Feedback and more feedback.*** Career planning advice and frequent performance appraisals are keys to holding on to young hires. Lehman Brothers provides new hires with two mentors—a slightly older peer to help them get settled and a senior employee to give long-term guidance.

- ***Giving back matters.*** Today's altruistic young graduates expect to have opportunities for community service. Wells Fargo encourages its employees to teach financial literacy classes in the community. Accenture and Bain allow employees to consult for nonprofits.

Some advice on how to get hired (based on Fortune's "100 Best Companies to Work For"):

- **It helps to know someone.** Almost all of the "Best Companies" rely extensively on employee referrals. Principal Financial Group and many others get about 40 percent of new hires this way.

- **Do creative research.** Know more about the place and the industry than your rivals. A Google search is not viewed as a form of "creative research." Said Jay Jones, a recruiting manager for Alcon Laboratories: "Detailed research, including talking to customers, is so rare it will almost guarantee you get hired."

- **Unleash your inner storyteller.** By far the most popular interview style is what's known as behavioral, meaning that you will be asked to describe troublesome situations in past jobs and tell exactly how you handled them.

- **No Lone Rangers need apply.** By and large, team players are wanted. "I actually count the number of times a candidate says 'I' in an interview," said Adobe's recruiting director, Jeff Vijungco. "We'd rather hear 'we.'"

- **Be open to learning new things.** Showing passion is a must, and most of the "100 Best" pride themselves on creating "learning environments." Thus, talk about the skills you'd like to acquire or polish. Declaring that you're already the best at what you do is a turnoff.

Source: Fisher, A. 2008. How to get hired by a "best" company. *Fortune*, February 4: 96; and, Gerdes, L. 2006. The top 50 employers for new college grads. *BusinessWeek*, September 18: 64–81.

Developing Human Capital

It is not enough to hire top-level talent and expect that the skills and capabilities of those employees will remain current throughout the duration of their employment. Rather, training and development must take place at all levels of the organization.[44] For example, Solectron assembles printed circuit boards and other components for its Silicon Valley clients.[45] Its employees receive an average of 95 hours of company-provided training each year. Chairman Winston Chen observed, "Technology changes so fast that we estimate 20 percent of an engineer's knowledge becomes obsolete each year. Training is an obligation we owe to our employees. If you want high growth and high quality, then training is a big part of the equation." Although the financial returns on training may be hard to calculate, most experts believe it is essential. One company that has calculated the benefit from training is Motorola. Every dollar spent on training returns $30 in productivity gains over the following three years.

In addition to training and developing human capital, firms must encourage widespread involvement, monitor and track employee development, and evaluate human capital.[46]

Encouraging Widespread Involvement   Developing human capital requires the active involvement of leaders at all levels. It won't be successful if it is viewed only as the responsibility of the human resources department. Each year at General Electric, 200 facilitators, 30 officers, 30 human resource executives, and many young managers actively participate in GE's orientation program at Crotonville, its training center outside New York City. Topics include global competition, winning on the global playing field, and personal examination of the new employee's core values vis-à-vis GE's values. As a senior manager once commented, "There is nothing like teaching Sunday school to force you to confront your own values."

Similarly, A. G. Lafley, Procter & Gamble's former CEO, claimed that he spent 40 percent of his time on personnel.[47] Andy Grove, who was previously Intel's CEO, required all senior people, including himself, to spend at least a week a year teaching high flyers. And Nitin Paranjpe, CEO of Hindustan Unilever, recruits people from campuses and regularly visits high-potential employees in the company's offices.

Transferring Knowledge   Often in our lives, we need to either transfer our knowledge to someone else (a child, a junior colleague, a peer) or access accumulated bits of wisdom—someone else's tacit knowledge.[48] This is a vital aspect of developing human capital.[49] However, before we can even begin to plan such a transfer, we need to understand how our brains process incoming information. According to Dorothy A. Leonard of Harvard University:

> Our existing tacit knowledge determines how we assimilate new experiences. Without receptors—hooks on which to hang new information—we may not be able to perceive and process the information. It is like being sent boxes of documents but having no idea how they could or should be organized.

This cognitive limitation also applies to the organizational level. When GE Healthcare sets up or transfers operations, it appoints an experienced manager as the "pitcher" and a team in the receiving plant as the "catcher." These two teams work together, often over a period of years—first at the pitcher's location and then at the catcher's. To ensure a smooth transition, the pitching team needs to be sensitive to the catching team's level of experience and familiarity with GE Healthcare procedures.

Strategy Spotlight 4.2 discusses an emerging trend in organizations—reverse mentoring. Here, tech-savvy new hires mentor seasoned executives.

Monitoring Progress and Tracking Development   Whether a firm uses on-site formal training, off-site training (e.g., universities), or on-the-job training, tracking

Reverse Mentoring at Godrej Group in India

Adi Godrej, chairman of Godrej Group, has direct experience with bottom-up feedback, or reverse mentoring. Starting in 2001, Godrej started taking lessons on information technology and sales and marketing from two young managers—Saugata Saha, an area sales manager with Godrej Consumer Products Ltd (GCPL), and Sheetal Shirke, a marketing manager with Godrej Sara Lee. The 20-something managers were chosen as mentors because of their front-line contact with customers, which kept them informed of current best practices. "While I have a lot of experience in marketing and sales over the years, I needed to understand what young people, who are hands-on, find in the market, what they are suggesting and what could be changed," Godrej said.

For two to four hours every month, Saha and Shirke offered Godrej feedback on various issues, from new ideas for existing processes to updates on the latest techniques in marketing, advertising, and market research. Some of the mentors' suggestions soon found a place among the group's best practices. Shirke's update on the latest market research techniques ensured that the group took market research more seriously, while Saha's suggestions on sales-related issues also found a positive response.

For instance, some changes in the Godrej distribution network can be linked to what transpired in the mentoring sessions. Other areas also benefited from the interaction, such as the management training program where employees from all functions are put on a forced job-rotation in sales; each employee has to perform a customer-facing job at some point in order to understand the system better.

Reverse mentoring doesn't preclude traditional mentoring. At the same time, Godrej mentored Saha and Shirke on leadership. "Reverse mentoring is an excellent process because senior managers need to learn certain aspects of business from young managers," Godrej said. "At the same time senior managers can impart a lot of knowledge and inspiration to young managers."

Source: Sangameshwaran, P. 2004. Strategy Speak: Reverse mentoring—when juniors know more than the boss. *www.business-standard.com/india/news/reverse-mentoring-when-juniors-know-more-thanboss/147491/*. March 30.

---

individual progress—and sharing this knowledge with both the employee and key managers—becomes essential. Like many leading-edge firms, GlaxoSmithKline (GSK) places strong emphasis on broader experiences over longer time periods. Dan Phelan, senior vice president and director of human resources, explained, "We ideally follow a two-plus-two-plus-two formula in developing people for top management positions." This reflects the belief that GSK's best people should gain experience in two business units, two functional units (such as finance and marketing), and two countries.

Evaluating Human Capital   In today's competitive environment, collaboration and interdependence are vital to organizational success. Individuals must share their knowledge and work constructively to achieve collective, not just individual, goals. However, traditional systems evaluate performance from a single perspective (i.e., "top down") and generally don't address the "softer" dimensions of communications and social skills, values, beliefs, and attitudes.[50]

To address the limitations of the traditional approach, many organizations use **360-degree evaluation and feedback systems**.[51] Here, superiors, direct reports, colleagues, and even internal and external customers rate a person's performance.[52] Managers rate themselves to have a personal benchmark. The 360-degree feedback system complements teamwork, employee involvement, and organizational flattening. As organizations continue to push responsibility downward, traditional top-down appraisal systems become insufficient.[53] For example, a manager who previously managed the performance of 3 supervisors might now be responsible for 10 and is less likely to have the in-depth knowledge needed to appraise and develop them adequately. Exhibit 4.4 provides a portion of Samsung's vision and key strategic strengths and approaches that are part of the company's overall evaluation system.

360-degree evaluation and feedback systems superiors, direct reports, colleagues, and even external and internal customers rate a person's performance.

- Company vision for the new decade is "Inspire the World, Create the Future."
- Reflects company's commitment to inspiring its communities by leveraging three key strengths: "New Technology," "Innovative Products," and "Creative Solutions."
- Strives to promote new value for Samsung's core networks: Industry, Partners, and Employees.
- Through these efforts, Samsung hopes to contribute to a better world and a richer experience for all.

As part of this vision, Samsung has mapped out a specific plan of reaching US$400 billion in revenue and becoming one of the world's top five brands by 2020. To this end, Samsung has also established three strategic approaches in its management: "Creativity," "Partnership," and "Talent."

Samsung is excited about the future. As we build on our previous accomplishments, we look forward to exploring new territories, including health, medicine, and biotechnology. Samsung is committed to being a creative leader in new markets and becoming a truly No. 1 business going forward.

Source: Samsung Electronics: Corporate profile, accessed at *www.samsung.com/ca/aboutsamsung/corporate profile/vision.html.*

Evaluation systems must also ensure that a manager's success does not come at the cost of compromising the organization's core values. Such behavior generally leads to only short-term wins for both the manager and the organization. The organization typically suffers long-term losses in terms of morale, turnover, productivity, and so on. Accordingly, Merck's former chairman, Ray Gilmartin, told his employees, "If someone is achieving results but not demonstrating the core values of the company, at the expense of our people, that manager does not have much of a career here."

Retaining Human Capital

It has been said that talented employees are like "frogs in a wheelbarrow."[54] They can jump out at any time! By analogy, the organization can either try to force employees to stay in the firm or try to keep them from jumping out by creating incentives.[55] In other words, today's leaders can either provide the work environment and incentives to keep productive employees and management from wanting to bail out, or they can use legal means such as employment contracts and noncompete clauses.[56] Firms must prevent the transfer of valuable and sensitive information outside the organization. Failure to do so would be the neglect of a leader's fiduciary responsibility to shareholders. However, greater efforts should be directed at the former (e.g., good work environment and incentives), but, as we all know, the latter (e.g., employment contracts and noncompete clauses) have their place.[57]

Identifying with an Organization's Mission and Values   People who identify with and are more committed to the core mission and values of the organization are less likely to stray or bolt to the competition. For example, take the perspective of the late Steve Jobs, Apple's widely admired CEO:[58]

> When I hire somebody really senior, competence is the ante. They have to be really smart. But the real issue for me is: Are they going to fall in love with Apple? Because if they fall in love with Apple, everything else will take care of itself. They'll want to do what's best for Apple, not what's best for them, what's best for Steve, or anyone else.

"Tribal loyalty" is another key factor that links people to the organization.[59] A tribe is not the organization as a whole (unless it is very small). Rather, it is teams, communities of practice, and other groups within an organization or occupation.

Brian Hall, CEO of Values Technology in Santa Cruz, California, documented a shift in people's emotional expectations from work. From the 1950s on, a "task first" relationship—"tell me what the job is, and let's get on with it"—dominated employee attitudes. Emotions and personal life were checked at the door. In the past few years, a "relationship-first" set of values has challenged the task orientation. Hall believes that it will become dominant. Employees want to share attitudes and beliefs as well as workspace.

Challenging Work and a Stimulating Environment Arthur Schawlow, winner of the 1981 Nobel Prize in physics, was asked what made the difference between highly creative and less creative scientists. His reply: "The labor of love aspect is very important. The most successful scientists often are not the most talented.[60] But they are the ones impelled by curiosity. They've got to know what the answer is."[61] Such insights highlight the importance of intrinsic motivation: the motivation to work on something because it is exciting, satisfying, or personally challenging.[62]

One way firms keep highly mobile employees motivated and challenged is through opportunities that lower barriers to an employee's mobility within a company. For example, Shell Oil Company has created an "open sourcing" model for talent. Jobs are listed on Shell's intranet, and, with a two-month notice, employees can go to work on anything that interests them. Monsanto[63] has developed a similar approach. According to one executive:

> Because we don't have a lot of structure, people will flow toward where success and innovation are taking place. We have a free-market system where people can move, so you have an outflow of people in areas where not much progress is being made. Before, the HR function ran processes like management development and performance evaluation. Now it also facilitates this movement of people.

Financial and Nonfinancial Rewards and Incentives Financial rewards are a vital organizational control mechanism (as we will discuss in Chapter 9). Money—whether in the form of salary, bonus, stock options, and so forth—can mean many different things to people. It might mean security, recognition, or a sense of freedom and independence.

Paying people more is seldom the most important factor in attracting and retaining human capital.[64] Most surveys show that money is not the most important reason why people take or leave jobs and that money, in some surveys, is not even in the top 10. Consistent with these findings, Tandem Computers (part of Hewlett-Packard) typically doesn't tell people being recruited what their salaries would be. People who asked were told that their salaries were competitive. If they persisted along this line of questioning, they would not be offered a position. Why? Tandem realized a rather simple idea: People who come for money will leave for money.

Another nonfinancial reward is accommodating working families with children. Balancing demands of family and work is a problem at some point for virtually all employees.

Exhibit 4.5 describes strategies used by three leading-edge firms to retain their key employees—even during difficult economic times.

Enhancing Human Capital: The Role of Diversity in the Workforce

A combination of demographic trends and accelerating globalization of business has made the management of cultural differences a critical issue.[65] Workforces, which reflect demographic changes in the overall population, will be increasingly heterogeneous along dimensions such as gender, race, ethnicity, and nationality.[66] Demographic trends in the United States indicate a growth in Hispanic Americans from 6.9 million in 1960 to over 35 million in 2000, an expected increase to over 59 million by 2020 and 102 million by 2050. Similarly, the Asian-American population should grow to 20 million in 2020 from 12 million in 2000 and only 1.5 million in 1970. And the African-American population is becoming

Start a Talent Agency: Yum Brands started a Talent Scout program to recruit outsiders. Selected top performers nominate at least 25 people, and they get cash when a recruit is hired. Global talent VP John Kurnick said 25 percent of the finance team's recent hires came from this program. Although it wasn't designed for retention, "it's been the most gratifying for the scout," said Kurnick, and it encourages the scout to stay with the company.

Change Up Bonus Time: Software maker Intuit moved its annual restricted stock grant up from July to February to address the economic uncertainties that the employees felt. Intuit's human resources team wanted the grant to make a big impact. Program manager Eileen Fagan claimed, "It took one more worry off people's plates. It was a huge incentive for feeling good about the company."

Send Them Abroad—If It Fits: During recessionary times, global opportunities can energize top performers, said Ari Bousbib, former executive VP of United Technologies. During the downturn, he said, the company offered more expatriate assignments (for those whose family situations allowed it) as bonuses came under pressure.

Source: McGregor, J. & Dubey, R. 2010. Giving back to your stars. *Fortune*, November 1: 53–54.

more ethnically heterogeneous. Census estimates project that in 2010 as many as 10 percent of Americans of African descent were immigrants from Africa or the Caribbean.[67]

The proportion of the world population that is from developing countries increased from 68 percent in 1950 to 82 percent in 2010. Areas that increased as a percentage of total world population: Asia, up slightly from 54 percent in 1950 to 56 percent in 2010; Sub-Saharan Africa, from 7 percent in 1950 to 12 percent in 2010; and Latin America and the Caribbean, from 6 percent in 1950 to 9 percent in 2010.[68]

Such demographic changes have implications not only for the labor pool but also for customer bases, which are also becoming more diverse.[69] This creates important organizational challenges and opportunities.

The effective management of diversity can enhance the social responsibility goals of an organization.[70] However, there are many other benefits as well. Six other areas where sound management of diverse workforces can improve an organization's effectiveness and competitive advantages are: (1) cost, (2) resource acquisition, (3) marketing, (4) creativity, (5) problem-solving, and (6) organizational flexibility.

- *Cost Argument.* As organizations become more diverse, firms effective in managing diversity will have a cost advantage over those that are not.
- *Resource Acquisition Argument.* Firms with excellent reputations as prospective employers for women and ethnic minorities will have an advantage in the competition for top talent. As labor pools shrink and change in composition, such advantages will become even more important.
- *Marketing Argument.* For multinational firms, the insight and cultural sensitivity that members with roots in other countries bring to marketing efforts will be very useful. A similar rationale applies to subpopulations within domestic operations.
- *Creativity Argument.* Less emphasis on conformity to norms of the past and a diversity of perspectives will improve the level of creativity.
- *Problem-Solving Argument.* Heterogeneity in decision-making and problem-solving groups typically produces better decisions because of a wider range of perspectives as well as more thorough analysis. Jim Schiro, former CEO of PriceWaterhouse Coopers, explained, "When you make a genuine commitment to diversity, you bring

a greater diversity of ideas, approaches, and experiences and abilities that can be applied to client problems. After all, six people with different perspectives have a better shot at solving complex problems than sixty people who all think alike."[71]

- ***Organizational Flexibility Argument.*** With effective programs to enhance workplace diversity, systems become less determinant, less standardized, and therefore more fluid. Such fluidity should lead to greater flexibility to react to environmental changes. Reactions should be faster and less costly.

Consider how Infosys has benefited from a diverse workforce. Addressing shareholders of Infosys' 27th annual general meeting, N. R. Narayana Murthy, chief mentor and chairman of Infosys Technologies' board, said:[72]

> With over 91,000 employees from 70 nationalities working in 90 countries, Infosys has built the base to grow in the future. We opened new centers in Monterrey, Mexico; Lodz, Poland; Bangkok, Thailand; and Manila, Philippines. . . . As corporations grow and globalize, I am more and more convinced that the greatest challenge they will face will be the creation of a diverse workforce.

The Vital Role of Social Capital

>LO4.3
The key role of social capital in leveraging human capital within and across the firm.

Successful firms are well aware that the attraction, development, and retention of talent *is a necessary but not sufficient condition* for creating competitive advantages.[73] In the knowledge economy, it is not the stock of human capital that is important, but the extent to which it is combined and leveraged.[74] In a sense, developing and retaining human capital becomes less important as key players (talented professionals, in particular) take the role of "free agents" and bring with them the requisite skill in many cases. Rather, the development of social capital (that is, the friendships and working relationships among talented individuals) gains importance, because it helps tie knowledge workers to a given firm.[75] Knowledge workers often exhibit greater loyalties to their colleagues and their profession than their employing organization, which may be "an amorphous, distant, and sometimes threatening entity."[76] Thus, a firm must find ways to create "ties" among its knowledge workers.

Let's look at a hypothetical example. Two pharmaceutical firms are fortunate enough to hire Nobel Prize–winning scientists.[77] In one case, the scientist is offered a very attractive salary and outstanding facilities and equipment, and told to "go to it!" In the second case, the scientist is offered approximately the same salary, facilities, and equipment plus one additional ingredient: working in a laboratory with 10 highly skilled and enthusiastic scientists. Part of the job is to collaborate with these peers and jointly develop promising drug compounds. There is little doubt as to which scenario will lead to a higher probability of retaining the scientist. The interaction, sharing, and collaboration will create a situation in which the scientist will develop firm-specific ties and be less likely to bolt for a higher salary offer. Such ties are critical because knowledge-based resources tend to be more tacit in nature, as we mentioned early in this chapter. Therefore, they are much more difficult to protect against loss (i.e., the individual quitting the organization) than other types of capital, such as equipment, machinery, and land.

Another way to view this situation is in terms of the resource-based view of the firm that we discussed in Chapter 3. That is, competitive advantages tend to be harder for competitors to copy if they are based on "unique bundles" of resources.[78] So, if employees are working effectively in teams and sharing their knowledge and learning from each other, not only will they be more likely to add value to the firm, but they also will be less likely to leave the organization, because of the loyalties and social ties that they develop over time.

How Social Capital Helps Attract and Retain Talent

The importance of social ties among talented professionals creates a significant challenge (and opportunity) for organizations. In *The Wall Street Journal,* Bernard Wysocki described the increase in a type of "Pied Piper Effect," in which teams or networks of people are leaving one company for another.[79] The trend is to recruit job candidates at the crux of social relationships in organizations, particularly if they are seen as having the potential to bring with them valuable colleagues.[80] This is a process that is referred to as "hiring via personal networks." Let's look at one instance of this practice.

> Gerald Eickhoff, founder of an electronic commerce company called Third Millennium Communications, tried for 15 years to hire Michael Reene. Why? Mr. Eickhoff says that he has "these Pied Piper skills." Mr. Reene was a star at Andersen Consulting in the 1980s and at IBM in the 1990s. He built his businesses and kept turning down overtures from Mr. Eickhoff.
>
> However, in early 2000, he joined Third Millennium as chief executive officer, with a salary of just $120,000 but with a 20 percent stake in the firm. Since then, he has brought in a raft of former IBM colleagues and Andersen subordinates. One protégé from his time at Andersen, Mary Goode, was brought on board as executive vice president. She promptly tapped her own network and brought along former colleagues.
>
> Wysocki considers the Pied Piper effect one of the underappreciated factors in the war for talent today. This is because one of the myths of the New Economy is rampant individualism, wherein individuals find jobs on the Internet career sites and go to work for complete strangers. Perhaps, instead of Me Inc., the truth is closer to We Inc.[81]

Another example of social relationships causing human capital mobility is the emigration of talent from an organization to form start-up ventures. Microsoft is perhaps the best-known example of this phenomenon.[82] Professionals frequently leave Microsoft en masse to form venture capital and technology start-ups, called "Baby Bills," built around teams of software developers. For example, Ignition Corporation, of Bellevue, Washington, was formed by Brad Silverberg, a former Microsoft senior vice president. Eight former Microsoft executives, among others, founded the company.

Social relationships can provide an important mechanism for obtaining both resources and information from individuals and organizations outside the boundary of a firm.[83] Strategy Spotlight 4.3 describes how alumni programs for recently laid-off employees benefit both the individuals and the firm.

Social Networks: Implications for Knowledge Management and Career Success

>LO4.4

The importance of social networks in knowledge management and in promoting career success.

Managers face many challenges driven by such factors as rapid changes in globalization and technology. Leading a successful company is more than a one-person job. As Tom Malone recently put it in *The Future of Work,* "As managers, we need to shift our thinking from command and control to coordinate and cultivate—the best way to gain power is sometimes to give it away."[84] The move away from top-down bureaucratic control to more open, decentralized network models makes it more difficult for managers to understand how work is actually getting done, who is interacting with whom both within and outside the organization, and the consequences of these interactions for the long-term health of the organization.[85] In short, coordination, cultivation, and collaboration are increasingly becoming the mode of work at every level.[86]

social network analysis analysis of the pattern of social interactions among individuals.

But how can this be done? **Social network analysis** depicts the pattern of interactions among individuals and helps to diagnose effective and ineffective patterns.[87] It helps identify groups or clusters of individuals that comprise the network, individuals who link the clusters, and other network members. It helps diagnose communication patterns and,

Don't Go Away Mad . . . Now You Are a Valued Alum!

Traditionally, when an employee is laid off, the relationship between the company and that person comes to a bitter end. Increasingly, leading-edge global companies such as Dow Chemical and JPMorgan Chase are trying to maintain ties with their "alumni," even if they are moving on to other companies. What benefits do these efforts provide to the company and its ex-employees?

Source: Baker, S. 2009. You're fired—but stay in touch. *BusinessWeek*, May 4: 53–55.

These alumni networks, which are often organized on Facebook or LinkedIn, offer their members valuable benefits such as free job ads and connections to others who might help them in finding new jobs or facilitating entrepreneurial opportunities. For the firm, these networks constitute a laboratory for learning. Former employees who have nice things to say about a company are essentially "brand ambassadors" who can help in future recruiting efforts. The companies can also track the discussions in the network to identify hot topics, companies, products, and technologies. Best of all, when the economy recovers, this is an enormous talent pool for recruiting workers who are already familiar with the company and socialized into its culture.

---

consequently, communication effectiveness.[88] Such analysis of communication patterns is helpful because the configuration of group members' social ties within and outside the group affects the extent to which members connect to individuals who:

- Convey needed resources,
- Have the opportunity to exchange information and support,
- Have the motivation to treat each other in positive ways, and
- Have the time to develop trusting relationships that might improve the groups' effectiveness.

However, such relationships don't "just happen."[89] Developing social capital requires interdependence among group members. Social capital erodes when people in the network become independent. And increased interactions between members aid in the development and maintenance of mutual obligations in a social network.[90] Social networks such as Facebook may facilitate increased interactions between members in a social network via Internet-based communications.

Let's take a brief look at a simplified network analysis to get a grasp of the key ideas. In Exhibit 4.6, the links are used to depict informal relationships among individuals involving communication flows, personal support, and advice networks. There may be some individuals with literally no linkages, such as Fred. These individuals are typically labeled "isolates." However, most people do have some linkages with others.

To simplify, there are two primary types of mechanisms through which social capital will flow: *closure relationships* (depicted by Bill, Frank, George, and Susan) and *bridging relationships* (depicted by Mary). As we can see, in the former relationships one member is central to the communication flows in a group. In contrast, in the latter relationship, one person "bridges" or brings together groups that would have been otherwise unconnected.

Both closure and bridging relationships have important implications for the effective flow of information in organizations and for the management of knowledge. We will now briefly discuss each of these types of relationships. We will also address some of the implications that understanding social networks has for one's career success.

Closure   With **closure,** many members have relationships (or ties) with other members. As indicated in Exhibit 4.6, Bill's group would have a higher level of closure than

> **closure** the degree to which all members of a social network have relationships (or ties) with other group members.

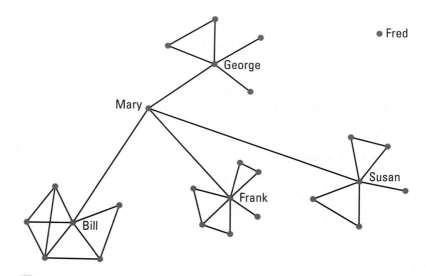

Exhibit 4.6 A Simplified Social Network

Frank, Susan, or George's groups because more group members are connected to each other. Through closure, group members develop strong relationships with each other, high levels of trust, and greater solidarity. High levels of trust help to ensure that informal norms in the group are easily enforced and there is less "free riding." Social pressure will prevent people from withholding effort or shirking their responsibilities. In addition, people in the network are more willing to extend favors and "go the extra mile" on a colleague's behalf because they are confident that their efforts will be reciprocated by another member in their group. Another benefit of a network with closure is the high level of emotional support. This becomes particularly valuable when setbacks occur that may destroy morale or an unexpected tragedy happens that might cause the group to lose its focus. Social support helps the group to rebound from misfortune and get back on track.

But high levels of closure often come with a price. Groups that become too closed can become insular. They cut themselves off from the rest of the organization and fail to share what they are learning from people outside their group. Research shows that while managers need to encourage closure up to a point, if there is too much closure, they need to encourage people to open up their groups and infuse new ideas through bridging relationships.[91]

bridging relationships relationships in a social network that connect otherwise disconnected people.

Bridging Relationships   The closure perspective rests on an assumption that there is a high level of similarity among group members. However, members can be quite heterogeneous with regard to their positions in either the formal or informal structures of the group or the organization. Such heterogeneity exists because of, for example, vertical boundaries (different levels in the hierarchy) and horizontal boundaries (different functional areas).

Bridging relationships, in contrast to closure, stress the importance of ties connecting people. Employees who bridge disconnected people tend to receive timely, diverse information because of their access to a wide range of heterogeneous information flows. Such bridging relationships span a number of different types of boundaries.

structural holes social gaps between groups in a social network where there are few relationships bridging the groups.

The University of Chicago's Ron Burt originally coined the term **"structural holes"** to refer to the social gap between two groups. Structural holes are common in organizations. When they occur in business, managers typically refer to them as "silos" or "stovepipes." Sales and engineering are a classic example of two groups whose members traditionally interact with their peers rather than across groups.

A study that Burt conducted at Raytheon, a $25 billion global electronics company and military contractor, provides further insight into the benefits of bridging.[92]

Burt studied several hundred managers in Raytheon's supply chain group and asked them to write down ideas to improve the company's supply chain management. Then he asked two Raytheon executives to rate the ideas. The conclusion: *The best suggestions consistently came from managers who discussed ideas outside their regular work group.*

Burt found that Raytheon managers were good at thinking of ideas but bad at developing them. Too often, Burt said, the managers discussed their ideas with colleagues already in their informal discussion network. Instead, he said, they should have had discussions outside their typical contacts, particularly with an informal boss, or someone with enough power to be an ally but not an actual supervisor.

Before we address how to overcome barriers to collaboration and the implications of social network theory for managers' career success, one might ask: Which is the more valuable mechanism to develop and nurture social capital—closure or bridging relationships? As with many aspects of strategic management, the answer becomes: "It all depends." So let's look at a few contingent issues.[93]

First, consider firms in competitive environments characterized by rapidly changing technologies and markets. Such firms should bridge relationships across networks because they need a wide variety of timely sources of information. Also, innovation is facilitated if there are multiple, interdisciplinary perspectives. On the other hand, firms competing in a stable environment would typically face less unpredictability. Thus, the cohesive ties associated with network closure would help to ensure the timely and effective implementation of strategies.

A second contingent factor would be the type of business strategies that a firm may choose to follow (a topic that we address next in Chapter 5). Managers with social networks characterized by closure would be in a preferred position if their firm is following an overall low-cost strategy.[94] Here, there is a need for control and coordination to implement strategies that are rather constrained by pressures to reduce costs. Alternatively, the uncertainties generally associated with differentiation strategies (i.e., creating products that are perceived by customers as unique and highly valued) would require a broad range of information sources and inputs. Social networks characterized by bridging relationships across groups would access the diverse informational sources needed to deal with more complex, multifaceted strategies.

A caveat: In both contingencies that we have discussed—competitive environment and business strategy—closure and bridging relationships across groups are necessary. Our purpose is to address where one type should be more dominant.

Developing Social Capital: Overcoming Barriers to Collaboration

Social capital within a group or organization develops through repeated interactions among its members and the resulting collaboration.[95] However, collaboration does not "just happen." People don't collaborate for various reasons. Effective collaboration requires overcoming four barriers:

- The not-invented-here barrier (people aren't willing to provide help)
- The hoarding barrier (people aren't willing to provide help)
- The search barrier (people are unable to find what they are looking for)
- The transfer barrier (people are unable to work with the people they don't know well)

All four barriers need to be low before effective collaboration can take place. Each one is enough to prevent people from collaborating well. The key is to identify which barriers are present in an organization and then to devise appropriate ways to overcome them.

Different barriers require different solutions. Motivational barriers require leaders to pull levers that make people more willing to collaborate. Ability barriers mean that leaders need to pull levers that enable motivated people to collaborate throughout the organization.

To be effective, leaders can choose a mix of three levers. First, when motivation is the problem, they can use the **unification lever,** wherein they craft compelling common

unification lever method for making people more willing to collaborate by crafting compelling common goals, articulating a strong value of cross-company teamwork, and encouraging collaboration in order to send strong signals to lift people's sights beyond their narrow interests toward a common goal.

goals, articulate a strong value of cross-company teamwork, and encourage collaboration in order to send strong signals to lift people's sights beyond their narrow interests toward a common goal.

Second, with the **people lever,** the emphasis isn't on getting people to collaborate more. Rather, it's on getting the right people to collaborate on the right projects. This means cultivating what may be called **T-shaped management:** people who simultaneously focus on the performance of their unit (the vertical part of the T) and across boundaries (the horizontal part of the T). People become able to collaborate when needed but are disciplined enough to say no when it's not required.

Third, by using the **network lever,** leaders can build nimble interpersonal networks across the company so that employees are better able to collaborate. Interpersonal networks are more effective than formal hierarchies. However, there is a dark side to networks: When people spend more time networking than getting work done, collaboration can adversely affect results.

Implications for Career Success   Let's go back in time in order to illustrate the value of social networks in one's career success. Consider two of the most celebrated artists of all time: Vincent van Gogh and Pablo Picasso. Strategy Spotlight 4.4 points out why these two artists enjoyed sharply contrasting levels of success during their lifetimes.

Effective social networks provide many advantages for the firm.[96] They can play a key role in an individual's career advancement and success. One's social network potentially can provide three unique advantages: private information, access to diverse skill sets, and power.[97] Managers see these advantages at work every day but might not consider how their networks regulate them.

Private Information   We make judgments, using both public and private information. Today, **public information** is available from many sources, including the Internet. However, since it is so accessible, public information offers less competitive advantage than it used to.

In contrast, **private information** from personal contacts can offer something not found in publicly available sources, such as the release date of a new product or knowledge about what a particular interviewer looks for in candidates. Private information can give managers an edge, though it is more subjective than public information since it cannot be easily verified by independent sources, such as Dunn & Bradstreet. Consequently the value of your private information to others—and the value of others' private information to you—depends on how much trust exists in the network of relationships.

Access to Diverse Skill Sets   Linus Pauling, one of only two people to win a Nobel Prize in two different areas and considered one of the towering geniuses of the 20th century, attributed his creative success not to his immense brainpower or luck but to his diverse contacts. He said, "The best way to have a good idea is to have a lot of ideas."

While expertise has become more specialized during the past 15 years, organizational, product, and marketing issues have become more interdisciplinary. This means that success is tied to the ability to transcend natural skill limitations through others. Highly diverse network relationships, therefore, can help you develop more complete, creative, and unbiased perspectives on issues. Trading information or skills with people whose experiences differ from your own provides you with unique, exceptionally valuable resources. It is common for people in relationships to share their problems. If you know enough people, you will begin to see how the problems that another person is struggling with can be solved by the solutions being developed by others. If you can bring together problems and solutions, it will greatly benefit your career.

Power   Traditionally, a manager's power was embedded in a firm's hierarchy. But, when corporate organizations became flatter, more like pancakes than pyramids, that power was repositioned in the network's brokers (people who bridged multiple networks), who could

---

people lever
method for making people more willing to collaborate by getting the right people to work on the right projects.

T-shaped management
people's dual focus on the performance of their unit (the vertical part of the T) and across boundaries (the horizontal part of the T).

network lever method for making people more willing to collaborate by building nimble interpersonal networks across the company.

public information
information that is available from public sources such as the internet.

private information
information that is not available from public sources, and is usually communicated in the context of personal relationships.

Picasso versus van Gogh: Who Was More Successful and Why?

Vincent van Gogh and Pablo Picasso are two of the most iconoclastic—and famous—artists of modern times. Paintings by both of them have fetched over $100 million. And both of them were responsible for some of the most iconic images in the art world: Van Gogh's *Self-Portrait* (the one sans the earlobe) and *Starry Night* and Picasso's *The Old Guitarist* and *Guernica.* However, there is an important difference between van Gogh and Picasso. Van Gogh died penniless. Picasso's estate was estimated at $750 million when he died in 1973. What was the difference?

Van Gogh's primary connection to the art world was through his brother. Unfortunately, this connection didn't feed directly into the money that could have turned him into a living success. In contrast, Picasso's myriad connections provided him with access to commercial riches. As noted by Gregory Berns in his book *Iconoclast: A Neuroscientist Reveals How to Think Differently,* "Picasso's wide ranging social network, which included artists, writers, and politicians, meant that he was never more than a few people away from anyone of importance in the world."

In effect, van Gogh was a loner, and the charismatic Picasso was an active member of multiple social circles. In social networking terms, van Gogh was a solitary "node" who had few connections. Picasso, on the other hand, was a "hub" who embedded himself in a vast network

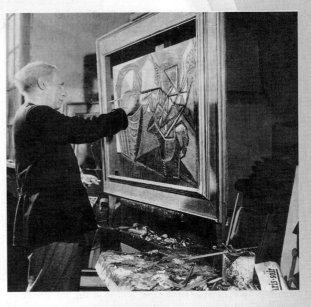

● Picasso was far more financially successful during his lifetime than van Gogh largely because of his extensive social network.

that stretched across various social lines. Where Picasso smoothly navigated multiple social circles, van Gogh had to struggle just to maintain connections with even those closest to him. Van Gogh inhabited an alien world, whereas Picasso was a social magnet. And because he knew so many people, the world was at Picasso's fingertips. From his perspective, the world was smaller.

Sources: Hayashi, A. M. 2008. Why Picasso out earned van Gogh. *MIT Sloan Management Review,* 50(1): 11–12; and, Berns, G. 2008. Iconoclast: *A neuroscientist reveals how to think differently.* Boston, MA: Harvard Business Press.

adapt to changes in the organization, develop clients, and synthesize opposing points of view. Such brokers weren't necessarily at the top of the hierarchy or experts in their fields, but they linked specialists in the firm with trustworthy and informative relationships.[98]

Most personal networks are highly clustered; that is, an individual's friends are likely to be friends with one another as well. Most corporate networks are made up of several clusters that have few links between them. Brokers are especially powerful because they connect separate clusters, thus stimulating collaboration among otherwise independent specialists.

Before moving on, Strategy Spotlight 4.5 discusses an interesting research study. It points out how women may differ from men in how they develop their social networks.

The Potential Downside of Social Capital

We'd like to close our discussion of social capital by addressing some of its limitations. First, some firms have been adversely affected by very high levels of social capital because it may breed **groupthink**—a tendency not to question shared beliefs.[99] Such thinking

groupthink a tendency in an organization for individuals not to question shared beliefs.

Developing Social Capital: Do Women and Men Differ?

Several years ago, Boris Groysberg conducted a study in which he warned managers about the risks associated with hiring star performers away from companies. His research investigated more than 1,000 star stock analysts, and he found that when one of them switches companies, not only does the star's performance plunge, but also the market value of the star's new company declines. In addition, the players don't tend to stay with their new firms very long—despite the generous pay packages that lured them in the first place. So everyone loses out.

However, when Groysberg further analyzed the data, he gained some new insights. One group of analysts maintained their stardom after changing employers: women. Unlike their male counterparts, female stars who switched firms performed just as well, in aggregate, as those who stayed put.

Why the gender discrepancy? There were two explanations. *First, the best female analysts appear to have built their franchises on portable, external relationships with clients and companies they covered—rather than on relationships within their firms.* In contrast, male analysts

Source: Groysberg, B. 2008. How star women build portable skills. *Harvard Business Review*, 86(2): 74–81.

built up greater firm- and team-specific human capital. That is, they invested more in internal networks and unique capabilities and resources of the firms where they worked.

Second, women took greater care when assessing a prospective employer. They evaluated their options more carefully and analyzed a wider range of factors than men did before deciding to uproot themselves from a firm where they had been successful. Female star analysts, it seems, take their work environment more seriously yet rely on it less than male stars do. And they tend to look for a firm that will allow them to keep building their successful franchise their own way.

There is a clear explanation as to why the female analysts spent more time developing their external networks. Most salespeople, traders, and investment bankers are men. And men tend to spend more time with other men. Not surprisingly, the star women in the study were generally thwarted in their efforts to integrate themselves into the existing power structure. Thus, they went to greater lengths to cultivate relationships with clients and contacts at the companies they covered. Their decision to maintain such an external focus rested on four main factors: uneasy in-house relationships, poor mentorships, neglect by colleagues, and a vulnerable position in the labor market.

---

may occur in networks with high levels of closure where there is little input from people outside of the network. In effect, too many warm and fuzzy feelings among group members prevent people from rigorously challenging each other. People are discouraged from engaging in the "creative abrasion" that Dorothy Leonard of Harvard University describes as a key source of innovation.[100] Two firms that were well known for their collegiality, strong sense of employee membership, and humane treatment—Digital Equipment (now part of Hewlett-Packard) and Polaroid—suffered greatly from market misjudgments and strategic errors. The aforementioned aspects of their culture contributed to their problems.

Second, if there are deep-rooted mind-sets, there would be a tendency to develop dysfunctional human resource practices. That is, the organization (or group) would continue to hire, reward, and promote like-minded people who tend to further intensify organizational inertia and erode innovation. Such homogeneity would increase over time and decrease the effectiveness of decision-making processes.

Third, the socialization processes (orientation, training, etc.) can be expensive in terms of both financial resources and managerial commitment. Such investments can represent a significant opportunity cost that should be evaluated in terms of the intended benefits. If such expenses become excessive, profitability would be adversely affected.

Finally, individuals may use the contacts they develop to pursue their own interests and agendas that may be inconsistent with the organization's goals and objectives. Thus, they may distort or selectively use information to favor their preferred courses of action or withhold information in their own self-interest to enhance their power to the detriment of the common good. Drawing on our discussion of social networks, this is particularly true in an organization that has too many bridging relationships but not enough closure relationships. In high closure groups, it is easier to watch each other to ensure that illegal or unethical acts don't occur. By contrast, bridging relationships make it easier for a person to play one group or individual off on another, with no one being the wiser.[101] We will discuss some behavioral control mechanisms in Chapter 9 (rewards, control, boundaries) that reduce such dysfunctional behaviors and actions.[102]

Using Technology to Leverage Human Capital and Knowledge

>LO4.5
The vital role of technology in leveraging knowledge and human capital.

Sharing knowledge and information throughout the organization can be a means of conserving resources, developing products and services, and creating new opportunities. In this section we will discuss how technology can be used to leverage human capital and knowledge within organizations as well as with customers and suppliers beyond their boundaries.

Using Networks to Share Information

As we all know, e-mail is an effective means of communicating a wide variety of information. It is quick, easy, and almost costless. Of course, it can become a problem when employees use it extensively for personal reasons. And we all know how fast jokes or rumors can spread within and across organizations!

Below is an example of how a CEO curbed what he felt was excessive e-mail use in his firm.[103]

> Scott Dockter, CEO of PBD Worldwide Fulfillment Services in Alpharetta, Georgia, launched "no e-mail Friday." Why? He suspected that overdependence on e-mail at PBD, which offers services such as call center management and distribution, was hurting productivity and, perhaps, sales. Accordingly, he instructed his 275 employees to pick up the phone or meet in person each Friday, and reduce e-mail use the rest of the time.
>
> That was tough to digest, especially for the younger staffers. "We discovered a lot of introverts . . . who had drifted into a pattern of communicating by e-mail," says Dockter. "However, in less than four months, the simple directive resulted in quicker problem-solving, better teamwork, and, best of all, happier customers."
>
> "Our relationship with PBD is much stronger," says Cynthia Fitzpatrick of Crown Financial Ministries. "You can't get to know someone through e-mail."

E-mail can also cause embarrassment if one is not careful. Consider the plight of a potential CEO—as recalled by Marshall Goldsmith, a well-known executive coach:[104]

> I witnessed a series of e-mails between a potential CEO and a friend inside the company. The first e-mail to the friend provided an elaborate description of "why the current CEO is an idiot." The friend sent a reply. Several rounds of e-mails followed. Then the friend sent an e-mail containing a funny joke. The potential CEO decided that the current CEO would love this joke and forwarded it to him. You can guess what happened next. The CEO scrolled down the e-mail chain and found the "idiot" message. The heir apparent was gone in a week.

E-mail can, however, be a means for top executives to communicate information efficiently. For example, Martin Sorrell, chairman of WPP Group PLC, a $2.4 billion advertising and public relations firm, is a strong believer in the use of e-mail.[105] He e-mails all of his employees once a month to discuss how the company is doing, address specific issues, and offer his perspectives on hot issues, such as new business models for the Internet. He believes that it keeps people abreast of what he is working on.

Technology can also enable much more sophisticated forms of communication in addition to knowledge sharing. Buckman Laboratories is a $505 million specialty chemicals company based in Memphis, Tennessee, with approximately 1,500 employees in over

100 countries. Buckman has successfully used its global knowledge-sharing network—known as K'Netix—to enhance its competitive advantages:[106]

> Here's an example of how the network can be applied. One of Buckman's paper customers in Michigan realized that the peroxide it was adding to remove ink from old magazines was no longer working. A Buckman sales manager presented this problem to the knowledge network. Within two days, salespeople from Belgium and Finland identified a likely cause: Bacteria in the paper slurry was producing an enzyme that broke down the peroxide. The sales manager recommended a chemical to control the bacteria, solving the problem. You can imagine how positive the customer felt about Buckman. And with the company and the customer co-creating knowledge, a new level of trust and value can emerge.

Technology can also help global companies help their employees share information in an internal online business network. In 2008, Germany's BASF, one of the world's biggest chemical companies, started connect.BASF, a social online platform for its employees. After several months of trials, the company officially launched the platform to the whole BASF group. Three months later, 11,000 employees had registered their profiles and more than 750 communities had been created. Some communities support the management of a specific project. Others gather experts in a given domain to discuss hot topics in their given field. Connect.BASF helps employees develop their personal brand within the company. The platform increases information sharing and makes the process more fluid. The experience at BASF seems promising for other multinational businesses as a way to bypass inner hyper-bureaucracy.[107]

Electronic Teams: Using Technology to Enhance Collaboration

>LO4.6
Why "electronic" or "virtual" teams are critical in combining and leveraging knowledge in organizations and how they can be made more effective.

Technology enables professionals to work as part of electronic, or virtual, teams to enhance the speed and effectiveness with which products are developed. For example, Microsoft has concentrated much of its development on **electronic teams** (or e-teams) that are networked together.[108] This helps to accelerate design and testing of new software modules that use the Windows-based framework as their central architecture. Microsoft is able to foster specialized technical expertise while sharing knowledge rapidly throughout the firm. This helps the firm learn how its new technologies can be applied rapidly to new business ventures such as cable television, broadcasting, travel services, and financial services.

What are electronic teams (or e-teams)? There are two key differences between e-teams and more traditional teams:[109]

electronic teams
a team of individuals that completes tasks primarily through e-mail communication.

- E-team members either work in geographically separated workplaces or they may work in the same space but at different times. E-teams may have members working in different spaces and time zones, as is the case with many multinational teams.
- Most of the interactions among members of e-teams occur through electronic communication channels such as fax machines and groupware tools such as e-mail, bulletin boards, chat, and videoconferencing.

E-teams have expanded exponentially in recent years.[110] Organizations face increasingly high levels of complex and dynamic change. E-teams are also effective in helping businesses cope with global challenges. Most e-teams perform very complex tasks and most knowledge-based teams are charged with developing new products, improving organizational processes, and satisfying challenging customer problems. For example, Eastman Kodak's e-teams design new products, Hewlett Packard's e-teams solve clients' computing problems, and Sun Microsystems' (part of Oracle) e-teams generate new business models.

Advantages   There are multiple advantages of e-teams.[111] In addition to the rather obvious use of technology to facilitate communications, the potential benefits parallel the other two major sections in this chapter—human capital and social capital.

First, e-teams are less restricted by the geographic constraints that are placed on face-to-face teams. Thus, e-teams have the potential to acquire a broader range of "human capital" or the skills and capacities that are necessary to complete complex assignments. So, e-team leaders can draw upon a greater pool of talent to address a wider range of problems since they are not constrained by geographic space. Once formed, e-teams can be more flexible in responding to unanticipated work challenges and opportunities because team members can be rotated out of projects when demands and contingencies alter the team's objectives.

Second, e-teams can be very effective in generating "social capital"—the quality of relationships and networks that form. Such capital is a key lubricant in work transactions and operations. Given the broader boundaries associated with e-teams, members and leaders generally have access to a wider range of social contacts than would be typically available in more traditional face-to-face teams. Such contacts are often connected to a broader scope of clients, customers, constituents, and other key stakeholders.

Challenges   However, there are challenges associated with making e-teams effective. Successful action by both traditional teams and e-teams requires that:

- Members *identify* who among them can provide the most appropriate knowledge and resources, and,
- E-team leaders and key members know how to *combine* individual contributions in the most effective manner for a coordinated and appropriate response.

Group psychologists have termed such activities "identification and combination" activities, and teams that fail to perform them face a "process loss."[112] Process losses prevent teams from reaching high levels of performance because of inefficient interaction dynamics among team members. Such poor dynamics require that some collective energy, time, and effort be devoted to dealing with team inefficiencies, thus diverting the team away from its objectives. For example, if a team member fails to communicate important information at critical phases of a project, other members may waste time and energy. This can lead to conflict and resentment as well as to decreased motivation to work hard to complete tasks.

The potential for process losses tends to be more prevalent in e-teams than in traditional teams because the geographical dispersion of members increases the complexity of establishing effective interaction and exchanges. Generally, teams suffer process loss because of low cohesion, low trust among members, a lack of appropriate norms or standard operating procedures, or a lack of shared understanding among team members about their tasks. With e-teams, members are more geographically or temporally dispersed, and the team becomes more susceptible to the risk factors that can create process loss. Such problems can be exacerbated when team members have less than ideal competencies and social skills. This can erode problem-solving capabilities as well as the effective functioning of the group as a social unit.

A variety of technologies, from e-mail and Internet groups to Skype (acquired by Microsoft in 2011) and Cisco's Umi TelePresence, have facilitated the formation and effective functioning of e-teams as well as a wide range of collaborations within companies. Strategy Spotlight 4.6 highlights Cisco's efforts to use technology to enable such communication. Such technologies greatly enhance the collaborative abilities of employees and managers within a company at a reasonable cost—despite the distances that separate them.

Codifying Knowledge for Competitive Advantage

There are two different kinds of knowledge. Tacit knowledge is embedded in personal experience and shared only with the consent and participation of the individual. Explicit (or codified) knowledge, on the other hand, is knowledge that can be documented, widely distributed, and easily replicated. One of the challenges of knowledge-intensive organizations is to capture and codify the knowledge and experience that, in effect, resides in the heads of its employees. Otherwise, they will have to constantly "reinvent the wheel," which is both expensive and inefficient. Also, the "new wheel" may not necessarily be superior to the "old wheel."[113]

Once a knowledge asset (e.g., a software code or processes) is developed and paid for, it can be reused many times at very low cost, assuming that it doesn't have to be

Videoconferencing: Allowing Employees to Communicate Face-to-Face over Long Distances

Cisco Systems has recognized that collaboration is the biggest technological trend of the next decade, driving productivity gains of 5 to 10 percent per year. It has created a strong portfolio of collaboration technologies, including TelePresence; WebEx; phones that run over the Internet; devices that produce, distribute, and archive videos; and hardware that can carry, distribute, and manage communications traffic no matter the origin or destination.

Internally, the use of these technologies has helped make Cisco's workforce one of the most distributed, connected, and productive in the world. Employees have experienced—and driven—a cultural revolution of not only information sharing, but also teamwork and transparency.

Cisco recently launched a new videoconferencing product, Umi TelePresence, that is aimed at the consumer

market. It costs $599 (for the camera, console, cables, and remote control that constitute the system) and comes with an unlimited calling plan that runs $25 a month. What makes the product more expensive is that you might have to purchase a second or third Umi for family members, simply because it takes at least "two to tango" when it comes to videoconferencing. However, corporations could also use such home systems to allow global employees to connect with headquarters during business hours. As noted by Srinath Narasimhan, CEO of Tata Communications, remote employees are loath to go to the office for a 3 a.m. call in a video "suite." However, with a home setup, these employees could stumble out of bed and into a meeting—as long as they remember to comb their hair first!

Cisco is not the only company making videoconferencing part of its daily routine. Samsung created a videoconference system called WhizMeeting to reduce meeting time and costs. Henkel of Germany, which recently acquired Dial, relies upon a highly effective videoconference system that enhances communications among diverse workforces scattered worldwide, resulting in substantial cost savings. Initially, Henkel started to invest in videoconferencing to reduce its worldwide carbon footprint.

Sources: *www.svconline.com and www.samsung.com,* accessed September 23, 2011; Copeland, M. V. 2010. The new global worker gadget: Videophones. *Fortune,* November 15: 36; Sidhu, I. 2010. *Doing both.* Boston: Harvard Business Press; and, Baig, E. C. 2010. Umi TelePresence brings videoconferencing home. *www.usatoday.com.* December 2: np.

---

substantially modified each time. Let's take the case of a consulting company, such as Accenture (formerly Andersen Consulting).[114] Since the knowledge of its consultants has been codified and stored in electronic repositories, it can be employed in many jobs by a huge number of consultants. Additionally, since the work has a high level of standardization (i.e., there are strong similarities across the numerous client engagements), there is a rather high ratio of consultants to partners. For example, the ratio of consultants to partners is roughly 30, which is quite high. As one might expect, there must be extensive training of the newly hired consultants for such an approach to work. The recruits are trained at Accenture's Center for Professional Education, a 150-acre campus in St. Charles, Illinois. Using the center's knowledge-management respository, the consultants work through many scenarios designed to improve business processes. In effect, the information technologies enable the consultants to be "implementers, not inventors."

Access Health, a call-in medical center, also uses technology to capture and share knowledge. When someone calls the center, a registered nurse uses the company's "clinical decision architecture" to assess the caller's symptoms, rule out possible conditions, and recommend a home remedy, doctor's visit, or trip to the emergency room. The company's knowledge repository contains algorithms of the symptoms of more than 500 illnesses. According to CEO Joseph Tallman, "We are not inventing a new way to cure disease. We are taking available knowledge and inventing processes to put it to better use." The software algorithms were very expensive to develop, but the investment has been repaid many times over. The first 300 algorithms that Access Health developed have each been used an average of 8,000 times a year. Further, the company's paying customers—insurance companies

Crowdsourcing: How SAP Taps Knowledge Well Beyond Its Boundaries

Traditionally, organizations built and protected their knowledge stocks—proprietary resources that no one else could access. However, the more the business environment changes, the faster the value of what you know at any point in time diminishes. In today's world, success hinges on the ability to access a growing variety of knowledge flows in order to rapidly replenish the firm's knowledge stocks. For example, when an organization tries to improve cycle times in a manufacturing process, it finds far more value in problem solving shaped by the diverse experiences, perspectives, and learning of a tightly knit team (shared through knowledge flows) than in a training manual (knowledge stocks) alone.

Knowledge flows can help companies gain competitive advantage in an age of near-constant disruption. The software company SAP, for example, routinely taps the more than 1.5 million participants in its Developer Network, which extends well beyond the boundaries of the firm. Those who post questions for the network community to address will receive a response in 17 minutes, on average, and 85 percent of all questions posted to date have been rated as "resolved." By providing a virtual platform for customers, developers, system integrators, and service vendors to create and exchange knowledge, SAP has significantly increased the productivity of all the participants in its ecosystem.

The site is open to everyone, regardless of whether you are an SAP customer, partner, or newcomer who needs to work with SAP technology. The site offers technical articles, web-based training, code samples, evaluation systems, discussion forums, and excellent blogs for community experts.

crowdsourcing

Sources: Hagel, J., III., Brown, J. S., & Davison, L. 2009. The big shift: Measuring the forces of change. *Harvard Business Review,* 87(4): 87; and, Anonymous. Undated. SAP Developer Network. *sap.sys-con.com.* np.

and provider groups—save money because many callers would have made expensive trips to the emergency room or the doctor's office had they not been diagnosed over the phone.

The user community can be a major source of knowledge creation for a firm. Strategy Spotlight 4.7 highlights how SAP, in an example of effective crowdsourcing, has been able to leverage the expertise and involvement of its users to develop new knowledge and transmit it to their entire user community.

We close this section with a series of questions managers should consider in determining (1) how effective their organization is in attracting, developing, and retaining human capital and (2) how effective they are in leveraging human capital through social capital and technology. These questions, included in Exhibit 4.7, summarize some of the key issues addressed in this chapter.

>LO4.7
The challenge of protecting intellectual property and the importance of a firm's dynamic capabilities.

Protecting the Intellectual Assets of the Organization: Intellectual Property and Dynamic Capabilities

In today's dynamic and turbulent world, unpredictability and fast change dominate the business environment. Firms can use technology, attract human capital, or tap into research and design networks to get access to pretty much the same information as their competitors. So what would give firms a sustainable competitive advantage?[115] Protecting a firm's intellectual property requires a concerted effort on the part of the company. After all, employees become disgruntled and patents expire. The management of **intellectual property (IP) rights** involves, besides patents, contracts with confidentiality and non-compete clauses, copyrights, and the development of trademarks. Moreover, developing dynamic capabilities is the only avenue providing firms with the ability to reconfigure their knowledge and activities to achieve a sustainable competitive advantage.

intellectual property rights intangible property owned by a firm in the forms of patents, copyrights, trademarks, or trade secrets.

Human Capital

Recruiting "Top-Notch" Human Capital

- Does the organization assess attitude and "general makeup" instead of focusing primarily on skills and background in selecting employees at all levels?
- How important are creativity and problem-solving ability? Are they properly considered in hiring decisions?
- Do people throughout the organization engage in effective networking activities to obtain a broad pool of worthy potential employees? Is the organization creative in such endeavors?

Enhancing Human Capital through Employee Development

- Does the development and training process inculcate an "organizationwide" perspective?
- Is there widespread involvement, including top executives, in the preparation and delivery of training and development programs?
- Is the development of human capital effectively tracked and monitored?
- Are there effective programs for succession at all levels of the organization, especially at the top-most levels?
- Does the firm effectively evaluate its human capital? Is a 360-degree evaluation used? Why? Why not?
- Are mechanisms in place to assure that a manager's success does not come at the cost of compromising the organization's core values?

Retaining the Best Employees

- Are there appropriate financial rewards to motivate employees at all levels?
- Do people throughout the organization strongly identify with the organization's mission?
- Are employees provided with a stimulating and challenging work environment that fosters professional growth?
- Are valued amenities provided (e.g., flex time, child-care facilities, telecommuting) that are appropriate given the organization's mission, strategy, and how work is accomplished?
- Is the organization continually devising strategies and mechanisms to retain top performers?

Social Capital

- Are there positive personal and professional relationships among employees?
- Is the organization benefiting (or being penalized) by hiring (or by voluntary turnover) en masse?
- Does an environment of caring and encouragement rather than competition enhance team performance?
- Do the social networks within the organization have the appropriate levels of closure and bridging relationships?
- Does the organization minimize the adverse effects of excessive social capital, such as excessive costs and groupthink?

Technology

- Has the organization used technologies such as e-mail and networks to develop products and services?
- Does the organization effectively use technology to transfer best practices across the organization?
- Does the organization use technology to leverage human capital and knowledge both within the boundaries of the organization and among its suppliers and customers?
- Has the organization effectively used technology to codify knowledge for competitive advantage?
- Does the organization try to retain some of the knowledge of employees when they decide to leave the firm?

Source: Adapted from Dess, G. G., & Picken, J. C. 1999. *Beyond productivity:* 63–64. New York: AMACON.

Intellectual Property Rights

Intellectual property rights are more difficult to define and protect than property rights for physical assets (e.g., plant, equipment, and land). However, if intellectual property rights are not reliably protected by the state, there will be no incentive to develop new products and services. Property rights have been enshrined in constitutions and rules of law in many countries. In the information era, though, adjustments need to be made to accommodate the new realities of knowledge. Knowledge and information are fundamentally different assets from the physical ones that property rights have been designed to protect.

The protection of intellectual rights raises unique issues, compared to physical property rights. IP is characterized by significant development costs and very low marginal costs. Indeed, it may take a substantial investment to develop a software program, an idea, or a digital music tune. Once developed, though, their reproduction and distribution cost may be almost zero, especially if the Internet is used. Effective protection of intellectual property is necessary before any investor will finance such an undertaking. Appropriation of their returns is harder to police since possession and deployment are not as readily observable. Unlike physical assets, intellectual property can be stolen by simply broadcasting it. Recall Napster's MP3 file sharing service as well as the debates about counterfeit software, music CDs, and DVDs coming from developing countries such as China. Part of the problem is that using an idea does not prevent others from simultaneously using it for their own benefit, which is typically impossible with physical assets. Moreover, new ideas are frequently built on old ideas and are not easily traceable.

Strategy Spotlight 4.8 describes the many legal battles fought by a Canadian firm, Research in Motion of Waterloo, the developer of the popular BlackBerry. This example illustrates the high stakes that ride on intellectual property rights.

Another intellectual property battle example is Apple's lawsuit against Samsung in June 2011, targeting the new Galaxy Tab 10.1 tablet. Samsung originally filed patent-infringement lawsuits against Apple in South Korea, Japan, and Germany in April 2011. Samsung was responding to Apple's filing with the U.S. District Court of Northern California, a 38-page lawsuit that claimed Samsung's smartphones and tablets closely copied the iPhone and iPad in look, packaging, and user interface. Apple also has patent-infringement suits lodged against HTC and Motorola, and recently settled a high-profile intellectual property dispute with Nokia. Under the terms of that agreement, Apple will pay Nokia a one-time fee in addition to royalties; neither company disclosed the amount of money at issue. Nokia and Apple had spent months trading brutally worded lawsuits, even taking complaints to the U.S. Federal Trade Commission. But Apple's probably hoping for a much more advantageous result with its Samsung lawsuit.[116]

Countries are attempting to pass new legislation to cope with developments in new pharmaceutical compounds, stem cell research, and biotechnology. However, a firm that is faced with this challenge today cannot wait for the legislation to catch up. New technological developments, software solutions, electronic games, online services, and other products and services contribute to our economic prosperity and the creation of wealth for those entrepreneurs who have the idea first and risk bringing it to the market.

Dynamic Capabilities

Dynamic capabilities entail the capacity to build and protect a competitive advantage.[117] This rests on knowledge, assets, competencies, and complementary assets and technologies as well as the ability to sense and seize new opportunities, generate new knowledge, and reconfigure existing assets and capabilities.[118] According to David Teece, an economist at the University of California at Berkeley, dynamic capabilities are related to the entrepreneurial side of the firm and are built within a firm through its environmental and technological "sensing" apparatus, its choices of organizational form, and its collective ability to strategize. Dynamic capabilities are about the ability of an organization to challenge the

dynamic capabilities a firm's capacity to build and protect a competitive advantage, which rests on knowledge, assets, competencies, complementary assets, and technologies. Dynamic capabilities include the ability to sense and seize new opportunities, generate new knowledge, and reconfigure existing assets and capabilities.

Research in Motion, Maker of the BlackBerry, Loses an Intellectual Property Lawsuit

Research in Motion (RIM) is a Waterloo, Ontario–based company that is best known for developing the Black-Berry, a wireless device that integrates the functionalities of a cell phone with the ability to receive e-mail messages. During its brief history, it has become one of the fastest growing companies in North America. Founded by Mike Lazaridis, a former University of Waterloo student in 1984, Research in Motion was a competent but obscure technology firm until 1999 when the first BlackBerry was released. Through the development of integrated hardware, software, and services that support multiple wireless network standards, the BlackBerry has enabled RIM to grow from less than $50 million in sales revenue in 1999 to $15 billion by 2010. Even more impressive, by early 2011 the company boasted a market capitalization in excess of $30 billion. RIM's commitment to its slogan "always on, always connected" has won it a legion of dedicated followers around the globe.

Interestingly, legal challenges have been the biggest obstacles that Research in Motion has faced in the eight years since the introduction of the first BlackBerry. In 2000, NTP, a pure patent-holding company, filed suit against RIM for violation of five of its patents and petitioned the court for an injunction on the sale and support of BlackBerry devices. The case dragged on for years, and RIM felt relatively secure that no injunction would be

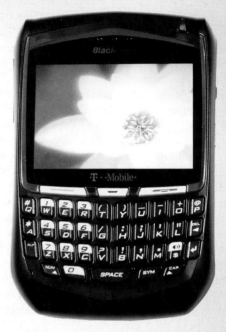

● Research in Motion (RIM) has faced litigation over its highly successful BlackBerry.

issued. On February 24, 2006, things dramatically changed. U.S. District Court Judge James Spencer indicated that he was inclined to grant the injunction and that his ruling was imminent. Faced with the acute risk of an unfavorable decision, RIM settled only one week later for $612.5 million. It wound up paying a fortune for rights that were dubious at best—given that all five NTP patents had already been preliminarily invalidated by the U.S. Patent and Trademark Office and that two of them then received a final rejection.

Sources: Henkel, J. & Reitzig, M. 2008. Patent sharks. *Harvard Business Review*, 86(6): 129–133; Hesseldahl, A. 2006. RIM's latest patent problem. *BusinessWeek Online*, May 2: np; Anonymous. 2006. Settlement reached in BlackBerry patent case. (The Associated Press) MSNBC.Com. March 3: np; Wolk, M . 2006. RIM pays up, taking "one for the team." MSNBC.Com. March 3; and, *finance.yahoo.com*.

conventional wisdom within its industry and market, learn and innovate, adapt to the changing world, and continuously adopt new ways to serve the evolving needs of the market.[119]

Examples of dynamic capabilities include product development, strategic decision making, alliances, and acquisitions.[120] Some firms have clearly developed internal processes and routines that make them superior in such activities. For example, 3M and Apple are ahead of their competitors in product development. Another example is Siemens, an international electrical engineering and electronics company employing more than 440,000 workers in more than 190 countries. Looking at Siemens from a dynamic capability perspective, the significance of its entrepreneurial venturing process stands out. The process created an interface between new product development and sales/operations and was divided into two phases: incubating and grafting. These phases play a fundamental role as dynamic capabilities, which allow rapidly changing innovations to be exploited by the existing sales network. These capabilities are closely related to Siemens' competitive advantage in the telecommunications industry.[121]

Cisco Systems has made numerous acquisitions over the years. It seems to have developed the capability to identify and evaluate potential acquisition candidates and seamlessly integrate them once the acquisition is completed. Other organizations can try to copy Cisco's practices. However, Cisco's combination of the resources of the acquired companies and their reconfiguration that Cisco has already achieved places it well ahead of its competitors. As markets become increasingly dynamic, traditional sources of long-term competitive advantage become less relevant. In such markets, all that a firm can strive for are a series of temporary advantages. Dynamic capabilities allow a firm to create this series of temporary advantages through new resource configurations.[122]

Reflecting on Career Implications . . .

- *Human Capital:* Does your organization effectively attract, develop, and retain talent? If not, you may have fewer career opportunities to enhance your human capital at your organization. Do you take advantage of your organization's human resource programs such as tuition reimbursement, mentoring, etc.?
- *Human Capital:* Does your organization value diversity? What kinds of diversity seem to be encouraged (e.g., age-based or ethnicity-based)? If not, there may be limited perspectives on strategic and operational issues, and a career at this organization may be less attractive to you.
- *Social Capital:* Does your organization have effective programs to build and develop social capital such that professionals develop strong ties to the organization? Alternatively, is social capital so strong that you see effects occur such as groupthink? From your perspective, how might you better leverage social capital towards pursuing other career opportunities?
- *Technology:* Does your organization provide and effectively use technology (e.g., groupware, knowledge management systems) to help you leverage your talents and expand your knowledge base?

Summary

Firms throughout the industrial world are recognizing that the knowledge worker is the key to success in the marketplace. However, we also recognize that human capital, although vital, is still only a necessary, but not a sufficient, condition for creating value. We began the first section of the chapter by addressing the importance of human capital and how it can be attracted, developed, and retained. Then we discussed the role of social capital and technology in leveraging human capital for competitive success. We pointed out that intellectual capital—the difference between a firm's market value and its book value—has increased significantly over the past few decades. This is particularly true for firms in knowledge-intensive industries, especially where there are relatively few tangible assets, such as software development.

The second section of the chapter addressed the attraction, development, and retention of human capital. We viewed these three activities as a "three-legged stool"—that is, it is difficult for firms to be successful if they ignore or are unsuccessful in any one of these activities. Among the issues we discussed in *attracting* human capital were "hiring for attitude, training for skill" and the value of using social networks to attract human capital. In particular, it is important to attract employees who can collaborate with others, given the importance of collective efforts such as teams and task forces. With regard to *developing* human capital, we discussed the need to encourage widespread involvement throughout the organization, monitor progress and track the development of human capital, and evaluate human capital. Among the issues that are widely practiced in evaluating human capital is the 360-degree evaluation system. Employees are evaluated by their superiors, peers, direct reports, and even internal and external customers. We also addressed the value of maintaining a diverse workforce. Finally, some mechanisms for retaining human capital are employees' identification with the organization's mission and values, providing challenging work and a stimulating environment, the importance of financial and nonfinancial rewards and incentives, and providing flexibility and amenities. A key issue here is that a firm should not overemphasize financial rewards. After all, if individuals join an organization for money, they also are likely to leave for money. With money as the primary motivator, there is little chance that employees will develop firm-specific ties to keep them with the organization.

The third section of the chapter discussed the importance of social capital in leveraging human capital. Social capital refers to the network of relationships that individuals have throughout the organization as well as with customers and suppliers. Such ties can be critical in obtaining both information and resources. With regard to recruiting, for example, we saw how some firms are able to hire en masse groups of individuals who are part of social networks. Social relationships can also be very important in the effective functioning of groups. Finally, we discussed some of the potential downsides of social capital. These include the expenses that firms may bear when promoting social and working relationships among individuals as well as the potential for groupthink, wherein individuals are reluctant to express divergent (or opposing) views on an issue because of social pressures to conform. We also introduced the concept of social networks. The relative advantages of being central in a network versus bridging multiple networks were discussed. We addressed the key role that social networks can play in both improving knowledge management and promoting career success.

The fourth section addressed the role of technology in leveraging human capital. We discussed relatively simple means of using technology, such as e-mail and networks where individuals can collaborate by way of personal computers. We provided suggestions and guidelines on how electronic teams can be effectively managed. We also addressed more sophisticated uses of technology, such as sophisticated management systems. Here knowledge can be codified and reused at very low cost, as we saw in the examples of firms in the consulting, health care, and high-technology industries.

In the last section we discussed the increasing importance of protecting a firm's intellectual property.

Although traditional approaches such as patents, copyrights, and trademarks are important, the development of dynamic capabilities may be the best protection in the long run.

Summary Review Questions

1. Explain the role of knowledge in today's competitive environment.

2. Why is it important for managers to recognize the interdependence in the attraction, development, and retention of talented professionals?

3. What are some of the potential downsides for firms that engage in a "war for talent"?

4. Discuss the need for managers to use social capital in leveraging their human capital both within and across their firm.

5. Discuss the key role of technology in leveraging knowledge and human capital.

Key Terms

knowledge economy,   165
intellectual capital,   166
human capital,   167
social capital,   167
explicit knowledge,   167
tacit knowledge,   167
360-degree evaluation and feedback systems,   173
social network analysis,   178
closure,   179
bridging relationships,   180

structural holes,   180
unification lever,   181
people lever,   182
T-shaped management,   182
network lever,   182
public information,   182
private information,   182
groupthink,   183
electronic teams,   186
intellectual property rights,   189
dynamic capabilities,   191

Experiential Exercise

Pfizer, a leading health care firm with $68 billion in revenues, is often rated as one of *Fortune*'s "Most Admired Firms." It is also considered an excellent place to work and has generated high return to shareholders. Clearly, the firm values its human capital. Using the Internet and/or library resources, identify some of the actions/strategies Pfizer has taken to attract, develop, and retain human capital. What are their implications?

Activity	Actions/Strategies	Implications
Attracting human capital		
Developing human capital		
Retaining human capital		

Application Questions & Exercises

1. Look up successful firms in a high-technology industry as well as two successful firms in more traditional industries such as automobile manufacturing and retailing. Compare their market values and book values. What are some implications of these differences?

2. Select a firm for which you believe its social capital— both within the firm and among its suppliers and customers—is vital to its competitive advantage. Support your arguments.

3. Choose a company with which you are familiar. What are some of the ways in which it uses technology to leverage its human capital?

4. Using the Internet, look up a company with which you are familiar. What are some of the policies and procedures that it uses to enhance the firm's human and social capital?

Ethics Questions

1. Recall an example of a firm that recently faced an ethical crisis. How do you feel the crisis and management's handling of it affected the firm's human capital and social capital?

2. Based on your experiences or what you have learned in your previous classes, are you familiar with any companies that used unethical practices to attract talented professionals? What do you feel were the short-term and long-term consequences of such practices?

References

1. Farmbrough, R. 2010. List of the largest global technology companies: Part 1. *www.wikipedia.org.* November 1: np; and Arai, H. 2000. *Intellectual property policies for the twenty-first century: The Japanese experience in wealth creation.* WIPO Publication No. 834 (E). We thank Pratik Kapadia for his valued contribution.

2. Parts of this chapter draw upon some of the ideas and examples from: Dess, G. G. & Picken, J. C. 1999. *Beyond productivity.* New York: AMACOM.

3. An acknowledged trend: The world economic survey. 1996. *The Economist,* September 2(8): 25–28.

4. Quinn, J. B., Anderson, P., & Finkelstein, S. 1996. Leveraging intellect. *Academy of Management Executive,* 10(3): 7–27; and *https://www.cia.gov/library/publications/the=world=factbook/geos/us.html.*

5. Schwab, K. 2011. The Global Competitiveness Report 2011–2012. World Economic Forum. Accessed at *www.3.weforum.org/docs/WEF_GCR_Report_2011-12.pdf.*

6. Hamel, G. & Prahalad, C. K. 1996. Competing in the new economy: Managing out of bounds. *Strategic Management Journal,* 17: 238.

7. Stewart, T. A. 1997. *Intellectual capital: The new wealth of organizations.* New York: Doubleday/Currency.

8. Leif Edvisson and Michael S. Malone have a similar, more detailed definition of *intellectual capital:* "the

combined knowledge, skill, innovativeness, and ability to meet the task at hand." They consider intellectual capital to equal human capital plus structural capital. *Structural capital is defined as* "the hardware, software, databases, organization structure, patents, trademarks, and everything else of organizational capability that supports those employees' productivity—in a word, everything left at the office when the employees go home." Edvisson, L. & Malone, M. S. 1997. *Intellectual capital: Realizing your company's true value by finding its hidden brainpower:* 10–14. New York: HarperBusiness.

9. Stewart, T. A. 2001. Accounting gets radical. *Fortune,* April 16: 184–194.

10. Adams, S. & Kichen, S. 2008. Ben Graham then and now. *Forbes,* November 10: 56.

11. An interesting discussion of Steve Jobs's impact on Apple's valuation is in: Lashinsky, A. 2009. Steve's leave—what does it really mean? *Fortune,* February 2: 96–102.

12. Anonymous. 2007. Intel opens first high volume 45 nm microprocessor manufacturing factory. *www.intel.com.* October 25: np.

13. Thomas Stewart has suggested this formula in his book *Intellectual Capital* (1997, op. cit.). He provides an insightful discussion on pages 224–225, including some of the limitations of this approach to measuring intellectual capital. We recognize, of course, that during the late 1990s and in early 2000, there were some excessive market valuations of high-technology and Internet firms. For an interesting discussion of the extraordinary market valuation of Yahoo!, an Internet company, refer to: Perkins, A. B. 2001. The Internet bubble encapsulated: Yahoo! *Red Herring,* April 15: 17–18.

14. Roberts, P. W. & Dowling, G. R. 2002. Corporate reputation and sustained superior financial performance. *Strategic Management Journal,* 23(12): 1077–1095.

15. For a recent study on the relationships between human capital, learning, and sustainable competitive advantage, read: Hatch, N. W. & Dyer, J. H.

2005. Human capital and learning as a source of sustainable competitive advantage. *Strategic Management Journal,* 25: 1155–1178.

16. One of the seminal contributions on knowledge management is: Becker, G. S. 1993. *Human capital: A theoretical and empirical analysis with special reference to education* (3rd ed.). Chicago: University of Chicago Press.

17. For an excellent overview of the topic of social capital, read: Baron, R. A. 2005. Social capital. In Hitt, M. A. & Ireland, R. D. (Eds.), *The Blackwell encyclopedia of management* (2nd ed.): 224–226. Malden, MA: Blackwell.

18. For an excellent discussion of social capital and its impact on organizational performance, refer to: Nahapiet, J. & Ghoshal, S. 1998. Social capital, intellectual capital, and the organizational advantage. *Academy of Management Review,* 23: 242–266.

19. An interesting discussion of how knowledge management (patents) can enhance organizational performance can be found in: Bogner, W. C. & Bansal, P. 2007. Knowledge management as the basis of sustained high performance. *Journal of Management Studies,* 44(1): 165–188.

20. Polanyi, M. 1967. *The tacit dimension.* Garden City, NY: Anchor Publishing.

21. Barney, J. B. 1991. Firm resources and sustained competitive advantage. *Journal of Management,* 17: 99–120.

22. For an interesting perspective of empirical research on how knowledge can adversely affect performance, read: Haas, M. R. & Hansen, M. T. 2005. When using knowledge can hurt performance: The value of organizational capabilities in a management consulting company. *Strategic Management Journal,* 26(1): 1–24.

23. New insights on managing talent are provided in: Cappelli, P. 2008. Talent management for the twenty-first century. *Harvard Business Review,* 66(3): 74–81.

24. Some of the notable books on this topic include: Edvisson & Malone, op. cit.; Stewart, 1997, op. cit.; and Nonaka, I. & Takeuchi, I. 1995. *The*

knowledge creating company. New York: Oxford University Press.

25. Segalla, M. & Felton, N. 2010. Find the real power in your organization. *Harvard Business Review,* 88(5): 34–35.

26. Stewart, T. A. 2000. Taking risk to the marketplace. *Fortune,* March 6: 424.

27. Insights on the Generation X's perspective on the workplace are in: Erickson, T. J. 2008. Task, not time: Profile of a Gen Y job. *Harvard Business Review,* 86(2): 19.

28. Pfeffer, J. 2010. Building sustainable organizations: The human factor. *Academy of Management Perspectives,* 24(1): 34–45.

29. Dutton, G. 1997. Are you technologically competent? *Management Review,* November: 54–58.

30. Some workplace implications for the aging workforce are addressed in: Strack, R., Baier, J., & Fahlander, A. 2008. Managing demographic risk. *Harvard Business Review,* 66(2): 119–128.

31. For a discussion of attracting, developing, and retaining top talent, refer to: Goffee, R. & Jones, G. 2007. Leading clever people. *Harvard Business Review,* 85(3): 72–89.

32. Dess & Picken, op. cit.: 34.

33. Webber, A. M. 1998. Danger: Toxic company. *Fast Company,* November: 152–161.

34. Martin, J. & Schmidt, C. 2010. How to keep your top talent. *Harvard Business Review,* 88(5): 54–61.

35. Some interesting insights on why home-grown American talent is going abroad are found in: Saffo, P. 2009. A looming American diaspora. *Harvard Business Review,* 87(2): 27.

36. Morris, B. 1997. Key to success: People, people, people. *Fortune,* October 27: 232.

37. Davenport, T. H., Harris, J. & Shapiro, J. 2010. Competing on talent analytics. *Harvard Business Review,* 88(10): 62–69.

38. Ployhart, R. E. & Moliterno, T. P. 2011. Emergence of the human capital resource: A multilevel model. *Academy of Management Review,* 36(1): 127–150.

39. For insights on management development and firm performance in several

countries, refer to: Mabey, C. 2008. Management development and firm performance in Germany, Norway, Spain, and the UK. *Journal of International Business Studies,* 39(8): 1327–1342.

40. Blau, J. 2003. Corporate strategy: At Nokia temperament is a core competence. *www.allbusiness.com/human-resources /employee-development/597569-1 .html#ixzz1YOclMXkq.*

41. Cardin, R. 1997. Make your own Bozo Filter. *Fast Company,* October–November: 56.

42. Saumya, B. 2011. Best companies to work for in 2011. *www.businesstoday .intoday.in/.* February 6; and, Karishma, V. 2006. Indian firms facing talent crunch. *http://news.bbc.co.uk /.* October 11.

43. Martin, J. 1998. So, you want to work for the best. . . . *Fortune,* January 12: 77; and, Henkoff, R. 1993. Companies that train best. *Fortune,* March 22: 53–60.

44. An interesting perspective on developing new talent rapidly when they join an organization can be found in: Rollag, K., Parise, S., & Cross, R. 2005. Getting new hires up to speed quickly. *MIT Sloan Management Review,* 46(2): 35–41.

45. Stewart, T. A. 1998. Gray flannel suit? Moi? *Fortune,* March 18: 80–82.

46. An interesting perspective on how Cisco Systems develops its talent can be found in Chatman, J., O'Reilly, C., & Chang, V. 2005. Cisco Systems: Developing a human capital strategy. *California Management Review,* 47(2): 137–166.

47. Anonymous. 2011. Schumpeter: The tussle for talent. *The Economist,* January 8: 68.

48. This section is based on: Leonard, D. A. & Swap, W. 2004. Deep smarts. *Harvard Business Review,* 82(9): 88–97.

49. Useful insights on coaching can be found in: Coutu, D. & Kauffman, C. 2009. What can coaches do for you? *Harvard Business Review,* 67(1): 91–97.

50. For an innovative perspective on the appropriateness of alternate approaches to evaluation and rewards, refer to Seijts, G. H. & Lathan, G. P.

2005. Learning versus performance goals: When should each be used? *Academy of Management Executive,* 19(1): 124–132.

51. The discussion of the 360-degree feedback system draws on: UPS. 1997. 360-degree feedback: Coming from all sides. *Vision* (a UPS Corporation internal company publication), March: 3; Slater, R. 1994. *Get better or get beaten: Thirty-one leadership secrets from Jack Welch.* Burr Ridge, IL: Irwin; Nexon, M. 1997. General Electric: The secrets of the finest company in the world. *L'Expansion,* July 23: 18–30; and, Smith, D. 1996. Bold new directions for human resources. *Merck World* (internal company publication), October: 8.

52. Interesting insights on 360-degree evaluation systems are discussed in: Barwise, P. & Meehan, Sean. 2008. So you think you're a good listener. *Harvard Business Review,* 66(4): 22–23.

53. Insights into the use of 360-degree evaluation are in: Kaplan, R. E. & Kaiser, R. B. 2009. Stop overdoing your strengths. *Harvard Business Review,* 87(2): 100–103.

54. Kets de Vries, M. F. R. 1998. Charisma in action: The transformational abilities of Virgin's Richard Branson and ABB's Percy Barnevik. *Organizational Dynamics,* Winter: 20.

55. For an interesting discussion on how organizational culture has helped Zappos become number one in *Fortune's* 2009 survey of the best companies to work for, see: O'Brien, J. M. 2009. Zappos knows how to kick it. *Fortune,* February 2: 54–58.

56. We have only to consider the most celebrated case of industrial espionage in recent years, wherein José Ignacio Lopez was indicted in a German court for stealing sensitive product planning documents from his former employer, General Motors, and sharing them with his executive colleagues at Volkswagen. The lawsuit was dismissed by the German courts, but Lopez and his colleagues were investigated by the U.S. Justice Department. Also consider the recent litigation involving noncompete employment contracts

and confidentiality clauses of *International Paper v. Louisiana-Pacific, Campbell Soup v. H. J. Heinz Co.,* and *PepsiCo v. Quaker Oats's Gatorade.* In addition to retaining valuable human resources and often their valuable network of customers, firms must also protect proprietary information and knowledge. For interesting insights, refer to: Carley, W. M. 1998. CEO gets hard lesson in how not to keep his lieutenants. *The Wall Street Journal,* February 11: A1, A10; and, Lenzner, R. & Shook, C. 1998. Whose Rolodex is it, anyway? *Forbes,* February 23: 100–103.

57. For an insightful discussion of retention of knowledge workers in today's economy, read: Davenport, T. H. 2005. *The care and feeding of the knowledge worker.* Boston, MA: Harvard Business School Press.

58. Fisher, A. 2008. America's most admired companies. *Fortune,* March 17: 74.

59. Stewart, T. A. 2001. *The wealth of knowledge.* New York: Currency.

60. For insights on fulfilling one's potential, refer to: Kaplan, R. S. 2008. Reaching your potential. *Harvard Business Review,* 66(7/8): 45–57.

61. Amabile, T. M. 1997. Motivating creativity in organizations: On doing what you love and loving what you do. *California Management Review,* Fall: 39–58.

62. For an insightful perspective on alternate types of employee–employer relationships, read: Erickson, T. J. & Gratton, L. 2007. What it means to work here. *Harvard Business Review,* 85(3): 104–112.

63. Monsanto has been part of Pharmacia since 2002. *Hoover's Handbook of Am. Bus.* 2004: 562.

64. Pfeffer, J. 2001. Fighting the war for talent is hazardous to your organization's health. *Organizational Dynamics,* 29(4): 248–259.

65. Cox, T. L. 1991. The multinational organization. *Academy of Management Executive,* 5(2): 34–47. Without doubt, a great deal has been written on the topic of creating and maintaining an effective diverse workforce. Some excellent, recent books include: Harvey, C. P. &

Allard, M. J. 2005. *Understanding and managing diversity: Readings, cases, and exercises* (3rd ed.). Upper Saddle River, NJ: Pearson Prentice-Hall; Miller, F. A. & Katz, J. H. 2002. *The inclusion breakthrough: Unleashing the real power of diversity.* San Francisco: Berrett Koehler; and, Williams, M. A. 2001. *The 10 lenses: Your guide to living and working in a multicultural world.* Sterling, VA: Capital Books.

66. For an interesting perspective on benefits and downsides of diversity in global consulting firms, refer to: Mors, M. L. 2010. Innovation in a global consulting firm: When the problem is too much diversity. *Strategic Management Journal,* 31(8): 841–872.

67. www.rand.org/publications/RB/RB/5050. U. S. Census Bureau. 1970, 1980, 1990, and 2000 decennial censuses. Population projections, July 1, 2000, to July 1, 2050.

68. Shackman, G., Xun, W., & Ya-Lin, L. 2011. Brief review of world population trends. *http://gsociology.icaap.org/report/demsum.html.*

69. Hewlett, S. A. & Rashid, R. 2010. The battle for female talent in emerging markets. *Harvard Business Review,* 88(5): 101–107.

70. This section, including the six potential benefits of a diverse workforce, draws on: Cox, T. H. & Blake, S. 1991. Managing cultural diversity: Implications for organizational competitiveness. *Academy of Management Executive,* 5(3): 45–56.

71. *www.pwcglobal.com/us/eng/careers/diversity/index.html.*

72. CyberMedia News. 2008. Creating diverse workforce a big challenge: Murthy. *www.ciol.com/News/News-Reports/Creating-diverse-workforce-a-big-challenge-Murthy/14608107076/0/.* June 14.

73. This discussion draws on: Dess, G. G. & Lumpkin, G. T. 2001. Emerging issues in strategy process research. In Hitt, M. A., Freeman, R. E., & Harrison, J. S. (Eds.). *Handbook of strategic management:* 3–34. Malden, MA: Blackwell.

74. Wong, S.-S. & Boh, W. F. 2010. Leveraging the ties of others to build a reputation for trustworthiness among peers. *Academy of Management Journal,* 53(1): 129–148.

75. Adler, P. S. & Kwon, S. W. 2002. Social capital: Prospects for a new concept. *Academy of Management Review,* 27(1): 17–40.

76. Capelli, P. 2000. A market-driven approach to retaining talent. *Harvard Business Review,* 78(1): 103–113.

77. This hypothetical example draws on: Peteraf, M. 1993. The cornerstones of competitive advantage. *Strategic Management Journal,* 14: 179–191.

78. Wernerfelt, B. 1984. A resource-based view of the firm. *Strategic Management Journal,* 5: 171–180.

79. Wysocki, B., Jr. 2000. Yet another hazard of the new economy: The Pied Piper Effect. *The Wall Street Journal,* March 20: A1–A16.

80. Ideas on how managers can more effectively use their social network are addressed in: McGrath, C. & Zell, D. 2009. Profiles of trust: Who to turn to, and for what. *MIT Sloan Management Review,* 50(2): 75–80.

81. Ibid.

82. Buckman, R. C. 2000. Tech defectors from Microsoft resettle together. *The Wall Street Journal,* October: B1–B6.

83. An insightful discussion of the interorganizational aspects of social capital can be found in: Dyer, J. H. & Singh, H. 1998. The relational view: Cooperative strategy and sources of interorganizational competitive advantage. *Academy of Management Review,* 23: 66–79.

84. A study of the relationship between social networks and performance in China is found in: Li, J. J., Poppo, L., & Zhou, K. Z. 2008. Do managerial ties in China always produce value? Competition, uncertainty, and domestic vs. foreign firms. *Strategic Management Journal,* 29(4): 383–400.

85. Aime, F., Johnson, S., Ridge, J. W., & Hill, A. D. 2010. The routine may be stable but the advantage is not: Competitive implications of key employee mobility. *Strategic Management Journal,* 31(1): 75–87.

86. Hoppe, B. 2005. Structural holes, Part one. *connectedness.blogspot.com.* January 18: np.

87. There has been a tremendous amount of theory building and empirical research in recent years in the area of social network analysis. Unquestionably, two of the major contributors to this domain have been Ronald Burt and J. S. Coleman. For excellent background discussions, refer to: Burt, R. S. 1992. *Structural holes: The social structure of competition.* Cambridge, MA: Harvard University Press; Coleman, J. S. 1990. *Foundations of social theory.* Cambridge, MA: Harvard University Press; and, Coleman, J. S. 1988. Social capital in the creation of human capital. *American Journal of Sociology,* 94: S95–S120. For a more recent review and integration of current thought on social network theory, consider: Burt, R. S. 2005. *Brokerage & closure: An introduction to social capital.* Oxford Press: New York.

88. Our discussion draws on the concepts developed by: Burt, 1992, op. cit.; Coleman, 1990, op. cit.; Coleman, 1988, op. cit.; and, Oh, H., Chung, M., & Labianca, G. 2004. Group social capital and group effectiveness: The role of informal socializing ties. *Academy of Management Journal,* 47(6): 860–875. We would like to thank Joe Labianca (University of Kentucky) for his helpful feedback and ideas in our discussion of social networks.

89. Arregle, J. L., Hitt, M. A., Sirmon, D. G., & Very, P. 2007. The development of organizational social capital: Attributes of family firms. *Journal of Management Studies,* 44(1): 73–95.

90. A novel perspective on social networks is in: Pentland, A. 2009. How social networks network best. *Harvard Business Review,* 87(2): 37.

91. Oh et al., op. cit.

92. Hoppe, op. cit.

93. The discussion of these two contingent factors draws on: Dess, G. G. & Shaw, J. D. 2001. Voluntary turnover, social capital, and organizational performance. *Academy of Management Review,* 26(3): 446–456.

94. The business-level strategies of overall low cost and differentiation draws upon Michael E. Porter's classic work and will be discussed in more detail in Chapter 5. Source: Porter, M. E. 1985. *Competitive advantage.* Free Press: New York.

95. This section draws on: Hansen, M. T. 2009. *Collaboration: How leaders avoid the traps, create unity, and reap big results.* Boston, MA: Harvard Business Press.

96. Perspectives on how to use and develop decision networks are discussed in: Cross, R., Thomas, R. J., & Light, D. A. 2009. How "who you know" affects what you decide. *MIT Sloan Management Review*, 50(2): 35–42.

97. Our discussion of the three advantages of social networks draws on Uzzi, B. & Dunlap. S. 2005. How to build your network. *Harvard Business Review*, 83(12): 53–60. For a recent, excellent review on the research exploring the relationship between social capital and managerial performance, read: Moran, P. 2005. Structural vs. relational embeddedness: Social capital and managerial performance. *Strategic Management Journal*, 26(12): 1129–1151.

98. A perspective on personal influence is in: Christakis, N. A. 2009. The dynamics of personal influence. *Harvard Business Review*, 87(2): 31.

99. Prusak, L. & Cohen, D. 2001. How to invest in social capital. *Harvard Business Review*, 79(6): 86–93.

100. Leonard, D. & Straus, S. 1997. Putting your company's whole brain to work. *Harvard Business Review*, 75(4): 110–122.

101. For an excellent discussion of public (i.e., the organization) versus private (i.e., the individual manager) benefits of social capital, refer to: Leana, C. R. & Van Buren, H. J. 1999. Organizational social capital and employment practices. *Academy of Management Review*, 24(3): 538–555.

102. The authors would like to thank Joe Labianca, University of Kentucky, and John Lin, University of Texas at Dallas, for their very helpful input in our discussion of social network theory and its practical implications.

103. Brady, D. 2006. !#?@ the e-mail. Can we talk? *BusinessWeek*, December 4: 109.

104. Goldsmith, M. 2009. How not to lose the top job. *Harvard Business Review*, 87(1): 74.

105. Taylor, W. C. 1999. Whatever happened to globalization? *Fast Company*, December: 228–236.

106. Prahalad, C. K. & Ramaswamy, V. 2004. *The future of competition: Co-creating value with customers.* Boston: Harvard Business School Press.

107. connect.BASF: Introducing an Internal Online Business Network. *www.slideshare.net/basf/connect-basf-onlinebusinessnetwork.*

108. Lei, D., Slocum, J., & Pitts, R. A. 1999. Designing organizations for competitive advantage: The power of unlearning and learning. *Organizational Dynamics*, Winter: 24–38.

109. This section draws upon Zaccaro, S. J. & Bader, P. 2003. E-leadership and the challenges of leading e-teams: Minimizing the bad and maximizing the good. *Organizational Dynamics*, 31(4): 377–387.

110. Kirkman, B. L., Rosen, B., Tesluk, P. E., & Gibson, C. B. 2004. The impact of team empowerment on virtual team performance: The moderating role of face-to-face interaction. *Academy of Management Journal*, 47(2): 175–192.

111. The discussion of the advantages and challenges associated with e-teams draws on Zaccaro & Bader, op. cit.

112. For a recent study exploring the relationship between team empowerment, face-to-face interaction, and performance in virtual teams, read Kirkman, et al., op. cit.

113. For an innovative study on how firms share knowledge with competitors and the performance implications, read: Spencer, J. W. 2003. Firms' knowledge-sharing strategies in the global innovation system: Empirical evidence from the flat panel display industry. *Strategic Management Journal*, 24(3): 217–235.

114. The examples of Andersen Consulting and Access Health draw upon Hansen, M. T., Nohria, N., & Tierney, T. 1999. What's your strategy for managing knowledge? *Harvard Business Review*, 77(2): 106–118.

115. This discussion draws on Conley, J. G. 2005. *Intellectual capital management.* Kellogg School of Management and Schulich School of Business, York University, Toronto, KS 2003; Conley, J. G. & Szobocsan, J. 2001. Snow White shows the way. *Managing Intellectual Property*, June: 15–25; Greenspan, A. 2004. Intellectual property rights. the Federal Reserve Board, remarks by the chairman, February 27; and, Teece, D. J. 1998. Capturing value from knowledge assets. *California Management Review*, 40(3): 54–79. The authors would like to thank Professor Theo Peridis, York University, for his contribution to this section.

116. Nicholas, K. 2011. Apple upgrades Samsung lawsuit, targets Galaxy Tab 10.1. *www.eweek.com.* June 18.

117. Danneels. E. 2011. Trying to become a different type of company: Dynamic capability at Smith Corona. *Strategic Management Journal*, 32(1): 1–31.

118. A study of the relationship between dynamic capabilities and related diversification is: Doving, E. & Gooderham, P. N. 2008. *Strategic Management Journal*, 29(8): 841–858.

119. A perspective on strategy in turbulent markets is in: Sull, D. 2009. How to thrive in turbulent markets. *Harvard Business Review*, 87(2): 78–88.

120. Lee, G. K. 2008. Relevance of organizational capabilities and its dynamics: What to learn from entrants' product portfolios about the determinants of entry timing. *Strategic Management Journal*, 29(12): 1257–1280.

121. Bernard, K., Marcel D., & Franziska, B. 2001. Dynamic capabilities for entrepreneurial venturing—the case of Siemens Enterprise Networks. IAMOT Conference Paper 2001, Lausanne, Switzerland, March 19.

122. Eisenhardt, K. M. & Martin, J. E. 2000. Dynamic capabilities: What are they? *Strategic Management Journal*, 21: 1105–1121.

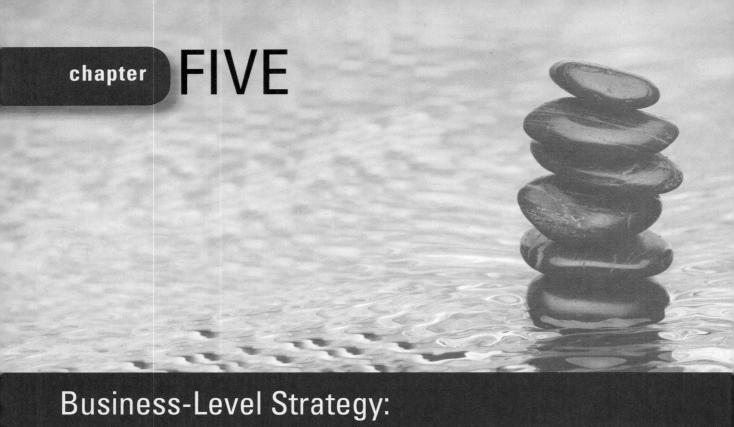

chapter FIVE

Business-Level Strategy:

Creating and Sustaining Competitive Advantages

After reading this chapter, you should have a good understanding of:

LO5.1 The central role of competitive advantage in the study of strategic management, and the three generic strategies: overall cost leadership, differentiation, and focus.

LO5.2 How the successful attainment of generic strategies can improve a firm's relative power vis-à-vis the five forces that determine an industry's average profitability.

LO5.3 The pitfalls managers must avoid in striving to attain generic strategies.

LO5.4 How firms can effectively combine the generic strategies of overall cost leadership and differentiation.

LO5.5 What factors determine the sustainability of a firm's competitive advantage.

LO5.6 How Internet-enabled business models are being used to improve strategic positioning.

LO5.7 The importance of considering the industry life cycle to determine a firm's business-level strategy and its relative emphasis on functional area strategies and value-creating activities.

LO5.8 The need for turnaround strategies that enable a firm to reposition its competitive position in an industry.

LEARNING OBJECTIVES

ow firms compete with each other and how they attain and sustain competitive advantages go to the heart of strategic management. In short, the key issue becomes: Why do some firms outperform others and enjoy such advantages over time? This subject, **business-level strategy,** is the focus of Chapter 5.

The first part of the chapter draws on Michael Porter's framework of generic strategies. He identifies three strategies—overall cost leadership, differentiation, and focus—that firms may apply to outperform their rivals in an industry. We begin by describing each of these strategies and providing examples of firms that have successfully attained them as a means of outperforming competitors in their industry. Next, we address how these strategies help a firm develop a favorable position vis-à-vis the "five forces," suggest some of the pitfalls that managers must avoid when pursuing these generic strategies, and discuss the conditions under which firms may effectively combine generic strategies to outperform rivals.

The second section discusses the factors that determine the sustainability of competitive advantages. Using an example from the manufacturing sector, we discuss whether or not a firm's competitive advantages may be sustained over a long period of time.

The third section addresses how competitive strategies should be revised and redeployed in light of the shifts in industry and competitive forces caused by Internet and digital strategies. Here, combination strategies are the most solid because they integrate the new capabilities with sound principles.

The fourth and final section discusses a vital consideration in the effective use of business-level strategies: industry life cycles. The four stages of the industry life cycle—introduction, growth, maturity, and decline—are indicative of an evolving management process that affects factors such as the market growth rate and the intensity of competition. Accordingly, the stages of an industry's life cycle are an important contingency that managers should take into account when making decisions concerning the optimal overall business-level strategies and the relative emphasis to place on functional capabilities and value-creating activities. At times, firms are faced with performance declines and must find ways to revitalize their competitive positions. The actions followed to do so are referred to as turnaround strategies, which may be needed at any stage of the industry life cycle. However, they occur more frequently during the maturity and decline stages.●

Recently, a battle over strategy divided top management and franchise owners at KFC.[1] Many franchise owners became upset with KFC's new strategy that moved away from its Southern fried heritage and moved toward promoting grilled chicken and sandwiches. In early 2009, CEO Roger Eaton introduced grilled chicken in a move to target health-conscious consumers in today's changing society. However, many franchise owners were disappointed with this strategy. Why? What went wrong?

On January 2010, the KFC National Council and Advertising Cooperative (which represents all U.S. franchises) sued KFC to gain control of their own ad strategy. This "civil war" erupted when the company introduced grilled chicken with the slogan "Unthink KFC." To make matters worse, after a year in the market, reports stated that grilled chicken accounted for only about 16 percent of all "on the bone" chicken sold. Also, an internal survey of 642 franchisees showed almost 50 percent of the stores' grilled chicken was thrown away!

One glaring example of miscommunication regarding business strategy between management and franchise owners occurred when KFC launched a grilled chicken giveaway on *Oprah,* a wildly popular television program, in May 2009. Management told franchisees to expect a couple hundred customers to redeem online coupons at each store. However, thousands showed up expecting free grilled chicken. One franchise owner said, "The cost to the franchisee was much larger than they said," and that the promotion cost her almost $15,000! This started a continued downfall in trust between management and owners. KFC canceled the promotion, and CEO Eaton apologized to customers in an online video.

Disagreements between KFC management and franchise owners over strategy led to decreased sales and store closings. KFC's franchisees were upset with the decision to push grilled chicken and claimed that it hurts the brand. They sued KFC and now do a lot of their own advertising to promote fried chicken at their stores.

business-level strategy a strategy designed for a firm or a division of a firm that competes within a single business.

generic strategies an analysis of business strategy into basic types based on breadth of target market (industrywide versus narrow market segment) and type of competitive advantage (low cost versus uniqueness).

In order to create and sustain a competitive advantage, companies such as KFC should analyze the value chains of their customers and suppliers to see where they can add value. They should not focus only on their internal operations. By not listening to and consulting with franchise owners, KFC has ignored and angered a large part of their extended value chain. The battle over ad strategy within the company has hurt the brand and eroded KFC's competitive advantage.

Types of Competitive Advantage and Sustainability

>LO5.1

The central role of competitive advantage in the study of strategic management, and the three generic strategies: overall cost leadership, differentiation, and focus.

Michael Porter presented three generic strategies that a firm can use to overcome the five forces and achieve competitive advantage.[2] Each of Porter's **generic strategies** has the potential to allow a firm to outperform rivals in its industry. The first, *overall cost leadership,* is based on creating a low-cost position. Here, a firm must manage the relationships throughout the value chain and lower costs throughout the entire chain. Second, *differentiation* requires a firm to create products and/or services that are unique and valued. Here, the primary emphasis is on "nonprice" attributes for which customers will gladly pay a premium.[3] Third, a *focus* strategy directs attention (or "focus") toward narrow product lines, buyer segments, or targeted geographic markets and firms must attain advantages either through differentiation or cost leadership.[4] Whereas the overall cost leadership and differentiation strategies strive to attain advantages industrywide, focusers have a narrow target market in mind. Exhibit 5.1 illustrates these three strategies on two dimensions: competitive advantage and strategic target.

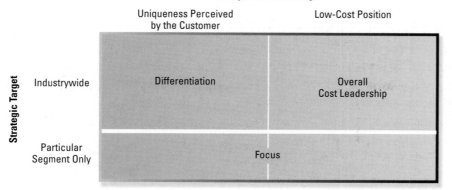

Exhibit 5.1 Three Generic Strategies

Source: Adapted and reprinted with the permission of The Free Press, a division of Simon & Schuster Inc. from *Competitive Strategy: Techniques for Analyzing Industries and Competitors* by Michael E. Porter. Copyright © 1980, 1998 by The Free Press. All rights reserved.

Both casual observation and research support the notion that firms that identify with one or more of the forms of competitive advantage outperform those that do not.[5] There has been a rich history of strategic management research addressing this topic. One study analyzed 1,789 strategic business units and found that businesses combining multiple forms of competitive advantage (differentiation and overall cost leadership) outperformed businesses that used only a single form. The lowest performers were those that did not identify with any type of advantage. They were classified as "stuck in the middle." Results of this study are presented in Exhibit 5.2.[6]

For an example of the dangers of being "stuck in the middle," consider Coach and Tiffany—two brands in the "affordable luxury" category.[7] Such brands target middle-class customers for whom a $300 bag is a splurge. After sales and stock declines, they are migrating away from the middle—and going either higher or lower:

In early 2008, Coach said that it would turn 40 of its nearly 300 stores into a more upscale format that will offer higher-end bags and concierge services. Tiffany, on the other hand, took

Exhibit 5.2 Competitive Advantage and Business Performance

	Competitive Advantage					
	Differentiation and Cost	Differentiation	Cost	Differentiation and Focus	Cost and Focus	Stuck in the Middle
Performance						
Return on investment (%)	35.5	32.9	30.2	17.0	23.7	17.8
Sales growth (%)	15.1	13.5	13.5	16.4	17.5	12.2
Gain in market share (%)	5.3	5.3	5.5	6.1	6.3	4.4
Sample size	123	160	100	141	86	105

the opposite tack. A new store opening in California will not sell any of its $148,000 diamond necklaces and instead focus on less expensive products like its $200-and-under silver jewelry. Claims Pat Conroy, head of Deloitte & Touche's consumer products sector: "Being in the middle is not a good place to be. You get assaulted from everyone."

overall cost leadership a firm's generic strategy based on appeal to the industrywide market using a competitive advantage based on low cost.

Overall Cost Leadership

The first generic strategy is **overall cost leadership.** Overall cost leadership requires a tight set of interrelated tactics that include:

- Aggressive construction of efficient-scale facilities.
- Vigorous pursuit of cost reductions from experience.
- Tight cost and overhead control.

Exhibit 5.3 Value-Chain Activities: Examples of Overall Cost Leadership

Support Activities
Firm Infrastructure
• Few management layers, to reduce overhead costs.
• Standardized accounting practices to minimize personnel required.
Human Resource Management
• Minimize costs associated with employee turnover through effective policies.
• Effective orientation and training programs to maximize employee productivity.
Technology Development
• Effective use of automated technology to reduce scrappage rates.
• Expertise in process engineering to reduce manufacturing costs.
Procurement
• Effective policy guidelines to ensure low-cost raw materials (with acceptable quality levels).
• Shared purchasing operations with other business units.

Primary Activities
Inbound Logistics
• Effective layout of receiving dock operations.
Operations
• Effective use of quality control inspectors to minimize rework.
Outbound Logistics
• Effective utilization of delivery fleets.
Marketing and Sales
• Purchase of media in large blocks.
• Sales force utilization maximized by territory management.
Service
• Thorough service repair guidelines to minimize repeat maintenance calls.
• Use of single type of vehicle to minimize repair costs.

Source: Adapted from: Porter, M.E. 1985. *Competitive advantage: Creating and sustaining superior performance.* New York: Free Press.

The Experience Curve

The experience curve, developed by Boston Consulting Group in 1968, is a way of looking at efficiencies developed through a firm's cumulative experience. In its basic form, the experience curve relates production costs to production output. As output doubles, costs decline by 10 percent to 30 percent. For example, if it costs $1 per unit to produce 100 units, the per unit cost will decline to between 70 and 90 cents as output increases to 200 units.

What factors account for this increased efficiency? First, the success of an experience curve strategy depends on the industry life cycle for the product. Early stages of a product's life cycle are typically characterized by rapid gains in technological advances in production efficiency. Most experience curve gains come early in the product life cycle.

Second, the inherent technology of the product offers opportunities for enhancement through gained experience. High-tech products give the best opportunity for gains in production efficiencies. As technology is developed, "value engineering" of innovative production processes is implemented, driving down the per unit costs of production.

Third, a product's sensitivity to price strongly affects a firm's ability to exploit the experience curve. Cutting the price of a product with high demand elasticity—where demand increases when price decreases—rapidly creates consumer purchases of the new product. By cutting prices, a firm can increase demand for its product. The increased demand in turn increases product manufacture, thus increasing the firm's experience in the manufacturing process. So by decreasing price and increasing demand, a firm gains manufacturing experience in that particular product, which drives down per unit production costs.

Fourth, the competitive landscape factors into whether or not a firm might benefit from an experience curve strategy. If other competitors are well positioned in the market,

Sources: Ghemawat, P. 1985. Building strategy on the experience curve. *Harvard Business Review*, March–April: 143–149; Porter, M. E. 1996. *On competition*. Boston: Harvard Business Review Press; and, Oster, S. M. 1994. *Modern competitive analysis* (2nd ed.). New York: Oxford University Press.

have strong capital resources, and are known to promote their product lines aggressively to gain market share, an experience curve strategy may lead to nothing more than a price war between two or more strong competitors. But if a company is the first to market with the product and has good financial backing, an experience curve strategy may be successful.

In an article in *Harvard Business Review*, Pankaj Ghemawat recommended answering several questions when considering an experience curve strategy:

- Does my industry exhibit a significant experience curve?
- Have I defined the industry broadly enough to take into account interrelated experience?
- What is the precise source of cost reduction?
- Can my company keep cost reductions proprietary?
- Is demand sufficiently stable to justify using the experience curve?
- Is cumulated output doubling fast enough for the experience curve to provide much strategic leverage?
- Do the returns from an experience curve strategy warrant the risks of technological obsolescence?
- Is demand price sensitive?
- Are there well-financed competitors who are already following an experience curve strategy or are likely to adopt one if my company does?

Michael Porter suggested, however, that the experience curve is not useful in all situations. Whether or not to base strategy on the experience curve depends on what specifically causes the decline in costs. For example, if costs drop from efficient production facilities and not necessarily from experience, the experience curve is not helpful. But as Sharon Oster pointed out in her book on competitive analysis, the experience curve can help managers analyze costs when efficient learning, rather than efficient machinery, is the source of cost savings.

- Avoidance of marginal customer accounts.
- Cost minimization in all activities in the firm's value chain, such as R&D, service, sales force, and advertising.

Exhibit 5.3 draws on the value-chain concept (see Chapter 3) to provide examples of how a firm can attain an overall cost leadership strategy in its primary and support activities.

Key to an overall cost leadership strategy is the **experience curve,** which refers to how business "learns" to lower costs as it gains experience with production processes. With experience, unit costs of production decline as output increases in most industries. The experience curve concept is discussed in Strategy Spotlight 5.1 and Exhibit 5.4.

> **experience curve**
> the decline in unit costs of production as cumulative output increases.

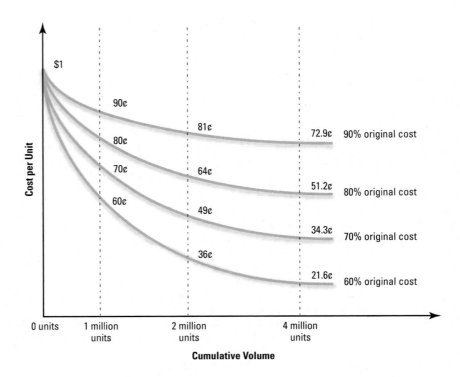

Exhibit 5.4 Comparing Experience Curve Effects

Cost per Unit

$1

90¢

81¢

72.9¢ · 90% original cost

80¢

80¢

70¢

64¢

51.2¢ · 80% original cost

60¢

70¢

49¢

34.3¢ · 70% original cost

60¢

36¢

21.6¢ · 60% original cost

0 units | 1 million units | 2 million units | 4 million units

Cumulative Volume

To generate above-average performance, a firm following an overall cost leadership position must attain **competitive parity** on the basis of differentiation relative to competitors.[8] In other words, a firm achieving parity is similar to its competitors, or "on par," with respect to differentiated products.[9] Competitive parity on the basis of differentiation permits a cost leader to translate cost advantages directly into higher profits than competitors. Thus, the cost leader earns above-average returns.[10]

The failure to attain parity on the basis of differentiation can be illustrated with an example from the automobile industry—the ill-fated Yugo. Below is an excerpt from a speech by J. W. Marriott Jr., chairman of Marriott Corporation:[11]

> . . . money is a big thing. But it's not the only thing. In the 1980s, a new automobile reached North America from behind the Iron Curtain. It was called the Yugo, and its main attraction was price. About $3,000 each. But the only way they caught on was as the butt of jokes. Remember the guy who told his mechanic, "I want a gas cap for my Yugo." "OK," the mechanic replied, "that sounds like a fair trade."

Yugo was offering a lousy value proposition. The cars literally fell apart before your eyes. And the lesson was simple. Price is just one component of value. No matter how good the price, the most cost-sensitive consumer won't buy a bad product.

Next, we discuss some examples of how firms enhance cost leadership position.

While other managed care providers were having a string of weak years, WellPoint, based in Thousand Oaks, California, had a number of banner years and enjoyed an annual profit growth of over 42 percent to $4.8 billion over the past three years.[12] Chairman Leonard Schaeffer credited the company's focus on innovation for both expanding revenues and cutting costs. For example, WellPoint asked the Food and Drug Administration (FDA) to make the allergy drug Claritin available over the counter. Surprisingly, this might have been the first time that an insurer approached the FDA with such a request. Schaeffer claimed, "They were kind of stunned," but the FDA agreed to consider it. It was a smart move for WellPoint. Now approved as an over-the-counter drug, Claritin reduces patient

Ryanair: A Highly Effective Overall Cost Leadership Strategy

Michael O'Leary, CEO of Ryanair Holdings PLC, makes no apologies for his penny-pinching. Want to check luggage? You'll pay up to US $9.50 per bag for the privilege. Expecting free drinks and snacks? You'll be disappointed. Even a bottle of water will cost you $3.40. And it is not just the passengers who are affected. Flight crews buy their own uniforms, and staff at Ryanair's Spartan Dublin Airport headquarters must supply their own pens. After a customer sued Ryanair for charging $34 for the use of a wheelchair, the company added a 63 cents "wheelchair levy" to every ticket!

Low-fare U.S. carriers have taken the opposite approach of Ryanair by adding perks such as leather seats, live television, and business class. "All of the low-cost carriers' costs have gotten a little out of control," said Tim Sieber, general manager of The Boyd Group, an Evergreen (Colorado) aviation consultant. Clearly Ryanair hasn't followed its industry peers.

Ryanair has been extremely successful. It recently became the first airline in Europe to carry more than 7 million passengers in one month. As of late 2010, the company had a market capitalization of $7.2 billion, dwarfing competitors easyJet ($2.3 billion) and Ireland's legacy airline, Aer Lingus ($612 million), but it is still a bit short of U.S. counterpart Southwest ($8.29 billion) and Delta ($8.22 billion). Over the past decade, at a time when the global airline industry collectively lost nearly $50 billion, Ryanair turned healthy net profits in 9 out of the 10 years—earning $431 million in the most recent year. In the process, O'Leary has become one of Ireland's wealthiest citizens—the value of his Ryanair shares is nearly $300 million.

What is O'Leary's secret? He thinks like a retailer and charges for every little thing. Imagine the seat as a cell

Sources: Gillete, F. 2010. The duke of discomfort. *Bloomberg Businessweek* September 12: 58–61; *Ryanair Annual Report*, 2008; Capell, K. 2006. Wal-Mart with wings. *BusinessWeek*. November 27: 44–45; Kumar, N. 2006. Strategies to fight low-cost rivals. *Harvard Business Review*, 84(12): 104–113; and, *Ryanair Annual Report*, 2006.

phone: It comes free, or nearly free, but its owner winds up spending money on all sorts of services.

However, what O'Leary loses in seat revenue he more than makes up by turning both his planes and the Ryanair website into stores brimming with irresistible goodies, even as he charges for such "perks" as priority boarding and assigned seating.

Sound outrageous? Probably so, but the strategy is clearly working. Although its average fare is $53, compared with $92 for Southwest Airlines, Ryanair's net margins are, at 18 percent, more than double the 7 percent achieved by Southwest. Said Nick van den Brul, an aviation analyst: "Ryanair is Walmart with wings." As O'Leary said, "You want luxury? Go somewhere else."

A few other Ryanair practices include:

- Flight attendants sell digital cameras ($137.50) and iPocket MP3 players ($165).

- The seats don't recline, seat-back pockets have been removed to cut cleaning time and speed turn-around of the planes, there's no entertainment, and seat-back trays will soon carry ads.

- Ryanair sells more than 98 percent of its tickets online. Its website offers insurance, hotels, car rentals, and more—even online bingo.

O'Leary is certainly a colorful person, and he has some "creative" or downright nutty ideas. Recently, he came up with the idea of replacing the last 10 rows with a standing cabin, outfitted with handrails, much like a New York City subway car, only without the benches and panhandlers. The increased capacity, he claimed, would lower fares by 20 percent to 25 percent. He said: "In no plane ever operated by Ryanair will it be all standing. You will always have the choice of paying for the seat. The argument against it is that if there's ever a crash, people will be injured. If there's ever a crash, the people in the sit-down seats will be injured, too."

visits to the doctor and eliminated the need for prescriptions—two reimbursable expenses for which WellPoint would otherwise have been responsible.

Stephen Sanger, CEO of General Mills, also came up with an idea that helped his firm cut costs.[13] To improve productivity, he sent technicians to watch pit crews during a NASCAR race. That experience inspired the techies to figure out how to reduce the time it takes to switch a plant line from five hours to 20 minutes. This provided an important lesson: Many interesting benchmarking examples can take place far outside of an industry. Often, process improvements involve identifying the best practices in other industries and adapting them for implementation in your own firm. After all, when firms benchmark competitors in their own industry, the end result is often copying and playing catch-up.[14]

A business that strives for a low-cost advantage must attain an absolute cost advantage relative to its rivals.[15] This is typically accomplished by offering a no-frills product or service to a broad target market using standardization to derive the greatest benefits from economies of scale and experience. However, such a strategy may fail if a firm is unable to attain parity on important dimensions of differentiation such as quick responses to customer requests for services or design changes. Strategy Spotlight 5.2 discusses Ryanair—a low-cost airline that has developed a very unique overall cost leadership strategy. One might say that it "one-upped" U.S.-based Southwest Airlines!

>LO5.2
How the successful attainment of generic strategies can improve a firm's relative power vis-à-vis the five forces that determine an industry's average profitability.

Overall Cost Leadership: Improving Competitive Position vis-à-vis the Five Forces An overall low-cost position enables a firm to achieve above-average returns despite strong competition. It protects a firm against rivalry from competitors, because lower costs allow a firm to earn returns even if its competitors eroded their profits through intense rivalry. A low-cost position also protects firms against powerful buyers. Buyers can exert power to drive down prices only to the level of the next most efficient producer. Also, a low-cost position provides more flexibility to cope with demands from powerful suppliers for input cost increases. The factors that lead to a low-cost position also provide substantial entry barriers from economies of scale and cost advantages. Finally, a low-cost position puts the firm in a favorable position with respect to substitute products introduced by new and existing competitors.[16]

A few examples will illustrate these points. Ryanair's close attention to costs helps to protect it from buyer power and intense rivalry from competitors. Thus, it is able to drive down costs and enjoy relatively high power over its customers. By increasing productivity and lowering unit costs, General Mills (and its competitors in that industry) enjoys greater scale economies and erects higher entry barriers for others. Having sufficient control over suppliers allows firms to lower costs. Walmart, with its economies of scale, exercises lots of bargaining power over its suppliers. An important aspect of the unique Toyota Production System is strong supplier relationships and their continuing development. Finally, as competitors such as WellPoint lower costs through means such as petitioning the FDA to make certain drugs available over the counter, they become less vulnerable to substitutes such as Internet-based competitors.

>LO5.3
The pitfalls managers must avoid in striving to attain generic strategies.

Potential Pitfalls of Overall Cost Leadership Strategies Potential pitfalls of overall cost leadership strategy include:

- *Too much focus on one or a few value-chain activities.* Would you consider a person to be astute if he cancelled his newspaper subscription and quit eating out to save money, but then "maxed out" several credit cards, requiring him to pay hundreds of dollars a month in interest charges? Of course not. Similarly, firms need to pay attention to all activities in the value chain.[17] Too often managers make big cuts in operating expenses, but don't question year-to-year spending on capital projects. Or managers may decide to cut selling and marketing expenses but ignore manufacturing expenses. Managers should explore *all* value-chain activities, including relationships among them, as candidates for cost reductions.
- *All rivals share a common input or raw material.* Here, firms are vulnerable to price increases in the factors of production. Since they're competing on costs, they are less able to pass on price increases, because customers can take their business to rivals who have lower prices. For example, consider manufacturing firms based in China that rely on a common input—low labor costs. Due to demographic factors, the supply of workers 16 to 24 years old has peaked and will drop by a third in the next 12 years, thanks to stringent family-planning policies that have sharply reduced China's population growth.[18] In one city, many factories are operating with vacancies of 15 to 20 percent, compelling some supervisors to cruise the streets in a desperate hiring quest during crunch times. Needless to say, there are strong demands for better working conditions and higher wages.

- **The strategy is imitated too easily.** One of the common pitfalls of a cost leadership strategy is that a firm's strategy may consist of value-creating activities that are easy to imitate.[19] Such was the case with online brokers in recent years.[20] As of early 2001, there were about 140 online brokers, hardly symbolic of an industry where imitation is extremely difficult. But according to Henry McVey, financial services analyst at Morgan Stanley, "We think you need five to ten" online brokers.

  What are some of the dynamics? First, although online brokers were geared up to handle 1.2 million trades a day, volume had shrunk to about 834,000—a 30 percent drop. Thus, competition for business intensified. Second, when the stock market is down, many investors trust their instincts less and seek professional guidance from brokerages that offer differentiated services. Eric Rajendra of A. T. Kearney, an international consulting company, claimed, "The current (online broker) model is inadequate for the pressures the industry is facing now."

- **A lack of parity on differentiation.** As noted earlier, firms striving to attain cost leadership advantages must obtain a level of parity on differentiation.[21] Firms providing online degree programs may offer low prices. However, they may not be successful unless they can offer instruction that is perceived as comparable to traditional providers. For them, parity can be achieved on differentiation dimensions such as reputation and quality and through signaling mechanisms such as accreditation agencies.

- **Erosion of cost advantages when the pricing information available to customers increases.** This is becoming a more significant challenge as the Internet dramatically increases both the quantity and volume of information available to consumers about pricing and cost structures. Life insurance firms offering whole life insurance provide an interesting example.[22] One study found that, for each 10 percent increase in consumer use of the Internet, there is a corresponding reduction in insurance prices to consumers of 3 to 5 percent. Recently, the nationwide savings (or, alternatively, reduced revenues to providers) was between $115 and $125 million annually.

Differentiation

As the name implies, a **differentiation strategy** consists of creating differences in the firm's product or service offering by creating something that is perceived *industrywide* as unique and valued by customers.[23] Differentiation can take many forms:

> **differentiation strategy** a firm's generic strategy based on creating differences in the firm's product or service offering by creating something that is perceived *industrywide* as unique and valued by customers.

- Prestige or brand image (Adam's Mark hotels, BMW automobiles, Rolex watches).[24]
- Technology (Martin guitars, Marantz stereo components, North Face camping equipment).
- Innovation (LG air conditioners, Apple's iPads).
- Features (Cannondale mountain bikes, Honda Goldwing motorcycles).
- Customer service (American Express, Sears lawn equipment retailing).
- Dealer network (Lexus automobiles, Caterpillar earthmoving equipment).
- Design (Bang & Olufsen audio systems, Diesel blue jeans).
- Materials and packaging (The Body Shop products, Nokia Chocolate phones).

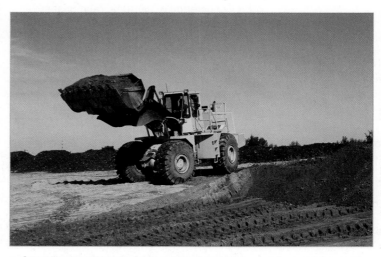

● Caterpillar is well known for its outstanding dealer network around the world.

Exhibit 5.5
**Value-Chain Activities:
Examples of
Differentiation**

Support Activities

Firm Infrastructure

- Superior MIS—to integrate value-creating activities to improve quality.
- Facilities that promote firm image.
- Widely respected CEO who enhances firm reputation.

Human Resource Management

- Programs to attract talented engineers and scientists.
- Training and incentives to ensure a strong customer service orientation.

Technology Development

- Superior material handling and sorting technology.
- Excellent applications engineering support.

Procurement

- Purchase of high-quality components to enhance product image.
- Use of most prestigious outlets.

Primary Activities

Inbound Logistics

- Superior material handling operations to minimize damage.
- Quick transfer of inputs to manufacturing process.

Operations

- Flexibility and speed in responding to changes in manufacturing specifications.
- Low defect rates to improve quality.

Outbound Logistics

- Accurate and responsive order processing.
- Effective product replenishment to reduce customer inventory.

Marketing and Sales

- Creative and innovative advertising programs.
- Fostering of personal relationship with key customers.

Service

- Rapid response to customer service requests.
- Complete inventory of replacement parts and supplies.

Source: Adapted from Porter, M.E. 1985. *Competitive advantage: Creating and sustaining superior performance*. New York: Free Press.

Exhibit 5.5 draws on the concept of the value chain as an example of how firms may differentiate themselves in primary and support activities.

Firms may differentiate themselves along several different dimensions at once.[25] For example, BMW is known for its high prestige, superior engineering, and high-quality automobiles. And Harley-Davidson differentiates on image and dealer services.[26]

Firms achieve and sustain differentiation advantages and attain above-average performance when their price premiums exceed the extra costs incurred in being unique.[27]

For example, both BMW and Harley-Davidson must increase consumer costs to offset added marketing expenses. Thus, a differentiator will always seek out ways of distinguishing itself from similar competitors to justify price premiums greater than the costs incurred by differentiating.[28] Clearly, a differentiator cannot ignore costs. After all, its premium prices would be eroded by a markedly inferior cost position. Therefore, it must attain a level of cost *parity* relative to competitors. Differentiators can do this by reducing costs in all areas that do not affect differentiation. Porsche, for example, invests heavily in engine design—an area in which its customers demand excellence—but it is less concerned and spends fewer resources in the design of the instrument panel or the arrangement of switches on the radio.[29]

Many companies successfully follow a differentiation strategy.[30] For example, John Mullen, CEO of DHL Express, noted that differentiation even for the world's largest expedited and express companies can come through size and strength:

> Differentiation is always a challenge. We all have our strengths. Obviously UPS is a powerful ground player in the United States. FedEx is extremely strong in the air. Our differentiation is that, while we are weak in the United States, we are the leader in the rest of the world. We have a full portfolio of products and a larger market share. That said, all of us are vulnerable.
>
> If a customer is in Hong Kong and all they do is send bank documents to London, there are lots of little players who will probably beat us on both speed and price since they've only got a couple of containers to put on a plane and take off on the other end. We have a whole aircraft to unload. But if the customer wants a Pan-Asian solution or a pan-global solution, with all sorts of complicated supply chain components and everything else, then obviously the small competitors can't play in that field at all. So, we have differentiation around the scale of our global network. It has size and strength. We offer full integration of everything from shipping to documents and the ability to provide that anywhere in the world.[31]

Lexus, a division of Toyota, provides an example of how a firm can strengthen its differentiation strategy by *achieving integration at multiple points along the value chain.*[32] Although the luxury car line was not introduced until the late 1980s, by the early 1990s the cars had already soared to the top of J. D. Power & Associates' customer satisfaction ratings.

> In the spirit of benchmarking, one of Lexus's competitors hired Custom Research Inc. (CRI), a marketing research firm, to find out why Lexus owners were so satisfied. CRI conducted a series of focus groups in which Lexus drivers eagerly offered anecdotes about the special care they experienced from their dealers. It became clear that, although Lexus was manufacturing cars with few mechanical defects, it was the extra care shown by the sales and service staff that resulted in satisfied customers. Such pampering is reflected in the feedback from one customer who claimed she never had a problem with her Lexus. However, upon further probing, she said, "Well, I suppose you could call the four times they had to replace the windshield a 'problem.' But frankly, they took care of it so well and always gave me a loaner car, so I never really considered it a problem until you mentioned it now." An insight gained in CRI's research is that perceptions of product quality (design, engineering, and manufacturing) can be strongly influenced by downstream activities in the value chain (marketing and sales, service).

Strategy Spotlight 5.3 addresses how Netflix, the successful Internet movie rental company, uses crowdsourcing to enhance its differentiation.

Differentiation: Improving Competitive Position vis-à-vis the Five Forces
Differentiation provides protection against rivalry since brand loyalty lowers customer sensitivity to price and raises customer switching costs.[33] By increasing a firm's margins, differentiation also avoids the need for a low-cost position. Higher entry barriers result because of customer loyalty and the firm's ability to provide uniqueness in its products or services.[34] Differentiation also provides higher margins that enable a firm to deal with supplier power.

Crowdsourcing: How Netflix Boosts Its Differentiation

Netflix is well-known for its inviting online presentation and efficient distribution system. However, this highly successful movie-rental company prides itself on its capability to offer subscribers a compact list of films that they are likely to enjoy watching. And it must be working: Netflix sends 35,000 titles a day to its 7.5 million subscribers.

"Imagine that our website [is] a brick-and-mortar store," said Netflix vice president, James Bennett. "When people walk through the door, they see DVDs rearrange themselves. The movies that might interest them fly onto the shelves, and all the rest go to the back room."

The movies, of course, don't do the rearranging—that is done by the customers themselves, with an assist from a computer program called Cinematch, which Netflix developed in 2000. Customers are invited to rate each film they watch on a 1 to 5 scale. Cinematch analyzes these ratings, searches through 80,000 titles in inventory, and determines the list of films tailored to the taste of each of the firm's subscribers. By enticing them to rate films, Netflix achieves the latest in business innovation—getting customers to serve themselves.

Netflix is not unique in its use of so-called recommenders. Consider other online retailers such as Amazon, Apple, eBay, and Overstock. All of these rely on their customers for a helping hand in predicting what products the customers will prefer—whether the product is bedding, books, CDs, or DVDs. Customer ratings are used to rank corporate service providers as well.

For all these companies, the recommender system provides more than a chance to create an extra service. It helps them to establish a stronger connection with their customers. And studies have shown that it can substantially increase online sales.

Sources: Copeland, M.V. 2009. Tapping tech's beautiful minds. *Fortune* October 12: 35–36; Libert, B. & Spector, J. 2008. *We are smarter than me*. Philadelphia: Wharton Publishing; and, Howe, J. 2008. *Crowdsourcing*. New York: Crown Business.

The extent of Netflix's commitment to personalized movie recommendations was made clear in 2006 when it offered a $1 million prize to anyone who could build a system that was at least 10 percent better than Cinematch. In late 2009, it awarded the prize to a seven-person team of computer scientists, mathematicians, and statisticians who were from New Jersey, Israel, Quebec, and Austria. They built a system that was 20 percent better than Cinematch.

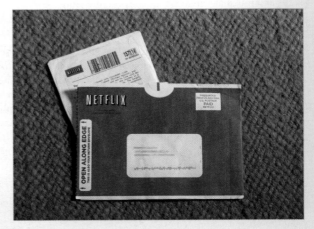

● Netflix generated a lot of favorable publicity with its $1 million prize competition.

Netflix has also developed another crowdsourcing feature called Friends. Here, subscribers see each other's list of films watched and compare the ratings they have awarded the films—in exchange for suggestions on other films to watch.

crowdsourcing

And it reduces buyer power, because buyers lack comparable alternatives and are therefore less price sensitive.[35] Supplier power is also decreased because there is a certain amount of prestige associated with being the supplier to a producer of highly differentiated products and services. Last, differentiation enhances customer loyalty, thus reducing the threat from substitutes.[36]

Our examples illustrate these points. Lexus has enjoyed enhanced power over buyers because its top J. D. Power ranking makes buyers more willing to pay a premium price. This lessens rivalry, since buyers become less price sensitive. The prestige associated with its brand name also lowers supplier power since margins are high. Suppliers would probably desire to be associated with prestige brands, thus lessening their incentives to drive up prices. Finally, the loyalty and "peace of mind" associated with a service provider such as FedEx makes such firms less vulnerable to rivalry or substitute products and services.

Potential Pitfalls of Differentiation Strategies   Potential pitfalls of a differentiation strategy include:

- *Uniqueness that is not valuable.* A differentiation strategy must provide unique bundles of products and/or services that customers value highly. It's not enough just to be "different." An example is Gibson's Dobro bass guitar. Gibson came up with a unique idea: Design and build an acoustic bass guitar with sufficient sound volume so that amplification wasn't necessary. The problem with other acoustic bass guitars was that they did not project enough volume because of the low-frequency bass notes. By adding a resonator plate on the body of the traditional acoustic bass, Gibson increased the sound volume. Gibson believed this product would serve a particular niche market—bluegrass and folk artists who played in small group "jams" with other acoustic musicians. Unfortunately, Gibson soon discovered that its targeted market was content with their existing options: an upright bass amplified with a microphone or an acoustic electric guitar. Thus, Gibson developed a unique product, but it was not perceived as valuable by its potential customers.[37]

- *Too much differentiation.* Firms may strive for quality or service that is higher than customers desire.[38] Thus, they become vulnerable to competitors who provide an appropriate level of quality at a lower price. For example, consider the expensive Mercedes-Benz S-Class, which ranges in price between $93,650 and $138,000 for the 2011 models.[39] *Consumer Reports* described it as "sumptuous," "quiet and luxurious," and a "delight to drive." The magazine also considered it to be the least reliable sedan available in the United States. According to David Champion, who runs *Consumer Reports'* testing program, the problems are electronic. "The engineers have gone a little wild," he said. "They've put every bell and whistle that they think of, and sometimes they don't have the attention to detail to make these systems work." Some features include: a computer-driven suspension that reduces body roll as the vehicle whips around a corner; cruise control that automatically slows the car down if it gets too close to another car; and seats that are adjustable 14 ways and that are ventilated by a system that uses eight fans.

- *Too high a price premium.* This pitfall is quite similar to too much differentiation. Customers may desire the product, but they are repelled by the price premium. For example, Duracell (a division of Gillette) recently charged too much for batteries.[40] The firm tried to sell consumers on its superior quality products, but the mass market wasn't convinced. Why? The price differential was simply too high. At a CVS drugstore just one block from Gillette's headquarters, a four-pack of Energizer AA batteries was on sale at $2.99 compared with a Duracell four-pack at $4.59. Duracell's market share dropped 2 percent in a recent period, and its profits declined over 30 percent. Clearly, the price/performance proposition Duracell offered customers was not accepted.

- *Differentiation that is easily imitated.* As we noted in Chapter 3, resources that are easily imitated cannot lead to sustainable advantages. For example, many of Singapore Airlines' physical assets (e.g., aircraft, spare parts, reservation systems) may be easily imitated. Competitors could match the physical assets required to run the company. However, the complexity of the interconnectedness of the company's history, culture, processes, and relationships with customers and suppliers worldwide has allowed it to be consistently rated as one of the world's best airlines. Similarly, firms may strive for, and even attain, a differentiation strategy that is successful for a time. However, the advantages are eroded through imitation. Consider Groupon, one of the most successful Internet coupon companies. As one would expect, once the Groupon idea proved successful, competitors entered the market because much of the initial risk had already been taken. As Groupon struggles to get its IPO (initial stock offering) off the ground, it remains to be seen whether the idea of coupon companies will last or fade from the Internet landscape.[41] One thing's for sure: There will continue to be many Groupon imitators around the globe.

- ***Dilution of brand identification through product-line extensions.*** Firms may erode their quality brand image by adding products or services with lower prices and less quality. Although this can increase short-term revenues, it may be detrimental in the long run. Consider Gucci.[42] In the 1980s Gucci wanted to capitalize on its prestigious brand name by launching an aggressive strategy of revenue growth. It added a set of lower-priced canvas goods to its product line. It also pushed goods heavily into department stores and duty-free channels and allowed its name to appear on a host of licensed items such as watches, eyeglasses, and perfumes. In the short term, this strategy worked. Sales soared. However, the strategy carried a high price. Gucci's indiscriminate approach to expanding its products and channels tarnished its sterling brand. Sales of its high-end goods (with higher profit margins) fell, causing profits to decline.

- ***Perceptions of differentiation may vary between buyers and sellers.*** The issue here is that "beauty is in the eye of the beholder." Companies must realize that although they may perceive their products and services as differentiated, their customers may view them as commodities. Indeed, in today's marketplace, many products and services have been reduced to commodities.[43] Thus, a firm could overprice its offerings and lose margins altogether if it has to lower prices to reflect market realities.

Exhibit 5.6 summarizes the pitfalls of overall cost leadership and differentiation strategies. In addressing the pitfalls associated with these two generic strategies there is one common, underlying theme. Managers must be aware of the dangers associated with concentrating so much on one strategy that they fail to attain parity on the other.

Exhibit 5.6 Potential Pitfalls of Overall Cost Leadership and Differentiation Strategies

Overall Cost Leadership:
- Too much focus on one or a few value-chain activities.
- All rivals share a common input or raw material.
- The strategy is imitated too easily.
- A lack of parity on differentiation.
- Erosion of cost advantages when the pricing information available to customers increases.

Differentiation:
- Uniqueness that is not valuable.
- Too much differentiation.
- The price premium is too high.
- Differentiation that is easily imitated.
- Dilution of brand identification through product-line extensions.
- Perceptions of differentiation may vary between buyers and sellers.

Focus

A **focus strategy** is based on the choice of a narrow competitive scope within an industry. A firm following this strategy selects a segment or group of segments and tailors its strategy to serve them. The essence of focus is the exploitation of a particular market niche. As you might expect, narrow focus itself (like merely "being different" as a differentiator) is simply not sufficient for above-average performance.

focus strategy a firm's generic strategy based on appeal to a narrow market segment within an industry.

The focus strategy, as indicated in Exhibit 5.1, has two variants. In a cost focus, a firm strives to create a cost advantage in its target segment. In a differentiation focus, a firm seeks to differentiate in its target market. Both variants of the focus strategy rely on providing better service than broad-based competitors who are trying to serve the focuser's target segment. Cost focus exploits differences in cost behavior in some segments, while differentiation focus exploits the special needs of buyers in other segments.

Let's look at examples of two firms that have successfully implemented focus strategies. Network Appliance (NA) has developed a more cost-effective way to store and distribute computer files.[44] Its larger rival, EMC, makes mainframe-style products priced over $1 million that store files and accommodate Internet traffic. NA makes devices that cost under $200,000 for particular storage jobs such as caching (temporary storage) of Internet content. Focusing on such narrow segments has certainly paid off for NA; it has posted a remarkable 20 straight quarters of revenue growth.

Paccar, an $8 billion Bellevue, Washington–based heavy-truck manufacturer, has chosen a differentiation focus strategy.[45] The firm targets one group of customers: owner-operators. These are the drivers who own their trucks and contract directly with shippers or serve as subcontractors to larger trucking companies.

Paccar has invested heavily to develop a variety of features with owner-operators in mind: luxurious sleeper cabins, plush leather seats, noise-insulated cabins, sleek exterior styling, and so forth. At Paccar's extensive network of dealers, prospective buyers use software to select among thousands of options to put their personal signature on their trucks. These customized trucks are built to order, not to stock, and are delivered in eight weeks. Not surprisingly, customers are happy to pay Paccar a 10 percent premium, and its Kenworth and Peterbilt brands are considered status symbols at truck stops.

Strategy Spotlight 5.4 illustrates that you can pay as much as you want for some products or services. Case in point: luxury car rentals around the world.

Focus: Improving Competitive Position vis-à-vis the Five Forces   Focus requires that a firm either have a low-cost position with its strategic target, high differentiation, or both. As we discussed with regard to cost and differentiation strategies, these positions provide defenses against each competitive force. Focus is also used to select niches that are least vulnerable to substitutes or where competitors are weakest.

Let's look at our examples to illustrate some of these points. First, Paccar experienced lower rivalry and greater bargaining power by providing products and services to a targeted market segment that was less price sensitive. New rivals have difficulty attracting customers away from Paccar based only on lower prices. Similarly, the brand image and quality that this brand evoked heightened rivals' entry barriers. With regard to the strategy of cost focus, Network Appliances, the successful rival to EMC in the computer storage industry, was better able to absorb pricing increases from suppliers as a result of its lower cost structure, reducing supplier power.

Potential Pitfalls of Focus Strategies   Potential pitfalls of focus strategies include:

- *Erosion of cost advantages within the narrow segment.* The advantages of a cost focus strategy may be fleeting if the cost advantages are eroded over time. For example, Dell's pioneering direct selling model in the personal computer industry has been eroded by rivals such as Hewlett-Packard as they gain experience with Dell's distribution method. Similarly, other firms have seen their profit margins drop as competitors enter their product segment.

- *Even product and service offerings that are highly focused are subject to competition from new entrants and from imitation.* Some firms adopting a focus strategy may enjoy temporary advantages because they select a small niche with few rivals. However, their advantages may be short-lived. A notable example is the multitude of dot-com firms that specialize in very narrow segments such as pet supplies, ethnic foods, and vintage automobile accessories. The entry barriers tend to be low, there is little buyer loyalty, and competition becomes intense. And since the marketing strategies and technologies employed by most rivals are largely nonproprietary, imitation is easy. Over time, revenues fall, profits margins are squeezed, and only the strongest players survive the shakeout.

- *Focusers can become too focused to satisfy buyer needs.* Some firms attempting to attain advantages through a focus strategy may have too narrow a product or service. Consider many retail firms. Hardware chains such as Ace and True Value are losing market share to rivals such as Lowe's and Home Depot that offer a full line of home and garden equipment and accessories. And given the enormous purchasing power of the national chains, it would be difficult for such specialty retailers to attain parity on costs.

> **>LO5.4**
> How firms can effectively combine the generic strategies of overall cost leadership and differentiation.

Combination Strategies: Integrating Overall Low Cost and Differentiation

Perhaps the primary benefit to firms that integrate low-cost and differentiation strategies is the difficulty for rivals to duplicate or imitate. This strategy enables a firm to provide two types of value to customers: differentiated attributes (e.g., high quality, brand identification, reputation) and lower prices (because of the firm's lower costs in value-creating activities). The goal is thus to provide unique value to customers in an efficient manner.[46] Some firms are able to attain both types of advantages simultaneously.[47] For example, superior quality can lead to lower costs because of less need for rework in manufacturing, fewer warranty claims, a reduced need for customer service personnel to resolve customer complaints, and so forth. Thus, the benefits of combining advantages, using **combination strategies,** can be additive, instead of merely involving trade-offs. Next, we consider three approaches to combining overall low cost and differentiation.

Automated and Flexible Manufacturing Systems   Given the advances in manufacturing technologies such as CAD/CAM (computer-aided design and computer-aided manufacturing) as well as information technologies, many firms have been able to manufacture unique products in relatively small quantities at lower costs—a concept known as **mass customization.**[48]

Let's consider Andersen Windows of Bayport, Minnesota in the United States—a $3 billion global manufacturer of windows for the building industry.[49] Until about 20 years ago, Andersen was a mass producer, in small batches, of a variety of standard windows. However, to meet changing customer needs, Andersen kept adding to its product line. The result was catalogs of ever-increasing size and a bewildering set of choices for both homeowners and contractors. Over a 6-year period, the number of products tripled, price quotes took several hours, and the error rate increased. This not only damaged the company's reputation, but also added to its manufacturing expenses.

To bring about a major change, Andersen developed an interactive computer version of its paper catalogs that it sold to distributors and retailers. Salespersons can now customize each window to meet the customer's needs, check the design for structural soundness, and provide a price quote. The system is virtually error free, customers get exactly what they want, and the time to develop the design and furnish a quotation has been cut by 75 percent. Each showroom computer is connected to the factory, and customers are assigned a code number that permits them to track the order. The manufacturing system has been developed to use some common finished parts, but it also allows considerable variation in the final products. Despite its huge investment, Andersen has been able to lower costs, enhance quality and variety, and improve its response time to customers.

Exhibit 5.7 provides other examples of how flexible production systems have enabled firms to successfully engage in mass customization for their customers.[50]

combination strategies firms' integrations of various strategies to provide multiple types of value to customers.

mass customization a firm's ability to manufacture unique products in small quantities at low cost.

- At Nikeid.com, customers can design an athletic or casual shoe to their specifications online, selecting almost every element of the shoe from the material of the sole to the color of the shoelace.

- Apf of France sells custom perfumes. Each product is created in response to a user profile constructed from responses to a survey about habits and preferences. Apf then provides a sample at modest cost to verify fit.

- Lands' End offers customized shirts and pants. Consumers specify style parameters, measurements, and fabrics through the firm's website. These settings are saved so that returning users can easily order a duplicate item.

- Cannondale permits consumers to specify the parameters that define a road bike frame, including custom colors and inscriptions. The user specifies the parameters on the firm's website and then arranges for delivery through a dealer.

- Kirby Allison's Hanger Project specializes in the development of unique luxury wooden hangers for men's and women's clothing. The hangers are created per the customer's style and requirements and finished to exacting specifications.

Exhibit 5.7 Effective Uses of Flexible Production Systems

Source: Randall, T., Terwiesch, C, & Ulrich, K. T. 2005. Principles for user design of customized products. *California Management Review,* 47(4): 68–85; and, Kirby Allison's hanger project, *www.hangerproject.com,* accessed October 4, 2011.

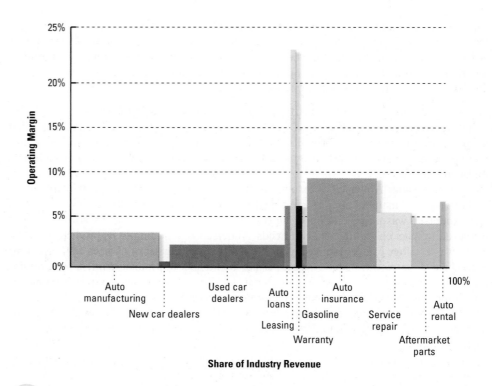

Exhibit 5.8 The U.S. Automobile Industry's Profit Pool

Source: Reprinted by permission of *Harvard Business Review,* Exhibit from "Profit Pools: A Fresh Look at Strategy," by O. Gadiesh and J. L. Gilbert, May–June 1999. Copyright © 1999 by the Harvard Business School Publishing Corporation; all rights reserved.

profit pool the total profits in an industry at all points along the industry's value chain.

Exploiting the Profit Pool Concept for Competitive Advantage A **profit pool** is defined as the total profits in an industry at all points along the industry's value chain.[51] Although the concept is relatively straightforward, the structure of the profit pool can be complex.[52] The potential pool of profits will be deeper in some segments of the value chain than in others, and the depths will vary within an individual segment. Segment profitability may vary widely by customer group, product category, geographic market, or distribution channel. Additionally, the pattern of profit concentration in an industry is very often different from the pattern of revenue generation.

Consider the automobile industry profit pool in Exhibit 5.8. Here we see little relationship between the generation of revenues and capturing of profits. While manufacturing generates most of the revenue, this value activity is far smaller profitwise than other value activities such as financing and extended warranty operations. So while a car manufacturer may be under tremendous pressure to produce cars efficiently, much of the profit (at least proportionately) can be captured in the aforementioned downstream operations. Thus, a carmaker would be ill-advised to focus solely on manufacturing and leave downstream operations to others through outsourcing.

Coordinating the "Extended" Value Chain by Way of Information Technology
Many firms have achieved success by integrating activities throughout the "extended value chain" by using information technology to link their own value chain with the value chains of their customers and suppliers. As noted in Chapter 3, this approach enables a firm to add value not only through its own value-creating activities, but also for its customers and suppliers.

Such a strategy often necessitates redefining the industry's value chain. A number of years ago, Walmart took a close look at its industry's value chain and decided to reframe the competitive challenge.[53] Although its competitors were primarily focused on retailing—merchandising and promotion—Walmart determined that it was not so much in the retailing industry as in the transportation logistics and communications industries. Here, linkages in the extended value chain became central. That became Walmart's chosen battleground. By redefining the rules of competition that played to its strengths, Walmart has attained competitive advantages and dominates its industry.

Integrated Overall Low-Cost and Differentiation Strategies: Improving Competitive Position vis-à-vis the Five Forces Firms that successfully integrate both differentiation and cost advantages create an enviable position. For example, Walmart's integration of information systems, logistics, and transportation helps it to drive down costs and provide outstanding product selection. This dominant competitive position serves to erect high entry barriers to potential competitors that have neither the financial nor physical resources to compete head-to-head. Walmart's size—over $400 billion in 2011 sales—provides the chain with enormous bargaining power over suppliers. Its low pricing and wide selection reduce the power of buyers (its customers), because there are relatively few competitors that can provide a comparable cost/value proposition. This reduces the possibility of intense head-to-head rivalry, such as protracted price wars. Finally, Walmart's overall value proposition makes potential substitute products (e.g., Internet competitors) a less viable threat.

Pitfalls of Integrated Overall Cost Leadership and Differentiation Strategies
The pitfalls of integrated overall cost leadership and differentiation include:

- *Firms that fail to attain both strategies may end up with neither and become "stuck in the middle."* A key issue in strategic management is the creation of competitive advantages that enable a firm to enjoy above-average returns. Some firms may become "stuck in the middle" if they try to attain both cost and differentiation advantages. An example that we are all familiar with would be the Big 3 U.S. automobile makers. They have been plagued by expensive "legacy costs" associated with pension and health care obligations—a central issue in 2008 federal bailout legislation. And they suffer from long-term customer perceptions of mediocre quality—inferior to their European and Japanese rivals. The troubling quality perceptions persist despite the fact that the Big 3 has attained approximate parity with their Japanese and European competitors in recent J. D. Power surveys.

- *Underestimating the challenges and expenses associated with coordinating value-creating activities in the extended value chain.* Integrating activities across a firm's value chain with the value chain of suppliers and customers involves a significant investment in financial and human resources. Firms must consider the expenses linked to technology investment, managerial time and commitment, and the involvement and investment required by the firm's customers and suppliers. The firm must be confident that it can generate a sufficient scale of operations and revenues to justify all associated expenses.

- *Miscalculating sources of revenue and profit pools in the firm's industry.* Firms may fail to accurately assess sources of revenue and profits in their value chain. This can occur for several reasons. For example, a manager may be biased due to his or her functional area background, work experiences, and educational background. If the manager's background is in engineering, he or she might perceive that proportionately greater revenue and margins were being created in manufacturing, product, and process design than a person whose background is in a "downstream" value-chain activity such as marketing and sales. Or politics could make managers "fudge" the numbers to favor their area of operations. This would make them responsible for a greater proportion of the firm's profits, thus improving their bargaining position.

A related problem is directing an overwhelming amount of managerial time, attention, and resources to value-creating activities that produce the greatest margins—to the detriment of other important, albeit less profitable, activities. For example, a car manufacturer may focus too much on downstream activities, such as warranty fulfillment and financing operations, to the detriment of differentiation and cost of the cars themselves.

>LO5.5
What factors determine the sustainability of a firm's competitive advantage.

Can Competitive Strategies Be Sustained? Integrating and Applying Strategic Management Concepts

Thus far this chapter has addressed how firms can attain competitive advantages in the marketplace. We discussed the three generic strategies—overall cost leadership, differentiation, and focus—as well as combination strategies. Next we discussed the importance of linking value-chain activities (both those within the firm and those linkages between the firm's suppliers and customers) to attain such advantages. We also showed how successful competitive strategies enable firms to strengthen their position vis-à-vis the five forces of industry competition as well as how to avoid the pitfalls associated with the strategies.

Competitive advantages are, however, often short-lived. As we discussed in the beginning of Chapter 1, the composition of the firms that constitute the Fortune 500 list has experienced significant turnover in its membership over the years—reflecting the temporary nature of competitive advantages. And recall Dell's fall from grace (Chapter 3). Here was a firm whose advantages in the marketplace seemed unassailable in the early 2000s. In fact, it was *Fortune*'s "Most Admired Firm" in 2005. However, cracks began to appear in 2007, and its competitive position has recently been severely eroded by rivals such as Hewlett-Packard. In short, Dell focused so much on operational efficiency and perfecting its "direct model" that it failed to deliver innovations that an increasingly sophisticated market demanded. Also, Dell continues to face further pricing pressures as a result of the commoditization of the personal computer industry.[54]

Clearly, "nothing is forever" when it comes to competitive advantages. Rapid changes in technology, globalization, and actions by rivals from within—as well as outside—the industry can quickly erode a firm's advantages. It is becoming increasingly important to recognize that the duration of competitive advantages is declining, especially in technology-intensive industries.[55] Even in industries that are normally viewed as "low tech," the increasing use of technology has suddenly made competitive advantages less sustainable.[56] Amazon's success in book retailing at the cost of Borders, the former industry leader, as well as Blockbuster's struggle against Netflix in the video rental industry serve to illustrate how difficult it has become for industry leaders to sustain competitive advantages that they once thought would last forever. Because of competition from other video rental companies, Blockbuster has seen significant revenue losses. The company filed for bankruptcy in September 2010, and in April 2011, it was won at auction by satellite provider Dish Network for $233 million (including the assumption of $87 million in liabilities and other obligations). Similarly, Borders filed bankruptcy in 2011 and had closed all stores by the end of the year.

In this section, we will discuss some factors that help determine whether a strategy is sustainable over a long period of time. We will draw on some strategic management concepts from the first five chapters. To illustrate our points, we will look at a company, Atlas Door, which created an innovative strategy in its industry and enjoyed superior performance for several years. Our discussion of Atlas Door draws on a *Harvard Business Review* article by George Stalk Jr.[57] It was published some time ago (1988), which provides us the benefit of hindsight to make our points about the sustainability of competitive advantage. After all, the strategic management concepts we have been addressing in the text are quite timeless in their relevance to practice. A brief summary follows:

Atlas Door: A Case Example

Atlas Door, a U.S.-based company, has enjoyed remarkable success. It has grown at an average annual rate of 15 percent in an industry with an overall annual growth rate of less than 5 percent. Recently, its pre-tax earnings were 20 percent of sales—about five times the industry average. Atlas is debt free and by its 10th year, the company achieved the number one competitive position in its industry.

Atlas produces industrial doors—a product with almost infinite variety, involving limitless choices of width and height and material. Given the importance of product variety, inventory is almost useless in meeting customer orders. Instead, most doors can be manufactured only after the order has been placed.

How Did Atlas Door Create Its Competitive Advantages in the Marketplace?

First, Atlas built just-in-time (JIT) factories. Although simple in concept, they require extra tooling and machinery to reduce changeover times. Further, the manufacturing process must be organized by product and scheduled to start and complete with all of the parts available at the same time.

Second, Atlas reduced the time to receive and process an order. Traditionally, when customers, distributors, or salespeople called a door manufacturer with a request for price and delivery, they would have to wait more than one week for a response. In contrast, Atlas first streamlined and then automated its entire order-entry, engineering, pricing, and scheduling process. Atlas can price and schedule 95 percent of its incoming orders while the callers are still on the telephone. It can quickly engineer new special orders because it has preserved on computer the design and production data of all previous special orders—which drastically reduces the amount of reengineering necessary.

Third, Atlas tightly controlled logistics so that it always shipped only fully complete orders to construction sites. Orders require many components, and gathering all of them at the factory and making sure that they are with the correct order can be a time-consuming task. Of course, it is even more time-consuming to get the correct parts to the job site after the order has been shipped! Atlas developed a system to track the parts in production and the purchased parts for each order. This helped to ensure the arrival of all necessary parts at the shipping dock in time—a just-in-time logistics operation.

The Result?   When Atlas began operations, distributors had little interest in its product. The established distributors already carried the door line of a much larger competitor and saw little to no reason to switch suppliers except, perhaps, for a major price concession. But as a startup, Atlas was too small to compete on price alone. Instead, it positioned itself as the door supplier of last resort—the company people came to if the established supplier could not deliver or missed a key date.

Of course, with an average industry order fulfillment time of almost four months, some calls inevitably came to Atlas. And when it did get the call, Atlas commanded a higher price because of its faster delivery. Atlas not only got a higher price, but its effective integration of value-creating activities saved time and lowered costs. Thus, it enjoyed the best of both worlds.

In 10 short years, the company replaced the leading door suppliers in 80 percent of the distributors in the United States. With its strategic advantage, the company could be selective—becoming the supplier for only the strongest distributors.

Are Atlas Door's Competitive Advantages Sustainable?

We will now take both the "pro" and "con" position as to whether or not Atlas Door's competitive advantages will be sustainable for a very long time. It is important, of course, to assume that Atlas Door's strategy is unique in the industry, and the central issue becomes whether or not rivals will be able to easily imitate its strategy or create a viable substitute strategy.

"Pro" Position: The Strategy Is Highly Sustainable   Drawing on Chapter 2, it is quite evident that Atlas Door has attained a very favorable position vis-á-vis the five forces of industry competition. For example, it is able to exert power over its customers (distributors) because of its ability to deliver a quality product in a short period of time. Also, its dominance in the industry creates high entry barriers for new entrants. It is also quite evident that Atlas Door has been able to successfully integrate many value-chain activities within the firm—a fact that is integral to its just-in-time strategy. As noted in Chapter 3, such integration of activities provides a strong basis for sustainability, because rivals would have difficulty in imitating this strategy due to causal ambiguity and path dependency (i.e., it is difficult to build up in a short period of time the resources that Atlas Door has accumulated and developed as well as disentangle the causes of what the valuable resources are or how they can be re-created). Further, as noted in Chapter 4, Atlas Door benefits from the social capital that it has developed with a wide range of key stakeholders (Chapter 1). These would include customers, employees, and managers (a reasonable assumption, given how smoothly the internal operations flow and their long-term relationships with distributors). It would be very difficult for a rival to replace Atlas Door as the supplier of last resort—given the reputation that it has earned over time for "coming through in the clutch" on time-sensitive orders. Finally, we can conclude that Atlas Door has created competitive advantages in both overall low cost and differentiation (Chapter 5). Its strong linkages among value-chain activities—a requirement for its just-in-time operations—not only lowers costs but enables the company to respond quickly to customer orders. As noted in Exhibit 5.5 (page 210), many of the value-chain activities associated with a differentiation strategy reflect the element of speed or quick response.

"Con" Position: The Strategy Can Be Easily Imitated or Substituted   An argument could be made that much of Atlas Door's strategy relies on technologies that are rather well known and nonproprietary. Over time, a well-financed rival could imitate its strategy (via trial and error), achieve a tight integration among its value-creating activities, and implement a just-in-time manufacturing process. Because human capital is highly mobile (Chapter 4), a rival could hire away Atlas Door's talent, and these individuals could aid the rival in transferring Atlas Door's best practices. A new rival could also enter the industry with a large resource base, which might enable it to price its doors well under Atlas Door to build market share (but this would likely involve pricing below cost and would be a risky and nonsustainable strategy). Finally, a rival could potentially "leapfrog" the technologies and processes that Atlas Door has employed and achieve competitive superiority. With the benefit of hindsight, it could use the Internet to further speed up the linkages among its value-creating activities and the order entry processes with its customers and suppliers. (But even this could prove to be a temporary advantage, since rivals could relatively easily do the same thing.)

What Is the Verdict?   Both positions have merit. Over time, it would be rather easy to see how a new rival could achieve parity with Atlas Door—or even create a superior competitive position with new technologies or innovative processes. However, two factors make it extremely difficult for a rival to challenge Atlas Door in the short term: (1) the success that Atlas Door has enjoyed with its just-in-time scheduling and production systems—which involve the successful integration of many value-creating activities—helps the firm not only lower costs but also respond quickly to customer needs, and (2) the strong, positive reputational effects that it has earned with multiple stakeholders—especially its customers.

Finally, it is important to also understand that it is Atlas Door's ability to appropriate most of the profits generated by its competitive advantages that make it a highly successful company. As we discussed in Chapter 3, profits generated by resources can be appropriated by a number of stakeholders such as suppliers, customers, employees, or rivals. The structure of the industrial door industry makes such value appropriation difficult: The suppliers provide generic parts, no one buyer is big enough to dictate prices, the tacit nature of the knowledge makes imitation difficult, and individual employees may be easily replaceable. Still, even with the advantages that Atlas Door enjoys, it needs to avoid becoming complacent or suffer the same fate as the dominant firm it replaced.

How the Internet and Digital Technologies Affect the Competitive Strategies

>LO5.6
How Internet-enabled business models are being used to improve strategic positioning.

Internet and digital technologies have swept across the economy and now have an impact on how nearly every company conducts its business. These changes have created new cost efficiencies and avenues for differentiation. However, the presence of these technologies is so widespread that it is questionable how any one firm can use them effectively in ways that genuinely set them apart from rivals. Thus, to stay competitive, firms must update their strategies to reflect the new possibilities and constraints that these phenomena represent. In this section, we address both the opportunities and the pitfalls that Internet and digital technologies offer to companies using overall cost leadership, differentiation, and focus strategies. We also briefly consider two major impacts that the Internet is having on business: lowering transaction costs and enabling mass customization.

Overall Cost Leadership

The Internet and **digital technologies** create new opportunities for firms to achieve low-cost advantages by enabling them to manage costs and achieve greater efficiencies. Managing costs, and even changing the cost structures of certain industries, is a key feature of the digital economy. Most analysts agree that the Internet's ability to lower transaction costs has transformed business. Broadly speaking, *transaction costs* refer to all the various expenses associated with conducting business. It applies not just to buy/sell transactions but to the costs of interacting with every part of a firm's value chain, within and outside the firm. Think about it. Hiring new employees, meeting with customers, ordering supplies, addressing government regulations—all of these exchanges have some costs associated with them. Because business can be conducted differently on the Internet, new ways of saving money are changing the competitive landscape.

digital technologies information that is in numerical form, which facilitates its storage, transmission, analysis, and manipulation.

Other factors also help to lower transaction costs. The process of **disintermediation** (in Chapter 2) has a similar effect. Each time intermediaries are used in a transaction, additional costs are added. Removing intermediaries lowers transaction costs. The Internet reduces the costs to search for a product or service, whether it is a retail outlet (as in the case of consumers) or a trade show (as in the case of business-to-business shoppers). Not only is the need for travel eliminated but so is the need to maintain a physical address, whether it's a permanent retail location or a temporary presence at a trade show.

disintermediation the process of bypassing buyer channel intermediaries such as wholesalers, distributors, and retailers.

Exhibit 5.9 identifies several types of cost leadership strategies that are made possible by Internet and digital technologies. These cost savings are available throughout a firm's value chain, in both primary and support activities.

Potential Internet-Related Pitfalls for Low-Cost Leaders One of the biggest threats to low-cost leaders is imitation. This problem is intensified for business done on the Internet. Most of the advantages associated with contacting customers directly, and even capabilities that are software driven (e.g., customized ordering systems or real-time access

Exhibit 5.9 Internet-Enabled Low-Cost Leader Strategies

- Online bidding and order processing eliminate the need for sales calls and minimize sales-force expenses.
- Online purchase orders have made many transactions paperless, thus reducing the costs of procurement and paper.
- Direct access to progress reports and the ability of customers to periodically check work in progress minimize rework.
- Collaborative design efforts using Internet technologies that link designers, materials suppliers, and manufacturers reduce the costs and speed the process of new product development.

to the status of work in progress), can be duplicated quickly and without threat of infringement on proprietary information. Another pitfall relates to companies that become overly enamored with using the Internet for cost-cutting and thus jeopardize customer relations or neglect other cost centers.

Differentiation

For many companies, Internet and digital technologies have enhanced their ability to build brand, offer quality products and services, and achieve other differentiation advantages.[58] Among the most striking trends are new ways to interact with consumers. In particular, the Internet has created new ways of differentiating by enabling *mass customization,* which improves the response to customer wishes.

Mass customization has changed how companies go to market and has challenged some of the tried-and-true techniques of differentiation. Traditionally, companies reached customers using high-end catalogs, the showroom floor, personal sales calls and products using prestige packaging, celebrity endorsements, and charity sponsorships. All of these avenues are still available and may still be effective, depending on a firm's competitive environment. But many customers now judge the quality and uniqueness of a product or service by their ability to be involved in its planning and design, combined with speed of delivery and reliable results. Internet and digitally based capabilities are thus changing the way differentiators make exceptional products and achieve superior service. Such improvements are being made at a reasonable cost, allowing firms to achieve parity on the basis of overall cost leadership.

Exhibit 5.10 identifies differentiation activities that are made possible by Internet and digital technologies. Opportunities to differentiate are available in all parts of a company's value chain—both primary and support activities.

Exhibit 5.10 Internet-Enabled Differentiation Strategies

- Personalized online access provides customers with their own "site within a site" in which their prior orders, status of current orders, and requests for future orders are processed directly on the supplier's website.
- Online access to real-time sales and service information is being used to empower the sales force and continually update R&D and technology development efforts.
- Internet-based knowledge management systems that link all parts of the organization are shortening response times and accelerating organization learning.
- Quick online responses to service requests and rapid feedback to customer surveys and product promotions are enhancing marketing efforts.

Potential Internet-Related Pitfalls for Differentiators   Traditional differentiation strategies such as building strong brand identity and prestige pricing have been undermined by Internet-enabled capabilities such as the ability to compare product features side-by-side or bid online for competing services. The sustainability of Internet-based gains from differentiation will deteriorate if companies offer differentiating features that customers don't want or create a sense of uniqueness that customers don't value. The result can be a failed value proposition—the value companies thought they were offering does not translate into sales.

Focus

A focus strategy targets a narrow market segment with customized products and/or services. With focus strategies, the Internet offers new avenues in which to compete because they can access markets less expensively (low cost) and provide more services and features (differentiation). Some claim that the Internet has opened up a new world of opportunities for niche players who seek to access small markets in a highly specialized fashion.[59] Niche businesses are among the most active users of digital technologies and e-business solutions. According to the ClickZ.com division of Jupitermedia Corporation, 77 percent of small businesses agree that a website is essential for small-business success. Small businesses also report that the Internet has helped them grow (58 percent), made them more profitable (51 percent), and helped reduce transaction costs (49 percent).[60] Clearly niche players and small businesses are using the Internet and digital technologies to create more viable focus strategies.

Many aspects of the Internet economy favor focus strategies because niche players and small firms have been able to extend their reach and effectively compete with larger competitors. For example, niche firms have been quicker than Fortune 1000 firms to adopt blogging as a way to create a community and gather customer feedback.[61] Effective use of blogs is an example of how focusers are using the new technology to provide the kinds of advantages that have been the hallmark of a focus strategy in the past—specialized knowledge, rapid response, and strong customer service. Thus, the Internet has provided many firms that pursue focus strategies with new tools for creating competitive advantages.

Exhibit 5.11 outlines several approaches to strategic focusing that are made possible by Internet and digital technologies. Both primary and support activities can be enhanced using the kind of singlemindedness that is characteristic of a focus strategy.

Potential Internet-Related Pitfalls for Focusers   A key danger for focusers using the Internet relates to correctly assessing the size of the online marketplace. Focusers can misread the scope and interests of their target markets. This can cause them to focus on segments that are too narrow to be profitable or to lose their uniqueness in overly broad niches, making them vulnerable to imitators or new entrants.

Exhibit 5.11 Internet-Enabled Focus Strategies

- Permission marketing techniques are focusing sales efforts on specific customers who opt to receive advertising notices.
- Niche portals that target specific groups are providing advertisers with access to viewers with specialized interests.
- Virtual organizing and online "officing" are being used to minimize firm infrastructure requirements.
- Procurement technologies that use Internet software to match buyers and sellers are highlighting specialized buyers and drawing attention to smaller suppliers.

What happens when an e-business focuser tries to overextend its niche? Efforts to appeal to a broader audience by carrying additional inventory, developing additional content, or offering additional services can cause it to lose the cost advantages associated with a limited product or service offering. Conversely, when focus strategies become too narrow, the e-business may have trouble generating enough activity to justify the expense of operating the website.

Are Combination Strategies the Key to E-business Success?

Because of the changing dynamics presented by digital and Internet-based technologies, new strategic combinations that make the best use of the competitive strategies may hold the greatest promise.[62] Many experts agree that the net effect of the digital economy is *fewer* rather than more opportunities for sustainable advantages.[63] This means strategic thinking becomes more important.

More specifically, the Internet has provided all companies with greater tools for managing costs. So it may be that cost management and control will become more important management tools. In general, this may be good if it leads to an economy that makes more efficient use of its scarce resources. However, for individual companies, it may shave critical percentage points off profit margins and create a climate that makes it impossible to survive, much less achieve sustainable above-average profits.

Many differentiation advantages are also diminished by the Internet. The ability to comparison shop—to check product reviews and inspect different choices with a few clicks of the mouse—is depriving some companies, such as auto dealers, of the unique advantages that were the hallmark of their prior success. Differentiating is still an important strategy, of course. But how firms achieve it may change, and the best approach may be to combine differentiation with other competitive strategies.

Perhaps the greatest beneficiaries are the focusers who can use the Internet to capture a niche that previously may have been inaccessible. However, because the same factors that make it possible for a small niche player to be a contender may make that same niche attractive to a big company. That is, an incumbent firm that previously thought a niche market was not worth the effort may use Internet technologies to enter that segment for a lower cost than in the past. The larger firm can then bring its market power and resources to bear in a way that a smaller competitor cannot match.

A combination strategy challenges a company to carefully blend alternative strategic approaches and remain mindful of the impact of different decisions on the firm's value-creating processes and its extended value-chain activities. Strong leadership is needed to maintain a bird's-eye perspective on a company's overall approach and to coordinate the multiple dimensions of a combination strategy.

Just-in-time (JIT) inventory systems can help reduce costs, as well as improve the quality and reliability of a company's products. This benefit is important to differentiated firms, for whom quality and reliability are essential ingredients of the product's appeal. Rolls-Royce automobiles, for example, are never supposed to break down. Improved quality control enhances a company's reputation and thus allows it to charge a premium price, which is one object of total quality management (TQM) programs.

Strategy Spotlight 5.5 describes the efforts of AirAsia, a company that used cost and differentiation strategies to its advantage.

Industry Life Cycle Stages: Strategic Implications

The **industry life cycle** refers to the stages of introduction, growth, maturity, and decline that occur over the life of an industry. In considering the industry life cycle, it is useful to think in terms of broad product lines such as personal computers, photocopiers, or long-distance telephone service. Yet the industry life cycle concept can be explored from several

industry life cycle the stages of introduction, growth, maturity, and decline that typically occur over the life of an industry.

>LO5.7
The importance of considering the industry life cycle to determine a firm's business-level strategy and its relative emphasis on functional area strategies and value-creating activities.

AirAsia: Flying Low Cost with High Hopes

AirAsia started out as a Malaysian government–controlled, full-service regional airline that offered lower fares than its number one competitor, Malaysian Airlines. In December 2001, private entrepreneur Tony Fernandez took over the debt-ridden airline and restructured AirAsia into the first no-frills, low-cost carrier (LCC) in Asia. Upon acquisition, he invited Conner McCarthy, former director of successful European LCC Ryanair, to join AirAsia's executive team. In mid-2008, amid surging oil prices and intense competition, AirAsia recorded its 25th consecutive quarter of profitability since 2002. How could AirAsia sustain its cost advantages and high-quality airline amid unstable oil prices and fierce competition among LCCs and full-service carriers?

AirAsia adopted the low-fare, no-frills business model and became the region's first airline operator to introduce fully ticketless travel and implement an unassigned seating policy. AirAsia offered only one standard-class cabin and did not provide in-flight entertainment or free meals. Under the tagline "Now Everyone Can Fly," it offered airfares that were 40 to 60 percent lower than those of its rivals. Many domestic leisure travelers were attracted to buy air tickets through its multiple websites. In line with the airline's "Easy to Book, Easy to Pay & Easy to Fly" approach, seats were also sold through a telephone booking center, sales offices, travel agents, and partnerships with local banks and post offices.

In 2007, AirAsia even made plans to pioneer a check-in service using customers' handheld devices. In spite of its unassigned-seat policy, the airline allowed a limited number of passengers who paid extra for its Xpress Boarding Service to board first in order to choose their seats with ease. AirAsia was also proud of its "Real 5 Star" offerings, such as its cozy leather seats and for-pay in-flight hot meals, which included a wide selection of popular Malaysian and Asian delicacies. Passengers could either buy the food on board or preorder meals on

Source: Ko, S. & Woo, C. H. L. 2009. AirAsia: Flying low cost with high hopes. *Harvard Business Review,* June 11.

the AirAsia website at a discounted rate. In response to passenger complaints about AirAsia's punctuality, passengers whose flight was delayed by more than three hours were awarded US$61 worth of AirAsia's e-gift vouchers.

AirAsia evolved from a classic LCC into an integrated service provider, offering not only no-frills air tickets but also financial services such as travel insurance and other holiday products. The company offered online booking services for hotels, hostels, car rentals, cruises, and medical care. AirAsia launched the co-branded Citibank–AirAsia credit card, which allowed eligible cardholders to earn free flights by accumulating reward points.

Having started as a three-aircraft operation in 2002, AirAsia owned 72 aircraft by 2008 and served more than 100 routes in the Asia-Pacific region. Its fast expansion from domestic routes to regional flights was supported by its cheeky advertising policy. For example, in 2004, when it began the route from Singapore to Bangkok, its full-page newspaper ad read, "There's a new girl in town: Twice the fun, half the price," poking fun at the iconic Singapore Airlines' female flight attendants, who were known widely as "Singapore girls" and had an elegant image. While all AirAsia ads focused on low fares, they also reflected the carrier's intention to be seen as high quality. With the ambition of being a low-cost but high-quality and innovative airline, it signed on to become the official airline sponsor of the world famous Manchester United football club and the AT&T Williams Formula One team, painting some of its aircraft with club colors and sports stars. Addressing global concern about carbon emissions, AirAsia's website illustrated how its operations help conserve the environment, such as through its ticketless system that reduced paper waste.

AirAsia's business model was initially based upon the potential for cost savings. But through differentiation via advertising, quality services, and innovation have provided the company with a fruitful combination of low-cost and differentiation advantages.

levels, from the life cycle of an entire industry to the life cycle of a single variation or model of a specific product or service.

Why are industry life cycles important?[64] The emphasis on various generic strategies, functional areas, value-creating activities, and overall objectives varies over the course of an industry life cycle. Managers must become even more aware of their firm's strengths and weaknesses in many areas to attain competitive advantages. For example, firms depend on their research and development (R&D) activities in the introductory stage. R&D is the source of new products and features that everyone hopes will appeal to customers. Firms develop products and services to stimulate consumer demand. Later, during the maturity phase, the functions of the product have been defined, more competitors have entered the market, and competition is intense. Managers then place greater emphasis on production efficiencies and process (as opposed to the product) engineering in order to lower manufacturing costs. This helps to protect the firm's market position and to extend the product life cycle because the firm's lower costs can be passed on to consumers in the form of lower prices, and price-sensitive customers will find the product more appealing.

Exhibit 5.12 illustrates the four stages of the industry life cycle and how factors such as generic strategies, market growth rate, intensity of competition, and overall objectives change over time. Managers must strive to emphasize the key functional areas during each

Exhibit 5.12 Stages of the Industry Life Cycle

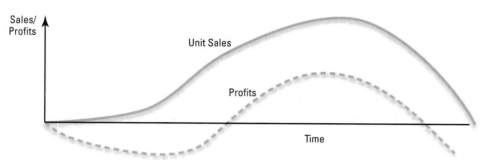

Stage Factor	Introduction	Growth	Maturity	Decline
Generic strategies	Differentiation	Differentiation	Differentiation Overall cost leadership	Overall cost leadership Focus
Market growth rate	Low	Very large	Low to moderate	Negative
Number of segments	Very few	Some	Many	Few
Intensity of competition	Low	Increasing	Very intense	Changing
Emphasis on product design	Very high	High	Low to moderate	Low
Emphasis on process design	Low	Low to moderate	High	Low
Major functional area(s) of concern	Research and development	Sales and marketing	Production	General management and finance
Overall objective	Increase market awareness	Create consumer demand	Defend market share and extend product life cycles	Consolidate, maintain, harvest, or exit

of the four stages and to attain a level of parity in all functional areas and value-creating activities. For example, although controlling production costs may be a primary concern during the maturity stage, managers should not totally ignore other functions such as marketing and R&D. If they do, they can become so focused on lowering costs that they miss market trends or fail to incorporate important product or process designs. Thus, the firm may attain low-cost products that have limited market appeal.

It is important to point out a caveat. While the life cycle idea is analogous to a living organism (i.e., birth, growth, maturity, and death), the comparison has limitations.[65] Products and services go through many cycles of innovation and renewal. Typically, only fad products have a single life cycle. Maturity stages of an industry can be "transformed" or followed by a stage of rapid growth if consumer tastes change, technological innovations take place, or new developments occur. The cereal industry is a good example. When medical research indicated that oat consumption reduced a person's cholesterol, sales of Quaker Oats increased dramatically.[66]

Strategies in the Introduction Stage

In the **introduction stage,** products are unfamiliar to consumers.[67] Market segments are not well defined, and product features are not clearly specified. The early development of an industry typically involves low sales growth, rapid technological change, operating losses, and the need for strong sources of cash to finance operations. Since there are few players and not much growth, competition tends to be limited.

introduction stage the first stage of the industry life cycle, characterized by (1) new products that are not known to customers, (2) poorly defined market segments, (3) unspecified product features, (4) low sales growth, (5) rapid technological change, (6) operating losses, and (7) a need for financial support.

Success requires an emphasis on research and development and marketing activities to enhance awareness. The challenge becomes one of (1) developing the product and finding a way to get users to try it, and (2) generating enough exposure so the product emerges as the "standard" by which all other rivals' products are evaluated.

There's an advantage to being the "first mover" in a market.[68] It led to Coca-Cola's success in becoming the first soft-drink company to build a recognizable global brand and enabled Caterpillar to get a lock on overseas sales channels and service capabilities.

However, there can also be a benefit to being a "late mover." Target carefully considered its decision to delay its Internet strategy. Compared to its competitors Walmart and Kmart, Target was definitely an industry laggard. But things certainly turned out well:[69]

> By waiting, Target gained a late mover advantage. The store was able to use competitors' mistakes as its own learning curve. This saved money, and customers didn't seem to mind the wait: When Target finally opened its website, it quickly captured market share from both Kmart and Walmart Internet shoppers. Forrester Research Internet analyst Stephen Zrike commented, "There's no question, in our mind, that Target has a far better understanding of how consumers buy online."

Examples of products currently in the introductory stages of the industry life cycle include electric vehicles, solar panels, and high-definition television (HDTV).

Strategies in the Growth Stage

The **growth stage** is characterized by strong increases in sales. Such potential attracts other rivals. In the growth stage, the primary key to success is to build consumer preferences for specific brands. This requires strong brand recognition, differentiated products, and the financial resources to support a variety of value-chain activities such as marketing and sales, and research and development. Whereas marketing and sales initiatives were mainly directed at spurring *aggregate* demand—that is, demand for all such products in the introduction stage—efforts in the growth stage are directed toward stimulating *selective* demand, in which a firm's product offerings are chosen instead of a rival's.

growth stage the second stage of the product life cycle, characterized by (1) strong increases in sales; (2) growing competition; (3) developing brand recognition; and (4) a need for financing complementary value-chain activities such as marketing, sales, customer service, and research and development.

Revenues increase at an accelerating rate because (1) new consumers are trying the product and (2) a growing proportion of satisfied consumers are making repeat purchases.[70]

In general, as a product moves through its life cycle, the proportion of repeat buyers to new purchasers increases. Conversely, new products and services often fail if there are relatively few repeat purchases. For example, Alberto-Culver introduced Mr. Culver's Sparklers, which were solid air fresheners that looked like stained glass. Although the product quickly went from the introductory to the growth stage, sales collapsed. Why? Unfortunately, there were few repeat purchasers because buyers treated them as inexpensive window decorations, left them there, and felt little need to purchase new ones. Examples of products currently in the growth stage include e-readers and smart phones.

Strategies in the Maturity Stage

In the **maturity stage** aggregate industry demand softens. As markets become saturated, there are few new adopters. It's no longer possible to "grow around" the competition, so direct competition becomes predominant.[71] With few attractive prospects, marginal competitors exit the market. At the same time, rivalry among existing rivals intensifies because of fierce price competition at the same time that expenses associated with attracting new buyers are rising. Advantages based on efficient manufacturing operations and process engineering become more important for keeping costs low as customers become more price sensitive. It also becomes more difficult for firms to differentiate their offerings, because users have a greater understanding of products and services.

An article in *Fortune* magazine that addressed the intensity of rivalry in mature markets was aptly titled "A Game of Inches." It stated, "Battling for market share in a slowing industry can be a mighty dirty business. Just ask laundry soap archrivals Unilever and Procter & Gamble."[72] These two firms have been locked in a battle for market share since 1965. Why is the competition so intense? There was not much territory to gain and industry sales were flat. An analyst noted, "People aren't getting any dirtier." Thus, the only way to win is to take market share from the competition. To increase its share, Procter & Gamble (P&G) spends $100 million a year promoting its Tide brand on television, billboards, buses, magazines, and the Internet. But Unilever isn't standing still. Armed with an $80 million budget, it launched a soap tablet product named Wisk Dual Action Tablets. For example, it delivered samples of this product to 24 million U.S. homes in Sunday newspapers, followed by a series of TV ads. P&G launched a counteroffensive with Tide Rapid Action Tablets ads showed in side-by-side comparisons of the two products dropped into beakers of water. In the promotion, P&G claimed that its product is superior because it dissolves faster than Unilever's product.

Although this is only one example, many product classes and industries, including consumer products such as beer, automobiles, and televisions, are in maturity.

Firms do not need to be "held hostage" to the life cycle curve. By positioning or repositioning their products in unexpected ways, firms can change how customers mentally categorize them. Thus, firms are able to rescue products floundering in the maturity phase of their life cycles and return them to the growth phase.

Two positioning strategies that managers can use to affect consumers' mental shifts are **reverse positioning,** which strips away "sacred" product attributes while adding new ones, and **breakaway positioning,** which associates the product with a radically different category.[73] We discuss each of these positioning strategies below and then provide an example of each in Strategy Spotlight 5.6.

Reverse Positioning   This assumes that although customers may desire more than the baseline product, they don't necessarily want an endless list of features. Such companies make the creative decision to step off the augmentation treadmill and shed product attributes that the rest of the industry considers sacred. Then, once a product is returned to its baseline state, the stripped-down product adds one or more carefully selected attributes that would usually be found only in a highly augmented product. Such an

Reverse and Breakaway Positioning: How to Avoid Being Held Hostage to the Life Cycle Curve

When firms adopt a reverse or breakaway positioning strategy, there is typically no pretense about what they are trying to accomplish. In essence, they subvert convention through unconventional promotions, prices, and attributes. That becomes a large part of their appeal—a cleverly positioned product offering. Next we discuss IKEA's reverse positioning and Swatch's breakaway positioning.

IKEA

Global furniture retailer IKEA has long been celebrated in the business press for its innovative marketing and phenomenal growth. There are plenty of good reasons for IKEA's success, not the least of which is its cheap but stylish inventory. But a key factor in the store's high performance is its brilliant reverse positioning.

Like most players in mature categories, furniture companies have steadily augmented their offerings. Today, top stores compete by carrying enormous and varied inventories, assuring not only that customers will find exactly what they want but that the couch they bring home will be the only one like it in the neighborhood. Sales consultants coddle customers, helping them measure furniture and visualize their options. Most retailers deliver new furniture to customers' homes and even truck away the old. And retailers work hard to instill the idea that furniture is designed to last forever.

Given this, IKEA's success is surprising. When consumers visit a typical IKEA store, they find there is no in-store sales assistance (though they will find disposable

Sources: Moon, Y. 2005. Break free from the product life cycle. *Harvard Business Review,* 83(5): 87–94; and, Swatch. *http://www.swatchgroup.com/en/group_profile/history/yesterday.*

measuring tapes so they can make their own measurements); the variety is limited (IKEA's furniture comes in a few basic styles); most of the furniture requires assembly; and durability is not to be expected (IKEA works to convince buyers that furniture should be replaced often).

Swatch

Interestingly, the name "Swatch" is often misconstrued as a contraction of the words *Swiss watch.* However, Nicholas Hayek, chairman, affirmed that the original contraction was "Second Watch"—the new watch was introduced as a new concept of watches as casual, fun, and relatively disposable accessories. And therein lies Swatch's *breakaway positioning.*

When Swatch was launched in 1983, Swiss watches were marketed as a form of jewelry. They were serious, expensive, enduring, and discreetly promoted. Once a customer purchased one, it lasted a lifetime. Swatch changed all of that by defining its watches as playful fashion accessories that were showily promoted. They inspired impulse buying—customers would often purchase half a dozen in different designs. Their price—$40 when the brand was introduced—expanded Swatch's reach beyond its default category (watches as high-end jewelry) and moved it into the fashion accessory category, where it had different customers and competitors. Swatch was the official timekeeper of the 1996, 2000, and 2004 Summer Olympics.

Today, Swatch Group is the largest watch company in the world. It has acquired many brands over the years including Omega, Longines, Calvin Klein, and Hamilton. Revenues have grown to $5.5 billion in 2009 and net income has increased to $753 million. These figures represent compound annual increases of 11 percent and 12 percent, respectively, over a four-year period.

---

unconventional combination of attributes allows the product to assume a new competitive position within the category and move backward from maturity into a growth position on the life cycle curve.

Breakaway Positioning As noted above, with reverse positioning, a product establishes a unique position in its category but retains a clear category membership. However, with breakaway positioning, a product escapes its category by deliberately associating with a different one. Thus, managers leverage the new category's conventions to change both how products are consumed and with whom they compete. Instead of merely seeing the breakaway product as simply an alternative to others in its category, consumers perceive it as altogether different.

When a breakaway product is successful in leaving its category and joining a new one, it is able to redefine its competition. Similar to reverse positioning, this strategy permits the product to shift backward on the life cycle curve, moving from the rather dismal maturity phase to a thriving growth opportunity.

Strategy Spotlight 5.6 provides examples of reverse and breakaway positioning.

Strategies in the Decline Stage

decline stage the fourth stage of the product life cycle, characterized by (1) falling sales and profits, (2) increasing price competition, and (3) industry consolidation.

Although all decisions in the phases of an industry life cycle are important, they become particularly difficult in the **decline stage.** Firms must face up to the fundamental strategic choices of either exiting or staying and attempting to consolidate their position in the industry.[74]

The decline stage occurs when industry sales and profits begin to fall. Typically, changes in the business environment are at the root of an industry or product group entering this stage.[75] Changes in consumer tastes or a technological innovation can push a product into decline. Typewriters entered into the decline stage because of the word processing capabilities of personal computers. Compact disks forced cassette tapes into decline in the prerecorded music industry, and digital video disks (DVDs) are replacing compact disks. About 30 years earlier, of course, cassette tapes had led to the demise of long-playing records (LPs).

Products in the decline stage often consume a large share of management time and financial resources relative to their potential worth. Sales and profits decline. Also, competitors may start drastically cutting their prices to raise cash and remain solvent. The situation is further aggravated by the liquidation of assets, including inventory, of some of the competitors that have failed. This further intensifies price competition.

In the decline stage, a firm's strategic options become dependent on the actions of rivals. If many competitors leave the market, sales and profit opportunities increase. On the other hand, prospects are limited if all competitors remain.[76] If some competitors merge, their increased market power may erode the opportunities for the remaining players. Managers must carefully monitor the actions and intentions of competitors before deciding on a course of action.

Four basic strategies are available in the decline phase: *maintaining, harvesting, exiting, or consolidating.*[77]

- *Maintaining* refers to keeping a product going without significantly reducing marketing support, technological development, or other investments, in the hope that competitors will eventually exit the market. Many offices, for example, still use typewriters for filling out forms and other purposes that cannot be completed on a PC. In some rural areas, rotary (or dial) telephones persist because of the older technology used in central switching offices. Thus, there may still be the potential for revenues and profits.

- *Harvesting* involves obtaining as much profit as possible and requires that costs be reduced quickly. Managers should consider the firm's value-creating activities and cut associated budgets. Value-chain activities to consider are primary (e.g., operations, sales and marketing) and support (e.g., procurement, technology development). The objective of a **harvesting strategy** is to wring out as much profit as possible.

harvesting strategy a strategy of wringing as much profit as possible out of a business in the short to medium term by reducing costs.

- *Exiting the market* involves dropping the product from a firm's portfolio. Since a residual core of consumers exist, eliminating it should be carefully considered. If the firm's exit involves product markets that affect important relationships with other product markets in the corporation's overall portfolio, an exit could have repercussions for the whole corporation. For example, it may involve the loss of valuable brand names or human capital with a broad variety of expertise in many value-creating activities such as marketing, technology, and operations.

- *Consolidating* involves one firm acquiring at a reasonable price the best of the surviving firms in an industry. This enables firms to enhance market power and acquire valuable assets. One example of a **consolidation strategy** took place in the defense industry in the early 1990s. As the cliché suggests, "peace broke out" at the end of the Cold War and overall U.S. defense spending levels plummeted.[78] Many companies that make up the defense industry saw more than 50 percent of their market disappear. Only one-quarter of the 120,000 companies that once supplied the Department of Defense still serve in that capacity; the others have shut down their defense business or dissolved altogether. But one key player, Lockheed Martin, became a dominant rival by pursuing an aggressive strategy of consolidation. During the 1990s, it purchased 17 independent entities, including General Dynamics' tactical aircraft and space systems divisions, GE Aerospace, Goodyear Aerospace, and Honeywell ElectroOptics. These combinations enabled Lockheed Martin to emerge as the top provider to three governmental customers: the Department of Defense, the Department of Energy, and NASA.

consolidation strategy a firm's acquiring or merging with other firms in an industry in order to enhance market power and gain valuable assets.

Examples of products currently in the decline stage of the industry life cycle include automotive spark plugs (replaced by electronic fuel ignition), videocassette recorders (replaced by digital video disk recorders), and personal computer zip drives (replaced by compact disk read-write drives). And, as we mentioned previously, compact disks are being replaced by digital video disks (DVDs) and Blu-ray disks.

The introduction of new technologies and associated products does not always mean that old technologies quickly fade away. Research shows that, in a number of cases, old technologies actually enjoy a very profitable "last gasp."[79] Examples include mainframe computers (versus minicomputers and PCs), coronary artery bypass graft surgery (versus angioplasty), and CISC (complex instruction set computing) architecture in computer processors versus RISC (reduced instruction set computing). In each case, the advent of new technology prompted predictions of the demise of the older technology, but each of these has proved to be resilient survivors. What accounts for their continued profitability and survival?

Retreating to more defensible ground is one strategy that firms specializing in technologies threatened with rapid obsolescence have followed. For example, while angioplasty may be appropriate for relatively healthier patients with blocked arteries, sicker, higher-risk patients seem to benefit more from coronary artery bypass graft surgery. This enabled the surgeons to concentrate on the more difficult cases and improve the technology itself. The advent of television unseated the radio as the major source of entertainment from American homes. However, the radio has survived and even thrived in venues where people are also engaged in other activities, such as driving.

Using the new to improve the old is a second approach. Carburetor manufacturers have improved the fuel efficiency of their product by incorporating electronic controls that were originally developed for electronic fuel injection systems. Similarly, CISC computer chip manufacturers have adopted many features from RISC chips.

Improving the price–performance trade-off is a third approach. IBM continues to make money selling mainframes long after their obituary was written. It retooled the technology using low-cost microprocessors and cut their prices drastically. Further, it invested and updated the software, enabling them to offer clients such as banks better performance and lower costs.

Clearly, "last gasps" may not necessarily translate into longer term gains, as the experience of the integrated steel mills suggests. When the first mini-mills appeared, integrated steel mills shifted to higher margin steel, but eventually mini-mills entered even the last strongholds of the integrated steel mills.

Turnaround Strategies

turnaround strategy a strategy that reverses a firm's decline in performance and returns it to growth and profitability.

A **turnaround strategy** involves reversing performance decline and reinvigorating growth toward profitability.[80] A need for turnaround may occur at any stage in the life cycle but is more likely to occur during maturity or decline. Most turnarounds require a firm to carefully analyze the external and internal environments.[81] The external analysis leads to identification of market segments or customer groups that may still find the product attractive.[82] Internal analysis results in actions aimed at reduced costs and higher efficiency. A firm needs to undertake a mix of both internally and externally oriented actions to effect a turnaround.[83] In effect, the cliché "you can't shrink yourself to greatness" applies.

A study of 260 mature businesses in need of a turnaround identified three strategies used by successful companies.[84]

>LO5.8
The need for turnaround strategies that enable a firm to reposition its competitive position in an industry.

- *Asset and cost surgery.* Very often, mature firms tend to have assets that do not produce any returns. Outright sales or sale and leaseback free up considerable cash and improve returns. Investment in new plants and equipment can be deferred. Firms in turnaround situations try to aggressively cut administrative expenses and inventories and speed up collection of receivables. Costs also can be reduced by outsourcing production of various inputs for which market prices may be cheaper than in-house production costs.
- *Selective product and market pruning.* Most mature or declining firms have many product lines that are losing money or are only marginally profitable. One strategy is to discontinue such product lines and focus all resources on a few core profitable areas. For example, in the early 1980s, faced with possible bankruptcy, Chrysler sold off all its nonautomotive businesses as well as all its production facilities abroad. Focus on the North American market and identification of a profitable niche—namely, minivans—were keys to its eventual successful turnaround.
- *Piecemeal productivity improvements.* There are many ways in which a firm can eliminate costs and improve productivity. Although individually these are small gains, they cumulate over time to substantial gains. Improving business processes by reengineering them, benchmarking specific activities against industry leaders, encouraging employee input to identify excess costs, increasing capacity utilization, and improving employee productivity lead to a significant overall gain.

Software maker Intuit is a case of a quick but well-implemented turnaround strategy. After stagnating and stumbling during the dot-com boom, Intuit, which is known for its QuickBooks and TurboTax software, hired Stephen M. Bennett, a 22-year GE veteran, in 1999. He immediately discontinued Intuit's online finance, insurance, and bill-paying operations that were losing money. Instead, he focused on software for small businesses that employ less than 250 people. He also instituted a performance-based reward system that greatly improved employee productivity. Within a few years, Intuit was once again making substantial profits and its stock was up 42 percent.[85]

Even when an industry is in overall decline, pockets of profitability remain. These are segments with customers who are relatively price insensitive. For example, the replacement demand for vacuum tubes affords its manufacturers an opportunity to earn above normal returns although the product itself is technologically obsolete. Surprisingly, within declining industries, there may still be segments that are either stable or growing. Although fountain pens ceased to be the writing instrument of choice a long time ago, the fountain pen industry has successfully reconceptualized the product as a high-margin luxury item that signals accomplishment and success. In the final analysis, every business has the potential for rejuvenation. But it takes creativity, persistence, and most of all a clear strategy to translate that potential into reality.

Strategy Spotlight 5.7 discusses Ford's remarkable global turnaround under the direction of CEO Alan Mulally.

Alan Mulally: Leading Ford's Extraordinary Global Turnaround

Shortly after Alan Mulally took over as Ford's CEO in September 2006, he organized a weekly meeting with his senior managers and asked them how things were going. Fine, fine, fine were the responses from around the table. To this, an incredulous Mulally exclaimed: "We are forecasting a $17 billion loss and no one has any problems!" Clearly, there were cultural issues at play (such as denial and executive rivalry) but also very serious strategic and financial problems as well.

What a change a few years can make! Ford's profits for 2010 were $6.6 billion and the firm has enjoyed seven straight quarters of profitability. This is quite a sharp contrast from its $14.7 billion loss in 2008—a time when high gasoline prices, bloated operations, and uncompetitive labor costs combined with the deep recession to create a perfect storm.

How did Mulally turn Ford around? It took many tough strategic decisions—involving not just company executives but Ford staff and the United Auto Workers (UAW). It involved downsizing, creating greater efficiency, improving quality, selling off the European luxury brands, and mortgaging assets to raise money. Ford's leaders and the United Auto Workers (UAW) also made transformational changes to lower the company's cost structure—a critical component to the company's long-term competitiveness.

Let's take a closer look at Mulally's strategic actions. We have to begin with the plan to undertake a dramatic refinancing of the business by raising bank loans secured against the company's assets. One of his first tasks was to finalize Ford's recovery plan and sell it to the banks. This financing enabled Ford to be the only major American automaker that avoided government-sponsored bankruptcy. And, as noted by Mulally, "The response that we received because we did not ask for the precious taxpayer's money has been tremendous." In fact, Jim Farley, head of marketing for Ford worldwide, estimates that Ford's standing on its own feet has been worth $1 billion in favorable publicity for the company and has attracted appreciative customers into its dealers' showrooms.

Second, he decided that the firm would concentrate resources on the Ford brand and sell off the Premier Automotive Group (PAG) businesses—even if it meant taking a loss. Mulally had ridiculed the idea that top management could focus on Jaguar before breakfast, attend to Volvo or Land Rover before lunch, and then consider Ford and its Lincoln offshoot in North America in the afternoon. Accordingly, in 2007, Aston Martin was sold to private investors; Jaguar and Land Rover were sold to India's Tata Group in 2008; and a Chinese carmaker, Geely, bought Volvo in 2010. Further, the Mercury brand is being phased out.

Third, Mulally realized that in addition to fewer brands, Ford needed a much narrower range of cars, albeit higher quality ones, carrying its familiar blue oval logo in all segments of the market. At one point Ford's designers had to deal with 97 different models—that was cut to 36 and may go lower.

Fourth, along with rationalizing the product range, Mulally insisted on raising the aspiration level with regard to quality. Although Ford used to talk about claiming parity with Toyota's Camry, Mulally shifted the emphasis to trying to make each car that Ford sells "best in class." A number of new cars being created under the One Ford policy are coming from Europe. Quality has improved dramatically according to some of the industry's outside arbiters, such as J. D. Power.

Fifth, to ensure that regional stars such as the Focus could become global successes, 8 of Ford's 10 platforms (the floor pan and its underpinnings) are now global platforms. More shared platforms enables Ford to build different models more quickly and economically to account for regional tastes in cars and variations in regulations. The company has been retooling its entire product creation process to develop and manufacture vehicles globally. The next-generation Ford Fiesta and Ford Focus are examples of cars the company has developed on global platforms. As part of Ford's emerging markets strategy, the redesigned four-door and five-door Fiesta was launched in China in 2009 before it was introduced in any other global market. Global manufacturing platforms allow Ford to take advantage of their unique resources around the world to meet the evolving needs of the global marketplace.

Sixth, Mulally had to make many painful restructuring decisions in order to match production to the number of cars that Ford could sell. Since 2006, Ford cut half of its shop-floor workforce in North America and a third of its office jobs. By the end of 2011, a total of 17 factories will have closed, and Ford's total employment will have fallen from 128,000 to 75,000. In addition, the number of dealers has been cut by a fifth. Helped by union concessions, Ford has shed about $14 billion in annual operational costs and now can compete with Japan's "transplant" factories in America.

(continued)

(continued)

Regarding Ford's successful transformation, Mulally claims: "While we still face a challenging road ahead, our transformation is working, and our underlying business continues to grow stronger. In the third quarter [of 2009], we made progress in all four areas of our plan, aggressively restructuring to operate profitably at the current demand and the changing model mix, accelerating development of new products our customers want, value financing our plan and strengthening our balance sheet, and working together effectively as one global team."

Sources: Ford Motor Company. Accessed at *www.fordahead.com/home/global-strategy*, October 20, 2011. Ford Motor Company Q3 2009 Earnings Call transcript. November 2, 2009. Accessed at *www.nasdaq.com*; Linn, A. 2010. For Ford's Mulally, big bets are paying off. *www.msnbc.com*. October 26: nd; Anonymous. 2010. Epiphany in Dearborn. *The Economist*. December 11: 83–85; Reagan, J. Ford Motor's extraordinary turnaround. December 10: np; and *www.finance.yahoo.com*.

Reflecting on Career Implications . . .

- ***Types of Competitive Advantage:*** Always be aware of your organization's business-level strategy. What do you do to help your firm either increase differentiation or lower costs? What are some ways that your role in the firm can help realize these outcomes?
- ***Combining Sources of Competitive Advantage:*** Are you engaged in activities that simultaneously help your organization increase differentiation and lower costs?
- ***Industry Life Cycle:*** If your firm is in the mature stage of the industry life cycle, can you think of ways to enhance your firm's level of differentiation in order to make customers less price sensitive to your organization's goods and services?
- ***Industry Life Cycle:*** If you sense that your career is maturing (or in the decline phase!), what actions can you take to restore career growth and momentum (e.g., training, mentoring, professional networking)? Should you actively consider professional opportunities in other industries?

Summary

How and why firms outperform each other goes to the heart of strategic management. In this chapter, we identified three generic strategies and discussed how firms are able not only to attain advantages over competitors, but also to sustain such advantages over time. Why do some advantages become long-lasting while others are quickly imitated by competitors?

The three generic strategies—overall cost leadership, differentiation, and focus—form the core of this chapter. We began by providing a brief description of each generic strategy (or competitive advantage) and furnished examples of firms that have successfully implemented these strategies. Successful generic strategies invariably enhance a firm's position vis-à-vis the five forces of that industry—a point that we stressed and illustrated with examples. However, as we pointed out, there are pitfalls to each of the generic strategies. Thus, the sustainability of a firm's advantage is always challenged because of imitation or substitution by new or existing rivals. Such competitor moves erode a firm's advantage over time.

We also discussed the viability of combining (or integrating) overall cost leadership and generic differentiation strategies. If successful, such integration can enable a firm to enjoy superior performance and improve its competitive position. However, this is challenging, and managers must be aware of the potential downside risks associated with such an initiative.

We addressed the challenges inherent in determining the sustainability of competitive advantages. Drawing on an example from a manufacturing industry, we discussed both the "pro" and "con" positions as to why competitive advantages are sustainable over a long period of time.

The way companies formulate and deploy strategies is changing because of the impact of the Internet and digital technologies in many industries. Further, Internet technologies are enabling the mass customization capabilities of greater numbers of competitors. Focus strategies are likely to increase in importance because the Internet provides highly targeted and lower-cost access to narrow or specialized markets. These strategies are not without their pitfalls, however, and firms need to understand the dangers as well as the potential benefits of Internet-based approaches.

The concept of the industry life cycle is a critical contingency that managers must take into account in striving to create and sustain competitive advantages. We identified the four stages of the industry life cycle—introduction, growth, maturity, and decline—and suggested how these stages can play a role in decisions that managers must make at the business level. These include overall strategies as well as the relative emphasis on functional areas and value—creating activities.

When a firm's performance severely erodes, turnaround strategies are needed to reverse its situation and enhance its competitive position. We have discussed three approaches—asset and cost surgery, selective product and market pruning, and piecemeal productivity improvements.

Summary Review Questions

1. Explain why the concept of competitive advantage is central to the study of strategic management.
2. Briefly describe the three generic strategies—overall cost leadership, differentiation, and focus.
3. Explain the relationship between the three generic strategies and the five forces that determine the average profitability within an industry.
4. What are some of the ways in which a firm can attain a successful turnaround strategy?
5. Describe some of the pitfalls associated with each of the three generic strategies.

6. Can firms combine the generic strategies of overall cost leadership and differentiation? Why or why not?
7. Explain why the industry life cycle concept is an important factor in determining a firm's business-level strategy.

Key Terms

Experiential Exercise

What are some examples of primary and support activities that enable Nucor, a $19 billion steel manufacturer, to achieve a low-cost strategy? (Fill in table on the following page.)

Application Questions Exercises

1. Go to the Internet and look up www.ikea.com. How has this firm been able to combine overall cost leadership and differentiation strategies?
2. Choose a firm with which you are familiar in your local business community. Is the firm successful in following one (or more) generic strategies? Why or why not? What do you think are some of the challenges it faces in implementing these strategies in an effective manner?
3. Think of a firm that has attained a differentiation focus or cost focus strategy. Are its advantages sustainable? Why? Why not? (*Hint:* Consider its position vis-à-vis Porter's five forces.)
4. Think of a firm that successfully achieved a combination overall cost leadership and differentiation strategy. What can be learned from this example? Are these advantages sustainable? Why? Why not? (*Hint:* Consider its competitive position vis-à-vis Porter's five forces.)

Value-Chain Activity	Yes/No	How Does Nucor Create Value for the Customer?
Primary:		
Inbound logistics		
Operations		
Outbound logistics		
Marketing and sales		
Service		
Support:		
Procurement		
Technology development		
Human resource management		
General administration		

Ethics Questions

1. Can you think of a company that suffered ethical consequences as a result of an overemphasis on a cost leadership strategy? What do you think were the financial and nonfinancial implications?

2. In the introductory stage of the product life cycle, what are some of the unethical practices that managers could engage in to enhance their firm's market position? What could be some of the long-term implications of such actions?

References

1. Helm, B. 2010. At KFC, a battle among the chicken-hearted. *Bloomberg Businessweek,* August 16: 19; De Nies, Y. & Acosta, C. 2010. Kentucky Fried fight. *www.abcnews.go.com.* August 17: np; and, Morran, C. 2010. Squabble between KFC & franchisees over advertising goes to court. *www.consumerist.com.* September 20: np. We thank Jason Hirsch for his valued contributions.

2. For a recent perspective by Porter on competitive strategy, refer to: Porter, M. E. 1996. What is strategy? *Harvard Business Review,* 74(6): 61–78.

3. For insights into how a start-up is using solar technology, see: Gimbel, B. 2009. Plastic power. *Fortune,* February 2: 34.

4. Useful insights on strategy in an economic downturn are in: Rhodes, D. & Stelter, D. 2009. Seize advantage in a downturn. *Harvard Business Review,* 87(2): 50–58.

5. Some useful ideas on maintaining competitive advantages can be found in: Ma, H. & Karri, R. 2005. Leaders beware: Some sure ways to lose your competitive advantage. *Organizational Dynamics,* 343(1): 63–76.

6. Miller, A. & Dess, G. G. 1993. Assessing Porter's model in terms of its generalizability, accuracy, and simplicity. *Journal of Management Studies,* 30(4): 553–585.

7. Cendrowski, S. 2008. Extreme retailing. *Fortune,* March 31: 14.

8. For insights on how discounting can erode a firm's performance, read: Stibel, J. M. & Delgrosso, P. 2008. Discounts can be dangerous. *Harvard Business Review,* 66(12): 31.

9. For a scholarly discussion and analysis of the concept of competitive parity, refer to: Powell, T. C. 2003. Varieties of competitive parity. *Strategic Management Journal,* 24(1): 61–86.

10. Rao, A. R., Bergen, M. E., & Davis, S. 2000. How to fight a price war. *Harvard Business Review,* 78(2): 107–120.

11. Marriot, J. W., Jr. Our competitive strength: Human capital. A speech given to the Detroit Economic Club on October 2, 2000.

12. Whalen, C. J., Pascual, A. M., Lowery, T., & Muller, J. 2001. The top 25 managers. *BusinessWeek,* January 8: 63.

13. Ibid.

14. For an interesting perspective on the need for creative strategies, refer to: Hamel, G. & Prahalad, C. K. 1994. *Competing for the future.* Boston: Harvard Business School Press.

15. Interesting insights on Walmart's effective cost leadership strategy are found in: Palmeri, C. 2008. Wal-Mart is up for this downturn. *BusinessWeek,* November 6: 34.

16. An interesting perspective on the dangers of price discounting is: Mohammad, R. 2011. Ditch the

discounts. *Harvard Business Review,* 89 (1/2): 23–25.

17. Dholakia, U. M. 2011. Why employees can wreck promotional offers. *Harvard Business Review,* 89(1/2): 28.

18. Jacobs, A. 2010. Workers in China voting with their feet. *International Herald Tribune,* July 13: 1, 14.

19. For a perspective on the sustainability of competitive advantages, refer to: Barney, J. 1995. Looking inside for competitive advantage. *Academy of Management Executive,* 9(4): 49–61.

20. Thornton, E. 2001. Why e-brokers are broker and broker. *BusinessWeek,* January 22: 94.

21. Mohammed, R. 2011. Ditch the discounts. *Harvard Business Review,* 89(1/2): 23–25.

22. Koretz, G. 2001. E-commerce: The buyer wins. *BusinessWeek,* January 8: 30.

23. For an "ultimate" in differentiated services, consider time shares in exotic automobiles such as Lamborghinis and Bentleys. Refer to: Stead, D. 2008. My Lamborghini—today, anyway. *BusinessWeek,* January 18:17.

24. For an interesting perspective on the value of corporate brands and how they may be leveraged, refer to: Aaker, D. A. 2004. *California Management Review,* 46(3): 6–18.

25. A unique perspective on differentiation strategies is: Austin, R. D. 2008. High margins and the quest for aesthetic coherence. *Harvard Business Review,* 86(1): 18–19.

26. MacMillan, I. & McGrath, R. 1997. Discovering new points of differentiation. *Harvard Business Review,* 75(4): 133–145; and, Wise, R. & Baumgarter, P. 1999. Beating the clock: Corporate responses to rapid change in the PC industry. *California Management Review,* 42(1): 8–36.

27. For a discussion on quality in terms of a company's software and information systems, refer to: Prahalad, C. K. & Krishnan, M. S. 1999. The new meaning of quality in the information age. *Harvard Business Review,* 77(5): 109–118.

28. The role of design in achieving differentiation is addressed in: Brown, T. 2008. Design thinking. *Harvard Business Review.* 86(6): 84–92.

29. Taylor, A., III. 2001. Can you believe Porsche is putting its badge on this car? *Fortune,* February 19: 168–172.

30. Ward, S., Light, L., & Goldstine, J. 1999. What high-tech managers need to know about brands. *Harvard Business Review,* 77(4): 85–95.

31. Morton, R. 2008. DHL plans to ease its $1.3 billion headache. *Outsourced Logistics,* July, Vol. 1, Issue 2: 20–30.

32. Markides, C. 1997. Strategic innovation. *Sloan Management Review,* 38(3): 9–23.

33. Bonnabeau, E., Bodick, N., & Armstrong, R. W. 2008. A more rational approach to new-product development. *Harvard Business Review,* 66(3): 96–102.

34. Insights on Google's innovation are in: Iyer, B. & Davenport, T. H. 2008. Reverse engineering Google's innovation machine. *Harvard Business Review,* 66(4): 58–68.

35. A discussion of how a firm used technology to create product differentiation is in: Mehta, S. N. 2009. Under Armour reboots. *Fortune.* February 2: 29–33 (5).

36. Bertini, M. & Wathieu, L. 2010. How to stop customers from fixating on price. *Harvard Business Review,* 88(5): 84–91.

37. The authors would like to thank Scott Droege, a faculty member at Western Kentucky University, for providing this example.

38. Dixon, M., Freeman, K., & Toman, N. 2010. Stop trying to delight your customers. *Harvard Business Review,* 88(7/8).

39. Flint, J. 2004. Stop the nerds. *Forbes,* July 5: 80; and, Fahey, E. 2004. Overengineering 101. *Forbes,* December 13: 62.

40. Symonds, W. C. 2000. Can Gillette regain its voltage? *BusinessWeek,* October 16: 102–104.

41. Anonymous. 2011. Groupon anxiety: The online-coupon firm will have to move fast to retain its impressive lead. *The Economist,* March 17; and, Anonymous. 2011. Internet coupon sites bad for business. Lee Law Firm PLLC, *www.leebankruptcy.com.* October 4.

42. Gadiesh, O. & Gilbert, J. L. 1998. Profit pools: A fresh look at strategy. *Harvard Business Review,* 76(3): 139–158.

43. Colvin, G. 2000. Beware: You could soon be selling soybeans. *Fortune,* November 13: 80.

44. Whalen et al., op. cit.: 63; Porter, M. E. 2008. The five competitive forces that shape strategy. *Harvard Business Review,* 86(1): 78–97; and, *www.finance.yahoo.com.*

45. Hall, W. K. 1980. Survival strategies in a hostile environment. *Harvard Business Review,* 58: 75–87; on the paint and allied products industry, see: Dess, G. G. & Davis, P. S. 1984. Porter's (1980) generic strategies as determinants of strategic group membership and organizational performance. *Academy of Management Journal,* 27: 467–488; for the Korean electronics industry, see: Kim, L. & Lim, Y. 1988. Environment, generic strategies, and performance in a rapidly developing country: A taxonomic approach. *Academy of Management Journal,* 31: 802–827; Wright, P., Hotard, D., Kroll, M., Chan, P., & Tanner, J. 1990. Performance and multiple strategies in a firm: Evidence from the apparel industry. In Dean, B. V. & Cassidy, J. C. (Eds.). *Strategic management: Methods and studies:* 93–110. Amsterdam: Elsevier-North Holland; and, Wright, P., Kroll, M., Tu, H., & Helms, M. 1991. Generic strategies and business performance: An empirical study of the screw machine products industry. *British Journal of Management,* 2: 1–9.

46. Gilmore, J. H. & Pine, B. J., II. 1997. The four faces of customization. *Harvard Business Review,* 75(1): 91–101.

47. Heracleous, L. & Wirtz, J. 2010. Singapore Airlines' balancing act. *Harvard Business Review,* 88(7/8): 145–149.

48. Gilmore & Pine, op. cit. For interesting insights on mass customization, refer to: Cattani, K., Dahan, E., &

Schmidt, G. 2005. Offshoring versus "spackling." *MIT Sloan Management Review,* 46(3): 6–7.

49. Goodstein, L. D. & Butz, H. E. 1998. Customer value: The linchpin of organizational change. *Organizational Dynamics,* Summer: 21–34.

50. Randall, T., Terwiesch, C., & Ulrich, K. T. 2005. Principles for user design of customized products. *California Management Review,* 47(4): 68–85.

51. Gadiesh & Gilbert, op. cit.: 139–158.

52. Insights on the profit pool concept are addressed in: Reinartz, W. & Ulaga, W. 2008. How to sell services more profitably. *Harvard Business Review,* 66(5): 90–96.

53. This example draws on: Dess & Picken. 1997, op. cit.

54. A rigorous and thorough discussion of the threats faced by industries due to the commoditization of products and services and what strategic actions firm should consider is found in: D'Aveni, R. A. 2010. *Beating the commodity trap.* Boston: Harvard Business Press.

55. For an insightful, recent discussion on the difficulties and challenges associated with creating advantages that are sustainable for any reasonable period of time and suggested strategies, refer to: D'Aveni, R. A., Dagnino, G. B., & Smith, K. G. 2010. The age of temporary advantage. *Strategic Management Journal,* 31(13): 1371–1385. This is the lead article in a special issue of this journal that provides many ideas that are useful to both academics and practicing managers. For an additional examination of declining advantage in technologically intensive industries, see: Vaaler, P. M. & McNamara, G. 2010. Are technology-intensive industries more dynamically competitive? No and yes. *Organization Science,* 21: 271–289.

56. Rita McGrath provides some interesting ideas on possible strategies for firms facing highly uncertain competitive environments: McGrath, R. G. 2011. When your business model is in trouble. *Harvard Business Review,* 89(1/2); 96–98.

57. The Atlas Door example draws on: Stalk, G., Jr. 1988. Time—the next source of competitive advantage. *Harvard Business Review,* 66(4): 41–51.

58. Edelman, D. C. 2010. Branding in the digital age. *Harvard Business Review,* 88(12): 62–69.

59. Seybold, P. 2000. Niches bring riches. *Business 2.0,* June 13: 135.

60. Greenspan, R. 2004. Net drives profits to small biz. ClickZ.com, March 25, *www.clickz.com;* and, Greenspan, R. 2002. Small biz benefits from Internet tools. ClickZ.com, March 28, *www.clickz.com.*

61. Burns, E. 2006. Executives slow to see value of corporate blogging. ClickZ .com, May 9, *www.clickz.com.*

62. Empirical support for the use of combination strategies in an e-business context can be found in: Kim, E., Nam, D., & Stimpert, J. L. 2004. The applicability of Porter's generic strategies in the Digital Age: Assumptions, conjectures, and suggestions. *Journal of Management,* 30(5): 569–589.

63. Porter, M. E. 2001. Strategy and the Internet. *Harvard Business Review,* 79: 63–78.

64. For an interesting perspective on the influence of the product life cycle and rate of technological change on competitive strategy, refer to Lei, D. & Slocum, J. W., Jr. 2005. Strategic and organizational requirements for competitive advantage. *Academy of Management Executive,* 19(1): 31–45.

65. Dickson, P. R. 1994. *Marketing management:* 293. Fort Worth, TX: Dryden Press; and, Day, G. S. 1981. The product life cycle: Analysis and application. *Journal of Marketing Research,* 45: 60–67.

66. Bearden, W. O., Ingram, T. N., & LaForge, R. W. 1995. *Marketing principles and practices.* Burr Ridge, IL: Irwin.

67. MacMillan, I. C. 1985. Preemptive strategies. In Guth, W. D. (Ed.). *Handbook of business strategy:* 9-1–9-22. Boston: Warren, Gorham & Lamont; Pearce, J. A. & Robinson, R. B. 2000. *Strategic management* (7th

ed.). New York: McGraw-Hill; and, Dickson, op. cit.: 295–296.

68. Bartlett, C. A. & Ghoshal, S. 2000. Going global: Lessons for late movers. *Harvard Business Review,* 78(2): 132–142.

69. Neuborne, E. 2000. E-tailers hit the relaunch key. *BusinessWeek,* October 17: 62.

70. Berkowitz, E. N., Kerin, R. A., & Hartley, S. W. 2000. *Marketing* (6th ed.). New York: McGraw-Hill.

71. MacMillan, op. cit.

72. Brooker, K. 2001. A game of inches. *Fortune,* February 5: 98–100.

73. Our discussion of reverse and breakaway positioning draws on: Moon, Y. 2005. Break free from the product life cycle. *Harvard Business Review,* 83(5): 87–94. This article also discusses stealth positioning as a means of overcoming consumer resistance and advancing a product from the introduction to the growth phase.

74. MacMillan, op. cit.

75. Berkowitz et al., op. cit.

76. Bearden et al., op. cit.

77. The discussion of these four strategies draws on MacMillan, op. cit.; Berkowitz et al., op. cit.; and, Bearden et al., op. cit.

78. Augustine, N. R. 1997. Reshaping an industry: Lockheed Martin's survival story. *Harvard Business Review,* 75(3): 83–94.

79. Snow, D. C. 2008. Beware of old technologies' last gasps. *Harvard Business Review,* January: 17–18; Lohr, S. 2008. Why old technologies are still kicking. *New York Times,* March 23: np; and, McGrath, R. G. 2008. Innovation and the last gasps of dying technologies. *ritamcgrath.com,* March 18: np.

80. Coyne, K. P., Coyne, S. T., & Coyne, E. J., Sr. 2010. When you've got to cut costs—now. *Harvard Business Review,* 88(5): 74–83.

81. A study that draws on the resource-based view of the firm to investigate successful turnaround strategies is: Morrow, J. S., Sirmon, D. G., Hitt, M. A., & Holcomb, T. R. 2007. *Strategic Management Journal,* 28(3): 271–284.

82. For a study investigating the relationship between organizational restructuring and acquisition performance, refer to: Barkema, H. G. & Schijven, M. Toward unlocking the full potential of acquisitions: The role of organizational restructuring. *Academy of Management Journal,* 51(4): 696–722.

83. For some useful ideas on effective turnarounds and handling downsizings, refer to: Marks, M. S. & De Meuse, K. P. 2005. Resizing the organization: Maximizing the gain while minimizing the pain of layoffs, divestitures and closings. *Organizational Dynamics,* 34(1): 19–36.

84. Hambrick, D. C. & Schecter, S. M. 1983. Turnaround strategies for mature industrial product business units. *Academy of Management Journal,* 26(2): 231–248.

85. Mullaney, T. J. 2002. The wizard of Intuit. *BusinessWeek,* October 28: 60–63.

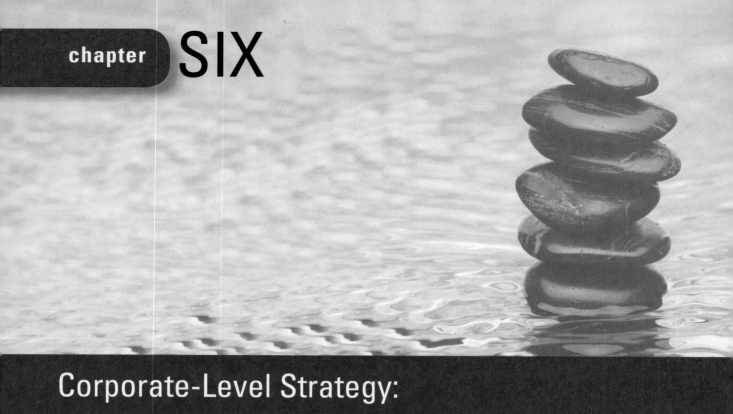

chapter SIX

Corporate-Level Strategy:

Creating Value through Diversification

After reading this chapter, you should have a good understanding of:

LO6.1   The reasons for the failure of many diversification efforts.

LO6.2   How managers can create value through diversification initiatives.

LO6.3   How corporations can use related diversification to achieve synergistic benefits through economies of scope and market power.

LO6.4   How corporations can use unrelated diversification to attain synergistic benefits through corporate restructuring, parenting, and portfolio analysis.

LO6.5   The various means of engaging in diversification—mergers and acquisitions, joint ventures/strategic alliances, and internal development.

LO6.6   Managerial behaviors that can erode the creation of value.

LEARNING OBJECTIVES

Corporate-level strategy addresses two related issues: (1) What businesses should a corporation compete in? and (2) how can these businesses be managed so they create "synergy"—that is, more value by working together than if they were freestanding units? As we will see, these questions present a key challenge for today's managers. Many diversification efforts fail or, in many cases, provide only marginal returns to shareholders. Thus, determining how to create value through entering new markets, introducing new products, or developing new technologies is a vital issue in strategic management.

We begin by discussing why diversification initiatives, in general, have not yielded the anticipated benefits. Then, in the next three sections of the chapter, we explore the two key alternative approaches: related and unrelated diversification. With related diversification, corporations strive to enter product markets that share some resources and capabilities with their existing business units or increase their market power. Here we suggest four means of creating value: leveraging core competencies, sharing activities, pooled negotiating power, and vertical integration. With unrelated diversification, there are few similarities in the resources and capabilities among the firm's business units, but value can be created in multiple ways. These include restructuring, corporate parenting, and portfolio analysis approaches. Whereas the synergies to be realized with related diversification come from *horizontal relationships* among the business units, the synergies from unrelated diversification are derived from *hierarchical relationships* between the corporate office and the business units.

The last two sections address (1) the various means that corporations can use to achieve diversification and (2) managerial behaviors (e.g., self-interest) that serve to erode shareholder value. We address mergers and acquisitions (M&A), divestitures, joint ventures/strategic alliances, and internal development. Each of these involves the evaluation of important trade-offs. Detrimental managerial behaviors, often guided by a manager's self-interest, are "growth for growth's sake," egotism, and antitakeover tactics. Some of these behaviors raise ethical issues because managers, in some cases, are not acting in the best interests of a firm's shareholders.

Learning from Mistakes

Internet company AOL purchased the social networking firm Bebo in early 2008 for $850 million. In June 2010, it sold Bebo for the fire-sale price of $10 million. What went wrong?[1]

AOL was one of the biggest stars of the dot-com era, but its traditional business, dial-up Internet services, has steadily declined since its peak in 2001. The company tried to reinvent itself in 2008 by entering the social networking market by acquiring Bebo; the acquisition came shortly before AOL demerged from Time Warner in 2009. But in the words of Jeff Bewkes, Time Warner CEO at the time, from the get-go Bebo was seen as the "riskiest acquisition" the company made that year.

AOL's original rationale in purchasing Bebo was to tap into the phenomenon of online social networking by acquiring a presence in the rapidly growing community. The deal was part of AOL's strategy to shift from a subscription-based service for Internet connectivity to one focused on generating ad revenue by providing online media. The acquisition of Bebo pulled AOL away from its core strength of providing Internet service and placed the company in direct competition with social networking firms, such as Facebook. Unfortunately, Bebo proved to be an ineffective means of entering the online media industry.

In 2008, Bebo was a thriving, mainly European online social network community that was popular among teens, with about 40 million users. AOL's purchase of Bebo was intended to further the community's expansion into the U.S. market. Quite the opposite happened. In May 2007, the firm had almost 9 million unique U.S. visitors, and a year later this number dropped to only 5 million unique visitors. (This was in contrast with its largest competitor in the social networking market, Facebook, which had 130.4 million unique U.S. visitors, showing continuous strong growth.)

One of the few actors that actually profited from Bebo was its founder, Michael Birch, who made $300 million from Bebo's original sale to AOL. According to Rory Cellan-Jones, BBC technology correspondent, AOL's decision to purchase Bebo was "one of the worst deals ever made in the dot-com era."

The acquisition was just one of a series of poor decisions that forced AOL to remove Randy Falco, the reigning CEO when the Bebo acquisition was made. It replaced him with Tim Armstrong, the one who divested it, in an effort to change strategies and bring the company back to profitability. According to Jim Clark, senior technology analyst at Mintel, the problems faced by AOL in integrating Bebo were a combination of paying too much in the first place as well as a lack of enough investment to make it profitable.*

* To make matters worse, in July 2010, AOL also sold ICQ instant messenger for $187.5 million, having purchased it for $400 million in 1998. The sales of Bebo and ICQ led to write-downs of $1.4 billion in the second quarter of 2010 and to a posted loss of $1.06 billion for the quarter.

>LO6.1
The reasons for the failure of many diversification efforts.

corporate-level strategy a strategy that focuses on gaining long-term revenue, profits, and market value through managing operations in multiple businesses.

AOL's experience with acquisitions is more the rule than the exception. Research shows that the vast majority of acquisitions result in value destruction rather than value creation. Many large multinational firms have also failed to effectively integrate their acquisitions, paid too high a premium for the target's common stock, or were unable to understand how the acquired firm's assets would fit with their own lines of business.[2] And, at times, top executives may not have acted in the best interests of shareholders. That is, the motive for the acquisition may have been to enhance the executives' power and prestige rather than to improve shareholder returns. At times, the only other people who may have benefited were the shareholders of the *acquired* firms—or the investment bankers who advise the acquiring firm, because they collect huge fees upfront regardless of what happens afterward![3]

Consider, for example, Pfizer's announcement on January 26, 2009, that it was acquiring Wyeth for $68 billion in cash and stock—which represented a 15 percent premium.[4] How did the market react? In rather typical fashion, Wyeth's stock went up 2 percent; Pfizer's went down 9 percent. And, interestingly, the shares of Crucell, a Dutch biotech company, sank 10 percent after Wyeth pulled out of talks to buy it.

There have been several studies that were conducted over a variety of time periods that show how disappointing acquisitions have typically turned out. For example:

- A study evaluated the stock market reaction of 600 acquisitions over the period between 1975 and 1991. The results indicated that the acquiring firms suffered an average 4 percent drop in market value (after adjusting for market movements) in the three months following the acquisitions announcement.[5]
- In a study by Solomon Smith Barney of U.S. companies acquired since 1997 in deals for $15 billion or more, the stocks of the acquiring firms have, on average, underperformed the S&P stock index by 14 percentage points and underperformed their peer group by 4 percentage points after the deals were announced.[6]
- A study investigated 270 mergers that took place between 2000 and 2003 in multiple countries and regions. It found that after a merger, sales growth decreased by 6 percent, earnings growth dropped 9.4 percent, and market valuations declined 2.5 percent (figures are adjusted for industry trends and refer to three years pre- or postmerger).[7]
- A study that investigated 86 completed takeover bids that took place between 1993 and 2008 noted a negative return of 2 percent per month in long-term performance for the 3-year postacquisition period.[8]

Exhibit 6.1 lists some well-known examples of failed acquisitions and mergers. Recently there have been several acquisitions—often at fire-sale prices—by financial services firms during the global financial crisis in 2008. For example, Bank of America bought Merrill Lynch, Wells Fargo purchased Wachovia, and JPMorgan acquired Washington Mutual. Only time will tell how well these turn out over the next few years.

Many acquisitions ultimately result in divestiture—an admission that things didn't work out as planned. In fact, some years ago, a writer for *Fortune* magazine lamented, "Studies show that 33 percent to 50 percent of acquisitions are later divested, giving corporate marriages a divorce rate roughly comparable to that of men and women."[9]

Admittedly, we have been rather pessimistic so far.[10] Clearly, many diversification efforts have worked out very well—whether through mergers and acquisitions, strategic

---

Exhibit 6.1
Some Well-Known M&A Blunders

Here are examples of some very expensive blunders:

- Sprint and Nextel merged in 2005. On January 31, 2008, the firm said it would take a merger-related charge of $31 billion. And, as of late January 2011, the stock had lost over 85 percent of its value since the merger.

- AOL paid $114 billion to acquire Time Warner in 2001. Over the next two years, AOL Time Warner lost $150 billion in market valuation.

- In October 2007, RBS (Royal Bank of Scotland), which led a consortium of Fortis Bank and Banco Santander, acquired ABN AMRO, a Dutch-owned state bank, for $100 billion. As a result of the subprime mortgage crisis, asset values crashed and credit markets tumbled. The crash in asset valuations led to huge write downs of more than 5.9 billion British pounds for RBS in 2008.

- Daimler Benz paid $36 billion to acquire Chrysler in 1998. After years of losses, it sold 80.1 percent of the unit to Cerberus Capital Management for $7.4 billion in 2007. And, as of 2009, Cerberus was trying to unload the unit.

- Quaker Oats' acquisition of the once high-flying Snapple for $1.8 billion in 1994 was followed by its divestment for $300 million three years later.

- AT&T bought computer equipment maker NCR for $7.4 billion in 1991, only to spin it off for $3.4 billion six years later.

- Sony acquired Columbia Pictures in 1989 for $4.8 billion although it had no competencies in movie production. Five years later, Sony was forced to take a $2.7 billion write-off on the acquisition.

Source: Ante, S.E. 2008. Sprint's wake-up call. *Businessweek.com*. February 21: np; Gupta, P. 2008. Daimler may sell remaining Chrysler stake. *www.reuters.com*. September 24: np; and, Tully, S. 2006. The (second) worst deal ever. *Fortune*, October 16: 102–119.

alliances and joint ventures, or internal development. We will discuss many success stories throughout this chapter. Next, we will discuss the primary rationales for diversification.

Making Diversification Work: An Overview

>LO6.2

How managers can create value through diversification initiatives.

Clearly, not all diversification moves, including those involving mergers and acquisitions, erode performance. For example, acquisitions in the oil industry, such as British Petroleum's purchases of Amoco and Arco, are performing well as is the Exxon-Mobil merger. In the automobile industry, the Renault-Nissan alliance, under CEO Carlos Ghosn's leadership, has led to a quadrupling of its collective market capitalization—from $20.4 billion to $84.9 billion—by the end of 2006.[11] Many leading high-tech firms such as Samsung, LG, and Intel have dramatically enhanced their revenues, profits, and market values through a wide variety of diversification initiatives, including acquisitions, strategic alliances, and joint ventures, as well as internal development.*

So the question becomes: Why do some diversification efforts pay off and others produce poor results? This chapter addresses two related issues: (1) What businesses should a corporation compete in? and (2) How should these businesses be managed to jointly create more value than if they were freestanding units?

diversification the process of firms expanding their operations by entering new businesses.

Diversification initiatives—whether through mergers and acquisitions, strategic alliances and joint ventures, or internal development—must be justified by the creation of value for shareholders.[12] But this is not always the case.[13] Acquiring firms typically pay high premiums when they acquire a target firm. For example, in 2008, Shire Ltd. acquired Jerini AG, a pharmaceutical company based in Berlin, Germany, for $518 million in another high-premium deal. The agreement regarding the strategic partnership provided for Shire to submit a voluntary public cash takeover offer at a price of 6.25 euros per share, through Maia Elfte Vermogensverwaltungs-GmbH (to be renamed Shire Deutschland Investments GmbH), to the shareholders of Jerini AG without a minimum acceptance threshold. The offer price corresponded to a premium of approximately 199 percent over the volume-weighted average stock price of 2.09 euros of Jerini AG's shares during the three months prior to the announcement of the offer.

Given the seemingly high inherent downside risks and uncertainties, one might ask: Why should companies even bother with diversification initiatives? The answer, in a word, is *synergy,* derived from the Greek word *synergos,* which means "working together." This can have two different, but not mutually exclusive, meanings.

First, a firm may diversify into *related* businesses. Here, the primary potential benefits to be derived come from *horizontal relationships;* that is, businesses sharing intangible resources (e.g., core competencies such as marketing) and tangible resources (e.g., production facilities, distribution channels).[14] Firms can also enhance their market power via pooled negotiating power and vertical integration. For example, Procter & Gamble enjoys many synergies from having businesses that share distribution resources.

Second, a corporation may diversify into *unrelated* businesses.[15] Here, the primary potential benefits are derived largely from *hierarchical relationships;* that is, value creation derived from the corporate office. Examples of the latter would include leveraging some of the support activities in the value chain that we discussed in Chapter 3, such as information systems or human resource practices. Cooper Industries has followed a successful strategy of unrelated diversification. There are few similarities in the products it

---

* Many high-tech firms, such as Motorola, IBM, Qualcomm, and Intel have also diversified through company-owned venture capital arms. Intel Capital, for example, has invested $4 billion in 1,000 companies over 15 years. Some 160 of those companies have been sold to other firms, while another 150 of them have been publicly listed. In 2006, Intel Capital's investments added $214 million to the parent company's net income. For an insightful discussion of how Apple might benefit from a venture capital initiative, refer to Hesseldahl, A. 2007. What to do with Apple's cash. *BusinessWeek,* March 19: 80.

makes or the industries in which it competes. However, the corporate office adds value through such activities as superb human resource practices and budgeting systems.

Please note that such benefits derived from horizontal (related diversification) and hierarchical (unrelated diversification) relationships are not mutually exclusive. Many firms that diversify into related areas benefit from information technology expertise in the corporate office. Similarly, unrelated diversifiers often benefit from the "best practices" of sister businesses even though their products, markets, and technologies may differ dramatically.

Exhibit 6.2 provides an overview of how we will address the various means by which firms create value through both related and unrelated diversification and also includes a summary of some examples that we will address in this chapter.[16]

Exhibit 6.2
Creating Value through Related and Unrelated Diversification

Related Diversification: Economies of Scope

Leveraging core competencies

- 3M leverages its competencies in adhesives technologies to many industries, including automotive, construction, and telecommunications.

Networking

- ANZ Bank achieves economies of scope from selling a range of products (banking services, insurance, superannuation, financial advice) through its branch network using the ANZ brand name.

Sharing activities

- McKesson, a large distribution company, sells many product lines, such as pharmaceuticals and liquor, through its superwarehouses.

Related Diversification: Market Power

Increasing market share

- Nestlé, which had a large baby-food position in emerging economies such as Brazil and China, lacked a presence in the United States. Thus, it acquired Gerber from Novartis AG, which had nearly an 80 percent share of the U. S. baby food market. After buying Gerber, Nestlé substantially increased its market power worldwide.

Pooled negotiating power

- Times Mirror Company increases its power over customers by providing "one-stop shopping" for advertisers to reach customers through multiple media—television and newspapers—in several huge markets such as New York and Chicago.

Vertical integration

- Shaw Industries, a giant carpet manufacturer, increases its control over raw materials by producing much of its own polypropylene fiber, a key input to its manufacturing process.

Unrelated Diversification: Parenting, Restructuring, and Financial Synergies

Corporate restructuring and parenting

- The corporate office of Samsung adds value by imposing tough standards of profitability and by disseminating knowledge and best practices quickly throughout the Samsung organization.

Portfolio management

- Novartis, formerly Ciba-Geigy, uses portfolio management to improve many key activities, including resource allocation and reward and evaluation systems.

related diversification a firm entering a different business in which it can benefit from leveraging core competencies, sharing activities, or building market power.

economies of scope cost savings from leveraging core competencies or sharing related activities among businesses in a corporation.

>LO6.3
How corporations can use related diversification to achieve synergistic benefits through economies of scope and market power.

core competencies a firm's strategic resources that reflect the collective learning in the organization.

Related Diversification: Economies of Scope and Revenue Enhancement

Related diversification enables a firm to benefit from horizontal relationships across different businesses in the diversified corporation by leveraging core competencies and sharing activities (e.g., production and distribution facilities). This enables a corporation to benefit from economies of scope. **Economies of scope** refers to cost savings from leveraging core competencies or sharing related activities among businesses in the corporation. A firm can also enjoy greater revenues if two businesses attain higher levels of sales growth combined than either company could attain independently.

For example, a sporting goods store with one or several locations may acquire retail stores carrying other product lines. This enables it to leverage, or reuse, many of its key resources—favorable reputation, expert staff and management skills, efficient purchasing operations—the basis of its competitive advantage(s), over a larger number of stores.[17]

Leveraging Core Competencies

The concept of core competencies can be illustrated by the imagery of the diversified corporation as a tree.[18] The trunk and major limbs represent core products; the smaller branches are business units; and the leaves, flowers, and fruit are end products. The core competencies are represented by the root system, which provides nourishment, sustenance, and stability. Managers often misread the strength of competitors by looking only at their end products, just as we can fail to appreciate the strength of a tree by looking only at its leaves. Core competencies may also be viewed as the "glue" that binds existing businesses together or as the engine that fuels new business growth.

Core competencies reflect the collective learning in organizations—how to coordinate diverse production skills, integrate multiple streams of technologies, and market diverse products and services.[19] The knowledge necessary to put a radio on a chip does not in itself assure a company of the skill needed to produce a miniature radio approximately the size of a business card. To accomplish this, Casio, a giant electronic products producer, must synthesize know-how in miniaturization, microprocessor design, material science, and ultrathin precision castings. These are the same skills that it applies in its miniature card calculators, pocket TVs, and digital watches.

For a core competence to create value and provide a viable basis for synergy among the businesses in a corporation, it must meet three criteria.[20]

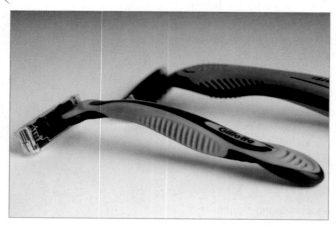

● Gillette's expertise in multiple competencies helps the company develop superior shaving products used worldwide.

- *The core competence must enhance competitive advantage(s) by creating superior customer value.* Every value-chain activity has the potential to provide a viable basis for building on a core competence.[21] At Gillette, for example, scientists developed the Fusion and Mach 3 after the introduction of the tremendously successful Sensor System because of a thorough understanding of several phenomena that underlie shaving. These include the physiology of facial hair and skin, the metallurgy of blade strength and sharpness, the dynamics of a cartridge moving across skin, and the physics of a razor blade severing hair. Such innovations are possible only with

Procter & Gamble Leverages Its Core Competence in Marketing and (Believe It or Not!) Franchising

Procter & Gamble, long dominant in detergents to wash clothes, wants to also dry clean them. The world's biggest consumer products company plans to roll out franchised Tide Dry Cleaners across America. P&G wants to put its brands to work selling services to boost U.S. revenue for its products.

Some think that its strategy could be a huge hit. For example, Andrew Cherng, founder of Panda Restaurant Group, which operates Chinese fast-food outlets in U.S. malls, plans to open around 150 Tide-branded dry cleaners over the next four years. He claimed: "I wasn't around when McDonald's was taking franchisees. I'm not going to miss this one."

In 2007, the firm launched Mr. Clean Car Wash. Nine franchises are now in operation. The following year, P&G opened three test Tide Dry Cleaners in Kansas City. Having fine-tuned the concept, the firm is now going national. According to Michael Stone, P&G is moving into services "that are virtually unbranded. One would think consumers would trust a Tide Dry Cleaners because they know P&G is behind it."

With more than 800,000 Facebook fans and legions of customers, P&G hopes that the Tide brand will draw people into franchise stores and that superior service—which includes drive-through service, 24-hour pickup, and cleaning methods it markets as environmentally safe—will keep them coming back. "The power of our brands represents disruptive innovation in these industries," said Nathan Estruth, vice president for FutureWorks, P&G's entrepreneurial arm. "Imagine getting to start my new business with the power of Tide."

But . . . it won't be easy. Competition is fierce, and customers can be prickly: Woe to the dry cleaner that ruins a favorite suit or dress—even if it was cheaply made and decades old. Sanjiv Mehra, who headed Unilever's attempt to break into the dry-cleaning business about a decade ago, says that the key to success is in figuring out a way to do it cheaper or much better than the mom-and-pop stores that dominate the industry. At the end of the day, Unilever realized that it couldn't do either. He said, "It comes back to, are you fundamentally changing the economics of the business?" adding that P&G's marketing muscle could turn out to be the difference. "That's where they will make a lot of money if they do it right."

Sources: Coleman-Lochner, L. & Clothier, M. 2010. P&G puts its big brands to work in franchises. *Bloomberg Businessweek.* September 6–12: 20; and, Martin, A. 2010. Smelling an opportunity. *www.nytimes.com.* December 8: np.

an understanding of such phenomena and the ability to combine such technologies into innovative products. Customers are willing to pay more for such technologically differentiated products.

- ***Different businesses in the corporation must be similar in at least one important way related to the core competence.*** It is not essential that the products or services themselves be similar. Rather, at least one element in the value chain must require similar skills in creating competitive advantage if the corporation is to capitalize on its core competence. At first glance you might think that cars and clothes have little in common. However, Strategy Spotlight 6.1 discusses how Procter & Gamble is leveraging its newfound competence in franchising to create a new revenue stream.

- ***The core competencies must be difficult for competitors to imitate or find substitutes for.*** As we discussed in Chapter 5, competitive advantages will not be sustainable if the competition can easily imitate or substitute them. Similarly, if the skills associated with a firm's core competencies are easily imitated or replicated, they are not a sound basis for sustainable advantages. Consider Sharp Corporation, a consumer electronics giant with 2010 revenues of $30 billion.[22] It has a set of specialized core competencies in optoelectronics technologies that are difficult to replicate and contribute to its competitive advantages in its core businesses. Its most successful technology has been liquid crystal displays (LCDs) that are critical components in nearly all of Sharp's products. Its expertise in this technology enabled Sharp to succeed in videocassette recorders (VCRs) with its innovative LCD viewfinder and led to the creation of its Wizard, a personal electronic organizer.

Before his death in October 2011, Steve Jobs provided insights on the importance of a firm's core competence. The Apple CEO was widely considered one of the world's most respected business leaders:[23]

> One of our biggest insights (years ago) was that we didn't want to get into any business where we didn't own or control the primary technology, because you'll get your head handed to you. We realized that for almost all future consumer electronics, the primary technology was going to be software. And we were pretty good at software. We could do the operating system software. We could write applications like iTunes on the Mac or even PC. And we could write the back-end software that runs on a cloud like iTunes. So we could write all these different kinds of software and tweed it all together and make it work seamlessly. And you ask yourself: What other companies can do that? It's a pretty short list.

Sharing Activities

As we saw above, leveraging core competencies involves transferring accumulated skills and expertise across business units in a corporation. Corporations also can achieve synergy by **sharing activities** across their business units. These include value-creating activities such as common manufacturing facilities, distribution channels, and sales forces. As we will see, sharing activities can potentially provide two primary payoffs: cost savings and revenue enhancements.

Deriving Cost Savings   Typically, this is the most common type of synergy and the easiest to estimate. Peter Shaw, head of mergers and acquisitions at the British chemical and pharmaceutical company ICI, refers to cost savings as "hard synergies" and contends that the level of certainty of their achievement is quite high. Cost savings come from many sources, including the elimination of jobs, facilities, and related expenses that are no longer needed when functions are consolidated, or from economies of scale in purchasing. Cost savings are generally highest when one company acquires another from the same industry in the same country. Shaw Industries, recently acquired by Berkshire Hathaway, is the nation's largest carpet producer. Over the years, it has dominated the competition through a strategy of acquisition which has enabled Shaw, among other things, to consolidate its manufacturing operations in a few, highly efficient plants and to lower costs through higher capacity utilization.

Sharing activities inevitably involve costs that the benefits must outweigh such as the greater coordination required to manage a shared activity. Even more important is the need to compromise on the design or performance of an activity so that it can be shared. For example, a salesperson handling the products of two business units must operate in a way that is usually not what either unit would choose if it were independent. If the compromise erodes the unit's effectiveness, then sharing may reduce rather than enhance competitive advantage.

Enhancing Revenue and Differentiation   Often an acquiring firm and its target may achieve a higher level of sales growth together than either company could on its own. Shortly after Gillette acquired Duracell, it confirmed its expectation that selling Duracell batteries through Gillette's existing channels for personal care products would increase sales, particularly internationally. Gillette sold Duracell products in 25 new markets in the first year after the acquisition and substantially increased sales in established international markets. Also, a target company's distribution channel can be used to escalate the sales of the acquiring company's product. Such was the case when Gillette acquired Parker Pen. Gillette estimated that it could gain an additional $25 million in sales of its own Waterman pens by taking advantage of Parker's distribution channels.

Firms also can enhance the effectiveness of their differentiation strategies by means of sharing activities among business units. A shared order-processing system, for example, may permit new features and services that a buyer will value. Also, sharing can reduce the cost of differentiation. For instance, a shared service network may make more advanced, remote service technology economically feasible. To illustrate the potential for enhanced differentiation through sharing, consider $7 billion VF Corporation—producer of such well-known brands as Lee, Wrangler, Vanity Fair, and Jantzen.

> VF's acquisition of Nutmeg Industries and H. H. Cutler provided it with several large customers that it didn't have before, increasing its plant utilization and productivity. But more importantly, Nutmeg designs and makes licensed apparel for sports teams and organizations, while Cutler manufactures licensed brand-name children's apparel, including Walt Disney kids' wear. Such brand labeling enhances the differentiation of VF's apparel products. According to VF President Mackey McDonald, "What we're doing is looking at value-added knitwear, taking our basic fleece from Basset-Walker [one of its divisions], embellishing it through Cutler and Nutmeg, and selling it as a value-added product." Additionally, Cutler's advanced high-speed printing technologies will enable VF to be more proactive in anticipating trends in the fashion-driven fleece market. Claims McDonald, "Rather than printing first and then trying to guess what the customer wants, we can see what's happening in the marketplace and then print it up."[24]

As a cautionary note, managers must keep in mind that sharing activities among businesses in a corporation can have a negative effect on a given business's differentiation. For example, with the merger of Chrysler and Daimler-Benz, many consumers may have lowered their perceptions of Mercedes's quality and prestige because they felt that common production components and processes were being used across the two divisions. And Ford's Jaguar division was adversely affected as consumers came to understand that it shared many components with its sister divisions at Ford, including Lincoln. Perhaps, it is not too surprising that both Chrysler and Jaguar were divested by their parent corporations.

Related Diversification: Market Power

We now discuss how companies achieve related diversification through **market power.** We also address the two principal means by which firms achieve synergy through market power: *pooled negotiating power* and *vertical integration.* Managers do, however, have limits on their ability to use market power for diversification, because government regulations can sometimes restrict the ability of a business to gain very large shares of a particular market. Consider GE's attempt to acquire Honeywell:

> When General Electric announced a $41 billion bid for Honeywell, the European Union stepped in. GE's market clout would have expanded significantly with the deal: GE would supply over one-half the parts needed to build several aircraft engines. The commission's concern, causing them to reject the acquisition, was that GE could use its increased market power to dominate the aircraft engine parts market and crowd out rivals.[25] Thus, while managers need to be aware of the strategic advantages of market power, they must at the same time be aware of regulations and legislation.

market power firms' abilities to profit through restricting or controlling supply to a market or coordinating with other firms to reduce investment.

Pooled Negotiating Power

Similar businesses working together or the affiliation of a business with a strong parent can strengthen an organization's bargaining position relative to suppliers and customers and enhance its position vis-à-vis competitors. Compare, for example, the position of an independent food manufacturer with the same business within Nestlé. Being part of Nestlé provides the business with significant clout—greater bargaining power with suppliers and customers—since it is part of a firm that makes large purchases from suppliers

pooled negotiating power the improvement in bargaining position relative to suppliers and customers.

and provides a wide variety of products. Access to the parent's deep pockets increases the business's strength, and the Nestlé unit enjoys greater protection from substitutes and new entrants. Not only would rivals perceive the unit as a more formidable opponent, but the unit's association with Nestlé would also provide greater visibility and improved image.

Consolidating an industry can also increase a firm's market power.[26] This is clearly an emerging trend in the multimedia industry.[27] All of these mergers and acquisitions have a common goal: to control and leverage as many news and entertainment channels as possible.

When acquiring related businesses, a firm's potential for pooled negotiating power vis-à-vis its customers and suppliers can be very enticing. However, managers must carefully evaluate how the combined businesses may affect relationships with actual and potential customers, suppliers, and competitors. For example, when PepsiCo diversified into the fast-food industry with its acquisitions of Kentucky Fried Chicken, Taco Bell, and Pizza Hut (now part of Yum! Brands), it clearly benefited from its position over these units that served as a captive market for its soft-drink products. However, many competitors, such as McDonald's, have refused to consider PepsiCo as a supplier of its own soft-drink needs because of competition with Pepsi's divisions in the fast-food industry. Simply put, McDonald's did not want to subsidize the enemy! Thus, although acquiring related businesses can enhance a corporation's bargaining power, it must be aware of the potential for retaliation.

Strategy Spotlight 6.2 discusses how 3M's actions to increase its market power led to a lawsuit (which 3M lost) by a competitor.

Vertical Integration

vertical integration an expansion or extension of the firm by integrating preceding or successive production processes.

Vertical integration occurs when a firm becomes its own supplier or distributor. That is, it represents an expansion or extension of the firm by integrating preceding or successive production processes.[28] The firm incorporates more processes toward the original source of raw materials (backward integration) or toward the ultimate consumer (forward integration). For example, a car manufacturer might supply its own parts or make its own engines to secure sources of supply or control its own system of dealerships to ensure retail outlets for its products. Similarly, an oil refinery might secure land leases and develop its own drilling capacity to ensure a constant supply of crude oil. Or it could expand into retail operations by owning or licensing gasoline stations to guarantee customers for its petroleum products.

Clearly, vertical integration can be a viable strategy for many firms. For example, Indian petrochemical giant Reliance Industries has made vertical integration a viable strategy. Initiated by the company's late founder, Dhirubhai Ambani, Reliance's backward integration into polyester fibers from textiles and then into petrochemicals now provides the company with a complete vertical product portfolio from oil and gas production, refining, petrochemicals, synthetic garments, and retail outlets.

Strategy Spotlight 6.3 discusses Shaw Industries, a carpet manufacturer that has attained a dominant position in the industry via a strategy of vertical integration. Shaw has successfully implemented strategies of both forward and backward integration. Exhibit 6.3 depicts the stages of Shaw's vertical integration.

Benefits and Risks of Vertical Integration Vertical integration is a means for an organization to reduce its dependence on suppliers or its channels of distribution to end users. However, the benefits associated with vertical integration—backward or forward—must be carefully weighed against the risks.[29]

The *benefits* of vertical integration include (1) a secure supply of raw materials or distribution channels that cannot be "held hostage" to external markets where costs can fluctuate over time, (2) protection and control over assets and services required to produce and deliver valuable products and services, (3) access to new business opportunities and new forms of technologies, and (4) simplified procurement and administrative procedures since key activities are brought inside the firm, eliminating the need to deal with a wide variety of suppliers and distributors.

How 3M's Efforts to Increase Its Market Power Backfired

In the spring and summer of 2006, 3M found itself in court facing three class-action lawsuits launched by consumers and retailers of transparent and invisible adhesive tape (often generically known as "Scotch tape"). The suits all alleged that 3M had unlawfully bullied its way into a monopoly position in the tape market and that, as a result, consumers had been deprived of their rightful amount of choice and often paid up to 40 percent too much for their tape.

One rival that was particularly interested in these cases is LePage's Inc. of North York, Ontario—3M's only significant competitor in the home and office adhesive tape market. LePage's has everything to gain from court penalties against 3M's selling practices. This includes greater access to the lucrative North American market. The Canadian company started 3M's legal travails in the first place; all of the current class-action suits were initiated by LePage's.

Back in 1997, LePage's (then based in Pittsburgh) filed a complaint in the Pennsylvania District Court against 3M's practice of selling its various tape products using what was called "bundled rebates." LePage's argued that it violated the Sherman Act, the century-old U.S. legislation that limited monopoly power. 3M's bundled rebate program offered significant rebates—sometimes in the millions of dollars—to retailers as a reward for selling targeted amounts of six product lines. LePage's claimed that such selling targets were so large that retailers could only meet them by excluding competing products—in this case LePage's tape—from store shelves. For example, LePage's argued that Kmart, which had constituted 10 percent of LePage's sales, dropped the account when 3M started offering the discount chain $1 million in rebates in return for selling more than $15 million worth of 3M products each year. Further, LePage's offered its own conspiracy theory: 3M introduced rebates not simply to grow its sales, but to eliminate LePage's—its only significant competitor.

A jury awarded LePage's $68.5 million in damages (the amount after trebling)—almost 15 percent of the 3M Consumer and Office Business unit's operating income in 2000. The Court of Appeals for the Third Circuit rejected 3M's appeal and upheld the judgment. It concluded that rebate bundling, even if above cost, may exclude equally efficient competitors from offering product (in this case, tape). In the ruling, Judge Dolores K. Sloviter wrote that "they may foreclose portions of the market to a potential competitor who does not manufacture an equally diverse group of products and who therefore cannot make a comparable offer." Therefore, the bundled rebates were judged to be an exploitation of 3M's monopoly power.

Sources: Bush, D. & Gelb, B. D. 2005. When marketing practices raise antitrust concerns. *MIT Sloan Management Review,* 46(4): 73–81; Campbell, C. 2006. Tale of the tape. *Canadian Business,* April 24: 39–40; and, Bergstrom, B. 2003. $68M jury award upheld against 3M in antitrust case. *The Associated Press,* March 26.

ethics

Winnebago, the leader in the market for drivable recreational vehicles with a 19.3 percent market share, illustrates some of vertical integration's benefits.[30] The word *Winnebago* means "big RV" to most Americans. And the firm has a sterling reputation for great quality. The firm's huge northern Iowa factories do everything from extruding aluminum for

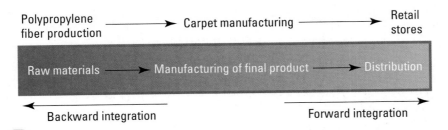

Exhibit 6.3 Simplified Stages of Vertical Integration: Shaw Industries

Vertical Integration at Shaw Industries

Shaw Industries (now part of Berkshire Hathaway) is an example of a firm that has followed a very successful strategy of vertical integration. By relentlessly pursuing both backward and forward integration, Shaw has become the dominant manufacturer of carpeting products in the United States. According to CEO Robert Shaw, "We want to be involved with as much of the process

of making and selling carpets as practical. That way, we're in charge of costs." For example, Shaw acquired Amoco's polypropylene fiber manufacturing facilities in Alabama and Georgia. These new plants provide carpet fibers for internal use and for sale to other manufacturers. With this backward integration, fully one-quarter of Shaw's carpet fiber needs are now met in-house. In early 1996 Shaw began to integrate forward, acquiring seven floor-covering retailers in a move that suggested a strategy to consolidate the fragmented industry and increase its influence over retail pricing. Exhibit 6.3 (on previous page) provides a simplified depiction of the stages of vertical integration for Shaw Industries.

Sources: White, J. 2003. Shaw to home in on more with Georgia Tufters deal. *HFN: The Weekly Newspaper for the Home Furnishing Network,* May 5: 32; Shaw Industries. 1993, 2000. Annual reports; and, Server, A. 1994. How to escape a price war. *Fortune,* June 13: 88.

body parts, to molding plastics for water and holding tanks, to dashboards. Such vertical integration at the factory may appear to be outdated and expensive, but it guarantees excellent quality. The Recreational Vehicle Dealer Association started giving a quality award in 1996, and Winnebago has won it every year.

The *risks* of vertical integration include (1) the costs and expenses associated with increased overhead and capital expenditures to provide facilities, raw material inputs, and distribution channels inside the organization; (2) a loss of flexibility resulting from the inability to respond quickly to changes in the external environment because of the huge investments in vertical integration activities that generally cannot be easily deployed elsewhere; (3) problems associated with unbalanced capacities or unfilled demand along the value chain; and (4) additional administrative costs associated with managing a more complex set of activities. Exhibit 6.4 summarizes the benefits and risks of vertical integration.

In making vertical integration decisions, five issues should be considered.[31]

Exhibit 6.4
Benefits and Risks of Vertical Integration

Benefits
• A secure source of raw materials or distribution channels.
• Protection of and control over valuable assets.
• Access to new business opportunities.
• Simplified procurement and administrative procedures.

Risks
• Costs and expenses associated with increased overhead and capital expenditures.
• Loss of flexibility resulting from large investments.
• Problems associated with unbalanced capacities along the value chain.
• Additional administrative costs associated with managing a more complex set of activities.

1. *Is the company satisfied with the quality of the value that its present suppliers and distributors are providing?* If the performance of organizations in the vertical chain—both suppliers and distributors—is satisfactory, it may not, in general, be appropriate for a company to perform these activities themselves. Nike and Reebok have outsourced the manufacture of their shoes to countries such as China and Indonesia where labor costs are low. Since the strengths of these companies are typically in design and marketing, it would be advisable to continue to outsource production operations and continue to focus on where they can add the most value.

2. *Are there activities in the industry value chain presently being outsourced or performed independently by others that are a viable source of future profits?* Even if a firm is outsourcing value-chain activities to companies that are doing a credible job, it may be missing out on substantial profit opportunities. To illustrate, consider the automobile industry's profit pool. As you may recall from Chapter 5, there is much more potential profit in many downstream activities (e.g., leasing, warranty, insurance, and service) than in the manufacture of automobiles. Not surprisingly, carmakers such as Toyota and Honda are undertaking forward integration strategies to become bigger players in these high-profit activities.

3. *Is there a high level of stability in the demand for the organization's products?* High demand or sales volatility is not conducive to vertical integration. With the high level of fixed costs in plant and equipment as well as operating costs that accompany endeavors toward vertical integration, widely fluctuating sales demand can either strain resources (in times of high demand) or result in unused capacity (in times of low demand). The cycles of "boom and bust" in the automobile industry are a key reason why the manufacturers have increased the amount of outsourced inputs.

4. *Does the company have the necessary competencies to execute the vertical integration strategies?* As many companies would attest, successfully executing strategies of vertical integration can be very difficult. For example, Unocal, a major petroleum refiner, which once owned retail gas stations, was slow to capture the potential grocery and merchandise side of the business that might have resulted from customer traffic to its service stations. Unocal lacked the competencies to develop a separate retail organization and culture. The company eventually sold the assets and brand.

5. *Will the vertical integration initiative have potential negative impacts on the firm's stakeholders?* Managers must carefully consider the impact that vertical integration may have on existing and future customers, suppliers, and competitors. After Lockheed Martin, a dominant defense contractor, acquired Loral Corporation, an electronics supplier, for $9.1 billion, it had an unpleasant and unanticipated surprise. Loral, as a captive supplier of Lockheed, is now viewed as a rival by many of its previous customers. Thus, before Lockheed Martin can realize any net synergies from this acquisition, it must make up for the substantial business that it has lost.

Analyzing Vertical Integration: The Transaction Cost Perspective Another approach that has proved very useful in understanding vertical integration is the **transaction cost perspective.**[32] According to this perspective, every market transaction involves some *transaction costs*. First, a decision to purchase an input from an outside source leads to *search* costs (e.g., the cost to find where it is available, the level of quality, etc.). Second, there are costs associated with *negotiating*. Third, a *contract* needs to be written spelling out future possible contingencies. Fourth, parties in a contract have to *monitor* each other. Finally, if a party does not comply with the terms of the contract, there are *enforcement* costs. Transaction costs are thus the sum of search costs, negotiation costs, contracting costs, monitoring costs, and enforcement costs. These transaction costs can be avoided by internalizing the activity—in other words, by producing the input in-house.

transaction cost perspective a perspective that the choice of a transaction's governance structure, such as vertical integration or market transaction, is influenced by transaction costs, including search, negotiating, contracting, monitoring, and enforcement costs, associated with each choice.

A related problem with purchasing a specialized input from outside is the issue of *transaction-specific investments.* For example, when an automobile company needs an input specifically designed for a particular car model, the supplier may be unwilling to make the investments in plant and machinery necessary to produce that component for two reasons. First, the investment may take many years to recover but there is no guarantee the automobile company will continue to buy from them after the contract expires, typically in one year. Second, once the investment is made, the supplier has no bargaining power. That is, the buyer knows that the supplier has no option but to supply at ever-lower prices because the investments were so specific that they cannot be used to produce alternative products. In such circumstances, again, vertical integration may be the only option.

Vertical integration, however, gives rise to a different set of costs. These costs are referred to as *administrative costs.* Coordinating different stages of the value chain now internalized within the firm causes administrative costs to go up. Decisions about vertical integration are, therefore, based on a comparison of transaction costs and administrative costs. If transaction costs are lower than administrative costs, it is best to resort to market transactions and avoid vertical integration. For example, McDonald's may be the world's biggest buyer of beef, but it does not raise cattle. The market for beef has low transaction costs and requires no transaction-specific investments. On the other hand, if transaction costs are higher than administrative costs, vertical integration becomes an attractive strategy. For example, Hyundai Motor Group was able to vertically integrate the production process for molten iron by creating Hyundai Steel and establishing the world's first resource circulating system with steel at the core.[33] Most automobile manufacturers produce their own engines because the market for engines involves high transaction costs and transaction-specific investments.

>LO6.4
How corporations can use unrelated diversification to attain synergistic benefits through corporate restructuring, parenting, and portfolio analysis.

Unrelated Diversification: Financial Synergies and Parenting

With **unrelated diversification,** unlike related diversification, few benefits are derived from *horizontal relationships*—that is, the leveraging of core competencies or the sharing of activities across business units within a corporation. Instead, potential benefits can be gained from *vertical (or hierarchical) relationships*—the creation of synergies from the interaction of the corporate office with the individual business units. There are two main sources of such synergies. First, the corporate office can contribute to "parenting" and restructuring of (often acquired) businesses. Second, the corporate office can add value by viewing the entire corporation as a family or "portfolio" of businesses and allocating resources to optimize corporate goals of profitability, cash flow, and growth. Additionally, the corporate office enhances value by establishing appropriate human resource practices and financial controls for each of its business units.

unrelated diversification a firm entering a different business that has little horizontal interaction with other businesses of a firm.

Corporate Parenting and Restructuring

We have discussed how firms can add value through related diversification by exploring sources of synergy *across* business units. Now, we discuss how value can be created *within* business units as a result of the expertise and support provided by the corporate office.

parenting advantage the positive contributions of the corporate office to a new business as a result of expertise and support provided and not as a result of substantial changes in assets, capital structure, or management.

Parenting   The positive contributions of the corporate office are called the **"parenting advantage."**[34] Many firms have successfully diversified their holdings without strong evidence of the more traditional sources of synergy (i.e., horizontally across business units). Diversified public corporations such as BTR, Emerson Electric, and Hanson and leveraged buyout firms such as Kohlberg, Kravis, Roberts & Company, and Clayton, Dublilier & Rice are a few examples.[35] Through its management processes, Wesfarmers in Australia appears to have created value across seemingly diverse businesses with no obvious synergy, but it has never set out to be an acquisition-and-restructure company like Hanson. These parent companies create value through management expertise. How? They improve plans and budgets and provide especially competent central functions such as legal, financial, human resource management, procurement, and the like. They also help subsidiaries make wise choices in their own acquisitions, divestitures, and new internal development decisions. Such contributions often help business units to substantially increase their revenues and profits. Consider Texas-based Cooper Industries' acquisition of Champion International, the spark plug company, as an example of corporate parenting:[36]

> Cooper applies a distinctive parenting approach designed to help its businesses improve their manufacturing performance. New acquisitions are "Cooperized"—Cooper audits their manufacturing operations; improves their cost accounting systems; makes their planning, budgeting, and human resource systems conform with its systems; and centralizes union negotiations. Excess cash is squeezed out through tighter controls and reinvested in productivity enhancements, which improve overall operating efficiency. As one manager observed, "When you get acquired by Cooper, one of the first things that happens is a truckload of policy manuals arrives at your door." Such active parenting has been effective in enhancing the competitive advantages of many kinds of manufacturing businesses.

Restructuring Restructuring is another means by which the corporate office can add value to a business.[37] The central idea can be captured in the real estate phrase "buy low and sell high." Here, the corporate office tries to find either poorly performing firms with unrealized potential or firms in industries on the threshold of significant, positive change. The parent intervenes, often selling off parts of the business; changing the management; reducing payroll and unnecessary sources of expenses; changing strategies; and infusing the company with new technologies, processes, reward systems, and so forth. When the restructuring is complete, the firm can either "sell high" and capture the added value or keep the business and enjoy financial and competitive benefits.[38]

Loews Corporation, a conglomerate with $15 billion in revenues, competes in such industries as oil and gas, tobacco, watches, insurance, and hotels. It provides an exemplary example of how firms can successfully "buy low and sell high" as part of their corporate strategy.[39]

> Energy accounts for 33 percent of Loews' $30 billion in total assets. In the 1980s it bought six oil tankers for only $5 million each during a sharp slide in oil prices. The downside was limited. After all these huge hulks could easily have been sold as scrap steel. However, that didn't have to happen. Eight years after Loews purchased the tankers, they sold them for $50 million each.
>
> Loews was also extremely successful with its next energy play—drilling equipment. Although wildcatting for oil is very risky, selling services to wildcatters is not, especially if the assets are bought during a down cycle. Loews did just that. It purchased 10 offshore drilling rigs for $50 million in 1989 and formed Diamond Offshore Drilling. In 1995 Loews received $338 million after taking a 30 percent piece of this operation public!

For the restructuring strategy to work, the corporate management must have the insight to detect undervalued companies (otherwise the cost of acquisition would be too high) or businesses competing in industries with a high potential for transformation.[40] Additionally, of course, they must have the requisite skills and resources to turn the businesses around, even if they may be in new and unfamiliar industries.

Restructuring can involve changes in assets, capital structure, or management.

- *Asset restructuring* involves the sale of unproductive assets, or even whole lines of businesses, that are peripheral. In some cases, it may even involve acquisitions that strengthen the core business.

restructuring the intervention of the corporate office in a new business that substantially changes the assets, capital structure, and/or management, including selling off parts of the business, changing the management, reducing payroll and unnecessary sources of expenses, changing strategies, and infusing the new business with new technologies, processes, and reward systems.

- *Capital restructuring* involves changing the debt-equity mix, or the mix between different classes of debt or equity. Although the substitution of equity with debt is more common in buyout situations, occasionally the parent may provide additional equity capital.
- *Management restructuring* typically involves changes in the composition of the top management team, organizational structure, and reporting relationships. Tight financial control, rewards based strictly on meeting short- to medium-term performance goals, and reduction in the number of middle-level managers are common steps in management restructuring. In some cases, parental intervention may even result in changes in strategy as well as infusion of new technologies and processes.

Hanson, plc, a British conglomerate, made numerous such acquisitions in the United States in the 1980s, often selling these firms at significant profits after a few years of successful restructuring efforts. Hanson's acquisition and subsequent restructuring of the SCM group is a classic example of the restructuring strategy. Hanson acquired SCM, a diversified manufacturer of industrial and consumer products (including Smith-Corona typewriters, Glidden paints, and Durkee Famous Foods), for $930 million in 1986 after a bitter takeover battle. In the next few months, Hanson sold SCM's paper and pulp operations for $160 million, the chemical division for $30 million, Glidden paints for $580 million, and Durkee Famous Foods for $120 million, virtually recovering the entire original investment. In addition, Hanson also sold the SCM headquarters in New York for $36 million and reduced the headquarters staff by 250. It still retained several profitable divisions, including the titanium dioxide operations and managed them with tight financial controls that led to increased returns.[41]

Exhibit 6.5 summarizes the three primary types of restructuring activities.

Portfolio Management

During the 1970s and early 1980s, several leading consulting firms developed the concept of **portfolio management** to achieve a better understanding of the competitive position of an overall portfolio (or family) of businesses, to suggest strategic alternatives for each of the businesses, and to identify priorities for the allocation of resources. Several studies have reported widespread use of these techniques among American firms.[42]

Description and Potential Benefits   The key purpose of portfolio models is to assist a firm in achieving a balanced portfolio of businesses.[43] This consists of businesses whose profitability, growth, and cash flow characteristics complement each other and adds up to a satisfactory overall corporate performance. Imbalance, for example, could be caused either by excessive cash generation with too few growth opportunities or by insufficient cash generation to fund the growth requirements in the portfolio. Chairman Alex Krauer decided to develop a customized portfolio planning concept for Ciba-Geigy, Switzerland's top chemical and pharmaceutical company. He enlisted the help of Hans-Jong Held as the head of corporate planning. In Held's words, their intention was "to improve the process of resource allocation and performance assessment. The main idea was to differentiate the business—to give us different objectives, different types of managers, and to allow us to

portfolio management a method of (a) assessing the competitive position of a portfolio of businesses within a corporation, (b) suggesting strategic alternatives for each business, and (c) identifying priorities for the allocation of resources across the businesses.

Exhibit 6.5
The Three Primary Types of Restructuring Activities

Asset Restructuring: The sale of unproductive assets, or even whole lines of businesses, that are peripheral.

Capital Restructuring: Changing the debt-equity mix, or the mix between different classes of debt or equity.

Management Restructuring: Changes in the composition of the top management team, organization structure, and reporting relationships.

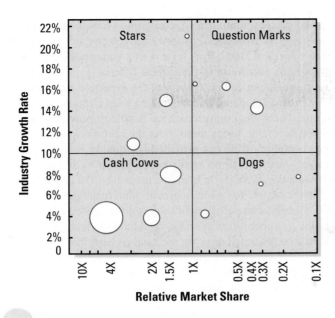

Exhibit 6.6 The Boston Consulting Group (BCG) Portfolio Matrix

adopt the organization structure that was appropriate for each business." He then added, "We needed a mental map with which to recognize diversity of our business in a rigorous, rather than intuitive, way."[44]

The Boston Consulting Group's (BCG) growth/share matrix is among the best known of these approaches.[45] In the BCG approach, each of the firm's strategic business units (SBUs) is plotted on a two-dimensional grid in which the axes are relative market share and industry growth rate. The grid is broken into four quadrants. Exhibit 6.6 depicts the BCG matrix. Following are a few clarifications:

1. Each circle represents one of the corporation's business units. The size of the circle represents the relative size of the business unit in terms of revenues.
2. Relative market share, measured by the ratio of the business unit's size to that of its largest competitor, is plotted along the horizontal axis.
3. Market share is central to the BCG matrix. This is because high relative market share leads to unit cost reduction due to experience and learning curve effects and, consequently, superior competitive position.

Each of the four quadrants of the grid has different implications for the SBUs that fall into the category:

- **Stars** are SBUs competing in high-growth industries with relatively high market shares. These firms have long-term growth potential and should continue to receive substantial investment funding.
- **Question Marks** are SBUs competing in high-growth industries but having relatively weak market shares. Resources should be invested in them to enhance their competitive positions.
- **Cash Cows** are SBUs with high market shares in low-growth industries. These units have limited long-run potential but represent a source of current cash flows to fund investments in "stars" and "question marks."
- **Dogs** are SBUs with weak market shares in low-growth industries. Because they have weak positions and limited potential, most analysts recommend that they be divested.

In using portfolio strategy approaches, a corporation tries to create shareholder value in a number of ways.[46] First, portfolio analysis provides a snapshot of the businesses in a corporation's portfolio. Therefore, the corporation is in a better position to allocate resources among the business units according to prescribed criteria (e.g., use cash flows from the "cash cows" to fund promising "stars"). Second, the expertise and analytical resources in the corporate office provide guidance in determining what firms may be attractive (or unattractive) acquisitions. Third, the corporate office is able to provide financial resources to the business units on favorable terms that reflect the corporation's overall ability to raise funds. Fourth, the corporate office can provide high-quality review and coaching for the individual businesses. Fifth, portfolio analysis provides a basis for developing strategic goals and reward/evaluation systems for business managers. For example, managers of cash cows would have lower targets for revenue growth than managers of stars, but the former would have higher threshold levels of profit targets on proposed projects than the managers of star businesses. Compensation systems would also reflect such realities. Cash cows understandably would be rewarded more on the basis of cash that their businesses generate than would managers of star businesses. Similarly, managers of star businesses would be held to higher standards for revenue growth than managers of cash cow businesses.

To see how companies can benefit from portfolio approaches, consider, again, Ciba-Geigy.

> In 1994 Ciba-Geigy adopted portfolio planning approaches to help it manage its business units, which competed in a wide variety of industries, including chemicals, dyes, pharmaceuticals, crop protection, and animal health.[47] It placed each business unit in a category corresponding to the BCG matrix. The business unit's goals, compensation programs, personnel selection, and resource allocation were strongly associated with the category within which the business was placed. For example, business units classified as "cash cows" had much higher hurdles for obtaining financial resources (from the corporate office) for expansion than "question marks" since the latter were businesses for which Ciba-Geigy had high hopes for accelerated future growth and profitability. Additionally, the compensation of a business unit manager in a cash cow would be strongly associated with its success in generating cash to fund other businesses, whereas a manager of a question mark business would be rewarded on his or her ability to increase revenue growth and market share. The portfolio planning approaches appear to be working. In 2010, Ciba-Geigy's (now Novartis) revenues and net income stood at $45 billion and $8.5 billion, respectively. This represents a 110 percent increase in revenues and a most impressive 49 percent growth in net income over a six-year period.

Limitations   Despite the potential benefits of portfolio models, there are also some notable downsides. First, they compare SBUs on only two dimensions, making the implicit but erroneous assumption that (1) those are the only factors that really matter and (2) every unit can be accurately compared on that basis. Second, the approach views each SBU as a stand-alone entity, ignoring common core business practices and value-creating activities that may hold promise for synergies across business units. Third, unless care is exercised, the process becomes largely mechanical, substituting an oversimplified graphical model for the important contributions of the CEO's (and other corporate managers') experience and judgment. Fourth, the reliance on "strict rules" regarding resource allocation across SBUs can be detrimental to a firm's long-term viability. For example, according to one study, over one-half of all the businesses that should have been cash users (based on the BCG matrix) were instead cash providers.[48] Finally, while colorful and easy to comprehend, the imagery of the BCG matrix can lead to some troublesome and overly simplistic prescriptions. According to one author:

> The dairying analogy is appropriate (for some cash cows), so long as we resist the urge to oversimplify it. On the farm, even the best-producing cows eventually begin to dry up. The farmer's solution to this is euphemistically called "freshening" the cow: The farmer

arranges a date for the cow with a bull, she has a calf, the milk begins flowing again. Cloistering the cow—isolating her from everything but the feed trough and the milking machines—assures that she will go dry.[49]

To see what can go wrong, consider Cabot Corporation.

Cabot Corporation supplies carbon black for the rubber, electronics, and plastics industries. Following the BCG matrix, Cabot moved away from its cash cow, carbon black, and diversified into stars such as ceramics and semiconductors in a seemingly overaggressive effort to create more revenue growth for the corporation. Predictably, Cabot's return on assets declined as the firm shifted away from its core competence to unrelated areas. The portfolio model failed by pointing the company in the wrong direction in an effort to spur growth—away from their core business. Recognizing its mistake, Cabot Corporation returned to its mainstay carbon black manufacturing and divested unrelated businesses. Today the company is a leader in its field with $3 billion in 2010 revenues.[50]

Exhibit 6.7 summarizes the limitations of portfolio model analysis.

Caveat: Is Risk Reduction a Viable Goal of Diversification?

One of the purposes of diversification is to reduce the risk that is inherent in a firm's variability in revenues and profits over time. That is, if a firm enters new products or markets that are affected differently by seasonal or economic cycles, its performance over time will be more stable. For example, a firm manufacturing lawn mowers may diversify into snow blowers to even out its annual sales. Or a firm manufacturing a luxury line of household furniture may introduce a lower-priced line since affluent and lower-income customers are affected differently by economic cycles.

Exhibit 6.7
Benefits and Limitations of Portfolio Models

Benefits

- The corporation is in a better position to allocate resources to businesses according to explicit criteria.
- The corporate office can provide guidance on what firms may be attractive acquisitions.
- The corporate office can provide financial resources to businesses on favorable terms (that reflect the corporation's ability to raise funds).
- The corporate office can provide high-quality review and coaching for the individual businesses.
- It provides a basis for developing strategic goals and evaluation/reward systems for businesses.

Limitations

- They are overly simplistic, consisting of only two dimensions (growth and market share).
- They view each business as separate, ignoring potential synergies across businesses.
- The process may become overly largely mechanical, minimizing the potential value of managers' judgment and experience.
- The reliance on strict rules for resource allocation across SBUs can be detrimental to a firm's long-term viability.
- The imagery (e.g., cash cows, dogs) while colorful, may lead to troublesome and overly simplistic prescriptions.

At first glance the above reasoning may make sense, but there are some problems with it. First, a firm's stockholders can diversify their portfolios at a much lower cost than a corporation, and they don't have to worry about integrating the acquisition into their portfolio. Second, economic cycles as well as their impact on a given industry (or firm) are difficult to predict with any degree of accuracy.

Notwithstanding the above, some firms have benefited from diversification by lowering the variability (or risk) in their performance over time. Consider Emerson Electronic.[51]

> Emerson Electronic is a $21 billion manufacturer that produces a wide variety of products, including measurement devices for heavy industry, temperature controls for heating and ventilation systems, and power tools sold at Home Depot. Recently, many analysts questioned Emerson's purchase of companies that sell power systems to the volatile telecommunications industry. Why? This industry is expected to experience, at best, minimal growth. However, CEO David Farr maintained that such assets could be acquired inexpensively because of the aggregate decline in demand in this industry. Additionally, he argued that the other business units, such as the sales of valves and regulators to the now-booming oil and natural gas companies, were able to pick up the slack. Therefore, while net profits in the electrical equipment sector (Emerson's core business) sharply decreased, Emerson's overall corporate profits increased 1.7 percent.

Risk reduction in and of itself is rarely viable as a means to create shareholder value. It must be undertaken with a view of a firm's overall diversification strategy.

The Means to Achieve Diversification

>LO6.5
The various means of engaging in diversification—mergers and acquisitions, joint ventures/strategic alliances, and internal development.

We have addressed the types of diversification (e.g., related and unrelated) that a firm may undertake to achieve synergies and create value for its shareholders. Now, we address the means by which a firm can go about achieving these desired benefits.

There are three basic means. First, through acquisitions or mergers, corporations can directly acquire a firm's assets and competencies. Although the terms *mergers* and *acquisitions* are used quite interchangeably, there are some key differences. With **acquisitions,** one firm buys another either through a stock purchase, cash, or the issuance of debt.[52] **Mergers,** on the other hand, entail a combination or consolidation of two firms to form a new legal entity. Mergers are relatively rare and entail a transaction among two firms on a relatively equal basis. Despite such differences, we consider both mergers and acquisitions to be quite similar in terms of their implications for a firm's corporate-level strategy.[53]

Second, corporations may agree to pool the resources of other companies with their resource base, commonly known as a joint venture or strategic alliance. Although these two forms of partnerships are similar in many ways, there is an important difference. Joint ventures involve the formation of a third-party legal entity where the two (or more) firms each contribute equity, whereas strategic alliances do not.

Third, corporations may diversify into new products, markets, and technologies through internal development. Called corporate entrepreneurship, it involves the leveraging and combining of a firm's own resources and competencies to create synergies and enhance shareholder value. We address this subject in greater length in Chapter 12.

acquisitions the incorporation of one firm into another through purchase.

mergers the combining of two or more firms into one new legal entity.

Mergers and Acquisitions

The rate of mergers and acquisitions (M&A) had dropped off beginning in 2001. This trend was largely a result of a recession, corporate scandals, and a declining stock market. However, the situation has changed dramatically. Over the past several years, several large mergers and acquisitions were announced. These include:[54]

- Vodafone AirTouch's merger with Mannesmann for $203 billion.
- InBev's acquisition of Anheuser-Busch for $52 billion.

- RFS Holdings' acquisition of ABN AMRO Holdings for $98 billion.
- Mittal Steel's acquisition of Arcelor for $33 billion.
- Royal Dutch Petrol's purchase of Shell Trans. & Trade for $80 billion.
- GlaxoWellcome's acquisition of SmithKline Beecham for $79 billion.
- Procter & Gamble's purchase of Gillette for $54 billion.
- Gaz de France's acquisition of Suez for $75 billion.

Exhibit 6.8 illustrates the dramatic increase in worldwide M&A activity in the U.S. up until 2008, when the global recession began. Several factors help to explain the rapid rise between 2002 and 2007. First, there was the robust economy and the increasing corporate profits that had boosted stock prices and cash. For example, the S&P 500 stock index companies, including financial companies, had a record of over $2 trillion in cash and other short-term assets.

Second, the weak U.S. dollar made U.S. assets less expensive relative to other countries. That is, from the perspective of a foreign acquirer, compared to any other period in recent memory, U.S. companies were "cheap." For example, a euro, which was worth only 80 cents in 1999, was worth $1.35 by mid-2007. This made U.S. companies a relative bargain for a European acquirer.

Third, stricter governance standards were requiring poorly performing CEOs and boards of directors to consider unsolicited offers. In essence, top executives and board members were less likely to be protected by antitakeover mechanisms such as greenmail, poison pills, and golden parachutes (discussed at the end of the chapter).

2009 was a bad year for M&A activities due to the global recession. However, with the economy improving in 2010, the pace picked up again. The total value for M&A activity in 2010 was $2.8 trillion—a 17 percent increase over the previous year. Further, in the United States, companies sought approval on 1,166 M&A transactions in 2010 compared to only 716 in 2009—reflecting a 63 percent increase. (U.S. merger approval is required by the Federal Trade Commission for any deal valued at $63 million or more.)[55] According to Andrew Gavil, an antitrust law professor at Howard University, "Merger activity is often

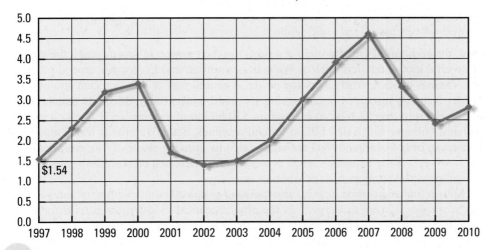

Global Value of Mergers and Acquisitions

Global mergers and acquisitions soared past their previous record and hit $4.6 trillion for the year 2007.

Exhibit 6.8 Global Value of Mergers and Acquisitions

Source: Bloomberg; Dealogic; personal communication with Meredith Leonard at Dealogic on January 27, 2009; and personal communication with Natalie Logan at Dealogic on January 27, 2011.

associated with optimism, willingness to spend cash on hand, availability of credit and general levels of economic activity," though it may also indicate how difficult the recovery has been for some businesses (that is, assets can be acquired quite cheaply).

Motives and Benefits   Growth through mergers and acquisitions has played a critical role in the success of many corporations in a wide variety of high-technology and knowledge-intensive industries. Here, market and technology changes can occur very quickly and unpredictably.[56] Speed—speed to market, speed to positioning, and speed to becoming a viable company—is critical in such industries. For example, Alex Mandl, then AT&T's president, was responsible for the acquisition of McCaw Cellular. Although many industry experts felt the price was too steep, he believed that cellular technology was a critical asset for the telecommunications business. Mandl claimed, "The plain fact is that acquiring is much faster than building."[57]

Mergers and acquisitions also can be a means of *obtaining valuable resources that can help an organization expand its product offerings and services.* For example, Cisco Systems, a dominant player in networking equipment, acquired more than 70 companies over a recent seven-year period.[58] This provides Cisco with access to the latest in networking equipment. Then it uses its excellent sales force to market the new technology to its corporate customers. Cisco also provides strong incentives to the staff of acquired companies to stay on. To realize the greatest value from its acquisitions, Cisco also has learned to integrate acquired companies efficiently and effectively.[59]

Mergers and acquisitions also can *provide the opportunity for firms to attain the three bases of synergy—leveraging core competencies, sharing activities, and building market power.* Consider Procter & Gamble's $57 billion acquisition of Gillette.[60] First, it helps Procter & Gamble to leverage its core competencies in marketing and product positioning in the area of grooming and personal care brands. For example, P&G has experience in repositioning brands such as Old Spice in this market (which recently passed Gillette's Right Guard brand to become No. 1 in the deodorant market). Gillette has very strong brands in razors and blades. Thus, P&G's marketing expertise enhances its market position. Second, there are opportunities to share value-creating activities. Gillette will benefit from P&G's stronger distribution network in developing countries where the potential growth rate for the industry's products remains higher than in the United States, Europe, or Japan. Consider the insight of A. F. Lafley, P&G's former CEO:

> When I was in Asia in the '90s, we had already gone beyond the top 500 cities in China. Today, we're way down into the rural areas. So we add three, four, five Gillette brands, and we don't even have to add a salesperson.

Third, the addition of Gillette increases P&G's market power. In recent years, the growth of powerful global retailers such as Walmart, Carrefour, and Costco has eroded much of the consumer goods industry's pricing power. A central part of P&G's recent strategy has been to focus its resources on enhancing its core brands. Today, 16 of its brands (each with revenues of over $1 billion) account for $30 billion of the firm's $51.4 billion in total revenues. Gillette, with $10.5 billion in total revenues, adds five brands which also have revenues of over $1 billion. P&G anticipates that its growing stable of "superbrands" will help it to weather the industry's tough pricing environment and enhance its power relative to large, powerful retailers such as Walmart and Target.

Merger and acquisition activity also can *lead to consolidation within an industry and can force other players to merge.*[61] In the pharmaceutical industry, the patents for many top-selling drugs are expiring and M&A activity is expected to heat up.[62] For example, many patents held by U.S. pharmaceutical companies (e.g., Pfizer's Lipitor) will expire in the next few years, which represents tens of billions of dollars in revenue. Clearly, this is an example of how the political–legal segment of the general environment (discussed in Chapter 2) can affect a corporation's strategy and performance. Although health care providers and patients are happy about the lower-cost generics that will arrive, drug firms are being pressed to make up for lost revenues. Combining top firms such as Glaxo Well-come and SmithKline Beecham has many potential long-term benefits. They not only promise significant postmerger cost savings, but also the increased size of the combined companies brings greater research and development possibilities.

Corporations can also *enter new market segments by way of acquisitions.* Although Charles Schwab & Co. is best known for providing discount trading services for middle America, it clearly is interested in other target markets.[63] In late 2000 Schwab surprised its rivals by paying $2.7 billion to acquire (divested in 2006) U.S. Trust Corporation, a 147-year-old financial services institution that is a top estate planner for the wealthy. However, Schwab is not ignoring its core market. The firm also purchased Cybercorp Inc., a Texas brokerage company, for $488 million. That firm offers active online traders sophisticated quotes and stock-screening tools. Exhibit 6.9 summarizes the benefits of mergers and acquisitions.

Potential Limitations   As noted in the previous section, mergers and acquisitions provide a firm with many potential benefits. However, at the same time, there are many potential drawbacks or limitations to such corporate activity.[64]

First, *the takeover premium that is paid for an acquisition typically is very high.* Two times out of three, the stock price of the acquiring company falls once the deal is made public. Since the acquiring firm often pays a 30 percent or higher premium for the target company, the acquirer must create synergies and scale economies that result in sales and market gains exceeding the premium price. Firms paying higher premiums set the performance hurdle even higher. For example, Household International paid an 82 percent premium to buy Beneficial, and Conseco paid an 83 percent premium to acquire Green Tree Financial. Historically, paying a high premium over the stock price has been a poor strategy.

Second, *competing firms often can imitate any advantages realized or copy synergies that result from the M&A.*[65] Thus, a firm can often see its advantages quickly erode. Unless the advantages are sustainable and difficult to copy, investors will not be willing to pay a high premium for the stock. Similarly, the time value of money must be factored into the stock price. M&A costs are paid up front. Conversely, firms pay for R&D, ongoing marketing, and capacity expansion over time. This stretches out the payments needed to gain new competencies. The M&A argument is that a large initial investment is worthwhile because it creates long-term advantages. However, stock analysts want to see immediate results from such a large cash outlay. If the acquired firm does not produce results quickly, investors often divest the stock, driving the price down.

Third, *managers' credibility and ego can sometimes get in the way of sound business decisions.* If the M&A does not perform as planned, managers who pushed for the deal find their reputation tarnished. This can lead them to protect their credibility by funneling more money, or escalating their commitment, into an inevitably doomed operation. Further, when a merger fails and a firm tries to unload the acquisition, they

---

- Obtain valuable resources that can help an organization expand its product offerings.
- Provide the opportunity for firms to attain three bases of synergy: leveraging core competencies, sharing activities, and building market power.
- Lead to consolidation within an industry and force other players to merge.
- Enter new market segments.

Exhibit 6.9
Benefits of Mergers and Acquisitions

Effectively Managing the Human Side of Acquisitions

When managing the human side of the mergers and acquisitions (M&A) process, firms face issues such as anxiety, employee shock, and protests. How companies manage such issues will reduce the volume of customer defections, supplier unrest, and government disapproval—as well as increase employee commitment.

In the follow-up to the P&G and Gillette merger, headhunters started targeting Gillette talent. P&G faced government disapproval and investigations in Gillette's home state of Massachusetts, as well as potential problems in India—where it intended to reduce the number of distributors. However, P&G was able to keep 90 percent of

Gillette employees who were offered jobs, which is much higher than the average in M&A situations.

P&G enlisted all Gillette employees in an active effort to keep customers, suppliers, and distributors happy, even employees who would eventually be let go. Former Gillette Chairman Jim Kilts said, "A lot of people who left were going to retire and leave anyway in the short term. And I think we seeded the company with some great talent down in the organization, so time will tell." In the instances when processes used by Gillette were deemed more efficient than P&G's, they were adopted. Overall, the company achieved its cost and revenue targets from the first year following the merger.

The best may be yet to come, as the company was able to make aggressive moves in key markets such as Brazil and India. In addition, there was a growing investment and expertise in sports marketing and faster internal decision making.

Source: Kanter, R. M. 2009. Mergers that stick. *Harvard Business Review,* 87(10): 121–125; and, Neff, J. 2010. Why P&G's $57 billion bet on Gillette hasn't paid off big—yet. *www.adage.com.* February 15: np.

often must sell at a huge discount. These problems further compound the costs and erode the stock price.

Fourth, *there can be many cultural issues that may doom the intended benefits from M&A endeavors.* Consider, the insights of Joanne Lawrence, who played an important role in the merger between SmithKline and the Beecham Group.[66]

> The key to a strategic merger is to create a new culture. This was a mammoth challenge during the SmithKline Beecham merger. We were working at so many different cultural levels, it was dizzying. We had two national cultures to blend—American and British— that compounded the challenge of selling the merger in two different markets with two different shareholder bases. There were also two different business cultures: One was very strong, scientific, and academic; the other was much more commercially oriented. And then we had to consider within both companies the individual businesses, each of which has its own little culture.

Exhibit 6.10 summarizes the limitations of mergers and acquisitions.

Strategy Spotlight 6.4 addresses the human side of M&A activity—how they may be successfully managed.

Divestment: The Other Side of the "M&A Coin"   When firms acquire other businesses, it typically generates quite a bit of "press" in business publications such as

Exhibit 6.10
Limitations of Mergers and Acquisitions

- Takeover premiums paid for acquisitions are typically very high.
- Competing firms often can imitate any advantages or copy synergies that result from the merger or acquisition.
- Managers' egos sometimes get in the way of sound business decisions.
- Cultural issues may doom the intended benefits from M&A endeavors.

Why Did Tyco International Sell a Majority Stake in One of Its Businesses?

Tyco International, with $17 billion in revenues, is the world's largest maker of security systems. On November 9, 2010, Tyco announced that it had agreed to sell a majority stake in its electrical and metal products unit to buyout firm Clayton Dubilier & Rice (CD&R) for $720 million. By taking this action, it withdrew its plans to spin off the division.

The proceeds from the sale of Tyco's 51 percent stake will help the firm accelerate its share buyback

program, which it had announced two months earlier. The unit, which had $1.4 billion in 2009 revenues, will operate as a standalone entity called Atkore International. It makes products such as metal-clad electrical cables and barbed razor ribbon. Tyco felt that it could profit more by selling the remaining 49 percent when markets improve.

The acquisition is very attractive to CD&R. According to Nathan K. Sleeper, a CD&R partner, "As a manufacturer and distributor of industrial products, Atkore is a leader in a market that CD&R knows very well. We look forward to working with the Atkore management team to build on the core strengths of the business—including an outstanding reputation, well-recognized brands, long-term customer relationships, and significant scale advantages—to create an even more successful independent enterprise."

Sources: Winter, C. 2010. Tyco International: Biding time in hope of better markets. *Bloomberg Businessweek.* November 15–22: 34; and, Franco, T. C. 2010. Clayton, Dubilier & Rice to acquire Tyco International's electrical and metal products business to be renamed Atkore International. *www.prnewswire.com.* November 9: np.

Financial Times, The Economist, and *The Wall Street Journal.* It makes for exciting news, and one thing is for sure—large acquiring firms automatically improve their standing in the Fortune 500 rankings (since it is based solely on total revenues). However, managers must also carefully consider the strategic implications of exiting businesses.

Divestments, the exit of a business from a firm's portfolio, are quite common. One study found that large, prestigious U.S. companies divested more acquisitions than they kept.[67] Well-known divestitures in business history include (1) Novell's purchase of WordPerfect for stock valued at $1.4 billion and later sold to Corel for $124 million, and (2) Quaker Oats' unloading of Snapple Beverage Company to Triarc for only $300 million in 1997—three years after it had bought it for $1.8 billion!

> **divestment** the exit of a business from a firm's portfolio.

Divesting a business can accomplish many different objectives.* As the examples above demonstrate, it can be used to help a firm reverse an earlier acquisition that didn't work out as planned. Often, this is simply to help "cut their losses." Other objectives include: (1) enabling managers to focus their efforts more directly on the firm's core businesses,[68] (2) providing the firm with more resources to spend on more attractive alternatives, and (3) raising cash to help fund existing businesses. Strategy Spotlight 6.5 discusses another reason for a divestiture. Here, Tyco International sold part of one of its businesses to raise cash for its share buyback.

---

*Firms can divest their businesses in a number of ways. Sell-offs, spin-offs, equity carve-outs, asset sales/ dissolution, and split-ups are some such modes of divestment. In a sell-off, the divesting firm privately negotiates with a third party to divest a unit/subsidiary for cash/stock. In a spin-off, a parent company distributes shares of the unit/subsidiary being divested pro-rata to its existing shareholders and a new company is formed. Equity carve-outs are similar to spin-offs except that shares in the unit/subsidiary being divested are offered to new shareholders. Dissolution involves sale of redundant assets, not necessarily as an entire unit/subsidiary as in sell-offs but a few bits at a time. A split-up, on the other hand, is an instance of divestiture where the parent company is split into two or more new companies and the parent ceases to exist. Shares in the parent company are exchanged for shares in new companies and the exact distribution varies case by case.

An example of divesting to raise funds for existing businesses, in 2008, FirstService Corporation, a Toronto-based company trading on the NASDAQ, sold its security guard and security systems integration business to ADT—a unit of Tyco International (NYSE). At the time of the sale, FirstService had total revenues exceeding $1.5 billion, and the guard and systems integration unit that was sold had revenues of around $200 million. Jay Hennick, CEO of FirstService, in announcing the sale, said, "FirstService will utilize the proceeds, together with existing funds and available capital, to drive global growth in its three core service platforms, commercial real estate, residential property management, and property improvement service."[69]

Divesting can enhance a firm's competitive position only to the extent that it reduces its tangible (e.g., maintenance, investments, etc.) or intangible (e.g., opportunity costs, managerial attention) costs without sacrificing a current competitive advantage or the seeds of future advantages.[70] To be effective, divesting requires a thorough understanding of a business unit's current ability and future potential to contribute to a firm's value creation. However, since such decisions involve a great deal of uncertainty, it is very difficult to make such evaluations. In addition, because of managerial self-interests and organizational inertia, firms often delay divestments of underperforming businesses.

Successful divestment involves establishing objective criteria for determining divestment candidates.[71] Clearly, firms should not panic and sell for a song in bad times. Private equity firms and conglomerates naturally place great emphasis on value when it comes to assessing which business units to keep. In identifying which assets to sell, the management committee of $10 billion Textron, for example, applies three tests of value to the firm's diverse portfolio—which is composed of some 12 divisions and 72 strategic business units (SBUs). For Textron to retain a business unit:

- The unit's long-term fundamentals must be sound. The team gauges this by assessing the attractiveness of each SBU's market and the unit's competitive strength within that market.
- Textron must be able to grow the unit's intrinsic value by 15 percent or more annually. The team applies this screen by carefully analyzing each SBU's business plan each year and challenging its divisional management teams to assess the value-growth potential of each business objectively.
- The unit's revenues must reach a certain threshold. Textron seeks to hold a portfolio of relevant businesses, each with at least $1 billion in revenue. Businesses that are not generating $1 billion or more in sales—and are not likely to reach this watershed within the foreseeable future—are targets for divestiture.

Strategic Alliances and Joint Ventures

strategic alliance a cooperative relationship between two or more firms.

A **strategic alliance** is a cooperative relationship between two (or more) firms.[72] Alliances may be either informal or formal—that is, involving a written contract. **Joint ventures** represent a special case of alliances, wherein two (or more) firms contribute equity to form a new legal entity.

Strategic alliances and joint ventures are assuming an increasingly prominent role in the strategy of leading firms, both large and small.[73] Such cooperative relationships have many potential advantages.[74] Among these are entering new markets, reducing manufacturing (or other) costs in the value chain, and developing and diffusing new technologies.[75]

joint ventures new entities formed within a strategic alliance in which two or more firms, the parents, contribute equity to form the new legal entity.

Entering New Markets Often a company that has a successful product or service wants to introduce it into a new market. However, it may not have the financial resources or the requisite marketing expertise because it does not understand customer needs, know how to promote the product, or have access to the proper distribution channels.[76]

The partnerships formed between Time Warner, Inc., and three African American–owned cable companies in New York City are examples of joint ventures created to serve a domestic market. Time Warner built a 185,000-home cable system in the city and asked the three cable companies to operate it. Time Warner supplied the product, and the cable companies supplied the knowledge of the community and the know-how to market the cable system. Joining with the local companies enabled Time Warner to win the acceptance of the cable customers and to benefit from an improved image in the black community.

Strategy Spotlight 6.6 discusses how a strategic alliance between two firms will help them crowdsource creative concepts.

Reducing Manufacturing (or Other) Costs in the Value Chain　Strategic alliances (or joint ventures) often enable firms to pool capital, value-creating activities, or facilities in order to reduce costs. For example, Molson Companies and Carling O'Keefe Breweries in Canada formed a joint venture to merge their brewing operations. Although Molson had a modern and efficient brewery in Montreal, Carling's was outdated. However, Carling had the better facilities in Toronto. In addition, Molson's Toronto brewery was located on the waterfront and had substantial real estate value. Overall, the synergies gained by using their combined facilities more efficiently added $150 million of pretax earnings during the initial year of the venture. Economies of scale were realized and facilities were better utilized.

Developing and Diffusing New Technologies　Strategic alliances also may be used to build jointly on the technological expertise of two or more companies. This may enable then to develop products technologically beyond the capability of the companies acting independently.[77]

STMicroelectronics (ST) is a high-tech company based in Geneva, Switzerland, that has thrived—largely due to the success of its strategic alliances.[78] The firm develops and manufactures computer chips for a variety of applications such as mobile phones, set-top boxes, smart cards, and flash memories. In 1995 it teamed up with Hewlett-Packard to develop powerful new processors for various digital applications. Another example was its strategic alliance with Nokia to develop a chip that would give Nokia's phones a longer battery life. Here, ST produced a chip that tripled standby time to 60 hours—a breakthough that gave Nokia a huge advantage in the marketplace.

The firm's CEO, Pasquale Pistorio, was among the first in the industry to form R&D alliances with other companies. Now ST's top 12 customers, including HP, Nokia, and Nortel, account for 45 percent of revenues. According to Pistorio, "Alliances are in our DNA." Such relationships help ST keep better-than-average growth rates, even in difficult times. That's because close partners are less likely to defect to other suppliers.

Potential Downsides　Despite their promise, many alliances and joint ventures fail to meet expectations for a variety of reasons.[79] First, without the proper partner, a firm should never consider undertaking an alliance, even for the best of reasons.[80] Each partner should bring the desired complementary strengths to the partnership. Ideally, the strengths contributed by the partners are unique; thus synergies created can be more easily sustained and defended over the longer term. The goal must be to develop synergies between the contributions of the partners, resulting in a win–win situation. Moreover, the partners must be compatible and willing to trust each other.[81] Unfortunately, often little attention is given to nurturing the close working relationships and interpersonal connections that bring together the partnering organizations.[82]

Internal Development

Firms can also diversify by means of corporate entrepreneurship and new venture development. In today's economy, **internal development** is such an important means by which companies expand their businesses that we have devoted a whole chapter to it (see Chapter 12). Sony and the Minnesota Mining & Manufacturing Co. (3M), for example, are known for

internal development entering a new business through investment in new facilities, often called corporate enterpreneurship and new venture development.

their dedication to innovation, R&D, and cutting-edge technologies. For example, 3M has developed its entire corporate culture to support its ongoing policy of generating at least 25 percent of total sales from products created within the most recent four-year period. During the 1990s, 3M exceeded this goal by achieving about 30 percent of sales per year from new internally developed products.

Zingerman's, a gourmet deli, has created a new business based on its core competence in human resource management. We discuss this new internal venture in Strategy Spotlight 6.7

Compared to mergers and acquisitions, firms that engage in internal development capture the value created by their own innovative activities without having to "share the wealth" with alliance partners or face the difficulties associated with combining activities across the value chains of several firms or merging corporate cultures.[83] Also, firms can often develop new products or services at a relatively lower cost and thus rely on their own resources rather than turning to external funding.[84]

There are also potential disadvantages. It may be time consuming; thus, firms may forfeit the benefits of speed that growth through mergers or acquisitions can provide. This may be especially important among high-tech or knowledge-based organizations in fast-paced environments where being an early mover is critical. Thus, firms that choose to diversify through internal development must develop capabilities that allow them to move quickly from initial opportunity recognition to market introduction.

>LO6.6
Managerial behaviors that can erode the creation of value.

How Managerial Motives Can Erode Value Creation

Thus far in the chapter, we have implicitly assumed that CEOs and top executives are "rational beings"; that is, they act in the best interests of shareholders to maximize long-term

A Gourmet Deli Firm Leverages Its Core Competence and Creates a New Business

In 1982, when Ari Weinzweig and Paul Saginaw opened Zingerman's Delicatessen in Ann Arbor, Michigan, their goal was to offer a world-class corned-beef sandwich. By 2003, Zingerman's was named "The Coolest Small Company in America" by *Inc.* magazine. Today, the Zingerman's Community of Businesses—including seven businesses—employs more than 500 people and generates annual sales of more than $35 million.

In 1994, the firm created a training arm, ZingTrain, to develop and deliver seminars on how to hire, fire, and inspire people. The program, mainly targeted at managers and small-business owners, promises "tips, tools, and techniques" to be more effective at every step—from hiring to the exit interview. At one session, the 15 participants included four managers from a pizza chain, a furniture store owner, two nonprofit executives, a co-owner of an Italian ice-cart business, and a journalist.

Source: Kanter, R. M. 2009. Mergers that stick. *Harvard Business Review,* 87(10): 121–125; O'Brien, C. 2008. ZingTrain keeps retail workers on the right track. *newhope360.com.* October 1: np; and, *www.zingtrain.com.*

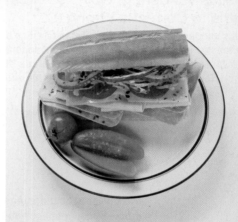

● Zingerman's, a delicatessen, leveraged its core competence in human resource management to create training programs.

During the session, the leaders drew on Zingerman's culture, discussing the "compact" in which employees take responsibility for their training's effectiveness. There were also tips for writing a great job description.

---

shareholder value. In the real world, however, they may often act in their own self-interest. We now address some **managerial motives** that can serve to erode, rather than enhance, value creation. These include "growth for growth's sake," excessive egotism, and the creation of a wide variety of antitakeover tactics.

managerial motives managers acting in their own self-interest rather than to maximize long-term shareholder value.

Growth for Growth's Sake

There are huge incentives for executives to increase the size of their firm. And these are not consistent with increasing shareholder wealth—in other words, **growth for growth's sake**. Top managers, including the CEO, of larger firms typically enjoy more prestige, higher rankings for their firms on the Fortune 500 list (based on revenues, *not* profits), greater incomes, more job security, and so on. There is also the excitement and associated recognition of making a major acquisition. As noted by Harvard's Michael Porter, "There's a tremendous allure to mergers and acquisitions. It's the big play, the dramatic gesture. With one stroke of the pen you can add billions to size, get a front-page story, and create excitement in markets.[85]

In recent years many high-tech firms have suffered from the negative impact of their uncontrolled growth. Consider, for example, Priceline.com's ill-fated venture into an online service to offer groceries and gasoline.[86] A myriad of problems—perhaps most importantly, a lack of participation by manufacturers—caused the firm to lose more than $5 million a

growth for growth's sake managers' actions to grow the size of their firms not to increase long-term profitability but to serve managerial self-interest.

Cornelius Vanderbilt: Going to Great Lengths to Correct a Wrong

Cornelius Vanderbilt's legendary ruthlessness set a bar for many titans to come. Back in 1853, the commodore took his first vacation, an extended voyage to Europe aboard his yacht. He was in for a big surprise when he returned.

Source: McGregor, J. 2007. Sweet revenge. *Business Week*, January 22: 64–70.

Two of his associates had taken the power of attorney that he had left them and sold his interest in his steamship concern, Accessory Transit Company, to themselves.

"Gentlemen," he wrote, in a classic battle cry, "you have undertaken to cheat me. I won't sue you for the law is too slow. I'll ruin you." He converted his yacht to a passenger ship to compete with them and added other vessels. He started a new line, appropriately named *Opposition*. Before long, he bought his way back in and regained control of the company.

---

week prior to abandoning these ventures. Such initiatives are often little more than desperate moves by top managers to satisfy investor demands for accelerating revenues. Unfortunately, the increased revenues often fail to materialize into a corresponding hike in earnings.

At times, executives' overemphasis on growth can result in a plethora of ethical lapses, which can have disastrous outcomes for their companies. A good example (of bad practice) is Joseph Bernardino's leadership at Andersen Worldwide. Bernardino had a chance early on to take a hard line on ethics and quality in the wake of earlier scandals at clients such as Waste Management and Sunbeam. Instead, according to former executives, he put too much emphasis on revenue growth. Consequently, the firm's reputation quickly eroded when it audited and signed off on the highly flawed financial statements of such infamous firms as Enron, Global Crossing, and WorldCom. Bernardino ultimately resigned in disgrace in March 2002, and his firm was dissolved later that year.[87]

egotism managers' actions to shape their firms' strategies to serve their selfish interests rather than to maximize long-term shareholder value.

Egotism

A healthy ego helps make a leader confident, clearheaded, and able to cope with change. CEOs, by their very nature, are intensely competitive people in the office as well as on the tennis court or golf course. But, sometimes when pride is at stake, individuals will go to great lengths to win. Such behavior, of course, is not a new phenomenon. We discuss the case of Cornelius Vanderbilt, one of the original Americans moguls, in Strategy Spotlight 6.8.

Egos can get in the way of a "synergistic" corporate marriage. Few executives (or lower-level managers) are exempt from the potential downside of excessive egos. Consider, for example, the reflections of General Electric's former CEO Jack Welch, considered by many to be the world's most admired executive. He admitted to a regrettable decision: "My hubris got in the way in the Kidder Peabody deal. [He was referring to GE's buyout of the soon-to-be-troubled Wall Street firm.] I got wise advice from Walter Wriston and other directors who said, 'Jack, don't do this.' But I was bully enough and on a run to do it. And I got whacked right in the head."[88] In addition to poor financial results, Kidder Peabody was wracked by a widely publicized trading scandal that tarnished the reputations of both GE and Kidder Peabody. Welch ended up selling Kidder in 1994.

The business press has included many stories of how egotism and greed have infiltrated organizations.[89] Some incidents are considered rather astonishing, such as Tyco's

How Antitakeover Measures May Benefit Multiple Stakeholders, Not Just Management

Antitakeover defenses represent a gray area, because management can often legitimately argue that such actions are not there solely to benefit themselves. Rather, they can benefit other stakeholders, such as employees, customers, and the community.

In the late 1980s, takeovers were very popular. Dayton Hudson Corporation (now Target) even appealed to the Minnesota legislature to pass an antitakeover bill to help Dayton Hudson in its struggle with Hafts—the former owners of Dart, a drug store chain on the East Coast. History had shown that the Dayton Hudson management in place at the time was much better able to manage Dayton Hudson in the long run. In addition to Minnesota, many states now have laws that allow firms to take the interests of all stakeholders into account when considering a takeover bid.

In the summer of 2003, Oracle launched a hostile bid for PeopleSoft. Many charged that the tactics of Oracle CEO Larry Ellison had been unfair, and many of PeopleSoft's customers took its side, indicating that Oracle ownership would not be of benefit to them. PeopleSoft was concerned that Oracle was merely seeking to buy PeopleSoft for its lucrative base of application software and was not interested in supporting the company's products. Oracle, on the other hand, sued PeopleSoft in an attempt to have the latter's so-called poison pill takeover defense removed.

In December 2004, Oracle struck a deal to buy PeopleSoft—ending a bitter 18-month hostile takeover battle. Oracle's $10.3 billion acquisition valued the firm at $26.50 a share—an increase of 66 percent over its initial offer of $16 a share. Noted analyst John DiFucci: "This is a financial acquisition primarily. Oracle is buying PeopleSoft for its maintenance stream." And, worth noting, PeopleSoft executives, including CEO and company founder David Duffield, did not join Oracle during the conference call announcing the acquisition. Oracle dropped its suit against PeopleSoft in which the former charged that PeopleSoft's "poison pill" takeover defense should be dismissed.

On moral grounds, some antitakeover defenses are not undertaken to entrench and protect management, but often they are. When such defenses are used simply to keep management in power, they are wrong. However, when they are used to defend the long-term financial health of the company and to protect broader stakeholder interests, they will be morally permissible.

Sources: Bowie, N. E. & Werhane, P. H. 2005. *Management ethics.* Malden, MA: Blackwell Publishing; and, La Monica, P. R. 2004. Finally, Oracle to buy PeopleSoft. *CNNMoney.com.* December 13: np.

former (and now convicted) CEO Dennis Kozlowski's well-chronicled purchase of a $6,000 shower curtain and vodka-spewing, full-size replica of Michaelangelo's David.[90] Other well-known examples of power grabs and extraordinary consumption of compensation and perks include executives at Enron, the Rigas family who were convicted of defrauding Adelphia of roughly $1 billion, former CEO Bernie Ebbers's $408 million loan from WorldCom, and so on.

A more recent example of excess and greed was exhibited by John Thain.[91] On January 22, 2009, he was ousted as head of Merrill Lynch by Bank of America's CEO, Ken Lewis:

> Thain embarrassingly doled out $4 billion in discretionary year-end bonuses to favored employees just before Bank of America's rescue purchase of failing Merrill. The bonuses amounted to about 10 percent of Merrill's 2008 losses.

> Obviously, John Thain believed that he was entitled. When he took over ailing Merrill in early 2008, he began planning major cuts, but he also ordered that his office be redecorated. He spent $1.22 million of company funds to make it "livable," which, in part, included $87,000 for a rug, $87,000 for a pair of guest chairs, $68,000 for a 19th-century credenza, and (what really got the attention of the press) $35,000 for a "commode with legs."

He later agreed to repay the decorating costs. However, one might still ask: What kind of person treats other people's money like this? And who needs a commode that costs as much as a new Lexus? Finally, a comment by Bob O'Brien, stock editor at Barrons.com clearly applies: "The sense of entitlement that's been engendered in this group of people has clearly not been beaten out of them by the brutal performance of the financial sector over the course of the last year."

Antitakeover Tactics

Unfriendly or hostile takeovers can occur when a company's stock becomes undervalued. A competing organization can buy the outstanding stock of a takeover candidate in sufficient quantity to become a large shareholder. Then it makes a tender offer to gain full control of the company. If the shareholders accept the offer, the hostile firm buys the target company and either fires the target firm's management team or strips them of their power. Thus, **antitakeover tactics** are common, including greenmail, golden parachutes, and poison pills.[92]

The first, **greenmail,** is an effort by the target firm to prevent an impending takeover. When a hostile firm buys a large block of outstanding target company stock and the target firm's management feels that a tender offer is impending, they offer to buy the stock back from the hostile company at a higher price than the unfriendly company paid for it. Although this often prevents a hostile takeover, the same price is not offered to preexisting shareholders. However, it protects the jobs of the target firm's management.

Second, a **golden parachute** is a prearranged contract with managers specifying that, in the event of a hostile takeover, the target firm's managers will be paid a significant severance package. Although top managers lose their jobs, the golden parachute provisions protect their income.

Third, **poison pills** are used by a company to give shareholders certain rights in the event of a takeover by another firm. They are also known as shareholder rights plans.

Clearly, antitakeover tactics can often raise some interesting ethical—and legal—issues. Strategy Spotlight 6.9 addresses how antitakeover measures can benefit multiple stakeholders—not just management.

Reflecting on Career Implications . . .

- *Corporate-Level Strategy:* Be aware of your firm's corporate-level strategy. Can you come up with an initiative that will create value both within and across business units?
- *Core Competencies:* What do you see as your core competencies? How can you leverage them both within your business unit as well as across other business units?
- *Sharing Infrastructures:* What infrastructure activities and resources (e.g., information systems, legal) are available in the corporate office that would help you add value for your business unit—or other business units?
- *Diversification:* From your career perspective, what actions can you take to diversify your employment risk (e.g., coursework at a local university, obtain professional certification such as a CPA, networking through professional affiliation, etc.)? For example, in periods of retrenchment, such actions will provide you with a greater number of career options.

Summary

A key challenge for today's managers is to create "synergy" when engaging in diversification activities. As we discussed in this chapter, corporate managers do not, in general, have a very good track record in creating value in such endeavors when it comes to mergers and acquisitions. Among the factors that serve to erode shareholder values are paying an excessive premium for the target firm, failing to integrate the activities of the newly acquired businesses into the corporate family, and undertaking diversification initiatives that are too easily imitated by the competition.

We addressed two major types of corporate-level strategy: related and unrelated diversification. With *related diversification* the corporation strives to enter into areas in which key resources and capabilities of the corporation can be shared or leveraged. Synergies come from horizontal relationships between business units. Cost savings and enhanced revenues can be derived from two major sources. First, economies of scope can be achieved from the leveraging of core competencies and the sharing of activities. Second, market power can be attained from greater, or pooled, negotiating power and from vertical integration.

When firms undergo *unrelated diversification* they enter product markets that are dissimilar to their present businesses. Thus, there is generally little opportunity to either leverage core competencies or share activities across business units. Here, synergies are created from vertical relationships between the corporate office and the individual business units. With unrelated diversification, the primary ways to create value are corporate restructuring and parenting, as well as the use of portfolio analysis techniques.

Corporations have three primary means of diversifying their product markets—mergers and acquisitions, joint ventures/strategic alliances, and internal development. There are key trade-offs associated with each of these. For example, mergers and acquisitions are typically the quickest means to enter new markets and provide the corporation with a high level of control over the acquired business. However, with the expensive premiums that often need to be paid to the shareholders of the target firm and the challenges associated with integrating acquisitions, they can also be quite expensive. Not surprisingly, many poorly performing acquisitions are subsequently divested. At times, however, divestitures can help firms refocus their efforts and generate resources. Strategic alliances and joint ventures between two or more firms, on the other hand, may be a means of reducing risk since they involve the sharing and combining of resources. But such joint initiatives also provide a firm with less control (than it would have with an acquisition) since governance is shared between two independent entities. Also, there is a limit to the potential upside for each partner because returns must be shared as well. Finally, with internal development, a firm is able to capture all of the value from its initiatives (as opposed to sharing it with a merger or alliance partner). However, diversification by means of internal development can be very time-consuming—a disadvantage that becomes even more important in fast-paced competitive environments.

Finally, some managerial behaviors may serve to erode shareholder returns. Among these are "growth for growth's sake," egotism, and antitakeover tactics. As we discussed, some of these issues—particularly antitakeover tactics—raise ethical considerations because the managers of the firm are not acting in the best interests of the shareholders.

Summary Review Questions

1. Discuss how managers can create value for their firm through diversification efforts.

2. What are some of the reasons that many diversification efforts fail to achieve desired outcomes?

3. How can companies benefit from related diversification? Unrelated diversification? What are some of the key concepts that can explain such success?

4. What are some of the important ways in which a firm can restructure a business?

5. Discuss some of the various means that firms can use to diversify. What are the pros and cons associated with each of these?

6. Discuss some of the actions that managers may engage in to erode shareholder value.

Key Terms

corporate-level
  strategy, 244
diversification, 246
related diversification, 248
economies of scope, 248
core competencies, 248
sharing activities, 250
market power, 251
pooled negotiating
  power, 251
vertical integration, 252
transaction cost
  perspective, 255

unrelated
  diversification, 256
parenting advantage, 256
restructuring, 257
portfolio
  management, 258
acquisitions, 262
mergers, 262
divestment, 267
strategic alliance, 268
joint ventures, 268
internal
  development, 269

diversification (e.g., leveraging core competencies, sharing infrastructures)?

Application Questions & Exercises

1. What were some of the largest mergers and acquisitions over the last two years? What was the rationale for these actions? Do you think they will be successful? Explain.

2. Discuss some examples from business practice in which an executive's actions appear to be in his or her self-interest rather than the corporation's well-being.

3. Discuss some of the challenges that managers must overcome in making strategic alliances successful. What are some strategic alliances with which you are familiar? Were they successful or not? Explain.

4. Use the Internet and select a company that has recently undertaken diversification into new product markets. What do you feel were some of the reasons for this

Ethics Questions

1. In recent years there has been a rash of corporate downsizing and layoffs. Do you feel that such actions raise ethical considerations? Why or why not?

2. What are some of the ethical issues that arise when managers act in a manner that is counter to their firm's best interests? What are the long-term implications for both the firms and the managers themselves?

Experiential Exercise

Time Warner (formerly AOL Time Warner) is a firm that follows a strategy of related diversification. Evaluate its success (or lack thereof) with regard to how well it has: (1) built on core competencies, (2) shared infrastructures, and (3) increased market power. (Fill answers in table below.)

Rationale for Related Diversification	Successful/Unsuccessful?	Why?
1. Build on core competencies		
2. Share infrastructures		
3. Increase market power		

References

1. Anonymous. 2010. Bebo sold by AOL after just two years. *www.bbc.co.uk.* June 17: np; Anonymous. 2010. AOL plans to sell or shut down Bebo. *www.bbc.co.uk.* April 7: np; Pimentel, B. 2008. AOL to buy Bebo for $850. *www.marketwatch.com.* October 25: np; Sarno, D. 2010. AOL posts loss but stock rises. *Los Angeles Times,* August 5: 3; Quinn, J. 2005. AOL losses top $1bn after writedowns. *The Daily Telegraph.* August 5: 3; Shearman, S. 2010. Returning to the fray. *Marketing,* October 13: 19; Steel, E. & Worthen, B. 2010 With Bebo a no-go, AOL will unload the social site. *The Wall Street Journal,* June 17: B1; and, Whitney, L. 2010. AOL sells off Bebo at last. *www.news.cnet.com.* October 25: np. We thank Ciprian Stan for his valued contribution.

2. Insights on measuring M&A performance are addressed in: Zollo, M. & Meier, D. 2008. What is M&A performance? *BusinessWeek,* 22(3): 55–77.

3. Insights on how and why firms may overpay for acquisitions are addressed in: Malhotra, D., Ku, G., & Murnighan, J. K. 2008. When winning is everything. *Harvard Business Review,* 66(5); 78–86.

4. Pfizer deal helps lift stocks. 2009. *online.wsy.com,* January 26: np.

5. Dr. G. William Schwert, University of Rochester study, cited in Pare, T. P. 1994. The new merger boom. *Fortune,* November 28: 96.

6. Lipin, S. & Deogun, N. 2000. Big mergers of the 1990s prove disappointing to shareholders. *The Wall Street Journal,* October 30: C1.

7. Rothenbuecher, J. & Schrottke, J. 2008. To get value from a merger, grow sales. *Harvard Business Review,* 86(5): 24–25; and, Rothenbuecher, J. 2008. Personal communication, October 1.

8. Kyriazis, D. 2010. The long-term post acquisition performance of Greek acquiring firms. *International Research Journal of Finance and Economics,* 43: 69–79.

9. Pare, T. P. 1994. The new merger boom. *Fortune,* November 28: 96.

10. A discussion of the effects of director experience and acquisition performance is in: McDonald, M. L. & Westphal, J. D. 2008. What do they know? The effects of outside director acquisition experience on firm acquisition performance. *Strategic Management Journal,* 29(11): 1155–1177.

11. Ghosn, C. 2006. Inside the alliance: The win–win nature of a unique business mode. *Address to the Detroit Economic Club,* November 16.

12. For a study that investigates several predictors of corporate diversification, read: Wiersema, M. F. & Bowen, H. P. 2008. Corporate diversification: The impact of foreign competition, industry globalization, and product diversification. *Strategic Management Journal,* 29(2): 114–132.

13. Kumar, M. V. S. 2011. Are joint ventures positive sum games? The relative effects of cooperative and non-cooperative behavior. *Strategic Management Journal,* 32(1): 32–54.

14. Makri, M., Hitt, M. A., & Lane, P. J. 2010. Complementary technologies, knowledge relatedness, and invention outcomes in high technology mergers and acquisitions. *Strategic Management Journal,* 31(6): 602–628.

15. A discussion of Tyco's unrelated diversification strategy is in: Hindo, B. 2008. Solving Tyco's identity crisis. *BusinessWeek,* February 18: 62.

16. Our framework draws upon a variety of sources, including: Goold, M. & Campbell, A. 1998. Desperately seeking synergy. *Harvard Business Review,* 76(5): 131–143; Porter, M. E. 1987. From advantage to corporate strategy. *Harvard Business Review,* 65(3): 43–59; and, Hitt, M. A., Ireland, R. D., & Hoskisson, R. E. 2001. *Strategic management: Competitiveness and globalization* (4th ed.). Cincinnati, OH: South-Western.

17. Collis, D. J. & Montgomery, C. A. 1987. *Corporate strategy: Resources and the scope of the firm.* New York: McGraw-Hill.

18. This imagery of the corporation as a tree and related discussion draws on: Prahalad, C. K. & Hamel, G. 1990. The core competence of the corporation. *Harvard Business Review,* 68(3): 79–91. Parts of this section also draw on Picken, J. C. & Dess, G. G. 1997. *Mission critical:* chap. 5. Burr Ridge, IL: Irwin Professional Publishing.

19. Graebner, M. E., Eisenhardt, K. M., & Roundy, P. T. 2010. Success and failure in technology acquisitions: Lessons for buyers and sellers. *The Academy of Management Perspectives,* 24(3): 73–92.

20. This section draws on Prahalad & Hamel, op. cit.; and Porter, op. cit.

21. A recent study that investigates the relationship between a firm's technology resources, diversification, and performance can be found in: Miller, D. J. 2004. Firms' technological resources and the performance effects of diversification. A longitudinal study. *Strategic Management Journal,* 25: 1097–1119.

22. Collis & Montgomery, op. cit.

23. Fisher, A. 2008. America's most admired companies. *Fortune,* March 17: 74.

24. Henricks, M. 1994. VF seeks global brand dominance. *Apparel Industry Magazine,* August: 21–40; and, VF Corporation. 1993. First quarter corporate summary report. *1993 VF Annual Report.*

25. Hill, A. & Hargreaves, D. 2001. Turbulent times for GE-Honeywell deal. *Financial Times,* February 28: 26.

26. An interesting discussion of a merger in the Russian mining industry is in: Bush, J. 2008. Welding a new metals giant. *BusinessWeek,* July 14 & 21: 56.

27. Lowry, T. 2001. Media. *BusinessWeek,* January 8: 100–101.

28. This section draws on Hrebiniak, L. G. & Joyce, W. F. 1984. *Implementing strategy.* New York: MacMillan; and, Oster, S. M. 1994. *Modern competitive analysis.* New York: Oxford University Press.

29. The discussion of the benefits and costs of vertical integration draws on: Hax, A. C. & Majluf, N. S. 1991. *The strategy concept and process: A pragmatic approach:* 139. Englewood Cliffs, NJ: Prentice Hall.

30. Fahey, J. 2005. Gray winds. *Forbes,* January 10: 143.

31. This discussion draws on: Oster, op. cit.; and, Harrigan, K. 1986. Matching vertical integration strategies to competitive conditions. *Strategic Management Journal,* 7(6): 535–556.

32. For a scholarly explanation on how transaction costs determine the boundaries of a firm, see: Oliver E. Williamson's pioneering books *Markets and Hierarchies: Analysis and Antitrust Implications* (New York: Free Press, 1975) and *The Economic Institutions of Capitalism* (New York: Free Press, 1985).

33. *www.hyundai-steel.com.* Accessed October 6, 2011.

34. Campbell, A., Goold, M., & Alexander, M. 1995. Corporate strategy: The quest for parenting advantage. *Harvard Business Review,* 73(2): 120–132; and Picken & Dess, op. cit.

35. Anslinger, P. A. & Copeland, T. E. 1996. Growth through acquisition: A fresh look. *Harvard Business Review,* 74(1): 126–135.

36. Campbell et al., op. cit.

37. This section draws on Porter, op. cit.; and, Hambrick, D. C. 1985. Turnaround strategies. In Guth, W. D. (Ed.). *Handbook of business strategy:* 10-1–10-32. Boston: Warren, Gorham & Lamont.

38. There is an important delineation between companies that are operated for a long-term profit and those that are bought and sold for short-term gains. The latter are sometimes referred to as "holding companies" and are generally more concerned about financial issues than strategic issues.

39. Lenzner, R. 2007. High on Loews. *Forbes,* February 26: 98–102.

40. Casico. W. F. 2002. Strategies for responsible restructuring. *Academy of*

Management Executive, 16(3): 80–91; and, Singh, H. 1993. Challenges in researching corporate restructuring. *Journal of Management Studies,* 30(1): 147–172.

41. Cusack, M. 1987. *Hanson Trust: A review of the company and its prospects.* London: Hoare Govett.

42. Hax & Majluf, op. cit. By 1979, 45 percent of Fortune 500 companies employed some form of portfolio analysis, according to Haspelagh, P. 1982. Portfolio planning: Uses and limits. *Harvard Busines Review,* 60: 58–73. A later study conducted in 1993 found that over 40 percent of the respondents used portfolio analysis techniques, but the level of usage was expected to increase to more than 60 percent in the near future: Rigby, D. K. 1994. Managing the management tools. *Planning Review,* September–October: 20–24.

43. Goold, M. & Luchs, K. 1993. Why diversify? Four decades of management thinking. *Academy of Management Executive,* 7(3): 7–25.

44. Collis, D. J. 1995. Portfolio planning at Ciba-Geigy and the Newport investment proposal. Harvard Business School Case No. 9-795-040, 17.

45. Other approaches include the industry attractiveness–business strength matrix developed jointly by General Electric and McKinsey and Company, the life cycle matrix developed by Arthur D. Little, and the profitability matrix proposed by Marakon. For an extensive review, refer to Hax & Majluf, op. cit.: 182–194.

46. Porter, op. cit.: 49–52.

47. Collis, op. cit. Novartis AG was created in 1996 by the merger of Ciba-Geigy and Sandoz.

48. Buzzell, R. D. & Gale, B. T. 1987. *The PIMS principles: Linking strategy to performance.* New York: Free Press; and, Miller, A. & Dess, G. G. 1996. *Strategic management* (2nd ed.). New York: McGraw-Hill.

49. Seeger, J. 1984. Reversing the images of BCG's growth share matrix. *Strategic Management Journal,* 5(1): 93–97.

50. Picken & Dess, op. cit.; and, Cabot Corporation. 2001. 10-Q filing, Securities and Exchange Commission, May 14.

51. Koudsi, S. 2001. Remedies for an economic hangover. *Fortune,* June 25: 130–139.

52. Insights on the performance of serial acquirers is found in: Laamanen, T. & Keil, T. 2008. Performance of serial acquirers: Toward an acquisition program perspective. *Strategic Management Journal,* 29(6): 663–672.

53. Some insights from Lazard's CEO on mergers and acquisitions are addressed in: Stewart, T. A. & Morse, G. 2008. Giving great advice. *Harvard Business Review,* 66(1): 106–113.

54. Coy, P., Thornton, E., Arndt, M., & Grow, B. 2005. Shake, rattle, and merge. *BusinessWeek,* January 10: 32–35; and, Anonymous. 2005. Love is in the air. *The Economist,* February 5: 9.

55. Silva, M. & Rovella, D. E. 2011. Intel is model to fight unfair competition, FTC chairman says. *www.bloomberg.com.* January 11: np.

56. For an interesting study of the relationship between mergers and a firm's product-market strategies, refer to: Krisnan, R. A., Joshi, S., & Krishnan, H. 2004. The influence of mergers on firms' product-mix strategies. *Strategic Management Journal,* 25: 587–611 and, Nash, M. B. 2010. The largest mergers and acquisitions in history. Accessed at *www.visualeconomics.com* and *www.thomsonreuters.com.*

57. Carey, D., moderator. 2000. A CEO roundtable on making mergers succeed. *Harvard Business Review,* 78(3): 146.

58. Shinal, J. 2001. Can Mike Volpi make Cisco sizzle again? *BusinessWeek,* February 26: 102–104; Kambil, A., Eselius, E. D., & Monteiro, K. A. 2000. Fast venturing: The quick way to start Web businesses. *Sloan Management Review,* 41(4): 55–67; and, Elstrom, P. 2001. Sorry, Cisco: The old answers won't work. *BusinessWeek,* April 30: 39.

59. Like many high-tech firms during the economic slump that began in mid-2000, Cisco Systems experienced declining performance. On April 16, 2001, it announced that its revenues for the quarter closing April 30 would drop 5 percent from a year earlier—and a stunning 30 percent from the previous three months—to about $4.7 billion. Furthermore, Cisco announced that it would lay off 8,500 employees and take an enormous $2.5 billion charge to write down inventory. By late October 2002, its stock was trading at around $10, down significantly from its 52-week high of $70. Elstrom, op. cit.: 39.

60. Coy, op. cit.; Anonymous. 2005. The rise of the superbrands. *The Economist.* February 5: 63–65; and, Sellers, P. 2005. It was a no-brainer. *Fortune,* February 21: 96–102.

61. For a discussion of the trend toward consolidation of the steel industry and how Lakshmi Mittal is becoming a dominant player, read: Reed, S. & Arndt, M. 2004. The Raja of steel. *BusinessWeek,* December 20: 50–52.

62. Barrett, A. 2001. Drugs. *BusinessWeek,* January 8: 112–113.

63. Whalen, C. J., Pascual, A. M., Lowery, T., & Muller, J. 2001. The top 25 managers. *BusinessWeek,* January 8: 63.

64. This discussion draws upon Rappaport, A. & Sirower, M. L. 1999. Stock or cash? The trade-offs for buyers and sellers in mergers and acquisitions. *Harvard Business Review,* 77(6): 147–158; and, Lipin, S. & Deogun, N. 2000. Big mergers of '90s prove disappointing to shareholders. *The Wall Street Journal,* October 30: C1.

65. The downside of mergers in the airline industry is found in: Gimbel, B. 2008. Why airline mergers don't fly. *BusinessWeek,* March 17: 26.

66. Mouio, A. (Ed.). 1998. Unit of one. *Fast Company,* September: 82.

67. Porter, op. cit.: 43.

68. The divestiture of a business which is undertaken in order to enable managers to better focus on its core business has been termed "downscoping." Refer to: Hitt, M. A., Harrison, J. S., & Ireland, R. D. 2001. *Mergers and acquisitions: A guide to creating value for stakeholders.* Oxford Press: New York.

69. Information accessed at *www.roberthperry.com/pubsarchiverequest.cfm.*

70. Sirmon, D. G., Hitt, M. A., & Ireland, R. D. 2007. Managing firm resources

in dynamic environments to create value: Looking inside the black box. *Academy of Management Review,* 32(1): 273–292.

71. This discussion draws on: Mankins, M. C., Harding, D., & Weddigne, R-M. 2008. How the best divest. *Harvard Business Review,* 86(1): 92–99.

72. A study that investigates alliance performance is: Lunnan, R. & Haugland, S. A. 2008. Predicting and measuring alliance performance: A multidimensional analysis. *Strategic Management Journal,* 29(5): 545–556.

73. For scholarly perspectives on the role of learning in creating value in strategic alliances, refer to: Anard, B. N. & Khanna, T. 2000. Do firms learn to create value? *Strategic Management Journal,* 12(3): 295–317; and, Vermeulen, F. & Barkema, H. P. 2001. Learning through acquisitions. *Academy of Management Journal,* 44(3): 457–476.

74. For a detailed discussion of transaction cost economics in strategic alliances, read: Reuer, J. J. & Arno, A. 2007. Strategic alliance contracts: Dimensions and determinants of contractual complexity. *Strategic Management Journal,* 28(3): 313–330.

75. This section draws on: Hutt, M. D., Stafford, E. R., Walker, B. A., & Reingen, P. H. 2000. Case study: Defining the strategic alliance. *Sloan Management Review,* 41(2): 51–62; and, Walters, B. A., Peters, S., & Dess, G. G. 1994. Strategic alliances and joint ventures: Making them work. *Business Horizons,* 4: 5–10.

76. A study that investigates strategic alliances and networks is: Tiwana, A.

2008. Do bridging ties complement strong ties? An empirical examination of alliance ambidexterity. *Strategic Management Journal,* 29(3): 251–272.

77. Phelps, C. 2010. A longitudinal study of the influence of alliance network structure and composition on firm exploratory innovation. *Academy of Management Journal,* 53(4): 890–913.

78. Edmondson, G. & Reinhardt, A. 2001. From niche player to Goliath. *BusinessWeek,* March 12: 94–96.

79. For an institutional theory perspective on strategic alliances, read: Dacin, M. T., Oliver, C., & Roy, J. P. 2007. The legitimacy of strategic alliances: An institutional perspective. *Strategic Management Journal,* 28(2): 169–187.

80. A study investigating factors that determine partner selection in strategic alliances is found in: Shah, R. H. & Swaminathan, V. 2008. *Strategic Management Journal,* 29(5): 471–494.

81. Arino, A. & Ring, P. S. 2010. The role of fairness in alliance formation. *Strategic Management Journal,* 31(6): 1054–1087.

82. Greve, H. R., Baum, J. A. C., Mitsuhashi, H., & Rowley, T. J. 2010. Built to last but falling apart: Cohesion, friction, and withdrawal from interfirm alliances. *Academy of Management Journal,* 53(4): 302–322.

83. For an insightful perspective on how to manage conflict between innovation and ongoing operations in an organization, read: Govindarajan, V. & Trimble, C. 2010. *The other side*

of innovation: Solving the execution challenge. Boston, MA: Harvard Business School Press.

84. Dunlap-Hinkler, D., Kotabe, M., & Mudambi, R. 2010. A story of breakthrough versus incremental innovation: Corporate entrepreneurship in the global pharmaceutical industry. *Strategic Entrepreneurship Journal,* 4(2): 106–127.

85. Porter, op. cit.: 43–59.

86. Angwin, J. S. & Wingfield, N. 2000. How Jay Walker built WebHouse on a theory that he couldn't prove. *The Wall Street Journal,* October 16: A1, A8.

87. The fallen. 2003. *BusinessWeek,* January 13: 80–82.

88. The Jack Welch example draws upon Sellers, P. 2001. Get over yourself. *Fortune,* April 30: 76–88.

89. Li, J. & Tang, Y. 2010. CEO hubris and firm risk taking in China: The moderating role of managerial discretion. *Academy of Management Journal,* 53(1): 45–68.

90. Polek, D. 2002. The rise and fall of Dennis Kozlowski. *BusinessWeek,* December 23: 64–77.

91. John Thain and his golden commode. 2009. Editorial. *Dallasnews .com.* January 26: np; Task, A. 2009. Wall Street's $18.4B bonus: The sense of entitlement has not been beaten out. *finance.yahoo.com* January 29: np; and, Exit Thain. 2009. *Newsfinancialcareers.com.* January 22: np.

92. This section draws on: Weston, J. F., Besley, S., & Brigham, E. F. 1996. *Essentials of managerial finance* (11th ed.): 18–20. Fort Worth, TX: Dryden Press, Harcourt Brace.

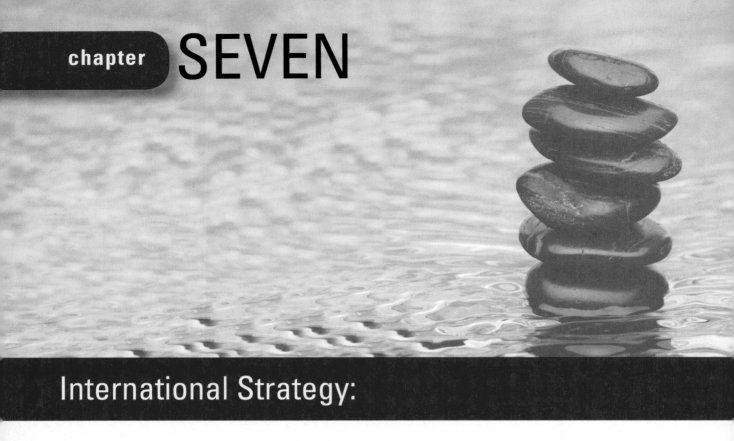

chapter SEVEN

International Strategy:

Creating Value in Global Markets

After reading this chapter, you should have a good understanding of:

LO7.1 The importance of international expansion as a viable diversification strategy.

LO7.2 The sources of national advantage; that is, why an industry in a given country is more (or less) successful than the same industry in another country.

LO7.3 The motivations (or benefits) and the risks associated with international expansion, including the emerging trend for greater offshoring and outsourcing activity.

LO7.4 The two opposing forces—cost reduction and adaptation to local markets—that firms face when entering international markets.

LO7.5 The advantages and disadvantages associated with each of the four basic strategies: international, global, multidomestic, and transnational.

LO7.6 The difference between regional companies and truly global companies.

LO7.7 The four basic types of entry strategies and the relative benefits and risks associated with each of them.

LEARNING OBJECTIVES

The global marketplace provides many opportunities for firms to increase their revenue base and their profitability. Furthermore, in today's knowledge-intensive economy, there is the potential to create advantages by leveraging firm knowledge when crossing national boundaries to do business. At the same time, however, there are pitfalls and risks that firms must avoid in order to be successful. In this chapter we will provide insights on how to be successful and create value when diversifying into global markets.

After some introductory comments on the global economy, we address the question: What explains the level of success of a given industry in a given country? To provide a framework for analysis, we draw on Michael Porter's "diamond of national advantage," in which he identified four factors that help to explain performance differences.

In the second section of the chapter, we shift our focus to the level of the firm and discuss some of the major motivations and risks associated with international expansion. Recognizing such potential benefits and risks enables managers to better assess the growth and profit potential in a given country. We also address important issues associated with a topic of growing interest in the international marketplace—offshoring and outsourcing.

Next, in the third section—the largest in this chapter—we address how firms can attain competitive advantages in the global marketplace. We discuss two opposing forces firms face when entering foreign markets: cost reduction and local adaptation. Depending on the intensity of each of these forces, they should select among four basic strategies: international, global, multidomestic, and transnational. We discuss both the strengths and limitations of each of these strategies. We also present a recent perspective which posits that even the largest multinational firms are more regional than global even today.

The final section addresses the four categories of entry strategies that firms may choose in entering foreign markets. These strategies vary along a continuum from low investment, low control (exporting) to high investment, high control (wholly owned subsidiaries and greenfield ventures). We discuss the pros and cons associated with each.

Learning from Mistakes

Carrefour is Europe's top retailer and ranks second in the world (behind Walmart). However, in late 2010, it decided to close up shop in much of Southeast Asia.[1] Its 44 stores in Thailand, 23 in Malaysia, and 2 in Singapore are up for sale. Potential buyers include Britain's Tesco, Japan's Aeon, and France's Casino.

Unfortunately, Carrefour's retreat may be ill-timed. Compared to Europe, the Southeast Asian economy is very strong. Thailand's modern retail sector is growing rapidly despite the country's political turmoil. Ditto for Malaysia. What went wrong?

Carrefour was one of the first foreign grocers to open shops in the region in the 1990s. However, Tesco, which arrived later, was far savvier in figuring out what consumers wanted. For example, when it found out that Thai shoppers traveled for miles to its "big-box" stores, it opened much smaller stores in rural towns. Carrefour, on the other hand, focused on Bangkok's big spenders and stuck to its hypermarket format. Toby Desforges, a marketing consultant, called this a "take it or leave it" approach. Unfortunately, Thai shoppers left it.

Another factor in Tesco's success in these markets was its choice of local partners. For example, in Thailand, it joined forces with CP Group, an agri-conglomerate, before going it alone. And its Malaysian partner, Sime Darby, was able to help it find properties that were suitable for its hypermarkets. Tesco also acquired eight stores in Malaysia from a rival in 2007. In contrast, Carrefour decided to go it alone in both markets and found itself boxed in by rivals.

Carrefour has operations in about 30 countries (twice as many as Tesco) and it may have overreached. In 2009, it pulled the plug on Russia—only months after opening its first store there. Tesco's outgoing chief executive, Sir Terry Leahy, felt that its rival entered emerging markets without a clear roadmap. He asserted, "Lots of retailers have begun international expansion, hit a problem, then retreated and lost market share." In the end, Carrefour ranked a distant fourth in Thailand and Malaysia; Tesco was first in both countries. Globally speaking, Carrefour still outranks Tesco in total revenues. But Tesco is more profitable.

In this chapter we discuss how firms create value and achieve competitive advantage in the global marketplace. Multinational firms are constantly faced with the dilemma of choosing between local adaptation—in product offerings, locations, advertising, and pricing—and global integration. We discuss how firms can avoid pitfalls such as those experienced by Carrefour in Southeast Asia. In addition, we address factors that can influence a nation's success in a particular industry. In our view, this is an important context in determining how well firms might eventually do when they compete beyond their nation's boundaries.

>LO7.1
The importance of international expansion as a viable diversification strategy.

The Global Economy: A Brief Overview

Managers face many opportunities and risks when they diversify abroad.[2] The trade among nations has increased dramatically in recent years and it is estimated that, by 2015, the trade *across* nations will exceed the trade within nations. In a variety of industries such as semiconductors, automobiles, commercial aircraft, telecommunications, computers, and consumer electronics, it is almost impossible to survive unless firms scan the world for competitors, customers, human resources, suppliers, and technology.[3]

GE's wind energy business benefits by tapping into talent around the world. The firm has built research centers in China, Germany, India, and the U.S. "We did it," said CEO Jeffrey Immelt, "to access the best brains everywhere in the world." All four centers have played a key role in GE's development of huge 92-ton turbines:[4]

- Chinese researchers in Shanghai designed the microprocessors that control the pitch of the blade.

- Mechanical engineers from India (Bangalore) devised mathematical models to maximize the efficiency of materials in the turbine.
- Power-systems experts in the U.S. (Niskayuna, New York), which has researchers from 55 countries, do the design work.
- Technicians in Munich, Germany, have created a "smart" turbine that can calculate wind speeds and signal sensors in other turbines to produce maximum electricity.

The rise of **globalization**—meaning the rise of market capitalism around the world—has undeniably contributed to the economic boom in America's New Economy and the overall global economy, where knowledge is the key source of competitive advantage and value creation.[5] It is estimated that it has brought phone service to about 300 million households in developing nations and a transfer of nearly $2 trillion from rich countries to poor countries through equity, bond investments, and commercial loans.[6]

There have been extremes in the effect of global capitalism on national economies and poverty levels around the world.[7] The economies of East Asia have attained rapid growth, but there has been comparatively little progress in other areas of the world.[8] For example, income in Latin America grew by only 6 percent in the past two decades when the continent was opening up to global capitalism. Average incomes in sub-Saharan Africa and the old Eastern European bloc have actually declined. The World Bank estimates that the number of people living on $1 per day has *increased* to 1.3 billion over the past decade.

Such disparities in wealth among nations raise an important question: Why do some countries and their citizens enjoy the fruits of global capitalism while others are mired in poverty? Or why do some governments make the best use of inflows of foreign investment and know-how and others do not? There are many explanations. Among these are the need of governments to have track records of business-friendly policies to attract multinationals and local entrepreneurs to train workers, invest in modern technology, and nurture local suppliers and managers. Also, it means carefully managing the broader economic factors in an economy, such as interest rates, inflation, and unemployment, as well as a good legal system that protects property rights, strong educational systems, and a society where prosperity is widely shared.

The above policies are the type that East Asia—in locations such as Hong Kong, Taiwan, South Korea, and Singapore—has employed to evolve from the sweatshop economies of the 1960s and 1970s to industrial powers today. On the other hand, many countries have moved in the other direction. For example, in Guatemala only 52.0 percent of males complete fifth grade and an astonishing 39.8 percent of the population subsists on less than $1 per day.[9] (By comparison, the corresponding numbers for South Korea are 98 percent and less than 2 percent, respectively.)

Strategy Spotlight 7.1 provides an interesting perspective on global trade—marketing to the "bottom of the pyramid."[10] This refers to the practice of a multinational firm targeting its goods and services to the nearly 5 billion poor people in the world who inhabit developing countries. Collectively, this represents a very large market with $14 trillion in purchasing power.

Next, we will address in more detail the question of why some nations and their industries are more competitive.[11] This establishes an important context or setting for the remainder of the chapter. After we discuss why some *nations and their industries* outperform others, we will be better able to address the various strategies that *firms* can take to create competitive advantage when they expand internationally.

globalization has two meanings. One is the increase in international exchange, including trade in goods and services as well as exchange of money, ideas, and information. Two is the growing similarity of laws, rules, norms, values, and ideas across countries.

Factors Affecting a Nation's Competitiveness

Michael Porter of Harvard University conducted a four-year study in which he and a team of 30 researchers looked at the patterns of competitive success in 10 leading trading

Marketing to the "Bottom of the Pyramid"

Many executives wrongly believe that profitable opportunities to sell consumer goods exist only in countries where income levels are high. Even when they expand internationally, they often tend to limit their marketing to only the affluent segments within the developing countries. Such narrow conceptualizations of the market cause them to ignore the vast opportunities that exist at "the bottom of the pyramid," according to University of Michigan professor C. K. Prahalad. The *bottom of the pyramid* refers to the nearly 5 billion poor people who inhabit the developing countries. Surprisingly, they represent $14 trillion in purchasing power! And they are looking for products and services that can improve the quality of their lives such as clean energy, personal-care products, lighting, and medicines. Multinationals are missing out on growth opportunities if they ignore this vast segment of the market.

Unilever, the Anglo-Dutch maker of such brands as Dove, Lipton, and Vaseline, built a following among the world's poorest consumers by upending some of the basic rules of marketing. Instead of focusing on value for money, it shrunk packages to set a price even consumers living on $2 a day could afford. It helped people make money to buy its products. "It's not about doing good," but about tapping new markets, said chief executive Patrick Cescau.

Sources: Reingold, J. 2011. Can P&G make money in places where people earn $2-a-day? *Fortune,* January 17: 86–91; McGregor, J. 2008. The world's most influential companies. *BusinessWeek,* December 22: 43–53; Miller, C. C. 2006. Easy money. *Forbes,* November 27: 134–138; and, Prahalad, C. K. 2005. *The fortune at the bottom of the pyramid: Eradicating poverty through profits.* Philadelphia: Wharton School Publishing.

The strategy was forged about 25 years ago when Indian subsidiary Hindustan Lever (HL) found its products out of reach for millions of Indians. HL came up with a strategy to lower the price while making a profit: single-use packets for everything from shampoo to laundry detergent, costing pennies a pack. A bargain? Maybe not. But it put marquee brands within reach.

It has trained rural women to sell products to their neighbors. "What Unilever does well is get inside these communities, understand their needs, and adapt its business model accordingly," noted a professor at Barcelona's IESE Business School.

Similarly, Procter & Gamble, with $79 billion in annual revenues, has launched a skunk works. It is staffed mostly by technical staff, rather than market researchers, to approach the $2-a-day consumer from a new perspective. Rather than try to invent products first or rely on market research alone, the group spends days or weeks in the field, visiting homes in Brazil, China, India, and elsewhere. It's the same approach the company uses in developed markets but requires much more effort, without the obvious potential payoff from consumers with disposable income. According to Robert McDonald, P&G's CEO and chairman: "Our innovation strategy is not just diluting the top-tier product for the lower-end consumer. You have to discretely innovate for every one of those consumers on that economic curve, and if you don't do that, you'll fail."

No one is helped by viewing the poor as the wretched of the earth. Instead, they are the latest frontier of opportunity for those who can meet their needs. A vast market that is barely tapped, the bottom of the pyramid offers enormous opportunities.

---

nations. He concluded that there are four broad attributes of nations that individually, and as a system, constitute what is termed "the diamond of national advantage." In effect, these attributes jointly determine the playing field that each nation establishes and operates for its industries. These factors are:

- *Factor endowments.* The nation's position in factors of production, such as skilled labor or infrastructure, necessary to compete in a given industry.
- *Demand conditions.* The nature of home-market demand for the industry's product or service.
- *Related and supporting industries.* The presence or absence in the nation of supplier industries and other related industries that are internationally competitive.
- *Firm strategy, structure, and rivalry.* The conditions in the nation governing how companies are created, organized, and managed, as well as the nature of domestic rivalry.

Factor Endowments[12,13]

Classical economics suggests that factors of production such as land, labor, and capital are the building blocks that create usable consumer goods and services.[14] However, companies in advanced nations seeking competitive advantage over firms in other nations *create* many of the factors of production. For example, a country or industry dependent on scientific innovation must have a skilled human resource pool to draw upon. This resource pool is not inherited; it is created through investment in industry-specific knowledge and talent. The supporting infrastructure of a country—that is, its transportation and communication systems as well as its banking system—are also critical.

Factors of production must be developed that are industry and firm specific. In addition, the pool of resources is less important than the speed and efficiency with which these resources are deployed. Thus, firm-specific knowledge and skills created within a country that are rare, valuable, difficult to imitate, and rapidly and efficiently deployed are the factors of production—**factor endowments**—that ultimately lead to a nation's competitive advantage.

For example, the island nation of Japan has little land mass, making the warehouse space needed to store inventory prohibitively expensive. But by pioneering just-in-time inventory management, Japanese companies managed to create a resource from which they gained advantage over companies in other nations that spent large sums to warehouse inventory.

Demand Conditions

Demand conditions refer to the demands that consumers place on an industry for goods and services. Consumers who demand highly specific, sophisticated products and services force firms to create innovative, advanced products and services to meet the demand. This consumer pressure presents challenges to a country's industries. But in response to these challenges, improvements to existing goods and services often result, creating conditions necessary for competitive advantage over firms in other countries.

Countries with demanding consumers drive firms in that country to meet high standards, upgrade existing products and services, and create innovative products and services. The conditions of consumer demand influence how firms view a market. This, in turn, helps a nation's industries to better anticipate future global demand conditions and proactively respond to product and service requirements.

Denmark, for instance, is known for its environmental awareness. Demand from consumers for environmentally safe products has spurred Danish manufacturers to become leaders in water pollution control equipment—products it successfully exported.

Related and Supporting Industries

Related and supporting industries enable firms to manage inputs more effectively. For example, countries with a strong supplier base benefit by adding efficiency to downstream activities. A competitive supplier base helps a firm obtain inputs using cost-effective, timely methods, thus reducing manufacturing costs. Also, close working relationships with suppliers provide the potential to develop competitive advantages through joint research and development and the ongoing exchange of knowledge.

Related industries offer similar opportunities through joint efforts among firms. In addition, related industries create the probability that new companies will enter the market, increasing competition and forcing existing firms to become more competitive through efforts such as cost control, product innovation, and novel approaches to distribution. Combined, these give the home country's industries a source of competitive advantage.

In the Italian footwear industry the supporting industries enhance national competitive advantage. In Italy, shoe manufacturers are geographically located near their suppliers. The manufacturers have ongoing interactions with leather suppliers and learn about new

> **>LO7.2**
> The sources of national advantage; that is, why an industry in a given country is more (or less) successful than the same industry in another country.

> **factor endowments (national advantage)** a nation's position in factors of production.

> **demand conditions (national advantage)** the nature of home-market demand for the industry's product or service.

> **related and supporting industries (national advantage)** the presence, absence, and quality in the nation of supplier industries and other related industries that supply services, support, or technology to firms in the industry value chain.

textures, colors, and manufacturing techniques while a shoe is still in the prototype stage. The manufacturers are able to project future demand and gear their factories for new products long before companies in other nations become aware of the new styles.

Firm Strategy, Structure, and Rivalry

Rivalry is particularly intense in nations with conditions of strong consumer demand, strong supplier bases, and high new entrant potential from related industries. This competitive rivalry in turn increases the efficiency with which firms develop, market, and distribute products and services within the home country. Domestic rivalry thus provides a strong impetus for firms to innovate and find new sources of competitive advantage.

This intense rivalry forces firms to look outside their national boundaries for new markets, setting up the conditions necessary for global competitiveness. Among all the points on Porter's diamond of national advantage, domestic rivalry is perhaps the strongest indicator of global competitive success. Firms that have experienced intense domestic competition are more likely to have designed **strategies and structures** that allow them to successfully compete in world markets.

In Japan, for example, intense rivalry has spurred companies such as Sony to find innovative ways to produce and distribute its digital camera products. This is largely a result of competition from Canon, Nikon, and Pentax.

Strategy Spotlight 7.2 discusses India's software industry. It provides an integrative example of how Porter's "diamond" can help to explain the relative degree of success of an industry in a given country. Exhibit 7.1 illustrates India's "software diamond."

Concluding Comment on Factors Affecting a Nation's Competitiveness

Porter drew his conclusions based on case histories of firms in more than 100 industries. Despite the differences in strategies employed by successful global competitors, a common theme emerged: Firms that succeeded in global markets had first succeeded in intensely competitive home markets. We can conclude that competitive advantage for global firms typically grows out of relentless, continuing improvement and innovation.[15]

International Expansion: A Company's Motivations and Risks

Motivations for International Expansion

Increase Market Size   There are many motivations for a company to pursue international expansion. The most obvious one is to *increase the size of potential markets* for a firm's products and services.[16] By early 2009, the world's population exceeded 6.9 billion, with the U.S. representing less than 5 percent. Exhibit 7.2 lists the population of the U.S. compared to other major markets abroad.

Many **multinational firms** are intensifying their efforts to market their products and services to countries such as India and China as the ranks of their middle class have increased over the past decade. These include Procter & Gamble's success in achieving a 50 percent share in China's shampoo market as well as PepsiCo's impressive inroads in the Indian soft-drink market.[17] Let's take a brief look at China's emerging middle class:[18]

- China's middle class has finally attained a critical mass—between 35 million and 200 million people, depending on what definition is used. The larger number is preferred by Fan Gong, director of China's National Economic Research Institute, who fixes the lower boundary of "middle" as a family income of $10,000.

India and the Diamond of National Advantage

Consider the following facts:

- SAP, the German software company, has developed new applications for notebook PCs at its 500-engineer Bangalore facility.

- General Electric plans to invest $100 million and hire 2,600 scientists to create the world's largest research and development lab in Bangalore, India.

- Microsoft plans to invest $400 million in new research partnerships in India.

- Over one-fifth of Fortune 1000 companies outsource their software requirements to firms in India.

- Indian software exports have soared from $5.9 billion in 2000 to $23.6 billion in 2005 to a predicted $68 to $70 billion by 2012.

- For the past decade, the Indian software industry has grown at a 25 percent annual rate.

- More than 800 firms in India are involved in software services as their primary activity.

- Software and information technology firms in India employed 2.3 million people in 2010.

- The information technology industry accounted for 6 percent of India's gross domestic product (GDP) in 2010—up from only 4.8 percent in 2007.

Sources: Sachitanand, R. 2010. The new face of IT. *Business Today,* 19:62; Anonymous. 2010. Training to lead. *www.Dqindia.com.* October 5: np; Nagaraju, B. 2011. India's software exports seen up 16–18 pct. in FY12. *www .reuters.com.* February 2: np; Ghemawat, P. & Hout, T. 2008. Tomorrow's global giants. *Harvard Business Review,* 86(11): 80–88; Mathur, S. K. 2007. Indian IT industry: A performance analysis and a model for possible adoption. *ideas.repec.org,* January 1: np; Kripalani, M. 2002. Calling Bangalore: Multinationals are making it a hub for high-tech research *BusinessWeek,* November 25: 52–54; Kapur, D. & Ramamurti, R. 2001. India's emerging competitive advantage in services. 2001. *Academy of Management Executive,* 15(2): 20–33; World Bank. *World development report:* 6. New York: Oxford University Press; and, Reuters. 2001. Oracle in India push, taps software talent. *Washington Post Online.* July 3.

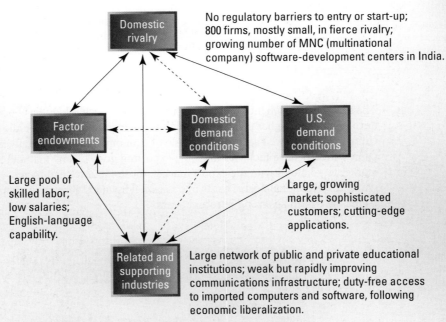

No regulatory barriers to entry or start-up; 800 firms, mostly small, in fierce rivalry; growing number of MNC (multinational company) software-development centers in India.

Large pool of skilled labor; low salaries; English-language capability.

Large, growing market; sophisticated customers; cutting-edge applications.

Large network of public and private educational institutions; weak but rapidly improving communications infrastructure; duty-free access to imported computers and software, following economic liberalization.

Note: Dashed lines represent weaker interactions.

Exhibit 7.1 India's Diamond in Software

Source: From Kampur D. and Ramamurti R., "India's Emerging Competition Advantage in Services," *Academy of Management Executive: The Thinking Manager's Source.* Copyright © 2001 by Academy of Management. Reproduced with permission of Academy of Management via Copyright Clearance Center.

(continued)

(continued)

What is causing such global interest in India's software services industry? Porter's diamond of national advantage helps clarify this question (see Exhibit 7.1).

First, *factor endowments* are conducive to the rise of India's software industry. Through investment in human resource development with a focus on industry-specific knowledge, India's universities and software firms have literally created this essential factor of production. For example, India produces the second largest annual output of scientists and engineers in the world, behind only the United States. In a knowledge-intensive industry such as software, development of human resources is fundamental to both domestic and global success.

Second, *demand conditions* require that software firms stay on the cutting edge of technological innovation. India has already moved toward globalization of its software industry; consumer demand conditions in developed nations such as Germany, Denmark, parts of Southeast Asia, and the United States created the consumer demand necessary to propel India's software makers toward sophisticated software solutions.*

Third, India has the *supplier base as well as the related industries* needed to drive competitive rivalry and

*Although India's success cannot be explained in terms of its home market demand (according to Porter's model), the nature of the industry enables software to be transferred among different locations simultaneously by way of communications links. Thus, competitiveness of markets outside India can be enhanced without a physical presence in those markets.

enhance competitiveness. In particular, information technology (IT) hardware prices declined rapidly in the 1990s. Furthermore, rapid technological change in IT hardware meant that latecomers like India were not locked into older-generation technologies. Thus, both the IT hardware and software industries could "leapfrog" older technologies. In addition, relationships among knowledge workers in these IT hardware and software industries offer the social structure for ongoing knowledge exchange, promoting further enhancement of existing products. Further infrastructure improvements are occurring rapidly.

Fourth, with over 800 firms in the software services industry in India, *intense rivalry forces firms to develop competitive strategies and structures.* Although firms like TCS, Infosys, and Wipro have become large, they were quite small less than a decade ago. And dozens of small and midsized companies are aspiring to catch up. This intense rivalry is one of the primary factors driving Indian software firms to develop overseas distribution channels, as predicted by Porter's diamond of national advantage.

It is interesting to note that the cost advantage of Indian firms may be eroding. For example, TCS's engineers' compensation has soared 13 percent in 2010. Other Asian companies are trying to steal its customers, and it is working hard to better understand overseas customers. Further, IBM and Accenture are aggressively building up their Indian operations, hiring tens of thousands of sought-after Indians by paying them more, thereby lowering their costs while raising those of TCS.

- The central government's emphasis on science and technology has boosted the rapid development of higher education, which is the incubator of the middle class.
- China may be viewed as a new example of economies of scale. Many American companies already have factories in China exporting goods. Now that there is a domestic market to go along with the export market, those factories can increase their output with little additional cost. That is one reason why many foreign companies' profits in China have been so strong in recent years.

Exhibit 7.2
Populations of Selected Nations and the World

Country	February 2011 (in est. millions)
China	1,334
India	1,182
United States	312
Japan	127
Germany	82
World Total	6,877

Source: *www.geohive.com/global/pop_data2.php.*

How Walmart Profits from Arbitrage

With sales of over $405 billion and net income of $14.8 billion, Walmart is considered one of the most successful companies in the world. In recent years, Walmart has embarked upon an ambitious international expansion agenda, opening stores in countries such as Mexico, China, Japan, and England. Walmart today has 4,122 stores outside the United States. Together they account for $100 billion in sales and $5 billion in operating income.

Walmart's above average industry profitability has been attributed to various factors, such as its superior logistics, strict control over overhead costs, and effective use of information systems. What is often lost sight of is that its "everyday low pricing" strategy cannot work successfully unless it is able to procure the thousands of items it carries in each of its stores at the lowest possible prices. This is where its expertise in arbitraging plays a critical role. In 2004, Walmart bought $18 billion worth of goods directly from China. By 2006, this had grown to $26.7 billion. If one considers indirect imports through its other suppliers as well, Walmart's total imports from China could be anywhere between $50 billion and $70 billion each year. At a conservative estimate, this represents cost savings of approximately $16 billion to $23 billion! (These savings represent how much more these goods would have likely cost Walmart had the firm purchased them from the United States.) Clearly, the core of Walmart's international strategy is not its international store expansion strategy but its pursuit of worldwide arbitrage opportunities.

Sources: 2010 Walmart annual report; Ghemawat, P. 2007. *Redefining global strategy.* Boston: Harvard Business School Press; Scott, R. E. 2007. The WalMart effect. *epi.org.* June 26: np; and, Basker, E. & Pham, V. H. 2008. WalMart as catalyst to U.S.-China trade. *ssrn.com*; np.

Expanding a firm's global presence also automatically increases its scale of operations, providing it with a larger revenue and asset base.[19] As we noted in Chapter 5 in discussing overall cost leadership strategies, such an increase in revenues and asset base potentially enables a firm to *attain economies of scale.* This provides multiple benefits. One advantage is the spreading of fixed costs such as R&D over a larger volume of production. Examples include the sale of Boeing's commercial aircraft and Microsoft's operating systems in many foreign countries.

Filmmaking is another industry in which international sales can help amortize huge developmental costs.[20] For example, Tom Cruise found foreign buyers for his "Valkyrie" in 2008 and the film ultimately got about 59 percent of its $200 million in ticket sales abroad. And Daniel Radcliffe, Rupert Grint, and Emma Watson's *Harry Potter and the Deathly Hallows: Part II*, as of July 31, 2011, had picked up $690 million or 70 percent of its $1.008 billion in total ticket sales from international markets.[21]

Take Advantage of Arbitrage   *Taking advantage of arbitrage opportunities* is a second advantage of international expansion. In its simplest form, **arbitrage opportunities** involve buying something from where it is cheap and selling it somewhere where it commands a higher price. A big part of Walmart's success can be attributed to the company's expertise in arbitrage (see Strategy Spotlight 7.3). The possibilities for arbitrage are not necessarily confined to simple trading opportunities. It can be applied to virtually any factor of production and every stage of the value chain. For example, a firm may locate its call centers in India, its manufacturing plants in China, and its R&D in Europe, where the specific types of talented personnel may be available at the lowest possible price. In today's integrated global financial markets, a firm can borrow anywhere in the world where capital is cheap and use it to fund a project in a country where capital is expensive. Such arbitrage opportunities are even more attractive to global corporations because their larger size enables them to buy in huge volume, thus increasing their bargaining power with suppliers.

Extend a Product's Life Cycle   *Extending the life cycle of a product* that is in its maturity stage in a firm's home country but that has greater demand potential elsewhere is

arbitrage opportunities an opportunity to profit by buying and selling the same good in different markets.

another benefit of international expansion. As we noted in Chapter 5, products (and industries) generally go through a four-stage life cycle of introduction, growth, maturity, and decline. In recent decades, Korean mobile phone producers such as Samsung and LG have aggressively pursued international markets to attain levels of growth that simply would not be available in Korea. Similarly, personal computer manufacturers such as Dell and Hewlett-Packard have sought out foreign markets to offset the growing saturation in the U.S. market.

Optimize the Location of Value-Chain Activities

Optimizing the physical location for every activity in its value chain is another benefit. Recall from our discussions in Chapters 3 and 5 that the value chain represents the various activities in which all firms must engage to produce products and services. They include primary activities, such as inbound logistics, operations, and marketing, as well as support activities, such as procurement, R&D, and human resource management. All firms have to make critical decisions as to where each activity will take place.[22] Optimizing the location for every activity in the value chain can yield one or more of three strategic advantages: performance enhancement, cost reduction, and risk reduction. We will now discuss each of these.

Performance Enhancement Microsoft's decision to establish a corporate research laboratory in Cambridge, England, is an example of a location decision that was guided mainly by the goal of building and sustaining world-class excellence in selected value-creating activities.[23] This strategic decision provided Microsoft with access to outstanding technical and professional talent. Location decisions can affect the quality with which any activity is performed in terms of the availability of needed talent, speed of learning, and the quality of external and internal coordination.

Cost Reduction Two location decisions founded largely on cost-reduction considerations are (1) Nike's decision to source the manufacture of athletic shoes from Asian countries such as China, Vietnam, and Indonesia, and (2) the decision of many multinational companies to set up production operations just south of the U.S.–Mexico border to access lower-cost labor. These operations are called *maquiladoras*. Such location decisions can affect the cost structure in terms of local manpower and other resources, transportation and logistics, and government incentives and the local tax structure.

Performance enhancement and cost-reduction benefits parallel the business-level strategies (discussed in Chapter 5) of differentiation and overall cost leadership. They can at times be attained simultaneously. Consider our example in the previous section on the Indian software industry. When Oracle set up a development operation in that country, the company benefited both from lower labor costs and operational expenses as well as from performance enhancements realized through the hiring of superbly talented professionals.

Risk Reduction Given the erratic swings in the exchange ratios between the U.S. dollar and the Japanese yen (in relation to each other and to other major currencies), an important basis for cost competition between Ford and Toyota has been their relative ingenuity at managing currency risks. One way for such rivals to manage currency risks has been to spread the high-cost elements of their manufacturing operations across a few select and carefully chosen locations around the world. Location decisions such as these can affect the overall risk profile of the firm with respect to currency, economic, and political risks.[24]

reverse innovation
new products developed by developed country multinational firms for emerging markets that have adequate functionality at a low cost.

Explore Reverse Innovation

Finally, *exploring possibilities for* **reverse innovation** has become a major motivation for international expansion. Many leading companies are discovering that developing products specifically for emerging markets can pay off in a big way. In the past, multinational companies typically developed products for their rich home markets and then tried to sell them in developing countries with minor adaptations.

However, as growth slows in rich nations and demand grows rapidly in developing countries such as India and China, this approach becomes increasingly inadequate. Instead, companies like GE have committed significant resources to developing products that meet the needs of developing nations, products that deliver adequate functionality at a fraction of the cost. Interestingly, these products have subsequently found considerable success in value segments in wealthy countries as well. Hence, this process is referred to as reverse innovation, a new motivation for international expansion.

As $3,000 cars, $300 computers, and $30 mobile phones bring what were previously considered as luxuries within the reach of the middle class of emerging markets, it is important to understand the motivations and implications of reverse innovation. *First,* it is impossible to sell first-world versions of products with minor adaptations in countries where average income per person is between $1,000 and $4,000, as is the case in most developing countries. To sell in these markets, entirely new products must be designed and developed by local technical talent and manufactured with local components. *Second,* although these countries are relatively poor, they are growing rapidly. For example, the Indian and Chinese economies are growing at double digit rates, and Brazil has achieved full employment. *Third,* if the innovation does not come from first-world multinationals, there are any number of local firms that are ready to grab the market with low-cost products. *Fourth,* as the consumers and governments of many first-world countries are rediscovering the virtues of frugality and are trying to cut down expenses, these products and services originally developed for the first world may gain significant market shares in developing countries as well.

Strategy Spotlight 7.4 describes several examples of reverse innovation.

Potential Risks of International Expansion

When a company expands its international operations, it does so to increase its profits or revenues. As with any other investment, however, there are also potential risks.[25] To help companies assess the risk of entering foreign markets, rating systems have been developed to evaluate political and economic, as well as financial and credit risks.[26] *Euromoney* magazine publishes a semiannual "Country Risk Rating" that evaluates political, economic, and other risks that entrants potentially face.[27] Exhibit 7.3 depicts a sample of country risk ratings, published by the World Bank, from the 178 countries that *Euromoney* evaluates. Note that the lower the score, the higher the country's expected level of risk.[28]

Next we will discuss the four main types of risk: political risk, economic risk, currency risk, and management risk.

Political and Economic Risk   Generally speaking, the business climate in the United States and Europe is very favorable. However, some countries around the globe may be hazardous to the health of corporate initiatives because of **political risk.**[29] Forces such as social unrest, military turmoil, demonstrations, and even violent conflict and terrorism can pose serious threats.[30] Consider, for example, the ongoing tension and violence in the Middle East between Israelis and Palestinians, and the social and political unrest in Indonesia.[31] Such conditions increase the likelihood of destruction of property and disruption of operations as well as nonpayment for goods and services. Thus, countries that are viewed as high risk are less attractive for most types of business.[32]

Another source of political risk in many countries is the absence of the **rule of law.** The absence of rules or the lack of uniform enforcement of existing rules leads to what might often seem to be arbitrary and inconsistent decisions by government officials. This can make it difficult for foreign firms to conduct business.

Consider Libya. The country has been noted for its capricious government under the leadership of its ruler, Muammar Qaddafi, who, until being deposed and his subsequent death in 2011, was in power for over 40 years. Here, business people often incur significant political risks. Let's look at a few examples:[33]

political risk potential threat to a firm's operations in a country due to ineffectiveness of the domestic political system.

rule of law a characteristic of legal systems where behavior is governed by rules that are uniformly enforced.

Reverse Innovation: How Developing Countries Are Becoming Hotbeds of Innovation

GE Healthcare's largest R&D facility is surprisingly located in Bangalore, India, thousands of miles away from its home country. Here, customers can hardly afford the sky-high prices of GE's medical devices. At 50,000 square feet and employing about 1,000 researchers and engineers, this facility recently developed a portable electrocardiogram machine that weighs only about two pounds, runs on batteries, and can do an electrocardiogram for 20 cents! Over the next six years, GE plans to spend $3 billion to create at least 100 health care innovations that would significantly lower costs, improve quality, increase access, and conquer the medical devices market in developing countries. Increasingly, many developing countries are becoming hotbeds of a new type of innovation often referred to as "reverse innovation" or "frugal innovation." Let us look at a few other examples of reverse innovation by GE as well as other companies:

- In the 1990s, GE attempted to sell ultrasound machines costing about $100,000 to high-end Chinese hospital imaging centers. But these expensive, bulky devices were poorly received by Chinese customers. Responding to this failure, a local GE team developed a cheap, portable ultrasound machine using a laptop computer enhanced with a probe that sold at a price between $30,000 and $40,000. By 2007, they were able to bring the price down to just $15,000. Today, these machines have found a worldwide market—both in developing economies as well as in the United States, where ambulance squads and emergency rooms are increasingly using them. Overall, sales of medical technology are exploding in China and India. China's market is expected to grow by 15 percent a year to 2015 and reach $43 billion by 2019. India's demand is growing at an even higher

rate, 23 percent, and should top $10 billion by 2020.

- Moline, Illinois–based Deere & Co. opened a center in Pune, India, almost a decade ago with the intention to penetrate the Indian market. Many observers were skeptical about the ability of a company known for its heavy-duty farm equipment and big construction gear to succeed in a market where the majority of the farmers still used oxen-pulled plows. However, Deere saw potential and its engineers in Pune responded with four no-frills models. Though lacking first-world features like GPS and air conditioning, they were sturdy enough to handle the rigors of commercial farming. The tractors cost between $8,400 and $11,600 in India. Subsequently, Deere targeted a segment of the home market that they had previously largely ignored—hobbyists as well as bargain hunters. These buyers do not care for advanced features but covet the same qualities as Indian farmers: affordability and maneuverability. Today, half of the no-frills models that Deere produces in India are exported to other countries. "These tractors are like Swiss Army knives. They get used for anything: mowing, transporting bales of hay, pushing dirt, and removing manure," claimed Mike Alvin, a product manager at Deere.

- Narayana Hrudayalaya Hospital in Bangalore performs open heart surgeries at about $2,000, which is a fraction of the $20,000 to $100,000 that it would cost in a U.S. hospital. How do they do it? By applying mass-production techniques pioneered by Henry Ford in the auto industry. The hospital has 1,000 beds, roughly eight times the size of an American hospital, and performs 600 operations a week. The large volume allows the hospital to benefit from both economies of scale (that reduce cost) and, even more importantly, experience curve effects that improve the success rate. Today the hospital has established video and Internet links with hospitals not only in India, but in countries in Africa as well as in Malaysia. As the need to contain health care costs becomes more pressing in developed countries like the United States, techniques pioneered by Narayana Hrudayalaya Hospital may find acceptance in these countries.

Sources: Anonymous. 2011. Frugal healing. *The Economist*, January 22: 73–74; Immelt, J. R., Govindarajan, V., & Trimble, C. 2009. How GE is disrupting itself. *Harvard Business Review*, 87 (10): 56–64; Chandran, R. 2010. Profiting from treating India's poor. *International Herald Tribune*, July 6: 17; Anonymous. 2010. The world turned upside down. *The Economist*, April 17: 3–17; Mero, J. 2008. John Deere's farm team. *Fortune*, April 14: 119–124; and, Anonymous. 2008. No-frills Indian tractors find favor with U.S. farmers. *www.theindian.com* April 29: np.

Exhibit 7.3   A Sample of International Country Risk Ratings: September 2010

Rank	Country	Overall Score (100)	Political Risk (30)	Economic Performance (30)	Infrastructure (10)	Total of Debt and Credit Indicators (20)	Access to Bank Finance/Capital Markets (10)
1	Norway	93.33	28.19	26.89	8.25	20.00	10.00
2	Switzerland	90.22	26.80	24.99	8.44	20.00	10.00
3	Sweden	88.93	28.04	22.65	8.24	20.00	10.00
4	Denmark	88.80	27.90	22.81	8.09	20.00	10.00
5	Finland	88.55	27.99	22.40	8.16	20.00	10.00
6	Luxembourg	88.27	27.54	21.71	9.03	20.00	10.00
7	Canada	88.26	27.80	22.12	8.34	20.00	10.00
8	Netherlands	88.20	27.71	22.85	7.64	20.00	10.00
9	Hong Kong	87.18	25.25	24.87	8.10	18.96	10.00
10	Australia	86.18	27.10	21.43	7.86	19.79	10.00
17	United States	82.10	26.26	17.91	7.92	20.00	10.00
36	China	72.60	17.37	22.31	6.81	17.45	8.67
110	Nigeria	37.80	11.25	12.12	5.25	2.19	7.00
120	Nicaragua	34.53	10.71	9.96	1.00	9.86	3.00
127	Iran	32.97	12.25	14.81	5.24	0.00	0.67
151	Afghanistan	20.95	8.26	8.31	3.38	0.00	1.00

Source: Country Risk September 2010: Full Results. *www.euromoney.com*.

- An Egyptian grocer spent years building a thriving business in Libya. Unfortunately, he made the mistake of going home during a holiday. Abrupt changes to visa rules meant that he could no longer return.
- The new manager of a hotel in Tripoli, an expatriate, fired some staff and switched suppliers. This prompted someone to make a telephone call. A sudden snap health inspection of the hotel revealed a few canned goods beyond their sell-by date. The manager was thrown in prison!
- A small Canadian oil firm, Verenex, joined the rush into Libya and struck an exciting find. Early in 2009, a Chinese company offered to buy Verenex, nearly all of whose assets are in Libya, for close to $450 million. The Libyan government blocked the sale but promised to match the price. After months of wrangling in the oil ministry, Libya's sovereign wealth fund slashed its offer to barely $300 million. Faced with further trouble if they failed to sell, Verenex shareholders reluctantly agreed.

The laws, and the enforcement of laws, associated with the protection of intellectual property rights can be a major potential **economic risk** in entering new countries.[34] Microsoft, for example, has lost billions of dollars in potential revenue through piracy of its software products in many countries, including China. Other areas of the globe, such as the former Soviet Union and some Eastern European nations, have piracy problems as well.[35] Firms rich in intellectual property have encountered financial losses as imitations of their products have grown due to a lack of law enforcement of intellectual property rights.[36]

economic risk potential threat to a firm's operations in a country due to economic policies and conditions, including property rights laws and enforcement of those laws.

Counterfeiting: A Worldwide Problem

Although counterfeiting used to be a luxury goods problem, people are now trying to counterfeit items that have a wider effect on the economy, such as pharmaceuticals and computer parts. A new study by the U.S. Department of Commerce shows that fake goods have been infiltrating the army. The number of counterfeit parts in military electronics systems more than doubled between 2005 and 2008, potentially damaging high-tech weapons.

Counterfeiting can have health and safety implications as well. The World Health Organization says that up to 10 percent of medicines worldwide are counterfeit—a deadly hazard that could be costing the pharmaceutical industry $46 billion a year. "You won't die from purchasing a pair of counterfeit blue jeans or a counterfeit golf club. You can die from taking counterfeit pharmaceutical products. And there's no doubt that people have died in China from bad medicine," said John Theirault, head of global security for American pharmaceutical giant Pfizer.

The International Anti-Counterfeiting Coalition (IACC), a Washington D.C.–based nonprofit organization, estimated that the true figure for counterfeit and pirated goods is close to $600 billion and makes up about 5–7 percent of world trade. Several factors have contributed to the increase in counterfeiting in recent years. The shift of much of the world's manufacturing to countries with poor protection of intellectual property rights has provided both technology and opportunity to make knock-offs. And the Internet and e-commerce sites like eBay have made it easier to distribute counterfeit goods. MarkMonitor, a firm that helps companies defend their brands online, estimates that sales of counterfeit goods via the Internet is about $135 billion.

The IACC provides some rather startling statistics relating to counterfeiting and its costs to business and society:

- Counterfeiting costs U.S. businesses $200 billion to $250 billion annually.

- Counterfeit merchandise is directly responsible for the loss of more than 750,000 American jobs.

- Since 1982, the global trade in illegitimate goods has increased from approximately $5.5 billion to $600 billion annually.

- U.S. companies suffer $9 billion in world trade losses due to international copyright piracy.

- Counterfeiting poses a threat to global health and safety.

The recent recession in the richer countries may have also given a boost to counterfeit goods. An anti-counterfeiting group has noticed a spike in knock-offs this recession, as consumers trade down from the real thing. Cost-cutting measures may have also made firms' supply chains more vulnerable to counterfeit parts. Lawsuits brought by companies are at an all-time high, said Kirsten Gilbert, a partner at a British law firm.

Source: Anonymous. 2010. Knock-offs catch on. *The Economist*, March 6: 81–82; Balfour, F. 2005. Fake! *BusinessWeek*, February 7: 54–64; and, Quinn, G. 2010. Counterfeiting costs businesses $200 billion annually. *www.ipwatchdog.com*, August 30: np.

---

counterfeiting selling of trademarked goods without the consent of the trademark holder.

Strategy Spotlight 7.5 discusses a problem that is a severe threat to global trade—**counterfeiting**. Estimates are that counterfeiting accounts for between 5 to 7 percent of global merchandise trade—the equivalent of as much as $600 billion a year. And the potential corrosive effects include health and safety, not just economic, damage.[37]

currency risk potential threat to a firm's operations in a country due to fluctuations in the local currency's exchange rate.

Currency Risks   Currency fluctuations can pose substantial risks. A company with operations in several countries must constantly monitor the exchange rate between its own currency and that of the host country to minimize **currency risks.** Even a small change in the exchange rate can result in a significant difference in the cost of production or net profit when doing business overseas. When the Japanese yen appreciates against other currencies, for example, Japanese goods can be more expensive to consumers in foreign countries. At the same time, however, appreciation of the Japanese yen can have negative implications for Japanese companies that have branch operations overseas. The reason for this is that profits from abroad must be exchanged for yen at a more expensive rate of exchange, reducing the amount of profit when measured in yen. For example, consider a British firm doing business in Italy. If this firm had a 20 percent profit in euros at its Italian center of operations, this profit would be totally wiped out when converted into British pounds if the euro had depreciated 20 percent against the British pound. (Global companies typically engage in sophisticated "hedging strategies" to minimize currency risk. The discussion of this is beyond the scope of this section.)

It is important to note that even when government intervention is well intended, the macroeconomic effects of such action can be very negative for multinational corporations. Such was the case in 1997 when Thailand suddenly chose to devalue its currency, the baht, after months of trying to support it at an artificially high level. This, in effect, made the baht nearly worthless compared to other currencies. And in 1998 Russia not only devalued its ruble but also elected not to honor its foreign debt obligations.

Below, we discuss how Israel's strong currency—the shekel—forced a firm to reevaluate its strategy.

> For years O.R.T. Technologies resisted moving any operations outside of Israel. However, when faced with a sharp rise in the value of the shekel, the maker of specialized software for managing gas stations froze all local hiring and decided to transfer some developmental work to Eastern Europe. Laments CEO Alex Milner, "I never thought I'd see the day when we would have to move R&D outside of Israel, but the strong shekel has forced us to do so."[38]

Management Risks   **Management risks** may be considered the challenges and risks that managers face when they must respond to the inevitable differences that they encounter in foreign markets. These take a variety of forms: culture, customs, language, income levels, customer preferences, distribution systems, and so on.[39] As we will note later in the chapter, even in the case of apparently standard products, some degree of local adaptation will become necessary.[40]

Differences in cultures across countries can also pose unique challenges for managers.[41] Cultural symbols can evoke deep feelings.[42] For example, in a series of advertisements aimed at Italian vacationers, Coca-Cola executives turned the Eiffel Tower, Empire State Building, and the Tower of Pisa into the familiar Coke bottle. So far, so good. However, when the white marble columns of the Parthenon that crowns the Acropolis in Athens were turned into Coke bottles, the Greeks became outraged. Why? Greeks refer to the Acropolis as the "holy rock," and a government official said the Parthenon is an "international symbol of excellence" and that "whoever insults the Parthenon insults international culture." Coca-Cola apologized. Below are some cultural tips for conducting business in Hong Kong:

- Handshakes when greeting and before leaving are customary.
- After the initial handshake, business cards are presented with both hands on the card. Carefully read the card before putting it away.
- In Hong Kong, Chinese people should be addressed by their professional title (or Mr., Mrs., Miss) followed by their surname.
- Appointments should be made as far in advance as possible.
- Punctuality is very important and demonstrates respect.

management risk potential threat to a firm's operations in a country due to the problems that managers have making decisions in the context of foreign markets.

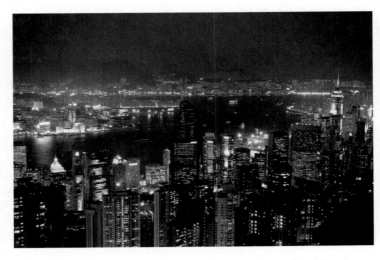

● Some of Hong Kong's customs are quite different from those of western countries.

- Negotiations in Hong Kong are normally very slow with much attention to detail. The same negotiating team should be kept throughout the proceedings.
- Tea will be served during the negotiations. Always accept and wait for the host to begin drinking before you partake.
- Be aware that "yes" may just be an indication that the person heard you rather than indicating agreement. A Hong Kong Chinese businessperson will have a difficult time saying "no" directly.

Below, we discuss a rather humorous example of how a local custom can affect operations at a manufacturing plant in Singapore.

> Larry Henderson, plant manager, and John Lichthental, manager of human resources, were faced with a rather unique problem. They were assigned by Celanese Chemical Corp. to build a plant in Singapore, and the plant was completed in July. However, according to local custom, a plant should only be christened on "lucky" days. Unfortunately, the next lucky day was not until September 3.
>
> The managers had to convince executives at Celanese's Dallas headquarters to delay the plant opening. As one might expect, it wasn't easy. But after many heated telephone conversations and flaming e-mails, the president agreed to open the new plant on a lucky day—September 3.[43]

Global Dispersion of Value Chains: Outsourcing and Offshoring

A major recent trend has been the dispersion of the value chains of multinational corporations across different countries; that is, the various activities that constitute the value chain of a firm are now spread across several countries and continents. Such dispersion of value occurs mainly through increasing offshoring and outsourcing.

A report issued by the World Trade Organization describes the production of a particular U.S. car as follows: "30 percent of the car's value goes to Korea for assembly, 17.5 percent to Japan for components and advanced technology, 7.5 percent to Germany for design, 4 percent to Taiwan and Singapore for minor parts, 2.5 percent to U.K. for advertising and marketing services, and 1.5 percent to Ireland and Barbados for data processing. This means that only 37 percent of the production value is generated in the U.S."[44] In today's economy, we are increasingly witnessing two interrelated trends: outsourcing and offshoring.

outsourcing using other firms to perform value-creating activities that were previously performed in-house.

Outsourcing occurs when a firm decides to utilize other firms to perform value-creating activities that were previously performed in-house.[45] It may be a new activity that the firm is perfectly capable of doing but chooses to have someone else perform for cost or quality reasons. Outsourcing can be to either a domestic or foreign firm.

offshoring shifting a value-creating activity from a domestic location to a foreign location.

Offshoring takes place when a firm decides to shift an activity that it was performing in a domestic location to a foreign location.[46] For example, both Microsoft and Intel now have R&D facilities in India, employing a large number of Indian scientists and engineers. Often, offshoring and outsourcing go together; that is, a firm may outsource an activity to a foreign supplier, thereby causing the work to be offshored as well.[47] Spending on offshore information technology will nearly triple between 2004 and 2010 to $60 billion, according to research firm Gartner.[48]

The recent explosion in the volume of outsourcing and offshoring is due to a variety of factors. Up until the 1960s, for most companies, the entire value chain was in one location. Further, the production took place close to where the customers were in order to keep transportation costs under control. In the case of service industries, it was generally believed that offshoring was not possible because the producer and consumer had to be present at the same place at the same time. After all, a haircut could not be performed if the barber and the client were separated!

For manufacturing industries, the rapid decline in transportation and coordination costs has enabled firms to disperse their value chains over different locations. For example, Nike's R&D takes place in the U.S., raw materials are procured from a multitude of countries, actual manufacturing takes place in China or Indonesia, advertising is produced in the U.S., and sales and service take place in practically all the countries. Each value-creating activity is performed in the location where the cost is the lowest or the quality is the best. Without finding optimal locations for each activity, Nike could not have attained its position as the world's largest shoe company.

The experience of the manufacturing sector was also repeated in the service sector by the mid-1990s. A trend that began with the outsourcing of low-level programming and data entry work to countries such as India and Ireland suddenly grew manyfold, encompassing a variety of white collar and professional activities ranging from call centers to R&D. The cost of a long-distance call from the U.S. to India has decreased from about $3 to $0.03 in the last 20 years, thereby making it possible to have call centers located in countries like India, where a combination of low labor costs and English proficiency presents an ideal mix of factor conditions.

Bangalore, India, in recent years, has emerged as a location where more and more U.S. tax returns are prepared. In India, U.S.–trained and licensed radiologists interpret chest X-rays and CT scans from U.S. hospitals for half the cost. The advantages from offshoring go beyond mere cost savings today. In many specialized occupations in science and engineering, there is a shortage of qualified professionals in developed countries, whereas countries like India, China, and Singapore have what seems like an inexhaustible supply.[49]

For most of the 20th century, domestic companies catered to the needs of local populations. However, with the increasing homogenization of customer needs around the world and the institutionalization of free trade and investment as a global ideology (especially after the creation of the WTO), competition has become truly global. Each company has to keep its costs low in order to survive.[50] They also must find the best suppliers and the most skilled workers as well as locate each stage of the value chain in places where factor conditions are most conducive. Thus, outsourcing and offshoring are no longer mere options to consider, but an imperative for competitive survival.

While there is a compelling logic for companies to engage in offshoring, there can be many pitfalls. This has spurred many companies to outsource tech services to low-cost locations within the United States, instead of offshoring to foreign countries. We discuss this trend in Strategy Spotlight 7.6.

Achieving Competitive Advantage in Global Markets

We now discuss the two opposing forces that firms face when they expand into global markets: cost reduction and adaptation to local markets. Then we address the four basic types of international strategies that they may pursue: international, global, multidomestic, and transnational. The selection of one of these four types of strategies is largely dependent on a firm's relative pressure to address each of the two forces.

Two Opposing Pressures: Reducing Costs and Adapting to Local Markets

Many years ago, the famed marketing strategist Theodore Levitt advocated strategies that favored global products and brands. He suggested that firms should standardize all of their products and services for all of their worldwide markets. Such an approach would help a firm lower its overall costs by spreading its investments over as large a market as possible. Levitt's approach rested on three key assumptions:

> **>LO7.4**
> The two opposing forces—cost reduction and adaptation to local markets—that firms face when entering international markets.

A Small-Town Alternative to Offshoring Tech Services Work

These are great times for Cayuse Technologies, a 200-employee tech outsourcing firm. It is owned by the Confederated Tribes of the Umatilla Indian Reservation in northeast Oregon. In 2009 it had $7.7 million in revenues—seven times what it had in 2007, its first year in operation. And with its business from corporate clients like Accenture expected to soar next year, Cayuse plans to hire another 75 workers. Said Marc Benoist, the firm's general manager, "We still have capacity here at our facility, so we have plenty of room for growth."

Cayuse is one of many information technology companies in remote areas of the United States that position themselves as alternatives to offshore outsourcing. And the economics seem to make sense. On an hourly basis, these "rural outsourcers" charge much more than their overseas rivals. But when factors such as oversight and quality control of the offshore work are factored in, their rates are competitive. Their rates are also much lower than their domestic counterparts located in big cities, because they operate in areas that have lower living costs. "Their value proposition is, 'We cost less than the East or West Coast, and we're easier to deal with than India,'" said Mary Lacity, a professor at the University of Missouri at St. Louis, who studies outsourcing. Cayuse Technologies develops software, provides outsourcing of business processes, and serves as a contact for Accenture's clients, for example, processing and adjusting insurance claims. "It makes much more sense for Cayuse to perform those activities," according to Randall Willis, managing director of Accenture.

Sources: Lieber, N. 2010. 'Rural outsourcers' vs. Bangalore. *Bloomberg Businessweek.* September 27–October 3: 52–53; Brickey, D. 2010. Rural outsourcing gains favor; Cayuse Technologies as a model. *www.eastoregonian.com.* October 13: np; and, Alsever, J. 2010. Forget India, outsource to Arkansas. *www.money.cnn.com.* July 8: np.

Consider the rationale behind Human Genome Sciences' (HGS) decision to use a rural outsourcing firm:

HGS, a Rockville, Maryland, biotech company with 900 employees, got bids from several outsourcers to handle the technical support for its back-office software. One of the bidders would have offshored the work to India. However, the idea of sending confidential company information overseas, outside the reach of the American intellectual property law, did not sit too well with David Evans, their IT director.

Instead, Evans hired Atlanta-based Rural Sourcing, Inc., and its team of software experts located in Jonesboro, Arkansas. HGS pays about $55 an hour for technical support from Rural Sourcing—a figure that is about 15 percent higher than the rates quoted by the Indian outsourcing firm that he considered. However, it is still about half of what it would cost for him to hire a software development firm located in the Washington, D.C., metro area.

Recently, IT research firm Gartner said in a report that while these firms make up a tiny portion of the market, they are an "attractive alternative" to offshore outsourcers because of language and other cultural factors. It is also easier for them to comply with U.S. data privacy regulations, according to the report.

Without a doubt, rural outsourcers won't replace the offshorers. After all, India has outsourcing revenues of about $50 billion, and that number is expected to triple by 2020, according to estimates by McKinsey & Company and an Indian trade group. In contrast, the rural outsourcing market is estimated to be less than $100 million. However, Lacity believes that this segment has growth potential—in part because of the efforts by federal policymakers to seek ways of creating jobs and as government outsourcing contracts increasingly require work to be done in the United States.

1. Customer needs and interests are becoming increasingly homogeneous worldwide.
2. People around the world are willing to sacrifice preferences in product features, functions, design, and the like for lower prices at high quality.
3. Substantial economies of scale in production and marketing can be achieved through supplying global markets.[51]

However, there is ample evidence to refute these assumptions.[52] Regarding the first assumption—the increasing worldwide homogeneity of customer needs and interests—consider the number of product markets, ranging from watches and handbags to soft drinks and fast foods. Companies have identified global customer segments and developed global products and brands targeted to those segments. Also, many other companies adapt lines to idiosyncratic country preferences and develop local brands targeted to local market segments. For example, Nestlé's line of pizzas marketed in the United Kingdom includes cheese with ham and pineapple topping on a French bread crust. Similarly, Coca-Cola in Japan markets Georgia (a tonic drink) as well as Classic Coke and Hi-C.

Consider the second assumption—the sacrifice of product attributes for lower prices. While there is invariably a price-sensitive segment in many product markets, there is no indication that this is increasing. In contrast, in many product and service markets—ranging from watches, personal computers, and household appliances, to banking and insurance—there is a growing interest in multiple product features, product quality, and service.

Finally, the third assumption is that significant economies of scale in production and marketing could be achieved for global products and services. Although standardization may lower manufacturing costs, such a perspective does not consider three critical and interrelated points. First, as we discussed in Chapter 5, technological developments in flexible factory automation enable economies of scale to be attained at lower levels of output and do not require production of a single standardized product. Second, the cost of production is only one component, and often not the critical one, in determining the total cost of a product. Third, a firm's strategy should not be product-driven. It should also consider other activities in the firm's value chain, such as marketing, sales, and distribution.

Based on the above, we would have a hard time arguing that it is wise to develop the same product or service for all markets throughout the world. While there are some exceptions, such as Harley-Davidson motorcycles and some of Coca-Cola's soft-drink products, managers must also strive to tailor their products to the culture of the country in which they are attempting to do business. Few would argue that "one size fits all" generally applies.

The opposing pressures that managers face place conflicting demands on firms as they strive to be competitive.[53] On the one hand, competitive pressures require that firms do what they can to *lower unit costs* so that consumers will not perceive their product and service offerings as too expensive. This may lead them to consider locating manufacturing facilities where labor costs are low, and developing products that are highly standardized across multiple countries.

In addition to responding to pressures to lower costs, managers also must strive to be *responsive to local pressures* in order to tailor their products to the demand of the local market in which they do business. This requires differentiating their offerings and strategies from country to country to reflect consumer tastes and preferences and making changes to reflect differences in distribution channels, human resource practices, and governmental regulations. However, since the strategies and tactics to differentiate products and services to local markets can involve additional expenses, a firm's costs will tend to rise.

The two opposing pressures result in four different basic strategies that companies can use to compete in the global marketplace: international, global, multidomestic, and transnational. The strategy that a firm selects depends on the degree of pressure that it is facing for cost reductions and the importance of adapting to local markets. Exhibit 7.4 shows the conditions under which each of these strategies would be most appropriate.

It is important to note that we consider these four strategies to be "basic" or "pure"; that is, in practice, all firms will tend to have some elements of each strategy.

International Strategy

There are a small number of industries in which pressures for both local adaptation and lowering costs are rather low. An extreme example of such an industry is the "orphan" drug industry. These are medicines for diseases that are severe but affect only a small number of people. Diseases such as the Gaucher disease and Fabry disease fit into this category. Companies such as Genzyme and Oxford GlycoSciences are active in this segment of the drug

> **>LO7.5**
> The advantages and disadvantages associated with each of the four basic strategies: international, global, multidomestic, and transnational.

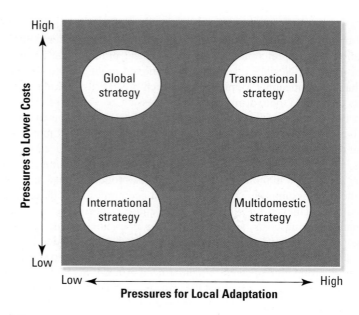

Exhibit 7.4 Opposing Pressures and Four Strategies

industry. There is virtually no need to adapt their products to the local markets. And the pressures to reduce costs are low; even though only a few thousand patients are affected, the revenues and margins are significant, because patients are charged up to $100,000 per year. Legislation has made this industry even more attractive. The 1983 Orphan Drug Act provides various tax credits and exclusive marketing rights for any drug developed to treat a disease that afflicts fewer than 200,000 patients. Since 1983, more than 280 orphan drugs have been licensed and used to treat 14 million patients.[54]

An **international strategy** is based on diffusion and adaptation of the parent company's knowledge and expertise to foreign markets. Country units are allowed to make some minor adaptations to products and ideas coming from the head office, but they have far less independence and autonomy compared to multidomestic companies. The primary goal of the strategy is worldwide exploitation of the parent firm's knowledge and capabilities. All sources of core competencies are centralized.

The majority of large U.S. multinationals pursued the international strategy in the decades following World War II. These companies centralized R&D and product development but established manufacturing facilities as well as marketing organizations abroad. Companies such as McDonald's and Kellogg are examples of firms following such a strategy. Although these companies do make some local adaptations, they are of a very limited nature. With increasing pressures to reduce costs due to global competition, especially from "low-cost" countries, opportunities to successfully employ international strategy are becoming more limited. This strategy is most suitable in situations where a firm has distinctive competencies that local companies in foreign markets lack.

Risks and Challenges Below, are some of the risks and challenges associated with an international strategy.

- Different activities in the value chain typically have different optimal locations. That is, R&D may be optimally located in a country with an abundant supply of scientists and engineers, whereas assembly may be better conducted in a low-cost location.

international strategy a strategy based on firms' diffusion and adaptation of the parent companies' knowledge and expertise to foreign markets, used in industries where the pressures for both local adaptation and lowering costs are low.

Nike, for example, designs its shoes in the United States, but all the manufacturing is done in countries like China or Thailand. The international strategy, with its tendency to concentrate most of its activities in one location, fails to take advantage of the benefits of an optimally distributed value chain.

- The lack of local responsiveness may result in the alienation of local customers. Worse still, the firm's inability to be receptive to new ideas and innovation from its foreign subsidiaries may lead to missed opportunities.

Exhibit 7.5 summarizes the strengths and weaknesses of international strategies in the global marketplace.

Global Strategy

As indicated in Exhibit 7.4, a firm whose emphasis is on lowering costs tends to follow a **global strategy**. Competitive strategy is centralized and controlled to a large extent by the corporate office. Since the primary emphasis is on controlling costs, the corporate office strives to achieve a strong level of coordination and integration across the various businesses.[55] Firms following a global strategy strive to offer standardized products and services as well as to locate manufacturing, R&D, and marketing activities in only a few locations.[56]

A global strategy emphasizes economies of scale due to the standardization of products and services, and the centralization of operations in a few locations. As such, one advantage may be that innovations that come about through efforts of either a business unit or the corporate office can be transferred more easily to other locations. Although costs may be lower, the firm following a global strategy may, in general, have to forgo opportunities for revenue growth since it does not invest extensive resources in adapting product offerings from one market to another.

A global strategy is most appropriate when there are strong pressures for reducing costs and comparatively weak pressures for adaptation to local markets. Economies of scale becomes an important consideration.[57] Advantages to increased volume may come from larger production plants or runs as well as from more efficient logistics and distribution networks. Worldwide volume is also especially important in supporting high levels of investment in research and development. As we would expect, many industries requiring high levels of R&D, such as pharmaceuticals, semiconductors, and jet aircraft, follow global strategies.

Another advantage of a global strategy is that it can enable a firm to create a standard level of quality throughout the world. Let's look at what Tom Siebel, former chairman of Siebel Systems (now part of Oracle), the $2 billion developer of e-business application software, had to say about global standardization.

> Our customers—global companies like IBM, Zurich Financial Services, and Citicorp—expect the same high level of service and quality, and the same licensing policies, no matter where we do business with them around the world. Our human resources and legal

global strategy a strategy based on firms' centralization and control by the corporate office, with the primary emphasis on controlling costs, and used in industries where the pressure for local adaptation is low and the pressure for lowering costs is high.

Strengths	Limitations
• Leverage and diffusion of a parent firm's knowledge and core competencies. • Lower costs because of less need to tailor products and services.	• Limited ability to adapt to local markets. • Inability to take advantage of new ideas and innovations occurring in local markets.

Exhibit 7.5
Strengths and Limitations of International Strategies in the Global Marketplace

departments help us create policies that respect local cultures and requirements worldwide, while at the same time maintaining the highest standards. We have one brand, one image, one set of corporate colors, and one set of messages, across every place on the planet. An organization needs central quality control to avoid surprises.[58]

Risks and Challenges   There are, of course, some risks associated with a global strategy.[59]

- A firm can enjoy scale economies only by concentrating scale-sensitive resources and activities in one or few locations. Such concentration, however, becomes a "double-edged sword." For example, if a firm has only one manufacturing facility, it must export its output (e.g., components, subsystems, or finished products) to other markets, some of which may be a great distance from the operation. Thus, decisions about locating facilities must weigh the potential benefits from concentrating operations in a single location against the higher transportation and tariff costs that result from such concentration.
- The geographic concentration of any activity may also tend to isolate that activity from the targeted markets. Such isolation may be risky since it may hamper the facility's ability to quickly respond to changes in market conditions and needs.
- Concentrating an activity in a single location also makes the rest of the firm dependent on that location. Such dependency implies that, unless the location has world-class competencies, the firm's competitive position can be eroded if problems arise. A European Ford executive, reflecting on the firm's concentration of activities during a global integration program in the mid-1990s, lamented, "Now if you misjudge the market, you are wrong in 15 countries rather than only one."

Many firms have learned through experience that products that work in one market may not be well received in other markets. Strategy Spotlight 7.7 describes the very different receptions that Pura, a cleaner-burning gasoline from Shell, received in Thailand and the Netherlands.

Exhibit 7.6 summarizes the strengths and weaknesses of global strategies.

Multidomestic Strategy

multidomestic strategy a strategy based on firms differentiating their products and services to adapt to local markets, used in industries where the pressure for local adaptation is high and the pressure for lowering costs is low.

According to Exhibit 7.4, a firm whose emphasis is on differentiating its product and service offerings to adapt to local markets follows a **multidomestic strategy**.[60] Decisions evolving from a multidomestic strategy tend to be decentralized to permit the firm to tailor its products and respond rapidly to changes in demand. This enables a firm to expand its market and to charge different prices in different markets. For firms following this strategy, differences in language, culture, income levels, customer preferences, and distribution systems are only a few of the many factors that must be considered. Even in the case of relatively standardized products, at least some level of local adaptation is often necessary. Consider, for example, Honda motorcycles.

> While Honda uses a common basic technology, it must develop different types of motorcycles for different regions of the world. For example, North Americans primarily use motorcycles for leisure and sports; thus aggressive looks and high horsepower are key. Southeast Asians provide a counterpoint. Here, motorcycles are a basic means of transportation. Thus, they require low cost and ease of maintenance. And in Australia and New Zealand, shepherds use motorcycles to herd sheep. Therefore, they demand low-speed torque, rather than high speed and horsepower.[61]

In addition to the products themselves, how they are packaged must sometimes be adapted to local market conditions. Some consumers in developing countries are likely to have packaging preferences very different from Western consumers. For example, single-serve packets, or sachets, are very popular in India.[62] They permit consumers to purchase

Why Shell's Innovative Gasoline Product Backfired in Holland

Not every consumer wants eco-friendly goods, and relatively few will pay more for them. However, every day more customers are including environmental factors in their buying decisions. But what "sells" in one place might not in another.

Consider, for example, Shell Oil's (part of the Royal Dutch/Shell Group) experience in marketing Pura, a new, cleaner-burning gasoline in two very different countries. According to Mark Weintraub, Shell's director of sustainable development strategy, the firm used a "sustainable development lens" to identify a need for cleaner fuels in Thailand. As is the case in much of Asia, the combination of dense cities and high traffic volume was damaging air quality in Bangkok and elsewhere. A cleaner-burning fuel such as Pura, which produced less sulfur and other harmful emissions, seemed like a winner.

In an example of superior eco-design, Shell developed just such a fuel by converting natural gas to a zero-sulfur liquid and then mixing it with regular diesel. Shell

Source: Esty, D. C., & Winston, A. S. 2009. *Green to gold.* Hoboken, NJ: Wiley; Peckham, J. 2002. Shell spots "premium diesel" opportunity for GTL blend. *Diesel Fuel News,* February 4: np; and, *www.showa-shell.co.jp.*

touted the blend as providing "more complete combustion to reduce smoke emissions and restore lost engine performance." Shell-Thailand Chairman Khun Vajrabhaya claimed, "Motorists should experience better performance of their vehicles within 2–3 tankfuls of Shell Pura diesel. From our road tests on diesel-engine vehicles in both Thailand and the U.K., black smoke was satisfactorily reduced." Even though Shell charged a 7.5 cent a gallon premium, Pura gained market share and sales have been very strong. In short, the launch was a complete success.

Shell assumed that it could use the same pitch when it rolled out Pura in other countries. However, the launch in the Netherlands fell flat. Why? Shell later realized that emphasizing how cleaner-burning fuel protects a car's engine was not resonating in Holland. The message was more important in Thailand, where people are much more concerned about gasoline quality and the effect of impurities on engine performance and quality of life.

Clearly, the "green pitch" never went over well in Holland—even though the country is full of customers who say that they will buy green. It is just that the need to clean the local city air is not as pressing a concern as it is in Asia. Eventually, Shell relaunched Pura in Holland under the name V-Power and marketed it by stressing enhanced engine power.

only what they need, experiment with new products, and conserve cash. Products as varied as detergents, shampoos, pickles, and cough syrup are sold in sachets in India. It is estimated that they make up 20 to 30 percent of the total sold in their categories. In China, sachets are spreading as a marketing device for such items as shampoos. This reminds us of the importance of considering all activities in a firm's value chain (discussed in Chapters 3 and 5) in determining where local adaptations may be required.

Cultural differences may also require a firm to adapt its personnel practices when it expands internationally.[63] For example, some facets of Walmart stores have been easily

Strengths	Limitations
• Strong integration across various businesses.	• Limited ability to adapt to local markets.
• Standardization leads to higher economies of scale, which lowers costs.	• Concentration of activities may increase dependence on a single facility.
• Helps create uniform standards of quality throughout the world.	• Single locations may lead to higher tariffs and transportation costs.

Exhibit 7.6
Strengths and Limitations of Global Strategies

Dealing with Bribery

Most multinational firms experience difficulty when it comes to the question of adapting rules and guidelines, both formal and informal, while operating in foreign countries. The Foreign Corrupt Practices Act of 1977 makes it illegal for U.S. companies to bribe foreign officials to gain business or facilitate approvals and permissions. In 1997, the trade and finance ministers from the Organization for Economic Cooperation and Development (OECD) followed the U.S. lead and adopted the *Convention on Combating Bribery of Foreign Public Officials in International Business Transactions*. Unfortunately, in many parts of the world, bribery is a way of life, with large payoffs to government officials and politicians the norm to win government contracts. At a lower level, goods won't clear customs

unless routine illegal, but well-accepted, payments are made to officials.

Bribery and corruption are serious risks in the oil and gas industry. BP is working to prevent and punish this behavior in its workforce. BP's code of conduct requires that its employees or others working on behalf of BP do not engage in bribery or corruption in any form in both the public and private sectors. In 2002, BP became one of the first companies to prohibit the use of facilitation payments in the course of doing business. Texas Instruments, on the other hand, follows a middle approach. It requires employees to "exercise good judgment" in questionable circumstances "by avoiding activities that could create even the appearance that our decisions could be compromised." And Analog Devices has set up a policy manager as a consultant to overseas operations. The policy manager does not make decisions for country managers. Instead, the policy manager helps country managers think through the issues and provides information on how the corporate office has handled similar situations in the past.

Information accessed at *www.oecd.org* and www.bp.com, October 6, 2011; and, Begley, T. M., & Boyd, D. P. 2003. The need for a corporate global mindset. *MIT Sloan Management Review*, Winter: 25–32.

"exported" to foreign operations, while others have required some modifications.[64] When the retailer entered the German market in 1997, it took along the company "cheer"—Give me a W! Give me an A! Give me an L! Who's Number One? The Customer!—which suited German employees. However, Walmart's 10-Foot Rule, which requires employees to greet any customer within a 10-foot radius, was not so well received in Germany, where employees and shoppers alike weren't comfortable with the custom.

Strategy Spotlight 7.8 describes how multinationals have adapted to the problem of bribery in various countries.

Risks and Challenges   As you might expect, there are some risks associated with a multidomestic strategy. Among these are the following:

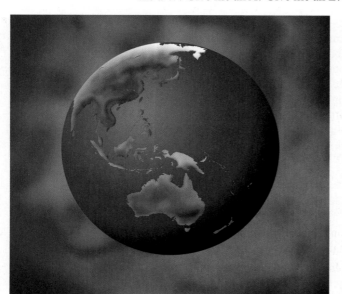

● Australia is geographically distant from the United States. However, it is much closer when other dimensions are considered, such as income levels, language, culture, and political/legal systems.

- Typically, local adaptation of products and services will increase a company's cost structure. In many industries, competition is so intense that most firms can ill afford any competitive disadvantages on the dimension of cost. A key challenge of managers is to determine the trade-off between local adaptation and its cost structure. For example, cost considerations led Procter & Gamble to standardize its diaper design across all European markets. This was done despite research data indicating that Italian mothers, unlike those in other countries, preferred diapers that covered the baby's navel. Later, however, P&G recognized that this feature was critical to these mothers, so the company decided to incorporate this feature for the Italian market despite its adverse cost implications.

- At times, local adaptations, even when well intentioned, may backfire. When the American restaurant chain TGI Friday's entered the South Korean market, it purposely incorporated many local dishes, such as kimchi (hot, spicy cabbage), in its menu. This responsiveness, however, was not well received. Company analysis of the weak market acceptance indicated that Korean customers anticipated a visit to TGI Friday's as a visit to America. Thus, finding Korean dishes was inconsistent with their expectations.

- The optimal degree of local adaptation evolves over time. In many industry segments, a variety of factors, such as the influence of global media, greater international travel, and declining income disparities across countries, may lead to increasing global standardization. On the other hand, in other industry segments, especially where the product or service can be delivered over the Internet (such as music), the need for even greater customization and local adaptation may increase over time. Firms must recalibrate the need for local adaptation on an ongoing basis; excessive adaptation extracts a price as surely as underadaptation.

Some films and TV programs may cross country boundaries rather successfully, while others are less successful. Let's consider an effort by Disney that fell far short:

> Remember *The Alamo,* not the nineteenth-century battle between Mexican forces and Texas rebels, but the 2004 movie? The film definitely met the big-budget criterion—it cost Disney nearly $100 million. It did not generate strong box-office receipts in English. But what was surprising was Disney's attempt to create crossover appeal to Latinos. These efforts included more balanced treatment of Anglos versus Mexicans, prominently featuring Tejano folk heroes in the film, and running a separate Spanish-language marketing effort. But such efforts were doomed to fail. Why? According to one authority, the Alamo is "such an open wound among American Hispanics."[65]

Exhibit 7.7 summarizes the strengths and limitations of multidomestic strategies.

Transnational Strategy

A **transnational strategy** strives to optimize the trade-offs associated with efficiency, local adaptation, and learning.[66] It seeks efficiency not for its own sake, but as a means to achieve global competitiveness.[67] It recognizes the importance of local responsiveness but as a tool for flexibility in international operations.[68] Innovations are regarded as an outcome of a larger process of organizational learning that includes the contributions of everyone in the firm.[69] Also, a core tenet of the transnational model is that a firm's assets and capabilities

transnational strategy a strategy based on firms optimizing the trade-offs associated with efficiency, local adaptation, and learning, used in industries where the pressures for both local adaptation and lowering costs are high.

Strengths	Limitations
• Ability to adapt products and services to local market conditions.	• Decreased ability to realize cost savings through scale economies.
• Ability to detect potential opportunities for attractive niches in a given market, enhancing revenue.	• Greater difficulty in transferring knowledge across countries.
	• May lead to "overadaptation" as conditions change.

Exhibit 7.7
Strengths and Limitations of Multidomestic Strategies

are dispersed according to the most beneficial location for each activity. Thus, managers avoid the tendency to either concentrate activities in a central location (a global strategy) or disperse them across many locations to enhance adaptation (a multidomestic strategy). Peter Brabeck, chairman of Nestlé, the giant food company, provides such a perspective.

> We believe strongly that there isn't a so-called global consumer, at least not when it comes to food and beverages. People have local tastes based on their unique cultures and traditions—a good candy bar in Brazil is not the same as a good candy bar in China. Therefore, decision making needs to be pushed down as low as possible in the organization, out close to the markets. Otherwise, how can you make good brand decisions? That said, decentralization has its limits. If you are too decentralized, you can become too complicated—you get too much complexity in your production system. The closer we come to the consumer, in branding, pricing, communication, and product adaptation, the more we decentralize. The more we are dealing with production, logistics, and supply-chain management, the more centralized decision making becomes. After all, we want to leverage Nestlé's size, not be hampered by it.[70]

The Nestlé example illustrates a common approach in determining whether or not to centralize or decentralize a value-chain activity. Typically, primary activities that are "downstream" (e.g., marketing and sales, and service), or closer to the customer, tend to require more decentralization in order to adapt to local market conditions. On the other hand, primary activities that are "upstream" (e.g., logistics and operations), or further away from the customer, tend to be centralized. This is because there is less need for adapting these activities to local markets and the firm can benefit from economies of scale. Additionally, many support activities, such as information systems and procurement, tend to be centralized in order to increase the potential for economies of scale.

A central philosophy of the transnational organization is enhanced adaptation to all competitive situations as well as flexibility by capitalizing on communication and knowledge flows throughout the organization.[71] A principal characteristic is the integration of unique contributions of all units into worldwide operations. Thus, a joint innovation by headquarters and by one of the overseas units can lead potentially to the development of relatively standardized and yet flexible products and services that are suitable for multiple markets.

Asea Brown Boveri (ABB) is a firm that successfully follows a transnational strategy. ABB, with its home bases in Sweden and Switzerland, illustrates the trend toward cross-national mergers that lead firms to consider multiple headquarters in the future. It is managed as a flexible network of units, and one of management's main functions is the facilitation of information and knowledge flows between units. ABB's subsidiaries have complete responsibility for product categories on a worldwide basis. Such a transnational strategy enables ABB to benefit from access to new markets and the opportunity to utilize and develop resources wherever they may be located.

Risks and Challenges As with the other strategies, there are some unique risks and challenges associated with a transnational strategy.

- *The choice of a seemingly optimal location cannot guarantee that the quality and cost of factor inputs (i.e., labor, materials) will be optimal.* Managers must ensure that the relative advantage of a location is actually realized, not squandered because of weaknesses in productivity and the quality of internal operations. Ford Motor Co., for example, has benefited from having some of its manufacturing operations in Mexico. While some have argued that the benefits of lower wage rates will be partly offset by lower productivity, this does not always have to be the case. Since unemployment in Mexico is higher than in the United States, Ford can be more selective in its hiring practices for its Mexican operations. And, given the lower turnover among its Mexican employees, Ford can justify a high level of investment in training and development. Thus, the net result can be not only lower wage rates but also higher productivity than in the United States.

- *Although knowledge transfer can be a key source of competitive advantage, it does not take place "automatically."* For knowledge transfer to take place from one subsidiary to another, it is important for the source of the knowledge, the target units, and the corporate headquarters to recognize the potential value of such unique know-how. Given that there can be significant geographic, linguistic, and cultural distances that typically separate subsidiaries, the potential for knowledge transfer can become very difficult to realize. Firms must create mechanisms to systematically and routinely uncover the opportunities for knowledge transfer.

Exhibit 7.8 summarizes the relative advantages and disadvantages of transnational strategies.

Global or Regional? A Second Look at Globalization

>LO7.6
The difference between regional companies and truly global companies.

Thus far, we have suggested four possible strategies from which a firm must choose once it has decided to compete in the global marketplace. In recent years, many writers have asserted that the process of globalization has caused national borders to become increasingly irrelevant.[72] However, some scholars have recently questioned this perspective, and they have argued that it is unwise for companies to rush into full-scale globalization.[73]

Before answering questions about the extent of firms' globalization, let's try to clarify what "globalization" means. Traditionally, a firm's globalization is measured in terms of its foreign sales as a percentage of total sales. However, this measure can be misleading. For example, consider a U.S. firm that has expanded its activities into Canada. Clearly, this initiative is qualitatively different from achieving the same sales volume in a distant country such as China. Similarly, if a Malaysian firm expands into Singapore or a German firm starts selling its products in Austria, this would represent an expansion into a geographically adjacent country. Such nearby countries would often share many common characteristics in terms of language, culture, infrastructure, and customer preferences. In other words, this is more a case of **regionalization** than globalization.

Extensive analysis of the distribution data of sales across different countries and regions led Alan Rugman and Alain Verbeke to conclude that there is a stronger case to be made in favor of regionalization than globalization. According to their study, a company would have to have at least 20 percent of its sales in each of the three major economic regions—North America, Europe, and Asia—to be considered a global firm. However, they found that only nine of the world's 500 largest firms met this standard! Even when they relaxed the criterion to 20 percent of sales each in at least two of the three regions, the number only increased to 25. *Thus, most companies are regional or, at best, biregional—not global—even today.* Exhibit 7.9 provides a listing of the large firms that met each of these two criteria.

regionalization
increasing international exchange of goods, services, money, people, ideas, and information; and the increasing similarity of culture, laws, rules, and norms within a region such as Europe, North America, or Asia.

Exhibit 7.8
Strengths and Limitations of Transnational Strategies

Strengths	Limitations
• Ability to attain economies of scale. • Ability to adapt to local markets. • Ability to locate activities in optimal locations. • Ability to increase knowledge flows and learning.	• Unique challenges in determining optimal locations of activities to ensure cost and quality. • Unique managerial challenges in fostering knowledge transfer.

Firms with at least 20 percent sales in Asia, Europe, and North America each but with less than 50 percent sales in any one region:

IBM	Nokia	Coca-Cola
Sony	Intel	Flextronics
Philips	Canon	LVMH

Firms with at least 20 percent sales in at least two of the three regions (Asia, Europe, North America) but with less than 50 percent sales in any one region:

BP Amoco	Alstom	Michelin
Toyota	Aventis	Kodak
Nissan	Daigeo	Electrolux
Unilever	Sun Microsystems	BAE
Motorola	Bridgestone	Alcan
GlaxoSmithKline	Roche	L'Oreal
EADS	3M	Lafarge
Bayer	Skanska	
Ericsson	McDonald's	

Firms with at least 50 percent of their sales in one of the three regions—other than their home region:

Daimler Chrysler	Santander	Sodexho Alliance
ING Group	Delhaize "Le Lion"	Manpower
Royal Ahold	Astra Zeneca	Wolseley
Honda	News Corporation	

Sources: Peng, M.W. 2010. *Global Strategy* (2nd ed.). Mason, OH: Thomson Southwestern; and, Rugman, A.M. & Verbeke, A. 2004. A perspective on regional and global strategies of multinational enterprises. *Journal of International Business Studies,* 35: 3–18.

In a world of instant communication, rapid transportation, and governments that are increasingly willing to open up their markets to trade and investment, why are so few firms "global"? The most obvious answer is that distance still matters. After all, it is easier to do business in a neighboring country than in a far away country, all else being equal. Distance, in the final analysis, may be viewed as a concept with many dimensions, not just a measure of geographical distance. For example, both Canada and Mexico are the same distance from the U.S. However, U.S. companies find it easier to expand operations into Canada than into Mexico. Why? Canada and the U.S. share many commonalities in terms of language, culture, economic development, legal and political systems, and infrastructure development. Thus, if we view distance as having many dimensions, the U.S. and Canada are very close, whereas there is greater distance between the U.S. and Mexico. Similarly, when we look at what we might call the "true" distance between the U.S. and China, the effects of geographic distance are multiplied by distance in terms of culture, language, religion, and legal and political systems between the two countries. On the other hand, although U.S. and Australia are geographically distant, the "true" distance is somewhat less when one considers distance along the other dimensions.

Another reason for regional expansion is the rise of the **trading blocs**. The European Union originally started in the 1950s as a regional trading bloc. However, recently it has

trading blocs groups of countries agreeing to increase trade between them by lowering trade barries.

achieved a large degree of economic and political integration in terms of common currency and common standards that many thought infeasible, if not impossible, only 20 years ago. The resulting economic benefits have led other regions also to consider similar moves. For example, the North American Free Trade Agreement (NAFTA) has the eventual abolition of all barriers to the free movement of goods and services among Canada, the U.S., and Mexico as its goal. Other regional trading blocks include MERCOSUR (consisting of Argentina, Brazil, Paraguay, and Uruguay) and the Association of Southeast Asian Nations (ASEAN) (consisting of about a dozen Southeast Asian countries).

Regional economic integration has progressed at a faster pace than global economic integration and the trade and investment patterns of the largest companies reflect this reality. After all, regions represent the outcomes of centuries of political and cultural history that results not only in commonalities but also mutual affinity. For example, stretching from Algeria and Morocco in the West to Oman and Yemen in the East, more than 30 countries share the Arabic language and the Muslim religion, making these countries a natural regional bloc. Similarly, the countries of South and Central America share the Spanish language (except Brazil), Catholic religion, and a shared history of Spanish colonialism. No wonder firms find it easier and less risky to expand within their region than to other regions.

Entry Modes of International Expansion

>LO7.7
The four basic types of entry strategies and the relative benefits and risks associated with each of them.

A firm has many options available to it when it decides to expand into international markets. Given the challenges associated with such entry, many firms first start on a small scale and then increase their level of investment and risk as they gain greater experience with the overseas market in question.[74]

Exhibit 7.10 illustrates a wide variety of modes of foreign entry, including exporting, licensing, franchising, joint ventures, strategic alliances, and wholly owned subsidiaries.[75] As the exhibit indicates, the various types of entry form a continuum ranging from exporting (low investment and risk, low control) to a wholly owned subsidiary (high investment and risk, high control).[76]

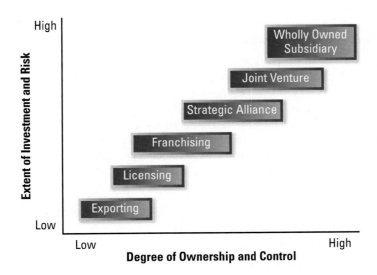

Exhibit 7.10 **Entry Modes for International Expansion**

There can be frustrations and setbacks as a firm evolves its international entry strategy from exporting to more expensive types, including wholly owned subsidiaries. For example, according to the CEO of a large U.S. specialty chemical company:

> In the end, we always do a better job with our own subsidiaries; sales improve, and we have greater control over the business. But we still need local distributors for entry, and we are still searching for strategies to get us through the transitions without battles over control and performance.[77]

Exporting

Exporting consists of producing goods in one country to sell in another.[78] This entry strategy enables a firm to invest the least amount of resources in terms of its product, its organization, and its overall corporate strategy. Many host countries dislike this entry strategy because it provides less local employment than other modes of entry.[79]

Multinationals often stumble onto a stepwise strategy for penetrating markets, beginning with the exporting of products. This often results in a series of unplanned actions to increase sales revenues. As the pattern recurs with entries into subsequent markets, this approach, named a "beachhead strategy," often becomes official policy.[80]

Benefits   Such an approach definitely has its advantages. After all, firms start from scratch in sales and distribution when they enter new markets. Because many foreign markets are nationally regulated and dominated by networks of local intermediaries, firms need to partner with local distributors to benefit from their valuable expertise and knowledge of their own markets. Multinationals, after all, recognize that they cannot master local business practices, meet regulatory requirements, hire and manage local personnel, or gain access to potential customers without some form of local partnership.

Multinationals also want to minimize their own risk. They do this by hiring local distributors and investing very little in the undertaking. In essence, the firm gives up control of strategic marketing decisions to the local partners—much more control than they would be willing to give up in their home market.

Risks and Limitations   Exporting is a relatively inexpensive way to enter foreign markets. However, it can still have significant downsides. In a study of 250 instances in which multinational firms used local distributors to implement their exporting entry strategy, the results were dismal. In the vast majority of the cases, the distributors were bought (to increase control) by the multinational firm or fired. In contrast, successful distributors shared two common characteristics:

- They carried product lines that complemented, rather than competed with, the multinational's products.
- They behaved as if they were business partners with the multinationals. They shared market information with the corporations, they initiated projects with distributors in neighboring countries, and they suggested initiatives in their own or nearby markets. Additionally, these distributors took on risk themselves by investing in areas such as training, information systems, and advertising and promotion in order to increase the business of their multinational partners.

The key point is the importance of developing collaborative, win–win relationships.

To ensure more control over operations without incurring significant risks, many firms have used licensing and franchising as a mode of entry. Let's now discuss these and their relative advantages and disadvantages.

Licensing and Franchising

Licensing and franchising are both forms of contractual arrangements. **Licensing** enables a company to receive a royalty or fee in exchange for the right to use its trademark, patent, trade secret, or other valuable item of intellectual property.[81]

Franchising contracts generally include a broader range of factors in an operation and have a longer time period during which the agreement is in effect. Franchising remains a primary form of American business. According to a recent survey, more than 400 U.S. franchisers have international exposure.[82] This is greater than the combined totals of the next four largest franchiser home countries—France, the United Kingdom, Mexico, and Austria.

Benefits In international markets, an advantage of licensing is that the firm granting a license incurs little risk, since it does not have to invest any significant resources in the country itself. In turn, the licensee (the firm receiving the license) gains access to the trademark, patent, and so on, and is able to potentially create competitive advantages. In many cases, the country also benefits from the product being manufactured locally. For example, Yoplait yogurt is licensed by General Mills from Sodima, a French cooperative, for sale in the United States. The logos of college and professional athletic teams in the United States are another source of trademarks that generate significant royalty income domestically and internationally.

> **franchising** a contractual arrangement in which a company receives a royalty or fee in exchange for the right to use its intellectual property; it usually involves a longer time period than licensing and includes other factors, such as monitoring of operations, training, and advertising.

Franchising has the advantage of limiting the risk exposure that a firm has in overseas markets. At the same time, the firm is able to expand the revenue base of the company.

Risks and Limitations The licensor gives up control of its product and forgoes potential revenues and profits. Furthermore, the licensee may eventually become so familiar with the patent and trade secrets that it may become a competitor; that is, the licensee may make some modifications to the product and manufacture and sell it independently of the licensor without having to pay a royalty fee. This potential situation is aggravated in countries that have relatively weak laws to protect intellectual property. Additionally, if the licensee selected by the multinational firm turns out to be a poor choice, the brand name and reputation of the product may be tarnished.[83]

With franchising, the multinational firm receives only a portion of the revenues, in the form of franchise fees. Had the firm set up the operation itself (e.g., a restaurant through direct investment), it would have had the entire revenue to itself.

Companies often desire a closer collaboration with other firms in order to increase revenue, reduce costs, and enhance their learning—often through the diffusion of technology. To achieve such objectives, they enter into strategic alliances or joint ventures, two entry modes we will discuss next.

Strategic Alliances and Joint Ventures

Joint ventures and strategic alliances have recently become increasingly popular.[84] These two forms of partnership differ in that joint ventures entail the creation of a third-party legal entity, whereas strategic alliances do not. In addition, strategic alliances generally focus on initiatives that are smaller in scope than joint ventures.[85]

Benefits As we discussed in Chapter 6, these strategies have been effective in helping firms increase revenues and reduce costs as well as enhance learning and diffuse technologies.[86] These partnerships enable firms to share the risks as well as the potential revenues and profits. Also, by gaining exposure to new sources of knowledge and technologies, such partnerships can help firms develop core competencies that can lead to competitive advantages in the marketplace.[87] Finally, entering into partnerships with host country firms can provide very useful information on local market tastes, competitive conditions, legal matters, and cultural nuances.[88]

Strategic alliances can be between firms in totally different industries. Strategy Spotlight 7.9 discusses a collaboration between the Italian automaker Lamborghini and Callaway, the U.S. golf equipment manufacturer.

Lamborghini and Callaway Form a High-Tech Alliance

Lamborghini's Sesto Elemento concept car was the hit at the 2010 Paris Auto Show. It would not seem to have much in common with Callaway's new Diablo Octane and Octane Tour drivers. However, both are made using an ingenious new material called forged composite that the companies developed together. The material is much stronger than titanium but weighs only one-third as much.

The partnership between Lamborghini and Callaway began in 2008. Researchers from the two companies met at a materials science conference and found that they had much in common. Said Callaway's CEO George Fellows, "The collaboration has been great. The DNA of both companies, pushing for a technological edge in performance-oriented consumer products, is very similar." In short, both firms are engaged in developing lighter and stronger composite materials for their products. And most would agree that the markets that they serve are dissimilar enough to make full cooperation feasible.

Source: Newport, J. P. 2010. Drive the ball like it's a Lamborghini, maybe. *The Wall Street Journal.* November 13–14: A14; *www.callaway.com*; and, Anonymous. 2010. Automobili Lamborghini and Callaway Golf form strategic partnership. *autonewscast.com* September 30: np.

Let's look at how each company has benefited from their joint development of forged composite.

The weight-savings in Callaway's new drivers, which deploy forged composite only in the crowns (the bottom half of the clubheads is still made of titanium), is only 10 grams. Although 10 grams might seem insignificant, such weight loss up top gives designers much more flexibility in how they distribute mass around the bottom. This helps to create more desirable ball flight characteristics and improve forgiveness on off-center hits.

For Lamborghini, forged composite enhances a car's power-to-weight ratio and acceleration capability. To illustrate, the Sesto Elemento can accelerate from 0 to 60 miles per hour in an astonishing 2.5 seconds. This is almost a full second faster than the Italian automaker's speed champ—the $240,000 Superleggera. The difference is entirely due to weight, in part because both cars use the same 570-horsepower, four-wheel-drivetrain. But by building the chassis almost entirely of forged composite, engineers were able to reduce the curb weight by nearly a third—to an anorexic 2,072 pounds. "The power-to-weight ratio is more like a motorcycle's," claimed Lamborghini's CEO Stephan Winkelmann. After further testing, he expected forged composite to begin working its way into production within a few years.

Risks and Limitations Managers must be aware of the risks associated with strategic alliances and joint ventures and how they can be minimized.[89] First, there needs to be a clearly defined strategy that is strongly supported by the organizations that are party to the partnership. Otherwise, the firms may work at cross-purposes and not achieve any of their goals. Second, and closely allied to the first issue, there must be a clear understanding of capabilities and resources that will be central to the partnership. Without such clarification, there will be fewer opportunities for learning and developing competencies that could lead to competitive advantages. Third, trust is a vital element. Phasing in the relationship between alliance partners permits them to get to know each other better and develop trust. Without trust, one party may take advantage of the other by, for example, withholding its fair share of resources and gaining access to privileged information through unethical (or illegal) means. Fourth, cultural issues that can potentially lead to conflict and dysfunctional behaviors need to be addressed. An organization's culture is the set of values, beliefs, and attitudes that influence the behavior and goals of its employees.[90] Thus, recognizing cultural differences as well as striving to develop elements of a "common culture" for the partnership is vital. Without a unifying culture, it will become difficult to combine and leverage resources that are increasingly important in knowledge-intensive organizations (discussed in Chapter 4).[91]

Finally, the success of a firm's alliance should not be left to chance.[92] To improve their odds of success, many companies have carefully documented alliance-management knowledge by creating guidelines and manuals to help them manage specific aspects of the entire alliance life cycle (e.g., partner selection and alliance negotiation and contracting). For example, Lotus Corp. (part of IBM) created what it calls its "35 rules of thumb" to manage each phase of an alliance from formation to termination. Hewlett-Packard developed 60 different tools and templates, which it placed in a 300-page manual for guiding decision making. The manual included such tools as a template for making the business case for an alliance, a partner evaluation form, a negotiation template outlining the roles and responsibilities of different departments, a list of the ways to measure alliance performance, and an alliance termination checklist.

When a firm desires the highest level of control, it develops wholly owned subsidiaries. Although wholly owned subsidiaries can generate the greatest returns, they also have the highest levels of investment and risk. We will now discuss them.

Wholly Owned Subsidiaries

A **wholly owned subsidiary** is a business in which a multinational company owns 100 percent of the stock. Two ways a firm can establish a wholly owned subsidiary are to (1) acquire an existing company in the home country or (2) develop a totally new operation (often referred to as a "greenfield venture").

wholly owned subsidiary a business in which a multinational company owns 100 percent of the stock.

Benefits   Establishing a wholly owned subsidiary is the most expensive and risky of the various entry modes. However, it can also yield the highest returns. In addition, it provides the multinational company with the greatest degree of control of all activities, including manufacturing, marketing, distribution, and technology development.[93]

Wholly owned subsidiaries are most appropriate where a firm already has the appropriate knowledge and capabilities that it can leverage rather easily through multiple locations. Examples range from restaurants to semiconductor manufacturers. To lower costs, for example, Intel Corporation builds semiconductor plants throughout the world—all of which use virtually the same blueprint. Knowledge can be further leveraged by hiring managers and professionals from the firm's home country, often through hiring talent from competitors.

Risks and Limitations   As noted, wholly owned subsidiaries are typically the most expensive and risky entry mode. With franchising, joint ventures, or strategic alliances, the risk is shared with the firm's partners. With wholly owned subsidiaries, the entire risk is assumed by the parent company. The risks associated with doing business in a new country (e.g., political, cultural, and legal) can be lessened by hiring local talent.

For example, Wendy's avoided committing two blunders in Germany by hiring locals to its advertising staff.[94] In one case, the firm wanted to promote its "old-fashioned" qualities. However, a literal translation would have resulted in the company promoting itself as "outdated." In another situation, Wendy's wanted to emphasize that its hamburgers could be prepared 256 ways. The problem? The German word that Wendy's wanted to use for "ways" usually meant "highways" or "roads." Although such errors may sometimes be entertaining to the public, it is certainly preferable to catch these mistakes before they confuse the consumer or embarrass the company.

We have addressed entry strategies as a progression from exporting through the creation of wholly owned subsidiaries. However, we must point out that many firms do not follow such an evolutionary approach. For example, because of political and regulatory reasons, Pepsi entered India through a joint venture with two Indian firms in 1998. As discussed in Strategy Spotlight 7.10, this provided Pepsi with a first-mover advantage within the Indian market, where it remains well ahead of its archrival, Coca-Cola.

Pepsi's First-Mover Advantage in India Has Paid Off

Pepsi (pronounced "Pay-psee") became a common synonym for cola in India's most widely spoken language after having the market to itself in the early 1990s. PepsiCo's linguistic advantage translates into higher sales for its namesake product. Although Atlanta-based Coke has larger total beverage sales in India because it owns several non-cola drink brands, Pepsi's 4.5 percent of the soft-drink market outshines Coke's 2.6 percent, according to Euromonitor. That's a notable exception to much of the rest of the world, where Coke's cola soundly beats its main rival.

What explains Pepsi's success in India? Coke pulled out of the market in 1977 after new government regulations forced it to partner with an Indian company and share the drink's secret formula. In contrast, Pepsi formed a joint venture in 1988 with two Indian companies and introduced products under the Lehar brand. (Lehar Pepsi was introduced in 1990.) Coke then re-entered the market in 1993 after Indian regulations were changed to permit foreign brands to operate without Indian partners.

Coke's time out of India cost it dearly. "Pepsi got here sooner, and got to India just as it was starting to engage with the West and with Western products," said Lalita Desai, a linguist at Jadavpur University who studies how English words enter Indian languages. "And with no real international competition, 'Pepsi' became the catchall for anything that was bottled, fizzy, and from abroad."

PepsiCo has also been very successful in promoting water conservation in India. Its Indian operation became the first of its global units (and probably the only one in the beverage industry) to conserve and replenish more water that it consumed in 2009. Its rival, Coca Cola, on the other hand, is facing a serious situation in India as it has been fined Rs 216 crore ($4.7 million) as compensation for groundwater pollution and depletion.

Today, PepsiCo is the fourth largest consumer products company in India. The firm also has invested more than $1 billion in India, created direct and indirect employment to 150,000 people in the country, and has 13 company-owned bottling plants.

Source: Srivastava, M. 2010. For India's consumers, Pepsi is the real thing. *Bloomberg Businessweek.* September 20–26: 26–27; Bhushan, R. 2010. Pepsi India touches eco watershed, first unit to achieve positive water balance. *www.indiatimes.com.* May 27: np; and, *www.pepsicoindia.*

Reflecting on Career Implications . . .

- *International Strategy:* Be aware of your organization's international strategy. What percentage of the total firm activity is international? What skills are needed to enhance your company's international efforts? How can you get more involved in your organization's international strategy? For your career, what conditions in your home country might cause you to seek careers abroad?
- *Outsourcing and Offshoring:* What activities in your organization can/should be outsourced or offshored? Be aware that you are competing in the global marketplace for employment and professional advancement. Continually take inventory of your talents, skills, and competencies.
- *International Career Opportunities:* Work assignments in other countries can often provide a career boost. Be proactive in pursuing promising career opportunities in other countries. Anticipate how such opportunities will advance your short- and long-term career aspirations.
- *Management Risks:* Develop cultural sensitivity. This applies, of course, to individuals from different cultures in your home-based organization as well as in your overseas experience.

Summary

We live in a highly interconnected global community where many of the best opportunities for growth and profitability lie beyond the boundaries of a company's home country. Along with the opportunities, of course, there are many risks associated with diversification into global markets.

The first section of the chapter addressed the factors that determine a nation's competitiveness in a particular industry. The framework was developed by Professor Michael Porter of Harvard University and was based on a four-year study that explored the competitive success of 10 leading trading nations. The four factors, collectively termed the "diamond of national advantage," were factor endowments, demand conditions, related and supporting industries, and firm strategy, structure, and rivalry.

The discussion of Porter's "diamond" helped, in essence, to set the broader context for exploring competitive advantage at the firm level. In the second section, we discussed the primary motivations and the potential risks associated with international expansion. The primary motivations included increasing the size of the potential market for the firm's products and services, achieving economies of scale, extending the life cycle of the firm's products, and optimizing the location for every activity in the value chain. On the other hand, the key risks included political and economic risks, currency risks, and management risks. Management risks are the challenges associated with responding to the inevitable differences that exist across countries such as customs, culture, language, customer preferences, and distribution systems. We also addressed some of the managerial challenges and opportunities associated with offshoring and outsourcing.

Next, we addressed how firms can go about attaining competitive advantage in global markets. We began by discussing the two opposing forces—cost reduction and adaptation to local markets—that managers must contend with when entering global markets. The relative importance of these two factors plays a major part in determining which of the four basic types of strategies to select: international, global, multidomestic, or transnational. The chapter covered the benefits and risks associated with each type of strategy. We also presented a recent perspective by Alan Rugman who argues that, despite all the talk of globalization, most of the large multinationals are regional or at best biregional (in terms of geographical diversification of sales) rather than global.

The final section discussed the four types of entry strategies that managers may undertake when entering international markets. The key trade-off in each of these strategies is the level of investment or risk versus the level of control. In order of their progressively greater investment/risk and control, the strategies range from exporting to licensing and franchising, to strategic alliances and joint ventures, to wholly owned subsidiaries. The relative benefits and risks associated with each of these strategies were addressed.

Summary Review Questions

1. What are some of the advantages and disadvantages associated with a firm's expansion into international markets?
2. What are the four factors described in Porter's diamond of national advantage? How do the four factors explain why some industries in a given country are more successful than others?
3. Explain the two opposing forces—cost reduction and adaptation to local markets—that firms must deal with when they go global.
4. There are four basic strategies—international, global, multidomestic, and transnational. What are the advantages and disadvantages associated with each?
5. What is the basis of Alan Rugman's argument that most multinationals are still more regional than global? What factors inhibit firms from becoming truly global?
6. Describe the basic entry strategies that firms have available when they enter international markets. What are the relative advantages and disadvantages of each?

Key Terms

globalization, 283
factor endowments (national advantage), 285
demand conditions (national advantage), 285
related and supporting industries (national advantage), 285
firm strategy, structure, and rivalry (national advantage), 286
multinational firms, 286
arbitrage opportunities, 289
reverse innovation, 290
political risk, 291
rule of law, 291
economic risk, 293
counterfeiting, 294
currency risk, 294
management risk, 295
outsourcing, 296
offshoring, 296
international strategy, 300
global strategy, 301
multidomestic strategy, 302
transnational strategy, 305
regionalization, 307
trading blocs, 308
exporting, 310
licensing, 310
franchising, 311
wholly owned subsidiary, 313

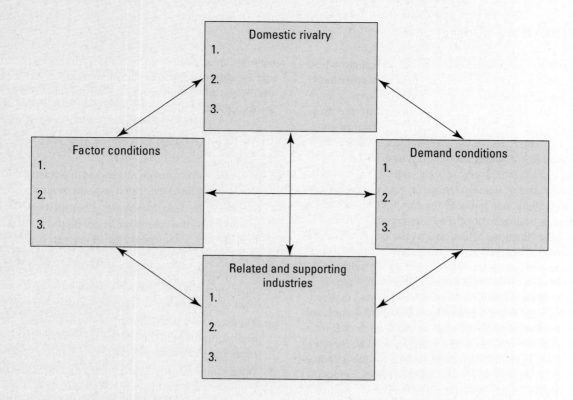

Domestic rivalry
1.
2.
3.

Factor conditions
1.
2.
3.

Demand conditions
1.
2.
3.

Related and supporting industries
1.
2.
3.

Experiential Exercise

The United States is considered a world leader in the motion picture industry. Using Porter's diamond framework for national competitiveness (provided above), explain the success of this industry.

Application Questions & Exercises

1. Data on the "competitiveness of nations" can be found at *www.imd.ch/wcy/ranking/*. This website provides a ranking on a 331 criteria for 59 countries. How might Porter's diamond of national advantage help to explain the rankings for some of these countries for certain industries that interest you?

2. The Internet has lowered the entry barriers for smaller firms that wish to diversify into international markets. Why is this so? Provide an example.

3. Many firms fail when they enter into strategic alliances with firms that link up with companies based in other countries. What are some reasons for this failure? Provide an example.

4. Many large U.S.–based management consulting companies such as McKinsey and Company and the BCG Group have been very successful in the international marketplace. How can Porter's diamond explain their success?

Ethics Questions

1. Over the past few decades, many American firms have relocated most or all of their operations from the United States to countries such as Mexico and China that pay lower wages. What are some of the ethical issues that such actions may raise?

2. Business practices and customs vary throughout the world. What are some of the ethical issues concerning payments that must be made in a foreign country to obtain business opportunities?

References

1. Anonymous. 2010. Exit Carrefour. *The Economist.* September 23: 77; Thomas, D. & Fuse, T. 2010. Retailers jump in for Carrefour SE Asia assets. *www.reuters.com.* September 1: np; and, Chan, C. 2010. Carrefour said to list Tesco, Casino as potential unit buyers. *www.businessweek.com.* September 9: np.

2. For a recent discussion on globalization by one of international business's most respected authors, read: Ohmae, K. 2005. *The next global stage: Challenges and opportunities in our borderless world.* Philadelphia: Wharton School Publishing.

3. Our discussion of globalization draws upon: Engardio, P. & Belton, C. 2000. Global capitalism: Can it be made to work better? *BusinessWeek,* November 6: 72–98.

4. Sellers, P. 2005. Blowing in the wind. *Fortune,* July 25: 63.

5. An interesting and balanced discussion on the merits of multinationals to the U.S. economy is found in: Mandel, M. 2008. Multinationals: Are they good for America? *BusinessWeek,* March 10: 41–64; and, trade statistics from World Trade Organization. Trade Expands by 9.5% in 2010 after Dismal 2009. WTO press release, March 26, 2010.

6. Engardio & Belton, op. cit.

7. For insightful perspectives on strategy in emerging economies, refer to: Wright, M., Filatotchev, I., Hoskisson, R. E., & Peng, M. W. 2005. Strategy research in emerging economies: Challenging the conventional wisdom. *Journal of Management Studies,* 42(1): 1–33.

8. Black, J. S. & Morrison, A. J. 2010. A cautionary tale for emerging market giants. *Harvard Business Review,* 88(9): 99–105.

9. The above discussion draws on: Clifford, M. L., Engardio, P., Malkin, E., Roberts, D., & Echikson, W. 2000. Up the ladder. *BusinessWeek,* November 6: 78–84.

10. A recent discussion of the "bottom of the pyramid" is: Akula, V. 2008. Business basics at the bottom of the pyramid. *Harvard Business Review,* 86(6): 53–59.

11. Some insights into how winners are evolving in emerging markets are addressed in: Ghemawat, P. & Hout, T. 2008. Tomorrow's global giants: Not the usual suspects. *Harvard Business Review,* 66(11): 80–88.

12. For another interesting discussion on a country perspective, refer to: Makino, S. 1999. MITI Minister Kaora Yosano on reviving Japan's competitive advantages. *Academy of Management Executive,* 13(4): 8–28.

13. The following discussion draws heavily upon: Porter, M. E. 1990. The competitive advantage of nations. *Harvard Business Review,* March–April: 73–93.

14. Landes, D. S. 1998. *The wealth and poverty of nations.* New York: W. W. Norton.

15. A recent study that investigates the relationship between international diversification and firm performance is: Lu, J. W. & Beamish, P. W. 2004. International diversification and firm performance: The s-curve hypothesis. *Academy of Management Journal,* 47(4): 598–609.

16. Part of our discussion of the motivations and risks of international expansion draws upon: Gregg, F. M. 1999. International strategy. In Helms, M. M. (Ed.). *Encyclopedia of management:* 434–438. Detroit: Gale Group.

17. These two examples are discussed, respectively, in: Dawar, N. & Frost, T. 1999. Competing with giants: Survival strategies for local companies in emerging markets. *Harvard Business Review,* 77(2): 119–129; and, Prahalad, C. K. & Lieberthal, K. 1998. The end of corporate imperialism. *Harvard Business Review,* 76(4): 68–79.

18. Meredith, R. 2004. Middle kingdom, middle class. *Forbes,* November 15: 188–192; and, Anonymous. 2004. Middle class becomes rising power in China. *www.Chinadaily.com.* November 6.

19. Eyring, M. J., Johnson, M. W., & Nair, H. 2011. New business models in emerging markets. *Harvard Business Review,* 89 (1/2): 88–98.

20. Cieply, M. & Barnes, B. 2010. After rants, skepticism over Gibson bankability grows in non-U.S. markets. *International Herald Tribune,* July 23: 1.

21. Information accessed at *www.boxoffice.com.*

22. This discussion draws upon: Gupta, A. K. & Govindarajan, V. 2001. Converting global presence into global competitive advantage. *Academy of Management Executive,* 15(2): 45–56.

23. Stross, R. E. 1997. Mr. Gates builds his brain trust. *Fortune,* December 8: 84–98.

24. For a good summary of the benefits and risks of international expansion, refer to: Bartlett, C. A. & Ghoshal, S. 1987. Managing across borders: New strategic responses. *Sloan Management Review,* 28(5): 45–53; and, Brown, R. H. 1994. *Competing to win in a global economy.* Washington, DC: U.S. Department of Commerce.

25. For an interesting insight into rivalry in global markets, refer to: MacMillan, I. C., van Putten, A. B., & McGrath, R. G. 2003. Global gamesmanship. *Harvard Business Review,* 81(5): 62–73.

26. It is important for firms to spread their foreign operations and outsourcing relationships with a broad, well-balanced mix of regions and countries to reduce risk and increase potential reward. For example, refer to: Vestring, T., Rouse, T., & Reinert, U. 2005. Hedge your offshoring bets. *MIT Sloan Management Review,* 46(3): 27–29.

27. An interesting discussion of risks faced by Lukoil, Russia's largest oil firm is in: Gimbel, B. 2009. Russia's king of crude. *Fortune,* February 2: 88–92.

28. Some insights on how Africa has improved as a potential source of investment is in: Collier, P. & Warnholz, J-L. 2009. Now's the time to invest in Africa. *Harvard Business Review,* 87(2): 23.

29. For a discussion of some of the challenges associated with government corruption regarding entry strategies in foreign markets, read: Rodriguez, P., Uhlenbruck, K., & Eden, L. 2005. Government corruption and entry strategies of multinationals. *Academy of Management Review,* 30(2): 383–396.

30. For a discussion of the political risks in China for United States companies, refer to: Garten, J. E. 1998. Opening the doors for business in China. *Harvard Business Review,* 76(3): 167–175.

31. Shari, M. 2001. Is a holy war brewing in Indonesia? *BusinessWeek,* October 15: 62.

32. Insights on how forensic economics can be used to investigate crimes and wrongdoing are in: Fisman, R. 2009. The rise of forensic economics. *Harvard Business Review,* 87(2): 26.

33. Anonymous. 2010. Libya: Why it is still stuck. *The Economist,* April 10: 49.

34. For an interesting perspective on the relationship between diversification and the development of a nation's institutional environment, read: Chakrabarti, A., Singh, K., & Mahmood, I. 2007. Diversification and performance: Evidence from East Asian firms. *Strategic Management Journal,* 28(2): 101–120.

35. A study looking into corruption and foreign direct investment is: Brouthers, L. E., Gao, Y., & McNicol, J. P. 2008. *Strategic Management Journal,* 29(6): 673–680.

36. Gikkas, N. S. 1996. International licensing of intellectual property: The promise and the peril. *Journal of Technology Law & Policy,* 1(1): 1–26.

37. Insights into bribery in the international context are addressed in: Martin, K. D., Cullen, J. B., Johnson, J. L., & Parboteeah, P. 2008. Deciding to bribe: A cross-level analysis of firm and home country influences on bribery activity. *Academy of Management Journal,* 50(6): 1401–1422.

38. Sandler, N. 2008. Israel: Attack of the super-shekel. *BusinessWeek,* February 25: 38.

39. For an excellent theoretical discussion of how cultural factors can affect knowledge transfer across national boundaries, refer to: Bhagat, R. S., Kedia, B. L., Harveston, P. D., & Triandis, H. C. 2002. Cultural variations in the cross-border transfer of organizational knowledge: An integrative framework. *Academy of Management Review,* 27(2): 204–221.

40. An interesting discussion on how local companies compete effectively with large multinationals is in: Bhattacharya, A. K. & Michael, D. C. 2008. How local companies keep multinationals at bay. *Harvard Business Review,* 66(3): 84–95.

41. To gain insights on the role of national and regional cultures on knowledge management models and frameworks, read: Pauleen, D. J. & Murphy, P. 2005. In praise of cultural bias. *MIT Sloan Management Review,* 46(2): 21–22.

42. Berkowitz, E. N. 2000. *Marketing* (6th ed.). New York: McGraw-Hill.

43. Harvey, M. & Buckley, M. R. 2002. Assessing the "conventional wisdoms" of management for the 21st century organization. *Organization Dynamics,* 30 (4): 368–378.

44. World Trade Organization. *Annual Report 1998.* Geneva: World Trade Organization.

45. Lei, D. 2005. Outsourcing. In Hitt, M. A. & Ireland, R. D. (Eds.). *The Blackwell encyclopedia of management.* Entrepreneurship: 196–199. Malden, MA: Blackwell.

46. Future trends in offshoring are addressed in: Manning, S., Massini, S., & Lewin, A. Y. 2008. A dynamic perspective on next-generation offshoring: The global sourcing of science and engineering talent. *Academy of Management Perspectives,* 22(3): 35–54.

47. An interesting perspective on the controversial issue regarding the offshoring of airplane maintenance is in: Smith, G. & Bachman, J. 2008. Flying in for a tune-up overseas. *Business Week,* April 21: 26–27.

48. Dolan, K.A. 2006. Offshoring the offshorers. *Forbes,* April 17: 74–78.

49. The discussion above draws from: Colvin, J. 2004. Think your job can't be sent to India? Just watch. *Fortune,* December 13: 80; Schwartz, N. D. 2004. Down and out in white collar America. *Fortune,* June 23: 321–325; and, Hagel, J. 2004. Outsourcing is not just about cost cutting. *The Wall Street Journal,* March 18: A3.

50. Insightful perspectives on the outsourcing of decision making are addressed in: Davenport, T. H. & Iyer, B. 2009. Should you outsource your brain? *Harvard Business Review,* 87 (2): 38.

51. Levitt, T. 1983. The globalization of markets. *Harvard Business Review,* 61(3): 92–102.

52. Our discussion of these assumptions draws upon: Douglas, S. P. & Wind, Y. 1987. The myth of globalization. *Columbia Journal of World Business,* Winter: 19–29.

53. Ghoshal, S. 1987. Global strategy: An organizing framework. *Strategic Management Journal,* 8: 425–440.

54. Huber, P. 2009. Who pays for a cancer drug? *Forbes,* January 12: 72.

55. For insights on global branding, refer to: Aaker, D. A. & Joachimsthaler, E. 1999. The lure of global branding. *Harvard Business Review,* 77(6): 137–146.

56. For an interesting perspective on how small firms can compete in their home markets, refer to: Dawar & Frost, op. cit.: 119–129.

57. Hout, T., Porter, M. E., & Rudden, E. 1982. How global companies win out. *Harvard Business Review,* 60(5): 98–107.

58. Fryer, B. 2001. Tom Siebel of Siebel Systems: High tech the old-fashioned way. *Harvard Business Review,* 79(3): 118–130.

59. The risks that are discussed for the global, multidomestic, and transnational strategies draw upon: Gupta & Govindarajan (2001), op. cit.

60. A discussion on how McDonald's adapts its products to overseas markets is in: Gumbel, P. 2008. Big Mac's local flavor. *Fortune,* May 5: 115–121.

61. Sigiura, H. 1990. How Honda localizes its global strategy. *Sloan Management Review,* 31: 77–82.

62. Prahalad & Lieberthal, op. cit.: 68–79. Their article also discusses how firms may have to reconsider their brand management, costs of market building, product design, and approaches to capital efficiency when entering foreign markets.

63. Hofstede, G. 1980. *Culture's consequences: International differences in work-related values.* Beverly Hills, CA: Sage; Hofstede, G. 1993. Cultural constraints in management theories. *Academy of Management Executive,* 7(1): 81–94; Kogut, B. & Singh, H. 1988. The effect of national culture on the choice of entry mode. *Journal of International Business Studies,* 19: 411–432; and, Usinier, J. C. 1996. *Marketing across cultures.* London: Prentice Hall.

64. McCune, J. C. 1999. Exporting corporate culture. *Management Review,* December: 53–56.

65. Ghemawat, P. 2007. *Redefining global strategy.* Boston: Harvard School Press.

66. Prahalad, C. K. & Doz, Y. L. 1987. *The multinational mission: Balancing local demands and global vision.* New York: Free Press.

67. For an insightful discussion on knowledge flows in multinational corporations, refer to: Yang, Q., Mudambi, R., & Meyer, K. E. 2008. Conventional and reverse knowledge flows in multinational corporations. *Journal of Management,* 34(5): 882–902.

68. Kidd, J. B. & Teramoto, Y. 1995. The learning organization: The case of Japanese RHQs in Europe. *Management International Review,* 35 (Special Issue): 39–56.

69. Gupta, A. K. & Govindarajan, V. 2000. Knowledge flows within multinational corporations. *Strategic Management Journal,* 21(4): 473–496.

70. Wetlaufer, S. 2001. The business case against revolution: An interview with Nestlé's Peter Brabeck. *Harvard Business Review,* 79(2): 112–121.

71. Nobel, R. & Birkinshaw, J. 1998. Innovation in multinational corporations: Control and communication patterns in international R&D operations. *Strategic Management Journal,* 19(5): 461–478.

72. Chan, C. M., Makino, S., & Isobe, T. 2010. Does subnational region matter? Foreign affiliate performance in the United States and China. *Strategic Management Journal,* 31 (11): 1226–1243.

73. This section draws upon: Ghemawat, P. 2005. Regional strategies for global leadership. *Harvard Business Review,* 84(12): 98–108; Ghemawat, P. 2006. Apocalypse now? *Harvard Business Review,* 84(12): 32; Ghemawat, P. 2001. Distance still matters: The hard reality of global expansion. *Harvard Business Review,* 79(8): 137–147; Peng, M.W. 2006. *Global strategy:* 387. Mason, OH: Thomson Southwestern; and, Rugman, A. M. & Verbeke, A. 2004. A perspective on regional and global strategies of multinational enterprises. *Journal of International Business Studies,* 35: 3–18.

74. For a rigorous analysis of performance implications of entry strategies, refer to: Zahra, S. A., Ireland, R. D., & Hitt, M. A. 2000. International expansion by new venture firms: International diversity, modes of entry, technological learning, and performance. *Academy of Management Journal,* 43(6): 925–950.

75. Li, J. T. 1995. Foreign entry and survival: The effects of strategic choices on performance in international markets. *Strategic Management Journal,* 16: 333–351.

76. For a discussion of how home-country environments can affect diversification strategies, refer to: Wan, W. P. & Hoskisson, R. E. 2003. Home country environments, corporate diversification strategies, and firm performance. *Academy of Management Journal,* 46(1): 27–45.

77. Arnold, D. 2000. Seven rules of international distribution. *Harvard Business Review,* 78(6): 131–137.

78. Sharma, A. 1998. Mode of entry and ex-post performance. *Strategic Management Journal,* 19(9): 879–900.

79. This section draws upon Arnold, op. cit.: 131–137; and, Berkowitz, op. cit.

80. Salomon, R. & Jin, B. 2010. Do leading or lagging firms learn more from exporting? *Strategic Management Journal,* 31(6): 1088–1113.

81. Kline, D. 2003. Strategic licensing. *MIT Sloan Management Review,* 44(3): 89–93.

82. Martin, J. 1999. Franchising in the Middle East. *Management Review,* June: 38–42.

83. Arnold, op. cit.; and, Berkowitz, op. cit.

84. An in-depth case study of alliance dynamics is found in: Faems, D., Janssens, M., Madhok, A., & Van Looy, B. 2008. Toward an integrative perspective on alliance governance: Connecting contract design, trust dynamics, and contract application. *Academy of Management Journal,* 51(6): 1053–1078.

85. Knowledge transfer in international joint ventures is addressed in: Inkpen, A. 2008. Knowledge transfer and international joint ventures. *Strategic Management Journal,* 29(4): 447–453.

86. Wen, S. H. & Chuang, C.-M. 2010. To teach or to compete? A strategic dilemma of knowledge owners in international alliances. *Asia Pacific Journal of Management,* 27(4): 697–726.

87. Manufacturer–supplier relationships can be very effective in global industries such as automobile manufacturing. Refer to: Kotabe, M., Martin, X., & Domoto, H. 2003. Gaining from vertical partnerships: Knowledge transfer, relationship duration, and supplier performance improvement in the U.S. and Japanese automotive industries. *Strategic Management Journal,* 24(4): 293–316.

88. For a good discussion, refer to: Merchant, H. & Schendel, D. 2000. How do international joint ventures create shareholder value? *Strategic Management Journal,* 21(7): 723–738.

89. This discussion draws upon: Walters, B. A., Peters, S., & Dess, G. G. 1994. Strategic alliances and joint ventures: Making them work. *Business Horizons,* 37(4): 5–11.

90. Some insights on partnering in the global area are discussed in: MacCormack, A. & Forbath, T. 2008. *Harvard Business Review,* 66(1): 24, 26.

91. For a rigorous discussion of the importance of information access in international joint ventures, refer to: Reuer, J. J. & Koza, M. P. 2000. Asymmetric information and joint venture performance: Theory and evidence for domestic and international joint ventures. *Strategic Management Journal,* 21(1): 81–88.

92. Dyer, J. H., Kale, P., & Singh, H. 2001. How to make strategic alliances work. *MIT Sloan Management Review,* 42(4): 37–43.

93. For a discussion of some of the challenges in managing subsidiaries, refer to: O'Donnell, S. W. 2000. Managing foreign subsidiaries: Agents of headquarters, or an independent network? *Strategic Management Journal,* 21(5): 525–548.

94. Ricks, D. 2006. *Blunders in international business* (4th ed.). Malden, MA: Blackwell Publishing.

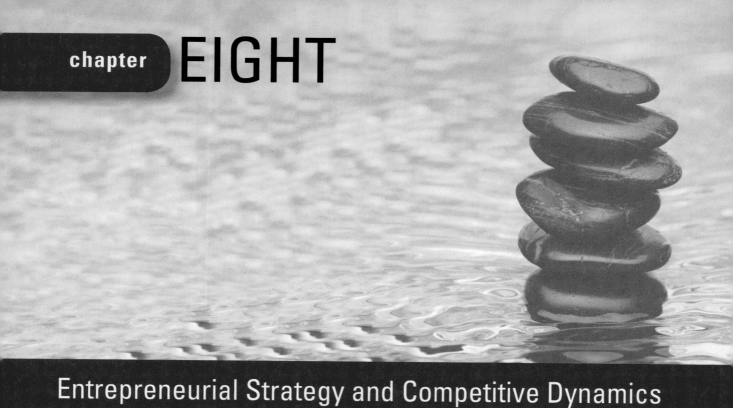

chapter EIGHT

Entrepreneurial Strategy and Competitive Dynamics

After reading this chapter, you should have a good understanding of:

LO8.1 The role of new ventures and small businesses in the U.S. and the global economy.

LO8.2 The role of opportunities, resources, and entrepreneurs in successfully pursuing new ventures.

LO8.3 Three types of entry strategies—pioneering, imitative, and adaptive—commonly used to launch a new venture.

LO8.4 How the generic strategies of overall cost leadership, differentiation, and focus are used by new ventures and small businesses.

LO8.5 How competitive actions, such as the entry of new competitors into a marketplace, may launch a cycle of actions and reactions among close competitors.

LO8.6 The components of competitive dynamics analysis—new competitive action, threat analysis, motivation and capability to respond, types of competitive actions, and likelihood of competitive reaction.

LEARNING OBJECTIVES

New technologies, shifting social and demographic trends, and sudden changes in the business environment create opportunities for entrepreneurship. New ventures, which often emerge under such conditions, face unique strategic challenges if they are going to survive and grow. Young and small businesses, which are a major engine of growth in the U.S. and the global economy because of their role in job creation and innovation, must rely on sound strategic principles to be successful.

This chapter addresses how new ventures and entrepreneurial firms can achieve competitive advantages. It also examines how entrepreneurial activity influences a firm's strategic priorities and intensifies the rivalry among an industry's close competitors.

In the first section, we discuss the role of opportunity recognition in the process of new venture creation. Three factors that are important in determining whether a value-creating opportunity should be pursued are highlighted—the nature of the opportunity, the resources available to undertake it, and the characteristics of the entrepreneur(s) pursuing it.

The second section addresses three different types of new entry strategies—pioneering, imitative, and adaptive. Then, the generic strategies (discussed in Chapter 5) as well as combination strategies are addressed in terms of how they apply to new ventures and entrepreneurial firms. Additionally, some of the pitfalls associated with each of these strategic approaches are presented.

In section three, we explain how new entrants and other competitors often set off a series of actions and reactions that affect the competitive dynamics of an industry. In determining how to react to a competitive action, firms must analyze whether they are seriously threatened by the action, how important it is for them to respond, and what resources they can muster to mount a response. They must also determine what type of action is appropriate—strategic or tactical—and whether their close competitors are likely to counterattack. Taken together, these actions often have a strong impact on the strategic choices and overall profitability of an industry •.

The wildly successful eBay concept allowed individuals to sell to the world.[1] Not surprisingly, the business of intermediating such sales quickly took off. It was even portrayed in the movie *The 40-Year-Old Virgin.* iSold It was one of the champions of this model and quickly gained popularity, as it made eBay access easier for people who did not want the hassle of researching prices, posting online, and collecting money. The company began in December 2003 by helping customers sell their unwanted stuff on eBay—basically acting as an intermediary and charging a percentage of the sales price. More recently, however, the company stopped selling franchises and is retracting many of the franchises already sold, because of financial losses. How did the company go from a top franchise pick by *Entrepreneur* magazine in 2006 to the firm in full retreat that we see today?

In 2005 the idea of a store helping customers sell their unwanted things on eBay was very popular, resulting in 7,000 of these types of stores opening around the United States. In June 2006, *Entrepreneur* magazine named iSold It "Hotter than hot" and ranked the firm 30th among other fastest-growing franchises. What is more, in 2007 iSold It earned the top spot in *Entrepreneur*'s new franchise rankings, listing a start-up cost of $105,000 per location! At the time, it seemed that selling other people's stuff online and collecting a fee had endless potential.

The firm researched the potential sale price, wrote the product description, posted the ads on eBay, monitored the auction, responded to any e-mails, collected the proceeds from the sale, and finally mailed the purchaser the product. The firm did not guarantee that the product would sell and had selection standards about what it tried to sell—it has to put in the same amount of effort whether the product sells for $75 or $1,000. If the advertised product did not sell, the firm still paid eBay's listing fee.

iSold It's founders realized that the firm was growing at a rate above their capabilities, so they stepped aside and hired outside help. In 2004 Ken Sully, a former vice president of Mail Boxes Etc., came on board as the new CEO. Ken standardized the firm's operations and made it possible for a store to be installed and set up in 48 hours. iSold It's founders saw no end in sight for the firm's growth, stating in 2006, "We've created this brick-and-mortar interface to the Internet" and stating that its firm was in a position to capitalize on the growth of Internet trade. In fact, by June 2006 the firm had already sold 800 franchises.

Although iSold It knew that people could sell their own merchandise online, they overestimated their willingness to pay an intermediary 20–30 percent of the sales price for the convenience of listing their products and collecting the money. *Entrepreneur* magazine in January 2010 called the eBay drop-off store concept "ridiculous," as customers quickly learned how to sell their stuff by themselves. With low barriers to entry in this industry, many copycat firms quickly entered the market. In early 2007, iSold It stopped selling new franchises and is quickly losing the ones it sold.

By offering a service tied to the rapid growth of eBay, iSold It seemed to have identified an attractive opportunity. But the start-up's failure shows what can go wrong when—even though a good opportunity, sufficient resources, and an experienced entrepreneurial team are brought together—a business opportunity disappears as quickly as it appeared.

The iSold It case illustrates how important it is for new entrepreneurial entrants—whether they are start-ups or incumbents—to think and act strategically. Even with a strong resource base and good track record, entrepreneurs are unlikely to succeed if their business ideas are easily imitated or substituted for.

In this chapter we address entrepreneurial strategies. The previous three chapters have focused primarily on the business-level, corporate-level, and international strategies of incumbent firms. Here we ask: What about the strategies of those entering into a market or industry for the first time? Whether it's a fast-growing start-up such as iSold It or an existing company seeking growth opportunities, new entrants need effective strategies.

Companies wishing to launch new ventures must also be aware that, consistent with the five-forces model in Chapter 2, new entrants are a threat to existing firms in an industry. Entry into a new market arena is intensely competitive from the perspective of incumbents in that arena. Therefore, new entrants can nearly always expect a competitive response from other companies in the industry it is entering. Knowledge of the competitive dynamics that are at work in the business environment is an aspect of entrepreneurial new entry that will be addressed later in this chapter.

Before moving on, it is important to highlight the role that entrepreneurial start-ups and small business play in entrepreneurial value creation. Young and small firms are responsible for more innovations and more new job creation than any other type of business.[2] For example, small and medium enterprises (SMEs) remain the backbone of the Europeon Union economy. Given that 99.8 percent of all enterprises are SMEs—a ratio that has been fairly stable over the past few years—the typical EU enterprise is an SME or, more specifically, a micro-enterprise with fewer than 10 employees. In 2010, 19.2 million micro-enterprises operated in the EU, comprising 92 percent of all European enterprises.[3] Strategy Spotlight 8.1 addresses some of the reasons why small business and entrepreneurship are viewed favorably in the United States.

Recognizing Entrepreneurial Opportunities

Defined broadly, **entrepreneurship** refers to new value creation. Even though entrepreneurial activity is usually associated with start-up companies, new value can be created in many different contexts including:

- Start-up ventures
- Major corporations
- Family-owned businesses
- Non-profit organizations
- Established institutions

For an entrepreneurial venture to create new value, three factors must be present—an entrepreneurial opportunity, the resources to pursue the opportunity, and an entrepreneur or entrepreneurial team willing and able to undertake the opportunity.[4] The entrepreneurial strategy that an organization uses will depend on these three factors. Thus, beyond merely identifying a venture concept, the opportunity recognition process also involves organizing the key people and resources that are needed to go forward. Exhibit 8.3 depicts the three factors that are needed to successfully proceed—opportunity, resources, and entrepreneur(s). In the sections that follow, we address each of these factors.

Entrepreneurial Opportunities

The starting point for any new venture is the presence of an entrepreneurial opportunity. Where do opportunities come from? For new business start-ups, opportunities come from many sources—current or past work experiences, hobbies that grow into businesses or lead to inventions, suggestions by friends or family, or a chance event that makes an entrepreneur aware of an unmet need. For established firms, new business opportunities come from the needs of existing customers, suggestions by suppliers, or technological developments that lead to new advances.[5] For all firms, there is a major, overarching factor behind all viable opportunities that emerge in the business landscape: change. Change creates opportunities. Entrepreneurial firms make the most of changes brought about by new technology, sociocultural trends, and shifts in consumer demand.

The Contribution of Small Businesses to the U.S. Economy

In the late 1970s, MIT professor David Birch launched a study to explore the sources of business growth. "I wasn't really looking for anything in particular," said Birch. But the findings surprised him: Small businesses create the most jobs. Since then, Birch and others have shown that it's not just big companies that power the economy. Small

Sources: Small Business Administration. 2009. *The small business economy.* Washington, DC: U.S. Government Printing Office; Small Business Administration. 2010. Small business by the numbers. *SBA Office of Advocacy,* June, *www.sba.gov/advo/*; Anonymous. 2001. Small business 2001: Where we are now. *Inc.,* May 29: 18–19; Minniti, M., & Bygrave, W. D. 2004. *Global entrepreneurship monitor—national entrepreneurship assessment: United States of America 2004, executive report.* Kansas City, MO: Kauffman Center for Entrepreneurial Leadership; and, Anonymous. 2001. The heroes: A portfolio. *Fortune,* October 4: 74.

business and entrepreneurship have become a major component of new job creation.

Here are the facts:

- In the United States, there are approximately 5.9 million companies with fewer than 100 employees. Another 88,586 companies have 100 to 500 employees. In addition, approximately 17.0 million individuals are nonemployer sole proprietors.

- Small businesses create the majority of new jobs. According to recent data, small business created 65 percent of U.S. net new jobs in a recent 17-year period. A small percentage of the fastest growing entrepreneurial firms (5 to 15 percent) account for a majority of the new jobs created.

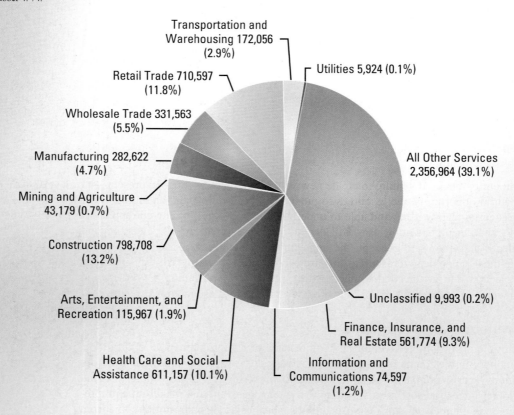

Exhibit 8.1 All U.S. Small Companies by Industry*

Businesses with 500 or fewer employees in 2007.

Source: Small Business Administration's Office of Advocacy, based on data provided by the U.S. Census Bureau, statistics of U.S. businesses.

(continued)

(continued)

- Small businesses (fewer than 500 employees) employ more than half of the private-sector workforce (59.9 million in 2007) and account for more than 50 percent of nonfarm private gross domestic product (GDP).
- Small firms produce 13 to 14 times more patents per employee than large patenting firms and employ 39 percent of high-tech workers (such as scientists and engineers). In addition, smaller entrepreneurial firms account for 55 percent of all innovations.

- Small businesses make up 97.5 percent of all U.S. exporters and accounted for 31 percent of known U.S. export value in 2008.

Exhibit 8.1 shows the number of small businesses in the United States and how they are distributed through different sectors of the economy.

There are also many types of small businesses. Exhibit 8.2 identifies three major categories that are often small and generally considered to be entrepreneurial—family businesses, franchises, and home-based businesses.

Type	Characteristics
Family Businesses	*Definition:* A family business, broadly defined, is a privately held firm in which family members have some degree of control over the strategic direction of the firm and intend for the business to remain within the family. *Scope:* According to the Family Firm Institute (FFI), family-owned businesses that meet the broad definition above comprise 80 to 90 percent of all business enterprises in the U.S., including 30 to 35 percent of the Fortune 500 companies. Further, 64 percent of the U.S. Gross Domestic Product (GDP) is generated by family-owned businesses.
Franchises	*Definition:* A franchise exists when a company that already has a successful product or service (franchisor) contracts with another business to be a dealer (franchisee) by using the franchisor's name, trademark, and business system in exchange for a fee. The most common type is the Business Format Franchise in which the franchisor provides a complete plan, or format, for managing the business. *Scope:* According to the International Franchise Association (IFA), franchises were the cause of $863 billion in annual output in the U.S. in 2010. There are over 900,000 franchise establishments employing more than 9.5 million people.
Home-Based Businesses	*Definition:* A home-based business, also referred to as SOHO (Small Office/Home Office), consists of companies with 20 or fewer employees, including the self-employed, freelancers, telecommuters, or other independent professionals working from a home-based setting. *Scope:* According to the National Association of Home-Based Businesses (NAHBB), approximately 20 million businesses are home-based. The U.S. Commerce Department estimates that more than half of all small businesses are home-based.

Sources: *www.ffi.org*; *www.franchise.org*; and *www.workingsolo.com*.

Exhibit 8.2 **Types of Entrepreneurial Ventures**

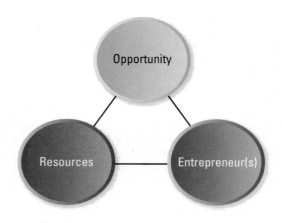

Exhibit 8.3 Opportunity Analysis Framework

Sources: Based on Timmons, J. A. & Spinelli, S. 2004.
New venture creation (6th ed.). New York: McGraw-Hill/
Irwin; and, Bygrave, W. D. 1997. The Entrepreneurial
Process. In Bygrave, W. D. (Ed.). *The portable MBA in
entrepreneurship* (2nd ed.). New York: Wiley.

How do changes in the external environment lead to new business creation? They spark creative new ideas and innovation. Businesspeople often have ideas for entrepreneurial ventures. However, not all such ideas are good ideas—that is, viable business opportunities. To determine which ideas are strong enough to become new ventures, entrepreneurs must go through a process of identifying, selecting, and developing potential opportunities. This is the process of **opportunity recognition.**[6]

Opportunity recognition refers to more than just the "Eureka!" feeling that people sometimes experience at the moment they identify a new idea. Although such insights are often very important, the opportunity recognition process involves two phases of activity—discovery and evaluation—that lead to viable new venture opportunities.[7]

The discovery phase refers to the process of becoming aware of a new business concept.[8] Many entrepreneurs report that their idea for a new venture occurred to them in an instant, as a sort of "Aha!" experience—that is, they had some insight or epiphany, often based on their prior knowledge, that gave them an idea for a new business. The discovery of new opportunities is often spontaneous and unexpected. For example, Howard Schultz, CEO of Starbucks, was in Milan, Italy, when he suddenly realized that the coffee-and-conversation café model that was common in Europe would work in the U.S. as well. According to Schultz, he didn't need to do research to find out if Americans would pay $3 for a cup of coffee—he just *knew.* Starbucks was just a small business at the time but Schultz began literally shaking with excitement about growing it into a bigger business.[9] Strategy Spotlight 8.2 tells how three entrepreneurs in the struggling city of Detroit identified their business opportunities.

Opportunity discovery also may occur as the result of a deliberate search for new venture opportunities or creative solutions to business problems. Viable opportunities often emerge only after a concerted effort. It is very similar to a creative process, which may be unstructured and "chaotic" at first but eventually leads to a practical solution or business innovation. To stimulate the discovery of new opportunities, companies often encourage creativity, out-of-the-box thinking, and brainstorming.

Opportunity evaluation, which occurs after an opportunity has been identified, involves analyzing an opportunity to determine whether it is viable and strong enough to

opportunity recognition the process of discovering and evaluating changes in the business environment, such as a new technology, sociocultural trends, or shifts in consumer demand, that can be exploited.

Entrepreneurial Vision to Revitalize Detroit

Detroit is the poorest major city in America. With an unemployment rate of 26 percent and a declining population, it would seem to be a nearly impossible place to start a new business. But challenging economic times are often the trigger for entrepreneurs to pursue their vision. Half the corporations listed on the *Fortune* 500 in 2010 were founded during challenging economic times, according to Dane Stangler, a senior analyst at the Kauffman Foundation. Individually and with the help of others, a range of entrepreneurs is striving to rejuvenate Detroit and realize their visions. Some of their businesses are the result of "Aha!" moments in which they envisioned bold new opportunities. Others are more modest traditional business ideas, but they all aim both to enrich the firms' founders and to improve the economic climate and the community of Detroit.

Daniel Gizaw, Founder of Danotek Motion Technologies

Rural Ethiopia is far from Detroit in more ways than one. Daniel Gizaw has taken the long journey from working on his father's farm in Ethiopia to founding a firm that produces products for the green energy business. He began by leaving home to study electrical engineering in Poland and Germany and later was part of the team designing the EV1, General Motor's first electric car. In order to follow his desire to pursue bold innovations and to exploit growing markets, he founded Danotek Motion Technologies, a firm that builds highly efficient turbines for the wind energy market as well as components for electric vehicles. To achieve his vision, he has recruited former colleagues, gotten support from Automation Alley (a consortium of business and government partners to improve the economic conditions of southeastern Michigan), and received governmental tax breaks to foster business growth. His firm plans to grow its business rapidly, keeping all its manufacturing in the greater Detroit area, as it creates over 350 new jobs. Daniel's advice to would-be entrepreneurs is clear: "Don't limit yourself to the sector you are in. Look into growing industries and ask, 'What can I offer?'"

Glenn Oliver, Founder of H2bid.com

Though he is an attorney by training and never ran a business prior to starting H2bid, Glenn Oliver inherited an entrepreneurial interest from his grandfather, who owned an appliance repair and installation business. Living in a state

Sources: Sohail, F. 2010. Alternative energy: Creating non-exportable jobs. *Forbes.com*. June 30: np; Easton, N. 2010. If you can remake yourself here. *Fortune*, November 1: 59–63; Gray, S. 2010. Where entrepreneurs Need nerves of steel. *Fortune*, October 18: 63–66; Saulny, S. 2010. Detroit entrepreneurs opt to look up. *The New York Times*, January 10: A18; Anonymous. 2010. Champions of the new economy, *dBusiness*, May/June: np; and, Whitford, D. 2010. Can farming save Detroit? *Fortune*, January 18: 78–84.

that is surrounded by the Great Lakes and having served as a member of the Detroit Water and Sewerage Board of Commissioners, Oliver appreciated the value of water as a critical resource needed for economic development. Fresh water is a commodity increasingly demanded around the globe. Oliver saw opportunity here and created H2bid .com, an online marketplace where contractors and suppliers can bid on water supply projects around the world. While he thinks the business will be profitable, he also believes his start-up will benefit the Detroit area. As he concludes, "Entrepreneurship is the largest creator of wealth." Others in the area are noting the potential with this business. Oliver received recognition as a "Champion of the New Economy," an award sponsored by *DBusiness,* WJR Radio, and Junior Achievement to recognize people whose businesses are helping to diversify Michigan's economy.

John Hantz, Founder of Hantz Farms

When many people drive through Detroit, they see a landscape of abandoned homes, empty commercial buildings, and vacant land. John Hantz sees opportunity. Already a successful entrepreneur, having founded Hantz Financial Services, a firm with 20 offices, 500 employees, and over $1.3 billion in assets under management, Hantz now has a new entrepreneurial vision. His vision grew out of his commuting across Detroit from his home to his office. Seeing all of the unused land and abandoned homes, he realized that he had to find a way to change the supply and demand relationship for land in Detroit. He sees urban farming as a partial solution to this issue. The farms he envisions are not the old style of farms growing crops in rows in large, open-air plots worked with large tractors. Instead, he plans to build compost-heated greenhouses and use hydroponic and aeroponic growing systems that don't rely on soil to grow crops. He is drawing on up to $30 million of his own financial resources to start the project and has tapped into expertise in the region, hiring Mike Score, an agricultural expert from Michigan State University to serve as president of the firm. He sees an economic opportunity here but also a chance to revitalize the area. His plan is to build small, visually attractive 300 to 1,000 acre farms or "pods" all across Detroit which will be surrounded by frontage property that could be developed for housing or commercial activity. Thus, he sees the farms as a way to reduce the supply of unused land while also stoking demand for redeveloped land surrounding the farms.

Although these businesses span a wide range of industries, they demonstrate that entrepreneurial vision often arises out of an individual's experiences and can encompass both a business idea as well as a vehicle with which to improve conditions in a larger community.

be developed into a full-fledged new venture. Ideas developed by new-product groups or in brainstorming sessions are tested by various methods, including talking to potential target customers and discussing operational requirements with production or logistics managers. A technique known as feasibility analysis is used to evaluate these and other critical success factors. This type of analysis often leads to the decision that a new venture project should be discontinued. If the venture concept continues to seem viable, a more formal business plan may be developed.[10]

Among the most important factors to evaluate is the market potential for the product or service. Established firms tend to operate in established markets. They have to adjust to market trends and to shifts in consumer demand, of course, but they usually have a customer base for which they are already filling a marketplace need. New ventures, in contrast, must first determine whether a market exists for the product or service they are contemplating. Thus, a critical element of opportunity recognition is assessing to what extent the opportunity is viable *in the marketplace.*

For an opportunity to be viable, it needs to have four qualities.[11]

- *Attractive.* The opportunity must be attractive in the marketplace; that is, there must be market demand for the new product or service.
- *Achievable.* The opportunity must be practical and physically possible.
- *Durable.* The opportunity must be attractive long enough for the development and deployment to be successful; that is, the window of opportunity must be open long enough for it to be worthwhile.
- *Value creating.* The opportunity must be potentially profitable; that is, the benefits must surpass the cost of development by a significant margin.

If a new business concept meets these criteria, two other factors must be considered before the opportunity is launched as a business: the resources available to undertake it, and the characteristics of the entrepreneur(s) pursuing it. In the next section, we address the issue of entrepreneurial resources; following that, we address the importance of entrepreneurial leaders and teams. But first, consider the opportunities that have been created by the recent surge in interest in environmental sustainability. Strategy Spotlight 8.3 discusses "green" plastics in the European community and highlights four global companies that began as small businesses and whose mission is to sustain environmental integrity through their products.

Entrepreneurial Resources

As Exhibit 8.3 indicates, resources are an essential component of a successful entrepreneurial launch. For start-ups, the most important resource is usually money because a new firm typically has to expend substantial sums just to start the business. However, financial resources are not the only kind of resource a new venture needs. Human capital and social capital are also important. Many firms also rely on government resources to help them thrive.[12]

Financial Resources   Hand-in-hand with the importance of markets (and marketing) to new venture creation, entrepreneurial firms must also have financing. In fact, the level of available financing is often a strong determinant of how the business is launched and its eventual success. Cash finances are, of course, highly important. But access to capital, such as a line of credit or favorable payment terms with a supplier, can also help a new venture succeed.

The types of financial resources that may be needed depend on two factors: the stage of venture development and the scale of the venture.[13] Entrepreneurial firms that are starting from scratch—start-ups—are at the earliest stage of development. Most start-ups also begin on a relatively small scale. The funding available to young and small firms tends to be quite limited. In fact, the majority of new firms are low-budget start-ups launched with personal savings and the contributions of family and friends.[14] Among firms included in

Green Plastics in Europe

The Association of Plastics Manufacturers in Europe reported that, in 2011, the Czech Republic had the highest recycling rate (48 percent) among European Union (EU) members. Recycling rates for packaging plastics are generally higher than the rates for plastics as a whole, exceeding 40 percent in the Czech Republic, Sweden, Germany, and Estonia. Switzerland, Germany, Austria, Belgium, the Netherlands, Norway, Italy, Slovakia, Latvia, the UK, Slovenia, and Lithuania have recycling rates between 30 and 40 percent; Denmark, Spain, Luxembourg, Finland, Hungary, Ireland, Poland, Romania, Greece, Bulgaria, and Portugal have mechanical recycling rates between 20 and 30 percent; and Cyprus and Malta have rates between 12 and 20 percent.

Four global, all of which began as start-up businesses in their respective countries, companies have voluntarily committed to using biodegradable and compostable polymers to manufacture packaging materials. A 10-year Environmental Agreement signed by the four companies and recognized by the European Commission includes a certification plan for ensuring quality control and a labeling plan to ensure ease of waste handling. The manufacturers that have signed the agreement are key players in the biodegradable plastics market: BASF of Germany, Cargill Dow of the United States, Novamont of Italy, and Rodenburg Biopolymers of the Netherlands.

BASF has been producing biodegradable products under the trade name Ecoflex since 1998. Under certain environmental conditions, such as those found in composting, the product degrades within a few weeks, leaving no harmful residues. Its properties guarantee a high strength when wet and a resistance to grease, so it is ideal for packaging that becomes highly contaminated with food residue after use—for example, wrapping paper, drink cartons, fast-food packaging, and drink cups. The combination of paper with fully biodegradable Ecoflex can be completely compostable. Ecoflex-coated food packaging made from renewable raw materials migrate to compost where they are completely biodegraded just like other materials (food, paper residues, etc.). In 2006, BASF introduced another biodegradable plastic, called Ecovio. This product is composed of biodegradable petrochemical-based plastic and polylactic acid, which is made from corn, another renewable raw material. This commitment to "going green" in plastic packaging not only preserves and protects food, it also helps reduce overall carbon emissions, an important component of sustaining the environment.

Sources: Osze, M. 2011. BASF also started as start up. European Entrepreneur Foundation. Accessed at *www.europreneurs.org*. Corporate websites: *www.basf.com/corporate/en/about-basf*; *www.cargill.com/company/history*; *www.novamont.com*; *www.biopolymers.nl/en/company/history*. Association of Plastics Manufacturers in Europe (APME). Plastics—the facts 2011. Brussels: APME; and, BASF. 2008. Biodegradable polymers—inspired by nature: Ecoflex and Ecovio. Accessed at *www.bioplastics.basf.com/ecoflex.html*.

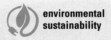
**environmental
sustainability**

---

the *Entrepreneur* list of the 100 fastest-growing new businesses in a recent year, 61 percent reported that their start-up funds came from personal savings.[15]

Although bank financing, public financing, and venture capital are important sources of small-business finance, these types of financial support are typically available only after a company has started to conduct business and generate sales. Even **angel investors**—private individuals who provide equity investments for seed capital during the early stages of a new venture—favor companies that already have a winning business model and dominance in a market niche.[16] According to Cal Simmons, coauthor of *Every Business Needs an Angel,* "I would much rather talk to an entrepreneur who has already put his money and his effort into proving the concept."[17] Peer-to-peer lending is a rapidly increasing Internet-based source of funding for entrepreneurs around the world. Strategy Spotlight 8.4 discusses Prosper.com, a peer-to-peer lending website that uses social affiliation to bring together entrepreneurs and potential lenders.

Once a venture has established itself as a going concern, other sources of financing become readily available. Banks, for example, are more likely to provide later-stage financing to companies with a track record of sales or other cash-generating activity. Start-ups that involve large capital investments or extensive development costs—such as

angel investors private individuals who provide equity investments for seed capital during the early stages of a new venture.

P2P Lending: Using the Power of the Social Group to Fund Entrepreneurs

Start-up entrepreneurs may need only a small amount of money to launch their ventures. However, if they have limited personal resources, they may never be able to turn their business ideas into operating enterprises. With lower credit limits and higher interest rates on credit cards and tougher standards for borrowers seeking bank loans, entrepreneurs are increasingly turning to other sources for seed capital. To fill this need, a new breed of lender has emerged online: peer-to-peer (P2P) lenders. This form of lending has taken off and was projected to involve over $5.8 billion in lending in 2010, according to the research firm Celent.

With P2P lending, borrowers seeking loans post descriptions of their business concepts, including the amount of funding they are seeking and personal information, such as their credit rating. Lenders, who are looking for opportunities to lend their money and make a decent return but who also often find satisfaction from helping out entrepreneurs, review business proposals and the borrowers' background information before making lending decisions. Depending on the rules of each P2P website, lenders either make a loan to borrowers at a preset interest rate or participate in an auction to "win" the opportunity to lend to the borrower. On the auction sites, lenders willing to lend at the lowest interest rates fund a borrower. Since the loans are unsecured, lenders are encouraged to spread their funds around, making small loans to a number of borrowers. As a result, a number of lenders typically provide small amounts of money that collectively meet the borrowing needs of an individual borrower.

There are many P2P lenders around the world. In Europe, for example, there are Babyloan and Veecus in France; Zopa and Funding Circle in the UK; Lubbus and Partizipa in Spain; Smava and Auxmoney in Germany; Kokos in Poland; Cashare in Switzerland; Noba in Hungary; and Fixura in Finland. P2P lenders in Asia include PPDai and CreditEase in China; AQUSH and Maneo in Japan; and Money Auction and Popfunding in Korea. In Oceania, there are IGrin, Peermint, and LendingHub in Australia and Nexx in New Zealand. Lastly, MyC4,

headquartered in Copenhagen, Demark, provides P2P lending to small businesses in Africa.

One of the largest P2P lending websites in the United States is Prosper.com. Launched in 2006, Prosper reports that investors lending through its website have provided over $214 million in loans to entrepreneurs and that it has over one million members. The root idea for Prosper.com came from the experience of Lyna Lam, the wife of Prosper's founder Chris Larsen. Lyna's family came to the United States as refugees from Vietnam in the early 1980s. Once they settled in San Jose, California, they joined a Vietnamese hui group, a group of individuals who make contributions to create a pool of money that one of the members can borrow to start or grow a business. Lyna Lam's family used money from the hui to start a landscaping business.

Larsen saw the group structure as a key strength of the hui. Hui groups tend to be successful because members of the group offer advice to each other but also feel strong social pressure from the group to work hard to repay the money borrowed from the group. This addresses one of the key weaknesses of P2P lending—the lack of trust that someone the lender doesn't know and never interacted with directly will repay the loan. Like most other P2P lending sites, Prosper collects factual information on the borrower and the business idea, runs a credit check on the borrower, and offers them scores that range from AA (the best rating) to HR (high risk) or NC (no credit history). But it also gives borrowers the opportunity to join a group. These groups are created and organized by a leader and bring together borrowers that share a common interest or identity, such as nationality, educational affiliation, religion, type of business, or hobby. Members of successful groups, those that have a strong repayment record, can attract more favorable interest terms from lenders. Thus, the group offers positive peer pressure to members to repay their loans. Members don't want to lose face by defaulting on their loan and tarnishing the group's reputation, resulting in financial consequences for all borrowers in the group. The group leader can also provide advice to the borrower and is rewarded when members of the group repay their loans. The system appears to work well, as 92 percent of loans were being repaid on schedule as of February 2010, according to Prosper.com's statistics.

Sources: *www.peer-lend.com/peer-to-peer-lending/p2p-lending-intl/* and *www.wiseclerk.com.* Accessed October 28, 2011; Libert, B. & Spector, J. 2008. *How to unleash the power of crowds in your business.* Philadelphia: Wharton School Publishing: 104–106; Dishman, L. 2009. Peer-to-peer lending explained: Brother, can you spare $100? *Fast Company,* November 11: np; *www.prosper.com*; *www.wikipedia.org*; and, *www.oneviet.com.*

crowdsourcing

manufacturing or engineering firms trying to commercialize an innovative product—may have high cash requirements soon after they are founded. Others need financing only when they are on the brink of rapid growth. To obtain such funding, entrepreneurial firms often seek venture capital.

Venture capital is a form of private equity financing through which entrepreneurs raise money by selling shares in the new venture. In contrast to angel investors, who invest their own money, venture capital companies are organized to place the funds of private investors into lucrative business opportunities. **Venture capitalists** nearly always have high performance expectations from the companies they invest in, but they also provide important managerial advice and links to key contacts in an industry.[18]

venture capitalists companies organized to place their investors' finds in lucrative business opportunities.

Despite the importance of venture capital to many fast-growing firms, the majority of external funding for young and small firms comes from informal sources such as family and friends. Based on a Kaufmann Foundation survey of entrepreneurial firms, Exhibit 8.4 identifies the source of funding used by start-up businesses and by ongoing firms that are five years old. The survey shows that most start-up funding, about 70 percent, comes from either equity investments by the entrepreneur and the entrepreneur's family and friends or personal loans taken out by the entrepreneur. After five years of operation, the largest source of funding is from loans taken out by the business. At both stages, 5 percent or less of the funding comes from outside investors, such as angel investors or venture capitalists. In fact, very few firms ever receive venture capital investments—only 7 of 2,606 firms in the Kaufmann study received money from outside investors. But when they do, these firms receive a substantial level of investment—over $1 million on average in the survey—because they tend to be the firms that are the most innovative and have the greatest growth potential. Regardless of their source, financial resources are essential for entrepreneurial ventures.[19]

Human Capital Bankers, venture capitalists, and angel investors agree that the most important asset an entrepreneurial firm can have is strong and skilled management.[20] According to Stephen Gaal, founding member of Walnut Venture Associates, venture investors do not invest in businesses; instead, "We invest in people . . . very smart people with very high integrity." Managers need to have a strong base of experience and extensive domain knowledge, as well as an ability to make rapid decisions and change direction as shifting circumstances may require. In the case of start-ups, more is better. New ventures

Exhibit 8.4
Sources of Capital for Start-Up Firms

	Capital Invested in Their First Year	Percentage of Capital Invested in Their First Year	Capital Invested in Their Fifth Year	Percentage of Capital Invested in Their Fifth Year
Insider equity	$33,034	41.1	$13,914	17.9
Investor equity	$4,108	5.1	$3,108	4.0
Personal debt of owners	$23,353	29.1	$21,754	28.0
Business debt	$19,867	24.7	$39,009	50.1
Total average capital invested	$80,362		$77,785	

Source: From Robb, A., Reedy, E. J., Ballou, J., DesRoches, D., Potter, F., & Zhao, A. 2010. An overview of the Kauffman Firm Survey. Reproduced with permission from the Ewing Marion Kauffman Foundation.

that are started by teams of three, four, or five entrepreneurs are more likely to succeed in the long run than are ventures launched by "lone wolf" entrepreneurs.[21]

Social Capital   New ventures founded by entrepreneurs who have extensive social contacts are more likely to succeed than are ventures started without the support of a social network.[22] Even though a venture may be new, if the founders have contacts who will vouch for them, they gain exposure and build legitimacy faster.[23] This support can come from several sources: prior jobs, industry organizations, and local business groups such as the chamber of commerce. These contacts can all contribute to a growing network that provides support for the entrepreneurial firm. Janina Pawlowski, co-founder of the online lending company E-Loan, attributes part of her success to the strong advisors she persuaded to serve on her board of directors, including Tim Koogle, former CEO of Yahoo![24]

Strategic alliances represent a type of social capital that can be especially important to young and small firms.[25] Strategy Spotlight 8.5 presents a few examples of alliances and some potential pitfalls of using alliances.[26]

Government Resources   Countries around the world support entrepreneurial firms in several ways. For example, in the UK, government supports financing for small and medium-sized enterprises (SMEs). There are a number of government-backed schemes designed to help SMEs access finance, be it loans or grants. In addition to the main two UK-wide initiatives—the Enterprise Finance Guarantee (EFG) plan and the Enterprise Capital Funds (ECFs)—there are separate programs in England, Wales, Scotland, and Northern Ireland. EFG was set up by the former Labour government to encourage more banks to lend to SMEs. Under the plan, the government guarantees 75 percent of an SME's bank loan, with the lenders covering the remaining 25 percent.[27]

In the U.S., the federal government provides support for entrepreneurial firms in two key arenas—financing and government contracting. The Small Business Administration (SBA) has several loan guarantee programs designed to support the growth and development of entrepreneurial firms. The government itself does not typically lend money but underwrites loans made by banks to small businesses, thus reducing the risk associated with lending to firms with unproven records. The SBA also offers training, counseling, and support services through its local offices and Small Business Development Centers.[28] State and local governments also have hundreds of programs to provide funding, contracts, and other support for new ventures and small businesses. These programs are often designed to grow the economy of a region, as seen with Danotek Motion Technologies in Strategy Spotlight 8.2.

Another key area of support is in government contracting. Programs sponsored by the SBA and other government agencies ensure that small businesses have the opportunity to bid on contracts to provide goods and services to the government. Although working with the government sometimes has its drawbacks in terms of issues of regulation and time-consuming decision making, programs to support small businesses and entrepreneurial activity constitute an important resource for entrepreneurial firms.

Entrepreneurial Leadership

entrepreneurial leadership
leadership appropriate for new ventures that requires courage, belief in one's convictions, and the energy to work hard even in difficult circumstances and that embodies vision, dedication and drive, and commitment to excellence.

Whether a venture is launched by an individual entrepreneur or an entrepreneurial team, effective leadership is needed. Launching a new venture requires a special kind of leadership.[29] **Entrepreneurial leadership** involves courage, belief in one's convictions, and the energy to work hard even in difficult circumstances. Yet these are the very challenges that motivate most business owners. Entrepreneurs put themselves to the test and get their satisfaction from acting independently, overcoming obstacles, and thriving financially. To do so, they must embody three characteristics of leadership—vision,

Strategic Alliances: A Key Entrepreneurial Resource

Strategic alliances provide a key avenue for growth by entrepreneurial firms. By partnering with other companies, young or small firms can expand or give the appearance of entering numerous markets and/or handling a range of operations. Here are several types of alliances that have been used to extend or strengthen entrepreneurial firms:

Technology Alliances

Tech-savvy entrepreneurial firms often benefit from forming alliances with older incumbents. The alliance allows the larger firm to enhance its technological capabilities and expands the revenue and reach of the smaller firm.

Manufacturing Alliances

The use of outsourcing and other manufacturing alliances by small firms has grown dramatically in recent years. Internet-enabled capabilities such as collaborating online

Sources: Copeland, M. V. & Tilin, A. 2005. Get someone to build it. *Business 2.0*, 6(5): 88–90; Misner, I. 2008. Use small actions to get big results. *www .entrepreneur.com*. December 3; Monahan, J. 2005. All systems grow. *Entrepreneur*, March: 78–82; Prince, C. J. 2005. Foreign affairs. *Entrepreneur*, March: 56; and, Weaver, K. M. & Dickson, P. 2004. Strategic alliances. In Dennis, W. J., Jr. (Ed.) *NFIB national small business poll*. Washington, DC: National Federation of Independent Business.

about delivery and design specifications has greatly simplified doing business, even with foreign manufacturers.

Retail Alliances

Licensing agreements allow one company to sell the products and services of another in different markets, including overseas. Specialty products—the types sometimes made by entrepreneurial firms—often seem more exotic when sold in another country.

According to the National Federation of Independent Business (NFIB), nearly two-thirds of small businesses currently hold or have held some type of alliance. Strategic alliances among entrepreneurial firms can take many different forms. Exhibit 8.5 shows the different types of partnering that small businesses and small manufacturers in the NFIB study often use.

Although such alliances often sound good, there are also potential pitfalls. Lack of oversight and control is one danger of partnering with foreign firms. Problems with product quality, timely delivery, and receiving payments can also sour an alliance relationship if it is not carefully managed. With technology alliances, there is a risk that big firms may take advantage of the technological know-how of their entrepreneurial partners. However, even with these potential problems, strategic alliances provide a good means for entrepreneurial firms to develop and grow.

Type of Alliance and/or Long-Term Agreement*	Small Manufacturers	Small Businesses
Licensing	20.0%	32.5%
Export/Import	14.4%	7.3%
Franchise	5.0%	5.3%
Marketing	18.0%	25.2%
Distribution	20.1%	20.5%
Production	26.5%	11.3%
Product/Services R&D	12.2%	12.6%
Process R&D	6.7%	5.3%
Purchaser/Supplier	23.5%	13.9%
Outside Contracting	23.2%	28.5%

Source: From Weaver, K. M. & Dickson, P. 2004. Strategic alliances. In Dennis, W. J., Jr. (Ed.) *NFIB National Small Business Poll.* Washington, DC: National Federation of Independent Business. Reprinted with permission.

* Columns add to over 100 percent because firms may use multiple alliances.

Exhibit 8.5　Use of Strategic Alliances by Small Businesses and Small Manufacturers

dedication and drive, and commitment to excellence—and pass these on to all those who work with them:

- **Vision.** This may be an entrepreneur's most important asset. Entrepreneurs envision realities that do not yet exist. But without a vision, most entrepreneurs would never even get their venture off the ground. With vision, entrepreneurs are able to exercise a kind of transformational leadership that creates something new and, in some way, changes the world. Just having a vision, however, is not enough. To develop support, get financial backing, and attract employees, entrepreneurial leaders must share their vision with others.

- **Dedication and drive.** Dedication and drive are reflected in hard work. Drive involves internal motivation; dedication calls for an intellectual commitment that keeps an entrepreneur going even in the face of bad news or poor luck. They both require patience, stamina, and a willingness to work long hours. However, a business built on the heroic efforts of one person may suffer in the long run. That's why the dedicated entrepreneur's enthusiasm is also important—like a magnet, it attracts others to the business to help with the work.[30]

- **Commitment to excellence.** Excellence requires entrepreneurs to commit to knowing the customer, providing quality goods and services, paying attention to details, and continuously learning. Entrepreneurs who achieve excellence are sensitive to how these factors work together. However, entrepreneurs may flounder if they think they are the only ones who can create excellent results. The most successful, by contrast, often report that they owe their success to hiring people smarter than themselves.

In his book *Good to Great,* Jim Collins makes another important point about entrepreneurial leadership: Ventures built on the charisma of a single person may have trouble growing "from good to great" once that person leaves.[31] Thus, the leadership that is needed to build a great organization is usually exercised by a team of dedicated people working together rather than a single leader. Another aspect of this team approach is attracting team members who fit with the company's culture, goals, and work ethic. Thus, for a venture's leadership to be a valuable resource and not a liability it must be cohesive in its vision, drive and dedication, and commitment to excellence.

Once an opportunity has been recognized, and an entrepreneurial team and resources have been assembled, a new venture must craft a strategy. Prior chapters have addressed the strategies of incumbent firms. In the next section, we highlight the types of strategies and strategic considerations faced by new entrants.

Entrepreneurial Strategy

entrepreneurial strategy a strategy that enables a skilled and dedicated entrepreneur, with a viable opportunity and access to sufficient resources, to successfully launch a new venture.

Successfully creating new ventures requires several ingredients. As indicated in Exhibit 8.3, three factors are necessary—a viable opportunity, sufficient resources, and a skilled and dedicated entrepreneur or entrepreneurial team. Once these elements are in place, the new venture needs a strategy—an **entrepreneurial strategy.** In this section, we consider several different strategic factors that are unique to new ventures and also how the generic strategies introduced in Chapter 5 can be applied to entrepreneurial firms. We also indicate how combination strategies might benefit entrepreneurial firms and address the potential pitfalls associated with launching new venture strategies.

To be successful, new ventures must evaluate industry conditions, the competitive environment, and market opportunities in order to position themselves strategically. However, a traditional strategic analysis may have to be altered somewhat to fit the entrepreneurial situation. For example, five-forces analysis (as discussed in Chapter 2) is typically used by established firms. It can also be applied to the analysis of new ventures to assess the impact of industry and competitive forces. But you may ask: How does a new entrant evaluate the threat of other new entrants?

First, the new entrant needs to examine barriers to entry. If the barriers are too high, the potential entrant may decide not to enter or to gather more resources before attempting to do so. Compared to an older firm with an established reputation and available resources, the barriers to entry may be insurmountable for an entrepreneurial start-up. Therefore, understanding the force of these barriers is critical in making a decision to launch.

A second factor that may be especially important to a young venture is the threat of retaliation by incumbents. In many cases, entrepreneurial ventures *are* the new entrants that pose a threat to incumbent firms. Therefore, in applying the five-forces model to new ventures, the threat of retaliation by established firms needs to be considered.

Part of any decision about what opportunity to pursue is a consideration of how a new entrant will actually enter a new market. The concept of entry strategies provides a useful means of addressing the types of choices that new ventures have.

Entry Strategies

One of the most challenging aspects of launching a new venture is finding a way to begin doing business that quickly generates cash flow, builds credibility, attracts good employees, and overcomes the liability of newness. The idea of an entry strategy or "entry wedge" describes several approaches that firms may take to get a foothold in a market.[32] Several factors will affect this decision.

>LO8.3
Three types of entry strategies—pioneering, imitative, and adaptive—commonly used to launch a new venture.

- Is the product/service high-tech or low-tech?
- What resources are available for the initial launch?
- What are the industry and competitive conditions?
- What is the overall market potential?
- Does the venture founder prefer to control the business or to grow it?

In some respects, any type of entry into a market for the first time may be considered entrepreneurial. But the entry strategy will vary depending on how risky and innovative the new business concept is.[33] New-entry strategies typically fall into one of three categories—pioneering new entry, imitative new entry, or adaptive new entry.[34]

Pioneering New Entry New entrants with a radical new product or highly innovative service may change the way business is conducted in an industry. This kind of breakthrough—creating new ways to solve old problems or meeting customers' needs in a unique new way—is referred to as a **pioneering new entry.** If the product or service is unique enough, a pioneering new entrant may actually have little direct competition. The first personal computer was a pioneering product; there had never been anything quite like it and it revolutionized computing. The first Internet browser provided a type of pioneering service. These breakthroughs created whole new industries and changed the competitive landscape. And breakthrough innovations continue to inspire pioneering entrepreneurial efforts. Strategy Spotlight 8.6 discusses Pandora, a firm that pioneered a new way to broadcast music in the United States.

pioneering new entry a firm's entry into an industry with a radical new product or highly innovative service that changes the way business is conducted.

In the UK, Last.fm is a music recommendation service founded in 2002. A European version of Pandora, it claimed 30 million active users in March 2009. CBS Interactive acquired Last.fm for $280 million in 2007. Using a music recommender system called Audioscrobbler, Last.fm builds a detailed profile of each user's musical taste by recording details of the songs the user listens to, from Internet radio stations, the user's computer, and many portable music devices. This information is transferred to Last.fm's database either via the music player itself (e.g., Rdio, Spotify, Amarok) or via a plug-in installed into the user's music player. The data is then displayed on the user's profile page and also compiled to create reference pages for individual artists. By April 2011, Last.fm reported more than

Pandora Rocks the Music Business

Whether the music was transmitted over FM radio signals, streamed over the web, or from a satellite, the musical choices radio listeners had were fairly standardized until Pandora arrived. Radio stations determined their play list based on a combination of interest evident in music sales and listener surveys along with the format of their stations. Listeners in a given market could decide if they wanted to listen to a top 40, adult contemporary, country, or classic rock station, but they couldn't custom design a station to meet their eclectic musical tastes.

Tim Westergren completely changed the radio business when he created Pandora. In 1999 he developed the Music Genome Project—a system that analyzes music for its underlying traits, including melody, rhythm, lyrics, instrumentation, and many other traits. Each song is measured on approximately 400 musical "genes" and given a vector or list of attributes. The vectors of multiple songs can be compared to assess the "distance" between the two songs. Using the Music Genome Project, Westergren launched Pandora in 2000. Users input bands or songs they like, and Pandora creates a customized station that plays music that meets the users' tastes. Users can then tweak the station by giving input on whether or not they like the songs Pandora plays for them.

Pandora radically changes the radio business in multiple ways. First, users create their own customized stations. Second, users can access their personal radio stations wherever they go through any Internet-connected device. Third, the playing of songs is driven by their musical traits, not how popular a band is. If an unsigned garage band has musical traits similar to Pearl Jam, their music will get play on a user's Pearl Jam station. This offers great exposure to aspiring musicians not available on commercial radio. It also offers an avenue for record labels to get exposure for newly signed bands that don't yet get air play on traditional radio.

Pandora has grown in 10 years from a boldly new idea to become the largest "radio" station in the world, with 65 million registered users. The next move is to dominate the location where Americans do most of their radio listening—their cars. Ford began offering a voice-activated Pandora system in its cars in early 2011. Other manufacturers are following suit. Pioneer is selling car stereos that support Pandora. In gaining control of music in cars, Pandora continues to rock the music business.

Sources: Copeland, M. V. 2010. Pandora's founder rocks the music business. *Fortune*, July 5: 27–28; Levy, A. 2010. Pandora's next frontier: Your wheels. *Bloomberg Businessweek*. October 14: np; and, www.pandora.com.

---

50 billion "scrobbles." The site offers numerous social networking features and can recommend and play artists similar to the user's favorites.[35]

The pitfalls associated with a pioneering new entry are numerous. For one thing, there is a strong risk that the product or service will not be accepted by consumers. The history of entrepreneurship is littered with new ideas that never got off the launching pad. Take, for example, Smell-O-Vision, an invention designed to pump odors into movie theatres from the projection room at preestablished moments in a film. It was tried only once (for the film *Scent of a Mystery*) before it was declared a major flop. Innovative? Definitely. But hardly a good idea at the time.[36]

A pioneering new entry is disruptive to the status quo of an industry. It is likely based on a technological breakthrough. If it is successful, other competitors will rush in to copy it. This can create issues of sustainability for an entrepreneurial firm, especially if a larger company with greater resources introduces a similar product. For a new entrant to sustain its pioneering advantage, it may be necessary to protect its intellectual property, advertise heavily to build brand recognition, form alliances with businesses that will adopt its products or services, and offer exceptional customer service.

Imitative New Entry   Whereas pioneers are often inventors or tinkerers with new technology, imitators usually have a strong marketing orientation. They look for opportunities to capitalize on proven market successes. An **imitative new entry** strategy is used by entrepreneurs who see products or business concepts that have been successful in one

imitative new entry a firm's entry into an industry with products or services that capitalize on proven market successes and that usually has a strong marketing orientation.

market niche or physical locale and introduce the same basic product or service in another segment of the market.

Sometimes the key to success with an imitative strategy is to fill a market space where the need had previously been filled inadequately. Entrepreneurs are also prompted to be imitators when they realize that they have the resources or skills to do a job better than an existing competitor. This can actually be a serious problem for entrepreneurial start-ups if the imitator is an established company. Consider the example of Tesla Motors. Founded in 2003, Tesla designs and manufactures electric cars. The average cost of a gallon of gasoline was about $1.50 when Tesla was incorporated, and the demand for alternative-fuel cars was not strong. Thus, it initially faced limited competition in this niche of the automotive market. However, by the time its first Tesla Roadster was ready for sale in 2008, rising gasoline prices and concerns about auto emissions had dramatically increased interest in electric cars. Tesla's success in winning design awards and car orders increased the profile of the firm and, more generally, electric cars. The major automakers are responding with their own models in this market. The Chevy Volt and Nissan Leaf both came on the market in 2010. Ford launched an electric version of the Ford Focus in 2011. Other major auto manufacturers are following suit. In spring 2012, Toyota, the world leader in selling hybrids, also planned to introduce a new battery–electric SUV—the RAV4EV—targeting a 100-mile range in a wide range of climates and conditions. While Tesla's original vehicle was a high-performance car that faced no direct competition, its goal was to expand into the mainstream market with an electric-powered sedan. With the fast response by major competitors, it is not clear that Tesla will be able to continue to grow its business.[37]

Adaptive New Entry   Most new entrants use a strategy somewhere between "pure" imitation and "pure" pioneering. That is, they offer a product or service that is somewhat new and sufficiently different to create new value for customers and capture market share. Such firms are adaptive in the sense that they are aware of marketplace conditions and conceive entry strategies to capitalize on current trends.

According to business creativity coach Tom Monahan, "Every new idea is merely a spin of an old idea. [Knowing that] takes the pressure off from thinking [you] have to be totally creative. You don't. Sometimes it's one slight twist to an old idea that makes all the difference."[38] An **adaptive new entry** approach does not involve "reinventing the wheel," nor is it merely imitative either. It involves taking an existing idea and adapting it to a particular situation. Exhibit 8.6 presents examples of four young companies that successfully modified or adapted existing products to create new value.

> **adaptive new entry** a firm's entry into an industry by offering a product or service that is somewhat new and sufficiently different to create value for customers by capitalizing on current market trends.

There are several pitfalls that might limit the success of an adaptive new entrant. First, the value proposition must be perceived as unique. Unless potential customers believe a new product or service does a superior job of meeting their needs, they will have little motivation to try it. Second, there is nothing to prevent a close competitor from mimicking the new firm's adaptation as a way to hold on to its customers. Third, once an adaptive entrant achieves initial success, the challenge is to keep the idea fresh. If the attractive features of the new business are copied, the entrepreneurial firm must find ways to adapt and improve the product or service offering.

Considering these choices, an entrepreneur or entrepreneurial team might ask, Which new entry strategy is best? The choice depends on many competitive, financial, and marketplace considerations. Nevertheless, research indicates that the greatest opportunities may stem from being willing to enter new markets rather than seeking growth only in existing markets. A recent study found that companies that ventured into arenas that were new to the world or new to the company earned total profits of 61 percent. In contrast, companies that made only incremental improvements, such as extending an existing product line, grew total profits by only 39 percent.[39]

Exhibit 8.6 Examples of Adaptive New Entrants

Company Name	Product	Adaptation	Result
HAAN Corporation Founded in 1999 (in Korea)	Steam cleaning machines and products	Used steam in cleaning machines and irons for sterilization.	HAAN Corporation is the top producer of steam cleaning products in Korea and plans to expand to global markets such as Japan, China, and the United States in the coming years. Its goal is to exceed $450 million in sales by 2015.
Under Armour, Inc. Founded in 1995	Undershirts and other athletic gear	Used moisture-wicking fabric to create better gear for sweaty sports.	Under Armour has 3,000 employees and 2010 sales in excess of $850 million.
Mint.com Founded in 2005	Comprehensive online money management	Created software that tells users what they are spending by aggregating financial information from online bank and credit card accounts.	Mint has over 4 million users and is tracking $200 billion in transactions.
Plum Organics Founded in 2005	Organic frozen baby food	Made convenient line of baby food using organic ingredients.	Added to Whole Foods product offering in 2006 and Babies 'R' Us in 2009.
Spanx Founded in 2000	Footless pantyhose and other undergarments for women	Combined nylon and Lycra® to create a new type of undergarment that is comfortable and eliminates panty lines.	Now produces over 200 products sold in 3,000 stores to over 6 million customers.

Sources: *www.ihaan.com/*, accessed October 28, 2011; Bryan, M. 2007. Spanx me, baby! *www.observer.com*, December 10, np.; Carey, J. 2006. Perspiration inspiration. *BusinessWeek,* June 5: 64; Palanjian, A. 2008. A planner plumbs for a niche. *www.wsj.com*. September 30, np.; Worrell, D. 2008. Making mint. *Entrepreneur,* September: 55; *www.mint.com*; *www.spanx.com*; *www.underarmour.com*; and, Buss, D. 2010. The mothers of invention. *The Wall Street Journal,* February 8: R7.

These findings led W. Chan Kim and Renee Mauborgne in their book *Blue Ocean Strategy* to conclude that companies that are willing to venture into market spaces where there is little or no competition—labeled "blue oceans"—will outperform those firms that limit growth to incremental improvements in competitively crowded industries—labeled "red oceans." Companies that identify and pursue blue ocean strategies follow somewhat different rules than those that are "bloodied" by the competitive practices in red oceans. Consider the following elements of a blue ocean strategy:

- *Create uncontested market space.* By seeking opportunities where they are not threatened by existing competitors, blue ocean firms can focus on customers rather than on competition.
- *Make the competition irrelevant.* Rather than using the competition as a benchmark, blue ocean firms cross industry boundaries to offer new and different products and services.

- **Create and capture new demand.** Rather than fighting over existing demand, blue ocean companies seek opportunities in uncharted territory.
- **Break the value/cost trade-off.** Blue ocean firms reject the idea that a trade-off between value and cost is inevitable and instead seek opportunities in areas that benefit both their cost structure and their value proposition to customers.
- **Pursue differentiation and low cost simultaneously.** By integrating the range of a firm's utility, price, and cost activities, blue ocean companies align their whole system to create sustainable strategies.

The essence of blue ocean strategy is not just to find an uncontested market, but to create one. Some blue oceans arise because new technologies create new possibilities, such as eBay's online auction business. Yet technological innovation is not a defining feature of a blue ocean strategy. Most blue oceans are created from within red oceans by companies that push beyond the existing industry boundaries. Any of the new entry strategies described earlier could be used to pursue a blue ocean strategy. Consider the example of Cirque du Soleil, which created a new market for circus entertainment by making traditional circus acts more like theatrical productions:

> By altering the industry boundaries that traditionally defined the circus concept, Cirque du Soleil created a new type of circus experience. Since the days of Ringling Bros. and Barnum & Bailey, the circus had consisted of animal acts, star performers, and Bozo-like clowns. Cirque questioned this formula and researched what audiences really wanted. It found that interest in animal acts was declining, in part because of public concerns over the treatment of circus animals. Because managing animals—and the celebrity trainers who performed with them—was costly, Cirque eliminated them.
>
> Instead, Cirque focused on three elements of the traditional circus tent event that still captivated audiences: acrobatic acts, clowns, and the tent itself. Elegant acrobatics became a central feature of its performances, and clown humor became more sophisticated and less slapstick. Cirque also preserved the image of the tent by creating exotic facades that captured the symbolic elements of the traditional tent. Finally, rather than displaying three different acts simultaneously, as in the classic three-ring circus, Cirque offers multiple productions with theatrical story lines, giving audiences a reason to go to the circus more often. Each production has a different theme and its own original musical score.
>
> Cirque's efforts to redefine the circus concept have paid off. Since 1984, Cirque's productions have been seen by over 90 million people in some 200 cities around the world.[40]

Once created, a blue ocean strategy is difficult to imitate. If customers flock to blue ocean creators, firms rapidly achieve economies of scale, learning advantages, and synergies across their organizational systems. The Body Shop, for example, chartered new territory by refusing to focus solely on beauty products. Traditional competitors such as Estee Lauder and L'Oreal, whose brands are based on promises of eternal youth and beauty, found it difficult to imitate this approach without repudiating their current images.

These factors suggest that blue ocean strategies provide an avenue by which firms can pursue an entrepreneurial new entry. Such strategies are not without risks, however. A new entrant must decide not only the best way to enter into business but also what type of strategic positioning will work best as the business goes forward. Those strategic choices can be informed by the guidelines suggested for the generic strategies. We turn to that subject next.

>LO8.4
How the generic strategies of overall cost leadership, differentiation, and focus are used by new ventures and small businesses.

Generic Strategies

Typically, a new entrant begins with a single business model that is equivalent in scope to a business-level strategy (Chapter 5). In this section we address how overall low cost, differentiation, and focus strategies can be used to achieve competitive advantages.

Overall Cost Leadership One of the ways entrepreneurial firms achieve success is by doing more with less. By holding down costs or making more efficient use of resources than larger competitors, new ventures are often able to offer lower prices and still be profitable. Thus, under the right circumstances, a low-cost leader strategy is a viable alternative for some new ventures. The way most companies achieve low-cost leadership, however, is typically different for young or small firms.

Recall from Chapter 5 that three of the features of a low-cost approach included operating at a large enough scale to spread costs over many units of production (economies of scale), making substantial capital investments in order to increase scale economies, and using knowledge gained from experience to make cost-saving improvements. These elements of a cost-leadership strategy may be unavailable to new ventures. Because new ventures are typically small, they usually don't have high economies of scale relative to competitors. Because they are usually cash strapped, they can't make large capital investments to increase their scale advantages. And because many are young, they often don't have a wealth of accumulated experience to draw on to achieve cost reductions.

Given these constraints, how can new ventures successfully deploy cost-leader strategies? Compared to large firms, new ventures often have simple organizational structures that make decision making both easier and faster. The smaller size also helps young firms change more quickly when upgrades in technology or feedback from the marketplace indicate that improvements are needed. They are also able to make decisions at the time they are founded that help them deal with the issue of controlling costs. For example, they may source materials from a supplier that provides them more cheaply or set up manufacturing facilities in another country where labor costs are especially low. Thus, new firms have several avenues for achieving low-cost leadership. Strategy Spotlight 8.7 highlights the success of Vizio, Inc., a new entrant with an overall cost leadership strategy. Whatever methods young firms use to achieve a low-cost advantage, this has always been a way that entrepreneurial firms take business away from incumbents—by offering a comparable product or service at a lower price.

Differentiation Both pioneering and adaptive entry strategies involve some degree of differentiation. That is, the new entry is based on being able to offer a differentiated value proposition. In the case of pioneers, the new venture is attempting to do something strikingly different, either by using a new technology or deploying resources in a way that radically alters the way business is conducted. Often, entrepreneurs do both.

Amazon founder Jeff Bezos set out to use Internet technology to revolutionize the way books are sold. He garnered the ire of other booksellers and the attention of the public by making bold claims about being the "earth's largest bookseller." As a bookseller, Bezos was not doing anything that had not been done before. But two key differentiating features—doing it on the Internet and offering extraordinary customer service—have made Amazon a differentiated success.

There are several factors that make it more difficult for new ventures to be successful as differentiators. For one thing, the strategy is generally thought to be expensive to enact. Differentiation is often associated with strong brand identity, and establishing a brand is usually considered to be expensive because of the cost of advertising and promotion, paid endorsements, exceptional customer service, etc. Differentiation successes are sometimes built on superior innovation or use of technology. These are also factors where it may be challenging for young firms to excel relative to established competitors.

Nevertheless all of these areas—innovation, technology, customer service, distinctive branding—are also arenas where new ventures have sometimes made a name for themselves even though they must operate with limited resources and experience. To be successful, according to Garry Ridge, CEO of the WD-40 Company, "You need to have a great product, make the end user aware of it, and make it easy to buy."[41] It sounds simple, but it is a difficult challenge for new ventures with differentiation strategies.

strategy spotlight

Low-Cost Imitator Vizio, Inc., Takes Off

The popularity of flat-panel TVs has grown rapidly since they were first introduced in the late 1990s—by 2012, it is estimated 85 percent of U.S households will have one. When first introduced, major manufacturers such as Samsung, Sony, and Matsushita (maker of Panasonic) made heavy investments in R&D in a competition for technological leadership. As a result, the early flat-panel TVs were expensive. Even as technological advances drove prices down, the TVs were growing larger and flatter, and they continued to command premium prices. By 2002, 50-inch plasma TVs were still selling for $8,000–$10,000. But by then, panel technology had also become somewhat commoditized. That's when William Wang, a former marketer of computer monitors, realized he could use existing technologies to create a high-quality TV. Wang discovered he could keep operations lean and outsource everything from tech support to R&D, so he founded Vizio, Inc.

In January 2003, Wang pitched Costco Wholesale Corp. on a 46-inch flat-panel plasma TV for $3,800—half the price of the competition. Although Costco executives laughed when Wang said he wanted to become the next Sony, they decided to give him a chance. By March 2003, the TVs were being offered in over 300 of Costco's U.S. warehouse stores. Today, Vizio is one of Costco's largest suppliers of TVs.

Vizio's success is due not only to enlightened imitation and low-cost operations, but also to Wang's unique approach to financing growth. Although he initially mortgaged his home and borrowed from family and friends, when he needed additional funding, he targeted the manufacturing partners who were supplying him parts. In 2004, Taiwan-based contract manufacturer AmTran Technology Co. purchased an 8 percent stake in Vizio for $1 million; today, AmTran owns 23 percent of Vizio and supplies over 80 percent of its TVs. "Unlike many PC companies who try to make their money by squeezing the vendor," says Wang, "we try to work with our vendor."

Although Vizio has a long way to go to be the next Sony, it has made remarkable progress. Vizio shipped 19.9 percent of the LCD TVs sold in the third quarter of 2010, leading the number two firm, Samsung, which had 17.7 percent of the market. Vizio expected to sell 6 million TVs in 2010, generating over $2.5 billion in sales. Vizio is now turning its attention to smaller electronic devices. Vizio recently announced it will introduce a line of cellphones and tablet computers. In extending its low-cost business model to these markets, it is taking one more step to being a full-range competitor to Sony, Samsung, and other major consumer electronics firms.

Sources: Lawton, C., Kane, Y. I., & Dean, J. 2008. U.S. upstart takes on TV giants in price war. *www.wsj.com*. April 15, np; Taub, E. A. 2008. Flat-panel TV prices plummet. *www.nytimes.com*. December 2, np; Wilson, S. 2008. Picture it. *Entrepreneur*, July: 43; *www.wikipedia.com*; Kane, Y. I. 2011. Vizio extends battle plan. *The Wall Street Journal*, January 3: B3; Edwards, C. 2010. How Vizio beat Sony in high-def TV. *Bloomberg Businessweek*. April 26: 51–52; and, *www.keloland.com*.

Focus   Focus strategies are often associated with small businesses because there is a natural fit between the narrow scope of the strategy and the small size of the firm. A focus strategy may include elements of differentiation and overall cost leadership, as well as combinations of these approaches. But to be successful within a market niche, the key strategic requirement is to stay focused. Here's why:

Despite all the attention given to fast-growing new industries, most start-ups enter industries that are mature.[42] In mature industries, growth in demand tends to be slow and there are often many competitors. Therefore, if a start-up wants to get a piece of the action, it often has to take business away from an existing competitor. If a start-up enters a market with a broad or aggressive strategy, it is likely to evoke retaliation from a more powerful competitor. Young firms can often succeed best by finding a market niche where they can get a foothold and make small advances that erode the position of existing competitors.[43] From this position, they can build a name for themselves and grow.

Consider, for example, the "Miniature Editions" line of books launched by Running Press, a small independent publisher in the U. S. city of Philadelphia. The books are palm-sized minibooks positioned at bookstore cash registers as point-of-sale impulse items costing about $4.95. Beginning with just 10 titles in 1993, Running Press grew rapidly and within 10 years had sold over 20 million copies. Even though these books represent just a tiny fraction of total sales in the $23 billion publishing industry, they have been a mainstay for Running Press.[44] As the Running Press example indicates, many new ventures are successful even though their share of the market is quite small.

Combination Strategies

One of the best ways for young and small businesses to achieve success is by pursuing combination strategies. By combining the best features of low-cost, differentiation, and focus strategies, new ventures can often achieve something truly distinctive.

Entrepreneurial firms are often in a strong position to offer a combination strategy because they have the flexibility to approach situations uniquely. For example, holding down expenses can be difficult for big firms because each layer of bureaucracy adds to the cost of doing business across the boundaries of a large organization.[45]

A similar argument could be made about entrepreneurial firms that differentiate. Large firms often find it difficult to offer highly specialized products or superior customer services. Entrepreneurial firms, by contrast, can often create high-value products and services through their unique differentiating efforts. Strategy Spotlight 8.8 shows how two entrepreneurs found a recipe to sell a common product line to a niche market while both cutting costs and offering a high service level.

For nearly all new entrants, one of the major dangers is that a large firm with more resources will copy what they are doing. Well-established incumbents that observe the success of a new entrant's product or service will copy it and use their market power to overwhelm the smaller firm. The threat may be lessened for firms that use combination strategies. Because of the flexibility of entrepreneurial firms, they can often enact combination strategies in ways that the large firms cannot copy. This makes the new entrant's strategies much more sustainable.

Perhaps more threatening than large competitors are close competitors, because they have similar structural features that help them adjust quickly and be flexible in decision making. Here again, a carefully crafted and executed combination strategy may be the best way for an entrepreneurial firm to thrive in a competitive environment. Nevertheless, competition among rivals is a key determinant of new venture success. To address this, we turn next to the topic of competitive dynamics.

>LO8.5
How competitive actions, such as the entry of new competitors into a marketplace, may launch a cycle of actions and reactions among close competitors.

Competitive Dynamics

New entry into markets, whether by start-ups or by incumbent firms, nearly always threatens existing competitors. This is true in part because, except in very new markets, nearly every market need is already being met, either directly or indirectly, by existing firms. As a result, the competitive actions of a new entrant are very likely to provoke a competitive response from companies that feel threatened. This, in turn, is likely to evoke a reaction to the response. As a result, a competitive dynamic—action and response—begins among the firms competing for the same customers in a given marketplace.

competitive dynamics intense rivalry, involving actions and responses, among similar competitors vying for the same customers in a marketplace.

Competitive dynamics—intense rivalry among similar competitors—has the potential to alter a company's strategy. New entrants may be forced to change their strategies or develop new ones to survive competitive challenges by incumbent rivals. New entry is among the most common reasons why a cycle of competitive actions and reactions gets started. It might also occur because of threatening actions among existing competitors, such as aggressive cost cutting. Thus, studying competitive dynamics helps explain why strategies evolve and reveals how, why, and when to respond to the actions of close competitors. Exhibit 8.7 identifies the factors that competitors need to consider when determining how to respond to a competitive act.

Diapers.com—Combining Focus, Low Cost, and Differentiation

Focusing on the needs of families with infants and toddlers, Marc Lore and Vinit Bharara turned a simple idea into a business worth $540 million in a matter of six years. Founded in January 2005, Diapers.com began by selling diapers out of a garage in Long Island, New York. Their business grew rapidly in geographic reach, products sold, and sales. But the firm's success relied on its ability to simultaneously focus on a particular market segment, offer a higher level of service, and maintain efficiency in operations. It now has a 30,000 square foot headquarters, over 500 employees, and over 600,000 square feet in warehouse space. In November 2010, at about the same time that it shipped their 500 millionth diaper, Diapers.com agreed to be acquired by Amazon.com for over a half billion dollars.

Diapers.com attracts customers by offering a high service level to busy parents who don't have the time to run out to Costco every time they need diapers and related baby care items. Over 70 percent of Diapers.com sales are to women, the majority of whom are in the 25–34 age range. Diapers.com sells 25,000 products, but they are high-use products for baby care, such as diapers, wipes,

Sources: Fowler, G. A. & Byron, L. 2010. Corporate news: Amazon to buy Diapers.com site. *The Wall Street Journal*, November 8: B4; Urstadt, B. 2010. Diapers vs. Goliath: Can two guys from Jersey outsell Amazon? *Bloomberg Businessweek*. October 11: 62–68; Birchall, J. 2010. Amazon aims to woo women with Quidsi acquisition. *Financial Times*, November 9: 23; and, Tiku, N. 2009. The way I work: Marc Lore of Diapers.com. *Inc.com*, September 1: np.

shampoo, and formula. In focusing on this limited range of products, Diapers.com is able to differentiate itself by offering a high level of service. Its website is simpler to navigate than broad Internet retailers. If customers need the help of knowledgeable customer service agents, Diapers.com has a staff of 85 agents to handle their inquiries. Meeting the needs of its customers, whom it refers to as Moms, is key. As co-founder Marc Lore commented, "The concept is just if Mom calls and there's an issue, do whatever is necessary to make her happy and really wow her." Diapers.com also delivers quickly, with nearly 75 percent of their shipments being overnight deliveries and free shipping for any order over $49. This has resulted in a loyal set of customers whose word-of-mouth advertising draws in new customers to the firm. Its focus allows the firm to be extremely efficient. Its advertising is focused in magazines targeted toward parents. Operationally, it has developed sophisticated algorithms to maintain the minimum inventory needed to insure it can fill customer orders 95 percent of the time and have a highly automated warehouse that relies on robots manufactured by Kiva Systems to quickly and efficiently fill orders. It also relies on a computer algorithm to pick out the smallest box possible for an order to minimize shipping costs. It also uses different shipping firms to ship to different regions, finding the lowest cost firm for that area. By meeting the needs of a narrow set of customers with a high service level and efficiency-oriented processes and resources, Diapers.com has excelled in a competitive, low-margin business.

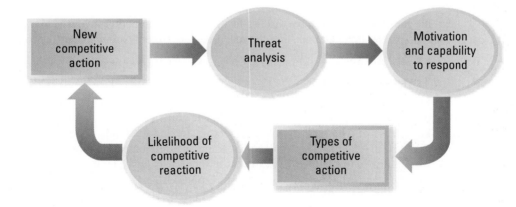

Exhibit 8.7 Model of Competitive Dynamics

Sources: Adapted from Chen, M. J. 1996. Competitor analysis and interfirm rivalry: Toward a theoretical integration. *Academy of Management Review*, 21(1): 100–134; Ketchen, D. J., Snow, C. C., & Hoover, V. L. 2004. Research on competitive dynamics: Recent accomplishments and future challenges. *Journal of Management*, 30(6): 779–804; and, Smith, K. G., Ferrier, W. J., & Grimm, C. M. 2001. King of the hill: Dethroning the industry leader. *Academy of Management Executive*, 15(2): 59–70.

New Competitive Action

Entry into a market by a new competitor is a good starting point to begin describing the cycle of actions and responses characteristic of a competitive dynamic process.[46] However, new entry is only one type of competitive action. Cutting prices, imitating successful products, or expanding production capacity are other examples of competitive acts that might provoke competitors to react.

Why do companies launch **new competitive actions**? There are several reasons:

- Improve market position
- Capitalize on growing demand
- Expand production capacity
- Provide an innovative new solution
- Obtain first mover advantages

new competitive action acts that might provoke competitors to react, such as new market entry, price cutting, imitation of successful products, and expansion of production capacity.

Underlying all of these reasons is a desire to strengthen financial outcomes, capture some of the extraordinary profits that industry leaders enjoy, and grow the business. Some companies are also motivated to launch competitive challenges because they want to build their reputation for innovativeness or efficiency. For example, Air Arabia of the United Arab Emirates was the first and largest low-cost airline in the Middle East. Once an upstart airline with only 15 destinations when it began to fly in 2003, Air Arabia has become extremely successful and an industry leader. However, Air Arabia's costs have increased in recent years, and now start-up airlines such as Flydubai are challenging industry leaders with their own low-cost strategies.[47] This is indicative of the competitive dynamic cycle. As former Intel Chairman Andy Grove stated, "Business success contains the seeds of its own destruction. The more successful you are, the more people want a chunk of your business and then another chunk and then another until there is nothing left."[48]

When a company enters into a market for the first time, it is an attack on existing competitors. As indicated earlier in the chapter, any of the entry strategies can be used to take competitive action. But competitive attacks come from many sources besides new entrants. Some of the most intense competition is among incumbent rivals intent on gaining strategic advantages. "Winners in business play rough and don't apologize for it," according to Boston Consulting Group authors George Stalk Jr. and Rob Lachenauer in their book *Hardball: Are You Playing to Play or Playing to Win?*[49] Exhibit 8.8 outlines their five strategies.

The likelihood that a competitor will launch an attack depends on many factors.[50] In the remaining sections, we discuss factors such as competitor analysis, market conditions, types of strategic actions, and the resource endowments and capabilities companies need to take competitive action.

Threat Analysis

threat analysis a firm's awareness of its closest competitors and the kinds of competitive actions they might be planning.

Prior to actually observing a competitive action, companies may need to become aware of potential competitive threats through **threat analysis**. That is, companies need to have a keen sense of who their closest competitors are and the kinds of competitive actions they might be planning.[51] This may require some environmental scanning and monitoring of the sort described in Chapter 2. Awareness of the threats posed by industry rivals allows a firm to understand what type of competitive response, if any, may be necessary.

For example, Netflix founder and CEO Reed Hastings has faced numerous competitive threats since launching the online movie rental company in 1997. According to Hastings, however, not all potential threats need to be taken seriously:

> We have to recognize that now there are tens and maybe hundreds of start-ups who think that they are going to eat Netflix's lunch. The challenge for a management team is to figure out which are real threats and which aren't. . . . It's conventional to say, "only the paranoid survive" but that's not true. The paranoid die because the paranoid take all threats as serious and get very distracted.

Exhibit 8.8 Five "Hardball" Strategies

Strategy	Description	Examples
Devastate rivals' profit sanctuaries	Not all business segments generate the same level of profits for a company. Through focused attacks on a rival's most profitable segments, a company can generate maximum leverage with relatively smaller-scale attacks. Recognize, however, that companies closely guard the information needed to determine just what their profit sanctuaries are.	In 2005, Walmart began offering low-priced extended warranties on home electronics after learning that its rivals such as Best Buy derived most of their profits from extended warranties.
Plagiarize with pride	Just because a close competitor comes up with an idea first does not mean it cannot be successfully imitated. Second movers, in fact, can see how customers respond, make improvements, and launch a better version without all the market development costs. Successful imitation is harder than it may appear and requires the imitating firm to keep its ego in check.	Blockbuster copied the online DVD rental strategy of its rival Netflix. Not only does Blockbuster continue to struggle even after this imitation, but also Netflix sued Blockbuster for patent violations.
Deceive the competition	A good gambit sends the competition off in the wrong direction. This may cause the rivals to miss strategic shifts, spend money pursuing dead ends, or slow their responses. Any of these outcomes support the deceiving firms' competitive advantage. Companies must be sure not to cross ethical lines during these actions.	Boeing spent several years touting its plans for a new high-speed airliner. After it became clear the customer valued efficiency over speed, Boeing quietly shifted its focus. When Boeing announced its new 7e7 (now 787) Dreamliner, its competitor, Airbus Industries, was surprised and caught without an adequate response, which helped the 787 set new sales records.
Unleash massive and overwhelming force	While many hardball strategies are subtle and indirect, this one is not. This is a full-frontal attack where a firm commits significant resources to a major campaign to weaken rivals' positions in certain markets. Firms must be sure they have the mass and stamina required to win before they declare war against a rival.	EasyJet took on British Airways (BA) in Northern Ireland and drove down BA's market share from 23 to 17 percent. EasyJet followed this up by flying to many short-haul markets—boosting its passenger numbers more than 7 percent to 49.7 million passengers in 2010—and extending its lead over BA in most European short-haul markets.
Raise competitors' costs	If a company has superior insight into the complex cost and profit structure of the industry, it can compete in a way that steers its rivals into relatively higher cost/lower profit arenas. This strategy uses deception to make the rivals think they are winning, when in fact they are not. Again, companies using this strategy must be confident that they understand the industry better than their rivals.	Ecolab, a company that sells cleaning supplies to businesses, encouraged a leading competitor, Diversity, to adopt a strategy to go after the low-volume, high-margin customers. What Ecolab knew that Diversity didn't is that the high servicing costs involved with this segment make the segment unprofitable—a situation Ecolab assured by bidding high enough to lose the contracts to Diversity but low enough to ensure the business lost money for Diversity.

Sources: Rothwell, S. 2011. EasyJet extends lead over British Airways in market for short-haul travel. *www.bloomberg.com/news/*. January 8; EasyJet overtakes British Airways in Northern Ireland, *www.easyjet.com/en/news/20010704_01.html*; Berner, R. 2005. Watch out, Best Buy and Circuit City. *BusinessWeek*, November 10; Halkias, M. 2006. Blockbuster strikes back at netflix suit. *Dallas Morning News*, June 14; Stalk, G., Jr. 2006. Curveball strategies to fool the competition. *Harvard Business Review*, 84(9): 114–121; and, Stalk, G., Jr. & Lachenauer, R. 2004. *Hardball: Are you playing to play or playing to win?* Cambridge, MA: Harvard Business School Press. Reprinted by permission of Harvard Business School Press from G. Stalk Jr. and R. Lachenauer. Copyright 2004 by the Harvard Business School Publishing Corporation; all rights reserved.

There are markets that aren't going to get very big, and then there are markets that are going to get big, but they're not directly in our path. In the first camp we have small companies like Movielink—a well-run company but not an attractive model for consumers, sort of a $4-download to watch a movie. We correctly guessed when it launched four years ago that this was not a threat and didn't react to it.

The other case I brought up is markets that are going to be very large markets, but we're just not the natural leader. Advertising supported online video, whether that's at CBS .com or YouTube—great market, kind of next door to us. But we don't do advertising-supported video, we do subscription, so it would be a huge competence expansion for us. And it's not a threat to movies.

Being aware of competitors and cognizant of whatever threats they might pose is the first step in assessing the level of competitive threat. Once a new competitive action becomes apparent, companies must determine how threatening it is to their business. Competitive dynamics are likely to be most intense among companies that are competing for the same customers or who have highly similar sets of resources.[52] Two factors are used to assess whether or not companies are close competitors:

- **Market commonality**—whether or not competitors are vying for the same customers and how many markets they share in common. For example, aircraft manufacturers Boeing and Airbus have a high degree of market commonality because they make very similar products and have many buyers in common.
- **Resource similarity**—the degree to which rivals draw on the same types of resources to compete. For example, the home pages of Baidu (China) and Naver and Daum (Korea) may look very different, but behind the scenes, they both rely on the talent pool of high-caliber software engineers to create the cutting-edge innovations that help them compete.

When any two firms have both a high degree of market commonality and highly similar resource bases, a stronger competitive threat is present. Such a threat, however, may not lead to competitive action. On the one hand, a market rival may be hesitant to attack a company that it shares a high degree of market commonality with because it could lead to an intense battle. On the other hand, once attacked, rivals with high market commonality will be much more motivated to launch a competitive response. This is especially true in cases where the shared market is an important part of a company's overall business.

How strong a response an attacked rival can mount will be determined by its strategic resource endowments. In general, the same set of conditions holds true with regard to resource similarity. Companies that have highly similar resource bases will be hesitant to launch an initial attack but pose a serious threat if required to mount a competitive response.[53] Greater strategic resources increase a firm's capability to respond.

Motivation and Capability to Respond

Once attacked, competitors are faced with deciding how to respond. Before deciding, however, they need to evaluate not only how they will respond, but also their reasons for responding and their capability to respond. Companies need to be clear about what problems a competitive response is expected to address and what types of problems it might create.[54] There are several factors to consider.

First, how serious is the impact of the competitive attack to which they are responding? For example, a large company with a strong reputation that is challenged by a small or unknown company may elect to simply keep an eye on the new competitor rather than quickly react or overreact. Part of the story of online retailer Amazon's early success is attributed to Barnes & Noble's overreaction to Amazon's claim that it was "earth's biggest bookstore." Because Barnes & Noble was already using the phrase "world's largest bookstore," it sued Amazon, but lost. The confrontation made it to the front pages of *The*

Wall Street Journal and Amazon was on its way to becoming a household name.[55]

Companies planning to respond to a competitive challenge must also understand their motivation for responding. What is the intent of the competitive response? Is it merely to blunt the attack of the competitor or is it an opportunity to enhance its competitive position? Sometimes the most a company can hope for is to minimize the damage caused by a competitive action.

A company that seeks to improve its competitive advantage may be motivated to launch an attack rather than merely respond to one. Strategy Spotlight 8.9 highlights how *The Wall Street Journal* saw an opportunity to improve its position by attacking a weakened *The New York Times*. A company must also assess its capability to respond. What strategic resources can be deployed to fend off a competitive attack? Does the company have an array of internal strengths it can draw on, or is it operating from a position of weakness?

Consider the role of firm age and size in calculating a company's ability to respond. Most entrepreneurial new ventures start out small. The smaller size makes them more nimble compared to large firms so they can respond quickly to competitive attacks. Because they are not well-known, start-ups also have the advantage of the element of surprise in how and when they attack. Innovative uses of technology, for example, allow small firms to deploy resources in unique ways.

Because they are young, however, start-ups may not have the financial resources needed to follow through with a competitive response.[56] In contrast, older and larger firms may have more resources and a repertoire of competitive techniques they can use in a counterattack. Large firms, however, tend to be slower to respond. Older firms tend to be predictable in their responses because they often lose touch with the competitive environment and rely on strategies and actions that have worked in the past.

Other resources may also play a role in whether a company is equipped to retaliate. For example, one avenue of counterattack may be launching product enhancements or new product/service innovations. For that approach to be successful, it requires a company to have both the intellectual capital to put forward viable innovations and the teamwork skills to prepare a new product or service and get it to market. Resources such as cross-functional teams and the social capital that makes teamwork production effective and efficient represent the type of human capital resources that enhance a company's capability to respond.

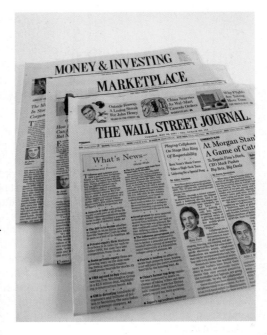

● *The Wall Street Journal* and *The New York Times* are engaged in an intense rivalry for market share.

Types of Competitive Actions

Once an organization determines whether it is willing and able to launch a competitive action, it must determine what type of action is appropriate. The actions taken will be determined by both its resource capabilities and its motivation for responding. There are also marketplace considerations. What types of actions are likely to be most effective given a company's internal strengths and weaknesses as well as market conditions?

Two broadly defined types of competitive action include strategic actions and tactical actions. **Strategic actions** represent major commitments of distinctive and specific resources. Examples include launching a breakthrough innovation, building a new production facility, or merging with another company. Such actions require significant planning and resources and, once initiated, are difficult to reverse.

Tactical actions include refinements or extensions of strategies. Examples of tactical actions include cutting prices, improving gaps in service, or strengthening marketing efforts. Such actions typically draw on general resources and can be implemented quickly.

strategic actions major commitments of distinctive and specific resources to strategic initiatives.

tactical actions refinements or extensions of strategies usually involving minor resource commitments.

The Wall Street Journal Challenges The New York Times

The newspaper business is an increasingly tough market. Circulation and advertising rates are dropping as news consumers move from traditional newspaper providers to online news services. In this difficult environment, newspapers have both increased motivation to take business from their remaining traditional competitors and reduced capability to respond to competitive attacks. These competing factors have resulted in an interesting competitive action in New York City. *The Wall Street Journal* (*WSJ*), a newspaper that has emphasized business and investing news since its inception in 1889, is taking on *The New York Times* (*Times*), a traditional city newspaper. The *WSJ* launched its Greater New York Edition in April 2010 to increase its base of affluent subscribers and female readers in the New York region, the core readers of the *Times.*

Why the *Times*, and why now? The *WSJ* has high motivation to act now. News Corp. purchased the *WSJ* in 2007 and brought with it an aggressive attitude that called for change at the *WSJ*. Rupert Murdoch, the chairman of News Corp., specifically stated at the time that he wanted to see the *WSJ* compete more directly with the *Times*. It is also motivated to act since the customers it is striving to attract make the *WSJ* more attractive to luxury product and service advertisers in the New York

area. The new edition has signed on luxury advertisers Saks Fifth Avenue, Bloomingdales, Cathay Pacific Airlines, Broadway's *Jersey Boys* musical, and the American Ballet Theatre. It also has the capability to act because the *WSJ* is one of the few traditional news providers with a growing number of readers. It also has the backing of News Corp., a major global media firm. Thus, it has the financial resources necessary to launch and sustain a competitive action against the *Times.*

But it is a different situation at the *Times*. While motivated to respond to the *WSJ*'s attack, it has limited resources to mount a major competitive response. It has experienced a significant decline in subscriptions, with the number of subscribers falling 8.5 percent in March 2010 compared to one year earlier. This has reduced the advertising rates it is able to charge. Also, the *Times* has limited cash resources. It is so strapped for cash that it was forced to borrow $250 million from Mexican industrialist Carlos Slim in 2009 at a 14 percent interest rate. When the *WSJ* launched its Greater New York Edition, the *Times* only had $36.5 million in cash on its balance sheet—not much of a war chest to take on News Corp. For Rupert Murdoch, the *Times*'s struggles are a signal to attack and an opportunity to cripple and potentially destroy *The New York Times*. As media investment expert Richard Dorfman stated, "This could be a money-losing venture for the *Journal*, but a potential big winner for Rupert if he's able to throw the *Times* over the edge of the abyss."

Other local papers should be wary. There are reports that, if successful with its Greater New York Edition, *The Wall Street Journal* will consider launching similar ventures in other major markets, including San Francisco, Los Angeles, and Washington, D.C.

Sources: Anonymous. 2010. Is the *Times* ready for a newspaper war? *Bloomberg Businessweek.* April 26: 30–31; Bensinger, G. 2010. *Wall Street Journal* circulation gains as new edition debuts. *Bloomberg Businessweek.* April 26: np; Anonymous. 2010. *Wall Street Journal* considers other local markets if NY edition a success. *Mediabuyerplanner.com.* April 18: np; and Sreenivasan, S. 2010. *The Wall Street Journal's* local edition launches. *Dnainfo.com.* April 26: np.

Exhibit 8.9 identifies several types of strategic and tactical competitive actions, and Strategy Spotlight 8.10 shows the range of actions that can occur in a rivalrous relationship.

Some competitive actions take the form of frontal assaults, that is, actions aimed directly at taking business from another company or capitalizing on industry weaknesses. This can be especially effective when firms use a low-cost strategy. The airline industry provides a good example of this head-on approach. When Southwest Airlines began its no-frills, no-meals strategy in the late-1960s, it represented a direct assault on the major carriers of the day. In Europe, Ryanair of Ireland has similarly directly challenged the traditional carriers with an overall cost leadership strategy. In Asia, AirAsia challenged traditional carrier Malaysian Airlines with an overall cost leadership strategy based on the low-fare, no-frills business model.

Guerilla offensives and selective attacks provide an alternative for firms with fewer resources.[57] These draw attention to products or services by creating buzz or generating

Exhibit 8.9   **Strategic and Tactical Competitive Actions**

	Actions	Examples
Strategic Actions	• Entrance into new markets	• Make geographical expansions • Expand into neglected markets • Target rivals' markets • Target new demographics
	• New product introductions	• Imitate rivals' products • Address gaps in quality • Leverage new technologies • Leverage brand name with related products • Protect innovation with patents
	• Changes in production capacity	• Create overcapacity • Tie up raw materials sources • Tie up preferred suppliers and distributors • Stimulate demand by limiting capacity
	• Mergers/Alliances	• Acquire/partner with competitors to reduce competition • Tie up key suppliers through alliances • Obtain new technology/intellectual property • Facilitate new market entry
Tactical Actions	• Price cutting (or increases)	• Maintain low price dominance • Offer discounts and rebates • Offer incentives (e.g., frequent flyer miles) • Enhance offering to move upscale
	• Product/service enhancements	• Address gaps in service • Expand warranties • Make incremental product improvements
	• Increased marketing efforts	• Use guerilla marketing • Conduct selective attacks • Change product packaging • Use new marketing channels
	• New distribution channels	• Access suppliers directly • Access customers directly • Develop multiple points of contact with customers • Expand Internet presence

Sources: Chen, M. J. & Hambrick, D. 1995. Speed, stealth, and selective attack: How small firms differ from large firms in competitive behavior. *Academy of Management Journal,* 38: 453–482; Davies, M. 1992. Sales promotions as a competitive strategy. *Management Decision,* 30(7): 5–10; Ferrier, W., Smith, K., & Grimm, C. 1999. The role of competitive action in market share erosion and industry dethronement: A study of industry leaders and challengers. *Academy of Management Journal,* 42(4): 372–388; and, Garda, R. A. 1991. Use tactical pricing to uncover hidden profits. *Journal of Business Strategy,* 12(5): 17–23.

enough shock value to get some free publicity. TOMS shoes has found a way to generate interest in its products without a large advertising budget to match Nike. Its policy of donating one pair of shoes to those in need for every pair of shoes purchased by customers has generated a lot of buzz on the Internet.[58] Over 700,000 people have given a "like" rating on TOMS's Facebook page. The policy has a real impact as well, with over 1,000,000 shoes donated as of September 2010.[59]

AMD and Intel: The Multiple Dimensions of Competitive Dynamics

Few business battles are as intense or as intensely reported as the one between chipmakers Intel and Advanced Micro Devices (AMD). These two firms have fought an intense competitive battle for over two decades. They started out on a much different footing. They were both founded in the late 1960s in Silicon Valley and were partners in their early years. But their history changed in 1986 after Intel cancelled a licensing agreement with AMD to manufacture microprocessors and refused to turn over technical details. Since that time, Intel has dominated the microprocessor market with approximately 80 percent market share but has regularly faced competitive initiatives from AMD and has as regularly taken competitive initiatives against AMD. As Intel Executive Vice President Sean Maloney stated, "We intend to energetically compete for every single microprocessor opportunity."

Their battle points out how highly competitive firms can take their competitive attacks to multiple battlefields. They have fought product design battles. Time and time again, they have aimed to pioneer new generations of chips. They fought over who would launch the first 64-bit processors. They competed in introducing

multiple-core chips. They competed in producing low-energy chips for laptops and notebooks. Currently, they are racing to launch chips that integrate graphics chip capabilities into the microprocessor. They have fought to build relationships with customers. According to governmental regulators, Intel locked in Dell and other PC manufacturers as exclusive customers by offering them rebates to use only Intel microprocessors. AMD fought back and won business supplying chips to Dell in 2006 and for Lenovo notebooks in 2009. They have developed aggressive marketing campaigns to promote their products. They have acquired other firms to pull in new technology to gain an advantage. For example, AMD bought ATI Technologies to gain access to graphics chip technology that it has integrated with the CPU in its latest generation of chips, the Fusion. They have fought legal battles. Both firms have sued each other over the right to technologies. Intel finally settled a multiyear legal battle with AMD for $1.25 billion in 2009.

This competitive battle shows how a long-standing competitive battle between firms can include a range of tactical and strategic actions as firms act to improve their own competitive position and unsettle the competitive position of their rival. This battle also demonstrates the potential benefits of high industry rivalry for consumers. The rivalry between AMD and Intel has led to tremendous improvements in microprocessor capabilities with declining prices over time. And there is no end in sight for these two pitched rivals.

Sources: Fortt, J. 2010. Intel vs. AMD gets interesting again. *CNNmoney.com.* May 12: np; Clark, D. 2010. AMD starts shipping new breed of chips. *The Wall Street Journal,* November 10: B7; Vance, A. 2010. Dell's trouble kicking the Intel habit. *The New York Times,* July 23; Parloff, R. 2010. What the Dell settlement means for Intel. *Fortune.com,* July 27: np; and, *www.wikipedia.org.*

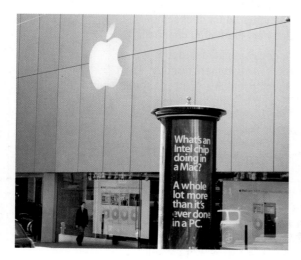

● Intel and AMD have had a fierce rivalry over the years.

Some companies limit their competitive response to defensive actions. Such actions rarely improve a company's competitive advantage, but a credible defensive action can lower the risk of being attacked and deter new entry. This may be especially effective during periods such as an industry shake-up, when pricing levels or future demand for a product line become highly uncertain. At such times, tactics such as lowering prices on products that are easily duplicated, buying up the available supply of goods or raw materials, or negotiating exclusive agreements with buyers and/or suppliers can insulate a company from a more serious attack.

Several of the factors discussed earlier in the chapter, such as types of entry strategies and the use of cost leadership versus differentiation strategies, can guide the decision about what types of competitive actions to take. Before launching a given strategy, however, assessing the likely response of competitors is a vital step.[60]

Likelihood of Competitive Reaction

The final step before initiating a competitive response is to evaluate what a competitor's reaction is likely to be. The logic of competitive dynamics suggests that once competitive actions are initiated, it is likely they will be met with competitive responses.[61] The last step before mounting an attack is to evaluate how competitors are likely to respond. Evaluating potential competitive reactions helps companies plan for future counterattacks. It may also lead to a decision to hold off—that is, not to take any competitive action at all because of the possibility that a misguided or poorly planned response will generate a devastating competitive reaction.

How a competitor is likely to respond will depend on three factors: market dependence, competitor's resources, and the reputation of the firm that initiates the action (actor's reputation). The implications of each of these is described briefly in the following sections.

Market Dependence   If a company has a high concentration of its business in a particular industry, it has more at stake because it must depend on that industry's market for its sales. Single-industry businesses or those where one industry dominates are more likely to mount a competitive response. Young and small firms with a high degree of **market dependence** may be limited in how they respond due to resource constraints. EasyJet, itself an aggressive competitor, is unable to match some of the perks its bigger rivals can offer, such as first-class seats or international travel benefits.

market dependence degree of concentration of a firm's business in a particular industry.

Competitor's Resources   Previously, we examined the internal resource endowments that a company must evaluate when assessing its capability to respond. Here, it is the competitor's resources that need to be considered. For example, a small firm may be unable to mount a serious attack due to lack of resources. Also, as we saw in Strategy Spotlight 8.9, a large but poorly performing firm may lack the resources to respond to an attack. As a result, it is more likely to react to tactical actions such as incentive pricing or enhanced service offerings because they are less costly to attack than large-scale strategic actions. In contrast, a firm with financial "deep pockets" may be able to mount and sustain a costly counterattack.

Actor's Reputation   Whether a company should respond to a competitive challenge will also depend on who launched the attack against it. Compared to relatively smaller firms with less market power, competitors are more likely to respond to competitive moves by market leaders. Another consideration is how successful prior attacks have been. For example, price-cutting by the big automakers usually has the desired result—increased sales to price-sensitive buyers—at least in the short run. Given that history, when GM offers discounts or incentives, rivals Ford and Chrysler cannot afford to ignore the challenge and quickly follow suit.

Choosing Not to React: Forbearance and Co-opetition

The above discussion suggests that there may be many circumstances in which the best reaction is no reaction at all. This is known as **forbearance**—refraining from reacting at all as well as holding back from initiating an attack. The decision of whether a firm should respond or show forbearance is not always clear. In Strategy Spotlight 8.11, we see the NFL and the UFL facing such a decision.

forbearance a firm's choice of not reacting to a rival's new competitive action.

Related to forbearance is the concept of **co-opetition.** This is a term that was coined by network software company Novell's founder and former CEO Raymond Noorda to suggest that companies often benefit most from a combination of competing and cooperating.[62] Close competitors that differentiate themselves in the eyes of consumers may work together behind the scenes to achieve industrywide efficiencies.[63] For example, breweries in Sweden cooperate in recycling used bottles but still compete for customers on the basis of taste and variety. As long as the benefits of cooperating are enjoyed by all participants in a co-opetition system, the practice can aid companies in avoiding intense and damaging competition.[64]

co-opetition a firm's strategy of both cooperating and competing with rival firms.

The UFL and the NFL: Cooperate or Compete?

If we look at the success and failure of professional football leagues from the past, the future for the United Football League (UFL) would not appear to be promising. Since the merger of the NFL with the AFL in the 1960s, several leagues trying to build a position in the American football market have failed. In the 1970s, it was the World Football League that rose and fell in a few years. In the 1980s, it was the United States Football league that followed the same pattern. In the 1990s, the Canadian Football League tried expanding south of the border, only to quickly retreat back north. The XFL lasted only a single year in 2001. Only the unique Arena Football League has lasted more than a few years, but its history has still been bumpy. The league went through bankruptcy in 2008 only to return in 2010.

The UFL is a new upstart football league trying to carve out a position in the professional football market. Unlike the Arena Football League, the UFL is playing a version of football that is almost identical to the NFL and plays during the traditional fall football season. The league began play in 2009 with four teams, expanded to five teams in 2010, and will play with six teams in 2012.

However, it is unclear at this point to what degree the UFL will compete with the NFL, and it is also unclear whether the NFL will act in a way to push the UFL out of the market or show forbearance and let it stay in the game. The UFL appears to be taking actions to avoid a direct confrontation with the NFL. It has placed its franchises in cities, such as Las Vegas, Omaha, and Orlando, that currently do not have NFL franchises. It also has not tried to compete with the NFL for players. It has made no effort to sign active NFL players. Instead, its rosters are a combination of former NFL players, such as JaMarcus Russell, hoping to revive their NFL careers and young players hoping to make an impression and move up to the NFL. However, the league appears reluctant to position itself simply as a minor or developmental league for the NFL. It requires the NFL to pay a $150,000 transfer fee to allow a UFL player to sign with an NFL team, limiting the willingness of NFL teams to sign UFL players. Also, they are looking to expand into markets that the NFL also sees as desirable. The UFL has announced an expansion into the Los Angeles market in either 2011 or 2012, but the NFL is working with potential owners interested in moving an NFL franchise into the LA market as well. The intentions of the NFL are also unclear. The NFL has not taken any direct actions against the UFL. But the NFL has also not pursued a cooperative relationship with the upstart league. According to ESPN, the UFL offered the NFL the opportunity to buy part of the league and set up consistent rules for players to move from one league to the other, but the NFL did not agree to make the investment. It may be that the NFL is focused on its unsettled labor contract with the players' union and, as a result, doesn't have the motivation to act either cooperatively or competitively with the UFL at this point in time.

Given the history of prior football leagues, the ability of the UFL to find a position where it doesn't directly compete with the NFL for ticket buyers, players, or TV placement would appear to be key to its viability. Thus, figuring out how to appear similar enough to the NFL to attract fans while also different enough to not trigger a competitive reaction by the NFL should be a primary factor driving the UFL's actions.

Sources: Brown, R. 2011. Rumor: Next UFL expansion team will be in the "southwest." December 21. www.uflaccess.com; Mortensen, C. 2010. UFL puts 30 percent offer on NFL's table. ESPN.com. March 19: np; Cohan, W. D. 2010. Football's new game in town. Fortune, October 18: 111–112; and, www.wikipedia.org.

Despite the potential benefits of co-opetition, companies need to guard against cooperating to such a great extent that their actions are perceived as collusion, a practice that has legal ramifications in many countries. Recently, Dell and other PC manufacturers in the United States have faced scrutiny due to their possible collusion with Intel.

Once a company has evaluated a competitor's likelihood of responding to a competitive challenge, it can decide what type of action is most appropriate. Competitive actions can take many forms: the entry of a start-up into a market for the first time, an attack by a lower-ranked incumbent on an industry leader, or the launch of a breakthrough innovation that disrupts the industry structure. Such actions forever change the competitive dynamics of a marketplace. Thus, the cycle of actions and reactions that occur in business every day is a vital aspect of entrepreneurial strategy that leads to continual new value creation and the ongoing advancement of economic well-being.

Reflecting on Career Implications . . .

- **Opportunity Recognition:** What ideas for new business activities are actively discussed in your work environment? Could you apply the four characteristics of an opportunity to determine whether they are viable opportunities?
- **Entrepreneurial New Entry:** Are there opportunities to launch new products or services that might add value to the organization? What are the best ways for you to bring these opportunities to the attention of key managers? Or might this provide an opportunity for you to launch your own entrepreneurial venture?
- **Entrepreneurial Strategy:** Does your organization face competition from new ventures? If so, how are those young firms competing: Low cost? Differentiation? Focus? What could you do to help your company to address those competitive challenges?
- **Competitive Dynamics:** Is your organization "on the offense" with its close competitors or "playing defense"? What types of strategic and/or tactical actions have been taken by your close rivals recently to gain competitive advantages?

Summary

New ventures and entrepreneurial firms that capitalize on marketplace opportunities make an important contribution to the U.S. economy. They are leaders in terms of implementing new technologies and introducing innovative products and services. Yet entrepreneurial firms face unique challenges if they are going to survive and grow.

To successfully launch new ventures or implement new technologies, three factors must be present: an entrepreneurial opportunity, the resources to pursue the opportunity, and an entrepreneur or entrepreneurial team willing and able to undertake the venture. Firms must develop a strong ability to recognize viable opportunities. Opportunity recognition is a process of determining which venture ideas are, in fact, promising business opportunities.

In addition to strong opportunities, entrepreneurial firms need resources and entrepreneurial leadership to thrive. The resources that start-ups need include financial resources as well as human and social capital. Many firms also benefit from government programs that support new venture development and growth. New ventures thrive best when they are led by founders or owners who have vision, drive and dedication, and a commitment to excellence.

Once the necessary opportunities, resources, and entrepreneur skills are in place, new ventures still face numerous strategic challenges. Decisions about the strategic positioning of new entrants can benefit from conducting strategic analyses and evaluating the requirements of niche markets. Entry strategies used by new ventures take several forms, including pioneering new entry, imitative new entry, and adaptive new entry.

Entrepreneurial firms can benefit from using overall low cost, differentiation, and focus strategies although each of these approaches has pitfalls that are unique to young and small firms. Entrepreneurial firms are also in a strong position to benefit from combination strategies.

The entry of a new company into a competitive arena is like a competitive attack on incumbents in that arena. Such actions often provoke a competitive response, which may, in turn, trigger a reaction to the response. As a result, a competitive dynamic—action and response—begins among close competitors. In deciding whether to attack or counterattack, companies must analyze the seriousness of the competitive threat, their ability to mount a competitive response, and the type of action—strategic or tactical—that the situation requires. At times, competitors find it is better not to respond at all or to find avenues to cooperate with, rather than challenge, close competitors.

Summary Review Questions

1. Explain how the combination of opportunities, resources, and entrepreneurs helps determine the character and strategic direction of an entrepreneurial firm.
2. What is the difference between discovery and evaluation in the process of opportunity recognition? Give an example of each.
3. Describe the three characteristics of entrepreneurial leadership: vision, dedication and drive, and commitment to excellence.

4. Briefly describe the three types of entrepreneurial entry strategies: pioneering, imitative, and adaptive.

5. Explain why entrepreneurial firms are often in a strong position to use combination strategies.

6. What does the term *competitive dynamics* mean?

7. Explain the difference between strategic actions and tactical actions and provide examples of each.

Key Terms

Applications Questions & Answers

1. Smava and Auxmoney in Germany are two entre-preneurial firms that offer lending services over the Internet. Evaluate the features of these two companies and, for each company (in the boxes provided):

   a. Evaluate their characteristics and assess the extent to which they are comparable in terms of market commonality and resource similarity.

   b. Based on your analysis, what strategic and/or tactical actions might these companies take to improve their competitive position? Could Smava and Aux-money improve their performance more through co-opetition rather than competition? Explain your rationale.

2. Using the Internet, research the European Commission's Small Business portal (*www.ec.europa.eu/small-business*). What different types of financing are available to small firms in the European community? Besides financing, what other programs are available to support the growth and development of small businesses?

3. Think of an entrepreneurial firm that has been successfully launched in the last 10 years. What kind of entry strategy did it use—pioneering, imitative, or adaptive? Since the firm's initial entry, how has it used or combined overall low-cost, differentiation, and/or focus strategies?

4. Select an entrepreneurial firm you are familiar with in your local community. Research the company and discuss how it has positioned itself relative to its close competitors. Does it have a unique strategic advantage? Disadvantage? Explain.

Company	Market Commonality	Resource Similarity
Smava		
Auxmoney		

Company	Strategic Actions	Tactical Actions
Smava		
Auxmoney		

Ethics Questions

1. Imitation strategies are based on the idea of copying another firm's idea and using it for your own purposes. Is this unethical or simply a smart business practice? Discuss the ethical implications of this practice (if any).

2. Intense competition such as price wars is an accepted business practice, but cooperation between companies has legal ramifications because of antitrust laws. Should price wars that drive small businesses or new entrants out of business be illegal? What ethical considerations are raised (if any)?

References

1. Anonymous. 2006. 2006 fastest-growing franchise rankings. *Entrepreneur. http://entrepreneur.com,* accessed October 2010: np; Anonymous, 2007. Rising stars. *Entrepreneur. http://entrepreneur.com,* accessed October 2010: np; Edersheim Kalb, P. 2009. Cranky consumer: Hiring middlemen to sell stuff on eBay. *The Wall Street Journal,* January 29: D2; Ohngren, K. 2010. Kaboom! A look back at the wacky franchise ideas that exploded (and imploded) in an instant. Meet you at the eBay store. *Entrepreneur,* January 38(1): 120–124; and, Wilson, S. 2006. Hotter than hot. *Entrepreneur,* June 34(6): 72–81; April 35(4): 108–111. We thank Ciprian Stan for his valued contribution.

2. Small Business Administration. 2004. *The small business economy.* Washington, D.C.: U.S. Government Printing Office.

3. Wymenga, P., Spanikova, V., Derbyshire, J., & Barker, A. 2011. Are EU SMEs recovering from the crisis? *Annual report on EU small- and medium-sized enterprises 2010/2011.* Rotterdam: Ecorys, and Cambridge: Cambridge Econometrics.

4. Timmons, J. A. & Spinelli, S. 2004. *New venture creation* (6th ed.). New York: McGraw-Hill/Irwin; and, Bygrave, W. D. 1997. The entrepreneurial process. In Bygrave, W. D. (Ed.) *The portable MBA in entrepreneurship* (2nd ed.). New York: Wiley.

5. Fromartz, S. 1998. How to get your first great idea. *Inc.,* April 1: 91–94; and, Vesper, K. H. 1990. *New venture strategies* (2nd ed.). Englewood Cliffs, NJ: Prentice-Hall.

6. For an interesting perspective on the nature of the opportunity recognition process, see: Baron, R. A. 2006. Opportunity recognition as pattern recognition: How entrepreneurs "connect the dots" to identify new business opportunities. *Academy of Management Perspectives,* February: 104–119.

7. Gaglio, C. M. 1997. Opportunity identification: Review, critique and suggested research directions. In Katz, J. A. (Ed.). *Advances in entrepreneurship, firm emergence and growth,* vol. 3. Greenwich, CT: JAI Press: 139–202; Lumpkin, G. T., Hills, G. E., & Shrader, R. C. 2004. Opportunity recognition. In Welsch, H. L. (Ed.). *Entrepreneurship: The road ahead:* 73–90. London: Routledge; and, Long, W. & McMullan, W. E. 1984. Mapping the new venture opportunity identification process. *Frontiers of entrepreneurship research, 1984.* Wellesley, MA: Babson College: 567–90.

8. For an interesting discussion of different aspects of opportunity discovery, see: Shepherd, D. A. & De Tienne, D. R. 2005. Prior knowledge, potential financial reward, and opportunity identification. *Entrepreneurship theory & practice,* 29(1): 91–112; and, Gaglio, C. M. 2004. The role of mental simulations and counterfactual thinking in the opportunity identification process. *Entrepreneurship Theory & Practice,* 28(6): 533–552.

9. Stewart, T. A. 2002. How to think with your gut. *Business 2.0,* November: 99–104.

10. For more on the opportunity recognition process, see: Smith, B. R., Matthews, C. H., & Schenkel, M. T. 2009. Differences in entrepreneurial opportunities: The role of tacitness and codification in opportunity identification. *Journal of Small Business Management,* 47(1): 38–57.

11. Timmons, J. A. 1997. Opportunity recognition. In Bygrave, W. D. (Ed.). *The portable MBA in entrepreneurship* (2nd ed.): 26–54. New York: John Wiley.

12. Social networking is also proving to be an increasingly important type of entrepreneurial resource. For an interesting discussion, see: Aldrich, H. E. & Kim, P. H. 2007. Small worlds, infinite possibilities? How social networks affect entrepreneurial team formation and search. *Strategic Entrepreneurship Journal,* 1(1): 147–166.

13. Bhide, A. V. 2000. *The origin and evolution of new businesses.* New York: Oxford University Press.

14. Small Business 2001: Where are we now? 2001. *Inc.,* May 29: 18–19; and, Zacharakis, A. L., Bygrave, W. D., & Shepherd, D. A. 2000. *Global entrepreneurship monitor—national entrepreneurship assessment: United States of America 2000 Executive Report.* Kansas City, MO: Kauffman Center for Entrepreneurial Leadership.

15. Cooper, S. 2003. Cash cows. *Entrepreneur,* June: 36.

16. Seglin, J. L. 1998. What angels want. *Inc.,* 20(7): 43–44.

17. Torres, N. L. 2002. Playing an angel. *Entrepreneur,* May: 130–138.

18. For an interesting discussion of how venture capital practices vary across different sectors of the economy, see: Gaba, V. & Meyer, A. D. 2008. Crossing the organizational species barrier: How venture capital practices infiltrated the information technology sector. *Academy of Management Journal,* 51(5): 391–412.

19. For more on how different forms of organizing entrepreneurial firms as well as different stages of new firm growth and development affect financing, see: Cassar, G. 2004. The

financing of business start-ups. *Journal of Business Venturing,* 19(2): 261–283.

20. Kroll, M., Walters, B., & Wright, P. 2010. The impact of insider control and environment on post-IPO performance. *Academy of Management Journal,* 53: 693–725.

21. Eisenhardt, K. M. & Schoonhoven, C. B. 1990. Organizational growth: Linking founding team, strategy, environment, and growth among U.S. semiconductor ventures, 1978–1988. *Administrative Science Quarterly,* 35: 504–529.

22. Dubini, P. & Aldrich, H. 1991. Personal and extended networks are central to the entrepreneurship process. *Journal of Business Venturing,* 6(5): 305–333.

23. For more on the role of social contacts in helping young firms build legitimacy, see: Chrisman, J. J. & McMullan, W. E. 2004. Outside assistance as a knowledge resource for new venture survival. *Journal of Small Business Management,* 42(3): 229–244.

24. Vogel, C. 2000. Janina Pawlowski. *Working Woman,* June: 70.

25. For a recent perspective on entrepreneurship and strategic alliances, see: Rothaermel, F. T. & Deeds, D. L. 2006. Alliance types, alliance experience and alliance management capability in high-technology ventures. *Journal of Business Venturing,* 21(4): 429–460; and, Lu, J. W. & Beamish, P. W. 2006. Partnering strategies and performance of SMEs' international joint ventures. *Journal of Business Venturing,* 21(4): 461–486.

26. For more on the role of alliances in creating competitive advantages, see: Wiklund, J. & Shepherd, D. A. 2009. The effectiveness of alliances and acquisitions: The role of resource combination activities. *Entrepreneurship Theory & Practice,* 33(1): 193–212.

27. BBC News. 2011. Government financial support for SMEs. *www.bbc.co.uk/news/business.* January 4.

28. For more information, go to the Small Business Administration website at *www.sba.gov.*

29. Simsek, Z., Heavey, C., & Veiga, J. 2009. The Impact of CEO core self-evaluations on entrepreneurial

orientation. *Strategic Management Journal,* 31: 110–119.

30. For an interesting study of the role of passion in entrepreneurial success, see: Chen, X-P., Yao, X., & Kotha, S. 2009. Entrepreneur passion and preparedness in business plan presentations: A persuasion analysis of venture capitalists' funding decisions. *Academy of Management Journal,* 52(1): 101–120.

31. Collins, J. 2001. *Good to great.* New York: HarperCollins.

32. The idea of entry wedges was discussed by: Vesper, K. 1990. *New venture strategies* (2nd ed.). Englewood Cliffs, NJ: Prentice-Hall; and, Drucker, P. F. 1985. *Innovation and entrepreneurship.* New York: HarperBusiness.

33. See Dowell, G. & Swaminathan, A. 2006. Entry timing, exploration, and firm survival in the early U.S. bicycle industry. *Strategic Management Journal,* 27: 1159–1182, for a recent study of the timing of entrepreneurial new entry.

34. Dunlap-Hinkler, D., Kotabe, M., & Mudambi, R. 2010. A story of breakthrough vs. incremental innovation: Corporate entrepreneurship in the global pharmaceutical industry. *Strategic Entrepreneurship Journal,* 4: 106–127.

35. *www.crunchbase.com/company/last-fm; www.last.fm/about;* and *en.wikipedia.org/wiki/Last.fm.*

36. Maiello, M. 2002. They almost changed the world. *Forbes,* December 22: 217–220.

37. Wilson, R. 2010. 7 electric cars you'll be able to buy very soon. *The Huffington Post,* November 17: np; and, *www.pluginamerica.org/vehicles/toyota-rav4-ev.*

38. Williams, G. 2002. Looks like rain. *Entrepreneur,* September: 104–111.

39. Pedroza, G. M. 2002. Tech tutors. *Entrepreneur,* September: 120.

40. Kim, W. C., and Mauborgne, R. 2004. Blue ocean strategy. *Harvard Business Review,* October: 76–84; and, *www.cirquedusoleil.com.*

41. Romanelli, E. 1989. Environments and strategies of organization start-up: Effects on early survival. *Administrative Science Quarterly,* 34(3): 369–87.

42. Wallace, B. 2000. Brothers. *Philadelphia Magazine,* April: 66–75.

43. Buchanan, L. 2003. The innovation factor: A field guide to innovation. *Forbes,* April 21, *www.forbes.com.*

44. Kim, W. C. & Mauborgne, R. 2005. *Blue ocean strategy.* Boston: Harvard Business School Press.

45. For more on how unique organizational combinations can contribute to competitive advantages of entrepreneurial firms, see: Steffens, P., Davidsson, P., & Fitzsimmons, J. Performance configurations over times: Implications for growth- and profit-oriented strategies. *Entrepreneurship Theory & Practice,* 33(1): 125–148.

46. Smith, K. G., Ferrier, W. J., & Grimm, C. M. 2001. King of the hill: Dethroning the industry leader. *Academy of Management Executive,* 15(2): 59–70.

47. *www.airarabia.com/ver_html/about-airarabia.html;* and, Flydubai: High-class, low-fare airline. April 27, 2011, *www.rusbiznews.com/news/n1035.html.*

48. Grove, A. 1999. *Only the paranoid survive: How to exploit the crises points that challenge every company.* New York: Random House.

49. Stalk, Jr., G. & Lachenauer, R. 2004. *Hardball: Are you playing to play or playing to win?* Cambridge, MA: Harvard Business School Press.

50. Chen, M. J., Lin, H. C, & Michel, J. G. 2010. Navigating in a hypercompetitive environment: The roles of action aggressiveness and TMT integration. *Strategic Management Journal,* 31: 1410–1430.

51. Peteraf, M. A. & Bergen, M. A. 2003. Scanning competitive landscapes: A market-based and resource-based framework. *Strategic Management Journal,* 24: 1027–1045.

52. Chen, M. J. 1996. Competitor analysis and interfirm rivalry: Toward a theoretical integration. *Academy of Management Review,* 21(1): 100–134.

53. Chen, 1996, op. cit.

54. Chen, M. J., Su, K. H, & Tsai, W. 2007. Competitive tension: The awareness-motivation-capability perspective. *Academy of Management Journal,* 50(1): 101–118.

55. St. John, W. 1999. Barnes & Noble's epiphany. *www.wired.com.* June.

56. Souder, D. & Shaver, J. M. 2010. Constraints and incentives for making

long horizon corporate investments. *Strategic Management Journal,* 31: 1316–1336.

57. Chen, M. J. & Hambrick, D. 1995. Speed, stealth, and selective attack: How small firms differ from large firms in competitive behavior. *Academy of Management Journal,* 38: 453–482.

58. Fenner, L. 2009. TOMS shoes donates one pair of shoes for every pair purchased. *America.gov.* October 19: np.

59. *www.facebook.com/tomsshoes.*

60. For a discussion of how the strategic actions of Apple Computer contribute to changes in the competitive dynamics in both the cellular phone and music industries, see: Burgelman, R. A. & Grove, A. S. 2008. Cross-boundary disruptors: Powerful inter-industry entrepreneurial change agents. *Strategic Entrepreneurship Journal,* 1(1): 315–327,

61. Smith, K. G., Ferrier, W. J., & Ndofor, H. 2001. Competitive dynamics research: Critique and future directions. In Hitt, M. A., Freeman, R. E., & Harrison, J. S. (Eds.). *The Blackwell handbook of strategic management:* 315–361. Oxford, UK: Blackwell.

62. Gee, P. 2000. Co-opetition: The new market milieu. *Journal of Healthcare Management,* 45: 359–363.

63. Ketchen, D. J., Snow, C. C., & Hoover, V. L. 2004, Research on competitive dynamics: Recent accomplishments and future challenges. *Journal of Management,* 30(6): 779–804.

64. Khanna, T., Gulati, R., & Nohria, N. 2000. The economic modeling of strategy process: Clean models and dirty hands. *Strategic Management Journal,* 21: 781–790.

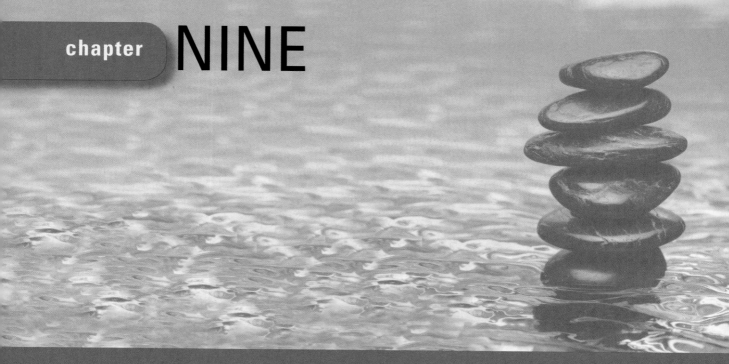

chapter NINE

Strategic Control and Corporate Governance

After reading this chapter, you should have a good understanding of:

LO9.1 The value of effective strategic control systems in strategy implementation.

LO9.2 The key difference between "traditional" and "contemporary" control systems.

LO9.3 The imperative for "contemporary" control systems in today's complex and rapidly changing competitive and general environments.

LO9.4 The benefits of having the proper balance among the three levers of behavioral control: culture; rewards and incentives; and, boundaries.

LO9.5 The three key participants in corporate governance: shareholders, management (led by the CEO), and the board of directors.

LO9.6 The role of corporate governance mechanisms in ensuring that the interests of managers are aligned with those of shareholders from both the United States and international perspectives.

LEARNING OBJECTIVES

Organizations must have effective strategic controls if they are to successfully implement their strategies. This includes systems that exercise both informational control and behavioral control. Controls must be consistent with the strategy that the firm is following. In addition, a firm must promote sound corporate governance to ensure that the interests of managers and shareholders are aligned.

In the first section, we address the need to have effective informational control, contrasting two approaches to informational control. The first approach, which we call "traditional," is highly sequential. Goals and objectives are set, then implemented, and after a set period of time, performance is compared to the desired standards. In contrast, the second approach, termed "contemporary," is much more interactive. Here, the internal and external environments are continually monitored, and managers determine whether the strategy itself needs to be modified. Today the contemporary approach is required, given the rapidly changing conditions in virtually all industries.

Next, we discuss behavioral control. Here the firm must strive to maintain a proper balance between culture, rewards, and boundaries. We also argue that organizations that have strong, positive cultures and reward systems can rely less on boundaries, such as rules, regulations, and procedures. When individuals in the firm internalize goals and strategies, there is less need for monitoring behavior, and efforts are focused more on important organizational goals and objectives.

The third section addresses the role of corporate governance in ensuring that managerial and shareholder interests are aligned. We provide examples of both effective and ineffective corporate governance practices. We discuss three governance mechanisms for aligning managerial and shareholder interests: a committed and involved board of directors, shareholder activism, and effective managerial rewards and incentives. Public companies are also subject to external control. We discuss several external control mechanisms, such as the market for corporate control, auditors, banks and analysts, the media, and public activists. We close with a discussion of corporate governance from an international perspective.

Learning from Mistakes

Chesapeake Energy had a terrible year in 2008. Its net income dropped about 50 percent from the previous year and its stock plummeted from 39 to 17 during the year—a loss of 56 percent.[1] Its board of directors, however, fared much better than its shareholders. In fact, its directors were among the highest paid corporate directors in 2008. For example, one of the eight "independent" directors, 80-year-old Breene Kerr, received $784,687 in total compensation. He's considered independent only because he is not a member of Chesapeake's management, but he just happens to be the cousin of the CEO, Aubrey McClendon. The other directors did almost as well, receiving an average of about $670,000 each. Let's take a look and see what possible reasons there may be for why the directors were compensated so well.

CEO Aubrey McClendon aggressively bought Chesapeake's stock in July 2008, mostly on margin, at prices as high as $72 a share. Unfortunately, the stock began to sharply drop. In September, margin calls forced McClendon to sell almost all of his position at a price between $13.60 and $24 a share, depleting his net worth.

The board rushed to the rescue! It promptly awarded McClendon a $75 million "special bonus" for 2008. As if such enormous (and undeserved) compensation were not sufficient, the board felt it necessary to justify another use of corporate funds. In December 2008, the company purchased McClendon's extensive collection of antique historic maps of the American Southwest for $12.1 million.

But that is not all. At a cost of $3.5 million, the company became a founding sponsor of the Oklahoma City Thunder, a National Basketball Association franchise owned and operated by The Professional Basketball Club, LLC ("PBC"). McClendon had a 19.2 percent equity interest in the franchise.

The company's compensation committee did provide a rationale for McClendon's huge bonus: It stressed the board's wish to keep him as CEO. And McClendon reciprocated when asked why Chesapeake pays its directors so much: "We have a very large and complex company and we value our directors' time."

---

strategic control the process of monitoring and correcting a firm's strategy and performance.

We first explore two central aspects of **strategic control:**[2] (1) *informational control,* which is the ability to respond effectively to environmental change, and (2) *behavioral control,* which is the appropriate balance and alignment among a firm's culture, rewards, and boundaries. In the final section of this chapter, we focus on strategic control from a much broader perspective—what is referred to as *corporate governance.*[3] Here, we direct our attention to the need for a firm's shareholders (the owners) and their elected representatives (the board of directors) to ensure that the firm's executives (the management team) strive to fulfill their fiduciary duty of maximizing long-term shareholder value. As we just saw in the Chesapeake Energy example, clearly there was a breakdown in corporate governance. This gave the CEO seemingly unlimited power at the expense of the shareholders.

>LO9.1
The value of effective strategic control systems in strategy implementation.

Ensuring Informational Control: Responding Effectively to Environmental Change

We discuss two broad types of control systems: "traditional" and "contemporary." As both general and competitive environments become more unpredictable and complex, the need for contemporary systems increases.

A Traditional Approach to Strategic Control

The **traditional approach to strategic control** is sequential: (1) strategies are formulated and top management sets goals, (2) strategies are implemented, and (3) performance is measured against the predetermined goal set, as illustrated in Exhibit 9.1.

Control is based on a feedback loop from performance measurement to strategy formulation. This process typically involves lengthy time lags, often tied to a firm's annual planning cycle. Such traditional control systems, termed "single-loop" learning by Harvard's Chris Argyris, simply compare actual performance to a predetermined goal.[4] They are most appropriate when the environment is stable and relatively simple, goals and objectives can be measured with a high level of certainty, and there is little need for complex measures of performance. Sales quotas, operating budgets, production schedules, and similar quantitative control mechanisms are typical. The appropriateness of the business strategy or standards of performance is seldom questioned.[5]

James Brian Quinn of Dartmouth College has argued that grand designs with precise and carefully integrated plans seldom work.[6] Rather, most strategic change proceeds incrementally—one step at a time. Leaders should introduce some sense of direction, some logic in incremental steps.[7] Similarly, McGill University's Henry Mintzberg has written about leaders "crafting" a strategy.[8] Drawing on the parallel between the potter at her wheel and the strategist, Mintzberg pointed out that the potter begins work with some general idea of the artifact she wishes to create, but the details of design—even possibilities for a different design—emerge as the work progresses. For businesses facing complex and turbulent business environments, the craftsperson's method helps us deal with the uncertainty about how a design will work out in practice and allows for a creative element.

Mintzberg's argument, like Quinn's, questions the value of rigid planning and goal-setting processes. Fixed strategic goals also become dysfunctional for firms competing in highly unpredictable competitive environments. Strategies need to change frequently and opportunistically. An inflexible commitment to predetermined goals and milestones can prevent the very adaptability that is required of a good strategy.

Even organizations that have been extremely successful in the past can become complacent or fail to adapt their goals and strategies to the new conditions. Nokia, the world's largest mobile phone maker by volume, is one such firm. Nokia has seen its market share plummet in recent years from increasing competition from Apple and Samsung. The company suffered from its failure in the smartphone business, which has also been affected by rising competition from Google's Android operating platform. Another example of such a firm is General Motors (GM). For many decades, it was the leading firm in the automotive industry. As recently as 2006, it was recognized by Morgan Stanley as the top car producer. However, GM suffered from many underlying problems that were aggravated by the recent worldwide recession, which eroded demand for automobiles. In Strategy Spotlight 9.1, we address what may be considered one of its key underlying problems—a lack of informational control.

A Contemporary Approach to Strategic Control

Adapting to and anticipating both internal and external environmental change is an integral part of strategic control. The relationships between strategy formulation, implementation, and control are highly interactive, as suggested by Exhibit 9.2. It also illustrates two different types of strategic control: informational control and behavioral control. **Informational control** is

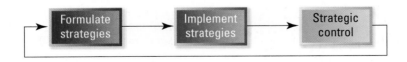

Exhibit 9.1 Traditional Approach to Strategic Control

traditional approach to strategic control a sequential method of organizational control in which (1) strategies are formulated and top management sets goals, (2) strategies are implemented, and (3) performance is measured against the predetermined goal set.

>LO9.2
The key difference between "traditional" and "contemporary" control systems.

>LO9.3
The imperative for "contemporary" control systems in today's complex and rapidly changing competitive and general environments.

informational control a method of organizational control in which a firm gathers and analyzes information from the internal and external environment in order to obtain the best fit between the organization's goals and strategies and the strategic environment.

strategy spotlight

What Did General Motors Do Wrong?

General Motors (GM), which was founded in 1908, had been ruling the automotive industry for more than half a century. GM provided a broad range of vehicles, reflecting the company's promise to offer "a car for every purse and purpose." As recently as 2007, its stock was trading above $40 a share. And then just a few months after celebrating its 100th anniversary in 2008, GM filed for bankruptcy. On May 29, 2009, GM's stock closed at 75 cents a share, which was a historic low for the company. The government funded a $50 billion bailout to save GM and took a 60 percent ownership stake in the company when it exited bankruptcy in 2010.

GM's market dominance grew out of its abilities to mass manufacture, market, and distribute cars for all customer types. While its advantage initially was based on automotive design and manufacturing prowess, over time, GM became rigid and lost its feel for reading the American car market that it helped create. It was not manufacturing competitive vehicles and increasingly relied on volume and the profits from financing auto sales for its success. At the same time, GM faced increasing competition from Japanese automakers, but it was slow to respond to this competitive entry due to its bureaucratic culture and complacency driven by the profitability of its financing operations. The Japanese competitors developed competencies to design world-class vehicles and produced them more efficiently than GM. As a result, they lured away many of GM's customers. GM's management failed to respond to changes in customer needs and automotive technologies as well as the evolving competitive landscape.

GM did have vast numbers of loyal buyers, but lost many of them through a series of strategic and cultural missteps. Trying to balance the competing needs of seven major brands, GM often resorted to a practice (sarcastically) called "launch and leave"—spending billions upfront to bring vehicles to market, but then failing to keep supporting them with sustained advertising. It also failed to differentiate the brands. Originally, each brand was designed to meet the needs of a different customer segment. However, GM's brand identities became muddled as it sold essentially the same car for different brands. According to Jim Wangers, a retired advertising

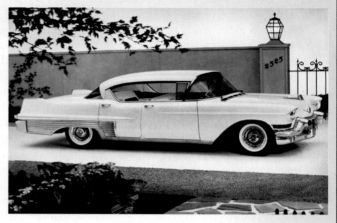

● A 1957 Cadillac—a successful product that reflects General Motors' glory days.

executive, "Nobody gave any respect to this thing called image because it wasn't in the business plan. It was all about, 'When is this going to earn a profit?'"

Faced with a declining market position, GM executives did not address the need for changes. Instead, they fell prey to two common biases. First, they exhibited *attribution bias*. When their performance started to fall, they attributed their struggles to outside forces, such as the weak Japanese yen, unfair trade practices, and higher costs from their unionized workers. In short, they became expert at the art of explaining away their problems, attributing blame to everyone but themselves. Second, they exhibited *confirmation bias*—the tendency of managers to filter out information that does not match up with their preconceived notions. GM rewarded people who followed the old way of doing things, and those who challenged that thinking were marginalized—causing them to lose opportunities for promotion. So the smart thing for those seeking promotion within GM was to praise the CEO's wisdom and carry out his orders. This confirmation bias syndrome kept GM from viewing the threat from Japanese automakers as significant, contributed to its decision to pull its electric car off the market, and more recently led it to ignore the effect of higher gas prices and a collapse in credit markets on consumers' willingness to buy profitable gas guzzlers like the Hummer or tricked-out Escalades and SUVs. In falling prey to these biases, GM's management failed to recognize the need for change in response to changes in the market, in technology, and in customers' demands.

Sources: Maynard, M. 2009. After many stumbles, the fall of a giant. *The New York Times*, June 1: A1; Smith, A. 2009. GM stock falls below $1. *money.cnn.com*. May 29: np; Maynard, M. 2009. After 93 years, GM shares go out on a low note. *dealbook.nytimes.com*. May 29: np; Holstein, W. J. 2009. Who's to blame for GM's bankruptcy? *www.businessweek.com*. June 1: np; and, Cohan, P. 2009. After 101 years, why GM failed. *www.dailyfinance.com*. May 31: np.

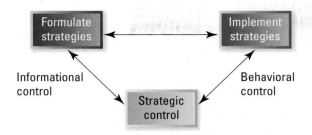

Exhibit 9.2 Contemporary Approach to Strategic Control

primarily concerned with whether or not the organization is "doing the right things." **Behavioral control,** on the other hand, asks if the organization is "doing things right" in the implementation of its strategy. Both the informational and behavioral components of strategic control are necessary, but not sufficient, conditions for success. What good is a well-conceived strategy that cannot be implemented? Or what use is an energetic and committed workforce if it is focused on the wrong strategic target?

> **behavioral control** a method of organizational control in which a firm influences the actions of employees through culture, rewards, and boundaries.

John Weston is the former CEO of ADP Corporation, the largest payroll and tax-filing processor in the world. He captures the essence of contemporary control systems:

> At ADP, 39 plus 1 adds up to more than 40 plus 0. The 40-plus-0 employee is the harried worker who at 40 hours a week just tries to keep up with what's in the "in" basket. . . . Because he works with his head down, he takes zero hours to think about what he's doing, why he's doing it, and how he's doing it. . . . On the other hand, the 39-plus-1 employee takes at least 1 of those 40 hours to think about what he's doing and why he's doing it. That's why the other 39 hours are far more productive.[9]

Informational control deals with the internal environment as well as the external strategic context. It addresses the assumptions and premises that provide the foundation for an organization's strategy. Do the organization's goals and strategies still "fit" within the context of the current strategic environment? Depending on the type of business, such assumptions may relate to changes in technology, customer tastes, government regulation, and industry competition.

This involves two key issues. First, managers must scan and monitor the external environment, as we discussed in Chapter 2. Also, conditions can change in the internal environment of the firm, as we discussed in Chapter 3, requiring changes in the strategic direction of the firm. These may include, for example, the resignation of key executives or delays in the completion of major production facilities.

In the contemporary approach, information control is part of an ongoing process of organizational learning that continuously updates and challenges the assumptions that underlie the organization's strategy. In such "double-loop" learning, the organization's assumptions, premises, goals, and strategies are continuously monitored, tested, and reviewed. The benefits of continuous monitoring are evident—time lags are dramatically shortened, changes in the competitive environment are detected earlier, and the organization's ability to respond with speed and flexibility is enhanced.

Contemporary control systems must have four characteristics to be effective.[10]

1. Focus on constantly changing information that has potential strategic importance.
2. The information is important enough to demand frequent and regular attention from all levels of the organization.
3. The data and information generated are best interpreted and discussed in face-to-face meetings.
4. The control system is a key catalyst for an ongoing debate about underlying data, assumptions, and action plans.

An executive's decision to use the control system interactively—in other words, to invest the time and attention to review and evaluate new information—sends a clear signal

Google's Interactive Control System

Google has tried typical hierarchical control systems typically found in large firms. However, the firm reverted to its interactive control system within weeks. All of Google's roughly 5,000 product developers work in teams of three engineers. Larger projects simply assemble several teams of three workers. Within teams, there is a rotating "über-tech leader" depending on the project. Engineers tend to work in more than one team and do not need permission to switch teams. According to Shona Brown, VP for operations, "If at all possible, we want people to commit to things rather than be assigned to things." At Google "employees don't need a lot of signoffs to try something new, but they won't get much in the way of resources until they've accumulated some positive user feedback."

Google's executives regularly review projects with project leaders and analyze data about projects. Google uses some of its own web page ranking technology in the review of software and other business projects. Using their own employees as mini test markets, managers often solicit employee opinions and analyze usage patterns of new product features and technologies. This interactive control of corporate information allows Google to make faster decisions about its business, including:

- Compare performance of customer usage and feedback among all components of the Google business in real time.

- Quickly discover shortfalls before major problems arise.

Sources: Hamel, G. 2007. Break free. *Fortune,* October 1, 156(7): 119–126; Iyer, B. & Davenport, T. 2008. Reverse engineering Google's innovation machine. *Harvard Business Review,* April: 59–68; Pham, A. 2008. Google to end virtual world, Lively, launched by the Internet giant less than five months ago. *Los Angeles Times,* November 21: C3; and, Helft, M. 2009. Google ends sale of ads in papers after 2 years. *The New York Times,* January 21: B3.

- Become aware of unexpected successes that have often led to innovations.

- Discontinue failing products and services in a timely manner to save the company money.

These manager meetings return significant rewards for Google. Innovations that have been implemented as a result of high information control include:

- Gmail, an e-mail system that utilizes Google's core search features to help users organize and find e-mail messages easily.

- Google News, a computer-generated news site that aggregates headlines from more than 4,500 English-language news sources worldwide, groups similar stories together, and displays them according to each reader's personalized interests.

- Google AdSense, a service that matches ads to a website's content and audience and operates on a revenue-sharing business model.

Google managers are able to quickly analyze user feedback and revenue data to discontinue projects that are not working out as originally intended. This information control allows managers to reallocate resources to more promising projects in a timely manner.

- Google Lively, a virtual world simulation, was launched and shut down after five months in 2008 after management determined that the service was not competitive.

- Google Print Ads, Google's automated method of selling ads through auctions to the newspaper industry, was terminated in early 2009 when managers analyzed the data and determined that the revenue stream was negligible compared to the costs of the program.

---

to the organization about what is important. The dialogue and debate that emerge from such an interactive process can often lead to new strategies and innovations. Strategy Spotlight 9.2 discusses how executives at Google use an interactive control process.

>LO9.4

The benefits of having the proper balance among the three levers of behavioral control: culture; rewards and incentives; and, boundaries.

Attaining Behavioral Control: Balancing Culture, Rewards, and Boundaries

Behavioral control is focused on implementation—doing things right. Effectively implementing strategy requires manipulating three key control "levers": culture, rewards, and boundaries (see Exhibit 9.3). There are two compelling reasons for an increased emphasis on culture and rewards in a system of behavioral controls.[11]

First, the competitive environment is increasingly complex and unpredictable, demanding both flexibility and quick response to its challenges. As firms simultaneously downsize and face the need for increased coordination across organizational boundaries, a control system based primarily on rigid strategies, rules, and regulations is dysfunctional. The use of rewards and culture to align individual and organizational goals becomes increasingly important.

Second, the implicit long-term contract between the organization and its key employees has been eroded.[12] Today's younger managers have been conditioned to see themselves as "free agents" and view a career as a series of opportunistic challenges. As managers are advised to "specialize, market yourself, and have work, if not a job," the importance of culture and rewards in building organizational loyalty claims greater importance.

Each of the three levers—culture, rewards, and boundaries—must work in a balanced and consistent manner. Let's consider the role of each.

Building a Strong and Effective Culture

Organizational culture is a system of shared values (what is important) and beliefs (how things work) that shape a company's people, organizational structures, and control systems to produce behavioral norms (the way we do things around here).[13] How important is culture? Very. Over the years, numerous best sellers, such as *Theory Z, Corporate Cultures, In Search of Excellence,* and *Good to Great,*[14] have emphasized the powerful influence of culture on what goes on within organizations and how they perform.

Collins and Porras argued in *Built to Last* that the key factor in sustained exceptional performance is a cultlike culture.[15] You can't touch it or write it down, but it's there in every organization; its influence is pervasive; and it can work for you or against you.[16] Effective leaders understand its importance and strive to shape and use it as one of their important levers of strategic control.[17]

> **organizational culture** a system of shared values and beliefs that shape a company's people, organizational structures, and control systems to produce behavioral norms.

The Role of Culture Culture wears many different hats, each woven from the fabric of those values that sustain the organization's primary source of competitive advantage. Some examples are:

- DHL and Singapore Airlines focus on customer service.
- Lexus (a division of Toyota) and Hewlett-Packard emphasize product quality.
- Apple and 3M place a high value on innovation.
- Nucor (steel) and Toyota are concerned, above all, with operational efficiency.

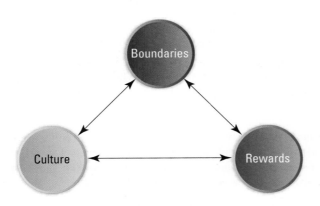

Exhibit 9.3 **Essential Elements of Behavioral Control**

Culture sets implicit boundaries—unwritten standards of acceptable behavior—in dress, ethical matters, and the way an organization conducts its business.[18] By creating a framework of shared values, culture encourages individual identification with the organization and its objectives. Culture acts as a means of reducing monitoring costs.[19]

Sustaining an Effective Culture   Powerful organizational cultures just don't happen overnight, and they don't remain in place without a strong commitment—both in terms of words and deeds—by leaders throughout the organization.[20] A viable and productive organizational culture can be strengthened and sustained. However, it cannot be "built" or "assembled"; instead, it must be cultivated, encouraged, and "fertilized."[21]

Storytelling is one way effective cultures are maintained. Many are familiar with the story of how Art Fry's failure to develop a strong adhesive led to 3M's enormously successful Post-it Notes. Perhaps less familiar is the story of Francis G. Okie.[22] In 1922 Okie came up with the idea of selling sandpaper to men as a replacement for razor blades. The idea obviously didn't pan out, but Okie was allowed to remain at 3M. Interestingly, the technology developed by Okie led 3M to develop its first blockbuster product: a waterproof sandpaper that became a staple of the automobile industry. Such stories foster the importance of risk taking, experimentation, freedom to fail, and innovation—all vital elements of 3M's culture.

Rallies or "pep talks" by top executives also serve to reinforce a firm's culture. The late Sam Walton was known for his pep rallies at local Walmart stores. Four times a year, the founders of Home Depot—former CEO Bernard Marcus and Arthur Blank—used to don orange aprons and stage Breakfast with Bernie and Arthur, a 6:30 a.m. pep rally, broadcast live over the firm's closed-circuit TV network to most of its 45,000 employees.[23]

In 2008, Ram Mynampati, interim CEO of Satyam Computer Services, a leading Indian company, also gave pep talks to his staff. The company's previous chairman admitted he had overstated the company's financial condition by more than $1 billion and resigned. When Mynampati took over the company, he addressed the company's situation in a letter he wrote to employees:

> Let us fight this battle together. I am confident that we will emerge stronger, together. We will be conducting "U Speak" (our Meet-the-Leadership sessions) in each city in India starting next week and will have numerous webinars to address associates in various countries. We will be meeting many of our customers in person over the next two weeks and will meet those of you on-site, at that time. In these sessions, we will explain to you what happened and articulate the actions that are being taken to retain your confidence in our company.[24]

Motivating with Rewards and Incentives

Reward and incentive systems represent a powerful means of influencing an organization's culture, focusing efforts on high-priority tasks, and motivating individual and collective task performance.[25] Just as culture deals with influencing beliefs, behaviors, and attitudes of people within an organization, the **reward system**—by specifying who gets rewarded and why—is an effective motivator and control mechanism.[26] Consider how Starbucks uses its stock option plan as an incentive to motivate its employees.[27] By introducing a stock option plan called "bean stock" to managers, baristas, and other employees, Starbucks has turned every employee into a partner. Starbucks' managers began referring to all employees as *partners,* an appropriate title because all staff, including part-timers working at least 20 hours per week, were eligible for stock options after six months with the company. By turning employees into partners, Starbucks gave them a chance to share in the success of the company and make the connection between their contributions and the company's market value very clear. There was a pronounced effect on the attitudes and performance of employees because of the bean stock program. They began coming up with many innovative ideas about how to cut costs, increase sales, and create value.

reward system
policies that specify who gets rewarded and why.

The Potential Downside   Generally speaking, people in organizations act rationally, each motivated by their personal best interest.[28] However, the collective sum of individual behaviors of an organization's employees does not always result in what is best for the organization; individual rationality is no guarantee of organizational rationality.

As corporations grow and evolve, they often develop different business units with multiple reward systems. They may differ based on industry contexts, business situations, stage of product life cycles, and so on. Subcultures within organizations may reflect differences among functional areas, products, services, and divisions. To the extent that reward systems reinforce such behavioral norms, attitudes, and belief systems, cohesiveness is reduced; important information is hoarded rather than shared, individuals begin working at cross-purposes, and they lose sight of overall goals.

Such conflicts are commonplace in many organizations. For example, sales and marketing personnel promise unrealistically quick delivery times to bring in business, much to the dismay of operations and logistics; overengineering by R&D creates headaches for manufacturing; and so on. Conflicts also arise across divisions when divisional profits become a key compensation criterion. As ill will and anger escalate, personal relationships and performance may suffer.

Creating Effective Reward and Incentive Programs To be effective, incentive and reward systems need to reinforce basic core values, enhance cohesion and commitment to goals and objectives, and meet with the organization's overall mission and purpose.[29]

At General Mills, to ensure a manager's interest in the overall performance of his or her unit, half of a manager's annual bonus is linked to business-unit results and half to individual performance.[30] For example, if a manager simply matches a rival manufacturer's performance, his or her salary is roughly 5 percent lower. However, if a manager's product ranks in the industry's top 10 percent in earnings growth and return on capital, the manager's total pay can rise to nearly 30 percent beyond the industry norm.

Effective reward and incentive systems share a number of common characteristics.[31] (see Exhibit 9.4). The perception that a plan is "fair and equitable" is critically important. The firm must have the flexibility to respond to changing requirements as its direction and objectives change. In recent years many companies have begun to place more emphasis on growth. Emerson Electric has shifted its emphasis from cost cutting to growth. To ensure that changes take hold, the management compensation formula has been changed from a largely bottom-line focus to one that emphasizes growth, new products, acquisitions, and international expansion. Discussions about profits are handled separately, and a culture of risk taking is encouraged.[32]

Setting Boundaries and Constraints

In an ideal world, a strong culture and effective rewards should be sufficient to ensure that all individuals and subunits work toward the common goals and objectives of the whole organization.[33] However, this is not usually the case. Counterproductive behavior can arise because of motivated self-interest, lack of a clear understanding of goals and objectives, or outright malfeasance. **Boundaries and constraints** can serve many useful purposes for organizations, including:

boundaries and constraints rules that specify behaviors that are acceptable and unacceptable.

- Objectives are clear, well understood, and broadly accepted.
- Rewards are clearly linked to performance and desired behaviors.
- Performance measures are clear and highly visible.
- Feedback is prompt, clear, and unambiguous.
- The compensation "system" is perceived as fair and equitable.
- The structure is flexible; it can adapt to changing circumstances.

Exhibit 9.4
Characteristics of Effective Reward and Evaluation Systems

- Focusing individual efforts on strategic priorities.
- Providing short-term objectives and action plans to channel efforts.
- Improving efficiency and effectiveness.
- Minimizing improper and unethical conduct.

Focusing Efforts on Strategic Priorities   Boundaries and constraints play a valuable role in focusing a company's strategic priorities. A well-known example of a strategic boundary is Jack Welch's (former CEO of General Electric) demand that any business in the corporate portfolio be ranked first or second in its industry. Similarly, Eli Lilly has reduced its research efforts to five broad areas of disease, down from eight or nine a decade ago.[34] This concentration of effort and resources provides the firm with greater strategic focus and the potential for stronger competitive advantages in the remaining areas.

Norman Augustine, Lockheed Martin's former chairman, provided four criteria for selecting candidates for diversification into "closely related" businesses.[35] They must (1) be high-tech, (2) be systems-oriented, (3) deal with large customers (either corporations or government) as opposed to consumers, and (4) be in growth businesses. Augustine said, "We have found that if we can meet most of those standards, then we can move into adjacent markets and grow."

Boundaries also have a place in the nonprofit sector. For example, a British relief organization uses a system to monitor strategic boundaries by maintaining a list of companies whose contributions it will neither solicit nor accept. Such boundaries are essential for maintaining legitimacy with existing and potential benefactors.

Providing Short-Term Objectives and Action Plans   In Chapter 1 we discussed the importance of a firm having a vision, mission, and strategic objectives that are internally consistent and that provide strategic direction. In addition, short-term objectives and action plans provide similar benefits. That is, they represent boundaries that help to allocate resources in an optimal manner and to channel the efforts of employees at all levels throughout the organization.[36] To be effective, short-term objectives must have several attributes. They should:

- Be specific and measurable.
- Include a specific time horizon for their attainment.
- Be achievable, yet challenging enough to motivate managers who must strive to accomplish them.

Research has found that performance is enhanced when individuals are encouraged to attain specific, difficult, yet achievable, goals (as opposed to vague "do your best" goals).[37]

Short-term objectives must provide proper direction and also provide enough flexibility for the firm to keep pace with and anticipate changes in the external environment, new government regulations, a competitor introducing a substitute product, or changes in consumer taste. Unexpected events within a firm may require a firm to make important adjustments in both strategic and short-term objectives. The emergence of new industries can have a drastic effect on the demand for products and services in more traditional industries.

Action plans are critical to the implementation of chosen strategies. Unless action plans are specific, there may be little assurance that managers have thought through all of the resource requirements for implementing their strategies. In addition, unless plans are specific, managers may not understand what needs to be implemented or have a clear time frame for completion. This is essential for the scheduling of key activities that must be implemented. Finally, individual managers must be held accountable for the implementation. This helps to provide the necessary motivation and "sense of ownership" to implement action plans on a timely basis. Strategy Spotlight 9.3 illustrates how action

Developing Meaningful Action Plans: Aircraft Interior Products, Inc.

MSA Aircraft Interior Products, Inc., is a manufacturing firm based in San Antonio, Texas, that was founded in 1983 by Mike Spraggins and Robert Plenge. The firm fills a small but highly profitable niche in the aviation industry with two key products. The Accordia line consists of patented, lightweight, self-contained window-shade assemblies. MSA's interior cabin shells are state-of-the-art assemblies that include window panels, side panels, headliners, and suspension system structures. MSA's products have been installed on a variety of aircraft, such as the Gulfstream series; the Cessna Citation; and Boeing's 727, 737, 757, and 707.

Much of MSA's success can be attributed to carefully articulated action plans consistent with the firm's mission and objectives. During the past five years, MSA has increased its sales at an annual rate of 15 to 18 percent. It has also succeeded in adding many prestigious companies to its customer base. Below are excerpts from MSA's mission statement and objectives as well as the action plans to achieve a 20 percent annual increase in sales.

Mission Statement

- Be recognized as an innovative and reliable supplier of quality interior products for the high-end, personalized transportation segments of the aviation, marine, and automotive industries.

- Design, develop, and manufacture interior fixtures and components that provide exceptional value to

Source: For purposes of confidentiality, some of the information presented in this spotlight has been disguised. We would like to thank company management and Joseph Picken, consultant, for providing us with the information used in this application.

the customer through the development of innovative designs in a manner that permits decorative design flexibility while retaining the superior functionality, reliability, and maintainability of well-engineered, factory-produced products.

- Grow, be profitable, and provide a fair return, commensurate with the degree of risk, for owners and stockholders.

Objectives

1. Achieve sustained and profitable growth over the next three years:
   - 20 percent annual growth in revenues.
   - 12 percent pretax profit margins.
   - 18 percent return on shareholder's equity.

2. Expand the company's revenues through the development and introduction of two or more new products capable of generating revenues in excess of $8 million a year by 2014.

3. Continue to aggressively expand market opportunities and applications for the Accordia line of window-shade assemblies, with the objective of sustaining or exceeding a 20 percent annual growth rate for at least the next three years.

Exhibit 9.5 details an "Action Plan" for Objective 3.

MSA's action plans are supported by detailed month-by-month budgets and strong financial incentives for its executives. Budgets are prepared by each individual department and include all revenue and cost items. Managers are motivated by their participation in a profit-sharing program, and the firm's two founders each receive a bonus equal to three percent of total sales.

	Description	Primary Responsibility	Target Date
1.	Develop and implement 2010 marketing plan, including specific plans for addressing Falcon 20 retrofit programs and expanded sales of cabin shells.	R. H. Plenge (V.P. Marketing)	December 15, 2011
2.	Negotiate new supplier agreement with Gulfstream Aerospace.	M. Spraggins (President)	March 1, 2012
3.	Continue and complete the development of the UltraSlim window and have a fully tested and documented design ready for production at a manufacturing cost of less than $900 per unit.	D. R. Pearson (V.P. Operations)	June 15, 2012
4.	Develop a window design suitable for L-1011 and similar wide-body aircraft and have a fully tested and documented design ready for production at a manufacturing cost comparable to the current Boeing window.	D. R. Pearson (V.P. Operations)	September 15, 2012

Exhibit 9.5   Action Plan for Objective Number 3

plans fit into the mission statement and objectives of a small manufacturer of aircraft interior components. Exhibit 9.5 provides details of an action plan to fulfill one of the firm's objectives.

Improving Operational Efficiency and Effectiveness Rule-based controls are most appropriate in organizations with the following characteristics:

- Environments are stable and predictable.
- Employees are largely unskilled and interchangeable.
- Consistency in product and service is critical.
- The risk of malfeasance is extremely high (e.g., in banking or casino operations).[38]

McDonald's Corp. has extensive rules and regulations that regulate the operation of its franchises.[39] Its policy manual states, "Cooks must turn, never flip, hamburgers. If they haven't been purchased, Big Macs must be discarded in 10 minutes after being cooked and French fries in 7 minutes. Cashiers must make eye contact with and smile at every customer."

Guidelines can also be effective in setting spending limits and the range of discretion for employees and managers, such as the $2,500 limit that hotelier Ritz-Carlton uses to empower employees to placate dissatisfied customers. Regulations also can be initiated to improve the use of an employee's time at work.[40] Computer Associates restricts the use of e-mail during the hours of 10 a.m. to noon and 2 p.m. to 4 p.m. each day.[41]

Minimizing Improper and Unethical Conduct Guidelines can be useful in specifying proper relationships with a company's customers and suppliers.[42] Many companies have explicit rules regarding commercial practices, including the prohibition of any form of payment, bribe, or kickback. Cadbury Schweppes has followed a simple but effective step in controlling the use of bribes by specifying that all payments, no matter how unusual, are recorded on the company's books. Its former chairman, Sir Adrian Cadbury, contended that such a practice causes managers to pause and consider whether a payment is simply a bribe or a necessary and standard cost of doing business.[43]

Regulations backed up with strong sanctions can also help an organization avoid conducting business in an unethical manner. After the passing of the Sarbanes-Oxley Act (which provides for stiffer penalties for financial reporting misdeeds), many chief financial officers (CFOs) have taken steps to ensure ethical behavior in the preparation of financial statements. For example, Home Depot's CFO, Carol B. Tome, strengthened the firm's code of ethics and developed stricter guidelines. Now all 25 of her subordinates must sign personal statements that all of their financial statements are correct—just as she and her CEO have to do now.[44]

● McDonald's relies on extensive rules and regulations to maintain efficient operations at its restaurants around the world.

Behavioral Control in Organizations: Situational Factors

Here, the focus is on ensuring that the behavior of individuals at all levels of an organization is directed toward achieving organizational goals and objectives. The three fundamental types of control are culture, rewards and incentives, and boundaries and constraints. An organization may pursue one or a combination of them on the basis of a variety of internal and external factors.

Not all organizations place the same emphasis on each type of control.[45] In high-technology firms engaged in basic research, members may work under high levels of autonomy. An individual's performance is generally quite difficult to measure accurately because of the long lead times involved in R&D activities. Thus, internalized norms and values become very important.

When the measurement of an individual's output or performance is quite straightforward, control depends primarily on granting or withholding rewards. Frequently, a sales manager's compensation is in the form of a commission and bonus tied directly to his or her sales volume, which is relatively easy to determine. Here, behavior is influenced more strongly by the attractiveness of the compensation than by the norms and values implicit in the organization's culture. The measurability of output precludes the need for an elaborate system of rules to control behavior.[46]

Control in bureaucratic organizations is dependent on members following a highly formalized set of rules and regulations. Most activities are routine and the desired behavior can be specified in a detailed manner because there is generally little need for innovative or creative activity. Managing an assembly plant requires strict adherence to many rules as well as exacting sequences of assembly operations. In the public sector, the Department of Motor Vehicles in most states must follow clearly prescribed procedures when issuing or renewing driver licenses.

Exhibit 9.6 provides alternate approaches to behavioral control and some of the situational factors associated with them.

Evolving from Boundaries to Rewards and Culture

In most environments, organizations should strive to provide a system of rewards and incentives, coupled with a culture strong enough that boundaries become internalized. This reduces the need for external controls such as rules and regulations.

First, hire the right people—individuals who already identify with the organization's dominant values and have attributes consistent with them. We addressed this issue in Chapter 4; recall the "Bozo Filter" developed by Cooper Software (page 170). Microsoft's David Pritchard is well aware of the consequences of failing to hire properly:

Exhibit 9.6
Organizational Control: Alternative Approaches

Approach	Some Situational Factors
Culture: A system of unwritten rules that forms an internalized influence over behavior.	• Often found in professional organizations. • Associated with high autonomy. • Norms are the basis for behavior.
Rules: Written and explicit guidelines that provide external constraints on behavior.	• Associated with standardized output. • Tasks are generally repetitive and routine. • Little need for innovation or creative activity.
Rewards: The use of performance-based incentive systems to motivate.	• Measurement of output and performance is rather straightforward. • Most appropriate in organizations pursuing unrelated diversification strategies. • Rewards may be used to reinforce other means of control.

If I hire a bunch of bozos, it will hurt us, because it takes time to get rid of them. They start infiltrating the organization and then they themselves start hiring people of lower quality. At Microsoft, we are always looking for people who are better than we are.

Second, training plays a key role. For example, in elite military units such as the Green Berets and Navy SEALs, the training regimen so thoroughly internalizes the culture that individuals, in effect, lose their identity. The group becomes the overriding concern and focal point of their energies. At firms such as DHL, training not only builds skills, but also plays a significant role in building a strong culture on the foundation of each organization's dominant values.

Third, managerial role models are vital. Andy Grove, former CEO and co-founder of Intel, didn't need (or want) a large number of bureaucratic rules to determine who was responsible for what, who was supposed to talk to whom, and who got to fly first class (no one). He encouraged openness by not having many of the trappings of success—he worked in a cubicle like all the other professionals. Can you imagine any new manager asking whether or not he can fly first class? Grove's personal example eliminated such a need.

Fourth, reward systems must be clearly aligned with the organizational goals and objectives. Where do you think rules and regulations are more important in controlling behavior—Home Depot, with its generous bonus and stock option plan, or Walmart, which does not provide the same level of rewards and incentives?

The Role of Corporate Governance

>LO9.5
The three key participants in corporate governance: shareholders, management (led by the CEO), and the board of directors.

corporate governance the relationship among various participants in determining the direction and performance of corporations. The primary participants are (1) the shareholders, (2) the management, and (3) the board of directors.

We now address the issue of strategic control in a broader perspective, typically referred to as "corporate governance." Here we focus on the need for both shareholders (the owners of the corporation) and their elected representatives, the board of directors, to actively ensure that management fulfills its overriding purpose of increasing long-term shareholder value.[47]

Robert Monks and Nell Minow, two leading scholars in **corporate governance,** define it as "the relationship among various participants in determining the direction and performance of corporations. The primary participants are (1) the shareholders, (2) the management (led by the CEO), and (3) the board of directors."* Our discussion will center on how corporations can succeed (or fail) in aligning managerial motives with the interests of the shareholders and their elected representatives, the board of directors.[48] As you will recall from Chapter 1, we discussed the important role of boards of directors and provided some examples of effective and ineffective boards.[49]

Good corporate governance plays an important role in the investment decisions of major institutions, and a premium is often reflected in the price of securities of companies that practice it. The corporate governance premium is larger for firms in countries with sound corporate governance practices compared to countries with weaker corporate governance standards.[50]

Sound governance practices often lead to superior financial performance. However, this is not always the case. For example, practices such as independent directors (directors who are not part of the firm's management) and stock options are generally assumed to result in

---

*Management cannot ignore the demands of other important firm stakeholders such as creditors, suppliers, customers, employees, and government regulators. In times of financial duress, powerful creditors can exert strong and legitimate pressures on managerial decisions. In general, however, the attention to stakeholders other than the owners of the corporation must be addressed in a manner that is still consistent with maximizing long-term shareholder returns. For a seminal discussion on stakeholder management, refer to Freeman, R. E. 1984. *Strategic management: A stakeholder approach.* Boston: Pitman.

The Relationship between Recommended Corporate Governance Practices and Firm Performance

A significant amount of research has examined the effect of corporate governance on firm performance. Some research has shown that implementing good corporate governance structures yields superior financial performance. Other research has not found a positive relationship between governance and performance. Results of a few of these studies are summarized below.

1. *A positive correlation between corporate governance and different measures of corporate performance.* Recent studies show that there is a strong positive correlation between effective corporate governance and different indicators of corporate performance such as growth, profitability, and customer satisfaction. Over a recent three-year period, the average return of large capitalized firms with the best governance practices was more than five times higher than the performance of firms in the bottom corporate governance quartile.

Sources: Dalton, D. R., Daily, C. M., Ellstrand, A. E., & Johnson, J. L., 1998. Meta-analytic reviews of board composition, leadership structure, and financial performance. *Strategic Management Journal*, 19(3): 269–290; Sanders, W. G. & Hambrick, D. C. 2007. Swinging for the fences: The effects of CEO stock options on company risk-taking and performance. *Academy of Management Journal*, 50(5): 1055–1078; Harris, J. & Bromiley, P. 2007. Incentives to cheat: The influence of executive compensation and firm performance on financial misrepresentation. *Organization Science*, 18(3): 350–367; Bauwhede, H. V. 2009. On the relation between corporate governance compliance and operating performance. *Accounting and Business Research*, 39(5): 497–513; Gill, A. 2001. Credit Lyonnais Securities (Asia). *Corporate governance in emerging markets: Saints and sinners*, April; and, Low, C. K. 2002. *Corporate governance: An Asia-Pacific critique*. Hong Kong: Sweet & Maxwell Asia.

2. *Compliance with international best practices leads to superior performance.* Studies of European companies show that greater compliance with international corporate governance best practices concerning board structure and function has significant and positive relationships with return on assets (ROA). In 10 of 11 Asian and Latin American markets, companies in the top corporate governance quartile for their respective regions averaged 10 percent greater return on capital employed (ROCE) than their peers. In a study of 12 emerging markets, companies in the lowest corporate governance quartile had a much lower ROCE than their peers.

3. *Many recommended corporate governance practices do not have a positive relationship with firm performance.* In contrast to these studies, there is also a body of research suggesting that corporate governance practices do not have a positive influence on firm performance. With corporate boards, there is no evidence that including more external directors on the board of directors of U.S. corporations has led to substantially higher firm performance. Also, giving more stock options to CEOs to align their interests with stakeholders may lead them to take high-risk bets in firm investments that have a low probability to improve firm performance. Rather than making good decisions, CEOs may "swing for the fences" with these high-risk investments. Additionally, motivating CEOs with large numbers of stock options appears to increase the likelihood of unethical accounting violations by the firm as the CEO tries to increase the firm's stock price.

ethics

---

better performance. But in many cases, independent directors may not have the necessary expertise or involvement, and the granting of stock options to the CEO may lead to decisions and actions calculated to prop up share price only in the short term. Strategy Spotlight 9.4 presents some research evidence on governance practices and firm performance.

At the same time, few topics in the business press are generating as much interest (and disdain!) as corporate governance.

Some recent notable examples of flawed corporate governance include:[51]

- Satyam Computer Services, a leading Indian outsourcing company that serves more than a third of the Fortune 500 companies, significantly inflated its earnings and assets for years. The chairman, Ramalinga Raju, resigned and admitted he had cooked the books. Raju said he had overstated cash on hand by $1 billion and inflated profits and revenues in the September 2008 quarter. Satyam shares sank 78 percent, and the benchmark Sensex index lost 7.3 percent that day (January 7, 2009).

- Former Brocade CEO Gregory Reyes was sentenced to 21 months in prison and fined $15 million for his involvement in backdating stock option grants. Reyes was the first executive to go on trial and be convicted over the improper dating of stock option awards, which dozens of companies have acknowledged since the practice came to light (January 17, 2008).
- In December 2010, Calisto Tanzi, founder and former chairman of Parmalat, one of Italy's largest companies, was sentenced to 10 years in prison for his involvement in an $18.5 billion fraud scandal that bankrupted the food giant in 2003. According to an independent auditor, Parmalat falsified its earnings reports for at least 13 years, losing almost $2.4 billion in that period and realizing only one profitable year. Tanzi took more than $1 billion from the company from 1990 to 2002, the period covered by the auditor's report.
- Bernard L. Madoff, a former stock broker, investment advisor, and nonexecutive chairman of the NASDAQ stock market, was sentenced to 150 years of prison in June 2009 for a massive Ponzi scheme that defrauded thousands of investors of billions of dollars. Madoff pleaded guilty to 11 felony counts and admitted to managing the largest Ponzi scheme in history and concealing it from federal authorities and investors for more than a decade.

Because of the many lapses in corporate governance, we can see the benefits associated with effective practices.[52] However, corporate managers may behave in their own self-interest, often to the detriment of shareholders. Next we address the implications of the separation of ownership and management in the modern corporation, and some mechanisms that can be used to ensure consistency (or alignment) between the interests of shareholders and those of the managers to minimize potential conflicts.

The Modern Corporation:
The Separation of Owners (Shareholders) and Management

Some of the proposed definitions for a *corporation* include:

- "The business corporation is an instrument through which capital is assembled for the activities of producing and distributing goods and services and making investments. Accordingly, a basic premise of corporation law is that a business corporation should have as its objective the conduct of such activities with a view to enhancing the corporation's profit and the gains of the corporation's owners, that is, the shareholders." (Melvin Aron Eisenberg, *The Structure of Corporation Law*)
- "A body of persons granted a charter legally recognizing them as a separate entity having its own rights, privileges, and liabilities distinct from those of its members." (*American Heritage Dictionary*)
- "An ingenious device for obtaining individual profit without individual responsibility." (Ambrose Bierce, *The Devil's Dictionary*)[53]

corporation a mechanism created to allow different parties to contribute capital, expertise, and labor for the maximum benefit of each party.

All of these definitions have some validity and each one reflects a key feature of the corporate form of business organization—its ability to draw resources from a variety of groups and establish and maintain its own persona that is separate from all of them. As Henry Ford once said, "A great business is really too big to be human."

Simply put, a **corporation** is a mechanism created to allow different parties to contribute capital, expertise, and labor for the maximum benefit of each party.[54] The shareholders (investors) are able to participate in the profits of the enterprise without taking direct responsibility for the operations. The management can run the company without the responsibility of personally providing the funds. The shareholders have limited liability as well as rather limited involvement in the company's affairs. However, they reserve the right to elect directors who have the fiduciary obligation to protect their interests.

Over 70 years ago, Columbia University professors Adolf Berle and Gardiner C. Means addressed the divergence of the interests of the owners of the corporation from the professional managers who are hired to run it. They warned that widely dispersed ownership "released management from the overriding requirement that it serve stockholders." The separation of ownership from management has given rise to a set of ideas called "agency theory." Central to agency theory is the relationship between two primary players—the *principals* who are the owners of the firm (stockholders) and the *agents,* who are the people paid by principals to perform a job on their behalf (management). The stockholders elect and are represented by a board of directors that has a fiduciary responsibility to ensure that management acts in the best interests of stockholders to ensure long-term financial returns for the firm.

Agency theory is concerned with resolving two problems that can occur in agency relationships.[55] *The first is the agency problem that arises (1) when the goals of the principals and agents conflict, and (2) when it is difficult or expensive for the principal to verify what the agent is actually doing.*[56] The board of directors would be unable to confirm that the managers were actually acting in the shareholders' interests because managers are "insiders" with regard to the businesses they operate and thus are better informed than the principals. Thus, managers may act "opportunistically" in pursuing their own interests—to the detriment of the corporation.[57] Managers may spend corporate funds on expensive perquisites (e.g., company jets and expensive art), devote time and resources to pet projects (initiatives in which they have a personal interest but that have limited market potential), engage in power struggles (where they may fight over resources for their own betterment and to the detriment of the firm), and negate (or sabotage) attractive merger offers because they may result in increased employment risk.[58]

The second issue is the problem of risk sharing. This arises when the principal and the agent have different attitudes and preferences toward risk. The executives in a firm may favor additional diversification initiatives because, by their very nature, they increase the size of the firm and thus the level of executive compensation.[59] At the same time, such diversification initiatives may erode shareholder value because they fail to achieve some synergies that we discussed in Chapter 6 (e.g., building on core competencies, sharing activities, or enhancing market power). Agents (executives) may have a stronger preference toward diversification than shareholders because it reduces their personal level of risk from potential loss of employment. Executives who have large holdings of stock in their firms are more likely to have diversification strategies that are more consistent with shareholder interests—increasing long-term returns.[60]

At times, top-level managers engage in actions that reflect their self-interest rather than the interests of shareholders. We provide two examples below:[61]

- Micky M. Arison is chief executive of Carnival, the big cruise line. He is also chief executive and owner of the Miami Heat of the National Basketball Association. Carnival paid the Heat $675,000 for sponsorship, advertising, and season tickets. Although that may be a rather small sum—given Carnival's $2.2 billion in net income for the period—we could still ask whether the money would have been spent on something else if Arison didn't own the team.
- In August 2011, Benjamin Koorbatoff, former CEO of Brink Energy Ltd. based in Calgary, Canada, was sent to prison for two years for misappropriating nearly $500,000 from the firm. He withdrew two bank drafts from a company account, made them out in his and his wife's name, then deposited them in a law firm's account for the purchase of a home. Also, he purchased a 1969 Chevrolet Camaro, worth nearly

agency theory
a theory of the relationship between principals and their agents, with emphasis on two problems: (1) the conflicting goals of principals and agents, along with the difficulty of principals to monitor the agents, and (2) the different attitudes and preferences toward risk of principals and agents.

$50,000 and made a loan for $100,000 from Brink to another employee to help him obtain a mortgage, with the loan to be secured by the employee's stock options.

Governance Mechanisms: Aligning the Interests of Owners and Managers

As noted above, a key characteristic of the modern corporation is the separation of ownership from control. To minimize the potential for managers to act in their own self-interest, or "opportunistically," the owners can implement some governance mechanisms.[62] First, there are two primary means of monitoring the behavior of managers. These include (1) a committed and involved *board of directors* that acts in the best interests of the shareholders to create long-term value and (2) *shareholder activism,* wherein the owners view themselves as share*owners* instead of share*holders* and become actively engaged in the governance of the corporation. Finally, there are managerial incentives, sometimes called "contract-based outcomes," which consist of *reward and compensation agreements.* Here the goal is to carefully craft managerial incentive packages to align the interests of management with those of the stockholders.[63]

We close this section with a brief discussion of one of the most controversial issues in corporate governance—duality. Here, the question becomes: Should the CEO also be chairperson of the board of directors? In many global Fortune 500 firms, the same individual serves in both roles. However, in recent years, we have seen a trend toward separating these two positions. The key issue is what implications CEO duality has for firm governance and performance.

A Committed and Involved Board of Directors   The **board of directors** acts as a fulcrum between the owners and controllers of a corporation. They are the intermediaries who provide a balance between a small group of key managers in the firm based at the corporate headquarters and a sometimes vast group of shareholders.[64] In the United States and other developed countries, the law imposes on the board a strict and absolute fiduciary duty to ensure that a company is run consistent with the long-term interests of the owners—the shareholders. The reality, as we have seen, is somewhat more ambiguous.[65]

The Business Roundtable, representing the largest U.S. corporations, describes the duties of the board as follows:

1. Select, regularly evaluate, and, if necessary, replace the CEO. Determine management compensation. Review succession planning.
2. Review and, where appropriate, approve the financial objectives, major strategies, and plans of the corporation.
3. Provide advice and counsel to top management.
4. Select and recommend to shareholders for election an appropriate slate of candidates for the board of directors; evaluate board processes and performance.
5. Review the adequacy of the systems to comply with all applicable laws/regulations.[66]

Given these principles, what makes for a good board of directors?[67] According to the Business Roundtable, the most important quality is a board of directors who are active, critical participants in determining a company's strategies.[68] That does not mean board members should micromanage or circumvent the CEO. Rather, they should provide strong oversight going beyond simply approving the CEO's plans. A board's primary responsibilities are to ensure that strategic plans undergo rigorous scrutiny, evaluate managers against high performance standards, and take control of the succession process.[69]

Although boards in the past were often dismissed as CEOs' rubber stamps, increasingly they are playing a more active role by forcing out CEOs who cannot deliver on performance.[70] According to the consulting firm Booz Allen Hamilton, the rate of CEO departures for performance reasons more than tripled, from 1.3 percent to 4.2 percent, between 1995 and 2002.[71] In August 2009, OC Oerlikon Corp., a Swiss textile machinery maker, fired Chief Executive Officer Uwe Krueger amid two years of losses and mounting debt.

The maker of spinning and embroidery machines was reeling from slumping demand for its equipment among cloth makers in Turkey, India, and China after consumer spending slowed and lenders stifled loans.[72]

Today's CEOs are not immune to termination. In September 2010, Jonathan Klein, the president of the CNN/U.S. cable channel, was fired because CNN's ratings had suffered.[73] Don Blankenship, CEO of coal mining giant Massey Energy, resigned in December 2010 after a deadly explosion in Massey's Upper Big Branch mine in West Virginia, a mine that had received numerous citations for safety violations in the last few years. The blast was the worst mining disaster in the United States in 40 years and resulted in criminal as well as civil investigations and lawsuits. Tony Hayward, CEO of oil and energy company British Petroleum (BP), was forced to step down in October 2010 after the Deepwater Horizon oil spill in the Gulf of Mexico led to an environmental disaster and a $20 billion recovery fund financed by BP.

Interestingly, CEO turnover declined during the recent financial crisis—going from 12.7 percent in 2007 to only 9.4 percent in 2010. One likely reason: Boards were reluctant to change leadership during the recession, concerned that if a CEO departed, investors might think that the company was coming unglued. However, with the economy recovering, Peter Crist, chairman of an executive search firm, predicts a return to double-digit turnover at big companies. He says, "We are going into a 24-month cycle of CEO volatility." "Deliver or depart" will clearly become a stronger message from boards.

Increasing CEO turnover could, however, pose a major problem for many organizations. Why? It appears that boards of directors are not typically engaged in effective succession planning. For example, only 35 percent of 1,318 executives surveyed by Korn/Ferry International in December 2010 said their companies had a succession plan. And 61 percent of respondents to a survey (conducted by Heidrick & Struggles and Stanford University's Rock Center for Corporate Governance) claimed their companies had *no* viable internal candidates.

Another key component of top-ranked boards is director independence.[74] Governance experts believe that a majority of directors should be free of all ties to either the CEO or the company.[75] That means a minimum of "insiders" (past or present members of the management team) should serve on the board, and that directors and their firms should be barred from doing consulting, legal, or other work for the company.[76] Interlocking directorships—in which CEOs and other top managers serve on each other's boards—are not desirable. But perhaps the best guarantee that directors act in the best interests of shareholders is the simplest: Most good companies now insist that directors own significant stock in the company they oversee.[77]

Such guidelines are not always followed. At times, the practices of the boards of directors are the antithesis of such guidelines. Consider Walt Disney Co. Over a five-year period, former CEO Michael Eisner pocketed an astonishing $531 million. He likely had very little resistance from his board of directors:

> Many investors view the Disney board as an anachronism. Among Disney's 16 directors is Eisner's personal attorney—who for several years was chairman of the company's compensation committee! There was also the architect who designed Eisner's Aspen home and his parents' apartment. Joining them are the principal of an elementary school once attended by his children and the president of a university to which Eisner donated $1 million. The board also includes the actor Sidney Poitier, seven current and former Disney executives, and an attorney who does business with Disney. Moreover, most of the outside directors own little or no Disney stock. "It is an egregiously bad board—a train wreck waiting to happen," warns Michael L. Useem, a management professor at the University of Pennsylvania's Wharton School.[78]

This example also shows that "outside directors" are only beneficial to strong corporate governance if they are vigilant in carrying out their responsibilities.[79] As humorously suggested by Warren Buffett, founder and chairman of Berkshire Hathaway: "The ratcheting up of compensation has been obscene. . . . There is a tendency to put cocker spaniels on compensation committees, not Doberman pinschers."[80]

Many firms do have exemplary board practices. Below we list some of the excellent practices at Intel Corp., the world's largest semiconductor chip manufacturer, with $35 billion in revenues:[81]

- **_Mix of inside and outside directors._** The board believes that there should be a majority of independent directors on the board. However, the board is willing to have members of management, in addition to the CEO, as directors.
- **_Board presentations and access to employees._** The board encourages management to schedule managers to be present at meetings who: (1) can provide additional insight into the items being discussed because of personal involvement in these areas, or (2) have future potential that management believes should be given exposure to the board.
- **_Formal evaluation of officers._** The Compensation Committee conducts, and reviews with the outside directors, an annual evaluation to help determine the salary and executive bonus of all officers, including the chief executive officer.

Exhibit 9.7 shows how boards of directors can improve their practices.

Shareholder Activism As a practical matter, there are so many owners of the largest American corporations that it makes little sense to refer to them as "owners" in the sense of

Exhibit 9.7 Best Practice Ideas: The New Rules for Directors

Issue	Suggestion
Pay	**Know the Math**
Companies will disclose full details of CEO payouts. Activist investors are already drawing up hit lists of companies where CEO paychecks are out of line with performance.	Before okaying any financial package, directors must make sure they can explain the numbers. They need to adopt the mindset of an activist investor and ask: What's the harshest criticism someone could make about this package?
Strategy	**Make It a Priority**
Boards have been so focused on compliance that duties like strategy and leadership oversight too often get ignored. Only 59 percent of directors in a recent study rated their board favorably on setting strategy.	To avoid spending too much time on compliance issues, move strategy up to the beginning of the meeting. Annual one-, two- or three-day offsite meetings on strategy alone are becoming standard for good boards.
Financials	**Put in the Time**
Although 95 percent of directors in the recent study said they were doing a good job of monitoring financials, the number of earnings restatements hit a new high in 2006, after breaking records in 2004 and 2005.	Even nonfinancial board members need to monitor the numbers and keep a close eye on cash flows. Audit committee members should prepare to spend 300 hours a year on committee responsibilities.
Crisis Management	**Dig in**
Some 120 companies are under scrutiny for options backdating, and the 100 largest companies have replaced 56 CEOs in the past five years—nearly double the terminations in the prior five years.	The increased scrutiny on boards means that a perfunctory review will not suffice if a scandal strikes. Directors can no longer afford to defer to management in a crisis. They must roll up their sleeves and move into watchdog mode.

Source: From Byrnes, N. & Sassen, J. 2007. Board of hard knocks: *BusinessWeek*, January 22, 36–39. Used with permission of *Bloomberg BusinessWeek*. Copyright © 2007. All rights reserved.

individuals becoming informed and involved in corporate affairs.[82] However, even an individual shareholder has several rights, including (1) the right to sell the stock, (2) the right to vote the proxy (which includes the election of board members), (3) the right to bring suit for damages if the corporation's directors or managers fail to meet their obligations, (4) the right to certain information from the company, and (5) certain residual rights following the company's liquidation (or its filing for reorganization under bankruptcy laws), once creditors and other claimants are paid off.[83]

Collectively, shareholders have the power to direct the course of corporations.[84] This may involve acts such as being party to shareholder action suits and demanding that key issues be brought up for proxy votes at annual board meetings.[85] The power of shareholders has intensified in recent years because of the increasing influence of large institutional investors such as mutual funds (e.g., T. Rowe Price and Fidelity Investments) and retirement systems such as TIAA-CREF (for university faculty members and school administrative staff).[86] Institutional investors hold approximately 50 percent of all listed corporate stock in the United States.[87]

Shareholder activism refers to actions by large shareholders, both institutions and individuals, to protect their interests when they feel that managerial actions diverge from shareholder value maximization.

shareholder activism actions by large shareholders to protect their interests when they feel that managerial actions of a corporation diverge from shareholder value maximization.

Many institutional investors are aggressive in protecting and enhancing their investments. They are shifting from traders to owners. They are assuming the role of permanent shareholders and rigorously analyzing issues of corporate governance. In the process they are reinventing systems of corporate monitoring and accountability.[88]

Consider the proactive behavior of CalPERS, the California Public Employees' Retirement System, which manages over $200 billion in assets and is the third largest pension fund in the world. Every year CalPERS reviews the performance of U.S. companies in its stock portfolio and identifies those that are among the lowest long-term relative performers and have governance structures that do not ensure full accountability to company owners. This generates a long list of companies, each of which may potentially be publicly identified as a CalPERS "Focus Company"—corporations to which CalPERS directs specific suggested governance reforms. CalPERS meets with the directors of each of these companies to discuss performance and governance issues. The CalPERS Focus List contains those companies that continue to merit public and market attention at the end of the process.

The 2009 CalPERS Focus List named four companies for poor economic and governance practices: *Eli Lilly* of Indianapolis, Indiana; *Hill-Rom Holdings* of Batesville, Indiana; *Hospitality Properties Trust* of Newton, Massachusetts; and *IMS Health* of Norwalk, Connecticut.[89] In addition to the four firms performing below their peer group for the past five years, CalPERS has expressed the following specific concerns about these firms:

- Eli Lilly, the big drug manufacturer, continues to deny shareowners any opportunity to amend bylaws.
- Hill-Rom Holdings, a medical technology provider, refuses to remove its staggered board structure and to allow shareowners to amend its bylaws.
- Hospitality Properties Trust, a real estate investment fund in hotels and trade centers, refuses to terminate its "classified" board, where directors serve staggered terms rather than standing for election each year.
- IMS Health, a provider of intelligence to the pharmaceutical and health care industries, denies the right of shareowners to call a special meeting or act by written consent and to adopt annual nonbinding advisory votes on executive compensation practices.

While appearing punitive to company management, such aggressive activism has paid significant returns for CalPERS (and other stockholders of the "Focused" companies). A Wilshire Associates study of the "CalPERS Effect" of corporate governance examined the performance of 62 targets over a five-year period: While the stock of these companies trailed the Standard & Poor's Index by 89 percent in the five-year period before CalPERS acted, the same stocks outperformed the index by 23 percent in the following five years, adding approximately $150 million annually in additional returns to the fund.

Perhaps no discussion of shareholder activism would be complete without mention of Carl Icahn, a famed activist with a personal net worth of about $13 billion:

> The bogeyman I am now chasing is the structure of American corporations, which permit managements and boards to rule arbitrarily and too often receive egregious compensation even after doing a subpar job. Yet they remain accountable to no one.[90]

Managerial Rewards and Incentives   As we discussed earlier in the chapter, incentive systems must be designed to help a company achieve its goals.[91] From the perspective of governance, one of the most critical roles of the board of directors is to create incentives that align the interests of the CEO and top executives with the interests of owners of the corporation—long-term shareholder returns.[92] Shareholders rely on CEOs to adopt policies and strategies that maximize the value of their shares.[93] A combination of three basic policies may create the right monetary incentives for CEOs to maximize the value of their companies:[94]

1. Boards can require that the CEOs become substantial owners of company stock.
2. Salaries, bonuses, and stock options can be structured so as to provide rewards for superior performance and penalties for poor performance.
3. Threat of dismissal for poor performance can be a realistic outcome.

In recent years the granting of stock options has enabled top executives of publicly held corporations to earn enormous levels of compensation. In 2007, the average CEO in the Standard & Poor's 500 stock index took home 433 times the pay of the average worker—up from 40 times the average in 1980. The counterargument, that the ratio is down from the 514 multiple in 2000, doesn't get much traction.[95] It has been estimated that there could be as many as 50 or more companies with CEO pay packages over $150 million.[96]

Many boards have awarded huge option grants despite poor executive performance, and others have made performance goals easier to reach. In 2002 nearly 200 companies swapped or repriced options—all to enrich wealthy executives who are already among the country's richest people. However, stock options can be a valuable governance mechanism to align the CEO's interests with those of the shareholders. The extraordinarily high level of compensation can, at times, be grounded in sound governance principles.[97] For example, Howard Solomon, CEO of Forest Laboratories, received total compensation of $148.5 million in 2001.[98] This represented $823,000 in salary, $400,000 in bonus, and $147.3 million in stock options that were exercised. However, shareholders also did well, receiving gains of 40 percent. The firm has enjoyed spectacular growth over the past 10 years, and Solomon has been CEO since 1977. Thus, huge income is attributed largely to gains that have built up over many years. As stated by compensation committee member Dan Goldwasser, "If a CEO is delivering substantial increases in shareholder value, . . . it's only appropriate that he be rewarded for it."

However, the "pay for performance" principle doesn't always hold.[99] In addition to the granting of stock options, boards of directors are often failing to fulfill their fiduciary responsibilities to shareholders when they lower the performance targets that executives need to meet in order to receive millions of dollars. At Ford, for example, its "profit" goal for 2007 was to *lose* $4.9 billion. Ford beat the target, however, and lost *only* $3.9 billion. CEO Alan Mulally was rewarded $12 million in compensation, including a $7 million bonus for exceeding the profit goal. Ford's stock price fell 10 percent in 2007.

TIAA-CREF has provided several principles of corporate governance with regard to executive compensation (see Exhibit 9.8).[100] These include the importance of aligning the rewards of all employees—rank and file as well as executives—to the long-term performance of the corporation; general guidelines on the role of cash compensation, stock, and "fringe benefits"; and the mission of a corporation's compensation committee.[101]

Exhibit 9.8
TIAA-CREF's Principles
on the Role of Stock in
Executive Compensation

Stock-based compensation plans are a critical element of most compensation programs and can provide opportunities for managers whose efforts contribute to the creation of shareholder wealth. In evaluating the suitability of these plans, considerations of reasonableness, scale, linkage to performance, and fairness to shareholders and all employees also apply. TIAA-CREF, the largest pension system in the world, has set forth the following guidelines for stock-based compensation. Proper stock-based plans should:

- Allow for creation of executive wealth that is reasonable in view of the creation of shareholder wealth. Management should not prosper through stock while shareholders suffer.

- Have measurable and predictable outcomes that are directly linked to the company's performance.

- Be market oriented, within levels of comparability for similar positions in companies of similar size and business focus.

- Be straightforward and clearly described so that investors and employees can understand them.

- Be fully disclosed to the investing public and be approved by shareholders.

Source: *www.tiaa-cref.org/pubs.*

CEO Duality: Is It Good or Bad?

CEO duality is one of the most controversial issues in corporate governance. It refers to the dual leadership structure where the CEO acts simultaneously as the chair of the board of directors.[102] Scholars, consultants, and executives who are interested in determining the best way to manage a corporation are divided on the issue of the roles and responsibilities of a CEO. Two schools of thought represent the alternative positions:

Unity of Command   Advocates of the unity of command perspective believe when one person holds both roles, he or she is able to act more efficiently and effectively. CEO duality provides firms with a clear focus on both objectives and operations as well as eliminates confusion and conflict between the CEO and the chair. Thus, it enables smoother, more effective strategic decision making. Holding dual roles as CEO/chair creates unity across a company's managers and board of directors and ultimately allows the CEO to serve the shareholders even better. Having leadership focused in a single individual also enhances a firm's responsiveness and ability to secure critical resources. This perspective maintains that separating the two jobs—that of a CEO and that of the chairperson of the board of directors—may produce all types of undesirable consequences. CEOs may find it harder to make quick decisions. Ego-driven chief executives and chairs may squabble over who is ultimately in charge. The shortage of first-class business talent may mean that bosses find themselves second-guessed by people who know little about the business.[103] Companies like Coca-Cola, JPMorgan Chase, and Time Warner have refused to divide the CEO's and chairperson's jobs and support this duality structure.

Agency Theory   Supporters of agency theory argue that the positions of CEO and chair should be separate. The case for separation is based on the simple principle of the separation of power. How can boards discharge their basic duty—monitoring the boss—if the boss is chairing its meetings and setting its agenda? How can a board act as a safeguard against corruption or incompetence when the possible source of that corruption and incompetence is sitting at the head of the table? CEO duality can create a conflict of interest that could negatively affect the interests of the shareholders.

Duality also complicates the issue of CEO succession. In some cases, a CEO/chairperson may choose to retire as CEO but keep his or her role as the chair. Although this splits up the roles, which appeases an agency perspective, it nonetheless puts the new CEO in a difficult position. The chair is bound to question some of the new changes put in place, and the board as a whole might take sides with the chairperson they trust and with whom they have a history. This conflict of interest would make it difficult for the new CEO to institute any changes, as the power and influence would still remain with the former CEO.[104]

Duality also serves to reinforce popular doubts about the legitimacy of the system as a whole and evokes images of bosses writing their own performance reviews and setting their own salaries. One of the first things that some of America's troubled banks, including Citigroup, Washington Mutual, Wachovia, and Wells Fargo, did when the financial crisis hit in 2007–2008 was to separate the two jobs. Firms like Siebel Systems, Disney, Oracle, and Microsoft have also decided to divide the roles between CEO and chairperson and eliminate duality.

The increasing pressures for effective corporate governance have led to a sharp decline in duality. Firms now routinely separate the jobs of chair and chief executive. For example, in 2009, fewer than 12 percent of incoming CEOs were also made chair—compared with 48 percent in 2002.

These same pressures have led to other changes in corporate governance practices. For example, the New York Stock Exchange and NASDAQ have demanded that companies should have a majority of independent directors. Also, CEOs are held accountable for their performance and tossed out if they fail to perform, with the average length of tenure dropping from 8.1 years in 2000 to 6.3 years in 2009. Finally, more than 90 percent of S&P 500 companies with CEOs who also serve as chair of the board have appointed "lead" or "presiding" directors to act as a counterweight to a combined chairperson and chief executive.

External Governance Control Mechanisms

Thus far, we've discussed internal governance mechanisms. Internal controls, however, are not always enough to ensure good governance. The separation of ownership and control that we discussed earlier requires multiple control mechanisms, some internal and some external, to ensure that managerial actions lead to shareholder value maximization. Further, society-at-large wants some assurance that this goal is met without harming other stakeholder groups. Now we discuss several **external governance control mechanisms** that have developed in most modern economies. These include the market for corporate control, auditors, banks and analysts, governmental regulatory bodies, media, and public activists.

external governance control mechanisms
methods that ensure that managerial actions lead to shareholder value maximization and do not harm other stakeholder groups that are outside the control of the corporate governance system.

The Market for Corporate Control Let us assume for a moment that internal control mechanisms in a company are failing. This means that the board is ineffective in monitoring managers and is not exercising the oversight required of it and that shareholders are passive and are not taking any actions to monitor or discipline managers. Under these circumstances managers may behave opportunistically.[105] Opportunistic behavior can take many forms. First, they can *shirk* their responsibilities. Shirking means that managers fail to exert themselves fully, as is required of them. Second, they can engage in *on-the-job consumption.* Examples of on-the-job consumption include private jets, club memberships, expensive artwork in the offices, and so on. Each of these represents consumption by managers that does not in any way increase shareholder value. Instead, they actually diminish shareholder value. Third, managers may engage in *excessive product-market diversification.*[106] As we discussed in Chapter 6, such diversification serves to reduce only the employment risk of the managers rather than the financial risk of the shareholders, who can more cheaply diversify their risk by owning a portfolio of investments. Is there any external mechanism to stop managers from shirking, consumption on the job, and excessive diversification?

The **market for corporate control** is one external mechanism that provides at least some partial solution to the problems described. If internal control mechanisms fail and the management is behaving opportunistically, the likely response of most shareholders will be to sell their stock rather than engage in activism.[107] As more stockholders vote with their feet, the value of the stock begins to decline. As the decline continues, at some point the market value of the firm becomes less than the book value. A corporate raider can take over the company for a price less than the book value of the assets of the company. The first thing that the raider may do on assuming control over the company will be to fire the underperforming management. The risk of being acquired by a hostile raider is often referred to as the **takeover constraint.** The takeover constraint deters management from engaging in opportunistic behavior.[108]

<aside>
market for corporate control an external control mechanism in which shareholders dissatisfied with a firm's management sell their shares.
</aside>

Although in theory the takeover constraint is supposed to limit managerial opportunism, in recent years its effectiveness has become diluted as a result of a number of defense tactics adopted by incumbent management (see Chapter 6). Foremost among them are poison pills, greenmail, and golden parachutes. Poison pills are provisions adopted by the company to reduce its worth to the acquirer. An example would be payment of a huge one-time dividend, typically financed by debt. Greenmail involves buying back the stock from the acquirer, usually at an attractive premium. Golden parachutes are employment contracts that cause the company to pay lucrative severance packages to top managers fired as a result of a takeover, often running to several million dollars.

<aside>
takeover constraint the risk to management of the firm being acquired by a hostile raider.
</aside>

Auditors Even when there are stringent disclosure requirements, there is no guarantee that the information disclosed will be accurate. Managers may deliberately disclose false information or withhold negative financial information as well as use accounting methods that distort results based on highly subjective interpretations. Therefore, all accounting statements are required to be audited and certified to be accurate by external auditors. These auditing firms are independent organizations staffed by certified professionals who verify the firm's books of accounts. Audits can unearth financial irregularities and ensure that financial reporting by the firm conforms to standard accounting practices.

Recent developments leading to the bankruptcy of firms such as Enron and WorldCom and a spate of earnings restatements raise questions about the failure of the auditing firms to act as effective external control mechanisms. Why did an auditing firm like Arthur Andersen, with decades of good reputation in the auditing profession at stake, fail to raise red flags about accounting irregularities? First, auditors are appointed by the firm being audited. The desire to continue that business relationship sometimes makes them overlook financial irregularities. Second, most auditing firms also do consulting work and often have lucrative consulting contracts with the firms that they audit. Understandably, some of them tend not to ask too many difficult questions, because they fear jeopardizing the consulting business, which is often more profitable than the auditing work.

The restatement of earnings by Xerox is an example of the lack of independence of auditing firms. The SEC filed a lawsuit against KPMG, the world's third largest accounting firm, in January 2003 for allowing Xerox to inflate its revenues by $3 billion between 1997 and 2000. Of the $82 million that Xerox paid KPMG during those four years, only $26 million was for auditing. The rest was for consulting services. When one of the auditors objected to Xerox's practice of booking revenues for equipment leases earlier than it should have, Xerox asked KPMG to replace him. It did.[109]

Banks and Analysts Commercial and investment banks have lent money to corporations and therefore have to ensure that the borrowing firm's finances are in order and that the loan covenants are being followed. Stock analysts conduct ongoing in-depth studies of the firms that they follow and make recommendations to their clients to buy, hold, or sell. Their rewards and reputation depend on the quality of these recommendations. Their access to information, knowledge of the industry and the firm, and the insights they gain from interactions with the management of the company enable them to alert the investing community of both positive and negative developments relating to a company.

It is generally observed that analyst recommendations are often more optimistic than warranted by facts. "Sell" recommendations tend to be exceptions rather than the norm. Many analysts failed to grasp the gravity of the problems surrounding failed companies such as Parmalat and Enron till the very end. Part of the explanation may lie in the fact that most analysts work for firms that also have investment banking relationships with the companies they follow. Negative recommendations by analysts can displease the management, who may decide to take their investment banking business to a rival firm. Otherwise independent and competent analysts may be pressured to overlook negative information or tone down their criticism. A settlement between the Securities and Exchange Commission and the New York State Attorney General with 10 banks required them to pay $1.4 billion in penalties and to fund independent research for investors.[110]

Regulatory Bodies   The extent of government regulation is often a function of the type of industry. Banks, utilities, and pharmaceuticals are subject to more regulatory oversight because of their importance to society. Public corporations are subject to more regulatory requirements than private corporations.[111]

All public corporations are required by bodies such as the Securities and Exchange Commission to disclose a substantial amount of financial information. These include quarterly and annual filings of financial performance, stock trading by insiders, and details of executive compensation packages. There are two primary reasons behind such requirements. First, markets can operate efficiently only when the investing public has faith in the market system. In the absence of disclosure requirements, the average investor suffers from a lack of reliable information and therefore may completely stay away from the capital market. This will negatively impact an economy's ability to grow. Second, disclosure of information such as insider trading protects the small investor to some extent from the negative consequences of information asymmetry. The insiders and large investors typically have more information than the small investor and can therefore use that information to buy or sell before the information becomes public knowledge.

The failure of a variety of external control mechanisms led the U.S. Congress to pass the Sarbanes-Oxley Act in 2002. This act calls for many stringent measures that would ensure better governance of U.S. corporations. Some of these measures include:[112]

- *Auditors* are barred from certain types of nonaudit work. They are not allowed to destroy records for five years. Lead partners auditing a client should be changed at least every five years.
- *CEOs* and *CFOs* must fully reveal off-balance-sheet finances and vouch for the accuracy of the information revealed.
- *Executives* must promptly reveal the sale of shares in firms they manage and are not allowed to sell when other employees cannot.
- *Corporate lawyers* must report to senior managers any violations of securities law lower down.

Strategy Spotlight 9.5 addresses one of the increased expenses that many companies now face in complying with the Sarbanes-Oxley Act—higher compensation for more involved and committed directors.

Media and Public Activists   The press is not usually recognized as an external control mechanism in the literature on corporate governance. There is no denying that in all developed capitalist economies, the financial press and media play an important indirect role in monitoring the management of public corporations. In the UK, business magazines such as *The Economist* and *Euromoney,* financial newspapers such as

The Impact of the 2002 Sarbanes-Oxley Act on Corporate Directors

The cost of outside directors has been rising. Not only are well-qualified directors in short supply but also the Sarbanes-Oxley Act has increased the demands of the job. According to compensation consultants Pearl Meyer & Partners, the typical director of a large corporation earned $216,000 in 2009, up from $129,667 in 2003. For some, total compensation, including cash payments, stock grants, and other perks, has climbed above seven figures. Even during the recession of 2008–2009, corporate directors' paychecks seemed to be soaring. For example, in 2008 Anthony P. Terracciano made $4.8 million as the chairman of student loan giant SLM and Jack P. Randall made $1.5 million from XTO Energy, an oil and natural gas producing company.

Directors can thank the Sarbanes-Oxley Act for the continuing generosity. The act was created to protect shareholders by restricting the power of corporate executives. In the past, many boards had become little more than rubber stamps for everything from merger strategy to executive compensation. This led to disaster in cases such as Enron, WorldCom, and Tyco. Sarbanes-Oxley and other regulatory efforts sought to protect shareholders by empowering directors and making them more accountable.

Following the Sarbanes-Oxley Act, there were several years of 20 percent to 30 percent annual increases as director compensation rose to reflect the new realities of expanded responsibilities for directors as well as the increased demand for directors who met independence rules. The pay increases came at a time when the supply of new directors was declining due to the additional risks—real or perceived—of serving as a director.

One consequence of Sarbanes-Oxley is that many directors work harder. A decade ago a typical director attended four board meetings a year and spent about 100 hours a year on board tasks, according to the National Association of Corporate Directors. Now, directors attend an average of six board meetings a year, spend an average of 225 hours a year on board duties, and convene at other times for committee meetings. In fact, corporate directors can log as many as 400 hours a year when corporations are financially distressed or reorganizing.

Sources: Byrnes, N. 2010. The gold-plated boardroom. *Bloomberg Businessweek.* February 22: 72–73; and, Hilburn, W. 2010. Trends in director compensation. *www.businessweek.com.* October 19: np.

The Financial Times and *The Guardian,* as well as television networks like the BBC are constantly reporting on companies. Public perceptions about a company's financial prospects and the quality of its management are greatly influenced by the media. Food Lion's reputation was sullied when ABC's *Prime Time Live* in 1992 charged the company with employee exploitation, false package dating, and unsanitary meat handling practices. Bethany McLean of *Fortune* magazine is often credited as the first to raise questions about Enron's long-term financial viability.[113]

Similarly, consumer groups and activist individuals often take a crusading role in exposing corporate malfeasance.[114] Well-known examples include Ralph Nader and Erin Brockovich, who played important roles in bringing to light the safety issues related to GM's Corvair and environmental pollution issues concerning Pacific Gas and Electric Company, respectively. Ralph Nader has created over 30 watchdog groups, including:[115]

- *Aviation Consumer Action Project.* Works to propose new rules to prevent flight delays, impose penalties for deceiving passengers about problems, and push for higher compensation for lost luggage.
- *Center for Auto Safety.* Helps consumers find plaintiff lawyers and agitate for vehicle recalls, increased highway safety standards, and lemon laws.
- *Center for Study of Responsive Law.* This is Nader's headquarters. Home of a consumer project on technology, this group sponsored seminars on Microsoft remedies and pushed for tougher Internet privacy rules. It also took on the drug industry over costs.
- *Pension Rights Center.* This center helped employees of IBM, General Electric, and other companies to organize themselves against cash-balance pension plans.

Two Examples of Powerful External Control Mechanisms

McDonald's

After years of fending off and ignoring critics, McDonald's has begun working with them. In 1999, People for the Ethical Treatment of Animals (PETA) launched its "McCruelty" campaign asking the company to take steps to alleviate the suffering of animals killed for its restaurants. Since then, PETA has switched tactics and is cooperating with the burger chain to modernize the company's animal welfare standards and make further improvements. Following pressure from PETA, McDonald's used its influence to force egg suppliers to improve the living conditions of hens and cease debeaking them. PETA has publicly lauded the company for its efforts. Recently, McDonald's also has required beef and pork processors to improve their handling of livestock prior to slaughter. The company conducts regular audits of the packing plants to determine whether the animals are being treated humanely and will suspend purchases from slaughterhouses that don't meet the company's standards. The company's overall image appears to have improved. According to the global consulting firm Reputation Institute, McDonald's score, on a scale of 100, has climbed 8 points to 63 since 2007—a dramatic improvement.

Sources: Kiley, D. & Helm, B. 2009. The great trust offensive. *Bloomberg Businessweek.* September 28: 38–42; Brasher, P. 2010. McDonald's orders improvements in treatment of hens. *abcnews.com.* August 23: np; Glover, K. 2009. PETA vs. McDonald's: The nicest way to kill a chicken. *www.bnet.com.* February 20: np; *www.mccruelty.com;* Greenhouse, S. 2010. Pressured, Nike to help workers in Honduras. *The New York Times,* July 27: B1; Padgett, T. 2010. Just pay it: Nike creates fund for Honduran workers. *www.time.com.* July 27: np; and, Bustillo, M. 2010. Nike to pay some $2 million to workers fired by subcontractors. *www.online.wsj.com.* July 26: np.

Nike

In January 2009, 1,800 laborers lost their jobs in Honduras when two local factories that made shirts for the U.S. sports-apparel giant Nike suddenly closed their doors and did not pay workers the $2 million in severance and other unemployment benefits they were due by law. Following pressure from U.S. universities and student groups, Nike announced that it was setting up a $1.5 million "workers' relief fund" to assist the workers. Nike also agreed to provide vocational training and finance health coverage for workers laid off by the two subcontractors.

The relief fund from Nike came after pressure by groups such as the Worker Rights Consortium, which informed Nike customers of the treatment of the workers. The Worker Rights Consortium also convinced scores of U.S. universities whose athletic programs and campus shops buy Nike shoes and clothes to threaten cancellation of those lucrative contracts unless Nike did something to address the plight of the Honduran workers. Another labor watchdog, United Students Against Sweatshops, staged demonstrations outside Nike shops while chanting "Just Pay It," a play on Nike's commercial slogan, "Just Do It." The University of Wisconsin cancelled its licensing agreement with the company over the matter, and other schools, including Cornell University and the University of Washington, indicated they were thinking of following suit. The agreement is the latest involving overseas apparel factories in which an image-conscious brand like Nike responded to campaigns led by college students, who often pressure universities to stand up to producers of college-logo apparel when workers' rights are threatened.

As we have noted above, some public activists and watchdog groups can exert a strong force on organizations and influence decisions that they may make. Strategy Spotlight 9.6 provides two examples of this phenomenon.

Corporate Governance: An International Perspective

The topic of corporate governance has long been dominated by agency theory and based on the explicit assumption of the separation of ownership and control.[116] The central conflicts are principal–agent conflicts between shareholders and management. However, such an underlying assumption seldom applies outside the United States and the United Kingdom. This is particularly true in emerging economies and continental Europe. Here, there is often concentrated ownership, along with extensive family ownership and control, business group structures, and weak legal protection for minority shareholders. Serious conflicts tend to exist between two classes of principals: controlling shareholders and minority shareholders. Such conflicts can be called **principal–principal (PP) conflicts,** as opposed to *principal–agent* conflicts (see Exhibits 9.9 and 9.10).

Strong family control is one of the leading indicators of concentrated ownership. In East Asia (excluding China), approximately 57 percent of the corporations have board chairs and CEOs from the controlling families. In continental Europe, this number is 68 percent. A very common practice is the appointment of family members as board chairs, CEOs, and other top executives. This happens because the families are controlling (not necessarily majority) shareholders. In 2003, 30-year-old James Murdoch was appointed CEO of British Sky Broadcasting (BSkyB), Europe's largest satellite broadcaster. There was very vocal resistance by minority shareholders. Why was he appointed in the first place? James's father just happened to be Rupert Murdoch, who controlled 35 percent of BSkyB and chaired the board. Clearly, this is a case of a PP conflict.

In general, three conditions must be met for PP conflicts to occur:

principal–principal (PP) conflicts conflicts between two classes of principals—controlling shareholders and minority shareholders—within the context of a corporate governance system.

- A dominant owner or group of owners who have interests that are distinct from minority shareholders.
- Motivation for the controlling shareholders to exercise their dominant positions to their advantage.
- Few formal (such as legislation or regulatory bodies) or informal constraints that would discourage or prevent the controlling shareholders from exploiting their advantageous positions.

Exhibit 9.9
Traditional Principal–Agent Conflicts versus Principal–Principal Conflicts: How They Differ along Dimensions

	Principal–Agent Conflicts	Principal–Principal Conflicts
Goal Incongruence	Between shareholders and professional managers who own a relatively small portion of the firm's equity.	Between controlling shareholders and minority shareholders.
Ownership Pattern	Dispersed—5%–20% is considered "concentrated ownership."	Concentrated—often greater than 50% of equity is controlled by controlling shareholders.
Manifestations	Strategies that benefit entrenched managers at the expense of shareholders in general (e.g., shirking, pet projects, excessive compensation, and empire building).	Strategies that benefit controlling shareholders at the expense of minority shareholders (e.g., minority shareholder expropriation, nepotism, and cronyism).
Institutional Protection of Minority Shareholders	Formal constraints (e.g., judicial reviews and courts) set an upper boundary on potential expropriation by majority shareholders. Informal norms generally adhere to shareholder wealth maximization.	Formal institutional protection is often lacking, corrupted, or unenforced. Informal norms are typically in favor of the interests of controlling shareholders ahead of those of minority investors.

Source: Adapted from Young, M., Peng, M. W., Ahlstrom, D., & Bruton, G. 2002. Governing the corporation in emerging economies: A principal–principal perspective. *Academy of Management Best Papers Proceedings,* Denver.

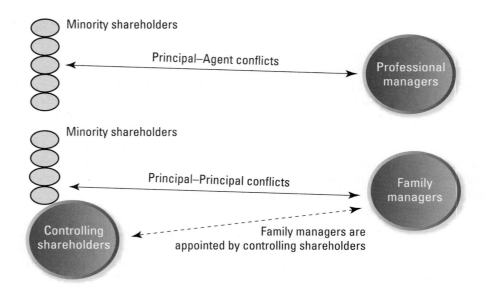

Exhibit 9.10 Principal–Agent Conflicts and Principal–Principal Conflicts: A Diagram

Source: Young, M. N., Peng, M. W., Ahlstrom, D., Bruton, G. D., & Jiang, Y. 2008. Principal–principal conflicts in corporate governance. *Journal of Management Studies* 45(1):196–220; and, Peng, M. V. 2006. *Global strategy.* Cincinnati: Thomson South-Western. We are very appreciative of the helpful comments of Mike Young of Hong Kong Baptist University and Mike Peng of the University of Texas at Dallas.

expropriation of minority shareholders
activities that enrich the controlling shareholders at the expense of the minority shareholders.

business group
a set of firms that, though legally independent, are bound together by a constellation of formal and informal ties and are accustomed to taking coordinated action.

The result is often that family managers, who represent (or actually are) the controlling shareholders, engage in **expropriation of minority shareholders,** which is defined as activities that enrich the controlling shareholders at the expense of minority shareholders. What is their motive? After all, controlling shareholders have incentives to maintain firm value. But controlling shareholders may take actions that decrease aggregate firm performance if their personal gains from expropriation exceed their personal losses from their firm's lowered performance.

Another ubiquitous feature of corporate life outside the United States and United Kingdom are *business groups* such as the keiretsus of Japan and the chaebols of South Korea. These are particularly dominant in emerging economies. A **business group** is "a set of firms that, though legally independent, are bound together by a constellation of formal and informal ties and are accustomed to taking coordinated action."[117] Business groups are especially common in emerging economies, and they differ from other organizational forms in that they are communities of firms without clear boundaries.

Business groups have many advantages that can enhance the value of a firm. They often facilitate technology transfer or intergroup capital allocation that otherwise might be impossible because of inadequate institutional infrastructure such as excellent financial services firms. On the other hand, informal ties—such as cross-holdings, board interlocks, and coordinated actions—can often result in intragroup activities and transactions, often at very favorable terms to member firms. Expropriation can be legally done through *related transactions,* which can occur when controlling owners sell firm assets to another firm they own at below market prices or spin off the most profitable part of a public firm and merge it with another of their private firms.

Strategy Spotlight 9.7 provides examples from Latin America of effective corporate governance.

Effective and Ineffective Corporate Governance among "Multilatinas"

Latin-owned companies, such as Mexico's Cemex, Argentina's Arcor, and Brazil's Embraer, have been successful in their home markets against U.S. and European competitors. Several of these companies have become "multilatinas," pursuing a strategy of regional and international expansion. Recently, 82 percent of merger and acquisition deals in Latin America were originated by Latin companies. However, while the rise of these Latin firms is promising, it is not enough to ensure they will be competitive globally against large industrialized multinational firms. Access to international capital markets necessary for the "multilatinas" to grow has created a need for a new openness in corporate governance and transparency for these firms.

There are three components emerging-market multinational firms need to implement to succeed:

Sources: Pigorini, P., Ramos, A., & de Souza, I. 2008. Pitting Latin multinationals against established giants. *Strategy + Business,* November 4: *www. strategy-business.com/media/file/leading_ideas-20081104.pdf*; Martinez, J., Esperanca, J., & de la Torre, J. 2005. Organizational change among emerging Latin American firms: From "multilatinas" to multinationals. *Management Research,* 3(3): 173–188; and, Krauss, C. 2007. Latin American companies make big U.S. gains. *The New York Times,* May 2: *www.nytimes.com/2007/05/02/-business/worldbusiness/02latin.html.*

- **Shareholder rights.** Minority shareholders must be protected through clear and fair dividend distribution and fair valuation in the event of mergers and acquisitions.
- **Compliance.** The audit committee of the board must be empowered to evaluate the financial statements of the firm and interact with both internal and external auditors.
- **Board and management composition.** Because many multilatinas are still in the process of building effective governance systems, it is important that the board members and top managers have credible professional backgrounds and experience.

These firms need to set up the right board and manager dynamics both to improve access to capital and to implement international management. Many multilatinas were or still are family-owned firms. Boards of these firms tend to be filled with members who have a strong loyalty to the controlling family, but not necessarily exposure to global strategic initiatives and strategies. Many of these firms still use centralized information control systems. In order to grow, some firms may have to consider giving local country managers more authority to make decisions.

Reflecting on Career Implications . . .

- *Behavioral Control:* What sources of behavioral control does your organization employ? In general, too much emphasis on rules and regulations may stifle initiative and be detrimental to your career opportunities.
- *Rewards and Incentives:* Is your organization's reward structure fair and equitable? Does it effectively reward outstanding performance? If not, there may be a long-term erosion of morale that may have long-term adverse career implications for you.
- *Culture:* Consider the type of organization culture that would provide the best work environment for your career goals. How does your organization's culture deviate from this concept? Does your organization have a strong and effective culture? If so, professionals are more likely to develop strong "firm-specific" ties, which further enhances collaboration.
- *Corporate Governance:* Does your organization practice effective corporate governance? Such practices will enhance a firm's culture and it will be easier to attract top talent. Operating within governance guidelines is usually a strong indicator of organizational citizenship, which, in turn, should be good for your career prospects.

Summary

For firms to be successful, they must practice effective strategic control and corporate governance. Without such controls, the firm will not be able to achieve competitive advantages and outperform rivals in the marketplace.

We began the chapter with the key role of informational control. We contrasted two types of control systems: what we termed "traditional" and "contemporary" information control systems. Whereas traditional control systems may have their place in placid, simple competitive environments, there are fewer of those in today's economy. Instead, we advocated the contemporary approach wherein the internal and external environment are constantly monitored so that, when surprises emerge, the firm can modify its strategies, goals, and objectives.

Behavioral controls are also a vital part of effective control systems. We argued that firms must develop the proper balance between culture, rewards and incentives, and boundaries and constraints. Where there are strong and positive cultures and rewards, employees tend to internalize the organization's strategies and objectives. This permits a firm to spend fewer resources on monitoring behavior, and assures the firm that the efforts and initiatives of employees are more consistent with the overall objectives of the organization.

In the final section of this chapter, we addressed corporate governance, which can be defined as the relationship between various participants in determining the direction and performance of the corporation. The primary participants include shareholders, management (led by the chief executive officer), and the board of directors. We reviewed studies that indicated a consistent relationship between effective corporate governance and financial performance. There are also several internal and external control mechanisms that can serve to align managerial interests and shareholder interests. The internal mechanisms include a committed and involved board of directors, shareholder activism, and effective managerial incentives and rewards. The external mechanisms include the market for corporate control, banks and analysts, regulators, the media, and public activists. We also addressed corporate governance from both a United States and an international perspective.

Summary Review Questions

1. Why are effective strategic control systems so important in today's economy?
2. What are the main advantages of "contemporary" control systems over "traditional" control systems? What are the main differences between these two systems?
3. Why is it important to have a balance between the three elements of behavioral control—culture, rewards and incentives, and boundaries?
4. Discuss the relationship between types of organizations and their primary means of behavioral control.
5. Boundaries become less important as a firm develops a strong culture and reward system. Explain.
6. Why is it important to avoid a "one best way" mentality concerning control systems? What are the consequences of applying the same type of control system to all types of environments?
7. What is the role of effective corporate governance in improving a firm's performance? What are some of the key governance mechanisms that are used to ensure that managerial and shareholder interests are aligned?
8. Define principal–principal (PP) conflicts. What are the implications for corporate governance?

Key Terms

strategic control, 360
traditional approach to
  strategic control, 361
informational
  control, 361
behavioral control, 363
organizational
  culture, 365
reward system, 366
boundaries and
  constraints, 367
corporate
  governance, 372
corporation, 374

agency theory, 375
board of directors, 376
shareholder
  activism, 379
external governance control
  mechanisms, 382
market for corporate
  control, 383
takeover constraint, 383
principal–principal (PP)
  conflicts, 387
expropriation of minority
  shareholders, 388
business group, 388

Experiential Exercise

McDonald's Corporation, the world's largest fast-food restaurant chain, with 2010 revenues of $24 billion, has recently been on a "roll." Its shareholder value has more than doubled between February 2006 and February 2011. Using the Internet or library sources, evaluate the quality of the corporation in terms of management, the board of directors, and shareholder activism. Are the issues you list (in the provided diagram, following) favorable or unfavorable for sound corporate governance?

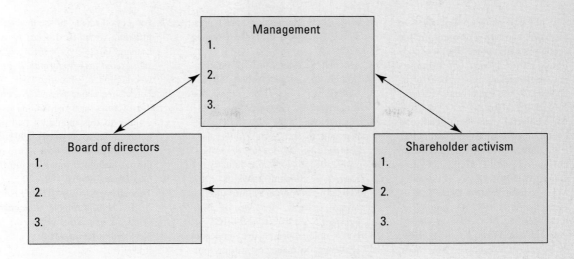

Application Questions & Exercises

1. The problems of many firms may be attributed to a "traditional" control system that failed to continuously monitor the environment and make necessary changes in their strategy and objectives. What companies are you familiar with that responded appropriately (or inappropriately) to environmental change?

2. How can a strong, positive culture enhance a firm's competitive advantage? How can a weak, negative culture erode competitive advantages? Explain and provide examples.

3. Use the Internet to research a firm that has an excellent culture and/or reward and incentive system. What are this firm's main financial and nonfinancial benefits?

4. Using the Internet, go to the website of a large, publicly held corporation in which you are interested. What evidence do you see of effective (or ineffective) corporate governance?

Ethics Questions

1. Strong cultures can have powerful effects on employee behavior. How does this create inadvertent control mechanisms? That is, are strong cultures an ethical way to control behavior?

2. Rules and regulations can help reduce unethical behavior in organizations. To be effective, however, what other systems, mechanisms, and processes are necessary?

References

1. Loomis, C. J. 2010. Directors: Feeding at the trough. *Fortune,* January 18: 20; Schonberger, J. 2009. Why you should care about corporate governance, *www.fool.com.* November 10: np; Hood, H. J. 2009. *Chesapeake Energy Corporation* Schedule 14A; and, *www.sec.gov.* November 10: np. We thank Zia Shakir for his valued contributions.

2. This chapter draws upon: Picken, J. C. & Dess, G. G. 1997. *Mission critical.* Burr Ridge, IL: Irwin Professional Publishing.

3. For a unique perspective on governance, refer to: Carmeli, A. & Markman, G. D. 2011. Capture, governance, and resilience: Strategy implications from the history of Rome. *Strategic Management Journal,* 32(3):332–341.

4. Argyris, C. 1977. Double-loop learning in organizations. *Harvard Business Review,* 55: 115–125.

5. Simons, R. 1995. Control in an age of empowerment. *Harvard Business Review,* 73: 80–88. This chapter draws on this source in the discussion of informational control.

6. Goold, M. & Quinn, J. B. 1990. The paradox of strategic controls. *Strategic Management Journal,* 11: 43–57.

7. Quinn, J. B. 1980. *Strategies for change.* Homewood, IL: Richard D. Irwin.

8. Mintzberg, H. 1987. Crafting strategy. *Harvard Business Review,* 65: 66–75.

9. Weston, J. S. 1992. Soft stuff matters. *Financial Executive,* July–August: 52–53.

10. This discussion of control systems draws upon Simons, op. cit.

11. Ryan, M. K., Haslam, S. A., & Renneboog, L. D. R. 2011. Who gets the carrot and who gets the stick? Evidence of gender discrimination in executive remuneration. *Strategic Management Journal,* 32(3): 301–321.

12. For an interesting perspective on this issue and how a downturn in the economy can reduce the tendency toward "free agency" by managers and professionals, refer to: Morris, B. 2001. White collar blues. *Fortune,* July 23: 98–110.

13. For a colorful example of behavioral control in an organization, see: Beller, P. C. 2009. Activision's unlikely hero. *Forbes,* February 2: 52–58.

14. Ouchi, W. 1981. *Theory Z.* Reading, MA: Addison-Wesley; Deal, T. E. & Kennedy, A. A. 1982. *Corporate cultures.* Reading, MA: Addison-Wesley; Peters, T. J. & Waterman, R. H. 1982. *In search of excellence.* New York: Random House; Collins, J. 2001. *Good to great.* New York: HarperCollins.

15. Collins, J. C. & Porras, J. I. 1994. *Built to last: Successful habits of visionary companies.* New York: Harper Business.

16. Lee, J. & Miller, D. 1999. People matter: Commitment to employees, strategy, and performance in Korean firms. *Strategic Management Journal,* 6: 579–594.

17. For an insightful discussion of IKEA's unique culture, see: Kling, K. & Goteman, I. 2003. IKEA CEO Anders Dahlvig on international growth and IKEA's unique corporate culture and brand identity. *Academy of Management Executive,* 17(1): 31–37.

18. For a discussion of how professionals inculcate values, refer to: Uhl-Bien, M. & Graen, G. B. 1998. Individual self-management: Analysis of professionals' self-managing activities in functional and cross-functional work teams. *Academy of Management Journal,* 41(3): 340–350.

19. A perspective on how antisocial behavior can erode a firm's culture can be found in Robinson, S. L. & O'Leary-Kelly, A. M. 1998. Monkey see, monkey do: The influence of work groups on the antisocial behavior of employees. *Academy of Management Journal,* 41(6): 658–672.

20. An interesting perspective on organizational culture is in: Mehta, S. N. 2009. Under Armour reboots. *Fortune,* February 2: 29–33.

21. For insights on social pressure as a means for control, refer to: Goldstein, N. J. 2009. Harnessing social pressure. *Harvard Business Review,* 87(2): 25.

22. Mitchell, R. 1989. Masters of innovation. *BusinessWeek,* April 10: 58–63.

23. Sellers, P. 1993. Companies that serve you best. *Fortune,* May 31: 88.

24. Anonymous. 2009. New CEO gives pep talk to staff. *The Hindu.* www.hindu.com/2009/01/08/stories/2009010859941500.htm. January 8.

25. Kerr, J. & Slocum, J. W., Jr. 1987. Managing corporate culture through reward systems. *Academy of Management Executive,* 1(2): 99–107.

26. For a unique perspective on leader challenges in managing wealthy professionals, refer to: Wetlaufer, S. 2000. Who wants to manage a millionaire? *Harvard Business Review,* 78(4): 53–60.

27. www.starbucks.com; Wood, Z. 2010. Starbucks' staff set to get free shares in incentive schemes. www.guardian.co.uk. December 19: np; and, Hammers, M. 2003. Starbucks is pleasing employees and pouring profits. *Workforce Management,* October: 58–59.

28. These next two subsections draw upon: Dess, G. G. & Picken, J. C. 1997. *Beyond productivity.* New York: AMACOM.

29. For a discussion of the benefits of stock options as executive compensation, refer to: Hall, B. J. 2000. What you need to know about stock options. *Harvard Business Review,* 78(2): 121–129.

30. Tully, S. 1993. Your paycheck gets exciting. *Fortune,* November 13: 89.

31. Carter, N. M. & Silva, C. 2010. Why men still get more promotions than women. *Harvard Business Review,* 88(9): 80–86.

32. Zellner, W., Hof, R. D., Brandt, R., Baker, S., & Greising, D. 1995. Go-go goliaths. *BusinessWeek,* February 13: 64–70.

33. This section draws on Dess & Picken, 1997, op. cit.: chap. 5.

34. Simons, op. cit.

35. Davis, E. 1997. Interview: Norman Augustine. *Management Review,* November: 11.

36. This section draws upon: Dess, G. G. & Miller, A. 1993. *Strategic management.* New York: McGraw-Hill.

37. For a good review of the goal-setting literature, refer to: Locke, E. A. & Latham, G. P. 1990. *A theory of goal setting and task performance.* Englewood Cliffs, NJ: Prentice Hall.

38. For an interesting perspective on the use of rules and regulations that is counter to this industry's (software) norms, refer to: Fryer, B. 2001. Tom Siebel of Siebel Systems: High tech the old-fashioned way. *Harvard Business Review,* 79(3): 118–130.

39. Thompson, A. A., Jr. & Strickland, A. J., III. 1998. *Strategic management: Concepts and cases* (10th ed.): 313. New York: McGraw-Hill.

40. Ibid.

41. Teitelbaum, R. 1997. Tough guys finish first. *Fortune,* July 21: 82–84.

42. Weaver, G. R., Trevino, L. K., & Cochran, P. L. 1999. Corporate ethics programs as control systems: Influences of executive commitment and environmental factors. *Academy of Management Journal,* 42(1): 41–57.

43. Cadbury, S. A. 1987. Ethical managers make their own rules. *Harvard Business Review,* 65: 3, 69–73.

44. Weber, J. 2003. CFOs on the hot seat. *BusinessWeek,* March 17: 66–70.

45. William Ouchi has written extensively about the use of clan control (which is viewed as an alternate to bureaucratic or market control). Here, a powerful culture results in people aligning their individual interests with those of the firm. Refer to Ouchi, op. cit. This section also draws on: Hall, R. H. 2002. *Organizations: Structures, processes, and outcomes* (8th ed.). Upper Saddle River, NJ: Prentice Hall.

46. Poundstone, W. 2003. *How would you move Mount Fuji?:* 59. New York: Little, Brown and Company.

47. Interesting insights on corporate governance are in: Kroll, M., Walters, B. A., & Wright, P. 2008. Board vigilance, director experience, and corporate outcomes. *Strategic Management Journal,* 29(4): 363–382.

48. For a brief review of some central issues in corporate governance research, see: Hambrick, D. C., Werder, A. V., & Zajac, E. J. 2008. New directions in corporate

governance research. *Organization Science,* 19(3): 381–385.

49. Monks, R. & Minow, N. 2001. *Corporate governance* (2nd ed.). Malden, MA: Blackwell.

50. Pound, J. 1995. The promise of the governed corporation. *Harvard Business Review,* 73(2): 89–98.

51. Maurer, H. & Linblad, C. 2009. Scandal at Satyam. *BusinessWeek,* January 19: 8; Scheck, J. & Stecklow, S. 2008. Brocade ex-CEO gets 21 months in prison. *The Wall Street Journal,* January 17: A3; Sylvers, E. 2004. International business; new audit details fall of Parmalat. *The New York Times,* April 17; Associated Press. 2010. Parmalat founder guilty of bankruptcy fraud. *The New York Times,* December 10; Frank, R., Efrati, A., Lucchetti, A., & Bray, C. 2009. Madoff jailed after admitting epic scam. *The Wall Street Journal.* March 13: A1; and, Henriques, D. B. 2009. Madoff is sentenced to 150 years for Ponzi scheme. *www.nytimes.com.* June 29: np.

52. Corporate governance and social networks are discussed in: McDonald, M. L., Khanna, P., & Westphal, J. D. 2008. *Academy of Management Journal,* 51(3): 453–475.

53. This discussion draws upon Monks & Minow, op. cit.

54. For an interesting perspective on the politicization of the corporation, read: Palazzo, G. & Scherer, A. G. 2008. Corporate social responsibility, democracy, and the politicization of the corporation. *Academy of Management Review,* 33(3): 773–774.

55. Eisenhardt, K. M. 1989. Agency theory: An assessment and review. *Academy of Management Review,* 14(1): 57–74. Some of the seminal contributions to agency theory include: Jensen, M. & Meckling, W. 1976. Theory of the firm: Managerial behavior, agency costs, and ownership structure. *Journal of Financial Economics,* 3: 305–360; Fama, E. & Jensen, M. 1983. Separation of ownership and control. *Journal of Law and Economics,* 26: 301, 325; and, Fama, E. 1980. Agency problems and the theory of the firm. *Journal of Political Economy,* 88: 288–307.

56. Nyberg, A. J., Fulmer, I. S., Gerhart, B., & Carpenter, M. 2010. Agency theory revisited: CEO return and shareholder interest alignment. *Academy of Management Journal,* 53(5): 1029–1049.

57. Managers may also engage in "shirking"—that is, reducing or withholding their efforts. See, for example, Kidwell, R. E., Jr. & Bennett, N. 1993. Employee propensity to withhold effort: A conceptual model to intersect three avenues of research. *Academy of Management Review,* 18(3): 429–456.

58. For an interesting perspective on agency and clarification of many related concepts and terms, visit *www.encycogov.com.*

59. The relationship between corporate ownership structure and export intensity in Chinese firms is discussed in: Filatotchev, I., Stephan, J., & Jindra, B. 2008. Ownership structure, strategic controls and export intensity of foreign-invested firms in transition economies. *Journal of International Business,* 39(7): 1133–1148.

60. Argawal, A. & Mandelker, G. 1987. Managerial incentives and corporate investment and financing decisions. *Journal of Finance,* 42: 823–837.

61. McDonald, E. 2004. Crony capitalism. *Forbes,* June 21: 140–146; and, Slade, D. 2011. Ex-Calgary oil CEO jailed for two years as judge cites Madoff case. *www.calgaryherald.com.* August 22.

62. For an insightful, recent discussion of the academic research on corporate governance, and in particular the role of boards of directors, refer to: Chatterjee, S. & Harrison, J. S. 2001. Corporate governance. In Hitt, M. A., Freeman, R. E., & Harrison, J. S. (Eds.). *Handbook of strategic management:* 543–563. Malden, MA: Blackwell.

63. For an interesting theoretical discussion on corporate governance in Russia, see: McCarthy, D. J. & Puffer, S. M. 2008. Interpreting the ethicality of corporate governance decisions in Russia: Utilizing integrative social contracts theory to evaluate the relevance of agency theory norms.

Academy of Management Review, 33(1): 11–31.

64. Haynes, K. T. & Hillman, A. 2010. The effect of board capital and CEO power on strategic change. *Strategic Management Journal,* 31(110): 1145–1163.

65. This opening discussion draws on: Monks & Minow, op. cit.: 164, 169; see also Pound, op. cit.

66. Business Roundtable. 1990. *Corporate governance and American competitiveness.* March: 7.

67. The director role in acquisition performance is addressed in: Westphal, J. D. & Graebner, M. E. 2008. What do they know? The effects of outside director acquisition experience on firm acquisition performance. *Strategic Management Journal,* 29(11): 1155–1178.

68. Byrne, J. A., Grover, R., & Melcher, R. A. 1997. The best and worst boards. *BusinessWeek,* November 26: 35–47. The three key roles of boards of directors are monitoring the actions of executives, providing advice, and providing links to the external environment to provide resources. See: Johnson, J. L., Daily, C. M., & Ellstrand, A. E. 1996. Boards of directors: A review and research agenda. *Academy of Management Review,* 37: 409–438.

69. Pozen, R. C. 2010. The case for professional boards. *Harvard Business Review,* 88(12): 50–58.

70. The role of outside directors is discussed in: Lester, R. H., Hillman, A., Zardkoohi, A., & Cannella, A. A., Jr. 2008. Former government officials as outside directors: The role of human and social capital. *Academy of Management Journal,* 51(5): 999–1013.

71. McGeehan, P. 2003. More chief executives shown the door, study says. *The New York Times,* May 12: C2.

72. Ligi, A. 2009. Oerlikon fires chief, seeks 'urgent' strategy fix. *www.bloomberg.com/apps/news?pid=newsarchive&sid=aF4JazjJVCAQ.* August 25.

73. The examples in this paragraph draw upon: Helyar, J. & Hymowitz, C. 2011. The recession is gone, and the CEO could be next. *Bloomberg*

Businessweek. Februrary 7–February 13: 24–26; Stelter, B. 2010. Jonathan Klein to leave CNN. *mediadecoder .blogs.nytimes.com.* September 24: np; Silver, A. 2010. Milestones. *TIME Magazine.* December 20: 28; *www .bp.com* and Mouawad, J. & Krauss, C. 2010. BP is expected to replace Hayward as chief with American. *The New York Times,* July 26: A1.

74. For an analysis of the effects of outside directors' compensation on acquisition decisions, refer to: Deutsch, T., Keil, T., & Laamanen, T. 2007. Decision making in acquisitions: The effect of outside directors' compensation on acquisition patterns. *Journal of Management,* 33(1): 30–56.

75. Director interlocks are addressed in: Kang, E. 2008. Director interlocks and spillover effects of reputational penalties from financial reporting fraud. *Academy of Management Journal,* 51(3): 537–556.

76. There are benefits, of course, to having some insiders on the board of directors. Inside directors would be more aware of the firm's strategies. Additionally, outsiders may rely too often on financial performance indicators because of information asymmetries. For an interesting discussion, see: Baysinger, B. D. & Hoskisson, R. E. 1990. The composition of boards of directors and strategic control: Effects on corporate strategy. *Academy of Management Review,* 15: 72–87.

77. Hambrick, D. C. & Jackson, E. M. 2000. Outside directors with a stake: The linchpin in improving governance. *California Management Review,* 42(4): 108–127.

78. Ibid.

79. Disney has begun to make many changes to improve its corporate governance, such as assigning only independent directors to important board committees, restricting directors from serving on more than three boards, and appointing a lead director who can convene the board without approval by the CEO. In recent years, Disney Co. has shown up on some "best" board lists. In addition Eisner has recently relinquished the chairman position.

80. Talk show. 2002. *BusinessWeek,* September 30: 14.

81. Ward, R. D. 2000. *Improving corporate boards.* New York: Wiley.

82. A discussion on the shareholder approval process in executive compensation is presented in: Brandes, P., Goranova, M., & Hall, S. 2008. Navigating shareholder influence: Compensation plans and the shareholder approval process. *Academy of Management Perspectives,* 22(1): 41–57.

83. Monks and Minow, op. cit.: 93.

84. A discussion of the factors that lead to shareholder activism is found in: Ryan, L. V. & Schneider, M. 2002. The antecedents of institutional investor activism. *Academy of Management Review,* 27(4): 554–573.

85. For an insightful discussion of investor activism, refer to: David, P., Bloom, M., & Hillman, A. 2007. Investor activism, managerial responsiveness, and corporate social performance. *Strategic Management Journal,* 28(1): 91–100.

86. There is strong research support for the idea that the presence of large block shareholders is associated with value-maximizing decisions. For example, refer to: Johnson, R. A., Hoskisson, R. E., & Hitt, M. A. 1993. Board of director involvement in restructuring: The effects of board versus managerial controls and characteristics. *Strategic Management Journal,* 14: 33–50.

87. For a discussion of institutional activism and its link to CEO compensation, refer to: Chowdhury, S. D. & Wang, E. Z. 2009. Institutional activism types and CEO compensation. *Journal of Management,* 35(1): 5–36.

88. For an interesting perspective on the impact of institutional ownership on a firm's innovation strategies, see: Hoskisson, R. E., Hitt, M. A., Johnson, R. A., & Grossman, W. 2002. *Academy of Management Journal,* 45(4): 697–716.

89. *www.calpers.ca.gov.*

90. Icahn, C. 2007. Icahn: On activist investors and private equity run wild. *BusinessWeek,* March 12: 21–22. For an interesting perspective on Carl Icahn's self-styled transition from corporate raider to shareholder activist, read: Grover, R. 2007. Just don't call him a raider. *BusinessWeek,* March 5: 68–69. The quote in the text is part of Icahn's response to the article by R. Grover.

91. For a study of the relationship between ownership and diversification, refer to: Goranova, M., Alessandri, T. M., Brandes, P., & Dharwadkar, R. 2007. Managerial ownership and corporate diversification: A longitudinal view. *Strategic Management Journal,* 28(3): 211–226.

92. Jensen, M. C. & Murphy, K. J. 1990. CEO incentives—it's not how much you pay, but how. *Harvard Business Review,* 68(3): 138–149.

93. For a perspective on the relative advantages and disadvantages of "duality"—that is, one individual serving as both chief executive officer and chairman of the board, see: Lorsch, J. W. & Zelleke, A. 2005. Should the CEO be the chairman? *MIT Sloan Management Review,* 46(2): 71–74.

94. A discussion of knowledge sharing is addressed in: Fey, C. F. & Furu, P. 2008. Top management incentive compensation and knowledge sharing in multinational corporations. *Strategic Management Journal,* 29(12): 1301–1324.

95. Sasseen, J. 2007. A better look at the boss's pay. *BusinessWeek,* February 26: 44–45; and, Weinberg, N., Maiello, M., & Randall, D. 2008. Paying for failure. *Forbes,* May 19: 114, 116.

96. Byrnes, N. & Sasseen, J. 2007. Board of hard knocks. *BusinessWeek,* January 22: 36–39.

97. Research has found that executive compensation is more closely aligned with firm performance in companies with compensation committees and boards dominated by outside directors. See, for example, Conyon, M. J. & Peck, S. I. 1998. Board control, remuneration committees, and top management compensation. *Academy of Management Journal,* 41: 146–157.

98. Lavelle, L., Jespersen, F. F., & Arndt, M. 2002. Executive pay. *BusinessWeek,* April 15: 66–72.

99. A perspective on whether or not CEOs are overpaid is provided in: Kaplan, S. N. 2008. Are U.S. CEOs overpaid? A response to Bogle and Walsh. *Academy of Management Perspectives.* 22(3): 28–34.

100. *www.tiaa-cref.org/pubs.*

101. Some insights on CEO compensation—and the importance of ethics—are addressed in: Heineman, B. W., Jr. 2008. The fatal flaw in pay for performance. *Harvard Business Review,* 86(6): 31, 34.

102. Chahine, S. & Tohme, N. S. 2009. Is CEO duality always negative? An exploration of CEO duality and ownership structure in the Arab IPO context. *Corporate Governance: An International Review,* 17(2): 123–141; and, McGrath, J. 2009. How CEOs work. *HowStuffWorks.com.* January 28: np.

103. Anonymous. 2009. Someone to watch over them. *The Economist,* October 17: 78; Anonymous. 2004. Splitting up the roles of CEO and chairman: Reform or red herring? *Knowledge@Wharton.* June 2: np; and, Kim, J. 2010. Shareholders reject split of CEO and chairman jobs at JPMorgan. *FierceFinance.com.* May 18: np.

104. Tuggle, C. S., Sirmon, D. G., Reutzel, C. R., & Bierman, L. 2010. Commanding board of director attention: Investigating how organizational performance and CEO duality affect board members' attention to monitoring. *Strategic Management Journal,* 31: 946–968; Weinberg, N. 2010. No more lapdogs. *Forbes,* May 10: 34–36; and, Anonymous. 2010. Corporate constitutions. *The Economist,* October 30: 74.

105. Such opportunistic behavior is common in all principal–agent relationships. For a description of agency problems, especially in the context of the relationship between shareholders and managers, see: Jensen, M. C. & Meckling, W. H. 1976. Theory of the firm: Managerial behavior, agency costs, and ownership structure. *Journal of Financial Economics,* 3: 305–360.

106. Hoskisson, R. E. & Turk, T. A. 1990. Corporate restructuring: Governance and control limits of the internal market. *Academy of Management Review,* 15: 459–477.

107. For an insightful perspective on the market for corporate control and how it is influenced by knowledge intensity, see: Coff, R. 2003. Bidding wars over R&D-intensive firms: Knowledge, opportunism, and the market for corporate control. *Academy of Management Journal,* 46(1): 74–85.

108. Walsh, J. P. & Kosnik, R. D. 1993. Corporate raiders and their disciplinary role in the market for corporate control. *Academy of Management Journal,* 36: 671–700.

109. Gunning for KPMG. 2003. *The Economist,* February 1: 63.

110. Timmons, H. 2003. Investment banks: Who will foot their bill? *BusinessWeek,* March 3: 116.

111. The role of regulatory bodies in the banking industry is addressed in: Bhide, A. 2009. Why bankers got so reckless. *BusinessWeek,* February 9: 30–31.

112. Wishy-washy: The SEC pulls its punches on corporate-governance rules. 2003. *The Economist,* February 1: 60.

113. McLean, B. 2001. Is Enron overpriced? *Fortune,* March 5: 122–125.

114. Swartz, J. 2010. Timberland's CEO on standing up to 65,000 angry activists. *Harvard Business Review,* 88 (9): 39–43.

115. Bernstein, A. 2000. Too much corporate power. *BusinessWeek,* September 11: 35–37.

116. This section draws upon Young, M. N., Peng, M. W., Ahlstrom, D., Bruton, G. D., & Jiang, Y. 2008. Principal–principal conflicts in corporate governance. *Journal of Management Studies* 45(1): 196–220; and, Peng, M. W. 2006. *Global strategy.* Cincinnati: Thomson South-Western. We appreciate the helpful comments of Mike Young of Hong Kong Baptist University and Mike Peng of the University of Texas at Dallas.

117. Khanna, T. & Rivkin, J. 2001. Estimating the performance effects of business groups in emerging markets. *Strategic Management Journal,* 22: 45–74.

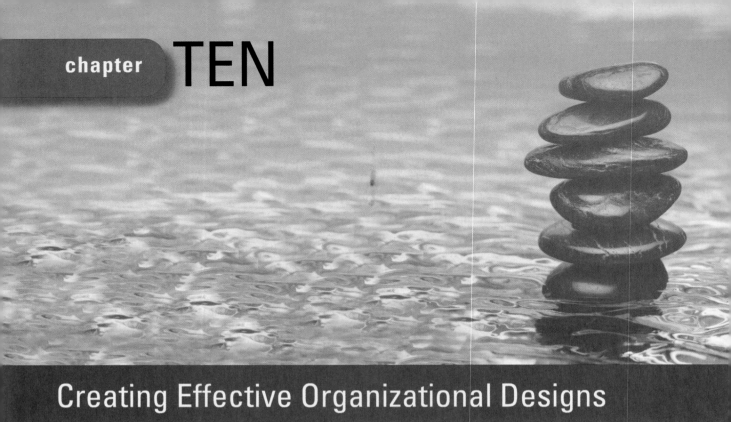

chapter TEN

Creating Effective Organizational Designs

After reading this chapter, you should have a good understanding of:

LO10.1 The growth patterns of major corporations and the relationship between a firm's strategy and its structure.

LO10.2 Each of the traditional types of organizational structure: simple, functional, divisional, and matrix.

LO10.3 The implications of a firm's international operations for organizational structure.

LO10.4 Why there is no "one best way" to design strategic reward and evaluation systems, and the important contingent roles of business- and corporate-level strategies.

LO10.5 The different types of boundaryless organizations—barrier-free, modular, and virtual—and their relative advantages and disadvantages.

LO10.6 The need for creating ambidextrous organizational designs that enable firms to explore new opportunities and effectively integrate existing operations.

LEARNING OBJECTIVES

To implement strategies successfully, firms must have appropriate organizational designs. These include the processes and integrating mechanisms necessary to ensure that boundaries among internal activities and external parties, such as suppliers, customers, and alliance partners, are flexible and permeable. A firm's performance will suffer if its managers don't carefully consider both of these organizational design attributes.

In the first section, we begin by discussing the growth patterns of large corporations to address the important relationships between the strategy that a firm follows and its corresponding structure. For example, as firms diversify into related product-market areas, they change their structure from functional to divisional. We then address the different types of traditional structures—simple, functional, divisional, and matrix—and their relative advantages and disadvantages. We close with a discussion of the implications of a firm's international operations for the structure of its organization.

The second section takes the perspective that there is no "one best way" to design an organization's strategic reward and evaluation system. Here we address two important contingencies: business- and corporate-level strategy. For example, when strategies require a great deal of collaboration, as well as resource and information sharing, there must be incentives and cultures that encourage and reward such initiatives.

The third section discusses the concept of the "boundaryless" organization. We do *not* argue that organizations should have no internal and external boundaries. Instead, we suggest that, in rapidly changing and unpredictable environments, organizations must strive to make their internal and external boundaries both flexible and permeable. We suggest three different types of boundaryless organizations: barrier-free, modular, and virtual.

The fourth section focuses on the need for managers to recognize that they typically face two opposing challenges: (1) being proactive in taking advantage of new opportunities and (2) ensuring the effective coordination and integration of existing operations. This suggests the need for ambidextrous organizations; that is, firms that can both be efficient in how they manage existing assets and competencies and take advantage of opportunities in rapidly changing and unpredictable environments—conditions that are becoming more pronounced in today's global markets. ●

▓▓ Learning from Mistakes

In mid-July 2010, Hong Kong's travel industry was reeling from a wild rant by a commission-based tour guide that was unfortunately captured on video.[1] The video went viral on the Internet and hit television screens across the mainland. More than a dozen television stations picked up the online video and played it constantly over a two-day period. What happened?

The seven-minute clip featured a female guide (nicknamed Ah Zhen) berating a group of mainland visitors and threatening to lock them out of their hotel rooms because they did not spend much at a jewelry store. In effect, this provided a shocking view of what Hong Kong can offer visitors. It followed a series of complaints about visitors being strong-armed by tour guides to go shopping and spend their money.

Ah Zhen is heard scolding the tourists in fluent Mandarin after they boarded their bus. "Don't tell me you don't need to shop," she said. "So later you are going to say you don't need to eat? I will lock you out of your hotel rooms. It's okay for you to stay poor at home, but when you travel outside, don't be like this. In this world there is no such thing as a free lunch."

She went on to talk about how the visitors found money for their airfares and then chides them: "We don't do this for charity. Let me be responsible for charity. I donated 10,500 yuan ($1,500) for Sichuan earthquake victims." She then pointed to shops offering top-quality goods, before adding, "Why did you bother to come to Hong Kong?" She lamented that the group did not look good compared with another group of tourists, who spent HKD137,000 ($17,000). "For a group of 24 people you only just spent HKD13,000 ($2,100). How can you just walk out of the shop like that?"

"It's you who owe me here, not me owing you," the guide continued. "I provided you with food and accommodations, but you people will not give. If you don't repay the debt in this life, you will have to repay it in your next life." She added, "Tonight I will lock all hotel room doors, because you don't need accommodations."

The clip sparked an outcry on the Internet. Some people said that they would no longer dare visit Hong Kong. Travel Industry Council Chairman Michael Wu Siu-ying said he had asked for the names of the travel agency and the tour agent from Guangdong, so that the council could take action.

When contacted, the tour guide became defensive and extremely vocal about mainland tourists condemning tour guides for forcing them to make purchases. "We don't force them to buy. When they sign up for the tour group, they should act responsibly. . . . You can see how much the tour group fees are. . . . You sign up for such a group, then you must do whatever is required. It is that simple. We did not force them to buy anything. We can't force them." She also said, "When they come, they know what they are doing. How much do they pay in fees? How many days are they staying?"

She further said, "Everybody has to earn a living. . . . I did this for the sake of surviving, just like you calling me in order for you to survive. . . . I have to eat. It is very normal for me to tell them about making purchases." Clearly, she was not happy about the media "hyping trivia" so that fewer mainland tour groups are coming. She also threatened the reporter not to write about her. "I will come and hold you accountable. I don't think there is anything wrong with what I did."

The government has given the Travel Industry Council three months to develop concrete measures to address the deteriorating image of Hong Kong as a tourist destination amid anger at the treatment of mainland tourists by commission-hungry guides. The council has set up a special task force to look into the issue.

One person's action has caused a chain reaction and tarnished the image of Hong Kong. One of the pitfalls of outsourcing is that the firm has less control. When companies outsource key activities, an inherent risk is that the quality of the performance of the contractors is not up to the standards of the firm. Further, at times, there are differences in cultural norms and insufficient training in place to ensure that contract employees adhere to standards and expectations.

One of the central concepts in this chapter is the importance of boundaryless organizations. Successful organizations create permeable boundaries among the internal activities as well as between the organization and its external customers, suppliers, and alliance partners. We introduced this idea in Chapter 3 in our discussion of the value-chain concept, which consisted of several primary (e.g., inbound logistics, marketing and sales) and support activities (e.g., procurement, human resource management). There are a number of possible benefits to outsourcing activities as part of becoming an effective boundaryless organization. However, outsourcing can also create challenges. As in the case of the tour operator in Hong Kong, the firm lost a certain amount of control by using independent contractors to provide services. Clearly, the outsourced tour guide was more focused on her personal financial incentives than the welfare of the travel firm or the tourists.

Today's managers are faced with two ongoing and vital activities in structuring and designing their organizations.[2] First, they must decide on the most appropriate type of organizational structure. Second, they need to assess what mechanisms, processes, and techniques are most helpful in enhancing the permeability of both internal and external boundaries.

Traditional Forms of Organizational Structure

Organizational structure refers to the formalized patterns of interactions that link a firm's tasks, technologies, and people.[3] Structures help to ensure that resources are used effectively in accomplishing an organization's mission. Structure provides a means of balancing two conflicting forces: a need for the division of tasks into meaningful groupings and the need to integrate such groupings in order to ensure efficiency and effectiveness.[4] Structure identifies the executive, managerial, and administrative organization of a firm and indicates responsibilities and hierarchical relationships. It also influences the flow of information as well as the context and nature of human interactions.[5]

> **organizational structure** the formalized patterns of interactions that link a firm's tasks, technologies, and people.

Most organizations begin very small and either die or remain small. Those that survive and prosper embark on strategies designed to increase the overall scope of operations and enable them to enter new product-market domains. Such growth places additional pressure on executives to control and coordinate the firm's increasing size and diversity. The most appropriate type of structure depends on the nature and magnitude of growth.

> **>LO10.1**
> The growth patterns of major corporations and the relationship between a firm's strategy and its structure.

Patterns of Growth of Large Corporations: Strategy—Structure Relationships

A firm's strategy and structure change as it increases in size, diversifies into new product markets, and expands its geographic scope.[6] Exhibit 10.1 illustrates common growth patterns of firms.

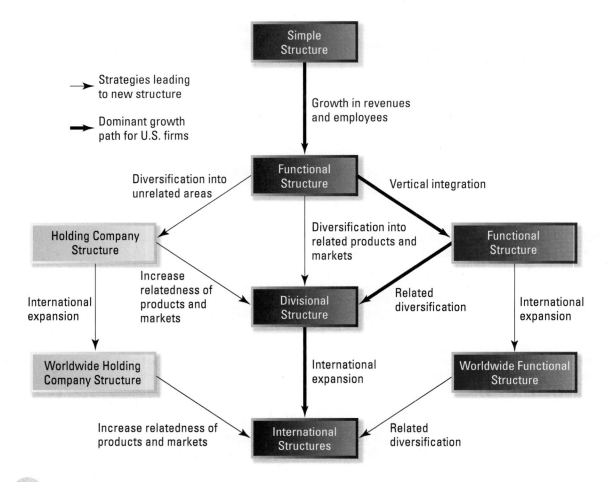

Exhibit 10.1   **Dominant Growth Patterns of Large Corporations**

Source: Adapted from J. R. Galbraith and R. K. Kazanjian. *Strategy Implementation: Structure, Systems and Process,* 2nd ed. Copyright © 1986.

A new firm with a *simple structure* typically increases its sales revenue and volume of outputs over time. It may also engage in some vertical integration to secure sources of supply (backward integration) as well as channels of distribution (forward integration). The simple-structure firm then implements a *functional structure* to concentrate efforts on both increasing efficiency and enhancing its operations and products. This structure enables the firm to group its operations into either functions, departments, or geographic areas. As its initial markets mature, a firm looks beyond its present products and markets for possible expansion.

A strategy of related diversification requires a need to reorganize around product lines or geographic markets. This leads to a *divisional structure.* As the business expands in terms of sales revenues, and domestic growth opportunities become somewhat limited, a firm may seek opportunities in international markets. A firm has a wide variety of structures to choose from. These include *international division, geographic-area division, worldwide product division, worldwide functional,* and *worldwide matrix.* Deciding upon the most appropriate structure when a firm has international operations depends on three primary factors: the extent of international expansion, type of strategy (global, multidomestic, or transnational), and the degree of product diversity.[7]

Some firms may find it advantageous to diversify into several product lines rather than focus their efforts on strengthening distributor and supplier relationships through vertical integration. They would organize themselves according to product lines by implementing a divisional structure. Also, some firms may choose to move into unrelated product areas, typically by acquiring existing businesses. Frequently, their rationale is that acquiring assets and competencies is more economical or expedient than developing them internally. Such an unrelated, or conglomerate, strategy requires relatively little integration across businesses and sharing of resources. Thus, a *holding company structure* becomes appropriate. There are many other growth patterns, but these are the most common.*

Now we will discuss some of the most common types of organizational structures—simple, functional, divisional (including two variants: *strategic business unit* and *holding company*), and matrix and their advantages and disadvantages. We will close the section with a discussion of the structural implications when a firm expands its operations into international markets.[8]

Simple Structure

The **simple organizational structure** is the oldest, and most common, organizational form. Most organizations are very small and have a single or very narrow product line in which the owner-manager (or top executive) makes most of the decisions. The owner-manager controls all activities, and the staff serves as an extension of the top executive.

Advantages   The simple structure is highly informal and the coordination of tasks is accomplished by direct supervision. Decision making is highly centralized, there is little specialization of tasks, few rules and regulations, and an informal evaluation and reward system. Although the owner-manager is intimately involved in almost all phases of the business, a manager is often employed to oversee day-to-day operations.

Disadvantages   A simple structure may foster creativity and individualism since there are generally few rules and regulations. However, such "informality" may lead to problems. Employees may not clearly understand their responsibilities, which can lead to conflict and confusion. Employees may take advantage of the lack of regulations, act in their own self-interest, which can erode motivation and satisfaction and lead to the possible misuse of organizational resources. Small organizations have flat structures that limit opportunities for upward mobility. Without the potential for future advancement, recruiting and retaining talent may become very difficult.

Functional Structure

When an organization is small (15 employees or less), it is not necessary to have a variety of formal arrangements and groupings of activities. However, as firms grow, excessive demands may be placed on the owner-manager in order to obtain and process all of the information necessary to run the business. Chances are the owner will not be skilled in all specialties (e.g., accounting, engineering, production, marketing). Thus, he or she will need to hire specialists in the various functional areas. Such growth in the overall scope and complexity of the business necessitates a **functional organizational structure** wherein the major functions of the firm are grouped internally. The coordination and integration of the functional areas become one of the most important responsibilities of the chief executive of the firm (see Exhibit 10.2).

* The lowering of transaction costs and globalization have led to some changes in the common historical patterns that we have discussed. Some firms are, in effect, bypassing the vertical integration stage. Instead, they focus on core competencies and outsource other value-creation activities. Also, even relatively young firms are going global early in their history because of lower communication and transportation costs. For an interesting perspective on global start-ups, see McDougall, P. P. & Oviatt, B. M. 1996. New venture internationalization, strategic change and performance: A follow-up study. *Journal of Business Venturing,* 11: 23–40; and, McDougall, P. P. & Oviatt, B. M. (Eds.). 2000. The Special Research Forum on International Entrepreneurship. *Academy of Management Journal,* October: 902–1003.

> **>LO10.2**
> Each of the traditional types of organizational structure: simple, functional, divisional, and matrix.

simple organizational structure an organizational form in which the owner-manager makes most of the decisions and controls activities, and the staff serves as an extension of the top executive.

functional organizational structure an organizational form in which the major functions of the firm, such as production, marketing, R&D, and accounting, are grouped internally.

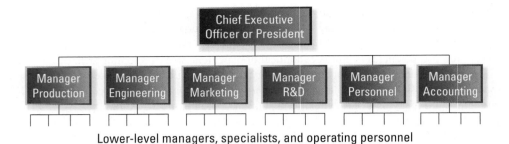

Lower-level managers, specialists, and operating personnel

Exhibit 10.2 Functional Organizational Structure

Functional structures are generally found in organizations in which there is a single or closely related product or service, high production volume, and some vertical integration. Initially, firms tend to expand the overall scope of their operations by penetrating existing markets, introducing similar products in additional markets, or increasing the level of vertical integration. Such expansion activities clearly increase the scope and complexity of the operations. The functional structure provides for a high level of centralization that helps to ensure integration and control over the related product-market activities or multiple primary activities (from inbound logistics to operations to marketing, sales, and service) in the value chain (addressed in Chapters 3 and 4). Strategy Spotlight 10.1 provides an example of an effective functional organization structure—DnB NOR of Norway.

Advantages   By bringing together specialists into functional departments, a firm is able to enhance its coordination and control within each of the functional areas. Decision making in the firm will be centralized at the top of the organization. This enhances the organizational-level (as opposed to functional area) perspective across the various functions in the organization. In addition, the functional structure provides for a more efficient use of managerial and technical talent since functional area expertise is pooled in a single department (e.g., marketing) instead of being spread across a variety of product-market areas. Finally, career paths and professional development in specialized areas are facilitated.

Disadvantages   The differences in values and orientations among functional areas may impede communication and coordination. Edgar Schein of MIT has argued that shared assumptions, often based on similar backgrounds and experiences of members, form around functional units in an organization. This leads to what are often called "stove pipes" or "silos," in which departments view themselves as isolated, self-contained units with little need for interaction and coordination with other departments. This erodes communication because functional groups may have not only different goals but also differing meanings of words and concepts. According to Schein:

> The word "marketing" will mean product development to the engineer, studying customers through market research to the product manager, merchandising to the salesperson, and constant change in design to the manufacturing manager. When they try to work together, they will often attribute disagreements to personalities and fail to notice the deeper, shared assumptions that color how each function thinks.[9]

Such narrow functional orientations also may lead to short-term thinking based largely upon what is best for the functional area, not the entire organization. In a manufacturing firm, sales may want to offer a wide range of customized products to appeal to the firm's customers; R&D may overdesign products and components to achieve technical elegance; and manufacturing may favor no-frills products that can be produced at low cost by means

DnB NOR: A Successful Functional Organizational Structure

In 2003, after a major banking crisis in Norway triggered a wave of bank consolidations, DnB and Gjensidige NOR merged to form DnB NOR. As part of the merger, senior management decided to change the company's organizational structure to a functional one. According to Olav Hytta, the group's chief executive at the time, "Our main priority has been to adapt the functional organization as far as possible to our customer activities, making sure that the chosen structure will enable us to realize potential synergies."

As economic and market conditions changed dramatically as a result of the global recession, DnB NOR continued to be involved in a number of bank mergers and acquisitions and has expanded its international activities, including a top spot in global financing for the shipping industry.

In the company's 2010 Business Review report, Rune Bjerke, the current group chief executive, described some of the changes the company implemented as a result of changing its organizational structure and weathering the global recession. He said the firm established common vision and values, leadership principles, strategic priorities, and a target position in the financial industry. As a result, financial losses were limited, existing customer relationships were cultivated, and new customer relationships were established. In 2011, the company simplified its brand structure, changed its name to DNB, and introduced a new corporate identity, to not only enhance the company's growing reputation in Norway but also signal its continuing efforts in the global arena.

Sources: Norway: Financial Services Report. March 16, 2011. Economist Intelligence Unit, accessed at *www.eiu.com*; DnB NOR Business Review 2010. Accessed at *www.dnbnor.no/portalfront/aarsrapoort/2010/eng-article-rapport.php*; Anonymous. 2003. DnB NOR: Organizational structure in place; future group management appointed. *Europe Intelligence Wire.* June 11.

of long production runs. Functional structures may overburden the top executives in the firm because conflicts have a tendency to be "pushed up" to the top of the organization since there are no managers who are responsible for the specific product lines. Functional structures make it difficult to establish uniform performance standards across the entire organization. It may be relatively easy to evaluate production managers on the basis of production volume and cost control, but establishing performance measures for engineering, R&D, and accounting become more problematic.

Divisional Structure

The **divisional organizational structure** (sometimes called the multidivisional structure or M-Form) is organized around products, projects, or markets. Each of the divisions, in turn, includes its own functional specialists who are typically organized into departments.[10] A divisional structure encompasses a set of relatively autonomous units governed by a central corporate office. The operating divisions are relatively independent and consist of products and services that are different from those of the other divisions.[11] Operational decision making in a large business places excessive demands on the firm's top management. In order to attend to broader, longer-term organizational issues, top-level managers must delegate decision making to lower-level managers. Divisional executives play a key role: They help to determine the product-market and financial objectives for the division as well as their division's contribution to overall corporate performance.[12] The rewards are based largely on measures of financial performance such as net income and revenue. Exhibit 10.3 illustrates a divisional structure.

General Motors was among the earliest firms to adopt the divisional organizational structure.[13] In the 1920s the company formed five major product divisions (Cadillac, Buick, Oldsmobile, Pontiac, and Chevrolet) as well as several industrial divisions. Since then, many firms have discovered that, as they diversified into new product-market activities, functional structures—with their emphasis on single functional departments—were unable to manage the increased complexity of the entire business.

> **divisional organizational structure** an organizational form in which products, projects, or product markets are grouped internally.

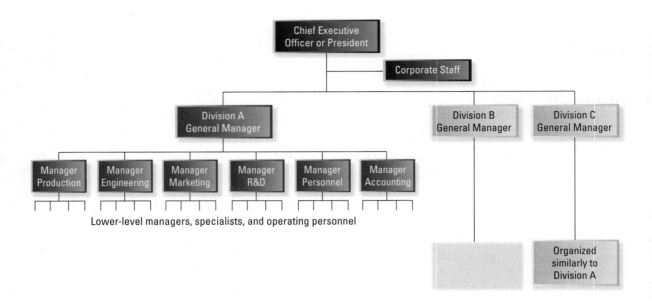

Exhibit 10.3 Divisional Organizational Structure

Advantages By creating separate divisions to manage individual product markets, there is a separation of strategic and operating control. Divisional managers can focus their efforts on improving operations in the product markets for which they are responsible, and corporate officers can devote their time to overall strategic issues for the entire corporation. The focus on a division's products and markets—by the divisional executives— provides the corporation with an enhanced ability to respond quickly to important changes. Since there are functional departments within each division of the corporation, the problems associated with sharing resources across functional departments are minimized. Because there are multiple levels of general managers (executives responsible for integrating and coordinating all functional areas), the development of general management talent is enhanced.

Disadvantages It can be very expensive; there can be increased costs due to the duplication of personnel, operations, and investment since each division must staff multiple functional departments. There also can be dysfunctional competition among divisions since each division tends to become concerned solely about its own operations. Divisional managers are often evaluated on common measures such as return on assets and sales growth. If goals are conflicting, there can be a sense of a "zero-sum" game that would discourage sharing ideas and resources among the divisions for the common good of the corporation. Ghoshal and Bartlett, two leading strategy scholars, note:

> As their label clearly warns, divisions divide. The divisional model fragmented companies' resources; it created vertical communication channels that insulated business units and prevented them from sharing their strengths with one another. Consequently, the whole of the corporation was often less than the sum of its parts.[14]

With many divisions providing different products and services, there is the chance that differences in image and quality may occur across divisions. One division may offer no-frills products of lower quality that may erode the brand reputation of another division that has top quality, highly differentiated offerings. Since each division is evaluated in terms of financial measures such as return on investment and revenue growth, there is often an urge

strategy spotlight

Why Sun Microsystems Experienced Major Problems When It Changed Its Organizational Structure

In general, organizational structures don't fail; managers fail at implementing them correctly. For example, in the 1990s, Sun Microsystems (acquired by Oracle in 2010) undertook a major corporate reorganization and changed from a functional structure to a divisional structure. At the time, the rationale seemed quite logical: Management wanted to create miniature Suns to provide autonomy, which would help restore the entrepreneurial spirit of the firm's start-up days.

Separate divisions were created for high-end servers, desktop computers, printers, software, services, and so on. In total, there were nine divisions. Such a configuration led them to call the structure "Sun and the nine planets." However, things certainly didn't work out as planned!

Sources: Galbraith, J. 2009. *Designing matrix organizations that actually work*. San Francisco: Jossey-Bass; Southwick, K. 1999. *High noon: The inside story of Scott McNealy and the rise of Sun Microsystems*. Hoboken, NJ: Wiley; and, Shankland, S. 2010. Oracle buys Sun, becomes hardware company. *www.news.cnet.com*. January 27: np.

Within a few years, Sun discovered the problems associated with this new structure. Management discovered that it wound up with nine different compensation plans, nine IT systems, nine sales forces calling on the same customers, and so on. In essence, it had nine of everything and, not surprisingly, escalating overhead expenses. As noted by Larry Hambly, Sun's chief quality officer and president of its customer service division, "The planets placed too much visibility on each entity." This resulted in the sales forces competing with each other, while people who were supposed to give customer service passed the buck. Lamented Hambly, "There was too much of, 'I don't know; that is somebody else's problem.'" In addition, it became almost impossible to move talent from one division to the next. As one would expect, Sun soon abandoned this highly autonomous structure and moved back to one similar to what it previously had.

Does this mean that autonomous divisional structures don't work? Of course not. Such a structure works well at diversified firms such as United Technologies and General Electric. Sun simply failed to implement the structure best suited to its particular situation.

---

to focus on short-term performance. If corporate management uses quarterly profits as the key performance indicator, divisional management may tend to put significant emphasis on "making the numbers" and minimizing activities, such as advertising, maintenance, and capital investments, which would detract from short-term performance measures.

When firms change their organization's structure, things don't always work out as planned. In Strategy Spotlight 10.2 we give one example—the problems that Sun Microsystems faced when the firm changed from a functional structure to a divisional structure.

We'll discuss two variations of the divisional form: the strategic business unit (SBU) and holding company structures.

Strategic Business Unit (SBU) Structure   Highly diversified corporations such as ConAgra, a $12 billion food producer, may consist of dozens of different divisions.[15] If ConAgra were to use a purely divisional structure, it would be nearly impossible for the corporate office to plan and coordinate activities, because the span of control would be too large. To attain synergies, ConAgra has put its diverse businesses into three primary SBUs: food service (restaurants), retail (grocery stores), and agricultural products.

With an **SBU structure,** divisions with similar products, markets, and/or technologies are grouped into homogeneous units to achieve some synergies. These include those discussed in Chapter 6 for related diversification, such as leveraging core competencies, sharing infrastructures, and market power. Generally the more related businesses are within a corporation, the fewer SBUs will be required. Each of the SBUs in the corporation operates as a profit center.

Advantages The SBU structure makes the task of planning and control by the corporate office more manageable. Also, with greater decentralization of authority, individual

> **strategic business unit (SBU) structure** an organizational form in which products, projects, or product-market divisions are grouped into homogeneous units.

businesses can react more quickly to important changes in the environment than if all divisions had to report directly to the corporate office.

Disadvantages Since the divisions are grouped into SBUs, it may become difficult to achieve synergies across SBUs. If divisions in different SBUs have potential sources of synergy, it may become difficult for them to be realized. The additional level of management increases the number of personnel and overhead expenses, while the additional hierarchical level removes the corporate office further from the individual divisions. The corporate office may become unaware of key developments that could have a major impact on the corporation.

Holding Company Structure   The **holding company structure** (sometimes referred to as a *conglomerate*) is also a variation of the divisional structure. Whereas the SBU structure is often used when similarities exist between the individual businesses (or divisions), the holding company structure is appropriate when the businesses in a corporation's portfolio do not have much in common. Thus, the potential for synergies is limited.

holding company structure an organizational form that is a variation of the divisional organizational structure in which the divisions have a high degree of autonomy both from other divisions and from corporate headquarters.

Holding company structures are most appropriate for firms with a strategy of unrelated diversification. Companies such as Hanson Trust, ITT, the CP Group of Thailand, and LG Group of Korea have used holding company structure to implement their unrelated diversification strategies. Since there are few similarities across the businesses, the corporate offices in these companies provide a great deal of autonomy to operating divisions and rely on financial controls and incentive programs to obtain high levels of performance from the individual businesses. Corporate staffs at these firms tend to be small because of their limited involvement in the overall operation of their various businesses.[16]

Advantages The holding company structure has the cost savings associated with fewer personnel and the lower overhead resulting from a small corporate office and fewer hierarchical levels. The autonomy of the holding company structure increases the motivational level of divisional executives and enables them to respond quickly to market opportunities and threats.

Disadvantages There is an inherent lack of control and dependence that corporate-level executives have on divisional executives. Major problems could arise if key divisional executives leave the firm, because the corporate office has very little "bench strength"—additional managerial talent ready to quickly fill key positions. If problems arise in a division, it may become very difficult to turn around individual businesses because of limited staff support in the corporate office.

Matrix Structure

matrix organizational structure an organizational form in which there are multiple lines of authority and some individuals report to at least two managers.

One approach that tries to overcome the inadequacies inherent in the other structures is the **matrix organizational structure.** It is a combination of the functional and divisional structures. Most commonly, functional departments are combined with product groups on a project basis. For example, a product group may want to develop a new addition to its line; for this project, it obtains personnel from functional departments such as marketing, production, and engineering. These personnel work under the manager of the product group for the duration of the project, which can vary from a few weeks to an open-ended period of time. The individuals who work in a matrix organization become responsible to two managers: the project manager and the manager of their functional area. Exhibit 10.4 illustrates a matrix structure.

Some large multinational corporations rely on a matrix structure to combine product groups and geographical units. Product managers have global responsibility for the development, manufacturing, and distribution of their own line, while managers of geographical regions have responsibility for the profitability of the businesses in their regions. In the mid-1990s, Caterpillar, Inc., implemented this type of structure.

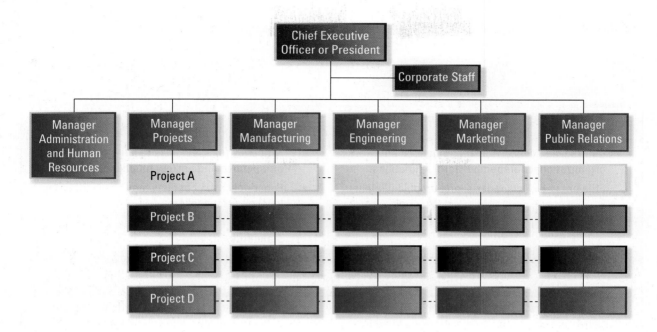

Exhibit 10.4 Matrix Organizational Structure

Advantages The matrix structure facilitates the use of specialized personnel, equipment, and facilities. Instead of duplicating functions, as would be the case in a divisional structure based on products, the resources are shared. Individuals with high expertise can divide their time among multiple projects. Such resource sharing and collaboration enable a firm to use resources more efficiently and to respond more quickly and effectively to changes in the competitive environment. The flexibility inherent in a matrix structure provides professionals with a broader range of responsibility. Such experience enables them to develop their skills and competencies.

Disadvantages The dual-reporting structures can result in uncertainty and lead to intense power struggles and conflict over the allocation of personnel and other resources. Working relationships become more complicated. This may result in excessive reliance on group processes and teamwork, along with a diffusion of responsibility, which in turn may erode timely decision making.

Let's look at Procter & Gamble (P&G) to see some of the disadvantages associated with a matrix structure:

> After 50 years with a divisional structure, P&G went to a matrix structure in 1987. In this structure, they had product categories, such as soaps and detergents, on one dimension and functional managers on the other dimension. Within each product category, country managers reported to regional managers who then reported to product managers. The structure became complex to manage, with 13 layers of management and significant power struggles as the functional managers developed their own strategic agendas that often were at odds with the product managers' agendas. After seeing their growth rate decline from 8.5 percent in the 1980s to 2.6 percent in the late 1990s, P&G scrapped the matrix structure to go to a global product structure with three major product categories to offer unity in direction and more responsive decision making.[17]

Exhibit 10.5 briefly summarizes the advantages and disadvantages of the functional, divisional, and matrix organizational structures.

Functional Structure

Advantages	Disadvantages
• Pooling of specialists enhances coordination and control.	• Differences in functional area orientation impede communication and coordination.
• Centralized decision making enhances an organizational perspective across functions.	• Tendency for specialists to develop short-term perspective and narrow functional orientation.
• Efficient use of managerial and technical talent.	• Functional area conflicts may overburden top-level decision makers.
• Facilitates career paths and professional development in specialized areas.	• Difficult to establish uniform performance standards.

Divisional Structure

Advantages	Disadvantages
• Increases strategic and operational control, permitting corporate-level executives to address strategic issues.	• Increased costs incurred through duplication of personnel, operations, and investment.
• Quick response to environmental changes.	• Dysfunctional competition among divisions may detract from overall corporate performance.
• Increases focus on products and markets.	• Difficult to maintain uniform corporate image.
• Minimizes problems associated with sharing resources across functional areas.	• Overemphasis on short-term performance.
• Facilitates development of general managers.	

Matrix Structure

Advantages	Disadvantages
• Increases market responsiveness through collaboration and synergies among professional colleagues.	• Dual-reporting relationships can result in uncertainty regarding accountability.
• Allows more efficient utilization of resources.	• Intense power struggles may lead to increased levels of conflict.
• Improves flexibility, coordination, and communication.	• Working relationships may be more complicated and human resources duplicated.
• Increases professional development through a broader range of responsibility.	• Excessive reliance on group processes and teamwork may impede timely decision making.

>LO10.3
The implications of a firm's international operations for organizational structure.

International Operations: Implications for Organizational Structure

Today's managers must maintain an international outlook on their firm's businesses and competitive strategies. In the global marketplace, managers must ensure consistency between their strategies (at the business, corporate, and international levels) and the structure of their organization. As firms expand into foreign markets, they generally follow a pattern of change in structure that parallels the changes in their strategies.[18] Three major contingencies that influence the chosen structure are (1) the type of strategy that is driving a firm's foreign operations, (2) product diversity, and (3) the extent to which a firm is dependent on foreign sales.[19]

As international operations become an important part of a firm's overall operations, managers must make changes that are consistent with their firm's structure. The primary types of structures used to manage a firm's international operations are:[20]

- International division
- Geographic-area division
- Worldwide matrix
- Worldwide functional
- Worldwide product division

Multidomestic strategies are driven by political and cultural imperatives requiring managers within each country to respond to local conditions. The structures consistent with such a strategic orientation are the **international division** and **geographic-area division structures.** Here local managers are provided with a high level of autonomy to manage their operations within the constraints and demands of their geographic market. As a firm's foreign sales increase as a percentage of its total sales, it will likely change from an international division to a geographic-area division structure. And, as a firm's product and/or market diversity becomes large, it is likely to benefit from a **worldwide matrix structure.**

Global strategies are driven by economic pressures that require managers to view operations in different geographic areas to be managed for overall efficiency. The structures consistent with the efficiency perspective are the **worldwide functional** and **worldwide product division structures.** Here, division managers view the marketplace as homogeneous and devote relatively little attention to local market, political, and economic factors. The choice between these two types of structures is guided largely by the extent of product diversity. Firms with relatively low levels of product diversity may opt for a worldwide product division structure. However, if significant product-market diversity results from highly unrelated international acquisitions, a worldwide holding company structure should be implemented. Such firms have very little commonality among products, markets, or technologies, and have little need for integration.

Global Start-Ups: A New Phenomenon

International expansion occurs rather late for most corporations, typically after possibilities of domestic growth are exhausted. Increasingly, we are seeing two interrelated phenomena. First, many firms now expand internationally relatively early in their history. Second, some firms are "born global"—that is, from the very beginning, many start-ups are global in their activities. For example, Logitech Inc., a leading producer of personal computer accessories, was global from day one. Founded in 1982 by a Swiss national and two Italians, the company was headquartered both in California and Switzerland. R&D and manufacturing were also conducted in both locations and, subsequently, in Taiwan and Ireland.[21]

The success of companies such as Logitech challenges the conventional wisdom that a company must first build up assets, internal processes, and experience before venturing into faraway lands. It also raises a number of questions: What exactly is a global start-up? Under what conditions should a company start out as a global start-up? What does it take to succeed as a global start-up?

A **global start-up** has been defined as a business organization that, from inception, seeks to derive significant competitive advantage from the use of resources and the sale of outputs in multiple countries. Right from the beginning, it uses inputs from around the world and sells its products and services to customers around the world. Geographical boundaries of nation-states are irrelevant for a global start-up.

There is no reason for every start-up to be global. Being global necessarily involves higher communication, coordination, and transportation costs. Therefore, it is important to

---

international division structure an organizational form in which international operations are in a separate, autonomous division. Most domestic operations are kept in other parts of the organization.

geographic-area division structure a type of divisional organizational structure in which operations in geographical regions are grouped internally.

worldwide matrix structure a type of matrix organizational structure that has one line of authority for geographic-area divisions and another line of authority for worldwide product divisions.

worldwide functional structure a functional structure in which all departments have worldwide reponsibilities.

worldwide product division structure a product division structure in which all divisions have worldwide responsibilities.

global start-up a business organization that, from inception, seeks to derive significant advantage from the use of resources and the sale of outputs in multiple countries.

identify the circumstances under which going global from the beginning is advantageous.[22] First, if the required human resources are globally dispersed, going global may be the best way to access those resources. For example, Italians are masters in fine leather and Europeans in ergonomics. Second, in many cases foreign financing may be easier to obtain and more suitable. Traditionally, U.S. venture capitalists have shown greater willingness to bear risk, but they have shorter time horizons in their expectations for return. If a U.S. start-up is looking for patient capital, it may be better off looking overseas. Third, the target customers in many specialized industries are located in other parts of the world. Fourth, in many industries a gradual move from domestic markets to foreign markets is no longer possible because, if a product is successful, foreign competitors may immediately imitate it. Therefore, preemptive entry into foreign markets may be the only option. Finally, because of high up-front development costs, a global market is often necessary to recover the costs. This is particularly true for start-ups from smaller nations that do not have access to large domestic markets.

Successful management of a global start-up presents many challenges. Communication and coordination across time zones and cultures are always problematic. Since most global start-ups have far less resources than well-established corporations, one key for success is to internalize few activities and outsource the rest. Managers of such firms must have considerable prior international experience so that they can successfully handle the inevitable communication problems and cultural conflicts. Another key for success is to keep the communication and coordination costs low. The only way to achieve this is by creating less costly administrative mechanisms. The boundaryless organizational designs that we discuss in the next section are particularly suitable for global start-ups because of their flexibility and low cost.

Strategy Spotlight 10.3 discusses three global start-ups.

How an Organization's Structure Can Influence Strategy Formulation

Discussions of the relationship between strategy and structure usually strongly imply that structure follows strategy. The strategy that a firm chooses (e.g., related diversification) dictates such structural elements as the division of tasks, the need for integration of activities, and authority relationships within the organization. However, an existing structure can influence strategy formulation. Once a firm's structure is in place, it is very difficult and expensive to change.[23] Executives may not be able to modify their duties and responsibilities greatly, or may not welcome the disruption associated with a transfer to a new location. There are costs associated with hiring, training, and replacing executive, managerial, and operating personnel. Strategy cannot be formulated without considering structural elements.

An organization's structure can also have an important influence on how it competes in the marketplace. It can also strongly influence a firm's strategy, day-to-day operations, and performance.[24] Brinker International, one of the world's leading casual dining restaurant companies with stores in more than 31 countries, changed its organizational structure from functional to divisional in an effort to organize its restaurant groups into different units to focus on market niches. The new structure enabled the company to adapt to change more rapidly and innovate more effectively with its various restaurant brands around the world. Brinker's management did not believe they were effective with their previous functional organizational structure.[25]

>LO10.4
Why there is no "one best way" to design strategic reward and evaluation systems, and the important contingent roles of business- and corporate-level strategies.

Linking Strategic Reward and Evaluation Systems to Business-Level and Corporate-Level Strategies

The effective use of reward and evaluation systems can play a critical role in motivating managers to conform to organizational strategies, achieve performance targets, and

Global on Day One

Conventional wisdom would suggest that a firm "get it right" in its home market before venturing abroad. Once established in the home market, a firm could consider the relatively risky move of selling in other countries. However, many new firms are turning conventional wisdom on its head.

More and more start-ups are being born global for two basic reasons. One reason is defensive: to be competitive, many new businesses need to globalize some parts of their business to control costs, access customers, or tap employees from day one. While this might seem an obviously logical choice, until recently many venture capital firms required companies to build locally first, gain a track record, and then branch out. The other reason firms are born global is offensive; many entrepreneurs find that new business opportunities span multiple countries. Going after opportunities in several countries simultaneously from the start can sometimes give firms the operating scope they need to thrive.

Going global is not without significant challenges. Coping with distance in terms of physical, time zone, and cultural dimensions is perhaps a larger hurdle for smaller organizations to tackle. However, start-ups that can articulate a global purpose tend to do better than those with weaker goal orientation toward a global strategy. The following three examples are of start-ups that thought global from day one:

- In 2008, Actavis Pharmaceuticals' revenues were over $2 billion. Robert Wessman took control of this small generic pharmaceutical maker in his native Iceland in 1999. Within weeks of taking over, he realized that to succeed in the generics market, a player had to globalize its core functions, including manufacturing and R&D. Actavis has since entered 60 countries to gain scale and develop a larger portfolio of drugs. In 2011, the company had more than 800 products on the market and over 330 products in development.

- Baradok Pridor, 38, and Yonatan Aumann, 42, Israeli founders of ClearForest, developed an innovative software product—a program that can analyze unstructured electronic data, such as a web page or a video clip, as if it were already in a spreadsheet or database. Instead of waiting for customers to show up, right from the beginning, they started sending their engineers to make presentations to potential clients around the world. Today, the company's customers include Dow Chemical, Thomson Financial, and the FBI! They have raised $33 million so far in three rounds of venture financing. Interestingly, the headquarters of the 83-person company is in Boston!

- HyperRoll, an Israeli company that makes software for analyzing massive databases, has raised $28 million in venture funding. Referring to the firm's hiring practices, Yossi Matias, founder of HyperRoll, said, "We build the strongest team possible, unconstrained by locality, affinity, or culture. It requires every employee to accept and support a multicultural environment." Although the firm is essentially an Israeli start-up, he even banned the use of Hebrew in the office to facilitate greater integration between the American and Israeli employees.

Sources: *www.actavis.com*; Isenberg, D. J. 2008. The global entrepreneur. *Harvard Business Review*, December: 107–111; Copeland, M. V. 2004. The start-up oasis. *Business 2.0*, August: 46–48.; and, Brown, E. 2004. Global start-up. *Forbes*, November 29: 150–161.

reduce the gap between organizational and individual goals. In contrast, reward systems, if improperly designed, can lead to behaviors that either are detrimental to organizational performance or can lower morale and cause employee dissatisfaction.

As we will see in this section, there is no "one best way" to design reward and evaluation systems. Instead, it is contingent on many factors. Two of the most important factors are a firm's business-level strategy (see Chapter 5) and its corporate-level strategy (see Chapter 6).

Business-Level Strategy: Reward and Evaluation Systems

In Chapter 5 we discussed two approaches that firms may take to secure competitive advantages: overall cost leadership and differentiation.[26] As we might expect, implementing these strategies requires fundamentally different organizational arrangements, approaches to control, and reward and incentive systems.

Overall Cost Leadership   This strategy requires that product lines remain rather stable and that innovations deal mostly with production processes. Given the emphasis on efficiency, costly changes even in production processes tend to be rare. Since products are quite standardized and change rather infrequently, procedures can be developed to divide work into its basic components—those that are routine, standardized, and ideal for semiskilled and unskilled employees. As such, firms competing on the basis of cost must implement tight cost controls, frequent and comprehensive reports to monitor the costs associated with outputs, and highly structured tasks and responsibilities. Incentives tend to be based on explicit financial targets since innovation and creativity are expensive and might tend to erode competitive advantages.

Nucor, a highly successful steel producer with $16 billion in revenues, competes primarily on the basis of cost and has a reward and incentive system that is largely based on financial outputs and financial measures.[27] Nucor uses four incentive compensation systems that correspond to the levels of management.

1. *Production incentive program.* Groups of 20 to 40 people are paid a weekly bonus based on either anticipated product time or tonnage produced. Each shift and production line is in a separate bonus group.
2. *Department managers.* Bonuses are based on divisional performance, primarily measured by return on assets.
3. *Employees not directly involved in production.* These include engineers, accountants, secretaries, receptionists, and others. Bonuses are based on two factors: divisional and corporate return on assets.
4. *Senior incentive programs.* Salaries are lower than comparable companies, but a significant portion of total compensation is based on return on stockholder equity. A portion of pretax earnings is placed in a pool and divided among officers as bonuses that are part cash and part stock.

The culture at Nucor reflects its reward and incentive system. Since incentive compensation can account for more than half of their paychecks, employees become nearly obsessed with productivity and apply a lot of pressure on each other. Ken Iverson, a former CEO, recalled an instance in which one employee arrived at work in sunglasses instead of safety glasses, preventing the team from doing any work. Furious, the other workers chased him around the plant with a piece of angle iron!

Differentiation   This strategy involves the development of innovative products and services that require experts who can identify the crucial elements of intricate, creative designs and marketing decisions. Highly trained professionals such as scientists and engineers are essential for devising, assessing, implementing, and continually changing complex product designs. This also requires extensive collaboration and cooperation among specialists and functional managers from different areas within a firm. They must evaluate and implement a new design, constantly bearing in mind marketing, financial, production, and engineering considerations.

Given the need for cooperation and coordination in many functional areas, it becomes difficult to evaluate individuals using set quantitative criteria. It also is difficult to measure specific outcomes of such efforts and attribute outcomes to specific individuals. More behavioral measures (how effectively employees collaborate and share information) and intangible incentives and rewards become necessary to support a strong culture and to motivate employees. Consider 3M, a highly innovative company whose core value is innovation.

> Rewards are tied closely to risk-taking and innovation-oriented behavior. Managers are not penalized for product failures. Instead, those same people are encouraged to work on another project that borrows from their shared experience and insight. A culture of creativity and "thinking out of the box" is reinforced by their well-known "15 percent rule," which

permits employees to set aside 15 percent of their work time to pursue personal research interests. And a familiar 3M homily, "Thou shall not kill new ideas for products," is known as the 11th commandment. It is the source of countless stories, including one that tells how L. D. DeSimone (3M's former CEO) tried five times (and failed) to kill the project that yielded the 3M blockbuster product, Thinsulate.[28]

Corporate-Level Strategy: Reward and Evaluation Systems

In Chapter 6 we discussed two broad types of diversification strategies: related and unrelated. The type of diversification strategy that a firm follows has important implications for the type of reward and evaluation systems that it should use.

Sharp Corporation, a $34 billion Japanese consumer electronics giant, follows a strategy of *related* diversification.[29] Its most successful technology has been liquid crystal displays (LCDs) that are critical components in nearly all of the firm's products. With its expertise in this area, it moved into high-end displays for cellular telephones, handheld computers, and digital computers.[30]

Given the need to leverage such technologies across multiple product lines, Sharp needs reward and evaluation systems that foster coordination and sharing. It must focus more on individuals' behavior rather than on short-term financial outcomes. Promotion is a powerful incentive, and it is generally based on seniority and subtle skills exhibited over time, such as teamwork and communication. It helps to ensure that the company's reward system will not reward short-term self-interested orientations.

Like many Japanese companies, Sharp's culture reinforces the view that the firm is a family whose members should cooperate for the greater good. With the policy of lifetime employment, turnover is low. This encourages employees to pursue what is best for the entire company. Such an outlook lessens the inevitable conflict over sharing important resources such as R&D knowledge.

In contrast to Sharp, Hanson PLC (a British conglomerate) followed a strategy of unrelated diversification for most of its history. At one time it owned as many as 150 operating companies in areas such as tobacco, footwear, building products, brewing, and food. There were limited product similarities across businesses and therefore little need for sharing of resources and knowledge across divisional boundaries. James Hanson and Gordon White, founders of the company, actually did not permit any sharing of resources between operating companies even if it was feasible!

Their reward and evaluation system placed such heavy emphasis on individual accountability that they viewed resource sharing, with its potential for mutual blaming, unacceptable. The operating managers had more than 60 percent of their compensation tied to annual financial performance of their subsidiaries. All decision making was decentralized so that subsidiary managers could be held responsible for the return on capital they employed. However, there was one area in which they had to obtain approval from the corporate office. No subsidiary manager was allowed to incur a capital expenditure greater than $3,000 without permission from the corporate office. Hanson managed to be successful with a very small corporate office because of its decentralized structure, tight financial controls, and an incentive system that motivated managers to meet financial goals. Gordon White was proud of claiming that he had never visited any of the operating companies that were part of the Hanson empire.[31]

The key issue becomes the need for *in*dependence versus *inter*dependence. With cost leadership strategies and unrelated diversification, there tends to be less need for interdependence. The reward and evaluation systems focus more on the use of financial indicators because unit costs, profits, and revenues can be rather easily attributed to a given business unit or division.

In contrast, firms that follow related diversification strategies have intense needs for tight interdependencies among the functional areas and business units. Sharing of resources, including raw materials, R&D knowledge, marketing information, and so on, is critical to organizational success. It is more important to achieve synergies with value-creating activities and business units than with cost leadership or unrelated strategies. Reward and evaluation systems tend to incorporate more behavioral indicators.

Although Exhibit 10.6 suggests guidelines on how an organization should match its strategies to its evaluation and reward systems, all organizations must have combinations of both financial and behavioral rewards. Both overall cost leadership and unrelated diversification strategies require a need for collaboration and the sharing of best practices across both value-creating activities and business units. General Electric has developed many integrating mechanisms to enhance sharing "best practices" across what would appear to be rather unrelated businesses such as jet engines, appliances, and network television. For both differentiation and related diversification strategies, financial indicators such as revenue growth and profitability should not be overlooked at both the business-unit and corporate levels.

Boundaryless Organizational Designs

>LO10.5
The different types of boundaryless organizations— barrier-free, modular, and virtual—and their relative advantages and disadvantages.

The term *boundaryless* may bring to mind a chaotic organizational reality in which "anything goes." This is not the case. As Jack Welch, GE's former CEO, has suggested, boundaryless does not imply that all internal and external boundaries vanish completely, but that they become more open and permeable.[32] Strategy Spotlight 10.4 discusses four types of boundaries.

We are not suggesting that **boundaryless organizational designs** replace the traditional forms of organizational structure, but they should complement them. Sharp Corp. has implemented a functional structure to attain economies of scale with its applied research and manufacturing skills. However, to bring about this key objective, Sharp has relied on several integrating mechanisms and processes:

boundaryless organizational designs
organizations in which the boundaries, including vertical, horizontal, external, and geographic boundaries, are permeable.

> To prevent functional groups from becoming vertical chimneys that obstruct product development, Sharp's product managers have responsibility—but not authority—for coordinating the entire set of value-chain activities. And the company convenes enormous numbers of cross-unit and corporate committees to ensure that shared activities, including the corporate R&D unit and sales forces, are optimally configured and allocated among the different product lines. Sharp invests in such time-intensive coordination to minimize the inevitable conflicts that arise when units share important activities.[33]

We will discuss three approaches to making boundaries more permeable, that help to facilitate the widespread sharing of knowledge and information across both the internal and external boundaries of the organization. The *barrier-free* type involves making all organizational boundaries—internal and external—more permeable. Teams are a central building block for implementing the boundaryless organization. The *modular* and *virtual* types of organizations focus on the need to create seamless relationships

Exhibit 10.6
Summary of Relationships between Reward and Evaluation Systems and Business-Level and Corporate-Level Strategies

Level of Strategy	Types of Strategy	Need for Interdependence	Primary Type of Reward and Evaluation System
Business-level	Overall cost leadership	Low	Financial
Business-level	Differentiation	High	Behavioral
Corporate-level	Related diversification	High	Behavioral
Corporate-level	Unrelated diversification	Low	Financial

Boundary Types

There are primarily four types of boundaries that place limits on organizations. In today's dynamic business environment, different types of boundaries are needed to foster high degrees of interaction with outside influences and varying levels of permeability.

1. *Vertical boundaries between levels in the organization's hierarchy.* SmithKline Beecham asks employees at different hierarchical levels to brainstorm ideas for managing clinical trial data. The ideas are incorporated into action plans that significantly cut the new product approval time of its pharmaceuticals. This would not have been possible if the barriers between levels of individuals in the organization had been too high.

2. *Horizontal boundaries between functional areas.* Fidelity Investments makes the functional barriers more porous and flexible among divisions, such as marketing, operations, and customer service, in order to offer customers a more integrated experience when conducting business with the company. Customers can take their questions to one person, reducing the chance that customers will "get the runaround" from employees who feel customer service is not their responsibility. At Fidelity, customer service is everyone's business, regardless of functional area.

3. *External boundaries between the firm and its customers, suppliers, and regulators.* GE Lighting, by working closely with retailers, functions throughout the value chain as a single operation. This allows GE to track point-of-sale purchases, giving it better control over inventory management.

4. *Geographic boundaries between locations, cultures, and markets.* The global nature of today's business environment spurred PricewaterhouseCoopers to use a global groupware system. This allows the company to instantly connect to its 26 worldwide offices.

Source: Ashkenas, R. 1997. The organization's New Clothes. In Hesselbein, F., Goldsmith, M., & Beckhard, R. (Eds.). *The organization of the future:* 104–106. San Francisco: Jossey Bass.

with external organizations such as customers or suppliers. While the modular type emphasizes the outsourcing of noncore activities, the virtual (or network) organization focuses on alliances among independent entities formed to exploit specific market opportunities.

The Barrier-Free Organization

The "boundary" mind-set is ingrained deeply into bureaucracies. It is evidenced by such clichés as "That's not my job," "I'm here from corporate to help," or endless battles over transfer pricing. In the traditional company, boundaries are clearly delineated in the design of an organization's structure. Their basic advantage is that the roles of managers and employees are simple, clear, well-defined, and long-lived. A major shortcoming was pointed out to the authors during an interview with a high-tech executive: "Structure tends to be divisive; it leads to territorial fights."

Such structures are being replaced by fluid, ambiguous, and deliberately ill-defined tasks and roles. Just because work roles are no longer clearly defined, however, does not mean that differences in skills, authority, and talent disappear. A **barrier-free organization** enables a firm to bridge real differences in culture, function, and goals to find common ground that facilitates information sharing and other forms of cooperative behavior. Eliminating the multiple boundaries that stifle productivity and innovation can enhance the potential of the entire organization.

Creating Permeable Internal Boundaries   For barrier-free organizations to work effectively, the level of trust and shared interests among all parts of the organization must be raised.[34] The organization needs to develop among its employees the skill level needed

barrier-free organization an organizational design in which firms bridge real differences in culture, function, and goals to find common ground that facilitates information sharing and other forms of cooperative behavior.

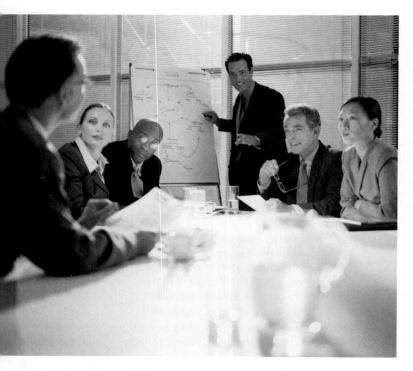

● Teams frequently develop more creative solutions to problems because they can share each individual's knowledge.

to work in a more democratic organization. Barrier-free organizations also require a shift in the organization's philosophy from executive to organizational development, and from investments in high-potential individuals to investments in leveraging the talents of all individuals.

Teams can be an important aspect of barrier-free structures.[35] Jeffrey Pfeffer, author of several insightful books, including *The Human Equation,* suggests that teams have three primary advantages.[36] First, teams substitute peer-based control for hierarchical control of work activities. Employees control themselves, reducing the time and energy management needs to devote to control. Second, teams frequently develop more creative solutions to problems because they encourage the sharing of the tacit knowledge held by individuals.[37] Brainstorming, or group problem solving, involves the pooling of ideas and expertise to enhance the chances that at least one group member will think of a way to solve the problems at hand. Third, by substituting peer control for hierarchical control, teams permit the removal of layers of hierarchy and absorption of administrative tasks previously performed by specialists. This avoids the costs of having people whose sole job is to watch the people who watch other people do the work.

Effective barrier-free organizations must go beyond achieving close integration and coordination within divisions in a corporation. Research on multidivisional organizations has stressed the importance of interdivisional coordination and resource sharing.[38] This requires interdivisional task forces and committees, reward and incentive systems that emphasize interdivisional cooperation, and common training programs.

Frank Carruba (former head of Hewlett-Packard's labs) found that the difference between mediocre teams and good teams was generally varying levels of motivation and talent.[39] But what explained the difference between good teams and truly superior teams? The key difference—and this explained a 40 percent overall difference in performance—was the way members treated each other: the degree to which they believed in one another and created an atmosphere of encouragement rather than competition. Vision, talent, and motivation could carry a team only so far. What clearly stood out in the "super" teams were higher levels of authenticity and caring, which allowed the full synergy of their individual talents, motivation, and vision.

Developing Effective Relationships with External Constituencies   In barrier-free organizations, managers must also create flexible, porous organizational boundaries and establish communication flows and mutually beneficial relationships with internal (e.g., employees) and external (e.g., customers) constituencies.[40] Michael Dell, founder and CEO of Dell Computer, is a strong believer in fostering close relationships with his customers:

> We're not going to be just your PC vendor anymore. We're going to be your IT department for PCs. Boeing, for example, has 100,000 Dell PCs, and we have 30 people that live at

The Business Roundtable: A Forum for Sharing Best Environmental Sustainability Practices

The Business Roundtable is a group of chief executive officers of major U.S. corporations that was created to promote pro-business public policy. It was formed in 1972 through the merger of three existing organizations: The March Group, the Construction Users Anti-Inflation Roundtable, and the Labor Law Study Committee. The group has been called President Obama's "closest ally in the business community."

The Business Roundtable became the first broad-based business group to agree on the need to address climate change through collective action, and it remains committed to limiting greenhouse gas emissions and setting the United States on a more sustainable path. The organization considers that threats to water quality and quantity, rising greenhouse gas emissions, and the risk of climate change—along with increasing energy prices and growing demand—are of great concern.

Its recent report, "Enhancing Our Commitment to a Sustainable Future 2010," provides best practices and metrics from Business Roundtable member companies that represent nearly all sectors of the economy with $6 trillion in annual revenues. CEOs from Walmart, FedEx, PepsiCo, Whirlpool, and Verizon are among the 97 executives from leading U.S. companies that shared some of their best sustainability initiatives in this report. These companies are committed to reducing emissions, increasing energy efficiency, and developing more sustainable business practices.

Let's look, for example, at some of Walmart's initiatives. The firm's CEO, Mike Duke, said it is working with suppliers, partners, and consumers to drive its sustainability program. It has helped establish the Sustainability Consortium to drive metrics for measuring the environmental effects of consumer products across their life cycle. The retailer also helped lead the creation of a Sustainable Product Index to provide product information to consumers about the environmental impact of the products they purchase.

There are many ways in which Walmart has increased the energy efficiency of its operations:

- It has 30 facilities in California and Hawaii with solar power installations, and it is purchasing 226 million kilowatt hours (kWh) of wind energy annually in Texas.
- It has an agreement in Japan to buy 1 million kWh of clean, renewable energy per year.
- Its trucking fleet in the United Kingdom has cut greenhouse gas (GHG) emissions by 40 percent through the use of new technology, consolidated supplier deliveries, and increased use of rail transportation.

Walmart has also significantly removed GHG emissions from the products that it sells:

- In February 2009, Walmart committed to eliminating 20 million metric tons of GHG emissions from the life cycle of the products it sells worldwide by 2015.
- In 2007, Walmart launched a pilot program to cut supply-chain emissions. Through this program, DVD suppliers reduced packaging and cut more than 28,000 metric tons of GHG.
- Walmart has sold more than 350 million compact fluorescent light bulbs in the United States alone. The firm estimates that, during the life of these bulbs, its customers will save more than $13 billion and avoid producing more than 65 million metric tons of GHG emissions.

Sources: Anonymous. 2010. Leading CEOs share best sustainability practices. *www.environmentalleader.com*. April 26: np; Hopkins, M. No date. Sustainable growth. *www.businessroundtable*. np; Castellani, J. J. 2010. Enhancing our commitment to a sustainable future report. *www.businessroundtable.org*. March 31: np; and Business Roundtable. *www.en.wikipedia.org*.

Boeing, and if you look at the things we're doing for them or for other customers, we don't look like a supplier, we look more like Boeing's PC department. We become intimately involved in planning their PC needs and the configuration of their network.

It's not that we make these decisions by ourselves. They're certainly using their own people to get the best answer for the company. But the people working on PCs together, from both Dell and Boeing, understand the needs in a very intimate way. They're right there living it and breathing it, as opposed to the typical vendor who says, "Here are your computers. See you later."[41]

Barrier-free organizations create successful relationships between both internal and external constituencies, but there is one additional constituency—competitors—with whom some organizations have benefited as they developed cooperative relationships. After years of seeing its empty trucks return from warehouses back to production facilities after deliveries, General Mills teamed up with 16 of its competitors. They formed an e-commerce business to help the firms find carriers with empty cargo trailers to piggyback freight loads to distributors near the production facilities.[42] This increases revenue for all network members and reduces fuel costs.

By joining and actively participating in the Business Roundtable—an organization consisting of CEOs of leading U.S. corporations—Walmart has been able to learn about cutting-edge sustainable initiatives of other major firms. This free flow of information has enabled Walmart to undertake a number of steps that increased the energy efficiency of its operations. These are described in Strategy Spotlight 10.5

CEO participation in business roundtables is not limited to companies in the United States. Consider the following examples of CEO business roundtables around the world:[43]

- The Canada Europe Roundtable for Business (CERT) is dedicated to creating business opportunities between Canada and the European Union. Founded in 1999, CERT develops company-member interests by contributing recommendations on trade and investment to government officials and hosting thematic, high-level meetings focused on developing strategic relationships between company executives and with government officials.
- The EU–Japan Business Round Table (BRT) is a forum that brings together CEOs and senior executives of more than 50 leading EU and Japanese companies. BRT members meet annually to review factors that affect all aspects of business between the EU and Japan and to suggest ways in which government action can improve the EU–Japan business environment and facilitate cross-investment. The BRT provides valuable business input and gives the European Commission a realistic overview of the practical problems that companies face in Europe and Japan.
- The EU–Russia Industrialists' Round Table (IRT) is a business-driven group that was originally endorsed by the EU–Russia Summit of July 1997. IRT's main objective is to provide a permanent forum for businesspeople to present joint recommendations to the European Commission and the Russian government with regard to business and investment conditions and promotion of industrial cooperation.

Risks, Challenges, and Potential Downsides   Many firms find that creating and managing a barrier-free organization can be frustrating.[44] Puritan-Bennett Corporation, a manufacturer of respiratory equipment, found that its product development time more than doubled after it adopted team management. Roger J. Dolida, director of R&D, attributed this failure to a lack of top management commitment, high turnover among team members, and infrequent meetings. Often, managers trained in rigid hierarchies find it difficult to make the transition to the more democratic, participative style that teamwork requires.

Christopher Barnes, a consultant with PricewaterhouseCoopers, previously worked as an industrial engineer for Challenger Electrical Distribution (a subsidiary of Westinghouse, now part of CBS) at a plant that produced circuit-breaker boxes. His assignment was to lead a team of workers from the plant's troubled final-assembly operation with the mission: "Make things better." That vague notion set the team up for failure. After a year of futility, the team was disbanded. In retrospect, Barnes identified several reasons for the debacle: (1) limited personal credibility—he was viewed as an "outsider"; (2) a lack of commitment to the team—everyone involved was forced to be on the team; (3) poor communications—nobody was told why the team was important; (4) limited autonomy—line managers refused to give up control over team members; and (5) misaligned incentives—the culture rewarded individual performance over team performance.

Pros	Cons
• Leverages the talents of all employees. • Enhances cooperation, coordination, and information sharing among functions, divisions, SBUs, and external constituencies. • Enables a quicker response to market changes through a single-goal focus. • Can lead to coordinated win–win initiatives with key suppliers, customers, and alliance partners.	• Difficult to overcome political and authority boundaries inside and outside the organization. • Lacks strong leadership and common vision, which can lead to coordination problems. • Time-consuming and difficult-to-manage democratic processes. • Lacks high levels of trust, which can impede performance.

Exhibit 10.7
Pros and Cons of Barrier-Free Structures

Barnes's experience has implications for all types of teams, whether they are composed of managerial, professional, clerical, or production personnel.[45] The pros and cons of barrier-free structures are summarized in Exhibit 10.7.

The Modular Organization

As Charles Handy, author of *The Age of Unreason,* has noted:

> While it may be convenient to have everyone around all the time, having all of your workforce's time at your command is an extravagant way of marshaling the necessary resources. It is cheaper to keep them outside the organization . . . and to buy their services when you need them.[46]

The **modular organization** outsources nonvital functions, tapping into the knowledge and expertise of "best in class" suppliers, but retains strategic control. Outsiders may be used to manufacture parts, handle logistics, or perform accounting activities.[47] The value chain can be used to identify the key primary and support activities performed by a firm to create value: Which activities do we keep "in-house" and which activities do we outsource to suppliers?[48] The organization becomes a central hub surrounded by networks of outside suppliers and specialists and parts can be added or taken away. Both manufacturing and service units may be modular.[49]

modular organization an organization in which nonvital functions are outsourced, which uses the knowledge and expertise of outside suppliers while retaining strategic control.

Apparel is an industry in which the modular type has been widely adopted. Nike and Reebok, for example, concentrate on their strengths: designing and marketing high-tech, fashionable footwear. Nike has few production facilities and Reebok owns no plants. These two companies contract virtually all their footwear production to suppliers in China, Vietnam, and other countries with low-cost labor. Avoiding large investments in fixed assets helps them derive large profits on minor sales increases. Nike and Reebok can keep pace with changing tastes in the marketplace because their suppliers have become expert at rapidly retooling to produce new products.[50]

In a modular company, outsourcing the noncore functions offers three advantages.

1. A firm can decrease overall costs, stimulate new product development by hiring suppliers with superior talent to that of in-house personnel, avoid idle capacity, reduce inventories, and avoid being locked into a particular technology.
2. A company can focus scarce resources on the areas where it holds a competitive advantage. These benefits can translate into more funding for R&D, hiring the best engineers, and providing continuous training for sales and service staff.
3. An organization can tap into the knowledge and expertise of its specialized supply-chain partners, adding critical skills and accelerating organizational learning.[51]

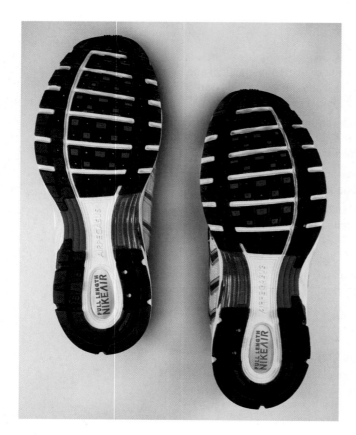

● Nike is one of many athletic shoe companies that have outsourced most of their production to low-cost-labor countries such as Indonesia and Vietnam.

The modular type enables a company to leverage relatively small amounts of capital and a small management team to achieve seemingly unattainable strategic objectives.[52] Certain preconditions are necessary before the modular approach can be successful. First, the company must work closely with suppliers to ensure that the interests of each party are being fulfilled. Companies need to find loyal, reliable vendors who can be trusted with trade secrets. They also need assurances that suppliers will dedicate their financial, physical, and human resources to satisfy strategic objectives such as lowering costs or being first to market.

Second, the modular company must be sure that it selects the proper competencies to keep in-house. For Nike and Reebok, the core competencies are design and marketing, not shoe manufacturing; for Honda, the core competence is engine technology. An organization must avoid outsourcing components that may compromise its long-term competitive advantages.

Strategic Risks of Outsourcing   The main strategic concerns are (1) loss of critical skills or developing the wrong skills, (2) loss of cross-functional skills, and (3) loss of control over a supplier.[53]

Too much outsourcing can result in a firm "giving away" too much skill and control.[54] Outsourcing relieves companies of the requirement to maintain skill levels needed to manufacture essential components.[55] At one time, semiconductor chips seemed like a simple technology to outsource, but they have now become a critical component of a wide variety of products. Companies that have outsourced the manufacture of these chips run the risk of losing the ability to manufacture them as the technology escalates. They become more dependent upon their suppliers. Lego, in an effort to reduce costs and avoid bankruptcy, outsourced certain production tasks to a company in Singapore with disastrous results. The company was forced to rethink its outsourcing strategies and brought jobs back to its homeland of Denmark.[56]

Cross-functional skills refer to the skills acquired through the interaction of individuals in various departments within a company.[57] Such interaction assists a department in solving problems as employees interface with others across functional units. However, if a firm outsources key functional responsibilities, such as manufacturing, communication across departments can become more difficult. A firm and its employees must now integrate their activities with a new, outside supplier.

The outsourced products may give suppliers too much power over the manufacturer. Suppliers that are key to a manufacturer's success can, in essence, hold the manufacturer "hostage." Nike manages this potential problem by sending full-time "product expatriates" to work at the plants of its suppliers. Also, Nike often brings top members of supplier management and technical teams to its headquarters. This way, Nike keeps close tabs on the pulse of new developments, builds rapport and trust with suppliers, and develops long-term relationships with suppliers to prevent hostage situations.

Strategy Spotlight 10.6 discusses Microsoft's effective outsourcing strategy for its video games. Exhibit 10.8 summarizes the pros and cons of modular structures.[58]

10.6

Video Games: Microsoft's Outsourcing Strategy

The convergence of Hollywood and Silicon Valley has led to the explosive growth of the worldwide video game industry, with revenues of $66.5 billion. In fact, it has recently overtaken the movie industry's box office receipts. While broadcast TV audiences dwindle and movie attendance stagnates, gaming is emerging as the newest and perhaps the strongest pillar in the media world. So it's no surprise that film studios, media giants, game creators, and Japanese electronics companies are all battling to win the "Game Wars."

Microsoft has dominated the market for computer software with its Windows operating system and its Office and Explorer application software. Seeing the growth in the gaming market, the company diversified into the video game industry with the Xbox and its successor, the Xbox 360. Microsoft faces tough competition from Sony Corp.'s PlayStation 3 and Nintendo Co.'s Wii in the video game industry. However, Microsoft's Xbox 360 beat Wii and PlayStation 3 in sales in the month of February 2010 to become the best-selling video game console in the United States for the first time in more than two years. Microsoft extended its advantage in November 2010 by introducing Kinect, the first motion-sensing system that doesn't require a remote.

Microsoft has a sophisticated approach to outsourcing video game software and hardware. On the software front, since the developmental phase of Xbox 360 in early 2003, Microsoft has reached out to developers by organizing events for the developers to recruit support for the system. Instead of limiting access to video game development software to those with big projects, big budgets, and the backing of the big game labels, Microsoft delivered the necessary tools of game development to hobbyists, students, indie developers, and studios alike. Knowing full well that great game ideas are brewing in the minds of students everywhere, Microsoft has targeted students at colleges, universities, and high schools as game developers. This practice helped bring creative game ideas to life while nurturing game development talent, a collaboration that benefited the entire industry.

For manufacturing the hardware of Xbox 360, Microsoft partnered with companies like Flextronics, Wistron, and Celestica, which produce the game system in their plants in China. According to Jim Sacherman, vice president of business development at Flextronics, "Our goal is to act as a true partner, not just a contractor." The firm showed a willingness to be a team player by collaborating with Microsoft on all aspects of the manufacturing and design process. From the beginning, Microsoft and Flextronics worked together to outline each company's roles and responsibilities and to ensure that all parties knew what was expected of them in all anticipated scenarios. The relationship between Microsoft and Flextronics quickly became a successful hybrid of the two most traditional outsourcing arrangements: Microsoft never turned over complete responsibility to Flextronics or passively waited to hear about progress. Neither did it act as a typical employer, dictating tasks and keeping Flextronics in the dark about its long-term plans for the product. Instead, the two companies worked together collaboratively from the beginning.

Sources: *www.microsoft.com*; Alpeyev, P. & Satariano, A. 2010. Microsoft's Xbox sales beat Wii, PS3 in February on "BioShock." *www.businessweek.com*. March 11: np; Grover, R., Edwards, C., Rowley, I., & Moon, I. 2005. Game wars. *BusinessWeek*, February 28: 35–40; Radd, D. 2005. Xbox 360 manufacturers revealed. *www.businessweek.com*. August 16: np; and, Anonymous. 2002. Outsourcing Xbox manufacturing: Microsoft shows the way for successful outsourcing relationships. *www.goliath.ecnext.com*. np.

The Virtual Organization

In contrast to the "self-reliant" thinking that guided traditional organizational designs, the strategic challenge today has become doing more with less and looking outside the firm for opportunities and solutions to problems. The virtual organization provides a new means of leveraging resources and exploiting opportunities.[59]

The **virtual organization** can be viewed as a continually evolving network of independent companies—suppliers, customers, even competitors—linked together to share skills, costs, and access to one another's markets.[60] The members of a virtual organization, by pooling and sharing the knowledge and expertise of each of the component organizations, simultaneously "know" more and can "do" more than any one member of the group

virtual organization a continually evolving network of independent companies that are linked together to share skills, costs, and access to one another's markets.

Exhibit 10.8
Pros and Cons of
Modular Structures

Pros	Cons
• Directs a firm's managerial and technical talent to the most critical activities.	• Inhibits common vision through reliance on outsiders.
• Maintains full strategic control over most critical activities—core competencies.	• Diminishes future competitive advantages if critical technologies or other competencies are outsourced.
• Achieves "best in class" performance at each link in the value chain.	• Increases the difficulty of bringing back into the firm activities that now add value due to market shifts.
• Leverages core competencies by outsourcing with smaller capital commitment.	• Leads to an erosion of cross-functional skills.
• Encourages information sharing and accelerates organizational learning.	• Decreases operational control and potential loss of control over a supplier.

could do alone. By working closely together, each gains in the long run from individual and organizational learning.[61] The term *virtual,* meaning "being in effect but not actually so," is commonly used in the computer industry. A computer's ability to appear to have more storage capacity than it really possesses is called virtual memory. Similarly, by assembling resources from a variety of entities, a virtual organization may seem to have more capabilities than it really possesses.[62]

The virtual organization is a grouping of units from different organizations that have joined in an alliance to exploit complementary skills in pursuing common strategic objectives. A case in point is Lockheed Martin's use of specialized coalitions between and among three entities—the company, academia, and government—to enhance competitiveness. According to former CEO Norman Augustine:

> The underlying beauty of this approach is that it forces us to reach outward. No matter what your size, you have to look broadly for new ideas, new approaches, new products. Lockheed Martin used this approach in a surprising manner when it set out during the height of the Cold War to make stealth aircraft and missiles. The technical idea came from research done at the Institute of Radio Engineering in Moscow in the 1960s that was published, and publicized, quite openly in the academic media.
>
> Despite the great contrasts among government, academia and private business, we have found ways to work together that have produced very positive results, not the least of which is our ability to compete on a global scale.[63]

Virtual organizations need not be permanent and participating firms may be involved in multiple alliances. Virtual organizations may involve different firms performing complementary value activities, or different firms involved jointly in the same value activities, such as production, R&D, and distribution. The percentage of activities that are jointly performed with partners may vary significantly from alliance to alliance.[64]

How does the virtual type of structure differ from the modular type? Unlike the modular type, in which the focal firm maintains full strategic control, the virtual organization is characterized by participating firms that give up part of their control and accept interdependent destinies. Participating firms pursue a collective strategy that enables them to cope with uncertainty through cooperative efforts. The benefit is that, just as virtual memory increases storage capacity, the virtual organizations enhance the capacity or competitive

How Eli Lilly Used the Collaborative Power of Internet-Based Collaboration to Foster Innovation

The e.Lilly division of pharmaceutical giant Eli Lilly was among the first to harness the collaborative power of the Internet when it launched Innocentive in 2001. Innocentive is the first online, incentive-based scientific network created specifically for the global research and development community. Innocentive's online platform enabled world-class scientists and R&D-based companies to collaborate to attain innovative solutions to complex challenges.

Innocentive offers "seeker companies" the opportunity to increase their R&D potential by posting challenges without violating their confidentiality and intellectual property interests. Seeker companies might be looking for a chemical to be used in art restoration, for example, or the efficient synthesis of butane tetracarboxylic acid. David Bradin, a patent attorney from Seattle, was recently paid $4,000 for his tetracarboxylic acid formula. And Procter & Gamble claims that Innocentive has increased its share of its new products originating outside the company from 20 to 35 percent.

Often individuals outside the seeker company find the best solutions to the company's problem. By using Innocentive to post their problems, companies do not have to admit publicly that they need help, yet they get access to a much broader range of ideas than can be generated inside the firm. Within firms, even those firms hiring the best and brightest scientists and engineers, ideas are tossed around by the same few people over and over. This situation can create a narrowing of the possible solutions to a problem (i.e., groupthink can occur) rather than searching over the broadest range of ideas. Anne Goldberg, technical knowledge manager at Solvay Pharmaceuticals, said, "The benefits [of Innocentive] are mainly in the simultaneous access to a lot of different scientific backgrounds that could bring new perspectives on sometimes old problems."

Sources: Libert, B. & Spector, J. 2008. *We are smarter than me.* Philadelphia: Wharton School Publishing: Lakhani, K. & Jeppesen, L. 2007. Getting unusual suspects to solve R&D puzzles. *Harvard Business Review,* 85(5): 30–32; and, Caldwell, T. 2007. R&D finds answers in the crowd. *Information World Review,* 236: 8.

crowdsourcing

---

advantage of participating firms. Strategy Spotlight 10.7 addresses the variety of collaborative relationships in the biotechnology industry.

Each company that links up with others to create a virtual organization contributes only what it considers its core competencies. It will mix and match what it does best with the best of other firms by identifying its critical capabilities and the necessary links to other capabilities.[65]

Challenges and Risks   Such alliances often fail to meet expectations: The alliance between IBM and Microsoft soured in early 1991 when Microsoft began shipping Windows in direct competition to OS/2, which they jointly developed. The runaway success of Windows frustrated IBM's ability to set an industry standard. In retaliation, IBM entered into an alliance with Microsoft's archrival, Novell, to develop network software to compete with Microsoft's LAN Manager.

The virtual organization demands that managers build relationships with other companies, negotiate win–win deals for all parties, find the right partners with compatible goals and values, and provide the right balance of freedom and control. Information systems must be designed and integrated to facilitate communication with current and potential partners.

Managers must be clear about the strategic objectives while forming alliances. Some objectives are time bound, and those alliances need to be dissolved once the objective is fulfilled. Some alliances may have relatively long-term objectives and will need to be clearly monitored and nurtured to produce mutual commitment and avoid bitter fights for control. The highly dynamic personal computer industry is characterized by multiple temporary alliances among hardware, operating systems, and

Exhibit 10.9

Pros and Cons of Virtual Structures

Pros	Cons
• Enables the sharing of costs and skills. • Enhances access to global markets. • Increases market responsiveness. • Creates a "best of everything" organization since each partner brings core competencies to the alliance. • Encourages both individual and organizational knowledge sharing and accelerates organizational learning.	• Harder to determine where one company ends and another begins, due to close interdependencies among players. • Leads to potential loss of operational control among partners. • Results in loss of strategic control over emerging technology. • Requires new and difficult-to-acquire managerial skills.

Source: Miles, R. E., & Snow, C. C. 1986. Organizations: New concepts for new forms. *California Management Review,* Spring: 62–73; Miles & Snow. 1999. Causes of failure in network organizations. *California Management Review,* Summer: 53–72; and, Bahrami, H. 1991. The emerging flexible organization: Perspectives from Silicon Valley. *California Management Review,* Summer: 33–52.

software producers.[66] But alliances in the more stable automobile industry, such as those involving Nissan and Volkswagen have long-term objectives and tend to be relatively stable.

The virtual organization is a logical culmination of joint-venture strategies of the past. Shared risks, costs, and rewards are the facts of life in a virtual organization.[67] When virtual organizations are formed, they involve tremendous challenges for strategic planning. As with the modular corporation, it is essential to identify core competencies. However, for virtual structures to be successful, a strategic plan is also needed to determine the effectiveness of combining core competencies.

The strategic plan must address the diminished operational control and overwhelming need for trust and common vision among the partners. This new structure may be appropriate for firms whose strategies require merging technologies (e.g., computing and communication) or for firms exploiting shrinking product life cycles that require simultaneous entry into multiple geographical markets. It may be effective for firms that desire to be quick to the market with a new product or service. The recent profusion of alliances among airlines was primarily motivated by the need to provide seamless travel demanded by the full-fare paying business traveler. Exhibit 10.9 summarizes the advantages and disadvantages.

Boundaryless Organizations: Making Them Work

Designing an organization that simultaneously supports the requirements of an organization's strategy, is consistent with the demands of the environment, and can be effectively implemented by the people around the manager is a tall order for any manager.[68] The most effective solution is usually a combination of organizational types. That is, a firm may outsource many parts of its value chain to reduce costs and increase quality, engage simultaneously in multiple alliances to take advantage of technological developments or penetrate new markets, and break down barriers within the organization to enhance flexibility.

When an organization faces external pressures, resource scarcity, and declining performance, it tends to become more internally focused, rather than directing its efforts toward managing and enhancing relationships with existing and potential external stakeholders. This may be the most opportune time for managers to carefully analyze their value-chain activities and evaluate the potential for adopting elements of modular, virtual, and barrier-free organizational types.

Achieving the coordination and integration necessary to maximize the potential of an organization's human capital involves much more than just creating a new structure. Techniques and processes to ensure the coordination and integration of an organization's key value-chain activities are critical. Teams are key building blocks of the new organizational forms, and teamwork requires new and flexible approaches to coordination and integration.

Managers trained in rigid hierarchies may find it difficult to make the transition to the more democratic, participative style that teamwork requires. As Douglas K. Smith, co-author of *The Wisdom of Teams,* pointed out, "A completely diverse group must agree on a goal, put the notion of individual accountability aside and figure out how to work with each other. Most of all, they must learn that if the team fails, it's everyone's fault."[69] Within the framework of an appropriate organizational design, managers must select a mix and balance of tools and techniques to facilitate the effective coordination and integration of key activities. Some of the factors that must be considered include:

- Common culture and shared values.
- Horizontal organizational structures.
- Horizontal systems and processes.
- Communications and information technologies.
- Human resource practices.

Common Culture and Shared Values   Shared goals, mutual objectives, and a high degree of trust are essential to the success of boundaryless organizations. In the fluid and flexible environments of the new organizational architectures, common cultures, shared values, and carefully aligned incentives are often less expensive to implement and are often a more effective means of strategic control than rules, boundaries, and formal procedures.

Horizontal Organizational Structures   **Horizontal organizational structures,** which group similar or related business units under common management control, facilitate sharing resources and infrastructures to exploit synergies among operating units and help to create a sense of common purpose. Consistency in training and the development of similar structures across business units facilitates job rotation and cross training and enhances understanding of common problems and opportunities. Cross-functional teams and interdivisional committees and task groups represent important opportunities to improve understanding and foster cooperation among operating units.

> **horizontal organizational structures** organizational forms that group similar or related business units under common management control and facilitate sharing resources and infrastructures to exploit synergies among operating units and help to create a sense of common purpose.

Horizontal Systems and Processes   Organizational systems, policies, and procedures are the traditional mechanisms for achieving integration among functional units. Existing policies and procedures often do little more than institutionalize the barriers that exist from years of managing within the framework of the traditional model. Beginning with an understanding of basic business processes in the context of "a collection of activities that takes one or more kinds of input and creates an output that is of value to the customer," Michael Hammer and James Champy's 1993 best-selling *Reengineering the Corporation* outlined a methodology for redesigning internal systems and procedures that has been embraced by many organizations.[70] Successful reengineering lowers costs, reduces inventories and cycle times, improves quality, speeds response times, and enhances organizational flexibility. Others advocate similar benefits through the reduction of cycle times, total quality management, and the like.

Communications and Information Technologies (IT)   The effective use of IT can play an important role in bridging gaps and breaking down barriers between organizations. Electronic mail and videoconferencing can improve lateral communications across long distances and multiple time zones and circumvent many of the barriers of the traditional model. IT can be a powerful ally in the redesign and streamlining of internal business processes and in improving coordination and integration between suppliers and customers. Internet technologies have eliminated the paperwork in many buyer–supplier relationships,

Crest's Whitestrips: An Example of How P&G Creates and Derives Benefits from a Boundaryless Organization

Given its breadth of products—soaps, diapers, toothpaste, potato chips, lotions, detergent—Procter & Gamble (P&G) has an enormous pool of resources it can integrate in various ways to launch exciting new products. For example, the company created a new category, teeth-whitening systems, with Crest Whitestrips. Teeth whitening done at a dentist's office can brighten one's smile in as little as one visit, but it can cost hundreds of dollars. On the other hand, over-the-counter home whitening kits like Crest Whitestrips cost far less and are nearly equally effective.

Whitestrip was created through a combined effort of product developers from three different units in P&G. People at the oral-care division provided teeth-whitening

expertise; experts from the fabric and home-care division supplied bleach expertise; and scientists at corporate research and development provided a novel film technology. Three separate units, by collaborating and combining their technologies, succeeded in developing an affordable product to brighten smiles and, according to the website, bring "greater success in work and love." With $300 million in annual retail sales, the launch of the Whitestrips product has been a big success for P&G, one that would not have been possible without the firm's collaborative ability.

Such collaborations are the outcome of well-established organizational mechanisms. P&G has created more than 20 communities of practice, with 8,000 participants. Each group comprises volunteers from different parts of the company and focuses on an area of expertise (fragrance, packaging, polymer chemistry, skin science, and so on). The groups solve specific problems that are brought to them, and they meet to share best practices. The company also has posted an "ask me" feature on its intranet, where employees can describe a business problem, which is directed to those people with appropriate expertise. At a more fundamental level, P&G promotes from within and rotates people across countries and business units. As a result, its employees build powerful cross-unit networks.

Sources: Hansen, M. T. 2009. *Collaboration: How leaders avoid the traps, create unity, and reap big results.* Boston: Harvard Business Press, 24–25; Anonymous. 2004. At P&G, it's 360-degree innovation. *www.businessweek.com*, October 11: np; *www.whitestrips.com*; Anonymous. 2009. The price of a whiter, brighter smile. *www.washingtonpost.com*. July 21: np; and, Hansen, M. T. & Birkinshaw, J. 2007. The innovation value chain. *Harvard Business Review*, June: 85(6): 121–130.

enabling cooperating organizations to reduce inventories, shorten delivery cycles, and reduce operating costs. IT must be viewed more as a prime component of an organization's overall strategy than simply in terms of administrative support.

Human Resource Practices   Change always involves and affects the human dimension of organizations. The attraction, development, and retention of human capital are vital to value creation. As boundaryless structures are implemented, processes are reengineered, and organizations become increasingly dependent on sophisticated IT, the skills of workers and managers alike must be upgraded to realize the full benefits.

Strategy Spotlight 10.8 discusses Procter & Gamble's successful introduction of Crest Whitestrips. This example shows how P&G's tools and techniques, such as communities of practice, information technology, and human resource practices, help to achieve effective collaboration and integration across the firm's different business units.

>LO10.6

The need for creating ambidextrous organizational designs that enable firms to explore new opportunities and effectively integrate existing operations.

Creating Ambidextrous Organizational Designs

In Chapter 1, we introduced the concept of "ambidexterity," which incorporates two contradictory challenges faced by today's managers.[71] First, managers must explore new opportunities and adjust to volatile markets in order to avoid complacency. They must ensure that they maintain **adaptability** and remain proactive in expanding and/or modifying their product-market scope to anticipate and satisfy market conditions. Such competencies are especially challenging when change is rapid and unpredictable.

Second, managers must also effectively exploit the value of their existing assets and competencies. They need to have **alignment,** which is a clear sense of how value is being created in the short term and how activities are integrated and properly coordinated. Firms that achieve both adaptability and alignment are considered *ambidextrous organizations—* aligned and efficient in how they manage today's business but flexible enough to changes in the environment so that they will prosper tomorrow.

Handling such opposing demands is difficult because there will always be some degree of conflict. Firms often suffer when they place too strong a priority on either adaptability or alignment. If it places too much focus on adaptability, the firm will suffer low profitability in the short term. If managers direct their efforts primarily at alignment, they will likely miss out on promising business opportunities.

Ambidextrous Organizations: Key Design Attributes

A recent study by Charles O'Reilly and Michael Tushman[72] provides some insights into how some firms were able to create successful **ambidextrous organizational designs.** They investigated companies that attempted to simultaneously pursue modest, incremental innovations as well as more dramatic, breakthrough innovations. The team investigated 35 attempts to launch breakthrough innovations undertaken by 15 business units in nine different industries. They studied the organizational designs and the processes, systems, and cultures associated with the breakthrough projects as well as their impact on the operations and performance of the traditional businesses.

Companies structured their breakthrough projects in one of four primary ways:

- Seven were carried out within existing *functional organizational structures.* The projects were completely integrated into the regular organizational and management structure.
- Nine were organized as *cross-functional teams.* The groups operated within the established organization but outside the existing management structure.
- Four were organized as *unsupported teams.* Here, they became independent units set up outside the established organization and management hierarchy.
- Fifteen were conducted within *ambidextrous organizations.* Here, the breakthrough efforts were organized within structurally independent units, each having its own processes, structures, and cultures. However, they were integrated into the existing senior management structure.

The performance results of the 35 initiatives were tracked along two dimensions:

- Their success in creating desired innovations was measured by either the actual commercial results of the new product or the application of practical market or technical learning.
- The performance of the existing business was evaluated.

The study found that the organizational structure and management practices employed had a direct and significant impact on the performance of both the breakthrough initiative and the traditional business. The ambidextrous organizational designs were more effective than the other three designs on both dimensions: launching breakthrough products or services (i.e., adaptation) and improving the performance of the existing business (i.e., alignment).

Why Was the Ambidextrous Organization the Most Effective Structure?

The study found that there were many factors. A clear and compelling vision, consistently communicated by the company's senior management team, was critical in building the

adaptibility
managers' exploration of new opportunities and adjustment to volatile markets in order to avoid complacency.

alignment
managers' clear sense of how value is being created in the short term and how activities are integrated and properly coordinated.

ambidextrous organizational designs
organizational designs that attempt to simultaneously pursue modest, incremental innovations as well as more dramatic, breakthrough innovations.

ambidextrous designs. The structure enabled cross-fertilization while avoiding cross-contamination. The tight coordination and integration at the managerial levels enabled the newer units to share important resources from the traditional units such as cash, talent, and expertise. Such sharing was encouraged and facilitated by effective reward systems that emphasized overall company goals. The organizational separation ensured that the new units' distinctive processes, structures, and cultures were not overwhelmed by the forces of "business as usual." The established units were shielded from the distractions of launching new businesses, and they continued to focus all of their attention and energy on refining their operations, enhancing their products, and serving their customers.

Reflecting on Career Implications . . .

- *Strategy–Structure:* Is there an effective "fit" between your organization's strategy and its structure? If not, there may be inconsistencies in how you are evaluated, which often leads to role ambiguity and confusion. A poor fit could also affect communication among departments as well as across the organization's hierarchy.
- *Matrix Structure:* If your organization employs elements of a matrix structure (e.g., dual reporting relationships), are there effective structural supporting elements (e.g., culture and rewards)? If not, there could be a high level of dysfunctional conflict among managers.
- *The "Fit" between Rewards and Incentives and "Levels of Strategy" (Business- and Corporate-Level):* What metrics are used to evaluate the performance of your work unit? Are there strictly financial measures of success or are you also rewarded for achieving competitive advantages (through effective innovation, organizational learning, or other activities that increase knowledge but may be costly in the short run)?
- *Boundaryless Organizational Designs:* Does your firm have structural mechanisms (e.g., culture, human resource practices) that facilitate sharing of information across boundaries? If so, you should be better able to enhance your human capital by leveraging your talents and competencies.

Summary

Successful organizations must ensure that they have the proper type of organizational structure. Furthermore, they must ensure that their firms incorporate the necessary integration and processes so that the internal and external boundaries of their firms are flexible and permeable. Such a need is increasingly important as the environments of firms become more complex, rapidly changing, and unpredictable.

In the first section of the chapter, we discussed the growth patterns of large corporations. Although most organizations remain small or die, some firms continue to grow in terms of revenues, vertical integration, and diversity of products and services. In addition, their geographical scope may increase to include international operations. We traced the dominant pattern of growth, which evolves from a simple structure to a functional structure as a firm grows in terms of size and increases

its level of vertical integration. After a firm expands into related products and services, its structure changes from a functional to a divisional form of organization. Finally, when the firm enters international markets, its structure again changes to accommodate the change in strategy.

We also addressed the different types of organizational structure—simple, functional, divisional (including two variations—strategic business unit and holding company), and matrix—as well as their relative advantages and disadvantages. We closed the section with a discussion of the implications for structure when a firm enters international markets. The three primary factors to take into account when determining the appropriate structure are type of international strategy, product diversity, and the extent to which a firm is dependent on foreign sales.

In the second section, we took a contingency approach to the design of reward and evaluation systems.

That is, we argued that there is no one best way to design such systems; rather, it is dependent on a variety of factors. The two that we discussed are business- and corporate-level strategies. With an overall cost leadership strategy and unrelated diversification, it is appropriate to rely primarily on cultures and reward systems that emphasize the production outcomes of the organization, because it is rather easy to quantify such indicators. In contrast, differentiation strategies and related diversification require cultures and incentive systems that encourage and reward creativity initiatives as well as the cooperation among professionals in many different functional areas. Here it becomes more difficult to measure accurately each individual's contribution, and more subjective indicators become essential.

The third section of the chapter introduced the concept of the boundaryless organization. We did not suggest that the concept of the boundaryless organization replaces the traditional forms of organizational structure. Rather, it should complement them. This is necessary to cope with the increasing complexity and change in the competitive environment. We addressed three types of boundaryless organizations. The barrier-free type focuses on the need for the internal and external boundaries of a firm to be more flexible and permeable. The modular type emphasizes the strategic outsourcing of noncore activities. The virtual type centers on the strategic benefits of alliances and the forming of network organizations. We discussed both the advantages and disadvantages of each type of boundaryless organization as well as suggested some techniques and processes that are necessary to successfully implement them. These are common culture and values, horizontal organizational structures, horizontal systems and processes, communications and information technologies, and human resource practices.

The final section addresses the need for managers to develop ambidextrous organizations. In today's rapidly changing global environment, managers must be responsive and proactive in order to take advantage of new opportunities. At the same time, they must effectively integrate and coordinate existing operations. Such requirements call for organizational designs that establish project teams that are structurally independent units, with each having its own processes, structures, and cultures. But, at the same time, each unit needs to be effectively integrated into the existing management hierarchy.

Summary Review Questions

1. Why is it important for managers to carefully consider the type of organizational structure that they use to implement their strategies?

2. Briefly trace the dominant growth pattern of major corporations from simple structure to functional structure to divisional structure. Discuss the relationship between a firm's strategy and its structure.

3. What are the relative advantages and disadvantages of the types of organizational structure—simple, functional, divisional, matrix—discussed in the chapter?

4. When a firm expands its operations into foreign markets, what are the three most important factors to take into account in deciding what type of structure is most appropriate? What are the types of international structures discussed in the text and what are the relationships between strategy and structure?

5. Briefly describe the three different types of boundaryless organizations: barrier-free, modular, and virtual.

6. What are some of the key attributes of effective groups? Ineffective groups?

7. What are the advantages and disadvantages of the three types of boundaryless organizations: barrier-free, modular, and virtual?

8. When are ambidextrous organizational designs necessary? What are some of their key attributes?

Key Terms

organizational structure, 399
simple organizational structure, 401
functional organizational structure, 401
divisional organizational structure, 403
strategic business unit (SBU) structure, 405
holding company structure, 406
matrix organizational structure, 406
international division structure, 409
geographic-area division structure, 409
worldwide matrix structure, 409

worldwide functional structure, 409
worldwide product division structure, 409
global start-up, 409
boundaryless organizational designs, 414
barrier-free organization, 415
modular organization, 419
virtual organization, 421
horizontal organizational structures, 425
adaptability, 427
alignment, 427
ambidextrous organizational designs, 427

Experiential Exercise

Many firms have recently moved toward a modular structure. For example, they have increasingly outsourced

	Firm	Rationale	Implication(s) for Performance
1.			
2.			
3.			

many of their information technology (IT) activities. Identify three such organizations. Using secondary sources, evaluate, in the above table, (1) the firm's rationale for IT outsourcing and (2) the implications for performance.

Application Questions & Exercises

1. Select an organization that competes in an industry in which you are particularly interested. Go on the Internet and determine what type of organizational structure this organization has. In your view, is it consistent with the strategy that it has chosen to implement? Why? Why not?

2. Choose an article from *The Economist, The Financial Times, Business Standard* of India, or any other well-known global publication that describes a company that has undergone a significant change in its strategic direction. What are the implications for the structure of this organization?

3. Go on the Internet and look up some of the public statements or speeches of an executive in a global corporation about a significant initiative such as entering into a joint venture or launching a new product line. What do you feel are the implications for making the internal and external barriers of the firm more flexible and permeable? Does the executive discuss processes, procedures, integrating mechanisms, or cultural issues that should serve this purpose? Or are other issues discussed that enable a firm to become more boundaryless?

4. Look up a recent article in the publications listed in question 2 that addresses a firm's involvement in outsourcing (modular organization) or in strategic alliance or network organizations (virtual organization). Was the firm successful or unsuccessful in this endeavor? Why? Why not?

Ethics Questions

1. If a firm has a divisional structure and places extreme pressures on its divisional executives to meet short-term profitability goals (e.g., quarterly income), could this raise some ethical considerations? Why? Why not?

2. If a firm enters into a strategic alliance but does not exercise appropriate behavioral control of its employees (in terms of culture, rewards and incentives, and boundaries—as discussed in Chapter 9) that are involved in the alliance, what ethical issues could arise? What could be the potential long-term and short-term downside for the firm?

References

1. Eng, D. 2010. Free tour, new steps to mend HK image. *South China Morning Post,* July 17: A2; Carothers, C. 2010. Hong Kong: Don't shop? Don't come. *blogs.wsj.com.* November 10: np; and, Xinhua, J. 2010. Authority issues travel advisory on trip to Hong Kong. *china.org.cn.* November 10: np. We thank Zia Shakir for his valued contributions.

2. For a unique perspective on organization design, see: Rao, R. 2010. What 17th century pirates can teach us about job design. *Harvard Business Review,* 88(10): 44.

3. This introductory discussion draws upon: Hall, R. H. 2002. *Organizations: Structures, processes, and*

outcomes (8th ed.). Upper Saddle River, NJ: Prentice Hall; and, Duncan, R. E. 1979. What is the right organization structure? Decision-tree analysis provides the right answer. *Organizational Dynamics,* 7(3): 59–80. For an insightful discussion of strategy–structure relationships in the organization theory and strategic management literatures, refer to: Keats, B. & O'Neill, H. M. 2001. Organization structure: Looking through a strategy lens. In Hitt, M. A., Freeman, R. E., & Harrison, J. S. 2001. *The Blackwell handbook of strategic management:* 520–542. Malden, MA: Blackwell.

4. Gratton, L. 2011. The end of the middle manager. *Harvard Business Review,* 89(1/2): 36.

5. An interesting discussion on the role of organizational design in strategy execution is in: Neilson, G. L., Martin, K. L., & Powers, E. 2009. The secrets to successful strategy execution. *Harvard Business Review,* 87(2): 60–70.

6. This discussion draws upon: Chandler, A. D. 1962. *Strategy and structure.* Cambridge, MA: MIT Press; Galbraith, J. R. & Kazanjian, R. K. 1986. *Strategy implementation: The role of structure and process.* St. Paul, MN: West Publishing; and, Scott, B. R. 1971. Stages of corporate development. Intercollegiate Case Clearing House, 9-371-294, BP 998. Harvard Business School.

7. Our discussion of the different types of organizational structures draws on a variety of sources, including: Galbraith & Kazanjian, op. cit.; Hrebiniak, L. G. & Joyce, W. F. 1984. *Implementing strategy.* New York: Macmillan; Distelzweig, H. 2000. Organizational structure. In Helms, M. M. (Ed.). *Encyclopedia of management:* 692–699. Farmington Hills, MI: Gale; and, Dess, G. G. & Miller, A. 1993. *Strategic management.* New York: McGraw-Hill.

8. A discussion of an innovative organizational design is in: Garvin, D. A. & Levesque, L. C. 2009. The multiunit enterprise. *Harvard Business Review,* 87(2): 106–117.

9. Schein, E. H. 1996. Three cultures of management: The key to organizational learning. *Sloan Management Review,* 38(1): 9–20.

10. Insights on governance implications for multidivisional forms are in: Verbeke, A. & Kenworthy, T. P. 2008. Multidivisional vs. metanational governance. *Journal of International Business,* 39(6): 940–956.

11. Martin, J. A. & Eisenhardt, K. 2010. Rewiring: Cross-business-unit collaborations in multibusiness organizations. *Academy of Management Journal,* 53(2): 265–301.

12. For a discussion of performance implications, refer to: Hoskisson, R. E. 1987. Multidivisional structure and performance: The contingency of diversification strategy. *Academy of Management Journal,* 29: 625–644.

13. For a thorough and seminal discussion of the evolution toward the divisional form of organizational structure in the United States, refer to: Chandler, op. cit. A rigorous empirical study of the strategy and structure relationship is found in: Rumelt, R. P. 1974. *Strategy, structure, and economic performance.* Cambridge, MA: Harvard Business School Press.

14. Ghoshal S. & Bartlett, C. A. 1995. Changing the role of management: Beyond structure to processes. *Harvard Business Review,* 73(1): 88.

15. Koppel, B. 2000. Synergy in ketchup? *Forbes,* February 7: 68–69; and, Hitt, M. A., Ireland, R. D., & Hoskisson, R. E. 2001. *Strategic management: Competitiveness and globalization* (4th ed.). Cincinnati, OH: Southwestern Publishing.

16. Pitts, R. A. 1977. Strategies and structures for diversification. *Academy of Management Journal,* 20(2): 197–208.

17. Andersen, M. M., Froholdt, M., Poulfelt, F. 2010. *Return on strategy: How to achieve it.* New York: Routledge.

18. Haas, M. R. 2010. The double-edged swords of autonomy and external knowledge: Analyzing team effectiveness in a multinational organization. *Academy of Management Journal,* 53(5): 989–1008.

19. Daniels, J. D., Pitts, R. A., & Tretter, M. J. 1984. Strategy and structure of U.S. multinationals: An exploratory study. *Academy of Management Journal,* 27(2): 292–307.

20. Habib, M. M. & Victor, B. 1991. Strategy, structure, and performance of U.S. manufacturing and service MNCs: A comparative analysis. *Strategic Management Journal,* 12(8): 589–606.

21. Our discussion of global start-ups draws from: Oviatt, B. M. & McDougall, P. P. 2005. The internationalization of entrepreneurship. *Journal of International Business Studies,* 36(1): 2–8; Oviatt, B. M. & McDougall, P. P. 1994. Toward a theory of international new ventures. *Journal of International Business Studies,* 25(1): 45–64; and, Oviatt, B. M. & McDougall, P. P. 1995. Global start-ups: Entrepreneurs on a worldwide stage. *Academy of Management Executive,* 9(2): 30–43.

22. Some useful guidelines for global start-ups are provided in:, Kuemmerle, W. 2005. The entrepreneur's path for global expansion. *MIT Sloan Management Review,* 46(2): 42–50.

23. See, for example, Miller, D. & Friesen, P. H. 1980. Momentum and revolution in organizational structure. *Administrative Science Quarterly,* 13: 65–91.

24. Many authors have argued that a firm's structure can influence its strategy and performance. These include: Amburgey, T. L. & Dacin, T. 1995. As the left foot follows the right? The dynamics of strategic and structural change. *Academy of Management Journal,* 37: 1427–1452; Dawn, K. & Amburgey, T. L. 1991. Organizational inertia and momentum: A dynamic model of strategic change. *Academy of Management Journal,* 34: 591–612; Fredrickson, J. W. 1986. The strategic decision process and organization structure. *Academy of Management Review,* 11: 280–297; Hall, D. J. & Saias, M. A. 1980. Strategy follows structure! *Strategic Management Journal,* 1: 149–164; and, Burgelman, R. A. 1983. A model of the interaction of

strategic behavior, corporate context, and the concept of strategy. *Academy of Management Review,* 8: 61–70.

25. *www.brinker.com,* accessed November 2, 2011; CEO interview: Ronald A. McDougall, Brinker International. 1999. *Wall Street Transcript,* January 20: 1–4.

26. This discussion of generic strategies and their relationship to organizational control draws upon: Porter, M. E. 1980. *Competitive strategy.* New York: Free Press; and, Miller, D. 1988. Relating Porter's business strategies to environment and structure: Analysis and performance implications. *Academy of Management Journal,* 31(2): 280–308.

27. Rodengen, J. L. 1997. *The legend of Nucor Corporation.* Fort Lauderdale, FL: Write Stuff Enterprises.

28. The 3M example draws upon: *Blueprints for service quality.* 1994. New York: American Management Association; personal communication with Katerine Hagmeier, program manager, external communications, 3M Corporation, March 26, 1998; Lei, D., Slocum, J. W., & Pitts, R. A. 1999. Designing organizations for competitive advantage: The power of unlearning and learning. *Organizational Dynamics,* 27(3): 24–38; and, Graham, A. B. & Pizzo, V. G. 1996. A question of balance: Case studies in strategic knowledge management. *European Management Journal,* 14(4): 338–346.

29. The Sharp Corporation and Hanson PLC examples are based on: Collis, D. J. & Montgomery, C. A. 1998. Creating corporate advantage. *Harvard Business Review,* 76(3): 70–83.

30. Kunii, I. 2002. Japanese companies' survival skills. *BusinessWeek,* November 18: 18.

31. White, G. 1988. How I turned $3,000 into $10 billion. *Fortune,* November 7: 80–89. After the death of the founders, the Hanson PLC conglomerate was found to be too unwieldy and was broken up into several separate, publicly traded corporations. For more on its more limited current scope of operations, see *www.hansonplc.com.*

32. An interesting discussion on how the Internet has affected the boundaries of firms can be found in: Afuah, A. 2003. Redefining firm boundaries in the face of the Internet: Are firms really shrinking? *Academy of Management Review,* 28(1): 34–53.

33. Collis & Montgomery, op. cit.

34. Govindarajan, V. G. & Trimble, C. 2010. Stop the innovation wars. *Harvard Business Review,* 88(7/8): 76–83.

35. For a discussion of the role of coaching on developing high performance teams, refer to: Kets de Vries, M. F. R. 2005. Leadership group coaching in action: The Zen of creating high performance teams. *Academy of Management Executive,* 19(1): 77–89.

36. Pfeffer, J. 1998. *The human equation: Building profits by putting people first.* Cambridge, MA: Harvard Business School Press.

37. For a discussion on how functional area diversity affects performance, see: Bunderson, J. S. & Sutcliffe, K. M. 2002. *Academy of Management Journal,* 45(5): 875–893.

38. See, for example, Hoskisson, R. E., Hill, C. W. L., & Kim, H. 1993. The multidivisional structure: Organizational fossil or source of value? *Journal of Management,* 19(2): 269–298.

39. Pottruck, D. A. 1997. Speech delivered by the co-CEO of Charles Schwab Co., Inc., to the Retail Leadership Meeting, San Francisco, CA, January 30; and, Miller, W. 1999. Building the ultimate resource. *Management Review,* January: 42–45.

40. Public–private partnerships are addressed in: Engardio, P. 2009. State capitalism. *BusinessWeek,* February 9: 38–43.

41. Magretta, J. 1998. The power of virtual integration: An interview with Dell Computer's Michael Dell. *Harvard Business Review,* 76(2): 75.

42. Forster, J. 2001. Networking for cash. *BusinessWeek,* January 8: 129.

43. *www.canada-europe.org/en/; www.eu-japan-brt.eu/index.php?content=round-table;* and, *http://ec.europa.eu/enterprise/policies/international/listening-stakeholders/round-tables/.*

44. Dess, G. G., Rasheed, A. M. A., McLaughlin, K. J., & Priem, R. 1995. The new corporate architecture. *Academy of Management Executive,* 9(3): 7–20.

45. Barnes, C. 1998. A fatal case. *Fast Company,* February–March: 173.

46. Handy, C. 1989. *The age of unreason.* Boston: Harvard Business School Press; Ramstead, E. 1997. APC maker's low-tech formula: Start with the box. *The Wall Street Journal,* December 29: B1; Mussberg, W. 1997. Thin screen PCs are looking good but still fall flat. *The Wall Street Journal,* January 2: 9; Brown, E. 1997. Monorail: Low cost PCs. *Fortune,* July 7: 106–108; and, Young, M. 1996. Ex-Compaq executives start new company. *Computer Reseller News,* November 11: 181.

47. An original discussion on how open-sourcing could help the Big 3 automobile companies is in: Jarvis, J. 2009. How the Google model could help Detroit. *BusinessWeek,* February 9: 32–36.

48. For a discussion of some of the downsides of outsourcing, refer to: Rossetti, C. & Choi, T. Y. 2005. On the dark side of strategic sourcing: Experiences from the aerospace industry. *Academy of Management Executive,* 19(1): 46–60.

49. Tully, S. 1993. The modular corporation. *Fortune,* February 8: 196.

50. Offshoring in manufacturing firms is addressed in: Coucke, K. & Sleuwaegen, L. 2008. Offshoring as a survival strategy: Evidence from manufacturing firms in Belgium. *Journal of International Business Studies,* 39(8): 1261–1277.

51. Quinn, J. B. 1992. *Intelligent enterprise: A knowledge and service based paradigm for industry.* New York: Free Press.

52. For an insightful perspective on outsourcing and its role in developing capabilities, read: Gottfredson, M., Puryear, R., & Phillips, C. 2005. Strategic sourcing: From periphery to the core. *Harvard Business Review,* 83(4): 132–139.

53. This discussion draws upon: Quinn, J. B. & Hilmer, F. C. 1994. Strategic

54. Reitzig, M. & Wagner, S. 2010. The hidden costs of outsourcing: Evidence from patent data. *Strategic Management Journal,* 31(11): 1183–1201.

55. Insights on outsourcing and private branding can be found in: Cehn, S-F. S. 2009. A transaction cost rationale for private branding and its implications for the choice of domestic vs. offshore outsourcing. *Journal of International Business Strategy,* 40(1): 156–175.

56. Larsen, M. M., Pedersen, T., & Slepniov, D. 2010. Lego Group: An outsourcing journey. *Harvard Business Review,* November 12; Meyer, K. 2009. Lego figures it out. March 10, 2009. Evolving excellence: Thoughts on lean enterprise leadership (blog), March 10, *www.evolvingexcellence .com/blog/2009/03/legos-newfound -love-of-insourcing.html.*

57. For an insightful perspective on the use of outsourcing for decision analysis, read: Davenport, T. H. & Iyer, B. 2009. Should you outsource your brain? *Harvard Business Review,* 87(2): 38.

58. See also Stuckey, J. & White, D.1993. When and when not to vertically integrate. *Sloan Management Review,* Spring: 71–81; Harrar, G. 1993. Outsource tales. *Forbes ASAP,* June 7: 37–39, 42; and, Davis, E. W. 1992. Global outsourcing: Have U.S. managers thrown the baby out with the bath water? *Business Horizons,* July–August: 58–64.

59. For a discussion of knowledge creation through alliances, refer to: Inkpen, A. C. 1996. Creating knowledge through collaboration. *California Management Review,* 39(1): 123–140; and, Mowery, D. C., Oxley, J. E., & Silverman, B. S. 1996. Strategic alliances and interfirm knowledge transfer. *Strategic Management Journal,* 17 (Special Issue, Winter): 77–92.

60. Doz, Y. & Hamel, G. 1998. *Alliance advantage: The art of creating value through partnering.* Boston: Harvard Business School Press.

61. DeSanctis, G., Glass, J. T., & Ensing, I. M. 2002. Organizational designs for R&D. *Academy of Management Executive,* 16(3): 55–66.

62. Barringer, B. R. & Harrison, J. S. 2000. Walking a tightrope: Creating value through interorganizational alliances. *Journal of Management,* 26: 367–403.

63. Davis, E. 1997. Interview: Norman Augustine. *Management Review,* November: 14.

64. One contemporary example of virtual organizations is R&D consortia. For an insightful discussion, refer to: Sakaibara, M. 2002. Formation of R&D consortia: Industry and company effects. *Strategic Management Journal,* 23(11): 1033–1050.

65. Bartness, A. & Cerny, K. 1993. Building competitive advantage through a global network of capabilities. *California Management Review,* Winter: 78–103. For an insightful historical discussion of the usefulness of alliances in the computer industry, see: Moore, J. F. 1993. Predators and prey: A new ecology of competition. *Harvard Business Review,* 71(3): 75–86.

66. See Lorange, P. & Roos, J. 1991. Why some strategic alliances succeed and others fail. *Journal of Business Strategy,* January–February: 25–30; and, Slowinski, G. 1992. The human touch in strategic alliances. *Mergers and Acquisitions,* July–August: 44–47. A compelling argument for strategic alliances is provided by Ohmae, K. 1989. The global logic of strategic alliances. *Harvard Business Review,* 67(2): 143–154.

67. Some of the downsides of alliances are discussed in: Das, T. K. & Teng, B. S. 2000. Instabilities of strategic alliances: An internal tensions perspective. *Organization Science,* 11: 77–106.

68. This section draws upon: Dess, G. G. & Picken, J. C. 1997. *Mission critical.* Burr Ridge, IL: Irwin Professional Publishing.

69. Katzenbach, J. R. & Smith, D. K. 1994. *The wisdom of teams: Creating the high performance organization.* New York: HarperBusiness.

70. Hammer, M. & Champy, J. 1993. *Reengineering the corporation: A manifesto for business revolution.* New York: HarperCollins.

71. This section draws on: Birkinshaw, J. & Gibson, C. 2004. Building ambidexterity into an organization. *MIT Sloan Management Review,* 45(4): 47–55; and, Gibson, C. B. & Birkinshaw, J. 2004. The antecedents, consequences, and mediating role of organizational ambidexterity. *Academy of Management Journal,* 47(2): 209–226. Robert Duncan is generally credited with being the first to coin the term "ambidextrous organizations" in his article entitled: Designing dual structures for innovation. In Kilmann, R. H., Pondy, L. R., & Slevin, D. (Eds.). 1976. *The management of organizations,* vol. 1: 167–188. For a seminal academic discussion of the concept of exploration and exploitation, which parallels adaptation and alignment, refer to: March, J. G. 1991. Exploration and exploitation in organizational learning. *Organization Science,* 2: 71–86.

72. This section is based on: O'Reilly, C. A. & Tushman, M. L. 2004. The ambidextrous organization. *Harvard Business Review,* 82(4): 74–81.

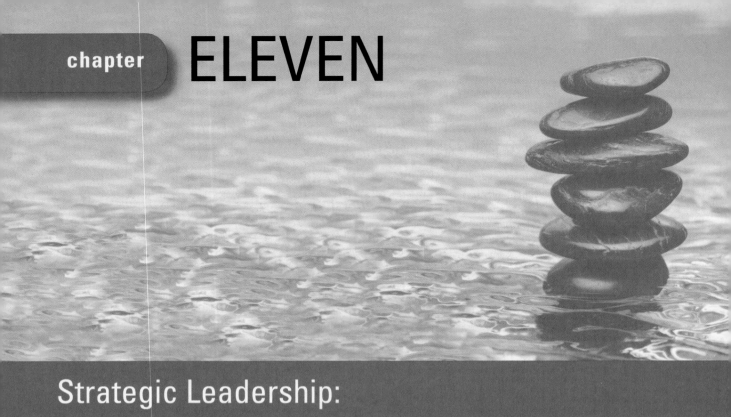

chapter ELEVEN

Strategic Leadership:

Creating a Learning Organization and an Ethical Organization

After reading this chapter, you should have a good understanding of:

LO11.1   The three key interdependent activities in which all successful leaders must be continually engaged.

LO11.2   Three elements of effective leadership: integrative thinking, overcoming barriers to change, and the effective use of power.

LO11.3   The crucial role of emotional intelligence (EI) in successful leadership as well as its potential drawbacks.

LO11.4   The value of creating and maintaining a learning organization in today's global marketplace.

LO11.5   The leader's role in establishing an ethical organization.

LO11.6   The difference between integrity-based and compliance-based approaches to organizational ethics.

LO11.7   Several key elements that organizations must have to become an ethical organization.

LEARNING OBJECTIVES

To compete in the global marketplace, organizations need to have strong and effective leadership. This involves the active process of both creating and implementing proper strategies. In this chapter we address key activities in which leaders throughout the organization must be involved to be successful in creating and sustaining competitive advantages.

In the first section, we provide a brief overview of the three key leadership activities. These are (1) setting a direction, (2) designing the organization, and (3) nurturing a culture committed to excellence and ethical behavior. Each of these activities is "necessary but not sufficient"; that is, to be effective, leaders must give proper attention to each of them.

Section two addresses practices and capabilities that enable executives to be effective as leaders. To be successful in a complex business environment, leaders must perform a variety of functions and exhibit key strengths. We focus on three capabilities that effective leaders often exhibit—integrative thinking, overcoming barriers to change, and the effective use of power.

The third section discusses the vital role of emotional intelligence (EI) in effective strategic leadership. EI refers to an individual's capacity for recognizing his or her emotions and those of others. It consists of five components: self-awareness, self-regulation, motivation, empathy, and social skills. We also address potential downsides or drawbacks that may result from the ineffective use of EI.

Next we address the important role of a leader in creating a learning organization. Here, leaders must strive to harness the individual and collective talents of individuals throughout the entire organization. Creating a learning organization is particularly important in today's competitive environment, which is increasingly unpredictable, dynamic, and interdependent. The key elements of a learning organization are inspiring and motivating people with a mission or purpose, empowering employees at all levels, accumulating and sharing internal and external information, and challenging the status quo to enable creativity.

The final section discusses a leader's challenge in creating and maintaining an ethical organization. There are many benefits of having an ethical organization. It can provide financial benefits, enhance human capital, and help to ensure positive relationships with suppliers, customers, society at large, and governmental agencies. By contrast failure to operate ethically leading to an ethical crisis can be very costly for many reasons. We address four key elements of an ethical organization: role models, corporate credos and codes of conduct, reward and evaluation systems, and policies and procedures.

Learning from Mistakes

Duke Energy appeared to be doing the right thing by investing in clean-coal technology. Through a state-of-the-art power plant, Duke Energy would convert coal to flammable gas, a move approved by state regulators, who allowed the firm to pass some of the costs on to consumers. The firm's CEO, Jim Rogers, had even been profiled by *The New York Times* in 2008 as a "green coal baron," who constantly lobbied for a national price on carbon output, seeking to move out of low-tech coal plants to cleaner, more expensive coal plants. Yet in December 2010, the firm was rocked by an ethics scandal caused by e-mail exchanges between some of its executives and state regulators who oversaw its operations, and who decided what rates the utility could charge its customers. What went wrong?[1]

An ethics investigation led to several resignations. These included James Turner (one of Duke Energy's top executives) and two other executives as well as a prominent Indiana state regulator. The press obtained several e-mail exchanges between the four men, relating to alcohol, cars, their wives, and the open mocking of state ethical standards. While the investigation focused on the e-mail exchanges, the main concern was the relationship between Duke and state regulators, raising the question of a possible revolving door between the two entities. The improper relationship between Duke and regulators might have been foreseeable, considering that most big players at Duke had at one point worked for the Indiana government and that the head of Indiana's utility commission had been a lawyer for a local utility acquired by Duke.

While working for Duke, Turner was the second highest paid executive in 2009, totaling $4.3 million in compensation. Even following his resignation, he received a severance and retirement package worth more than $10 million. Turner had frequent e-mail exchanges with the head of Indiana's Utility Regulatory Commission, David Hardy, at times trading up to 10 messages a day. The men frequently ridiculed state ethics rules that were enacted to prevent state-regulated utilities from exerting undue influence on their regulators. In an e-mail, Turner wondered whether the "ethics police would have a cow" if he was visited at his weekend home by a top state regulator. In another published e-mail, Hardy brags about relaxing by the pool in the morning and inquiring about a good breakfast wine, and in reply Turner wrote, "Does anyone know if a desire to 'bitch slap a chairman' violates any state's hate crime laws?" Other e-mails addressed the hiring process of Scott Storm and Mike Reed, as they sought and then obtained jobs with Duke, with Hardy, their former boss, constantly demanding reports on the hiring process and inquiring whether he should try to influence Duke's CEO's decision.

The relationship with state regulators is an important one for Duke, as it invests heavily in the state in an attempt to position itself to prosper in the age of climate politics by investing in a first-of-its-kind clean-coal power plant. Duke received approval from a state commission to raise its rates for Indiana customers by approximately 16 percent, passing on to them costs of almost $2.9 billion when the plant is completed in 2012. Considering that the firm is $1 billion over its previous budget estimates, critics point out that there are cheaper ways to produce energy to meet the state's needs. Some of the matters related to the approval of the clean-coal plant had been overseen by Scott Storm, who was hired by Duke in September 2010.

Storm was a lawyer who had, until then, worked for the Indiana Utility Regulatory Commission as an administrative law judge, as their top legal officer. In that position he had worked on several Duke cases, but there was no indication that he had provided special treatment to the firm. He received an ethics waiver from a state panel to forgo a one-year cooling-off period after leaving state service prior to accepting employment with a company that he had helped regulate. This decision outraged consumer advocates and finally led to the firing of the commission's head, Hardy, by the governor of Indiana and to the reopening of the decision regarding Duke. Both Storm and the Duke executive that hired him, Mike Reed, resigned from the company. Reed had taken the position at Duke as its president for Indiana 16 months after he had himself been the executive director of the Indiana Utility Regulatory Commission. Even after leaving Duke, Storm faced a state ethics panel hearing claiming that he did not recuse himself from cases related to Duke while considering employment with the company.

In response, Duke has drafted new employment guidelines to ensure that it only hires from "regulatory and oversight groups" with no prior affairs related to Duke Energy. However, this seems to be too little, too late.

Clearly, many of the decisions and actions of Duke Energy's top executives were not in the best interests of the firm and its shareholders and were not consistent with norms of ethical behavior. In contrast, effective leaders play an important and often pivotal role in creating and implementing strategies.

This chapter provides insights into the role of strategic leadership in managing, adapting, and coping in the face of increased environmental complexity and uncertainty. First, we define leadership and its components. Then, we identify three elements of leadership that contribute to success—integrative thinking, overcoming barriers to change, and the effective use of power. The third section focuses on emotional intelligence, a trait that is increasingly acknowledged to be critical to successful leadership. Next, we emphasize the importance of developing a learning organization and how leaders can help their firms learn and proactively adapt in the face of accelerating change. Here, we focus on empowerment wherein employees and managers throughout an organization develop a sense of self-determination, competence, meaning, and impact that is centrally important to learning. Finally, we address the leader's role in building an ethical organization and the elements of an ethical culture that contribute to firm effectiveness.

Leadership: Three Interdependent Activities

In today's chaotic world, few would argue against the need for leadership, but how do we go about encouraging it? Is it enough to merely keep an organization afloat, or is it essential to make steady progress toward some well-defined objective? We believe custodial management is not leadership. Leadership is proactive, goal-oriented, and focused on the creation and implementation of a creative vision. **Leadership** is the process of transforming organizations from what they are to what the leader would have them become. This definition implies a lot: *dissatisfaction* with the status quo, a *vision* of what should be, and a *process* for bringing about change. An insurance company executive shared the following insight: "I lead by the Noah Principle: It's all right to know when it's going to rain, but, by God, you had better build the ark."

leadership the process of transforming organizations from what they are to what the leader would have them become.

Doing the right thing is becoming increasingly important. Many industries are declining; the global village is becoming increasingly complex, interconnected, and unpredictable; and product and market life cycles are becoming increasingly compressed. When asked to describe the life cycle of his company's products, the CEO of a supplier of computer components replied, "Seven months from cradle to grave—and that includes three months to design the product and get it into production!" Richard D'Aveni, author of *Hypercompetition,* argued that, in a world where all dimensions of competition appear to be compressed in time and heightened in complexity, *sustainable* competitive advantages are no longer possible.

Despite the importance of doing the "right thing," leaders must also be concerned about "doing things right." Charan and Colvin strongly believe that execution, that is, the implementation of strategy, is also essential to success:

> Mastering execution turns out to be the odds-on best way for a CEO to keep his job. So what's the right way to think about that sexier obsession, strategy? It's vitally important— obviously. The problem is that our age's fascination feeds the mistaken belief that developing exactly the right strategy will enable a company to rocket past competitors. In reality, that's less than half the battle.[2]

Thus, leaders are change agents whose success is measured by how effectively they formulate *and* implement a strategic vision and mission.[3]

Many authors contend that successful leaders must recognize three interdependent activities that must be continually reassessed for organizations to succeed. As shown in Exhibit 11.1, these are: (1) setting a direction, (2) designing the organization, and (3) nurturing a culture dedicated to excellence and ethical behavior.[4]

The interdependent nature of these three activities is self-evident. Consider an organization with a great mission and a superb organizational structure, but a culture that implicitly encourages shirking and unethical behavior. Or one with a sound direction and strong culture, but counterproductive teams and a "zero-sum" reward system that leads to the dysfunctional situation in which one party's gain is viewed as another party's loss, and collaboration and sharing are severely hampered. Clearly, such combinations would be ineffective.

A new approach on leadership highlights the importance of being "ambicultural," which emphasizes taking the best elements of the philosophies and practices from multiple cultures while avoiding their negative aspects. Such an approach can be highly effective in performing the three leadership activities in today's increasingly global economy.

>LO11.1

The three key interdependent activities in which all successful leaders must be continually engaged.

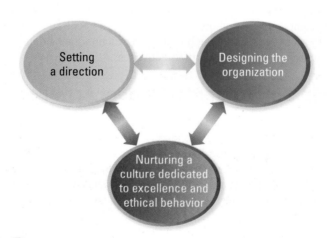

Exhibit 11.1 **Three Interdependent Leadership Activities**

Julie Gilbert Sets a New Direction for Best Buy

Julie Gilbert is evidence that significant and creative change can be brought about by people who do not happen to be at the very top of an organization. As a senior VP at retailer Best Buy from 2000 to early 2009, she saw a looming crisis in the firm's failure to profit from the greater involvement of women in the male-oriented world of consumer electronics. Women were becoming more influential in purchasing decisions, directly and indirectly. But capitalizing on this trend would require something beyond a smart marketing plan. It would demand a change in the company's orientation.

Getting an organization to adapt to changes in the environment is not easy. You need to confront loyalty to legacy practices and understand that your desire to change them makes you a target of attack. Gilbert believed that instead of simply selling technology products to mostly male customers, Best Buy needed to appeal to women by reflecting the increasing integration of consumer electronics into family life. So Gilbert headed up an initiative to establish in-store boutiques that sold home theater systems along with coordinated furniture and accessories. Stores set up living-room displays to showcase not just electronics but also the entertainment environment. Salespeople were trained to interact with the previously ignored female customers who came in with men to look at systems.

Source: Heifetz, R., Grashow, A., & Linsky, M. 2009. Leadership in a (permanent) crisis. *Harvard Business Review*, 87 (7/8): 62–69; and, Bustillo, M. & Lloyd, M. 2010. Best Buy tests new appeals to women. *www.wsj.com*. June 16: np.

Gilbert says that championing this approach subjected her to some nasty criticism from managers who viewed Best Buy as a retailer of technology *products,* not experiences. However, focusing on the female purchaser when a man and a woman walked into the store—making eye contact and greeting her, asking about her favorite movies, and demonstrating them on the systems—often resulted in the couple's purchasing a higher-end product than they had originally considered. According to Gilbert, returns and exchanges of purchases made by couples were 60 percent lower than those made by men. With the rethinking of traditional practices, Best Buy's home theater business flourished, growing from two pilot in-store boutiques in mid-2004 to more than 350 five years later.

Such success does not appear to just happen by chance at Best Buy. Consider:

- Best Buy is empowering female workers and consulting teenage girls to suggest new ways to sell to women. The move reflects that women are becoming the most coveted customers in some of the hottest areas of electronic retailing in stores—smart phones and other mobile services.

- Executives say that the best insights on expanding the female customer base come from the company's "Women Leadership Forums," a loose-knit group of female workers and customers that meet around the country. The groups helped increase appliance sales, for example, by suggesting that showrooms be redesigned to resemble kitchens.

Often, failure of today's organizations can be attributed to a lack of equal consideration of these three activities. The imagery of a three-legged stool is instructive: It will collapse if one leg is missing or broken. Let's briefly look at each of these activities as well as the value of an ambicultural approach to leadership.

Setting a Direction

A holistic understanding of an organization's stakeholders requires an ability to scan the environment to develop a knowledge of all of the company's stakeholders and other salient environmental trends and events. Managers must integrate this knowledge into a vision of what the organization could become.[5] It necessitates the capacity to solve increasingly complex problems, become proactive in approach, and develop viable strategic options. A strategic vision provides many benefits: a clear future direction; a framework for the organization's mission and goals; and enhanced employee communication, participation, and commitment.

setting a direction
a strategic leadership activity of strategy analysis and strategy formulation.

At times the creative process involves what the CEO of Yokogawa, GE's Japanese partner in the Medical Systems business, called "bullet train" thinking.[6] That is, if you want to increase the speed by 10 miles per hour, you look for incremental advances. However, if you want to double the speed, you've got to think "out of the box" (e.g., widen the track, change the overall suspension system). Leaders need more creative solutions than just keeping the same train with a few minor tweaks. Instead, they must come up with more revolutionary visions.

The experience of Julie Gilbert, VP of electronics global retailer Best Buy, in changing the orientation of the company to attract more female shoppers, is an excellent example of how leaders can overcome resistance and set new directions for their organizations. Strategy Spotlight 11.1 describes her initiatives.

Designing the Organization

designing the organization a strategic leadership activity of building structures, teams, systems, and organizational processes that facilitate the implementation of the leader's vision and strategies.

At times, almost all leaders have difficulty implementing their vision and strategies.[7] Such problems may stem from a variety of sources:

- Lack of understanding of responsibility and accountability among managers.
- Reward systems that do not motivate individuals (or collectives such as groups and divisions) toward desired organizational goals.
- Inadequate or inappropriate budgeting and control systems.
- Insufficient mechanisms to integrate activities across the organization.

Successful leaders are actively involved in building structures, teams, systems, and organizational processes that facilitate the implementation of their vision and strategies. We discussed the necessity for consistency between business-level and corporate-level strategies and organizational control in Chapter 9. Without appropriately structuring organizational activities, a firm would generally be unable to attain an overall low-cost advantage by closely monitoring its costs through detailed and formalized cost and financial control procedures. With regard to corporate-level strategy, a related diversification strategy would necessitate reward systems that emphasize behavioral measures, whereas an unrelated strategy should rely more on financial (or objective) indicators of performance.

These examples illustrate the important role of leadership in creating systems and structures to achieve desired ends. As Jim Collins says about the importance of **designing the organization**, "Along with figuring out what the company stands for and pushing it to understand what it's really good at, building mechanisms is the CEO's role—the leader as architect."[8]

Nurturing an Excellent and Ethical Culture

excellent and ethical organizational culture an organizational culture focused on core competencies and high ethical standards.

Excellent and ethical organizational culture can be an effective means of organizational control.[9] Leaders play a key role in changing, developing, and sustaining an organization's culture. Consider a Chinese firm, Huawei, a highly successful producer of communication network solutions and services.[10] In 2009, it achieved revenues of $21.8 billion and net profits of $2.7 billion. Its strong culture can be attributed to its founder, Ren Zhengfei, and his background in the People's Liberation Army. It is a culture which eliminates individualism and promotes collectivism and the idea of hunting in packs. It is the "wolf culture" of Huawei:

The culture of Huawei is built on a sense of patriotism, with Mr. Zhengfei frequently citing Mao Zedong's thoughts in his speeches and internal publications such as the employee magazine "Huawei People." Sales teams are referred to as "Market Guerrillas," and battlefield tactics, such as "occupy rural areas first to surround cities," are used internally. In addition to Mao Zedong, Mr. Zhengfei has urged his employees to look to the Japanese and Germans for inspiration on how to conduct themselves. This is exemplified by the words written in a letter to new hires that states, "I hope you abandon the mentality of achieving

IKEA's Founder: "Low Prices—But Not at Any Price"

IKEA's founder, Ingvar Kamprad, although believed to be one of the world's top 10 richest men, is leading his company by example. He flies coach, drives an aging Volvo, and stays in cheap hotels when traveling. Early in his career, Kamprad recognized that promoting a double standard between him and his employees would be detrimental to the health and wealth of the entire company. He contended, "It's a question of good leadership."

His money-pinching habits are thus exemplified and reinforced in the company he founded. As an example of his thriftiness: Upon seeing some small pencils in a pile of debris on the floor, Kamprad sent the store manager to recover the pencils, even though their value was less than a penny.

Even though the company is usually tight-fisted, when it comes to environmental issues, IKEA spends millions of dollars in sorting and recycling the various types of plastic, metal, and wood used in packaging its products. Clearly, taking the time to sort the various materials entails significant costs and slows down the replenishment process. However, the processes are considered highly relevant to

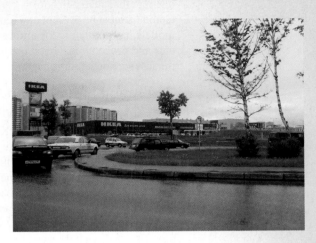

● Swedish retailer IKEA is well-known for its inexpensive but stylish furniture as well as its concern for the environment.

the firm's spirit of leadership. It is worth mentioning that none of these steps are a regulatory requirement, but are voluntary.

An explanation for IKEA's actions can be found in the company's slogan that is often observed in its offices: "Low prices—but not at any price." For IKEA this is not just another slogan but is reflected in its employees' everyday actions.

Source: Esty, D. C. & Winston, A. S. 2009. *Green to gold*. Hoboken, NJ: Wiley; and, Carmichael, E. Undated. Lesson #2: The best leadership is by example. *www.evancarmichael.com*, np.

quick results, learn from the Japanese down-to-earth attitude and the German's spirit of being scrupulous to every detail."

The notion of "wolf culture" stems from the fact that Huawei workers are encouraged to learn from the behavior of wolves, which have a keen sense of smell, are aggressive, and, most important of all, hunt in packs. It is this collective and aggressive spirit that is the center of the Huawei culture. Combining the behavior of wolves with military-style training has been instrumental in building the culture of the company, which, in turn, is widely thought to be instrumental in the company's success.

In sharp contrast, leaders can also have a very detrimental effect on a firm's culture and ethics. Imagine the negative impact that Todd Berman's illegal activities have had on a firm that he cofounded—New York's private equity firm Chartwell Investments.[11] He stole more than $3.6 million from the firm and its investors. Berman pleaded guilty to fraud charges brought by the Justice Department. For 18 months he misled Chartwell's investors concerning the financial condition of one of the firm's portfolio companies by falsely claiming it needed to borrow funds to meet operating expenses. Instead, Berman transferred the money to his personal bank account, along with fees paid by portfolio companies.

Clearly, a leader's behavior and values can make a strong impact on an organization—for good or for bad. Strategy Spotlight 11.2 provides a positive example. It discusses how the values and behavior of Ingvar Kamprad, founder of Swedish furniture retailer IKEA, have resulted in a culture of frugality and environmental consciousness within the company.

Managers and top executives must accept personal responsibility for developing and strengthening ethical behavior throughout the organization. They must consistently demonstrate that such behavior is central to the vision and mission of the organization. Several elements must be present and reinforced for a firm to become highly ethical, including role models, corporate credos and codes of conduct, reward and evaluation systems, and policies and procedures. Given the importance of these elements, we address them in detail in the last section of this chapter.

The Ambicultural Approach: A Key to Successfully Fulfilling the Three Leadership Activities

Highly successful leaders don't rely strictly on one philosophy and its associated set of business practices and apply them to every decision they face. Rather, they endeavor to merge the best from different approaches. For example, leaders can benefit by taking the best of different philosophies and business practices while avoiding the negatives. This is called an "ambicultural" perspective on leadership.[12] For example, a company can try to combine the best of Chinese and Western practices to create a truly ambicultural organization.

Each society has particular strengths and weaknesses as they apply to business practice. The challenge for managers is to utilize the thinking and orientations of both cultures in order to understand, identify with, and benefit from each of them. And we will see that it has important implications for setting an organization's direction and its designing structures and processes, as well as instilling a strong culture.

Stan Shih, the legendary founder of Acer Group, personifies the ambicultural perspective on leadership. Acer is the second-largest computer maker in the world, with revenues for the firm and its sister businesses, BenQ and Winstron, totaling $52 billion. Shih's overall orientation might be best described as a long-term view that values benefits not only for all company stakeholders but the entire global community.[13]

His major influence from the Chinese culture is a patient, holistic, community-driven orientation. From the Western perspective, he has taken a more decentralized and empowering management philosophy. At the same time, he has striven to avoid the mistrust, secrecy, and authoritarian paternalism that have sometimes characterized Eastern practices, and to avoid the short-term, bottom-line-driven focus and grandiosity of some Western companies.

Let's take a closer look at some Western practices that Shih has avoided and some that he has adopted. Most of all, he has avoided short-termism and narrow individualism and its corresponding intolerant, money-driven, up-or-out culture. His concern has never been with short-term profits or kill-or-be-killed competitive reasoning. He has avoided corporate cultures that lavishly reward the very few at the expense of the many. Nor has he focused exclusively on owners at the expense of other stakeholders or society as a whole. In these respects, he has much in common with enduring great Western family businesses.

At the same time, Shih has not universally ignored or dismissed aspects of American or Western management. He has been a strong proponent of decentralization, flat structures, and employee discretion. He has been quick to give up power to the next generations, and he has appreciated the value of brands, branding, and globalization. Unlike most Chinese firms, Acer did not pursue a typical cost-driven strategy or focus on low-end manufacturing. Theirs was more of a Western approach to branding and selling higher-end products. However, Shih did take note of the mistake of so many Western firms of outsourcing too many functions and thereby letting the outsourcers move up the value chain and steal their business. Acer kept total control of the value chain by employing different companies belonging to the same corporate group.

Elements of Effective Leadership

The demands on leaders in today's business environment require them to perform a variety of functions. The success of their organizations often depends on how they as individuals meet challenges and deliver on promises. What practices and skills are needed to get the job done effectively? In this section, we focus on three capabilities that are marks of successful leadership—integrative thinking, overcoming barriers to change, and the effective use of power. Then, in the next section, we will examine an important human trait that helps leaders be more effective—emotional intelligence.

Integrative Thinking

The challenges facing today's leaders require them to confront a host of opposing forces. As the previous section indicated, maintaining consistency across a company's culture, vision, and organizational design can be difficult, especially if the three activities are out of alignment.

>LO11.2
Three elements of effective leadership: integrative thinking, overcoming barriers to change, and the effective use of power.

How does a leader make good strategic decisions in the face of multiple contingencies and diverse opportunities? A recent study by Roger L. Martin revealed that executives who have a capability known as "integrative thinking" are among the most effective leaders. In his book *The Opposable Mind,* Martin contends that people who can consider two conflicting ideas simultaneously, without dismissing one of the ideas or becoming discouraged about reconciling them, often make the best problem solvers because of their ability to creatively synthesize the opposing thoughts. In explaining the source of his title, Martin quotes F. Scott Fitzgerald, who observed, "The test of a first-rate intelligence is the ability to hold two opposing ideas in mind at the same time and still retain the ability to function. One should, for example, be able to see that things are hopeless yet be determined to make them otherwise."[14]

In contrast to conventional thinking, which tends to focus on making choices between competing ideas from a limited set of alternatives, **integrative thinking** is the process by which people reconcile opposing thoughts to identify creative solutions that provide them with more options and new alternatives. Exhibit 11.2 outlines the four stages of the integrative thinking and deciding process. Martin uses the admittedly simple example of deciding where to go on vacation to illustrate the stages:

integrative thinking a process of reconciling opposing thoughts by generating new alternatives and creative solutions rather than rejecting one thought in favor of another.

- *Salience*—Take stock of what features of the decision you consider relevant and important. For example: Where will you go? What will you see? Where will you stay? What will it cost? Is it safe? Other features may be less important, but try to think of everything that may matter.
- *Causality*—Make a mental map of the causal relationships between the features, that is, how the various features are related to one another. For example, is it worth it to invite friends to share expenses? Will an exotic destination be less safe?
- *Architecture*—Use the mental map to arrange a sequence of decisions that will lead to a specific outcome. For example, will you make the hotel and flight arrangements first, or focus on which sightseeing tours are available? No particular decision path is right or wrong, but considering multiple options simultaneously may lead to a better decision.
- *Resolution*—Make your selection. For example, choose which destination, which flight, and so forth. You final resolution is linked to how you evaluated the first three stages; if you are dissatisfied with your choices, the dotted arrows in the diagram (Exhibit 11.2) suggest you can go back through the process and revisit your assumptions.

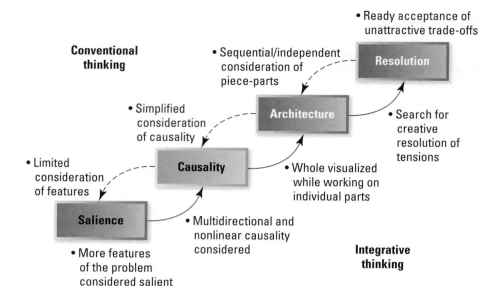

Conventional thinking

- Ready acceptance of unattractive trade-offs
- Sequential/independent consideration of piece-parts
- Simplified consideration of causality
- Limited consideration of features

Resolution

Architecture

Causality

Salience

- Search for creative resolution of tensions
- Whole visualized while working on individual parts
- Multidirectional and nonlinear causality considered
- More features of the problem considered salient

Integrative thinking

Exhibit 11.2 Integrative Thinking: The Process of Thinking and Deciding

Source: Reprinted by permission of Harvard Business School Press from R. L. Martin. *The Opposable Mind*, 2007. Copyright 2007 by the Harvard Business School Publishing Corporation; all rights reserved.

Applied to business, an integrative thinking approach enables decision makers to consider situations not as forced trade-offs—either decrease costs or invest more; either satisfy shareholders or please the community—but as a method for synthesizing opposing ideas into a creative solution. The key is to think in terms of "both-and" rather than "either-or." "Integrative thinking," said Martin, "shows us that there's a way to integrate the advantages of one solution without canceling out the advantages of an alternative solution."

Although Martin found that integrative thinking comes naturally to some people, he also believes it can be taught. But it may be difficult to learn, in part because it requires people to *un*learn old patterns and become aware of how they think. For executives willing to take a deep look at their habits of thought, integrative thinking can be developed into a valuable skill. Strategy Spotlight 11.3 tells how Red Hat cofounder Bob Young made his company a market leader by using integrative thinking to resolve a major problem in the domain of open-source software.

Overcoming Barriers to Change

What are the **barriers to change** that leaders often encounter, and how can they best bring about organizational change?[15] After all, people generally have some level of choice about how strongly they support or resist a leader's change initiatives. Why is there often so much resistance? Organizations at all levels are prone to inertia and are slow to learn, adapt, and change because:

1. Many people have **vested interests in the status quo.** People tend to be risk averse and resistant to change. There is a broad stream of research on "escalation," wherein certain individuals continue to throw "good money at bad decisions" despite negative performance feedback.[16]

2. There are **systemic barriers.** The design of the organization's structure, information processing, reporting relationships, and so forth impede the proper flow and

barriers to change
characteristics of individuals and organizations that prevent a leader from transforming an organization.

vested interests in the status quo barriers to change that stem from people's risk aversion.

systemic barriers
barriers to change that stem from an organizational design that impedes the proper flow and evaluation of information.

Integrative Thinking at Red Hat

How can a software developer make money giving away free software? That was the dilemma Red Hat founder Bob Young was facing during the early days of the open-source software movement. A Finnish developer named Linus Torvalds, using freely available UNIX software, had developed an operating system dubbed "Linux" that was being widely circulated in the freeware community. The software was intended specifically as an alternative to the pricey proprietary systems sold by Microsoft and Oracle. To use proprietary software, corporations had to pay hefty installation fees and were required to call Microsoft or Oracle engineers to fix it when anything went wrong. In Young's view it was a flawed and unsustainable business model.

But the free model was flawed as well. Although several companies had sprung up to help companies use Linux, there were few opportunities to profit from using it. As Young said, "You couldn't make any money selling [the Linux] operating system because all this stuff was free, and if you started to charge money for it, someone else would come in and price it lower. It was a commodity in the truest sense of the word." To complicate matters, hundreds of developers were part of the software community that was constantly modifying and debugging Linux—at a rate equivalent to three updates per day. As a result, systems administrators at corporations that tried to adopt the software spent so much time keeping track of updates that they didn't enjoy the savings they expected from using free software.

Source: Martin, R. L. 2007. *The opposable mind.* Boston: Harvard Business School Press; *www.finance.yahoo.com*; and, *www.redhat.com/about/companyprofile/facts/.*

Young saw the appeal of both approaches but also realized a new model was needed. While contemplating the dilemma, he realized a salient feature that others had overlooked—because most major corporations have to live with software decisions for at least 10 years, they will nearly always choose to do business with the industry leader. Young realized he had to position Red Hat as the top provider of Linux software. To do that, he proposed a radical solution: provide the authoritative version of Linux and deliver it in a new way—as a download rather than on CD. He hired programmers to create a downloadable version—still free—and promised, in essence, to maintain its quality (for a fee, of course) by dealing with all the open-source programmers who were continually suggesting changes. In the process, he created a product companies could trust and then profited by establishing ongoing service relationships with customers. Red Hat's version of Linux became the de facto standard. By 2000, Linux was installed in 25 percent of server operating systems worldwide and Red Hat had captured over 50 percent of the global market for Linux systems.

By recognizing that a synthesis of two flawed business models could provide the best of both worlds, Young exhibited the traits of integrative thinking. He pinpointed the causal relationships between the salient features of the marketplace and Red Hat's path to prosperity. He then crafted an approach that integrated aspects of the two existing approaches into a new alternative. By resolving to provide a free downloadable version, Young also took responsibility for creating his own path to success. The payoff was substantial: when Red Hat went public in 1999, Young became a billionaire on the first day of trading. And by February 2011 Red Hat had over $850 million in annual revenues and a market capitalization of nearly $9 billion.

evaluation of information. A bureaucratic structure with multiple layers, onerous requirements for documentation, and rigid rules and procedures will often "inoculate" the organization against change.

3. **Behavioral barriers** cause managers to look at issues from a biased or limited perspective due to their education, training, work experiences, and so forth. Consider an incident shared by David Lieberman, marketing director at GVO, an innovation consulting firm:

A company's creative type had come up with a great idea for a new product. Nearly everybody loved it. However, it was shot down by a high-ranking manufacturing representative who exploded: "A new color? Do you have any idea of the spare-parts problem that it will

behavioral barriers
barriers to change associated with the tendency for managers to look at issues from a biased or limited perspective based on their prior education and experience.

create?" This was not a dimwit exasperated at having to build a few storage racks at the warehouse. He'd been hearing for years about cost cutting, lean inventories, and "focus." Lieberman's comment: "Good concepts, but not always good for innovation."

4. **Political barriers** refer to conflicts arising from power relationships. This can be the outcome of a myriad of symptoms such as vested interests, refusal to share information, conflicts over resources, conflicts between departments and divisions, and petty interpersonal differences.

5. **Personal time constraints** bring to mind the old saying about "not having enough time to drain the swamp when you are up to your neck in alligators." Gresham's law of planning states that operational decisions will drive out the time necessary for strategic thinking and reflection. This tendency is accentuated in organizations experiencing severe price competition or retrenchment wherein managers and employees are spread rather thin.

Leaders must draw on a range of personal skills as well as organizational mechanisms to move their organizations forward in the face of such barriers. Integrative thinking provides one avenue by equipping leaders with an ability to consider creative alternatives to the kind of resistance and doubt that cause many barriers. Two factors mentioned earlier—building a learning organization and ethical organization—provide the kind of climate within which a leader can advance the organization's aims and make progress toward its goals.

One of the most important tools a leader has for overcoming barriers to change is his or her personal and organizational power. On the one hand, good leaders must be on guard not to abuse power. On the other hand, successful leadership requires the measured exercise of power. We turn to that topic next.

The Effective Use of Power

Successful leadership requires effective use of power in overcoming barriers to change.[17] As humorously noted by Mark Twain, "I'm all for progress. It's change I object to." **Power** refers to a leader's ability to get things done in a way he or she wants them to be done. It is the ability to influence other people's behavior, to persuade them to do things that they otherwise would not do, and to overcome resistance and opposition to changing direction. Effective exercise of power is essential for successful leadership.[18]

A leader derives his or her power from several sources or bases. The simplest way to understand the bases of power is by classifying them as organizational and personal, as shown in Exhibit 11.3.

Organizational bases of power refer to the power that a person wields because of holding a formal management position.[19] These include legitimate power, reward power, coercive power, and information power. *Legitimate power* is derived from organizationally conferred decision-making authority and is exercised by virtue of a manager's position in the organization. *Reward power* depends on the ability of the leader or manager to confer rewards for positive behaviors or outcomes. *Coercive power* is the power a manager exercises over employees using fear of punishment for errors of omission or commission. *Information power* arises from a manager's access, control, and distribution of information that is not freely available to everyone in an organization.

A leader might also be able to influence subordinates because of his or her personality characteristics and behavior. These would be considered the **personal bases of power,** including referent power and expert power. The source of *referent power* is a subordinate's identification with the leader. A leader's personal attributes or charisma might influence subordinates and make them devoted to that leader. The source of

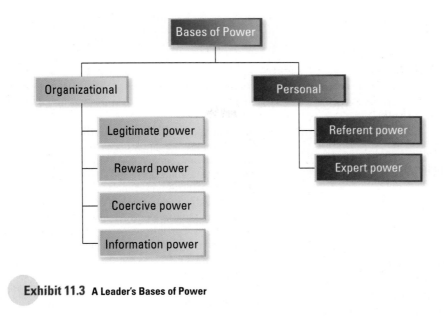

Exhibit 11.3 A Leader's Bases of Power

expert power is the leader's expertise and knowledge in a particular field. The leader is the expert on whom subordinates depend for information that they need to do their jobs successfully.

Successful leaders use the different bases of power, and often a combination of them, as appropriate to meet the demands of a situation, such as the nature of the task, the personality characteristics of the subordinates, the urgency of the issue, and other factors.[20] Leaders must recognize that persuasion and developing consensus are often essential, but so is pressing for action. At some point stragglers must be prodded into line.[21] Peter Georgescu, who recently retired as CEO of Young & Rubicam (an advertising and media subsidiary of the UK-based WPP Group), summarized a leader's dilemma brilliantly (and humorously), "I have knee pads and a .45. I get down and beg a lot, but I shoot people too."[22]

Strategy Spotlight 11.4 addresses some of the subtleties of power. It focuses on William Bratton, Chief of the Los Angeles Police Department, who has enjoyed a very successful career in law enforcement.

Emotional Intelligence: A Key Leadership Trait

>LO11.3
The crucial role of emotional intelligence (EI) in successful leadership as well as its potential drawbacks.

In the previous sections, we discussed skills and activities of strategic leadership. The focus was on "what leaders do and how they do it." Now, the issue becomes "who leaders *are,*" that is, what leadership traits are the most important. Clearly, these two issues are related, because successful leaders possess the valuable traits that enable them to perform effectively in order to create value for their organization.[23]

There has been a vast amount of literature on the successful traits of leaders.[24] These traits include integrity, maturity, energy, judgment, motivation, intelligence, expertise, and so on. For simplicity, these traits may be grouped into three broad sets of capabilities:

- Purely technical skills (like accounting or operations research).
- Cognitive abilities (like analytical reasoning or quantitative analysis).
- Emotional intelligence (like self-management and managing relationships).

William Bratton: Using Multiple Bases of Power

William Bratton, Chief of the Los Angeles Police Department, has an enviable track record in turning around police departments in crime-ridden cities. First, while running the police division of the Massachusetts Bay Transit Authority (MBTA) in Boston, then as police commissioner of New York in the mid-1990s, and with Los Angeles from 2002 to late 2009, Chief Bratton is credited with reducing crime and improving police morale in record time. An analysis of his success at each of these organizations reveals similar patterns both in terms of the problems he faced and the many ways in which he used the different bases of power to engineer a rapid turnaround.

In Boston, New York, and Los Angeles, Chief Bratton faced similar hurdles: organizations wedded to the status quo, limited resources, demotivated staffs, and opposition from powerful vested interests. But he does not give up in the face of these seemingly insurmountable problems. He is persuasive in calls for change, capable of mobilizing the commitment of key players, silencing vocal naysayers, and building rapport with superiors and subordinates while building bridges with external constituencies.

Chief Bratton's persuasion tactics are unconventional, yet effective. When he was running the MBTA police, the Transit Authority decided to buy small squad cars, which are cheaper to buy and to run, but inadequate for the police officer's task. Instead of arguing, Bratton invited the general manager for a tour of the city. He rode with the general manager in exactly the same type of car that was ordered for ordinary officers, and drove over every pothole on the road. He moved the seats forward so that the general manager could feel how little leg room was there. And he put on his belt, cuffs, and gun so that the general manager could understand how limited the space was. After two hours in the cramped car, the general manager was ready to change the order and get more suitable cars for the officers!

Another tactic Bratton used effectively was insisting on community meetings between police officers and citizens. This went against the long-standing practice of detachment between police and community to decrease the chances of corruption. The result was that his department had a better understanding of public concerns and rearranged their priorities, which in turn led to better community relations. For internal communications, he relied mainly on professionally produced videos instead of long, boring memos.

Chief Bratton also shows a remarkable talent for building political bridges and silencing naysayers. As he was introducing his zero-tolerance policing approach that aggressively targets "quality of life" crimes such as panhandling, drunkenness, and prostitution, opposition came from the city's courts, which feared being inundated by a large number of small-crimes cases. Bratton enlisted the support of Rudolph Giuliani, the mayor of New York, who had considerable influence over the district attorneys, the courts, and the city jail. He also took the case to *The New York Times* and managed to get the issue of zero-tolerance on the front pages of the newspaper. The courts were left with no alternative but to cooperate.

To a great extent, Bratton's success can be attributed to his understanding of the subtleties of power, including persuasion, motivation, coalition building, empathy for subordinates, and a focus on goals.

Let's take a quick look at his success during his tenure as Los Angeles's chief of police. Crime dropped significantly: Violent crimes were down 53 percent; property crimes were down 33 percent, and gang-related crimes were cut by 34 percent. Connie Rice, a prominent civil-rights lawyer, feels that Bratton's biggest achievement was turning the LAPD's old "warrior culture" into "policing as something not done to people but with people." She says, "Little old ladies who used to shake their head when the cops came around are now calling them about somebody doing crack." This is quite a strong endorsement coming from someone who *The Economist* says "spent much of her career suing the Los Angeles Police Department."

Sources: Exit Bratton. 2009. *The Economist*, October 31:42; Kim, W. C. & Mauborgne, R. A. 2003. Tipping point leadership. *Harvard Business Review*, 81(4): 60–69; and, McCarthy, T. 2004. The gang buster. *Time*, January 19: 56–58.

"Emotional intelligence (EI)" has become popular in both the literature and management practice in recent years.[25] *Harvard Business Review* articles published in 1998 and 2000 by psychologist/journalist Daniel Goleman, who is most closely associated with the concept, have become *HBR*'s most highly requested reprint articles. And two of Goleman's recent books, *Emotional Intelligence* and *Working with Emotional Intelligence,* were both on *The New York Times*'s best-seller lists. Goleman defines **emotional intelligence** as the capacity for recognizing one's own emotions and those of others.[26]

Recent studies of successful managers have found that effective leaders consistently have a high level of EI.[27] Findings indicate that EI is a better predictor of life success (economic well-being, satisfaction with life, friendship, family life), including occupational attainments, than IQ. Such evidence has been extrapolated to the catchy phrase: "IQ gets you hired, but EQ (Emotional Quotient) gets you promoted." Human resource managers believe this statement to be true, even for highly technical jobs such as those of scientists and engineers.

This is not to say that IQ and technical skills are irrelevant, but they become "threshold capabilities." They are the necessary requirements for attaining higher-level managerial positions. EI, on the other hand, is essential for leadership success. Without it, Goleman claims, a manager can have excellent training, an incisive analytical mind, and many smart ideas but will still not be a great leader.

Exhibit 11.4 identifies the five components of EI: self-awareness, self-regulation, motivation, empathy, and social skill.

> **emotional intelligence (EI)**
> an individual's capacity for recognizing his or her own emotions and those of others, including the five components of self-awareness, self-regulation, motivation, empathy, and social skill.

Exhibit 11.4   The Five Components of Emotional Intelligence at Work

	Definition	Hallmarks
Self-management skills:		
Self-awareness	• The ability to recognize and understand your moods, emotions, and drives, as well as their effect on others.	• Self-confidence • Realistic self-assessment • Self-deprecating sense of humor
Self-regulation	• The ability to control or redirect disruptive impulses and moods. • The propensity to suspend judgment—to think before acting.	• Trustworthiness and integrity • Comfort with ambiguity • Openness to change
Motivation	• A passion to work for reasons that go beyond money or status. • A propensity to pursue goals with energy and persistence.	• Strong drive to achieve • Optimism, even in the face of failure • Organizational commitment
Managing relationships:		
Empathy	• The ability to understand the emotional makeup of other people. • Skill in treating people according to their emotional reactions.	• Expertise in building and retaining talent • Cross-cultural sensitivity • Service to clients and customers
Social skill	• Proficiency in managing relationships and building networks. • An ability to find common ground and build rapport.	• Effectiveness in leading change • Persuasiveness • Expertise in building and leading teams

Source: Reprinted by permission of *Harvard Business Review*. Exhibit from "What Makes a Leader," by D. Goleman, January 2004. Copyright © 2004 by the Harvard Business School Publishing Corporation; all rights reserved.

Self-Awareness

Self-awareness is the first component of EI and brings to mind that Delphic oracle who gave the advice "know thyself" thousands of years ago. Self-awareness involves a person having a deep understanding of his or her emotions, strengths, weaknesses, and drives. People with strong self-awareness are neither overly critical nor unrealistically optimistic. Instead, they are honest with themselves and others.

People generally admire and respect candor. Leaders are constantly required to make judgment calls that require a candid assessment of capabilities—their own and those of others. People who assess themselves honestly (i.e., self-aware people) are well suited to do the same for the organizations they run.[28]

Self-Regulation

Biological impulses drive our emotions. Although we cannot do away with them, we can strive to manage them. Self-regulation, which is akin to an ongoing inner conversation, frees us from being prisoners of our feelings.[29] People engaged in such conversation feel bad moods and emotional impulses just as everyone else does. However, they find ways to control them and even channel them in useful ways.

Self-regulated people are able to create an environment of trust and fairness where political behavior and infighting are sharply reduced and productivity tends to be high. People who have mastered their emotions are better able to bring about and implement change in an organization. When a new initiative is announced, they are less likely to panic; they are able to suspend judgment, seek out information, and listen to executives explain the new program.

Motivation

Successful executives are driven to achieve beyond expectations—their own and everyone else's. Although many people are driven by external factors, such as money and prestige, those with leadership potential are driven by a deeply embedded desire to achieve for the sake of achievement.

Motivated people show a passion for the work itself, such as seeking out creative challenges, a love of learning, and taking pride in a job well done. They also have a high level of energy to do things better as well as a restlessness with the status quo. They are eager to explore new approaches to their work.

Empathy

Empathy is probably the most easily recognized component of EI. Empathy means thoughtfully considering an employee's feelings, along with other factors, in the process of making intelligent decisions. Empathy is particularly important in today's business environment for at least three reasons: the increasing use of teams, the rapid pace of globalization, and the growing need to retain talent.[30]

When leading a team, a manager is often charged with arriving at a consensus—often in the face of a high level of emotions. Empathy enables a manager to sense and understand the viewpoints of everyone around the table.

Globalization typically involves cross-cultural dialogue that can easily lead to miscues. Empathetic people are attuned to the subtleties of body language; they can hear the message beneath the words being spoken. They have a deep understanding of the existence and importance of cultural and ethnic differences.

Empathy also plays a key role in retaining talent. Human capital is particularly important to a firm in the knowledge economy when it comes to creating advantages that are sustainable. Leaders need empathy to develop and keep top talent, because when high performers leave, they take their tacit knowledge with them.

Social Skill

While the first three components of EI are all self-management skills, the last two—empathy and social skill—concern a person's ability to manage relationships with others. Social skill may be viewed as friendliness with a purpose: moving people in the direction you desire, whether that's agreement on a new marketing strategy or enthusiasm about a new product.

Socially skilled people tend to have a wide circle of acquaintances as well as a knack for finding common ground and building rapport. They recognize that nothing gets done alone, and they have a network in place when the time for action comes.

Social skill can be viewed as the culmination of the other dimensions of EI. People will be effective at managing relationships when they can understand and control their own emotions and empathize with others' feelings. Motivation also contributes to social skill. People who are driven to achieve tend to be optimistic, even when confronted with setbacks. And when people are upbeat, their "glow" is cast upon conversations and other social encounters. They are popular, and for good reason.

Bert Pijls, CEO of Egg Banking, a British Internet banking firm, provides some insights into the importance of emotional intelligence in successfully leading an organization:[31]

> Emotional intelligence really means for me two things. It means how you relate to other people and, as a result, how other people feel about you. Second thing is how you deal emotionally with setbacks yourself. So part of emotional intelligence is internal; things don't always go the way you planned. And you have two options. Either you complain about that and get depressed about it, or you use it as an opportunity to re-energize yourself and keep going nonetheless. People who have great emotional intelligence are able to make the people who work with them feel totally free to express themselves, feel almost fearless, and, as a result, do things they thought they couldn't do.

Emotional Intelligence: Some Potential Drawbacks and Cautionary Notes

Many great leaders have great reserves of empathy, interpersonal astuteness, awareness of their own feelings, and an awareness of their impact on others.[32] More importantly, they know how to apply these capabilities judiciously as best benefits the situation. Having some minimum level of EI will help a person be effective as a leader as long as it is channeled appropriately. However, if a person has a high level of these capabilities it may become "too much of a good thing" if he or she is allowed to drive inappropriate behaviors. Some additional potential drawbacks of EI can be gleaned by considering the flip side of its benefits.

Effective Leaders Have Empathy for Others However, they also must be able to make the "tough decisions." Leaders must be able to appeal to logic and reason and acknowledge others' feelings so that people feel the decisions are correct. However, it is easy to overidentify with others or confuse empathy with sympathy. This can make it more difficult to make the tough decisions.

Effective Leaders Are Astute Judges of People A danger is that leaders may become judgmental and overly critical about the shortcomings they perceive in others. They are likely to dismiss other people's insights, making them feel undervalued.

Effective Leaders Are Passionate about What They Do, and They Show It This doesn't mean that they are always cheerleaders. Rather, they may express their passion as persistence in pursuing an objective or a relentless focus on a valued principle. However, there is a fine line between being excited about something and letting your passion close your mind to other possibilities or cause you to ignore realities that others may see.

Effective Leaders Create Personal Connections with Their People   Most effective leaders take time to engage employees individually and in groups, listening to their ideas, suggestions and concerns, and responding in ways that make people feel that their ideas are respected and appreciated. However, if the leader makes too many unannounced visits, it may create a culture of fear and micromanagement. Clearly, striking a correct balance is essential.

From a moral standpoint, emotional leadership is neither good nor bad. On the one hand, emotional leaders can be altruistic, focused on the general welfare of the company and its employees, and highly principled. On the other hand, they can be manipulative, selfish, and dishonest. For example, if a person is using leadership solely to gain power, that is not leadership at all.[33] Rather, that person is using his or her EI to grasp what people want and pander to those desires in order to gain authority and influence. After all, easy answers sell.

Next, we turn to guidelines for developing a "learning organization." In today's competitive environment, the old saying that "a chain is only as strong as the weakest link" applies more than ever before. To learn and adapt proactively, firms need "eyes, ears, and brains" throughout all parts of the organization. One person, or a small group of individuals, can no longer think and learn for the entire entity.

>LO11.4
The value of creating and maintaining a learning organization in today's global marketplace.

Developing a Learning Organization

Charles Handy, author of *The Age of Unreason* and *The Age of Paradox* and one of today's most respected business visionaries, shared an amusing story several years ago:

> The other day, a courier could not find my family's remote cottage. He called his base on his radio, and the base called us to ask directions. He was just around the corner, but his base managed to omit a vital part of the directions. So he called them again, and they called us again. Then the courier repeated the cycle a third time to ask whether we had a dangerous dog. When he eventually arrived, we asked whether it would not have been simpler and less aggravating to everyone if he had called us directly from the roadside telephone booth where he had been parked. "I can't do that," he said, "because they won't refund any money I spend." "But it's only pennies!" I exclaimed. "I know," he said, "but that only shows how little they trust us!"[34]

At first glance, it would appear that the story epitomizes the lack of empowerment and trust granted to the hapless courier: Don't ask questions! Do as you're told![35] However, implicit in this scenario is also the message that learning, information sharing, adaptation, decision making, and so on are *not* shared throughout the organization. In contrast, leading-edge organizations recognize the importance of having everyone involved in the process of actively learning and adapting. As noted by today's leading expert on learning organizations, MIT's Peter Senge, the days when Henry Ford, Alfred Sloan, and Tom Watson *"learned **for** the organization"* are gone.

> In an increasingly dynamic, interdependent, and unpredictable world, it is simply no longer possible for anyone to "figure it all out at the top." The old model, "the top thinks and the local acts," must now give way to integrating thinking and acting at all levels. While the challenge is great, so is the potential payoff. "The person who figures out how to harness the collective genius of the people in his or her organization," according to former Citibank CEO Walter Wriston, "is going to blow the competition away."[36]

Learning and change typically involve the ongoing questioning of an organization's status quo or method of procedure. This means that all individuals throughout the organization must be reflective.[37] Many organizations get so caught up in carrying out their day-to-day work that they rarely, if ever, stop to think objectively about themselves and their businesses. They often fail to ask the probing questions that might lead them to call into question their basic assumptions, to refresh their strategies, or to reengineer their work processes. According to Michael Hammer and Steven Stanton, the pioneer consultants who touched off the reengineering movement:

> Reflection entails awareness of self, of competitors, of customers. It means thinking without preconception. It means questioning cherished assumptions and replacing them with new approaches. It is the only way in which a winning company can maintain its leadership position, by which a company with great assets can ensure that they continue to be well deployed.[38]

To adapt to change, foster creativity, and remain competitive, leaders must build learning organizations. Exhibit 11.5 lists the five elements of a learning organization.

Inspiring and Motivating People with a Mission or Purpose

Successful **learning organizations** create a proactive, creative approach to the unknown, actively solicit the involvement of employees at all levels, and enable all employees to use their intelligence and apply their imagination. Higher-level skills are required of everyone, not just those at the top.[39] A learning environment involves organizationwide commitment to change, an action orientation, and applicable tools and methods.[40] It must be viewed by everyone as a guiding philosophy and not simply as another change program.

A critical requirement of all learning organizations is that everyone feels and supports a compelling purpose. In the words of William O'Brien, CEO of Hanover Insurance, "Before there can be meaningful participation, people must share certain values and pictures about where we are trying to go. We discovered that people have a real need to feel that they're part of an enabling mission."[41] Such a perspective is consistent with an intensive study by Kouzes and Posner, authors of *The Leadership Challenge*.[42] They recently analyzed data from nearly 1 million respondents who were leaders at various levels in many organizations throughout the world. A major finding was that what leaders struggle with most is communicating an image of the future that draws others in, that is, it speaks to what others see and feel. To illustrate:

> Buddy Blanton, a principal program manager at Rockwell Collins, learned this lesson firsthand. He asked his team for feedback on his leadership, and the vast majority of it was positive. However, he got some strong advice from his team about how he could be more effective in inspiring a shared vision. "You would benefit by helping us, as a team, to understand how you go to your vision. We want to walk with you while you create the goals and vision, so we all get to the end of the vision together."[43]

Inspiring and motivating people with a mission or purpose is a necessary but not sufficient condition for developing an organization that can learn and adapt to a rapidly changing, complex, and interconnected environment.

learning organizations organizations that create a proactive, creative approach to the unknown, characterized by (1) inspiring and motivating people with a mission and purpose, (2) empowering employees at all levels, (3) accumulating and sharing internal knowledge, (4) gathering and integrating external information, and (5) challenging the status quo and enabling creativity.

These are the five key elements of a learning organization. Each of these items should be viewed as *necessary, but not sufficient*. That is, successful learning organizations need all five elements.

1. Inspiring and motivating people with a mission or purpose.
2. Empowering employees at all levels.
3. Accumulating and sharing internal knowledge.
4. Gathering and integrating external information.
5. Challenging the status quo and enabling creativity.

Exhibit 11.5 Key Elements of a Learning Organization

Empowering Employees at All Levels

"The great leader is a great servant," asserted Ken Melrose, CEO of Toro Company and author of *Making the Grass Greener on Your Side.*[44] A manager's role becomes one of creating an environment where employees can achieve their potential as they help move the organization toward its goals. Instead of viewing themselves as resource controllers and power brokers, leaders must envision themselves as flexible resources willing to assume numerous roles as coaches, information providers, teachers, decision makers, facilitators, supporters, or listeners, depending on the needs of their employees.[45]

The central key to empowerment is effective leadership. Empowerment can't occur in a leadership vacuum. According to Melrose, "You best lead by serving the needs of your people. You don't do their jobs for them; you enable them to learn and progress on the job." Robert Quinn and Gretchen Spreitzer made an interesting point about two diametrically opposite perspectives on empowerment—top-down and bottom-up.[46]

In the top-down perspective, empowerment is about delegation and accountability—senior management has developed a clear vision and has communicated specific plans to the rest of the organization.[47] This strategy for empowerment encompasses the following:

- Start at the top.
- Clarify the organization's mission, vision, and values.
- Clearly specify the tasks, roles, and rewards for employees.
- Delegate responsibility.
- Hold people accountable for results.

By contrast, the bottom-up view looks at empowerment as concerned with risk taking, growth, and change. It involves trusting people to "do the right thing" and having a tolerance for failure. It encourages employees to act with a sense of ownership and typically "ask for forgiveness rather than permission." Here the salient elements of empowerment are:

- Start at the bottom by understanding the needs of employees.
- Teach employees self-management skills and model desired behavior.
- Build teams to encourage cooperative behavior.
- Encourage intelligent risk taking.
- Trust people to perform.

These two perspectives draw a sharp contrast in assumptions that people make about trust and control. Quinn and Spreitzer recently shared these contrasting views of empowerment with a senior management team. After an initial heavy silence, someone from the first group voiced a concern about the second group's perspective, "We can't afford loose cannons around here." A person in the second group retorted, "When was the last time you saw a cannon of any kind around here?"

Many leading-edge organizations are moving in the direction of the second perspective—recognizing the need for trust, cultural control, and expertise at all levels instead of the extensive and cumbersome rules and regulations inherent in hierarchical control.[48] Some have argued that too often organizations fall prey to the "heroes-and-drones syndrome," wherein the value of those in powerful positions is exalted and the value of those who fail to achieve top rank is diminished. Such an attitude is implicit in phrases such as "Lead, follow, or get out of the way" or, even less appealing, "Unless you're the lead horse, the view never changes." Few will ever reach the top hierarchical positions in organizations, but in the information economy, the strongest organizations are those that effectively use the talents of all the players on the team.

Empowering individuals by soliciting their input helps an organization to enjoy better employee morale. It also may help to create a culture of shared sacrifice, which may be critical during difficult economic times, as described in Strategy Spotlight 11.5.

A Hospital's Unique Approach to Empowerment

Beth Israel Deaconess is a medical center formed by the merger of two Harvard teaching hospitals. Early in 2009, it was facing a projected $20 million annual loss after several years of profitability. CEO Paul Levy held a meeting to discuss layoffs.

He expressed concern that cutbacks would affect low-wage employees, such as housekeepers, and he floated what he thought would be an unpopular idea: protecting some of those low-paying jobs by reducing the salary and benefits of higher-paid employees—including many sitting in the auditorium. To his surprise, the room erupted in applause!

His candid request for help led to countless suggestions for cost savings. This included an offer by the 13 medical department heads to save 10 jobs through personal donations totaling $350,000. In addition, the plan for reducing layoffs included a combination of delayed raises and a temporary reduction in benefits. Such efforts ultimately reduced the number of planned layoffs by 75 percent.

In the end, the low-wage workers were really taken care of. They were exempt from the salary cuts and even received 3 percent raises.

Sources: Heifetz, R., Grashow, A., & Linsky, M. 2009. Leadership in a (permanent) crisis. *Harvard Business Review*, 87(4): 67; and, Cooney, E. 2009. Beth Israel pares its plan for layoffs. *www.bostonglobe.com*. March 25: np.

Accumulating and Sharing Internal Knowledge

Effective organizations must also *redistribute information, knowledge* (skills to act on the information), and *rewards*.[49] A company might give frontline employees the power to act as "customer advocates," doing whatever is necessary to satisfy customers. The company needs to disseminate information by sharing customer expectations and feedback as well as financial information. The employees must know about the goals of the business as well as how key value-creating activities in the organization are related to each other. Finally, organizations should allocate rewards on how effectively employees use information, knowledge, and power to improve customer service quality and the company's overall performance.[50]

Let's take a look at Whole Foods Market, Inc., the largest natural foods grocer in the United States with stores in Canada and the UK.[51] An important benefit of the sharing of internal information at Whole Foods becomes the active process of *internal benchmarking.* Competition is intense at Whole Foods. Teams compete against their own goals for sales, growth, and productivity; they compete against different teams in their stores; and they compete against similar teams at different stores and regions. There is an elaborate system of peer reviews through which teams benchmark each other. The "Store Tour" is the most intense. On a periodic schedule, each Whole Foods store is toured by a group of as many as 40 visitors from another region. Lateral learning—discovering what your colleagues are doing right and carrying those practices into your organization—has become a driving force at Whole Foods.

In addition to enhancing the sharing of company information both up and down as well as across the organization, leaders also have to develop means to tap into some of the more informal sources of internal information. In a recent survey of presidents, CEOs, board members, and top executives in a variety of nonprofit organizations, respondents were asked what differentiated the successful candidates for promotion. The consensus: The executive was seen as a person who listens. According to Peter Meyer, the author of the study, "The value of listening is clear: You cannot succeed in running a company if you do not hear what your people, customers, and suppliers are telling you. . . . Listening and understanding well are key to making good decisions."[52]

Gathering and Integrating External Information

Recognizing opportunities, as well as threats, in the external environment is vital to a firm's success. As organizations *and* environments become more complex and evolve rapidly, it is far more critical for employees and managers to become more aware of environmental trends and events—both general and industry-specific—and more knowledgeable about their firm's competitors and customers. Next, we will discuss some ideas on how to do it.

First, the Internet has dramatically accelerated the speed with which anyone can track down useful information or locate people who might have useful information. Prior to the Net, locating someone who used to work at a company—always a good source of information—was quite a challenge. However, today people post their résumés on the web; they participate in discussion groups and talk openly about where they work.

Marc Friedman, manager of market research at $1 billion Andrew Corporation, a fast-growing global manufacturer of wireless communications products, provides an example of effective Internet use.[53] One of Friedman's preferred sites to visit is Corptech's website, which provides information on 45,000 high-tech companies and more than 170,000 executives. One of his firm's product lines consisted of antennae for air-traffic control systems. He got a request to provide a country-by-country breakdown of upgrade plans for various airports. He knew nothing about air-traffic control at the time. However, he found a site on the Internet for the International Civil Aviation Organization. Fortunately, it had a great deal of useful data, including several research companies working in his area of interest.

Second, company employees at all levels can use "garden variety" traditional sources to acquire external information. Much can be gleaned by reading trade and professional journals, books, and popular business magazines. Other venues for gathering external information include membership in professional or trade organizations, attendance at meetings and conventions, and networking among colleagues inside and outside your industry. Intel's former CEO Andy Grove gathered information from people like DreamWorks SKG's Steven Spielberg and Tele-Communications Inc.'s John Malone.[54] He believed that such interaction provided insights into how to make personal computers more entertaining and better at communicating. Internally, Grove spent time with the young engineers who ran Intel Architecture labs, an Oregon-based facility that Grove hoped would become the de facto R&D lab for the entire PC industry.

Third, **benchmarking** *can be a useful means of employing external information.* Here managers seek out the best examples of a particular practice as part of an ongoing effort to improve the corresponding practice in their own organization.[55] There are two primary types of benchmarking. **Competitive benchmarking** restricts the search for best practices to competitors, while **functional benchmarking** endeavors to determine best practices regardless of industry. Industry-specific standards (e.g., response times required to repair power outages in the electric utility industry) are typically best handled through competitive benchmarking, whereas more generic processes (e.g., answering 1-800 calls) lend themselves to functional benchmarking because the function is essentially the same in any industry.

Ford Motor Company used benchmarking to study Mazda's accounts payable operations.[56] Its initial goal of a 20 percent cut in its 500-employee accounts payable staff was ratcheted up to 75 percent—and met. Ford found that staff spent most of their time trying to match conflicting data in a mass of paper, including purchase orders, invoices, and receipts. Following Mazda's example, Ford created an "invoiceless system" in which invoices no longer trigger payments to suppliers. The receipt does the job.

Another classic benchmarking example involves Canon and Xerox. In 1979, Canon introduced a midsize copier for less than $10,000. Xerox, which could not manufacture or retail a similar machine for that price, initially assumed that Canon was deliberately underpricing its product to buy market share. Over time, however, as Canon's copier sales continued without a price increase, Xerox engineers determined that Canon's more efficient production methods enabled it to sell profitably at lower prices. As a result, Xerox decided to benchmark Canon's processes with the objective of reducing its own costs. From 1980 to 1985, Xerox adapted Japanese business techniques, which enabled the company to cut unit production costs by half and reduce inventory costs by more than 60 percent. This remarkable turnaround by Xerox launched benchmarking as a popular new management movement in the United States.[57]

Fourth, focus directly on customers for information. For example, William McKnight, head of 3M's Chicago sales office, required that salesmen of abrasives products talk directly to the workers in the shop to find out what they needed, instead of calling on only front-office executives. [58] This was very innovative at the time—1909! But it illustrates the need to get to the end user of a product or service. (McKnight went on to become 3M's president from 1929 to 1949 and chairman from 1949 to 1969.) James Taylor, former senior vice president for global marketing at Gateway 2000 (since acquired by Acer), discussed the value of customer input in reducing response time, a critical success factor in the PC industry.

> We talk to 100,000 people a day—people calling to order a computer, shopping around, looking for tech support. Our website gets 1.1 million hits per day. The time it takes for an idea to enter this organization, get processed, and then go to customers for feedback is down to minutes. We've designed the company around speed and feedback.[59]

Challenging the Status Quo and Enabling Creativity

Earlier in this chapter we discussed some of the barriers that leaders face when trying to bring about change in an organization: vested interests in the status quo, systemic barriers, behavioral barriers, political barriers, and personal time constraints. For a firm to become a learning organization, it must overcome such barriers in order to foster creativity and enable it to permeate the firm. This becomes quite a challenge if the firm is entrenched in a status quo mentality.

Perhaps the best way to challenge the status quo is for the leader to forcefully create a sense of urgency. For example, Paul Clark, CEO of Charter UK, a company that produces customer feedback management software, said one way to initiate change is to focus on the overall importance of retaining customers:

> People need to spend their money wisely. In good times, they want a good deal, from a trustworthy supplier; in tough times, they really need one. That's why now, more than ever, customer service is so important. Woe betide the business that doesn't listen to its customers, respond to their needs, react to their complaints, resolve their issues. Our business is all about managing and handling complaints and feedback, right across an enterprise. It's about using this feedback better to understand customers. What's more, it's about doing it cost-effectively—because we know times are tough for business, too.[60]

Such initiative, if sincere and credible, establishes a shared mission and the need for major transformations. It can channel energies to bring about both change and creative endeavors.

Establishing a "culture of dissent" can be another effective means of questioning the status quo and serving as a spur toward creativity. Here norms are established whereby dissenters can openly question a superior's perspective without fear of retaliation or retribution. Consider the perspective of Steven Ballmer, Microsoft's CEO.

> Bill [Gates] brings to the company the idea that conflict can be a good thing. . . . Bill knows it's important to avoid that gentle civility that keeps you from getting to the heart of an issue quickly. He likes it when anyone, even a junior employee, challenges him, and you know he respects you when he starts shouting back.[61]

Motorola has gone a step further and institutionalized its culture of dissent.[62] By filing a "minority report," an employee can go above his or her immediate supervisor's head and officially lodge a different point of view on a business decision. According to former

CEO George Fisher, "I'd call it a healthy spirit of discontent and a freedom by and large to express your discontent around here or to disagree with whoever it is in the company, me or anybody else."

Closely related to the culture of dissent is the fostering of a culture that encourages risk taking. "If you're not making mistakes, you're not taking risks, and that means you're not going anywhere," claimed John Holt, coauthor of *Celebrate Your Mistakes*.[63] "The key is to make errors faster than the competition, so you have more chances to learn and win."

Companies that cultivate cultures of experimentation and curiosity make sure that *failure* is not, in essence, an obscene word. They encourage mistakes as a key part of their competitive advantage. This philosophy was shared by Stan Shih, CEO of Acer, a Taiwan-based computer company. If a manager at Acer took an intelligent risk and made a mistake—even a costly one—Shih wrote off the loss as tuition payment for the manager's education. Such a culture must permeate the entire organization. As a high-tech executive told us during an interview: "Every person has a freedom to fail."

Exhibit 11.6 has insights on how organizations can both embrace risk and learn from failure.

Exhibit 11.6   Best Practices: Learning from Failures

It's innovation's great paradox: Success—that is, true breakthroughs—usually comes through failure. Here are some ideas on how to help your team get comfortable with taking risks and learning from mistakes:

- **Formalize Forums for Failure**
  To keep failures and the valuable lessons they offer from getting swept under the rug, *carve out time for reflection.* GE recently began sharing lessons from failures by bringing together managers whose "Imagination Breakthrough" efforts are put on the shelf.

- **Move the Goalposts**
  Innovation requires flexibility in meeting goals, since early predictions are often little more than educated guesses. Intuit's Scott Cook even suggests that teams developing new products ignore forecasts in the early days. "For every one of our failures, we had spreadsheets that looked awesome," he said.

- **Share Personal Stories**
  If employees hear leaders discussing their own failures, *they'll feel more comfortable talking about their own.* But it's not just the CEO's job. Front-line leaders are even more important, said Harvard Business School professor Amy Edmondson. "That person needs to be inviting, curious, and the first to say: 'I made a mistake.'"

- **Bring in Outsiders**
  Outsiders can *help neutralize the emotions and biases that prop up a flop.* Customers can be the most valuable. After its DNA chip failed, Corning brought pharmaceutical companies in early to test its new drug-discovery technology, Epic.

- **Prove Yourself Wrong, Not Right**
  Development teams tend to look for supporting, rather than countervailing, evidence. "You have to reframe what you're seeking in the early days," said Innosight's Scott Anthony. *"You're not really seeking proof that you have the right answer.* It's more about testing to prove yourself wrong."

- **Celebrate Smart Failures**
  Managers should design performance-management systems that reward risk taking and foster a long-term view. But they should also *celebrate failures that teach something new,* energizing people to try again and offering them closure.

Source: From J. McGregor, "How Failure Breeds Success," *Bloomberg BusinessWeek*, July 10, 2006, pp. 42–52 used with permission of *Bloomberg BusinessWeek*. Copyright © 2006. All rights reserved.

Creating an Ethical Organization

>LO11.5
The leader's role in establishing an ethical organization.

Ethics may be defined as a system of right and wrong.[64] Ethics assists individuals in deciding when an act is moral or immoral, socially desirable or not. The sources for an individual's ethics include religious beliefs, national and ethnic heritage, family practices, community standards, educational experiences, and friends and neighbors. Business ethics is the application of ethical standards to commercial enterprise.

ethics a system of right and wrong that assists individuals in deciding when an act is moral or immoral and/or socially desirable or not.

Individual Ethics versus Organizational Ethics

Many leaders think of ethics as a question of personal scruples, a confidential matter between employees and their consciences. Such leaders are quick to describe any wrong-doing as an isolated incident, the work of a rogue employee. They assume the company should not bear any responsibility for individual misdeeds. In their view, ethics has nothing to do with leadership.

Ethics has everything to do with leadership. Seldom does the character flaw of a lone actor completely explain corporate misconduct. Instead, unethical business practices typically involve the tacit, if not explicit, cooperation of others and reflect the values, attitudes, and behavior patterns that define an organization's operating culture. Ethics is as much an organizational as a personal issue. Leaders who fail to provide proper leadership to institute proper systems and controls that facilitate ethical conduct share responsibility with those who conceive, execute, and knowingly benefit from corporate misdeeds.[65]

The **ethical orientation** of a leader is a key factor in promoting ethical behavior. Ethical leaders must take personal, ethical responsibility for their actions and decision making. Leaders who exhibit high ethical standards become role models for others and raise an organization's overall level of ethical behavior. Ethical behavior must start with the leader before the employees can be expected to perform accordingly.

ethical orientation the practices that firms use to promote an ethical business culture, including ethical role models, corporate credos and codes of conduct, ethically based reward and evaluation systems, and consistently enforced ethical policies and procedures.

There has been a growing interest in corporate ethical performance. Some reasons for this trend may be the increasing lack of confidence regarding corporate activities, the growing emphasis on quality of life issues, and a spate of recent corporate scandals. Without a strong ethical culture, the chance of ethical crises occurring is enhanced. Ethical crises can be very expensive—both in terms of financial costs and in the erosion of human capital and overall firm reputation. Merely adhering to the minimum regulatory standards may not be enough to remain competitive in a world that is becoming more socially conscious. Strategy Spotlight 11.6 highlights potential ethical problems at utility companies that are trying to capitalize on consumers' desire to participate in efforts to curb global warming.

Potential ethical problems in corporate performance are not limited to any one country. Consider Denmark and its green power program. On Earth Day in April 2010, President Obama praised Denmark as a great green power model, telling a U.S. audience, "America produces less than 3 percent of our electricity through renewable sources like wind and solar—less than 3 percent. Now, in comparison, Denmark produces almost 20 percent of their electricity through wind power." Yet a 2009 report issued by CEPOS, a Danish think tank, told a far different story. Its study found that, while wind provided 19 percent of Denmark's electricity generation, it only met an average 9.7 percent of the demand over a five-year period, and a mere 5 percent during 2006. Since it can't use all the electricity it produces, Denmark exports about half of its extra supply to Norway and Sweden where hydroelectric power can be switched on and off to balance their electrical grids. Despite export sales to other countries, government wind subsidies cause Danish customers to pay the highest electricity rates in Europe.[66]

The past several years have been characterized by numerous examples of unethical and illegal behavior by many top-level corporate executives. These include executives of firms such as Enron, Tyco, and WorldCom in the United States; Parmalat of Italy; and

Green Energy: Real or Just a Marketing Ploy?

Many consumers want to "go green" and are looking for opportunities to do so. Utility companies that provide heat and electricity are one of the most obvious places to turn, because they often use fossil fuels that could be saved through energy conservation or replaced by using alternative energy sources. In fact, some consumers are willing to pay a premium to contribute to environmental sustainability efforts if paying a little more will help curb global warming. Knowing this, many power companies in many countries have developed alternative energy programs and appealed to customers to help pay for them.

Unfortunately, many of the power companies that are offering eco-friendly options are falling short on delivering them. Some utilities have simply gotten off to a slow start or found it difficult to profitably offer alternative power. Others, however, are suspected of committing a new type of fraud—"greenwashing." This refers to companies that make unsubstantiated claims about how environmentally friendly their products or services really are. In the case of many power companies, their claims of "green power" are empty promises. Instead of actually generating additional renewable energy, most of the premiums are going for marketing costs. "They are preying on people's goodwill," says Stephen Smith, executive director of the Southern Alliance for Clean Energy, an advocacy group in Knoxville, Tennessee.

Exhibit 11.7 shows what three power companies offered and how the money was actually spent. Unfortunately, utilities that spend only a fraction of voluntary energy premiums on renewable energy are becoming more rather than less common. It will likely be up to consumers or public service commissions to hold the utilities to a higher ethical standard—either by making power companies' advertising more truthful or, better still, by insisting that they deliver on their renewable energy promises. Either way, the idea of defrauding customers who are trying to "do the right thing" makes the utilities' unethical decision even more dishonorable.

Sources: Elgin, B. & Holden, D. 2008. Green power: Buyers beware. *BusinessWeek*, September 29: 68–70; and, *www.cleanenergy.org*.

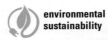 **environmental sustainability**

Exhibit 11.7 How "Green" Utilities Actually Used Customer Payments

Company/Program	What Customers Were Told	What Really Happened
Duke Energy of Indiana GoGreen Power	Pay a green energy premium and a specified amount of electricity will be obtained from renewable sources.	Less than 18 percent of voluntary customer contributions in a recent year went to renewable energy development.
Alliant Energy of Iowa Second Nature™	"Support the growth of earth-friendly 'green power' created by wind and biomass."	More than 56 percent of expenditures went to marketing and administrative costs, not green energy development.
Georgia Power Green Energy®	Paying the premium "is equivalent to planting 125 trees or not driving 2,000 miles" and will "help bring more renewable power to Georgia."	Customers pay an annual $54 premium, but green energy is actually cheaper to provide than electricity from conventional sources.

Sources: Elgin, B. & Holden, D. 2008. Green power: Buyers beware. *BusinessWeek*, September 29: 68–70; *www.alliantenergy.com; www.duke-energy.com;* and, *www.georgiapower.com*.

Brink Energy in Canada, who were all forced to resign and are facing (or have been convicted of) criminal charges. Perhaps the most glaring example is Bernie Madoff, whose Ponzi scheme, which unraveled in 2008, defrauded investors of $50 billion in assets they had set aside for retirement and charitable donations.

The ethical organization is characterized by a conception of ethical values and integrity as a driving force of the enterprise.[67] Ethical values shape the search for opportunities, the design of organizational systems, and the decision-making process used by individuals and groups. They provide a common frame of reference that serves as a unifying force across different functions, lines of business, and employee groups. **Organizational ethics** helps to define what a company is and what it stands for.

There are many potential benefits of an ethical organization, but they are often indirect. Research has found somewhat inconsistent results concerning the overall relationship between ethical performance and measures of financial performance.[68] However, positive relationships have generally been found between ethical performance and strong organizational culture, increased employee efforts, lower turnover, higher organizational commitment, and enhanced social responsibility.

The advantages of a strong ethical orientation can have a positive effect on employee commitment and motivation to excel. This is particularly important in today's knowledge-intensive organizations, where human capital is critical in creating value and competitive advantages. Positive, constructive relationships among individuals (i.e., social capital) are vital in leveraging human capital and other resources in an organization. Drawing on the concept of stakeholder management, an ethically sound organization can also strengthen its bonds among its suppliers, customers, and governmental agencies.

Integrity-Based versus Compliance-Based Approaches to Organizational Ethics

Before discussing the key elements of an ethical organization, one must understand the links between organizational integrity and the personal integrity of an organization's members.[69] There cannot be high-integrity organizations without high-integrity individuals. However, individual integrity is rarely self-sustaining. Even good people can lose their bearings when faced with pressures, temptations, and heightened performance expectations in the absence of organizational support systems and ethical boundaries. Organizational integrity rests on a concept of purpose, responsibility, and ideals for an organization as a whole. An important responsibility of leadership is to create this ethical framework and develop the organizational capabilities to make it operational.[70]

Lynn Paine, an ethics scholar at Harvard, identifies two approaches: the compliance-based approach and the integrity-based approach. (See Exhibit 11.8 for a comparison of compliance-based and integrity-based strategies.) Faced with the prospect of litigation, several organizations reactively implement **compliance-based ethics programs.** Such programs are typically designed by a corporate counsel with the goal of preventing, detecting, and punishing legal violations. But being ethical is much more than being legal, and an integrity-based approach addresses the issue of ethics in a more comprehensive manner.

Integrity-based ethics programs combine a concern for law with an emphasis on managerial responsibility for ethical behavior. It is broader, deeper, and more demanding than a legal compliance initiative. It is broader in that it seeks to enable responsible conduct. It is deeper in that it cuts to the ethos and operating systems of an organization and its members, their core guiding values, thoughts, and actions. It is more demanding because it requires an active effort to define the responsibilities that constitute an organization's ethical compass. Most importantly, organizational ethics is seen as the responsibility of management.

A corporate counsel may play a role in designing and implementing integrity strategies, but it is managers at all levels and across all functions that are involved in the process. Once

organizational ethics the values, attitudes, and behavioral patterns that define an organization's operating culture and that determine what an organization holds as acceptable behavior.

>LO11.6
The difference between integrity-based and compliance-based approaches to organizational ethics.

compliance-based ethics programs programs for building ethical organizations that have the goal of preventing, detecting, and punishing legal violations.

integrity-based ethics programs programs for building ethical organizations that combine a concern for law with an emphasis on managerial responsibility for ethical behavior, including (1) enabling ethical conduct; (2) examining the organization's and members' core guiding values, thoughts, and actions; and (3) defining the responsibilities and aspirations that constitute an organization's ethical compass.

Exhibit 11.8 Approaches to Ethics Management

Characteristics	Compliance-Based Approach	Integrity-Based Approach
Ethos	Conformity with externally imposed standards	Self-governance according to chosen standards
Objective	Prevent criminal misconduct	Enable responsible conduct
Leadership	Lawyer-driven	Management-driven with aid of lawyers, HR, and others
Methods	Education, reduced discretion, auditing and controls, penalties	Education, leadership, accountability, organizational systems and decision processes, auditing and controls, penalties
Behavioral Assumptions	Autonomous beings guided by material self-interest	Social beings guided by material self-interest, values, ideals, peers

Source: Reprinted by permission of *Harvard Business Review*. Exhibit from "Managing Organizational Integrity," by L. S. Paine. Copyright © 1994 by the Harvard Business School Publishing Corporation; all rights reserved.

integrated into the day-to-day operations, such strategies can prevent damaging ethical lapses, while tapping into powerful human impulses for moral thought and action. Ethics becomes the governing ethos of an organization and not burdensome constraints.

> KPMG is one of the world's largest professional services firms. In July 2010, KPMG launched a web-based training course called the Ethics Factor for all partners and employees around the world. Designed in a reality game-show format, the course allows the learner to play a judge who provides feedback to contestants trying to show how to do the right thing, in the right way, and have a positive impact on the company's ethical culture.
>
> Using two main themes—Stay Informed (know the rules and the risks) and Raise Your Hand (recognize and raise issues)—learners use their knowledge of relevant firm policies to judge whether contestants have that extra "something" demonstrating they not only know how to do the right thing in the right way but also how to set a stellar example for everyone around them in the organization.
>
> Within six weeks, more than 99 percent of the firm had completed the training, and the feedback was overall positive. The goal was to provide an interactive self-study lesson that reinforced firm policies and standards of behavior set forth in the Code of Conduct in a manner that was fun and informative, and most learners felt the course met that goal.[71]

Compliance-based approaches are externally motivated—that is, based on the fear of punishment for doing something unlawful. On the other hand, integrity-based approaches are driven by a personal and organizational commitment to ethical behavior.

A firm must have several key elements to become a highly ethical organization:

- Role models.
- Corporate credos and codes of conduct.
- Reward and evaluation systems.
- Policies and procedures.

>LO11.7
Several key elements that organizations must have to become an ethical organization.

These elements are highly interrelated. Reward structures and policies will be useless if leaders are not sound role models. That is, leaders who implicitly say, "Do as I say, not as I do," will quickly have their credibility eroded and such actions will sabotage other elements that are essential to building an ethical organization.

Role Models

For good or for bad, leaders are role models in their organizations. Leaders must "walk the talk"; they must be consistent in their words and deeds. The values as well as the character of leaders become transparent to an organization's employees through their behaviors. When leaders do not believe in the ethical standards that they are trying to inspire, they will not be effective as good role models. Being an effective leader often includes taking responsibility for ethical lapses within the organization—even though the executives themselves are not directly involved. Consider the perspective of Dennis Bakke, CEO of AES, the $14 billion global electricity company based in Arlington, Virginia.

> There was a major breach (in 1992) of the AES values. Nine members of the water treatment team in Oklahoma lied to the EPA about water quality at the plant. There was no environmental damage, but they lied about the test results. A new, young chemist at the plant discovered it, told a team leader, and we then were notified. Now, you could argue that the people who lied were responsible and were accountable, but the senior management team also took responsibility by taking pay cuts. My reduction was about 30 percent.[72]

Such action enhances the loyalty and commitment of employees throughout the organization. Many would believe that it would have been much easier (and personally less expensive!) for Bakke and his management team to merely take strong punitive action against the nine individuals who were acting contrary to the behavior expected in AES's ethical culture. However, by taking responsibility for the misdeeds, the top executives—through their highly visible action—made it clear that responsibility and penalties for ethical lapses go well beyond the "guilty" parties. Such courageous behavior by leaders helps to strengthen an organization's ethical environment.

Corporate Credos and Codes of Conduct

Corporate credos and codes of conduct are mechanisms that provide statements of norms and beliefs as well as guidelines for decision making. They provide employees with a clear understanding of the organization's policies and ethical position. Such guidelines also provide the basis for employees to refuse to commit unethical acts and help to make them aware of issues before they are faced with the situation. For such codes to be truly effective, organization members must be aware of them and what behavioral guidelines they contain.[73] Consider, for example, the Dutch retail chain HEMA. The company has stores in several European countries and buys products from around the globe. In June 2011, HEMA issued a code of conduct, which clearly specifies the code of conduct it expects not only from employees at all levels but from its global suppliers. Company departments may augment the code of conduct with additional guidelines or rules regarding the way in which the employees, suppliers, and other stakeholders should behave if they work for or do business with HEMA.[74] Strategy Spotlight 11.7 identifies four key reasons why codes of conduct support organizational efforts to maintain a safe and ethical workplace.

corporate credo a statement of the beliefs typically held by managers in a corporation.

Large corporations are not the only ones to develop and use codes of conduct. Consider the example of Wetherill Associates (WAI), a small, privately held supplier of electrical parts to the automotive market.

> Rather than a conventional code of conduct, WAI has a Quality Assurance Manual—a combination of philosophy text, conduct guide, technical manual, and company profile—that describes the company's commitment to honesty, ethical action, and integrity. WAI doesn't have a corporate ethics officer, because the company's corporate ethics officer is Marie Bothe, WAI's CEO. She sees her main function as keeping the 350-employee company on the path of ethical behavior and looking for opportunities to help the community. She delegates the "technical" aspects of the business—marketing, finance, personnel, and operations—to other members of the organization.[75]

Elements of a Corporate Code

Corporate codes are not simply useful for conveying organizational norms and policies, but they also serve to legitimize an organization in the eyes of others. In the United States, federal guidelines advise judges, when determining how to sentence a company convicted of a crime, to consider whether it had a written code and was out of compliance with its own ethical guidelines. The United Nations and countries around the world have endorsed codes as a way to promote corporate social responsibility. As such, a code provides an increasingly important corporate social contract that signals a company's willingness to act ethically.

For employees, codes of conduct serve four key purposes:

Sources: Paine, L., Deshpande, R., Margolis, J. D., & Bettcher, K. E. 2005. Up to code: Does your company's conduct meet world class standards? *Harvard Business Review*, 82(12): 122–126; and, Stone, A. 2004. Putting teeth in corporate ethics codes. *www.businessweek.com*. February 19.

1. Help employees from diverse backgrounds work more effectively across cultural backgrounds.

2. Provide a reference point for decision making.

3. Help attract individuals who want to work for a business that embraces high standards.

4. Help a company to manage risk by reducing the likelihood of damaging misconduct.

With recent scandals on Wall Street, many corporations are trying to put more teeth into their codes of conduct. NASDAQ now requires that listed companies distribute a code to all employees. German software giant SAP's code informs employees that violations of the code "can result in consequences that affect employment, and could possibly lead to external investigation, civil law proceedings, or criminal charges." Clearly, codes of conduct are an important part of maintaining an ethical organization.

Perhaps the best-known credo is that of Johnson & Johnson (J&J). It is reprinted in Exhibit 11.9. The credo stresses honesty, integrity, superior products, and putting people before profits. What distinguishes the J&J credo from others is the amount of energy the company's top managers devote to ensuring that employees live by its precepts:

> Over a recent three-year period, Johnson & Johnson undertook a massive effort to assure that its original credo, already decades old, was still valid. More than 1,200 managers attended two-day seminars in groups of 25, with explicit instructions to challenge the credo. The president or CEO of the firm presided over each session. The company came out of the process believing that its original document was still valid. However, the questioning process continues. Such "challenge meetings" are still replicated every other year for all new managers. These efforts force J&J to question, internalize, and then implement its credo. Such investments have paid off handsomely many times—most notably in 1982, when eight people died from swallowing capsules of Tylenol, one of its flagship products, that someone had laced with cyanide. Leaders such as James Burke, who without hesitation made an across-the-board recall of the product even though it affected only a limited number of untraceable units, send a strong message throughout the firm.

Reward and Evaluation Systems

It is entirely possible for a highly ethical leader to preside over an organization that commits several unethical acts. How? A flaw in the organization's reward structure may inadvertently cause individuals to act in an inappropriate manner if rewards are seen as being distributed on the basis of outcomes rather than the means by which goals and objectives are achieved.[76]

Consider the example of Sears, Roebuck & Co.'s automotive operations. Here, unethical behavior, rooted in a faulty reward system, took place primarily at the operations level: its automobile repair facilities.[77]

Exhibit 11.9
Johnson & Johnson's
Credo

We believe our first responsibility is to the doctors, nurses, and patients, to mothers and fathers and all others who use our products and services. In meeting their needs everything we do must be of high quality. We must constantly strive to reduce our costs in order to maintain reasonable prices. Customers' orders must be serviced promptly and accurately. Our suppliers and distributors must have an opportunity to make a fair profit.

We are responsible to our employees, the men and women who work with us throughout the world. Everyone must be considered as an individual. We must respect their dignity and recognize their merit. They must have a sense of security in their jobs. Compensation must be fair and adequate, and working conditions clean, orderly, and safe. We must be mindful of ways to help our employees fulfill their family responsibilities. Employees must feel free to make suggestions and complaints. There must be equal opportunity for employment, development, and advancement for those qualified. We must provide competent management, and their actions must be just and ethical.

We are responsible to the communities in which we live and work and to the world community as well. We must be good citizens—support good works and charities and bear our fair share of taxes. We must encourage civic improvements and better health and education. We must maintain in good order the property we are privileged to use, protecting the environment and natural resources

Our final responsibility is to our stockholders. Business must make a sound profit. We must experiment with new ideas. Research must be carried on, innovative programs developed, and mistakes paid for. New equipment must be purchased, new facilities provided, and new products launched. Reserves must be created to provide for adverse times. When we operate according to these principles, the stockholders should realize a fair return.

Source: Reprinted with permission of Johnson & Johnson Co.

In 1992 Sears was flooded with complaints about its automotive service business. Consumers and attorneys general in more than 40 states accused the firm of misleading customers and selling them unnecessary parts and services, from brake jobs to front-end alignments.

In the face of declining revenues and eroding market share, Sears's management had attempted to spur the performance of its auto centers by introducing new goals and incentives for mechanics. Automotive service advisers were given product-specific quotas for a variety of parts and repairs. Failure to meet the quotas could lead to transfers and reduced hours. Many employees spoke of "pressure, pressure, pressure" to bring in sales.

Not too surprisingly, the judgment of many employees suffered. In essence, employees were left to chart their own course, given the lack of management guidance and customer ignorance. The bottom line: In settling the spate of lawsuits, Sears offered coupons to customers who had purchased certain auto services over the most recent two-year period. The total cost of the settlement, including potential customer refunds, was estimated to be $60 million. The cost in terms of damaged reputation? Difficult to assess, but certainly not trivial.

This example makes two points. First, inappropriate reward systems may cause individuals at all levels throughout an organization to commit unethical acts that they might not otherwise commit. Second, the penalties in terms of damage to reputations, human capital erosion, and financial loss—in the short run and long run—are typically much higher than any gains that could be obtained through such unethical behavior.

Many companies have developed reward and evaluation systems that evaluate whether a manager is acting in an ethical manner. For example, Raytheon, a $20 billion defense contractor, incorporates the following items in its "Leadership Assessment Instrument":[78]

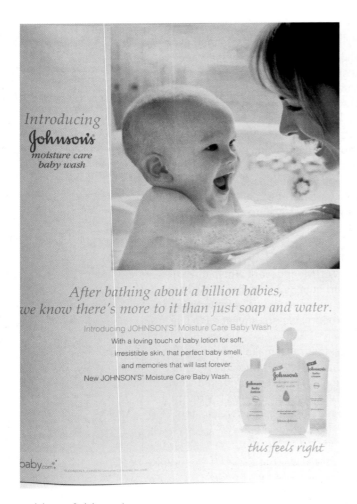

● Johnson & Johnson is well-known for its credo, which stresses honesty, integrity, superior products, and putting people before profits.

- Maintains unequivocal commitment to honesty, truth, and ethics in every facet of behavior.
- Conforms with the letter and intent of company policies while working to affect any necessary policy changes.
- Actions are consistent with words; follows through on commitments; readily admits mistakes.
- Is trusted and inspires others to be trusted.

As noted by Dan Burnham, Raytheon's former CEO: "What do we look for in a leadership candidate with respect to integrity? What we're really looking for are people who have developed an inner gyroscope of ethical principles. We look for people for whom ethical thinking is part of what they do—no different from 'strategic thinking' or 'tactical thinking.'"

Policies and Procedures

Many situations that a firm faces have regular, identifiable patterns. Leaders tend to handle such routine by establishing a policy or procedure to be followed that can be applied uniformly to each occurrence. Such guidelines can be useful in specifying the proper relationships with a firm's customers and suppliers. For example, Levi Strauss has developed stringent global sourcing guidelines and Chemical Bank (part of J.P. Morgan Chase Bank) has a policy of forbidding any review that would determine if suppliers are Chemical customers when the bank awards contracts.

Carefully developed policies and procedures guide behavior so that all employees will be encouraged to behave in an ethical manner. However, they must be reinforced with effective communication, enforcement, and monitoring, as well as sound corporate governance practices. In addition, corporate governance reforms such as the Sarbanes-Oxley Act of 2002 in the United States and the revised Combined Code on Corporate Governance of 2010 in the UK provide considerable legal protection to employees of publicly traded companies who report unethical or illegal practices. Provisions in the Sarbanes-Oxley Act include:[79]

- Make it unlawful to "discharge, demote, suspend, threaten, harass, or in any manner discriminate against 'a whistle-blower.'"
- Establish criminal penalties of up to 10 years in jail for executives who retaliate against whistle-blowers.
- Require board audit committees to establish procedures for hearing whistle-blower complaints.
- Allow the Secretary of Labor to order a company to rehire a terminated whistle-blower with no court hearings whatsoever.
- Give a whistle-blower the right to a jury trial, bypassing months or years of cumbersome administrative hearings.

Reflecting on Career Implications . . .

- *Strategic Leadership:* Do managers in your firm effectively set the direction, design the organization, and instill a culture committed to excellence and ethical behavior? If you are in a position of leadership, do you practice all of these three elements effectively?
- *Power:* What sources of power do managers in your organization use? For example, if there is an overemphasis on organizational sources of power (e.g., position power), there could be negative implications for creativity, morale, and turnover among professionals. How much power do you have? What is the basis of it? How might it be used to both advance your career goals and benefit the firm?
- *Emotional Intelligence:* Do leaders of your firm have sufficient levels of EI? Alternatively, are there excessive levels of EI present that have negative implications for your organization? Is your level of EI sufficient to allow you to have effective interpersonal and judgment skills in order to enhance your career success?
- *Learning Organization:* Does your firm effectively practice all five elements of the learning organization? If one or more elements are absent, adaptability and change will be compromised. What can you do to enhance any of the elements that might be lacking?
- *Ethics:* Does your organization practice a compliance-based or integrity-based ethical culture? Integrity-based cultures can enhance your personal growth. In addition, such cultures foster greater loyalty and commitment among all employees.

Summary

Strategic leadership is vital in ensuring that strategies are formulated and implemented in an effective manner. Leaders must play a central role in performing three critical and interdependent activities: setting the direction, designing the organization, and nurturing a culture committed to excellence and ethical behavior. If leaders ignore or are ineffective at performing any one of the three, the organization will not be very successful. We also identified three elements of leadership that contribute to success—integrative thinking, overcoming barriers to change, and the effective use of power.

For leaders to effectively fulfill their activities, emotional intelligence (EI) is very important. Five elements that contribute to EI are self-awareness, self-regulation, motivation, empathy, and social skill. The first three elements pertain to self-management skills, whereas the last two are associated with a person's ability to manage relationships with others. We also addressed some of the potential drawbacks from the ineffective use of EI. These include the dysfunctional use of power as well as a tendency to become overly empathetic, which may result in unreasonably lowered performance expectations.

Leaders must also play a central role in creating a learning organization. Gone are the days when the top-level managers "think" and everyone else in the organization "does." With the rapidly changing, unpredictable, and complex competitive environments that characterize most industries, leaders must engage everyone in the ideas and energies of people throughout the organization. Great ideas can come from anywhere in the organization—from the executive suite to the factory floor. The five elements that we discussed as central to a learning organization are inspiring and motivating people with a mission or purpose, empowering people at all levels throughout the organization, accumulating and sharing internal knowledge, gathering external information, and challenging the status quo to stimulate creativity.

In the final section of the chapter, we addressed a leader's central role in instilling ethical behavior in the organization. We discussed the enormous costs that firms face when ethical crises arise—costs in terms of financial and reputational loss as well as the erosion of human capital and relationships with suppliers, customers, society at large, and governmental agencies. And, as we would expect, the benefits of having a strong ethical organization are also numerous. We contrasted compliance-based and integrity-based approaches to organizational ethics. Compliance-based approaches are largely externally motivated; that is, they are motivated by the fear of punishment for doing something that is unlawful. Integrity-based approaches, on the other hand, are driven by a personal and organizational commitment to ethical behavior. We also addressed the four key elements of an ethical organization: role models, corporate credos and codes of conduct, reward and evaluation systems, and policies and procedures.

Summary Review Questions

1. Three key activities—setting a direction, designing the organization, and nurturing a culture and ethics—are all part of what effective leaders do on a regular basis. Explain how these three activities are interrelated.

2. Define emotional intelligence (EI). What are the key elements of EI? Why is EI so important to successful strategic leadership? Address potential "downsides."

3. The knowledge a firm possesses can be a source of competitive advantage. Describe ways that a firm can continuously learn to maintain its competitive position.

4. How can the five central elements of "learning organizations" be incorporated into global companies?

5. What are the benefits to firms and their shareholders of conducting business in an ethical manner?

6. Firms that fail to behave in an ethical manner can incur high costs. What are these costs and what is their source?

7. What are the most important differences between an "integrity organization" and a "compliance organization" in a firm's approach to organizational ethics?

8. What are some of the important mechanisms for promoting ethics in a firm?

Key Terms

leadership, 437
setting a direction, 439
designing the
  organization, 440
excellent and ethical
  organizational
  culture, 440
integrative thinking, 443
barriers to change, 444
vested interests in
  the status quo, 444
systemic barriers, 444
behavioral barriers, 445
political barriers, 446
personal time
  constraints, 446
power, 446
organizational bases of
  power, 446
personal bases of
  power, 446

emotional intelligence
  (EI), 449
learning
  organizations, 453
benchmarking, 456
competitive
  benchmarking, 456
functional
  benchmarking, 456
ethics, 459
ethical
  orientation, 459
organizational
  ethics, 461
compliance-based
  ethics programs, 461
integrity-based
  ethics programs, 461
corporate credo, 463

Experiential Exercise

Select two well-known business leaders—one you admire and one you do not. Evaluate each of them on the five characteristics of emotional intelligence listed below.

Emotional Intelligence Characteristics	Admired Leader	Leader Not Admired
Self-awareness		
Self-regulation		
Motivation		
Empathy		
Social skills		

Application Questions & Exercises

1. Identify two CEOs of global organizations whose leadership you admire. What is it about their skills, attributes, and effective use of power that causes you to admire them?

2. Founders have an important role in developing their organization's culture and values. At times, their influence persists for many years. Identify and describe two global organizations in which the cultures and values established by the founder(s) continue to flourish. You may find research on the Internet helpful in answering these questions.

3. Some leaders place a great emphasis on developing superior human capital. In what ways does this help a firm to develop and sustain competitive advantages?

4. In this chapter we discussed the five elements of a "learning organization." Select a firm with which you are familiar and discuss whether or not it epitomizes some (or all) of these elements.

Ethics Questions

1. Sometimes organizations must go outside the firm to hire talent, thus bypassing employees already working for the firm. Are there conditions under which this might raise ethical considerations?

2. Ethical crises can occur in virtually any organization. Describe some of the systems, procedures, and processes that can help to prevent such crises.

References

1. Smith, R. 2010. Another Duke exit amid inquiry. *The Wall Street Journal,* December 7: B3; Smith R. 2010. Corporate news: Indiana panel finds Duke wasn't favored. *The Wall Street Journal,* December 9: B4; O'Malley, C. 2010. Scandal rocks IURC, Duke. *Indianapolis Business Journal,* December 27: 13A; Jenkins, H. W. 2010. A fine clean coal mess. *The Wall Street Journal,* December 15: A19; Anonymous. 2010. Top Duke executive who resigned after ethics flap gets $10 million severance retirement deal. *Associated Press Newswires,* December 10, 11: 11; and, Henderson, B. 2010. Duke Energy executive resigns over e-mails. *The Herald,* December 7: 11. We thank Ciprian Stan for his valued contribution.

2. Charan, R. & Colvin, G. 1999. Why CEOs fail. *Fortune,* June 21: 68–78.

3. Yukl, G. 2008. How leaders influence organizational effectiveness. *Leadership Quarterly,* 19(6): 708–722.

4. These three activities and our discussion draw from: Kotter, J. P. 1990. What leaders really do. *Harvard Business Review,* 68(3): 103–111; Pearson, A. E. 1990. Six basics for general managers. *Harvard Business Review,* 67(4): 94–101; and, Covey, S. R. 1996. Three roles of the leader in the new paradigm. In Hesselbein,

F., Goldsmith, M., & Beckhard, R. (Eds.). *The leader of the future:* 149–160. San Francisco: Jossey-Bass. Some of the discussion of each of the three leadership activity concepts draws on: Dess, G. G. & Miller, A. 1993. *Strategic management:* 320–325. New York: McGraw-Hill.

5. García-Morales, V. J., Lloréns-Montes, F. J., & Verdú-Jover, A. J. 2008. The effects of transformational leadership on organizational performance through knowledge and innovation. *British Journal of Management,* 19(4): 299–319.

6. Day, C., Jr. & LaBarre, P. 1994. GE: Just your average everyday $60 billion family grocery store. *Industry Week,* May 2: 13–18.

7. Martin, R. 2010. The execution trap. *Harvard Business Review,* 88(7/8): 64–71.

8. Collins, J. 1997. What comes next? *Inc. Magazine.* October: 34–45.

9. Hsieh, T. 2010. Zappos's CEO on going to extremes for customers. *Harvard Business Review,* 88(7/8): 41–44.

10. Andersen, M. M., Froholdt, M., & Poulfelt, F. 2010. *Return on strategy.* New York: Routledge; and, 2009 Huawei Annual Report.

11. Anonymous. 2006. Looking out for number one. *BusinessWeek,* October 30: 66.

12. This section draws on: Chen, M.-J. & Miller, D. 2010. West meets East: Toward an ambicultural approach to management. *Academy of Management Perspectives,* 24(4): 17–24.

13. For an interesting, in-depth interview with Stan Shih, read: Lin, H.-C. & Hou, S. T. 2010. Managerial lessons from the East: An interview with Acer's Stan Shih. *Academy of Management Perspectives,* 24(4): 6–16.

14. Evans, R. 2007. The either/or dilemma. *www.ft.com,* December 19; and, Martin, R. L. 2007. *The opposable mind.* Boston: Harvard Business School Press.

15. Schaffer, R. H. 2010. Mistakes leaders keep making. *Harvard Business Review,* 88(9): 86–91.

16. For insightful perspectives on escalation, refer to: Brockner, J. 1992. The escalation of commitment to a failing course of action. *Academy of Management Review,* 17(1): 39–61; and, Staw, B. M. 1976. Knee-deep in the big muddy: A study of commitment to a chosen course of action. *Organizational Behavior and Human Decision Processes,* 16: 27–44. The discussion of systemic, behavioral, and political barriers draws on: Lorange, P. & Murphy, D. 1984. Considerations in implementing strategic control. *Journal of Business Strategy,* 5: 27–35. In a similar vein, Noel M.

Tichy has addressed three types of resistance to change in the context of General Electric: technical resistance, political resistance, and cultural resistance. See Tichy, N. M. 1993. Revolutionalize your company. *Fortune,* December 13: 114–118. Examples draw from: O'Reilly, B. 1997. The secrets of America's most admired corporations: New ideas and new products. *Fortune,* March 3: 60–64.

17. This section draws on: Champoux, J. E. 2000. *Organizational behavior: Essential tenets for a new millennium.* London: South-Western; and, The mature use of power in organizations. 2003. *RHR International-Executive Insights,* May 29, *12.19.168.197/ execinsights/8-3.htm.*

18. An insightful perspective on the role of power and politics in organizations is provided in: Ciampa, K. 2005. Almost ready: How leaders move up. *Harvard Business Review,* 83(1): 46–53.

19. Pfeffer, J. 2010. Power play. *Harvard Business Review,* 88(7/8): 84–92.

20. Westphal, J. D., & Graebner, M. E. 2010. A matter of appearances: How corporate leaders manage the impressions of financial analysts about the conduct of their boards. *Academy of Management Journal,* 53(4): 15–44.

21. A discussion of the importance of persuasion in bringing about change can be found in: Garvin, D. A. & Roberto, M. A. 2005. Change through persuasion. *Harvard Business Review,* 83(4): 104–113.

22. Lorsch, J. W. & Tierney, T. J. 2002. *Aligning the stars: How to succeed when professionals drive results.* Boston: Harvard Business School Press.

23. Some consider EI to be a "trait," that is, an attribute that is stable over time. However, many authors, including Daniel Goleman, have argued that it can be developed through motivation, extended practice, and feedback. For example, in Goleman. D. 1998. What makes a leader? *Harvard Business Review,* 76(5): 97, Goleman addresses this issue in a sidebar: "Can emotional intelligence be learned?"

24. For a review of this literature, see: Daft, R. 1999. *Leadership: Theory and practice.* Fort Worth, TX: Dryden Press.

25. This section draws on: Luthans, F. 2002. Positive organizational behavior: Developing and managing psychological strengths. *Academy of Management Executive,* 16(1): 57–72; and, Goleman, D. 1998. What makes a leader? *Harvard Business Review,* 76(6): 92–105.

26. EI has its roots in the concept of "social intelligence" that was first identified by E. L. Thorndike in 1920 (Intelligence and its uses. *Harper's Magazine,* 140: 227–235). Psychologists have been uncovering other intelligences for some time now and have grouped them into such clusters as abstract intelligence (the ability to understand and manipulate verbal and mathematical symbols), concrete intelligence (the ability to understand and manipulate objects), and social intelligence (the ability to understand and relate to people). See Ruisel, I. 1992. Social intelligence: Conception and methodological problems. *Studia Psychologica,* 34(4–5): 281–296. Refer to *trochim.human.cornell.edu/gallery.*

27. See, for example, Luthans, op. cit.; Mayer, J. D., Salvoney, P., & Caruso, D. 2000. Models of emotional intelligence. In Sternberg, R. J. (Ed.). *Handbook of intelligence.* Cambridge, UK: Cambridge University Press; and, Cameron, K. 1999. Developing emotional intelligence at the Weatherhead School of Management. *Strategy: The Magazine of the Weatherhead School of Management,* Winter: 2–3.

28. Tate, B. 2008. A longitudinal study of the relationships among self-monitoring, authentic leadership, and perceptions of leadership. *Journal of Leadership & Organizational Studies,* 15(1): 16–29.

29. Moss, S. A., Dowling, N., & Callanan, J. 2009. Towards an integrated model of leadership and self-regulation. *Leadership Quarterly,* 20(2): 162–176.

30. An insightful perspective on leadership, which involves discovering, developing and celebrating what is unique about each individual, is found in: Buckingham, M. 2005. What great managers do. *Harvard Business Review,* 83(3): 70–79.

31. Lewis, N. 2010. Interview with Bert Pijls, CEO of Egg Banking. September 4. *http://vimeo.com/14703400;* and, Reuters. 2011. Yorkshire Building Society to buy Egg. *www .telegraph.co.uk/finance/newsbysector/ banksandfinance/8659091/Yorkshire-Building-Society-to-buy-Egg.html.*

32. This section draws upon: Klemp, G. 2005. *Emotional intelligence and leadership: What really matters.* Cambria Consulting, Inc. *www .cambriaconsulting.com.*

33. Heifetz, R. 2004. Question authority. *Harvard Business Review,* 82(1): 37.

34. Handy, C. 1995. Trust and the virtual organization. *Harvard Business Review,* 73(3): 40–50.

35. This section draws upon: Dess, G. G. & Picken, J. C. 1999. *Beyond productivity.* New York: AMACOM. The elements of the learning organization in this section are consistent with the work of Dorothy Leonard-Barton. See, for example, Leonard-Barton, D. 1992. The factory as a learning laboratory. *Sloan Management Review,* 11: 23–38.

36. Senge, P. M. 1990. The leader's new work: Building learning organizations. *Sloan Management Review,* 32(1): 7–23.

37. Bernoff, J. & Schandler, T. 2010. Empowered. *Harvard Business Review,* 88(7/8): 94–101.

38. Hammer, M. & Stanton, S. A. 1997. The power of reflection. *Fortune,* November 24: 291–296.

39. Hannah, S. T. & Lester, P. B. 2009. A multilevel approach to building and leading learning organizations. *Leadership Quarterly,* 20(1): 34–48.

40. For some guidance on how to effectively bring about change in organizations, refer to: Wall, S. J. 2005. The protean organization: Learning to love change. *Organizational Dynamics,* 34(1): 37–46.

41. Covey, S. R. 1989. *The seven habits of highly effective people: Powerful lessons in personal change.* New York: Simon & Schuster.

42. Kouzes, J. M. & Posner, B. Z. 2009. To lead, create a shared vision. *Harvard Business Review,* 87(1): 20–21.

43. Kouzes and Posner, op. cit.

44. Melrose, K. 1995. *Making the grass greener on your side: A CEO's*

journey to leading by servicing. San Francisco: Barrett-Koehler.

45. Tekleab, A. G., Sims Jr., H. P., Yun, S., Tesluk, P. E., & Cox, J. 2008. Are we on the same page? Effects of self-awareness of empowering and transformational leadership. *Journal of Leadership & Organizational Studies,* 14(3): 185–201.

46. Quinn, R. C. & Spreitzer, G. M. 1997. The road to empowerment: Seven questions every leader should consider. *Organizational Dynamics,* 25: 37–49.

47. For an interesting perspective on top-down approaches to leadership, see: Pellegrini, E. K. & Scandura, T. A. 2008. Paternalistic leadership: A review and agenda for future research. *Journal of Management,* 34(3): 566–593.

48. Helgesen, S. 1996. Leading from the grass roots. In Hesselbein et al., op. cit.: 19–24.

49. Bowen, D. E. & Lawler, E. E., III. 1995. Empowering service employees. *Sloan Management Review,* 37: 73–84.

50. Easterby-Smith, M. & Prieto, I. M. 2008. Dynamic capabilities and knowledge management: An integrative role for learning? *British Journal of Management,* 19(3): 235–249.

51. Schafer, S. 1997. Battling a labor shortage? It's all in your imagination. *Inc.,* August: 24.

52. Meyer, P. 1998. So you want the president's job . . . *Business Horizons,* January–February: 2–8.

53. Imperato, G. 1998. Competitive intelligence: Get smart! *Fast Company,* May: 268–279.

54. Novicki, C. 1998. The best brains in business. *Fast Company,* April: 125.

55. The introductory discussion of benchmarking draws on: Miller, A. 1998. *Strategic management:* 142–143. New York: McGraw-Hill.

56. Port, O. & Smith, G. 1992. Beg, borrow—and benchmark. *Business-Week,* November 30: 74–75.

57. Patterson, J. G. 1995. Benchmarking basics: Looking for a better way.

Mississauga, Ontario, Canada: Crisp Learning.

58. Main, J. 1992. How to steal the best ideas around. *Fortune,* October 19: 102–106.

59. Taylor, J. T. 1997. What happens after what comes next? *Fast Company,* December–January: 84–85.

60. Charter UK corporate website. 2011. Customer service more important than ever, says Charter UK CEO. June 30. *www.charter-uk.com/customer-service-important.php.*

61. Isaacson, W. 1997. In search of the real Bill Gates. *Time,* January 13: 44–57.

62. Baatz, E. B. 1993. Motorola's secret weapon. *Electronic Business,* April: 51–53.

63. Holt, J. W. 1996. *Celebrate your mistakes.* New York: McGraw-Hill.

64. This opening discussion draws upon: Conley, J. H. 2000. Ethics in business. In Helms, M. M. (Ed.). *Encyclopedia of management* (4th ed.): 281–285. Farmington Hills, MI: Gale Group; Paine, L. S. 1994. Managing for organizational integrity. *Harvard Business Review,* 72(2): 106–117; and, Carlson, D. S. & Perrewe, P. L. 1995. Institutionalization of organizational ethics through transformational leadership. *Journal of Business Ethics,* 14: 829–838.

65. Pinto, J., Leana, C. R., & Pil, F. K. 2008. Corrupt organizations or organizations of corrupt individuals? Two types of organization-level corruption. *Academy of Management Review,* 33(3): 685–709.

66. Bell, L. 2011. Lessons from lemmings: The EU's green power folly. October 4. *www.forbes.com;* and, CEPOS (Center for Politiske Studier). 2009. Wind energy: The case of Denmark. *www.scribd.com/doc/24197996/Wind-Energy-The-Case-of-Denmark.*

67. Soule, E. 2002. Managerial moral strategies—in search of a few good principles. *Academy of Management Review,* 27(1): 114–124.

68. Carlson & Perrewe, op. cit.

69. This discussion is based upon: Paine, 1994, op. cit.; Paine, L. S. 1997. *Cases in leadership, ethics, and organizational integrity: A strategic approach.* Burr Ridge, IL: Irwin; and, Fontrodona, J. 2002. Business ethics across the Atlantic. Business Ethics Direct, *www.ethicsa.org/BED_art_fontrodone.html.*

70. For more on operationalizing capabilities to sustain an ethical framework, see: Largay III, J. A. & Zhang, R. 2008. Do CEOs worry about being fired when making investment decisions? *Academy of Management Perspectives,* 22(1): 60–61.

71. KPMG: The 2010 ethics and compliance report 2011. *www.kpmg.com/us/en/issuesandinsights/articlespublications/pages/ethics-and-compliance-report-2010.aspx.*

72. Wetlaufer, S. 1999. Organizing for empowerment: An interview with AES's Roger Sant and Dennis Bakke. *Harvard Business Review,* 77(1): 110–126.

73. For an insightful, academic perspective on the impact of ethics codes on executive decision making, refer to: Stevens, J. M., Steensma, H. K., Harrison, D. A., & Cochran, P. S. 2005. Symbolic or substantive document? The influence of ethics code on financial executives' decisions. *Strategic Management Journal,* 26(2): 181–195.

74. HEMA Code of Conduct. 2011. *www.hema.nl/SiteCollectionDocuments/OndernemingscodeEngelsejuni2011.pdf.*

75. Paine, 1994, op. cit.

76. For a recent study on the effects of goal setting on unethical behavior, read: Schweitzer, M. E., Ordonez, L., & Douma, B. 2004. Goal setting as a motivator of unethical behavior. *Academy of Management Journal,* 47(3): 422–432.

77. Paine, 1994, op. cit.

78. Fulmer, R. M. 2004. The challenge of ethical leadership. *Organizational Dynamics,* 33 (3): 307–317.

79. *www.sarbanes-oxley.com.*

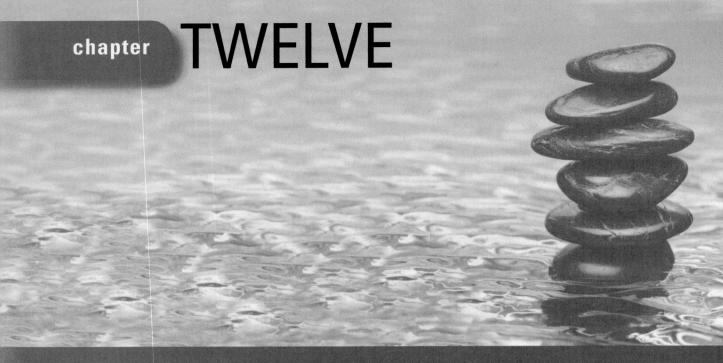

chapter TWELVE

Managing Innovation and Fostering Corporate Entrepreneurship

After reading this chapter, you should have a good understanding of:

LO12.1 The importance of implementing strategies and practices that foster innovation.

LO12.2 The challenges and pitfalls of managing corporate innovation processes.

LO12.3 How corporations use new venture teams, business incubators, and product champions to create an internal environment and culture that promote entrepreneurial development.

LO12.4 How corporate entrepreneurship achieves both financial goals and strategic goals.

LO12.5 The benefits and potential drawbacks of real options analysis in making resource deployment decisions in corporate entrepreneurship contexts.

LO12.6 How an entrepreneurial orientation can enhance a firm's efforts to develop promising corporate venture initiatives.

LEARNING OBJECTIVES

To remain competitive, established firms must continually seek out opportunities for growth and new methods for strategically renewing their performance. Changes in customer needs, new technologies, and shifts in the competitive landscape require that companies continually innovate and initiate corporate ventures in order to compete effectively. This chapter addresses how entrepreneurial activities can be an avenue for achieving competitive advantages.

In the first section, we address the importance of innovation in identifying venture opportunities and strategic renewal. Innovations can take many forms, including radical breakthroughs, incremental improvements, and disruptive innovations. Innovations often create new markets, update products or services, and help renew organizational processes. We discuss how firms can successfully manage the innovation process. Impediments and challenges to effective innovation are discussed, and examples of good innovation practices are presented.

We discuss the unique role of corporate entrepreneurship in the strategic management process in the second section. Here we highlight two types of activities corporations use to remain competitive—focused and dispersed. New venture groups and business incubators are often used to focus a firm's entrepreneurial activities. In other corporations, the entrepreneurial spirit is dispersed throughout the organization and gives rise to product champions and other autonomous strategic behaviors that organizational members engage in to foster internal corporate venturing. We also discuss the benefits and potential drawbacks of real options analysis in making decisions about which venture activities merit additional investment and which should be abandoned.

In the final section we describe how a firm's entrepreneurial orientation can contribute to its growth and renewal as well as enhance the methods and processes strategic managers use to recognize opportunities and develop initiatives for internal growth and development. The chapter also evaluates the pitfalls that firms may encounter when implementing entrepreneurial strategies. ●

Learning from Mistakes

In April 2006, *Bloomberg Businessweek* described HTC as "the hottest tech outfit you never heard of," but oh how the times have changed.[1]

Founded in 1997 as a contract manufacturer, the company has long been the world's top maker of mobile handsets using Microsoft's Windows Mobile operating system. HTC has several strategic partnerships, including partners such as Intel, Texas Instruments, and Qualcomm. HTC is known for its innovation and is consistently highly ranked by insiders and consumers alike. It is constantly broadening the range of devices it offers—introducing devices to support specific applications that meet the increasingly diverse needs of its customers and partners. Currently *Bloomberg Businessweek* lists HTC as number 47 of the Most Innovative Companies. HTC Chief Executive Peter Chou said, "Innovation is not a one-time job—innovation is a journey. . . . Hardware innovation is less than half the battle," when it comes to the handheld market.

Let's take a look at what happens when corporate entrepreneurship fails to add value through innovation.

> HTC paired its proprietary intuitive user interface, Sense, with Windows Mobile version 6.5, Microsoft's mobile operating system, to create the HD2 Smartphone available through T-Mobile. It features a luxurious 4.3-inch touch screen, Qualcomm Snapdragon processor (the same one that powers Google's Nexus One), 5-megapixel camera with flash, and all in sleek design that fits in a shirt pocket! Just one catch, Microsoft's operating system is soon to be obsolete, and its new Windows Mobile 7 is not backward compatible. Bottom line: Consumers are spending $199 on two-year contracts with T-Mobile to have a phone that won't work! What went wrong?
>
> Although Microsoft was one of the first to recognize the power of handhelds, it struggled to look past its ideas of a handheld computer to a more intuitive smartphone. This allowed Microsoft to slip in the market as it attempted to perfect its software. Microsoft—as first mover—was the market leader. However, Blackberry followed and took over the corporate market, while Apple's iPhone ruled the consumer market. In three months, Microsoft smartphone subscribers slipped down to 15.7 percent of the smartphone market by January 2010, according to comScore. HTC has a long history of pairing with Microsoft to innovate in the handheld market. Unfortunately, this partnership of corporate entrepreneurs could not overcome the poor mix of Microsoft's baffling software with HTC's elegant hardware. All of this reinforces the fact that, according to *Bloomberg Businessweek,* "even innovative companies can be hobbled by suppliers peddling out-of-date technology."

>LO12.1

The importance of implementing strategies and practices that foster innovation.

Managing change is one of the most important functions performed by strategic leaders. There are two major avenues through which companies can expand or improve their business—innovation and corporate entrepreneurship. These two activities go hand-in-hand because they both have similar aims. The first is strategic renewal. Innovations help an organization stay fresh and reinvent itself as conditions in the business environment change. This is why managing innovation is such an important strategic implementation issue. The second is the pursuit of venture opportunities. Innovative breakthroughs, as well as new product concepts, evolving technologies, and shifting demand, create opportunities for corporate venturing. In this chapter we will explore these topics—how change and innovation can stimulate strategic renewal and foster corporate entrepreneurship.

Managing Innovation

One of the most important sources of growth opportunities is innovation. **Innovation** involves using new knowledge to transform organizational processes or create commercially viable products and services. The sources of new knowledge may include the latest technology, the results of experiments, creative insights, or competitive information. However it comes about, innovation occurs when new combinations of ideas and information bring about positive change.

The emphasis on newness is a key point. For example, for a patent application to have any chance of success, one of the most important attributes it must possess is novelty. You can't patent an idea that has been copied. This is a central idea. In fact, the root of the word *innovation* is the Latin *novus,* which means new. Innovation involves introducing or changing to something new.[2]

Among the most important sources of new ideas is new technology. Technology creates new possibilities. Technology provides the raw material that firms use to make innovative products and services. But technology is not the only source of innovations. There can be innovations in human resources, firm infrastructure, marketing, service, or in many other value-adding areas that have little to do with anything "high-tech." Strategy Spotlight 12.1 highlights a simple but effective innovation by James Dyson. As the Dyson Air Multiplier example suggests, innovation can take many forms.

> **innovation** the use of new knowledge to transform organizational processes or create commercially viable products and services.

Types of Innovation

Although innovations are not always high-tech, changes in technology can be an important source of change and growth. When an innovation is based on a sweeping new technology, it often has a more far-reaching impact. Sometimes even a small innovation can add value and create competitive advantages. Innovation can and should occur throughout an organization—in every department and all aspects of the value chain.

One distinction that is often used when discussing innovation is between process innovation and product innovation.[3] **Product innovation** refers to efforts to create product designs and applications of technology to develop new products for end users. Recall from Chapter 5 how generic strategies were typically different depending on the stage of the industry life cycle. Product innovations tend to be more common during the earlier stages of an industry's life cycle. Product innovations are also commonly associated with a differentiation strategy. Firms that differentiate by providing customers with new products or services that offer unique features or quality enhancements often engage in product innovation.

Process innovation, by contrast, is typically associated with improving the efficiency of an organizational process, especially manufacturing systems and operations. By drawing on new technologies and an organization's accumulated experience (Chapter 5), firms can often improve materials utilization, shorten cycle time, and increase quality. Process innovations are more likely to occur in the later stages of an industry's life cycle as companies seek ways to remain viable in markets where demand has flattened out and competition is more intense. As a result, process innovations are often associated with overall cost leader strategies, because the aim of many process improvements is to lower the costs of operations.

Another way to view the impact of an innovation is in terms of its degree of innovativeness, which falls somewhere on a continuum that extends from incremental to radical.[4]

> **product innovation** efforts to create product designs and applications of technology to develop new products for end users.

> **process innovation** efforts to improve the efficiency of organizational processes, especially manufacturing systems and operations.

- **Radical innovations** produce fundamental changes by evoking major departures from existing practices. These breakthrough innovations usually occur because of technological change. They tend to be highly disruptive and can transform a company or even revolutionize a whole industry. They may lead to products or processes that can be patented, giving a firm a strong competitive advantage. Examples include

> **radical innovation** an innovation that fundamentally changes existing practices.

Dyson's Simple Innovation

People around the world are accustomed to fans that consist of a motor and blades, which, through their circular motion and shapes, suck up air from behind them and push it forward. But British inventor James Dyson created a new, groundbreaking type of fan, which has no blades. It sports a very simple, circular design, with nothing in the middle. However, it can push a massive amount of air forward every second and ensures a smooth airflow within the room, *LiveScience* reported. It's one of the latest innovations from Dyson and is called the Air Multiplier.

Sources: Good Housekeeping Research Institute. 2011. Third Annual VIP (Very Innovative Products) Awards: Dyson Air Multiplier. *www.goodhousekeeping.com/product-reviews/innovative-products-awards-2011#slide-2;* Red Dot Award: Product Design, Best of the Best. 2010. *en.reddot.org/2775.html?&cHash=3fcf27cd82ca6ad36490dc5c67719268&detail=7583&year=1;* and, Vieru, T. 2009. New, bladeless fan uses "Air Multiplier" technology. *http://news.softpedia.com. October 14.*

Since the first fan appeared more than 200 years ago, few changes have been made to its base design because people thought the device could not be improved. But Dyson thought differently and invented the Air Multiplier technology, which allows the bladeless fan to push as much as 119 gallons of air every second. Manufactured in Malaysia, the fan is a massive improvement when compared with 19th-century Middle Eastern fans, which were powered by streaming water and a system of belts.

As a result of his innovative thinking, Dyson has achieved much success with his new invention and the fan has won several international awards, including the Red Dot: Best of the Best 2010, which is one of the leading and largest international design competitions in the world; a 2010 Australian International Design Award; and a 2011 Third Annual VIP (Very Innovative Product) Award by the Good Housekeeping Research Institute, which commemorates the most innovative products from the past decade.

electricity, the telephone, the transistor, desktop computers, fiber optics, artificial intelligence, and genetically engineered drugs.

incremental innovation an innovation that enhances existing practices or makes small improvements in products and processes.

- **Incremental innovations** enhance existing practices or make small improvements in products and processes. They may represent evolutionary applications within existing paradigms of earlier, more radical innovations. Because they often sustain a company by extending or expanding its product line or manufacturing skills, incremental innovations can be a source of competitive advantage by providing new capabilities that minimize expenses or speed productivity. Examples include frozen food, sports drinks, steel-belted radial tires, electronic bookkeeping, shatterproof glass, and digital telephones.

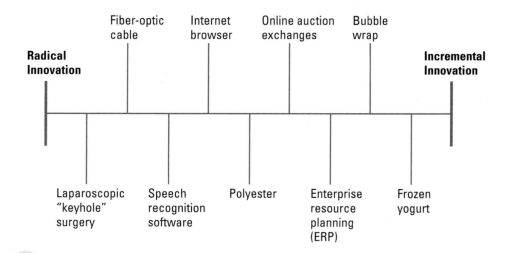

Exhibit 12.1 Continuum of Radical and Incremental Innovations

Some innovations are highly radical; others are only slightly incremental. But most innovations fall somewhere between these two extremes (see Exhibit 12.1).

Harvard Business School Professor Clayton M. Christensen identified another useful approach to characterize types of innovations.[5] Christensen draws a distinction between sustaining and disruptive innovations. *Sustaining innovations* are those that extend sales in an existing market, usually by enabling new products or services to be sold at higher margins. Such innovations may include either incremental or radical innovations. For example, the Internet was a breakthrough technology that transformed retail selling. But rather than disrupting the activities of catalog companies such as Lands' End and L.L. Bean, the Internet energized their existing business by extending their reach and making their operations more efficient.

By contrast, *disruptive innovations* are those that overturn markets by providing an altogether new approach to meeting customer needs. The features of a disruptive innovation make it somewhat counterintuitive. Disruptive innovations:

- Are technologically simpler and less sophisticated than currently available products or services.
- Appeal to less demanding customers who are seeking more convenient, less expensive solutions.
- Take time to take effect and only become disruptive once they have taken root in a new market or low-end part of an existing market.

Christensen cites Walmart and Southwest Airlines as two disruptive examples. Walmart started with a single store, Southwest with a few flights. But because they both represented major departures from existing practices and tapped into unmet needs, they steadily grew into ventures that appealed to a new category of customers and eventually overturned the status quo. "Instead of sustaining the trajectory of improvement that has been established in a market," said Christensen, a disruptive innovation "disrupts it and redefines it by bringing to the market something that is simpler."[6]

The Linux operating system provides a more recent example. When it first became available, few systems administrators used the open-source operating system even though it was free. However, problems with more expensive proprietary operating systems, such as Microsoft Windows, have made Linux increasingly popular. By 2008, the majority of Internet hosting companies and supercomputer operating systems were Linux-based. In addition to being relatively more convenient to use, it is supported by a community of developers.

Seeing the unmet needs of others can also trigger the development of potentially disruptive innovations. For example, Nintendo saw the need to fill a niche in the video game market for non-gamers. Strategy Spotlight 12.2 describes how the company created an innovative product for consumers who wanted to play games with a simple wand-like controller.

Innovation is a force in both the external environment (technology, competition) and also a factor affecting a firm's internal choices (generic strategy, value-adding activities).[7] Nevertheless, innovation can be quite difficult for some firms to manage, especially those that have become comfortable with the status quo.

Challenges of Innovation

>LO12.2
The challenges and pitfalls of managing corporate innovation processes.

Innovation is essential to sustaining competitive advantages. Recall from Chapter 3 that one of the four elements of the balanced scorecard is the innovation and learning perspective. The extent and success of a company's innovation efforts are indicators of its overall performance. As management guru Peter Drucker warned, "An established company which, in an age demanding innovation, is not capable of innovation is doomed to decline

A Disruptive Innovation: Nintendo's Wii

How can companies enter markets with strong competitors and still experience substantial growth? Disruptive innovation is an important tool to achieve such growth. Fusajiro Yamauchi ventured into the business of playing cards in 1889. He founded a Japanese company that would eventually evolve into Nintendo long after he was gone. When the organization began making video games and electronic toys, it entered the United States market, making and marketing video games and enhancements.

The year 2000 was a landmark year for the video game industry, given that all three major players launched new products. Previously, Nintendo was the market leader in video gaming. However, with the launch of Sony's PlayStation2 (PS2), Nintendo lost this coveted position. PS2 outsold its competitors, including Microsoft's Xbox and Nintendo's GameCube. Sony and Microsoft continued to enhance their products by adding new features, but with the appointment of Satoru Iwata as Nintendo's president in 2002, the organization decided to take a very different route to growth.

Nintendo observed that the customer base in video games was in decline. This could have been attributed to customers believing that new versions of video products were too complicated and included features that they just didn't want. Nintendo decided to try a different path altogether. It realized that there was a huge market for non-gamers that had not been tapped—segments of the existing customer base that slowly ceased to buy video games, the products with increased features as well as higher prices. Nintendo decided to target these two segments. There was definite uncertainty, as introducing new products was not the sure answer for success. Also, since this would be an emerging market, traditional performance measures might paint a gloomy picture. Despite these obstacles, Nintendo launched the Wii—a revolutionary video game system played with a simple wand-like controller. No complex wiring or controls gamers were needed to understand or maneuver. The wand's movement was detected by the screen's motion detectors, translating these motions into gaming actions. Wii was an instant hit, and within a year of the product's launch, Nintendo's market value tripled.

Sources: Ghosh, A. 2010. Growth through disruptive innovation. *www.business-standard.com. www.business-standard.com/india/news/growth-through-disruptive-innovation/414790/*. November 15; and, Cohen, D. S. nd. Fusajiro Yamauchi—founder of Nintendo, classic video games. *http://classicgames.about.com/od/classicvideogames101/p/FusajiroYamauch.htm.*

and extinction."[8] In today's competitive environment, most firms have only one choice: "Innovate or die."

As with change, however, firms are often resistant to innovation. Only those companies that actively pursue innovation, even though it is often difficult and uncertain, will get a payoff from their innovation efforts. But managing innovation is challenging.[9] As former Pfizer chairman and CEO William Steere put it: "In some ways, managing innovation is analogous to breaking in a spirited horse. You are never sure of success until you achieve your goal. In the meantime, everyone takes a few lumps."[10]

What is it that makes innovation so difficult? The uncertainty about outcomes is one factor. Companies are often reluctant to invest time and resources into activities with an unknown future. Another factor is that the innovation process involves so many choices. These choices present five dilemmas that companies must wrestle with when pursuing innovation.[11]

- *Seeds versus Weeds.* Most companies have an abundance of innovative ideas. They must decide which of these is most likely to bear fruit—the "Seeds"—and which should be cast aside—the "Weeds." This is complicated by the fact that some innovation projects require a considerable level of investment before a firm can fully evaluate whether they are worth pursuing. Firms need a mechanism with which they can choose among various innovation projects.

- ***Experience versus Initiative.*** Companies must decide who will lead an innovation project. Senior managers may have experience and credibility but tend to be more risk averse. Midlevel employees, who may be the innovators themselves, may have more enthusiasm because they can see firsthand how an innovation would address specific problems. Firms need to support and reward organizational members who bring new ideas to light.

- ***Internal versus External Staffing.*** Innovation projects need competent staffs to succeed. People drawn from inside the company may have greater social capital and know the organization's culture and routines. But this knowledge may actually inhibit them from thinking outside the box. Staffing innovation projects with external personnel requires that project managers justify the hiring and spend time recruiting, training, and relationship building. Firms need to streamline and support the process of staffing innovation efforts.

- ***Building Capabilities versus Collaborating.*** Innovation projects often require new sets of skills. Firms can seek help from other departments and/or partner with other companies that bring resources and experience as well as share costs of development. However, such arrangements can create dependencies and inhibit internal skills development. Further, struggles over who contributed the most or how the benefits of the project are to be allocated may arise. Firms need a mechanism for forging links with outside parties to the innovation process.

- ***Incremental versus Preemptive Launch.*** Companies must manage the timing and scale of new innovation projects. An incremental launch is less risky because it requires fewer resources and serves as a market test. But a launch that is too tentative can undermine the project's credibility. It also opens the door for a competitive response. A large-scale launch requires more resources, but it can effectively preempt a competitive response. Firms need to make funding and management arrangements that allow for projects to hit the ground running and be responsive to market feedback.

These dilemmas highlight why the innovation process can be daunting even for highly successful firms. Next, we consider five steps that firms can take to improve the innovation process within the firm.[12]

Cultivating Innovation Skills

Some firms, such as Apple, Google, and Amazon, regularly produce innovative products and services, while other firms struggle to generate new, marketable products. What separates these innovative firms from the rest of the pack? Jeff Dyer, Hal Gregersen, and Clayton Christensen argue it is the innovative DNA of the leaders of these firms.[13] The leaders of these firms have exhibited "discovery skills" that allow them to see the potential in innovations and to move the organization forward in leveraging the value of those innovations.[14] These leaders spend 50 percent more time on these discovery activities than the leaders of less innovative firms. To improve their innovative processes, firms need to cultivate the innovation skills of their managers.

The key attribute that firms need to develop in their managers in order to improve their innovative potential is creative intelligence. Creative intelligence is driven by a core skill of associating—the ability to see patterns in data and integrating different questions, information, and insights—and four patterns of action: questioning, observing, experimenting, and networking. As managers practice the four patterns of action, they will begin to develop the skill of association. Dyer and his colleagues offer the following illustration to demonstrate that individuals using these skills are going to develop more creative, higher-potential innovations.

> Imagine that you have an identical twin, endowed with the same brains and natural talents that you have. You're both given one week to come up with a creative new business-venture

idea. During that week, you come up with ideas alone in your room. In contrast, your twin (1) talks with 10 people—including an engineer, a musician, a stay-at-home dad, and a designer—about the venture, (2) visits three innovative start-ups to observe what they do, (3) samples five "new to the market" products, (4) shows a prototype he's built to five people, and (5) asks the questions "What if I tried this?" and "Why do you do that?" at least 10 times each day during these networking, observing, and experimenting activities. Who do you bet will come up with the more innovative (and doable) ideas?

The point is that by questioning, observing, experimenting, and networking as part of the innovative process, managers will both make better innovation decisions now but, more importantly, start to build the innovative DNA needed to be more successful innovators in the future. As they get into the practice of these habits, decision makers will see opportunities and be more creative as they associate information from different parts of their life, different people they come in contact with, and different parts of their organizations. The ability to innovate is not hardwired into our brains at birth. Research suggests that only one-third of our ability to think creatively is genetic. The other two-thirds is developed over time. Neuroscience research indicates that the brain is "plastic," meaning it changes over time due to experiences. As managers build up the ability to ask creative questions, develop a wealth of experiences from diverse settings, and link together insights from different arenas of their lives, their brains will follow suit and will build the ability to easily see situations creatively and draw upon a wide range of experiences and knowledge to identify creative solutions. The five traits of the effective innovator are described and examples of each trait are presented in Exhibit 12.2.

Defining the Scope of Innovation

strategic
envelope a firm-specific view of innovation that defines how a firm can create new knowledge and learn from an innovation initiative even if the project fails.

Firms must have a means to focus their innovation efforts. By defining the **strategic envelope**—the scope of a firm's innovation efforts—firms ensure that their innovation efforts are not wasted on projects that are outside the firm's domain of interest. Strategic enveloping defines the range of acceptable projects. As Alistair Corbett, an innovation expert with the global consulting firm Bain & Company, said, "One man's radical innovation is another man's incremental innovation."[15] A strategic envelope creates a firm-specific view of innovation that defines how a firm can create new knowledge and learn from an innovation initiative even if the project fails. It also gives direction to a firm's innovation efforts, which helps separate seeds from weeds and builds internal capabilities.

One way to determine which projects to work on is to focus on a common technology. Then, innovation efforts across the firm can aim at developing skills and expertise in a given technical area. Another potential focus is on a market theme. Consider how Teijin of Japan responded to a growing concern for environmentally sensitive products:

> Demand for biodegradable resins has grown rapidly in the last decade, as people have become increasingly aware of the need to preserve the environment. Teijin Ltd., a leading Japanese manufacturer of fibers, plastics, and pharmaceuticals, announced in September 2004 that it had successfully developed a plastic that was both photodegradable and biodegradable. Teijin's plastic was certified as a biodegradable plastic by the Biodegradable Plastics Society, a private organization for promoting the practical application of biodegradable plastics in Japan. The company now uses this plastic for various products, such as food containers and farming materials.[16]

Companies must be clear not only about the kinds of innovation they are looking for but also the expected results. Each company needs to develop a set of questions to ask itself about its innovation efforts:

- How much will the innovation initiative cost?
- How likely is it to actually become commercially viable?

Exhibit 12.2   The Innovator's DNA

Trait	Description	Example
Associating	Innovators have the ability to connect seemingly unrelated questions, problems, and ideas from different fields. This allows them to creatively see opportunities that others miss.	Pierre Omidyar saw the opportunity that led to eBay when he linked three items: (1) a personal fascination with creating more efficient markets, (2) his fiancee's desire to locate hard to find collectible Pez dispensers, and (3) the ineffectiveness of local classified ads in locating such items.
Questioning	Innovators constantly ask questions that challenge common wisdom. Rather than accept the status quo, they ask "Why not?" or "What if?" This gets others around them to challenge the assumptions that limit the possible range of actions the firm can take.	After witnessing the emergence of eBay and Amazon, Marc Benioff questioned why computer software was still sold in boxes rather than leased with a subscription and downloaded through the Internet. This was the genesis of Salesforce.com, a firm with over $1.3 billion in sales in 2010.
Observing	Discovery-driven executives produce innovative business ideas by observing regular behavior of individuals, especially customers and potential customers. Such observations often identify challenges customers face and previously unidentified opportunities.	From watching his wife struggle to keep track of the family's finances, Intuit founder Scott Cook identified the need for easy-to-use financial software that provided a single place for managing bills, bank accounts, and investments.
Experimenting	Thomas Edison once said, "I haven't failed. I've simply found 10,000 ways that do not work." Innovators regularly experiment with new possibilities, accepting that many of their ideas will fail. Experimentation can include new jobs, living in different countries, and new ideas for their businesses.	Founders Larry Page and Sergey Brin provide time and resources for Google employees to experiment. Some, such as the Android cell phone platform, have been big winners. Others, such as the Orkut and Buzz social networking systems, have failed. But Google will continue to experiment with new products and services.
Networking	Innovators develop broad personal networks. They use this diverse set of individuals to find and test radical ideas. This can be done by developing a diverse set of friends. It can also be done by attending idea conferences where individuals from a broad set of backgrounds come together to share their perspectives and ideas, such as the Technology, Entertainment, and Design (TED) Conference or the Aspen Ideas Festival.	Michael Lazaridis got the idea for a wireless e-mail device that led him to found Research in Motion from a conference he attended. At the conference, a speaker was discussing a wireless system Coca-Cola was using that allowed vending machines to send a signal when they needed refilling. Lazaridis saw the opportunity to use the same concept with e-mail communications, and the idea for the Blackberry was hatched.

Source: Reprinted by permission of Harvard Business Review. Exhibit from "The Innovator's DNA," by J. H. Dyer, H. G. Gregerson, & C. M. Christensen. Copyright 2009 by The Harvard Business School Publishing Corporation; all rights reserved.

- How much value will it add; that is, what will it be worth if it works?
- What will be learned if it does not pan out?

However a firm envisions its innovation goals, it needs to develop a systematic approach to evaluating its results and learning from its innovation initiatives. Viewing innovation from this perspective helps firms manage the process.[17]

Managing the Pace of Innovation

Along with clarifying the scope of an innovation by defining a strategic envelope, firms also need to regulate the pace of innovation. How long will it take for an innovation initiative to realistically come to fruition? The project time line of an incremental innovation may be 6 months to 2 years, whereas a more radical innovation is typically long term—10 years or more.[18] Radical innovations often begin with a long period of exploration in which experimentation makes strict timelines unrealistic. In contrast, firms that are innovating incrementally in order to exploit a window of opportunity may use a milestone approach that is more stringently driven by goals and deadlines. This kind of sensitivity to realistic time frames helps companies separate dilemmas temporally so they are easier to manage.

Time pacing can also be a source of competitive advantage because it helps a company manage transitions and develop an internal rhythm.[19] Time pacing does not mean the company ignores the demands of market timing; instead, companies have a sense of their own internal clock in a way that allows them to thwart competitors by controlling the innovation process.

Not all innovation lends itself to speedy development, however. Radical innovation often involves open-ended experimentation and time-consuming mistakes. The creative aspects of innovation are often difficult to time. When software maker Intuit's new CEO, Steve Bennett, began to turn around that troubled business, he required every department to implement Six Sigma, a quality control management technique that focuses on being responsive to customer needs. Everybody, that is, but the techies.

> "We're not GE, we're not a company where Jack says 'Do it,' and everyone salutes," says Bill Hensler, Intuit's vice president for process excellence. That's because software development, according to many, is more of an art than a science. At the Six Sigma Academy, president of operations Phil Samuel says even companies that have embraced Six Sigma across every other aspect of their organization usually maintain a hands-off policy when it comes to software developers. Techies, it turns out, like to go at their own pace.[20]

Some projects can't be rushed. Companies that hurry up their research efforts or go to market before they are ready can damage their ability to innovate—and their reputation. Thus, managing the pace of innovation can be an important factor in long-term success.

Staffing to Capture Value from Innovation

People are central to the processes of identifying, developing, and commercializing innovations effectively. They need broad sets of skills as well as experience—experience working with teams and experience working on successful innovation projects. To capture value from innovation activities, companies must provide strategic decision makers with staff members who make it possible.

This insight led strategy experts Rita Gunther McGrath and Thomas Keil to research the types of human resource management practices that effective firms use to capture value from their innovation efforts.[21] Four practices are especially important:

- Create innovation teams with experienced players who know what it is like to deal with uncertainty and can help new staff members learn venture management skills.

- Require that employees seeking to advance their career with the organization serve in the new venture group as part of their career climb.
- Once people have experience with the new venture group, transfer them to mainstream management positions where they can use their skills and knowledge to revitalize the company's core business.
- Separate the performance of individuals from the performance of the innovation. Otherwise, strong players may feel stigmatized if the innovation effort they worked on fails.

There are other staffing practices that may sound as if they would benefit a firm's innovation activities but may, in fact, be counterproductive:

- Creating a staff that consists only of strong players whose primary experience is related to the company's core business. This provides too few people to deal with the uncertainty of innovation projects and may cause good ideas to be dismissed because they do not appear to fit with the core business.
- Creating a staff that consists only of volunteers who want to work on projects they find interesting. Such players are often overzealous about new technologies or overly attached to product concepts, which can lead to poor decisions about which projects to pursue or drop.
- Creating a climate where innovation team members are considered second-class citizens. In companies where achievements are rewarded, the brightest and most ambitious players may avoid innovation projects with uncertain outcomes.

Unless an organization can align its key players into effective new venture teams, it is unlikely to create any differentiating advantages from its innovation efforts.[22] An enlightened approach to staffing a company's innovation efforts provides one of the best ways to ensure that the challenges of innovation will be effectively met. Strategy Spotlight 12.3 describes the approach. Samsung Electronics used to enhance its innovation efforts.

Collaborating with Innovation Partners

It is rare for any one organization to have all the information it needs to carry an innovation from concept to commercialization. Even a company that is highly competent with its current operations usually needs new capabilities to achieve new results. Innovation partners provide the skills and insights that are needed to make innovation projects succeed.[23]

Innovation partners may come from many sources, including research universities and the federal government. Each year the federal government issues requests for proposals (RFPs) asking private companies for assistance in improving services or finding solutions to public problems. Universities are another type of innovation partner. Chip-maker Intel, for example, has benefited from underwriting substantial amounts of university research. Rather than hand universities a blank check, Intel bargains for rights to patents that emerge from Intel-sponsored research. The university retains ownership of the patent, but Intel gets royalty-free use of it.[24]

Strategic partnering requires firms to identify their strengths and weaknesses and make choices about which capabilities to leverage, which need further development, and which are outside the firm's current or projected scope of operations.

To choose partners, firms need to ask what competencies they are looking for and what the innovation partner will contribute.[25] These might include knowledge of markets, technology expertise, or contacts with key players in an industry. Innovation partnerships also typically need to specify how the rewards of the innovation will be shared and who will own the intellectual property that is developed.[26]

Innovation efforts that involve multiple partners and the speed and ease with which partners can network and collaborate are changing the way innovation is conducted.[27]

Samsung's VIP Center

When it comes to implementing innovation efforts, Samsung Electronics recognizes the importance of staff for achieving success. Headquartered in Seoul, South Korea, Samsung has annual sales of about $137 billion, business operations in over 50 countries, and 170,000 employees worldwide. The company has a strong reputation for effectively embedding innovation into its culture through its unique employee engagement processes. Samsung's Value Innovation Program (VIP) Center continues to be a crucial weapon in the company's strategy for ensuring future innovation and growth. The center was created more than a decade ago after company executives concluded

that as much as 80 percent of cost and quality are determined in the initial stages of product development. By bringing together everyone at the very beginning to hash out differences, Samsung aimed to streamline its operations and make better gadgets. Specifically, the VIP Center brings together engineers, designers, product planners, and marketers early in a product's development to brainstorm ideas for making gadgets more user friendly and to trim inefficiencies in the manufacturing and development process. The center was set up to create quality products that could compete effectively in the cutthroat electronics market, but in recent years it has shifted its focus to creating products that offer "new value" for customers.

The company's goal is to rival the likes of Microsoft Corp. and IBM as a key shaper of information technology around the globe. Although the Korean giant still isn't an innovation leader on the order of Apple, Samsung hopes to transform itself into the most successful electronics company in Asia.

Sources: Hansen, M. T., Ibarra, H., & Peyer, U. 2010. The best-performing CEOs in the world. *Harvard Business Review, http://hbr.org/2010/01/the-best-performing-ceos-in-the-world/ar/1.* January 2010; and, Camp Samsung. Camp Samsung. 2006. *Bloomberg Businessweek, www.businessweek.com/magazine/content/06_27/b3991052.htm.* July 3.

Strategy Spotlight 12.4 outlines how IBM is using crowdsourcing technologies to foster collaboration between employees, customers, suppliers, and other stakeholders to enhance its innovation efforts.

Successful innovation involves a companywide commitment because the results of innovation affect every part of the organization. Innovation also requires an entrepreneurial spirit and skill set to be effective. Few companies have a more exemplary reputation than W. L. Gore. Exhibit 12.3 highlights the policies that help make Gore an innovation leader. One of the most important ways that companies improve and grow is when innovation is put to the task of creating new corporate ventures.

Corporate Entrepreneurship

corporate entrepreneurship
the creation of new value for a corporation, through investments that create either new sources of competitive advantage or renewal of the value proposition.

Corporate entrepreneurship (CE) has two primary aims: the pursuit of new venture opportunities and strategic renewal.[28] The innovation process keeps firms alert by exposing them to new technologies, making them aware of marketplace trends, and helping them evaluate new possibilities. CE uses the fruits of the innovation process to help firms build new sources of competitive advantage and renew their value propositions. Just as the innovation process helps firms to make positive improvements, corporate entrepreneurship helps firms identify opportunities and launch new ventures. Strategy Spotlight 12.5 outlines how Cisco is being entrepreneurial by expanding into new, growing product segments.

Corporate new venture creation was labeled "intrapreneuring" by Gifford Pinchot because it refers to building entrepreneurial businesses within existing corporations.[29] However, to engage in corporate entrepreneurship that yields above-average returns and contributes to sustainable advantages, it must be done effectively. In this section we will

Crowdsourcing: IBM's Innovation Jam

IBM is one of the best known corporations in the world, but its CEO, Samuel Palmisano, saw a major challenge for the firm. Though IBM had great ability to do basic scientific research and owned the rights to over 40,000 patents, it had struggled to translate its patented knowledge into marketable products. Also, it had built a reputation with investors as a firm with incremental product development, not the reputation needed in dynamic technological markets. Palmisano saw crowdsourcing as a means to move IBM forward in a bold way.

In 2006, IBM hosted an Innovation Jam, an open event that involved 150,000 IBM employees, family members, business partners, clients, and university researchers. The jam took place over two 72-hour sessions. Participants from over 100 countries jammed for 24 hours a day over three days. The discussions were organized around 25 technologies in six broad categories. While the jam discussions were rich in content, it was a challenge for IBM to pull meaningful data from them. The 24-hour format meant that no single moderator could follow any discussion, and the volume of posts to the discussion threads left IBM with a huge amount of data to wade through. The discussions yielded 46,000 potential business ideas. To make sense of the data, IBM organized the discussion threads using sophisticated text analysis software and had a team of 50 managers read through the organized data. Using data from the first session, the managers identified 31 "big ideas." They further explored these 31 ideas in the second jam session. IBM then used another set of 50 global managers to review the discussions from the jam. Teams

Sources: Bjelland, O. M. & Wood, R. C. 2008. An inside view of IBM's Innovation Jam. *Sloan Management Review.* Fall: 32–40; Hempel, J. 2006. Big Blue brainstorm. *BusinessWeek,* August 7: 70; and, Takahashi, D. 2008. IBM's Innovation Jam 2008 shows how far crowdsourcing has come. *Businessweek. com.* October 9: np.

of managers focused on related groups of ideas, such as health care and the environment.

IBM's managers saw the jam as serving three purposes. First, it gave individuals both inside and outside IBM who already had big ideas a forum in which to share their vision with top managers. Second, it gave individuals with smaller ideas a venue to link up with others with related ideas, resulting in larger major initiatives. For example, individuals who had ideas about better local weather forecasting, sensing devices for water utilities, and long-term climate forecasting came together to create "Predictive Water Management," a comprehensive solution for water authorities to manage their resources, a business solution no one at IBM had thought of before the jam. Third, the global structure of the jam allowed IBM, early on, to see how employees, partners, and customers from different regions had different goals and concerns about possible new businesses. For example, what customers wanted from systems to manage health care records varied greatly across regions.

Based on the jam sessions, IBM launched 10 new businesses using $100 million in funding. One, the Intelligent Transportation System, a system that gathers, manages, and disseminates real-time information about metropolitan transportation systems to optimize traffic flow, has been sold to transportation authorities in Sweden, the UK, Singapore, Dubai, and Australia. Another, Intelligent Utility Networks, became a core product in IBM's public utility business. A third, Big Green, became part of the largest initiative in IBM's history, a billion-dollar project on better managing energy and other resources.

crowdsourcing

examine the sources of entrepreneurial activity within established firms and the methods large corporations use to stimulate entrepreneurial behavior.

In a typical corporation, what determines how entrepreneurial projects will be pursued? That depends on many factors, including:

- Corporate culture.
- Leadership.
- Structural features that guide and constrain action.
- Organizational systems that foster learning and manage rewards.

All of the factors that influence the strategy implementation process will also shape how corporations engage in internal venturing.

Exhibit 12.3
W. L. Gore's New Rules
for Fostering Innovation

Rule	Implications
The power of small teams	Gore believes that small teams promote familiarity and autonomy. Even its manufacturing plants are capped at just 200 people. That way everyone can get to know one another on a first-name basis and work together with minimal rules. This also helps to cultivate "an environment where creativity can flourish," according to CEO Chuck Carroll.
No ranks, no titles, no bosses	Because Gore believes in maximizing individual potential, employees, dubbed "associates," decide for themselves what new commitments to take on. Associates have "sponsors," rather than bosses, and there are no standardized job descriptions or categories. Everyone is supposed to take on a unique role. Committees of co-workers evaluate each team member's contribution and decide on compensation.
Take the long view	Although impatient about the status quo, Gore exhibits great patience with the time—often years, sometimes decades—it takes to nurture and develop breakthrough products and bring them to market.
Make time for face time	Gore avoids the traditional hierarchical chain of command, opting instead for a team-based environment that fosters personal initiative. Gore also discourages memos and e-mail and promotes direct, person-to-person communication among all associates—anyone in the company can talk to anyone else.
Lead by leading	Associates are encouraged to spend about 10 percent of their time pursuing speculative new ideas. Anyone is free to champion products, as long as they have the passion and ideas to attract followers. Many of Gore's breakthroughs started with one person acting on his or her own initiative and developed as colleagues helped in their spare time.
Celebrate failure	When a project doesn't work out and the team decides to kill it, they celebrate just as they would if it had been a success— with some beer and maybe a glass of champagne. Rather than condemning failure, Gore figures that celebrating it encourages experimentation and risk taking.

Source: Deutschman, A. 2004. The fabric of creativity. *Fast Company,* 89: 54–62; Levering, R. & Moskowitz, M. 2006. The 100 best companies to work for. *Fortune, www.fortune.com*, January; and, *www.gore.com*.

Other factors will also affect how entrepreneurial ventures will be pursued.

- The use of teams in strategic decision making.
- Whether the company is product or service oriented.
- Whether its innovation efforts are aimed at product or process improvements.
- The extent to which it is high-tech or low-tech.

Cisco Looks to Video to Spur Demand

Cisco produces both hardware and software used to manage network and communication systems. Cisco, which was founded in San Francisco in 1984, began by manufacturing routers to manage Internet communications. It has expanded from its original market position in computer routers by acquiring firms that make network switches, voice over Internet protocol (VOIP) systems, home networking equipment, and other information technology products and services. Today, Cisco dominates the market for Internet protocol–based networking equipment and provides routers and switches used to direct data, voice, and video traffic. Cisco has had a nice run over the last 10 years, with sales growing from $19 billion in 2001 to $40 billion in 2010 and net income growing from $2.7 billion to $7.8 billion over the same period.

Even with this success, Cisco is not one to rest on its laurels. Managers at Cisco retain an entrepreneurial orientation and look to expand their product portfolio to meet where the market is going. A few years ago, Cisco introduced Teleprescence, an Internet-based videoconference technology. This has been a winning product during the recent recessionary years, since many corporations have turned to videoconferencing as a means to host meetings without the travel expense of bringing employees together. From this experience, John Chambers, the firm's CEO, began to believe that the Internet's primary payload going forward will be video and has placed a big bet on Internet video.

As the Internet moves toward being primarily a video-based medium, communications hardware and software to manage video traffic will be valued resources, because HD video takes about 50 times as much Internet bandwidth as audio data. To meet the challenge of this new Internet era, Cisco has developed a technology, called Medianet, that facilitates the flow of video media across all devices transferring, delivering, or receiving Internet-based videos. For example, a smartphone could tell a Medianet-enabled network the phone's screen size and connection speed. The network would then tailor how it delivered the media to the phone to optimize the transfer and to use the network hardware as efficiently as possible.

Sources: Fortt, J. 2010. Cisco's online video gamble. *Fortune,* November 1: 43; Lawson, S. 2008. Cisco plays up video for business, carriers. *IDG News Service,* September 16: np; *www.hoovers.com;* and, *www.cisco.com.*

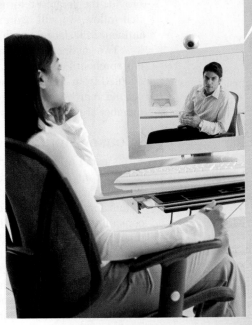

● Cisco Systems continues to develop its Internet-based video media products.

Cisco's ultimate objective with this new product is to extend its dominance in the network business. As Cisco develops systems that increase the use of Internet-based video, it stokes up demand for its core products. Telecommunication service providers and corporations will need to ramp up their investment in network gear to meet the growing demand for Internet video. These firms will likely turn to Cisco to purchase Medianet-enabled network gear as they expand their network systems. As Robert Hagerty, the former CEO of Polycom, a competitor of Cisco, commented that Cisco's "real motivation is to sell more routers and switches on the enterprise side." In line with this, Procter & Gamble has expanded its purchasing of Cisco's network equipment as it has worked to double its network capacity in 2010 in anticipation of greater video traffic. Thus, Cisco's entrepreneurial entry into the Internet-video business has fostered growth in the value of its core markets.

Because these factors are different in every organization, some companies may be more involved than others in identifying and developing new venture opportunities.[30] These factors will also influence the nature of the CE process.

Successful CE typically requires firms to reach beyond their current operations and markets in the pursuit of new opportunities. It is often the breakthrough opportunities that provide the greatest returns. Such strategies are not without risks, however. In the sections that follow, we will address some of the strategic choice and implementation issues that influence the success or failure of CE activities.

Two distinct approaches to corporate venturing are found among firms that pursue entrepreneurial aims. The first is *focused* corporate venturing, in which CE activities are isolated from a firm's existing operations and worked on by independent work units. The second approach is *dispersed,* in which all parts of the organization and every organization member are engaged in intrapreneurial activities.

Focused Approaches to Corporate Entrepreneurship

Firms using a focused approach typically separate the corporate venturing activity from the other ongoing operations of the firm. CE is usually the domain of autonomous work groups that pursue entrepreneurial aims independent of the rest of the firm. The advantage of this approach is that it frees entrepreneurial team members to think and act without the constraints imposed by existing organizational norms and routines. This independence is often necessary for the kind of open-minded creativity that leads to strategic breakthroughs. The disadvantage is that, because of their isolation from the corporate mainstream, the work groups that concentrate on internal ventures may fail to obtain the resources or support needed to carry an entrepreneurial project through to completion. Two forms—new venture groups (NVGs) and business incubators—are among the most common types of **focused approaches to corporate entrepreneurship**.

New Venture Groups (NVGs) Corporations often form NVGs whose goal is to identify, evaluate, and cultivate venture opportunities. These groups typically function as semiautonomous units with little formal structure. The **new venture group** may simply be a committee that reports to the president on potential new ventures. Or it may be organized as a corporate division with its own staff and budget. The aims of the NVG may be open-ended in terms of what ventures it may consider. Alternatively, some corporations use them to promote concentrated effort on a specific problem. In both cases, they usually have a substantial amount of freedom to take risks and a supply of resources to do it with.[31]

NVGs usually have a larger mandate than a typical R&D department. Their involvement extends beyond innovation and experimentation to coordinating with other corporate divisions, identifying potential venture partners, gathering resources, and actually launching the venture. Strategy Spotlight 12.6 shows how WD-40 has used an NVG to improve its CE efforts.

Business Incubators The term *incubator* was originally used to describe a device in which eggs are hatched. **Business incubators** are designed to "hatch" new businesses. They are a type of corporate NVG with a somewhat more specialized purpose—to support and nurture fledgling entrepreneurial ventures until they can thrive on their own as stand-alone businesses. Corporations use incubators as a way to grow businesses identified by the NVG. Although they often receive support from many parts of the corporation, they still operate independently until they are strong enough to go it alone. Depending on the type of business, they are either integrated into an existing corporate division or continue to operate as a subsidiary of the parent firm.

focused approches to corporate entrepreneurship corporate entrepreneurship in which the venturing entity is separated from the other ongoing operations of the firm.

new venture group a group of individuals, or a division within a corporation, that identifies, evaluates, and cultivates venture opportunities.

business incubator a corporate new venture group that supports and nurtures fledgling entrepreneurial ventures until they can thrive on their own as stand-alone businesses.

Using Team Tomorrow to Grow WD-40

When a hinge squeaks, most people reach for a can of WD-40. The iconic lubricant in the blue cans has been around for over 50 years and commands a 70 percent market share in the spray lubricant business. Garry Ridge, the CEO of WD-40, quipped that "more people use WD-40 every day than use dental floss." Still, Ridge wanted the firm to look forward, searching for growth opportunities. Historically, WD-40's marketing team was responsible for new product development, but this typically involved minor product changes or new packaging for existing products.

Knowing the incremental focus of the current structure and wanting to get WD-40 focused on bolder new product opportunities, Ridge created a multifunctional team, dubbed Team Tomorrow, to manage its global CE efforts. This team includes members from marketing, research, supply chain, purchasing, and distribution. To head the team, Ridge tapped an experienced executive, Graham Milner, who thought globally and had a marketing background. There was some resistance from the marketing staff, because they lost power in the new product-development process. Ridge overcame this in a number of ways. He was active in forming the team, got involved during times of conflict between Team Tomorrow and other groups in the organization, and carried around an early prototype of the team's first product, the No Mess Pen, to show how interested he was in the new product. His involvement signaled the importance of the team to WD-40. By placing a marketing executive in charge of Team Tomorrow, he signaled the importance of marketing to the organization. Milner and the other team leader, Stephanie Barry, worked collaboratively with the head of marketing, instituted an open-door policy, and shared information with marketing. Collectively, these actions broke down resistance to Team Tomorrow.

Ridge also gave the team a bold goal. He charged the team to create new products that would generate $100 million in sales per year from products developed and launched within the previous three years. As of 2010, the team had created products that generate $165 million in sales. Ridge also sees a large change in the rest of the firm as a result of this effort. He sees the firm's employees as being members of a "tribe" and the organization as a "living learning laboratory."

Sources: Ferrarini, E. 2010. WD-40 Company CEO talks about rebuilding an innovative brand and taking it global. *Enterprise Leadership,* February 27: np; Bounds, G. 2006. WD-40 CEO repackages a core product. *Pittsburgh Post Gazette,* May 23: np; Govindarajan, V. & Trimble, D. 2010. Stop the innovation wars. *Harvard Business Review,* July–August: 76–83; and, www.intheboardroom.com.

Incubators typically provide some or all of the following five functions.[32]

- **Funding.** Includes capital investments as well as in-kind investments and loans.
- **Physical space.** Incubators in which several start-ups share space often provide fertile ground for new ideas and collaboration.
- **Business services.** Along with office space, young ventures need basic services and infrastructure; may include anything from phone systems and computer networks to public relations and personnel management.
- **Mentoring.** Senior executives and skilled technical personnel often provide coaching and experience-based advice.
- **Networking.** Contact with other parts of the firm and external resources such as suppliers, industry experts, and potential customers facilitates problem solving and knowledge sharing.

The risks associated with incubating ventures should not be overlooked. Companies have at times spent millions on new ideas with very little to show for it. Major corporations such as Vodafone Group, British Airways, and Hewlett-Packard deactivated their incubators and scaled back new venture portfolios after experiencing major declines in value during recent financial downturns.[33]

To encourage entrepreneurship, corporations sometimes need to do more than create independent work groups or venture incubators to generate new enterprises. In some firms, the entrepreneurial spirit is spread throughout the organization.

Dispersed Approaches to Corporate Entrepreneurship

dispersed approaches to corporate entrepreneurship corporate entrepreunership in which a dedication to the principles and policies of entrepreunership is spread throughout the organization.

The second type of CE is **dispersed approaches to corporate entrepreneurship**. For some companies, a dedication to the principles and practices of entrepreneurship is spread throughout the organization. One advantage of this approach is that organizational members don't have to be reminded to think entrepreneurially or be willing to change. The ability to change is considered to be a core capability. This leads to a second advantage: Because of the firm's entrepreneurial reputation, stakeholders such as vendors, customers, or alliance partners can bring new ideas or venture opportunities to anyone in the organization and expect them to be well-received. Such opportunities make it possible for the firm to stay ahead of the competition. However, there are disadvantages as well. Firms that are overzealous about CE sometimes feel they must change for the sake of change, causing them to lose vital competencies or spend heavily on R&D and innovation to the detriment of the bottom line. Two related aspects of dispersed entrepreneurship include entrepreneurial cultures that have an overarching commitment to CE activities and the use of product champions in promoting entrepreneurial behaviors.

Entrepreneurial Culture In some large corporations, the corporate culture embodies the spirit of entrepreneurship. A culture of entrepreneurship is one in which the search for venture opportunities permeates every part of the organization. The key to creating value successfully is viewing every value-chain activity as a source of competitive advantage. The effect of CE on a firm's strategic success is strongest when it animates all parts of an organization. It is found in companies where the strategic leaders and the culture together generate a strong impetus to innovate, take risks, and seek out new venture opportunities.[34]

entrepreneurial culture corpotate culture in which change and renewal are a constant focus of attention.

In companies with an **entrepreneurial culture**, everyone in the organization is attuned to opportunities to help create new businesses. Many such firms use a top-down approach to stimulate entrepreneurial activity. The top leaders of the organization support programs and incentives that foster a climate of entrepreneurship. Many of the best ideas for new corporate ventures, however, come from the bottom up. Here's what Martin Sorrell, CEO of the WPP Group, a London-based global communication services group, said about drawing on the talents of lower-level employees:

> The people at the so-called bottom of an organization know more about what's going on than the people at the top. The people in the trenches are the ones in the best position to make critical decisions. It's up to the leaders to give those people the freedom and the resources they need.[35]

product champion an individual working within a corporation who brings entrepreneurial ideas forward, identifies what kind of market exists for the product or service, finds resources to support the venture, and promotes the venture concept to upper management.

An entrepreneurial culture is one in which change and renewal are on everybody's mind. Sony, 3M, Intel, and Cisco are among the corporations best known for their corporate venturing activities. Many fast-growing young corporations also attribute much of their success to an entrepreneurial culture. But other successful firms struggle in their efforts to remain entrepreneurial. Strategy Spotlight 12.7 describes Microsoft's struggles with its CE efforts.

Product Champions CE does not always involve making large investments in start-ups or establishing incubators to spawn new divisions. Often, innovative ideas emerge in the normal course of business and are brought forth and become part of the way of doing business. Entrepreneurial champions are often needed to take charge of internally

Microsoft's Struggles with Corporate Entrepreneurship

Microsoft generated $62 billion in sales and nearly $19 billion in profits in 2010 and dominates the market for PC operating system and office suite application software, yet its stock languishes at a price lower than it was 10 years ago. Why is this the case? Investors have little confidence that Microsoft will produce blockbuster products that will replace its core PC software products as the information technology market moves into the post-PC phase.

It isn't that Microsoft has failed to generate innovative ideas. The firm spends $9 billion a year on R&D. Over 10 years ago, engineers at Microsoft developed a tablet PC and an e-book system, two of the hottest technology products today. They also pioneered Web-TV. But they failed to turn these pioneering efforts into marketable products. In other markets, they have not pioneered, but have seen limited success with products they've designed to meet emerging challengers. The Zune music player was supposed to challenge the iPod but was a flop in the market. Recently, it introduced the Kin One and Kin Two, smartphones with flashy designs and social networking capabilities, but it pulled the phones from the market within two months. The Xbox 360 has arguably been Microsoft's most successful product launch designed to take on a pioneering rival, but even there, the firm is competitive but not dominating the market.

With all of its resources, why has Microsoft struggled to translate its innovations into market successes? Let's look at three reasons that have been talked about in the business press.

First, the dominance of the Windows and Office software has made it difficult to launch new products. Developers of new products have, at times, had to justify how their new product fit into the core Microsoft product line. Dick Brass, a former VP at Microsoft, stated, "The company routinely manages to frustrate the efforts of its visionary leaders." For example, when Brass and his team developed an innovative technology to display text on a screen, called ClearType, engineers in the Windows group hampered the product by falsely arguing it had bugs and wouldn't display some colors properly. Others in the firm stated they would support the technology only if they could control it. In the end, it took 10 years to get ClearType integrated into Windows.

Second, Microsoft has a difficult time attracting the top software designers. The firm is not seen as a hip place to work. It is seen by developers as too bureaucratic. And their flat stock price makes it hard to entice top designers with promises of wealth from rising stock options—a common compensation element for technology talent.

Third, great innovations are increasingly the output of collaborative, open-source design, but Microsoft is reluctant to fully embrace the open-source development model. It developed a system where start-up firms can sign onto a program to gain access to free Microsoft software and provide development ideas to Microsoft and has signed up 35,000 firms, but its system is still more bureaucratic than those of its competitors. As one entrepreneur commented about working with Microsoft, "We got introduced to Microsoft through our investors. They don't do this for just anybody." As a result, Microsoft has lost those "anybodies" as development partners and future customers.

Sources: Vance, A. 2010. At top of business but just not cool. *International Herald Tribune*, July 6: 2; Clarke, G. 2010. Inside Microsoft's innovation crisis. *Theregister.co.uk*. February 5: np; and, Brass, D. 2010. Microsoft's creative destruction. *NYTimes.com*. February 4: np.

generated ventures. **Product** (or project) **champions** are those individuals working within a corporation who bring entrepreneurial ideas forward, identify what kind of market exists for the product or service, find resources to support the venture, and promote the venture concept to upper management.[36]

When lower-level employees identify a product idea or novel solution, they will take it to their supervisor or someone in authority. A new idea that is generated in a technology lab may be introduced to others by its inventor. If the idea has merit, it gains support and builds momentum across the organization.[37] Even though the corporation may not be looking for new ideas or have a program for cultivating internal ventures, the independent behaviors of a few organizational members can have important strategic consequences.

No matter how an entrepreneurial idea comes to light, however, a new venture concept must pass through two critical stages or it may never get off the ground:

1. **Project definition.** An opportunity has to be justified in terms of its attractiveness in the marketplace and how well it fits with the corporation's other strategic objectives.
2. **Project impetus.** For a project to gain impetus, its strategic and economic impact must be supported by senior managers who have experience with similar projects. It then becomes an embryonic business with its own organization and budget.

For a project to advance through these stages of definition and impetus, a product champion is often needed to generate support and encouragement. Champions are especially important during the time after a new project has been defined but before it gains momentum. They form a link between the definition and impetus stages of internal development, which they do by procuring resources and stimulating interest for the product among potential customers.[38] Often, they must work quietly and alone. Consider the example of Ken Kutaragi, the Sony engineer who championed the PlayStation.

> Even though Sony had made the processor that powered the first Nintendo video games, no one at Sony in the mid-1980s saw any future in such products. "It was a kind of snobbery," Kutaragi recalled. "For Sony people, the Nintendo product would have been very embarrassing to make because it was only a toy." But Kutaragi was convinced he could make a better product. He began working secretly on a video game. Kutaragi said, "I realized that if it was visible, it would be killed." He quietly began enlisting the support of senior executives, such as the head of R&D. He made a case that Sony could use his project to develop capabilities in digital technologies that would be important in the future. It was not until 1994, after years of "underground" development and quiet building of support, that Sony introduced the PlayStation. By the year 2000, Sony had sold 55 million of them, and Kutaragi became CEO of Sony Computer Entertainment. By 2005, Kutagari was Sony's Chief Operating Officer, and was supervising efforts to launch PS3, the next generation version of the market-leading PlayStation video game console.[39]

Product champions play an important entrepreneurial role in a corporate setting by encouraging others to take a chance on promising new ideas.[40]

Measuring the Success of Corporate Entrepreneurship Activities

At this point in the discussion, it is reasonable to ask whether CE is successful. Corporate venturing, like the innovation process, usually requires a tremendous effort. Is it worth it? We consider factors that corporations need to take into consideration when evaluating the success of CE programs. We also examine techniques that companies can use to limit the expense of venturing or to cut their losses when CE initiatives appear doomed.

>LO12.4
How corporate entrepreneurship achieves both financial goals and strategic goals.

Comparing Strategic and Financial CE Goals   Not all corporate venturing efforts are financially rewarding. In terms of financial performance, slightly more than 50 percent of corporate venturing efforts reach profitability (measured by ROI) within six years of their launch.[41] If this were the only criterion for success, it would seem to be a rather poor return. On the one hand, these results should be expected, because CE is riskier than other investments such as expanding ongoing operations. On the other hand, corporations expect a higher return from corporate venturing projects than from normal operations. Thus, in terms of the risk–return trade-off, it seems that CE often falls short of expectations.[42]

There are several other important criteria, however, for judging the success of a corporate venture initiative. Most CE programs have strategic goals.[43] The strategic reasons for undertaking a corporate venture include strengthening competitive position, entering into new markets, expanding capabilities by learning and acquiring new knowledge, and building the corporation's base of resources and experience. Three questions should be used to assess the effectiveness of a corporation's venturing initiatives:[44]

1. *Are the products or services offered by the venture accepted in the marketplace?* Is the venture considered to be a market success? If so, the financial returns are likely to be satisfactory. The venture may also open doors into other markets and suggest avenues for other venture projects.

2. *Are the contributions of the venture to the corporation's internal competencies and experience valuable?* Does the venture add to the worth of the firm internally? If so, strategic goals such as leveraging existing assets, building new knowledge, and enhancing firm capabilities are likely to be met.[45]

3. *Is the venture able to sustain its basis of competitive advantage?* Does the value proposition offered by the venture insulate it from competitive attack? If so, it is likely to place the corporation in a stronger position relative to competitors and provide a base from which to build other advantages.

These criteria include both strategic and financial goals of CE. Another way to evaluate a corporate venture is in terms of the four criteria from the balanced scorecard (Chapter 3). In a successful venture, not only are financial and market acceptance (customer) goals met but so are the internal business and innovation and learning goals. Thus, when assessing the success of corporate venturing, it is important to look beyond simple financial returns and consider a well-rounded set of criteria.[46]

Exit Champions Although a culture of championing venture projects is advantageous for stimulating an ongoing stream of entrepreneurial initiatives, many—in fact, most—of the ideas will not work out. At some point in the process, a majority of initiatives will be abandoned. Sometimes, however, companies wait too long to terminate a new venture and do so only after large sums of resources are used up or, worse, result in a marketplace failure. Motorola's costly global satellite telecom project known as Iridium provides a useful illustration. Even though problems with the project existed during the lengthy development process, Motorola refused to pull the plug. Only after investing $5 billion and years of effort was the project abandoned.[47]

One way to avoid these costly and discouraging defeats is to support a key role in the CE process: **exit champions.** In contrast to product champions and other entrepreneurial enthusiasts within the corporation, exit champions are willing to question the viability of a venture project.[48] By demanding hard evidence and challenging the belief system that is carrying an idea forward, exit champions hold the line on ventures that appear shaky.

Both product champions and exit champions must be willing to energetically stand up for what they believe. Both put their reputations on the line. But they also differ in important ways.[49] Product champions deal in uncertainty and ambiguity. Exit champions reduce ambiguity by gathering hard data and developing a strong case for why a project should be killed. Product champions are often thought to be willing to violate procedures and operate outside normal channels. Exit champions often have to reinstate procedures and re-assert the decision-making criteria that are supposed to guide venture decisions. Whereas product champions often emerge as heroes, exit champions run the risk of losing status by opposing popular projects.

The role of exit champion may seem unappealing. But it is one that could save a corporation both financially and in terms of its reputation in the marketplace. It is especially important because one measure of the success of a firm's CE efforts is the extent to which it knows when to cut its losses and move on.

exit champion an individual working within a corporation who is willing to question the viability of a venture project by demanding hard evidence of venture success and challenging the belief system that carries a venture forward.

real options analysis an investment analysis tool that looks at an investment or activity as a series of sequential steps, and for each step the investor has the option of (a) investing additional funds to grow or accelerate, (b) delaying, (c) shrinking the scale of, or (d) abandoning the activity.

Real Options Analysis: A Useful Tool

One way firms can minimize failure and avoid losses from pursuing faulty ideas is to apply the logic of real options. **Real options analysis** (ROA) is an investment analysis tool from the field of finance. It has been slowly, but increasingly, adopted by consultants and executives to support strategic decision making in firms. What does ROA consist of and how can it be appropriately applied to the investments required to initiate strategic decisions? To understand *real* options it is first necessary to have a basic understanding of what *options* are.

Options exist when the owner of the option has the right but not the obligation to engage in certain types of transactions. The most common are stock options. A stock option grants the holder the right to buy (call option) or sell (put option) shares of the stock at a fixed price (strike price) at some time in the future.[50] The investment to be made immediately is small, whereas the investment to be made in the future is generally larger. An option to buy a rapidly rising stock currently priced at $50 might cost as little as $.50.[51] Owners of such a stock option have limited their losses to $.50 per share, while the upside potential is unlimited. This aspect of options is attractive, because options offer the prospect of high gains with relatively small up-front investments that represent limited losses.

The phrase "real options" applies to situations where options theory and valuation techniques are applied to real assets or physical things as opposed to financial assets. Applied to entrepreneurship, real options suggest a path that companies can use to manage the uncertainty associated with launching new ventures. Some of the most common applications of real options are with property and insurance. A real estate option grants the holder the right to buy or sell a piece of property at an established price some time in the future. The actual market price of the property may rise above the established (or strike) price—or the market value may sink below the strike price. If the price of the property goes up, the owner of the option is likely to buy it. If the market value of the property drops below the strike price, the option holder is unlikely to execute the purchase. In the latter circumstance, the option holder has limited his or her loss to the cost of the option, but during the life of the option retains the right to participate in whatever the upside potential might be.

Applications of Real Options Analysis to Strategic Decisions

The concept of options can also be applied to strategic decisions where management has flexibility. Situations arise where management must decide whether to invest additional funds to grow or accelerate the activity, perhaps delay in order to learn more, shrink the scale of the activity, or even abandon it. Decisions to invest in new ventures or other business activities such as R&D, motion pictures, exploration and production of oil wells, and the opening and closing of copper mines often have this flexibility.[52] Important issues to note are:

- ROA is appropriate to use when investments can be staged; a smaller investment up-front can be followed by subsequent investments. Real options can be applied to an investment decision that gives the company the right, but not the obligation, to make follow-on investments.
- Strategic decision makers have "tollgates," or key points at which they can decide whether to continue, delay, or abandon the project. Executives have flexibility. There are opportunities to make other go or no-go decisions associated with each phase.
- It is expected that there will be increased knowledge about outcomes at the time of the next investment and that additional knowledge will help inform the decision makers about whether to make additional investments (i.e., whether the option is in the money or out of the money).

Many strategic decisions have the characteristic of containing a series of options. The phenomenon is called "embedded options," a series of investments in which at each stage of the investment there is a go/no-go decision. Consider the real options logic that Johnson

Controls, a maker of car seats, instrument panels, and interior control systems uses to advance or eliminate entrepreneurial ideas.[53] Johnson options each new innovative idea by making a small investment in it. To decide whether to exercise an option, the idea must continue to prove itself at each stage of development. Here's how Jim Geschke, vice president and general manager of electronics integration at Johnson, described the process:

> Think of Johnson as an innovation machine. The front end has a robust series of gates that each idea must pass through. Early on, we'll have many ideas and spend a little money on each of them. As they get more fleshed out, the ideas go through a gate where a go or no-go decision is made. A lot of ideas get filtered out, so there are far fewer items, and the spending on each goes up. . . . Several months later each idea will face another gate. If it passes, that means it's a serious idea that we are going to develop. Then the spending goes way up, and the number of ideas goes way down. By the time you reach the final gate, you need to have a credible business case in order to be accepted. At a certain point in the development process, we take our idea to customers and ask them what they think. Sometimes they say, "That's a terrible idea. Forget it." Other times they say, "That's fabulous. I want a million of them."

This process of evaluating ideas by separating winning ideas from losing ones in a way that keeps investments low has helped Johnson Controls grow its revenues to over $34 billion a year. Using real options logic to advance the development process is a key way that firms reduce uncertainty and minimize innovation-related failures.[54]

Potential Pitfalls of Real Options Analysis

Despite the many benefits that can be gained from using ROA, managers must be aware of its potential limitations or pitfalls. Below we will address three major issues.[55]

Agency Theory and the Back-Solver Dilemma   Let's assume that companies adopting a real options perspective invest heavily in training and that their people understand how to effectively estimate variance—the amount of dispersion or range that is estimated for potential outcomes. Such training can help them use ROA. However, it does not solve another inherent problem: Managers may have an incentive and the know-how to "game the system." Most electronic spreadsheets permit users to simply back-solve any formula; that is, you can type in the answer you want and ask what values are needed in a formula to get that answer. If managers know that a certain option value must be met in order for the proposal to get approved, they can back-solve the model to find a variance estimate needed to arrive at the answer that upper management desires.

Agency problems are typically inherent in investment decisions. They may occur when the managers of a firm are separated from its owners—when managers act as "agents" rather than "principals" (owners). A manager may have something to gain by not acting in the owner's best interests, or the interests of managers and owners are not co-aligned. Agency theory suggests that as managerial and owner interests diverge, managers will follow the path of their own self-interests. Sometimes this is to secure better compensation: Managers who propose projects may believe that if their projects are approved, they stand a much better chance of getting promoted. So while managers have an incentive to propose projects that *should* be successful, they also have an incentive to propose projects that *might* be successful—the **back-solver dilemma**. And because of the subjectivity involved in formally modeling a real option, managers may have an incentive to choose variance values that increase the likelihood of approval.

back-solver dilemma problem with investment decisions in which managers scheme to have a project meet investment approval criteria, even though the investment may not enhance firm value.

Managerial Conceit: Overconfidence and the Illusion of Control   Often, poor decisions are the result of such traps as biases, blind spots, and other human frailties. Much of this literature falls under the concept of **managerial conceit**.[56]

First, managerial conceit occurs when decision makers who have made successful choices in the past come to believe that they possess superior expertise for managing uncertainty. They believe that their abilities can reduce the risks inherent in decision

managerial conceit biases, blind spots, and other human frailties that lead to poor managerial decisions.

making to a much greater extent than they actually can. Such managers are more likely to shift away from analysis to trusting their own judgment. In the case of real options, they can simply declare that any given decision is a real option and proceed as before. If asked to formally model their decision, they are more likely to employ variance estimates that support their viewpoint.

Second, employing the real options perspective can encourage decision makers toward a bias for action. Such a bias may lead to carelessness. Managerial conceit is as much a problem (if not more so) for small decisions as for big ones. Why? The cost to write the first stage of an option is much smaller than the cost of full commitment, and managers pay less attention to small decisions than to large ones. Because real options are designed to minimize potential losses while preserving potential gains, any problems that arise are likely to be smaller at first, causing less concern for the manager. Managerial conceit could suggest that managers will assume that those problems are the easiest to solve and control—a concern referred to as the illusion of control. Managers may fail to respond appropriately because they overlook the problem or believe that, since it is small, they can easily resolve it. Thus, managers may approach each real option decision with less care and diligence than if they had made a full commitment to a larger investment.

Managerial Conceit: Irrational Escalation of Commitment   A strength of a real options perspective is also one of its Achilles heels. Both real options and decisions involving **escalation of commitment** require specific environments with sequential decisions.[57] As the escalation-of-commitment literature indicates, simply separating a decision into multiple parts does not guarantee that decisions made will turn out well. This condition is potentially present whenever the exercise decision retains some uncertainty, which most still do. The decision to abandon also has strong psychological factors associated with it that affect the ability of managers to make correct exercise decisions.[58]

An option to exit requires reversing an initial decision made by someone in the organization. Organizations typically encourage managers to "own their decisions" in order to motivate them. As managers invest themselves in their decision, it proves harder for them to lose face by reversing course. For managers making the decision, it feels as if they made the wrong decision in the first place, even if it was initially a good decision. The more specific the manager's human capital becomes, the harder it is to transfer it to other organizations. Hence, there is a greater likelihood that managers will stick around and try to make an existing decision work. They are more likely to continue an existing project even if it should perhaps be ended.[59]

Despite the potential pitfalls of a real options approach, many of the strategic decisions that product champions and top managers must make are enhanced when decision makers have an entrepreneurial mind-set.

Entrepreneurial Orientation

Firms that want to engage in successful CE need to have an entrepreneurial orientation (EO).[60] EO refers to the strategy-making practices that businesses use in identifying and launching corporate ventures. It represents a frame of mind and a perspective toward entrepreneurship that is reflected in a firm's ongoing processes and corporate culture.[61]

An EO has five dimensions that permeate the decision-making styles and practices of the firm's members: autonomy, innovativeness, proactiveness, competitive aggressiveness, and risk taking. These factors work together to enhance a firm's entrepreneurial performance. But even those firms that are strong in only a few aspects of EO can be very successful.[62] Exhibit 12.4 summarizes the dimensions of **entrepreneurial orientation.** Below, we discuss the five dimensions of EO and how they have been used to enhance internal venture development.

Exhibit 12.4
Dimensions of
Entrepreneurial
Orientation

Dimension	Definition
Autonomy	Independent action by an individual or team aimed at bringing forth a business concept or vision and carrying it through to completion.
Innovativeness	A willingness to introduce novelty through experimentation and creative processes aimed at developing new products and services as well as new processes.
Proactiveness	A forward-looking perspective characteristic of a marketplace leader that has the foresight to seize opportunities in anticipation of future demand.
Competitive aggressiveness	An intense effort to outperform industry rivals characterized by a combative posture or an aggressive response aimed at improving position or overcoming a threat in a competitive marketplace.
Risk taking	Making decisions and taking action without certain knowledge of probable outcomes; some undertakings may also involve making substantial resource commitments in the process of venturing forward.

Sources: Dess, G. G. & Lumpkin, G. T. 2005. The role of entrepreneurial orientation in stimulating effective corporate entrepreneurship. *Academy of Management Executive,* 19(1): 147–156; Covin, J. G. & Slevin, D. P. 1991. A conceptual model of entrepreneurship as firm behavior. *Entrepreneurship Theory & Practice,* Fall: 7–25; Lumpkin, G. T. & Dess, G. G. 1996. Clarifying the entrepreneurial orientation construct and linking it to performance. *Academy of Management Review,* 21: 135–172; and, Miller, D. 1983. The correlates of entrepreneurship in three types of firms. *Management Science,* 29: 770–791.

Autonomy

Autonomy refers to a willingness to act independently in order to carry forward an entrepreneurial vision or opportunity. It applies to both individuals and teams that operate outside an organization's existing norms and strategies. In the context of corporate entrepreneurship, autonomous work units are often used to leverage existing strengths in new arenas, identify opportunities that are beyond the organization's current capabilities, and encourage development of new ventures or improved business practices.[63]

The need for autonomy may apply to either dispersed or focused entrepreneurial efforts. Because of the emphasis on venture projects that are being developed outside the normal flow of business, a focused approach suggests a working environment that is relatively autonomous. But autonomy may also be important in an organization where entrepreneurship is part of the corporate culture. Everything from the methods of group interaction to the firm's reward system must make organizational members feel as if they can think freely about venture opportunities, take time to investigate them, and act without fear of condemnation. This implies a respect for the autonomy of each individual and an openness to the independent thinking that goes into championing a corporate venture idea. Thus, autonomy represents a type of empowerment (see Chapter 11) that is directed at identifying and leveraging entrepreneurial opportunities. Exhibit 12.5 identifies two techniques that organizations often use to promote autonomy.

autonomy
independent action by an individual or team aimed at bringing forth a business concept or vision and carrying it through to completion.

Exhibit 12.5 Autonomy Techniques

	Autonomy	
Technique	**Description/Purpose**	**Example**
Use skunkworks to foster entrepreneurial thinking.	Skunkworks are independent work units, often physically separate from corporate headquarters. They allow employees to get out from under the pressures of their daily routines to engage in creative problem solving.	Malaysia Airlines set up what it calls "laboratories," or skunkworks, small groups of people brought together on an ad hoc basis to address specific issues. A group stays together for a month or so, until it has fulfilled its agreed-upon "exit criteria."
Design organizational structures that support independent action.	Established companies with traditional structures often need to break out of such old forms to compete more effectively.	Deloitte Consulting, a division of Deloitte Touche Tohmatsu, found it difficult to compete against young agile firms. So it broke the firm into small autonomous units called "chip-aways" that operate with the flexibility of a start-up. In its first year, revenues were $40 million—10 percent higher than its projections.

Sources: Idea: Skunkworks. 2008. *The Economist, http://dr.economist.com/node/11993055*. August 25; Conlin, M. 2006. Square feet. oh how square! *BusinessWeek, www.businessweek.com*. July 3; Cross, K. 2001. Bang the drum quickly. *Business 2.0*, May: 28–30; Sweeney, J. 2004. A firm for all reasons. *Consulting Magazine, www.consultingmag.com*; and, Wagner, M. 2005. Out of the skunkworks. *Internet Retailer, www.internetretailer.com*. January.

Creating autonomous work units and encouraging independent action may have pitfalls that can jeopardize their effectiveness. Autonomous teams often lack coordination. Excessive decentralization has a strong potential to create inefficiencies, such as duplication of effort and wasting resources on projects with questionable feasibility. For example, Chris Galvin, former CEO of Motorola, scrapped the skunkworks approach the company had been using to develop new wireless phones. Fifteen teams had created 128 different phones, which led to spiraling costs and overly complex operations.[64]

For autonomous work units and independent projects to be effective, such efforts have to be measured and monitored. This requires a delicate balance: Companies must have the patience and budget to tolerate the explorations of autonomous groups and the strength to cut back efforts that are not bearing fruit. It must be undertaken with a clear sense of purpose—namely, to generate new sources of competitive advantage.

Innovativeness

innovativeness a willingness to introduce novelty through experimentation and creative processes aimed at developing new products and services as well as new processes.

Innovativeness refers to a firm's efforts to find new opportunities and novel solutions. In the beginning of this chapter we discussed innovation; here the focus is on innovativeness—a firm's attitude toward innovation and willingness to innovate. It involves creativity and experimentation that result in new products, new services, or improved technological processes.[65] Innovativeness is one of the major components of an entrepreneurial strategy. As indicated at the beginning of the chapter, however, the job of managing innovativeness can be very challenging.

Innovativeness requires that firms depart from existing technologies and practices and venture beyond the current state of the art. Inventions and new ideas need to be nurtured

The Body Shop Finds Social Responsibility Drives Business

Multinational corporations are among the most controversial organizations in modern times. An oft-repeated critique claims they exploit disadvantaged people and developing countries. But The Body Shop has deliberately chosen a different approach since its beginnings in the mid-1970s, becoming an international proponent of the view that corporations can and should make helpful contributions to the developing world.

The Body Shop was founded in 1976 by UK businesswoman and environmental activist Dame Anita Roddick. Today, as part of the L'Oréal Corporate Group, the chain does business in more than 45 countries and continues to be widely known as a pioneer for its staunch commitment to social and environmental concerns. In 1994, it formalized its conviction by modifying its mission statement to "help achieve positive social and environmental change by informing, inspiring, involving, and empowering employees, customers, and the community." The Body Shop is also regarded as a pioneer of modern corporate social responsibility (CSR) as one of the first companies to publish the Values Report. This was the precursor to all subsequent annual CSR reporting and the first time a company felt compelled to state not only its financial performance but also the nonfinancial impacts its operations had on the communities and the environment in which the company operated.

The Body Shop produces biodegradable products, promotes recycling, and requires each of its stores to get involved in community projects. At the 2002 World Summit on Sustainable Development, campaign members presented a petition with over 1.6 million signatures, calling on governments to get serious about climate change and to set a timetable as well as targets for renewable energy use. As part of The Body Shop's Trade Not Aid Project, a number of micro-enterprise initiatives were launched, illustrating the potential of fair trading practices. The project established direct trading links with producer communities in developing countries so that they can sustainably finance their own social and economic development. It also strives to protect a community's traditional way of life as well as the environment.

Sources: Unruh, G. 2010. Part I in a CSR series: Corporate citizenship in a global economy. *www.forbes.com*. May 7; The Body Shop: Living our values: The Values Report 2009, accessed at *www.thebodyshop.com/_en/_ww/services/aboutus_values.aspx;* and, Corporate responsibility at the Body Shop. 2003. *https://docs.google.com/viewer?a=v&q=cache:vaxj1Y0r3nsJ:lencd.com/data/docs/225-Bk3PartB_GLOBAL%2520body%2520shop.pdf+&hl=en&gl=us&pid=bl&srcid=ADGEESj9k-gNJm1jEA-S4G2c9mpc-RfiWSUhk0UyFKzjgHICGnAEtjwsVeyKvvWGgZv1l39k62nRbiktruFxcwePY-acGDOvQqUJFxGhucGsbTUDPspvE_a5zoZGMPS4a7JrmyPMsOB0a&sig=AHIEtbQs93lrypxCOPk8Cqf9omdd_TgLRQ.*

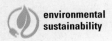

● The Body Shop, a global cosmetics retailer, has integrated social responsibility into all aspects of its value chain.

The aim of another Body Shop program—on community trade—is to support sustainable development by sourcing ingredients and accessories from disadvantaged communities around the world. One such example is henna, used in the hair color products the company introduced back in 2000. Henna is gathered by nomadic people in Somalia and supplied by Asli Mills, the trading arm of Candlelight for Health and Education, an NGO. Candlelight's initiative has given some 70 nomadic people an additional income as well as access to education and health programs, from which they would not normally benefit. Henna leaves are collected from trees that grow wild in mountainous regions, and Candlelight/Asli Mills monitors the harvest to ensure that the trees and local environment are not damaged.

The Body Shop's corporate purchasing policy includes an environmental checklist that employees consult for these kinds of issues when buying new supplies. It looks at ecological life-cycle assessments that take into account the waste impacts of raw material sourcing on biodiversity, human and animal rights, and endangered species. The company has also been a lead innovator in corporate auditing, which assesses a firm's environmental and social impacts in order to improve its practices. In a survey published in December 2001 by the *Financial Times,* media and non-governmental organizations ranked The Body Shop second among the world's best companies for managing environmental resources. Roddick's support of sustainable development was recognized with the United Nations' "Global 500" environmental award.

environmental sustainability

 ethics

even when their benefits are unclear. However, in today's climate of rapid change, effectively producing, assimilating, and exploiting innovations can be an important avenue for achieving competitive advantages. Interest in global warming and other ecological concerns has led many corporations to focus their innovativeness efforts on solving environmental problems. Strategy Spotlight 12.8 describes how The Body Shop uses entrepreneurial thinking and innovative practices to deliver socially responsible solutions.

As our earlier discussion of CE indicated, many corporations owe their success to an active program of innovation-based corporate venturing.[66] Exhibit 12.6 highlights two of the methods companies can use to enhance their competitive position through innovativeness.

Innovativeness can be a source of great progress and strong corporate growth, but there are also major pitfalls for firms that invest in innovation. Expenditures on R&D aimed at identifying new products or processes can be a waste of resources if the effort does not yield results. Another danger is related to the competitive climate. Even if a company innovates a new capability or successfully applies a technological breakthrough, another company may develop a similar innovation or find a use for it that is more profitable. Finally R&D and other innovation efforts are among the first to be cut back during an economic downturn.

Even though innovativeness is an important means of internal corporate venturing, it also involves major risks, because investments in innovations may not pay off. For strategic managers of entrepreneurial firms, successfully developing and adopting innovations can generate competitive advantages and provide a major source of growth for the firm.

proactiveness a forward-looking perspective characteristic of a marketplace leader that has the foresight to seize opportunities in anticipation of future demand.

Proactiveness

Proactiveness refers to a firm's efforts to seize new opportunities. Proactive organizations monitor trends, identify the future needs of existing customers, and anticipate changes

Exhibit 12.6 Innovativeness Techniques

Innovativeness		
Technique	**Description/Purpose**	**Example**
Foster creativity and experimentation.	Companies that support idea exploration and allow employees to express themselves creatively enhance innovation outcomes.	To tap into its reserves of innovative talent, Royal Dutch/Shell created "GameChanger" to help employees develop promising ideas. The process provides funding up to $600,000 for would-be entrepreneurs to pursue innovative projects and conduct experiments.
Invest in new technology, R&D, and continuous improvement.	The latest technologies often provide sources of new competitive advantages. To extract value from a new technology, companies must invest in it.	Dell Computer Corporation's new OptiPlex manufacturing system revolutionized the traditional assembly line. Hundreds of custom-built computers can be made in an eight-hour shift using state-of-the-art automation techniques that have increased productivity per person by 160 percent.

Sources: Breen, B. 2004. Living in Dell time. *Fast Company*, November: 88–92: Hammonds, K. H. 2002. Size is not a strategy. *Fast Company*, August: 78–83; Perman, S. 2001. Automate or die. *eCompanyNow.com*. July; Dell, M. 1999. *Direct from Dell*. New York: HarperBusiness; and Watson, R. 2006. Expand your innovation horizons. *Fast Company, www.fastcompany.com*. May.

in demand or emerging problems that can lead to new venture opportunities. Proactiveness involves not only recognizing changes but also being willing to act on those insights ahead of the competition.[67] Strategic managers who practice proactiveness have their eye on the future in a search for new possibilities for growth and development. Such a forward-looking perspective is important for companies that seek to be industry leaders. Many proactive firms seek out ways not only to be future oriented but also to change the very nature of competition in their industry.

Proactiveness puts competitors in the position of having to respond to successful initiatives. The benefit gained by firms that are the first to enter new markets, establish brand identity, implement administrative techniques, or adopt new operating technologies in an industry is called first mover advantage.[68]

First movers usually have several advantages. First, industry pioneers, especially in new industries, often capture unusually high profits because there are no competitors to drive prices down. Second, first movers that establish brand recognition are usually able to retain their image and hold on to the market share gains they earned by being first. Sometimes these benefits also accrue to other early movers in an industry, but, generally speaking, first movers have an advantage that can be sustained until firms enter the maturity phase of an industry's life cycle.[69]

First movers are not always successful. The customers of companies that introduce novel products or embrace breakthrough technologies may be reluctant to commit to a new way of doing things. In his book *Crossing the Chasm,* Geoffrey A. Moore noted that most firms seek evolution, not revolution, in their operations. This makes it difficult for a first mover to sell promising new technologies.[70]

Even with these caveats, however, companies that are first movers can enhance their competitive position. Exhibit 12.7 illustrates two methods firms can use to act proactively.

Exhibit 12.7 **Proactiveness Techniques**

Proactiveness		
Technique	**Description/Purpose**	**Example**
Introduce new products or technological capabilities ahead of the competition.	Being a first mover provides companies with an ability to shape the playing field and shift competitive advantages in their favor.	Sony's mission states, "We should always be the pioneers with our products—out front leading the market." This philosophy has made Sony technologically strong with industry-leading products such as the PlayStation and Vaio laptop computers.
Continuously seek out new product or service offerings.	Firms that provide new resources or sources of supply can benefit from a proactive stance.	Costco seized a chance to leverage its success as a warehouse club that sells premium brands when it introduced Costco Home Stores. The home stores are usually located near its warehouse stores and its rapid inventory turnover gives it a cost advantage of 15 to 25 percent over close competitors such as Bassett Furniture and Bombay Company.

Sources: Bryce, D. J. & Dyer, J. H. 2007. Strategies to crack well-guarded markets. *Harvard Business Review,* May: 84–92; Collins, J. C. & Porras, J. I. 1997. *Built to last.* New York: HarperBusiness; Robinson, D. 2005. Sony pushes reliability in Vaio laptops. *IT Week, www.itweek.co.uk.* October 12; and, *www.sony.com.*

Being an industry leader does not always lead to competitive advantages. Some firms that have launched pioneering new products or staked their reputation on new brands have failed to get the hoped-for payoff. Coca-Cola and PepsiCo invested $75 million to launch sodas that would capitalize on the low-carb diet trend. But with half the carbohydrates taken out, neither *C2,* Coke's entry, nor *Pepsi Edge* tasted very good. The two new brands combined never achieved more than 1 percent market share. PepsiCo halted production in 2005 and Coca-Cola followed suit in 2007.[71] Such missteps are indicative of the dangers of trying to proactively anticipate demand. Another danger for opportunity-seeking companies is that they will take their proactiveness efforts too far. For example, Porsche has tried to extend its brand images outside the automotive arena. While some efforts have worked, such as Porsche-designed T-shirts and sunglasses, other efforts have failed, such as the Porsche-branded golf clubs.

Careful monitoring and scanning of the environment, as well as extensive feasibility research, are needed for a proactive strategy to lead to competitive advantages. Firms that do it well usually have substantial growth and internal development to show for it. Many of them have been able to sustain the advantages of proactiveness for years.

Competitive Aggressiveness

competitive aggressiveness an intense effort to outperform industry rivals characterized by a combative posture or an aggressive response aimed at improving position or overcoming a threat in a competitive marketplace.

Competitive aggressiveness refers to a firm's efforts to outperform its industry rivals. Companies with an aggressive orientation are willing to "do battle" with competitors. They might slash prices and sacrifice profitability to gain market share or spend aggressively to obtain manufacturing capacity. As an avenue of firm development and growth, competitive aggressiveness may involve being very assertive in leveraging the results of other entrepreneurial activities such as innovativeness or proactiveness.

Competitive aggressiveness is directed toward competitors. The SWOT analysis discussed in Chapters 2 and 3 provides a useful way to distinguish between these different approaches to CE. Proactiveness, as we saw in the last section, is a response to opportunities—the O in SWOT. Competitive aggressiveness, by contrast, is a response to threats—the T in SWOT. A competitively aggressive posture is important for firms that seek to enter new markets in the face of intense rivalry.

Strategic managers can use competitive aggressiveness to combat industry trends that threaten their survival or market position. Sometimes firms need to be forceful in defending the competitive position that has made them an industry leader. Firms often need to be aggressive to ensure their advantage by capitalizing on new technologies or serving new market needs. Exhibit 12.8 suggests two of the ways competitively aggressive firms enhance their entrepreneurial position.

Another practice companies use to overcome the competition is to make preannouncements of new products or technologies. This type of signaling is aimed not only at potential customers but also at competitors to see how they will react or to discourage them from launching similar initiatives. Sometimes the preannouncements are made just to scare off competitors, an action that has potential ethical implications.

Competitive aggressiveness may not always lead to competitive advantages. Some companies (or their CEOs) have severely damaged their reputations by being overly aggressive. Although it continues to be a dominant player, Microsoft's highly aggressive profile makes it the subject of scorn by some businesses and individuals. Efforts to find viable replacements for the Microsoft products have helped fuel interest in alternative options provided by Google, Apple, and the open-source software movement.[72]

Competitive aggressiveness is a strategy that is best used in moderation. Companies that aggressively establish their competitive position and vigorously exploit opportunities to achieve profitability may, over the long run, be better able to sustain their competitive advantages if their goal is to defeat, rather than decimate, their competitors.

Exhibit 12.8 Competitive Aggressiveness Techniques

Competitive Aggressiveness		
Technique	**Description/Purpose**	**Example**
Enter markets with drastically lower prices.	Narrow operating margins make companies vulnerable to extended price competition.	HEATTECH is a highly functional line of innerwear from Japan that offers amazing comfort at a low price, which has won over a multitude of customers. In the 2010 fall/winter season, 80 million HEATTECH items were sold worldwide.
Find successful business models and copy them.	As long as a practice is not protected by intellectual property laws, it's probably okay to imitate it. Finding solutions to existing problems is generally quicker and cheaper than inventing them.	With annual revenues in excess of $89 million and over 400 stores, South Korea's fastest-growing coffee chain, Cafe Bene, received best reviews in a recent consumer survey as compared to international coffee chains such as Starbucks. The business model for selling not just coffee but also the entire space where coffee can be enjoyed has successfully appealed to Korean consumers.

Sources: Guth, R. A. 2006. Trolling the web for free labor, software upstarts are new force. *The Wall Street Journal,* November 12: 1; Mochari, I. 2001. Steal this strategy. *Inc.,* July: 62–67; *www.best-in-class.com*; and *www.zimbra.com*; UNIQLO Business Strategy. 2011. *www.fastretailing.com/eng/*; and, Lee, J. Y. 2011. Cafe Bene favored most among specialty coffee brands: Survey. *www.koreaherald.com/*. August 24.

Risk Taking

Risk taking refers to a firm's willingness to seize a venture opportunity even though it does not know whether the venture will be successful—to act boldly without knowing the consequences. To be successful through corporate entrepreneurship, firms usually have to take on riskier alternatives, even if it means forgoing the methods or products that have worked in the past. To obtain high financial returns, firms take such risks as assuming high levels of debt, committing large amounts of firm resources, introducing new products into new markets, and investing in unexplored technologies.

risk taking making decisions and taking action without certain knowledge of probable outcomes. Some undertakings may also involve making substantial resource commitments in the process of venturing forward.

All of the approaches to internal development that we have discussed are potentially risky. Whether they are being aggressive, proactive, or innovative, firms on the path of CE must act without knowing how their actions will turn out. Before launching their strategies, corporate entrepreneurs must know their firm's appetite for risk.[73]

Three types of risk that organizations and their executives face are business risk, financial risk, and personal risk:

- *Business risk taking* involves venturing into the unknown without knowing the probability of success. This is the risk associated with entering untested markets or committing to unproven technologies.
- *Financial risk taking* requires that a company borrow heavily or commit a large portion of its resources in order to grow. In this context, risk is used to refer to the risk/return trade-off that is familiar in financial analysis.
- *Personal risk taking* refers to the risks that an executive assumes in taking a stand in favor of a strategic course of action. Executives who take such risks stand to

Exhibit 12.9 Risk-Taking Techniques

Risk Taking		
Technique	**Description/Purpose**	**Example**
Research and assess risk factors to minimize uncertainty.	Companies that "do their homework"—that is, carefully evaluate the implications of bold actions—reduce the likelihood of failure.	Graybar Electric Co. took a risk when it invested $144 million to revamp its distribution system. It consolidated 231 small centers into 16 supply warehouses and installed the latest communications network. Graybar is now considered a leader in facility redesign and its sales have increased steadily since the consolidation, topping $5 billion in sales in a recent year.
Use techniques that have worked in other domains.	Risky methods that other companies have tried may provide an avenue for advancing company goals.	Teva, an international pharmaceutical company in Israel, advertised "Optalgin Pain Relief" during the UEFA Champions League final in 2010. Each time a player from Barcelona or Manchester United hit the ground after a foul, the Optalgin ad appeared at the bottom of the TV screen stating, "Optalgin. Strong for strong pain." Its ads made a big impression on spectators watching the match.

Sources: Anonymous. 2006. Graybar offers data center redesign seminars. *Cabling Installation and Maintenance, www.cim.pennnet.com* September 1; Keenan, F. & Mullaney, T. J. 2001. Clicking at Graybar. *BusinessWeek,* June 18: 132–34; Weintraub, A. 2001. Make or break for Autobytel. *BusinessWeek e.biz,* July 9: EB30-EB32; *www.autobytel.com*; *www.graybar.com*; and, *http://wn.com/Optalgin.*

influence the course of their whole company, and their decisions also can have significant implications for their careers.

Even though risk taking involves taking chances, it is not gambling. The best-run companies investigate the consequences of various opportunities and create scenarios of likely outcomes. A key to managing entrepreneurial risks is to evaluate new venture opportunities thoroughly enough to reduce the uncertainty surrounding them. Exhibit 12.9 indicates two methods companies can use to strengthen their competitive position through risk taking.

Risk taking, by its nature, involves potential dangers and pitfalls. Only carefully managed risk is likely to lead to competitive advantages. Actions that are taken without sufficient forethought, research, and planning may prove to be very costly. Therefore, strategic managers must always remain mindful of potential risks. In his book *Innovation and Entrepreneurship,* Peter Drucker argued that successful entrepreneurs are typically not risk takers. Instead, they take steps to minimize risks by carefully understanding them. That is how they avoid focusing on risk and remain focused on opportunity.[74] Risk taking is a good place to close this chapter on corporate entrepreneurship. Companies that choose to grow through internal corporate venturing must remember that entrepreneurship always involves embracing what is new and uncertain.

Reflecting on Career Implications . . .

- *Innovation:* Look around at the types of innovations being pursued by your company. Do they tend to be incremental or radical? Product-related or process-related? What new types of innovations might benefit your organization? How can you add value to such innovations?
- *Managing Innovation:* How might your organization's chances of a successful innovation increase through collaboration with innovation partners? Your ability to collaborate with individuals from other departments and firms will make you more receptive to and capable of innovation initiatives and enhance your career opportunities.
- *Corporate Entrepreneurship:* Do you consider the company you work for to be entrepreneurial? If not, what actions might you take to enhance its entrepreneurial spirit? If so, what have been the keys to its entrepreneurial success? Can these practices be repeated to achieve future successes?
- *Entrepreneurial Orientation:* Consider the five dimensions of entrepreneurial orientation. Is your organization especially strong at any of these? Especially weak? What are the career implications of your company's entrepreneurial strengths or weaknesses?

Summary

To remain competitive in today's economy, established firms must find new avenues for development and growth. This chapter has addressed how innovation and corporate entrepreneurship can be a means of internal venture creation and strategic renewal, and how an entrepreneurial orientation can help corporations enhance their competitive position.

Innovation is one of the primary means by which corporations grow and strengthen their strategic position. Innovations can take several forms, ranging from radical breakthrough innovations to incremental improvement innovations. Innovations are often used to update products and services or for improving organizational processes. Managing the innovation process is often challenging, because it involves a great deal of uncertainty and there are many choices to be made about the extent and type of innovations to pursue. By cultivating innovation skills, defining the scope of innovation, managing the pace of innovation, staffing to capture value from innovation, and collaborating with innovation partners, firms can more effectively manage the innovation process.

We also discussed the role of corporate entrepreneurship in venture development and strategic renewal. Corporations usually take either a focused or dispersed approach to corporate venturing. Firms with a focused approach usually separate the corporate venturing activity from the ongoing operations of the firm in order to foster independent thinking and encourage entrepreneurial team members to think and act without the constraints imposed by the corporation. In corporations where venturing activities are dispersed, a culture of entrepreneurship permeates all parts of the company in order to induce strategic behaviors by all organizational members. In measuring the success of corporate venturing activities, both financial and strategic objectives should be considered. Real options analysis is often used to make better quality decisions in uncertain entrepreneurial situations. However, a real options approach has potential drawbacks.

Most entrepreneurial firms need to have an entrepreneurial orientation: the methods, practices, and decision-making styles that strategic managers use to act entrepreneurially. Five dimensions of entrepreneurial orientation are found in firms that pursue corporate venture strategies. Autonomy, innovativeness, proactiveness, competitive aggressiveness, and risk taking each make a unique contribution to the pursuit of new opportunities. When deployed effectively, the methods and practices of an entrepreneurial orientation can be used to engage successfully in corporate entrepreneurship and new venture creation. However, strategic managers must remain mindful of the pitfalls associated with each of these approaches.

Summary Review Questions

1. What is meant by the concept of a continuum of radical and incremental innovations?

2. What are the dilemmas that organizations face when deciding what innovation projects to pursue? What steps can organizations take to effectively manage the innovation process?

3. What is the difference between focused and dispersed approaches to corporate entrepreneurship?

4. How are business incubators used to foster internal corporate venturing?

5. What is the role of the product champion in bringing a new product or service into existence in a corporation? How can companies use product champions to enhance their venture development efforts?

6. Explain the difference between proactiveness and competitive aggressiveness in terms of achieving and sustaining competitive advantage.

7. Describe how the entrepreneurial orientation (EO) dimensions of innovativeness, proactiveness, and risk taking can be combined to create competitive advantages for entrepreneurial firms.

Key Terms

innovation, 475
product innovation, 475
process innovation, 475
radical innovation, 475
incremental innovation, 476
strategic envelope, 480
corporate entrepreneurship, 484
focused approaches to corporate entrepreneurship, 488
new venture group, 488
business incubator, 488
dispersed approaches to corporate entrepreneurship, 490
entrepreneurial culture, 490
product champion, 490
exit champion, 493
real options analysis, 494
back-solver dilemma, 495
managerial conceit, 495
escalation of commitment, 496
entrepreneurial orientation, 496
autonomy, 497
innovativeness, 498
proactiveness, 500
competitive aggressiveness, 502
risk taking, 503

Entrepreneurial Orientation	Company A	Company B
Autonomy		
Innovativeness		
Proactiveness		
Competitive Aggressiveness		
Risk Taking		

Experiential Exercise

Select two different global corporations from two different industries (you might use Fortune 500 companies to make your selection). Compare and contrast these organizations in terms of their entrepreneurial orientation (using the above table).

Based on Your Comparison:

1. How is the corporation's entrepreneurial orientation reflected in its strategy?

2. Which corporation would you say has the stronger entrepreneurial orientation?

3. Is the corporation with the stronger entrepreneurial orientation also stronger in terms of financial performance?

Application Questions & Exercises

1. Select a firm known for its corporate entrepreneurship activities. Research the company and discuss how it has positioned itself relative to its close competitors.

Does it have a unique strategic advantage? Disadvantage? Explain.

2. Explain the difference between product innovations and process innovations. Provide examples of firms that have recently introduced each type of innovation. What are the types of innovations related to the strategies of each firm?

3. Using the Internet, select a company that is listed on the NASDAQ or London Stock Exchange. Research the extent to which the company has an entrepreneurial culture. Does the company use product champions? Does it have a corporate venture capital fund? Do you believe its entrepreneurial efforts are sufficient to generate sustainable advantages?

4. How can an established firm use an entrepreneurial orientation to enhance its overall strategic position? Provide examples.

Ethics Questions

1. Innovation activities are often aimed at making a discovery or commercializing a technology ahead of the competition. What are some of the unethical practices that companies could engage in during the innovation process? What are the potential long-term consequences of such actions?

2. Discuss the ethical implications of using entrepreneurial policies and practices to pursue corporate social responsibility goals. Are these efforts authentic and genuine or just an attempt to attract more customers?

References

1. HTC. 2010. About HTC. *HTC.com*, np; Einhorn, M. & Arndt, B. 2010. The 50 most innovative companies. *Bloomberg Businessweek,* April 25: 34–40; and, Jaroslovsky, R. 2010. HTC's elegant dead-end phone. *Bloomberg Businessweek,* April 25: 42. We thank Kimberly Kentfield for her valued contributions.

2. For an interesting discussion, see: Johannessen, J. A., Olsen, B., & Lumpkin, G. T. 2001. Innovation as newness: What is new, how new, and new to whom? *European Journal of Innovation Management,* 4(1): 20–31.

3. The discussion of product and process innovation is based on: Roberts, E. B. (Ed.). 2002. *Innovation: Driving product, process, and market change.* San Francisco: Jossey-Bass; Hayes, R. & Wheelwright, S. 1985. Competing through manufacturing. *Harvard Business Review,* 63(1): 99–109; and, Hayes, R. & Wheelwright, S. 1979. Dynamics of product–process life cycles. *Harvard Business Review,* 57(2): 127–136.

4. The discussion of radical and incremental innovations draws from: Leifer, R., McDermott, C. M., Colarelli, G., O'Connor, G. C., Peters, L. S., Rice, M. P., & Veryzer, R. W. 2000. *Radical innovation: How mature companies can outsmart upstarts.* Boston: Harvard Business School Press; Damanpour, F. 1996. Organizational complexity and innovation: Developing and testing multiple contingency models. *Management Science,* 42(5): 693–716; and, Hage, J. 1980. *Theories of organizations.* New York: Wiley.

5. Christensen, C. M. & Raynor, M. E. 2003. *The innovator's solution.* Boston: Harvard Business School Press.

6. Dressner, H. 2004. The Gartner Fellows interview: Clayton M. Christensen. *www.gartner.com.* April 26.

7. For another perspective on how different types of innovation affect organizational choices, see: Wolter, C. & Veloso, F. M. 2008. The effects of innovation on vertical structure: Perspectives on transactions costs and competences. *Academy of Management Review,* 33(3): 586–605.

8. Drucker, P. F. 1985. *Innovation and entrepreneurship: 2000.* New York: Harper & Row.

9. Birkinshaw, J., Hamel, G., & Mol, M. J. 2008. Management innovation. *Academy of Management Review,* 33(4): 825–845.

10. Steere, W. C., Jr. & Niblack, J. 1997. Pfizer, Inc. In Kanter, R. M., Kao, J., & Wiersema, F. (Eds.) *Innovation: Breakthrough thinking at 3M, DuPont, GE, Pfizer, and Rubbermaid:* 123–145. New York: HarperCollins.

11. Morrissey, C. A. 2000. Managing innovation through corporate venturing. *Graziadio Business Report,* Spring, *gbr.pepperdine.edu;* and, Sharma, A. 1999. Central dilemmas of managing innovation in large firms. *California Management Review,* 41(3): 147–164.

12. Sharma, op. cit.

13. Dyer, J. H., Gregerson, H. B., & Christensen, C. M. 2009. The innovator's DNA. *Harvard Business Review,* December: 61-67.

14. Eggers, J. P. & Kaplan, S. 2009. Cognition and renewal: Comparing CEO and organizational effects on incumbent adaptation to technical change. *Organization Science,* 20: 461–477.

15. Canabou, C. 2003. Fast ideas for slow times. *Fast Company,* May: 52.

16. Japan for Sustainability corporate website. 2005. Teijin develops photodegradable, biodegradable plastic. *www.japanfs.org/en/pages/025799.html.* January 9; and, Teijin corporate website. 2011. *www.teijin.co.jp/english/index.html.*

17. For more on defining the scope of innovation, see: Valikangas, L. & Gibbert, M. 2005. Boundary-setting strategies for escaping innovation traps. *MIT Sloan Management Review,* 46(3): 58–65.

18. Leifer et al., op. cit.

19. Bhide, A. V. 2000. *The origin and evolution of new businesses.* New York: Oxford University Press; and, Brown, S. L. & Eisenhardt, K. M. 1998. *Competing on the edge: Strategy as structured chaos.* Cambridge, MA: Harvard Business School Press.

20. Caulfield, B. 2003. Why techies don't get Six Sigma. *Business 2.0,* June: 90.

21. McGrath, R. G. & Keil, T. 2007. The value captor's process: Getting the most out of your new business ventures. *Harvard Business Review,* May: 128–136.

22. For an interesting discussion of how sharing technology knowledge with different divisions in an organization can contribute to innovation processes, see: Miller, D. J., Fern, M. J., & Cardinal, L. B. 2007. The use of knowledge for technological innovation within diversified firms. *Academy of Management Journal,* 50(2): 308–326.

23. Ketchen, D. J. Jr., Ireland, R. D., & Snow, C. C. 2007 Strategic entrepreneurship, collaborative innovation, and wealth creation. *Strategic Entrepreneurship Journal,* 1(3–4): 371–385.

24. Chesbrough, H. 2003. *Open innovation: The new imperative for creating and profiting from technology.* Boston: Harvard Business School Press.

25. For a recent study of what makes alliance partnerships successful, see: Sampson, R. C. 2007. R&D alliances and firm performance: The impact of technological diversity and alliance organization on innovation. *Academy of Management Journal,* 50(2): 364–386.

26. For an interesting perspective on the role of collaboration among multinational corporations, see: Hansen, M. T. & Nohria, N. 2004. How to build collaborative advantage. *MIT Sloan Management Review,* 46(1): 22–30.

27. Wells, R. M. J. 2008. The product innovation process: Are managing information flows and cross-functional collaboration key? *Academy of Management Perspectives,* 22(1): 58–60; Dougherty, D., & Dunne, D. D. 2011. Organizing ecologies of complex innovation. *Organization Science,* forthcoming. Kim, H. E. & Pennings, J. M. 2009. Innovation and strategic renewal in mature markets: A study of the tennis racket industry. *Organization Science,* 20: 368–383.

28. Guth, W. D. & Ginsberg, A. 1990. Guest editor's introduction: Corporate entrepreneurship. *Strategic Management Journal,* 11: 5–15.

29. Pinchot, G. 1985. *Intrapreneuring.* New York: Harper & Row.

30. For an interesting perspective on the role of context on the discovery and creation of opportunities, see: Zahra, S. A. 2008. The virtuous cycle of discovery and creation of entrepreneurial opportunities. *Strategic Entrepreneurship Journal,* 2(3): 243–257.

31. Birkinshaw, J. 1997. Entrepreneurship in multinational corporations: The characteristics of subsidiary initiatives. *Strategic Management Journal,* 18(3): 207–229; and, Kanter, R. M. 1985. *The change masters.* New York: Simon & Schuster.

32. Hansen, M. T., Chesbrough, H. W., Nohria, N., & Sull, D. 2000. Networked incubators: Hothouses of the new economy. *Harvard Business Review,* 78(5): 74–84.

33. Stein, T. 2002. Corporate venture investors are bailing out. *Red Herring,* December: 74–75.

34. For more on the importance of leadership in fostering a climate of entrepreneurship, see: Ling, Y., Simsek, Z., Lubatkin, M. H., & Veiga, J. F. 2008. Transformational leadership's role in promoting corporate entrepreneurship: Examining the CEO-TMT interface. *Academy of Management Journal,* 51(3): 557–576.

35. Is your company up to speed? 2003. *Fast Company,* June: 86.

36. For an interesting discussion, see: Davenport, T. H., Prusak, L., & Wilson, H. J. 2003. Who's bringing you hot ideas and how are you responding? *Harvard Business Review,* 80(1): 58–64.

37. Howell, J. M. 2005. The right stuff. Identifying and developing effective champions of innovation. *Academy of Management Executive,* 19(2): 108–119. See also Greene, P., Brush, C., & Hart, M. 1999. The corporate venture champion: A resource-based approach to role and process. *Entrepreneurship Theory & Practice,* 23(3): 103–122; and, Markham, S. K. & Aiman-Smith, L. 2001. Product champions: Truths, myths and management. *Research Technology Management,* May–June: 44–50.

38. Burgelman, R. A. 1983. A process model of internal corporate venturing in the diversified major firm. *Administrative Science Quarterly,* 28: 223–244.

39. Hamel, G. 2000. *Leading the revolution.* Boston: Harvard Business School Press.

40. Greene, Brush, & Hart, op. cit.; and, Shane, S. 1994. Are champions different from non-champions? *Journal of Business Venturing,* 9(5): 397–421.

41. Block, Z. & MacMillan, I. C. 1993. *Corporate venturing—creating new businesses with the firm.* Cambridge, MA: Harvard Business School Press.

42. For an interesting discussion of these trade-offs, see: Stringer, R. 2000. How to manage radical innovation. *California Management Review,* 42(4): 70–88; and, Gompers, P. A. & Lerner, J. 1999. *The venture capital cycle.* Cambridge, MA: MIT Press.

43. Cardinal, L. B., Turner, S. F., Fern, M. J., & Burton, R. M. 2011. Organizing for product development across technological environments: Performance trade-offs and priorities. *Organization Science,* forthcoming.

44. Albrinck, J., Hornery, J., Kletter, D., & Neilson, G. 2001. Adventures in corporate venturing. *Strategy + Business,* 22: 119–129; and, McGrath, R. G. & MacMillan, I. C. 2000. *The entrepreneurial mind-set.* Cambridge, MA: Harvard Business School Press.

45. Kiel, T., McGrath, R. G., Tukiainen, T., 2009. Gems from the ashes: Capability creation and transforming in internal corporate venturing. *Organization Science,* 20: 601–620.

46. For an interesting discussion of how different outcome goals affect organizational learning and employee motivation, see: Seijts, G. H. & Latham, G. P. 2005. Learning versus performance goals: When should each be used? *Academy of Management Executive,* 19(1): 124–131.

47. Crockett, R. O. 2001. Motorola. *BusinessWeek,* July 15: 72–78.

48. The ideas in this section are drawn from: Royer, I. 2003. Why bad projects are so hard to kill. *Harvard Business Review,* 81(2): 48–56.

49. For an interesting perspective on the different roles that individuals play in the entrepreneurial process, see: Baron, R. A. 2008. The role of affect in the entrepreneurial process. *Academy of Management Review,* 33(2): 328–340.

50. Hoskin, R. E. 1994. *Financial accounting*. New York: Wiley.

51. We know stock options as derivative assets—that is, "an asset whose value depends on or is derived from the value of another, the underlying asset": Amram, M. & Kulatilaka, N. 1999. *Real options: Managing strategic investment in an uncertain world: 34*. Boston: Harvard Business School Press.

52. For an interesting discussion on why it is difficult to "kill options," refer to: Royer, op. cit.

53. Slywotzky, A. & Wise, R. 2003. Double-digit growth in no-growth times. *Fast Company,* April: 66–72; *www.hoovers.com;* and, *www.johnsoncontrols.com.*

54. For more on the role of real options in entrepreneurial decision making, see: Folta, T. B. & O'Brien, J. P. 2004. Entry in the presence of dueling options. *Strategic Management Journal,* 25: 121–138.

55. This section draws on: Janney, J. J. & Dess, G. G. 2004. Can real options analysis improve decision-making? Promises and pitfalls. *Academy of Management Executive,* 18(4): 60–75. For additional insights on pitfalls of real options, consider: McGrath, R. G. 1997. A real options logic for initiating technology positioning investment. *Academy of Management Review,* 22(4): 974–994; Coff, R. W. & Laverty, K. J. 2001. Real options on knowledge assets: Panacea or Pandora's box? *Business Horizons,* 73: 79; McGrath, R. G. 1999. Falling forward: Real options reasoning and entrepreneurial failure. *Academy of Management Review,* 24(1): 13–30; and, Zardkoohi, A. 2004. Do Real Options Lead to Escalation of Commitment? *Academy of Management Review,* 29(1): 111–119.

56. For an understanding of the differences between how managers say they approach decisions and how they actually do, March and Shapira's discussion is perhaps the best: March, J. G. & Shapira, Z. 1987. Managerial perspectives on risk and risk-taking. *Management Science,* 33(11): 1404–1418.

57. A discussion of some factors that may lead to escalation in decision making is included in: Choo, C. W. 2005. Information failures and organizational disasters. *MIT Sloan Management Review,* 46(3): 8–10.

58. For an interesting discussion of the use of real options analysis in the application of wireless communications, which helped to lower the potential for escalation, refer to: McGrath, R. G., Ferrier, W. J., & Mendelow, A. L. 2004. Real options as engines of choice and heterogeneity. *Academy of Management Review,* 29(1): 86–101.

59. One very useful solution for reducing the effects of managerial conceit is to incorporate an "exit champion" into the decision process. Exit champions provide arguments for killing off the firm's commitment to a decision. For a very insightful discussion on exit champions, refer to: Royer, op. cit.

60. For more on how entrepreneurial orientation influences organizational performance, see: Wang, L. 2008. Entrepreneurial orientation, learning orientation, and firm performance. *Entrepreneurship Theory & Practice,* 32(4): 635–657; and, Runyan, R., Droge, C., & Swinney, J. 2008. Entrepreneurial orientation versus small business orientation: What are their relationships to firm performance? *Journal of Small Business Management,* 46(4): 567–588.

61. Covin, J. G. & Slevin, D. P. 1991. A conceptual model of entrepreneurship as firm behavior. *Entrepreneurship Theory and Practice,* 16(1): 7–24; Lumpkin, G. T. & Dess, G. G. 1996. Clarifying the entrepreneurial orientation construct and linking it to performance. *Academy of Management Review,* 21(1): 135–172; and, McGrath, R. G. & MacMillan, I. C. 2000. *The entrepreneurial mind-set.* Cambridge, MA: Harvard Business School Press.

62. Lumpkin, G. T. & Dess, G. G. 2001. Linking two dimensions of entrepreneurial orientation to firm performance: The moderating role of environment and life cycle. *Journal of Business Venturing,* 16: 429–451.

63. For an interesting discussion, see: Day, J. D., Mang, P. Y., Richter, A., & Roberts, J. 2001. The innovative organization: Why new ventures need more than a room of their own. *McKinsey Quarterly,* 2: 21–31.

64. Crockett, R. O. 2001. Chris Galvin shakes things up—again. *BusinessWeek,* May 28: 38–39.

65. For insights into the role of information technology in innovativeness, see: Dibrell, C., Davis, P. S., & Craig, J. 2008. Fueling innovation through information technology in SMEs. *Journal of Small Business Management,* 46(2): 203–218.

66. For an interesting discussion of the impact of innovativeness on organizational outcomes, see: Cho, H. J. & Pucik, V. 2005. Relationship between innovativeness, quality, growth, profitability, and market value. *Strategic Management Journal,* 26(6): 555–575.

67. Danneels, E., & Sethi, R. 2011. New product exploration under environmental turbulence. *Organization Science,* forthcoming.

68. Lieberman, M. B. & Montgomery, D. B. 1988. First mover advantages. *Strategic Management Journal,* 9 (Special Issue): 41–58.

69. The discussion of first mover advantages is based on several articles, including: Lambkin, M. 1988. Order of entry and performance in new markets. *Strategic Management Journal,* 9: 127–140; Lieberman & Montgomery, op. cit.: 41–58; and, Miller, A. & Camp, B. 1985. Exploring determinants of success in corporate ventures. *Journal of Business Venturing,* 1(2): 87–105.

70. Moore, G. A. 1999. *Crossing the chasm* (2nd ed.). New York: HarperBusiness.

71. Mallas, S. 2005. PepsiCo loses its Edge. *Motley Fool, www.fool.com.* June 1.

72. Lyons, D. 2006. The cheap revolution. *Forbes,* September 18: 102–111.

73. Miller, K. D. 2007. Risk and rationality in entrepreneurial processes. *Strategic Entrepreneurship Journal,* 1(1–2): 57–74.

74. Drucker, op. cit., pp. 109–110.

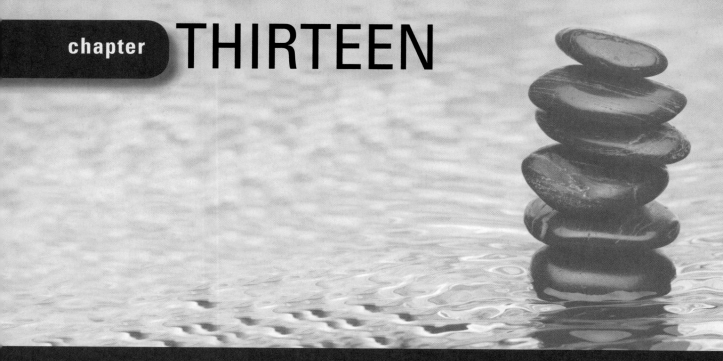

After reading this chapter, you should have a good understanding of:

LO13.1   How strategic case analysis is used to simulate real-world experiences.

LO13.2   How analyzing strategic management cases can help develop the ability to differentiate, speculate, and integrate when evaluating complex business problems.

LO13.3   The steps involved in conducting a strategic management case analysis.

LO13.4   How to get the most out of case analysis.

LO13.5   How conflict-inducing discussion techniques can lead to better decisions.

LO13.6   How to use the strategic insights and material from each of the 12 previous chapters in the text to analyze issues posed by strategic management cases.

LEARNING OBJECTIVES

Case analysis is one of the most effective ways to learn strategic management. It provides a complement to other methods of instruction by asking you to use the tools and techniques of strategic management to deal with an actual business situation. Strategy cases include detailed descriptions of management challenges faced by executives and business owners. By studying the background and analyzing the strategic predicaments posed by a case, you first see that the circumstances businesses confront are often difficult and complex. Then you are asked what decisions you would make to address the situation in the case and how the actions you recommend will affect the company. Thus, the processes of analysis, formulation, and implementation that have been addressed in this textbook can be applied in a real-life situation.

In this chapter we will discuss the role of case analysis as a learning tool in both the classroom and the real world. One of the benefits of strategic case analysis is to develop the ability to differentiate, speculate, and integrate. We will also describe how to conduct a case analysis and address techniques for deriving the greatest benefit from the process, including the effective use of conflict-inducing decision techniques. Finally, we will discuss how case analysis in a classroom setting can enhance the process of analyzing, making decisions, and taking action in real-world strategic situations.

Why Analyze Strategic Management Cases?

>LO13.1

How strategic case analysis is used to simulate real-world experiences.

It is often said that the key to finding good answers is to ask good questions. Strategic managers and business leaders are required to evaluate options, make choices, and find solutions to the challenges they face every day. To do so, they must learn to ask the right questions. The study of strategic management poses the same challenge. The process of analyzing, decision making, and implementing strategic actions raises many good questions.

- Why do some firms succeed and others fail?
- Why are some companies higher performers than others?
- What information is needed in the strategic planning process?
- How do competing values and beliefs affect strategic decision making?
- What skills and capabilities are needed to implement a strategy effectively?

case analysis a method of learning complex strategic management concepts—such as environmental analysis, the process of decision making, and implementing strategic actions—through placing students in the middle of an actual situation and challenging them to figure out what to do.

How does a student of strategic management answer these questions? By strategic case analysis. **Case analysis** simulates the real-world experience that strategic managers and company leaders face as they try to determine how best to run their companies. It places students in the middle of an actual situation and challenges them to figure out what to do.[1]

Asking the right questions is just the beginning of case analysis. In the previous chapters we have discussed issues and challenges that managers face and provided analytical frameworks for understanding the situation. But once the analysis is complete, decisions have to be made. Case analysis forces you to choose among different options and set forth a plan of action based on your choices. But even then the job is not done. Strategic case analysis also requires that you address how you will implement the plan and the implications of choosing one course of action over another.

A strategic management case is a detailed description of a challenging situation faced by an organization.[2] It usually includes a chronology of events and extensive support materials, such as financial statements, product lists, and transcripts of interviews with employees. Although names or locations are sometimes changed to provide anonymity, cases usually report the facts of a situation as authentically as possible.

One of the main reasons to analyze strategic management cases is to develop an ability to evaluate business situations critically. In case analysis, memorizing key terms and conceptual frameworks is not enough. To analyze a case, it is important that you go beyond textbook prescriptions and quick answers. It requires you to look deeply into the information that is provided and root out the essential issues and causes of a company's problems.

>LO13.2

How analyzing strategic management cases can help develop the ability to differentiate, speculate, and integrate when evaluating complex business problems.

The types of skills that are required to prepare an effective strategic case analysis can benefit you in actual business situations. Case analysis adds to the overall learning experience by helping you acquire or improve skills that may not be taught in a typical lecture course. Three capabilities that can be learned by conducting case analysis are especially useful to strategic managers—the ability to differentiate, speculate, and integrate.[3] Here's how case analysis can enhance those skills.

1. **Differentiate.** Effective strategic management requires that many different elements of a situation be evaluated at once. This is also true in case analysis. When analyzing cases, it is important to isolate critical facts, evaluate whether assumptions are useful or faulty, and distinguish between good and bad information. Differentiating between the factors that are influencing the situation presented by a case is necessary for making a good analysis. Strategic management also involves understanding that problems are often complex and multilayered. This applies to case analysis as well. Ask whether the case deals with operational, business-level, or corporate issues. Do the problems stem from weaknesses in the internal value chain or threats in

the external environment? Dig deep. Being too quick to accept the easiest or least controversial answer will usually fail to get to the heart of the problem.

2. *Speculate.* Strategic managers need to be able to use their imagination to envision an explanation or solution that might not readily be apparent. The same is true with case analysis. Being able to imagine different scenarios or contemplate the outcome of a decision can aid the analysis. Managers also have to deal with uncertainty since most decisions are made without complete knowledge of the circumstances. This is also true in case analysis. Case materials often seem to be missing data or the information provided is contradictory. The ability to speculate about details that are unknown or the consequences of an action can be helpful.

3. *Integrate.* Strategy involves looking at the big picture and having an organization-wide perspective. Strategic case analysis is no different. Even though the chapters in this textbook divide the material into various topics that may apply to different parts of an organization, all of this information must be integrated into one set of recommendations that will affect the whole company. A strategic manager needs to comprehend how all the factors that influence the organization will interact. This also applies to case analysis. Changes made in one part of the organization affect other parts. Thus, a holistic perspective that integrates the impact of various decisions and environmental influences on all parts of the organization is needed.

In business, these three activities sometimes "compete" with each other for your attention. For example, some decision makers may have a natural ability to differentiate among elements of a problem but are not able to integrate them very well. Others have enough innate creativity to imagine solutions or fill in the blanks when information is missing. But they may have a difficult time when faced with hard numbers or cold facts. Even so, each of these skills is important. The mark of a good strategic manager is the ability to simultaneously make distinctions and envision the whole, and to imagine a future scenario while staying focused on the present. Thus, another reason to conduct case analysis is to help you develop and exercise your ability to differentiate, speculate, and integrate.

Case analysis takes the student through the whole cycle of activity that a manager would face. Beyond the textbook descriptions of concepts and examples, case analysis asks you to "walk a mile in the shoes" of the strategic decision maker and learn to evaluate situations critically. Executives and owners must make decisions every day with limited information and a swirl of business activity going on around them. Consider the example of Sapient Health Network, an Internet start-up that had to undergo some analysis and problem solving just to survive. Strategy Spotlight 13.1 describes how this company transformed itself after a serious self-examination during a time of crisis.

As you can see from the experience of Sapient Health Network, businesses are often faced with immediate challenges that threaten their lives. The Sapient case illustrates how the strategic management process helped it survive. First, the company realistically assessed the environment, evaluated the marketplace, and analyzed its resources. Then it made tough decisions, which included shifting its market focus, hiring and firing, and redeploying its assets. Finally, it took action. The result was not only firm survival, but also a quick turnaround leading to rapid success.

How to Conduct a Case Analysis

>LO13.3
The steps involved in conducting a strategic management case analysis.

The process of analyzing strategic management cases involves several steps. In this section we will review the mechanics of preparing a case analysis. Before beginning, there are two things to keep in mind that will clarify your understanding of the process and make the results of the process more meaningful.

Analysis, Decision Making, and Change at Sapient Health Network

Sapient Health Network (SHN) had gotten off to a good start. CEO Jim Kean and his two cofounders had raised $5 million in investor capital to launch their vision: an Internet-based health care information subscription service. The idea was to create an Internet community for people suffering from chronic diseases. It would provide members with expert information, resources, a message board, and chat rooms so that people suffering from the same ailments could provide each other with information and support. "Who would be more voracious consumers of information than people who are faced with life-changing, life-threatening illnesses?" thought Bill Kelly, one of SHN's cofounders. Initial market research and beta tests had supported that view.

During the beta tests, however, the service had been offered for free. The troubles began when SHN tried to convert its trial subscribers into paying ones. Fewer than 5 percent signed on, far less than the 15 percent the company had projected. Sapient hired a vice president of marketing who launched an aggressive promotion, but after three months of campaigning SHN still had only 500 members. SHN was now burning through $400,000 per month, with little revenue to show for it.

At that point, according to SHN board member Susan Clymer, "there was a lot of scrambling around trying to figure out how we could wring value out of what we'd already accomplished." One thing SHN had created was

an expert software system which had two components: an "intelligent profile engine" (IPE) and an "intelligent query engine" (IQE). SHN used this system to collect detailed information from its subscribers.

SHN was sure that the expert system was its biggest selling point. But how could the service use it? Then the founders remembered that the original business plan had suggested there might be a market for aggregate data about patient populations gathered from the website. Could they turn the business around by selling patient data? To analyze the possibility, Kean tried out the idea on the market research arm of a huge East Coast health care conglomerate. The officials were intrigued. SHN realized that its expert system could become a market research tool.

Once the analysis was completed, the founders made the decision: They would still create Internet communities for chronically ill patients, but the service would be free. And they would transform SHN from a company that processed subscriptions to one that sold market research.

Finally, they enacted the changes. Some of it was painful, including laying off 18 employees. Instead, SHN needed more health care industry expertise. It even hired an interim CEO, Craig Davenport, a 25-year veteran of the industry, to steer the company in its new direction. Finally, SHN had to communicate a new message to its members. It began by reimbursing the $10,000 of subscription fees they had paid.

All of this paid off dramatically in a matter of just two years. Revenues jumped to $1.9 million and early in the third year, SHN was purchased by WebMD. Less than a year after that, WebMD merged with Healtheon. The combined company still operates a thriving office out of SHN's original location in Portland, Oregon.

Sources: Ferguson, S. 2007. Health care gets a better IT prescription. *Baseline,* www.baselinemag.com. May 24; Brenneman, K. 2000. Healtheon/WebMD's local office is thriving. *Business Journal of Portland,* June 2; and, Raths, D. 1998. Reversal of Fortune. *Inc. Technology,* 2: 52–62.

First, unless you prepare for a case discussion, there is little you can gain from the discussion and even less that you can offer. Effective strategic managers don't enter into problem-solving situations without doing some homework—investigating the situation, analyzing and researching possible solutions, and sometimes gathering the advice of others. Good problem solving often requires that decision makers be immersed in the facts, options, and implications surrounding the problem. In case analysis, this means reading and thoroughly comprehending the case materials before trying to make an analysis.

The second point is related to the first. To get the most out of a case analysis you must place yourself "inside" the case—that is, think like an actual participant in the case situation. However, there are several positions you can take. These are discussed in the following paragraphs:

- **Strategic decision maker.** This is the position of the senior executive responsible for resolving the situation described in the case. It may be the CEO, the business owner, or a strategic manager in a key executive position.

- **Board of directors.** Since the board of directors represents the owners of a corporation, it has a responsibility to step in when a management crisis threatens the company. As a board member, you may be in a unique position to solve problems.
- **Outside consultant.** Either the board or top management may decide to bring in outsiders. Consultants often have an advantage because they can look at a situation objectively. But they also may be at a disadvantage since they have no power to enforce changes.

Before beginning the analysis, it may be helpful to envision yourself assuming one of these roles. Then, as you study and analyze the case materials, you can make a diagnosis and recommend solutions in a way that is consistent with your position. Try different perspectives. You may find that your view of the situation changes depending on the role you play. As an outside consultant, for example, it may be easy for you to conclude that certain individuals should be replaced in order to solve a problem presented in the case. However, if you take the role of the CEO who knows the individuals and the challenges they have been facing, you may be reluctant to fire them and will seek another solution instead.

The idea of assuming a particular role is similar to the real world in various ways. In your career, you may work in an organization where outside accountants, bankers, lawyers, or other professionals are advising you about how to resolve business situations or improve your practices. Their perspective will be different from yours but it is useful to understand things from their point of view. Conversely, you may work as a member of the audit team of an accounting firm or the loan committee of a bank. In those situations, it would be helpful if you understood the situation from the perspective of the business leader who must weigh your views against all the other advice that he or she receives. Case analysis can help develop an ability to appreciate such multiple perspectives.

One of the most challenging roles to play in business is as a business founder or owner. For small businesses or entrepreneurial start-ups, the founder may wear all hats at once—key decision maker, primary stockholder, and CEO. Hiring an outside consultant may not be an option. However, the issues faced by young firms and established firms are often not that different, especially when it comes to formulating a plan of action. Business plans that entrepreneurial firms use to raise money or propose a business expansion typically revolve around a few key issues that must be addressed no matter what the size or age of the business. Strategy Spotlight 13.2 reviews business planning issues that are most important to consider when evaluating any case, especially from the perspective of the business founder or owner.

Next we will review five steps to follow when conducting a strategic management case analysis: becoming familiar with the material, identifying the problems, analyzing the strategic issues using the tools and insights of strategic management, proposing alternative solutions, and making recommendations.[4]

Become Familiar with the Material

Written cases often include a lot of material. They may be complex and include detailed financials or long passages. Even so, to understand a case and its implications, you must become familiar with its content. Sometimes key information is not immediately apparent. It may be contained in the footnotes to an exhibit or an interview with a lower-level employee. In other cases the important points may be difficult to grasp because the subject matter is so unfamiliar. When you approach a strategic case try the following technique to enhance comprehension:

- Read quickly through the case one time to get an overall sense of the material.
- Use the initial read-through to assess possible links to strategic concepts.
- Read through the case again, in depth. Make written notes as you read.

Using a Business Plan Framework to Analyze Strategic Cases

Established businesses often have to change what they are doing in order to improve their competitive position or sometimes simply to survive. To make the changes effectively, businesses usually need a plan. Business plans are no longer just for entrepreneurs. The kind of market analysis, decision making, and action planning that is considered standard practice among new ventures can also benefit going concerns that want to make changes, seize an opportunity, or head in a new direction.

The best business plans, however, are not those loaded with decades of month-by-month financial projections or that depend on rigid adherence to a schedule of events that is impossible to predict. The good ones are focused on four factors that are critical to new-venture success. These same factors are important in case analysis as well because they get to the heart of many of the problems found in strategic cases.

1. *The People.* "When I receive a business plan, I always read the résumé section first," said Harvard Professor William Sahlman. The people questions that are critically important to investors include: What are their skills? How much experience do they have? What is their reputation? Have they worked together as a team? These same questions also may be used in case analysis to evaluate the role of individuals in the strategic case.

2. *The Opportunity.* Business opportunities come in many forms. They are not limited to new ventures.

The chance to enter new markets, introduce new products, or merge with a competitor provides many of the challenges that are found in strategic management cases. What are the consequences of such actions? Will the proposed changes affect the firm's business concept? What factors might stand in the way of success? The same issues are also present in most strategic cases.

3. *The Context.* Things happen in contexts that cannot be controlled by a firm's managers. This is particularly true of the general environment where social trends, economic changes, or events such as the September 11, 2001, terrorist attacks can change business overnight. When evaluating strategic cases, ask: Is the company aware of the impact of context on the business? What will it do if the context changes? Can it influence the context in a way that favors the company?

4. *Risk and Reward.* With a new venture, the entrepreneurs and investors take the risks and get the rewards. In strategic cases, the risks and rewards often extend to many other stakeholders, such as employees, customers, and suppliers. When analyzing a case, ask: Are the managers making choices that will pay off in the future? Are the rewards evenly distributed? Will some stakeholders be put at risk if the situation in the case changes? What if the situation remains the same? Could that be even riskier?

Whether a business is growing or shrinking, large or small, industrial or service oriented, the issues of people, opportunities, context, and risks and rewards will have a large impact on its performance. Therefore, you should always consider these four factors when evaluating strategic management cases.

Sources: Wasserman, E. 2003. A simple plan. *MBA Jungle*, February: 50–55; DeKluyver, C. A. 2000. *Strategic thinking: An executive perspective.* Upper Saddle River, NJ: Prentice Hall; and, Sahlman, W. A. 1997. How to write a great business plan. *Harvard Business Review,* 75(4): 98–108.

- Evaluate how strategic concepts might inform key decisions or suggest alternative solutions.
- After formulating an initial recommendation, thumb through the case again quickly to help assess the consequences of the actions you propose.

Identify Problems

When conducting case analysis, one of your most important tasks is to identify the problem. Earlier we noted that one of the main reasons to conduct case analysis was to find solutions. But you cannot find a solution unless you know the problem. Another saying you may have heard is, "A good diagnosis is half the cure." In other words, once you have determined what the problem is, you are well on your way to identifying a reasonable solution.

Some cases have more than one problem. But the problems are usually related. For a hypothetical example, consider the following: Company A was losing customers to a new competitor. Upon analysis, it was determined that the competitor had a 50 percent faster delivery time even though its product was of lower quality. The managers of company A could not understand why customers would settle for an inferior product. It turns out that no one was marketing to company A's customers that its product was superior. A second problem was that falling sales resulted in cuts in company A's sales force. Thus, there were two related problems: inferior delivery technology and insufficient sales effort.

When trying to determine the problem, avoid getting hung up on **case symptoms**. Zero in on the problem. For example, in the company A example above, the symptom was losing customers. But the problems were an underfunded, understaffed sales force combined with an outdated delivery technology. Try to see beyond the immediate symptoms to the more fundamental **case problems**.

case symptoms
observable and concrete information in a case analysis that indicates an undesirable state of affairs.

Another tip when preparing a case analysis is to articulate the problem.[5] Writing down a problem statement gives you a reference point to turn to as you proceed through the case analysis. This is important because the process of formulating strategies or evaluating implementation methods may lead you away from the initial problem. Make sure your recommendation actually addresses the problems you have identified.

case problems
inferred causes of case symptoms.

One more thing about identifying problems: Sometimes problems are not apparent until *after* you do the analysis. In some cases the problem will be presented plainly, perhaps in the opening paragraph or on the last page of the case. But in other cases the problem does not emerge until after the issues in the case have been analyzed. We turn next to the subject of strategic case analysis.

Conduct Strategic Analyses

This textbook has presented numerous analytical tools (e.g., five-forces analysis and value-chain analysis), contingency frameworks (e.g., when to use related rather than unrelated diversification strategies), and other techniques that can be used to evaluate strategic situations. The previous 12 chapters have addressed practices that are common in strategic management, but only so much can be learned by studying the practices and concepts. The best way to understand these methods is to apply them by conducting analyses of specific cases.

The first step is to determine which strategic issues are involved. Is there a problem in the company's competitive environment? Or is it an internal problem? If it is internal, does it have to do with organizational structure? Strategic controls? Uses of technology? Or perhaps the company has overworked its employees or underutilized its intellectual capital. Has the company mishandled a merger? Chosen the wrong diversification strategy? Botched a new product introduction? Each of these issues is linked to one or more of the concepts discussed earlier in the text. Determine what strategic issues are associated with the problems you have identified. Remember also that most real-life case situations involve issues that are highly interrelated. Even in cases where there is only one major problem, the strategic processes required to solve it may involve several parts of the organization.

Once you have identified the issues that apply to the case, conduct the analysis. For example, you may need to conduct a five-forces analysis or dissect the company's competitive strategy. Perhaps you need to evaluate whether its resources are rare, valuable, difficult to imitate, or difficult to substitute. Financial analysis may be needed to assess the company's economic prospects. Perhaps the international entry mode needs to be reevaluated because of changing conditions in the host country. Employee empowerment techniques may need to be improved to enhance organizational learning. Whatever the case, all the strategic concepts introduced in the text include insights for assessing their effectiveness. Determining how well a company is doing these things is central to the case analysis process.

financial ratio analysis a method of evaluating a company's performance and financial well-being through ratios of accounting values, including short-term solvency, long-term solvency, asset utilization, profitability, and market value ratios.

Financial ratio analysis is one of the primary tools used to conduct case analysis. Appendix 1 to Chapter 13 includes a discussion and examples of the financial ratios that are often used to evaluate a company's performance and financial well-being. Exhibit 13.1 provides a summary of the financial ratios presented in Appendix 1 to this chapter.

In this part of the overall strategic analysis process, it is also important to test your own assumptions about the case.[6] First, what assumptions are you making about the case materials? It may be that you have interpreted the case content differently than your team members or classmates. Being clear about these assumptions will be important in determining how to analyze the case. Second, what assumptions have you made about the best way to resolve the problems? Ask yourself why you have chosen one type of analysis over another. This process of assumption checking can also help determine if you have gotten to the heart of the problem or are still just dealing with symptoms.

Exhibit 13.1   Summary of Financial Ratio Analysis Techniques

Ratio	What It Measures
Short-term solvency, or liquidity, ratios:	
Current ratio	Ability to use assets to pay off liabilities.
Quick ratio	Ability to use liquid assets to pay off liabilities quickly.
Cash ratio	Ability to pay off liabilities with cash on hand.
Long-term solvency, or financial leverage, ratios:	
Total debt ratio	How much of a company's total assets are financed by debt.
Debt-equity ratio	Compares how much a company is financed by debt with how much it is financed by equity.
Equity multiplier	How much debt is being used to finance assets.
Times interest earned ratio	How well a company has its interest obligations covered.
Cash coverage ratio	A company's ability to generate cash from operations.
Asset utilization, or turnover, ratios:	
Inventory turnover	How many times each year a company sells its entire inventory.
Days' sales in inventory	How many days on average inventory is on hand before it is sold.
Receivables turnover	How frequently each year a company collects on its credit sales.
Days' sales in receivables	How many days on average it takes to collect on credit sales (average collection period).
Total asset turnover	How much of sales is generated for every dollar in assets.
Capital intensity	The dollar investment in assets needed to generate $1 in sales.
Profitability ratios:	
Profit margin	How much profit is generated by every dollar of sales.
Return on assets (ROA)	How effectively assets are being used to generate a return.
Return on equity (ROE)	How effectively amounts invested in the business by its owners are being used to generate a return.
Market value ratios:	
Price-earnings ratio	How much investors are willing to pay per dollar of current earnings.
Market-to-book ratio	Compares market value of the company's investments to the cost of those investments.

As mentioned earlier, sometimes the critical diagnosis in a case can only be made after the analysis is conducted. However, by the end of this stage in the process, you should know the problems and have completed a thorough analysis of them. You can now move to the next step: finding solutions.

Propose Alternative Solutions

It is important to remember that in strategic management case analysis, there is rarely one right answer or one best way. Even when members of a class or a team agree on what the problem is, they may not agree upon how to solve the problem. Therefore, it is helpful to consider several different solutions.

After conducting strategic analysis and identifying the problem, develop a list of options. What are the possible solutions? What are the alternatives? First, generate a list of all the options you can think of without prejudging any one of them. Remember that not all cases call for dramatic decisions or sweeping changes. Some companies just need to make small adjustments. In fact, "Do nothing" may be a reasonable alternative in some cases. Although that is rare, it might be useful to consider what will happen if the company does nothing. This point illustrates the purpose of developing alternatives: to evaluate what will happen if a company chooses one solution over another.

Thus, during this step of a case analysis, you will evaluate choices and the implications of those choices. One aspect of any business that is likely to be highlighted in this part of the analysis is strategy implementation. Ask how the choices made will be implemented. It may be that what seems like an obvious choice for solving a problem creates an even bigger problem when implemented. But remember also that no strategy or strategic "fix" is going to work if it cannot be implemented. Once a list of alternatives is generated, ask:

- Can the company afford it? How will it affect the bottom line?
- Is the solution likely to evoke a competitive response?
- Will employees throughout the company accept the changes? What impact will the solution have on morale?
- How will the decision affect other stakeholders? Will customers, suppliers, and others buy into it?
- How does this solution fit with the company's vision, mission, and objectives?
- Will the culture or values of the company be changed by the solution? Is it a positive change?

The point of this step in the case analysis process is to find a solution that both solves the problem and is realistic. A consideration of the implications of various alternative solutions will generally lead you to a final recommendation that is more thoughtful and complete.

Make Recommendations

The basic aim of case analysis is to find solutions. Your analysis is not complete until you have recommended a course of action. In this step the task is to make a set of recommendations that your analysis supports. Describe exactly what needs to be done. Explain why this course of action will solve the problem. The recommendation should also include suggestions for how best to implement the proposed solution because the recommended actions and their implications for the performance and future of the firm are interrelated.

Recall that the solution you propose must solve the problem you identified. This point cannot be overemphasized; too often students make recommendations that treat only symptoms or fail to tackle the central problems in the case. Make a logical argument that shows how the problem led to the analysis and the analysis led to the recommendations you are proposing. Remember, an analysis is not an end in itself; it is useful only if it leads to a solution.

The actions you propose should describe the very next steps that the company needs to take. Don't say, for example, "If the company does more market research, then I would recommend the following course of action. . . ." Instead, make conducting the research part of your recommendation. Taking the example a step further, if you also want to suggest subsequent actions that may be different *depending* on the outcome of the market research, that's OK. But don't make your initial recommendation conditional on actions the company may or may not take.

In summary, case analysis can be a very rewarding process but, as you might imagine, it can also be frustrating and challenging. If you will follow the steps described above, you will address the different elements of a thorough analysis. This approach can give your analysis a solid footing. Then, even if there are differences of opinion about how to interpret the facts, analyze the situation, or solve the problems, you can feel confident that you have not missed any important steps in finding the best course of action.

Students are often asked to prepare oral presentations of the information in a case and their analysis of the best remedies. This is frequently assigned as a group project. Or you may be called upon in class to present your ideas about the circumstances or solutions for a case the class is discussing. Exhibit 13.2 provides some tips for preparing an oral case presentation.

How to Get the Most from Case Analysis

> **>LO13.4**
> How to get the most out of case analysis.

One of the reasons case analysis is so enriching as a learning tool is that it draws on many resources and skills besides just what is in the textbook. This is especially true in the study of strategy. Why? Because strategic management itself is a highly integrative task that draws on many areas of specialization at several levels, from the individual to the whole of society. Therefore, to get the most out of case analysis, expand your horizons beyond the concepts in this text and seek insights from your own reservoir of knowledge. Here are some tips for how to do that.[7]

- *Keep an open mind.* Like any good discussion, a case analysis discussion often evokes strong opinions and high emotions. But it's the variety of perspectives that makes case analysis so valuable: Many viewpoints usually lead to a more complete analysis. Therefore, avoid letting an emotional response to another person's style or opinion keep you from hearing what he or she has to say. Once you evaluate what is said, you may disagree with it or dismiss it as faulty. But unless you keep an open mind in the first place, you may miss the importance of the other person's contribution. Also, people often place a higher value on the opinions of those they consider to be good listeners.
- *Take a stand for what you believe.* Although it is vital to keep an open mind, it is also important to state your views proactively. Don't try to figure out what your friends or the instructor wants to hear. Analyze the case from the perspective of your own background and belief system. For example, perhaps you feel that a decision is unethical or that the managers in a case have misinterpreted the facts. Don't be afraid to assert that in the discussion. For one thing, when a person takes a strong stand, it often encourages others to evaluate the issues more closely. This can lead to a more thorough investigation and a more meaningful class discussion.
- *Draw on your personal experience.* You may have experiences from work or as a customer that shed light on some of the issues in a case. Even though one of the purposes of case analysis is to apply the analytical tools from this text, you may be able to add to the discussion by drawing on your outside experiences and background. Of course, you need to guard against carrying that to extremes. In other words, don't think that your perspective is the only viewpoint that matters! Simply recognize that

Exhibit 13.2   Preparing an Oral Case Presentation

Rule	Description
Organize your thoughts.	Begin by becoming familiar with the material. If you are working with a team, compare notes about the key points of the case and share insights that other team members may have gleaned from tables and exhibits. Then make an outline. This is one of the best ways to organize the flow and content of the presentation.
Emphasize strategic analysis.	The purpose of case analysis is to diagnose problems and find solutions. In the process, you may need to unravel the case material as presented and reconfigure it in a fashion that can be more effectively analyzed. Present the material in a way that lends itself to analysis—don't simply restate what is in the case. This involves three major categories with the following emphasis:
	Background/Problem Statement 10– 20% Strategic Analysis/Options 60–75% Recommendations/Action Plan 10–20%
	As you can see, the emphasis of your presentation should be on analysis. This will probably require you to reorganize the material so that the tools of strategic analysis can be applied.
Be logical and consistent.	A presentation that is rambling and hard to follow may confuse the listener and fail to evoke a good discussion. Present your arguments and explanations in a logical sequence. Support your claims with facts. Include financial analysis where appropriate. Be sure that the solutions you recommend address the problems you have identified.
Defend your position.	Usually an oral presentation is followed by a class discussion. Anticipate what others might disagree with and be prepared to defend your views. This means being aware of the choices you made and the implications of your recommendations. Be clear about your assumptions. Be able to expand on your analysis.
Share presentation responsibilities.	Strategic management case analyses are often conducted by teams. Each member of the team should have a clear role in the oral presentation, preferably a speaking role. It's also important to coordinate the different parts of the presentation into a logical, smooth-flowing whole. How well a team works together is usually very apparent during an oral presentation.

firsthand experience usually represents a welcome contribution to the overall quality of case discussions.

- *Participate and persuade.* Have you heard the phrase, "Vote early . . . and often"? Among loyal members of certain political parties, it has become rather a joke. Why? Because a democratic system is built on the concept of one person, one vote. Even though some voters may want to vote often enough to get their candidate elected, it is against the law. Not so in a case discussion. People who are persuasive and speak their mind can often influence the views of others. But to do so, you have to be prepared and convincing. Being persuasive is more than being loud or long-winded. It involves understanding all sides of an argument and being able to overcome objections to your own point of view. These efforts can make a case discussion more lively. And they parallel what happens in the real world; in business, people frequently share their opinions and attempt to persuade others to see things their way.

- *Be concise and to the point.* In the previous point, we encouraged you to speak up and "sell" your ideas to others in a case discussion. But you must be clear about what you are selling. Make your arguments in a way that is explicit and direct. Zero in on the most important points. Be brief. Don't try to make a lot of points at once by jumping around between topics. Avoid trying to explain the whole case situation at once. Remember, other students usually resent classmates who go on and on, take up a lot of "airtime," or repeat themselves unnecessarily. The best way to avoid this is to stay focused and be specific.

- *Think out of the box.* It's OK to be a little provocative; sometimes that is the consequence of taking a stand on issues. But it may be equally important to be imaginative and creative when making a recommendation or determining how to implement a solution. Albert Einstein once stated, "Imagination is more important than knowledge." The reason is that managing strategically requires more than memorizing concepts. Strategic management insights must be applied to each case differently—just knowing the principles is not enough. Imagination and out-of-the-box thinking help to apply strategic knowledge in novel and unique ways.

- *Learn from the insights of others.* Before you make up your mind about a case, hear what other students have to say. Get a second opinion, and a third, and so forth. Of course, in a situation where you have to put your analysis in writing, you may not be able to learn from others ahead of time. But in a case discussion, observe how various students attack the issues and engage in problem solving. Such observation skills also may be a key to finding answers within the case. For example, people tend to believe authority figures, so they would place a higher value on what a company president says. In some cases, however, the statements of middle managers may represent a point of view that is even more helpful for finding a solution to the problems presented by the case.

- *Apply insights from other case analyses.* Throughout the text, we have used examples of actual businesses to illustrate strategy concepts. The aim has been to show you how firms think about and deal with business problems. During the course, you may be asked to conduct several case analyses as part of the learning experience. Once you have performed a few case analyses, you will see how the concepts from the text apply in real-life business situations. Incorporate the insights learned from the text examples and your own previous case discussions into each new case that you analyze.

- *Critically analyze your own performance.* Performance appraisals are a standard part of many workplace situations. They are used to determine promotions, raises, and work assignments. In some organizations, everyone from the top executive down is subject to such reviews. Even in situations where the owner or CEO is not evaluated by others, they often find it useful to ask themselves regularly, Am I being effective? The same can be applied to your performance in a case analysis situation. Ask yourself, Were my comments insightful? Did I make a good contribution? How might I improve next time? Use the same criteria on yourself that you use to evaluate others. What grade would you give yourself? This technique will not only make you more fair in your assessment of others but also will indicate how your own performance can improve.

- *Conduct outside research.* Many times, you can enhance your understanding of a case situation by investigating sources outside the case materials. For example, you may want to study an industry more closely or research a company's close competitors. Recent moves such as mergers and acquisitions or product introductions may be reported in the business press. The company itself may provide useful information on its website or in its annual reports. Such information can usually spur additional discussion and enrich the case analysis. (*Caution:* It is best to check with your instructor in advance to be sure this kind of additional research is encouraged. Bringing in outside research may conflict with the instructor's learning objectives.)

Several of the points suggested above for how to get the most out of case analysis apply only to an open discussion of a case, like that in a classroom setting. Exhibit 13.3 provides some additional guidelines for preparing a written case analysis.

Using Conflict-Inducing Decision-Making Techniques in Case Analysis

>LO13.5
How conflict-inducing discussion techniques can lead to better decisions.

Next we address some techniques often used to improve case analyses that involve the constructive use of conflict. In the classroom—as well as in the business world—you will

Exhibit 13.3   **Preparing a Written Case Analysis**

Rule	Description
Be thorough.	Many of the ideas presented in Exhibit 13.2 about oral presentations also apply to written case analysis. However, a written analysis typically has to be more complete. This means writing out the problem statement and articulating assumptions. It is also important to provide support for your arguments and reference case materials or other facts more specifically.
Coordinate team efforts.	Written cases are often prepared by small groups. Within a group, just as in a class discussion, you may disagree about the diagnosis or the recommended plan of action. This can be healthy if it leads to a richer understanding of the case material. But before committing your ideas to writing, make sure you have coordinated your responses. Don't prepare a written analysis that appears contradictory or looks like a patchwork of disconnected thoughts.
Avoid restating the obvious.	There is no reason to restate material that everyone is familiar with already, namely, the case content. It is too easy for students to use up space in a written analysis with a recapitulation of the details of the case—this accomplishes very little. Stay focused on the key points. Only restate the information that is most central to your analysis.
Present information graphically.	Tables, graphs, and other exhibits are usually one of the best ways to present factual material that supports your arguments. For example, financial calculations such as break-even analysis, sensitivity analysis, or return on investment are best presented graphically. Even qualitative information such as product lists or rosters of employees can be summarized effectively and viewed quickly by using a table or graph.
Exercise quality control.	When presenting a case analysis in writing, it is especially important to use good grammar, avoid misspelling words, and eliminate typos and other visual distractions. Mistakes that can be glossed over in an oral presentation or class discussion are often highlighted when they appear in writing. Make your written presentation appear as professional as possible. Don't let the appearance of your written case keep the reader from recognizing the importance and quality of your analysis.

frequently be analyzing cases or solving problems in groups. While the word *conflict* often has a negative connotation (e.g., rude behavior, personal affronts), it can be very helpful in arriving at better solutions to cases. It can provide an effective means for new insights as well as for rigorously questioning and analyzing assumptions and strategic alternatives. In fact, if you don't have constructive conflict, you may only get consensus. When this happens, decisions tend to be based on compromise rather than collaboration.

In your organizational behavior classes, you probably learned the concept of "groupthink."[8] Groupthink, a term coined by Irving Janis after he conducted numerous studies on executive decision making, is a condition in which group members strive to reach agreement or consensus without realistically considering other viable alternatives. In effect, group norms bolster morale at the expense of critical thinking, and decision making is impaired.[9]

Many of us have probably been "victims" of groupthink at one time or another in our life. We may be confronted with situations when social pressure, politics, or "not wanting to stand out" may prevent us from voicing our concerns about a chosen course of action. Nevertheless, decision making in groups is a common practice in the management of many businesses. Most companies, especially large ones, rely on input from various top managers to provide valuable information and experience from their specialty area as well as their unique perspectives. Chapter 11 emphasized the importance of empowering individuals at all levels to participate in decision-making processes. In terms of this course, case analysis involves a type of decision making that is often conducted in groups. Strategy Spotlight 13.3 provides guidelines for making team-based approaches to case analysis more effective.

Clearly, understanding how to work in groups and the potential problems associated with group decision processes can benefit the case analysis process. Therefore, let's first look at some of the symptoms of groupthink and suggest ways of preventing it. Then, we will suggest some conflict-inducing decision-making techniques—devil's advocacy and dialectical inquiry—that can help to prevent groupthink and lead to better decisions.

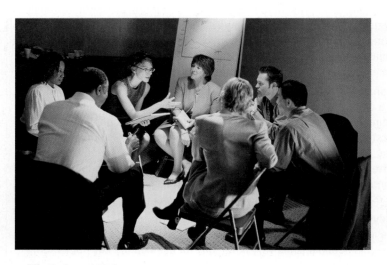

● Effectively working in teams is a critical skill—both in the classroom and in business organizations.

Symptoms of Groupthink and How to Prevent It

Irving Janis identified several symptoms of groupthink, including:

- *An illusion of invulnerability.* This reassures people about possible dangers and leads to overoptimism and failure to heed warnings of danger.
- *A belief in the inherent morality of the group.* Because individuals think that what they are doing is right, they tend to ignore ethical or moral consequences of their decisions.
- *Stereotyped views of members of opposing groups.* Members of other groups are viewed as weak or not intelligent.
- *The application of pressure to members who express doubts about the group's shared illusions or question the validity of arguments proposed.*
- *The practice of self-censorship.* Members keep silent about their opposing views and downplay to themselves the value of their perspectives.

Making Case Analysis Teams More Effective

Working in teams can be very challenging. Not all team members have the same skills, interests, or motivations. Some team members just want to get the work done. Others see teams as an opportunity to socialize. Occasionally, there are team members who think they should be in charge and make all the decisions; other teams have freeloaders—team members who don't want to do anything except get credit for the team's work.

One consequence of these various styles is that team meetings can become time wasters. Disagreements about how to proceed, how to share the work, or what to do at the next meeting tend to slow down teams and impede progress toward the goal. While the dynamics of case analysis teams are likely to always be challenging depending on the personalities involved, one thing nearly all members realize is that, ultimately, the team's work must be completed. Most team members also aim to do the highest quality work possible. The following guidelines provide some useful insights about how to get the work of a team done more effectively.

Spend More Time Together

One of the factors that prevents teams from doing a good job with case analysis is their failure to put in the necessary time. Unless teams really tackle the issues surrounding case analysis—both the issues in the case itself and organizing how the work is to be conducted—the end result will probably be lacking because decisions that are made too quickly are unlikely to get to the heart of the problem(s) in the case. "Meetings should be a precious resource, but they're treated like a necessary evil," says Kenneth Sole, a consultant who specializes in organizational behavior. As a result, teams that care more about finishing the analysis than getting the analysis right often make poor decisions.

Therefore, expect to have a few meetings that run long, especially at the beginning of the project when the work is being organized and the issues in the case are being sorted out, and again at the end when the team must coordinate the components of the case analysis that will be presented. Without spending this kind of time together, it is doubtful that the analysis will be comprehensive and the presentation is likely to be choppy and incomplete.

Make a Focused and Disciplined Agenda

To complete tasks and avoid wasting time, meetings need to have a clear purpose. To accomplish this at Roche, the Swiss drug and diagnostic product maker, CEO Franz Humer implemented a "decision agenda." The agenda focuses only on Roche's highest value issues and discussions are limited to these major topics. In terms of case analysis, the major topics include sorting out the issues of the case, linking elements of the case to the strategic issues presented in class or the text, and assigning roles to various team members. Such objectives help keep team members on track.

Agendas also can be used to address issues such as the time line for accomplishing work. Otherwise the purpose of meetings may only be to manage the "crisis" of getting the case analysis finished on time. One solution is to assign a team member to manage the agenda. That person could make sure the team stays focused on the tasks at hand and remains mindful of time constraints. Another role could be to link the team's efforts to the steps presented in Exhibits 13.2 and Exhibit 13.3 on how to prepare a case analysis.

Pay More Attention to Strategy

Teams often waste time by focusing on unimportant aspects of a case. These may include details that are interesting but irrelevant or operational issues rather than strategic issues. It is true that useful clues to the issues in the case are sometimes embedded in the conversations of key managers or the trends evident in a financial statement. But once such insights are discovered, teams need to focus on the underlying strategic problems in the case. To solve such problems, major corporations such as Cadbury Schweppes and Boeing hold meetings just to generate strategic alternatives for solving their problems. This gives managers time to consider the implications of various courses of action. Separate meetings are held to evaluate alternatives, make strategic decisions, and approve an action plan.

Once the strategic solutions or "course corrections" are identified—as is common in most cases assigned—the operational implications and details of implementation will flow from the strategic decisions that companies make. Therefore, focusing primarily on strategic issues will provide teams with insights for making recommendations that are based on a deeper understanding of the issues in the case.

Produce Real Decisions

Too often, meetings are about discussing rather than deciding. Teams often spend a lot of time talking without reaching any conclusions. As Raymond Sanchez, CEO of Florida-based Security Mortgage Group, said, meetings are often used to "rehash the hash that's already been hashed." To be efficient and productive, team meetings

(continued)

(continued)

need to be about more than just information sharing and group input. For example, an initial meeting may result in the team realizing that it needs to study the case in greater depth and examine links to strategic issues more carefully. Once more analysis is conducted, the team needs to reach a consensus so that the decisions that are made will last once the meeting is over. Lasting decisions are more actionable because it frees team members to take the next steps.

One technique for making progress in this way is recapping each meeting with a five-minute synthesis report. According to Pamela Schindler, director of the

Sources: Mankins, M. C. 2004. Stop wasting valuable time. *Harvard Business Review,* September: 58–65; and, Sauer, P. J. 2004. Escape from meeting hell. *Inc. Magazine, www.inc.com.* May.

Center for Applied Management at Wittenberg University, it's important to think through the implications of the meeting before ending it. "The real joy of synthesis," said Schindler, "is realizing how many meetings you won't need."

Not only are these guidelines useful for helping teams finish their work, but they can also help resolve some of the difficulties that teams often face. By involving every team member, using a meeting agenda, and focusing on the strategic issues that are critical to nearly every case, the discussion is limited and the criteria for making decisions become clearer. This allows the task to dominate rather than any one personality. And if the team finishes its work faster, this frees up time to focus on other projects or put the finishing touches on a case analysis presentation.

- *An illusion of unanimity.* People assume that judgments expressed by members are shared by all.
- *The appointment of mindguards.* People sometimes appoint themselves as mindguards to protect the group from adverse information that might break the climate of consensus (or agreement).

Clearly, groupthink is an undesirable and negative phenomenon that can lead to poor decisions. Irving Janis considers it to be a key contributor to such faulty decisions as the failure to prepare for the attack on Pearl Harbor, the escalation of the Vietnam conflict, and the failure to prepare for the consequences of the Iraqi invasion. Many of the same sorts of flawed decision making occur in business organizations. Janis has provided several suggestions for preventing groupthink that can be used as valuable guides in decision making and problem solving:

- Leaders must encourage group members to address their concerns and objectives.
- When higher-level managers assign a problem for a group to solve, they should adopt an impartial stance and not mention their preferences.
- Before a group reaches its final decision, the leader should encourage members to discuss their deliberations with trusted associates and then report the perspectives back to the group.
- The group should invite outside experts and encourage them to challenge the group's viewpoints and positions.
- The group should divide into subgroups, meet at various times under different chairpersons, and then get together to resolve differences.
- After reaching a preliminary agreement, the group should hold a "second chance" meeting, which provides members a forum to express any remaining concerns and rethink the issue prior to making a final decision.

Using Conflict to Improve Decision Making

In addition to the above suggestions, the effective use of conflict can be a means of improving decision making. Although conflict can have negative outcomes, such as ill will, anger, tension, and lowered motivation, both leaders and group members must strive to assure that it is managed properly and used in a constructive manner.

Two conflict-inducing decision-making approaches that have become quite popular are *devil's advocacy* and *dialectical inquiry*. Both approaches incorporate conflict into the decision-making process through formalized debate. A group charged with making a decision or solving a problem is divided into two subgroups and each will be involved in the analysis and solution.

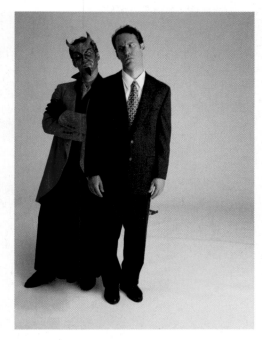

Devil's Advocacy   With the devil's advocate approach, one of the groups (or individuals) acts as a critic to the plan. The devil's advocate tries to come up with problems with the proposed alternative and suggest reasons why it should not be adopted. The role of **devil's advocacy** is to create dissonance. This ensures that the group will take a hard look at its original proposal or alternative. By having a group (or individual) assigned the role of devil's advocate, it becomes clear that such an adversarial stance is legitimized. It brings out criticisms that might otherwise not be made.

Some authors have suggested that the use of a devil's advocate can be very helpful in helping boards of directors to ensure that decisions are addressed comprehensively and to avoid groupthink.[10] And Michael Woodford, former president of Olympus—a Japanese manufacturer of cameras and medical equipment—has pointed out:

> Harmony and consensus have their place and time but scrutiny and challenging—devil's advocacy—leads to better decision making. You have to be able to confront and to say "Oi" [hey!] too, because much of your management is going to be outside of Japan.[11]

As one might expect, there can be some potential problems with using the devil's advocate approach. If one's views are constantly criticized, one may become demoralized. Thus, that person may come up with "safe solutions" in order to minimize embarrassment or personal risk and become less subject to criticism. Additionally, even if the devil's advocate is successful with finding problems with the proposed course of action, there may be no new ideas or counterproposals to take its place. Thus, the approach sometimes may simply focus on what is wrong without suggesting other ideas.

Dialectical Inquiry   **Dialectical inquiry** attempts to accomplish the goals of the devil's advocate in a more constructive manner. It is a technique whereby a problem is approached from two alternative points of view. The idea is that out of a critique of the opposing perspectives—a thesis and an antithesis—a creative synthesis will occur. Dialectical inquiry involves the following steps:

1. Identify a proposal and the information that was used to derive it.
2. State the underlying assumptions of the proposal.
3. Identify a counterplan (antithesis) that is believed to be feasible, politically viable, and generally credible. However, it rests on assumptions that are opposite to the original proposal.
4. Engage in a debate in which individuals favoring each plan provide their arguments and support.
5. Identify a synthesis that, hopefully, includes the best components of each alternative.

There are some potential downsides associated with dialectical inquiry. It can be quite time consuming and involve a good deal of training. Further, it may result in a series of compromises between the initial proposal and the counterplan. In cases where the original proposal was the best approach, this would be unfortunate.

● Conflict-inducing decision-making techniques, such as devil's advocacy, can be very effective.

devil's advocacy a method of introducing conflict into a decision-making process by having specific individuals or groups act as a critic to an analysis or planned solution.

dialectical inquiry a method of introducing conflict into a decision-making process by devising different proposals that are feasible, politically viable, and credible, but rely on different assumptions; and debating the merits of each.

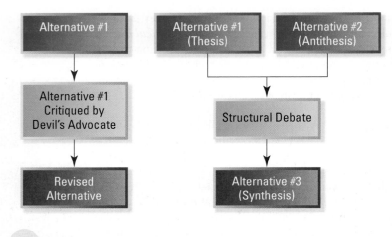

Exhibit 13.4 Two Conflict-Inducing Decision-Making Processes

Despite some possible limitations associated with these conflict-inducing decision-making techniques, they have many benefits. Both techniques force debate about underlying assumptions, data, and recommendations between subgroups. Such debate tends to prevent the uncritical acceptance of a plan that may seem to be satisfactory after a cursory analysis. The approach serves to tap the knowledge and perspectives of group members and continues until group members agree on both assumptions and recommended actions. Given that both approaches serve to use, rather than minimize or suppress, conflict, higher quality decisions should result. Exhibit 13.4 briefly summarizes these techniques.

Following the Analysis-Decision-Action Cycle in Case Analysis

In Chapter 1 we defined strategic management as the analysis, decisions, and actions that organizations undertake to create and sustain competitive advantages. It is no accident that we chose that sequence of words because it corresponds to the sequence of events that typically occurs in the strategic management process. In case analysis, as in the real world, this cycle of events can provide a useful framework. First, an analysis of the case in terms of the business environment and current events is needed. To make such an analysis, the case background must be considered. Next, based on that analysis, decisions must be made. This may involve formulating a strategy, choosing between difficult options, moving forward aggressively, or retreating from a bad situation. There are many possible decisions, depending on the case situation. Finally, action is required. Once decisions are made and plans are set, the action begins. The recommended action steps and the consequences of implementing these actions are the final stage.

Each of the previous 12 chapters of this book includes techniques and information that may be useful in a case analysis. However, not all of the issues presented will be important in every case. As noted earlier, one of the challenges of case analysis is to identify the most critical points and sort through material that may be ambiguous or unimportant.

In this section we draw on the material presented in each of the 12 chapters to show how it informs the case analysis process. The ideas are linked sequentially and in terms of an overarching strategic perspective. One of your jobs when conducting case analysis is to see how the parts of a case fit together and how the insights from the study of strategy can help you understand the case situation.

>LO13.6

How to use the strategic insights and material from each of the 12 previous chapters in the text to analyze issues posed by strategic management cases.

1. *Analyzing organizational goals and objectives.* A company's vision, mission, and objectives keep organization members focused on a common purpose. They also influence how an organization deploys its resources, relates to its stakeholders, and matches its short-term objectives with its long-term goals. The goals may even impact how a company formulates and implements strategies. When exploring issues of goals and objectives, you might ask:

   • Has the company developed short-term objectives that are inconsistent with its long-term mission? If so, how can management realign its vision, mission, and objectives?

   • Has the company considered all of its stakeholders equally in making critical decisions? If not, should the views of all stakeholders be treated the same or are some stakeholders more important than others?

   • Is the company being faced with an issue that conflicts with one of its long-standing policies? If so, how should it compare its existing policies to the potential new situation?

2. *Analyzing the external environment.* The business environment has two components. The general environment consists of demographic, sociocultural, political/legal, technological, economic, and global conditions. The competitive environment includes rivals, suppliers, customers, and other factors that may directly affect a company's success. Strategic managers must monitor the environment to identify opportunities and threats that may have an impact on performance. When investigating a firm's external environment, you might ask:

   • Does the company follow trends and events in the general environment? If not, how can these influences be made part of the company's strategic analysis process?

   • Is the company effectively scanning and monitoring the competitive environment? If so, how is it using the competitive intelligence it is gathering to enhance its competitive advantage?

   • Has the company correctly analyzed the impact of the competitive forces in its industry on profitability? If so, how can it improve its competitive position relative to these forces?

3. *Analyzing the internal environment.* A firm's internal environment consists of its resources and other value-adding capabilities. Value-chain analysis and a resource-based approach to analysis can be used to identify a company's strengths and weaknesses and determine how they are contributing to its competitive advantages. Evaluating firm performance can also help make meaningful comparisons with competitors. When researching a company's internal analysis, you might ask:

   • Does the company know how the various components of its value chain are adding value to the firm? If not, what internal analysis is needed to determine its strengths and weakness?

   • Has the company accurately analyzed the source and vitality of its resources? If so, is it deploying its resources in a way that contributes to competitive advantages?

   • Is the company's financial performance as good as or better than that of its close competitors? If so, has it balanced its financial success with the performance criteria of other stakeholders such as customers and employees?

4. *Assessing a firm's intellectual assets.* Human capital is a major resource in today's knowledge economy. As a result, attracting, developing, and retaining talented workers is a key strategic challenge. Other assets such as patents and trademarks are also critical. How companies leverage their intellectual assets through social networks and strategic alliances, and how technology is used to manage knowledge may be a major

influence on a firm's competitive advantage. When analyzing a firm's intellectual assets, you might ask:

- Does the company have underutilized human capital? If so, what steps are needed to develop and leverage its intellectual assets?
- Is the company missing opportunities to forge strategic alliances? If so, how can it use its social capital to network more effectively?
- Has the company developed knowledge-management systems that capture what it learns? If not, what technologies can it employ to retain new knowledge?

5. ***Formulating business-level strategies.*** Firms use the competitive strategies of differentiation, focus, and overall cost leadership as a basis for overcoming the five competitive forces and developing sustainable competitive advantages. Combinations of these strategies may work best in some competitive environments. Additionally, an industry's life cycle is an important contingency that may affect a company's choice of business-level strategies. When assessing business-level strategies, you might ask:

- Has the company chosen the correct competitive strategy given its industry environment and competitive situation? If not, how should it use its strengths and resources to improve its performance?
- Does the company use combination strategies effectively? If so, what capabilities can it cultivate to further enhance profitability?
- Is the company using a strategy that is appropriate for the industry life cycle in which it is competing? If not, how can it realign itself to match its efforts to the current stage of industry growth?

6. ***Formulating corporate-level strategies.*** Large firms often own and manage portfolios of businesses. Corporate strategies address methods for achieving synergies among these businesses. Related and unrelated diversification techniques are alternative approaches to deciding which business should be added to or removed from a portfolio. Companies can diversify by means of mergers, acquisitions, joint ventures, strategic alliances, and internal development. When analyzing corporate-level strategies, you might ask:

- Is the company competing in the right businesses given the opportunities and threats that are present in the environment? If not, how can it realign its diversification strategy to achieve competitive advantages?
- Is the corporation managing its portfolio of businesses in a way that creates synergies among the businesses? If so, what additional business should it consider adding to its portfolio?
- Are the motives of the top corporate executives who are pushing diversification strategies appropriate? If not, what action can be taken to curb their activities or align them with the best interests of all stakeholders?

7. ***Formulating international-level strategies.*** Foreign markets provide both opportunities and potential dangers for companies that want to expand globally. To decide which entry strategy is most appropriate, companies have to evaluate the trade-offs between two factors that firms face when entering foreign markets: cost reduction and local adaptation. To achieve competitive advantages, firms will typically choose one of three strategies: global, multidomestic, or transnational. When evaluating international-level strategies, you might ask:

- Is the company's entry into an international marketplace threatened by the actions of local competitors? If so, how can cultural differences be minimized to give the firm a better chance of succeeding?
- Has the company made the appropriate choices between cost reduction and local adaptation to foreign markets? If not, how can it adjust its strategy to achieve competitive advantages?

- Can the company improve its effectiveness by embracing one international strategy over another? If so, how should it choose between a global, multidomestic, or transnational strategy?

8. *Formulating entrepreneurial strategies.* New ventures add jobs and create new wealth. To do so, they must identify opportunities that will be viable in the marketplace as well as gather resources and assemble an entrepreneurial team to enact the opportunity. New entrants often evoke a strong competitive response from incumbent firms in a given marketplace. When examining the role of strategic thinking on the success of entrepreneurial ventures and the role of competitive dynamics, you might ask:

   - Is the company engaged in an ongoing process of opportunity recognition? If not, how can it enhance its ability to recognize opportunities?
   - Do the entrepreneurs who are launching new ventures have vision, dedication and drive, and a commitment to excellence? If so, how have these affected the performance and dedication of other employees involved in the venture?
   - Have strategic principles been used in the process of developing strategies to pursue the entrepreneurial opportunity? If not, how can the venture apply tools such as five-forces analysis and value-chain analysis to improve its competitive position and performance?

9. *Achieving effective strategic control.* Strategic controls enable a firm to implement strategies effectively. Informational controls involve comparing performance to stated goals and scanning, monitoring, and being responsive to the environment. Behavioral controls emerge from a company's culture, reward systems, and organizational boundaries. When assessing the impact of strategic controls on implementation, you might ask:

   - Is the company employing the appropriate informational control systems? If not, how can it implement a more interactive approach to enhance learning and minimize response times?
   - Does the company have a strong and effective culture? If not, what steps can it take to align its values and rewards system with its goals and objectives?
   - Has the company implemented control systems that match its strategies? If so, what additional steps can be taken to improve performance?

10. *Creating effective organizational designs.* Organizational designs that align with competitive strategies can enhance performance. As companies grow and change, their structures must also evolve to meet new demands. In today's economy, firm boundaries must be flexible and permeable to facilitate smoother interactions with external parties such as customers, suppliers, and alliance partners. New forms of organizing are becoming more common. When evaluating the role of organizational structure on strategy implementation, you might ask:

    - Has the company implemented organizational structures that are suited to the type of business it is in? If not, how can it alter the design in ways that enhance its competitiveness?
    - Is the company employing boundaryless organizational designs where appropriate? If so, how are senior managers maintaining control of lower-level employees?
    - Does the company use outsourcing to achieve the best possible results? If not, what criteria should it use to decide which functions can be outsourced?

11. *Creating a learning organization and an ethical organization.* Strong leadership is essential for achieving competitive advantages. Two leadership roles are especially important. The first is creating a learning organization by harnessing talent and encouraging the development of new knowledge. Second, leaders play a vital role in

motivating employees to excellence and inspiring ethical behavior. When exploring the impact of effective strategic leadership, you might ask:

- Do company leaders promote excellence as part of the overall culture? If so, how has this influenced the performance of the firm and the individuals in it?
- Is the company committed to being a learning organization? If not, what can it do to capitalize on the individual and collective talents of organizational members?
- Have company leaders exhibited an ethical attitude in their own behavior? If not, how has their behavior influenced the actions of other employees?

12. ***Fostering corporate entrepreneurship.*** Many firms continually seek new growth opportunities and avenues for strategic renewal. In some corporations, autonomous work units such as business incubators and new-venture groups are used to focus corporate venturing activities. In other corporate settings, product champions and other firm members provide companies with the impetus to expand into new areas. When investigating the impact of entrepreneurship on strategic effectiveness, you might ask:

- Has the company resolved the dilemmas associated with managing innovation? If so, is it effectively defining and pacing its innovation efforts?
- Has the company developed autonomous work units that have the freedom to bring forth new product ideas? If so, has it used product champions to implement new venture initiatives?
- Does the company have an entrepreneurial orientation? If not, what can it do to encourage entrepreneurial attitudes in the strategic behavior of its organizational members?

Summary

Strategic management case analysis provides an effective method of learning how companies analyze problems, make decisions, and resolve challenges. Strategic cases include detailed accounts of actual business situations. The purpose of analyzing such cases is to gain exposure to a wide variety of organizational and managerial situations. By putting yourself in the place of a strategic decision maker, you can gain an appreciation of the difficulty and complexity of many strategic situations. In the process you can learn how to ask good strategic questions and enhance your analytical skills. Presenting case analyses can also help develop oral and written communication skills.

In this chapter we have discussed the importance of strategic case analysis and described the five steps involved in conducting a case analysis: becoming familiar with the material, identifying problems, analyzing strategic issues, proposing alternative solutions, and making recommendations. We have also discussed how to get the most from case analysis. Finally, we have described how the case analysis process follows the analysis-decision-action cycle of strategic management and outlined issues and questions that are associated with each of the previous 12 chapters of the text.

Key Terms

case analysis, 512
case symptoms, 517
case problems, 517
financial ratio
  analysis, 518
devil's
  advocacy, 527
dialectical
  inquiry, 527

References

1. The material in this chapter is based on several sources, including: Barnes, L. A., Nelson, A. J., & Christensen, C. R. 1994. *Teaching and the case method: Text, cases and readings.* Boston: Harvard Business School Press; Guth, W. D. 1985. Central concepts of business unit and corporate strategy. In Guth, W. D. (Ed.). *Handbook of business strategy:* 1–9. Boston: Warren, Gorham & Lamont; Lundberg, C. C. & Enz, C. 1993. A framework for student case preparation. *Case Research Journal,* 13 (Summer): 129–140; and, Ronstadt, R. 1980. *The art of case analysis: A guide to the diagnosis of business situations.* Dover, MA: Lord Publishing.

2. Edge, A. G. & Coleman, D. R. 1986. *The guide to case analysis and reporting* (3rd ed.). Honolulu, HI: System Logistics.

3. Morris, E. 1987. Vision and strategy: A focus for the future. *Journal of Business Strategy,* 8: 51–58.

4. This section is based on Lundberg & Enz, op. cit., and Ronstadt, op. cit.

5. The importance of problem definition was emphasized in: Mintzberg, H., Raisinghani, D., & Theoret, A. 1976. The structure of "unstructured" decision processes. *Administrative Science Quarterly,* 21(2): 246–275.

6. Drucker, P. F. 1994. The theory of the business. *Harvard Business Review,* 72(5): 95–104.

7. This section draws on Edge & Coleman, op. cit.

8. Irving Janis is credited with coining the term *groupthink,* and he applied it primarily to fiascos in government (such as the Bay of Pigs incident in 1961). Refer to: Janis, I. L. 1982. *Victims of groupthink* (2nd ed.). Boston: Houghton Mifflin.

9. Much of our discussion is based upon: Finkelstein, S. & Mooney, A. C. 2003. Not the usual suspects: How to use board process to make boards better. *Academy of Management Executive,* 17(2): 101–113; Schweiger, D. M., Sandberg, W. R., & Rechner, P. L. 1989. Experiential effects of dialectical inquiry, devil's advocacy, and consensus approaches to strategic decision making. *Academy of Management Journal,* 32(4): 745–772; and, Aldag, R. J. & Stearns, T. M. 1987. *Management.* Cincinnati: South-Western Publishing.

10. Finkelstein and Mooney, op. cit.

11. Soble, J. 2011. Japan's changing "gaijin" CEOs. *Financial Times, www.ft.com/intl/cms/s/0/239aeec8-a666-11e0-ae9c-00144feabdc0.html#axzz1dgra6l75.* July 4 ; and, Tabuchi, H. 2012. Former Chief Ends His Bid to Overhaul Olympus. January 6.

Appendix 1 to Chapter 13

Financial Ratio Analysis*

Standard Financial Statements

One obvious thing we might want to do with a company's financial statements is to compare them to those of other, similar companies. We would immediately have a problem, however. It's almost impossible to directly compare the financial statements for two companies because of differences in size.

For example, Oracle and IBM are obviously serious rivals in the computer software market, but IBM is much larger (in terms of assets), so it is difficult to compare them directly. For that matter, it's difficult to even compare financial statements from different points in time for the same company if the company's size has changed. The size problem is compounded if we try to compare IBM and, say, SAP (of Germany). If SAP's financial statements are denominated in euros, then we have a size *and* a currency difference.

To start making comparisons, one obvious thing we might try to do is to somehow standardize the financial statements. One very common and useful way of doing this is to work with percentages instead of total dollars. The resulting financial statements are called *common-size statements.* We consider these next.

Common-Size Balance Sheets

For easy reference, Prufrock Corporation's 2010 and 2011 balance sheets are provided in Exhibit 13A.1. Using these, we construct common-size balance sheets by expressing each item as a percentage of total assets. Prufrock's 2010 and 2011 common-size balance sheets are shown in Exhibit 13A.2.

---

*This entire Appendix is adapted from Rows, S. A., Westerfield, R. W., & Jordan, B. D. 1999. *Essentials of corporate finance* (2nd ed.): chap. 3. New York: McGraw-Hill.

Exhibit 13A.1

Prufrock Corporation

Balance Sheets as of December 31, 2010 and 2011 ($ in millions)

	2010	2011
Assets		
Current assets		
Cash	$ 84	$ 98
Accounts receivable	165	188
Inventory	393	422
Total	$ 642	$ 708
Fixed assets		
Net plant and equipment	$2,731	$2,880
Total assets	$3,373	$3,588
Liabilities and Owners' Equity		
Current liabilities		
Accounts payable	$ 312	$ 344
Notes payable	231	196
Total	$ 543	$ 540
Long-term debt	$ 531	$ 457
Owners' equity		
Common stock and paid-in surplus	$ 500	$ 550
Retained earnings	1,799	2,041
Total	$2,299	$2,591
Total liabilities and owners' equity	$3,373	$3,588

Notice that some of the totals don't check exactly because of rounding errors. Also notice that the total change has to be zero since the beginning and ending numbers must add up to 100 percent.

In this form, financial statements are relatively easy to read and compare. For example, just looking at the two balance sheets for Prufrock, we see that current assets were 19.7 percent of total assets in 2011, up from 19.1 percent in 2010. Current liabilities declined from 16.0 percent to 15.1 percent of total liabilities and equity over that same time. Similarly, total equity rose from 68.1 percent of total liabilities and equity to 72.2 percent.

Overall, Prufrock's liquidity, as measured by current assets compared to current liabilities, increased over the year. Simultaneously, Prufrock's indebtedness diminished as a percentage of total assets. We might be tempted to conclude that the balance sheet has grown "stronger."

Common-Size Income Statements

A useful way of standardizing the income statement, shown in Exhibit 13A.3, is to express each item as a percentage of total sales, as illustrated for Prufrock in Exhibit 13A.4.

This income statement tells us what happens to each dollar in sales. For Prufrock, interest expense eats up $.061 out of every sales dollar and taxes take another $.081. When all is said and done, $.157 of each dollar flows through to the bottom line (net income), and that amount is split into $.105 retained in the business and $.052 paid out in dividends.

Exhibit 13A.2
Prufrock Corporation
Common-Size
Balance Sheets as of
December 31, 2010
and 2011 (%)

	2010	2011	Change
Assets			
Current assets			
Cash	2.5%	2.7%	+ .2%
Accounts receivable	4.9	5.2	+ .3
Inventory	11.7	11.8	+ .1
Total	19.1	19.7	+ .6
Fixed assets			
Net plant and equipment	80.9	80.3	− .6
Total assets	100.0%	100.0%	.0%
Liabilities and Owners' Equity			
Current liabilities			
Accounts payable	9.2%	9.6%	+ .4%
Notes payable	6.8	5.5	−1.3
Total	16.0	15.1	− .9
Long-term debt	15.7	12.7	−3.0
Owners' equity			
Common stock and paid-in surplus	14.8	15.3	+ .5
Retained earnings	53.3	56.9	+3.6
Total	68.1	72.2	+4.1
Total liabilities and owners' equities	100.0%	100.0%	.0%

Note: Numbers may not add up to 100.0% due to rounding.

These percentages are very useful in comparisons. For example, a relevant figure is the cost percentage. For Prufrock, $.582 of each $1.00 in sales goes to pay for goods sold. It would be interesting to compute the same percentage for Prufrock's main competitors to see how Prufrock stacks up in terms of cost control.

Ratio Analysis

Another way of avoiding the problems involved in comparing companies of different sizes is to calculate and compare *financial ratios*. Such ratios are ways of comparing and investigating the relationships between different pieces of financial information. We cover some of the more common ratios next, but there are many others that we don't touch on.

One problem with ratios is that different people and different sources frequently don't compute them in exactly the same way, and this leads to much confusion. The specific definitions we use here may or may not be the same as others you have seen or will see elsewhere. If you ever use ratios as a tool for analysis, you should be careful to document how you calculate each one, and, if you are comparing your numbers to those of another source, be sure you know how its numbers are computed.

For each of the ratios we discuss, several questions come to mind:

1. How is it computed?
2. What is it intended to measure, and why might we be interested?
3. What is the unit of measurement?

Exhibit 13A.3

Prufrock Corporation

2011 Income Statement
($ in millions)

Sales		$2,311
Cost of goods sold		1,344
Depreciation		276
Earnings before interest and taxes		$ 691
Interest paid		141
Taxable income		$ 550
Taxes (34%)		187
Net income		$ 363
Dividends	$121	
Addition to retained earnings	242	

Exhibit 13A.4

Prufrock Corporation

2011 Common-Size
Income Statement (%)

Sales		100.0%
Cost of goods sold		58.2
Depreciation		11.9
Earnings before interest and taxes		29.9
Interest paid		6.1
Taxable income		23.8
Taxes (34%)		8.1
Net income		15.7%
Dividends	5.2%	
Addition to retained earnings	10.5	

4. What might a high or low value be telling us? How might such values be misleading?

5. How could this measure be improved?

Financial ratios are traditionally grouped into the following categories:

1. Short-term solvency, or liquidity, ratios.

2. Long-term solvency, or financial leverage, ratios.

3. Asset management, or turnover, ratios.

4. Profitability ratios.

5. Market value ratios.

We will consider each of these in turn. In calculating these numbers for Prufrock, we will use the ending balance sheet (2011) figures unless we explicitly say otherwise. The numbers for the various ratios come from the income statement and the balance sheet.

Short-Term Solvency, or Liquidity, Measures

As the name suggests, short-term solvency ratios as a group are intended to provide information about a firm's liquidity, and these ratios are sometimes called *liquidity measures*. The primary concern is the firm's ability to pay its bills over the short run without undue stress. Consequently, these ratios focus on current assets and current liabilities.

For obvious reasons, liquidity ratios are particularly interesting to short-term creditors. Since financial managers are constantly working with banks and other short-term lenders, an understanding of these ratios is essential.

One advantage of looking at current assets and liabilities is that their book values and market values are likely to be similar. Often (though not always), these assets and liabilities just don't live long enough for the two to get seriously out of step. On the other hand, like any type of near cash, current assets and liabilities can and do change fairly rapidly, so today's amounts may not be a reliable guide to the future.

Current Ratio   One of the best-known and most widely used ratios is the *current ratio*. As you might guess, the current ratio is defined as:

$$\text{Current ratio} = \frac{\text{Current assets}}{\text{Current liabilities}}$$

For Prufrock, the 2011 current ratio is:

$$\text{Current ratio} = \frac{\$708}{\$540} = 1.31 \text{ times}$$

Because current assets and liabilities are, in principle, converted to cash over the following 12 months, the current ratio is a measure of short-term liquidity. The unit of measurement is either dollars or times. So, we could say Prufrock has $1.31 in current assets for every $1 in current liabilities, or we could say Prufrock has its current liabilities covered 1.31 times over.

To a creditor, particularly a short-term creditor such as a supplier, the higher the current ratio, the better. To the firm, a high current ratio indicates liquidity, but it also may indicate an inefficient use of cash and other short-term assets. Absent some extraordinary circumstances, we would expect to see a current ratio of at least 1, because a current ratio of less than 1 would mean that net working capital (current assets less current liabilities) is negative. This would be unusual in a healthy firm, at least for most types of businesses.

The current ratio, like any ratio, is affected by various types of transactions. For example, suppose the firm borrows over the long term to raise money. The short-run effect would be an increase in cash from the issue proceeds and an increase in long-term debt. Current liabilities would not be affected, so the current ratio would rise.

Finally, note that an apparently low current ratio may not be a bad sign for a company with a large reserve of untapped borrowing power.

Quick (or Acid-Test) Ratio   Inventory is often the least liquid current asset. It's also the one for which the book values are least reliable as measures of market value, since the quality of the inventory isn't considered. Some of the inventory may later turn out to be damaged, obsolete, or lost.

More to the point, relatively large inventories are often a sign of short-term trouble. The firm may have overestimated sales and overbought or overproduced as a result. In this case, the firm may have a substantial portion of its liquidity tied up in slow-moving inventory.

To further evaluate liquidity, the *quick,* or *acid-test, ratio* is computed just like the current ratio, except inventory is omitted:

$$\text{Quick ratio} = \frac{\text{Current assets} - \text{Inventory}}{\text{Current liabilities}}$$

Notice that using cash to buy inventory does not affect the current ratio, but it reduces the quick ratio. Again, the idea is that inventory is relatively illiquid compared to cash.

For Prufrock, this ratio in 2011 was:

$$\text{Quick ratio} = \frac{\$708 - 422}{\$540} = .53 \text{ times}$$

The quick ratio here tells a somewhat different story than the current ratio, because inventory accounts for more than half of Prufrock's current assets. To exaggerate the point, if this inventory consisted of, say, unsold nuclear power plants, then this would be a cause for concern.

Cash Ratio A very short-term creditor might be interested in the *cash ratio:*

$$\text{Cash ratio} = \frac{\text{Cash}}{\text{Current liabilities}}$$

You can verify that this works out to be .18 times for Prufrock.

Long-Term Solvency Measures

Long-term solvency ratios are intended to address the firm's long-run ability to meet its obligations, or, more generally, its financial leverage. These ratios are sometimes called *financial leverage ratios* or just *leverage ratios.* We consider three commonly used measures and some variations.

Total Debt Ratio The *total debt ratio* takes into account all debts of all maturities to all creditors. It can be defined in several ways, the easiest of which is:

$$\text{Total debt ratio} = \frac{\text{Total assets} - \text{Total equity}}{\text{Total assets}}$$

$$= \frac{\$3,588 - 2,591}{\$3,588} = .28 \text{ times}$$

In this case, an analyst might say that Prufrock uses 28 percent debt.[1] Whether this is high or low or whether it even makes any difference depends on whether or not capital structure matters.

Prufrock has $.28 in debt for every $1 in assets. Therefore, there is $.72 in equity ($1 − .28) for every $.28 in debt. With this in mind, we can define two useful variations on the total debt ratio, the *debt-equity ratio* and the *equity multiplier:*

$$\text{Debt-equity ratio} = \text{Total debt/Total equity}$$
$$= \$.28/\$.72 = .39 \text{ times}$$
$$\text{Equity multiplier} = \text{Total assets/Total equity}$$
$$= \$1/\$.72 = 1.39 \text{ times}$$

The fact that the equity multiplier is 1 plus the debt-equity ratio is not a coincidence:

$$\text{Equity multiplier} = \text{Total assets/Total equity} = \$1/\$.72 = 1.39$$
$$= (\text{Total equity} + \text{Total debt})/\text{Total equity}$$
$$= 1 + \text{Debt-equity ratio} = 1.39 \text{ times}$$

The thing to notice here is that given any one of these three ratios, you can immediately calculate the other two, so they all say exactly the same thing.

Times Interest Earned Another common measure of long-term solvency is the *times interest earned* (TIE) *ratio.* Once again, there are several possible (and common) definitions, but we'll stick with the most traditional:

$$\text{Times interest earned ratio} = \frac{\text{EBIT}}{\text{Interest}}$$

$$= \frac{\$691}{\$141} = 4.9 \text{ times}$$

As the name suggests, this ratio measures how well a company has its interest obligations covered, and it is often called the interest coverage ratio. For Prufrock, the interest bill is covered 4.9 times over.

Cash Coverage A problem with the TIE ratio is that it is based on earnings before interest and taxes (EBIT), which is not really a measure of cash available to pay interest. The reason is that

---

[1] Total equity here includes preferred stock, if there is any. An equivalent numerator in this ratio would be (Current liabilities + Long-term debt).

depreciation, a noncash expense, has been deducted. Since interest is most definitely a cash outflow (to creditors), one way to define the *cash coverage ratio* is:

$$\text{Cash coverage ratio} = \frac{\text{EBIT} + \text{Depreciation}}{\text{Interest}}$$

$$= \frac{\$691 + 276}{\$141} = \frac{\$967}{\$141} = 6.9 \text{ times}$$

The numerator here, EBIT plus depreciation, is often abbreviated EBDIT (earnings before depreciation, interest, and taxes). It is a basic measure of the firm's ability to generate cash from operations, and it is frequently used as a measure of cash flow available to meet financial obligations.

Asset Management, or Turnover, Measures

We next turn our attention to the efficiency with which Prufrock uses its assets. The measures in this section are sometimes called *asset utilization ratios*. The specific ratios we discuss can all be interpreted as measures of turnover. What they are intended to describe is how efficiently, or intensively, a firm uses its assets to generate sales. We first look at two important current assets: inventory and receivables.

Inventory Turnover and Days' Sales in Inventory   During the year, Prufrock had a cost of goods sold of $1,344. Inventory at the end of the year was $422. With these numbers, *inventory turnover* can be calculated as:

$$\text{Inventory turnover} = \frac{\text{Cost of goods sold}}{\text{Inventory}}$$

$$= \frac{\$1,344}{\$422} = 3.2 \text{ times}$$

In a sense, we sold off, or turned over, the entire inventory 3.2 times. As long as we are not running out of stock and thereby forgoing sales, the higher this ratio is, the more efficiently we are managing inventory.

If we know that we turned our inventory over 3.2 times during the year, then we can immediately figure out how long it took us to turn it over on average. The result is the average *days' sales in inventory*:

$$\text{Days' sales in inventory} = \frac{365 \text{ days}}{\text{Inventory turnover}}$$

$$= \frac{365}{3.2} = 114 \text{ days}$$

This tells us that, on average, inventory sits 114 days before it is sold. Alternatively, assuming we used the most recent inventory and cost figures, it will take about 114 days to work off our current inventory.

For example, we frequently hear things like "Majestic Motors has a 60 days' supply of cars." This means that, at current daily sales, it would take 60 days to deplete the available inventory. We could also say that Majestic has 60 days of sales in inventory.

Receivables Turnover and Days' Sales in Receivables   Our inventory measures give some indication of how fast we can sell products. We now look at how fast we collect on those sales. The *receivables turnover* is defined in the same way as inventory turnover:

$$\text{Receivables turnover} = \frac{\text{Sales}}{\text{Accounts receivable}}$$

$$= \frac{\$2,311}{\$188} = 12.3 \text{ times}$$

Loosely speaking, we collected our outstanding credit accounts and reloaned the money 12.3 times during the year.[2]

This ratio makes more sense if we convert it to days, so the *days' sales in receivables* is:

$$\text{Days' sales in receivables} = \frac{365 \text{ days}}{\text{Receivables turnover}}$$

$$= \frac{365}{12.3} = 30 \text{ days}$$

Therefore, on average, we collect on our credit sales in 30 days. For obvious reasons, this ratio is very frequently called the *average collection period* (ACP).

Also note that if we are using the most recent figures, we can also say that we have 30 days' worth of sales currently uncollected.

Total Asset Turnover   Moving away from specific accounts like inventory or receivables, we can consider an important "big picture" ratio, the *total asset turnover ratio*. As the name suggests, total asset turnover is:

$$\text{Total asset turnover} = \frac{\text{Sales}}{\text{Total assets}}$$

$$= \frac{\$2,311}{\$3,588} = .64 \text{ times}$$

In other words, for every dollar in assets, we generated $.64 in sales.

A closely related ratio, the *capital intensity ratio,* is simply the reciprocal of (i.e., 1 divided by) total asset turnover. It can be interpreted as the dollar investment in assets needed to generate $1 in sales. High values correspond to capital-intensive industries (e.g., public utilities). For Prufrock, total asset turnover is .64, so, if we flip this over, we get that capital intensity is $1/.64 = $1.56. That is, it takes Prufrock $1.56 in assets to create $1 in sales.

Profitability Measures

The three measures we discuss in this section are probably the best known and most widely used of all financial ratios. In one form or another, they are intended to measure how efficiently the firm uses its assets and how efficiently the firm manages its operations. The focus in this group is on the bottom line, net income.

Profit Margin   Companies pay a great deal of attention to their *profit margin:*

$$\text{Profit margin} = \frac{\text{Net income}}{\text{Sales}}$$

$$= \frac{\$363}{\$2,311} = 15.7\%$$

This tells us that Prufrock, in an accounting sense, generates a little less than 16 cents in profit for every dollar in sales.

All other things being equal, a relatively high profit margin is obviously desirable. This situation corresponds to low expense ratios relative to sales. However, we hasten to add that other things are often not equal.

For example, lowering our sales price will usually increase unit volume, but will normally cause profit margins to shrink. Total profit (or, more importantly, operating cash flow) may go up or down; so the fact that margins are smaller isn't necessarily bad. After all, isn't it possible that, as the saying goes, "Our prices are so low that we lose money on everything we sell, but we make it up in volume!"[3]

---

[2] Here we have implicitly assumed that all sales are credit sales. If they were not, then we would simply use total credit sales in these calculations, not total sales.

[3] No, it's not; margins can be small, but they do need to be positive!

Return on Assets *Return on assets* (ROA) is a measure of profit per dollar of assets. It can be defined several ways, but the most common is:

$$\text{Return on assets} = \frac{\text{Net income}}{\text{Total assets}}$$

$$= \frac{\$363}{\$3,588} = 10.12\%$$

Return on Equity *Return on equity* (ROE) is a measure of how the stockholders fared during the year. Since benefiting shareholders is our goal, ROE is, in an accounting sense, the true bottom-line measure of performance. ROE is usually measured as:

$$\text{Return on equity} = \frac{\text{Net income}}{\text{Total equity}}$$

$$= \frac{\$363}{\$2,591} = 14\%$$

For every dollar in equity, therefore, Prufrock generated 14 cents in profit, but, again, this is only correct in accounting terms.

Because ROA and ROE are such commonly cited numbers, we stress that it is important to remember they are accounting rates of return. For this reason, these measures should properly be called *return on book assets* and *return on book equity*. In addition, ROE is sometimes called *return on net worth*. Whatever it's called, it would be inappropriate to compare the results to, for example, an interest rate observed in the financial markets.

The fact that ROE exceeds ROA reflects Prufrock's use of financial leverage. We will examine the relationship between these two measures in more detail below.

Market Value Measures

Our final group of measures is based, in part, on information not necessarily contained in financial statements—the market price per share of the stock. Obviously, these measures can only be calculated directly for publicly traded companies.

We assume that Prufrock has 33 million shares outstanding and the stock sold for $88 per share at the end of the year. If we recall that Prufrock's net income was $363 million, then we can calculate that its earnings per share were:

$$\text{EPS} = \frac{\text{Net income}}{\text{Shares outstanding}} = \frac{\$363}{33} = \$11$$

Price-Earnings Ratio The first of our market value measures, the *price-earnings,* or PE, *ratio* (or multiple), is defined as:

$$\text{PE ratio} = \frac{\text{Price per share}}{\text{Earnings per share}}$$

$$= \frac{\$88}{\$11} = 8 \text{ times}$$

In the vernacular, we would say that Prufrock shares sell for eight times earnings, or we might say that Prufrock shares have, or "carry," a PE multiple of 8.

Since the PE ratio measures how much investors are willing to pay per dollar of current earnings, higher PEs are often taken to mean that the firm has significant prospects for future growth. Of course, if a firm had no or almost no earnings, its PE would probably be quite large; so, as always, be careful when interpreting this ratio.

Market-to-Book Ratio   A second commonly quoted measure is the *market-to-book ratio:*

$$\text{Market-to-book ratio} = \frac{\text{Market value per share}}{\text{Book value per share}}$$

$$= \frac{\$88}{(\$2,591/33)} = \frac{\$88}{\$78.5} = 1.12 \text{ times}$$

Notice that book value per share is total equity (not just common stock) divided by the number of shares outstanding.

Since book value per share is an accounting number, it reflects historical costs. In a loose sense, the market-to-book ratio therefore compares the market value of the firm's investments to their cost. A value less than 1 could mean that the firm has not been successful overall in creating value for its stockholders.

Conclusion

This completes our definition of some common ratios. Exhibit 13A.5 summarizes the ratios we've discussed.

I. Short-term solvency, or liquidity, ratios

$$\text{Current ratio} = \frac{\text{Current assets}}{\text{Current liabilities}}$$

$$\text{Quick ratio} = \frac{\text{Current assets} - \text{Inventory}}{\text{Current liabilities}}$$

$$\text{Cash ratio} = \frac{\text{Cash}}{\text{Current liabilities}}$$

II. Long-term solvency, or financial leverage, ratios

$$\text{Total debt ratio} = \frac{\text{Total assets} - \text{Total equity}}{\text{Total assets}}$$

$$\text{Debt-equity ratio} = \text{Total debt/Total equity}$$

$$\text{Equity multiplier} = \text{Total assets/Total equity}$$

$$\text{Times interest earned ratio} = \frac{\text{EBIT}}{\text{Interest}}$$

$$\text{Cash coverage ratio} = \frac{\text{EBIT} + \text{Depreciation}}{\text{Interest}}$$

III. Asset utilization, or turnover, ratios

$$\text{Inventory turnover} = \frac{\text{Cost of goods sold}}{\text{Inventory}}$$

$$\text{Days' sales in inventory} = \frac{365 \text{ days}}{\text{Inventory turnover}}$$

$$\text{Receivables turnover} = \frac{\text{Sales}}{\text{Accounts receivable}}$$

$$\text{Days' sales in receivables} = \frac{365 \text{ days}}{\text{Receivables turnover}}$$

$$\text{Total asset turnover} = \frac{\text{Sales}}{\text{Total assets}}$$

$$\text{Capital intensity} = \frac{\text{Total assets}}{\text{Sales}}$$

IV. Profitability ratios

$$\text{Profit margin} = \frac{\text{Net income}}{\text{Sales}}$$

$$\text{Return on assets (ROA)} = \frac{\text{Net income}}{\text{Total assets}}$$

$$\text{Return on equity (ROE)} = \frac{\text{Net income}}{\text{Total equity}}$$

$$\text{ROE} = \frac{\text{Net income}}{\text{Sales}} \times \frac{\text{Sales}}{\text{Assets}} \times \frac{\text{Assets}}{\text{Equity}}$$

V. Market value ratios

$$\text{Price-earnings ratio} = \frac{\text{Price per share}}{\text{Earnings per share}}$$

$$\text{Market-to-book ratio} = \frac{\text{Market value per share}}{\text{Book value per share}}$$

Exhibit 13A.5   **A Summary of Five Types of Financial Ratios**

APPENDIX 2 TO CHAPTER 13

Sources of Company and Industry Information*

In order for business executives to make the best decisions when developing corporate strategy, it is critical for them to be knowledgeable about their competitors and about the industries in which they compete. The process used by corporations to learn as much as possible about competitors is often called "competitive intelligence." This appendix provides an overview of important and widely available sources of information that may be useful in conducting basic competitive intelligence. Much information of this nature is available in libraries in article databases, in business reference books, and on websites. This list will recommend a variety of them. Ask a librarian for assistance, because library collections and resources vary.

The information sources are organized into 10 categories:

Competitive Intelligence

Public or Private, Subsidiary or Division, U.S. or Foreign?

Annual Report Collections—Public Companies

Guides and Tutorials

SEC Filings/EDGAR—Company Disclosure Reports

Company Rankings

Business Websites

Strategic and Competitive Analysis—Information Sources

Sources for Industry Research and Analysis

Search Engines

Competitive Intelligence

Students and other researchers who want to learn more about the value and process of competitive intelligence should see four recent books on this subject.

Mike Biere. *The New Era of Enterprise Business Intelligence: Using Analytics to Achieve a Global Competitive Advantage.* Upper Saddle River, NJ: IBM Press/Pearson, 2011.

Seena Sharp. *Competitive Intelligence Advantage: How to Minimize Risk, Avoid Surprises, and Grow Your Business in a Changing World.* Hoboken, NJ: Wiley, 2009.

T. J. Waters. *Hyperformance: Using Competitive Intelligence for Better Strategy and Execution.* San Francisco: Jossey-Bass, 2010.

Benjamin Gilad. *Early Warning: Using Competitive Intelligence to Anticipate Market Shifts, Control Risk, and Create Powerful Strategies.* New York: American Management Association, 2004.

Public or Private, Subsidiary or Division, U.S. or Foreign?

Companies traded on stock exchanges in the United States are required to file a variety of reports that disclose information about the company. This begins the process that produces a wealth of data on public companies and at the same time distinguishes them from private companies, which often lack available data. Similarly, financial data of subsidiaries and divisions are typically filed in a

---

* This information was compiled by Ruthie Brock and Carol Byrne, business librarians at The University of Texas at Arlington. We greatly appreciate their valuable contribution.

consolidated financial statement by the parent company, rather than treated independently, thus limiting the kind of data available on them. On the other hand, foreign companies that trade on U.S. stock exchanges are required to file 20F reports, similar to the 10-K for U.S. companies, the most comprehensive of the required reports. The following directories provide brief facts about companies, including whether they are public or private, subsidiary or division, U.S. or foreign.

Corporate Directory of U.S. Public Companies. San Mateo, CA: Walker's Research, LLC, 2010.
The *Corporate Directory* provides company profiles of more than 9,000 publicly traded companies in the United States, including foreign companies trading on the U.S. exchanges (ADRs). Some libraries may subscribe to an alternative online version at *www.walkersresearch.com.*

Corporate Affiliations. New Providence, NJ: LexisNexis, 2010.
This 8-volume directory features brief profiles of major U.S. and foreign corporations, both public and private, as well as their subsidiaries, divisions, and affiliates. The directory also indicates hierarchies of corporate relationships. An online version of the directory allows retrieval of a list of companies that meet specific criteria. Results can be downloaded to a spreadsheet. The online version requires a subscription, available in some libraries.

ReferenceUSA. Omaha, NE: Infogroup. Inc.
ReferenceUSA is an online directory of more than 14 million businesses located in the United States. One of the unique features is that it includes public and private companies, both large and small. Custom and Guided search tabs are available. Also, results can be analyzed using Quick, the data summary feature, which allows for a snapshot of how the industry breaks down by size, geographic location, etc. Other subscription options are available using the ReferenceUSA interface and may be available in some libraries.

Ward's Business Directory of U.S. Private and Public Companies. Farmington Hills, MI: Gale CENGAGE Learning, 2010. 8 vols.
Ward's Business Directory lists brief profiles on more than 112,000 public and private companies and indicates whether they are public or private, a subsidiary or division. Two volumes of the set are arranged using the Standard Industrial Classifications (SIC) and the North American Industry Classification System (NAICS) and feature company rankings within industries. Some libraries may offer this business directory as part of a database called *Gale Directory Library.*

Finding Public Company Information

Most companies have their annual report to shareholders and other financial reports available on their corporate website. Note that some companies use a variation of their company name in their web address, such as Procter & Gamble: *www.pg.com.* A few "aggregators" have also conveniently provided an accumulation of links to many reports of U.S. and international corporations or include a PDF document as part of their database, although these generally do not attempt to be comprehensive.

The Public Register Online. Woodstock Valley, CT: Bay Tact Corp.
Public Register Online includes over 5,000 public company shareholder annual reports and 10-K filings for online viewing. Links are provided to reports on individual companies' websites, official filings from the Securities and Exchange Commission website, stock information from the NYSE Euronext exchange, or some combination of these sources. A link is also provided on this website for ordering personal copies of hard copy annual reports. *www.annualreportservice.com/*

Mergent Online. New York: Mergent, Inc.
Mergent Online is a database that provides company reports and financial statements for both U.S. and foreign public companies. Mergent's database has up to 25 years of quarterly and annual financial data that can be downloaded into a spreadsheet for analysis across time or across companies. Students should check with a librarian to determine the availability of this database at their college or university library.
http://mergentonline.com

Guides and Tutorials for Researching Companies and Industries

Researching Companies Online. Fort Lauderdale, FL: Debbie Flanagan
This site provides a step-by-step process for finding free company and industry information on the web.
www.learnwebskills.com/company/

Guide to Financial Statements and *How to Read Annual Reports.* Armonk, NY: IBM
These two educational guides, located on IBM's website, provide basic information on how to read and make sense of financial statements and other information in 10-K and shareholder annual reports for companies in general, not IBM specifically.
www.ibm.com/investor/help/guide/introduction.wss
www.ibm.com/investor/help/reports/introduction.wss

EDGAR Full-Text Search Frequently Asked Questions (FAQ). Washington, DC: U.S. Securities and Exchange Commission
The capability to search full-text SEC filings (popularly known as EDGAR filings) was vastly improved when the SEC launched its new search form in late 2006. Features are explained at the FAQ page.
www.sec.gov/edgar/searchedgar/edgarfulltextfaq.htm

Locating Company Information. Tutorial. William and Joan Schreyer Business Library, Penn State University, University Park, PA
Created by librarians at Penn State, this outstanding tutorial provides suggestions for online and print resources for company information. Click on "how to" links for each item to view a brief instruction vignette.
www.libraries.psu.edu/psul/researchguides/business.html

Ten Steps to Industry Intelligence. Industry Tutorial. George A. Smathers Libraries, University of Florida, Gainesville, FL
Provides a step-by-step approach for finding information about industries, with embedded links to recommended sources.
http://businesslibrary.uflib.ufl.edu/industryresearch

SEC Filings/EDGAR—Company Disclosure Reports

SEC filings are the various reports that publicly traded companies must file with the Securities and Exchange Commission to disclose information about their corporation. These are often referred to as "EDGAR" filings, an acronym for the Electronic Data Gathering, Analysis and Retrieval System. Some websites and commercial databases improve access to these reports by offering additional retrieval features not available on the official (*www.sec.gov*) website.

EDGAR Database Full-Text Search. U.S. Securities and Exchange Commission (SEC), Washington, DC
10-K reports and other required corporate documents are made available in the SEC's EDGAR database within 24 hours after being filed. Annual reports, on the other hand, are typically sent directly to shareholders and are not required as part of EDGAR by the SEC, although some companies voluntarily include them. Both 10-Ks and shareholders' annual reports are considered basic sources of company research. The SEC offers a search interface for full-text searching of the content and exhibits of EDGAR SEC filings. The advanced search is recommended to locate "hard-to-find" information within documents filed by corporations and their competitors. Searches for specific types of reports or certain industries can also be performed.
http://searchwww.sec.gov/EDGARFSClient/jsp/EDGAR_MainAccess.jsp

LexisNexis Academic—SEC Filings & Reports. Bethesda, MD: LexisNexis.
Company Securities Exchange Commission filings and reports are available through a database called LexisNexis Academic. These reports and filings can be retrieved by company name, industry code, or ticker symbol for a particular time period or by a specific report. Proxy, 10-Ks, prospectus, and registration filings are also available.

Mergent Online—EDGAR Search. New York: Mergent, Inc.

As an alternative to *sec.gov,* the Securities and Exchange Commission website, it is possible to use the *Mergent Online* database to search for official company filings. Check to be sure if your library subscribes to the *Mergent Online* database. Select the "Filings" tab and then click on the "EDGAR Search" link. Next, Mergent's Government Filings search allows searching by company name, ticker, CIK (Central Index Key) number, or industry SIC number. The search can be limited by date and by type of SEC filing. The URL below should also work if your library subscribes to the Mergent Online database.

http://www.mergentonline.com/filingsearch.php?type=edgar&criteriatype=findall& submitvalues

Company Rankings

Fortune 500. New York: Time Inc.

The *Fortune 500* list and other company rankings are published in the printed edition of *Fortune* magazine and are also available online.

http://money.cnn.com/magazines/fortune/fortune500/2008/full_list/index.html

Forbes Global 2000. Forbes, Inc.

The companies listed on The Forbes Global 2000 are the biggest and most powerful in the world.

www.forbes.com/lists

Ward's Business Directory of U.S. Private and Public Companies. Farmington Hills, MI: Gale CENGAGE Learning, 2008, 8 vols.

Ward's Business Directory is one of the few directories to rank both public and private companies together by sales within an industry, using both the Standard Industrial Classification system (in vol. 5 only) and the North American Industry Classification System (in vol. 8 only). With this information, it is easy to spot who the big "players" are in a particular product or industry category. Market share within an industry group can be calculated by determining what percentage a company's sales figure is of the total given by Ward's for that industry group. Some libraries may offer this business directory as part of a database called *Gale Directory Library.*

Business Websites

Big Charts. San Francisco: MarketWatch, Inc.

BigCharts is a comprehensive and easy-to-use investment research website, providing access to professional-level research tools such as interactive charts, current and historical quotes, industry analysis, and intraday stock screeners, as well as market news and commentary. MarketWatch operates this website, a service of Dow Jones & Company. Supported by site sponsors, it is free to self-directed investors.

http://bigcharts.marketwatch.com/

GlobalEdge. East Lansing, MI: Michigan State University

GlobalEdge is a web portal providing a significant amount of information about international business, countries around the globe, the U.S. states, industries, and news.

http://globaledge.msu.edu/

Hoover's Online. Hoover's, Inc. Short Hills, NJ: Dun & Bradstreet Corp.

Hoover's includes a limited amount of free information on companies and industries. The subscribers' edition provides more in-depth information, especially for competitors and industries.

www.hoovers.com

Yahoo Finance. Sunnyvale, CA: Yahoo! Inc.

This website links to information on U.S. markets, world markets, data sources, finance references, investment editorials, financial news, and other helpful websites.

http://finance.yahoo.com

Strategic and Competitive Analysis—Information Sources

Analyzing a company can take the form of examining its internal and external environment. In the process, it is useful to identify the company's strengths, weaknesses, opportunities and threats (SWOT). Sources for this kind of analysis are varied, but perhaps the best would be to locate articles from *The Wall Street Journal,* business magazines and industry trade publications. Publications such as these can be found in the following databases available at many public and academic libraries. When using a database that is structured to allow it, try searching the company name combined with one or more keywords, such as "IBM and competition" or "Microsoft and lawsuits" or "AMR and fuel costs" to retrieve articles relating to the external environment.

ABI/Inform Complete. Ann Arbor, MI: ProQuest LLC
ABI/Inform Complete provides abstracts and full-text articles covering management, law, taxation, human resources, and company and industry information from more than 5,400 business and management journals. *ABI/Inform* includes market condition reports, corporate strategies, case studies, executive profiles, and global industry conditions.

Business & Company Resource Center. Farmington Hills, MI: Gale CENGAGE Learning
Business & Company Resource Center provides company and industry intelligence for a selection of public and private companies. Company profiles include parent-subsidiary relationships, industry rankings, products and brands, investment reports, industry statistics, and financial ratios. A selection of full-text investment reports and SWOT analysis reports are also available.

Business Source Complete. Ipswich, MA: EBSCO Publishing
Business Source Complete is a full-text database with over 3,800 scholarly business journals covering management, economics, finance, accounting, international business, and more. The database also includes detailed company profiles for the world's 10,000 largest companies, as well as selected country economic reports provided by the Economist Intelligence Unit (EIU). The database includes case studies, investment and market research reports, SWOT analyses, and more. *Business Source Complete* contains over 1,850 peer-reviewed business journals.

Investext Research Reports. Detroit, MI: Thomson Reuters Corp.
Investext Research Reports offer full-text analytical reports on more than 65,000 companies worldwide. The research reports are excellent sources for strategic and financial profiles of a company and its competitors and of industry trends. Developed by a global roster of brokerage, investment banking, and research firms, these full-text investment reports include a wealth of current and historical information useful for evaluating a company or industry over time.

International Directory of Company Histories. Detroit, MI: St. James Press, 1988–present, 120 volumes to date.
This directory covers more than 11,000 multinational companies, and the series is still adding volumes. Each company history is approximately three to five pages in length and provides a summary of the company's mission, goals, and ideals, followed by company milestones, principal subsidiaries, and competitors. Strategic decisions made during the company's period of existence are usually noted. This series covers public and private companies and nonprofit entities. Entry information includes a company's legal name, headquarters information, URL, incorporation date, ticker symbol, stock exchange, sales figures, and the primary North American Industry Classification System (NAICS) code. Further reading selections complete the entry information. Volume 59 to current date is available electronically in the Gale Virtual Reference Library database from Gale CENCAGE Learning.

LexisNexis Academic. Bethesda, MD: LexisNexis
The "business" category in *LexisNexis Academic* provides access to timely business articles from newspapers, magazines, journals, wires, and broadcast transcripts. Other information available in this section includes detailed company financials, company comparisons, and database industry and market information for over 25 industries. The Company Dossier research tool allows a researcher to compare up to five companies' financial statements at one time with download capabilities.

The Wall Street Journal. New York: Dow Jones & Co.

This respected business newspaper is available in searchable full text from 1984 to the present in the *Factiva* database. The "News Pages" link provides access to current articles and issues of *The Wall Street Journal.* Dow Jones, publisher of the print version of *The Wall Street Journal,* also has an online subscription available at wsj.com. Some libraries provide access to *The Wall Street Journal* through the ProQuest Newspapers database.

Sources for Industry Research and Analysis

Factiva. New York: Dow Jones & Co.

The *Factiva* database has several options for researching an industry. One would be to search the database for articles in the business magazines and industry trade publications. A second option in *Factiva* would be to search in the Companies/Markets category for company/industry comparison reports.

Mergent Online. New York: Mergent Inc.

Mergent Online is a searchable database of over 60,000 global public companies. The database offers worldwide industry reports, U.S. and global competitors, and executive biographical information. *Mergent*'s Basic Search option permits searching by primary industry codes (either SIC or NAICS). Once the search is executed, companies in that industry should be listed. A comparison or standard peer group analysis can be created to analyze companies in the same industry on various criteria. The Advanced Search allows the user to search a wider range of financial and textual information. Results, including ratios for a company and its competitors, can be downloaded to a spreadsheet.

North American Industry Classification System (NAICS)

The North American Industry Classification System has officially replaced the Standard Industrial Classification (SIC) as the numerical structure used to define and analyze industries, although some publications and databases offer both classification systems. The NAICS codes are used in Canada, the United States, and Mexico. In the United States, the NAICS codes are used to conduct an Economic Census every five years, providing a snapshot of the U.S. economy at a given moment in time.

NAICS: *www.census.gov/eos/www/naics/*

Economic Census: *www.census.gov/econ/census07/*

NetAdvantage. New York: Standard & Poor's

The database includes company, financial, and investment information as well as the well-known publication called *Industry Surveys.* Each industry report includes information on the current environment, industry trends, key industry ratios and statistics, and comparative company financial analysis. Available in HTML, PDF, or Excel formats.

Search Engines

Google. Mountain View, CA: Google, Inc.

Recognized for its advanced technology, quality of results, and simplicity, the search engine Google is highly recommended by librarians and other expert web surfers.

www.google.com

Dogpile. Bellevue, WA: InfoSpace, Inc.

Dogpile is a metasearch engine that searches and compiles the most relevant results from more than 12 individual search engines.

www.dogpile.com/

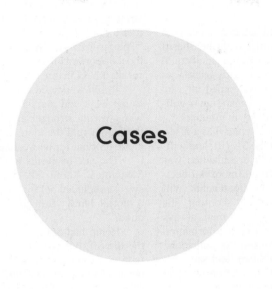

Cases

Case 1 Robin Hood*

It was in the spring of the second year of his insurrection against the High Sheriff of Nottingham that Robin Hood took a walk in Sherwood Forest. As he walked he pondered the progress of the campaign, the disposition of his forces, the Sheriff's recent moves, and the options that confronted him.

The revolt against the Sheriff had begun as a personal crusade, erupting out of Robin's conflict with the Sheriff and his administration. Alone, however, Robin Hood could do little. He therefore sought allies, men with grievances and a deep sense of justice. Later he welcomed all who came, asking few questions, and only demanding a willingness to serve. Strength, he believed, lay in numbers.

He spent the first year forging the group into a disciplined band, united in enmity against the Sheriff, and willing to live outside the law. The band's organization was simple. Robin ruled supreme, making all important decisions. He delegated specific tasks to his lieutenants. Will Scarlett was in charge of intelligence and scouting. His main job was to shadow the Sheriff and his men, always alert to their next move. He also collected information on the travel plans of rich merchants and tax collectors. Little John kept discipline among the men, and saw to it that their archery was at the high peak that their profession demanded. Scarlock took care of the finances, converting loot into cash, paying shares of the take, and finding suitable hiding places for the surplus. Finally, Much the Miller's son had the difficult task of provisioning the ever-increasing band of Merrymen.

The increasing size of the band was a source of satisfaction for Robin, but also a source of concern. The fame of his Merrymen was spreading, and new recruits poured in from every corner of England. As the band grew larger, their small bivouac became a major encampment. Between raids the men milled about, talking and playing games. Vigilance was in decline, and discipline was becoming harder to enforce. "Why," Robin reflected, "I don't know half the men I run into these days."

The growing band was also beginning to exceed the food capacity of the forest. Game was becoming scarce, and supplies had to be obtained from outlying villages. The cost of buying food was beginning to drain the band's financial reserves at the very moment when revenues were in decline. Travelers, especially those with the most to lose, were now giving the forest a wide berth. This was costly and inconvenient to them, but it was preferable to having all their goods confiscated.

Robin believed that the time had come for the Merrymen to change their policy of outright confiscation of goods to one of a fixed transit tax. His lieutenants strongly resisted this idea. They were proud of the Merrymen's famous motto: "Rob the rich and give to the poor." "The farmers and the townspeople," they argued, "are our most important allies. How can we tax them, and still hope for their help in our fight against the Sheriff?"

Robin wondered how long the Merrymen could keep to the ways and methods of their early days. The Sheriff was growing stronger and better organized. He now had the money and the men, and was beginning to harass the band, probing for its weaknesses.

The tide of events was beginning to turn against the Merrymen. Robin felt that the campaign must be decisively concluded before the Sheriff had a chance to deliver a mortal blow. "But how," he wondered, "could this be done?"

Robin had often entertained the possibility of killing the Sheriff, but the chances for this seemed increasingly remote. Besides, while killing the Sheriff might satisfy his personal thirst for revenge, it would not improve the situation. Robin had hoped that the perpetual state of unrest, and the Sheriff's failure to collect taxes, would lead to his removal from office. Instead, the Sheriff used his political connections to obtain reinforcement. He had powerful friends at court, and was well regarded by the regent, Prince John.

Prince John was vicious and volatile. He was consumed by his unpopularity among the people, who wanted the imprisoned King Richard back. He also lived in constant fear of the barons, who had first given him the regency, but were now beginning to dispute his claim to the throne. Several of these barons had set out to collect the ransom that would release King Richard the Lionheart from his jail in Austria. Robin was invited to join the conspiracy in return for future amnesty. It was a dangerous proposition. Provincial banditry was one thing, court intrigue another. Prince John's spies were everywhere. If the plan failed, the pursuit would be relentless and retribution swift.

The sound of the supper horn startled Robin from his thoughts. There was the smell of roasting venison in the air. Nothing was resolved or settled. Robin headed for camp promising himself that he would give these problems his utmost attention after tomorrow's raid.

* Prepared by Joseph Lampel, City University, London. Copyright Joseph Lampel © 1985, revised 1991. Reprinted with permission.

Case 2 — Crown Cork & Seal in 1989*

John F. Connelly, Crown Cork & Seal's ailing octogenarian chairman, stepped down and appointed his long-time disciple, William J. Avery, chief executive officer of the Philadelphia can manufacturer in May 1989. Avery had been president of Crown Cork & Seal since 1981, but had spent the duration of his career in Connelly's shadow. As Crown's new CEO, Avery planned to review Connelly's long-followed strategy in light of the changing industry outlook.

The metal container industry had changed considerably since Connelly took over Crown's reins in 1957. American National had just been acquired by France's state-owned Pechiney International, making it the world's largest beverage can producer. Continental Can, another long-standing rival, was now owned by Peter Kiewit Sons, a privately held construction firm. In 1989, all or part of Continental's can-making operations appeared to be for sale. Reynolds Metals, a traditional supplier of aluminum to can makers, was now also a formidable competitor in cans. The moves by both suppliers and customers of can makers to integrate into can manufacturing themselves had profoundly redefined the metal can industry since John Connelly's arrival.

Reflecting on these dramatic changes, Avery wondered whether Crown, with $1.8 billion in sales, should consider bidding for all or part of Continental Can. Avery also wondered whether Crown should break with tradition and expand its product line beyond the manufacture of metal cans and closures. For 30 years Crown had stuck to its core business, metal can making, but analysts saw little growth potential for metal cans in the 1990s. Industry observers forecast plastics as the growth segment for containers. As Avery mulled over his options, he asked: Was it finally time for a change?

The Metal Container Industry

The metal container industry, representing 61% of all packaged products in the United States in 1989, produced metal cans, crowns (bottle caps), and closures (screw caps, bottle lids) to hold or seal an almost endless variety of consumer and industrial goods. Glass and plastic containers split the balance of the container market with shares of 21% and 18%, respectively. Metal cans served the beverage, food, and general packaging industries.

Metal cans were made of aluminum, steel, or a combination of both. Three-piece cans were formed by rolling a sheet of metal, soldering it, cutting it to size, and attaching two ends, thereby creating a three-piece, seamed can. Steel was the primary raw material of three-piece cans, which were most popular in the food and general packaging industries. Two-piece cans, developed in the 1960s, were formed by pushing a flat blank of metal into a deep cup, eliminating a separate bottom, a molding process termed "drawn and ironed." While aluminum companies developed the original technology for the two-piece can, steel companies ultimately followed suit with a thin-walled steel version. By 1983, two-piece cans dominated the beverage industry where they were the can of choice for beer and soft drink makers. Of the 120 billion cans produced in 1989, 80% were two-piece cans.

Throughout the decade of the 1980s, the number of metal cans shipped grew by an annual average of 3.7%. Aluminum can growth averaged 8% annually, while steel can shipments fell by an average of 3.1% per year. The number of aluminum cans produced increased by almost 200% during the period 1980–1989, reaching a high of 85 billion, while steel can production dropped by 22% to 35 billion for the same period (see Exhibit 1).

Industry Structure Five firms dominated the $12.2 billion U.S. metal can industry in 1989, with an aggregate 61% market share. The country's largest manufacturer—American National Can—held a 25% market share. The four firms trailing American National in sales were Continental Can (18% market share), Reynolds Metals (7%), Crown Cork & Seal (7%), and Ball Corporation (4%). Approximately 100 firms served the balance of the market.

Pricing Pricing in the can industry was very competitive. To lower costs, managers sought long runs of standard items, which increased capacity utilization and reduced the need for costly changeovers. As a result, most companies offered volume discounts to encourage large orders. Despite persistent metal can demand, industry operating margins fell approximately 7% to roughly 4% between 1986 and 1989. Industry analysts attributed the drop in operating margins to (1) a 15% increase in aluminum can sheet prices at a time when most can makers had guaranteed volume prices that did not incorporate substantial cost increases; (2) a 7% increase in beverage can production capacity between 1987 and 1989; (3) an increasing number of the nation's major brewers producing containers in house; and (4) the consolidation of soft drink bottlers throughout the decade. Forced to economize following

* Professor Stephen P. Bradley and Research Associate Sheila M. Cavanaugh prepared this case. Harvard Business School cases are developed solely as the basis for class discussion. Cases are not intended to serve as endorsements, sources of primary data, or illustrations of effective or ineffective management.

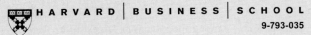

9-793-035

Exhibit 1   Metal Can Shipments by Market and Product, 1981–1989 (millions of cans)

	1981	%	1983	%	1985	%	1987	%	(Est.) 1989	%
Total Metal Cans Shipped	88,810		92,394		101,899		109,214		120,795	
By Market										
For sale:	59,433	67	61,907	67	69,810	69	81,204	74	91,305	76
Beverage	42,192		45,167		52,017		62,002		69,218	
Food	13,094		12,914		13,974		15,214		18,162	
General packaging	4,147		3,826		3,819		3,988		3,925	
For own use:	29,377	33	31,039	33	32,089	31	28,010	26	29,490	24
Beverage	14,134		16,289		18,160		14,771		17,477	
Food	15,054		14,579		13,870		13,167		11,944	
General packaging	189		171		59		72		69	
By Product										
Beverage:	56,326	63	61,456	67	70,177	69	76,773	70	86,695	72
Beer	30,901		33,135		35,614		36,480		37,276	
Soft drinks	25,425		28,321		34,563		40,293		49,419	
Food:	28,148	32	26,941	29	27,844	27	28,381	26	30,106	25
Dairy products	854		927		1,246		1,188		1,304	
Juices	13,494		11,954		11,385		11,565		12,557	
Meat, poultry, seafood	2,804		3,019		3,373		3,530		3,456	
Pet food	3,663		3,571		4,069		4,543		5,130	
Other	7,333		7,470		7,771		7,555		7,659	
General packaging:	4,336	5	3,997	4	3,878	4	4,060	4	3,994	3
Aerosol	2,059		2,144		2,277		2,508		2,716	
Paint: varnish	813		817		830		842		710	
Automotive products	601		229		168		128		65	
Other nonfoods	863		807		603		582		503	
By Materials Used										
Steel	45,386	52	40,116	45	34,316	37	34,559	34	35,318	29
Aluminum	42,561	48	48,694	55	58,078	63	67,340	66	85,477	71

Source: Can Shipment Report, Can Manufacturers Institute, 1981–1989.

costly battles for market share, soft drink bottlers used their leverage to obtain packaging price discounts.[1] Over-capacity and a shrinking customer base contributed to an unprecedented squeeze on manufacturers' margins, and the can manufacturers themselves contributed to the margin deterioration by aggressively discounting to protect market share. As one manufacturer confessed, "When you look at the beverage can industry, it's no secret that we are selling at a lower price today than we were 10 years ago."

Customers   Among the industry's largest users were the Coca-Cola Company, Anheuser-Busch Companies, Inc., PepsiCo Inc., and Coca-Cola Enterprises Inc. (see Exhibit 2). Consolidation within the soft drink segment of the bottling industry reduced the number of bottlers from approximately 8,000 in 1980 to about 800 in 1989 and placed a significant amount of beverage volume in the hands of a few large companies.[2] Since the can constituted about 45% of the total cost of a packaged beverage, soft drink bottlers

Exhibit 2 Top U.S. Users of Containers, 1989

Rank	Company	Soft Drink/ Beverage Sales ($000)	Principal Product Categories
1	The Coca-Cola Company[a] (Atlanta, GA)	$8,965,800	Soft drinks, citrus juices, fruit drinks
2	Anheuser-Busch Companies, Inc.[b] (St. Louis, MO)	7,550,000	Beer, beer imports
3	PepsiCo Inc. (Purchase, NY)	5,777,000	Soft drinks, bottled water
4	The Seagram Company, Ltd. (Montreal, Quebec, Canada)	5,581,779	Distilled spirits, wine coolers, mixers, juices
5	Coca-Cola Enterprises, Inc.[a] (Atlanta, GA)	3,881,947	Soft drinks
6	Philip Morris Companies, Inc. (New York, NY)	3,435,000	Beer
7	The Molson Companies, Ltd. (Toronto, Ontario, Canada)	1,871,394	Beer, coolers, beer imports
8	John Labatt, Ltd. (London, Ontario, Canada)	1,818,100	Beer, wine
9	The Stroh Brewery Company[c] (Detroit, MI)	1,500,000	Beer, coolers, soft drinks
10	Adolph Coors Company[d] (Golden, CO)	1,366,108	Beer, bottled water

Source: Beverage World, 1990–1991 Databank.

[a]The Coca-Cola Company and Coca-Cola Enterprises purchased (versus in-house manufacture) all of its cans in 1989. Coca-Cola owned 49% of Coca-Cola Enterprises—the largest Coca-Cola bottler in the United States.

[b]In addition to in-house manufacturing at its wholly owned subsidiary (Metal Container Corporation), Anheuser-Busch Companies purchased its cans from four manufacturers. The percentage of cans manufactured by Anheuser-Busch was not publicly disclosed.

[c]Of the 4 to 5 billion cans used by The Stroh Brewery in 1989, 39% were purchased and 61% were manufactured in-house.

[d]Adolph Coors Company manufactured all of its cans, producing approximately 10 to 12 million cans per day, five days per week.

and brewers usually maintained relationships with more than one can supplier. Poor service and uncompetitive prices could be punished by cuts in order size.

Distribution   Due to the bulky nature of cans, manufacturers located their plants close to customers to minimize transportation costs. The primary cost components of the metal can included (1) raw materials at 65%; (2) direct labor at 12%; and (3) transportation at roughly 7.5%. Various estimates placed the radius of economical distribution for a plant at between 150 and 300 miles. Beverage can producers preferred aluminum to steel because of aluminum's lighter weight and lower shipping costs. In 1988, steel cans weighed more than twice as much as aluminum.[3] The costs incurred in transporting cans to overseas markets made international trade uneconomical. Foreign

markets were served by joint ventures, foreign subsidiaries, affiliates of U.S. can manufacturers, and local overseas firms.

Manufacturing   Two-piece can lines cost approximately $16 million, and the investment in peripheral equipment raised the per-line cost to $20–$25 million. The minimum efficient plant size was one line and installations ranged from one to five lines. While two-piece can lines achieved quick and persistent popularity, they did not completely replace their antecedents—the three-piece can lines. The food and general packaging segment—representing 28% of the metal container industry in 1989—continued using three-piece cans throughout the 1980s. The beverage segment, however, had made a complete switch from three-piece to two-piece cans by 1983.

Exhibit 3 **Comparative Performance of Major Aluminum Suppliers, 1988** (dollars in millions)

	Sales	Net Income	Net Profit Margin %	Long-Term Debt	Net Worth	Earnings Per Share
Alcan Aluminum						
1988	$8,529.0	$931.0	10.9%	$1,199.0	$4,320.0	$3.85
1987	6,797.0	445.0	6.5	1,336.0	3,970.0	1.73
1986	5,956.0	177.0	3.0	1,366.0	3,116.0	.79
1985	5,718.0	25.8	0.5	1,600.0	2,746.0	.12
1984	5,467.0	221.0	4.0	1,350.0	2,916.0	1.00
Alcoa						
1988	9,795.3	861.4	8.8	1,524.7	4,635.5	9.74
1987	7,767.0	365.8	4.7	2,457.6	3,910.7	4.14
1986	4,667.2	125.0	2.7	1,325.6	3,721.6	1.45
1985	5,162.7	107.4	2.1	1,553.5	3,307.9	1.32
1984	5,750.8	278.7	4.8	1,586.5	3,343.6	3.41
Reynolds Metals[a]						
1988	5,567.1	482.0	8.7	1,280.0	2,040.1	9.01
1987	4,283.8	200.7	4.7	1,567.7	1,599.6	3.95
1986	3,638.9	50.3	1.4	1,190.8	1,342.0	.86
1985	3,415.6	24.5	0.7	1,215.0	1,151.7	.46
1984	3,728.3	133.3	3.6	1,146.1	1,341.1	3.09

Source: *Value Line.*

[a]Reynolds Metals Company was the second-largest aluminum producer in the United States. The company was also the third-largest manufacturer of metal cans, with a 7% market share.

A typical three-piece can production line cost between $1.5 and $2 million and required expensive seaming, end-making, and finishing equipment. Since each finishing line could handle the output of three or four can-forming lines, the minimum efficient plant required at least $7 million in basic equipment. Most plants had 12 to 15 lines for the increased flexibility of handling more than one type of can at once. However, any more than 15 lines became unwieldy because of the need for duplication of set-up crews, maintenance, and supervision. The beverage industry's switch from three- to two-piece lines prompted many manufacturers to sell complete, fully operational three-piece lines "as is" for $175,000 to $200,000. Some firms shipped their old lines overseas to their foreign operations where growth potential was great, there were few entrenched firms, and canning technology was not well understood.

Suppliers Since the invention of the aluminum can in 1958, steel had fought a losing battle against aluminum. In 1970, steel accounted for 88% of metal cans, but by 1989

had dropped to 29%. In addition to being lighter, of higher, more consistent quality, and more economical to recycle, aluminum was also friendlier to the taste and offered superior lithography qualities. By 1989, aluminum accounted for 99% of the beer and 94% of the soft drink metal container businesses, respectively.

The country's three largest aluminum producers supplied the metal can industry. Alcoa, the world's largest aluminum producer, with 1988 sales of $9.8 billion, and Alcan, the world's largest marketer of primary aluminum, with 1988 sales of $8.5 billion, supplied over 65% of the domestic can sheet requirements. Reynolds Metals, the second-largest aluminum producer in the United States, with 1988 sales of $5.6 billion, supplied aluminum sheet to the industry and also produced about 11 billion cans itself.[4] Reynolds Metals was the only aluminum company in the United States that produced cans (see Exhibit 3).

Steel's consistent advantage over aluminum was price. According to The American Iron and Steel Institute in 1988, steel represented a savings of from $5 to $7 for every thousand cans produced, or an estimated savings of $500 million a year for can manufacturers. In 1988, aluminum prices increased an estimated 15%, while the lower steel prices increased by only 5% to 7%. According to a representative of Alcoa, the decision on behalf of the firm to limit aluminum price increases was attributed to the threat of possible inroads by steel.[5]

Industry Trends The major trends characterizing the metal container industry during the 1980s included (1) the continuing threat of in-house manufacture; (2) the emergence of plastics as a viable packaging material; (3) the steady competition from glass as a substitute for aluminum in the beer market; (4) the emergence of the soft drink industry as the largest end-user of packaging, with aluminum as the primary beneficiary; and (5) the diversification of, and consolidation among, packaging producers.

In-House Manufacture Production of cans at "captive" plants—those producing cans for their own company use—accounted for approximately 25% of the total can output in 1989. Much of the expansion in in-house manufactured cans, which persisted throughout the 1980s, occurred at plants owned by the nation's major food producers and brewers. Many large brewers moved to hold can costs down by developing their own manufacturing capability. Brewers found it advantageous to invest in captive manufacture because of high-volume, single-label production runs. Adolph Coors took this to the extreme by producing all their cans in-house and supplying almost all of their own aluminum requirements from their 130-million-pound sheet rolling mill in San Antonio, Texas.[6] By the end of the 1980s, the beer industry had the capacity to supply about 55% of its beverage can needs.[7]

Captive manufacturing was not widespread in the soft drink industry, where many small bottlers and franchise operations were generally more dispersed geographically compared with the brewing industry. Soft drink bottlers were also geared to low-volume, multilabel output, which was not as economically suitable for the in-house can manufacturing process.

Plastics Throughout the 1980s, plastics was the growth leader in the container industry with its share growing from 9% in 1980 to 18% in 1989. Plastic bottle sales in the United States were estimated to reach $3.5 billion in 1989, with food and beverage—buoyed by soft drinks sales—accounting for 50% of the total. Plastic bottles accounted for 11% of domestic soft drink sales, with most of its penetration coming at the expense of glass. Plastic's light weight and convenient handling contributed to widespread consumer acceptance. The greatest challenge facing plastics, however, was the need to produce a material that simultaneously retained carbonation and prevented infiltration of oxygen. The plastic bottle often allowed carbonation to escape in less than 4 months, while aluminum cans held carbonation for more than 16 months. Anheuser-Busch claimed that U.S. brewers expected beer containers to have at least a 90-day shelf-life, a requirement that had not been met by any plastic can or bottle.[8] Additionally, standard production lines that filled 2,400 beer cans per minute required containers with perfectly flat bottoms, a feature difficult to achieve using plastic.[9] Since 1987, the growth of plastics had slowed somewhat apparently due to the impact on the environment of plastic packaging. Unlike glass and aluminum, plastics recycling was not a "closed loop" system.[10]

There were many small players producing plastic containers in 1988, often specializing by end-use or geographic region. However, only seven companies had sales of over $100 million. Owens-Illinois, the largest producer of plastic containers, specialized in custom-made bottles and closures for food, health and beauty, and pharmaceutical products. It was the leading supplier of prescription containers, sold primarily to drug wholesalers, major drug chains, and the government. Constar, the second-largest domestic producer of plastic containers, acquired its plastic bottle operation from Owens-Illinois, and relied on plastic soft drink bottles for about two-thirds of its sales. Johnson Controls produced bottles for the soft drink industry from 17 U.S. plants and six non-U.S. plants, and was the largest producer of plastic bottles for water and liquor. American National and Continental Can both produced plastic bottles for food, beverages, and other products such as tennis balls (see Exhibit 4 for information on competitors).

Glass Glass bottles accounted for only 14% of domestic soft drink sales, trailing metal cans at 75%. The cost advantage that glass once had relative to plastic in the popular 16-ounce bottle size disappeared by the mid-1980s because of consistently declining resin prices. Moreover, soft drink bottlers preferred the metal can to glass because of a variety of logistical and economic benefits: faster filling speeds, lighter weight, compactness for inventory, and transportation efficiency. In 1989, the delivered cost (including closure and label) of a 12-ounce can (the most popular size) was about 15% less than that of glass or plastic 16-ounce bottles (the most popular size).[11] The area in which glass continued to outperform metal, however, was the beer category where consumers seemed to have a love affair with the "long neck" bottle that would work to its advantage in the coming years.[12]

Soft Drinks and Aluminum Cans Throughout the 1980s, the soft drink industry emerged as the largest end-user of packaging. In 1989, soft drinks captured more than 50% of the total beverage market. The soft drink industry accounted for 42% of metal cans shipped in 1989—up from 29% in 1980. The major beneficiary of this trend was the aluminum can. In addition to the industry's continued commitment to advanced technology and innovation, aluminum's penetration could be traced to several factors: (1) aluminum's weight advantage over glass and steel; (2) aluminum's ease of handling; (3) a wider variety of graphics options provided by multipack can containers; and (4) consumer preference.[13] Aluminum's growth was also

Exhibit 4 Major U.S. Producers of Blow-Molded Plastic Bottles, 1989 (dollars in millions)

Company	Total Sales	Net Income	Plastic Sales	Product Code	Major Market
Owens-Illinois	$3,280	$ (57)	$754	1,3,4,6	Food, health and beauty, pharmaceutical
American National	4,336	52	566	1,2,3,6	Beverage, household, personal care, pharmaceutical
Constar	544	12	544	1,2,3,4,6	Soft drink, milk, food
Johnson Controls	3,100	104	465	2	Soft drink, beverages
Continental Can	3,332	18	353	1,2,3,4,5,6	Food, beverage, household, industrial
Silgan Plastics	415	96	100	1,2,3,4,6	Food, beverage, household, pharmaceutical, personal care
Sonoco Products Co.	1,600	96	N/A	1,3,4,6	Motor oil, industrial

Source: *The Rauch Guide to the U.S. Plastics Industry.* 1991; company annual reports.

Product code: (1) HDPE; (2) PET; (3) PP; (4) PVC; (5) PC; (6) multilayer.

supported by the vending machine market, which was built around cans and dispensed approximately 20% of all soft drinks in 1989. An estimated 60% of Coca-Cola's and 50% of Pepsi's beverages were packaged in metal cans. Coca-Cola Enterprises and Pepsi Cola Bottling Group together accounted for 22% of all soft drink cans shipped in 1989.[14] In 1980, the industry shipped 15.9 billion aluminum soft drink cans. By 1989, that figure had increased to 49.2 billion cans. This increase, representing a 12% average annual growth rate, was achieved during a decade that experienced a 3.6% average annual increase in total gallons of soft drinks consumed.

Diversification and Consolidation Low profit margins, excess capacity, and rising material and labor costs prompted a number of corporate diversifications and subsequent consolidations throughout the 1970s and 1980s. While many can manufacturers diversified across the spectrum of rigid containers to supply all major end-use markets (food, beverages, and general packaging), others diversified into nonpackaging businesses such as energy (oil and gas) and financial services.

Over a 20-year period, for example, American Can reduced its dependence on domestic can manufacturing, moving into totally unrelated fields, such as insurance. Between 1981 and 1986 the company invested $940 million to acquire all or part of six insurance companies. Ultimately, the packaging businesses of American Can were acquired by Triangle Industries in 1986, while the financial services businesses re-emerged as Primerica. Similarly, Continental Can broadly diversified its holdings, changing its name to Continental Group in 1976 when can

sales dropped to 38% of total sales. In the 1980s, Continental Group invested heavily in energy exploration, research, and transportation, but profits were weak and they were ultimately taken over by Peter Kiewit Sons in 1984.

While National Can stuck broadly to containers, it diversified through acquisition into glass containers, food canning, pet foods, bottle closures, and plastic containers. However, instead of generating future growth opportunities, the expansion into food products proved a drag on company earnings.

Under the leadership of John W. Fisher, Ball Corporation, a leading glass bottle and can maker, expanded into the high-technology market and by 1987 had procured $180 million in defense contracts. Fisher directed Ball into such fields as petroleum engineering equipment, and photo-engraving and plastics, and established the company as a leading manufacturer of computer components.

Major Competitors in 1989 For over 30 years, three of the current five top competitors in can manufacturing dominated the metal can industry. Since the early 1950s, American Can, Continental Can, Crown Cork & Seal, and National Can held the top four rankings in can manufacturing. A series of dramatic mergers and acquisitions among several of the country's leading manufacturers throughout the 1980s served to shift as well as consolidate power at the top. Management at fourth-ranked Crown Cork & Seal viewed the following four firms as constituting its primary competition in 1989: American National Can, Continental Can, Reynolds Metals, and Ball Corporation. Two smaller companies—Van Dorn Company and Heekin Can—were strong competitors regionally (see Exhibit 5).

Exhibit 5   **Comparative Performance of Major Metal Can Manufacturers** (dollars in millions)

Company[a]	Net Sales	SG&A as a % of Sales	Gross Margin	Operating Income	Net Profit	Return on Sales	Return on Average Assets	Return on Average Equity
Ball Corporation								
1988	$1,073.0	8.1%	$161.7	$113.0	$47.7	4.4%	5.7%	11.6%
1987	1,054.1	8.5	195.4	147.6	59.8	5.7	7.8	15.7
1986	1,060.1	8.2	168.0	150.5	52.8	5.0	7.6	15.2
1985	1,106.2	7.5	140.7	140.5	51.2	4.6	8.1	16.4
1984	1,050.7	7.9	174.1	123.9	46.3	4.4	7.8	16.6
1983	909.5	8.2	158.2	114.6	39.0	4.3	7.3	15.6
1982	889.1	8.4	147.4	100.5	34.5	3.9	6.9	15.8
Crown Cork & Seal								
1988	1,834.1	2.8	264.6	212.7	93.4	5.1	8.6	14.5
1987	1,717.9	2.9	261.3	223.3	88.3	5.1	8.7	14.5
1986	1,618.9	2.9	235.3	202.4	79.4	4.9	8.8	14.3
1985	1,487.1	2.9	216.4	184.4	71.7	4.8	8.6	13.9
1984	1,370.0	3.1	186.6	154.8	59.5	4.4	7.3	11.4
1983	1,298.0	3.3	182.0	138.9	51.5	4.0	6.2	9.3
1982	1,351.8	3.3	176.2	132.5	44.7	3.3	5.2	7.9
Heekin Can, Inc.								
1988	275.8	3.7	38.9	36.4	9.6	3.5	4.8	22.6
1987	230.4	4.0	33.6	30.2	8.8	3.8	5.8	26.3
1986	207.6	4.1	31.1	28.0	7.0	3.4	5.4	27.5
1985	221.8	3.2	31.8	29.0	6.8	3.1	5.2	42.5
1984	215.4	2.7	28.4	26.5	5.5	2.6	4.3	79.7
1983	181.6	3.2	24.4	22.8	3.8	2.1	3.3	102.7
1982[b]	—							
Van Dorn Company								
1988	333.5	16.5	75.3	26.7	11.7	3.5	6.6	12.2
1987	330.0	15.7	73.6	28.4	12.3	3.7	7.7	12.7
1986	305.1	16.3	70.4	26.5	11.7	3.8	7.7	12.9
1985	314.3	15.1	75.6	33.6	15.4	4.9	10.6	19.0
1984	296.4	14.7	74.9	36.5	16.8	5.7	12.9	24.9
1983	225.9	14.8	48.5	20.1	7.4	3.3	6.8	12.8
1982	184.3	16.1	37.7	12.7	3.6	2.0	3.5	6.6
American Can Company[c]								
1985	2,854.9	22.6	813.4	1670.0	149.1	5.2	5.2	10.9
1984	3,177.9	18.0	740.8	168.3	132.4	4.2	4.9	11.2
1983	3,346.4	15.0	625.4	123.6	94.9	2.8	3.5	9.7

(*continued*)

Exhibit 5 *(continued)*

Company[a]	Net Sales	SG&A as a % of Sales	Gross Margin	Operating Income	Net Profit	Return on Sales	Return on Average Assets	Return on Average Equity
American Can Company[c]								
1982	$4,063.4	16.1%	$766.3	$113.4	$23.0	0.6%	0.8%	2.4%
1981	4,836.4	15.0	949.6	223.0	76.7	1.2	2.7	7.2
1980	4,812.2	15.8	919.5	128.1	85.7	1.8	3.1	8.0
National Can Company[d]								
1983	1,647.5	5.1	215.3	93.5	22.1	1.3	2.7	6.3
1982	1,541.5	4.6	206.3	100.7	34.1	2.2	4.4	10.0
1981	1,533.9	4.6	191.7	86.3	24.7	1.6	3.1	7.5
1980	1,550.9	5.4	233.7	55.0	50.6	3.3	6.4	16.7
The Continental Group, Inc.[e]								
1983	4,942.0	6.3	568.0	157.0	173.5	3.5	4.4	9.4
1982	5,089.0	6.4	662.0	217.0	180.2	3.5	4.3	9.6
1981	5,291.0	7.2	747.0	261.0	242.2	4.6	5.9	13.6
1980	5,171.0	7.2	700.0	201.0	224.8	4.3	5.5	13.7
1979	4,544.0	6.5	573.0	171.0	189.2	4.2	5.3	13.1

Source: *Value Line* and company annual reports (for SGA, COGS, and Asset figures).

[a]Refer to Exhibit 3 for Reynolds Metals Company.

[b]Figures not disclosed for 1982.

[c]In 1985, packaging made up 60% of total sales at American Can, with the remainder in specialty retailing. In 1986 Triangle Industries purchased the U.S. packaging business of American Can. In 1987, American National Can was formed through the merger of American Can Packaging and National Can Corporation. In 1989, Triangle sold American National Can to Pechiney, SA.

[d]In 1985, Triangle Industries bought National Can.

[e]In 1984, Peter Kiewit Sons purchased The Continental Group. SG&A as a percentage of sales for Continental Can hovered around 6.5% through the late 1980s.

American National Can Representing the merger of two former, long-established competitors, American National—a wholly-owned subsidiary of the Pechiney International Group—generated sales revenues of $4.4 billion in 1988. In 1985, Triangle Industries, a New Jersey–based maker of video games, vending machines, and jukeboxes, bought National Can for $421 million. In 1986, Triangle bought the U.S. packaging businesses of American Can for $550 million. In 1988, Triangle sold American National Can (ANC) to Pechiney, SA, the French state-owned industrial concern, for $3.5 billion. Pechiney was the world's third-largest producer of aluminum and, through its Cebal Group, a major European manufacturer of packaging. A member of the Pechiney International Group, ANC was the largest beverage can maker in the world—producing more than 30 billion cans annually. With more than 100 facilities in 12 countries, ANC's product line of aluminum and steel cans, glass containers, and caps and closures served the major beverage, food, pharmaceuticals, and cosmetics markets.

Continental Can Continental Can had long been a financially stable container company; its revenues increased every year without interruption from 1923 through the mid-1980s. By the 1970s, Continental had surpassed American Can as the largest container company in the United States. The year 1984, however, represented a turning point in Continental's history when the company became an attractive takeover target. Peter Kiewit Sons Inc., a private construction firm in Omaha, Nebraska, purchased Continental Group for $2.75 billion in 1984. Under the direction of Vice Chairman Donald Strum, Kiewit dismantled Continental Group in an effort to make the operation more profitable. Within a year, Strum had sold $1.6 billion worth of insurance, gas pipelines, and oil and gas reserves. Staff at Continental's Connecticut headquarters was reduced from 500 to 40. Continental Can generated sales revenues of $3.3 billion in 1988, ranking it second behind American National. By the late 1980s, management at Kiewit considered divesting—in whole or in part—Continental Can's packaging operations, which included Continental Can USA, Europe, and Canada, as well as metal packaging operations in Latin America, Asia, and the Middle East.

Reynolds Metals   Based in Richmond, Virginia, Reynolds Metals was the only domestic company integrated from aluminum ingot through aluminum cans. With 1988 sales revenues of $5.6 billion and net income of $482 million, Reynolds served the following principal markets: packaging and containers; distributors and fabricators; building and construction; aircraft and automotive; and electrical. Reynolds' packaging and container revenue amounted to $2.4 billion in 1988. As one of the industry's leading can makers, Reynolds was instrumental in establishing new uses for the aluminum can and was a world leader in can-making technology. Reynolds' developments included high-speed can-forming machinery with capabilities in excess of 400 cans per minute, faster inspection equipment (operating at speeds of up to 2,000 cans per minute), and spun aluminum tops which contained less material. The company's next generation of can end-making technology was scheduled for installation in the early 1990s.

Ball Corporation   Founded in 1880 in Muncie, Indiana, Ball Corporation generated operating income of $113 million on sales revenues of $1 billion in 1988. Considered one of the industry's low-cost producers, Ball was the fifth-largest manufacturer of metal containers as well as the third-largest glass container manufacturer in the United States. Ball's packaging businesses accounted for 82.5% of total sales and 77.6% of consolidated operating earnings in 1988. Ball's can-making technology and manufacturing flexibility allowed the company to make shorter runs in the production of customized, higher-margin products designed to meet customers' specifications and needs. In 1988, beverage can sales accounted for 62% of total sales. Anheuser-Busch, Ball's largest customer, accounted for 14% of sales that year. In 1989, Ball was rumored to be planning to purchase the balance of its 50%-owned joint venture, Ball Packaging Products Canada, Inc. The acquisition would make Ball the number two producer of metal beverage and food containers in the Canadian market.

Van Dorn Company   The industry's next two largest competitors, with a combined market share of 3%, were Van Dorn Company and Heekin Can, Inc. Founded in 1872 in Cleveland, Ohio, Van Dorn manufactured two product lines: containers and plastic injection molding equipment. Van Dorn was one of the world's largest producers of drawn aluminum containers for processed foods, and a major manufacturer of metal, plastic, and composite containers for the paint, petroleum, chemical, automotive, food, and pharmaceutical industries. Van Dorn was also a leading manufacturer of injection molding equipment for the plastics industry. The company's Davies Can Division, founded in 1922, was a regional manufacturer of metal and plastic containers. In 1988, Davies planned to build two new can manufacturing plants at a cost of about $20 million each. These facilities would each produce about 40 million cans annually. Van Dorn's consolidated can sales of $334 million in 1988 ranked it sixth overall among the country's leading can manufacturers.

Heekin Can   James Heekin, a Cincinnati coffee merchant, founded Heekin Can in 1901 as a way to package his own products. The company experienced rapid growth and soon contained one of the country's largest metal lithography plants under one roof. Three generations of the Heekin family built Heekin into a strong regional force in the packaging industry. The family sold the business to Diamond International Corporation, a large, diversified publicly held company, in 1965. Diamond operated Heekin as a subsidiary until 1982 when it was sold to its operating management and a group of private investors. Heekin went public in 1985. With 1988 sales revenues of $275.8 million, seventh-ranked Heekin primarily manufactured steel cans for processors, packagers, and distributors of food and pet food. Heekin represented the country's largest regional can maker.

Crown Cork & Seal Company

Company History   In August 1891, a foreman in a Baltimore machine shop hit upon an idea for a better bottle cap—a piece of tin-coated steel with a flanged edge and an insert of natural cork. Soon this crown-cork cap became the hit product of a new venture, Crown Cork & Seal Company. When the patents ran out, however, competition became severe and nearly bankrupted the company in the 1920s. The faltering Crown was bought in 1927 by a competitor, Charles McManus.[15]

Under the paternalistic leadership of McManus, Crown prospered in the 1930s, selling more than half of the United States and world supply of bottle caps. He then correctly anticipated the success of the beer can and diversified into can making, building one of the world's largest plants in Philadelphia. However, at one million square feet and containing as many as 52 lines, it was a nightmare of inefficiency and experienced substantial losses. Although McManus was an energetic leader, he engaged in nepotism and never developed an organization that could run without him. Following his death in 1946, the company ran on momentum, maintaining dividends at the expense of investment in new plants. Following a disastrous attempt to expand into plastics and a ludicrous diversification into metal bird cages, Crown reorganized along the lines of the much larger Continental Can, incurring additional personnel and expense that again brought the company near to bankruptcy.

At the time, John Connelly was just a fellow on the outside, looking to Crown as a prospective customer and getting nowhere. The son of a Philadelphia blacksmith, Connelly had begun in a paperbox factory at 15 and worked his way up to become eastern sales manager of the Container Corporation of America. When he founded his own company, Connelly Containers, Inc., in 1946, Crown promised him some business. That promise was forgotten by the post-McManus regime, which loftily refused to "take a chance" on a small supplier like Connelly. By 1955, when Crown's distress became evident, Connelly began buying stock and in November 1956 was asked to be an outside director—a desperate move by the ailing company.[16]

In April 1957, Crown Cork & Seal teetered on the verge of bankruptcy. Bankers Trust Company withdrew Crown's line of credit; it seemed that all that was left was to write the company's obituary when John Connelly took over the presidency. His rescue plan was simple—as he called it, "just common sense." Connelly's first move was to pare down the organization. Paternalism ended in a blizzard of pink slips. Connelly moved quickly to cut headquarters staff by half to reach a lean force of 80. The company returned to a simple functional organization. In 20 months Crown had eliminated 1,647 jobs or 24% of the payroll. As part of the company's reorganization, Connelly discarded divisional accounting practices; at the same time he eliminated the divisional line and staff concept. Except for one accountant maintained at each plant location, all accounting and cost control was performed at the corporate level; the corporate accounting staff occupied one-half the space used by the headquarters group. In addition, Connelly disbanded Crown's central research and development facility.

The second step was to institute the concept of accountability. Connelly aimed to instill a deep-rooted pride of workmanship throughout the company by establishing Crown managers as "owner-operators" of their individual businesses. Connelly gave each plant manager responsibility for plant profitability, including any allocated costs. (All company overhead, estimated at 5% of sales, was allocated to the plant level.) Previously, plant managers had been responsible only for controllable expenses at the plant level. Although the plant managers' compensation was not tied to profit performance, one senior executive pointed out that the managers were "certainly rewarded on the basis of that figure." Connelly also held plant managers responsible for quality and customer service.

The next step was to slow production to a halt and liquidate $7 million in inventory. By mid-July Crown paid off the banks. Connelly introduced sales forecasting dovetailed with new production and inventory controls. This move put pressure on the plant managers, who were no longer able to avoid layoffs by dumping excess products into inventory.

By the end of 1957, Crown had, in one observer's words, "climbed out of the coffin and was sprinting." Between 1956 and 1961, sales increased from $115 million to $176 million and profits soared. Throughout the 1960s, the company averaged an annual 15.5% increase in sales and 14% in profits. Connelly, not satisfied simply with short-term reorganizations of the existing company, developed a strategy that would become its hallmark for the next three decades.

Connelly's Strategy

According to William Avery, "From his first day on the job, Mr. Connelly structured the company to be successful. He took control of costs and did a wonderful job taking us in the direction of becoming owner-operators." But what truly separated Connelly from his counterparts, Avery explained, was that while he was continually looking for new ways of controlling costs, he was equally hell-bent on improving quality. Connelly, described by *Forbes* as an individual with a "scrooge-like aversion to fanfare and overhead," emphasized cost efficiency, quality, and customer service as the essential ingredients for Crown's strategy in the decades ahead.

Products and Markets Recognizing Crown's position as a small producer in an industry dominated by American Can and Continental Can, Connelly sought to develop a product line built around Crown's traditional strengths in metal forming and fabrication. He chose to emphasize the areas Crown knew best—tin-plated cans and crowns—and to concentrate on specialized uses and international markets.

A dramatic illustration of Connelly's commitment to this strategy occurred in the early 1960s. In 1960, Crown held over 50% of the market for motor oil cans. In 1962, R. C. Can and Anaconda Aluminum jointly developed fiber-foil cans for motor oil, which were approximately 20% lighter and 15% cheaper than the metal cans then in use. Despite the loss of sales, management decided that it had other more profitable opportunities and that new materials, such as fiber-foil, provided too great a threat in the motor oil can business. Crown's management decided to exit from the oil can market.

In the early 1960s Connelly singled out two specific applications in the domestic market: beverage cans and the growing aerosol market. These applications were called "hard to hold" because cans required special characteristics to either contain the product under pressure or to avoid affecting taste. Connelly led Crown directly from a soldered can into the manufacture of two-piece steel cans in the 1960s. Recognizing the enormous potential of the soft drink business, Crown began designing its equipment specifically to meet the needs of soft drink producers, with innovations such as two printers in one line and conversion printers that allowed for rapid design changeover to accommodate just-in-time delivery.[17] After producing exclusively steel cans through the late 1970s, Connelly spearheaded Crown's conversion from steel to aluminum cans in the early 1980s.

In addition to the specialized product line, Connelly's strategy was based on two geographic thrusts: expand to national distribution in the United States and invest heavily abroad. Connelly linked domestic expansion to

Crown's manufacturing reorganization; plants were spread out across the country to reduce transportation costs and to be nearer customers. Crown was unusual in that it did not set up plants to service a single customer. Instead, Crown concentrated on providing products for a number of customers near their plants. In international markets, Crown invested heavily in developing nations, first with crowns and then with cans as packaged foods became more widely accepted. Metal containers generated 65% of Crown's $1.8 billion 1988 sales, while closures generated 30% and packaging equipment 5%.

Manufacturing   When Connelly took over in 1957, Crown had perhaps the most outmoded and inefficient production facilities in the industry. Dividends had taken precedence over new investment, and old machinery combined with the cumbersome Philadelphia plant had generated very high production and transportation costs. Soon after he gained control, Connelly took drastic action, closing down the Philadelphia facility and investing heavily in new and geographically dispersed plants. From 1958 to 1963, the company spent almost $82 million on relocation and new facilities. From 1976 through 1989, Crown had 26 domestic plant locations versus 9 in 1955. The plants were small (usually 2 to 3 lines for two-piece cans) and were located close to the customer rather than the raw material source. Crown operated its plants 24 hours a day with unique 12-hour shifts. Employees had two days on followed by two days off and then three days on followed by three days off.

Crown emphasized quality, flexibility, and quick response to customer needs. One officer claimed that the key to the can industry was "the fact that nobody stores cans" and when customers need them "they want them in a hurry and on time. . . . Fast answers get customers." To accommodate customer demands, some of Crown's plants kept more than a month's inventory on hand. Crown also instituted a total quality improvement process to refine its manufacturing processes and gain greater control. According to a Crown spokesperson, "The objective of this quality improvement process is to make the best possible can at the lowest possible cost. You lower the cost of doing business not by the wholesale elimination of people, but by reducing mistakes in order to improve efficiency. And you do that by making everybody in the company accountable."

Recycling   In 1970, Crown formed Nationwide Recyclers, Inc., as a wholly owned subsidiary. By 1989, Crown believed Nationwide was one of the top four or five aluminum can recyclers in the country. While Nationwide was only marginally profitable, Crown had invested in the neighborhood of $10 million in its recycling arm.

Research and Development (R&D)   Crown's technology strategy focused on enhancing the existing product line. As one executive noted, "We are not truly pioneers. Our philosophy is not to spend a great deal of money for basic research. However, we do have tremendous skills in die forming and metal fabrication, and we can move to

adapt to the customer's needs faster than anyone else in the industry."[18] For instance, Crown worked closely with large breweries in the development of the two-piece drawn-and-ironed cans for the beverage industry. Crown also made an explicit decision to stay away from basic research. According to one executive, Crown was not interested in "all the frills of an R&D section of high-class, ivory-towered scientists. . . . There is a tremendous asset inherent in being second, especially in the face of the ever-changing state of flux you find in this industry. You try to let others take the risks and make the mistakes. . . ."

This philosophy did not mean that Crown never innovated. For instance, Crown was able to beat its competitors into two-piece can production. Approximately $120 million in new equipment was installed from 1972 through 1975, and by 1976 Crown had 22 two-piece lines in production—more than any other competitor.[19] Crown's research teams also worked closely with customers on specific customer requests. For example, a study of the most efficient plant layout for a food packer or the redesign of a dust cap for the aerosol packager were not unusual projects.

Marketing and Customer Service   The cornerstone of Crown's marketing strategy was, in John Connelly's words, the philosophy that "you can't just increase efficiency to succeed; you must at the same time improve quality." In conjunction with its R&D strategy, the company's sales force maintained close ties with customers and emphasized Crown's ability to provide technical assistance and specific problem solving at the customer's plant. Crown's manufacturing emphasis on flexibility and quick response to customers' needs supported its marketing emphasis on putting the customer first. Michael J. McKenna, president of Crown's North American Division, insisted, "We have always been and always will be extremely customer driven."[20]

Competing cans were made of identical materials to identical specifications on practically identical machinery, and sold at almost identical prices in a given market. At Crown, all customers' gripes went to John Connelly, who was the company's best salesman. A visitor recalled being in his office when a complaint came through from the manager of a Florida citrus-packing plant. Connelly assured him the problem would be taken care of immediately, then casually remarked that he would be in Florida the next day. Would the plant manager join him for dinner? He would indeed. As Crown's president put the telephone down, his visitor said that he hadn't realized Connelly was planning to go to Florida. "Neither did I," confessed Connelly, "until I began talking."[21]

Financing   After he took over in 1957, Connelly applied the first receipts from the sale of inventory to get out from under Crown's short-term bank obligations. He then steadily reduced the debt/equity ratio from 42% in 1956 to 18.2% in 1976 and 5% in 1986. By the end of 1988, Crown's debt represented less than 2% of total capital. Connelly discontinued cash dividends in 1956, and in

1970 repurchased the last of the preferred stock, eliminating preferred dividends as a cash drain. From 1970 forward, management applied excess cash to the repurchase of stock. Connelly set ambitious earnings goals and most years he achieved them. In the 1976 annual report he wrote, "A long time ago we made a prediction that some day our sales would exceed $1 billion and profits of $60.00 per share. Since then, the stock has been split 20-for-1 so this means $3.00 per share." Crown Cork & Seal's revenues reached $1 billion in 1977 and earnings per share reached $3.46. Earnings per share reached $10.11 in 1988 adjusted for a 3-for-1 stock split in September 1988.

International A significant dimension of Connelly's strategy focused on international growth, particularly in developing countries. Between 1955 and 1960, Crown received what were called "pioneer rights" from many foreign governments aiming to build up the industrial sectors of their countries. These "rights" gave Crown first chance at any new can or closure business introduced into these developing countries. Mark W. Hartman, president of Crown's International Division, described Connelly as "a Johnny Appleseed with respect to the international marketplace. When the new countries of Africa were emerging, for example, John was there offering crown-making capabilities to help them in their industrialization, while at the same time getting a foothold for Crown. John's true love was international business."[22] By 1988, Crown's 62 foreign plants generated 44% of sales and 54% of operating profits. John Connelly visited each of Crown's overseas plants. (See Exhibit 6 for map of plant locations.)

Crown emphasized national management wherever possible. Local people, Crown asserted, understood the local marketplace: the suppliers, the customers, and the unique conditions that drove supply and demand. Crown's overseas investment also offered opportunities to recycle equipment that was, by U.S. standards, less sophisticated. Because can manufacturing was new to many regions of the world, Crown's older equipment met the needs of what was still a developing industry overseas.

Performance Connelly's strategy met with substantial success throughout his tenure at Crown. With stock splits and price appreciation, $100 invested in Crown stock in 1957 would be worth approximately $30,000 in 1989. After restructuring the company in his first three years, revenues grew at 12.2% per year while income grew at 14.0% over the next two decades (see Exhibit 7). Return on equity averaged 15.8% for much of the 1970s, while Continental Can and American Can lagged far behind at 10.3% and 7.1%, respectively. Over the period 1968–1978 Crown's total return to shareholders ranked 114 out of the Fortune 500, well ahead of IBM (183) and Xerox (374).

In the early 1980s, flat industry sales, combined with an increasingly strong dollar overseas, unrelenting penetration by plastics, and overcapacity in can manufacturing at home, led to declining sales revenues at Crown. Crown's sales dropped from $1.46 billion in 1980 to $1.37 billion by 1984. However, by 1985 Crown had rebounded and annual sales growth averaged 7.6% from 1984 through 1988 while profit growth averaged 12% (see Exhibits 8 and 9). Over the period 1978–1988 Crown's total return to shareholders was 18.6% per year, ranking 146 out of the Fortune 500. In 1988, *BusinessWeek* noted that Connelly—earning a total of only $663,000 in the three years ending in 1987—garnered shareholders the best returns for the least executive pay in the United States. As an industry analyst observed, "Crown's strategy is a no-nonsense, back-to-basics strategy—except they never left the basics."[23]

John Connelly's Contribution to Success Customers, employees, competitors, and Wall Street analysts attributed Crown's sustained success to the unique leadership of John Connelly. He arrived at Crown as it headed into bankruptcy in 1957, achieved a 1,646% increase in profits on a relatively insignificant sales increase by 1961, and proceeded to outperform the industry's giants throughout the next three decades. A young employee expressed the loyalty created by Connelly: "If John told me to jump out the window, I'd jump—and be sure he'd catch me at the bottom with a stock option in his hand."

Yet Connelly was not an easy man to please. Crown's employees had to get used to Connelly's tough, straight-line management. *Fortune* credited Crown's success to Connelly, "whose genial Irish grin masks a sober salesman executive who believes in the eighty-hour week and in traveling while competitors sleep." He went to meetings uninvited, and expected the same devotion to Crown of his employees as he demanded of himself. As one observer remembered:

> The Saturday morning meeting is standard operating procedure. Crown's executives travel and confer only at night and on weekends. William D. Wallace, vice president for operations, travels 100,000 miles a year, often in the company plane. But Connelly sets the pace. An associate recalls driving to his home in the predawn blackness to pick him up for a flight to a distant plant. The Connelly house was dark, but he spotted a figure sitting on the curb under a street light, engrossed in a loose-leaf book. Connelly's greeting, as he jumped into the car: "I want to talk to you about last month's variances."[24]

Avery's Challenge in 1989 Avery thought long and hard about the options available to him in 1989. He considered the growing opportunities in plastic closures and containers, as well as glass containers. With growth slowing in metal containers, plastics was the only container segment that held much promise. However, the possibility of diversifying beyond the manufacture of containers altogether had some appeal, although the appropriate opportunity was not at hand. While Crown's competitors had aggressively expanded in a variety of directions, Connelly had been cautious, and had prospered. Avery wondered if now was the time for a change at Crown.

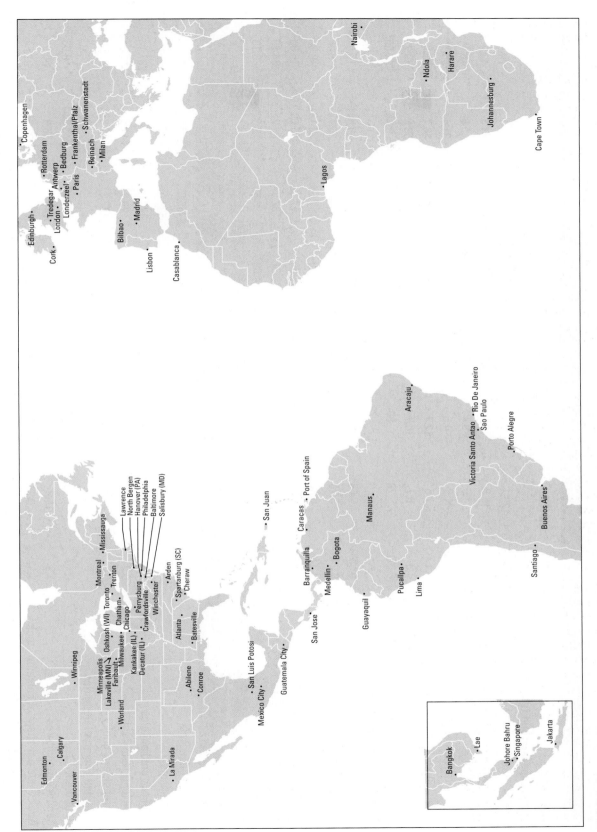

Exhibit 6 Crown Cork & Seal Facilities, 1989

Exhibit 7 Crown Cork & Seal Company Consolidated Statement of Income (dollars in millions, year-end December 31)

	1956	1961	1966	1971	1973	1975	1977	1979
Net Sales	$115.1	$177.0	$279.8	$448.4	$571.8	$825.0	$1,049.1	$1,402.4
Costs, Expenses and Other Income								
Cost of products sold	95.8	139.1	217.2	350.9	459.2	683.7	874.1	1,179.3
Sales and administration	13.5	15.8	18.4	21.1	23.4	30.1	34.8	43.9
Depreciation	2.6	4.6	9.4	17.0	20.9	25.4	5.6	16.4
Net interest expense	1.2	1.3	4.6	5.1	4.4	7.4	31.7	40.1
Provision for taxes on income	.1	7.6	12.7	24.6	26.7	34.9	48.7	51.8
Net income	.3	6.7	16.7	28.5	34.3	41.6	53.8	70.2
Earnings per common share (actual)	(6.01)	.28	.80	1.41	1.81	2.24	3.46	4.65
Selected Financial Statistics								
Return on average equity	0.55%	9.66%	16.44%	14.05%	14.46%	15.20%	15.88%	15.57%
Return on sales	0.24	3.76	5.99	6.35	6.00	5.04	5.13	5.00
Return on average assets	0.32	6.00	6.76	7.25	8.00	7.69	9.13	8.93
Gross profit margin	16.76	21.43	22.37	21.76	19.69	17.13	16.68	15.90
Cost of goods sold/sales	83.24	78.57	77.63	78.24	80.31	82.87	83.32	84.29
SGA/sales	11.73	8.65	6.56	4.70	4.09	3.65	3.32	3.13

Crown Cork & Seal Company Consolidated Statement of Financial Position (dollars in millions, year-end December 31)

	1956	1961	1966	1971	1973	1975	1977	1979
Total current assets	$50.2	$66.3	$109.4	$172.3	$223.4	$265.0	$340.7	$463.3
Total assets	86.5	129.2	269.5	398.1	457.5	539.0	631.1	828.2
Total current liabilities	15.8	24.8	75.3	110.2	139.6	170.0	210.8	287.1
Total long-term debt	20.2	17.7	57.9	41.7	37.9	29.7	12.8	12.2
Shareholders' equity	50.3	77.5	110.8	211.8	243.9	292.7	361.8	481.0
Selected Financial Statistics								
Debt/equity	0.40	0.23	0.52	0.20	0.16	0.10	0.04	0.03
Capital expenditures	1.9	11.8	32.7	33.1	40.4	49.0	58.9	55.9
Book value per share of common stock	1.57	2.74	5.19	10.62	13.13	16.64	23.54	31.84

Source: Adapted from Annual Reports.

Exhibit 8 Crown Cork & Seal Company Consolidated Statement of Income (dollars in millions except earnings per share, year-end December 31)

	1981	1982	1983	1984	1985	1986	1987	1988
Net Sales	$1,373.9	$1,351.9	$1,298.0	$1,369.6	$1,487.1	$1,618.9	$1,717.9	$1,834.1
Costs, Expenses, and Other Income:								
Cost of products sold	1,170.4	1,175.6	1,116.0	1,172.5	1,260.3	1,370.2	1,456.6	1,569.5
Sales and administrative	45.3	44.2	42.9	42.1	43.0	46.7	49.6	50.9
Depreciation	38.0	39.9	38.4	40.2	43.7	47.2	56.9	57.2
Interest expense	12.3	9.0	9.0	8.9	12.2	6.2	8.9	10.0
Interest income	—	—	—	—	—	—	(15.2)	(14.8)
Total Expenses	1,266.1	1,268.6	1,206.2	1,263.6	1,359.2	1,470.3	1,556.8	1,672.9
Income before taxes	107.8	83.2	91.8	105.9	127.9	148.6	161.1	161.2
Provision for taxes on income	43.0	38.5	40.2	46.4	56.2	69.2	72.7	67.8
Net income	64.8	44.7	51.5	59.5	71.7	79.4	88.3	93.4
Earnings per common share	1.48	1.05	1.27	1.59	2.17	2.48	2.86	3.37

Note: Earnings per common share have been restated to reflect a 3-for-1 stock split on September 12, 1988.

Selected Financial Statistics								
	1981	1982	1983	1984	1985	1986	1987	1988
Return on Average Equity (%):	11.72%	7.94%	9.34%	11.42%	13.94%	14.34%	14.46%	14.45%
Return on sales	4.72	3.31	3.97	4.35	4.82	4.91	5.14	5.09
Return on average assets	7.38	5.19	6.20	7.31	8.58	8.80	8.67	8.61
Gross profit margin	14.81	13.04	14.03	14.39	15.25	15.36	15.21	14.42
Cost of goods sold/sales	85.19	86.96	85.97	85.61	84.75	84.64	84.79	85.58
SGA/sales	3.30	3.27	3.30	3.07	2.89	2.88	2.89	2.78
Net Sales ($):								
United States	775.0	781.0	749.9	844.5	945.3	1,010.3	985.5	1,062.5
Europe	324.0	304.4	298.7	283.0	282.8	365.6	415.6	444.2
All others	283.6	273.1	259.1	261.3	269.3	269.0	342.5	368.6
Operating Profit ($):								
United States	62.8	58.9	55.0	67.1	88.9	92.8	95.4	70.6
Europe	20.6	19.0	24.0	17.2	17.0	21.9	22.4	33.4
All others	40.0	37.3	33.1	38.3	40.6	39.6	64.9	66.1
Operating Ratio (%):								
United States	8.1	7.5	7.3	7.9	9.4	9.7	9.6	6.6
Europe	6.3	6.2	8.0	6.0	6.0	5.9	5.4	7.5
All others	14.1	13.6	12.7	14.6	15.0	14.7	18.9	17.9

Source: Adapted from Annual Reports.

Note: The above sales figures are before the deduction of intracompany sales.

Exhibit 9 Crown Cork & Seal Company Consolidated Statement of Financial Position (dollars in millions, year-end December 31)

	1981	1982	1983	1984	1985	1986	1987	1988
Current Assets:								
Cash	$21.5	$15.8	$21.0	$ 7.0	$14.8	$16.5	$27.6	$ 18.0
Accounts receivable	262.8	257.1	240.6	237.6	279.0	270.4	280.7	248.1
Inventory	206.2	184.4	170.2	174.6	171.9	190.1	228.1	237.6
Total Current Assets	490.6	457.3	431.7	419.2	465.6	477.0	536.4	503.8
Investments	12.4	14.6	26.7	28.8	41.5	43.7	NA	NA
Goodwill	11.2	10.8	9.6	10.3	11.8	14.1	16.7	16.5
Property, plant and equipment	368.4	357.8	353.7	348.0	346.9	404.0	465.7	495.9
Other noncurrent assets	NA	NA	NA	NA	NA	NA	79.1	57.0
Total Assets	882.6	840.6	821.7	806.4	865.8	938.8	1,097.9	1,073.2
Current Liabilities:								
Short-term debt	22.7	21.6	24.4	42.0	16.3	17.2	44.0	20.2
Accounts payable	193.0	165.6	163.1	177.9	197.1	220.1	265.9	277.6
U.S. and foreign taxes	17.3	4.7	11.4	6.0	11.4	11.3	28.4	23.3
Total Current Liabilities	233.0	191.9	198.8	225.8	224.8	248.5	338.2	321.2
Long-term debt	5.8	5.6	2.8	2.7	2.2	1.4	19.7	9.4
Other	14.5	18.5	12.8	15.8	31.2	29.3	0.0	0.0
Total Long-term Debt	20.3	24.1	15.6	18.5	33.5	30.7	19.7	9.4
Deferred income taxes	55.5	57.7	57.8	60.7	71.3	79.2	89.4	93.7
Minority equity in subsidiaries	7.2	7.2	5.2	3.7	4.7	3.8	5.0	0.9
Shareholders' equity	566.7	559.8	544.3	497.8	531.5	576.6	645.6	648.0
Liability and owners' equity	882.6	840.6	821.7	806.4	865.8	938.8	1,097.9	1,073.2

Selected Financial Statistics

	1981	1982	1983	1984	1985	1986	1987	1988
Debt/equity	1.02%	0.99%	0.51%	0.54%	0.42%	0.24%	3.06%	1.45%
Debt/(debt + equity)	3.5%	4.1%	2.7%	3.5%	6.0%	5.0%	3.0%	1.4%
Shares outstanding at year end (M)	14.5	14.0	13.2	11.5	10.5	10.0	9.5	27.0
Capital expenditures ($M)	$63.8	$50.3	$55.5	$53.8	$50.9	$94.0	$99.5	$102.6
Shares repurchased (000)	75.4	528.3	863.1	1,694.5	1,006.0	677.1	638.7	2,242.9
Stock price: High[a]	$12.00	$10.00	$13.00	$15.75	$29.62	$38.25	$46.87	$ 46.72
Stock price: Low[a]	$ 8.00	$ 7.00	$10.00	$11.75	$15.12	$25.25	$28.00	$ 30.00

Source: Adapted from Annual Reports.

[a]Restated for 9/1988 stock split.

Within the traditional metal can business, Avery had to decide whether or not to get involved in the bidding for Continental Can. The acquisition of Continental Can Canada (CCC)—with sales of roughly $400 million—would make Canada Crown's largest single presence outside of the United States. Continental's USA business—with estimated revenues of $1.3 billion in 1989—would double the size of Crown's domestic operations. Continental's Latin American, Asian, and Middle Eastern operations were rumored to be priced in the range of $100 million to $150 million. Continental's European operations generated estimated sales of $1.5 billion in 1989 and included a work force of 10,000 at 30 production sites. Potential bidders for all, or part of Continental's operations, included many of Crown's U.S. rivals in addition to European competition: Pechiney International of France, Metal Box of Great Britain (which had recently acquired Carnaud SA), and VIAG AG, a German trading group, among others.

Avery knew that most mergers in this industry had not worked out well. He also thought about the challenge of taking two companies that come from completely different cultures and bringing them together. There would be inevitable emotional and attitudinal changes, particularly for Continental's salaried managers and Crown's "owner-operators." Avery also knew that the merger of American Can and National Can had its difficulties. That consolidation was taking longer than expected and, according to one observer, "American Can would be literally wiped out in the end."

Avery found himself challenging Crown's traditional strategies and thought seriously of drafting a new blueprint for the future.

Endnotes

1. Salomon Brothers. 1990. *Beverage Cans Industry Report,* March 1.
2. Davis T. 1990. Can do: A metal container update. *Beverage World,* June: 34.
3. Sheehan J. J. 1988. Nothing succeeds like success. *Beverage World,* November: 82.
4. Until 1985, aluminum cans were restricted to carbonated beverages because it was the carbonation that prevented the can from collapsing. Reynolds discovered that by adding liquid nitrogen to the can's contents, aluminum containers could hold noncarbonated beverages and still retain their shape. The liquid nitrogen made it possible for Reynolds to make cans for liquor, chocolate drinks, and fruit juices.
5. Sly, J. 1988. A "can-do crusade" by steel industry. *Chicago Tribune,* July 3: 1.
6. Merrill Lynch Capital Markets. 1991. *Containers and Packaging Industry Report.* March 21.
7. Salomon Brothers Inc. 1991. *Containers/Packaging: Beverage Cans Industry Report,* April 3.
8. Agoos, A. 1985. Aluminum girds for the plastic can bid. *Chemical Week,* January 16: 18.
9. Oman, B. 1990. A clear choice? *Beverage World,* June: 78.
10. In response to public concern, the container industry developed highly efficient "closed loop" recycling systems. Containers flowed from the manufacturer, through the wholesaler/distributor, to the retailer, to the consumer, and back to the manufacturer or material supplier for recycling. Aluminum's high recycling value permitted can manufacturers to sell cans at a lower cost to beverage producers. The reclamation of steel cans lagged that of aluminum because collection and recycling did not result in significant energy or material cost advantages.
11. Lang, N. 1990. A touch of glass. *Beverage World,* June: 36.
12. Ibid.
13. U.S. Industrial Outlook, 1984–1990.
14. The First Boston Corporation. 1990. *Packaging Industry Report,* April 4.
15. Whalen, R. J. 1962. The unoriginal ideas that rebuilt Crown Cork. *Fortune,* October.
16. Ibid.: 156.
17. In the mid-1960s, growth in demand for soft drink and beer cans was more than triple that for traditional food cans.
18. Hamermesh, R. G., Anderson, M. J., Jr., and Harris, J. E. 1978. Strategies for low market share business. *Harvard Business Review,* May–June: 99.
19. In 1976, there were 47 two-piece tinplate and 130 two-piece aluminum lines in the United States.
20. *One Hundred Years.* Crown Cork & Seal Company, Inc.
21. Whalen, The unoriginal ideas that rebuilt Crown Cork.
22. *One Hundred Years.* Crown Cork & Seal Company, Inc.
23. *BusinessWeek.* 1987. These penny-pinchers deliver a big bang for their bucks. May 4.
24. Whalen, The unoriginal ideas that rebuilt Crown Cork.

Case 3   Pixar*

When *Wall-E* won the Academy Award for best animated feature in February 2009, it hardly took anyone by surprise. The latest offering from Pixar Animation Studios had already been heralded by almost all the critics as soon as it was released during the prior summer. It went on to gross $533 million in theaters worldwide, landing among the top 10 animated films of all time (see Exhibit 1). *Wall-E* managed to achieve this success in spite of its challenging theme: It centered on robots and had little dialogue. Moreover, with this win, Pixar claimed its fourth feature-length animation Oscar, which represented half of the eight trophies that had been handed out since the category was added in 2001.

The recent string of successful releases—*Cars, Ratatouille,* and *Wall-E*—suggests that Pixar has continued to flourish despite its 2006 acquisition by the Walt Disney Company for the hefty sum of $7.4 billion. The deal was finalized by Steve Jobs, the Apple Computer chief executive, who also heads the computer animation firm. Jobs had developed a production and distribution pact with Disney, under which the two firms split the profits that Pixar films generated from ticket sales, video sales, and merchandising royalties. But the deal was set to expire after the release of *Cars* in summer 2006. Disney CEO Bob Iger worked hard to clinch the deal to acquire Pixar, whose track record has made it one of the world's most successful animation companies.

Both Jobs and Iger realized, however, that they must try to protect Pixar's creative culture while also trying to carry some of it over to Disney's animation efforts. Even though Pixar has continued to operate independently of Disney's own animation studios, its key talent has overseen the combined activities of both Pixar and Disney. As part of the deal, Jobs gained considerable influence over Disney by assuming the position of a nonindependent director and becoming its largest individual stockholder.

In order to ensure that Pixar manages to preserve its freewheeling entrepreneurial culture, Jobs sits on a committee that includes other top talent from the animation studio whose key task is to protect its unique approach to making movies. Pixar's lengthy process of crafting a film stands in stark contrast to the production-line approach pursued by Disney. This contrast in culture is best reflected in the Oscars which the employees at Pixar have displayed proudly but which have been painstakingly dressed in Barbie-doll clothing.

Above all, everyone at Pixar remains committed to making films that are original in concept and execution, despite the risks involved. All of the studio's films have been based on original stories, and apart from *Toy Story,* Pixar has resisted the temptation to make sequels. On behalf of Disney, Iger has reinforced the importance of maintaining the formula that was responsible for Pixar's string of successful animated films. He has pledged that he will do whatever he can to make sure "that the Pixar culture be protected and allowed to continue."[1]

Pushing for Computer Animated Films

The roots of Pixar stretch back to 1975 with the founding of a vocational school in Old Westbury, New York, called the New York Institute of Technology. It was there that Edwin E. Catmull, a straitlaced Mormon from Salt Lake City who loved animation but couldn't draw, teamed up with the people who would later form the core of Pixar. "It was artists and technologists from the very start," recalled Alvy Ray Smith, who worked with Catmull during those years. "It was like a fairy tale."[2]

By 1979, Catmull and his team decided to join forces with famous Hollywood director George W. Lucas, Jr. They were hopeful that this would allow them to pursue their dream of making animated films. As part of Lucas's filmmaking facility in San Rafael, California, Catmull's group of aspiring animators was able to make substantial progress in the art of computer animation. But the unit was not able to generate any profits, and Lucas was not willing to let it grow beyond using computer animation for special effects.

In 1985, Catmull finally turned to Jobs, who had just been ousted from Apple. Jobs was reluctant to invest in a firm that wanted to make full-length feature films using computer animation. But a year later, Jobs did decide to buy Catmull's unit for just $10 million, which was one-third of Lucas's asking price. While the newly named Pixar Animation Studios tried to push the boundaries of computer animation over the next five years, Jobs ended up having to invest an additional $50 million—more than 25 percent of his total wealth at the time. "There were times that we all despaired, but fortunately not all at the same time," said Jobs.[3]

Still, Catmull's team did continue to make substantial breakthroughs in the development of computer-generated full-length feature films (see Exhibit 2). In 1991, Disney ended up giving Pixar a three-film contract that started with *Toy Story.* When the movie was finally released in 1995, its success surprised everyone in the film industry. Rather than the nice little film Disney had expected, *Toy Story* became the sensation of 1995. It rose to the rank of third-highest-grossing animated film of all time, earning $362 million in worldwide box office revenues.

Within days, Jobs decided to take Pixar public. When the shares, initially priced at $22, shot past $33, Jobs called his best friend, Oracle CEO Lawrence J. Ellison,

* This case was developed by Professor Jamal Shamsie, Michigan State University, with the assistance of Professor Alan B. Eisner, Pace University. Material has been drawn from published sources to be used for class discussion. Copyright © 2009 Jamal Shamsie and Alan B. Eisner.

Exhibit 1   **Leading Animated Films** (in millions of U.S. dollars)

All nine of Pixar's films released to date have ended up among the top animated films of all time, based on worldwide box office revenues.

	Title	Year	Revenues	Studio
1.	Shrek 2	2004	$881	Dreamworks
2.	Finding Nemo	2003	865	Pixar
3.	Shrek 3	2007	791	Dreamworks
4.	The Lion King	1994	783	Disney
5.	Kung Fu Panda	2008	633	Dreamworks
6.	The Incredibles	2004	624	Pixar
7.	Ice Age: The Meltdown	2006	623	Fox
8.	Ratatouille	2007	616	Pixar
9.	Madagascar: Escape 2 Africa	2008	581	Dreamworks
10.	Wall-E	2008	533	Pixar
11.	Monsters, Inc.	2001	529	Pixar
12.	The Simpsons Movie	2007	526	Fox
13.	Aladdin	1992	502	Disney
14.	Toy Story 2	1999	486	Pixar
15.	Shrek	2001	455	Dreamworks
16.	Cars	2006	454	Pixar
17.	Tarzan	1999	435	Disney
18.	Madagascar	2005	407	Dreamworks
19.	Happy Feet	2006	379	Warner
20.	Beauty and the Beast	1991	378	Disney
21.	Ice Age	2002	377	Fox
22.	Toy Story	1995	359	Pixar
23.	A Bug's Life	1998	358	Pixar
24.	Dinosaur	2000	348	Disney
25.	Pocahontas	1995	347	Disney

Source: IMDB, *Variety.*

to tell him he had company in the billionaire's club. With Pixar's sudden success, Jobs returned to strike a new deal with Disney. Early in 1996, at a lunch with Walt Disney chief Michael D. Eisner, Jobs made his demands: an equal share of the profits, equal billing on merchandise and on-screen credits, and guarantees that Disney would market Pixar films as it did its own.

Boosting the Creative Component

With the success of *Toy Story,* Jobs realized that he had hit something big. He had obviously tapped into his Silicon Valley roots and turned to computers to forge a unique style of creative moviemaking. In each of its subsequent films, Pixar continued to develop computer animation that allowed for more lifelike backgrounds, texture, and movement than ever before. For example, since real leaves are translucent, Pixar's engineers developed special software algorithms that both reflect and absorb light, creating luminous scenes among jungles of clover.

In spite of the significance of these advancements in computer animation, Jobs was well aware that successful feature films would require a strong creative spark. He understood that it would be the marriage of technology and creativity that would allow Pixar to rise above most of

Exhibit 2 Milestones

1986	Steve Jobs buys Lucas's computer group and christens it Pixar. The firm completes a short film, *Luxo Jr.,* which is nominated for an Oscar.
1988	Pixar adds computer-animated ads to its repertoire, making spots for Listerine, Lifesavers, and Tropicana. Another short, *Tin Toy,* wins an Oscar.
1991	Pixar signs a production agreement with Disney. Disney is to invest $26 million; Pixar is to deliver at least three full-length, computer-animated feature films.
1995	Pixar releases *Toy Story,* the first fully digital feature film, which becomes the top-grossing movie of the year and wins an Oscar. A week after release, the company goes public.
1997	Pixar and Disney negotiate a new agreement: a 50-50 split of the development costs and profits of five feature-length movies. Short *Geri's Game* wins an Oscar.
1998–99	*A Bug's Life* and *Toy Story 2* are released, together pulling in $1.3 billion in box office and video revenues.
2001–04	Pixar releases a string of hits: *Monsters Inc., Finding Nemo,* and *The Incredibles.*
2006	Disney acquires Pixar and assigns responsibilities for its own animation unit to Pixar's creative brass. *Cars* is released and becomes another box office hit.
2009	*Wall-E* becomes the fourth film from Pixar to receive the Oscar for a feature-length animated film.

Source: Pixar.

its competition. To achieve that, Jobs fostered a campus-like environment within the newly formed outfit similar to the freewheeling, charged atmosphere in the early days of his beloved Apple, where he also returned as acting CEO. "It's not simply the technology that makes Pixar," said Dick Cook, president of Walt Disney Studios.[4]

Even though Jobs has played a crucial supportive role, it is Catmull, now elevated to the position of Pixar's president, who has been mainly responsible for ensuring that the firm's technological achievements help pump up the firm's creative efforts. He has been the keeper of the company's unique innovative culture, which blends Silicon Valley techies, Hollywood production honchos, and artsy animation experts. In the pursuit of Catmull's vision, this eclectic group has transformed office cubicles into tiki huts, circus tents, and cardboard castles with bookshelves that are stuffed with toys and desks that are adorned with colorful iMac computers.

Catmull has also been working hard to build on this pursuit of creative innovation by creating programs to develop the employees. Employees are encouraged to devote up to four hours a week, every week, to furthering their education at Pixar University. The in-house training program offers 110 different courses that cover subjects such as live improvisation, creative writing, painting, drawing, sculpting, and cinematography. The school's dean is Randall E. Nelson, a former juggler who has been known to perform his act using chain saws so that students in animation classes have something compelling to draw.

It is this emphasis on the creative use of technology that has kept Pixar on the cutting edge. The firm has turned out ever more lifelike short films, including 1998's Oscar-winning *Geri's Game,* which used a technology called *subdivision surfaces.* This makes the realistic simulation of human skin and clothing possible. "They're absolute geniuses," gushed Jules Roman, cofounder and CEO of rival Tippett Studio, when speaking of Pixar's staff. "They're the people who created computer animation really."[5]

Becoming Accomplished Storytellers

A considerable part of the creative energy at Pixar goes into story development. Jobs understands that a film works only if its story can move the hearts and minds of families around the world. His goal is to develop Pixar into an animated movie studio that is known for the quality of its storytelling above everything else. "We want to create some great stories and characters that endure with each generation," Jobs recently stated.[6]

For story development, Pixar relies heavily on 43-year-old John Lasseter, who goes by the title of vice president of the creative. Known for his Hawaiian shirts and irrepressible playfulness, Lasseter has been the key to the appeal of all of Pixar's films. Lasseter gets very passionate about developing great stories and then harnessing computers to tell those stories. Most of Pixar's employees believe that it is this passion that has enabled the studio to ensure that each of its films has been a commercial hit. In fact, Lasseter is being regarded as the Walt Disney of the 21st century.

When it's time to start a project, Lasseter isolates a group of eight or so writers and directs them to forget about the constraints of technology. While many studios try to rush from script to production, Lasseter takes up to two years just to develop the story. Once the script has been developed, artists create storyboards and copy them onto videotapes called *reels.* Even computer-animated films must begin with pencil sketches that are viewed on tape. "You can't really shortchange the story development," Lasseter has emphasized.[7]

Only after the basic story is set does Lasseter begin to think about what he'll need from Pixar's technologists, and it's always more than the computer animators expect. Lasseter, for example, demanded that the crowds of ants in *A Bug's Life* not be a single mass of look-alike faces. To solve the problem, computer expert William T. Reeves developed software that randomly applied physical and emotional characteristics to each ant. In another instance, writers brought a model of a butterfly named Gypsy to researchers, asking them to write code so that when she rubs her antennas, viewers can see the hairs press down and pop back up.

At any stage during the process, Lasseter may go back to potential problems that he might see with the story. In *A Bug's Life,* for example, the story was totally revamped after more than a year of work had been completed. Originally, it was about a troupe of circus bugs run by P. T. Flea that tries to rescue a colony of ants from marauding grasshoppers. But because of a flaw in the story—why would the circus bugs risk their lives to save stranger ants?—codirector Andrew Stanton recast the story to be about Flik, the heroic ant who recruits Flea's troupe to fight the grasshoppers. "You have to rework and rework it," explained Lasseter. "It is not rare for a scene to be rewritten as much as 30 times."[8]

Pumping Out the Hits

In spite of its formidable string of hits, Pixar has had difficulty in stepping up its pace of production. Although they may cost 30 percent less than nonanimated films, computer-generated animated films take considerable time to develop. Furthermore, because of the emphasis on every single detail, Pixar used to complete most of the work on a film before moving on to the next one. Catmull and Lasseter have since decided to work on several projects at the same time, but the firm has not been able to release more than one movie in a year.

To push for an increase in production, Pixar has more than doubled its number of employees over the last decade. It is also turning to a stable of directors to oversee its movies. Lasseter, who directed Pixar's first three films, is supervising other directors who are taking the helm of various films that the studio chooses to develop. *Monsters, Inc., Finding Nemo, The Incredibles,* and *Ratatouille* were directed by some of this new talent. But there are concerns about the number of directors that Pixar can rely on to turn out high-quality animated films. Michael Savner of Bank of America Securities commented: "You can't simply double production. There is a finite amount of talent."[9]

To meet the faster production pace, Catmull has added new divisions, including one to help with the development of new movies and one to oversee movie development shot by shot. The eight-person development team has helped generate more ideas for new films. "Once more ideas are percolating, we have more options to choose from so no one artist is feeling the weight of the world on their shoulders," said Sarah McArthur, Pixar's vice president of production.[10]

Finally, Catmull is turning to new technology to help ramp up production. His goal is to reduce the number of animators to no more than 100 per film. Toward this end, Catmull has been overseeing the development of new animation software called Luxo, which enables fewer people to do more work. While the firm's old system allowed animators to easily make a change to a specific character, Luxo adjusts the environment as well (see Exhibit 3). For example, if an animator adds a new head to a monster, the system would automatically cast the proper shadow.

Catmull is well aware of the dangers of growth for a studio whose successes came out of a lean structure that wagered everything on each film. It remains to be seen whether Pixar can keep drawing on its talent to increase production without compromising the high standards that have been set by Catmull and Lasseter. Jobs has been keen to maintain the quality of every one of Pixar's films by ensuring that each one gets the best efforts of the firm's animators, storytellers, and technologists. "Quality is more important than quantity," he recently emphasized. "One home run is better than two doubles."[11]

To preserve the studio's high standards, Catmull has been working hard to retain Pixar's commitment to quality even as the studio grows. He has been using Pixar University to encourage collaboration among all employees so that they can develop and retain the key values that are tied to their success. In addition, he has helped devise ways to avoid collective burnout. A masseuse and a doctor come to Pixar's campus each week, and animators must get permission from their supervisors if they want to work more than 50 hours a week.

To Infinity and Beyond?

The ongoing success of Pixar's films clearly indicates that the studio continued to turn out quality films even after it was acquired by Disney in 2006. This has settled some

---

Exhibit 3 **Proprietary Software**

Marionette: An animation software system used for modeling, animating, and lighting.

Ringmaster: A production management software system for scheduling, coordinating, and tracking a computer-animation project.

Renderman: A rendering software system for high-quality, photo-realistic image synthesis.

Source: Pixar.

of the concerns that arose at the time of the acquisition about its possible effect on Pixar's rather unique creative culture. David Price, author of a recent book on the animation firm, stated, "Most acquisitions, particularly in media, are value-destroying as opposed to value-creating and that certainly has not turned out to be the case here."[12]

Along the same lines, Jobs recently expressed his satisfaction with the close relationship that the two animation studios have developed with each other: "Disney is the only company with animation in their DNA."[13] In fact, the acquisition of Pixar was viewed as an attempt by Disney to acquire a group in which the talent of the individuals and the quality of the finished product are valued above everything else. Disney CEO Iger has been hoping that his firm will not only be able to preserve the culture of Pixar but also be able to import parts of it into Disney's own animation unit, whose greatest successes, *The Lion King* and *Aladdin,* date back to 1994 and 1992.

To ensure this goal, Pixar president Ed Catmull was given charge of the combined animation business of both Pixar and Disney. Apart from continuing to manage Pixar, Catmull has been working hard to get Disney's animated film division back into space after a long run of lackluster movies. Disney Studios chairman Dick Cook referred to Catmull as one of the fathers of computer-generated animation, adding: "Ed sets the tone in the way he works, his accessibility and willingness to look at things."[14]

More significantly, Pixar's creative force, John Lasseter, was saddled with the role of chief creative officer of the combined company as well as the role of adviser for Disney's Imagineering division, which designs attractions for the theme parks. In an unusual arrangement within a hierarchical firm such as Disney, Lasseter reports directly to Iger. For Lasseter, his new responsibilities for Disney represent a return to his roots. He had been inspired by Disney films as a kid, and he started his career at Disney before being lured away to Pixar by Catmull. "For many of us at Pixar, it was the magic of Disney that influenced us to pursue our dreams of becoming animators, artists, storytellers and filmmakers," Lasseter recently stated.[15]

Catmull and Lasseter continue to face a challenging task. They must ensure that they keep developing hits for Pixar even as they try to turn things around at Disney. In particular, there are concerns about the ability of Pixar to hold on to the creative talent behind its recent hits. But both Catmull and Lasseter are confident that they can maintain their group while being part of Disney. "We created the studio we want to work in," Lasseter remarked recently. "We have an environment that's wacky. It's a creative brain trust: It's not a place where I make my movies—it's a place where a group of people make movies."[16]

Endnotes

1. Laura M. Holson. Disney Agrees to Acquire Pixar in a $7.4 Billion Deal. *The New York Times,* January 25, 2006, p. C6.
2. Peter Burrows and Ronald Grover. Steve Jobs: Movie Mogul. *BusinessWeek,* November 23, 1998, p. 150.
3. Ibid.
4. Ibid., p. 146.
5. Ibid.
6. Marc Graser. Pixar Run by Focused Group. *Variety,* December 20, 1999, p. 74.
7. Ibid.
8. Burrows and Grover, November 23, 1998, p. 146.
9. Andrew Bary. Coy Story. *Barron's,* October 13, 2003, p. 21.
10. Pui-Wing Tam. Will Quantity Hurt Pixar's Quality? *The Wall Street Journal,* February 15, 2001, p. B4.
11. Peter Burrows and Ronald Grover. Steve Jobs' Magic Kingdom. *BusinessWeek,* February 6, 2006, p. 66.
12. Brooks Barnes. For Disney and Pixar, a Smooth (So Far) Ride. *International Herald Tribune,* June 2, 2008, p. 9.
13. Holson, 2006, p. C6.
14. Nick Wingfield and Merissa Marr. A Techie's Task: Drawing Pixar's Magic to Disney. *The Wall Street Journal,* January 30, 2006, p. B7.
15. Charles Solomon. Pixar Creative Chief to Seek to Restore the Disney Magic. *The New York Times,* January 25, 2006.
16. Bary, 2003.

Case 4 Nintendo's Wii*

Not only did Nintendo sit behind Sony and Microsoft in terms of overall sales, but it also derived most of its revenue from the video game business. Sony had more than 180,500 employees, and its 2008 revenues were over $88 billion.[1] Microsoft had more than 81,000 employees, and its 2008 revenues were $60 billion.[2] Nintendo was founded in 1889 but had roughly only 3,000 employees and 2008 revenues of $16.4 billion.[3] Thus, Nintendo sat in the middle of two potentially dominating firms. Yet Nintendo was in the lead in video console sales growth and second, to Microsoft, in overall units sold (Microsoft had shipped its product a year ahead of Nintendo and Sony). Sales continued to soar, and within two years of its release, Nintendo Wii became the market leader of the generation. However, some observers questioned whether Nintendo's CEO Iwata would manage to keep the Wii momentum rolling into the next generation of gaming systems.

Nintendo's all-conquering Wii game console is showing its first signs of weakness, with Japanese sales falling below those of Sony's PlayStation 3 during March 2009.[4] However, Nintendo was less than frightened, since the Wii outsold the PS3 by almost three to one in the larger U.S. market in February 2009, selling 750,000 units.

Background

Although Nintendo dates back to 1889 as a playing-card maker, Nintendo's first video game systems were developed in 1979 and were known as TV Game 15 and TV Game 6.[5] In 1980 Nintendo developed the first portable LCD video game with a microprocessor. In 1985 Nintendo created the Nintendo Entertainment System (NES), an 8-bit video game console. The original NES was very successful, as its graphics were superior to any home-based console that was available at the time, and as a result more than 60 million units were sold worldwide.[6] The NES set the bar for subsequent consoles in platform design, as well as for accepting games that were manufactured by third-party developers. As competitors began developing 16-bit devices, such as Sega's Genesis system or NEC's PC Engine, Nintendo knew that it had to respond and develop its own 16-bit system.

The Super Nintendo Entertainment System (SNES) was developed to stay current with the competitors. The Super Nintendo was released in 1991 and, when purchased, came with one game, Super Mario World. This was the successor to the previous Mario Brothers games that were played on the original 8-bit NES. In 1996 Nintendo released Nintendo 64, which caused the popularity of the

Super Nintendo to decline. The Nintendo 64 is Nintendo's third-generation video game console and was named after the 64-bit processor. During its product lifetime, more than 30 million Nintendo 64 units were sold worldwide.[7]

The Nintendo 64, like its predecessors, used cartridges to play its games, but at the time, the competing systems of Sony and Sega were using CDs for game storage. Cartridges could store 64 megabytes of data, while CDs could store around 700 megabytes of data. Also, CDs were much cheaper to manufacture, distribute, and create; thus many game developers that traditionally supported Nintendo platforms began creating games that would support the other platforms to increase profits.[8] At the time, the average cost of producing a Nintendo 64 cartridge was cited as $25, compared to 10 cents to produce a CD. Therefore, game producers passed the higher expense to the consumer, which explains why Nintendo 64 games tended to sell for higher prices than Sony PlayStation games. While most Sony PlayStation games rarely exceeded $50, Nintendo 64 titles could reach $70.[9] Third-party developers naturally switched to the systems that used a less expensive CD platform (such as the PlayStation).

In 2001 Nintendo released its GameCube, which was part of the sixth-generation era of video game systems. These systems included Sony's PlayStation 2, Microsoft's Xbox, and Sega's Dreamcast. Although the GameCube did not use cartridges, Nintendo began producing its games using a proprietary optical-disk technology. This technology, while similar in appearance to CDs, was actually several inches smaller in diameter and was unable to be played using a standard CD player.

Genyo Takeda, general manager of Integrated Research and Development for Nintendo, explained that innovation and creativity were fostered by giving several different development teams "free rein to couple a dedicated controller or peripheral with a GameCube title, and then see whether or not the end result was marketable. This project gave rise not only to the Donkey Kong Bongos and the Dancing Stage Mario Mix Action Pad, but also to a number of ideas and designs that would find their way into the Wii Remote."[10]

When Nintendo released the Wii video game console in 2006, it was already in the midst of a very competitive market. The previous generation of video game consoles consisted of the Sega Dreamcast, Sony PlayStation 2, Nintendo GameCube, and Microsoft Xbox. These systems were all released between 1999 and 2001 in the United States, and although the GameCube sold more systems than the Sega Dreamcast, it fell into third place behind the PlayStation 2 and the Xbox. The PlayStation 2 sold more than 115 million units worldwide, more than twice the combined unit sales of the GameCube and Xbox (21 million and 24 million, respectively). The next generation of video game consoles was about to become even more competitors.

* This case was prepared by graduate student Eshai J. Gorshein and Professor Alan B. Eisner of Pace University. This case was based solely on library research and was developed for class discussion rather than to illustrate either effective or ineffective handling of an administrative situation. Copyright © 2007, 2009 Alan B. Eisner.

As of 2008, Nintendo's revenues and income were on attractive upward trajectories (see Exhibits 1 and 2). Exhibit 3 shows that Nintendo's stock price was soaring, despite the recession, relative to that of its larger competitors.

The Launch of the Wii

In 2006 Nintendo released its direct successor to the GameCube, the Wii (pronounced "we"). There were many reasons cited as to why the name *Wii* was chosen, but perhaps the most compelling reason was that "'Wii' sounded like 'we,' which emphasized that the console was for everyone. Wii could be remembered easily by people around the world, no matter what language they spoke. No confusion."[11] Initially the system was known by its code name, Revolution, but later the name was changed to Wii. Nintendo stated that it wanted to make the Wii a system that would make anyone who tried it talk to his or her friends and neighbors about it.[12]

The Wii was created to establish a new standard in game control, using an innovative and unprecedented interface, the Wii Remote.[13] The Wii Remote was what made the Wii a unique home console. The remote acted as the primary controller for the Wii. Its motion-sensor capabilities allowed the user to interact and manipulate objects on the screen by moving and pointing the remote in various directions.[14] The Wii Remote was the size of a traditional remote control, and it was "limited only by the game designer's imagination."[15] For example, in a game of tennis it served as the racket when the user swung his or her arm, or in a shooting game it served as the user's gun. Not only did the remote serve as a controller, but it also had a built-in speaker and a rumble feature for even greater tactile feedback and game involvement.

The Wii remote came with an arm strap that could be tied to the user's wrist so that the remote couldn't fly away when being used. The remote was powered by two AA batteries, which could power it for approximately 30 to 60 hours.[16] Exhibit 4 shows the Wii and Wii Remote.

The second part of the Wii remote innovation was the Wii Nunchuk. The Nunchuk was designed to perfectly fit the user's hand, and it connected to the remote at its expansion port. The Nunchuk had the same motion-sensing

Exhibit 1 Income Statements (in millions of yen, except per-share items; year-end March 31)

	2008	2007	2006	2005	2004
Revenue	1,672,420	966,534	509,249	515,292	514,805
Cost of revenue, total	972,362	568,722	294,133	298,115	307,233
Gross profit	700,061	397,812	215,116	217,177	207,572
Selling, general, and administrative expenses, total	172,433	131,414	92,410	83,524	82,218
Research and development	37,000	37,706	30,588	20,505	15,820
Depreciation/amortization	3,405	2,664	1,764	1,621	1,846
Unusual expense (income)	10,740	(3)	(2,227)	(123)	(2,065)
Total operating expense	1,195,940	740,503	416,668	403,642	405,052
Operating income	476,483	226,031	92,581	111,650	109,753
Interest/investment income, nonoperating	(48,151)	60,619	71,514	31,846	(58,877)
Interest income(expense), net nonoperating	(48,151)	60,619	71,513	31,846	(58,877)
Gain (loss) on sale of assets	3,671	(132)	(20)	(13)	761
Other, net	1,777	3,087	2,398	1,924	1,335
Net income before taxes	433,780	289,605	166,472	145,407	52,972
Provision for income taxes	176,532	115,348	68,138	57,962	19,692
Net income after taxes	257,248	174,257	98,334	87,445	33,280
Minority interest	99	37	46	(24)	(79)
Net income	**257,347**	**174,294**	**98,380**	**87,421**	**33,201**

Source: reuters.com.

Exhibit 2 Balance Sheets (in millions of yen, except for per-share items; year-end March 31)

	2008	2007	2006	2005	2004
Cash and equivalents	899,251	962,197	812,064	826,653	767,270
Short-term investments	353,070	115,971	64,287	20,485	17,375
Cash and short-term investments	1,252,320	1,078,170	876,351	847,138	784,645
Accounts receivable—trade, net	145,611	87,780	42,312	49,263	25,465
Total receivables, net	145,611	87,780	42,312	49,263	25,465
Total inventory	104,842	88,609	30,835	49,758	30,955
Other current assets, total	144,060	140,114	69,231	47,730	49,695
Total current assets	1,646,830	1,394,670	1,018,730	993,889	890,760
Property, plant, and equipment, total—gross	30,559	32,812	32,645	32,479	31,925
Property, plant, and equipment, total—net	55,149	57,597	55,968	54,417	55,083
Intangibles, net	2,009	505	319	354	245
Long-term investments	73,756	92,412	60,213	73,393	53,866
Other long-term assets, total	24,737	30,405	25,470	10,432	10,072
Total assets	**1,802,480**	**1,575,590**	**1,160,700**	**1,132,480**	**1,010,030**
Accounts payable	335,820	301,080	83,817	111,045	57,945
Accrued expenses	1,848	1,779	1,732	1,650	1,712
Other current liabilities, total	229,553	165,576	96,724	92,752	53,588
Total current liabilities	567,221	468,435	182,273	205,447	113,245
Minority interest	98	138	176	222	232
Other liabilities, total	5,292	5,141	4,160	5,351	6,303
Total liabilities	**572,611**	**473,714**	**186,609**	**211,020**	**119,780**
Common stock, total	10,065	10,065	10,065	10,065	10,065
Additional paid-in capital	11,640	11,586	11,585	11,584	11,584
Retained earnings (accumulated deficit)	1,380,430	1,220,290	1,096,070	1,032,830	964,524
Treasury stock—common	(156,184)	(155,396)	(155,112)	(129,896)	(86,898)
Unrealized gain (loss)	5,418	8,898	10,717	7,194	6,650
Other equity, total	(21,495)	6,432	762	(10,315)	(15,677)
Total equity	**1,229,870**	**1,101,880**	**974,090**	**921,466**	**890,248**
Total liabilities and shareholders' equity	**1,802,480**	**1,575,590**	**1,160,700**	**1,132,490**	**1,010,030**

Source: reuters.com.

capabilities that the remote had, but it also had an analog stick to help the user move his or her characters. In addition to the analog stick, the Nunchuk had two buttons that gave the user quick access to other game functions. Thus the Nunchuk offered some of the benefits of a standard game controller coupled with the high-technology motion sensors of the remote. Users could hold a Nunchuk in one hand and the Wii remote in the other while playing the Wii Sports Boxing game and be transformed into the boxing ring with on-screen opponents. The game controls were intuitive for jabs and punches; however, a missed block did not hurt as much as if one were really in the boxing ring.

The ambidextrous nature of the Wii controllers was something seldom seen in other game controllers; the Wii controllers permitted the user to hold the remote and Nunchuk whichever way felt most comfortable.[17]

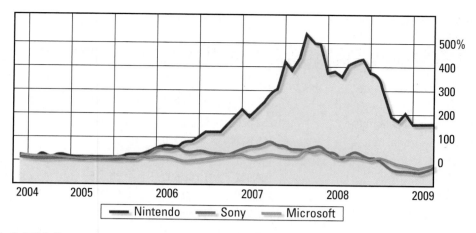

Exhibit 3 **Five-Year Stock Chart of Nintendo, Sony, and Microsoft, 2004–2009**
Source: reuters.com.

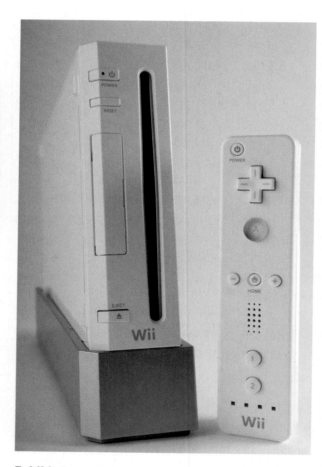

Exhibit 4 **Wii Game Console and Remote**

Features

In addition to the Wii Remote, there were other features unique to the Wii. One was the Wii Menu, which was the first screen that appeared on the television when the Wii was turned on. According to Nintendo, the Wii Menu easily integrated itself into the everyday lives of its users.[18]

The menu displayed several different icons; one of them was the Mii Channel (pronounced "me"). This channel gave the users the ability to create and personalize a 3-D caricature of themselves. Another icon was the Everybody Votes Channel, which permitted individuals to vote in national and worldwide polls on a variety of topics. There was also the New Channel, which gave the individual up-to-date breaking news from around the world, organized into a variety of topics. The Forecast Channel was another icon displayed on the Wii Menu. This allowed the individual to view weather reports from anywhere around the world. Users had the ability to download older Nintendo games from the Wii Shopping Channel. A Wii Message Board allowed users to leave messages on the Wii for other users of the same console or leave reminders for themselves. The Internet Channel allowed individuals to surf the Internet from their Wii. The Photo Channel allowed the user to view photos stored on a standard SD memory card. And lastly there was the Disc Channel, which gave the user the ability to play Wii games or Nintendo GameCube disks.[19] The Wii was backward-compatible with the Nintendo GameCube's games, memory cards, and controllers.

Online Capabilities

Nintendo's Wii was the first Nintendo console that had online capabilities. The Wii could connect to the Internet in several different ways. One way was via a standard wireless protocol—a consumer's home high-speed Internet hookup (usually from a cable TV service or telephone company DSL). Another way the Wii could connect to the Internet was via the Nintendo DS, which had wireless capability built in. The Wii could also be connected to the Internet via an optional wired USB–Ethernet adapter.

According to Nintendo of America's president and COO, Reggie Fils-Aime, the Wii would "offer online-enabled games that consumers will not have to pay a subscription fee for. They'll be able to play right out of the box. . . . It will not have any hidden fees or costs."[20] However as of mid-2007, no such games existed. So far, the only consoles to allow an individual to play games interactively with other users online were the competing products: Microsoft Xbox 360 and Sony PlayStation 3.

The Wii was released in North America on November 19, 2006, and worldwide cumulative sales as of September 30, 2008, were in excess of 34 million units (see Exhibit 5).[21] In 2006, Wii units were simultaneously released in Japan, the Americas, Oceania, Asia, and Europe. Two years later, Nintendo expanded the Wii market to South Korea and Taiwan.[22]

However, although the sales numbers were quite large, Nintendo had been experiencing production problems with the Wii. Nintendo was unable to meet demand during 2007 and also struggled throughout 2008. In an interview on the Web site Game Theory, Perrin Kapaln, Nintendo vice president of marketing and corporate affairs, suggested that shortages were expected for some time. "We are at absolute maximum production and doing everything we can . . . but demand continues to be really high."[23]

Demographics

According to Nintendo, one of the key differences between the Wii and the competitors' systems was the broad audience that the Wii targeted.[24] Many of the Wii games were able to be played by people of all ages, and they were easier to control than the complicated controllers of the Sony PlayStation 3 or Microsoft Xbox 360. Nintendo's TV commercials of the Wii showed people of different ages and social classes playing the Wii. According to Nintendo, the Wii remote allowed people of all ages to enjoy its use. Nintendo wanted to create a controller that was "as inviting as it was sophisticated."[25] Nintendo's goal was to create games that everyone could play and a system that would appeal to women and people who had never played video games in the past. Shigeru Miyamoto, a senior director at Nintendo, explained, "Most of the game business is going down a similar path toward hyperrealistic graphics which re-create sports or movies. . . . We want to put a little more art into it in a way that casual consumers can enjoy the game."[26] The Wii offered something for both the advanced gamer and the person who had never played a video game before. The advanced gamer would enjoy the remote's unique features, whereas the novice gamer could use the remote as his or her hand and wouldn't need elaborate instructions on how to play a new game straight out of the box. Although the Nintendo games were easily played by a greater range of ages, the graphics were undoubtedly a relative weakness of the product.

Although Nintendo had been able to target a large range of age groups, it seemed to lack the lineup of games offered by other systems. Nintendo had focused on its proprietary Mario Brothers series games, as well as low-graphic, low-complexity games that could be played by people in a wide range of age levels. PlayStation 3's top-selling game was Resistance: Fall of Man, which had won many awards; but more important, it had a rating of *Mature* (a rating given by the Entertainment Software Rating Board), which meant that it was suitable for audiences of 17 and older only. Xbox's best-selling game was Gears of War, which also had a rating of *Mature*. The Wii's best-selling games were The Legend of Zelda: Twilight Princess, which had a rating of *Teen,* which meant it was suitable for ages 13 and up, and Wii Sports, which was rated *Everyone,* suitable for all audiences. One of the Wii's shortcomings was obviously its graphics.[27] It was widely believed that the Wii had 2.5 times the power of the GameCube but hardly enough to compete with the Xbox 360 or PlayStation 3.

Although Nintendo hoped to target people of all ages, it had long been seen as a system that made video games for children, as evident from its Mario, Zelda, and Donkey Kong series. It was going to be difficult for Nintendo to position itself as a console for gamers of all ages and tastes.

Gaining the Interest of Game Developers

As evident from the history of game consoles, game developers have tried to make games more and more complex with each new generation of systems. This meant that more money was invested in the production of each subsequent generation of games. Because game developers were spending more money on developing games, they were at great financial risk if games did not succeed. Thus, many developers felt more secure in simply creating sequels to existing games, which in turn restricted innovation. The Wii's innovative controller, the Wii remote, required a rethinking and reengineering of the human interface for game developers and programmers. Another issue with developing games for the Wii was that its graphics were not quite as good as those of the PlayStation 3 and Xbox 360, and therefore game developers were required to be more creative and develop special Wii editions of their games.

Many game developers used virtual-machine software in developing new games. It was believed that game developers could develop games for the Wii and then make them for other platforms on the basis of the same programming, thereby reducing production costs. However, while the Wii remote distinguished itself from its competitors, it

Exhibit 5 Wii Cumulative Unit Sales

Region	Units Sold	First Available
The Americas	15,190,000	11/19/06
Japan	6,100,000	12/2/06
Other Regions	12,450,000	12/8/06
Total	**34,550,000**	

Source: Nintendo.

created a hurdle for developers. When a developer created a game for the PlayStation 3, she could create the same game for the Xbox 360 and vice versa, whereas when a developer created a game for the Wii, it required significant rework to deploy the title for the other platforms. Converting a title from the Xbox 360 or PlayStation 3 also required significant work to modify the game to incorporate code for the Wii Remote's special features.

The Competition

The launches of the Wii and the PlayStation 3 in November 2006 were the beginning of the battle for market share in the fierce competition of the seventh generation of video game consoles (see Exhibit 6). Although the Xbox 360 was released a year earlier, Microsoft intended to relaunch the Xbox 360 after some minor enhancements.

The price of $249 for the Wii included the Wii Remote, the Nunchuk attachment, the sensor bar, and the Wii Sports software title. The Wii sports title included tennis, baseball, golf, bowling, and boxing games. This retail price was much less than the prices of the PlayStation 3 and Xbox 360, possibly due to the fact that the Wii did not have as advanced a central processor unit or a high-definition video player.

Xbox 360

The Xbox 360 by Microsoft was released in November 2005, giving it a year lead over Nintendo's and Sony's new systems. While the configurations were changed several times, the Xbox 360 came in three different versions: Elite ($399 retail), Premium System ($299 retail), and Core System ($199 retail) as of 2009.

Although the prices were quite expensive to the retail consumer, in reality Microsoft was losing money on each sale. Take, for example, Microsoft's cost of producing the Premium System. It cost Microsoft $470 before assembly and an additional $55 for the cost of the cables, power cord, and controllers, bringing Microsoft's cost to $526. Thus, Microsoft was losing $227 on the sale of each system. This was the case not only with the Xbox 360 but also with its predecessor, the Xbox. There, too, Microsoft was selling a system for $299 that cost Microsoft $323 to produce.

One of the important features of the Xbox 360 was Xbox Live. According to Microsoft, Xbox Live was the "premier online gaming and entertainment service that enables you to connect your Xbox to the Internet and play games online."[28] This feature allowed individuals to play online against other users from around the world. Thus Microsoft had created a community of individuals who were able to communicate with one another by voice chats and/or play against each other in a video game. It even allowed users to "see what their friends are up to at any time" and to look not only at their friends' lists but also their friends' friends lists.[29] Another service offered by Xbox Live was the Xbox Live Marketplace, which enabled users to download movies, game trailers, game demos, and

Exhibit 6   Game Systems Comparison, 2009

	Nintendo	Sony	Microsoft
Console name	Wii	PlayStation 3	Xbox 360
Game format	12-cm Wii optical disk	Blu-Ray disc, DVD-Rom, CD-Rom	HD DVD, DVD, DVD-DL
Hard drive	None	80 GB or 160 GB	60 GB, or 120 GB
Price	$249	$399 (80 GB) or $499 (160 GB)	$199, $299, $399
Ethernet	Wi-fi standard	Wi-fi optional	Wi-fi optional
Online services	WiiConnect24, Wii Channels, no online game play	PlayStation Network, has online game play	Xbox live, has online game play
Controller	Wii remote (wireless, motion sensing)	Max 7 SixAxis (wireless)	Wired or wireless
Backward compatibility	Yes (Nintendo GameCube)	Yes (PlayStation 2)	Yes (certain Xbox games)
Game count	532	354	470*

*As of April 2009, there were 470 games specifically designed for the Xbox360. However, there were an additional 500+ games from the previous version of the Xbox that function on the Xbox360.

Source: Company reports, gamestop.com, and author estimates.

arcade games. It was estimated that more than 70 percent of connected Xbox users were downloading content from the Xbox Live Marketplace, totaling more than 8 million members.[30] According to Microsoft, there were more than 12 million downloads in less than a year and, due to this popularity, major publishers and other independent gamers had submitted more than 1,000 Xbox Live games.[31] Similar to the Wii, the Xbox 360 had a dashboard that showed up when the system was powered up. This gave the user the ability to play either DVDs or games.

The Xbox 360 had the capability to play high-definition DVDs.[32] The CPU of the Xbox 360 was a custom triple-core PowerPC-based design manufactured by IBM and known as the Xenon. The Xbox 360 played all its games in 5.1-channel Dolby Digital surround sound, and along with the HD display, the Xbox 360 could truly display excellent picture and sound quality. However, a consumer who did not have a high-definition-enabled television set was not able to enjoy the high-definition features of the system. The Xbox 360 played all its games on dual-layer DVDs, which could store up to 8.5 GB per disc but also had the ability to play many other formats.[33] The system had an Ethernet port and three USB ports but could also connect to the Internet via a wireless network.

Microsoft began production of the Xbox 360 only 69 days before the launch date.[34] As a result, Microsoft was unable to supply enough systems to meet the initial demand, and therefore many potential customers were not able to purchase a console at launch.[35] However, according to Bill Gates, Microsoft had over 10 million units out in the market by the time Sony and Nintendo launched their systems.[36]

Sony PlayStation 3

The PlayStation 3 was Sony's seventh-generation video game console. The PlayStation 3 had many advanced features, including a Cell Broadband Engine 64-bit processor that features a main power-processing element and up to eight parallel-processing elements. This was a multiprocessing unit that provided advanced support for graphics-intense games. Another notable feature of the PlayStation 3 was its ability to play Blu-Ray discs. Blu-Ray was a form of high-definition video, which enabled game developers to create games of higher sophistication.[37] Another key feature of the PlayStation 3 was the SixAxis wireless controller. This controller had sensors that could determine when a player maneuvered or angled his or her controller to allow game play to become a "natural extension of the player's body."[38] Although this was a more advanced remote than a standard wired remote, it lacked the true motion-sensing capabilities of the Wii Remote in its first version.[39]

The PlayStation 3 could play music CDs, connect to the Internet, copy CDs directly to its hard drive, play Blu-Ray discs and DVDs, connect to a digital camera, view photos, and more. However, a consumer who did not have a high-definition-enabled television set was not able to enjoy the high-definition features of the system.

Sales in North America were initially strong but tapered off rapidly, with 1.3 million units sold during the first six months of sales.[40] The United Kingdom also saw record-breaking sales of PlayStation 3, with more than 165,000 units (through heavy preordering) in its first two days on the shelves,[41] although the total European sales for the first six months of availability were only 920,000 units.[42] Sony CEO Howard Stringer attributed the slowing sales to a lack of software titles and said that Sony expected at least 380 new PlayStation 3 games to hit the market by 2008.[43] However, halfway into 2009, there were only 354 titles available for the PlayStation 3. Sony introduced new 40GB and 80 GB versions of PlayStation 3, and thanks to new features cumulative sales rose to 9.2 million units by March 2008.[44]

Part of the PlayStation Network's success was the ability to play games online. This allowed individuals to play with other players who were located in other parts of the world. The PlayStation Network allowed users to download games, view movie and game trailers, and text-message and chat with friends. Users were also able to browse the Internet and open up to six windows at once.[45]

Since the launch of the PlayStation 3, there have been mixed reports about it. On the positive note, MSN stated that the PlayStation 3 was a "versatile and impressive piece of home-entertainment equipment that lives up to the hype . . . the PS3 is well worth its hefty price tag."[46] However, *PC World* magazine ranked the PlayStation 3 eighth out of the Top-21 Tech Screw-Ups of 2006.[47]

While Sony and Microsoft envisioned long-term profits on software sales of PlayStation 3 and Xbox 360, both companies experienced losses producing their seventh-generation consoles. Among the three rivals, Nintendo was the only one earning a significant profit margin on each Wii unit sold. According to David Gibson at Macquarie Securities, sales of Nintendo Wii bring $6 of operating profit per console. [48]

Supply and Demand

When the Xbox 360 hit stores in November 2005, thousands of video game fans waited outside stores (some even in freezing weather) to be the first to purchase the console. And although the console quickly sold out, it became available several months later and there have not been problems purchasing one since. The same held true with the release of the PlayStation 3. Although it quickly sold out in stores, it was available thereafter, and anyone willing to spend the money is able to purchase it. However, Nintendo fans have had problems finding a Wii to purchase since its launch in November 2006. Lucky customers might have walked into a retailer at the moment the latest Wii shipment arrived or might have waited in lines for hours for the privilege of paying the retail price of only $249. The unlucky customers had to search various auction Web sites such as eBay and pay premiums of double to triple the retail price.

There had been a great deal of speculation regarding the production problems with the Wii. Several analysts had argued that lack of availability of the Wii was a marketing ploy to create hype and increase demand. However, others have hypothesized that Nintendo was having production problems and was unable to meet the huge demand for the Wii. The predictions of Billy Pidgeon, program manager for IDC's Consumers Markets, that consumers would have a difficult time purchasing the Wii through late 2008 proved right. Pidgeon stated that he believed that the Wii would continue to be a successful force in the gaming industry and that Nintendo needed to start shipping out more consoles. Furthermore, he said that he didn't believe "supply will meet demand for the Wii until 2009."[49]

The supply problem was confirmed by Nintendo CEO Satoru Iwata during a company financial briefing and later on a Web site question–and-answer session in May 2007. Iwata said, "We are currently facing product shortages . . . we have been running short of inventories, and [the retailers] are getting after us."[50] Iwata said further, "Making a significant volume of the high-tech hardware, and making an additional volume, is not an easy task at all. In fact, when we clear one bottleneck for a production increase, we will face another one."[51] The supply shortage first hit the United Kingdom in 2006 and quickly spread to North America by the end of 2007. Demand for Wii units outpaced supply in the U.S. market, and as of July 2008, Nintendo was still having a hard time restocking its retail shelves on time.[52]

There were 235 games for the Nintendo Wii by the end of its release year. By 2009, however, the total number of games for the Wii (532 games) exceeded the total number of games available for its main competitor, Xbox 360 (470 games), depending on whether one counted backward compatibility with previous-generation games. The number of games indicates that the Wii was obviously a successful system—one that had drawn a good amount of interest from game developers and gamers around the world. The production problem, then, was augmented because there was great interest in the Wii. However, if Nintendo did not meet the hardware demand, game developers could simply begin developing software for systems that were available to consumers.

CEO Iwata claimed that "shipments will increase and that we are trying to increase the shipments in order to comply with the needs of patiently waiting customers," as well as increase the number of software titles available for the system from Nintendo and third-party software developers.[53] Iwata's plan and strategic management helped to achieve record sales for Nintendo Wii within 2 years of its launch. With more than 40 million (including software) units sold worldwide by January 2009,[54] Nintendo Wii claimed first place in the game industry; its main competitor, Xbox 360, was far behind, with only 28 million units.[55] However, the question remained as to whether Nintendo's Iwata could manage to keep the Wii momentum rolling into the next generation of gaming systems.

Endnotes

1. Sony. Annual Report, March 31, 2008.
2. Microsoft. Annual Report, June 30, 2008.
3. Nintendo. Annual Report, March 31, 2008.
4. Robin Harding and Chris Nuttall. Nintendo plays it cool as Sony's PS3 dents Wii's Japanese sales. *Financial Times,* April 7, 2009.
5. Nintendo. Annual Report, March 31, 2008.
6. *www.nintendo.com/systemsclassic?type=nes.*
7. Nintendo. Annual Report, March 31, 2008.
8. C. Bacani and M. Mutsuko. Nintendo's new 64-bit platform sets off a scramble for market share. *AsiaWeek,* April 18, 1997, *www.asiaweek.com/asiaweek/97/0418/cs1.html.*
9. Biggest blunders. *GamePro,* May 2005, p. 45.
10. *http://wii.nintendo.com/iwata_asks_vol2_p1.jsp.*
11. Chris Moriss. "Nintendo goes Wii . . ." April 2006, *http:// money.cnn.com/2006/04/27/commentary/game_over/ nintendo/index.htm.*
12. T. Surette. Nintendo exec talks Wii Online marketing. *GameSpot.com.* August 17, 2006,. *www.cnet.com.au/ games/wii/0,239036428,240091920,00.htm.*
13. Nintendo. Annual Report, 2006.
14. See *http://wii.nintendo.com.*
15. *http://wii.nintendo.com/controller.jsp.*
16. *http://wii.ign.com/articles/718/718946p1.html.*
17. *http://wii.nintendo.com/controller.jsp.*
18. See *http://wii.Nintendo.com.*
19. See *http://wii.nintendo.com*
20. Surette. Nintendo exec talks Wii online.
21. Nintendo. Consolidated Financial Statements, October 30, 2008.
22. See *http://wii.Nintendo.com.*
23. *http://livenintendo.com/2007/04/12/ more-supply-problems-for-the-wii.*
24. Nintendo. Annual Report, March 31, 2007.
25. *http://wii.nintendo.com/controller.jsp.*
26. En garde! Fight foes using a controller like a sword. *The New York Times,* October 30, 2006, *www.nytimes .com/2006/10/30/technology/30nintendo.html?ex=131986 4400&en=135a11a72ad4a4f7&ei=5088&partner=rssny t&emc=rss.*
27. *www.pcmag.com/article2/0,1895,2058406,00.asp.*
28. *www.Xbox.com/en-US.*
29. *www.xbox.com/en-US/live/globalcommunity/ fosteringcommunity.htm.*
30. *www.microsoft.com/Presspass/press/2007/nov07/ 11-13XboxLIVEFivePR.mspx.*
31. Ibid.
32. *www.microsoft.com/Presspass/press/2007/jul07/ 07-26ComicConXboxHDDVDPR.mspx.*
33. *www.xbox.com/en-AU/support/xbox360/manuals/ xbox360specs.htm.*
34. money.cnn.com/2006/07/05/commentary/-column_gaming/ index.htm?section=money_latest.
35. news.bbc.co.uk/2/hi/technology/4491804.stm.
36. *www.microsoft.com/presspass/press/2006/may06/ 05-09E32006BriefingPR.mspx.*
37. *www.us.playstation.com/PS3/About/BluRay.*

38. *www.us.playstation.com/PS3/About/WirelessController.*
39. *www.scei.co.jp/corporate/release/pdf/060509be.pdf.*
40. *www.cbsnews.com/stories/2007/01/07/ap/business/ -mainD8MGN9J80.shtml.*
41. *news.bbc.co.uk/1/hi/technology/6499841.stm.*
42. *news.bbc.co.uk/2/hi/technology/6499841.stm.*
43. N. Layne and K. Hamada. Sony promises more games to boost PS3 demand. *reuters.com,* June 21, 2007, *http://www .reuters.com/article/-technologyNews/idUST28081120070 621?sp=true.*
44. Sony. Annual Report, March 31, 2008.
45. *www.us.playstation.com/PS3/Network.*
46. tech.uk.msn.com/features/article.aspx?cp-documentid= 4370234.
47. *www.pcworld.com/article/id,128265-page,4-c,industrynews/ article.html.*
48. Chana R.Schoenberger. "Wii's future in motion." *Forbes,* December 12, 2008, *www.forbes.com/2008/11/28/nintendo- wii-wii2-tech-personal-cz-cs-1201wii.html.*
49. *http://news.teamxbox.com/xbox/13335/Analyst- Supply-Wont-Meet-Demand-for-the-Wii-Until-2009.*
50. *Nintendo Investor Relations, www.nintendo.co.jp/ir/en/ library/events/070427qa/02.html.*
51. E. Boyes. Nintendo: Wii have a supply problem. *CNET .News.com,*2007, *http://news.com.com/Nintendo+ Wii+have +a+supply+problem/2100-1043_ 3-6181842.html.*
52. *www.npd.com.*
53. *Nintendo Investor Relations, www.nintendo.co.jp/ir/en/ library/events/070427qa/02.html.*
54. Ibid.
55. *www.microsoft.com.* Press release, January 6, 2009.

Case 5 McDonald's*

Even in the midst of a global economic slowdown, McDonald's reported strong results for the fourth quarter of 2008 and announced plans to add 650 more outlets by the end of 2009 (see Exhibits 1 and 2). The fast-food chain's performance was particularly impressive as rivals such as KFC and Wendy's had not managed to cope as well with the spending downturn. Same-store sales, a key indicator of the firm's health, actually rose by 7.2 percent during the last quarter from the figures reported a year earlier. Responding to McDonald's performance, CEO Jim Skinner remarked: "We continue to be recession-resistant."[1]

Analysts attribute the continued success of McDonald's to its "Plan to Win" strategy, which was first outlined by James R. Cantalupo over six years ago after overexpansion caused the chain to lose focus. The core of the plan was to increase sales at existing locations by improving the menu, refurbishing the outlets, and extending hours. The firm also added snacks and drinks, two of the few

*This case was developed by Professor Jamal Shamsie, Michigan State University, with the assistance of Professor Alan B. Eisner, Pace University. Material has been drawn from published sources to be used for class discussion. Copyright © 2009 Jamal Shamsie and Alan B. Eisner.

areas where restaurant sales are still growing. "We do so well because our strategies have been so well planned out," said Skinner in a recent interview.[2]

At the same time, Skinner has been monitoring pricing in order to make sure the menu stays affordable without hurting the firm's profit margins. Even as it continues to wrestle with cost increases, McDonald's has maintained the pricing on its Dollar Menu, which generates almost 15 percent of total sales. In December 2008, McDonald's did decide to replace its $1 double cheeseburger with the McDouble, a similar burger that is less expensive to make because it has less cheese. Steven Kron, an analyst with Goldman Sachs, emphasized the attractiveness of the firm's affordable Dollar Menu: "When people are seeking value, these guys have a very powerful component."[3]

Nevertheless, there are strong concerns that McDonald's will continue to be squeezed by long-term trends that are threatening to leave it marginalized. The chain is facing a rapidly fragmenting market, where changes in the tastes of consumers have made once-exotic foods like sushi and burritos everyday options. Many of its fast-food customers continue to switch to food that is

Exhibit 1 Income Statement (in thousands of dollars)

	2008	2007	2006
Total revenue	23,522,400	22,786,600	21,586,400
Cost of revenue	14,883,200	9,819,000	14,602,100
Gross profit	8,639,200	12,967,600	6,984,300
Operating expenses:			
Selling, general, and administrative	2,355,500	7,429,400	2,405,000
Nonrecurring	(48,500)	1,774,800	134,200
Operating income or loss	6,332,200	3,763,400	4,445,100
Income from continuing operations:			
Total other income/expenses net	237,700	103,200	123,300
Earnings before interest and taxes	6,680,600	3,982,200	4,568,400
Interest expense	522,600	410,100	402,000
Income before tax	6,158,000	3,572,100	4,166,400
Income tax expense	1,844,800	1,237,100	1,293,400
Net income from continuing ops	4,313,200	2,335,000	2,873,000
Nonrecurring events:			
Discontinued operations	—	60,100	671,200
Net income	4,313,200	2,395,100	3,544,200

Source: McDonald's.

Exhibit 2 **Balance Sheet** (in thousands of dollars)

	2008	2007	2006
Assets			
Current assets:			
Cash and cash equivalents	2,063,400	1,981,300	2,136,400
Net receivables	931,200	1,053,800	904,200
Inventory	111,500	125,300	149,000
Other current assets	411,500	421,500	435,700
Total current assets	**3,517,600**	**3,581,900**	**3,625,300**
Long-term investments	1,222,300	1,156,400	1,036,200
Property, plant, and equipment	20,254,500	20,984,700	20,845,700
Goodwill	2,237,400	2,301,300	2,209,200
Other assets	1,229,700	1,367,400	1,307,400
Total assets	**28,461,500**	**29,391,700**	**29,023,800**
Liabilities and Equity			
Current liabilities:			
Accounts payable	2,506,100	3,634,000	2,739,000
Short/current long-term debt	31,800	864,500	17,700
Other current liabilities	—	—	251,400
Total current liabilities	**2,537,900**	**4,498,500**	**3,008,100**
Long-term debt	10,186,000	7,310,000	8,416,500
Other liabilities	1,410,100	1,342,500	1,074,900
Deferred long-term liability charges	944,900	960,900	1,066,000
Total liabilities	**15,078,900**	**14,111,900**	**13,565,500**
Stockholders' equity:			
Common stock	16,600	16,600	16,600
Retained earnings	28,953,900	26,461,500	25,845,600
Treasury stock	(20,289,400)	(16,762,400)	(13,552,200)
Capital surplus	4,600,200	4,226,700	3,445,000
Other stockholders' equity	101,300	1,337,400	(296,700)
Total stockholders' equity	**13,382,600**	**15,279,800**	**15,458,300**
Net tangible assets	**$11,145,200**	**$12,978,500**	**$13,249,100**

Source: McDonald's.

much healthier and better tasting. Furthermore, competition has been coming from quick meals of all sorts that can be found in supermarkets, convenience stores, and even vending machines.

Many analysts believe that McDonald's must continue to work on its turnaround strategy in order to meet these challenges. But they acknowledge that the firm has pushed hard to transform itself, and they are encouraged by the results that it has achieved over the last six years. Even during the past year, the chain registered growth in the number of customers served, from 56 million to 58 million a day. "They have experienced a comeback the likes of which have been pretty unprecedented," said Bob Golden, executive vice president of Technomic, a food service consultancy. "When restaurants start to slide, it really takes a lot to turn them around."[4]

Experiencing a Downward Spiral

Since it was founded, more than 50 years ago, McDonald's has been defining the fast-food business. It provided millions of Americans their first jobs even as it changed their eating habits. It rose from a single outlet in a nondescript Chicago suburb to one of the largest chain of outlets spread around the globe. But it was stumbling during the past decade (see Exhibit 3).

The decline in McDonald's once-vaunted service and quality can be traced to its expansion in the 1990s, when headquarters stopped grading franchises for cleanliness, speed, and service. By the end of the decade, the chain ran into more problems because of the tighter labor market. McDonald's began to cut back on training as it struggled hard to find new recruits, a policy that led to a dramatic falloff in the skills of its employees. According to a 2002 survey by market researcher Global Growth Group, McDonald's came in third in average service time behind Wendy's and sandwich shop Chick-fil-A Inc.

McDonald's also began to fail consistently with its new product introductions, such as the low-fat McLean Deluxe and Arch Deluxe burgers, both of which were meant to appeal to adults. It did no better with its attempts to diversify beyond burgers, often because of problems with the product development process. Consultant Michael Seid, who manages a franchise consulting firm in West Hartford, pointed out that McDonald's offered a pizza that didn't fit through the drive-through window and salad shakers that were packed so tightly that dressing couldn't flow through them.

In 1998, after McDonald's posted its first-ever decline in annual earnings, CEO Michael R. Quinlan was forced out and replaced by Jack M. Greenberg, a 16-year veteran of the firm. Greenberg did try to cut back on McDonald's expansion as he tried to deal with some of the growing problems. But his efforts to deal with the decline of McDonald's were slowed down by his acquisition of other fast-food chains such as Chipotle Mexican Grill and Boston Market.

On December 5, 2002, after watching McDonald's stock slide 60 percent in three years, the board ousted Greenberg. He had lasted little more than two years. His short tenure had been marked by the introduction of 40 new menu items, none of which caught on big, and the purchase of a handful of nonburger chains, none of which helped the firm to sell more burgers. Indeed, his critics say that by trying so many different things and executing them poorly, Greenberg allowed the burger business to continue declining. According to Los Angeles franchisee Reggie

Webb: "We would have been better off trying fewer things and making them work."[5]

Pinning Hopes on a New Leader

By the beginning of 2003, consumer surveys were indicating that McDonald's was headed for serious trouble. Measures of the service and quality of the chain were continuing to fall, dropping far behind those of its rivals. To deal with its deteriorating performance, the firm decided to bring back retired vice chairman James R. Cantalupo, 59, who had overseen McDonald's successful international expansion in the 1980s and 1990s. Cantalupo, who had retired only a year earlier, was perceived to be the only candidate with the necessary qualifications, despite shareholder sentiment for an outsider. The board felt that it needed someone who knew the company well and could move quickly to turn things around.

Cantalupo realized that McDonald's often tended to miss the mark on delivering the critical aspects of consistent, fast, friendly service and an all-around enjoyable experience for the whole family. He understood that its franchisees and employees alike needed to be inspired as well as retrained in their role of putting the smile back into the McDonald's experience. When Cantalupo and his team laid out their turnaround plan in 2003, they stressed getting the basics of service and quality right, in part by reinstituting a tough "up or out" grading system that would kick out underperforming franchisees. "We have to rebuild the foundation. It's fruitless to add growth if the foundation is weak," said Cantalupo.[6]

To begin with, Cantalupo cut back on the opening of new outlets, focusing instead on generating more sales from the chain's existing outlets. In fact, he shifted his emphasis to obtaining most of the growth in future revenues from an increase in sales in the over 30,000 outlets that were already operating around the world (see Exhibits 4 through 6). In part, McDonalds tried to draw more customers through the introduction of new products. The chain has had a positive response to its increased emphasis on healthier foods, led by a revamped line of fancier salads. The revamped menu was promoted through a new worldwide ad slogan, "I'm loving it," which was delivered by pop idol Justin Timberlake through a set of MTV-style commercials.

But the biggest success for the firm came in the form of the McGriddles breakfast sandwich, which was launched nationwide in June 2003. The popular new offering consisted of a couple of syrup-drenched pancakes, stamped with the Golden Arches, which acted as the top and bottom of a sandwich filled with eggs, cheese, sausage, and bacon in three different combinations. McDonald's estimated that the new breakfast addition has been bringing in about 1 million new customers every day.

With his efforts largely directed at a turnaround strategy for McDonald's, Cantalupo decided to divest the nonburger chains that his predecessor had acquired. Collectively lumped under the Partner Brands, these chains

Exhibit 3   **McDonald's Milestones**

1948	Brothers Richard and Maurice McDonald open the first restaurant in San Bernadino, California, that sells hamburgers, fries, and milk shakes.
1955	Ray A. Kroc, 52, opens his first McDonald's in Des Plaines, Illinois. Kroc, a distributor of milk-shake mixers, figures he can sell a bundle of them if he franchises the McDonalds' business and installs his mixers in the new stores.
1961	Six years later, Kroc buys out the McDonald brothers for $2.7 million.
1963	Ronald McDonald makes his debut as corporate spokesclown using future NBC-TV weatherman Willard Scott. During the year, the company also sells its 1 billionth burger.
1965	McDonald's stock goes public at $22.50 a share. It will split 12 times in the next 35 years.
1967	The first McDonald's restaurant outside the United States opens in Richmond, British Columbia. Today there are 31,108 McDonald's in 118 countries.
1968	The Big Mac, the first extension of McDonald's basic burger, makes its debut and is an immediate hit.
1972	McDonald's switches to the frozen variety for its successful french fries.
1974	Fred L. Turner succeeds Kroc as CEO. In the midst of a recession, the minimum wage rises to $2 per hour, a big cost increase for McDonald's, which is built around a model of young, low-wage workers.
1975	The first drive-through window is opened in Sierra Vista, Arizona.
1979	McDonald's responds to the needs of working women by introducing Happy Meals. A burger, some fries, a soda, and a toy give working moms a break.
1987	Michael R. Quinlan becomes chief executive.
1991	Responding to the public's desire for healthier foods, McDonald's introduces the low-fat McLean Deluxe burger. It flops and is withdrawn from the market. Over the next few years, the chain will stumble several times trying to spruce up its menu.
1992	The company sells its 90 billionth burger, and stops counting.
1996	In order to attract more adult customers, the company launches its Arch Deluxe, a "grown-up" burger with an idiosyncratic taste. Like the low-fat burger, it also falls flat.
1997	McDonald's launches Campaign 55, which cuts the cost of a Big Mac to $0.55. It is a response to discounting by Burger King and Taco Bell. The move, which prefigures similar price wars in 2002, is widely considered a failure.
1998	Jack M. Greenberg becomes McDonald's fourth chief executive. A 16-year company veteran, he vows to spruce up the restaurants and their menu.
1999	For the first time, sales from international operations outstrip domestic revenues. In search of other concepts, the company acquires Aroma Cafe, Chipotle, Donatos, and, later, Boston Market.
2000	McDonald's sales in the United States peak at an average of $1.6 million annually per restaurant, a figure that has not changed since. It is, however, still more than sales at any other fast-food chain.
2001	Subway surpasses McDonald's as the fast-food chain with the most U.S. outlets. At the end of the year it had 13,247 stores, 148 more than McDonald's.
2002	McDonald's posts its first-ever quarterly loss, of $343.8 million. The stock drops to around $13.50, down 40% from five years ago.
2003	James R. Cantalupo returns to McDonald's in January as CEO. He immediately pulls back from the company's 10% to 15% forecast for per-share earnings growth.
2004	Charles H. Bell takes over the firm after the sudden death of Cantalupo. He states he will continue with the strategies that have been developed by his predecessor.
2005	Jim Skinner takes over as CEO after Bell announces retirement for health reasons.
2006	McDonald's launches specialty beverages, including coffee-based drinks.

Source: McDonald's.

were Chipotle Mexican Grill and Boston Market. The purpose of these acquisitions had been to find new growth and to offer the best franchises new expansion opportunities. But the acquired businesses had not fueled much growth and had actually posted considerable losses in recent years.

Striving for Healthier Offerings

As Skinner took over the reins of McDonald's in late 2004, he expressed his commitment to Cantalupo's plans to pursue various avenues for growth. But Skinner felt that one of his top priorities was to deal with growing concerns about the unhealthy image of McDonald's, given the rise of obesity in the United States. These concerns had recently been highlighted by the release of a popular documentary, *Super Size Me,* made by Morgan Spurlock. Spurlock vividly displayed the health risks that were posed by a steady diet of food from the fast-food chain. With a rise in awareness of the high fat content of most of the products offered by McDonald's, the firm was also beginning to face lawsuits from some of its loyal customers.

In response to the growing health concerns, one of the first steps taken by McDonald's was to phase out supersizing by the end of 2004. The supersizing option allowed customers to get a larger order of french fries and a bigger soft drink by paying a little extra. McDonald's also announced that it intends to start providing nutrition information on the packaging of its products. The information will be easy to read and will tell customers about the calories, fat, protein, carbohydrates, and sodium that are in each product. Finally, McDonald's pledged to gradually remove the artery-clogging trans-fatty acids from the oil that it uses to make its french fries.

Skinner was also trying to provide more offerings that were likely to be perceived by customers as being healthier. McDonald's continued to build on its chicken offerings, using white meat with products such as Chicken Selects. It also placed a great deal of emphasis on its new salad

Exhibit 4   Number of Outlets

	Total	Company Owned	Franchised
2008	31,967	6,502	25,465
2007	31,377	6,906	24,471
2006	31,046	8,166	22,880
2005	30,766	8,173	22,593
2004	30,496	8,179	22,317

Source: McDonald's.

Exhibit 5   Distribution of Outlets

	2008	2007	2006	2005	2004
United States	13,918	13,862	13,774	13,727	13,673
Europe	6,628	6,480	6,403	6,352	6,287
Asia Pacific	8,255	7,938	7,822	7,692	7,567
Americas*	3,166	3,097	3,047	2,995	2,969

* Canada and Latin America.

Source: McDonald's.

Exhibit 6   Breakdown of Revenues (in millions of dollars)

	2008	2007	2006	2005	2004
United States	8,078	7,906	7,464	6,955	6,525
Europe	9,923	8,926	7,638	7,072	6,737
Asia Pacific	4,231	3,599	3,053	2,815	2,721
Americas*	1,290	2,356	2,740	2,275	1,906

* Canada and Latin America.

Source: McDonald's.

offerings. Although the firm had failed to attract many customers in the past with its salads, McDonald's carried out extensive experiments and tests with its new, premium versions. It chose higher-quality ingredients, from a variety of lettuces and tasty cherry tomatoes to sharper cheeses and better cuts of meat. It offered a choice of Newman's Own dressings, a well-known higher-end brand.

McDonald's has also been trying to include more fruits and vegetables in its well-known and popular Happy Meals. In many locations, the firm is offering apple slices called Apple Dippers in place of french fries in the children's Happy Meal. The addition of fruits and vegetables has raised the firm's operating costs because the perishable nature of produce makes it more expensive to ship and store. But Skinner believes that the firm had to push more heavily on fruits and salads. "Salads have changed the way people think of our brand," said Wade Thoma, vice president for menu development in the United States. "It tells people that we are very serious about offering things people feel comfortable eating."[7]

The current rollout of new beverages, highlighted by new coffee-based drinks, represents the chain's biggest menu expansion in almost three decades. Under a plan to add a McCafe section to all of its nearly 14,000 United States outlets, McDonald's has been offering lattes, cappuccinos, ice-blended frappes, and fruit-based smoothies to its customers. "In many cases, they're now coming for the beverage, whereas before they were coming for the meal," said Lee Renz, the firm's vice president, who is responsible for the rollout.[8]

Revamping the Outlets

As part of its turnaround strategy, McDonald's has been selling off the outlets that it owned. More than 75 percent of its outlets are now in the hands of franchisees and other affiliates. Skinner is working with the franchisees to address the look and feel of many of the chain's aging stores. Without any changes to their décor, the firm is likely to be left behind by other, more savvy fast-food and drink retailers. The firm is in the midst of pushing harder to refurbish—or reimage—all of its outlets around the world. "This is all part of becoming more relevant to our consumers," said company spokesman Walt Riker. "When a customer enters our restaurant, they enter our brand."[9]

The reimaging concept was first tried in France in 1996 by Dennis Hennequin, now president of McDonald's Europe, who felt that the effort was essential to revive the firm's sagging sales. "We were hip 15 years ago, but I think we lost that," he said.[10] McDonald's is now applying the reimaging concept to its outlets around the world, with a budget of more than half of its total annual capital expenditures. In the United States, the changes cost an average of $150,000 per restaurant, a cost that is shared with the franchisees when the outlet is not company-owned.

One of the prototype interiors being tested out by McDonald's has curved counters with surfaces painted in bright colors. In one corner, a touch-activated screen allows customers to punch in orders without queuing. The interiors can feature armchairs and sofas, modern lighting, large television screens, and even wireless Internet access. The firm is also trying to develop new features for its drive-through customers, who account for 65 percent of all transactions in the United States. The features include music aimed at queuing vehicles and a wall of windows on the drive-through side of the restaurant, allowing customers to see meals being prepared from their cars.

The chain has even been developing McCafes inside its outlets next to the usual fast-food counter. The McCafe concept originated in Australia in 1993 and has been rolled out in many restaurants around the world. McDonald's has just begun to introduce the concept in the United States as it refurbishes many of its existing outlets. In fact, part of the refurbishment has focused on the installation of a specialty beverage platform across all U.S. outlets. The cost of installing this equipment is running at about $100,000 per outlet, with McDonald's subsidizing part of the expense.

Eventually, all McCafes will offer espresso-based coffee, gourmet coffee blends, fresh baked muffins, and high-end desserts. Customers will be able to consume these products while they relax in soft leather chairs listening to jazz, big-band, or blues music. Commenting on this significant expansion of offerings, Marty Brochstein, executive editor of *The Licensing Letter,* said: "McDonald's wants to be seen as a lifestyle brand, not just a place to go to have a burger."[11]

A New and Improved McDonalds?

Even though Skinner's efforts to transform McDonald's have led to improvements in its sales and profits, there are questions about the future of the fast-food chain. The firm is trying out a variety of strategies in order to increase its appeal to different segments of the market. Through the adoption of a mix of outlet décor and menu items, McDonald's is trying to target young adults, teenagers, children, and families. In so doing, it must ensure that it does not alienate any one of these groups in its efforts to reach out to the others. Its new marketing campaign, anchored around the catchy phase "I'm loving it," takes on different forms in order to target each of the groups that it is seeking.

Larry Light, the head of global marketing at McDonald's since 2002, insists that the firm has to exploit its brand by pushing it in many different directions. The brand can be positioned differently in different locations, at different times of the day, and for different targeted customer segments. In large urban centers, for instance, McDonald's can target young adults for breakfast with its gourmet coffee, egg sandwiches, and fat-free muffins. Light explains the adoption of this approach as multiformat strategy: "The days of mass-media marketing are over."[12]

As McDonald's expands on its concept of fast food, it is moving beyond its staple of burgers and fries to a wider variety of offerings. In particular, many analysts are questioning the decision to invest in specialty beverages during a period when consumers are cutting back on spending. In fact, there are indications that the initial sales of lattes and frappes have not met expectations. Skinner recently denied that beverage addition may not have been successful. "You have to remember that everything we do at McDonald's is for the long term," he responded.[13]

Nevertheless, the additional offerings do raise some fundamental questions. Most significantly, it is not clear just how far McDonald's can stretch its brand while keeping all of its outlets under the traditional symbol of its golden arches. Chief Financial Officer Paull acknowledged that burgers continued to be the main draw for McDonald's. "There is no question that we make more money from selling hamburgers and cheeseburgers," he recently stated.[14]

Above all, Skinner is convinced that McDonald's must do whatever it can to make sure that it keeps its established customer base from bolting to the growing number of competitors such as the California-based In-N-Out chain. The long-term success of the firm may well depend on its ability to compete with rival burger chains. "The burger category has great strength," added David C. Novak, chairman and CEO of Yum! Brands, parent of KFC and Taco Bell. "That's America's food. People love hamburgers."[15]

Endnotes

1. Carolyn Walkup. McD Scores Amid Downturn, but Doubts Persist about Espresso, Dollar Menu Plans. *Nation's Restaurant News,* November 3, 2008, p. 4.
2. Janet Adamy. McDonald's to Expand, Posting Strong Results. *The Wall Street Journal,* January 27, 2009, p. B1.
3. Ibid.
4. Neil Buckley. McDonald's Shares Survive Resignation. November 24, 2004, p. 18.
5. Pallavi Gogoi and Michael Arndt. Hamburger Hell. *BusinessWeek,* March 3, 2003, p. 106.
6. Ibid.
7. Melanie Warner. You Want Any Fruit with That Big Mac? *The New York Times,* February 20, 2005, p. 8.
8. Janet Adamy. McDonald's Coffee Strategy Is Tough Sell. *The Wall Street Journal,* October 27, 2008, p. B3.
9. Bruce Horovitz. You Want Ambiance with That? *USA Today,* October 30, 2003, p. 3B.
10. Jeremy Grant. McDonald's to Revamp UK Outlets. *Financial Times,* February 2, 2006, p. 14.
11. Bruce Horovitz. McDonald's Ventures beyond Burgers to Duds, Toys. *USA Today,* November 14, 2003, p. 6B.
12. Big Mac's Makeover. *The Economist,* October 16, 2004, p. 65.
13. *The Wall Street Journal,* January 27, 2009, p. B1.
14. *The Economist,* Big Mac's Makeover, 2004, p. 64.
15. *BusinessWeek,* Hamburger Hell, 2003, p. 108.

Case 6   Apple Inc.: Taking a Bite Out of the Competition*

In September 2008, after announcing record year-end results, Steve Jobs, Apple Inc.'s CEO, commented, "We don't yet know how this economic downturn will affect Apple. But we're armed with the strongest product line in our history, the most talented employees and the best customers in our industry. And $25 billion of cash safely in the bank with zero debt."[1] Then, in January 2009, in the midst of the economic downturn that had seen most of its competitors reporting reduced results, Apple reported one of its best quarters, surpassing $10 billion in quarterly revenue for the first time in its history[2] (see Exhibits 1 and 2).

Also in January came the news that Apple's visionary leader and CEO, Steve Jobs, would be taking a medical leave of absence until the end of June. Although Jobs, then 53 years old, had appeared to be completely cured of the pancreatic cancer that sidelined him in 2004, he had lost considerable weight during 2008, causing speculation that his cancer had returned. Jobs's physicians found that a hormone imbalance, a side effect of the cancer treatment, was creating a nutritional problem that needed monitoring and treatment.[3] Stating that his "health-related issues are more complex than I originally thought," Jobs asked COO Tim Cook to be responsible for Apple's day-to-day operations, while Jobs remained "involved in major strategic decisions."[4] This news caused Apple shares to drop 7.56 percent on that day and prompted the Securities and Exchange Commission to wonder whether the Apple board of directors (which included former U.S. Vice President Al Gore and Google's CEO, Dr. Eric Schmidt, among others) "was as forthcoming about [Jobs's] illness as it should have been."[5]

For market watchers, Apple investors, and the sometimes cultlike Apple users, the possibility that CEO Steve Jobs might finally depart from the company he helped found in 1976 was unsettling news. One analyst said that an Apple without Jobs "would still be a remarkable company, but with less of the competitive edge that Jobs helped create. . . . If he isn't able to return, I think you'd see a high-functioning company, but one without the lightning strike of genius. [Apple would] have a human batting average."[6]

Apple, at the top of *BusinessWeek*'s Most Innovative Companies list since 2004,[7] had distinguished itself by excelling over the years not only in product innovation but also in revenue and margins (since 2006 Apple had consistently reported gross margins of around 30 percent). Founded as a computer company in 1976, and known initially for its intuitive adaptation of the "graphical user interface" or GUI (via the first mouse and the first onscreen

"windows"),[8] Apple had dropped the word *computer* from its corporate name in 2007. Apple Inc. in 2009 was known for having top-selling products not only in desktop (iMac) and notebook (MacBook) personal computers but also in portable digital music players (iPod), online music services (iTunes), mobile communication devices (iPhone), digital consumer entertainment (Apple TV), and handheld devices able to download third-party applications, including games (iPod Touch via the App Store). (See Exhibit 3.)

Although most of those innovations occurred after 1998, when Apple was under Steve Jobs's leadership, there was a 12-year period in which Jobs was not in charge. The company's ongoing stated strategy had been to leverage "its unique ability to design and develop its own operations system, hardware, application software, and services to provide its customers new products and solutions with superior ease-of-use, seamless integration and innovative industrial design."[9] This strategy required not only product design and marketing expertise but also scrupulous attention to operational details. Given Apple's global growth in multiple product categories, and the associated complexity in strategic execution, would the potential loss of one man be sufficient to prevent the company from sustaining its competitive advantage? Was Steve Jobs essential to Apple's success?

Company Background

Founder Steve Jobs   Apple Computer was founded in Mountain View, California, on April 1, 1976, by Steve Jobs and Steve Wozniak. Jobs was the visionary and marketer, Wozniak was the technical genius, and A. C. "Mike" Markkula, Jr., who had joined the team several months earlier, was the businessman. Jobs set the mission of empowering individuals, one person–one computer, and doing so with elegance of design and fierce attention to detail. In 1977 the first version of the Apple II became the first computer ordinary people could use right out of the box, and its instant success in the home market caused a computing revolution, essentially creating the personal computer industry. By 1980 Apple was the industry leader and went public in December of that year.

In 1983, Wozniak left the firm and Jobs hired John Sculley away from PepsiCo to take the role of CEO at Apple, citing the need for someone to spearhead marketing and operations while Jobs worked on technology. The result of Jobs's creative focus on personal computing was the Macintosh. Introduced in 1984, with the now-famous Super Bowl television ad based on George Orwell's novel,[10] the Macintosh was a breakthrough in terms of elegant design and ease of use. Its ability to handle large graphic files quickly made it a favorite with graphic designers, but it had slow performance and limited compatible software was available, so the product was unable to significantly help Apple's failing bottom line. In addition, Jobs had given

* This case was prepared by Professor Alan B. Eisner of Pace University and Professor Pauline Assenza of Manhattanville College. This case was solely based on library research and was developed for class discussion rather than to illustrate either effective or ineffective handling of an administrative situation. Copyright © 2009 Alan B. Eisner and Pauline Assenza.

Exhibit 1   Apple Sales

	2008 (in millions)	Change	2007 (in millions)	Change	2006 (in millions)
Product Net Sales					
Desktops	$ 5,603	39%	$ 4,020	21%	$ 3,319
Portables	8,673	38	6,294	55	4,056
iPod	9,153	10	8,305	8	7,676
Music	3,340	34	2,496	32	1,885
iPhone*	1,844	N/A	123	N/A	—
Peripherals	1,659	32	1,260	15	1,100
Software, services	2,207	46	1,508	18	1,279
Total net sales	**$32,479**	**35%**	**$24,006**	**24%**	**$19,315**
Cost of sales	21,334		15,852		13,717
Gross margin	**$11,145**		**$ 8,154**		**$ 5,598**
Gross margin %	34.4%		34%		29%
Research and development	$ 1,109		$ 782		$ 712
Percent of net sales	3.4%		3.3%		3.7%
Selling, general, and administrative	$ 3,761		$ 2,963		$ 2,433
Percent of net sales	11.6%		12.3%		12.6%
Total operating expenses	**$ 4,870**		**$ 3,745**		**$ 3,145**
Net income†	**$ 4,834**		**$ 3,496**		**$ 1,989**
Region Net Sales					
Americas	$14,573	26%	$11,596	23%	$ 9,415
Europe	7,622	40	5,460	33	4,096
Japan	1,509	39	1,082	(11)	1,211
Retail	6,315	53	4,115	27	3,246
Other	2,460	40	1,753	30	1,347

*iPhone sales derived from handset sales, carrier agreements, and Apple-branded and third-party iPhone accessories. Total revenue reported for iPhone in 2007 represented only one fiscal quarter.

†Net income reflects other income and expense, plus provision for income taxes.

Source: Apple 10K SEC filing.

Bill Gates at Microsoft some Macintosh prototypes to use to develop software, and in 1985 Microsoft subsequently came out with the Windows operating system, a version of GUI for use on IBM PCs.

Steve Jobs's famous volatility led to his resignation from Apple in 1985. Jobs then founded NeXT Computer; the NeXT Cube computer proved too costly for the business to become commercially profitable, but its technological contributions could not be ignored. In 1997, then–Apple CEO Gilbert Amelio bought out NeXT, hoping to use its Rhapsody, a version of the NeXTStep operating system, to

jump-start the Mac OS development, and Jobs was brought back as a part-time adviser.

Under CEOs Sculley, Spindler, and Amelio

John Sculley tried to take advantage of Apple's unique capabilities. Because of this, Macintosh computers were easy to use, with seamless integration (the original plug-and-play) and reliable performance. This premium performance meant Apple could charge a premium price. However, with the price of IBM compatibles dropping, and Apple's costs, especially R&D, way above industry averages (in

Exhibit 2 Apple First Quarter 2009 Sales

	1st Quarter 2009 (in millions)	1st Quarter 2008 (in millions)	Percent Change
Product Net Sales			
Desktops	$ 1,043	$1,515	(31%)
Portables	2,511	2,037	23
iPod	3,371	3,997	(16)
Music	1,011	808	25
iPhone*	1,247	241	417
Peripherals	378	382	(1)
Software, services	606	628	(4)
Total net sales	**$10,167**	**$9,608**	**6%**
Region Net Sales			
Americas	$ 4,501	$4,298	5%
Europe	2,771	2,471	12
Japan	481	400	20
Retail	1,740	1,701	2
Other	674	738	(9)

*iPhone sales derived from handset sales, carrier agreements, and Apple-branded and third-party iPhone accessories. Total revenue reported for iPhone in 2007 represented only one fiscal quarter.

Source: Apple 10Q SEC filing.

1990 Apple spent 9 percent of sales on R&D, compared to 5 percent at Compaq and 1 percent at many manufacturers of IBM clones),[11] this was not a sustainable scenario.

All Sculley's innovative efforts were not enough to substantially improve Apple's bottom line, and he was replaced as CEO in 1993 by company president Michael Spindler. Spindler continued the focus on innovation, producing the PowerMac, based on the PowerPC microprocessor, in 1994. Even though this combination produced a significant price-performance edge over both previous Macs and Intel-based machines, the IBM clones continued to undercut Apple's prices. Spindler's response was to allow other companies to manufacture Mac clones, a strategy that ultimately led to clones stealing 20 percent of Macintosh unit sales.

Gilbert Amelio, an Apple director and former semiconductor turnaround expert, was asked to reverse the company's financial direction. Amelio intended to reposition Apple as a premium brand, but his extensive reorganizations and cost-cutting strategies couldn't prevent Apple's stock price from slipping to a new low. However, Amelio's decision to stop work on a brand-new operating system and try to jump-start development by using NeXTStep brought Steve Jobs back to Apple in 1997.

Steve Jobs's Return   One of Jobs's first strategies on his return was to strengthen Apple's relationships with third-party software developers, including Microsoft. In 1997, Jobs announced an alliance with Microsoft that would allow for the creation of a Mac version of the popular Microsoft Office software. He also made a concerted effort to woo other developers, such as Adobe, to continue to produce Mac-compatible programs.

In late October 2001, Apple released its first major noncomputer product, the iPod. This device was an MP3 music player that packed up to 1,000 CD-quality songs into an ultraportable, 6.5-ounce design: "With iPod, Apple has invented a whole new category of digital music player that lets you put your entire music collection in your pocket and listen to it wherever you go," said Steve Jobs. "With iPod, listening to music will never be the same again."[12]

This prediction became even truer in 2002 when Apple introduced an iPod that would download from Windows—its first product that didn't require a Macintosh computer and thus opened up the Apple "magic" to everyone. In 2003 all iPod products were sold with a Windows version of iTunes, making it even easier to use the device regardless of computer platform.

Exhibit 3 **Apple Innovation Time Line**

Date	Product	Events
1976	Apple I	Steve Jobs, Steve Wozniak, and Ronald Wayne found Apple Computer.
1977	Apple II	Apple logo first used.
1979	Apple II +	Apple employs 250 people; the first personal computer spreadsheet software, VisiCalc, is written by Dan Bricklin on an Apple II.
1980	Apple III	Apple goes public with 4.6 million shares; IBM personal computer announced.
1983	Lisa	John Sculley becomes CEO.
1984	Mac 128K, Apple IIc	Super Bowl ad introduces the Mac desktop computer.
1985		**Jobs resigns** and forms NeXT Software; Windows 1.01 released.
1986	Mac Plus	Jobs establishes Pixar.
1987	Mac II, Mac SE	Apple sues Microsoft over GUI.
1989	Mac Portable	Apple sued by Xerox over GUI.
1990	Mac LC	Apple listed on Tokyo Stock Exchange.
1991	Powerbook 100, System 7	System 7 operating-system upgrade released, the first Mac OS to support PowerPC-based computers.
1993	Newton Message Pad (one of the first PDAs)	Sculley resigns; Spindler becomes CEO; PowerBook sales reach 1 million units.
1996		Spindler is out; Amelio becomes CEO; Apple acquires NeXT Software, with Jobs as adviser.
1997		Amelio is out; **Jobs returns** as interim CEO; online retail Apple Store opened.
1998	iMac	iMac colorful design introduced, including USB interface; Newton scrapped.
1999	iMovie, Final Cut Pro video editing software	iBook (part of Powerbook line) becomes best-selling retail notebook in October; Apple has 11% share of notebook market.
2000	G4Cube	**Jobs becomes permanent CEO.**
2001	iPod, OS X	First retail store opens, in Virginia.
2002	iMac G4	Apple releases iLife software suite.
2003	iTunes	Apple reaches 25 million iTunes downloads.
2004	iMac G5	**Jobs undergoes successful surgery for pancreatic cancer.**
2005	iPod Nano, iPod Shuffle, Mac Mini	First video iPod released; video downloads available from iTunes.
2006	MacBook Pro	Apple computers use Intel's Core Duo CPU and can run Windows software; iWork software competes with Microsoft Office.
2007	iPhone, Apple TV, iPod Touch	Apple Computer changes name to Apple Inc.; Microsoft Vista released.
2008	iPhone 3G, MacBook Air	App Store launched for third-party applications for iPhone and iPod Touch and brings in $1 million in one day.
2009	17-inch MacBook Pro, iLife, iWork '09	iTunes Plus provides DRM-free music, with variable pricing; **Jobs takes medical leave.**

Source: Apple.com; CNET News, "Apple Turns 30," *http://news.cnet.com/2009-1041-6053869.html?tag=txt:* Wikipedia, "Apple Inc." entry.

In April 2003, Apple opened the online iTunes Music Store to everyone. This software, downloadable on any computer platform, sold individual songs through the iTunes application for 99 cents each. When announced, the iTunes Music Store already had the backing of five major record labels and a catalog of 200,000 songs. Later that year, the iTunes Music Store was selling roughly 500,000 songs a day. In 2003, the iPod was the only portable digital player that could play music purchased from iTunes, and this intended exclusivity helped both products become dominant.

After 30 years of carving a niche for itself as the premier provider of technology solutions for graphic artists, Web designers, and educators, Apple appeared to be reinventing itself as a digital entertainment company, moving beyond the personal computer industry. The announcement in 2007 of the iPhone, a product incorporating a wireless phone, a music and video player, and a mobile Internet browsing device, meant Apple was also competing in the cell phone/smartphone industry. Steve Jobs subsequently announced on January 9, 2007, that Apple Computer would become Apple Inc. This name change confirmed for many commentators that Apple had made the shift from being a computer company to being an integrated digital consumer electronics company. Jobs said, "Apple's name change doesn't have any direct impact on the business, but it does accomplish the following—it signals to employees the company's long-term strategy, it clarifies the marketing message and it prods investors to compare Apple to consumer electronics firms rather than just computer makers." It also meant that Apple was now "much more diversified, so you don't compare it by peer group as much as by product line."[13]

In 2008, Apple expanded the iPhone to operate on AT&T's 3G network, and it introduced the iPod Touch, a portable media player and Wi-Fi Internet device that allowed users to purchase and download music directly from iTunes without a computer. Then, in July 2008, Apple opened the App Store. Users could now purchase applications written by third-party developers specifically for the iPhone and iPod Touch. These applications included games, prompting analysts to wonder whether Apple was now becoming a competitor in the gaming market.

Apple was becoming a diversified digital entertainment corporation (see Exhibit 4). Apple also had not abandoned its computing roots. Even with the growth of the iPod/iTunes and iPhone categories, computer sales, especially the portable category, continued to see substantial growth (see Exhibit 5).

Analysts had already believed Apple had "changed the rules of the game for three industries—PCs, consumer electronics, and music . . . and appears to have nothing to fear from major rivals."[14] Apple was now taking bites out of the competition on all fronts (see Exhibit 6).

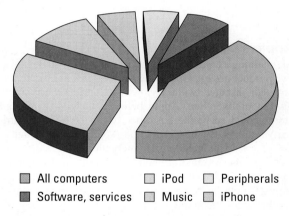

■ All computers   □ iPod   □ Peripherals
■ Software, services   □ Music   □ iPhone

Exhibit 4 **Apple Product Sales, 2008**

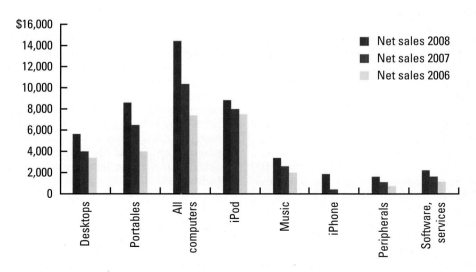

Exhibit 5 **Apple Product Sales, 2006–2008**

Exhibit 6 Apple's Product Lines and Major Competitors

Product Category	Apple Products	Major Competitors
Computers	iMac, Mac Pro, Mac Mini, MacBook, MacBook Pro, MacBook Air	HP, Dell, Toshiba in the laptop, Acer in the netbook form factor
Portable music/media players	iPod Shuffle, iPod Nano, iPod Classic, iPod Touch	Creative Zen, SanDisk Sansa, Archos, Microsoft Zune
Smartphones	iPhone	Nokia, RIM, Samsung, LG, Sony Ericsson, HTC
Music/media downloads	iTunes, the App Store	Amazon, MySpace
Handheld gaming devices	iPod Touch, iPhone	Nintendo, Sony
Software*	Safari Web browser, QuickTime	Microsoft IE, Mozilla Firefox, Google Chrome, Windows Media Player, RealNetworks
Home theater downloads	Apple TV	Possibly Tivo

*Includes only the software that is sold separately to use on either Windows or Mac computers.

Apple's Operations

Maintaining a competitive edge required more than innovative product design. Operational execution was also important. For instance, while trying to market its increasingly diverse product line, Apple believed that its own retail stores could serve the customer better than could third-party retailers. By the end of 2008, Apple had an average of 247 stores open, including 19 international locations, with average store revenue of about $29.9 million. In addition to the "Genius Bars" Apple had installed in its own retail stores, Apple had also invested in programs to enhance reseller sales, including the placement of Apple employees and knowledgeable contractors at selected third-party reseller locations, explaining that it "believes providing direct contact with its targeted customers is an efficient way to demonstrate the advantages of its . . . products over those of its competitors."[15]

In further operational matters, regarding a head-to-head competition against Dell in the computer market, for instance, Steve Jobs was quick to point out that market share wasn't everything. While Dell's perceived dominance might have been partly the result of its efficient supply chain management, Apple had outperformed Dell in inventory and other metrics since 2001.[16] In addition, Apple had the best margins, partly because of its simpler product line, leading to cheaper manufacturing costs.[17] In 2008, Apple beat Dell and HP (as well as Nokia, IBM, Samsung, and Sony Ericsson) and took the number-one spot on AMR Research's Supply Chain Top 25.[18]

Regarding suppliers of components for Apple's diverse products, Apple had entered into certain multiyear agreements with suppliers of key components, including microprocessors, NAND flash memory, dynamic random access memory (DRAM), and LCD displays. Some of these long-term supplier-agreement partners included

Hynix Semiconductor, Intel Corporation, Micron Technology, Samsung Electronics, and Toshiba Corporation. Also, in addition to using its own manufacturing facilities in Ireland, Apple had been outsourcing manufacturing and final assembly of iMacs, iPods, and iPhones to partners in Asia, paying close attention to scheduling and quality issues.

Supply chain and product design and manufacturing efficiencies were not the only measures of potential competitive superiority. Apple had also historically paid attention to research and development, increasing its R&D investment year after year. In 2008, Apple spent $1.1 billion on R&D, a 42 percent increase from the previous year and more than twice what was spent in 2005.[19] On the basis of 2007 numbers, among its current rivals, Apple's R&D investment was beaten only by Microsoft, Hewlett-Packard, and Google.[20]

Status of Apple's Business Units in 2008

The Apple Computer Business In the computer market, Apple had always refused to compete on price, relying instead on its reliability, design elegance, ease of use, and integrated features to win customers. Some analysts believed Apple had the opportunity to steal PC market share as long as its system was compatible, and no longer exclusively proprietary, and offered upgrades at a reasonable cost.[21] But the real opportunity for increased market share was the Intel-based iMac desktop and the MacBook/MacBook Pro portable, both using the Intel Core Duo processor. The only part of the computer system not designed and manufactured by Apple was this processor and the memory.

In 2008, Apple introduced its newest computer product, the MacBook Air, the "world's thinnest notebook."[22] Although the design was considered "revolutionary," the stripped-down product did not have an optical drive except

Exhibit 7 Domestic PC Market Share, Fourth Quarter 2008

Company	4Q08 Shipments (thousands of units)	4Q08 Market Share (%)	4Q07 Shipments (thousands of units)	4Q07 Market Share (%)	4Q08–4Q07 Growth (%)
Dell	4,465.8	28.6	5,344.6	30.8	−16.4
Hewlett-Packard	4,288.3	27.5	4,439.5	25.6	−3.4
Acer	2,373.9	15.2	1,527.3	8.8	55.4
Apple	1,255.0	8.0	1,159.3	6.7	8.3
Toshiba	1,002.7	6.5	900.0	5.2	12.0
Others	2,219.2	14.2	3,992.6	23.0	−44.0
Total	**15,609.8**	**100.0**	**17,363.3**	**100.0**	**−10.1**

Note: Data include desk-based PCs, mobile PCs (notebooks and netbooks), and X86 servers.

Source: Gartner, January 2009, as reported at *http://apple20.blogs.fortune.cnn.com/2009/01/16/despite-everything-mac-sales-grew-year-to-year*.

as a separate external purchase, had limited connectivity with only one USB port, and had a battery that was not user-replaceable. Even so, with its aluminum construction, it was perceived to be sturdy and much easier to carry than other full-size notebooks and therefore most appropriate for travelers in Wi-Fi hotspot areas.[23]

The continuing push to convert customers to the Macintosh computing products saw Apple sell 2,524,000 Mac computers, both desktops and laptops, worldwide during the first quarter of 2009, an increase of almost 9 percent over the same quarter in the previous year, in spite of the worldwide economic decline.[24] Sales of Apple computers in the United States did see a decline over the previous quarter, but not as much as the yearly domestic shipments of Dell (down 16.4 percent) and HP (down 3.4 percent).[25] According to market analysis done by Gartner, the Mac's domestic market share slipped from 9.5 to 8 percent in October, moving Apple from third to fourth place in Gartner's survey of PC vendor units shipped in 4Q08 (see Exhibit 7).

The Personal Digital Entertainment Devices: iPod

Although many analysts felt the MP3 player market was oversaturated, Apple introduced the iPod Touch in 2007, intending it to be "an iPhone without the phone," a portable media player and Wi-Fi Internet device without the AT&T phone bill.[26] The iPod Touch borrowed most of its features from the iPhone, including the finger-touch interface, but it remained mainly an iPod, with a larger viewing area for videos. Apple released the second-generation iPod Touch in 2008, with upgraded features that turned it into "more pocket PC than MP3 player"[27] and allowed it to download programs such as games from Apple's new App Store. Both the iPhone and the iPod Touch were positioned as "viable devices in the mobile games market" during fall 2008, subsequently producing a significant jump in application downloads on Christmas Day 2008.

Exhibit 8 Portable Music Player (MP3) Worldwide Market Share, 2008 (in percent)

Company	July 2008	1Q08	1Q07	2Q06
Apple (iPod)*	73.4	71	70	75
SanDisk (Sansa)	8.6	11	10	10
Microsoft (Zune)	2.6	4	3	—[†]
Other	15.4	—	—	Samsung: 2.5
				Sony: 2
Creative (Zen)	—[‡]	2	4	5

*As of September 2008, Apple reported over 160 million iPods sold; iTunes as the number-one distributor of music in any format in the U.S., with a catalog of 8.5 million songs, over 30,000 TV episodes, and over 2,500 films including 600 in high-definition video; and over 100 million applications downloaded from the App Store since its launch in July 2008.

[†]Released in 2006.

[‡]Included in other.

Source: NPD data, as reported at *www.manifest-tech.com/ce_gallery/portable_gallery_players.htm*.

Apple reported selling a record 22,727,000 iPod units during the first quarter of 2009, a growth of 3 percent over the same period in the previous year.[28] This contributed to Apple's extending its lead over rivals (see Exhibit 8).

Mobile Communication Devices: iPhone

In 2007, further competition came from the blurring of lines between the digital music player and other consumer electronic devices: The telecom players wanted to join the digital music market. While others may have seen the computer as central to the future of digital music, the telecom companies thought the mobile phone could become a center of this emerging world. Apple's entry, the new iPhone device, combined an Internet-enabled smartphone and video iPod. The iPhone allowed users to access all iPod content and play music and video content purchased from iTunes. Apple made an exclusive arrangement with AT&T's Cingular Wireless network to provide cellular service.

The iPhone debuted with a 4-GB model for $499 and an 8-GB model for $599, and estimates from component manufacturers suggested it would cost between $230 and $265 to make, yielding Apple's preferred gross margin of about 50 percent.[29] This would allow room for price adjustments based on component or customer demand. The smartphone market in 2007 was estimated at 10 percent of all mobile phone sales, or 100 million devices a year. Steve Jobs said he "would like to see the iPhone represent 1 percent of all mobile phone sales by the end of 2008."[30] This proved to be a conservative estimate.

In July 2008, Apple began selling iPhone 3G, the second-generation of the iPhone product. The 3G service upgrade accompanied expanded worldwide distribution, through carrier relationships in over 70 countries. Either because of the increased access or because of Apple's marketing push, 6.9 million iPhone 3Gs were sold in the first quarter of its availability, compared to "6.1 first-generation iPhone units sold in the prior five quarters combined."[31] As one analyst commented, "When Steve Jobs first introduced the iPhone in 2007, he pointed out that

the market for cell phones worldwide was far greater than the market for any other type of consumer electronic device."[32] Worldwide appeal for the iPhone was growing: The iPhone was launched in Saudi Arabia and the UAE in February 2009, through Mobily and Etisalat, and got 25,000 subscribers in the first few hours of its availability.[33] Now it appeared that Jobs was correct: He had forecast a 1 percent market share of the cell phone market in 2008 and had achieved 1.1 percent (see Exhibit 9).

Going into 2009, it appeared that the cell phone landscape was changing yet again, with smartphones becoming the device of choice for most manufacturers—smartphones with multiple features, including cameras. New cell phones with megapixel cameras debuted at Barcelona's 2009 Mobile World Congress from Sony Ericsson and Samsung: "What's behind the megapixel marathon? It's no secret that the iPhone's camera is one of its weakest points. Seems to me the competition is looking for vulnerabilities and has identified imaging capability as something they can deliver that the iPhone so far hasn't."[34] Along with Sony Ericsson and Samsung, other cell phone makers, LG and Taiwanese manufacturer High Tech Computers (HTC), offered new phones with touch screens in an attempt to compete with the iPhone.[35]

Part of the popularity of the iPhone during the 2008 holiday season was explained by analysts as being the result of the highly prolific output of third-party software developers, whose applications were available via Apple's App Store, where they could be downloaded to

Exhibit 9   Worldwide Market Share—Cell Phones, 2008

Manufacturer	Percent Market Share	Percent Increase over 2007	Comments
Nokia	38.6	1.8	2008 4th-quarter growth stalled.
Samsung	16.2	2.7	Strong 4th quarter; new products 1Q09.
LG	8.3	1.5	North America grew; new products 1Q09.
Sony Ericsson	8.0	(0.7)	2008 3d-quarter stalled; new products 1Q09.
Motorola	8.3	(5.1)	Nothing new in the pipeline.
Research in Motion	1.9	0.9	New products; good growth potential.
Kyocera	1.4	—	
Apple iPhone	1.1	0.8	First released in mid-2007; strong 4Q08.
HTC	1.1	—	New to market; new products 1Q09.
Sharp	1.0	—	
Other	14.1	—	Expect handset shipment contraction in 2009 to be down 5%–10%, due to worldwide economic conditions; smartphones may prosper.

Source: From ABIresearch, January 29, 2009, *www.abiresearch.com/press/1357-Enter+the+Year+of+the+Smartphone%3A+171+Million+and+Rising.*

the iPhone, either increasing its capability or allowing users to play games and otherwise entertain themselves. This prompted these analysts to wonder whether gaming companies such as Nintendo and Sony would have to pay attention to Apple as a competitor in the gaming market. The analysts quoted one iPhone customer who said he had sold his Sony PSP and might get rid of his Nintendo DS, since "the short amount of time I've had the iPhone, I've played more games on that than on my PSP and DS combined."[36] Regarding additional upgrades to the iPhone, or to other products in the smartphone group, CEO Steve Jobs agreed that Apple's iPhone business "had become too big to ignore" and that the iPhone had accounted for 39 percent of Apple's business in 2008.

However, analysts believed that the idea of Apple transforming the smartphone industry as it had the MP3 player market might require that Apple broaden its market even more. New offerings might include cell phone products that could compete with the new netbook PCs: a portable book reader to compete with Amazon's new Kindle reader, a portable movie player, and even a low-cost, entry-level phone—and all should provide services and add-ons through the App Store so that "average users can clearly see that there are enough high-quality services on offer to justify spending $30 per month [for a] mobile broadband subscription."[37]

Responding to a rumor of the possible release of a low-end $99 iPhone by summer 2009, Apple's acting-CEO Tim Cook said, "We're not going to play in the low-end voice phone business. That's not who we are, that's not why we're here. [Our] goal is not to lead unit sales, but to build the world's best phone."[38]

Digital Entertainment Solutions: Apple TV

In 2007, CEO Steve Jobs had considered the Apple TV product to be a "hobby" device, rather than a core business such as computers, music, or phones, saying, "A lot of people have tried and failed to make it a business."[39] In 2009, analysts were wondering whether the product was "at a crossroads," particularly since Apple sold more than three times the number of units it had sold in 2007.[40] Apple had not made any major changes to the hardware, but it had updated the software in 2008, allowing movie fans to rent DVD-quality or HD movies from the iTunes Store directly via their widescreen TV for $2.99 to $3.99 depending on the movie release dates. All audio or video purchases from iTunes downloaded to Apple TV could also be synced back to the user's computer, iPod, or iPhone.[41]

In 2009, Apple announced it had signed a $500 million five-year contract with South Korean LCD panel maker LG Display Co. Since Apple uses the LCD flat-panel display in the MacBook Pro laptop, this was likely a move to ensure manufacturing capacity to meet Apple's demand.[42] However, analysts wondered whether this deal, plus Apple's recent patent filings, also might help Apple develop DVR (digital video recorder) as well as iTunes functionality into a networked HDTV; they pointed out

that such a device could "replace most, if not all, of the other living room set top boxes."[43]

The Software Market

Although Apple had always created innovative hardware, software development was also an important goal, with implications for long-term sales growth. Software was increasingly becoming Apple's core strength.[44] The premier piece of Apple software was the operating system. OS X allowed Apple to develop software applications such as Final Cut Pro, a video-editing program for professionals' digital camcorders, and the simplified version for regular consumers, called iMovie. The iLife software provided five integrated applications allowing the computer to become a home studio: iMovie; iDVD, for recording photos, movies, and music onto DVDs; iPhoto, for touching up digital photos; Garage-Band, for making and mixing personally created music; and the iTunes digital music jukebox. Also available was iWork, containing a PowerPoint-type program called Keynote and a word-processor/page-layout program called Pages. Both iLife and iWork underwent major upgrades in 2009, further increasing their respective abilities to compete with Microsoft applications.

Apple's Web browser Safari was upgraded in 2009 to further compete with Windows Internet Explorer, Mozilla Firefox and the new entrant Chrome from Google. Apple announced, "Safari 4 was the world's fastest and most innovative browser,"[45] but analysts were quick to point out that Google's Chrome, which debuted six months earlier, was perhaps the first to take the browser interface in a new direction. One commentator called Chrome "a wake-up call for the Safari UI guys. . . . It's not that any particular feature of Chrome is so wonderful, or even that the sum of those features puts Safari back on its heels in the browser wars. It's the idea that someone other than Apple has taken such clear leadership in this area. Google Chrome makes Safari's user interface look conservative; it makes Apple look timid. And when it comes to innovation, overall daring counts for a lot more than individual successes or failures on the long-term graph."[46] Reviews of Apple's Safari upgrade noted, "Whether or not the individual features of Chrome inspired Apple, it's clear that Apple isn't going to let Google have the lead in browser innovation without a fight. And the more innovation that happens, the better it will be for users of Web browsers—which at this point is pretty much everybody with a computer!"[47]

Operating Systems

Further opportunity for software development came from the Mac's new ability to run Windows. This meant that software such as iWorks could now convert Microsoft Office files to run on a Mac. In the past, third-party software developers such as Adobe always had to make a sometimes risky decision to create Mac OS versions of their popular products. Now that the Macs were using Intel Core Duo chips, much more versatility and cross-platform compatibility made it more profitable to design and develop for the Mac market.

An additional opportunity for operating-system competition opened up in 2007 with the introduction of the "netbook" category of portable computers. Smaller and cheaper than a regular laptop or notebook, these machines didn't have the computing power to run the full version of either Windows XP or Mac OS X, so most manufacturers used the Linux operating system.[48] Microsoft announced in late 2008 that its new operating system, Windows 7, the replacement for Vista, would be capable of running on a netbook. However, according to CEO Steve Jobs, Apple did not have any plans for producing a netbook product.[49] Since the Apple operating system, designed to run only on Apple computers, was not available for independent sale, the new Windows operating system might gain traction in another computing category once again.

iTunes Arguably, Apple's most innovative software product was iTunes, a free downloadable software program for consumers running either newer Mac or Windows operating systems. It was bundled with all Mac computers and iPods and connected with the iTunes Music Store for purchase of digital music and movie files that could be played by iPods and the iPhone and by iTunes on PCs.

Although the volume was there, iTunes had not necessarily been a profitable venture. Out of the 99 cents Apple charged for a song, about 65 cents went to the music label; 25 cents went for distribution costs, including credit card charges, servers, and bandwidth; and the balance went to marketing, promotion, and the amortized cost of developing the iTunes software.[50]

Several competitors had tried to compete with the iTunes service. RealNetworks' Rhapsody subscription service, Yahoo MusicMatch, and AOL music downloads all had competed for the remaining market share, using the potentially buggy Microsoft Windows Media format.[51] Even though one commentator had said in 2004 that "ultimately someone will build a piece of software that matches iTunes,"[52] as of 2008 the only serious competition was from Amazon and My Space.

Making it potentially worse for Apple's competitors, music artists were overwhelmingly supportive of Apple, since, as Jobs reported, "almost every song and CD is made on a Mac, it's recorded on a Mac, it's mixed on a Mac. The artwork's done on a Mac. Almost every artist I've met has an iPod, and most of the music execs now have iPods. And one of the reasons Apple was able to do what we did was because we are perceived by the music industry as the most creative technology company."[53]

Steve Jobs had negotiated a deal with the Big Five record companies (Sony Music Entertainment, BMG, EMI, Universal, and Warner) to sell songs on iTunes. In 2007 Jobs asked the music labels to stop requiring that digital music distributors such as iTunes use copyright protection. By taking the lead in this, Apple could potentially come out ahead of the game again: If copyright protection was not required, iTunes songs could be played on non-iPod music players, and music purchased on other services could be played on the iPod. In what might have been perceived as a PR ploy, Jobs said that allowing music to be sold online without digital rights management (DRM) technology would "create a truly interoperable music marketplace— one that Apple would embrace 'wholeheartedly.'"[54]

In January 2009, Apple subsequently announced that "all four major music labels—Universal Music Group, Sony BMG, Warner Music Group, and EMI, along with thousands of independent labels, are now offering their music in iTunes Plus, Apple's DRM (digital rights management)-free format with higher-quality 256 kbps ACC encoding for audio quality virtually indistinguishable from the original recordings."[55] This made iTunes, with its 10 million DRM-free tracks, "the largest music store library on Earth."[56] In addition, iPhone 3G customers could download music directly onto their phone for the same price as downloading to their computer, the price having changed to include three price points, $0.69, $0.99, or $1.29, depending on what the music labels charged Apple. This tiered pricing was supposedly adopted in response to potential competition from other download sites such as Amazon and MySpace, although analysts pointed out that the music labels had previously demanded variable pricing and that Apple needed this cooperation from the content providers.[57] As of 2009, the iTunes Store had sold over 6 billion songs, and analysts projected that by 2012 it could "well account for a staggering 28 percent of *all* music sold worldwide."[58]

The App Store In March 2008, Apple announced that it was releasing the iPhone software development kit (SDK), allowing developers to create applications for the iPhone and iPod Touch and sell these third-party applications via the Apple App Store. The App Store was made available on version 7.7 of iTunes, and it was directly available from the iPhone and iPod Touch products. This opened the window for another group of Apple customers, the application developers, to collaborate with Apple. Developers could purchase the iPhone Developer Program from Apple for $99, create either free or commercial applications for the iPhone and iPod Touch, and then submit these applications to be sold in the App Store. Developers would be paid 70 percent of the download fee iPhone or iPod Touch customers paid to the App Store, and Apple would get 30 percent of the revenue. The applications ranged from simple audio files that were available for free (e.g., ringtones), to straightforward programs that sold for 99 cents (e.g., a program that turned the iPhone into a simple voice recorder), to full-featured applications that retailed for up to $69.99 (e.g., ForeFlight Mobile, which allowed pilots to get weather and airport information).

The App Store opened in July 2008, at the same time as the introduction of the iPhone 3G, and as of February 2009, over 15,000 programs had been offered for sale, creating 500 million downloads, and millions of dollars in revenue, collectively, for developers.[59] The success of this distribution channel for smartphone add-ons had Microsoft and other manufacturers, such as Nokia and

Blackberry maker Research in Motion, rushing to open their own mobile software stores, hoping to follow Apple's "runaway success"[60] in yet another category.

The Future of Apple Although Steve Jobs was credited with Apple's ability to innovate and to appeal especially to a certain type of consumer (Jobs estimated Apple's market share in the creative-professional marketplace as over 50 percent),[61] Jobs himself credited his people:

> We hire people who want to make the best things in the world . . . our primary goal is to make the world's best PCs—not to be the biggest or the richest. We have a second goal, which is to always make a profit—both to make some money but also so we can keep making those great products. . . . [regarding the systemization of innovation] the system is that there is no system. That doesn't mean we don't have process. Apple is a very disciplined company, and we have great processes. But that's not what it's about. Process makes you more efficient . . . but innovation . . . comes from saying no to 1,000 things to make sure we don't get on the wrong track or try to do too much. We're always thinking about new markets we could enter, but it's only by saying no that you can concentrate on the things that are really important.[62]

Given Steve Jobs's announced medical leave, the media was particularly interested in the rest of Apple's management team. In late 2008, Tony Fadell, Apple's senior vice president of the iPod Division, and his wife Danielle Lambert, vice president of Human Resources, had announced that they were reducing their roles within the company to devote more time to their young family.[63] Sometimes credited as the "father of the iPod" and part of the team involved in the development of the iPhone,[64] Fadell would remain with the company as an adviser to the CEO. Fadell would be replaced by Mark Papermaster, in the position of senior vice president of Devices Hardware Engineering. Papermaster would lead Apple's iPod and iPhone hardware engineering teams and would report directly to Steve Jobs. Papermaster was previously a vice president at IBM and had played a major role in IBM's PowerPC chip design. This role led IBM to hold up Papermaster's move to Apple for several months while it worked out a noncompete agreement.[65]

With the exception of Fadell's reduced role, Apple's upper management had been stable since 1999. This stability among the nine executive officers had relieved some analysts as they contemplated what might happen to Apple if Steve Jobs did not return from his medical leave of absence.[66] In fact, COO Tim Cook, designated to take over Apple operations during Jobs's absence, had run Apple operations in 2004 while Jobs recovered from his pancreatic cancer. Since his arrival in 1998, Cook had been called the "genius behind Steve" because of his handling of the day-to-day business at Apple.[67]

Most analysts had no doubt that Apple had many top-notch executives, but there was no evidence of a clear succession plan, nor was there a history of nurturing top performers to "broaden their skills and groom them for bigger jobs."[68] This was a problem, as Apple had gotten larger over time, with multiple product lines, critical supplier alliances, diverse distribution outlets, and an increasingly global market. However, while agreeing that it would be very difficult to replace Steve Jobs's visionary product design and marketing skills, analysts pointed out that Jobs had been "on a creative tear" since the introduction of the iPod in 2001—and since Apple had traditionally maintained a "top-secret pipeline of products" ready to roll out in "the next few years," it was possible that "were Jobs no longer around, Apple could live off those products for some time."[69]

During the 2009 first-quarter conference call, Apple presenter and COO Tim Cook was asked whether he felt he was a "de facto successor" in the event Steve Jobs did not return from his medical leave in July. Cook responded, "There is an extraordinary breadth and depth and tenure to Apple's executive team . . . they manage 35,000 employees, all of whom are wicked smart. . . . I strongly believe that Apple is doing the best work in its history."[70] The rest of the executive management team agreed. However, at the time, Steve Jobs was still CEO of the company.

Editor's Note: Since this case was written, Steve Jobs passed away in October 2011.

Endnotes

1. "Apple reports fourth quarter results," October 21, 2008, from *www.apple.com/pr/library/2008/10/21 results.html*.
2. "Apple reports first quarter results," January 21, 2009, from *www.apple.com/pr/library/2009/01/21results.html*.
3. "Letter from Apple CEO Steve Jobs," January 5, 2009, from *www.apple.com/pr/library/2009/01/05sjletter.html*
4. "Apple Media Advisory," January 14, 2009, from *www.apple.com/pr/library/2009/01/14advisory.html*
5. A. Hesseldahl, "Apple's impressive quarterly numbers," *BusinessWeek,* January 22, 2009, from *www.businessweek.com/technology/content/jan2009/tc20090121_101972.htm?link_position=link5*.
6. G. Keizer, "Apple can still thrive, sans Job," *Computerworld,* January 15, 2009, from *www.pcworld.com/article/157735/jobs.html?loomia_ow=t0:a16:g12:r2:c0.240847:b21196707*.
7. See *www.businessweek.com/magazine/content/08_17/b4081062882948.htm*.
8. Apple was the first firm to have commercial success selling GUI systems, but Xerox developed the first systems in 1973. Xerox PARC researchers built a single-user computer called the Alto that featured a bit-mapped display and a mouse and the world's first what-you-see-is-what-you-get (WYSIWYG) editor. From *www.parc.xerox.com/about/history/default.html*.
9. From the Apple Inc. 2008 Annual Report, 10-K filing, available at *www.apple.com/investor*.
10. January 24, 2009, is the 25th anniversary of the Macintosh, unveiled by Apple in the "Big Brother" Super

Bowl ad in 1984. Watch via YouTube: *www.youtube.com/watch?v=OYecfV3ubP8*. See also the 1983 Apple keynote speech by a young Steve Jobs, introducing this ad: *www.youtube.com/watch?v=lSiQA6KKyJo*.

11. See D. A. Mank and H. E. Nystrom, "The relationship between R&D spending and shareholder returns in the computer industry," *Engineering Management Society, Proceedings of the 2000 IEEE,* 2000, pp. 501–504.

12. "Ultra-portable MP3 music player puts 1,000 songs in your pocket," October 23, 2001, from *www.apple.com/pr/library/2001/oct/23ipod.html*.

13. "What's in a name? For Apple, a focus on the digital living room," *Knowledge@Wharton,* January 24, 2007, from *http://knowledge.wharton.upenn.edu/article.cfm?articleid=1641*.

14. B. Schlender, "How big can Apple get?" *Fortune,* February 21, 2005, from *http://money.cnn.com/magazines/fortune/-fortune_archive/2005/02/21/8251769/index.htm*.

15. From the Apple Inc. 2008 Annual Report, 10-K filing, available at */www.apple.com/investor*.

16. P. Burrows, "The seed of Apple's innovation," *BusinessWeek Online,* October 12, 2004, from *www.businessweek.com/bwdaily/dnflash/oct2004/nf20041012_4018_db083.htm?chan=search*.

17. F. Fox, "Mac Pro beats HP and Dell at their own game: Price," *lowendmac.com,* May 16, 2008, from *http://lowendmac.com/ed/fox/08ff/mac-pro-vs-dell-hp.html*.

18. "AMR Research Supply Chain Top 25, 2008," from *www.amrresearch.com/supplychaintop25*.

19. P. McLean, "Apple outlines shift in strategy, rise in R&D spending, more," *AppleInsider,* November 5, 2008, from *www.appleinsider.com/articles/08/11/05/apple_outlines_shift_in_strategy_rise_in_rd_spending_more*.

20. R. Hertzberg, "Top 50 technology R&D spenders," *CIO Zone,* 2008, from *www.ciozone.com/index.php/Editorial-Research/Top-50-Technology-R&D-Spenders/50-Biggest-R.html*.

21. "Growing market share—branding in the computer industry 2006," from *www.stealingshare.com/content/1137644625875.htm*.

22. "Apple introduces MacBook Air—the world's thinnest notebook," January 15, 2008, from *www.apple.com/pr/library/2008/01/15mbair.html*.

23. "Apple MacBook Air (80GB)," *CNET Review,* January 25, 2008, from *http://reviews.cnet.com/laptops/apple-macbook-air-80gb/4505-3121_7-32818756.html*.

24. "Apple reports first-quarter results," January 21, 2009, from *www.apple.com/pr/library/2009/01/21results.html*.

25. P. Elmer-DeWitt, "Despite everything, Mac sales grew year-to-year," *Apple 2.0—Blogs,* January 16, 2009, from *http://apple20.blogs.fortune.cnn.com/2009/01/16/despite-everything-mac-sales-grew-year-to-year*.

26. P. Elmer-DeWitt, "Apple challenges Sony and Nintendo," *Apple 2.0—Blogs,* December 13, 2008, from *http://apple20.blogs.fortune.cnn.com/2008/12/13/apple-challenges-sony-and-nintendo*.

27. D. Bell, "Apple iPod Touch (second generation, 16GB)," *CNET Review,* September 11, 2008, from *http://reviews.cnet.com/portable-video-players-pvps/apple-ipod-touch-second/4505-6499_7-33248627.html?tag=mncol;txt*.

28. "Apple reports first-quarter results," January 21, 2009, from *www.apple.com/pr/library/2009/01/21results.html*.

29. A. Hesseldahl, "What the iPhone will cost to make," *BusinessWeek Online,* January 18, 2007, from *www.businessweek.com/technology/content/jan2007/tc20070118_961148.htm*.

30. E. Zemen, "Ballmer says iPhone won't succeed. Has Windows mobile?" *Information Week,* May 1, 2007, from *www.informationweek.com/blog/main/archives/2007/05/ballmer_says_ip.html*.

31. "Apple reports fourth-quarter results," October 21, 2008, from *www.apple.com/pr/library/2008/10/21results.html*.

32. "Phone reaches 1% market share in worldwide cellphone market," *Edible Apple,* February 1, 2009, from *www.edibleapple.com/iphone-reaches-1-market-share-in-worldwide-cellphone-market*.

33. A. Sambridge, "25,000 Saudi iPhone subscribers within hours of launch," *ArabianBusiness.com,* February 23, 2009, from *www.arabianbusiness.com/547625-25000-saudi-iphone-subscribers-within-hours-of-launch*.

34. Y. Arar, "Sony Ericsson, Samsung duke it out for mega-pixel supremacy," *PC World,* February 15, 2009, from *www.pcworld.com/article/159579/article.html?tk=nl_cxanws*.

35. Y. Arar, "Next-gen cell phone stars shine in Barcelona," *PC World,* February 17, 2009, from *www.pcworld.com/article/159659-6/nextgen_cell_phone_stars_shine_in_barcelona.html*.

36. N. Wingfield and C. Lawton, "Apple's iPhone faces off with the game champs," *Wall Street Journal: Personal Technology,* November 12, 2008, from *http://online.wsj.com/article/SB122644912858819085.html*.

37. Ibid.

38. A. Kim, "Analyst speculation on $99 iPhone and higher resolution iPhone 3G," *MacRumors.com,* February 11, 2009, from *www.macrumors.com/2009/02/11/analyst-speculation-on-99-iphone-and-higher-resolution-iphone-3g*.

39. R. Block, "Steve Jobs live from D 2007," *engadget,* May 30, 2007, from *www.engadget.com/2007/05/30/steve-jobs-live-from-d-2007*.

40. M. G. Siegler, "Hobby turning serious? Apple TV gets a survey, Valentine's promotion," *VentureBeat DigitalMedia,* February 9, 2009, from *http://venturebeat.com/2009/02/09/hobby-turning-serious-apple-tv-gets-a-survey-valentines-promotion*.

41. "Apple introduces new Apple TV software & lowers price to $229," January 15, 2008, from *www.apple.com/pr/library/2008/01/15appletv.html*

42. C. Foresman, "LG Display deal could mean impending Cinema Display refresh," *ars technica,* January 12, 2009, from *http://arstechnica.com/apple/news/2009/01/lg-display-deal-could-mean-impending-cinema-display-refresh.ars*.

43. D. Chartier, "Rumors return of Apple's living room device to rule them all," *ars technica,* February 5, 2009, from *http://arstechnica.com/apple/news/2009/02/rumors-return-of-apples-living-room-device-to-rule-them-all.ars*.

44. Schlender, "How big can Apple get?"

45. "Apple Announces Safari 4—the world's fastest and most innovative browser," February 24, 2009, from *www.apple.com/pr/library/2009/02/24safari.html*.

46. J. Siracusa, "Straight out of Compton: Google Chrome as a paragon of ambition, if not necessarily execution," *ars technica,* September 2, 2008, from *http://arstechnica.com/staff/fatbits/2008/09/straight-out-of-compton.ars.*

47. J. Snell, "Google Chrome: A wake-up call for Safari," *PC World,* February 24, 2009, from *www.pcworld.com/businesscenter/article/160129/google_chrome_a_wakeup_call_for_safari.html?loomia_ow=t0:a16:g12:r4:c0.334067:b22235984.*

48. M. Horowitz, "What is a netbook computer?" *CNET News,* October 12, 2008, from *http://news.cnet.com/what-is-a-netbook-computer.*

49. E. Ogg, "Three things Apple won't do," *CNET News,* October 15, 2008, from *http://news.cnet.com/8301-13579_3-10066317-37.html.*

50. S. Cherry, "Selling music for a song," *Spectrum Online,* December 2004, from *www.spectrum.ieee.org/dec04/3857.*

51. D. Leonard, "The player," *Fortune,* March 8, 2006, from *http://money.cnn.com/magazines/fortune/fortune_archive/2006/03/20/8371750/index.htm.*

52. A. Salkever, "It's time for an iPod IPO," *BusinessWeek,* May 5, 2004, from *www.businessweek.com/technology/content/may2004/tc2004055_8689_tc056.htm.*

53. J. Goodell, "Steve Jobs: The *Rolling Stone* interview," *Rolling Stone,* December 3, 2003, from *www.rollingstone.com/news/story/5939600/steve_jobs_the_rolling_stone_interview.*

54. A. Hesseldahl, "Steve Jobs' music manifesto," *Business-Week Online,* February 7, 2007, from *www.businessweek.com/technology/content/feb2007/tc20070206_576721.htm?chan=search,*

55. "Changes coming to the iTunes Store," January 6, 2009, from *www.apple.com/pr/library/2009/01/06itunes.html.*

56. Ibid.

57. C. Breen, "Variable iTunes pricing and the future," *Macworld,* January 13, 2009, from *www.macworld.com/article/138173/itunesvariablepricing.html?loomia_ow=t0:a16:g2:r6:c0.0465853:b20601077.*

58. E. Van Buskirk, "iTunes Store may capture one-quarter of worldwide music by 2012," *Wired.com,* April 27, 2008, from *www.wired.com/entertainment/music/news/2008/04/itunes_birthday.*

59. R. Kim, "Apple App Store developers look to next level," *SFGate.com,* February 9, 2009, from */www.sfgate.com/cgi-bin/article.cgi?f=/c/a/2009/02/08/BU8U15ADEB.DTL.*

60. Reuters, 2009. "Microsoft, Nokia gun for Apple's App Store," *internetnews.com,* February 17, 2009, from *www.internetnews.com/breakingnews/article.php/3803411.*

61. Goodell, "Steve Jobs: The *Rolling Stone* interview."

62. Burrows, "The seed of Apple's innovation."

63. "Mark Papermaster joins Apple as senior vice president of Devices Hardware Engineering," November 4, 2008, in "Apple reports first quarter results," January 21, 2009, from *www.apple.com/pr/library/2009/01/21results.html.*

64. A. Kim, "Tony Fadell ('father of the iPod') leaves Apple," *MacRumors.com,* November 4, 2008, from *www.macrumors.com/2008/11/04/tony-fadell-father-of-ipod-leaves-apple.*

65. S. Weintraub, "Why did Apple hire away IBM's Mark Papermaster?" *Computerworld Blogs,* November 1, 2008, from *http://blogs.computerworld.com/why_did_apple_hire_away_ibms_mark_papermaster.*

66. G. Keizer, "Apple can still thrive, sans Jobs," *PCWorld,* January 15, 2009, from *www.pcworld.com/article/157735/jobs.html?loomia_ow=t0:a16:g12:r2:c0.240847:b21196707.*

67. A. Lashinsky, "The genius behind Steve," *Fortune,* November 10, 2008, from *http://money.cnn.com/2008/11/09/technology/cook_apple.fortune/index.htm?postversion=2008111010.*

68. P. Burrows, "What Fadell's departure means for Apple," *BusinessWeek,* November 5, 2008, from *www.businessweek.com/technology/content/nov2008/tc2008115_625046.htm?chan=technology_technology+index+page_computers.*

69. Lashinsky, "The genius behind Steve."

70. Hesseldahl, "Apple's impressive quarterly numbers."

Case 7   Gazprom: The Evolution of a Giant in the Global Oil and Gas Industry*

Today Gazprom is a modern, open, dynamic company. In just the last five years, the amount of tax it pays has more than doubled, and it accounts for nearly 20 percent of the country's budget. Gazprom's capitalisation has reached a new historic high, surpassing the 350 billion dollar mark. It is one of the largest companies in the world.

Obviously, the success of the company has been in large part due to intelligent and flexible policies, not only Gazprom's but also those of the government and the state. Such close cooperation is in full accord with the current trends in the global oil and gas industry. Moreover, it provides the company, the industry, and the entire economy with additional opportunities for long-term development. Given Gazprom's strategic importance for Russia, the state will continue to keep the situation under its direct control.

–Vladimir Putin, then-president of Russia, Speech Commemorating 15th Anniversary of Gazprom, *www.gazprom.ru/eng/articles/article27020.shtml.*

Alexei Miller had been a key architect in the emergence of Gazprom as a global player. In seven short years, he had been largely responsible for engineering the global rise of the Russian gas superpower that was sure to dominate the industry for decades to come. Gazprom had been launched as a joint stock company in 1993 when the Russian government decided to spin off the administrative arm that was managing gas assets in the country. By early 2008, the company had increased gas reserves to some 4.3 tcm (trillion cubic meters), the largest in the world, had about 22,000 km of gas trunk lines reaching out into Eastern and Central Europe, as well as points along the Caspian Sea, and a market capitalization that had grown 200-fold since inception. Western Europe was increasingly dependent on gas supplied by Gazprom, as were other former Soviet Union countries such as Ukraine and Belarus. It was the largest employer in Russia, the largest exporter, and accounted for roughly 20 percent of the country's tax base—a leviathan by all accounts. Despite Gazprom's dominant position, especially at a time when the world's energy resources were becoming scarce, there were some critical challenges that cast a long shadow over its future. (See Appendix 1 for key statistics on Gazprom, and Appendix 2 for comparisons with competitors.)

The company had been unable to increase its production significantly despite its command over vast reserves.

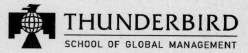

THUNDERBIRD
SCHOOL OF GLOBAL MANAGEMENT

Many Russian analysts believed that without substantial investments in new projects, Gazprom could soon find itself unable to honor its mandatory commitments even to the domestic market. However, many of Gazprom's reserves were located in very challenging environments such as the Arctic shelf and Siberia. These projects required fairly sophisticated levels of technical expertise and huge amounts of capital. In the recent past, the company had, surprisingly, spent much of its capital budget on large acquisitions of new reserves and forays into unrelated sectors of the economy, such as media and banking. It remained to be seen whether the company would have the skills and resources to execute these crucial projects.

In the global arena, Gazprom was still dependent on western European sales for much of its lucrative overseas revenues. It realized roughly five to ten times the price for its gas in Western Europe compared to its domestic market. However, in the next decade, Europe seemed likely to welcome other suppliers from North Africa, Central Asia, and the Middle East. The competition was also bound to intensify with rapid changes wrought by liquified natural gas (LNG) technology, a technically complex field where Gazprom did not have much experience. These nettlesome issues were sure to undermine the unassailable image that Gazprom was projecting.

The Genesis of Gazprom

Gazprom is a mutant. People need to be aware of what kind of animal it is. It doesn't follow business logic or political logic. It's a mixture of a business empire and a presidential administration.

–Russian Analyst Pavel Baev, "How Gazprom Turned Up the Heat on the West," *The Independent,* September 3, 2007.

Gazprom traced its origins to the USSR Ministry of Oil and Gas Industry. In 1989, the Soviet government, under Victor Chernomyrdin, reorganized this administrative arm and named it Gazprom. In 1993, Gazprom was given further autonomy and constituted as a joint stock company by the Boris Yeltsin government.

Russia had chosen to adopt completely different approaches to its assets in the oil sector and gas sector. While it had encouraged foreign investors to participate in the privatization of oil assets, no such invitation was extended with respect to gas assets. The privatization of oil occurred at a particularly trying economic period for Russia and seemed to be a quick way to overcome some of the financial distress. At the end of this process, Russia was left with effective control over the main arterial pipelines that were used to export oil, but the base assets themselves had been sold to Russian and foreign interests.

This process allowed those close to the Kremlin to make enormous profits. Many Russian oligarchs, such as Oleg Deripaska, Vladimir Potanin, Roman Abramovich, Mikhail Fridman, and others, built huge empires almost overnight.

In contrast, when it came time to set forth a strategy for gas assets, Russia retained effective control over vast reserves by using Gazprom as the entity responsible for the majority of the country's gas assets. The company was listed on European and U.S. stock exchanges via GDRs (Global Depository Receipts) and ADRs (American Depository Receipts) in 1996. However, the Russian government always held significant control in the company, either financially or politically, alongside private and institutional investors. The chairman of the board had traditionally been a government appointee with management control vested in the hands of a handpicked technocrat. For example, Victor Zubkov, the current chairman of Gazprom, was originally the prime minister of Russia under Vladimir Putin. He relinquished his post to make way for Putin when Putin's term of office as president of Russia expired. Dmitri Medvedev, who was elected to succeed Putin as president, was the previous chairman of Gazprom. The nexus between the government and Gazprom had been a source of some advantage for the company both at home and abroad.

Gazprom had managed to marshal very significant land tracts all across Russia bearing rich deposits of gas, and government patronage surely helped it along the way. Combined with a far-reaching network of gas transportation pipelines, Gazprom evolved to become the largest and most widely known Russian company and its most widely known globally. It had the rather unique distinction of being perhaps the only gas company in the world that was permitted to maintain its own standing army, ostensibly for defending its vast reserves and production assets.[1] It employed more than 430,000 people, making it the country's largest single employer in the industrial sector. Representing 20 percent of tax inflows into the Russian exchequer, it was also no doubt one of the Russian government's most favored companies.[2] Over the years, Gazprom had diversified into a host of related and unrelated areas, both of its own volition and also at the prodding of the Russian government. This unwieldy portfolio included significant assets in AB Gazprombank, a significant power in domestic banking; NPF Gazfund, Russia's biggest nongovernmental pension fund; insurance company Sogaz; and a media giant, Gazprom Media.[3]

Organized along global functional lines, by 2008 Gazprom had moved from a geographic approach to managing its assets to a more functional approach. This structure, it was believed, offered the potential for leveraging knowledge assets, especially in the areas of prospecting and development. It also offered the prospect of leveraging some scale economies. Gazprom had developed a two-stage plan to reorganize the company's seven subsidiaries, spread over 11 geographic regions, into six business divisions overseeing production, maintenance, and transportation.

Starting with a stronghold in gas, Gazprom had expanded to other areas within the realm of energy. In 2005, it acquired most of Sibneft, the country's fifth largest oil company, in a buyout that was then the biggest ever in Russian history. Gazprom also had a 10 percent interest in RAO UES, Russia's largest electricity provider, and 25 percent of Mosenergo, Moscow's utility services company. These holdings cemented Gazprom's position as the leading energy company in the country. It was this dominant position combined with opaque relationships with the power brokers in the Kremlin that worried competitors and customers both within and outside Russia. (Appendix 3 shows the holdings portfolio of Gazprom.)

The Domestic Market for Gas in Russia

Price controls and government supply mandates were two of the most crucial features that had come to characterize the market for energy in Russia. Although Russia was adopting a more modern approach to its enterprises by encouraging their globalization, allowing their listing on foreign exchanges, and helping them forge alliances and joint ventures with western firms, it still had to contend with its legacy under communism when collective good outweighed all else. In the energy sector, this translated into crippling controls on pricing. For example, Gazprom was able to earn only about 20 percent of the revenues in its home market of what it could earn in foreign markets. Russian law mandated that Gazprom sell gas domestically at a controlled price, about $50/thousand cubic meters (including taxes and excise duties), although the government, despite widespread discontent, was committed to raising the floor prices. The Russian government had committed to wholesale deregulation of gas prices by 2011 when Gazprom would be permitted to charge market-based prices to its industrial customers. However, prices for domestic consumers, who constituted 15.7 percent of Gazprom's sales in 2007, were not expected to be deregulated.

Domestic consumption in Russia was increasing significantly at a time when production was declining in three of Gazprom's biggest fields. The West Siberian fields of Urengoy, Yamburg, and Medvezhye had all fallen close to 50 percent below their original production levels. To compensate for these aging fields, Gazprom had set forth a plan to accelerate development of many smaller fields, but it was believed that even with these new fields coming online, there would still be a supply shortfall. Domestic consumption growth was partly attributed to the overall growth of the economy itself. This growth pressure was also accentuated by some of the realities of the local gas distribution system. For example, most buildings designed during the Soviet era did not have the necessary infrastructure to monitor gas usage. Individual meters for customers were unheard of and retrofits almost impossible. Thus, customers did not know how much gas they were using, making it impossible to institute any energy savings plans. To complicate matters further, it was even difficult to get a clear idea of how much they were paying for gas on an individual basis. Payments were possible in a wide range of options from cash to barter arrangements.[4] It was widely believed that Russia was the only country in the world where gas was cheaper than coal, making it difficult to rein in consumption. In keeping with national plans for both rural and urban development, more and more parts of the country were coming under the gas infrastructure. Roughly 62 percent of the homes in Russia had begun to use gas, a 20 percent increase since 1993 when Gazprom was privatized. This trend was expected to continue with the government's ambitious plan to bring the eastern regions of the country under a gas infrastructure.

Gazprom's Gas Fields—The Crown Jewels

Gazprom controlled the vast majority of Russia's gas resources, a pre-eminent position considering the fact that Russia was also the single largest holder of gas reserves worldwide. Many of the reserves were located in the challenging Siberian regions of the country that were characterized by very short periods that allowed for exploration, followed by long periods of harsh winter conditions. The largest remaining untapped fields were in the Yamal-Nenets region, onshore as well as offshore. These fields included Shtokman and Bovanenkov, both of which were considered gas giants. Much of the production, about 70 percent of Gazprom's total output, was occurring in the Urengoy, Yamburg, and Medvezhye fields, all of which had seen brighter days with respect to yields.

In the near term, Gazprom's four largest fields were expected to suffer production declines of around 50.4 bcm/y.[5] Although there were new fields awaiting investments for commercialization, Gazprom had competing priorities. The last field to come online was the huge Zapolyarnoe field with a yield of about 100 bcm/y. The Yuzhno-Russkoye field was also brought online in late

December of 2007. A joint venture with BASF, this field was expected to reach its designed production capacity of 25 bcm by 2011. Despite these new additions, the amount of new gas being brought online was believed to be incapable of stemming Gazprom's production declines. It is worth noting that prior to the Zapolyarnoe and Yuzhno fields coming online, the last previous addition to the capacity had occurred in 1991.

In addition to the new fields, there were three more that had come under Gazprom's sphere of influence. At the behest of the Russian government, Gazprom had obtained a controlling interest in the Sakhalin II project, developed by Shell and its consortium of Japanese partners in 2007. One of the largest of its kind in the world, this project was expected to yield 643 bcm of gas and 173.4 million tons of oil and condensate. The project was in advanced stages of commissioning when Gazprom bought a controlling interest for $7.45 billion. (Appendix 4 provides a brief history of Sakhalin II and the assumption of control by Gazprom.)

The second major field awaiting development was the massive Shtokman field in the Barents Sea. Gazprom had originally intended to use a consortium of contractors to develop the field instead of partnering with IOCs, who were clamoring for the opportunity. Subsequently, a partnership deal was struck between Gazprom, Total of France, and StatoilHydro of Norway. In a departure from the standard practice of offering the IOC partners an equity stake in the field, Gazprom constituted a wholly owned subsidiary that would hold the lease and title to Shtokman. Total and StatoilHydro would function as contractors to the company and own 25 percent and 24 percent, respectively, of the company's equity, albeit one step removed from the title holder.

The third major field that had emerged was Kovykta, originally discovered in 1987. BP and its partner had held it for a considerable period of time. Alleging production delays at the field, BP and its partner, TNK, were

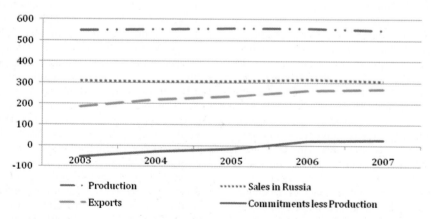

Exhibit 1 Gazprom's Supply v. Sales (data in billion cubic meters—bcm)

Source: Gazprom

sidelined to make way for Gazprom to take it over. TNK-BP agreed to sell the field to Gazprom in 2007 for between $700–$900 million. Analysts had estimated the value of the property at $3 billion, making the deal a very good one for Gazprom. Kovykta was thought to contain 2 tcm of gas, making it one of the largest fields in the world. However, as of October 2008, the transaction had not been completed. Given the very long-term development horizon and the cost involved, Gazprom had even observed that the property was "worthless."[6]

A confluence of likely scenarios included spiraling domestic demand, a decline in domestic production, ever-increasing costs to bring new capacity on stream, and an increase in prices demanded by FSU (Former Soviet Union) suppliers that fell within the Gazprom sphere of influence. In assuaging some of the fears expressed by foreign buyers in Western Europe, Alexei Miller had observed, "Our international business ties and our joint projects have turned Gazprom into a global company. We will rigorously abide by all of our long-term contract obligations. The size of our reserves permits us to confidently state that Gazprom is able to meet any solvent consumers' demand for gas, in domestic and foreign markets alike."[7]

The Power of the Pipeline

There was perhaps no bigger asset that Gazprom inherited at its creation than the network of pipelines to transport gas. Called the Unified Gas Supply System of Russia (UGSS), the network was the largest in the world, built to withstand challenging environments. It spanned 157,000 km (97,500 miles), enough to circle the world more than 24 times. Although it had achieved a throughput of 717 bcm by 2007,

it was already far below the capacity needed. Of this capacity, roughly 22 percent was used to carry gas produced by independent producers, both within and outside Russia—for example, from fields in Central Asia. This network provided Gazprom significant power to dictate the strategy of many independent producers, both local and foreign. Exhibit 3 shows a map of Gazprom's UGSS network.

In the face of rocketing demand and declining gas yields, Gazprom had resorted to importing gas from friendly FSU countries, such as Turkmenistan. While some of the domestic oil producers did indeed have the ability to produce gas from their operations, there was little incentive for them to do so since Gazprom virtually controlled the entire domestic transmission system. The company had been very careful in allowing transmission from other producers, sometimes claiming that specifications of their production were not within the tolerances allowed by its network or that no spare capacity was available. However, it did stand to benefit significantly by tapping other independent producers to transport gas to locations where it could make a trading gain. Most independent producers had to sell to Gazprom at wellhead prices that were below even domestic prices. For example, Lukoil was selling gas under long-term contract from its Yamal-Nenets field to Gazprom at $22 per thousand cubic meters, when Gazprom itself was charging more than $36 even in nearby domestic markets. This also had the important benefit of strengthening its supply position by augmenting its own production and making it even more powerful.

The UGSS infrastructure was also a tool of political influence used by the Russian government. This was illustrated most notably in 2006 when Gazprom decided to

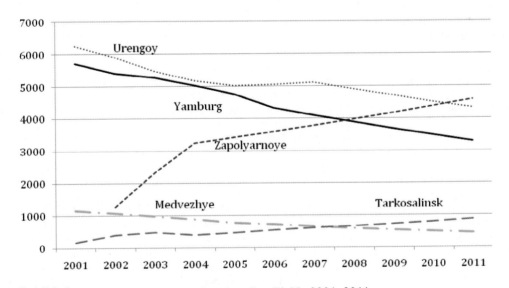

Exhibit 2 Production in Major Russian Gas Fields 2001–2011
Source: "Russia," *Country Analysis Brief*, Energy Information Administration, 2008. 2008–2011 are estimates.

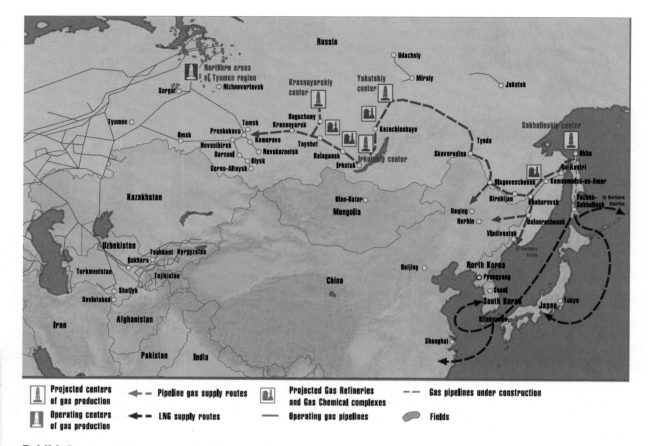

Exhibit 3 The Unified Gas Supply System of Russia

Source: Gazprom.

shut off gas supplies to Ukraine. The shutdown was ostensibly meant to force Ukraine to settle its bills for the gas it had already received, and also to enforce a higher price for future supplies. Russia had always provided subsidized gas to the FSU republics, but the cost of such a subsidy had risen significantly. The closure of the pipeline coincided with the Orange Revolution in Ukraine when the newly elected democratic government there started moving closer to Western powers. Thus, it was unclear whether political priorities superseded business interests, or vice versa. The effects of this closure continued to linger in the EU countries that were importing Russian gas. Many of these countries were aggressively pursuing alternatives so that they could reduce their dependence on Gazprom supplies.[8] (Appendix 5 provides data on the proportion of market shares controlled by Gazprom in Europe.)

By 2008, there were many serious questions about the continued viability of the transmission network. First, there was the issue of increasing demand on the one hand, and the pipeline capacity bottleneck on the other. It was estimated that by 2020 the network would need additional capacity of 170 bcm, an increase of roughly 24 percent over its installed capacity as of 2008. Second, it was believed that much of the UGSS infrastructure had to be significantly upgraded. It was reported that roughly 60 percent of the pipelines were more than 20 years old,[9] and about 14 percent were being operated well beyond their expected life.[10] Upgrading these assets required very significant investment—around $2 billion annually. Gazprom was in the process of strengthening the network, although most of its focus was on international transmission. There was feverish activity to build new trunk lines that would enable Gazprom to reach deeper into Europe and ports along the Caspian Sea to tap into export markets.

The Foray into the Oil Business

The purchase of Sibneft in 2005 was Gazprom's most significant oil investment. While some, including Dmitri Medvedev, the current president of Russia, then chairman of Gazprom, presented the Sibneft acquisition as a fairly common one that occurred in all free markets globally, others believed that there was much more to it. This was seen as a vital piece of Russia's strategy to bring back oil resources that had been privatized. Rosneft, the Russian oil giant, had already acquired Yukos, originally one of Russia's leading oil producers. Yukos had been decimated by a tax charge that many believed was payback for Yukos CEO Mikhail Khodorkhovsky's political ambitions that crossed Putin's path. Thus, the acquisition of Sibneft by Gazprom, a friendly ally of the government, was considered a good step to effectively rein in a significant part of Russia's oil assets.

Describing the Sibneft acquisition, Russian Natural Resources Minister Yuri Trutnev said, "On the one hand, this makes Gazprom the world's largest energy company, which positively influences the investment attractiveness of both the firm and also of Russia. On the other hand, the transaction arouses certain fears as to the efficiency of managing the new oil assets and the possibility of monopolizing the market."[11]

Roman Abramovich, who bought the company via a privatization plan in 1995, paid $100 million for Sibneft. Barely ten years later, Gazprom paid $13 billion to acquire the company from Abramovich. At the time, Sibneft was the fifth largest oil company in Russia with a production of 650,000 barrels (88,400 tons) a day. The company came with healthy reserves estimated at four billion barrels. It also had a very large refining capacity in Omsk, believed to be among the biggest in Russia. This was indeed a crucial piece of Gazprom's vertical integration strategy in oil, given that the refinery was linked to all its major fields via pipeline networks. The company leveraged this close proximity to its Siberian fields as a source of significant cost advantage over other producers.

Gazprom's oil interests were also consolidated through a joint venture with TNK-BP for a 50 percent interest in Slavneft. Through this venture, Gazprom had access to more refining capacity. There had been rumors of a forced sell-off of TNK-BP's interests in the venture to Gazprom, but this had not materialized. The company also owned a retail network that was strong in Western Siberia, where many of its oil fields were located.

Gazprom intended to leverage its position in the oil business and expand operations to cover parts of Central Asia and beyond. By 2008, it was already operating a small network of retail outlets in Kyrgyzstan. The immediate priorities, however, were related to bringing more of its fields online and increasing its prospecting activities so that it could book more reserves. Its reserves to production ratio stood at 23 years. A significant proportion of the company's projects were considered to be early in the cycle of production development, however. Although mostly limited to Russia, Sibneft's portfolio of exploration leases was quite large. The service operations of its oil business were carried out by 17 service affiliates, all owned by Gazprom. These companies alone employed 20,000 people. They carried out the basic service functions, such as seismic surveys, drilling rigs construction, well drilling, and other related activities. The oil interests ensured synergies in strategic thinking and execution. The service companies were managed as a consolidated entity named Gazprom Neft–Neft'eservice.

Gazprom had built an advantageous position in the petrochemicals segment as well by moving quickly to capitalize on an opportunity that emerged in 2001. Through its banking arm Gazprombank, it was able to gain control of 70 percent of SIBUR Holding, Russia's largest petrochemical company. Gazfond, Russia's largest pension fund, controlled 25 percent, and the rest were in the hands of company management. This move proved to be a crucial one in that it cemented Gazprom's position as a fully integrated company spanning both upstream and downstream segments, including the lucrative petrochemicals segments. Of particular relevance was the dry gas processing facilities that SIBUR operated. Between Gazprom's own gas refineries and those of SIBUR, Gazprom essentially controlled almost the entire gas processing market in the country.

Global Ambitions: "Near" Abroad and "Far" Abroad

Global challenges require global efforts for their resolution. For this reason, the sphere of our interests is not limited to the European continent. It is well known that gas production has been steadily dropping in the United States in recent years (by more than 30 billion cubic meters between 2001

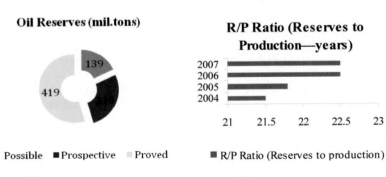

Oil Reserves (mil.tons)

Possible ■ Prospective ▪ Proved

R/P Ratio (Reserves to Production—years)

■ R/P Ratio (Reserves to production)

Exhibit 4 **Prospects in Oil for Gazprom Neft'**

Source: Gazprom Neft.

and 2006), while Russia over the same period has been able to boost production by 70 billion cubic meters. Gazprom has unique experience, know-how, and modern technologies, and is the world's most advanced company in the field of gas transmission via high-pressure gas pipelines.

Alexei Miller, Chairman, OAO Gazprom, XII St. Petersburg International Economic Forum, June 2008.

Gazprom was conceived within an international context. The breakup of the Soviet Union resulted in a set of self-governing republics that became independent countries in their own right. Although they parted ways with central-ized Soviet control, the gas infrastructure that was built to supply many of these former republics was still very much in use. Countries like Turkmenistan, Kazakhstan, and others along the Caspian Sea who were producers used the UGSS operated by Gazprom. Countries such as Belarus and Ukraine were dependent on Russian gas carried through Gazprom pipelines. Referred to as the "near abroad" by Russians, these countries belonged to the Soviet Union. *Near abroad* also signified close links that had been fostered over the decades when they were politically connected to the Soviet Union's sphere of influ-ence. Leveraging these connections was indeed a natural avenue for Gazprom to capitalize on as it set its sights on crafting a global strategy. The first step was essentially to entrench itself in the near abroad so that it could retain crucial transit rights for its pipelines that would eventually target Western European markets while at the same time help monetize gas production in the former Soviet Union countries.

Gazprom also exerted significant influence over those near abroad countries that either did not have energy reserves or were otherwise unable to access them. Coun-tries such as Armenia, Belarus, Moldova, to name a few, were supplied fully by Russia through Gazprom pipelines. These relationships were also a throwback to the Soviet days. The pricing structure for many of these countries was a fraction of free-market prices, thus ensuring that their governments were indeed beholden to Russia in a variety of foreign policy matters.

Although the near abroad had become Gazprom's fiefdom, there were periodic difficulties in enforcing con-trol over its pipeline networks, especially when the repub-lics involved were being wooed by Western powers that had their own designs. The Baku-Tbilisi-Ceyhan pipeline, from Baku in Azerbaijan to Ceyhan on the Turkish Medi-terranean coast, was a prime example of the jostling for influence by major political powers. While Russia wanted to ensure continued control over the near-abroad coun-tries, far-abroad powers were exploring ways in which they could create alternatives to Russian dominance in the region. With the patronage of the Russian government, Gazprom had managed to navigate these choppy waters and maintain its position as either a premier supplier of gas or a partner of choice for producing countries in the region. Many of the countries, such as Macedonia and Belarus,

Exhibit 5 **Russian Gas Supply Prices for Near-Abroad Countries (2008)**

Destination	Price in $ per thousand cubic meters
Lithuania	280.00
Latvia	280.00
Estonia	280.00
Georgia	230.00
Moldova	191.25
Ukraine	179.50
Belarus	119.00
Armenia	110.00
Western Europe	370.00

Source: "Russia," *Country Analysis Brief*, Energy Information Administration, 2008.

were dependent on Russian supplies for almost 100 percent of their needs. In 2007, Russia exported 191 bcm (billion cubic meters) of natural gas, of which roughly 37 bcm went to the near-abroad countries. Although these coun-tries constituted only 22 percent of Russian gas exports, their importance was far more strategic when it came to ensuring transit access to the more lucrative European mar-kets to the west. For example, 80 percent of all Russian gas exports had to flow through pipelines located in Ukraine. Thus, while Ukraine itself had no natural gas deposits, its position on the transit route gave it unique leverage that had been used to keep gas prices low in that country.

First, producer countries in the near-abroad region—such as Turkmenistan—did not have alternative routes to monetize their energy reserves. Gazprom, under the aus-pices of the Russian government, was able to persuade these countries to link to its extensive network as a means of commercializing the gas that they produced. These deals were inked at very low prices, giving Gazprom the ability to sell the same gas to Western European buyers at much higher prices. For example, Turkmenistan signed a 25-year deal with Gazprom at $44 per thousand cubic meters to be paid in cash and commodities. Gazprom was selling the same gas to Western Europe at three times the price,[12] making an easy transactional profit that would continue for years to come. Second, the augmentation of supplies from the near abroad ensured not just continued Russian control, but also offered Gazprom an easy way to overcome the supply shortfalls it had in its domestic and/or export markets. Within Russia, the government had decreed that Gazprom would be the only legal channel for gas exports, thus giving it a wide berth to articulate a global approach to its business.

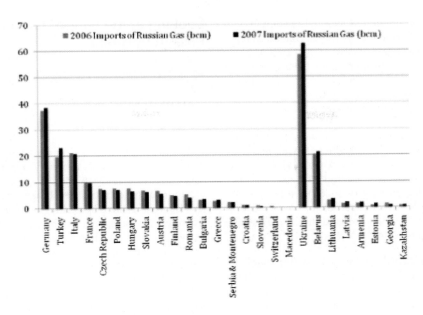

Exhibit 6 **Major Destinations for Russian Gas**

Sources: "Domestic Consumption," EIA International Energy Annual, 2007; "Exports 2006 and 2007," Gazexport as cited by *Energy Intelligence*, March 2008.

Gazprom in Western Europe

Gazprom was able to leverage the export channels to reach customer markets in countries such as Germany, Italy, France, and Austria. Gazprom's predecessor (the Ministry of Oil and Gas Industry) had been exporting gas to Austria since 1968. By 2008, Gazprom was supplying roughly one third of total gas consumed in Western Europe. For example, Germany was dependent on Russian gas for nearly 39 percent of its consumption, and Italy was dependent to the tune of 31 percent. Starting with an approach of selling gas only at the border of its customer countries, Gazprom had become a participant in the entire delivery chain at the local level in some places. One of the key examples of such vertical integration was the joint venture forged with Wintershall, a German oil and gas company owned by BASF, to create a new venture named Wingas in 1993. Gazprom held 50 percent minus one share in the enterprise. Wingas owned 2,000 km of distribution pipelines in Germany, and Europe's largest underground storage facility. The venture offered Gazprom its first local access in a Western European market. (Appendix 6 shows a schematic of Gazprom pipelines in Europe.)

Gazprom sold its gas primarily on long-term contracts, typically over a 25-year period. These contracts also contained "take-or-pay" clauses that reduced the risks that Gazprom would otherwise have to carry. Going forward, these contracts seemed to be crucial to Gazprom because Western European buyers were evaluating potential alternatives that had appeared over the horizon. North Africa and the Middle East seemed to be two viable provider regions, but it was premature to determine their viability in the near term. Many of the European oil and gas companies were engaged in alliances and joint ventures with Gazprom as a possible foil to the perceived imbalance in the relationship between the provider and buyers. Companies such as Eni of Italy, E.ON of Germany, and Gaz de France (GDF) were all associated with Gazprom on a range of projects from exploration to pipeline construction. Besides the obvious benefits of an assured market for its gas, Gazprom was focused on Western Europe because of the higher prices it was able to realize there. Three major projects were in various stages of approvals and execution to cement these links. The Blue Stream, Nord Stream, and South Stream projects were primarily pipeline projects that were targeted to carry gas to markets in Western Europe. The company expected to grow its Western European market faster than its domestic and near-abroad markets.

Gazprom had set up operations in the U.K. in 2006 at a time when the relationship between Russia and the U.K. was at a low point following allegations of espionage and murder involving KGB agents and Russian oligarchs domiciled in the U.K. Gazprom had bought a fairly small British gas supply business, Pennine Natural Gas, a company that supplied gas mostly to small- and medium-scale enterprises. By 2008, it had grown its customer base to about 5,000. However, these moves were being watched very closely. *The Wall Street Journal* reported that the EU was seriously contemplating how such moves could be stopped. "Gazprom embodies everything the EU is trying to change—vertically integrated national champion with a monopoly on exports and that owns gas fields and pipelines. In a preemptive move against Gazprom, the EU is mulling a plan to stop such companies from controlling EU distribution networks."[13] The company did point out that much of the gas that it was selling in the U.K. came from swaps and not from its fields in Siberia, more than 7,000 miles away.

Gazprom also did have its supporters. Reflecting a widespread sentiment among U.K. brokers who had done business with Gazprom, Michael Abbot of Inenco, an energy consulting company, observed, "Gazprom is new to the market, so they're fleet of foot and innovative."[14] Building on this U.K. experience, Gazprom intended to move into France, although it believed that the legislative barriers could be more formidable there.

Going to America: The Very Far Abroad

The promise of America was indeed a strong pull on Gazprom's global intentions. In 2005, the company had delivered LNG to the Cove Point regasification terminal in Maryland under contract with British Gas and Shell. Although there had been some talk about shipping LNG from its Sakhalin II project with Shell to Baja California, it was unclear whether the plans for exports to the U.S. market would ever take flight. The U.S. was one of the largest consumers of gas by a wide margin, and Gazprom was keen to establish a foothold there. The company was examining several possible avenues to achieve this goal, including acquisitions. Vitaly Vasiliev, the CEO of Gazprom marketing and trading, observed, "We can build organically; we can do it with a partnership to build an outlet for us in the U.S., or the third option would be acquisition."[15] Gazprom had already signed a deal with a consortium of French and Canadian partners to set up an LNG regasification terminal in Quebec, Canada. The intent was to bring gas from Gazprom's Shtokman field to North America. It was also in discussions with BP and ConocoPhillips on participating in the Alaskan gas pipeline that had been planned. "It is important that we have a position in the most liquid gas market, which is in Houston for Henry Hub," said Vasiliev, in describing Gazprom's desire to anchor its U.S. operations in America's oil country.[16]

The more Gazprom had pushed into Western markets, the more it realized that it would have to go beyond its delivery-at-the-border approach. Many of the buyers, it found, were trading its gas in markets where price margins were a lot higher, distributing themselves, converting it to electricity, and in general making a lot more money than Gazprom did. In capturing additional value for itself, Gazprom had sought to bolster its own marketing and trading operations. It was with that end in mind that it targeted Houston. It had already captured 8 percent of the wholesale market in the U.K. and 1.5 percent of the retail market as well. Its customer base had doubled in a year. Similar results were expected in France. Success in the U.S. would complete that strategy of capturing value for itself.

Looking at the Future: An Ambitious Project Portfolio

Because you are Gazprom, everybody wants to talk to you. There are so many opportunities; the idea is to choose the best.

Vitaly Vasiliev, quoted in "Russian Unit Heads in New Direction," *Financial Times*, June 11, 2008.

Gazprom appeared to be in an enviable position in mid-2008. However, it was also very apparent that it would have to move quickly to address some strategic priorities methodically. Hostilities had broken out between Russia and Georgia in the disputed region of South Ossetia. The fighting had also spread to Abkhazia, another nearby disputed region on the Black Sea. Although a hasty cease-fire had been called, there was a real danger that the Baku-Tbilisi-Ceyhan (BTC) pipeline could be damaged. The BTC represented the first tangible achievement of Western Europe's desire to seek alternatives to Russian gas. It brought Azeri gas from Baku to the Turkish port city of Ceyhan and well into the sphere of EU influence. Apart from a gentle condemnation of the conflict, Western Europe did not appear to have much to say about Russia's role. Gazprom had won friends through the pipeline after all. Of course, it was also in Gazprom's best interests to help keep those friends.

While the key components of Gazprom's global strategy had focused largely on Europe, eyeing the rise of India and China, Gazprom had started looking East. It had already entered into a joint exploration program with the Gas Authority of India Ltd. (GAIL). It was also prospecting in Vietnam in some of the prime targets for gas deposits. It had cast its net quite wide to also include Venezuela, where it held prospecting licenses. Libya and Nigeria were possibilities as well, and some high-level talks had been conducted at an intergovernmental level. Gazprom had set out an agenda to first capture gas that was being flared in Nigeria, and had also made a statement that it could easily replace Shell in that country should there be a meeting of the minds. These were indeed ominous signs that created concern among EU countries and U.S. IOCs that were among the first to commercialize Nigeria's energy resources. Gazprom had also signed exploration deals with Libya and, in 2007, struck a downstream deal as well. Under terms of the agreement, Libya's National Oil Corporation (NOC) would form an alliance with Gazprom to set up a refining plant in Libya. Gazprom had also offered to buy all Libyan oil and gas exports, an offer that was reportedly well received by the Libyan government.[17] U.S. officials, who feared a loss of control and influence over future energy supplies, also did not welcome this move. U.S. Deputy Assistant Secretary of Eurasian Affairs Matthew Bryza observed, "The monopolist Gazprom is behaving like a monopolist does. It tries to gain control of the market as much as possible and to stifle competition. And that's clearly what's going on."[18]

Gazprom had risen on the wave of success in exploiting gas resources within its own borders and the near-abroad countries. Its future, at least in part, seemed to be tied to that of Central Asia. A significant portion of Gazprom's gas exports came from supplies that it had contracted for in Turkmenistan, Uzbekistan, and Kazakhstan. These three countries accounted for roughly 54.4 bcm/y against Russia's exports of 191 bcm/y. Turkmenistan and Uzbekistan were already exploring other routes to commercialize their gas outside the Central Asia center pipeline that Gazprom operated. Gazprom was developing projects in Tajikistan and Kazakhstan, countries that seemed friendlier than some others. Access and transit rights depended on pricing and the ability to lock in long-term contracts. It remained to be seen whether some of these markets would turn liquid and favor spot trading with the advent of more transportation options. The pricing for gas from these countries had already started to trend upwards.

At home, Gazprom was looking to become far more active in the Yamal-Nenets region, where several new finds had been made. The region comprised 26 fields that had not yet been harnessed, a process that would considerably ease the strains and stresses of declining yields in Russian fields. However, it was estimated that this process would cost roughly $160 billion to accomplish.[19] It was toward this end that the company had announced its intent to increase capital expenditure by 40 percent in 2009, to $65 billion. Although this appeared like a fairly steep increase, some analysts opined that the figures were inflated largely by rising service costs rather than true investments. Gazprom planned to spend $20.4 billion in natural gas production and transportation, of which $8.7 billion had been earmarked for production in 2008.

On the anvil for Gazprom were some large-scale pipeline projects that had the ability to either solidify its reach or weaken it beyond repair. The Nord Stream and the South Stream projects were two that seemed to have both a strong economic and political dimension. The Nord Stream pipeline was a joint partnership between Gazprom (51 percent), BASF (24.5 percent), and E.ON (24.5 percent). It planned to link production from the Russian gas main at Gyrasovez to the Baltic Sea at Vyborg, and with the gas distribution system of Germany, without transiting any other countries. More than 1,200 km of the pipeline would run under the Baltic Sea. While the first segment was expected to become operational in 2010, it would reach its capacity by 2016. It was estimated to cost around $7.4 billion. By mid-2008, the project had been delayed by Sweden, a Baltic neighbor, as the government did not appear satisfied with the environmental impact assessment of the project. While this project would certainly help German consumers, it did pose a challenge to the EU because it wanted to speak with one voice regarding gas distribution among EU member states and relationships with Gazprom. The South Stream was a similar venture seeking to establish a direct line between Russia and Italy.

There were additional projects on the drawing board to connect Russia with China via the Eastern route from Sakhalin, and via a Western route from Western Siberia. Gazprom had been exploring the feasibility of these lines with China National Petroleum Corporation (CNPC). The ambitious projects would drain much of Gazprom's capital budgets, leaving very little for augmenting production. Many of its customers felt that while the pipelines to carry the gas might eventually become a reality, there was less certainty about Gazprom's ability to increase its gas production in parallel to keep the pipeline stocked and flowing. This greatly influenced Gazprom's perceptions of energy security.

Storm Clouds over the Horizon

Gazprom had indeed become a major force to contend with on the world scene by 2008. It seemed to be poised to become a premier player in some areas, but in many ways these were both the best of times and the worst of times. There were several critical issues that had to be sorted out, both internally and externally.

In late 2007, Gazprom had clearly signaled its intent to use the production of gas from the Sakhalin I project owned by a consortium of partners that included Exxon-Mobil, Russia's Rosneft, Japan's Sakhalin Oil and Gas Development Company, and India's ONGC Videsh. Gazprom had unveiled its Eastern Strategy calling for gas fields in that region to contribute 30 percent of all Russian energy exports, a ten-fold increase, by 2030. The major point of concern was the mandate that Gazprom had been given by the Russian government to gasify the Russian Far East. Gazprom expected help to come from two sources: Kovytka and Sakhalin. Under the watchful eyes of the Russian government, TNK-BP was engulfed in a crisis over its Kovytka fields. The government alleged that the project was set back because of undue delays, thus limiting the prospects of a fair return to the Russians anytime soon. This gave the government the leverage to inject Gazprom into the equation as a potential buyout partner for Kovykta. TNK-BP appeared willing to go along, although progress was slow and protracted. BP contended that the fields had become uneconomical because the government had decreed that it could sell its output only in the domestic market where prices were controlled. Along similar lines, it was quite possible that ExxonMobil and its partners in the Sakhalin I project would also be called upon to sell gas domestically. It appeared that ExxonMobil would not entertain such a stipulation because the economics of the project would be in jeopardy, given the paltry prices that prevailed in the Russian Far East.

The EU was unhappy over the turn of events over the last decade that had seen the rise of Gazprom as the key gas supplier to Western Europe. The precarious dependence seemed to be accentuated by the fact that Gazprom seemed able to strike separate deals with EU countries and also venture forward with integration into distribution systems in some of these countries. The EU wanted to bring Russia under the rules of its energy charter so that Gazprom would not exercise undue leverage, given its pre-eminent position as a supplier to Western Europe. Fifty-one countries had signed the charter in 1990 as a prelude to energy cooperation in Europe. Russia had refused to sign on given obvious differences.

Gazprom had become quite dependent on its European portfolio just as its customers had become reliant on Gazprom for stable supplies. (See Appendix 7 for an analysis of Gazprom sales and destinations.) Thus, diversifying away its dependence seemed an urgent priority. Money for expansion and diversification projects was sure to be in short supply. By early October 2008, the global financial crisis that was rocking key markets had begun impacting Russia as well. The price of oil had dropped from its highs of $146 per barrel to below $70 dollars, drying up potential sources of capital funds for many of the energy companies such as Gazprom. In 2007, Gazprom already had a debt load of $61 billion, of which $21 billion was short term. (See Appendices 8–11 for data on Gazprom's finances.) With local sources of capital drying up, it appeared that Gazprom would be forced to seek capital in foreign markets, a proposition that would be far more expensive.

The stance with European and U.S. IOCs had also become quite hardened. Medvedev, in an interview with the *Financial Times*, had remarked, "Gazprom's strategy calls for the formation of complete-cycle 'production-sales' transnational chains. Therefore, while discussing the possibility of access for foreign partners to the development of our reserves, we want to understand what the deal will give Gazprom from the point of view of the development of our production chain abroad. We do not need assets as such; we need a synergy with existing business and enhanced positions of a global player in the energy market."[20] Eni of Italy had been a notable partner for Gazprom, and had shown a willingness to join hands with the company under these terms of complementary access to reserves and markets. It had signed on as a key partner on the South Stream project to carry Russian gas to Italy. Gazprom had also been promised downstream participation in the domestic Italian market, plus a variety of other projects under the aegis of Eni, such as in Libya and, jointly, in Venezuela.

In the middle of a frigid winter in early 2009, Gazprom once again shut off gas supplies to Ukraine. Citing the very same reasons of low prices and unpaid bills, Prime Minister Putin personally ordered the shutoff. Western European nations were up in arms because of the uncertainty surrounding continued supplies of gas, especially because of the importance of Ukraine in the transit routes. This once again demonstrated the unreliability of Russia as a supplier, they said. Buyers who argued that Gazprom had violated their contracts were contemplating legal action. In turn, Gazprom used the occasion to underscore the need for immediate action on the Nord Stream pipeline that would bypass Ukraine. Tensions flared on all sides before a resolution was hastily crafted. Ukraine would pay off unpaid bills and agree to higher gas prices. The effect of this sudden closure left Western European buyers deeply disturbed because they believed this could happen all over again, and they might eventually suffer the consequences of a loss in supply.

Would Gazprom ever be a reliable partner? Would it ever be able to realize its full potential in the global gas business? With declining prices on the horizon, the once rosy future now seemed a bit hazy. Alexei Miller had much to contemplate as he thought about the challenges ahead. He did appear positively ebullient despite the formidable tasks that lay ahead. In an interview with the *Financial Times*, Miller had observed, "We think the price of oil will reach $250 per barrel in 2009. The competition for resources is growing and the tendency is very noticeable."[21] Whether this was indeed a realistic possibility or just wishful thinking, only time would tell.

Endnotes

1. Mortished, Carl, "Gazprom to Raise Its Own Private Army to Protect Oil Installations," *The Times*, July 5, 2007.
2. Kramer, Andrew, "As Gazprom Goes, So Goes Russia," *The New York Times*, May 11, 2008.
3. Victor, Nadejda Makarova, "Gazprom: Gas Giant under Strain," Working Paper 71, Program on Energy and Sustainable Development, Stanford University, 2008.
4. Ibid.
5. "Russia," *Country Analysis Brief*, U.S Energy Information Administration, *www.eia.doe.gov/emeu/cabs/Russia/NaturalGas.html, 2008.*
6. Crooks, E., and Belton, C., "Stake in TNK-BP Labeled 'Worthless,' " *Financial Times*, October 17, 2008.
7. Miller, Alexei, "Energy—Global Players and Referees (Interdependence, Partnership and Competition)," XII St Petersburg International Economic Forum, St Petersburg, Russia, June 6–9, 2008.
8. Mitrova, T., "Gazprom's Perspective on International Markets," *Russian Analytical Digest*, Vol 42, pp 2–16.
9. *http://eng.gazpromquestions.ru/index.php?id=6.*
10. Fredholm, M., "Strategy and Energy Policy: Pipeline Diplomacy or Mutual Dependence?" Conflict Studies Research Centre, UK Defence Academy, Russian Series, 05/41, 2005.
11. "Gazprom-Sibneft: A Transaction with Many Dimensions," Hermitage Capital Management, November 8, 2005, pp 10–16.
12. Smith, K. C., "Russian Energy Politics in the Baltics, Poland, and Ukraine," Center for Strategic and International Studies, Washington, D.C., 2004.
13. Chazan, Guy, "Gazprom Eyes UK as Foothold into Consumer Market," *The Wall Street Journal*, January 28, 2008.
14. Ibid.
15. Crooks, E., and Politi, J., "Gazprom Looks at Acquisitions for US Toehold," *Financial Times*, June 11, 2008.
16. Ibid.
17. Murina, E., and Pedersen, J., "Gazprom, Libya to Form Refining JV," *www.downstreamtoday.com/News/*

Articles/200807/gazprom_Libya_To_Form_Refining_
JV_11786.aspx, 2008.

18. "Gazprom Libya Bid Imperils Moves to Curb Russia's
    Energy Clout," *Tehran Times*, July 12, 2008.
19. "Russia Gazprom Investment," Oxford Analytics,
    International Herald Tribune, April 23, 2008.

20. Belton, C., Hoyos, C., and Crooks, E., "Transcript:
    Interview with Gazprom Chief," *Financial Times*, *www
    .ft.com*, June 26 2008.
21. Hoyos, C., and Blas, J., "Gazprom Predicts Oil Will Reach
    $250," *Financial Times*, June 10, 2008.

Appendix 1   Gazprom Key Statistics

	2007	2006	2005	2004	2003
Share of global natural gas proved reserves %	16.30	16.02	16.10	15.77	15.93
Share of Russian national gas reserves %	62.3	62.4	61.0	60.5	58.3
Share of global natural gas production %	17.37	18.05	18.52	18.59	19.02
Share of Russian national natural gas production %	84.27	84.72	86.61	87.33	88.29
Pipeline infrastructure ('000 Km)	545	514	485	463	428
Size of retail customer network (million homes)	25.9	26.1	25.6	25.1	22.8
Total Natural Gas Reserves tcm	20.82	20.73	20.66	20.9	18.5
Gas condensate reserves (million tons)	686.1	658.99	692.60	654.4	588.2
Crude oil (million tons)	1132.5	1066.48	1231.7	235.96	132.5

Source: "Gazprom: What Is the Nature of Monopoly's Income Growth?" Bloomberg and Veles Capital, July 11, 2008.

Appendix 2   Gazprom and Competitors—Financial Comparisons

Company	Country	Market Cap. Mn $	P/E ratio	ROE%	ROA%	ROIC%
Gazprom	Russia	317,462	11.60	15.30	9.70	13.20
Lukoil	Russia	77,869	6.66	25.67	17.63	22.46
Gazprom Neft	Russia	35,607	9.55	40.69	26.98	33.44
Surgutneftegas	Russia	41,176	10.86	9.83	9.15	9.71
TNK-BP	Russia	33.912	5.01	73.96	31.86	60.87
Rosneft	Russia	112,447	14.03	51.13	21.16	29.45
Novatek	Russia	26,112	24.18	25.04	19.90	23.62
PetroChina	China	389,842	10.75	22.06	15.07	20.44
Petrobras	Brazil	250,332	14.66	20.35	9.74	16.07
BP	UK	200,450	8.53	23.39	9.19	18.64
Chevron Texaco	USA	194,242	10.30	25.60	13.28	23.11
ConocoPhillips	USA	135,273	8.34	13.86	6.94	11.33
ExxonMobil	USA	445.468	10.96	34.47	17.61	32.47
Royal Dutch Shell	Netherlands	238,571	7.20	27.28	12.41	23.75
GLOBAL MEAN			9.26	27.98	13.15	24.38

Source: "Gazprom: What Is the Nature of Monopoly's Income Growth?" Bloomberg and Veles Capital, July 11, 2008.

Appendix 3 The Portfolio of Ownership and Holdings of OAO Gazprom

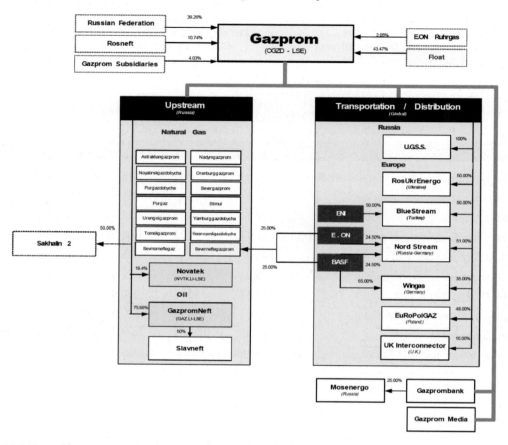

Source: "OAO Gazprom: Taming the Lion," Bear Stearns, March 13, 2007.

Appendix 4 The Sakhalin II Saga

The Sakhalin fields in the Russian Far East were opened for development through PSA arrangements in the early 1990s to reach the booming economies in the Asia Pacific region. There were six different Sakhalin projects created for this purpose. Much of the gas in this region is found under deep water several miles beyond the Sakhalin Island coast. Thus, Russia did not have either the technology or the capital outlays needed to bring the gas to market. Realizing these critical shortcomings, the country opened bids for allotting acreages to international oil companies such as ExxonMobil, Shell, and others.

In May 1991, just before the collapse of the Soviet Union, Marathon, McDermott, and Mitsui were awarded a contract to examine the feasibility of producing gas and crude oil from two fields off the Northeastern coast of Sakhalin. In 1992, Royal Dutch Shell and Mitsubishi joined the consortium as partners to establish the Sakhalin Energy Investment Company (SEIC), and signed a Production Sharing Agreement (PSA) with the Russian government in 1994 to produce both crude oil and gas from the fields they had leased. It was then estimated that the region comprised 4.6 billion barrels of crude and 24 tcf of natural gas. This marked the point at which Shell played out a series of strategies to gain a stronger foothold in the project and consolidate its ownership interests. McDermott sold out its share (20 percent) to Shell, and subsequently Shell was able to convince Marathon to also sell them its share. These negotiations were protracted but did serve Shell's intent to gain a majority position in SEIC. By December 2000, Shell had a 55 percent share of the project with Mitsui and Mitsubishi evenly splitting the remaining equity. The Sakhalin II projects were covered by a PSA that established the following broad conditions:

- SEIC would have the right to 100 percent cost recovery before allocating profits to the federal and provincial governments
- Best effort to achieve 70 percent Russian content measured in labor and materials

(*continued*)

- 6 percent royalty on oil and gas produced for the life of the project
- Exemption from VAT, customs duties, and certain road taxes
- Title on assets held by SEIC until full cost recovery has been obtained, after which it would be transferred to the Russian government. SEIC would retain the rights to exclusive use for as long as it is viable.

The first phase, Russia's first offshore oil project, involved development of the Piltun oil field. This $1.9 billion project came online in 1999 and produced oil for six months of the year. The other half of the year, the platforms were frozen solid and hence could not produce. The second phase of the project was by far more expensive and complex. Expected to cost $10 billion, the project was expected to bring gas from the Lunskoe field off the northeastern coast of the island, which would be piped to land and then delivered by a pipeline running the entire length of the island to an LNG terminal at the southern end.

The project ran into trouble almost from the beginning. The political climate in the country had changed, and the Russian parliament was unwilling to resolve conflicting laws that impacted the project. Public sentiment had also turned against foreign investors. The Putin government was recentralizing power at the federal level with distinct nationalistic overtones. Four of the Sakhalin projects were mothballed, and future PSAs became almost impossible to obtain. Around this time, Gazprom appeared keenly interested in joining the consortium, a prospect that it had not found very appealing when Shell had approached the company earlier. The Russian government also filed charges of environmental non-compliance, and a failure to follow local content and employment guidelines. By that time, project costs had doubled to $20 billion. The project was also faced with external pressures since ExxonMobil and partners appeared to be ahead of the race in their Sakhalin I venture close by. Long-term contracts with Japanese and Korean buyers were delayed because of the uncertainties surrounding the project, thus making it difficult for SEIC to capture the value of its first mover advantage over Sakhalin I.

In 2005, Shell and its partners agreed to a new deal that allowed Gazprom to take a majority stake in the project. Shell agreed to continue as the operator. Gazprom paid roughly $7.5 billion for a 50 percent stake plus one share in the project. The Russian government decided to drop all charges. As of early 2008, the project had yet to come online.

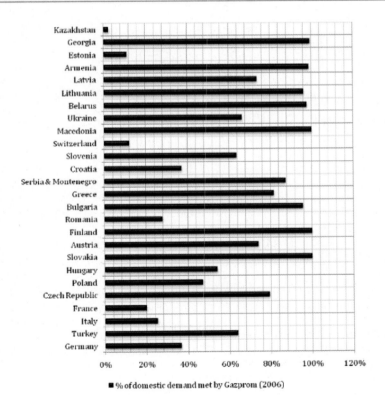

■ % of domestic demand met by Gazprom (2006)

Appendix 5 Gazprom's Share of Domestic Consumption in European Markets

Sources: "Domestic Consumption," EIA International Energy Annual, 2007; "Exports 2006 and 2007," Gazexport as cited by *Energy Intelligence*, March 2008.

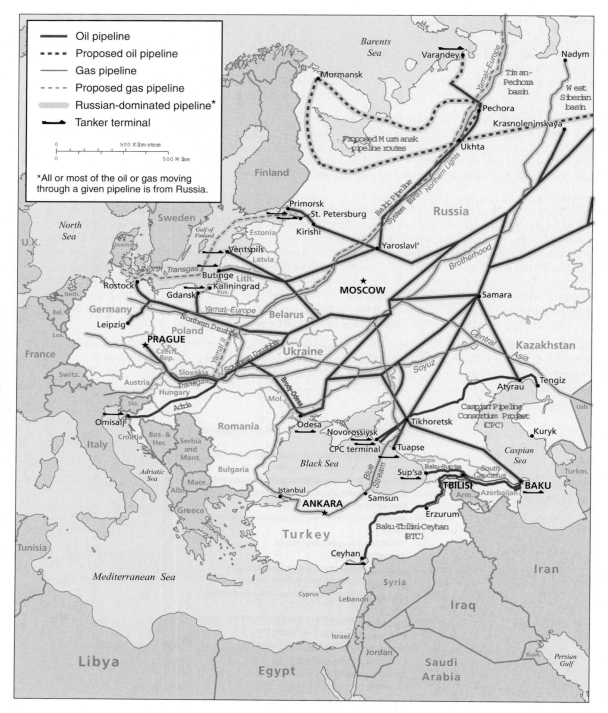

Appendix 6   **Russia's European Network Access**

Source: U.S. Department of Energy, Energy Information Administration, "Russia," *Country Analysis Brief*, April 2007, p. 11, *www.eia.doe.gov/emeu/cabs/Russia/pdf*.pdf (August 20, 2007).

	2007	2006	2005	2004	2003
Gas Sales					
Russian Federation	399,452	357,274	311,336	252,552	207,056
Former Soviet Union	273,550	243,133	131,393	88,440	58,945
Far Abroad	1,161,549	1,149,582	850,017	607,695	567,855
Gross Sales of Gas					
Refined Products	1,834,551	1,749,989	1,292,746	948,687	833,856
Russian Federation	268,278	233,044	123,565		
Former Soviet Union	42,181	29,776	14,414		
Far Abroad	181,979	172,165	64,891		
Total Sales of Refined Products					
Crude Oil and Condensate	492,438	434,985	202,870		
Russian Federation	31,024	26,737	17,376		
Former Soviet Union	19,586	19,213	4,793		
Far Abroad	117,148	125,759	30,422		
Total Crude Oil and Condensate Sales	167,758	171,709	52,591	122,248	92,180
Gas Transportation					
Russian Federation	41,252	34,468			
Former Soviet Union	488	32			
Total Transportation Revenues	41,740	34,500	65,559	29,027	28,226
Total Sales	**2,390,467**	**2,152,111**	**1,383,545**	**976,776**	**954,262**
Gas	76.74%	81.31%	93.43%	97.12%	87.38%
Refined Products	20.60%	20.21%	14.66%		
Crude Oil & Condensate	7.01%	7.98%	3.80%	12.50%	9.65%
Gas Transportation	1.75%	1.60%	4.73%	2.97%	2.96%

Source: Gazprom Annual Reports, 2003–2007.

Destination Analysis

	2007	2006	2005	2004	2003
Gas Sales					
Russian Federation %	21.77	20.42	24.08	26.62	24.83
Former Soviet Union %	14.91	13.89	10.16	9.32	7.07
Far Abroad %	63.32	65.69	65.75	64.06	68.10
Refined Products					
Russian Federation %	54.48	53.58	60.91		
Former Soviet Union %	8.57	6.85	7.11		
Far Abroad %	36.95	39.58	31.99		
Crude Oil and Condensate					
Russian Federation %	18.49	15.57	33.04		
Former Soviet Union %	11.68	11.19	9.11		
Far Abroad %	69.83	73.24	57.85		

Source: Author's analysis.

Appendix 8   Gazprom's Balance Sheet 2003–2007 (*in Million Russian rubles*)

	2003	2004	2005	2006	2007
Current Assets					
Cash and cash equivalents	71,396	106,157	146,866	269,224	279,109
Restricted cash	33,743	16,861	18,040	12,356	12,025
Short term financial assets	57,069	40,428	79,001	106,574	113,911
A/c receivables and prepayments	234,929	316,709	394,659	662,040	697,464
Inventories	111,330	130,400	169,121	207,459	245,406
VAT recoverable	85,909	94,863	145,484	140,305	122,558
Other current assets	6,086	21,262	48,282	84,347	95,944
	485,159	**726,680**	**1,001,453**	**1,482,305**	**1,566,417**
Non-Current Assets					
Property, plant and equipment	1,973,781	2,183,084	2,791,011	3,034,968	3,490,477
Investment in associated firms	58,939	81,783	233,782	318,142	670,403
Long term accounts receivables	93,769	6,302	179,187	251,123	402,382
Available for-sale long term financial assets	8,178	28,710	67,847	150,874	256,210
Other non-current assets	28,958	39,230	65,814	72,513	406,667
	2,163,625	2,479,109	3,337,641	3,827,620	5,226,139
Total Assets	**2,764,087**	**3,205,789**	**4,339,094**	**5,309,925**	**6,792,556**
Current Liabilities					
Accounts payables and accrued charges	124,273	174,433	219,983	398,126	485,466
Taxes payable	103,799	84,977	104,817	68,380	73,563
Short-term borrowings	170,622	156,172	180,959	290,705	504,070
Short-term promissory notes payable	27,433	20,845	20,710	102,859	21,455
	426,127	**436,427**	**526,469**	**860,070**	**1,084,554**
Non-Current Liabilities					
Long term borrowings	303,755	427,086	741,849	668,343	98,1406
Long term promissory notes payable	13,715	11,640	10,639	17,186	3,555
Restructured tax liabilities	6,111	1,829	1,128	822	0
Provisions for liabilities and charges	34,880	44,275	83,794	119,578	79,213
Deferred tax liabilities	96,823	137,062	251,868	275,508	308,353
Other non-current liabilities	12,573	9,446	4,613	18,598	22,376
	468,037	**631,338**	**1,093,891**	**1,100,035**	**1,394,905**
Total Liabilities	**894,164**	**1,067,765**	**1,620,360**	**1,960,105**	**2,479,459**
Equity					
Share capital	325,194	325,194	325,194	325,194	325,194
Treasury shares	−33,889	−41,586	−19,504	−41,801	−20,801
Retained earnings and reserves	1,563,825	1,808,865	2,270,277	2,905,065	3,646,396
	1,855,130	**2,092,473**	**2,576,417**	**3,188,458**	**3,950,789**
Minority interest	14,793	45,551	142,317	161,362	362,308
Total Equity	**1,869,923**	**2,138,024**	**2,718,734**	**3,349,820**	**4,313,097**
Total Liability and Equity	**2,764,087**	**3,205,789**	**4,339,094**	**5,309,925**	**6,792,556**

Source: Gazprom's IFRS Consolidated Financial Statements, 2003-2007.

Appendix 9 Gazprom's Income Statement, 2003–2007 (*in Million Russian Rubles*)

	2003	2004	2005	2006	2007
Sales	819,753	976,776	1,383,545	215,2111	2,390,467
Less Operating Expenses	563,415	714,165	929,561	1,363,923	1,688,689
Operating Profit	226,338	262,611	453,984	788,188	701,778
Gain from sale of interest in a subsidiary	..	..	..	..	50,853
Gain from change in fair value of call option	..	..	..	..	50,738
Deconsolidation of NPF-Gazfund	..	..	..	..	44,692
Finance Income	74,866	69,332	53,890	97,923	159,380
Less Finance Expense	72,725	53,482	69,926	65,220	132,573
Share of income from jointly controlled entities	3,478	8,151	11,782	26,363	24,234
Gains from sale of available for sale financial assets	5,017	5,018	385	8,811	25,102
Profit before profit tax	236,974	291,630	450,115	856,065	924,204
Current profit tax expense	42,368	57,949	118,028	213,844	218,266
Deferred profit tax expense	32,449	21,939	16,156	5,760	10,953
Profit tax expense	74,817	79,888	134,184	219,604	229,219
Profit for the period	162,157	211,742	315,931	636,461	694,985
Attributable to					
Equity Holders of OAO Gazprom	159,095	209,449	311,125	613,345	658,038
Minority Interests	3,062	2,293	4,806	23,116	36,947
	162,157	211,742	315,931	636,461	694,985
Diluted earnings per share of OAO Gazprom (Russian Rubles)	8.02	10.44	14.55	26.90	28.07

Source: Gazprom's IFRS Consolidated Financial Statements from 2003 to 2007.

Appendix 10 Operating Expenses Structure (*Selected elements only. In Million Russian Rubles*)

	2003	2004	2005	2006	2007
Purchased Oil and Gas	25,666	66,546	87,723	280,062	382,054
Staff Costs	100,122	122,853	168,076	199,588	248,894
Transit Fees for Gas and Refined Products	108,711	103,853	110,863	156,489	152,093
Social Expenses	11,724	13,335	15,674	18,563	16,343
Research and Development	6,083	5,845	6,544	13,123	15,486

Source: Gazprom Annual Reports, 2003–2007. Appendix 11. Gazprom's Financial Ratios 2003–2007.

Appendix 11 Gazprom's Financial Ratios 2003–2007

	2003	2004	2005	2006	2007
Return on equity %	7.60	8.70	6.08	9.40	9.11
Return on assets %	5.65	6.41	4.79	7.55	6.90
Return on sales %	26.59	23.85	29.09	30.87	27.41
Debt to capital ratio %	22.40	23.70	20.23	16.90	23.39
P/E for domestic market	6.30	11.29	22.65	20.83	23.61
P/E for external market	12.67	14.49	24.06	20.83	23.61
Market capitalization $ billion	26.99	54.24	91.13	239.33	259.00

Source: Gazprom in figures, 2003–2007.

Case 8   Ryanair: Flying High in a Competitive Atmosphere*

"Can we do what we are doing at a reduced cost? Can we achieve what we want to achieve a different way? How can we hand on those cost savings to the customer?"[1]

Michael Cawley, Commercial Director and CFO, Ryanair

The airline industry in Europe was flooded with around 50 low cost carriers leading to severe competition among them. In fact the low cost carriers simplified airline travel by reducing luxury services thereby focusing on cheaper rates for air travel. They were exploiting the demand for cheap travel by saving on services, operations and overhead. To achieve this, they increased seats in their aircraft compared to full service airlines. Snacks served during flights and other auxiliary services were charged for and made optional. They reduced operating costs through low wages, low costs for maintenance, simple boarding processes and ticket sales through their websites. Many corporations who focused on reducing their air travel expenses shifted to low cost carrier services and saved 3–5% of costs in air travel. Through innovative branding and pricing strategies, they tapped the available opportunities in "seat only" and charter traffic segments. The full service airlines could not reach the load factor[2] and operational margins of low cost carriers like Ryanair.

Ryanair was aggressively promoted as a low cost airline company with cheaper flights. It had become the leading low cost carrier in Ireland and the UK. It accounted for 30% of seat capacity in Europe's low cost segment. It had an average load factor of 83% and it flew 35 million passengers in 2005. What were the strategies followed by Ryanair in cost cutting and branding to remain the leader among the European low cost airlines?

Low Cost Airline Industry in Europe

Low cost carriers (LCCs) in Europe emerged during the post liberalization era in the 1990s. A single European Aviation Market was created in 1993 which led to the growth in intra-European air travel. Their share of capacity increased from 1.4% in 1996 to 20.2% in 2003. Ryanair and easyJet[3] in Europe operated on similar lines as Southwest Airlines[4] in the US.[5] Although the market share growth of low cost carriers in Europe stabilized at 9.1% in 2003, it grew to 18% of all flights in September 2006 (Exhibit 1). The countries in which they had the greatest presence were Ireland (42%), Slovakia (41.4%) and the UK (31.6%) as of May 2006 (Exhibit 2).

www.ibscdc.org

IBS CDC

* This case was written by Dileep, R. Warrier under the direction of Saravanan I B, IBSCDC. It is intended to be used as the basis for class discussion rather than to illustrate either effective or ineffective handling of a management situation. This case was compiled from published sources.

©2007, IBSCDC

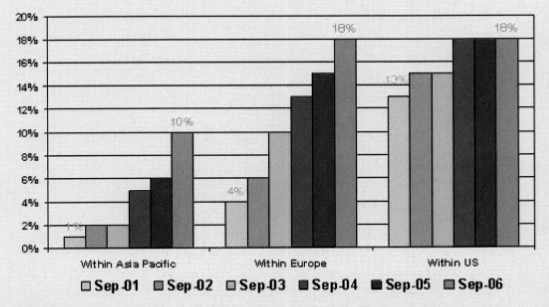

Exhibit 1 Growth in Share of Low Cost Carriers in US, Europe and Asia Pacific
Source: *http://www.oag.com/*

Exhibit 2 Low Cost Carrier—Market Share in Different States in Europe

Annex 1. Low-cost market share per state

Traffic Zone	Low-Cost Market Share: all IFR movements					Local Low-Cost Market Share: excluding overflights				
	2005 Jan-May		2006 Jan-May		Share Growth (% points)	2005 Jan-May		2006 Jan-May		Share Growth (% points)
	Daily Mvts	Share	Daily Mvts	Share		Daily Mvts	Share	Daily Mvts	Share	
Albania	21	8.0%	18	7.4%	-0.5%	.	.	0	0.7%	.
Austria	329	12.7%	369	13.8%	1.1%	85	9.5%	88	9.7%	0.2%
Belarus	5	1.6%	7	2.0%	0.5%	.	.	.	.	.
Belgium/Luxembourg	416	15.7%	458	16.7%	1.0%	87	8.8%	93	9.3%	0.5%
Bosnia-Herzegovina	23	6.5%	37	10.2%	3.7%	1	1.8%	0	0.8%	-1.0%
Bulgaria	60	7.0%	94	10.8%	3.8%	0	0.3%	4	2.9%	2.6%
Canary Islands	40	5.1%	56	6.8%	1.7%	40	5.9%	56	7.8%	2.0%
Croatia	55	7.3%	72	9.9%	2.6%	6	4.2%	12	8.0%	3.8%
Cyprus	8	1.4%	11	2.0%	0.5%	0	0.3%	2	1.8%	1.4%
Czech Republic	223	14.8%	257	16.9%	2.1%	46	11.1%	55	12.7%	1.7%
Denmark	139	8.8%	242	15.3%	6.5%	52	6.2%	115	14.6%	8.4%
Estonia	8	1.2%	14	4.4%	3.2%	5	2.3%	5	5.8%	3.5%
FYROM	22	9.3%	21	8.6%	-0.7%	3	9.1%	2	5.8%	-3.3%
Finland	22	3.3%	121	17.7%	14%	11	1.9%	111	19.1%	17%
France	1125	15.8%	1338	18.3%	2.5%	292	7.5%	373	9.2%	1.8%
Georgia	0	0.2%	0	0.2%	0.0%	0	1.1%	0	1.8%	0.7%
Germany	1112	15.0%	1391	18.2%	3.1%	775	15.7%	935	18.5%	2.9%
Greece	57	4.6%	69	5.6%	1.0%	38	5.6%	36	5.1%	-0.4%
Hungary	129	9.7%	156	10.9%	1.2%	58	18.0%	52	15.7%	-2.2%
Ireland	270	19.7%	310	21.5%	1.8%	263	39.9%	293	42.0%	2.1%
Italy	522	13.2%	613	15.1%	1.9%	384	13.0%	474	15.5%	2.4%
Latvia	14	3.5%	26	6.3%	2.7%	9	10.2%	16	18.3%	8.1%
Lisbon FIR	88	8.8%	127	12.0%	3.3%	56	10.5%	80	13.9%	3.3%
Lithuania	10	2.3%	23	5.5%	3.2%	0	0.0%	4	4.1%	4.0%
Malta	3	1.4%	2	1.3%	-0.1%	2	3.4%	2	3.1%	-0.4%
Moldova	0	0.6%	0	0.2%	-0.3%	.	.	.	.	.
Netherlands	409	15.6%	527	19.3%	3.8%	175	13.5%	210	15.7%	2.2%
Norway	104	8.1%	151	11.1%	3.0%	99	8.3%	147	11.6%	3.3%
Poland	88	8.4%	162	13.3%	4.9%	63	13.0%	125	21.4%	8.4%
Romania	61	6.4%	69	7.1%	0.7%	10	4.3%	16	6.2%	2.0%
Santa Maria FIR	0	0.1%	3	1.1%	1.0%	.	.	1	1.0%	.
Serbia&Montenegro	45	5.7%	78	9.2%	3.5%	6	4.2%	4	2.9%	-1.3%
Slovakia	109	14.8%	124	16.1%	1.2%	32	36.7%	37	41.4%	4.7%
Slovenia	47	8.0%	65	11.2%	3.2%	4	4.8%	3	3.8%	-1.0%
Spain	710	17.9%	830	19.9%	2.1%	602	19.5%	691	21.4%	1.9%
Sweden	215	11.9%	310	17.0%	5.1%	177	15.2%	213	18.8%	3.6%
Switzerland	401	15.1%	480	17.8%	2.7%	134	11.3%	147	12.5%	1.2%
Turkey	96	6.4%	137	8.4%	1.9%	89	10.1%	127	12.9%	2.8%
Ukraine	5	0.6%	4	0.4%	-0.2%	0	0.0%	.	.	.
United Kingdom	1530	24.8%	1818	28.4%	3.6%	1488	27.7%	1752	31.6%	3.9%
ESRA	**3053**	**12.9%**	**3744**	**15.3%**	**2.4%**	**3051**	**13.0%**	**3741**	**15.4%**	**2.4%**

Source: Low Cost Carrier Market Update May 2006, Eurocontrol.

The low cost carriers attracted people who traveled through charter airlines without an accompanying tour package and those who traveled to holiday homes. The passengers who traveled weekly and the cost conscious business passengers planned ahead and flew in low cost airlines. There was huge competition among low cost carriers, and as a consequence their number in Europe decreased to 50 in 2006. From among them, there were 15 low cost carriers which had more than 50 flights/day compared to 13 (out of 100) in 2005.[6] But they added 2.4% to their market share during 2005-2006 (Exhibit 3). Major development and growth for LCCs were happening in the UK, Denmark

Exhibit 3   Low Cost Carrier Performance—Jan–May 2006

Period	LCC	Others	Total	Share
Jan – May 2005	3,053	20,561	23,614	12.9%
Jan – May 2006	3,744	20,702	24,447	15.3%
Net Additional Movements	691	141	833	2.4%
% of all net additional movements	83%	17%		

Source: Low Cost Carrier Market Update May 2006, Eurocontrol.

and Finland (Exhibit 4). Ten of the top 25 low cost country-pair[7] flows involved the United Kingdom, and these ten flows had 42% of all low cost flight movements. There was 17% growth in market share of low cost carriers in Finland and they had 9% growth in Denmark and Poland. The frequency of low cost carriers between Finland and Sweden had grown to 13% of all country-pair flights. The low cost carriers accounted for 28% of passenger traffic in 2005. Their share was expected to grow to 37% by 2012 as they were in expansion mode and building brand popularity. The major low cost carriers were Ryanair, easyJet and Virgin Express, and there were emerging low cost carriers like Wizz Air,[8] Czech Airlines[9] and Air Berlin.[10]

Background

Ryanair[11] was founded in 1985 by Christy Ryan, Liam Lonergan and Tony Ryan. Its initial flight was between Waterford in the southeast of Ireland to London Gatwick,

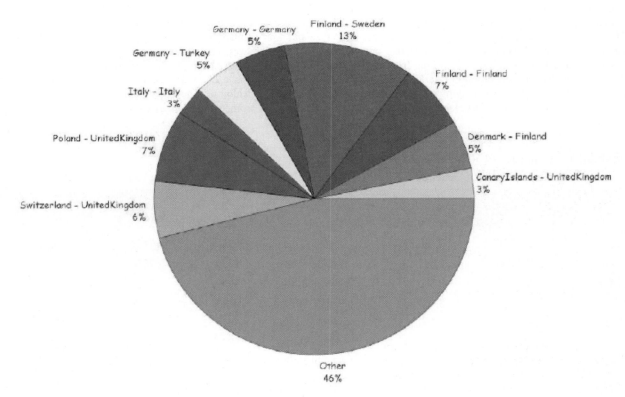

Exhibit 4   Country-Pair Traffic of Low Cost Carriers in Europe
Source: Low Cost Carrier Market Update May 2006, Eurocontrol.

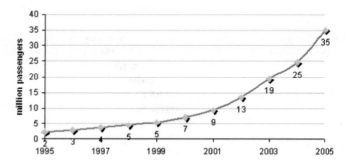

Exhibit 5 Passenger Traffic Ryanair 1995–2005

Source: *www.wikipedia.com.*

using a 15 seat Embraer turboprop aircraft. Ryanair obtained permission in 1986 from regulatory authorities to operate between Dublin and London. The flights between the two airports were at a rate of just 99 British pounds, but it broke the duopoly of British Airways[12] and Aer Lingus.[13] With two routes in operation, Ryanair carried 82,000 passengers in 1986. In 1987, Ryanair increased its network with other flight routes from Dublin to Liverpool, Manchester, Glasgow and Cardiff and also from Luton to Cork, Shannon, Galway and Waterford.

In 1990, Ryanair decided to extend itself to the rest of Europe. Due to intense price competition from British Airways and Aer Lingus, Ryanair accumulated £20 million in losses. The Ryan family invested £20 million further and made many strategic decisions to reduce operational expenses and work as a low cost airline. In 2001, Ryanair added a new base for operation in Charleroi in South Brussels. In 2002, Ryanair began flying to 26 new routes and established a hub[14] at Frankfurt-Hahn airport. In April 2003,

Ryanair acquired Buzz[15] from KLM.[16] The revenue of Ryanair increased from 231 million euros in 1998 to 843 million euros in 2003 and its net profit was 239 million euros in 2003.The airline flew 127 routes and operated from 11 hubs, including two more bases Rome and Barcelona in 2004. After 1 May 2004, Ryanair opened new routes to six new European Union member states. The company ordered 70 more Boeing aircraft in 2005 hoping that there would be greater demand with increase in number of routes.

Ryanair had sales growth of 28.3% between 2000 and 2005. It was reporting profit when other low cost airlines were struggling in bankruptcy and quitting the industry. It recorded a market capitalization of 11.82 billion euros and a profit margin of 20.09% in the first quarter of 2006. The passengers carried by Ryanair increased to 35 million in 2005 from 25 million in 2004 (Exhibit 5). It had a load factor of 84% in 2006 and the average fare for travel was 46 euros (Exhibit 6). The Profit after Tax (PAT) of Ryanair increased from 64 million euros in 2005 to 116 million

Exhibit 6   Load Factor Pattern of Ryanair

	2005	2006	Rolling 12 months	2005	2006	Rolling 12 months
Jan	2,041,575	2,538,371	33,865,381	74%	74%	83%
Feb	2,123,896	2,592,133	34,333,618	79%	78%	83%
Mar	2,565,706	3,000,901	34,768,813	80%	79%	83%
Apr	2,656,855	3,439,009	35,550,967	81%	85%	83%
May	2,904,939	3,556,113	36,202,141	82%	82%	83%
Jun	2,988,075	3,670,542	36,884,608	87%	87%	83%
Jul	3,198,977	3,940,792	37,626,423	90%	90%	83%
Aug	3,257,009	4,002,358	38,371,772	91%	91%	84%

Source: *www.ryanair.com*

	Mar 06 €'M	Jun 06 €'M
Aircraft (incl Deposits)	2,676.0	2,647.4
Cash	1,972.0	2,184.4
Total	4,649.0	4,831.8
	Net Cash €294m	Net Cash €543m
Liabilities	979.3	1,080.5
Debt	1,677.7	1,641.4
Shareholders Funds	1,992.0	2,109.9
Total	4,649.0	4,831.8

'Ms (IFRS)	Jun 05	Jun 06	Change
Passenger Numbers	8.5m	10.7m	+25%
Load Factor	83%	84%	+1pt
Average Fare	€41	€46	+13%
Revenue Per Pax	€47	€53	+12%
Revenues	€405m	€567m	+40%
Profit after Tax	€64m	€116m	+80%
Net Margin	16%	20%	+4pts

Exhibit 7 **Financial Data of Ryanair**

Source: 3rd Quarter Financial Results, *www.ryanair.com*.

euros in 2006 (Exhibit 7). It had the highest operating margin among low cost airlines like Southwest Airlines and easyJet.[17] It was expanding to new airport bases to cover the European continent and worked at minimal operating costs and fares (Exhibit 8).

Ryanair's Strategies

Ryanair, positioned aggressively as a low cost airline, had shown a profitable performance by implementing innovative strategies like common aircraft fleet, contracting, online ticket booking and network expansion to secondary airports. Their strategies resulted in better operating margins, the U.S. increase in load factor, on time flight movements and fewer passenger complaints. Like Southwest Airlines in the U.S., it had only point to point flights,[18] normal seats without pillows and no frills during flight. It also had the first mover advantage in the Irish and European markets.

In spite of increasing competition, it had attracted attention through its advertising strategies which focused on promoting "value for money" as the major advantage

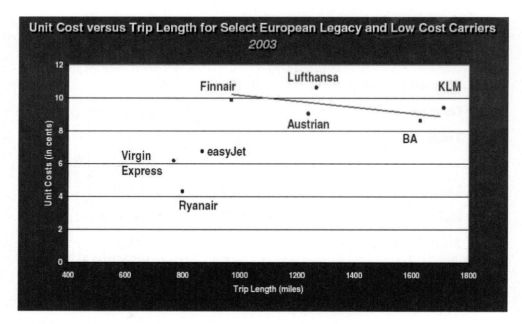

Exhibit 8 Unit Cost—Trip Length Graph of Selected Airlines in Europe

Source: Growth of Low Cost Carriers in Europe and Asia, Eighteenth Annual Aircraft Finance Conference, S, H&E Inc., 2004.

in comparison with other airlines. Its customers booked tickets online and rented apartments through its website without the help of travel agents. It acquired Buzz, one of its competitors in 2002 to expand its network and increase market share. Its strategies to retain and develop loyal customers had been successful.

Marketing and Branding Ryanair focused on spreading the idea of widely available lower fares on various routes. It advertised its services in national and regional newspapers in Ireland and the UK. Press conferences, publicity stunts, billboards and the local media were also utilized for promotional activities. The advertisements featured the slogan "Ryanair.com, Fly Cheaper" to build a brand identity as the leading low cost carrier in Europe. The company conducted cooperative advertising campaigns with other travel agents and local tourist boards also. While it entered into new markets and inaugurated new services, Ryanair launched special advertising campaigns in the local media and its sales team visited pubs, shopping malls, factories, offices and universities to increase consumer awareness about the company (Exhibit 9).

Ryanair travel fares were lower and it hoped to attract price conscious passengers and business travelers who often used alternative transportation (Exhibit 10). It sold airline tickets on a one-way basis which eliminated minimum stay requirements and did not compel the customer to book to and fro flights. The fares were set according to the demand for particular flights and although 70% of occupied seats were sold at a particular rate, the fares charged were higher if booking dates were closer to time of departure. On an average 130 passengers were carried in a flight using Boeing 737 aircraft and the load factor for flights was more than 80%. Ryanair's Dublin to London (Stansted) route had the largest passenger volume and the fare range was 0.99 to 199.9 euros.[19] It had point to point flights which had better punctuality and reported fewer cases of lost bags and cancellations according to the reports of Association of European Airlines.

Secondary Airports and Third Party Contracts Ryanair focused on airports like Barcelona in Spain, Pisa and Milan in Italy and London (Stansted), Luton and Glasgow in the UK (Exhibit 11). These short haul routes were convenient for Ryanair to offer frequent service and avoid frills during travel. The concept of point to point flying allowed direct nonstop routes leading to lower turnaround times and increased frequency of flights. It focused on secondary[20] and regional airports which resulted in less congestion, fewer terminal delays, easy airport access and lower handling costs and shorter turnaround times[21] compared to major airports. Secondary and regional airports often had lesser operating restrictions and slot requirements which would not limit the number of allowed take offs and landings.

Ryanair entered into agreements with third parties at airports for passenger and aircraft handling, ticketing and other services. The company negotiated with them for competitive rates and multiyear contracts. This way,

Criteria	Ryanair	easyJet	Go	Buzz	Virgin Express	Debonair[1]
Simple product ("no frills")	■ Genuine no-frills offerings	■ Genuine no-frills offerings	■ Genuine no-frills offerings	■ Use of KLM lounges, reservations possible	■ Hybrid business design (low-cost, charter, wet lease)	■ Two-class product ■ Frequent flyer program ■ "High frills"
Low operating costs	■ Sec. airports ■ Homog. fleet ■ Minimum cost base	■ Services major airports, hence higher turnaround times and fees	■ Services major airports, hence higher turnaround times and fees	■ Major airports: higher turnaround times and fees ■ 2 types of plane	■ Services major airports, hence higher turnaround times and fees	■ Complex processes ■ No cost advantages
Positioning	■ Straightforward, aggressive low-cost positioning	■ Low-cost position except for major airports	■ Low-cost position except for major airports	■ Major airports ■ Bulk customers ■ Business focus	■ Unclear position (low cost, code share SN, charter)	■ Unclear position with "low cost, high frills"

Exhibit 9 Ryanair and Other Low Cost Carriers—Branding

Source: Mercer Management Consulting, *www.mercermc.com*.

Ryanair reduced the need for additional staff and eliminated difficulties in luggage and traffic handling. Its engineering staff carried out routine maintenance and repair of aircraft, but heavy maintenance was done through third party contracts. Ryanair staff supervised the operations of third parties to ensure the safety and quality of its operations.

Common Fleet   Ryanair had initially decided to buy used aircraft of a single type to reduce aircraft buying

		Av. Fare	% > Ryanair
Low	Ryanair	€41	
High	easyJet	€62	52%
	Air Berlin	€87	113%
	Iberia	€141	244%
	Alitalia	€186	353%
	Air France	€220	437%
	Lufthansa	€220	437%
	British Airways	€268	553%

Ryanair Investor Day – 4 October 2005

Exhibit 10 Comparison of Ryanair Fare with Other LCCs and Scheduled Airlines

Source: *www.ryanair.com*

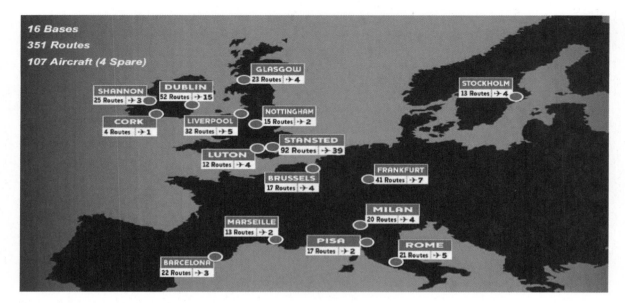

Exhibit 11 Major Bases of Ryanair

Source: Full Report, 31 March 2006, Ryanair.

costs. From 1994 to 1998, it purchased Boeing 737–200 aircraft which were 11 to 17 years old and its fleet had an average age of 23 years as of March 31, 2004. It changed this policy in 1998 and decided to buy Boeing 737–800s because used aircraft for sale were scarce. The fleet of Boeing 737–800s had many common characteristics similar to the used aircraft fleet. It had placed an order for 100 Boeing 737-800 aircraft in 2002 expecting to expand its network and capacity. The idea of having a common fleet enabled it to limit costs associated with training of personnel, purchasing and replacement of spare parts and ensured flexibility in scheduling of crews and equipment. There were 107 aircraft with 189 seat capacity with Ryanair in 2006.

Increasing Productivity For reduction in labor costs and improved productivity, Ryanair emphasized productivity-based pay incentives and a salary structure based on working hours and encouraged the labor force to join stock option programs. Ryanair's pilots flew more hours and the cabin crew served more people compared to those in the traditional airlines. It imposed strict rules like banning the use of personal mobile phones and negotiated with employees regarding wages, work practices and conditions of employment in order to maintain employee productivity.

Ryanair changed its reservation system from the British Airways Booking System (BABS) to a new system called 'Flightspeed' by forming an agreement with Accenture Open Skies for ten years. An internet booking facility called 'Skylight' was developed with the help of Accenture.[22] The Skylight system allowed Internet users to access Ryanair's reservation system to book, pay and confirm reservations in real time. As a result, 99% of all daily reservations were carried out through Internet bookings in September 2006. In March 2006, Ryanair introduced "Check 'N' Go" web based check-in service for passengers with EU passports traveling with hand luggage only, reducing the time for checking in before a flight. It also added online gaming and offers to attract more customers to book through the site directly.

Providing Ancillary Services for Additional Revenue Ryanair provided several ancillary services like beverages, food and merchandise, hotel booking and vehicle rentals for its passengers. It sold bus and air tickets in its aircraft as well as through its websites. It had a contract with the Hertz Corporation for automobile related services and car rentals. It charged a fixed fee from passengers for usage of credit and debit cards for payments for its services. In September 2006, it entered into a letter of intent with On Air, a provider for mobile voice communication services for aircraft. Ryanair had to bear the cost for equipment and its installation. It had also made a five year agreement with Inviseo Media to install seatback advertising in current and new fleets. The "Inviseo Table" was a custom-made, personal backrest tray-table which had an integrated advertising panel for printed advertisements. This gave an on-board advertising medium for the advertisers to attract mobile consumers in Europe. They also allowed advertisements on the wings and the body of the aircraft and promotions inside the airplane during flights.

Challenges

There were several challenges faced by low cost carriers in Europe like rising aviation fuel costs, ensuring staff productivity and maintaining a large fleet for expansion. As there were many low cost carriers in the European continent, the regional airports had become demanding in nature and gained more bargaining power. It would result in an increase in air traffic control charges. The customers had become price sensitive and Ryanair and easyJet were competing with each other on common routes. Although Ryanair maintained cheaper air fares, the increase in fuel costs and cost of expansion made its position more risky.

Fuel Costs   The aviation turbine fuel costs fluctuated owing to economic and political changes and increase in demand. The fuel charges were usually paid in US dollars and fluctuation in exchange rates caused subsequent variation in fuel costs. The fuel costs also fluctuated with the changing political scenario and the hostility between nations in the Middle East region. Ryanair's fuel prices during the year which ended in March 31, 2006 increased by 74.3% compared to that of 2005. The fuel costs accounted for 34.5% of Ryanair's total operating expenses compared to 26.3% in 2005. The fuel and oil costs included the direct cost of fuel, cost of delivering fuel to aircraft and aircraft de- icing[23] costs. These costs had increased from just 17% of total operating costs in 2001 to 35% in 2006.[24] Ryanair had not added surcharges like other airlines so that it could maintain the low fares. But the rising fuel costs made it more risky for the company to operate at lower fares.

Competition   Ryanair faced stiff competition from other low cost carriers in Europe. Low cost airlines competed with each other with respect to fare levels, frequency and dependability of services and name recognition (Exhibit 12). The state owned carriers could pose a threat to Ryanair because they would also fly at lower rates if they were provided government aid and subsidies. The major competitors of Ryanair were easyJet, bmibaby,[25] Air Berlin, SkyEurope[26] and Wizz Air. Aer Lingus which moved to the low fares strategy in 2002 became a competitor on Irish routes. Go, a low cost carrier attempted to compete with Ryanair by starting services from Dublin to Glasgow and Edinburgh. After a fierce battle for market share Go finally withdrew its services. EasyJet and Ryanair had also cancelled services from Gatwick out of competition from regional players. Ryanair had acquired Buzz, another low cost carrier in 2002 and was negotiating with Aer Lingus to buy its shares in 2006. The airlines in the charter flight segment had entered into the low fares market. There were other low cost substitutes like train and tram services in some regions of Europe.

Risks of Expansion   Ryanair was looking forward to expanding in the European continent as it was becoming a popular tourist destination. It was planning to expand its network to North Africa also. The network expansion it had planned would require more aircraft, human resources

Exhibit 12   **Ryanair versus easyJet–2005**

Parameter	Ryanair	easyJet
Average fare	41 €	62 €
Total revenue per pax	48 €	72 €
Load factor	86.40%	84%
Fleet	Airbus-87	Boeing 737-200-9
	Boeing 737-800-32	Boeing 737-800-98
Seats per plane	189	130

Source: Compiled by the author referring to *www.ryanair.com, www.easyJet.com.*

and agreements with airport authorities and governments. The incidents of terrorism in UK and Europe resulted in increased security measures on all UK outbound flights in 2006. It cancelled 279 flights and refunded 2.7 million euros. The September 2001 terrorist attacks in the U.S. also had severe impacts on the airline industry in Europe. It faced threats from airports in case they increased the rates for airport access and included policies like slot allocations. Each slot needed authorization to take off and land at particular airports at specific time periods. It would not be able to fly to those regions where it did not have the slot rights.

The Road Ahead

Ryanair added three more bases, namely, Madrid, Bremen and Marseille with direct routes to airports at London, Frankfurt, Dublin and Rome. It expanded its network to 20 new routes touching Dublin and was expecting to add 113 new routes in 2007. In total, it had 16 bases, 351 routes and 107 aircraft as of September 2006.[27] In order to become the leading airline in Ireland, it had acquired 19.2% share of Aer Lingus for 254 million euros. It had a traffic growth of 22% and passenger traffic of 42.5 million as of September 2006. It was using fuel hedging practices to reduce fuel costs. As it had resorted to buying new Boeing aircraft which had better fuel efficiency and lower pollution levels, it complied with EU regulations of pollution control. Its operational efficiency and cost cutting strategies had been phenomenal and it was able to record profits when other low cost carriers were struggling to become financially feasible with rising fuel costs. It was the leader in Dublin–London (45% market share) and other routes like Rome–London (34%), London–Barcelona (30%) and Stockholm–Milan (50%). It was expecting a 35% increase in passenger traffic in the UK, 15% in Italy and 12% in Ireland by 2007.[28]

After the liberalization in air travel in Europe, the traditional airlines had become slower and many low cost carriers began flooding the continent with attractive packages. The passengers began to fly for leisure and business activities in and around Europe as the European Union opened up for intra-European business with a common currency.[29] The flights between the UK and U.S., the UK and UAE, and Germany and the UK had grown significantly. Liberalization resulted in 44 million additional passengers and an increase of 33% in total passenger traffic in Europe. The European GDP had grown by 85 billion US$ and added 1.4 million jobs. The European airports contributed 2.6% of Europe's GDP as of 2005. Liberalization resulted in favorable regulations for the growth of tourism and business not only in the European continent, but also between Europe, the Middle East and Africa. The expansion of Ryanair's network to North Africa and other European continents would augur well because there were many unexplored opportunities for flight development between Europe and Africa. Ryanair CEO Michael O'Leary summed it up, *"Our strategy is like Wal-Mart: We pile it high and sell it cheap."*

Endnotes

1. 'The Ryanair Success story: Price as Brand', *http://www.ericsson.com/telecomreport/article.asp?aid=10&tid=85&ma=1&msa=3.*
2. Load factor: The percentage of passengers who had traveled to total number of available seats.
3. easyJet is a low cost airline officially known as easyJet Airline Company Limited, based at London Luton Airport. The airline operates frequent scheduled services for leisure and business passengers and serves more than 200 routes between more than 65 European airports.
4. Southwest Airlines, Inc. based in Dallas, Texas, is a low-fare airline in the United States. It is the third-largest airline in the world by number of passengers carried and the largest in the United States by number of passengers carried domestically.
5. Hyped Hopes for Europe, Binggeli Urs, Pompeo Luceo, *The Economist,* 2002.
6. Low Cost Carrier Market Update, May 2006, Eurocontrol.
7. Country-pair: Agreement between two countries to allow aircraft flights between them.
8. Wizz Air is a Polish/Hungarian low-cost airline focusing on the markets of Central Europe.
9. CSA Czech Airlines is the Czech national airline company, and former carrier of Czechoslovakia based at Ruzyně International Airport, Prague. The airline connects to most major European destinations and to transit points in North America, Asia, Middle East and North Africa.
10. Air Berlin is Europe's third largest low-cost airline based in Berlin, Germany. It operates scheduled services from a range of European airports.
11. *www.wikipedia.com.*
12. British Airways is the largest airline of the United Kingdom and the third largest in Europe with flights from Europe across the Atlantic. Its main hubs are London Heathrow and London Gatwick, with wide-reaching European and domestic shorthaul networks, including smaller hubs at other UK airports including Manchester, from which some longer-haul flights are also operated.
13. Aer Lingus is the national airline of Ireland. Based in Dublin, it operates over 30 aircraft serving Europe, the United States and recently Dubai, United Arab Emirates.
14. Airline hub: An airport that serves as the base of operations for an airline.
15. Buzz was a low-cost airline based at London Stansted operating within Europe.
16. KLM: (in full: Koninklijke Luchtvaart Maatschappij, literally *Royal Aviation Company*; usual English: Royal Dutch Airlines) is a subsidiary of Air France-KLM. Before its merger with Air France, KLM was the national airline of the Netherlands.
17. Airline Business, Association of European Airlines, U.S. Department of Transportation, McKinsey Analysis, 2002.
18. Point to point fight: The flights are arranged from one airport to another directly without landing and taking off from a hub. This reduces waiting time at a hub. But it is more suitable for short haul routes.
19. *www.ryanair.com.*
20. Secondary airports: They are the regional airports which are second to major airports in a particular area.
21. Turnaround time: The time taken by a flight to land, unload passengers and take off.
22. Accenture is a global management, consulting, technology services and outsourcing company.
23. De-icing: De-icing is the process of removing ice from a surface. De-icing can be accomplished by mechanical methods (scraping), through the application of heat, by use of chemicals designed to lower the freezing point of water (various salts or alcohols), or a combination of these different techniques.
24. Ryanair Annual Report & Financial Statements 2001 to 2006, *www.ryanair.com.*
25. bmibaby is the low-cost airline subsidiary of bmi. It flies to destinations in Europe from its main bases at East Midlands, Manchester, Cardiff, and Birmingham International.
26. SkyEurope Airlines is a low-cost airline with its main base at M. R. Stefanik Airport (BTS) in Bratislava, Slovakia, and other bases in Kraków, Prague, Warsaw and Budapest.
27. Ryanair's Annual Report 2006, *www.ryanair.com.*
28. Ibid.
29. "The Economic Impact of Air Service Liberalisation," InterVISTAS-ga Consulting Inc, *www.intervistas.us.*

Case 9   DeBeers's Diamond Dilemma*

The mystique of natural diamonds has been built by the industry. One hundred fifty million carats of mined diamonds are produced every year, so they are really not that special if you look at those terms.[1]

—CEO of Gemesis Corporation

We don't see synthetic diamonds as a threat, but you cannot ignore it completely.[2]

—Stuart Brown, Finance Director, De Beers

It was early summer 2007 and Lee Mandell decided that the time was right to propose to Diane, his girlfriend of four years. Being the romantic he was, Lee wanted to pop the question over a candle light dinner that included an exceptional bottle of Bordeaux. Logistical details of where to buy the special ring and what type of diamond, however, were less certain in his mind.

Lee and Diane had recently rented the movie Blood *Diamond*, set in Sierra Leone in the 1990s when a civil war was raging and the rebel group, the Revolutionary United Front, relied on proceeds from smuggled diamonds to finance its military operation. The 11-year war, which ended in 2002, resulted in the deaths of tens of thousands and the displacement of more than 2 million people, nearly one-third of the country's population. Both Diane and Lee had been disturbed by the story the movie told, the hardship and violence, the children who were forcibly recruited to fight, and the lives that were destroyed all over gems that were worn by hundreds of millions of people, men and women alike, throughout the world.

As he thought about his options, Lee recalled a magazine article he had recently read about the growing market for synthetic diamonds. The article described the process by which diamonds could be grown in a laboratory environment, far from the war torn lands of Africa. Chemically, lab-grown diamonds were identical to diamonds that were extracted from the ground. Instead of taking millions or billions of years to form, hundreds of miles underground, however, a laboratory environment could produce a flawless diamond within days.

Lee was starting to think that a synthetic diamond was a great alternative. But how would Diane react upon learning he had bought her a diamond that was made in a laboratory just outside of Boston? Would she be relieved

and touched by his humanitarian and eco-friendly purchase or would she wonder if the 20% to 40% he would save by buying a synthetic diamond was an indication of the depth of his love?

For producers of synthetic diamonds, it was consumers like Lee Mandell that proved there was a market demand for an alternative to the natural diamond. But for South Africa–based DeBeers, which up until the late 1990s single-handedly controlled the world's supply of diamonds, Lee's rationale was misguided and he was giving his girlfriend nothing more than costume jewelry. Nevertheless, the fact of the matter was that people were buying lab-produced diamonds and the number doing so was growing at a faster rate than those buying those extracted from the ground.

The dilemma that DeBeers faced came down to whether it should enter the market with its own synthetic diamonds or whether it should have faith that synthetics would be a passing fad and that, at the end of the day, consumers would always prefer buying what, in DeBeers's mind, was the real thing. Complicating the company's dilemma, however, was the fact that it was in the midst of trying to remake its image, tarnished from decades of anti-competitive business practices, to one that was demand driven and focused on brand development. While DeBeers at one time produced 45% of the world's rough diamonds and sold 80% of total supply, by 2007 it was producing 40% and selling just 45%.[3]

Did synthetic diamonds in fact pose a threat to the diamond industry and if so, what should DeBeers's response be if any?

The Diamond Industry

Natural diamonds, the hardest, most transparent material in existence, were made of carbon atoms that over the course of millions of years and with tremendous heat and pressure deep under the earth's surface bonded into a cubic structure.[4] Due to their heterogeneity, unlike gold or silver, diamonds were not considered a commodity. As one diamond trader explained, "When you talk about commodities, you know that a ton of copper is worth this much, and an ounce of gold is worth this much because they are homogenous. But diamonds are not homogenous."[5]

Supply   The global diamond industry produced an estimated $13 billion of rough stones and $62 billion in jewelry annually. Between 2000 and 2005, world production of diamond rough grew 31% by volume and 70% by value, highlighting the upward trend of diamond prices (Figures 1 and 2).

Seven countries—Angola, Australia, Botswana, Canada, the Democratic Republic of the Congo, Russia, and South Africa—represented 88% of the value of diamond production and 96% of global production volume.[6] As depicted in Figure 3, for some producers, there was great disparity in the relationship between the volume and value

* This case was prepared by Cate Reavis under the supervision of Professor David McAdams. Professor McAdams is the Cecil and Ida Green Career Development Professor.

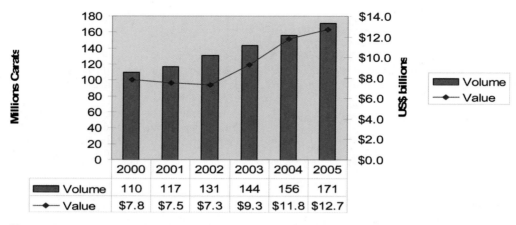

Figure 1 Diamond Rough Production by Volume and Value (2000–2005)

Source: "The Global Gems and Jewelry Industry: Vision 2015; Transforming for Growth," KPMG, December 2006.

of production. While the Congo and Australia were significant producers on a volume basis, the value of their production was quite low. Angola presented the reverse scenario.

Change in Industry Structure The $19 billion processing industry (which involved the cutting and polishing of diamonds) was dominated by India. The 1 million people employed by India's processing industry processed more than half of the world's diamonds in value terms, at costs significantly lower than other processing countries—$10 per carat as opposed to $17/carat in China, $40/carat in South Africa and Israel, and $70/carat in Belgium. Israel and China were the second and third largest processors with 15% and 10% of the market, respectively.[7] But this part of the value chain, at one time dominated almost exclusively by Belgium and Israel, was undergoing significant changes.[8]

Since the late 1990s, empowered by DeBeers's shrinking market position, the voices from Southern African

countries to keep more of the value added activities such as cutting and polishing in-country had become noticeably louder and a number of countries were amending their diamond laws to support and build local diamond-related industries. In 1999, Namibia inserted a clause in a new law permitting the government to force miners to sell a percentage of their diamonds to local polishers,[9] and in 2004, Lev Leviev, an Israeli of Uzbek decent who was one of Israel's largest manufacturers of polished stones, opened the country's first cutting and polishing factory. At the opening of the new factory, Namibia's president was quoted as saying, "To our brothers and sisters of neighboring states, Angola, Botswana, South Africa, I hope that this gives you inspiration to try to imitate what we have here."[10] In 2005, South Africa passed the Diamonds Amendment Act establishing a State Diamond Trader as well as a Diamonds and Precious Metals Regulator. Under the new legislation, scheduled to take effect in 2007, producers would be hit with duties on exported rough diamonds.[11] In response to Southern Africa's attempts to enter into more downstream

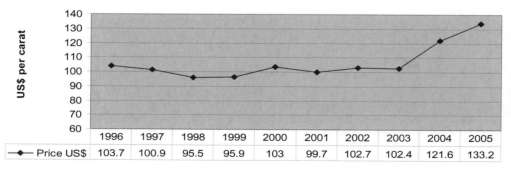

Figure 2 Diamond Rough Prices, 1996-2005

Source: "The Global Gems and Jewelry Industry: Vision 2015; Transforming for Growth," KPMG, December 2006.

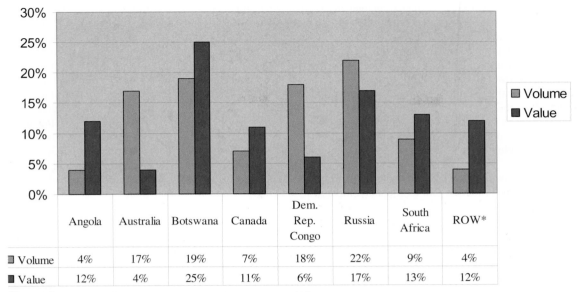

	Angola	Australia	Botswana	Canada	Dem. Rep. Congo	Russia	South Africa	ROW*
Volume	4%	17%	19%	7%	18%	22%	9%	4%
Value	12%	4%	25%	11%	6%	17%	13%	12%

Figure 3 **Top Diamond Producers by Volume and Value**

Source: "The Global Gems and Jewelry Industry: Vision 2015; Transforming for Growth," KPMG, December 2006.

*ROW: Rest of world.

activities, one industry expert remarked, "There's a political and an emotional point. [Africa] is saying, 'We have these resources as Africans, why are we not able to capitalize on the beneficiation on these resources in our possession? Why are Indians cutting African diamonds?'"[12]

Alongside shifts in the value chain, the industry was experiencing an increasing level of forward and backward integration: mines were integrating forward into retail and retail outlets were integrating backward by investing in mines. In 1999, high-end jeweler Tiffany & Co. announced that it was buying a stake in a Canadian mining concern for $104 million and would no longer source its diamonds through DeBeers. In 2003, Aber Diamond, a Canadian mining group, purchased U.S. luxury jewelry retailer Harry Winston giving it storefronts in the United States, Japan and Switzerland.[13] In 2005, Russia's mining giant Alrosa opened up a diamond retail store in a shopping complex off Red Square.[14] As DeBeers's CEO remarked, "The verticalization of the industry is clearly its long-term trend; it's absolutely the way to grow a business and build a brand. Retail clearly adds value. But there are several different kinds of know-how involved in the different levels of the chain and you have to respect, and learn, all of them."[15]

Demand The United States was far and away the world's biggest purchaser of diamonds accounting for 46% of total demand followed by the Middle East with 12% and Japan with 9% (Figure 4). However, demand, particularly for diamonds over 2 carats (worth $15,000 or more), was soaring in India and China[16] in concert with increasing disposable incomes and a growing middle class. India was the fastest growing diamond jewelry market with a growth rate of 19% in 2005.

While at one time the diamond industry was supply-side driven, with little attention given to the end consumer, by the late 1990s the industry began focusing more on the demand side. The main catalyst for this shift was DeBeers's decision to conduct business in a whole new way.

DeBeers Under Attack

In the early 1990s DeBeers ruled the diamond industry. While it only produced 45% of the world's rough diamonds, it sold 80% of the total supply from its marketing

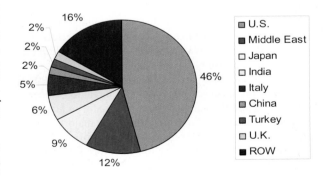

Figure 4 **World Sales of Diamonds, 2005 (polished wholesale price)**

Source: "The Global Gems and Jewelry Industry: Vision 2015; Transforming for Growth," KPMG, December 2006.

unit in London. Its market dominance enabled its Central Selling Organization to choose whom to sell to, how much to sell, and at what price. Buyers who turned down an offer to purchase a parcel of diamonds might not be invited to purchase from DeBeers again. Meanwhile, buyers who strayed from DeBeers's selling arm and purchased directly from a mine would be dropped by the company or financially punished.[17] In 1981, after Zaire decided to stop selling its industrial-grade diamonds to the syndicate, DeBeers dipped into its stockpile and flooded the market bringing down the price of Zairian diamonds by 40%.[18]

DeBeers's monopoly was shaken in the 1990s from the emergence of three producers that fell outside of its grasp, making its strategy of controlling supply costly both financially and legally. The first big hit came shortly after the collapse of the Soviet Union in 1991. Through a marketing agreement that dated back to the late 1950s when diamond deposits were first discovered in Siberia, the Soviets had sold their entire diamond production to DeBeers's Central Selling Organization. Once the Soviet system disintegrated, however, DeBeers was unable to enforce contracts and Russian diamonds were soon being smuggled onto the international market causing prices to fall.

But DeBeers' challenges in Russia could not be blamed solely on the country's economic and political upheaval. Lev Leviev, one of Israel's largest manufacturers of polished stones, was making his move in Russia where he was well connected politically. In 1989, two years after Leviev became a sightholder for DeBeers, Russia's state-run diamond mining and trading group, now known as Alrosa, entered into a joint venture with Leviev to establish the country's first cutting factory, the stones of which would be supplied directly by Russian mines, not through DeBeers.[19] The partnership marked the first time in which rough diamonds were cut in their country of origin. Over the next five years, Leviev's position in the Russian diamond industry grew to the point where, in 1995, DeBeers terminated his sightholder status.[20]

The second jolt to DeBeers's position came in 1996 with the decision by Australia's Argyle diamond mine, which produced low quality diamonds suitable for inexpensive jewelry, to terminate its contract with DeBeers and begin marketing its own diamonds. It sold 42 million carats directly to polishers in Antwerp that year.[21]

Finally, the emergence of Canada in the early 1990s as a diamond producer served as a further threat to DeBeers's position. While the company was successful in acquiring stakes in a couple of Canadian mines, the majority of the country's production fell outside of its control.

In order to keep prices high, therefore safeguard its market dominance, DeBeers was forced to both hold back a large portion of its diamonds from the market and purchase much of the excess supply from these producing countries often at inflated prices. By the end of the 1990s, DeBeers's market share had fallen from 85% to 65% while its diamond stockpile had grown from $2.5 billion to $5 billion. Between December 1989 and 1998 DeBeers's share price fell from $17 to $12, a nearly 30% drop.[22]

In addition to the financial sting DeBeers was feeling resulting from its supply-side strategy, antitrust regulators in the United States and the European Union were becoming increasingly aggressive in their attempts to formally end the company's price control practices. In a 1994 indictment, the United States accused DeBeers of violating the Sherman Antitrust Act by fixing the price of industrial diamonds. The government contended that a subsidiary of DeBeers conspired with General Electric, another producer of industrial diamond products, to fix the world prices of industrial diamonds in 1991 and 1992. While the United States Justice Department was unable to prosecute DeBeers because its operations were overseas and it refused to subject itself to the jurisdiction of an American court, the company was prohibited from conducting business in the United States.

On a completely different front, DeBeers faced yet another threat, which was quickly turning into a public relations nightmare for the entire diamond industry. In the mid-1990s, Angola, the world's third largest producer of rough diamonds, was overrun by rebel forces opposed to President Dos Santos. Gaining control of the country's diamond supplies, the rebels flooded the market with up to $1.2 billion worth of rough diamonds. To maintain control over supply, therefore prices, DeBeers had little choice but to buy what were becoming known as "blood diamonds," the proceeds of which went toward financing the armed conflict. Angola was not a lone participant in the blood diamond trade. Rebel forces in Sierra Leone, Liberia, and the Democratic Republic of the Congo were also using the illicit diamond trade to finance their respective armed conflicts.

DeBeers's involvement in the "blood diamond" trade was exposed in a 1998 report by Global Witness which accused the company of "operat[ing] with an extraordinary lack of accountability."[23] As Martin Rapaport, publisher of the diamond industry pricing guide, asked rhetorically, "How can it be that tens of millions of dollars are exported from diamond areas and yet there is no electricity, no plumbing, no wells, no improvement in the lives of the people?" Rapaport went on to ask the more complicated question of, "Do we owe anything to the people of Africa just because we buy their diamonds? Are we responsible for what we buy?"[24]

For DeBeers, these challenges and threats in aggregate were creating a "*perfect storm*" of sorts. Significant changes to the company's strategy that had served it well for decades had to be made.

A New Direction   In 1998, on the advice of U.S. consulting firm Bain and Company, DeBeers decided to "ditch its role of buyer of last resort" and develop a strategy that was demand-driven and brand-focused whereby profits were more important than market share.[25] When explaining its strategic shift, DeBeers's Managing Director stated,

"We don't have to go rushing about the world trying to buy every diamond. What is the point of us buying diamonds close to or over our selling prices? It's silly. I'm perfectly happy to market 60%. What I want to do is differentiate the portion that does come to us and create value on those goods . . . in order to sell them first, more advantageously, and at better prices."[26]

As a part of its strategy, DeBeers ended its practice of stockpiling diamonds, stopped buying diamonds on the open market, and began only selling diamonds from its own operations which enabled it to guarantee that its supply was "conflict free." The company promised the European Union it would stop buying diamonds from Alrosa, the state-owned Russian firm that accounted for 20% of global production by 2009 to promote competition.[27] The promise was formalized in a 2006 agreement with Russia.

A new demand-centered strategy required that DeBeers build new relationships with its suppliers. This came about in what was dubbed the "Supplier of Choice" program, the goal of which was to make DeBeers the supplier of choice in the eyes of its customers, in lieu of the buyer of last resort. DeBeers scaled down the number of its sightholders from 120 to 80 and formalized business relationships with those that were chosen with a written contract.[28] Sightholders were no longer expected to purchase whatever stones DeBeers offered to them. Rather, they requested a specific package of stones based on sales and marketing strategies they had created.[29] The criteria to being a sightholder were no longer based on financial strength and manufacturing capabilities but rather marketing savvy.

Under the new arrangement, sightholders were entitled to use DeBeers's Forevermark, a tiny logo that was etched into natural diamonds which guaranteed the polished diamonds were natural, ethically traded and non-treated. (The Forevermark diamond was sold in Hong Kong, China, Japan, and India.) Sightholders also benefited from DeBeers's marketing data including consumer buying habits and patterns and the number of engagements worldwide. Those sightholders that successfully built strong brands were partially reimbursed for the money they spent on advertising and marketing efforts. As Nicky Oppenheimer, DeBeers's chairman, explained, "We want people to say, 'While I can get diamonds from people other than DeBeers, the package DeBeers gives me is so valuable, I get a better return from them."[30] Accompanying DeBeers' efforts at building a new identity, the company's Central Selling Organization was renamed the Diamond Trading Company (DTC).

In step with the Supplier of Choice Program, DeBeers developed a marketing and retail strategy to position its diamonds as a branded luxury item. Unlike other luxury brand producers, diamond producers had suffered from poor financial performance over the years due to the lack of branding. In fact, many in the industry lamented that although not traded as one, diamonds had become a commodity of sorts. Lev Leviev implied that DeBeers was largely responsible: "There are two main reasons why diamond retailers fail. Lack of innovation—they have the same stones in the same settings in the window year after year—and dependence on one supplier for their stones. You can never plan your sales even one year ahead, because you can only work with what they give you, and they decide."[31]

A Boston-based diamond wholesaler, however, had proven that branding diamonds could work, especially since the market was shifting to a demand-driven model. In 1997, the wholesaler, who sourced his raw stones from DeBeers sightholders and others, began selling a branded diamond called Hearts on Fire which was differentiated by its cut. Marketed as "the world's most perfectly cut diamond," the diamonds were cut by hand in Antwerp, Belgium in a pattern known as "hearts and arrows." When viewed under magnification, each diamond revealed a symmetrical ring of hearts and eight pointed arrows.[32] The brand produced $40 million in sales each year. In 1999, DeBeers entered into the brand world by marketing a limited-edition (20,000 stones) Millennium diamond, engraved with the company's logo and the year 2000. The Millennuim diamond's campaign came with a tag line of, "Show her you'll love her for the next thousand years."

DeBeers's brand positioning was accompanied by attempts to widen its customer base. A number of non-wedding advertisement campaigns were launched including the "Celebrate Her" campaign which urged men to show their love for their significant other by buying her a three-stone diamond ring. The campaign's advertisement pictured a middle aged man on bended knee asking, "Will you marry me again?" There was the "Women of the World Raise Your Right Hand" campaign which encouraged women to indulge in a diamond ring to be worn on their right hand as an expression of personal style.[33] In addition to new messages enticing consumers to buy diamonds for purposes other than engagements, in 2001, DeBeers entered into a joint venture with LVMH to open up a series of retail stores. Diamond jewelry was sold under the DeBeers name. By early 2007, DeBeers had 22 stores spanning the United States (3), Europe (4), the Middle East (1), and Asia (14).

From Public to Private At the same time the new strategy was being rolled out, DeBeers delisted from the Johannesburg Stock Exchange where it had traded since 1893. Purchased by a consortium that included the Oppenheimer family, Anglo American plc, and Debswana Diamond Co. (Pty) Ltd, DeBeers became the world's largest private diamond mining company. The privatization, which cost $17.6 billion (a 31% premium)[34] left DeBeers heavily in debt. Ironically, the terrorist attacks in the United States on September 11, 2001 helped alleviate the company's debt. As DeBeers's Chairman Nicky Oppenheimer explained, "Sentiment changed dramatically after September 11, though we did not realize it at the time. There was a swing back to traditional values such as family and all the sorts of things that diamond jewelry plays into."[35]

One of DeBeers's first major media grabbing acts as a private company came in 2004 when it pleaded guilty to charges of price-fixing of industrial diamonds and agreed to pay a $10 million fine. Settling the 10-year-old charges meant that DeBeers executives could visit and conduct business in the United States. In 2005, the company agreed to pay $250 million to settle a class action suit by diamond consumers who accused the company of monopolizing the international diamond business through its control of mines and agreements with diamond suppliers around the world.

In 2006, DeBeers made another surprising move when it signed an agreement with the Botswana government to establish the Diamond Trading Company Botswana. The 50:50 joint venture would start sorting and valuing all of the diamond production of Debswana (50:50 partnership between DeBeers and the Botswana government) likely at the end of 2007 or early 2008 upon completion of a $83 million complex near the capital's airport. From 2009, the partnership would take over aggregation duties (mixing of diamonds from different countries into similar assortments) of DeBeers's entire aggregation operation, currently carried out by DeBeers's DTC in London. As a result of the deal, Botswana had moved up the value chain from mining and sorting to sales and marketing.[36] As of 2006, four international diamond businesses had cutting factories and 11 new licenses had been issued. By some estimates, 3,500 new jobs would be created. Costs of cutting and polishing, however, would likely be significantly higher than they were in India and China.[37]

In early 2007, DeBeers signed a similar agreement with the Namibian government. All diamonds produced by their joint venture, Namdeb, would be sorted in Namibia and just under 50% of output, worth $300 million, would be sold locally.[38]

While DeBeers was reorganizing its traditional operations and making various amends, a new potential competitor to the natural diamond quietly began to emerge: laboratory-grown or, as DeBeers would call them, "synthetic" diamonds.

Enter Synthetic Diamonds

Unlike a cubic zirconium which was altogether a different chemical substance, synthetic diamonds were chemically identical to the mined variety.[39] Nearly $50 million worth of synthetic diamonds were sold each year and analysts predicted the market would grow at a CAGR of 45% until 2015, by which time sales would exceed $2 billion.[40] In 2006, 400,000 synthetic diamond carats were produced in the United States and prices rose 20%. "We are selling all that we can produce," admitted one synthetic producer.[41]

There were a handful of synthetic diamond producers in the United States including Adia Diamonds (Michigan/Ontario), Gemesis (Sarasota, Florida), Apollo (Boston,

Massachusetts), Chatham Created Gems (San Francisco, California), and an outfit called Life Gem (Chicago, Illinois) that created lab-grown diamonds with the carbon from a person's ashes. The company's slogan was "Love knows no boundaries; love knows no end." A 1-carat diamond from Gem Life sold for $13,000.[42] Producers typically retailed their collections through a wide variety of jewelers spread mainly throughout the United States. Apollo was scheduled to begin selling its diamonds via its website sometime in 2007.

While there was no disagreement over the fact that, chemically speaking, synthetic diamonds were equal to their natural counterparts, there was disagreement within the industry over what to call them. Preferring the term "cultured," synthetic manufacturers objected to the term synthetic, used by various industry groups including the European Gemological Laboratories, as consumers could very well associate it with imitation stones. The Gemological Institute of America, the organization responsible for developing the color, cut, clarity and carat standards for diamonds back in the late 1950s, used terms synthetic, man-made and laboratory grown interchangeably.

The diamond industry was appealing to the U.S. Federal Trade Commission to prohibit laboratory diamond producers from calling their products "cultured," suggesting that synthetic be the formal descriptor. Their fear was that the natural diamond industry could suffer the same fate as natural pearls did as a result of the introduction of cultured pearls in the early 1900s. According to Gem World International, cultured pearls accounted for more than 95% of all pearls sold globally.[43] "It's essential that synthetics are readily detectable from diamonds and that clear, unequivocal language is used to describe these man-made products," noted a DeBeers spokeswoman.[44]

Process The technology used to make lab-grown diamonds had been around since 1955 when General Electric began making industrial diamonds used to cut hard substances such as stones, ceramics, metals, and concrete.[45] DeBeers followed suit and also began making industrial diamonds and in the late 1950s, DeBeers's Chairman Harry Oppenheimer let it be known that the company would not produce synthetic stones unless it became economically necessary.

There were two types of processes for producing synthetic diamonds. The first process, called high pressure high temperature (HPHT), involved mixing a microscopic diamond grain with graphite and metal and placing the mixture into a 4,000-pound machine the size of a kitchen oven. The grain, put under pressure equal to 58,000 atmospheres and exposed to 2,300 degrees Fahrenheit (close to the melting point of steel), would then grow one atom at a time.[46] It typically took four days to grow a 2.5 carat diamond and approximately 20 kilowatts of energy was used per carat.[47] HPHT was the process General Electric used starting in the 1950s to manufacture industrial diamonds.

The second process was known as chemical vapor deposition (CVD). A more modern and delicate process than HPHT, CVD used a combination of carbon gases, temperature and pressure that replicated conditions present at the beginning of the universe. Atoms from the vapor landed on a tiny diamond chip placed in the chamber. Then the vapor particles took on the structure of that diamond—growing the diamond, atom by atom, into a much bigger diamond. The process could be tweaked to produce diamonds other than those used for jewerly. For instance, by adding enough boron to allow the diamond to conduct a current, the CVD process could turn a diamond into a semiconductor.[48] In 1996, Robert Linares, founder of Apollo Diamond Inc., received a patent for the CVD process he had developed for producing flawless diamonds. As one diamond scientist exclaimed upon putting a CVD diamond under a microscope, "It's too perfect to be natural. Things in nature have flaws. The growth and structure of this diamond is flawless."[49]

Unlike their natural counterparts, the majority of synthetic diamonds came in colors—yellow, green, pink, orange, and blue—filling a market niche. Colored natural diamonds, formed by impurities in the earth (e.g., nitrogen-yellow, boron-blue, natural radiation-green[50]) were rare and therefore prohibitively expensive for most consumers. "The market wants more fancy [colored] diamonds, so this is what we've decided to concentrate on," explained the CEO of Gemesis.[51] Although possible, manufacturing colorless diamonds (a process that entailed removing the nitrogen from yellow stones) was an expensive process.

One challenge the industry faced was that none of the synthetic manufacturers had found a way to produce a synthetic diamond bigger than 1 carat for the jewelry market.

Why Buy Synthetic? Laboratory diamond producers focused on the financial, environmental and political advantages that their product had over natural diamonds. Synthetic diamonds cost anywhere from 15% to 40% less than naturally mined diamonds and sometimes considerably less for colored stones. As Table 1 below shows, a one-carat natural pink diamond could cost upwards of $100,000, while its synthetic counterpart would retail for around $4,000.

Environmentally, compared to a natural diamond, which required several hundred tons of earth be extracted for each carat[52] often at the expense of both human and animal habitats, lab-grown diamonds were considerably more eco-friendly. According to the Canadian Arctic Resources Committee, as far as 200 kilometers downstream from the lake where Canada's Ekati diamond mine sat, environmental destruction, particularly of fish habitats, was seen in numerous lakes and streams. Diamond mining had also taken a toll on land-based widlife habitats. Scientists had observed that caribou and grizzly bears were spending far less time feeding in areas around the mines. Meanwhile diamond mines required the use of diesel fuel to operate, adding to the production of greenhouse gases.[53]

More than their financial and environmental advantages, lab-grown diamond producers emphasized the political advantages of buying a synthetic diamond, namely that consumers would in no way be at risk of acquiring a "blood diamond." A growing number of customers wanted to know where their diamonds came from and wanted a guarantee that they were clean. Once cut and polished, however, it was impossible for consumers to tell which diamonds were blood diamonds. All distinguishing characteristics which identified a diamond's country of origin were washed away with the polishing process.[54]

Measures had been taken by the diamond industry and various governments to assuage agitated consumers and curtail the number of blood diamonds that circulated on the open market and by 2006 blood diamonds made up a mere 1% of the overall diamond trade.[55] Much of this success was attributed to the Kimberley Process Certification Scheme, introduced in 2002, as an attempt by the industry to monitor its own abuses, and as a way to avoid a widespread consumer boycott. The 70 countries that participated in the Kimberley process could only trade with other participants who met the minimum standards. Each participant pledged to prevent the trade of conflict diamonds by implementing stricter monitoring practices which included shipping all diamonds in tamperproof containers with certificates verifying they came from a legitimate source. (Exhibit 1 provides more details on requirements.) Everyone who handled a diamond was responsible for maintaining an identity tag affixed to the stone from the time it was extracted from the ground.[56] Non-compliers were punished. The Democratic Republic of the Congo was ousted in 2004 and Venezuela was threatened with suspension in 2006 after reporting that

Table 1 Natural vs. Lab-Made Diamond Price Comparisons

	Natural	Lab-Made	Cubic Zirconia
Colorless Stones	1 carat = $6,800–$9,100	½ carat = $900–$2,500	1 carat = $5–$15
Colored Stones	1 carat = $9,000 (yellows)–$100,000 (pinks)	1 carat = $2,000–$7,000	1 carat = $10–$15

Source: Vanessa O'Connell, "Gem War," *The Wall Street Journal*, January 13, 2007.

Exhibit 1 **The Kimberley Process Certificate**

Each Participant should ensure that:

(a) a Kimberley Process Certificate (hereafter referred to as the Certificate) accompanies each shipment of rough diamonds on export;

(b) its processes for issuing Certificates meet the minimum standards of the Kimberley Process as set out in Section IV;

(c) Certificates meet the minimum requirements set out in Annex I. As long as these requirements are met, Participants may at their discretion establish additional characteristics for their own Certificates, for example their form, additional data or security elements;

(d) it notifies all other Participants through the Chair of the features of its Certificate as specified in Annex I, for purposes of validation.

Undertakings in respect of the international trade in rough diamonds

Each Participant should:

(a) with regard to shipments of rough diamonds exported to a Participant, require that each such shipment is accompanied by a duly validated Certificate;

(b) with regard to shipments of rough diamonds imported from a Participant: require a duly validated Certificate; ensure that confirmation of receipt is sent expeditiously to the relevant Exporting Authority. The confirmation should as a minimum refer to the Certificate number, the number of parcels, the carat weight and the details of the importer and exporter; require that the original of the Certificate be readily accessible for a period of no less than three years;

(c) ensure that no shipment of rough diamonds is imported from or exported to a non-Participant;

(d) recognise that Participants through whose territory shipments transit are not required to meet the requirement of paragraphs (a) and (b) above, and of Section II (a) provided that the designated authorities of the Participant through whose territory a shipment passes, ensure that the shipment leaves its territory in an identical state as it entered its territory (i.e., unopened and not tampered with).

Minimum requirements for Certificates

A Certificate is to meet the following minimum requirements:

- Each Certificate should bear the title "Kimberley Process Certificate" and the following statement: "The rough diamonds in this shipment have been handled in accordance with the provisions of the Kimberley Process Certification Scheme for rough diamonds"
- Country of origin for shipment of parcels of unmixed (i.e., from the same) origin
- Certificates may be issued in any language, provided that an English translation is incorporated
- Unique numbering with the Alpha 2 country code, according to ISO 3166-1
- Tamper and forgery resistant
- Date of issuance
- Date of expiry
- Issuing authority
- Identification of exporter and importer
- Carat weight/mass
- Value in US$
- Number of parcels in shipment
- Relevant Harmonised Commodity Description and Coding System
- Validation of Certificate by the Exporting Authority

it had no diamond exports for 2005. The process, however, was far from perfect and enforcement was proving to be next to impossible. As one example, Sierra Leone, which accounted for up to 33% of the world's smuggled diamonds, had a mere 200 monitors for the entire country sharing 10 USAID-donated motorcycles.[57]

However, some in the industry felt the Kimberley process was working and that the human rights argument could in fact hurt those it intended to help. As one industry observer stated, "When you're buying mined diamonds, you're helping communities in Africa. When you're buying them made from a machine, you're helping 20 guys in Florida."[58] One international diamond trader took issue with this sentiment stating that working conditions for many Africans involved in the mining business remained appalling, opining, "Conflict-free diamonds should not be confused with ethical diamonds."[59]

A new selling point for the synthetic diamond industry came in early 2007 when the Gemological Institute of America's Synthetic Diamond Report began grading the quality of lab-grown diamonds using the same 4-Cs (cut, carat, color, clarity) rating system used for natural diamonds. Certification papers would now accompany synthetic diamonds just as they did natural stones and would include a note stating, "This is a man-made diamond and has been produced in a laboratory."[60] GIA's public benefit mission required it to "describe and report on synthetics so that consumers can rely on full and proper disclosure" upon entering the marketplace.[61]

Beyond Jewelry Whether or not synthetic diamonds would make a significant dent in the natural diamond market was still unclear. But, many in the industry believed that due to the chemical composition of the diamond and its ability to be used in a wide array of industries, synthetics would inevitably have a bright future beyond the jewelry industry. As microprocessors became hotter, faster, and smaller in accordance with Moore's law, diamonds could be used as a substitute to heat sensitive silicon. Diamond microchips could handle extreme temperatures allowing them to run at speeds that would liquefy ordinary silicon. As a professor of materials science from MIT explained, "If Moore's law is going to be maintained, processors are going to get hotter and hotter. Eventually silicon is just going to turn into a puddle. Diamond is the solution to that problem."[62]

Up until the recent improvements in laboratory technology, there had been three main barriers to using diamonds as an input to semiconductors. First, diamonds had always been viewed as too expensive to use in such a scaled up way. Synthetic diamonds helped address that problem. Second, there had never been a steady and consistent supply of large pure diamonds. One mined diamond did not necessarily have the same electrical properties as the next. CVD produced diamonds solved that problem. Finally, prior to the new processes used for lab created diamonds,

no company or individual had been able to manufacture a negative charged diamond with sufficient conductivity needed to form microchip circuits.[63]

Alongside their use in the semiconductor industry, the thermal conductivity, hardness and transparency of diamonds made them an attractive component for next-generation optics, digital data storage,[64] as well as for biological purposes including skin implanted electrodes due to their ability to resist corrosion from acids and other organic compounds.[65]

The market for industrial diamonds was growing at 10% to 15% a year.[66] Synthetic diamonds accounted for 90% of the industrial market.[67] As the CEO of synthetic diamond manufacturer Apollo remarked, "Man-made diamonds will be with us in many different ways that we can only begin to imagine right now that will materially affect everybody on the planet."[68]

DeBeers Responds

Although DeBeers maintained a fairly nonchalant attitude about the emergence of jewelry-grade synthetic diamonds, there were two ways in which the company was attempting to protect the future of the natural diamond. One way was through its Gem Defensive Programme. In the early years, DeBeers warned jewelers about the arrival of synthetic stones and in 2000, the company began supplying gem labs, at no charge, with machinery designed to distinguish man-made from natural stones. Many synthetic manufacturers, however, were proactively supporting DeBeers's detection efforts by lasering the words "lab-created" on their diamonds. DeBeers had spent $17 million on research to differentiate natural and synthetic diamonds.[69]

A second defensive strategy focused on consumer education. In anticipation of the movie "Blood Diamond," DeBeers launched a completely different kind of diamond advertisement campaign than those of the past. In lieu of the glitzy pictures of model-esque women donning the perfect sparkler, the ads focused on how the industry provided mining communities with access to employment opportunities, schools for its children, and access to anti-HIV drugs for its mine workers, giving off the general sentiment that buying a diamond from Southern Africa was "an act of altruism."[70]

For the most part, however, DeBeers was fairly quiet about the potential threat posed by synthetic diamonds. As a DeBeers spokesperson put it, "Synthetics and diamonds are very different products. Diamonds are unique, ancient, natural treasures—the youngest diamond is 900 million years old."[71] Believing that the "real thing" would trump synthetics, the company was actively searching out new supplies of natural diamonds. In 2004, the company discovered 39 new diamond deposits and signed marketing agreements with producers in Canada, Botswana, India, Democratic Republic of the Congo, the Central African Republic, Russia, Australia, Brazil, and Madagascar.[72]

Conclusion

Lee Mandell walked up to the counter in one of the more reputable jewelry stores in Boston. The salesman asked if he would like some help. Lee responded that he was shopping for an engagement ring but was uncertain as to whether he was in the market for a natural or a synthetic diamond. With a look of utter horror on his face, the salesman said, "You simply can not give your girlfriend a synthetic. I won't let you. The appeal of a diamond is its age and where and how it was created. Where is the romance in something created in a lab by a cold, metallic machine? Besides, the synthetics don't come in sizes larger than 1 carat and I can tell that you want something grander for your loved one."

The jeweler's response was not totally convincing to Lee. His mind kept drifting back to that article he had read about the emerging synthetic diamond industry and the rationale one distributor gave for buying a lab-made diamond: "If you go into a florist and buy a beautiful orchid, it's not grown in some steamy hot jungle in Central America. It's grown in a hothouse somewhere in California. But that doesn't change the fact that it's a beautiful orchid."[73]

Endnotes

1. Karen Goldberg Goff, "Cultivated Carats," *The Washington Times*, February 4, 2007.
2. Danielle Rossingh, "DeBeers Says It Can't Ignore Synthetic Diamonds," *Bloomberg*, May 17, 2007.
3. "Diamonds: Changing Facets," *Economist Intelligence Unit*, February 26, 2007.
4. Karen Goldberg Goff, "Cultivated Carats," *The Washington Times*, February 4, 2007.
5. James Dunn, "Glittering Prizes," *The Australian*, October 4, 2006.
6. "The Global Gems and Jewelry Industry: Vision 2015; Transforming for Growth," *KPMG*, December 2006.
7. Ibid.
8. Ibid.
9. Nicole Itano, "Looking to Africa to Polish Its Diamonds," *The New York Times*, September 17, 2004.
10. "The Cartel Isn't For Ever," *The Economist*, July 17, 2004.
11. John Reed and David White, "Beneficiation: A Chance to Spread Southern African Wealth," *Financial Times*, July 14, 2006.
12. Nicole Itano, "Looking to Africa to Polish Its Diamonds," *The New York Times*, September 17, 2004.
13. Danielle Cadieux, "DeBeers and the Global Diamond Industry," *Ivey Case Study No. 9B05M040*, 2005.
14. Ben Aris, "A Diamond in the Rough," *The Moscow Times*, September 11, 2001.
15. Vanessa Friedman, "The New Rocks on the Block," *Financial Times*, May 10, 2006.
16. James Dunn, "Glittering Prizes," *The Australian*, October 4, 2006.
17. Danielle Cadieux, "DeBeers and the Global Diamond Industry," *Ivey Case Study No. 9B05M040*, 2005.
18. Debora L. Spar, "Continuity and Change in the International Diamond Market," *Journal of Economic Perspectives*, Volume 20, Number 3, Summer 2006.
19. "The Cartel Isn't Forever," *The Economist*, July 17, 2004.
20. Phyllis Berman and Lea Goldman, "Cracked DeBeers," *Forbes.com*, September 15, 2003.
21. Ibid.
22. Nicholas Stein, "The DeBeers Story: A New Cut On An Old Monopoly," *Fortune*, February 19, 2001.
23. Phyllis Berman and Lea Goldman, "Cracked DeBeers," *Forbes.com*, Spetember 15, 2003.
24. Kate Reardon, "Guilt Free Diamonds Sparkle Brighter for Ethical Shoppers," *The Times*, June 17, 2006.
25. "The Cartel Isn't For Ever," *The Economist*, July 17, 2004.
26. Nicholas Stein, "The DeBeers Story: A New Cut On An Old Monopoly," *Fortune*, February 19, 2001.
27. "Diamonds Get Their Sparkle Back," *New Zealand*, February 26, 2007.
28. Danielle Cadieux, "DeBeers and the Global Diamond Industry," *Ivey Case Study No. 9B05M040*, 2005.
29. Debora L. Spar, "Continuity and Change in the International Diamond Market," *Journal of Economic Perspectives*, Volume 20, Number 3, Summer 2006.
30. Nicholas Stein, "The DeBeers Story: A New Cut On An Old Monopoly," *Fortune*, February 19, 2001.
31. Vanessa Friedman, "The New Rocks on the Block," *Financial Times*, May 10, 2006.
32. Greg Gatlin, "Branding Becomes Gem of an Idea," *Boston Herald*, February 11, 2001.
33. Danielle Cadieux, "DeBeers and the Global Diamond Industry," *Ivey Case Study No. 9B05M040*, 2005.
34. David McKay, "A Private Life: Oppenheimer at 60," *miningmx.com*, July 4, 2005.
35. Brendan Ryan, "Nicky Oppenheimer, Private Treasure," *Financial Mail*, August 30, 2002.
36. John Reed and David White, "Beneficiation: A chance to spread southern African wealth," *Financial Times*, July 14, 2006.
37. David White, "A Question of Profile Image and Status," *Financial Times*, June 20, 2006.
38. "Diamonds Get Their Sparkle Back," *New Zealand Herald*, February 26, 2007.
39. Elsa Wenzel, "Synthetic Diamonds Are Still a Rough Cut," *CNET News.com*, February 14, 2007.
40. Melvyn Thomas, "Lab Tag for Synthetic Diamonds," *The Economic Times*, May 19, 2007.
41. Karen Goldberg Goff, "Cultivated Carats," *The Washington Times*, February 4, 2007.
42. Ibid.
43. Vanessa O'Connell, "Gem War," *The Wall Street Journal*, January 13, 2007.
44. Ibid.
45. Ibid.
46. Danielle Rossingh, "Diamonds by Linares," *Bloomberg.com*, July 5, 2007.
47. Elsa Wenzel, "Synthetic Diamonds Are Still a Rough Cut," *CNET News.com*, February 14, 2007.
48. Kevin Maney, "Man Made Diamonds Sparkle with Potential," *USA Today*, October 6, 2005.

49. Joshua Davis, "The New Diamond Age," *Wired*, September 2003.

50. "Diamonddaze," *South China Morning Post*, November 19, 2004.

51. Victoria Finlay, "Diamonds Are No Longer a Girl's Best Friend," *The Daily Telegraph*, December 22, 2006.

52. Elsa Wenzel, "Synthetic Diamonds Are Still a Rough Cut," *CNET News.com*, February 14, 2007.

53. *http://www.carc.org/mining_sustain/diamonds_arent.php.*

54. Sharon Barker, "Diamonds in the Rough," *The Jerusalem Post*, April 6, 2001.

55. Vivienne Walt, "Diamonds Aren't Forever," *Fortune*, December 11, 2006.

56. Debora L. Spar, "Continuity and Change in the International Diamond Market," *Journal of Economic Perspectives*, Volume 20, Number 3, Summer 2006.

57. Vivienne Walt, "Diamonds Aren't Forever," *Fortune*, December 11, 2006.

58. Elsa Wenzel, "Synthetic Diamonds Are Still a Rough Cut," *CNET News.com*, February 14, 2007.

59. "Diamonds: Changing Facets," *Economist Intelligence Unit*, February 26, 2007.

60. "GIA Launches Synthetic Grading Report," *Modern Jeweler*, January 1, 2007.

61. Ibid.

62. Joshua Davis, "The New Diamond Age," *Wired*, September 2003.

63. Ibid.

64. Elsa Wenzel, "Synthetic Diamonds Are Still a Rough Cut," *CNET News.com*, February 14, 2007.

65. Alice Park, "Diamonds De Novo," *Time*, February 12, 2007.

66. Ibid.

67. "Diamonds: Changing Facets," *Economist Intelligence Unit*, February 26, 2007.

68. Elsa Wenzel, "Synthetic Diamonds Are Still a Rough Cut," *CNET News.com*, February 14, 2007.

69. Danielle Rossingh, "DeBeers Says it Can't Ignore Synthetic Diamonds," *Bloomberg*, May 17, 2007.

70. Victoria Finlay, "Diamonds Are No Longer a Girl's Best Friend," *The Daily Telegraph*, December 22, 2006.

71. Amy Keller, "Carat Factory," *Florida Trend*, August 1, 2007.

72. Debora L. Spar, "Continuity and Change in the International Diamond Market," *Journal of Economic Perspectives*, Volume 20, Number 3, Summer 2006.

73. Joshua Davis, "The New Diamond Age," *Wired*, September 2003.

Case 10   World Wrestling Entertainment*

For World Wrestling Entertainment (WWE), 2009 looked like it was going to be another good year. The firm had just signed a deal with WGN America, Tribune Broadcasting's national superstation, which was to run a new program called *WWE Superstars*. The hour-long action-packed weekly show would be produced by WWE and would feature superstars and divas from the entire WWE roster. "WWE programming has a tremendous track record of consistently delivering a diverse and advertiser friendly audience. We fully anticipate that *WWE Superstars* will be a ratings winner for WGN America," said Kevin Dunn, WWE executive vice president of television production.[1]

This was followed by a distribution deal with Eurosport, Europe's leading sports and entertainment group, which would distribute two weekly WWE shows. Under the terms of the two-year agreement, Eurosport would broadcast *This Week in WWE* and *WWE Vintage Collection* in all of its European territories excluding the United Kingdom, delivering WWE programming to over 200 million viewers and 58 countries across the continent. *Vintage Collection* would feature WWE legends such as Stone Cold Steve Austin, The Rock, Hulk Hogan, and Bret 'The Hitman' Hart.

These deals clearly indicate that WWE has moved out of a slump that it endured between 2001 and 2005. During the 1990s, WWE's potent mix—shaved, pierced, and pumped-up muscled hunks; buxom, scantily-clad, and sometimes cosmetically enhanced beauties; and body-bashing clashes of good versus evil—resulted in an empire that claimed over 35 million fans. Furthermore, the vast majority of these fans were males between the ages of 12 and 34, the demographic segment that makes most advertisers drool.

Just when it looked like everything was going well, WWE hit a rough patch. During 2001 the firm experienced failure with a football league, which folded after just one season, and this was followed by a drop in revenues from its core wrestling businesses. WWE was struggling with its efforts to build new wrestling stars and to introduce new characters into its shows. Some of its most valuable younger viewers were turning to new reality-based shows on television, such as *Survivor, Fear Factor* and *Jackass.*

Since 2005, however, WWE has been winning fans back around the world. It has been rebuilding its fan base through live shows, television programming, consumer products, and Internet sales (see Exhibits 1 and 2). In fact, the firm was recently named as one of the top 200 Best Small Companies by *Forbes* magazine. WWE has been turning pro wrestling into a perpetual road show

that makes millions of fans pass through turnstiles worldwide. Its three television programs, *Raw, Smackdown,* and *Extreme Championship Wrestling,* have become the leading shows among male viewers on the nights that they are broadcast. Finally, WWE has been signing pacts with dozens of licensees to sell DVDs, video games, toys, and trading cards (see Exhibits 3 to 5). "We continue to see the distribution of our creative content through various emerging channels," stated WWE's president and CEO, Linda McMahon.[2]

Developing a Wrestling Empire

Most of the success of WWE can be attributed to the persistent efforts of Vince McMahon. He was a self-described juvenile delinquent who went to military school as a teenager to avoid being sent to a reformatory institution. Around 1970, Vince joined his father's wrestling company, Capital Wrestling Corporation. He did on-air commentary, developed scripts, and otherwise promoted wrestling matches. Vince bought Capital Wrestling from his father in 1982, eventually renaming it World Wrestling Federation (WWF). At that time, wrestling was managed by regional fiefdoms, and everyone avoided encroaching on anyone else's territory. Vince began to change all that by paying local television stations around the country to broadcast his matches. His aggressive pursuit of audiences across the country gradually squeezed out most of the rivals. "I banked on the fact that they were behind the times, and they were," said McMahon.[3]

Soon after, Vince broke another taboo by admitting to the public that wrestling matches were scripted. Although he made this admission in order to avoid the scrutiny of state athletic commissions, wrestling fans appreciated the honesty. The WWF began to draw in more fans through the elaborate story lines and the captivating characters of its wrestling matches. The firm turned wrestlers such as Hulk Hogan and Andre the Giant into mainstream icons of pop culture. By the late 1980s, the WWF's *Raw is War* had become a top-rated show on cable and the firm had also begun to offer pay-per-view shows.

Vince faced his most formidable competition after 1988, when Ted Turner bought out World Championship Wrestling (WCW), one of the few major rivals that was still operating. Turner spent millions luring away WWF stars such as Hulk Hogan and Macho Man Randy Savage. He used these stars to launch a show on his own TNT channel that went up against the WWF's major show, *Raw is War.* Although Turner's new show caused a temporary dip in the ratings of the WWF's shows, Vince fought back with pumped-up scripts, mouthy muscle-men, and Lycra-clad women. "Ted Turner decided to come after me and all of my talent," growled Vince, "and now he's where he should be."[4]

In 2001, Vince was finally able to acquire WCW from Turner's parent firm, AOL Time Warner, for a bargain

*This case was developed by Professor Jamal Shamsie, Michigan State University, with the assistance of Professor Alan B. Eisner, Pace University. Material has been drawn from published sources to be used for class discussion. Copyright © 2009 Jamal Shamsie and Alan B. Eisner.

Exhibit 1 **Income Statements** (in millions of dollars)

Period End Date: Period Length:	2008 12/31/08 12 Months	2007 12/31/07 12 Months	2006 12/31/06 8 Months	2006 04/30/06 12 Months	2005 04/30/05 12 Months
Revenue	526.46	485.66	262.94	400.05	366.43
Total revenue	**526.46**	**485.66**	**262.94**	**400.05**	**366.43**
Cost of revenue, total	311.78	298.77	157.09	227.17	213.29
Gross profit	**214.67**	**186.89**	**105.84**	**172.88**	**153.14**
Selling, general, administrative expenses, total	131.3	109.13	61.04	91.87	90.98
Research and development	0.0	0.0	0.0	0.0	0.0
Depreciation/amortization	13.08	9.32	5.56	10.47	11.87
Operating income	**70.29**	**68.43**	**39.24**	**70.54**	**50.29**
Other, net	−6.38	−0.52	0.88	0.55	1.35
Income before tax	**69.36**	**76.47**	**46.15**	**77.9**	**56.36**
Income tax, total	23.94	24.34	14.53	30.88	18.58
Income after tax	**45.42**	**52.14**	**31.62**	**47.01**	**37.78**
Discontinued operations	0.0	0.0	0.0	0.04	1.37
Net income	**45.42**	**52.14**	**31.62**	**47.05**	**39.15**

Source: moneycentral.msn.com and WWE.

price of $5 million. Because of the manner in which he eliminated most of his rivals, Vince has earned a reputation for being as aggressive and ambitious as any character in the ring. Paul MacArthur, publisher of *Wrestling Perspective,* an industry newsletter, praised his accomplishments: "McMahon understands the wrestling business better than anyone else. He's considered by most in the business to be brilliant."[5]

In 2002, the WWF was hit by a British court ruling which held that the firm's *WWF* acronym belonged to the World Wildlife Fund. The firm had to undergo a major branding transition, changing its well-known name and triple logo from WWF to WWE. Although the change in name has been costly, it is not clear that this will hurt the firm in the long run. "Their product is really the entertainment. It's the stars. It's the bodies," said Larry McNaughton, managing director and principal of CoreBrand, a branding consultancy.[6] Linda McMahon stated that the new name might actually be beneficial for the firm. "Our new name puts the emphasis on the 'E' for entertainment," she commented.[7]

Creating a Script for Success

After taking over the firm, Vince began to change the entire focus of the wrestling shows. He looked to television soap operas for ways of enhancing the entertainment value of his live events. Vince reduced the amount of actual wrestling and replaced it with wacky, yet somewhat compelling, story lines. He began to develop interesting characters and create compelling story lines by employing techniques that were quite similar to those being used by many successful television shows. There was a great deal of reliance on the "good versus evil" or the "settling the score" themes in the development of the plots for his wrestling matches. The plots and subplots ended up providing viewers with a mix of romance, sex, sports, comedy, and violence against a backdrop of pyrotechnics.

Over time, the scripts for the matches became tighter, with increasingly intricate story lines, plots, and dialogue. All the details of every match were worked out well in advance, leaving the wrestlers themselves to decide only the manner in which they would dispatch their opponents to the mat. Vince's use of characters was well thought out, and he began to refer to his wrestlers as "athletic performers" who were selected on the basis of their acting ability in addition to their physical stamina. Vince also ensured that his firm owned the rights to the characters that were played by his wrestlers. This would allow him to continue to exploit the characters that he developed for his television shows, even after the wrestler who played a particular character had left his firm.

Exhibit 2 **Balance Sheets** (in millions of dollars, except per-share items)

Period End Date:	2008 12/31/08	2007 12/31/07	2006 12/31/06	2006 04/30/06	2005 04/30/05
Assets					
Cash and short-term investments	177.34	266.35	248.16	280.86	258.06
Cash and equivalents	119.66	135.81	86.27	175.2	56.57
Short-term investments	57.69	130.55	161.89	105.66	201.49
Total receivables, net	60.13	56.6	52.11	67.78	61.9
Accounts receivable—trade, net	60.13	56.6	52.11	67.78	61.9
Accounts receivable—trade, gross	64.85	57.96	54.2	71.48	65.2
Provision for doubtful accounts	−4.72	−1.36	−2.08	−3.7	−3.3
Total inventory	4.96	4.72	3.05	1.79	1.06
Prepaid expenses	37.6	20.05	13.33	11.14	15.19
Total current assets	**280.03**	**347.72**	**317.12**	**362.02**	**336.75**
Property, plant, equipment, total—net	92.37	77.77	67.97	67.57	66.64
Intangibles, net	1.18	2.3	3.33	1.46	2.61
Long-term investments	22.3	0.0	0.0	0.0	0.0
Other long-term assets, total	33.53	42.26	64.86	48.34	35.41
Total assets	**429.41**	**470.06**	**453.29**	**479.39**	**441.41**
Liabilities and Shareholders' Equity					
Accounts payable	18.33	21.95	14.91	19.83	15.67
Accrued expenses	27.12	30.68	25.54	28.6	21.15
Current portion of long-term debt/capital leases	1.0	0.93	0.86	0.82	0.76
Other current liabilities, total	11.88	18.01	20.47	27.59	21.1
Total current liabilities	**58.33**	**71.57**	**61.77**	**76.83**	**58.67**
Total long-term debt	3.87	4.88	5.8	6.38	7.2
Long-term debt	3.87	4.88	5.8	6.38	7.2
Deferred income tax	7.23	10.23	0.0	0.0	0.0
Total liabilities	**69.44**	**86.68**	**67.57**	**83.21**	**65.87**
Common stock	0.73	0.72	0.71	0.71	0.69
Additional paid-in capital	317.11	301.33	286.99	277.69	254.72
Retained earnings (accumulated deficit)	40.97	78.44	97.35	117.43	121.04
Other equity, total	1.17	2.89	0.67	0.36	−0.91
Total equity	**359.97**	**383.38**	**385.71**	**396.18**	**375.53**
Total liabilities and shareholders' equity	**429.41**	**470.06**	**453.29**	**479.39**	**441.41**
Total common shares outstanding	72.79	71.79	71.0	70.56	68.88

Source: moneycentral.msn.com and WWE.

Exhibit 3   **Breakdown of Net Revenues** (in millions of dollars)

	Dec. 31, 2008	Dec. 31, 2007	Dec. 31, 2006	Apr. 30, 2006
Live and televised entertainment	331.5	316.8	183.0	290.8
Consumer products	135.7	118.1	59.2	86.4
Digital media	34.8	34.8	20.7	22.9
WWE films	24.5	16.0	—	—
Total	526.5	485.7	262.9	400.1

Source: WWE.

Exhibit 4   **Breakdown of Operating Income** (in millions of dollars)

	Dec. 31, 2007	Dec. 31, 2006	Apr. 30, 2006
Live and televised entertainment	100.2	57.0	93.9
Consumer products	68.6	26.9	46.4
Digital media	6.3	3.8	2.9
WWE films	(14.8)	(1.1)	(1.3)

Source: WWE.

Exhibit 5   **Percentage Breakdown of Net Revenues**

	Dec. 31, 2008	Dec. 31, 2007	Dec. 31, 2006
Live and televised entertainment:			
Live events	21%	21%	20%
Venue merchandise sales	4	4	5
Television	20	19	22
Pay-per-view	18	20	20
Video on demand	1	1	1
Consumer products:			
Licensing	12	10	6
Home video	12	11	13
Magazine publishing	3	4	3
Digital media:			
WWE.com	3	4	3
WWEShop	4	4	5

Source: WWE.

By the late 1990s Vince had two weekly shows on television. Besides the original flagship program on the USA cable channel, WWE had added the *Smackdown* show on the UPN broadcast channel. Vince developed a continuous story line using the same characters so that his audience would be driven to both shows. But the acquisition of WCW resulted in a significant increase in the number of wrestling stars under contract. Trying to incorporate more than 150 characters into the story lines for WWE's shows proved to be a challenging task. At the same time, the move of *Raw* to the Spike TV channel resulted in a loss of viewers.

In October 2005, WWE signed a new agreement with NBC that moved *Raw* back to its USA channel and gave the firm a new show called *Extreme Championship Wrestling* on the Sci-Fi channel. Its other show, *Smackdown,* was later picked up by the new MyNetworkTV channel, which has been attracting a younger audience. All of these programs have been at the top of the ratings charts, particularly for male viewers, because of the growth in popularity of a new breed of characters such as John Cena and Chris Benoit. The recently completed deal with Eurosport has provided WWE with two new shows that air throughout Europe and feature clips from the three different U.S. programs.

Managing a Road Show

A typical workweek for WWE can be grueling for the McMahons, for the talent, and for the crew. The organization is now putting on more than 300 live shows a year, requiring that everyone be on the road most days of the week. The touring crew includes over 200 members, including stagehands. All of WWE's live events, including those that are used for its two long-standing weekly shows *Raw* and *Smackdown,* as well as the newer ones, are held in different cities. Consequently, the crew is always packing up a dozen 18-wheelers and driving hundreds of miles to get from one performance to the next. Since there are no repeats of any WWE shows, the live performances must be held all year round.

In fact, the live shows form the core of all of WWE's businesses (see Exhibit 6). They give the firm a big advantage in the entertainment world. Most of the crowd shows up wearing WWE merchandise and screams throughout the show. Vince and his crew pay special attention to the response of the audience to different parts of the show. The script for each performance is not set until the day of the show, and sometimes changes are even made in the middle of a show. Vince boasted: "We're in contact with the public more than any entertainment company in the world."[8]

Although the live shows usually fill up, the attendance fee—running on average around $40—barely covers the cost of the production. But these live performances provide content for nine hours of original television programming as well as for the growing list of pay-per-view programming. Much of the footage from these live shows is also being used on the WWE Web site, which is the growth engine for the organization's new digital media business. The shows also create strong demand for WWE

merchandise, ranging from video games and toys to home videos and magazines.

The whole endeavor is managed not only by Vince but by all of his family. Vince's efforts notwithstanding, the development of WWE has turned into a family affair. While the slick and highly toned Vince could be regarded as the creative muscle behind the growing sports entertainment empire, his wife, Linda, began to quietly manage its day-to-day operations. Throughout its existence, she helped to balance the books, do the deals, and handle the details that were necessary for the growth and development of the WWE franchise.

One of Vince and Linda's greatest pleasures has been to see their children move into the business. Their son, Shane, became executive vice president, Global Media and their daughter, Stephanie, moved from being a member of the creative writing team to executive vice president, Creative. "This business is my heart and soul and passion and always has been," Stephanie commented.[9] The family's devotion lies behind much of the success of WWE. "If they are out there giving 110 percent, it's a lot easier to get it from everyone else," said wrestler Steve Blackman.[10]

Pursuing New Opportunities

In 1999, shortly after going public, WWE launched an eight-team football league called XFL. Promising full competitive sport, unlike the heavily scripted wrestling matches, Vince tried to make the XFL a faster-paced, more fan-friendly form of football than the NFL's brand. Vince was able to partner with NBC, which was looking for a lower-priced alternative to the NFL televised games. The XFL kicked off with great fanfare in February 2001. Although the games drew good attendance, television ratings dropped steeply after the first week. The football venture folded after just one season, resulting in a $57 million loss for WWF. Both Vince and Linda insisted that the venture could have paid off if it had been given enough time. Vince commented: "I think our pals at the NFL went out of their way to make sure this was not a successful venture."[11]

Since then, the firm has tried to seek growth opportunities that are driven by its core wrestling business. With more characters at its disposal and different characters being used in each of its shows, WWE has been ramping up the number of live shows, including more in overseas locations. An increase in the number of shows around the globe has been helping to boost the worldwide revenues that the firm is able to generate from its merchandise. International revenue nearly trebled from $45 million in 2002 to $120 million in 2007. The company has opened offices in six cities around the world to manage its overseas operations. "While it is based in America, the themes are worldwide: sibling rivalry, jealousy. We have had no pushback on the fact it was an American product," said Linda.[12]

There has also been considerable excitement generated by the launch of WWE 24/7, a subscriber video-on-demand service. The new service allows the firm to

Exhibit 6　**WrestleMania's Classic Bouts**

Andre the Giant vs. Hulk Hogan

WrestleMania III, March 29, 1987

- **The Lowdown:** A record crowd of 93,173 witnessed Andre the Giant, undefeated for 15 years, versus Hulk Hogan, wrestling's golden boy.
- **The Payoff:** Hogan body-slammed the 500-pound Giant, becoming the sport's biggest star and jump-starting wrestling's first big boom.

The Rock vs. Stone Cold Steve Austin

WrestleMania X-7, April 1, 2001

- **The Lowdown:** The two biggest stars of wrestling's modern era went toe-to-toe in the culmination of a two-year-long feud.
- **The Payoff:** Good-guy Austin aligned with "evil" WWE owner Vince McMahon and decimated the Rock to win the title in front of a shocked crowd.

Hulk Hogan vs. The Ultimate Warrior

WrestleMania VI, April 1, 1990

- **The Lowdown:** The most divisive feud ever—fan favorite Hulk Hogan defended his title against up-and-coming phenom the Ultimate Warrior.
- **The Payoff:** Half the crowd went into cardiac arrest (the other half were in tears) when Hogan missed his patented leg drop and the Warrior won.

Bret Hart vs. Shawn Michaels

WrestleMania XII, March 31, 1996

- **The Lowdown:** Two men who didn't like each other outside the ring locked up in a 60-minute Iron Man match for the title.
- **The Payoff:** After an hour, neither man had scored a pinfall. Finally, Michaels, aka the Heartbreak Kid, pinned Hart in overtime to win the belt.

Kurt Angle vs. Brock Lesnar

WrestleMania XIX, March 30, 2003

- **The Lowdown:** Olympic medalist Angle squared off against former NCAA wrestling champ Lesnar in a punishing bout.
- **The Payoff:** The 295-pound Lesnar landed on his head after attempting a high-flying attack. But he recovered to pin Angle and capture the championship.

Source: TV Guide.

distribute for a fee thousands of content hours consisting of highlights from old shows as well as exclusive new programming. Within a couple of years, WWE 24/7 has shown considerable growth, generating nearly $5 million in revenue.

WWE is also pushing into a new area of digital media, building an e-commerce site that offers broadband and mobile services. The site offers a broad range of content and wide range of merchandise. In a recent tally, it was attracting more than 16 million unique users each month. But the firm has barely tapped into the online ad market, with digital media revenue accounting for less than 10 percent of its total revenue. "The real value creation and growth will come from monetizing the presence on the Internet, where the company has a fanatic and loyal fan base," said Bobby Melnick, general partner with Terrier Partners, a New York money management firm that owns WWE stock.[13]

Finally, WWE has also become involved with movie production, using its wrestling stars and releasing a few films over the last five years. Recent releases included Steve Austin's *The Condemned* and John Cena's

The Marine. Though the films generated only a small amount of revenue in theaters, Linda believes that the movies will earn additional profit from home video markets, distribution on premium channels, and offerings on pay-per-view. In fact, *The Marine* debuted in January 2007 as the top DVD rental.

Reclaiming the Championship?

In spite of the growth of WWE in many forms, Vince and Linda have had to deal with serious challenges. In June 2007, the firm received word that Chris Benoit, one of its most popular wrestlers, had committed suicide after killing his wife and child. This was followed by news that steroids had been found in Benoit's home. Vince went on a public relations blitz to highlight WWE's steroid policy, which the company then bolstered with the suspension of at least 10 performers over the next few months. The firm's revenues dipped slightly, while the value of its stock dropped by 17 percent over the next six months.

More recently, Vince's wrestling empire has been facing a challenge from mixed martial arts (MMA), a growing form of combat sport that combines kickboxing and grappling. Because of its similarity to wrestling, this new combat sport is expected to pull away some of WWE's fans. Although MMA started in Japan and Brazil, the Ultimate Fighting Championship and the International Fight League are promoting it as a new type of spectator sport in the United States. But Dana White, president of the UFC, said: "People have been trying to count the WWE out for years. They are a powerhouse."[14]

The interest in wrestling is most evident each year with the frenzy that is created by WrestleMania, the annual pop culture extravaganza that began at New York's Madison Square Garden in 1985. Since then, it has become an almost weeklong celebration of everything wrestling. No wrestler becomes a true star until his or her performance is featured at WrestleMania, and any true fan must make the pilgrimage at least once in his or her life. Linda points to the continued popularity of this event to reject any suggestion that the fortunes of WWE may be driven by a fad that is unlikely to last. She maintains that the interest in WWE shows will survive in spite of growing competition from all other newer sources of entertainment.

Furthermore, Vince and Linda McMahon claim that their attempts to diversify were never meant to convey any loss of interest in wrestling. In fact, they believe that it was their experience with staging wrestling shows over the years that provided them with the foundation for moving into other areas of entertainment. After all, it was their ability to use wrestling to create a form of mass entertainment that made the WWE such a phenomenal success. In response to critics who question the value of wrestling

matches whose outcomes are rigged, James F. Byrne, senior vice president for marketing, stated: "Wrestling is 100 percent entertainment. There's no such thing as fake entertainment."[15]

Analysts have been impressed by WWE's recent performance. Its stock has done better than most others in its particular category. They also note that the firm has little debt and considerable cash flow, making it a relatively good investment over the longer term. Six out of ten analysts who cover the stock recently rated it as a buy, while the other four said it is a hold. "For long term investors, WWE is very interesting" remarked Michael Kelman, an analyst with Susquehanna Financial Group. "We make money when we are not hot," explained Vince. "When we are hot, its off the charts."[16]

Those who understand don't need an explanation. Those who need an explanation will never understand.

—**Marty,** a 19-year-old wrestling addict, quoted in *Fortune,* October 6, 2000

Endnotes

1. Anonymous. WGN America Enters WWE Ring with WWE Superstars. PR Newswire, January 5, 2009.
2. WWE. World Wrestling Entertainment, Inc., Reports Q3 Results. Press Release, February 23, 2005.
3. Bethany McLean. Inside the World's Weirdest Family Business. *Fortune,* October 16, 2000, p. 298.
4. Diane Bradley. Wrestling's Real Grudge Match. *BusinessWeek,* January 24, 2000, p.164.
5. Don Mooradian. WWF Gets a Grip after Acquisition. *Amusement Business,* June 4, 2001, p. 20.
6. Dwight Oestricher and Brian Steinberg. WW . . . E It Is, after Fight for F Nets New Name. *The Wall Street Journal,* May 7, 2002, p. B2.
7. David Finnigan. Down but Not Out, WWE Is Using a Rebranding Effort to Gain Strength. *Brandweek,* June 3, 2002, p. 12.
8. *Fortune,* October 16, 2000, p. 304.
9. Ibid., p. 302.
10. Ibid.
11. Diane Bradley. Rousing Itself Off the Mat? *BusinessWeek,* February 2, 2004, p. 73.
12. Brooke Masters. Wrestling's Bottom Line Is No Soap Opera. *Financial Times,* August 25, 2008, p. 15.
13. Paul R. La Monica. Wrestling's "Trump" Card. CNN Money.com, March 30, 2007.
14. R. M. Schneiderman. Better Days, and Even the Candidates, Are Coming to WWE. *The New York Times,* April 28, 2008, p. B3.
15. Edward Wyatt. Pro Wrestling Tries to Pin Down a Share Value. *The New York Times,* August 4, 1999, p. C11.
16. *BusinessWeek,* February 2, 2004, p. 74.

Case 11   What's Driving Porsche?*

There are some customers who love the idea that an engineer working on their project in the afternoon was the same guy working on a 911 motor in the morning.

—Managing Director, Porsche Engineering Group[1]

We were working with Volkswagen on the next generation of the Cayenne (which shared its structure with the VW Touareg and Audi Q7) and I wanted a clear connection to safeguard Porsche's interests. We could not do this alone.

—Porsche CEO Wendelin Wiedeking, on decision to acquire VW[2]

In early March 2008, Porsche's supervisory board, which included the chairman of the Volkswagen Group, Ferdinand Piëch, agreed to raise its holding in Volkswagen from 31% to 50% giving it a majority stake.

Porsche's takeover of VW was seen by many as a wise move for the small, independent car company that, unlike rival brands Jaguar, Ferrari, Lamborghini, and Lotus, had managed to avoid being gobbled up by the auto industry's behemoths the likes of General Motors, Chrysler and Ford. There was, however, a key strategic question about Porsche's acquisition of VW that was not receiving a lot of press: Would the long-term stability of Porsche's engineering and design prowess be at risk by bringing VW "in-house"?

Engineering and design were considered the hallmarks of Porsche's competitive advantage, and rather than keeping its R&D under tight wraps, Porsche shared its R&D team of 2,300 engineers with outside companies, and had built a lucrative engineering services business based on this model. Through its 100% wholly-owned customer engineering development company, the Porsche Engineering Group (PEG), Porsche made its wide-ranging expertise in the development and production of vehicles available to clients from a variety of industries. PEG was considered Porsche's "secret weapon, enabling it to employ more engineers than if it worked alone, giving it an edge in product development."[3] Porsche's small size and market niche made it easier for other auto manufacturers to trust that Porsche would not use the technology knowledge

* This case was prepared from published sources by Cate Reavis under the supervision of Professor Rebecca M. Henderson. Professor Henderson is the Eastman Kodak Leaders for Manufacturing Professor of Management. This case is based on research conducted by Julien Heider, Jody Muehlegger and Konrad Haunit (MIT Sloan MBAs, Class of 2008).

attained through its engineering services division to compete head-to-head.

Bringing the R&D functions of the two firms too close together could potentially weaken Porsche engineers' sense of belonging and demotivate them. While Porsche was a company that thrived on healthy profit margins, VW's business model was all about volume. Furthermore, if Porsche engineering was too closely associated with the entire VW portfolio, the company could lose its ability to sell external engineering to other OEMs concerned that Porsche would be sharing strategies and innovations with VW. The question facing Porsche's senior leadership was how to ensure that the integration of VW did not negatively affect Porsche's outside engineering business.

Porsche

Porsche was founded in 1931 by Ferdinand Porsche, along with his son and son-in-law, Anton Piëch, father of VW Chairman Ferdinand Piëch. Known in its early days as the Porsche Engineering Office, Porsche did not start off as an automaker, but rather a firm that sold design and engineering services to other carmakers. In 1934, Adolf Hitler commissioned Porsche to make a "people's car" or "volkswagen." The forerunner to the VW Beetle, the VW Type 60 hit the roads in the mid-1930s, and in 1938 the first plant dedicated to the manufacturing of the VW was opened. It wasn't until 1948, three years after the end of World War II, that Porsche produced its first branded sports car. Within two years, the Porsche 356 series rolled off the production lines.[4]

By 2007, Porsche was the world's most profitable automaker on a per unit basis,[5] a feat that was especially impressive considering it produced just over 100,000 automobiles annually. The company's recorded average revenue per car of €62,568 ($91,974) dwarfed that of Mercedes's €40,445 ($59,454), BMW's €34,766 ($51,106) and was nearly 2.5 times Audi's €27,500 ($40,425).[6] In an industry where scale was usually considered a prerequisite for reducing production costs, the company's operating margins of nearly 20%, double those of Toyota,[7] made Porsche an exception to the rule. In 2007, Porsche's income topped $9.4 billion on revenue of $10 billion. (See Exhibit 1 for select financials of Porsche and the top automakers.) Ironically, over 60% of Porsche's pre-tax earnings came from trading derivatives. All of the options trading Porsche was involved in pertained to its stake in VW. Porsche used the options to hedge against the likelihood that VW's shares would rise after its interest was made public.[8]

Porsche was renowned for the quality of its products. For three consecutive years (2006–2008), Porsche was the top ranking brand in J.D. Power and Associates "Initial Quality Study" (IQS). The study ranked brands by the fewest problems per 100 vehicles. Porsche spent about 12% of revenue on R&D compared to an industry average of

Exhibit 1   **Selected Financials for Carmakers, 2007** (revenue and net income in US$ millions)

	Toyota	GM (automotive)	VW	Ford (automotive)	Honda	Nissan	Fiat Group Automobiles	Porsche
Revenue	262,394	180,000	160,285	154,400	121,200	108,242	39,433	10,060
Net Income	17,146	−39	6,030	−5	6,060	4,823	1,181	9,400
% on R&D	3.6	4.5	4.2	4.9	4.9	4.8	2.8	11.8
Unit Sales	8,900,000	9,286,000	6,191,618	6,553,000	3,652,000	3,700,000	2,233,800	98,652
# Employees	299,394	266,000	329,305	246,000	179,000	180,535	50,542	12,202

Source: Annual Reports.

4% to 6%. (See Figure 1.) Approximately 19% of Porsche employees worked in its R&D facility compared to 6.6% at Volkswagen.

Turnaround   Porsche hit a speed bump in the early 1990s when production processes described as "fat and wasteful"[9] and a weak U.S. economy sent orders plummeting. Between 1986 and 1993 Porsche's sales had fallen from more than 50,000 units to 14,000 units.[10] The company was teetering on the verge of bankruptcy, and there were whispers about a possible takeover.

Newly named Porsche CEO Wendelin Wiedeking orchestrated a turnaround focused on building new core competencies in lean manufacturing and synchronized engineering. In the past, Porsche's celebration of craftwork encouraged individuals to work on their own processes rather than collaborating with the entire production line.

But this soon became a significant handicap for the company. Engineers were tempted to ignore the need for cross-department cooperation on Porsche's own car designs while making handsome profits for Porsche on outside sales of engineering services.[11] As one industry observer put it, "Porsche didn't have a full-fledged, adult-rated simultaneous engineering process in place. It was still struggling to completely shed the rigid, sequential system upon which it had relied for decades."[12] Wiedeking introduced lean manufacturing and the team concepts and processes followed by industry giants Toyota, Nissan and BMW.

Part of the turnaround included the decision to extend Porsche's product line beyond the sports car niche it had dominated for many decades. As Wiedeking explained, "Our strategy is to go beyond the one-dimensional product range we have had so far."[13] As Figure 2 shows, Porsche's

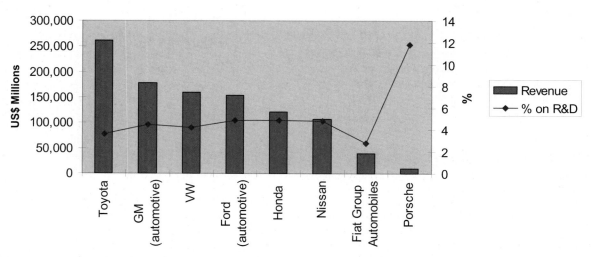

Figure 1 **R&D Expenditure as % of Revenue for Select Automakers (2007)**

Source: Annual Reports.

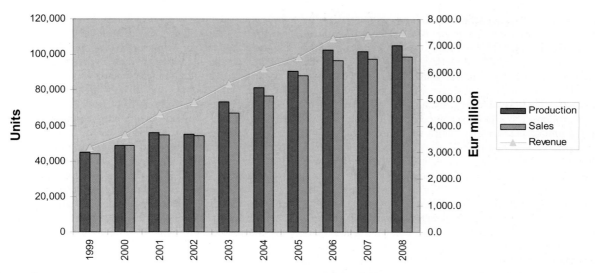

Figure 2 Porsche Sales, Production and Revenue Results (1999–2008)

Source: Porsche Annual Report.

production and sales doubled in just six years as did its revenue through organic growth.

In 2003 Porsche introduced the Cayenne, an SUV which was entering into a crowded field of competitors inhabited by Acura, Audi, BMW, Mercedes, Land Rover, Volkswagen, Volvo, Lexus, and Infiniti. The year the Cayenne was introduced, Porsche's vehicle production shot up from 50,000 to 75,000 units a year.[14] The Cayenne, produced in collaboration with VW at VW's factory in Slovakia and which shared the same frame and doors as VW's Touareg, was derided by many as a "corruption of the brand."[15] In fact the day after Porsche unveiled the first Cayenne prototype, the company's share price fell more than 4%.[16] Porsche CEO Wiedeking was aware of the risk the company was taking in being so closely associated with a mass production carmaker that produced a cheaper SUV.[17] It was a risk he believed would pay off down the road.

Porsche's first foray outside of its sports car market was not an immediate hit. The early version of the Cayenne was plagued with quality problems earning it the least reliable rating from *Consumer Reports* magazine. In its efforts to correct problems with the Cayenne, the company went through a cultural alignment of sorts. As one industry observer noted, "Sports car engineers didn't quite understand the demands of the many female buyers who ended up making the Cayenne their daily runabout."[18] One of those demands was having the capability to unlock the Cayenne from a much further distance. Porsche key fobs were originally designed to unlock sports cars at a very close distance. Porsche went to work to fix this defect and other more serious problems, and by 2006 the Cayenne occupied the No. 1 spot in the IQS

which measured buyer satisfaction in the first 90 days of ownership.[19]

In 2005, Porsche announced that it would be making another move outside its sports car niche. In partnership with VW, Porsche would produce a luxury sedan called the Panamera (named after a Mexican long-distance car race[20]) which would compete against models produced by Mercedes, Aston Martin, and Audi. The Panamera was being built in a low-cost part of East Germany and was scheduled to launch in 2010.[21]

Despite the significant changes to the company's product line, Porsche's outside engineering business, PEG, remained focused on selling services based on Porsche's strength in engineering.

Outside Engineering at Porsche

Providing outside engineering services for carmakers had always been an important part of Porsche's business model. While clients owned the research that Porsche conducted on their behalf, Porsche reserved the right to use the research if the client chose not to, with the understanding that it would not be sold to anyone else. Porsche could test or develop ideas that the company would not have been able to fund on its own.[22]

For several decades VW had been Porsche's main client. In 1949, Porsche and VW signed an agreement under which Porsche was forbidden to design a car for any other company with an engine between 1.0 and 1.3 liters through 1974.[23] The formality of this agreement, however, was in dispute with others characterizing the contract as a "loose agreement" between Ferdinand Porsche and VW's chairman in which about 40% of Porsche's development capacity belonged to VW over a certain number of years.[24]

By the 1980s Porsche was working with a variety of carmakers as well as motorcycle producer Harley-Davidson. In 1991, the company founded Porsche Engineering Services Inc. based outside of Detroit, Michigan, to serve the growing engineering demands of the North American market. As a wholly-owned subsidiary of Porsche AG, PES was able to work with a wide array of carmakers. As the CEO of PES explained, "We're not a competitor to automakers, due to the limited number of vehicles we produce. But we try to convince them that two OEMs working together, rather than one OEM and supporters, makes a difference. We understand the fundamentals of automaking."[25]

In 2001, PES became the North American arm of the Porsche Engineering Group. With 400 employees, PEG was based out of Porsche's R&D center in Weissach, a town of 7,000, 23 kilometers from Porsche's sales, marketing and production activities. PEG engineers had direct access to Porsche's entire engineering team of 2,300 which was also based at Weissach. To reassure clients that their projects would remain confidential, Porsche required all visitors to sign a confidentiality agreement, making them liable if any secrets learned at the Weissach complex were revealed.[26] In addition, the company not only kept the names of its clients confidential, but it also disguised the vehicles tested on its private racing track.

PEG worked with virtually every auto maker in the world, with the exception of those that produced luxury sports cars, and was also involved in projects involving elevators, forklifts, earthmovers, and artificial knees.[27] While revenues of PEG were not disclosed in Porsche's annual report, one source indicated it accounted for 3% of turnover.[28]

Of significant help to PEG engineers was a pool of nearly 600 graduate student interns who worked alongside Porsche's staff engineers. A budget of $30 million was allocated to finance paid internships for the students as well as university or institute-based research studies conducted exclusively for Porsche. Porsche offered its top interns (typically about 10%) full-time jobs, and those students who did not get a job offer became part of an alumni network that would be called on to provide advice on research and technology. A student intern cost 15% of what a full-time employee would cost.[29]

Competitors and Market   The outsourcing of engineering services for carmakers was a growing industry. Some of the big players for the automotive industry included Italy's Stola and U.K.-based Hawtal Whiting and the two U.S. automotive engineering companies MSX International Inc. and Modern Engineering Inc., each of which posted revenues between $100 and $500 million. Lotus Engineering was the only carmaker with whom Porsche competed for outsourced engineering business.

These firms had seen their share of hard times. In the economic downturns of the early 1990s and 2000s, a lot of outsourced activities were brought in-house again. But by the mid-2000s, many of these firms had their sights set on the U.S. auto industry where demand for outsourced engineering was growing in spades due to production challenges and increased market segmentation. Between 1995 and 2005, the number of new car models produced by U.S. automakers grew 50% while the annual sales per model dropped from 100,000 to 75,000 units.[30] As a CEO of a U.S.-based outside engineering firm opined: "Outside engineering is a permanent change in the way business is done. There's no manufacturing business that needs to be vertically integrated anymore. It just costs too much."[31] The CEO of PES echoed this sentiment in 2005: "We're following our customers' changes. The (automakers) have so many niche vehicles, it really compounds their resources. The downsizing and reduction of engineering means there are gaps in some engineering programs. There are opportunities for companies like us to provide that support."[32] As one industry observer noted, globalization was forcing many automakers to make the difficult decision of "entrust[ing] core engineering services, and even the complete end-to-end design and development of a vehicle, to firms with the experience, expertise and sheer innovative talent to help create better products, faster and at lower cost."[33]

Despite the uptick in demand in the U.S. market, PEG sold PES to automotive supplier Magna International in 2006 for an undisclosed sum. In commenting on the transaction, a Porsche executive simply stated, "In the future, we will center all development activities for external customers in our development centre in Weissach for efficiency reasons."[34]

VW Takeover

Porsche made its first move towards VW in 2005 when it acquired a 20% stake, igniting a rumor that its eventual takeover of VW was not an "if" but a "when." After all, it was no secret that VW was an important partner and supplier to Porsche. In March 2007, Porsche upped its stake to 31% by paying €5 billion ($6.6 billion),[35] an investment that was worth €16-17 billion ($23.4 billion)[36] by October of that same year.[37]

On the surface, it appeared as if Porsche and Volkswagen had little, if anything, in common. With 12,000 employees, Porsche was a small independent player in the auto industry focused on the performance sports car market. It typically sold about 100,000 cars a year at prices that ranged from $50,000 to more than $150,000. Historically, it had had few if any direct competitors. Other high-end sports car manufacturers like Ferrari, Maserati and Lamborghini never had the production numbers to threaten Porsche's sales. Companies like Mercedes Benz, BMW and Audi each produced more than 10 times the number Porsche did but for a wide range of vehicles outside the sports car market.

The Volkswagen Group sold more than 6 million cars a year. With 2007 revenue topping $160 billion (Figure 3)

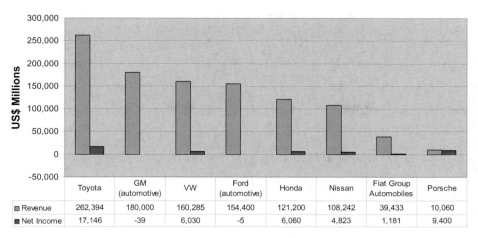

	Toyota	GM (automotive)	VW	Ford (automotive)	Honda	Nissan	Fiat Group Automobiles	Porsche
▥ Revenue	262,394	180,000	160,285	154,400	121,200	108,242	39,433	10,060
▪ Net Income	17,146	-39	6,030	-5	6,060	4,823	1,181	9,400

Figure 3 **Revenue and Net Income for Select Automakers, 2007 (US$ millions)**

Source: Annual Reports.

and 340,000 employees, it was the world's fourth largest carmaker (based on units sold) with a portfolio of eight brands that included Audi, Bentley, Lamborghini, and truck manufacturer Scania, with prices ranging from $18,000 to $250,000. It wasn't until the late 1990s that VW began moving upmarket purchasing Rolls-Royce and Italian sports carmakers Lamborghini and Bugatti all in one year.[38]

Despite their differences, VW and Porsche's histories were intimately intertwined. It was Ferdinand Porsche's engineering company that, in the 1930s, designed the first Volkswagen which later became known as the VW Beetle. A few years later, the first Porsche debuted with some of the same components used on the VW Beetle. More recently, Porsche and VW had built cars that shared platforms and components. In addition to sharing research and development, the two companies' leadership shared familial bonds. Legendary German-Austrian engineer Ferdinand Karl Piëch, the grandson of Ferdinand Porsche, was the chairman of Volkswagen's supervisory board and the Porsche and Piëch families together owned 50% of Porsche's shares and 100% of its voting stock.[39] Their alliance based on old family relationships allowed both companies to develop technology jointly without concern for confidentiality.

The ability to scale and create synergies across a number of areas were two driving forces that led Porsche to secure its partnership with VW. As Wiedeking explained, electronics was one area of particular interest: "Electronics account for 30% to 35% of our development costs. Spreading this investment over 2 million cars instead of Porsche's 100,000 will make a big difference and the components will be cheaper."[40] Furthermore, the capital intensity of R&D and required fixed assets in new technologies would be increasing, making it increasingly difficult for a premium-only OEM to survive unless operating in the context

of a larger OEM. Forming closer ties with VW would also enable Porsche to benefit from VW's more fuel-efficient technologies at a time when new emissions regulations would come into effect.

On a more macro level, by acquiring VW, Porsche was helping protect itself from the ups and downs of the auto sector. As one industry observer wrote, "A huge mainstream global car company like VW was in a better position to weather any marketplace vagaries than a luxury brand like Porsche."[41]

While Porsche looked at the VW takeover as a way to leverage synergies, Porsche and VW would exist as two separate companies that would sit under a new holding company called Porsche SE. (See Exhibit 2.)

A Repeat of Daimler-Chrysler?

While many in the industry believed that Porsche's acquisition of VW was a wise move, others expressed concern that VW would prove to be a distraction for Porsche, particularly at a time when the company was about to enter another new car market with its luxury sedan the Panamera. As one industry observer wrote, "As we've seen at Daimler-Chrysler, when cultural issues are in play, the products can suffer and when the products suffer, so does everything else at a car company."[42]

However, Wiedeking was adamant that the Porsche brand and culture would remain well protected: "Believe me, if you mix the Porsche guys with the Audi guys and VW guys you will have trouble. Each is proud to belong to his own company. My Porsche people are very proud of what they have achieved. They don't want to build a bastard in the future. They want to build a Porsche."[43]

But whether keeping Porsche and VW as separate operations under a Porsche holding company would adequately protect the engineering and design talents that Porsche was known for was not certain. And whether the

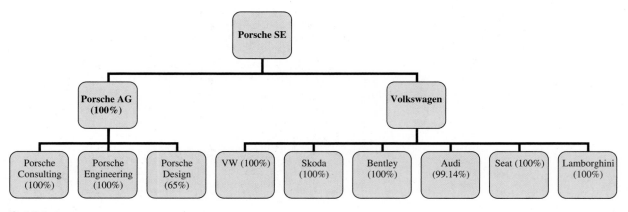

Exhibit 2 **Porsche SE**

Source: Porsche Annual Report.

carmakers that PEG had provided services to in the past would rethink their relationship with Porsche now that it would be producing a number of competing car models was also not certain. What was certain was that Porsche was no longer a small, nimble, carmaker focused solely on the luxury sports car market. With VW now under its wing, Porsche would soon be everywhere.

Endnotes

1. Scott Miller, "Road More Traveled," *The Wall Street Journal*, August 21, 2002.
2. Ray Hutton, "Porsche Set to Take the Wheel at VW," *The Sunday Times*, October 14, 2007.
3. Bret Orekson, "Engineering Is Porsche's Secret Weapon," *Automotive News*, January 15, 2001.
4. Adler, Dennis, *Porsche: The Road from Zuffenhausen*, 2003, p. 76.
5. Jeremy Cato, "Porsche Revs Up for Explosive Growth," *The Globe and Mail*, February 22, 2007.
6. €1 = US$1.47 (December 31, 2007)
7. Gail Edmondson, "Pedal to the Metal," *BusinessWeek*, September 3, 2007.
8. Richard Milne, "Share Options Put Porsche on a Faster Path to Profit," *Financial Times*, November 12, 2007.
9. Tom Mudd, "Back in High Gear," *Industry Week*, February 21, 2000.
10. Ibid.
11. Womack, James and Daniel Jones, *Lean Thinking: Banish Waste and Create Wealth in your Corporation*, 1996, p. 192.
12. Christopher Jensen and Don Sherman, "The Porsche Process," *Automotive Industries*, November 1, 1997.
13. Brandon Mitchener, "Rebounding Porsche Seeks to Shift More Output Abroad," *The Wall Street Journal Europe*, December 6, 1995.
14. Bret Okeson, "Engineering is Porsche's Secret Weapon," *Automotive News*, January 15, 2001.
15. Jeremy Cato, "Porsche Revs Up for Explosive Growth," *The Globe and Mail*, February 22, 2007.
16. Scott Miller, "Road More Traveled," *The Wall Street Journal*, August 21, 2002.
17. Jeffrey Fear and Carin-Isabel Knoop, "Dr. INg. H.c. F. Porsche AG (A): True to Brand?" HBS Case No. 9-706-018, *Harvard Business School Publishing*, 2006.
18. Jeremy Cato, "Porsche Revs Up for Explosive Growth," *The Globe and Mail*, February 22, 2007.
19. Ibid.
20. Stephen Power, "The Family Porsche," *The Wall Street Journal*, July 28, 2005.
21. Jeremy Cato, "Porsche Revs Up for Explosive Growth," *The Globe and Mail*, February 22, 2007.
22. Jeff Daniels, *Porsche: The Engineering Story*, (Somerset, UK: Haynes, 2007), p. 129–131.
23. Randy Leffingwell, *Porsche 911: Perfection by Design*," (Osceola, WI: Motorbooks, 2007), p. 68.
24. Ibid.
25. Gary Kobe and Lindsay Brooke, "How's Outside Engineering," *Automotive Industries*, September 1, 1994.
26. Bret Okeson, "Engineering Is Porsche's Secret Weapon," *Automotive News*, January 15, 2001.
27. Ibid.
28. Scott Miller, "Road More Traveled," *The Wall Street Journal*, August 21, 2002.
29. Sigvald Harryson and Peter Lorange, "Bringing the College Inside," *Harvard Business Review*, December 2005.
30. Terry Kosdrosky, "Switching Gears Pays Off," *Crain's Detroit Business*, October 10, 2005.
31. Stuart F. Brown, "New Products From Rented Brains," *Fortune*, September 4, 2000.
32. Terry Kosdrosky, "Switching Gears Pays Off," *Crain's Detroit Business*, October 10, 2005.
33. Warren Harris, "Engineering Services Outsourcing," *PR Newswire*, January 13, 2009.
34. "Magna Buys Porsche's North American Engineering Services Unit," *Austria Today*, August 10, 2006.
35. €1 = US$1.32 (March 1, 2007)
36. €1 = US$1.42 (October 1, 2007)

37. Ray Hutton, "Porsche Set to Take the Wheel at VW," *The Sunday Times*, October 14, 2007.

38. Jon Ashworth, "Porsche's New Empire," *The Business*, March 31, 2007.

39. Michael Connolly, "Porsche Tightens Grip on VW," *The Wall Street Journal*, November 15, 2006.

40. Ray Hutton, "Porsche Set to Take the Wheel at VW," *The Sunday Times*, October 14, 2007.

41. Jeremy Cato, "Porsche Revs Up for Explosive Growth," *The Globe and Mail*, February 22, 2007.

42. Mark Landler, "Porsche and VW: One Happy Family?" *The New York Times*, December 23, 2007.

43. Ray Hutton, "Porsche Set to Take the Wheel at VW," *The Sunday Times*, October 14, 2007.

Case 12   One Ford: The Shape of Ford Motor Company to Come?*

Despite joining GM and Chrysler in a request for emergency loans from Washington to avoid filing for bankruptcy, Ford had so far been determined not to actually seek use of its portion. Instead, Ford would tap credit lines it had the foresight to establish before credit markets dried up in order to bolster its cash position.[1] Ford might be facing the most challenging times of its history. Low sales had been hurting the company for years, and now macroeconomic issues such as a weak economy, volatile financial markets, and lack of liquidity in the market were adding complications for the already troubled firm. Jim Farley, Ford group vice president for marketing and communications, talking about low sales, said that "consumers and businesses are in a very fragile place. An already weak economy compounded by very tight credit conditions has created an atmosphere of caution."[2]

In January 2009, the struggling automaker posted a full-year net loss of $14.6 billion for 2008, the largest single-year loss in the company's history.[3] Attempts at restructuring Ford had been under way for years. Former CEO Jacques Nasser emphasized acquisitions to reshape Ford, but day-to-day business activities were ignored in the process. When he left in October 2001, Bill Ford took over and emphasized innovation as a core strategy to reshape Ford. Although "morale improved, still U.S. market share continued its decade-long-slide from 25 percent in 1997 to 13.7 percent in January 2009."[4] In an attempt to stem the downward slide at Ford, and perhaps to jump-start a turnaround, Alan Mulally was elected as president and chief executive officer of Ford on September 5, 2006. Mulally, former head of commercial airplanes at Boeing, was expected to steer the struggling automaker out of the problems of falling market share and serious financial losses (see Exhibit 1). Mulally was emphasizing his vision of "One Ford" to reshape the company, which claimed "to remain on track for both its overall and North American Automotive pre-tax results to be breakeven or profitable in 2011."[5] But could Mulally do it?

Why Would Ford Invite In an Outsider?

The Ford empire had been around for over a century, and the company had not gone outside its ranks for a top executive since hiring Ernest Breech away from General Motors Corporation in 1946 (see Exhibit 2).[6] Since taking the CEO position in 2001, Bill Ford had tried several times to find a qualified successor, "going after such

industry luminaries as Renault-Nissan CEO Carlos Ghosn and DaimlerChrysler chairman Dieter Zetsche."[7] Now Mulally had been selected and was expected to accomplish "nothing less than undoing a strongly entrenched management system put into place by Henry Ford II almost 40 years ago"—a system of regional fiefdoms around the world that had sapped the company's ability to compete in today's global industry and one that Chairman Bill Ford couldn't or wouldn't unwind.[8]

It had become more common to hire a CEO from outside the family or board. According to Joseph Bower from Harvard Business School, around one-third of the time at S&P 500 firms, and around 40 percent of the time at companies that were struggling with problems in operations or financial distress, an outsider was appointed as CEO. The reason might be to get a fresh point of view or to get the support of the board. "Results suggest that forced turnover followed by outsider succession, on average, improves firm performance."[9] Bill Ford claimed that to undertake major changes in Ford's dysfunctional culture, an outsider was more qualified than even the most proficient auto industry insider.[10]

An outsider CEO might also help restore faith in Ford management among investors, who had been discontented with the Ford family's high dividends and extravagant lifestyle. The Ford family controlled about 40 percent of the company's voting shares through their ownership of all its class B stock and holdings of common stock. The class B family shares had almost the same market value as that of common stock, but the voting rights of the family shares were exceptionally high by industry standards (see Exhibits 3 and 4). The dividend stream had been an annuity, which over the years had enabled various family members to own a football team, fund museums and philanthropic causes, and even promote the Hare Krishna movement. Given that the company was experiencing serious financial problems, these activities had raised stockholder dissent, as the annual retained earnings in the past had been dissipated as dividends instead of reinvested in firm operations or acquisitions to increase the net value of the firm.

Mulally—The New Savior

Alan Mulally came from a metal-bending business that, like automaking, was influenced by global competition, had a unionized workforce, and was subject to complex regulations and rapidly changing technologies.[11] Although he was not an auto guy, he had a proven record in an industry that faced issues similar to those faced by the automobile industry, and a lot of his expertise and management techniques were highly transferable. In his own words, "Everybody says, well, I'm not a car guy, so you couldn't make a contribution here. But I'm a product (guy) and I'm a designer."[12]

* This case study was prepared by Professor Helaine J. Korn of Baruch College, City University of New York; Professor Naga Lakshmi Damaraju of the Indian School of Business; and Professor Alan B. Eisner of Pace University. The purpose of the case is to stimulate class discussion rather than to illustrate effective or ineffective handling of a business situation. Copyright © 2009 Helaine Korn, Naga Damaraju, and Alan Eisner.

Exhibit 1 Ford Motor Company and Subsidiaries: Income Statements (in millions, except per-share amounts; year-end December 31)

	2008	2007	2006
Sales and revenues			
Automotive sales	$129,166	$154,379	$143,249
Financial Services revenues	17,111	18,076	16,816
Total sales and revenues	146,277	172,455	160,065
Costs and expenses			
Automotive cost of sales	127,103	142,587	148,866
Selling, administrative and other expenses	21,430	21,169	19,148
Goodwill impairment	—	2,400	—
Interest expense	9,682	10,927	8,783
Financial Services provision for credit and insurance losses	1,874	668	241
Total costs and expenses	160,089	177,751	177,038
Automotive interest income and other non-operating income/(expense), net	(755)	1,161	1,478
Automotive equity in net income/(loss) of affiliated companies	163	389	421
Income/(Loss) before income taxes	(14,404)	(3,746)	(15,074)
Provision for/(Benefit from) income taxes	63	(1,294)	(2,655)
Income/(Loss) before minority interests	(14,467)	(2,452)	(12,419)
Minority interests in net income/(loss) of subsidiaries	214	312	210
Income/(Loss) from continuing operations	(14,681)	(2,764)	(12,629)
Income/(Loss) from discontinued operations	9	41	16
Net Income/(loss)	$(14,672)	$ (2,723)	$(12,613)
Average number of shares of Common and Class B Stock outstanding	2,273	1,979	1,879
Amounts per share of common and class B stock			
Basic income/(loss)			
Income/(Loss) from continuing operations	$ (6.46)	$ (1.40)	$ (6.73)
Income/(Loss) from discontinued operations	—	0.02	0.01
Net income/(loss)	$ (6.46)	$ (1.38)	$ (6.72)
Diluted Income/(loss)			
Income/(Loss) from continuing operations	$ (6.46)	$ (1.40)	$ (6.73)
Income/(Loss) from discontinued operations	—	0.02	0.01
Net income/(loss)	$ (6.46)	$ (1.38)	$ (6.72)
Cash dividends	$ —	$ —	$ 0.25

Source: Ford Motor Company.

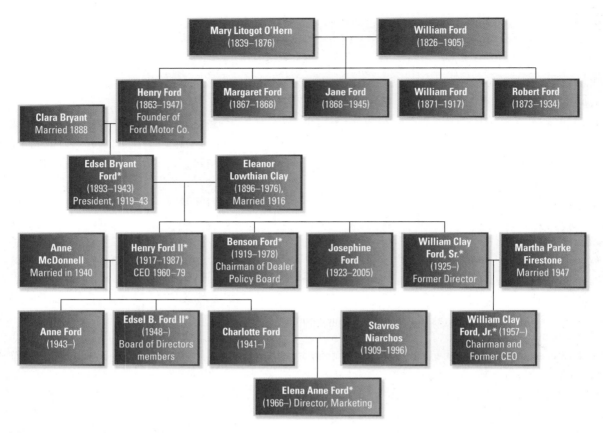

Exhibit 2 Ford Family Tree

Note: Family tree includes descendants of Henry Ford who worked at Ford Motor Co. and their children.

*Ford Family members who have worked at Ford Motor Co.
Source: Benson Ford Research Center, WSJ research.

Prior to joining Ford, Mulally served as executive vice president of the Boeing Company and as president and chief executive officer of Boeing Commercial Airplanes. In those roles, he was responsible for all the Boeing Company's commercial airplane programs and related services.[13] The advanced 777 aircraft, which Mulally led the development of in the early 1990s, became the most popular twin-engine jet in its class and was a testimony of Mulally's product and technology ingenuity. Under his leadership, Boeing regained its market leadership from Airbus. The appointment of Mulally at Ford was seen by the market as a move to utilize his experience and success in managing manufacturing and assembly lines to help shape the future of Ford.

Bill Ford praised Mulally as "an outstanding leader and a man of great character."[14] He noted that Mulally had applied many of the lessons from Ford's success in developing the Taurus to Boeing's creation of the revolutionary Boeing 777 airliner. "Clearly, the challenges Boeing faced in recent years have many parallels to our own," said Bill Ford about Mulally's appropriateness for the top position at Ford.[15] In his e-mail to Ford employees announcing the appointment of Mulally, Bill Ford wrote, "Alan has deep experience in customer satisfaction, manufacturing, supplier relations and labor relations, all of which have applications to the challenges of Ford. He also has the personality and team-building skills that will help guide our Company in the right direction."[16]

Nonetheless, when Mulally took over the steering wheel, Ford was already poised to make significant structural changes as the company announced details of its accelerated "Way Forward" plan. Moreover, the company seemed to indicate that Mulally's appointment would not change the timelines and decisions associated with the restructuring actions, according to analyst Himanshu Patel of J. P. Morgan. This indicated that in spite of the appointment of Mulally as CEO, much of the decision making still remained with Bill Ford, who said he would remain "extremely active" in the business.

What Changes Did the New CEO Bring In?

In his effort to point Ford in the right direction, Mulally flew to Japan in January 2007 to meet with top executives of Ford's toughest competitor, Toyota, to seek their advice.[17]

Exhibit 3 Ford Motor Company and Subsidiaries: Sector Balance Sheets (in millions)

	December 31, 2008	December 31, 2007
Assets		
Automotive		
Cash and cash equivalents	$ 6,377	$ 20,678
Marketable securities	9,296	2,092
Loaned securities	—	10,267
Total cash, marketable and loaned securities	15,673	33,037
Receivables, less allowances of $221 and $197	3,464	4,530
Inventories	8,618	10,121
Deferred income taxes	302	532
Other current assets	4,032	5,514
Current receivable from Financial Services	2,035	509
Total current assets	34,124	54,243
Equity in net assets of affiliated companies	1,069	2,283
Net property	28,352	35,979
Deferred income taxes	7,204	9,268
Goodwill and other net intangible assets	1,584	2,051
Assets of discontinued/held-for-sale operations	—	7,537
Other assets	1,512	5,614
Non-current receivable from Financial Services	—	1,514
Total Automotive assets	73,845	118,489
Financial Services		
Cash and cash equivalents	15,672	14,605
Marketable securities	8,607	3,156
Finance receivables, net	96,101	112,733
Net investment in operating leases	23,120	30,309
Retained interest in sold receivables	92	653
Equity in net assets of affiliated companies	523	570
Goodwill and other net intangible assets	9	18
Assets of discontinued/held-for-sale operations	198	—
Other assets	7,345	7,217
Total Financial Services assets	151,667	169,261
Intersector elimination	(2,535)	(2,023)
Total assets	$222,977	$285,727

(*continued*)

Exhibit 3 Ford Motor Company and Subsidiaries: Sector Balance Sheets (in millions) (*continued*)

	December 31, 2008	December 31, 2007
Liabilities and stockholders' equity		
Automotive		
Trade payables	$ 10,635	$ 15,718
Other payables	2,167	3,237
Accrued liabilites and deferred revenue	32,395	27,672
Deferred income taxes	2,790	2,671
Debt payable within one year	1,191	1,175
Total current liabilities	49,178	50,473
Long-term debt	24,655	25,779
Other liabilities	24,815	41,676
Deferred income taxes	614	783
Liabilities of discontinued/held-for-sale operations	—	4,824
Total Automotive liabilities	99,262	123,535
Financial Services		
Payables	1,970	1,877
Debt	128,842	141,833
Deferred income taxes	3,280	6,043
Other liabilities and deferred income	6,184	5,390
Liabilities of discontinued/held-for-sale operations	55	—
Payable to Automotive	2,035	2,023
Total Financial Services liabilities	142,366	157,166
Minority interests	1,195	1,421
Stockholders' equity		
Capital stock		
Common Stock, par value $0.01 per share (2,341 million shares issued of 6 billion authorized)	23	21
Class B Stock, par value $0.01 per share (71 million shares issued of 530 million authorized)	1	1
Capital in excess of par value of stock	9,076	7,834
Accumulated other comprehensive income/(loss)	(10,085)	(558)
Treasury stock	(181)	(185)
Retained earnings/(Accumulated deficit)	(16,145)	(1,485)
Total stockholders' equity	(17,311)	5,628
Intersector elimination	(2,535)	(2,023)
Total liabilities and stockholders' equity	**$222,977**	**$285,727**

Source: Ford Motor Company.

Exhibit 4 Ford Motor Company and Subsidiaries: Sector Statements of Cash Flows (in millions, year-end December 31)

	2008		2007		2006	
	Automotive	Financial Services	Automotive	Financial Services	Automotive	Financial Services
Cash flows from operating activities of continuing operations						
Net cash flows from operating activities	$(12,440)	$9,107	$8,725	$6,402	$(4,172)	$7,316
Cash flows from investing activities of continuing operations						
Capital expenditures	(6,620)	(76)	(5,971)	(51)	(6,809)	(39)
Acquisitions of retail and other finance receivables and operating leases	—	(44,562)	—	(55,681)	—	(59,793)
Collections of retail and other finance receivables and operating leases	—	42,479	—	45,518	—	41,867
Net (increase)/decrease in wholesale receivables	—	2,736	—	1,927	—	6,113
Purchases of securities	(41,347)	(23,831)	(2,628)	(8,795)	(4,068)	(19,610)
Sales and maturities of securities	43,617	18,429	2,686	15,974	4,865	13,591
Settlements of derivatives	1,157	1,376	1,051	(190)	308	178
Proceeds from sales of retail and other finance receivables and operating leases	—	—	—	708	—	5,120
Proceeds from sale of businesses	3,156	3,698	1,079	157	56	—
Cash paid for acquisitions	(13)	—	—	—	—	—
Transfer of cash balances upon disposition of discontinued/held-for-sale operations	(928)	—	(83)	—	(4)	—
Investing activity from Financial Services	9	—	—	—	1,185	—
Investing activity to Financial Services	—	—	(18)	—	(1,400)	—
Other	40	276	19	(230)	(290)	129
Net cash (used in)/Provided by investing activities	(929)	525	(3,865)	(663)	(6,157)	(12,444)
Cash flows from financing activities of continuing operations						
Cash dividends	—	—	—	—	(468)	—
Sales of Common Stock	756	—	250	—	431	—
Purchases of Common Stock	—	—	(31)	—	(183)	—

(continued)

Exhibit 4 Ford Motor Company and Subsidiaries: Sector Statements of Cash Flows (in millions, year-end December 31) *(continued)*

	2008		2007		2006	
	Automotive	Financial Services	Automotive	Financial Services	Automotive	Financial Services
Changes in short-term debt	104	(5,224)	(90)	1,009	414	(6,239)
Proceeds from issuance of other debt	203	41,960	240	32,873	12,254	46,004
Principal payments on other debt	(594)	(45,281)	(837)	(38,594)	(758)	(35,843)
Financing activity from Automotive	—	—	—	18	—	1,400
Financing activity to Automotive	—	(9)	—	—	—	(1,185)
Other	(252)	(352)	35	(123)	(147)	(192)
Net cash (used in)/provided by financing activities	217	(8,906)	(433)	(4,817)	11,543	3,945
Effect of exchange rate changes on cash	(309)	(499)	506	508	104	360
Net change in intersector receivables/payables and other liabilities	(840)	840	(291)	291	1,321	(1,321)
Net increase/(decrease) in cash and cash equivalents from continuing operations	(14,301)	1,067	4,642	1,721	2,639	(2,144)
Cash flows from discontinued operations						
Cash flows from operating activities of discontinued operations	—	—	16	10	(11)	—
Cash flows from investing activities of discontinued operations	—	—	—	—	—	—
Cash flows from financing activities of discontinued operations	—	—	—	—	—	—
Net increase/(decrease) in cash and cash equivalents	$(14,301)	$ 1,067	$ 4,658	$ 1,731	$ 2,628	$(2,144)
Cash and cash equivalents at January 1	$ 20,678	$ 14,605	$16,022	$12,874	$13,373	$15,018
Cash and cash equivalents of discontinued/held-for-sale operations at January 1	—	—	(2)	—	19	—
Net increase/(decrease) in cash and cash equivalents	(14,301)	1,067	4,658	1,731	2,628	(2,144)
Less: Cash and cash equivalents of discontinued/held-for-sale operations at December 31	—	—	—	—	2	—
Cash and cash equivalents at December 31	$ 6,377	$ 15,672	$20,678	$14,605	$16,022	$12,874

Source: Ford Motor Company.

This was a huge break from the Ford tradition, and only an outsider CEO would have the courage and imagination to openly try to learn from foreign competitors.

Mulally had set his own priorities for fixing Ford: "At the top of the list, I would put dealing with reality."[18] The newly elected CEO signaled that "the bigger-is-better worldview that has defined Ford for decades was being replaced with a new approach: Less is More."[19] Ford needed to pay more attention to cutting costs and transforming the way it did business than to traditional measurements such as market share.[20] The vision was to have a smaller and more profitable Ford. There were echoes in Detroit of Mulally's smaller-is-better thinking. GM was in the middle of its own revamping plan, and Chrysler was also preparing a plan of cutbacks.[21] "Less is More" could be a new trend in the auto industry.

Mulally's cutback plan built on the 14 plant closures and 30,000-plus job cuts announced by Ford in January 2007. Ford's new plan added two more North American plants to the closure list and exceeded the targeted $5 billion in cost cuts by the end of 2008,[22] but it pushed back a target for North American profitability by one year to 2009 and then again to 2011.[23] The company targeted seven vehicle manufacturing sites for closure and planned to have optimum capacity at that point. At the same time, it also planned to increase the plant utilization and production levels in each production unit, while focusing more on larger, more fuel-efficient vehicles. The overall strategy seemed to be toward restructuring as a tool to obtain operating profitability at lower volume and with a changing mix of products that better appealed to the market.

Mulally also refocused the company on the Ford brand when he announced a formal review of Volvo in July 2007 as the first step to putting the division up for sale. Volvo had been acquired eight years earlier to be part of the Premier Automotive Group of Ford, among Jaguar, Aston Martin, and Land Rover.[24] However, Volvo's primary selling point of superior safety had been challenged as other manufacturers made advances in safety technologies in their own brands. Ford was also reviewing bids for Jaguar and Land Rover, both of which had lost money in four out of the five previous years. Mulally said that the "real opportunity going forward is to integrate and leverage our Ford assets around the world" and decide on the best mix of brands in the company's portfolio.[25]

Since his appointment, Mulally had made some structural and procedural changes in the company. For instance, instead of discussing business plans monthly or semiannually as they used to do at Ford, executives now met with Mulally weekly. The in-depth sessions were a contrast to executives' previous efforts to explain away bad news, said Donat R. Leclair, Ford's chief financial officer. "The difference I see now is that we're actually committed to hitting the numbers. Before, it was a culture of trying to explain why we were off the plan. The more eloquently you could explain why you were off the plan, the more easy it was to change the plan."[26]

Mulally also did some senior executive reorganization at Ford, and many of the newly appointed executives reported to him directly, including a global head of product development. In addition, the head of worldwide purchasing, the chief of quality and advanced manufacturing, the head of information technology, the chief technical officer, and the leaders of Ford's European division, its Asia, Pacific, and Africa units, and its Americas unit all reported directly to him.[27]

A Shift toward Smaller and More Fuel-Efficient Cars

The global economic downturn and financial crisis had a significant impact on the global sales volumes in the auto industry, which were likely to decline over 10 percent in 2009.[28] See Exhibit 5 for weakening vehicle sales figures in the U.S. market. Mulally clearly understood that the once profitable business of manufacturing and selling trucks and SUVs was history. Oil prices had been persistently increasing over the last few years. This caused a dramatic change in consumers' car buying habits, reducing the demand for large vehicles. And that was not all: The diminished demand for SUVs resulted in a situation in which leased cars returned at the end of the lease period were being sold for much less than their residual values. Adjusting these residual values to their fair values

Exhibit 5 **Vehicle Sales by Segment, January 2009**

	January 2009	% Change from January 2008
Cars	315,863	−36.3
Midsize	143,726	−39.7
Small	112,073	−30.7
Luxury	54,934	−35.1
Large	5,130	−54.3
Light-duty trucks	341,113	−37.8
Pickup	100,500	−38.3
Crossover	129,820	−27.5
Minivan	34,102	−48.1
Midsize SUV	36,423	−52.6
Large SUV	15,935	−46.8
Small SUV	16,004	−12.5
Luxury SUV	8,329	−47.4
Total SUV/Crossover	206,511	−35.4
Total SUV	76,691	−45.6
Total Crossover	129,820	−27.5

Source: *www.motorintelligence.com.*

contributed to the losses.[29] Brenda Hines, spokeswoman for Ford Credit, said that "about 85 percent of the impaired vehicles were trucks and SUVs".[30]

The core strategy at Ford centered around a change in products, shifting to smaller and more fuel-efficient cars. Ford would import European-made small vehicles, the European Focus and Fiesta, into North America. It also planned to convert three truck-manufacturing plants to small-car production.[31] The Ford, Lincoln, and Mercury lines would all be upgraded, emphasizing fuel-economy improvement and the introduction of hybrid cars. By the end of 2010, two-thirds of spending would be on cars and crossovers–up from one-half in 2009.[32]

In 2009, the first applications of Ford's EcoBoost engines were introduced. EcoBoost used direct-injection technology for up to 20 percent better fuel economy, up to 15 percent fewer CO_2 emissions, and superior driving performance. The goal was to offer this engine on more than 80 percent of the North American–manufactured cars by the end of 2012.[33]

Globalizing the Ford Brand

In the auto industry it was common practice that different regions cooperated and companies basically sold the same cars around the world. This was not the case at Ford. Since it had set up its European operations, Ford Europe and Ford North America had gone separate ways. Moreover, due to Ford Europe's relative success while Ford North America was faltering, Ford Europe was reluctant to cooperate with changes that would bring the two into greater alignment. Nonetheless, Mulally was committed to making this happen.[34]

Under the One Ford vision, Mulally intended to globalize the Ford brand, meaning that all Ford vehicles competing in global segments would be the same in North America, Europe, and Asia within the next five years.[35] The company was looking for a reduction of complexity, and thus costs, in the purchasing and manufacturing processes. The idea was to deliver more vehicles worldwide from fewer platforms

and to maximize the use of common parts and systems. Ford was uniquely positioned to take advantage of its scale, global products, and brand to respond to the changing marketplace.[36] "We grew up regionally, Toyota grew up globally, essentially, and so we are going to try to use the best of those worlds going forward,"[37] said Mulally.

About the Ford Motor Company

Ford Motor had been sinking since 1999, when profits reached a remarkable $7.2 billion ($5.86 per share) and pretax income was $11 billion. At that time people even speculated that Ford would soon overtake General Motors as the world's number-one automobile manufacturer.[38] But soon Toyota, through its innovative technology, management philosophy of continuous improvement, and cost arbitrage due to its presence in multiple geographic locations, overtook the giants—GM and Ford. Compounding this were Ford's internal organizational problems and a failed diversification strategy led by Jacques Nasser, the CEO at that time. Ford's market share began to drop—from 25 percent in 1999 to 13.7 percent in 2009 (see Exhibits 6 and 7),[39] with major blows to market share in the light-vehicle segment. Moreover, Ford's stock prices decreased significantly over the last decade. While stocks traded at close to $60 in February 1999, prices in February 2009 were as low as $1.58.[40] See Exhibit 8 for Ford's stock performance compared to that of General Motors and the Standard & Poor's (S&P) 500.

In 2006, Chevrolet outsold Ford for the first time since 1986 in the sport utility vehicle market. Despite an extensive mechanical update, the much-improved Ford Explorer, which had been the world's best-selling sport utility vehicle, fell behind the dated Chevy TrailBlazer in sales. It did not help that the new Explorer looked just like the model it replaced. The long-neglected Ford Ranger, which had been the top-selling small pickup, fell behind competing models from both Toyota Motor and Chevrolet, and despite 20 years of trying, Ford had never been able to build a competitive minivan. Ford's most successful

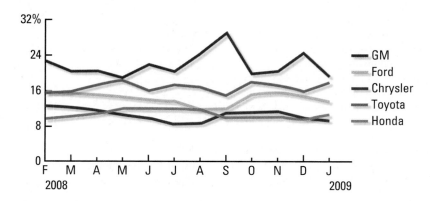

Exhibit 6 U.S. Market Share, 2008–2009

Source: *www.motorintelligence.com.*

Exhibit 7 Sales and Share of Total Market, by Manufacturer

	Sales			Market Share	
	Jan. 2009	Jan. 2008	% Chg	Jan. 2009	Jan. 2008
General Motors Corp.	127,243	249,154	−48.9	19.4	23.9
Total Cars	43,319	103,006	−57.9	6.6	9.9
Domestic Car	41,724	97,686	−57.3	6.4	9.4
Import Car	1,595	5,320	−70.0	0.2	0.5
Total Light Trucks	83,924	146,148	−42.6	12.8	14.0
Domestic Truck	83,924	146,148	−42.6	12.8	14.0
Import Truck	. . .	. . .	n.a.	. . .	. . .
Ford Motor Company	90,131	147,717	−39.0	13.7	14.1
Total Cars	28,707	44,259	−35.1	4.4	4.2
Domestic Car	28,707	44,259	−35.1	4.4	4.2
Import Car	. . .	. . .	n.a.	. . .	. . .
Total Light Trucks	61,424	103,458	−40.6	9.3	9.9
Domestic Truck	61,424	103,458	−40.6	9.3	9.9
Import Truck	. . .	. . .	n.a.	. . .	. . .
Chrysler LLC	62,157	137,392	−54.8	9.5	13.2
Total Cars	15,719	43,167	−63.6	2.4	4.1
Domestic Car	15,676	43,043	−63.6	2.4	4.1
Import Car	43	124	−65.3	. . .	. . .
Total Light Trucks	46,438	94,225	−50.7	7.1	9.0
Domestic Truck	46,438	94,225	−50.7	7.1	9.0
Import Truck	. . .	. . .	n.a.	. . .	. . .
Toyota Motor Sales USA Inc.	117,287	171,849	−31.7	17.9	16.5
Total Cars	67,263	94,586	−28.9	10.2	9.1
Domestic Car	38,277	55,438	−31.0	5.8	5.3
Import Car	28,986	39,148	−26.0	4.4	3.7
Total Light Trucks	50,024	77,263	−35.3	7.6	7.4
Domestic Truck	27,985	40,607	−31.1	4.3	3.9
Import Truck	22,039	36,656	−39.9	3.4	3.5
American Honda Motor Co Inc.	71,031	98,511	−27.9	10.8	9.4
Total Cars	40,532	55,345	−26.8	6.2	5.3
Domestic Car	30,562	40,632	−24.8	4.7	3.9
Import Car	9,970	14,713	−32.2	1.5	1.4
Total Light Trucks	30,499	43,166	−29.3	4.6	4.1
Domestic Truck	26,089	30,817	−15.3	4.0	2.9
Import Truck	4,410	12,349	−64.3	0.7	1.2
Totals:					
Total Car	315,863	496,067	−36.3	48.1	47.5
Domestic Car	87,745	190,432	−53.9	13.4	18.2
Import Car	228,118	305,635	−25.4	34.7	29.3
Total Truck	341,113	548,587	−37.8	51.9	52.5
Domestic Truck	191,786	343,831	−44.2	29.2	32.9
Import Truck	149,327	204,756	−27.1	22.7	19.6
Total Light Vehicle Sales	656,976	1,044,654	−37.1	100.0	100.0

Source: *www.motorintelligence.com*

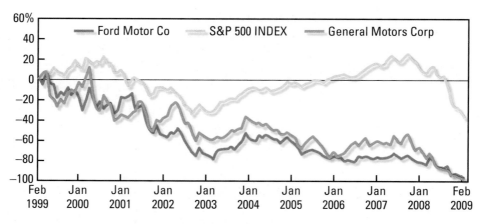

Exhibit 8 **Ford 10-Year Stock Price History**

Source: MSN Money.

vehicles were the F-series pickup trucks (see Exhibits 9 and 10). In 2008, for the 27th consecutive year, Ford F-series was ranked as America's top-selling vehicle.[41]

The company also experienced serious financial problems. Ford's turnaround plan aimed to cut $5 billion in costs by the end of 2008 by slashing 10,000 white-collar workers and offering buyouts to all of its 75,000 unionized employees. The loss, including restructuring costs, was Ford's largest quarterly loss since the first quarter of 1992, when the company lost $6.7 billion due mainly to accounting changes. "Ford and the entire auto industry faced an extraordinary slowdown in all major global markets in the fourth quarter that clearly had an impact on our results,"[42] commented Mullaly.

Automobile Industry in the United States

The automotive industry in the United States was a highly competitive, cyclical business. The number of cars and trucks sold to retail buyers, or "industry demand," varied substantially from year to year depending on "general economic situations, the cost of purchasing and operating cars and trucks, the availability of credit and fuel." Because cars and trucks were durable items, consumers could wait to replace them; industry demand reflected this factor (see Exhibit 11).

Competition in the United States intensified in the last few decades with Japanese carmakers gaining a foothold in the market. To counter the problem of being viewed as foreign, Japanese companies had set up production facilities in the United States and thus gained acceptance from American consumers. Production quality and lean production were judged to be the major weapons that Japanese carmakers used to gain an advantage over American carmakers. "The Toyota Motor Company of Japan issued a 2007 forecast that would make it first in global sales, ahead of General Motors, which has been the world's biggest auto company since 1931."[43] For American consumers, Toyota vehicles have been "a better value proposition"

than Detroit's products, said Mulally, who was the first Detroit leader who readily said he was an avid student of Toyota.[44] However, even Toyota's sales were hurt by the weakened economy, and the Japanese carmaker cut its annual profit forecast by half in November 2008.[45]

While there was a glut in the U.S. automobile market, the markets of Asia, Central and South America, and central and Eastern Europe all showed increasing promise for automobiles, and the automobile industry entered into an era of "global motorization."

Challenges Mulally and Ford Continue to Face

Mulally was faced with a lot of challenges. He had considerable experience dealing with manufacturing and labor relations issues, but he did not have much background in finance. Given the cash drain at Ford due to restructuring costs and product development, and the B + junk credit rating of Ford stock, cash was crucial to keep the company afloat, and Mulally's abilities would be tested.[46]

> Mulally's fearlessness was well suited to pushing through projects at Boeing, but its suitability to Ford's culture remained to be seen. Like every new leader, he had to move with confidence in his early days, but as an industry outsider, he would have to take care to avoid violating the long-standing industry norms.[47]

"Mulally's approach to management and communication hasn't been seen before in the halls of Ford, which have historically been the atmosphere of a kingdom with competing dukes."[48] Mulally was still in the honeymoon period, but already clashes had surfaced between his management style and the "Ford way."

Mulally busied himself breaking down a global structure in which Ford Europe, Ford Asia, Ford North America, Ford Australia, and Ford South America had long created redundancies of efforts, products, engineering platforms, engines, and the like as a way of perpetuating each

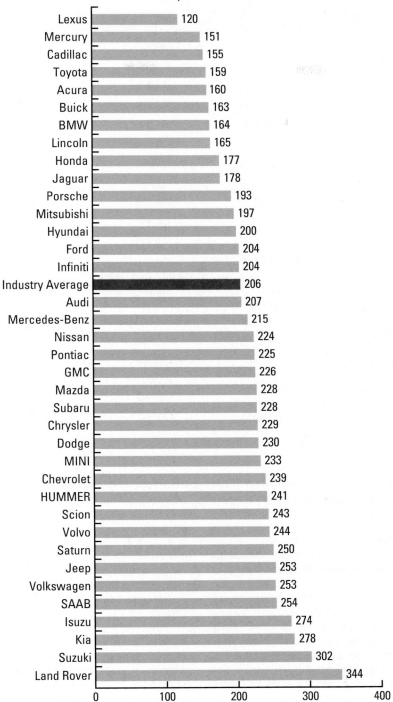

2008 Nameplate Ranking
Problems per 100 Vehicles

Lexus	120
Mercury	151
Cadillac	155
Toyota	159
Acura	160
Buick	163
BMW	164
Lincoln	165
Honda	177
Jaguar	178
Porsche	193
Mitsubishi	197
Hyundai	200
Ford	204
Infiniti	204
Industry Average	206
Audi	207
Mercedes-Benz	215
Nissan	224
Pontiac	225
GMC	226
Mazda	228
Subaru	228
Chrysler	229
Dodge	230
MINI	233
Chevrolet	239
HUMMER	241
Scion	243
Volvo	244
Saturn	250
Jeep	253
Volkswagen	253
SAAB	254
Isuzu	274
Kia	278
Suzuki	302
Land Rover	344

Exhibit 9 Vehicle Dependability Rankings, 2008

Source: J.D. Power and Associates, 2008 Vehicle Dependability Study.

Exhibit 10 Top-Selling Vehicles in the United States, 2008 (ranked by total units)

Rank Vehicle	2008	2007	2007 RANK	%Change
1 Ford F-Series P/U	515,513	690,589	1	−25.4
2 Chevy Silverado-C/K P/U	465,065	618,257	2	−24.8
3 Toyota Camry	436,617	473,108	3	−7.7
4 Honda Accord	372,789	392,231	6	−5.0
5 Toyota Corolla	351,007	371,390	4	−5.5
6 Honda Civic	339,289	331,095	8	+2.5
7 Nissan Altima	269,668	284,762	9	−5.3
8 Chevrolet Impala	265,840	311,128	7	−14.6
9 Dodge Ram P/U	245,840	358,295	5	−31.4
10 Honda CR-V	197,279	219,160	11	−10.0
11 Ford Focus	195,823	173,213	15	+13.1
12 Chevrolet Cobalt	188,045	200,620	14	−6.3
13 Chevrolet Malibu	178,253	128,312	26	+38.9
14 GMC Sierra P/U	168,544	208,243	12	−19.1
15 Toyota Prius	158,884	181,221	16	−12.3
16 Ford Escape	156,544	165,596	17	−5.5
17 Ford Fusion	147,569	149,552	20	−1.3
18 GM Pontiac G6	140,240	150,001	28	−6.5
19 Toyota Tundra	137,249	196,555	23	−30.2
20 Toyota RAV4	137,020	172,752	18	−20.7

Source: *www.reuters.com*.

division's independence.[49] Since the initial purpose of having an outsider CEO was to break the dysfunctional Ford culture, the clashes were expected and generally viewed as constructive.

However, the clashes also had their drawbacks. Unable to accept the Mulally management approach, some senior executives left Ford. The international chief of the company, Mark A. Schulz, was one of them. "He had decided to retire this year after working for more than three decades at the company. Mr. Schulz is just the latest in a string of senior executives to leave since Mulally took over. Ford's second-ranking North American executive, its North American manufacturing chief and its chief of staff also all announced their departures after Mulally's hiring."[50] Ford had lost some of its most experienced leaders because of the outsider CEO.

Despite his rich experience and proven success in turning around the manufacturing operations at Boeing, Mulally was still not completely qualified or accepted as an auto guy. "He recently had to ask what the name of the auto industry's lobby group is (Alliance of Automobile Manufacturers) and what NADA stands for (National Automobile Dealers Assn.)."[51] He had to learn the business and its unique terms on the fly. Speaking the auto language was still critical for an outsider CEO to be accepted in a giant company such as Ford, which had a long and distinct tradition of promoting insider leaders.

Nonetheless, Mulally was confident that his years of experience running a big manufacturer and his technical background had prepared him for the challenges facing Ford.[52]

Looking Ahead

The 2008 year-end earnings report was not without some good news. Ford had reduced automotive costs by $1.4 billion in the fourth quarter and $4.4 billion in 2008 versus costs in 2007. Global dealer stocks were reduced by more than 50,000 vehicles, compared with the third quarter, and Ford now had among the lowest days' supply in the industry. According to Mulally, "The progress we continued to make in the fourth quarter gives us great confidence that we have the right plan, the right people and the right

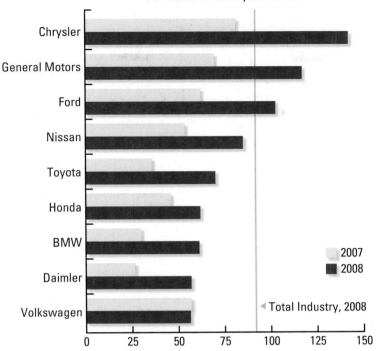

Average number of days a vehicle sits on the lot before being sold, December of each year shown

Legend:
- 2007 (light)
- 2008 (dark)
- ◄ Total Industry, 2008

Exhibit 11 **Dealer Turnover**

Note: Includes data from all brands sold by that manufacturer in the U.S.

Source: J.D. Power.

products to create a viable, profitably growing Ford for all of our stakeholders."[53] He added, "Our market share growth in the fourth quarter in the U.S. and Europe is a positive sign that customers recognize the value of our new products and understand that a new and different Ford is emerging."[54] However, Ford continued to face tough times and a treacherous business environment: A deeper economic and industry slowdown was projected, industry volumes were expected to decline even more in 2009, and market share was expected to remain low. Only time would tell whether the smaller-is-better strategy was the lifesaver for Ford and whether it was the right time to apply it or was too late.

Endnotes

1. B. Vlasic. After record loss, Ford will tap lines of credit to bolster cash. *New York Times,* January 30, 2009, p. B3.
2. M. Dolan, J. D. Stoll, and S. Terlep. Auto sales succumb as credit grows tight. *Wall Street Journal,* October 2, 2008, p. B1.
3. Vlasic. After record loss, Ford will tap lines of credit.
4. Autodata Corp.
5. Ford Motor Company. *http://media.ford.com/article_display.cfm?article_id=29746.*
6. F. Knowles. Boeing exec flies the coop: Ford hires Mulally to turn things. *Chicago Sun-Times,* September 6, 2006.
7. D. Welch, D. Kiley, and S. Holmes. Alan Mulally: A plan to make Ford fly. *BusinessWeek,* 2006.
8. D. Kiley. Mulally: Ford's most important new model. *BusinessWeek Online,* January 9, 2007, *www.businessweek.com.*
9. K. Rakesh. The changing of the guard: Causes, process and consequences of CEO turnover. 1998.
10. S. Berfield. The best leaders. *BusinessWeek Online,* December 18, 2006, *www.businessweek.com.*
11. D. Levin. Mulally's hire by Ford may be too late. Bloomberg.com, 2006.
12. K. Crain. Mulally wants fewer platforms, fewer dealers. *New York Times,* November 20, 2006.
13. Ford Motor Company. *http://media.ford.com/article_display.cfm?article_id=24203.*
14. Ibid.
15. Ibid.
16. Ibid.
17. M. Maynard. Ford chief sees small as virtue and necessity. *New York Times,* January 25, 2007, *www.nytimes.com.*
18. Ibid.
19. Ibid.
20. M. Maynard. Ford expects to fall soon to no. 3 spot. *New York Times,* December 21, 2006, *www.nytimes.com.*
21. Maynard. Ford chief sees small as virtue and necessity.
22. Ford Motor Company. Press release, January 29, 2009, *http://media.ford.com/images/10031/4Qfinancials.pdf.*

23. John Stoll. Ford looks to reshape business model, executive says. *Dow Jones Newswires,* September 18, 2006.

24. Micheline Maynard. Ford seeks a future by going backward. *New York Times,* July 17, 2007, p. C1.

25. Nick Bunkley and Micheline Maynard. Ford breaks string of losing quarters, but says respite will be brief. *New York Times,* July 27, 2007, p. C3.

26. Maynard. Ford chief sees small as virtue and necessity.

27. Bloomberg News. Ford reorganizes executives. *New York Times,* December 15, 2006, *www.nytimes.com.*

28. Ford Motor Company. Press release, January 29, 2009, *http://media.ford.com/images/10031/4Qfinancials.pdf.*

29. P. Ingrassia. Can America's auto makers survive? *Wall Street Journal Europe.* August 8, 2008, p. 13.

30. B. Vlasik and N. Bunkley. At Ford, end of era takes a toll. *New York Times,* July 27, 2008, p. C1.

31. N. Van Praet. US$8.7B loss turns Ford. *Financial Post,* July 25, 2008.

32. Ford Motor Company. *http://media.ford.com/article_display.cfm?article_id=28660.*

33. Ibid.

34. A. Taylor III. Can this car save Ford? *Fortune,* May 5, 2008.

35. Ford Motor Company. *http://media.ford.com/article_display.cfm?article_id=29746.*

36. Ford Motor Company. *http://media.ford.com/article_display.cfm?article_id=28660.*

37. B. Pope. That's why they call it earnings. *WARD'S DealerBusiness,* January 2008.

38. Autodata Corp.

39. *www.motorintelligence.com.*

40. Yahoo Finance. Ford Historical Prices.

41. P. Valdes-Dapena. Autos: 2008 Winners and Losers. *CNNMoney.com,* January 2008.

42. Ford Motor Company. Press release, January 29, 2009, *http://media.ford.com/images/10031/4Qfinancials.pdf.*

43. M. Maynard and M. Fackler. Toyota is poised to supplant GM as world's largest carmaker. *New York Times,* December 22, 2006, *www.nytimes.com.*

44. Ibid.

45. Martin Fackler. Wary of global downturn, Toyota cuts profit forecast by more than half. *New York Times,* November 4, 2008, *www.nytimes.com.*

46. Welch, Kiley, and Holmes. Alan Mulally.

47. Ibid.

48. Kiley. Mulally.

49. D. Kiley. The record year Ford hopes to shake off. *BusinessWeek Online,* January 26, 2007, *www.businessweek.com.*

50. Bloomberg News. Ford reorganizes executives.

51. Kiley. Mulally.

52. Maynard. Ford chief sees small as virtue and necessity.

53. Ford Motor Company. *http://media.ford.com/article_display.cfm?article_id=29746.*

54. Ibid.

Case 13   HTC Corporation: A Smartphone Pioneer From Taiwan*

In February 2010, Peter Chou, chief executive officer (CEO) of HTC Corporation, the pioneer of smartphone manufacturing in Taiwan, was attending an annual industry festival, the Mobile World Congress in Barcelona. At a press conference at the event, at which members of his global team were also present, Chou unveiled the company's "quietly brilliant" advertising campaign, aimed at reinforcing the spirit of the HTC brand. He also introduced three new smartphone models made by the company—of which two were based on the Android platform of Google Inc. (Google) and one on the Windows Mobile 6.5 platform of Microsoft Corporation (Microsoft). Although HTC products had gained credibility among mobile phone subscribers worldwide, Chou and his team faced a rapidly changing competitive landscape, in which the smartphone segment was getting more crowded and new categories (such as e-reader and tablet devices) were also emerging.

Company Background

HTC Corporation (known as High Tech Computer Corporation before 2008) was founded in Taiwan in May 1997 by two entrepreneurs: Cher Wang and H T Cho. Wang, who was from a well-known business family in Taiwan, had ventured out on her own path at a young age to create a successful enterprise that made computer chipsets. Cho was an engineer with Digital Equipment Corp (DEC), a U.S. mini-computer manufacturer that had a plant in Taiwan. HTC's start-up team also consisted of nine other engineers, including Chou, who joined HTC as vice president of Research and Development (R&D) and was named its CEO in 2004.

HTC was created on an investment of NT$5 million (roughly US$172,000) as a subcontractor of hand-held

* Professor Lien-Ti Bei (College of Commerce, National Chengchi University) and Professor Shih-Fen Chen (Richard Ivey School of Business, University of Western Ontario) co-authored this case solely to provide material for class discussion. The authors do not intend to illustrate either effective or ineffective handling of a managerial situation. The authors may have disguised certain names and other identifying information to protect confidentiality.

devices for Western buyers. The company's first client was Compaq Computers (Compaq) which, in January 1998, acquired DEC in what was considered a blockbuster deal, worth $9.6 billion.[1] Compaq was searching for a product to compete with the Palm Pilot, a personal data assistant (PDA) launched by Palm Computing Inc. (Palm) in 1996. Within weeks of launch in the United States, the Palm Pilot had sparked a mobile-computing revolution.

Chou, as vice president of HTC's R&D, had heard about the nascent mobile technology as early as February 1998, at the 3GSM World Congress in Cannes. After joining HTC, he formed a team to work on the idea of combining the data-processing ability of a PDA and the communication ability of a mobile phone.

HTC developed a PDA prototype for Compaq based on two innovations: a coloured screen (in 1999) and a Windows software platform (in 2000). This PDA was the only coloured handheld personal computer (PC) at that time—the first successful innovation by the fledgling startup. The software platform, called Windows CE, was originally developed by Microsoft for large consumer electronic products. HTC paid a licence fee of over US$1 million for the right to adapt it to PDA. This adaptation allowed HTC's PDA to communicate with PCs and run other Windows applications.

After signing up HTC as an original design manufacturer (ODM), Compaq marketed the new PDA under its own brand, iPAQ, which was introduced in April 2000. This pocket device caught on with business professionals because it used the Windows CE operating system and could run Microsoft Pocket Office applications. Eventually, HTC made 2.5 million PDAs per annum for Compaq and also supplied it under the ODM arrangement for other computer companies like HP and Dell.

In 2002, HTC expanded its ability to make white-label PDAs to two new customer segments: mobile phone manufacturers and mobile network operators. The trigger was provided by the close partnership HTC had fostered with Microsoft. Gaining early access to Microsoft's mobile platform technologies, HTC had eventually developed a smartphone using Windows compatible applications.

HTC's smartphone was marketed by O2 (a British network operator) under its XDA brand, by Orange (a French network operator) under its SPV name and by T-Mobile under its Pocket PC Phone label, all in 2002. All these network operators saw an increase in their average revenue per subscriber. This introduction of the smartphone line opened up an opportunity for HTC to become an ODM not only for other network operators (like Vodafone) but also for branded handset makers (such as Palm). Chou described the move from PDA to smartphone for the company: "Switching our business to smartphone starts a new era for HTC. We used to focus on cost-cutting, but now we have to be innovative. We hope that one day, when people think about Taiwan, they think about HTC."

In 2006, HTC launched a new smartphone line under its own name (see Exhibit 1). The company was now firmly on the path to becoming an own-brand manufacture (OBM) company. Up to the end of 2010, it had developed more than 50 models of smartphones. Each was a world-class product designed to deliver a unique and customized wireless telecommunication solution to the customer. Such a smooth transition from a subcontractor to a brand marketer surprised many investors, given that the initial launch of the HTC brand triggered a sharp drop in its stock price by approximately US$1 billion in total value.

For the year ending December 2009, HTC had revenues of NT$144.5 billion and a gross profit of NT$24.62 billion (see Exhibits 2A and 2B). HTC sold 24.7 million devices in 2010, up from 10.8 million smartphones in 2009. Its 2010 annual sales were NT$275 billion (about US$9.49 billion), which nearly doubled the figure of 2009. HTC was ranked fifth among smartphone manufacturers worldwide and ninth in the overall mobile market by share in 2010.

Mobile Telecom Industry

Globally, there were 4.9 billion mobile subscribers at the end of 2009. The number was forecasted to reach 5.3 billion by the end of 2010.[2] The year 2009 had, however, witnessed a 4.8 percent fall over the previous year in the total sales of mobile phones (regular and smart).[3] The fall was largely due to recessionary trends worldwide.

Contrastingly, the global sales of smartphones grew by 14.6 percent over 2008, topping 173.5 million units in 2009. Recession had not affected the appeal of smartphones, which acquired, in a short span, the status of a lifestyle accessory. The product life cycle was becoming shorter, between six and nine months, creating its own demand.

The smartphone had its origins at IBM, which showcased it as a concept in 1992.[4] While the mobile phone provided voice communications and text messaging through the wireless medium, a smartphone integrated mobile phone capabilities with the more advanced features of a handheld computer. It enabled web browsing and e-mail.

The technology of smartphones was Internet compatible. It was evolving even while incorporating progressively more advanced features like high-speed data transfer and directional services through GPS. Consumers saw the smartphone as both a productivity enhancement and entertainment tool, beyond the basic function of voice communication provided by the regular mobile phone.

Mobile Phone History The concept of a mobile phone was a century old. It had its tentative beginnings in the concept of a "car phone" as early as 1910 when Lars Magnus Ericsson, the founder of the eponymous Swedish telephone company, attempted to build a telephone into his vehicle and connect it to the overhead telephone lines. The technology was based on the idea that the voice of the speaker at either end could be transformed into radio waves, which could journey through the air; once they hit a receiver at a nearby base station, the latter used the mainline telephone network to re-route the call. However, the major requirement for this transmission was the radio spectrum, which was limited. As a result, there was no further development of the concept for the next four decades.

In 1947, Bell Laboratories in the United States devised a system by which a particular geographic territory could be divided into a number of cells, each serving as a base station with its own transmitter and receiver. The application ensured that the spectrum was not wasted. This was the beginning of modern cellular technology. In 1973, Motorola displayed the first portable phone, which weighed two kilograms. In 1979, NTT launched car phones on a pilot commercial scale in Tokyo.

The technology platform of the mobile phone went through three sequential phases. The first phase was known as 1G (first generation), characterized by analog transmission of voice communication. It was launched by Nordic Mobile Telephone (NMT) in 1981 in four countries simultaneously: Denmark, Finland, Norway and Sweden. The major limitations of 1G were low transmission capacity and poor quality of voice flow.[5]

Exhibit 1   HTC – Timeline

- 1997: HTC established
- 1998: First Windows PDA
- 1999: First colour palm-size PC
- 2000: First Microsoft Pocket PC
- 2002: First Microsoft wireless Pocket PC
- 2002: First Microsoft-powered smartphone
- 2004: First Microsoft Smart Music Phone—Large 2.8" TFT touch-screen LCD display
- 2005: First Microsoft 3G Phone
- 2005: First Microsoft Windows Mobile 5.0 Platform Phone
- 2005: First tri-band UMTS 3G device on the Microsoft Windows Mobile platform
- 2006: First Microsoft Windows 5.0 smartphone
- 2007: First tri-band UMTS PDA; first intuitive touch screen to allow finger tip navigation
- 2008: First Google Android smartphone
- 2010: First Nexus One smartphone for Google

Source: HTC company records.

Exhibit 2A HTC – Income Statement

	2010	2009	2008	2007	2006	2005	2004	2003	2002	2001
Operating revenues	275,046,954	144,880,715	152,558,766	118,579,958	104,816,548	72,768,522	36,397,166	21,821,605	20,644,316	15,550,363
Cost of sales	(195,489,982)	(99,018,232)	(101,916,912)	(72,880,172)	(70,779,066)	(54,758,040)	(28,493,144)	(17,938,644)	(17,041,738)	(13,429,918)
Gross profit	79,556,972	45,862,483	50,641,854	45,699,786	34,037,482	18,010,482	7,904,022	3,882,961	3,602,578	2,120,445
Operating expenses	(37,024,324)	(21,713,430)	(20,426,453)	(14,665,297)	(7,336,582)	(5,161,215)	(3,594,554)	(2,056,260)	(1,484,059)	(935,505)
Operating income	42,295,343	24,174,994	30,256,385	31,023,425	26,551,966	12,840,479	4,310,420	1,819,460	2,118,519	1,184,940
Non-operating income	2,536,080	1,623,362	2,300,018	1,810,908	1,234,336	217,975	312,956	482,678	421,980	255,943
Non-operating expenses	(340,114)	(585,892)	(965,924)	(683,036)	(828,424)	(902,515)	(662,848)	(342,293)	(1,032,470)	(450,632)
Income before income tax	44,491,309	25,212,464	31,590,479	32,151,297	26,957,878	12,155,939	3,960,528	1,959,845	1,508,029	990,251
Income tax expense	(4,957,709)	(2,603,562)	(2,955,130)	(3,212,435)	(1,710,551)	(373,995)	(105,182)	(109,113)	(43,575)	(27,523)
Net income	39,533,600	22,608,902	28,635,349	28,938,862	25,247,327	11,781,944	3,855,346	1,850,732	1,464,454	962,728

Note 1. All figures are in thousand NT dollars.

Note 2. US$1 is equal to NT$29 by the end of 2010.

Exhibit 2B HTC – Balance Sheet

	2010	2009	2008	2007	2006	2005	2004	2003	2002	2001	2000
Assets											
Current assets	156,908,107	101,503,673	101,271,990	83,172,719	61,810,772	36,616,174	19,391,836	13,118,636	6,787,550	4,402,907	3,369,442
Long-term investment	10,708,420	6,506,194	5,160,891	2,899,109	824,481	325,533	352,000	111,187	88,169	9,007	11,126
Fixed assets	10,941,230	8,314,177	7,375,651	3,715,901	2,909,624	2,495,256	2,518,942	2,234,005	2,288,487	2,220,442	1,005,116
Other assets	5,284,115	3,297,898	1,417,830	656,817	449,300	484,309	278,298	398,343	376,172	419,127	92,444
Total	184,050,453	119,621,942	115,226,362	90,444,546	65,994,177	39,921,272	22,541,076	15,862,171	9,540,378	7,051,483	4,478,128
Liabilities and Stockholders' Equity											
Current liabilities	109,335,331	53,980,282	54,558,470	34,368,139	23,421,319	16,935,170	9,421,405	8,184,249	5,097,949	3,877,586	2,660,285
Long-term liabilities	0	0	0	0	0	0	1,477,171	0	57,164	87,638	120,859
Other liabilities	628	1,210	6,406	628	640	561	273,078	32,174	19,835	12,675	13,294
Total liabilities	109,335,959	53,981,492	54,564,876	34,368,767	23,421,959	16,935,731	11,171,654	8,216,423	5,174,948	3,977,899	2,794,438
Stockholders' equity	74,714,494	65,640,450	60,661,486	56,075,779	42,572,218	22,985,541	11,369,422	7,645,748	4,365,430	3,073,584	1,683,690
Total	184,050,453	119,621,942	115,226,362	90,444,546	65,994,177	39,921,272	22,541,076	15,862,171	9,540,378	7,051,483	4,478,128

Note 1. All figures are in thousand NT dollars.

Note 2. US$1 is equal to NT$29 by the end of 2010.

The second phase was known as 2G (second generation). The transmission of voice was digital, which was a technological leap. 2G was available in several countries during the early 1990s. The medium of communication was clearer than 1G, the transmission had fewer interruptions and the transmission capacity was also higher. The global system for mobile communication (GSM) deployed by 2G went on to become a popular mobile digital standard in subsequent years.

The third phase was known as 3G (third generation), characterized by digital transmission of both voice and data through the medium of the Internet. The technology was pioneered by NTT DoCoMo in 2001. 3G facilitated applications requiring higher bandwidth, such as video-conferencing. The 3G market did not grow as quickly as system operators expected because handset makers could not keep pace with the progress in technology. By 2009, the penetration of 3G handsets was still only 15 percent.[6]

Even though 3G had still not covered all the markets, 4G was being developed simultaneously. The chief improvements of 4G over 3G were mobile ultra-broadband access (gigabit speed) and multi-carrier transmission.

Market Growth   The mobile market exploded in the 1990s largely because of two factors: the operators were awarded licences by their governments and the mobile phone became portable. Until 2008, the penetration rate of mobile phones was 42 percent worldwide (see Exhibit 3). The penetration rate in Europe was the highest, exceeding 100 percent in countries such as Greece. In North and South America, the rate was 90 percent in Argentina, Bahamas, Brazil, Chile, Jamaica and the United States. Both Canada and Mexico had a penetration rate of 60 percent.

The mobile communication markets in Australia and New Zealand were also mature, with penetration rates of 100.8 percent and 94 percent, respectively, in 2008. Countries in the Asia-Pacific region such as Hong Kong, Macau, Malaysia, Singapore and Taiwan had a penetration rate of 100 percent, and in Indonesia, Japan and South Korea, it was over 90 percent. China and India were two big markets with tremendous growth potential, where the penetration rate was about 50 percent. With their enormous populations, the two markets had become hot spots for both operators and manufacturers.

The African market was still under-developed. Nigeria had 16.5 percent penetration, making it the largest single market in Africa. Egypt (14.15 percent) and South Africa (13 percent) were in second and third place, respectively.

Worldwide, the mobile telecom industry consisted of two players: network operators and handset makers, which were sharply differentiated.

Network Operators   The world's largest network operator was China Mobile. It had 500 million mobile phone subscribers in 2009. More than 50 mobile operators in the world had 10 million plus subscribers each. More than 150 mobile operators had at least one million subscribers by the end of 2009.

The business of networks was characterized by scale and consolidation. Customers did not have a wide choice as far as network operators were concerned. In the United States, for example, over 90 percent of the networks market was confined to four major players: Verizon, AT&T, Sprint and Deutsche Telekom (now T-Mobile). In Canada, the market was also divided among four operators (Rogers Wireless, Bell Mobility, TELUS Mobility and Wind

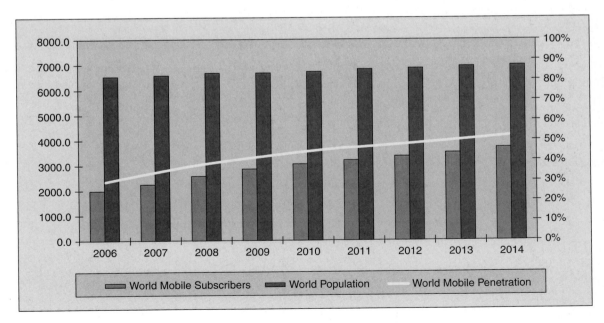

Exhibit 3 **Worldwide Mobile Subscription Penetration – Actuals & Forecast**

Source: Frost & Sullivan (*http://www.frost.com/prod/servlet/frost-home.pag*).

Mobile). Vodafone, Orange, Telefónica, Deutsche Telekom and O2 were the major European players. Another major market, Japan, had only three players (NTT DoCoMo, KDDI and Softbank Mobile). Other key operators in Asia included CMCC (China), China Unicom, China Telecom and CSL (Hong Kong). The primary operator in Australia was Telstra.

The networks business had high entry barriers because investments in fixed assets like cables, stations and towers were capital-intensive. Entry was also restricted to those holding a licence issued by the government. A licence was considered an asset in its own right. In each country, the telecom industry had a designated official regulator exercising control over competitive conduct.

In spite of the national level consolidation, the networks market was fragmented by region (e.g., Asia, Europe, etc.). National players competed in each country as a distinct market within the region. They also cooperated with their counterparts in other nations inside or outside the same region so that home consumers could make calls via international roaming while traveling to other countries.

Network operators wielded strong power over phone makers because they influenced the choice of handsets by customers. This was particularly true in the United States. A Verizon subscriber, for example, could buy only a handset that was approved by Verizon. Carriers subsidized the purchase of a handset as an incentive to subscribers.

Europe was an exception to this rule, where carriers did not usually lock in their handset providers.

Handset Makers   By 2010, the top five handset makers were Nokia, Samsung, LG, Research in Motion (RIM) and Apple (see Exhibit 4). Motorola lost its first mover advantage to Nokia during the 3G era, as did Sony Ericsson. The maturity of 3G devices reshuffled the ranks of mobile phone makers and pushed RIM and Apple into the top five list.

Nokia, a Finnish multinational, was driven by the vision of connecting people. Its competitive advantages included brand equity, scale, distribution capability, product portfolio and leadership in many individual markets. Its mobile devices covered many segments and price points. In its global expansion, the company was customizing its products to suit local conditions, as in emerging markets like India.

Samsung and LG were multinational conglomerates headquartered in South Korea. They both had a strong foundation in electronics on which they built their mobile phones business. Samsung's focus was on simplifying the way consumers work and play, while LG focused on manufacturing mobile phones that consumers would want to take everywhere, matching style with function.

Sony Ericsson was a 50/50 joint venture, established in 2001, by the Japanese consumer electronics company Sony and the Swedish telecommunications company

Exhibit 4   Worldwide Top Mobile Devices: Unit Sales and Market Share

Company Name	Rank	2010		Rank	2009	
		Sales	Share		Sales	Share
Nokia	1	461,318.20	28.89%	1	440,881.60	36.40%
Samsung	2	281,065.80	17.60	2	235,772.00	19.47
LG	3	114,154.60	9.42	3	121,972.10	10.07
Research In Motion	4	47,451.60	2.97	6	34,346.60	2.84
Apple	5	46,598.30	2.92	7	24,889.70	2.05
Sony Ericsson	6	41,819.20	2.62	5	54,956.60	4.54
Motorola	7	38,553.70	2.41	4	58,475.20	4.83
ZTE	8	28,768.70	1.80	8	16,026.10	1.32
HTC	9	24,688.40	1.55	10	10,811.90	0.89
Huawei Technologies	10	23,814.70	1.49	9	13,490.60	1.11
Others		488,569.33	30.60		199,617.20	16.48
Total		1,596,802.40			1,211,239.60	

Note 1: Sales unit in thousands.

Source: Gartner, (February 2011).

Exhibit 5   **Smartphone Operation System Vendors – Global Market Shares**

OS vendor	2010		2009		2008	
	Shipments	Share	Shipments	Share	Shipments	Share
Symbian	112,918,570	37.7%	78,511,980	47.2%	74,926,550	52.4%
RIM	48,897,460	16.3	34,544,100	20.8	23,562,650	16.5
Apple	47,506,160	15.9	25,103,770	15.1	13,727,740	9.6
Microsoft	12,310,150	4.1	14,679,720	8.8	19,945,530	13.9
Google (Android)	69,102,300	23.4	7,786,870	4.7	663,550	0.5
Others	7,984,440	2.7	5,644,610	3.4	10,241,510	7.2
Total	299,716,880	100.0	166,271,050	100.0	143,067,530	100.0

Source: Canalys estimates, May 2011.

Ericsson. Combining Sony's consumer electronics expertise with Ericsson's communication technology, this venture was aimed at providing experiences that blurred the lines between communication and entertainment.

Many players, like Sanyo, Siemens, Sagem, NEC, Sharp and Alcatel, owned less than one percent of the market. Over a dozen players held less than 0.1 percent of the global share. Mobile operators, such as T-Mobile and mmO2, also bought mobile phones from subcontractors and sold them under their own brand name. Some were co-branding with the manufacturer's brand.

Unlike network operators who operated locally, major mobile phone manufacturers usually shipped their products to the global market. For example, Nokia mobile phones were available in more than 160 countries. Handset makers produced mobile phones that could generally fit operators with GSM 900 MHz or 1800 MHz systems in most areas of the world before the 3G era.

The Rise of Smartphones   The main technological milestone that distinguished 2G from 3G environments was the use of packet-switching rather than circuit-switching for data transmission. The advanced development of data transmission allowed new application services, such as mobile Internet access, video calls and mobile television, plus traditional wireless voice telephone.

These new applications required technologies related to computers and the Internet. This suggested that new phones had to combine a phone and a hand-held computer into a single portable device—a device that was later dubbed the smartphone. Until the early 2000s, all major handset makers did not have enough technological ability to integrate the two functions, which opened a window for new players, such as RIM, HTC and Apple.

The key to the function of a smartphone was its operating system. The top five operating systems included BlackBerry (used by RIM), Windows mobile (introduced by Microsoft), Symbian (used by Nokia), iOS (used by Apple) and Android (introduced by Google).

Android, released in 2008, had originally been developed by Android Inc., a firm acquired by Google. The Android team at Google went on to create the Open Handset Alliance, a group of 79 handset makers and mobile network operators committed to an open source platform and to "accelerating innovation in mobile and offering consumers a richer, less expensive and a better mobile experience."[7]

The major smartphone manufacturers were HTC, Apple and RIM. As a member of the Android alliance, HTC was the first handset maker to use the Android system in its HTC Dream, a smartphone line distributed by T-Mobile in 2008. Unlike RIM, which incorporated a keyboard into its phones, HTC and Apple both pursued the development of finger-optimized touch screens, which was considered the trend of the future (see Exhibit 6).

Apple was a relative late-comer to the smartphone market but had quickly seized the initiative to lead the smartphone segment. In 2007, the company introduced its first iPhone, which had a touch screen. Customers who were familiar with the brand and its Macintosh range of computers had been highly anticipating the new features promised by the iPhone.

Under the 3G system, the software in smartphones needed to be customized to fit each operator's system in order to deliver Internet-related services and videos. Because manufacturers needed the assistance of operators to design and test new smartphones, the entry barriers for developing and making smartphones were higher than for designing a PC or other information technology products.

Network-Handset Interactions   Consumers had to buy a mobile phone and also subscribe to a system in order to use the mobile medium. The mobile phone was a one-time purchase, but the subscription would extend for

Exhibit 6   Touch-Screen Smartphones – Global Market Shares

| Vendor | 2009 | | 2008 | | Growth |
	Shipments	Share	Shipments	Share	2009/2008
Apple	25,103,770	33.1%	13,727,740	37.8%	82.9%
Nokia	22,364,000	29.5%	536,210	1.5%	4,070.8%
HTC	7,726,770	10.2%	7,270,630	20.0%	6.3%
Samsung	4,840,750	6.4%	2,290,110	6.3%	111.4%
Others	15,815,510	20.9%	12,484,660	34.4%	26.7%
Total	75,850,800	100.0%	36,309,350	100.0%	108.9%

Source: Press release by Canalys estimates, February 8, 2010, *http://www.canalys.com/pr/2010/r2010021.html.*

the period of contract. The two were commonly bundled together as a promotional package to attract consumers. The bundle was usually provided by the network operator who was the retail face of handsets to the customer. A lock-in operator would buy phones in bulk from handset makers at a discount and offer a package, at a bargain price, to the end-user.

A network operator would also try to entice end-users to switch from competitors. There were often switching costs to the customer (i.e., a locked-up handset), which were subsidized by the operator in some form. The switches would happen with the launch of a new phone model or the introduction of a new variant of the existing model. A network operator would provide special deals wherein end-users could own the most advanced phone with almost zero payment, for example. In this way, mobile phones were a promotional tool for network operators.

The nature of network-handset interactions might lead to some confusion over who was accountable for the ultimate quality of mobile phone service. Consumers had no information about who, between two vendors, played what role over a wide range of issues that mattered to them most, such as speed of transmission, quality of communication, connectivity, access to multimedia and the functionality of the mobile device.

Network-Handset Gaps in Technology   Network operators and mobile phone manufacturers had to work in harmony to deliver full service to consumers; however, there was a performance gap between the two in terms of technological development, where handset makers tended to fall behind network operators. While the latter had developed 3G technologies, for instance, the former were not keeping up. Their products could not upload, download or display pictures or video smoothly or quickly enough to fulfill consumers' needs.

There were several reasons for this dissonance. Most governments issued 1G, 2G and 3G licences separately.

Network operators would wait until the government issued the licence to establish their operating systems, followed by manufacturers introducing a new model to meet operators' needs. Additionally, 3G models had to be altered model by model and operator by operator. Manufacturers were unwilling to undertake small orders of customized phones for each operator in each market. To gain the benefits of scale, they would wait to identify the operators who would attract enough subscribers.

Furthermore, phone makers of the 2G era were not adept at digital information processing. For example, Motorola, Nokia and Ericsson were voice communication players with R&D ability in communication, not in data transmission. Initially, the content and applications for 3G phones were insufficient and consumers had reservations about buying the new 3G phones. Eventually, it was the popularity of the iPhone that attracted the attention of software developers who quickly provided application programs for iPhones and, subsequently, for other smartphones.

HTC Smartphone

The growth of HTC's smartphone business could be divided into three phases: ODM of PDA, ODM of mobile phones and own-brand manufacture (OBM) of smartphones.

ODM of PDA

The first phase of HTC's growth, as mentioned earlier, consisted of making PDAs as a subcontractor for computer manufacturers. Like most high-tech startups in Taiwan at the time, HTC sought subcontracting opportunities where its team had the necessary R&D experience and was confident of delivering end products with a reasonable value-to-price ratio to clients. Designing handheld devices was one of the areas of competence of its founding team of engineers, which could be traced to their days at DEC where they had worked together. Between 2000 and 2002, the PDA business was HTC's primary source of income, generating 13.64 percent of gross profits in 2001 and 17.45 percent in 2002.

The flipside of HTC's ODM business strategy was that the client seemed to have an inordinate amount of control. Even if Compaq accounted for 86 percent of HTC's revenue—and the iPAQs made by HTC accounted for 80 percent of Compaq's annual shipments—Compaq had no hesitation in looking for alternate sources of supply, such as LG Electronics. HTC had to diversify its revenue streams.

ODM of Mobile Phones

The second phase of HTC's growth was triggered by a collaboration opportunity with Palm to manufacture wireless PDAs: Palm VII in 1999. This gave HTC an opportunity to develop competencies in wireless technology, which would later provide growth momentum.

As a late-comer in handset design and manufacture, HTC faced barriers in securing subcontracting orders from established mobile phone makers (such as Nokia, Motorola and Sony Ericsson). These phone makers already had long-term subcontracting partners that competed with one another based largely on price. However, HTC was able to secure business from network operators and its mobile phone business was able to begin after obtaining an ODM order from O2. The focal handset in this deal had a touch colour screen and was sold under the XDA label, a brand name owned by O2.

Later, XDA was remodeled as the T-Mobile Pocket PC Phone Edition for introduction in the U.S. market. In seeking business from network operators, HTC was also fulfilling a market segment that had been under-served. Major handset manufacturers were less willing to supply phones to network operators because the order size was invariably small in relation to their global sales.

It was also in 2002 that HTC decided to gradually give up its PDA ODM business and concentrate on designing and producing smartphones. Chou explained this decision by saying:

> The decision did not go well with our investors. However, we, at the management, had two strong grounds. First, we knew that we simply didn't have enough resources to handle both businesses. Second, the PDA business was becoming competitive because there were too many new entrants. We wanted to move on to the next-generation product. We had set our minds on a business that could not be easily replicated by others. The business of smartphones seemed logical.

The success of XDA, which was HTC's first 2.5G mobile phone, had attracted the attention of other network operators like AT&T, Rogers, France Telecom and Deutsche Telekom AG. In early 2005, HTC started supplying 3G phones to British Telecom (BT), as a direct result of a joint development project initiated by the parties to bridge the network-handset gaps in technology. This joint project represented a milestone in the second phase of HTC's mobile phone business.

British Telecom Project

Being an ODM of mobile phones differed from being an ODM of PDAs in certain aspects. Subcontractors of smartphones not only designed and built the phones based on customer specifications but also tested them in a live operating environment. For instance, the data transmission function of a phone (such as email, instant news, word processing, etc.) had to be customized before delivery. There were incentive misalignments between handset makers and network operators on grounds of technology gaps and order sizes.

British Telecom (BT), a network operator in the United Kingdom, found a willing partner in HTC to bridge the network-handset gap. As an ODM supplier of wireless PDAs, HTC had established a relationship with BT, which was eager to demonstrate its leadership in 3G technologies in Europe. In 1998, Chou presented his idea of combining wireless and computing technologies together for the 2.5G mobile phones to BT. It was a fresh idea to BT, which had already spent over £5 billion (about US$3 billion) on 2.5G and 3G technologies but had yet to make any major breakthroughs. BT appreciated the idea of allying with a supplier that was adept at wireless data transmission in order to break the technological barrier and quickly offered HTC a platform to "co-develop" a smartphone.

HTC secured this co-development project partly because the opportunity was less attractive to major phone manufacturers. The initial order size from BT was relatively small, which did not appeal to major handset manufacturers such as Nokia and Motorola. Furthermore, traditional handset makers, like Nokia, did not seriously consider the offer from Microsoft to promote its platform for smartphones.

HTC's first joint research project with BT began in 1999 and lasted for three and half years, during which the R&D teams of both sides worked in close proximity. BT invested almost US$20 million in the joint project, which involved six sites in three continents, including HTC in Taiwan, BT in London, Microsoft in Seattle and several offices of Texas Instruments (TI) in the United States, France and Germany. BT promised to buy a minimum of 500,000 smartphones from HTC upon its launch.

HTC's relationship with BT had given it the credibility and momentum that would take the company to a premier market position in smartphones. It soon established subcontracting relationships with major network operators worldwide, including the five leading players in Europe (Orange, mmO2, T-Mobile, TeliaSonera and Vodafone), the top four in the United States (AT&T, Sprint, T-Mobile and Verizon) and many Asian operators (such as NTT DoCoMo of Japan). An increase in its customer base gave HTC a greater organizational focus on developing smartphones.

Limits of Subcontracting

Throughout its history, HTC developed products based on extensive R&D but without its own brand name. The company was therefore unable to communicate the attributes of its products directly to end-users. Simultaneously, ODM clients (network operators) were unlikely to emphasize the role of HTC as a designer and manufacturer of a brand that they owned.

Another problem that HTC faced as a subcontractor was that it did not have sufficient protection for its innovation. Some network operators would transfer HTC's designs to other subcontractors without compensating HTC. This issue had troubled HTC since its beginnings in selling PDAs to Compaq, which had once transferred the manufacturing of a model developed by HTC to LG Electronics, a leading South Korean company. "We can't blame Compaq for seeking more subcontractors," recalled Chou, "If I were to put myself in their shoes, I would make the same decision."

Subcontracting had its limits for network operators as well. Some were discovering that selling mobile phones with their own private brand had a negative side. They had to take responsibility for after-sales and repair services, which was costly. Indeed, some of them did not mind letting HTC co-brand the product and share part of the burden. BT, for example, allowed HTC to co-brand its first clamshell smartphone with a new label called Qtek. Consumers selected HTC's Qtek line largely due to BT's endorsement, which helped the brand to be recognized by the end-users in its own right.

In spite of launching the Qtek line in the European market, the management team at HTC believed that in order to support its corporate brand, the company must build a reservoir of capabilities in product design and brand marketing. HTC did not complete the last mile on the branding road until 2006, eight years after its founding as a PDA subcontractor. The year 2006 marked the beginning of the third phase of growth for HTC.

The HTC Brand

HTC had long known that the company should have its own brand; it was only a matter of time before the company began to move in that direction. When HTC made the first coloured screen smartphone for O2 in February 2002, O2 encouraged HTC to use its own brand but Chou did not think the timing was right. Although HTC had invested in Qtek in Europe in 2001, this line was only a small test of running a brand.

The HTC management team carefully evaluated the branding decision for five years and the board of directors discussed it for three years. In the middle of its internal deliberations over introducing its own brand, HTC established an R&D team in 2005 to develop a finger-optimized touch-screen smartphone. This initiative was unknown to anyone outside the company.

The right time for OBM came in 2006, when the secretive touch-screen project had reached major breakthroughs. In the meantime, HTC's revenue, margin and net profit all reached record highs. The arrival of this new generation of smartphones with an innovative touch-screen experience seemed like the perfect product with which to go solo. In 2006, the company formally triggered the process of launching a new mobile phone line under the HTC brand. "We should now be the one making the call and no longer the one waiting for the call," Chou stated.

Chou persuaded the board of directors at HTC to accept the branding idea by pointing out the nature of its ODM business, where profits would be vanishing eventually. Most investors and financial analysts, however, were not supportive because of apprehensions about the financial outlay. Furthermore, they felt that the branding decision might endanger the ODM business, where current clients might retaliate. Given the technological advantage that HTC enjoyed at the time, Chou firmly believed that the company should take the branding road. "We wanted to control our own destiny and we had the advantage to build a brand," said Chou, "HTC was the leader in many communication technologies. We had the technological advantage to support the brand."

Chou learned from earlier brand marketers in Asia (Acer Group in Taiwan, Samsung Electronics in Korea and Sony Corporation in Japan) that global marketing expertise was critical to the success of the HTC brand worldwide. Nevertheless, global managers were hesitant to work for unknown Asian companies. HTC would have to reshape its internal culture in order to project a successful global working environment and attract and keep managers recruited outside Taiwan.

It took HTC a year to shape an international culture for its new branding strategy. The company's management team carefully reexamined and rebuilt every step of its internal communications channels so that no cultural barriers would hinder information flow across managers of different nationalities. It sent engineers abroad to work with top-tier R&D teams worldwide. These efforts transformed HTC from a local Taiwanese firm into a multinational enterprise, which allowed Chou to persuade a variety of talents in hardware and software design to join the company.

The Brand The introduction of the HTC brand to the world finally came in 2006. The first popular model line sold under the new HTC logo was the HTC Touch (June 2007), the first smartphone with a touch-screen experience that preempted the need for a keyboard.

Before choosing HTC as the new brand name, the company considered using Qtek, the existing brand introduced earlier in Europe, or Dopod, another established trademark that was relatively recognizable in Asia. However, neither brand had premium and high-technology appeal that could compete effectively with major players in the global market. Chou believed that the HTC brand would best symbolize all that the company stood for. "We thought about Qtek or Dopod," said Chou, "They had enough brand awareness in certain regional markets but a local image was also tied to the names. We needed a fresh start even though it meant that we had to invest in rebuilding brand awareness and brand image."

Following the introduction of the HTC brand, Chou made the surprising decision to drop the ODM business altogether. This decision caused some internal and external debates. Many people suggested that HTC should keep both the ODM and branded businesses simultaneously and perhaps assign them to two separate companies. The ODM business represented easy money and constituted a large segment of the company's profit before 2006. Nevertheless, limited resources did not allow HTC to cover both businesses and Chou argued that if branding was the company's future, then all resources should be devoted to it.

A Distraction on the Branding Road

HTC initially planned to launch the new phone line during 2007, after more than two years of development and preparation. In January 2007, however, Apple made a dramatic announcement that necessitated immediate reaction from HTC.

On June 12, 2007, the HTC Touch, as the new brand was called, was formally launched in Asia and Europe—17 days before Apple shipped out its first iPhone in the United States. HTC intentionally held the announcement until the shipping day to attract the attention of venders and consumers. Following the introduction of the HTC Touch, the company launched another new product in May 2008, the HTC Touch Diamond.

From 2007 to 2008, HTC and Apple were the only two companies in the world selling smartphones with a finger-optimized touch screen. Based on their experience with PDAs, major handset makers (e.g., Nokia, Motorola, Samsung, LG and Sony Ericsson) believed that touch-screens were not on the right track, since consumers did not prefer to write directly on the screen. The iPhone's popularity threw other handset makers off balance, opening a window for HTC. In the United States, for example, HTC was happy to align with Verizon, T-Mobile and Sprint, while iPhone was bundled exclusively with AT&T's services.

Reactions of ODM Clients

One major concern for many ODM subcontractors who introduced their own brands was that their current clients might retaliate. Before the introduction of its own brand name, HTC estimated that most network operators would not object to its new branding strategy. Focusing on a particular geographic area, network operators were not competing with HTC in the handset market.

HTC launched its brand softly in that it did not insist on attaching the HTC logo to its products. The HTC brand was only an option for its operator clients. HTC's strategy was to promote the brand value to the consumer. Once the value of the HTC brand was recognized by the market, its operator clients would have no hesitation in accepting the logo and co-branding with it.

Before mid-2007, few operator customers had enough confidence in the HTC logo to display it on the product. For example, T-Mobile would rather use its own "T-Mobile MDA Touch" logo without showing the HTC label and Sprint called the model "Sprint Touch by HTC." Operator customers did not believe that the HTC logo could

provide add-on value for the phone. Their attitude towards the brand changed only after the HTC Touch became a hit product that was heavily discussed in trade magazines and on the Internet. From that point, more operator customers allowed HTC to co-brand its products.

However, some handset makers that were subcontracting to HTC remained concerned about the introduction of the HTC brand. For instance, a firm called i-mate (based in Dubai) shifted part of its orders to Inventec Corporation, a Taiwanese competitor of HTC, although i-mate used to outsource handsets exclusively from HTC for sales in Armenia, Australia, Italy, India, South Africa, and the United Kingdom, etc. Arguably, HTC might have lost these orders even if it did not take the branding road, since placing orders with multiple subcontractors to reduce risk was a general policy among many ODM clients.

Brand Performance

HTC continued to co-brand with network operators. In 2010, over 90 percent of HTC smartphones were sold via operators' stores, such as Verizon and AT&T stores in the United States. In Europe, more than half of its products were distributed through stores owned by network operators, including Vodafone, T-Mobile and Orange. In addition, HTC began to distribute its branded products through retail chains, such as Best Buy and Radio Shack in the United States and Carphone Warehouse in Europe. In Asia, most HTC smartphones were distributed through retail stores with the HTC logo on the products

Since 2007, HTC has released over 100 smartphone models under the HTC logo. The market response has been very positive. HTC also launched co-branded products with its network operator customers. In 2010, for example, it had designed the Nexus One for Google and co-branded this new line. It also sold a few models under private brands owned by network operators.

The new branding strategy had led to some changes in HTC's operations—particularly the reduction in its ODM business. In 2003, for instance, HP was the dominant client, constituting 90 percent of the ODM business. In 2007, however, subcontract orders accounted for only 10 percent of HTC's revenue, with the HTC brand making up the remaining 90 percent. By the end of 2009, the company's subcontracting business had dropped almost to zero. The last regular ODM order was placed by T-Mobile in 2009. Since then, HTC chose to work only on special ODM projects (e.g., developing a digital mobile television project for Qualcomm).

In July 2006 (prior to the introduction of its HTC brand), HTC had secured the third spot in *BusinessWeek's* list of InfoTech-100 companies in Asia. In August 2007, it was rated second-best among the magazine's list of top-performing technology companies. In 2008, HTC was the first handset maker that used Google's Android operating system to develop a smartphone. It was named the 2010 Technology Brand of the Year at T3's prestigious Gadget

Awards. The award was given to the most innovative, functional, visible and stylish gadgets and technology of the past 12 months by more than 750,000 readers and a panel of expert judges.

More Developments

The transformation of HTC's business from PDAs to smartphones might have seemed smooth to outsiders but those who were involved knew that it was not an easy task. After the transformation, HTC had built a strong management team at the strategy and execution levels. It had also built an impressive R&D group. Yet the move from contractual manufacturing to brand marketing posed new challenges. Both brand building and global marketing were new territory for the company.

The Quietly Brilliant Campaign   In late 2009, HTC debuted its first global advertising campaign: "quietly brilliant." In the campaign, HTC was portrayed as a company that did "great things in a humble way with the belief that the best things in life are experienced, not explained." This brand positioning not only fit its corporate culture very well but also reflected the shared personality of its employees (see Exhibit 7).

Compared to the other tag lines under consideration by HTC, "quietly brilliant" was not a brand position that was easy to explain or understand, yet the management team at HTC believed that the company embodied the attitude expressed in the slogan and could own the "quietly brilliant" position exclusively. Results of an internal survey revealed that the tag line was ownable, inspirational and honest. Since the fundamental attitude of humility behind this position fit HTC well, the marketing team did not need to make significant extra efforts to communicate this brand concept to its employees.

Initially, HTC was not sure whether this "quietly brilliant" concept, which seemed to work well in the Asian context, would succeed in the global arena. The company ran focus groups in major markets and the conclusion was that many individuals around the world had some friends who were "quietly brilliant." The tagline was culturally universal and was expected to connect well with the target audience.

The main theme of this global advertising campaign was expressed as: "You don't need to get a phone. You need a phone that gets you." The brand promise was, "It's all about YOU, the consumer, not the device." The "YOU"

in HTC's "quietly brilliant" campaign emphasized that HTC put the user at the centre of its focus (see Exhibit 8).

R&D Ability   HTC had set aside sufficient funds for R&D since day one. Financial support from Chairwoman Wang and other investors was unwavering. The company made a strong commitment to the spirit of innovation among its employees. "Innovation is the value of HTC," Chou stated repeatedly.

In 2005, HTC set up an R&D team dubbed MAGIC Labs, aimed at generating novel product concepts and breakthrough ideas. MAGIC stood for Mobility Advancement Group & Innovation Centre and consisted of a group of labs working together to ensure that new products launched by HTC would precede a competitor launch by 6 to 12 months. The members of the MAGIC Labs had various backgrounds, ranging from electronic engineering to psychology to jewelry design. One of the MAGIC Labs' early projects was the touch-screen phone.

HTC also established a design centre in Seattle, focusing on user interface design. It had also acquired a design company in San Francisco. One of the cornerstones of its R&D strategy was the concurrent execution of multiple projects. While ongoing projects were still being executed,

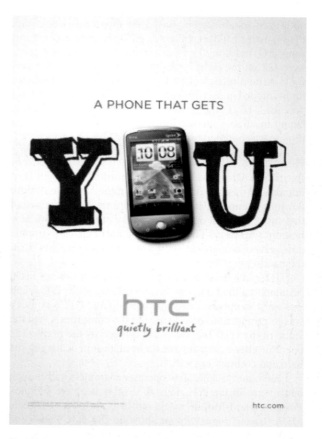

Exhibit 8   Advertisement Sample

hTC
quietly brilliant

Exhibit 7   The HTC Logo and Tag Line

Exhibit 9   HTC – R&D Intensity

Year	R&D Expenditure (1,000 billion NT$)	Revenue (1,000 billion NT$)	R&D Intensity (%)	R&D People
1998	1.49	3.62	41.20	119
1999	1.94	14.89	13.00	154
2000	3.11	43.35	7.20	222
2001	4.84	151.18	3.20	330
2002	6.99	199.74	3.50	424
2003	10.48	211.35	5.00	600
2004	19.94	355.98	5.60	840
2005	23.99	731.45	3.30	950
2006	29.74	1,053.58	2.80	1,140
2007	37.05	1,182.18	3.10	2,342
2008	93.51	1,523.53	6.10	2,718
2009	83.73	1,444.93	5.80	2,732
2010	129.40	2,787.61	4.60	2,978

Note 1. R&D Intensity equals R&D Expenditure divided by Revenue.

Note 2. US$1 is equal to NT$29 by the end of 2010.

dedicated teams would be working on future ideas. The company's R&D team had grown from 70 engineers in 1999 to 1,800 in 2010, accounting for 25 percent of HTC's total employee base. HTC had so far obtained more than 800 patents worldwide (see Exhibit 9).

Next Step   The competitive context for HTC was changing. Chou estimated that 3G products would continuously and quickly expand in 2011, while 4G products would be ready by 2011 and popular in 2012. At the same time, the smartphone segment would be getting more and more crowded. The company had to move faster than competitors, including Apple, which was seeing HTC as a threat. In addition, more traditional handset makers such as Samsung had invaded its territory by launching smartphones based on Windows Mobile.

Another notable development was the emergence of new product categories (e.g., e-readers and tablet devices). By the end of 2009, Amazon's Kindle and Barnes & Noble's Nook were both available with wireless Internet capacity. Apple had also embedded wireless Internet on its iPad, whose introduction in early 2010 caught the attention of the worldwide market. HTC had considered several projects on e-readers and tablet PCs and determined its product concepts had to be just as innovative as the current offerings by competitors.

"No me-too products" was one ground rule at HTC since its founding. The founding team had refused to introduce "me-too products" and be part of the price war in the PC market, which was why HTC had turned to handheld devices in the early days of the company. In response to the emerging trend of mobile computing a decade later, it had to join the tablet PC bandwagon. The question at hand was whether or not HTC could sustain this "no me-too" rule in an ever-evolving competitive landscape.

Endnotes

1. Randy Schultz, "Compaq to Buy DEC," CNNMoney, January 26, 1998.
2. www.itu.int/ITU-D/ict/statistics/material/graphs/2010/Global_mobile_cellular_00-10.jpg, accessed November 20, 2010.
3. HTC annual report for the year ending December 2009, p. 32.
4. J. Schneidawind, "Big Blue Unveiling," USA Today, November 23, 1992, p. 2B.
5. www.westlake.co.uk/Mobile_Phone_Glossary.htm, accessed October 26, 2010.
6. www.morganstanley.com/institutional/techresearch, accessed November 20, 2010.
7. www.openhandsetalliance.com/, accessed November 20, 2010.

Case 14 Microfinance

Going Global . . . and Going Public?*

In the world of development, if one mixes the poor and nonpoor in a program, the nonpoor will always drive out the poor, and the less poor will drive out the more poor, unless protective measures are instituted right at the beginning.

–**Dr. Muhammad Yunus,** founder of the Grameen Bank[1]

More than 2.5 billion people in the world earn less than $2.50 a day. None of the developmental economics theories have helped change this situation. Less than $2.50 a day means that these unfortunate people have been living without clean water, sanitation, or sufficient food to eat, or a proper place to sleep. In Southeast Asia alone, more than 500 million people live under these circumstances. In the past, almost every effort to help the very poor has been either a complete failure or at best partially successful. As Dr. Yunus argues, in every one of these instances, the poor will push the very poor out!

In 1972 Dr. Muhammad Yunus, a young economics professor trained at Vanderbilt, returned home to Bangladesh to take a position at Chittagong University. Upon his arrival, he was struck by the stark contrast between the developmental economics he taught in the classroom and the abject poverty of the villages surrounding the university. Dr. Yunus witnessed more suffering of the poor when, in 1974, inclement weather wiped out food crops and resulted in a widespread and prolonged famine. The theories of developmental economics and the traditional banking institutions, he concluded, were completely ineffectual for lessening the hunger and homelessness among the very poor of that region.

In 1976 Dr. Yunus and his students were visiting the poorest people in the village of Jobra to see whether they could directly help them in any way. They met a group of craftswomen making simple bamboo stools. After paying for their raw materials and financing, the women were left with a profit of just two cents per day. From his own pocket, Dr. Yunus gave $27 to be distributed among 42 craftswomen and *rickshaw* (human-driven transport) drivers. Little did he know that this simple act of generosity was the beginning of a global revolution in microfinance that would eventually help millions of impoverished and poor begin a transition from destitution to economic self-sufficiency. Dr. Yunus was convinced that a nontraditional approach to financing is the only way to help the very poor to help themselves.

* This case was developed by Brian C. Pinkham, LL.M., and Dr. Padmakumar Nair, both from the University of Texas at Dallas. Material has been drawn from published sources to be used for class discussion. Copyright © 2011 Brian C. Pinkham and Padmakumar Nair.

The Grameen Project would soon follow—it officially became a bank under the law in 1983. The poor borrowers own 95 percent of the bank, and the rest is owned by the Bangladeshi government. Loans are financed through deposits only, and there are 8.35 million borrowers, of which 97 percent are women. There are over 2,500 branches serving around 81,000 villages in Bangladesh with a staff of more than 22,000 people. Since its inception, the bank has dispersed more than $10 billion, with a cumulative loan recovery rate of 97.38 percent. The Grameen Bank has been profitable every year since 1976 except three years and pays returns on deposits up to 100 percent to its members.[2] In 2006 Dr. Yunus and the Grameen Bank shared the Nobel Peace Prize for the concept and methodology of microfinance, also known as microcredit or microloans.[3]

What Is Microfinance?

Microfinance involves a small loan (US $20–$750) with a high rate of interest (0 to 200 percent), typically provided to poor or destitute entrepreneurs without collateral.[4] A traditional loan has two basic components captured by interest rates: (1) risk of future payment, and (2) present value (given the time value of money). Risk of future payments is particularly high when dealing with the poor, who are unlikely to have familiarity with credit. To reduce this uncertainty, many microfinance banks refuse to lend to individuals and only lend to groups. Groups have proven to be an effective source of "social collateral" in the microloan process.

In addition to the risk and time value of money, the value of a loan must also include the transaction costs associated with administering the loan. A transaction cost is the cost associated with an economic exchange and is often considered the cost of doing business.[5] For banks like the Grameen Bank, the cost of administering ($125) a small loan may exceed the amount of the small loan itself ($120). These transaction costs have been one of the major deterrents for traditional banks.

Consider a bank with $10,000 to lend. If broken into small loans ($120), the available $10,000 can provide about 83 transactions. If the cost to administer a small loan ($120) is $125, its cost per unit is about 104 percent (!), while the cost of one $10,000 loan is only 1.25 percent. Because of the high cost per unit and the high risk of future payment, the rate of interest assigned to the smaller loan is much higher than the larger loan.

Finally, after these costs are accounted for, there must be some margin (or profit). In the case of microfinance banks, these margins are split between funding the growth of the bank (adding extra branches) and returns on deposits for bank members. This provides even the poorest bank member a feeling of "ownership."

Microfinance and Initial Public Offerings

With the global success of the microfinance concept, the number of private microfinance institutions exploded. Today there are more than 7,000 microfinance institutions, and their profitability has led many of the larger institutions to consider whether or not to "go public." Many microfinance banks redistribute profits to bank members (the poor) through returns on deposits. Once the bank goes public through an initial public offering (IPO), however, there is a transfer of control to public buyers (typically investors from developed economies). This transfer creates a fiduciary duty of the bank's management to maximize value for the shareholders.[6]

For example, Banco Compartamos (Banco) of Mexico raised $467 million in its IPO in 2007. The majority of buyers were leading investment companies from the United States and United Kingdom—the geographic breakdown of the investors was 52 percent U.S., 33 percent Europe, 5 percent Mexico, and 10 percent other Latin American countries. Similarly, Bank Rakyat Indonesia (BRI) raised $480 million in its IPO by listing on multiple stock exchanges in 2003; the majority of investors who purchased the available 30 percent interest in the bank were from the United States and United Kingdom. The Indonesian government controls the remaining 70 percent stake in BRI. In Kenya, Equity Bank raised $88 million in its IPO in late 2006. Because of the small scale of Equity Bank's initial listing on the Nairobi Stock Exchange, the majority of the investors were from Eastern Africa.[7] About one-third of the investors were from the European Union and United States.[8]

Banco Compartamos[9]

Banco started in 1990 as a nongovernmental organization (NGO). At the time, population growth in Latin America and Mexico outpaced job growth. This left few job opportunities within the largest population group in Mexico— the low-income. Banco recognized that the payoffs for high-income opportunities were much larger (dollars a day), relative to low-income opportunities that may only return pennies a day. Over the next 10 years, Banco offered larger loans to groups and individuals to help bridge the gap between these low-income and high-income opportunities. However, their focus is to serve low-income individuals and groups, particularly the women who make up 98 percent of Banco's members.

The bank offers two microfinance options available to women only. The first is the *credito mujer* (women's credit). This loan ranges from $115–$2,075, available to groups (12–50) of women. Maturity is four months, and payments are weekly or biweekly.

If a group of women demonstrates the ability to manage credit through the *credito mujer,* they have access to *credito mejora tu casa* (home-improvement loans). This loan ranges from $230–$2,300 with a 6- to 24-month maturity. Payments are either biweekly or monthly.

The average interest rate on these loans is 80 percent. Banco focuses on loans to *groups* of women and requires the guarantee of the group—*every* individual in the group is held liable for the payment of the loan. This provides a social reinforcement mechanism for loan payments typically absent in traditional loans. The bank also prefers groups because they are more likely to take larger loans. This has proven effective even in times of economic downturn, when banks typically expect higher demand for loans and lower recovery of loans.

In 2009, with Mexico still reeling from the economic recession of 2008, Banco provided financing to 1.5 million Mexican households. This represented a growth of 30 percent from 2008. The core of the financing was *credito mujer,* emphasizing the bank's focus on providing services for the low-income groups. The average loan was 4.6 percent of GDP per capita ($440), compared with an average loan of 54 percent of GDP per capita ($347) at the Grameen Bank in Bangladesh.[10] With pressure from the economic downturn, Banco also reduced its cost per client by more than 5 percent, and continues (in late 2010) to have a cost per client under $125.

Consider two examples of how these microloans are used. Julia González Cueto, who started selling candy door-to-door in 1983, used her first loan to purchase accessories to broaden the image of her business. This provided a stepping stone for her decision to cultivate mushrooms and *nopales* (prickly pear leaves) to supplement her candy business. She now exports wild mushrooms to an Italian restaurant chain. Leocadia Cruz Gómez has had 16 loans, the first in April 2006. She invested in looms and thread to expand her textile business. Today, her workshop has grown, she is able to travel and give classes, and her work is widely recognized.

Beyond the Grameen Bank

These are just a few examples of how capitalistic free-market enterprises have helped the world to progress. It is generally accepted that charitable contributions and government programs alone cannot alleviate poverty. More resources and professional management are essential for microfinance institutions to grow further and sustain their mission. An IPO is one way to achieve this goal when deposits alone cannot sustain the demand for loans. At the same time, investors expect a decent return on their investment, and this expectation might work against the most important goal of microfinancing, namely, to help the very poor. Dr. Yunus has recently reemphasized his concern of the nonpoor driving out the poor, and talks about microfinance institutions seeking investments from "social-objective-driven" investors with a need to create a separate "social stock market."[11]

The Grameen Bank story, and that of microfinancing, and the current enthusiasm in going public raise several concerns. Institutions like the Grameen Bank have to grow and sustain a long-run perspective. The Grameen Bank has not accepted donor money since 1998 and does not foresee a need for donor money or other sources of external capital. The Grameen Bank charges four interest rates, depending on who is borrowing and for what purpose the money is being used: 20 percent for income-generating loans, 8 percent for housing loans, 5 percent for student loans, and *interest-free* loans for struggling members (unsympathetically called beggars). (Although these rates would appear to be close to what U.S. banks charge, we must point out that the terms of these loans are typically three or four months. Thus, the annualized interest rates would be four or five times the aforementioned rates.)

The Grameen Bank's "Beggars-As-Members" program is a stark contrast to what has been theorized and practiced in contemporary financial markets—traditional banking would assign high-risk borrowers (like beggars) the highest interest rate compared to more reliable borrowers who are using the borrowed money for generating income. Interestingly, the loan recovery rate is 79 percent from the "Beggars-As-Members" program, and about 20,000 members (out of 110,000) have left begging completely.[12] However, it is difficult to predict the future, and it is possible that the Grameen Bank might consider expanding its capital base by going public just like its Mexican counterpart.

Most developmental economists question the wisdom of going public, because publicly traded enterprises are likely to struggle to find a balance between fiduciary responsibilities and social good.[13] The three large IPOs mentioned above (Banco, BRI, and Equity First) all resulted in improved transparency and reporting for stockholders. However, the profits, which were originally distributed to bank members as returns on deposits, are now split between bank members (poor) and stockholders (made up of mostly EU and U.S. investors). Many of these microfinance banks are feeling the pressure of NGOs and bank members requesting lower interest rates.[14] This trend could potentially erode the large profit margins these banks currently enjoy. When faced with falling profits, publicly traded microfinance institutions will have to decide how best to provide financial services for the very poor and struggling members of the society without undermining their fiduciary duties to stockholders.

Endnotes

1. Yunus, M. 2007. *Banker to the poor: Micro-lending and the battle against world poverty.* New York: PublicAffairs.
2. The Grameen Bank removes funding for administration and branch growth from the initial profits and redistributes the remaining profits to bank members. This means that a poor bank member who deposits $1 *in* January may receive up to $1 on December 31! Grameen Bank, *www.grameen-info.org.*
3. Grameen Bank, *www.grameen-info.org.*
4. Microfinance banks vary to the extent that the rates of interest are annualized or specified to the term. Grameen Bank, for instance, annualizes the interest on its microloans. However, many other banks set a periodic rate where, in extreme cases, interest may accrue daily. Grameen Bank, *www.grameen-info.org.*
5. Chapter 6, pages 255–256.
6. Khavul, S. 2010. Microfinance: Creating opportunities for the poor? *Academy of Management Perspectives,* 24(3): 58–72.
7. Equity Bank, *www.equitybank.co.ke.*
8. Rhyne, E., & Guimon, A. 2007. The Banco Compartamos initial public offering, *Accion: InSight,* no. 23: 1–17. *resources.centerforfinancialinclusion.org/insight/IS23en .pdf.*
9. Unless otherwise noted, this section uses information from Banco Compartamos, *www.compartamos.com.*
10. We calculated all GDP per capita information as normalized to current (as of 2010) U.S. dollars using the International Monetary Fund (IMF) website, *www.imf.org.* The estimated percentages are from Banco Compartamos, *www.compartamos.com.*
11. Yunus. 2007. *Banker to the poor.*
12. Grameen Bank, *www.grameen-info.org.*
13. Khavul. 2010. Microfinance.
14. Rhyne & Guimon. 2007. The Banco Compartamos initial public offering.

Case 15   Johnson & Johnson*

On January 23, 2009, health care conglomerate Johnson & Johnson announced the completion of its $1.1 billion acquisition of Mentor Corporation, a leading supplier of medical products for the global aesthetic market. J&J was the first major U.S. drug company to get into the cosmetic medicine market, doing so with the launch of its injectable wrinkle-filler Evolence during the previous year. The $4.6 billion market for such products is expected to grow to $6.7 billion by 2012. "It's a natural extension of where J&J would want to go," said Michael Weinstein, an analyst at JPMorgan Chase & Company.[1]

J&J has used such acquisitions to grow over the years. Just two years ago, the firm bought the consumer health unit of Pfizer for $16.6 billion, the biggest acquisition in its 120-year history. William C. Weldon, the firm's chief executive, is aware that it is getting much harder for J&J to spot smaller firms with promising drugs and to avoid running

* This case was developed by Professor Jamal Shamsie, Michigan State University, with the assistance of Professor Alan B. Eisner, Pace University. Material has been drawn from published sources to be used for class discussion. Copyright © 2009 Jamal Shamsie and Alan B. Eisner.

up against other firms that want to make the same kinds of deals. "You get to a point where finding acquisitions that fit the mold and make a contribution becomes increasingly difficult," warned UBS Warburg analyst David Lothson.[2]

Weldon recently told investors that his firm would search for other avenues for growth: "We'll come at it from a variety of different ways, to accelerate top- and bottom-line growth."[3] Given the scope of the businesses that J&J manages, he believes that the best opportunities may come from increased collaboration between its different units. The firm has the ability to develop new products by combining its strengths across pharmaceutical products, medical devices and diagnostics, and consumer products.

J&J desperately needs to find new avenues for growth. It was already alerting investors that its revenue for 2009 would show a drop from the previous year, the first decline the firm has experienced in its 120-year history (see Exhibits 1 and 2). Sales of its consumer products were slowing as a result of a decrease in the disposable income of its customers. Its pharmaceutical business was being affected by the expiration of patents on some of its best-selling drugs and by the growth of competition from

Exhibit 1   Income Statement (in thousands of dollars)

Period Ending:	2008	2007	2006
Total revenue	63,747,000	61,095,000	53,324,000
Cost of revenue	18,511,000	17,751,000	15,057,000
Gross profit	45,236,000	43,344,000	38,267,000
Operating expenses:			
Research and development	7,577,000	7,680,000	7,125,000
Selling, general, and administrative	21,490,000	20,451,000	17,433,000
Nonrecurring	181,000	1,552,000	559,000
Operating income or loss	15,988,000	13,661,000	13,150,000
Income from continuing operations:			
Total other income/expenses net	1,376,000	(82,000)	1,500,000
Earnings before interest and taxes	17,364,000	13,579,000	14,650,000
Interest expense	435,000	296,000	63,000
Income before tax	16,929,000	13,283,000	14,587,000
Income tax expense	3,980,000	2,707,000	3,534,000
Net income from continuing ops	12,949,000	10,576,000	11,053,000
Net income	12,949,000	10,576,000	11,053,000

Source: J&J.

Exhibit 2   **Balance Sheet** (in thousands of dollars)

Period Ending:	2008	2007	2006
Assets			
Current assets:			
Cash and cash equivalents	10,768,000	7,770,000	4,083,000
Short-term investments	2,041,000	1,545,000	1,000
Net receivables	13,149,000	12,053,000	10,806,000
Inventory	5,052,000	5,110,000	4,889,000
Other current assets	3,367,000	3,467,000	3,196,000
Total current assets	**34,377,000**	**29,945,000**	**22,975,000**
Long-term investments	4,000	2,000	16,000
Property, plant, and equipment	14,365,000	14,185,000	13,044,000
Goodwill	13,719,000	14,123,000	13,340,000
Intangible assets	13,976,000	14,640,000	15,348,000
Other assets	2,630,000	3,170,000	2,623,000
Deferred long-term asset charges	5,841,000	4,889,000	3,210,000
Total assets	**84,912,000**	**80,954,000**	**70,556,000**
Liabilities and Equity			
Current liabilities:			
Accounts payable	17,120,000	17,374,000	14,582,000
Short/current long-term debt	3,732,000	2,463,000	4,579,000
Other current liabilities	—	—	—
Total current liabilities	**20,852,000**	**19,837,000**	**19,161,000**
Long-term debt	8,120,000	7,074,000	2,014,000
Other liabilities	11,997,000	9,231,000	8,744,000
Deferred long-term liability charges	1,432,000	1,493,000	1,319,000
Total liabilities	**42,401,000**	**37,635,000**	**31,238,000**
Stockholders' equity:			
Common stock	3,120,000	3,120,000	3,120,000
Retained earnings	63,379,000	55,280,000	49,290,000
Treasury stock	(19,033,000)	(14,388,000)	(10,974,000)
Other stockholders' equity	(4,955,000)	(693,000)	(2,118,000)
Total stockholders' equity	**42,511,000**	**43,319,000**	**39,318,000**
Net tangible assets	**14,816,000**	**14,556,000**	**10,630,000**

Source: J&J.

generic drugs. "We are seeing some signs that consumers and patients are becoming more frugal," said Weldon. "There is downward pressure in lots of areas of health care."[4]

In fact, J&J is embarking on its biggest shake-up since Weldon took charge of the firm in 2002. It is elevating one of its rising stars, Nicholas Valeriani, to lead an office that will push for greater interaction between J&J's 250 different operating companies to squeeze more value from areas where they overlap. But Weldon is also acutely aware that much of the success of J&J over the years has been based on the relative autonomy and independence that it has accorded its various business units. Any push for greater collaboration must not threaten the strong entrepreneurial spirit that has been fostered through the firm's reliance on this type of organization.

Fostering Entrepreneurship

J&J has relied heavily on acquisitions to enter into and expand into a wide range of businesses that fall broadly under the category of health care. Over the last decade alone, the firm has spent nearly $50 billion on 70 different purchases. In the last few months of 2008, J&J made two small acquisitions to move into the area of wellness and protection, which has been growing in the United States and Europe. Firms in this business focus on creating systems to foster and monitor healthy behavior among employees.

As it has grown, J&J has developed into an astonishingly complex enterprise, made up of over 250 different businesses organized into three different divisions. The most widely known of these is the division that makes consumer products such as Johnson & Johnson baby care products, Band-Aid adhesive strips, and Listerine mouthwash. The consumer products division has provided the firm with several strong brands that have generated a steady stream of revenue. "You don't have to deal with the volatility that you have in pharmaceuticals and devices," explained Weldon.[5] But pharmaceutical products and medical devices have allowed the firm to reap huge profits from blockbuster drugs such as anemia drug Procrit, schizophrenia drug Risperdal, and Cypher coronary stents. Such products generally provide operating profit margins of around 30 percent, almost double those generated by the consumer business.

To a large extent, however, J&J's success across its three divisions and many different businesses has hinged on its unique structure and culture. Most of its far-flung business units were acquired because of the potential demonstrated by some promising new products in their pipelines. Each of these units was therefore granted nearly total autonomy to develop and expand on its best-selling products (see Exhibit 3). That independence has fostered an entrepreneurial attitude that has kept J&J intensely competitive as others around it have faltered. The relative autonomy that is accorded to the business units has also

provided the firm with the ability to respond swiftly to emerging opportunities.

In other words, the business units have been given considerable freedom to develop and execute their own strategies. In addition, these units have been allowed to work with their own resources. Many of the businesses even have their own finance and human resource departments. While this degree of decentralization entails relatively high overhead costs, none of the executives who have run J&J, Weldon included, has ever thought that this was too high a price to pay. "The company really operates more like a mutual fund than anything else," commented Pat Dorsey, director of equity research at Morningstar.[6]

In spite of the benefits that J&J has derived from giving its various enterprises considerable autonomy, there is a growing feeling that these businesses can no longer operate in near isolation. Weldon has begun to realize, as do most others in the industry, that some of the most important breakthroughs in 21st-century medicine are likely to come from the ability to apply scientific advances in one discipline to another. J&J should therefore be in a strong position to exploit new opportunities by drawing on the diverse skills of its various business units across the three divisions.

Restructuring for Synergies

Weldon strongly believes that J&J is perfectly positioned to profit from the shift toward combining drugs, devices, and diagnostics, since few companies can match its reach and strength in these basic areas. Indeed, J&J has top-notch products in each of those categories (see Exhibit 4). It has been boosting its research and development budget by more than 10 percent annually for the past few years, which puts it among the top spenders (see Exhibit 5). It now spends about 13 percent of its sales, over $7 billion, on more than 9,000 scientists working in research laboratories around the world.

Weldon believes, however, that J&J can profit from convergence by finding ways to make its fiercely independent businesses work together. In his own words, "There is a convergence that will allow us to do things we haven't done before."[7] Through pushing the various far-flung units of the firm to pool their resources, Weldon believes that the firm could become one of the few that may actually be able to attain that often-promised, rarely delivered idea of synergy.

In November 2007, J&J announced that it was breaking up its medical devices division into two groups, surgery and comprehensive care. The surgery unit will continue to work on its lucrative hip and knee replacement products, while the comprehensive unit will focus on diseases such as diabetes with a more integrated approach. For example, it will harness expertise from J&J's diagnostic tests to catch diabetes earlier and from its glucose monitoring arm to help patients living with the disease.

Exhibit 3   Segment Information

Johnson & Johnson is made up of over 250 different companies, many of which it has acquired over the years. These individual companies have been assigned to three different divisions:

	Pharmaceuticals	Medical Devices	Consumer Products
Share of firm's sales:			
2008	39%	36%	25%
2007	41	36	24
2004	47	36	18
2001	46	35	20
Share of firm's operating profits:			
2008	43	41	15
2007	48	35	17
2004	60	31	11
2001	63	25	12

Sales by Segment (in billions of dollars)

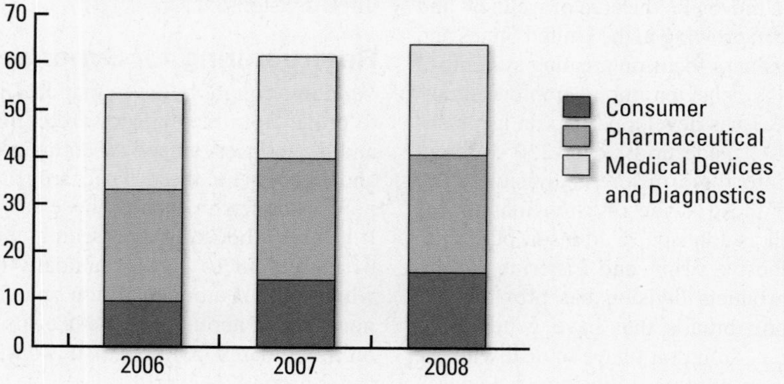

Legend:
- Consumer
- Pharmaceutical
- Medical Devices and Diagnostics

Source: J&J.

Although J&J is breaking up one of its divisions, Weldon views this as an opportunity to have the firm's various units working with one another to address different health problems. He has appointed Valeriani to head the new Office of Strategy and Growth that will attempt to get business units to work together on promising new opportunities. "It's a recognition that there's a way to treat disease that's not in silos," Weldon stated, referring to J&J's largely independent businesses.[8]

Such a push for communication and coordination will allow J&J to develop the synergy that Weldon has been seeking. But any effort to get the different business units to collaborate must not quash the entrepreneurial spirit that has spearheaded most of the growth of the firm to date. Jerry Caccott, managing director of consulting firm Strategic Decisions Group, emphasized that cultivating those alliances "would be challenging in any organization, but particularly in an organization that has been so successful because of its decentralized culture."[9]

Benefiting from Collaboration

Weldon, like every other leader in the company's history, has worked his way up through the ranks. His long tenure within the firm has turned him into a true believer in the J&J system. He certainly does not want to undermine the entrepreneurial spirit that has resulted from the autonomy that has been given to each of the businesses. Consequently, even though Weldon may talk incessantly about synergy and convergence, he has been cautious in the actual steps he has taken to push J&J's units to collaborate with each other.

Exhibit 4 **Key Brands**

Pharmaceuticals
Risperdal for schizophrenia
Procrit for anemia
Remicade for rheumatoid arthritis
Topamax for epilepsy
Duragesic for chronic pain
Doxil for ovarian cancer

Medical Devices
Depuy orthopedic joint reconstruction products
Cordis Cypher stents
Ethicon surgery products

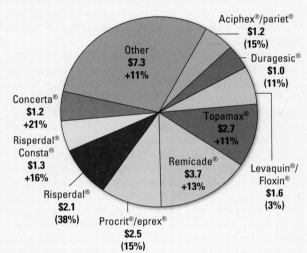

Pharmaceutical Segment Sales
Sales by Major Product
(in billions of dollars)*
2008 Sales: $24.6 billion   Growth Rate: (1.2%)

*Includes rounding.

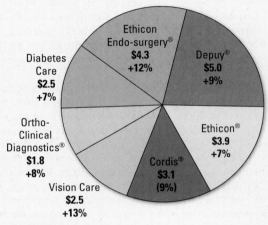

Medical Devices & Diagnostics Segment Sales
Sales by Major Franchise
(in billions of dollars)*
2008 Sales: $23.1 billion   Growth Rate: 6.4%

*Includes rounding.

Consumer Products
Band-Aid bandages
Johnson & Johnson baby care products
Neutrogena skin and hair care products
Listerine oral health care products
Tylenol pain killers
Rolaids antacids
Benadryl cold and cough syrups
Bengay pain relief ointments
Tuck's hemorrhoidal ointments
Visine eye drops
Rogaine hair regrowth treatments
Stayfree women's health products
Splenda sweeteners

Source: J&J.

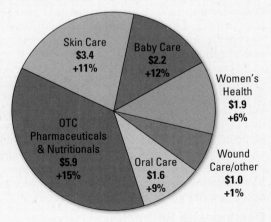

Consumer Segment Sales
Sales by Major Franchise
(in billions of dollars)*
2008 Sales: $16.0 billion   Growth Rate: 10.8%

*Includes rounding.

Exhibit 5   Research Expenditures
(in millions of dollars)

Year	Amount
2008	7,577
2007	7,680
2006	7,125
2005	6,462

Source: J&J.

For the most part, Weldon has confined himself to taking steps that foster better communication and more frequent collaboration among J&J's disparate operations. Besides appointing Valeriani, he has worked with James T. Lenehan, vice chairman and president of J&J, to set up groups that draw people from across the firm to focus their efforts on specific diseases. Each of the groups has been reporting every six months on potential strategies and projects.

Perhaps the most promising result of this new collaborative approach has been J&J's drug-coated stent, called Cypher. The highly successful new addition to the firm's lineup was a result of the efforts of teams that combined people from the drug business with others from the device business. They collaborated on manufacturing the stent, which props open arteries after angioplasty. Weldon claims that if J&J had not been able to bring together people with different types of expertise, it could not have developed the stent without getting assistance from outside the firm.

Even the company's fabled consumer brands have been starting to show growth as a result of increased collaboration between the consumer products and pharmaceutical divisions. Its new liquid Band-Aid is based on a material used in a wound-closing product sold by one of J&J's hospital-supply businesses, and J&J has used its prescription antifungal treatment, Nizoral, to develop a dandruff shampoo. In fact, products that have developed in large part out of such business-unit cross-fertilization have allowed the firm's consumer business to experience considerable internal growth.

Some of the projects that J&J is currently working on could produce even more significant results. Researchers working on genomic studies in the firm's labs were building a massive database using gene patterns that correlate to a certain disease or to someone's likely response to a particular drug. Weldon encouraged them to share this data with the various business units. As a result, the diagnostics team has been working on a test that the researchers in the pharmaceutical division could use to predict which patients would benefit from an experimental cancer therapy.

Dealing with Setbacks

Even as Weldon moves carefully to encourage collaboration between the business units, he has continued to push for the highest possible levels of performance. Those who know him well would say that he is compulsively competitive. Weldon has been known to state on more than one occasion that "it's no fun to be second."[10] He is such an intense athlete that he was just a sprint away from ruining his knee altogether when he finally decided to give up playing basketball.

For the most part, however, Weldon is known for letting his managers, working across J&J's units, make their own decisions on various projects. He usually likes to get briefed once a month on the progress that is being made on these projects. Beyond that, Weldon claims that he likes to trust his people. "They are the experts who know the marketplace, know the hospitals, and know the cardiologists," he once said about the team that worked on the Cypher stent. "I have the utmost confidence in them."[11] But for those executives who may fall short, Weldon does not usually have any difficulty in making it clear that he does not like to be disappointed.

Above all, Weldon is not discouraged by setbacks, such as those J&J has been facing in its pharmaceutical business, which has accounted for more than 40 percent of the firm's revenue. At this point, several of J&J's important drugs are under assault from competitors. Its well-known anemia drug Procrit has been dealing with rising competition and with growing safety concerns. Top-selling Risperdal, Duragesic, and Topamax drugs will start facing generic rivals in 2009. Furthermore, a new antipsychosis drug called Invega, recently launched to replace Risperdal, has not been able to meet sales expectations.

J&J has also been facing some challenges with sales of its medical devices. It has been losing sales on its well-selling Cypher stents because of concerns over their safety that have been raised in several studies. Additionally, these drug-coated stents have been facing growing competition from other strong rivals. To make things worse, J&J had to withdraw a promising new stent from Connor Medsystems, a recent acquisition, after it failed in trials in early summer 2007.

However, analysts believe that J&J has been working hard on developing new pharmaceutical drugs and medical devices. "We think they have a pretty good pipeline," remarked Jason Napodano, an analyst with Zacks.[12] J&J has stated that it is on target to seek regulatory approval for up to 10 new drugs, including treatments for cancer, autoimmune diseases, and HIV. One of its promising new drugs for rheumatoid arthritis could be approved within a few months. "We're optimistic about our short and long term prospects," said Christine Poon, the head of the firm's pharmaceutical division, who has announced she will be retiring soon.[13]

Is There a Cure Ahead?

Weldon realizes that J&J may face a few challenges over the next couple of years as it tries to push out new products in a tough economic environment. But the firm's diversified portfolio of products spread across various areas of health care has helped it to weather the economic downturn with few problems. In particular, J&J has managed to offset its loss of sales in pharmaceuticals and devices with relatively stable earnings from its consumer products. "With interests spread out all over the health-care industry, J&J does not live or die by any one product," remarked Herman Saftlas, a pharmaceutical analyst for Standard & Poor's.[14]

However, Weldon is aware that he needs to keep pushing his firm to find new opportunities to expand across various areas of health care. Even as he seeks growth, Weldon is also trying to move J&J away from its pattern of heavy reliance on acquisitions. With fewer and smaller acquisitions, he will need to find ways to get the various business units to come up with sufficient new ideas to maintain his firm's growth trajectory. His decisions to break up the medical devices unit and to appoint Valeriani have been designed to generate more internal growth as a result of greater interaction between the different units.

The moves that Weldon has made may generate more collaboration between the different business units of J&J. At the same time, it is not clear that the recent changes will be enough to produce the growth that he desires. Catherine Arnold, a drug industry analyst at Credit Suisse, feels that J&J may have to push harder. "Just making these management changes is not enough," she stated. "I'd see this as a step among many to face a more challenging business environment. It's a way to eliminate some of the obstacles that their structure creates."[15]

Weldon is aware that he can maintain J&J's record growth only by finding ways to encourage its businesses to work more closely together than they ever did in the past. The firm can tap into many more opportunities when it brings together the various skills that it has developed across different divisions. At the same time, Weldon is acutely aware that much of the firm's success has resulted from the relative autonomy that it has granted to each of its business units. Even as he strives to push for more collaborative effort, Weldon does not want to threaten the entrepreneurial spirit that has served J&J so well.

Endnotes

1. Shirley S. Wang & Rhonda L. Rundle. J&J to Acquire Breast-Implant Maker. *The Wall Street Journal,* December 2, 2008, p. B1.
2. Amy Barrett. Staying on Top. *BusinessWeek,* May 5, 2003, p. 61.
3. Christopher Bowe. J&J Reveals Its Guidant Motive. *Financial Times,* January 25, 2006, p. 17.
4. Peter Loftus & Shirley S. Wang. J&J Sales Show Health Care Feels the Pinch. *The Wall Street Journal,* January 21, 2009, p. B1.
5. Avery Johnson. J&J's Consumer Play Paces Growth. *The Wall Street Journal,* January 24, 2007, p. A3.
6. Holly Hubbard Preston. Drug Giant Provides a Model of Consistency. *Herald Tribune,* March 12–13, 2005, p. 12.
7. Barrett. Staying on Top. 2003, p. 62.
8. Avery Johnson. J&J Realigns Managers, Revamps Units. *The Wall Street Journal,* November 16, 2007, p. A10.
9. Barrett. Staying on Top. 2003, p. 62.
10. Ibid.
11. Ibid. p. 66.
12. Johanna Bennett. J&J: A Balm for Your Portfolio. *Barron's,* October 27, 2008, p. 39.
13. Jonathan D. Rockoff. J&J Profit Rises; Firm Boosts Its Forecast. *The Wall Street Journal,* October 15, 2008, p. B5.
14. Bennett. J&J. 2008.
15. Johnson. J&J Realigns Managers. 2007.

Case 16   Innovative Tata Inc.—India's Pride!

"The world will always need innovators and innovations; it is not a destination but an endless journey and the spirit of entrepreneurship will continue to be a great enabler." [1]

—**Syamal Gupta,** Director, Tata Sons.

"If you can imagine it, you can do it." [2]

—**Walt Disney,** Visionary Filmmaker.

"We are very pleased at the prospect of Jaguar and Land Rover being a significant part of our automotive business." [3]

—**Ratan Tata,** Chairman of Tata Sons and Tata Motors.

Companies across the globe are emerging as top-notch innovators. Tata Motors' innovation metrics not only include a number of patents, but also importance to increase their revenue and something valuable for the betterment of the society. The Tata Group has once again proved its determination as it ranked sixth on the list of top 25 'most innovative' companies of the world.[4] Tata has earned this position for designing the common man's car 'Nano' at an extremely affordable price. Apart from this, Tata's acquisition of the Anglo-Dutch steelmaker 'Corus' is considered as the largest Indian takeover of a foreign company and created the world's fifth-largest steel group. Another strategic and innovative move from Tata was the acquisition of the Jaguar and the Land Rover. This initiative is expected to give Tata the opportunity to expand its presence in the passenger car market beyond India and give it the clout necessary to compete with international players.

Tata Inc.: Growth through Innovation

The Tata Company was founded by Jamsetji Tata in 1868; the Tata Group's ventures in its early years were marked by the spirit of nationalism. The Tata Group pioneered a number of industries of national importance in India—like steel, power, hospitality and airlines. Tata is a rapidly growing business group based in India with significant international operations. It is one of India's oldest, largest and most respected business conglomerates. The Group's businesses are spread over seven business sectors (Annexure I). Revenues in 2007–2008 are estimated in excess of $55 billion,[5] of which 65% is from business outside India. It's comprised of 98 companies and operates

in six continents.[6] Tata Group's pioneering spirit has been showcased by companies like Tata Consultancy Services, India's first software company,[7] which pioneered the international delivery model, Tata Steel, Tata Power, Tata Chemicals, Tata Tea, Indian Hotels and Tata Communications. The group employs around 350,000 people worldwide.[8] The Tata name has earned respect for its devotion to strong values and business ethics and maintained its image for the last 140 years in India. The business operations of the Tata Group are divided into seven sectors: communications and information technology, engineering, materials, services, energy, consumer products and chemicals. As of July 3, 2008, Tata Group's 27 publicly listed ventures are among the most valued Indian business houses; they have a collective market capitalisation of $49.56 billion and a shareholder base of 2.9 million.[9]

Internationally, the Tata Group is recognised as a major player after their acquisition of Corus, the largest acquisition abroad by an Indian company.[10] This acquisition was a turning point for Tata Steel, after which it became the fifth largest steel maker in the world.[11] Corus was Europe's second largest steel producer with revenue of 9.2 billion in 2005,[12] and crude steel production of 18.2 million[13] tons primarily in the UK and Netherlands. This company was primarily engaged in the manufacture of semi-finished and finished carbon steel products. Its activities are divided into three main divisions: strip products, and the distribution and building systems division, which operates as a link between Corus's manufacturing operation and its customers. It has a global network of sales offices and service centers. The acquisition was made by Tata Steel UK, a wholly owned indirect subsidiary[14] of Tata Steel, incorporated in the UK for the purpose of completing the acquisition. The acquisition was funded through its own cash resources and loans raised by Tata Steel and its subsidiary companies formed for the purpose of this acquisition.

The acquisition of Corus by Tata Steel is in consonance with Tata Steel's stated objective of growth and globalisation. Growth at Tata Steel is focusing towards new, higher end-markets and a more sophisticated customer base. Tata Steel saw a number of prospects behind the acquisition of Corus. Its improved scale positioned the combined group as the sixth largest steel company in the world by production, with a presence in both Europe and Asia. The powerful combination of low cost upstream production in India with the high end downstream processing facilities of Corus improved the competitiveness of the European operations of Corus significantly. This combination of both the companies allows the cross-fertilisation of research and development capabilities in the automotive, packaging and construction sectors and there is a transfer of technology, best practices and expertise of senior Corus

www.ibscdc.org

* This case was written by Ravi, L, Acharya, S, and Syed, A, IBS Research Center. It is intended to be used as the basis for class discussion rather than to illustrate either effective or ineffective handling of a management situation. The case was compiled from published sources.

sl. No	Business Ventures	Details of the Business
1	Engineering	**Automotive** Tata AutoComp Systems-Subsidiaries / associates / joint ventures: Automotive Composite Systems International, Automotive Stampings and Assemblies, JBM Sung woo, Knorr-Bremse Systems for Commercial Vehicles, TACO Faurecia Design Center, TACO MobiApps Telematics, Tata Autoplastic Systems, Tata Ficosa, Tata Johnson Controls, Tata Nifco Fasteners, Tata Toyo Radiator, Tata Yazaki AutoComp, Tata Yutaka, TC Springs **Tata Motors** Subsidiaries / associates / joint ventures: Concorde Motors, HV Axels, HV Transmissions, Nita Company, TAL Manufacturing Solutions, Tata Cummins, Tata Daewoo Commercial Vehicles Company, Tata Engineering Services, Tata Finance, Tata Holset, Tata Precision Industries, Tata Technologies, Telco Construction Equipment Company **Engineering Services** Tata Projects, TCE Consulting Engineers, Voltas **Engineering Products** TAL Manufacturing Solutions, Telco Construction Equipment Company, TRF
2	Materials	**Composites** Tata Advanced Materials **Metals** **Tata Steel** Subsidiaries / associates / joint ventures: Jamshedpur Injection Powder (Jamipol), Lanka Special Steel, Metaljunction Services Ltd., Sila Eastern Company, Tata Metaliks, Tata Pigments, Tata Ryerson, Tata Sponge Iron, The Tinplate Company of India, Tata Refractories, Tayo Rolls, The Indian Steel and Wire Products, Wires Division
3	Energy	Transmission Tower **Power** **Tata BP Solar India, Tata Power** Subsidiaries / associates / joint ventures: Tata Ceramics, Tata Power Trading, Tata Petrodyne
4	Chemicals	Rallis India, Tata Chemicals, Tata Pigments
5	Services	**Hotels and Realty** **Indian Hotels (Taj group)** Subsidiaries / associates / joint ventures: Taj Air **THDC** **Financial Services** Tata-AIG General Insurance, Tata-AIG Life Insurance, Tata Asset Management, Tata Financial Services, Tata Investment Corporation, Tata Share Registry **Other Services** Tata Economic Consultancy Services, Tata Quality Management Services, Tata Services, Tata Strategic Management Group
6	Consumer Products	**Tata Tea** Subsidiaries / associates / joint ventures: Tetley Group, Tata Coffee, Tata Tetley, Tata Tea Inc. **Tata Ceramics, Tata McGraw-Hill Publishing Company, Titan Industries, Trent**

(*continued*)

Sl. No	Business Ventures	Details of the Business
7	Information Systems And Communications	**Information Systems** **Nelito Systems,** **Tata Consultancy Services** Subsidiaries / associates / joint ventures: APONLINE, Airline Financial Support Services, Aviation Software Development Consultancy, CMC, CMC Americas Inc., Conscripti, HOTV, TCS Business Transformation Solutions, Tata America International Corporation, TCS Business Transformation Solutions, WTI Advanced Technology. Tata Elxsi, Tata InfoTech, Tata Interactive Systems, Tata Technologies **Communications** **Idea Cellular, Tata Teleservices** Subsidiaries / associates / joint ventures: Tata Teleservices (Maharashtra), Tata Internet Services **VSNL, Tatanet** **Industrial Automation** **Nelco** Subsidiaries / associates / joint ventures: Tatanet

Compiled by the authors from: "Tata Group," http://www.managementparadise.com/forums/archive/index.php/t-153.html, August 23, 2005.

management, from Europe to India. In addition, Tata Steel retained access to low cost raw materials and slabs for the enlarged group, and exposure to high growth in emerging markets, whilst gaining price stability in developed markets. Between the two companies, there exists a high degree of cultural compatibility, which would facilitate an effective integration of the businesses. Tata Steel leads the enlarged group with a combined management team. Manufacturing will be organised so as to produce slabs/primary steel in low-cost facilities and produce high end products in proximity to client bases—in both Europe and India.

Tata Motors is India's largest automobile company, with revenues of $8.8 billion in 2007–2008.[15] This company is among the top five[16] commercial vehicle manufacturers and top three[17] in passenger vehicles manufacturers in the world. It is the world's fourth largest[18] truck manufacturer and the second largest[19] bus manufacturer. Tata cars, buses and trucks are being marketed in several countries in Europe, Africa, the Middle East, South Asia, South East Asia and South America. Tata Motors operates in South Korea, Thailand and Spain through its subsidiaries and associate companies. It also has a strategic alliance with Fiat for creation and establishment of an industrial joint venture in India. Tata Motors acquired Jaguar and Land Rover for $2.3 billion.[20] The main motive behind this acquisition is to own Jaguar and Land Rover for perpetual royalty-free licenses of all necessary Intellectual Property

Rights, manufacturing plants, two advanced design centers in the UK, and worldwide network of National Sales Companies. Ratan Tata stated that, "Jaguar and Land Rover are two iconic British brands with worldwide growth prospects. Tata is looking forward to extending their full support to the Jaguar Land Rover team to realise their competitive potential. Jaguar and Land Rover will retain their distinctive identities and continue to pursue their respective business plans as before. Tata Motors recognises the significant improvement in the performance of the two brands and looks forward to this trend continuing in the coming years too (Exhibit 1). It is their intention to work closely to support the Jaguar Land Rover team in building the success and supremacy of the two brands."[21]

The latest to strike the ever-growing Asian and European markets is the sensational Tata Nano, the no-fuss, fuel-efficient energy car that has fueled every Indian's dream to own a car. The Nano, the prototype of which was launched in January 2008, is the biggest innovation from Tata Motors (Exhibit 2). In India, this car is labeled as the "People's Car."[22] The manner in which the Nano has been built and the features that are included, for the declared price, show Tata's innovative strategy and vision.

According to the analysts, the impact of this venture is huge, and everyone is excited at the prospect of owning a car that is only INR 1 lakh ($2500).[23] The car is the result of about five years of research and input from designers across the world. But it is considered by industry watchers

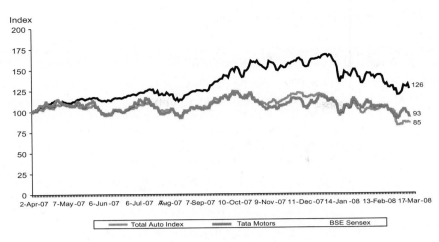

Exhibit 1 **Performance of Tata Motors from April–March 2008**

Source: "Annual Report of Tata Motors," *http://ir.tatamotors.com/performance/a_reports/pdf/2008/TML-2007-08.pdf.*

Note: All figures rebased to April 2, 2007 = 10.

Exhibit 2   **Tata Nano "People's Car" and Its Features**

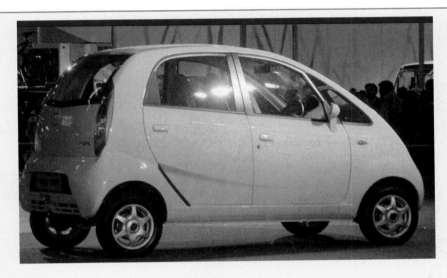

Features of this car:

- Affordable for all income groups
- Four-seater capacity designed to meet the need of a small family
- Meets safety requirements and emission norms
- Is fuel efficient
- Uniquely combines space and maneuverability on busy Indian roads
- First car in the world which uses two-cylinder gasoline engine with single balancer shaft
- Its performance is controlled by a specially designed electronic engine management system aimed at delivering high fuel efficiency.
- Safety features of the Nano's performance are expected to exceed modern regulatory requirements
- Offering the double benefits of an inexpensive transportation solution with a low carbon footprint

Compiled by the authors from: "Nano Car," http://www.mytatanano.co.in/nano-car-pic.html.

Exhibit 3   Innovative / Novel Endeavor by the Tata Group

Sl.No	Company Name	Innovation
1	Tata Motors	• An exciting project is the 'People's Car,' which would sell for around $2,200 (about Rs 1 lakh). A number of incremental innovations mark the project, like the possible use of bolted or glued panels instead of welded bodies. • Indigo—the first sedan designed and manufactured in India. This technology (as is used the world over) allows Tata Motors to meet customer needs in different segments with a single base model.
2	Titan	• Edge from Titan—the ultra slim wristwatch that is only 3.5mm thick and 30mm water-resistant is a path-breaking design concept. No other company selling mass produced watch is slimmer than this.
3	Tata Steel	• Developed low phosphorus steel from high phosphorus ore.
4	Tata BP Solar	• The sun, sand and sea (water) are all inexhaustible sources of renewable and clean energy. It will play a significant role in the years ahead in terms of innovative harnessing and applications of solar energy for the benefit of the larger mankind.

Compiled by the authors from: Gupta Syamal, "Innovation and entrepreneurship," http://www.tata.com/0_media/features/speakers_forum/20060321_syamal_gupta.htm.

as a step ahead in innovation—right from using aerospace adhesives instead of welding, and a clean and efficient fuel-burning technology, to the concept, distribution strategy and marketing—and has succeeded in catching the attention of the world.

TATA: The Pride of India

The founder of Tata Group Jamsetji Tata's creative thinking and foresight were established way back in the 19th century. He imagined hydroelectric power as a clean source of energy; a hundred years on, the world continues its debate on the Kyoto protocol sustainable development and clean development mechanism. His concept of welfare and community development around a steel plant was far ahead of his times. The Tata Group has raised innovative ideas and displayed entrepreneurial spirit in venturing into new geographies, market segments, and product areas (Exhibit 3).

BUSINESSWEEK magazine, issue dated April 28, 2008 has published its list of the world's 50 most innovative companies. The two Indian industrial groups, included in the list for the first time, are the Tatas and the Mukesh Ambani's Reliance Group (Exhibit 4), where the Tata Group is ranked 6th and Reliance bagged the 19th position (Annexure II). To achieve this position the Tata Group has taken up this challenge of innovation anticipating the need of the Indian community. Tata has faced challenges in many of its innovations but yet has been able to overcome those successfully. For instance, when Tata Indica was launched, it did not take off and was touted as a failure but after a thorough analysis of the cause for failure, Tata

Motors was able to put the car on the right path. According to the Boston Consulting Group (BCG) list, this group ranks well above IBM, BMW, Honda Motor, General Motors, Boeing, Audi and Daimler.

Exhibit 4   Top Most 50 Innovative Countries in the World (As per BCG Listing 2008)

Country	Number of Innovative Companies
USA	31
Britain	4
Germany	4
Japan	4
India	2
Canada	1
Finland	1
Netherlands	1
Singapore	1
South Korea	1
Total	50

Compiled by the authors from: "SAJA FORUM," http://www.sajaforum.org/2008/04/index.html, April 30, 2008.

Rank	Company	HQ Country	HQ Continent	Revenue Growth 2004-07* (in %)	Margin Growth 2004-07* (in %)	Stock Returns 2004-07** (in %)	Most Known for Its Innovative ... (% who think so)
1	Apple	USA	North America	47	69	83	Products (52%)
2	Google	USA	North America	73	5	53	Customer Experience (26%)
3	Toyota Motor	Japan	Asia	12	1	15	Processes (36%)
4	General Electric	USA	North America	9	1	3	Processes (43%)
5	Microsoft	USA	North America	16	8	12	Products (26%)
6	Tata Group	India	Asia	Private	Private	Private	Products (58%)
7	Nintendo	Japan	Asia	37	4	77	Products (63%)
8	Procter & Gamble	USA	North America	16	4	12	Processes (30%)
9	Sony	Japan	Asia	8	13	17	Products (56%)
10	Nokia	Finland	Europe	20	2	35	Products (36%)
11	Amazon.com	USA	North America	29	−11	28	Customer Experience (33%)
12	IBM	USA	North America	1	11	4	Processes (31%)
13	Research In Motion	Canada	North America	56	−1	51	Products (37%)
14	BMW	Germany	Europe	6	−5	11	Customer Experience (40%)
15	Hewlett-Packard	USA	North America	10	17	35	Processes, Business Models, and Customer Experience (27% each)
16	Honda Motor	Japan	Asia	12	6	14	Products (40%)
17	Walt Disney	USA	North America	6	14	7	Customer Experience (63%)
18	General Motors	USA	North America	−2	NA***	−11	Products (55%)
19	Reliance Industries	India	Asia	31	−7	94	Business Models (31%)
20	Boeing	USA	North America	9	32	21	Products (63%)

(*continued*)

Rank	Company	HQ Country	HQ Continent	Revenue Growth 2004-07* (in %)	Margin Growth 2004-07* (in %)	Stock Returns 2004-07** (in %)	Most Known for Its Innovative … (% who think so)
21	Goldman Sachs Group	USA	North America	30	6	28	Processes and Business Models (33% each)
22	3M	USA	North America	7	5	3	Products (45%)
23	Wal-Mart Stores	USA	North America	10	−2	−2	Processes (48%)
24	Target	USA	North America	11	3	0	Customer Experience (67%)
25	Facebook	USA	North America	Private	Private	Private	Customer Experience (51%)
26	Samsung Electronics	South Korea	Asia	2	−14	8	Products (42%)
27	AT&T	USA	North America	43	6	23	Customer Experience (33%)
28	Virgin Group	Britain	Europe	Private	Private	Private	Customer Experience (47%)
29	Audi	Germany	Europe	11	11	41	Products (50%)
30	McDonald's	USA	North America	7	−7	25	Customer Experience (42%)
31	Daimler	Germany	Europe	−11	37	28	Products (35%)
32	Starbucks	USA	North America	23	−2	−13	Customer Experience (60%)
33	Ebay	USA	North America	33	−37	−17	Business Models (28%)
34	Verizon Communications	USA	North America	12	0	9	Services (41%)
35	Cisco Systems	USA	North America	20	−5	12	Products (35%)
36	Ing Group	Netherlands	Europe	7	4	11	Services (41%)
37	Singapore Airlines	Singapore	Asia	9	5	20	Customer Experience (55%)

(*continued*)

Rank	Company	HQ Country	HQ Continent	Revenue Growth 2004-07* (in %)	Margin Growth 2004-07* (in %)	Stock Returns 2004-07** (in %)	Most Known for Its Innovative … (% who think so)
38	Siemens	Germany	Europe	1	21	22	Products (41%)
39	Costco Wholesale	USA	North America	11	−5	14	Customer Experience (46%)
40	HSBC	Britain	Europe	12	−1	4	Services (39%)
41	Bank of America	USA	North America	12	0	0	Customer Experience and Services (23% each)
42	Exxon Mobil	USA	North America	11	7	25	Processes (50%)
43	News Corp.	USA	North America	4	4	4	Business Models (47%)
44	BP	Britain	Europe	14	−5	11	Processes (42%)
45	Nike	USA	North America	8	−1	14	Customer Experience (43%)
46	Dell	USA	North America	7	−12	−17	Business Models (37%)
47	Vodafone Group	Britain	Europe	7	−21	15	Business Models (33%)
48	Intel	USA	North America	4	−10	6	Products (53%)
49	Southwest Airlines	USA	North America	15	9	−9	Customer Experience (50%)
50	American Express	USA	North America	3	1	3	Customer Experience (35%)

Source: "The World's 50 Most Innovative Companies," http://bwnt.businessweek.com/interactive_reports/innovative_companies/.

Notes: Analysis and data provided in collaboration with the innovation practice of the Boston Consulting Group and BCG-ValueScience. Reuters and Compustat were used for financial and industry data and Bloomberg for total shareholder returns.

*Compound growth rates for revenue and operating margins are based on 2004–07 fiscal year data as originally stated. Operating margin is earnings before interest and taxes, as a percentage of revenue. Where possible, quarterly and semiannual data were used to bring performance for pre-June year-ends closer to December, 2007. Financial figures were calculated in local currency.

**Stock returns are annualized, 12/31/04 to 12/31/07, and account for price appreciation and dividends.

***Calculating three-year compound annual growth rate for operating margins was not possible when either figure was negative.

The group is focusing on new technologies and innovation to drive its business in India and around the globe. Nano is one such example, which ranked the world's fourth fastest,[24] developed by one of its companies. The group aims to build a series of world class, world scale businesses in selected sectors. Headquartered in India and linked to its traditional values and strong ethics, the group is building a multinational business which will achieve growth through excellence and innovation with corresponding benefits to its shareholders, its employees and wider society.

Tata Group has accelerated its R&D, as many executives of the company continue to believe that enhanced innovation is required to fuel their future growth. R&D spending by Tata Group in the country is very huge and growing rapidly. The ongoing innovation in their products helps them gain competitive advantage. Tata Group is opening up a new era to develop and promote new business models in response to emerging market needs. A post of 'Chief Innovation Officer' was created to guide and promote the group's overall R&D strategy while working closely with each business group. Tata has taken steps to evaluate new opportunities and to bring about a match between innovation and market needs.

Tata is facing a challenging task ahead of becoming globally competitive in terms of cost and quality. They realise the need of the hour is to recognise and pursue innovation as a tool for sustainable advantage in products, processes, business models and organisations. They believe that innovation has to be integrally woven into a firm's strategy and has to drive and sustain competitiveness. Entrepreneurs are first and foremost change makers, achievers and not just visionaries. This thought has been echoed by visionaries such as Mahatma Gandhi[25] and J. R. D. Tata, who were enterprising in all their efforts and approaches. Tata BP Solar, a division of Tata Group, has developed various novel applications of solar photovoltaic and thermals with a view to serving the larger community and rural needs. The impact of innovative applications has a great role to play in enhancing the quality of life of the people in a developing country like India.

For instance, Tata Steel's acquisition of Corus has changed the steel industry, presenting a greater need for technically trained employees and engineers. The deal, which analysts say could still face a counter bid from rival steelmakers, illustrates the drive by low-cost producers to expand their global reach and add more high-technology products. Tata Group has a lot of challenges to face in the post-acquisition period of Corus. Their primary concern was to pay no more than reasonable compensation for Corus in order to result in a profitable combination. Second was to deal with the successful integration between the companies, timely execution of Greenfield projects in India and securing quality raw materials. Though Tata Steel's indigenous iron ore mines in India may be sufficient to meet the current requirements of its Indian operations at Jamshedpur (a city in India), Tata imports about 40% of the coal requirement for its Jamshedpur operations. Finally, it has started evaluating the strategic options for iron ore and coal to vertically integrate their operations and maintain profitability.

Another major challenge in the integration process is the cultural difference. But Tata Group has managed this situation by sharing very similar work ethics and culture, which is basic to the success of any post-acquisition integration process. They opted for a coordinated solution through collaboration which has led to the potential for greater gains for both. Tata Steel's integration process puts pressure on constant and seamless communication between not only the top management of both the companies but also between the operating units, to inculcate respect for each other's culture. This strategy will help in developing appropriate 'performance culture' and 'operating models' of the enlarged entity. Tata has retained the management structure in all their group of companies. The task that lies ahead of them is to continue to successfully execute the integration of operations. Tata stated that, "Together we will be even better equipped to remain at the leading edge of the fast changing steel industry."[26] Tata took extreme care and consideration to ensure that they fully understand the national and corporate cultures of the companies they have bought. At the time of the Jaguar acquisition, Tata also had issues of cultural and communication barriers. Tata was familiar with British business culture following the recent acquisition of steel producer Corus, but here also Tata worked hard to understand Jaguar and Land Rover's unique motoring heritage and business culture. Key to their success was their ability to maintain clear and open channels of communication with all Jaguar and Land Rover employees.

In the making of Nano, Tata is faced with challenges in meeting cost and time targets. The Nano is being produced entirely at Tata's Singur plant, West Bengal (a state in India), which is to have an annual capacity of 250,000–350,000 units. As part of the cost-cutting exercise, 35 parts suppliers have moved into the same complex, reducing transport costs and time delays dramatically. Some of the other challenges are from the rise in the fuel price and Singur being in a flood-prone area. At this stage, Tata has had to work on new variants of the world's cheapest car Nano, to overcome the challenge posed by high fuel prices, which could negatively impact vehicle sales. Tata Motors has also started developing alternative models of Nano to meet environmental and fuel price challenges, as well as market requirements of several international markets. Though fraught with a lot of challenges in achieving a place in the list of topmost innovative companies in the world, at the time of launch of Nano in January 2008, Ratan Tata stated that "The year ahead will be no more daunting than the challenges [we] have faced in difficult years in the past."[27]

Endnotes

1. "The world will always need innovators and innovations," *http://www.tata.com/media/Speeches/inside.aspx?artid=rp1fqgVFrmg=*, March 21, 2006.
2. Gupta, Syamal, "Innovation and entrepreneurship," *http://www.tata.com/0_media/features/speakers_forum/20060321_syamal_gupta.htm*.
3. "Tata buys Jaguar in £1.15bn deal," *http://news.bbc.co.uk/2/hi/business/7313380.stm*, March 26, 2008.
4. Nussbaum, Bruce, "50 of the Most Innovative Companies in the World. Tata, General Motors, Facebook Are Big Surprises," *http://www.businessweek.com/innovate/NussbaumOnDesign/archives/2008/04/50_most_innovat.html*, April 18, 2008.
5. "Tata Group profile," *http://www.tata.com/0_about_us/group_profile.htm*.
6. Ibid.
7. "Tata Consultancy Services—India's first global billion-dollar software organisation," *http://goliath.ecnext.com/coms2/gi_0199-2894756/Tata-Consultancy-Services-Indias.html*.
8. "Tata Group profile," op. cit.
9. "Tata Group profile," op. cit.
10. "Tata's 100 years of steeling the thunder," *http://www.tata.com/tata_steel/media/20070827_3.htm*, August 26, 2007.
11. Ibid.
12. "Tata Steel completes £6.2bn acquisition of Corus Group plc," *http://www.corusgroup.com/en/company/financial_information/tata_steel_offer/2007_tata_steel_acquisition_complete*, April 2, 2007.
13. Ibid.
14. Wholly owned subsidiaries are indirectly controlled by the parent company e.g. the parent company has a significant share/stake in the company to influence decision-making but they do not wholly own or directly control the company. A joint ventures is a good example of an indirect subsidiary.
15. "Tata Motors completes acquisition of Jaguar Land Rover," *http://www.tatamotors.com/our_world/press_releases.php?ID=370&action=Pull*.
16. Ibid.
17. Ibid.
18. Ibid.
19. Ibid.
20. "Tata acquires Jaguar, Land Rover for $2.30 bn," *http://timesofindia.indiatimes.com/Business/India_Business/Tata_acquires_Jaguar_Land_Rover_for_230_bn/rssarticleshow/2902216.cms*, March 26, 2008.
21. "Tata Motors completes acquisition of Jaguar Land Rover," op. cit.
22. "Tata Motors unveils the People's Car," *http://www.tatamotors.com/our_world/press_releases.php?ID=340&action=Pull*, January 10, 2008.
23. Ibid.
24. "Tata Group profile," op. cit.
25. Mohandas Karamchand Gandhi, commonly known around the world as Mahatma Gandhi, was a major political and spiritual leader of India and the Indian independence movement, which led India to independence and inspired movements for civil rights and freedom across the world. He is officially honoured in India as the 'Father of the Nation.'
26. "Tata to take over Corus," *http://www.financialexpress.com/old/latest_full_story.php?content_id=144037*, October 20, 2006.
27. "New Nano model underway to mitigate fuel price challenges: Tata," *http://economictimes.indiatimes.com/News/News_By_Industry/Auto/Automobiles/New_Nano_model_underway_to_mitigate_fuel_price_challengesTata/rssarticleshow/3184422.cms*, July 1, 2008.

Case 17   eBay: Expanding into Asia*

On March 31, 2008, eBay welcomed a new president and CEO, John Donahoe. Donahoe joined the company in 2005 as president of eBay Marketplaces and within three years managed to double the revenues and profits for that division. The new CEO replaced Meg Whitman, who had served as the president of the company for a decade and led eBay to become one of the fastest-growing companies in history. "eBay and its millions of users are in great hands as they head into the future," said Whitman, confident in Donahoe's capabilities.[1] Donahoe was set on improving overall customer satisfaction and protection, and shortly after his election he introduced significant changes to fee structure, seller standards, and feedback at eBay.[2] However, despite Donahoe's strategic management, eBay still faced challenges in its Asia Pacific market.

On August 14, 2008, eBay was granted approval by the South Korea's Fair Trade Commission to buy a combined 36.6 percent stake in Gmarket from the company's largest shareholder, Interpark Corp., and Interpark's chairman Ki Hyung Lee. Partly owned by Yahoo, Gmarket was one of the leading online auctioneers and shopping malls in South Korea.[3] The news suggested that eBay was once again struggling to compete in the Asian market. eBay followed the same strategy in December 2006 when it shut down its existing site in China and bought 49 percent of a joint venture with Beijing-based Tom Online. The move was expected to give eBay some of the local expertise it desperately needed to compete with China's top auction site, Taobao. Despite Meg Whitman calling the deal an evolution of the company's China strategy and not a failure, analysts viewed it as an indication that U.S. Web players were still lacking success with their strategy in Asia.[4] With Asia's population exceeding 3.7 billion, more than half the world's population, and Internet usage in the region skyrocketing at 406 percent, eBay needed to develop a strategy that would successfully adapt to Asian local markets and compete with Taobao and other major local competitors.

eBay

Since its inception in 1995, eBay enjoyed strong revenue growth and was a dominant player in the online auction industry. The company posted net income of $1.78 billion and revenue of $8.54 billion for 2008, up dramatically from 2007's net income of $0.35 billion and revenue of $7.62 billion. (See Exhibit 1.) "Despite the extremely challenging economic environment in 2008—including a slowdown in global e-commerce, a strengthening dollar, and declining interest rates—we delivered . . . an

11 percent increase from the prior year, and . . . a solid operating margin of 24 percent," commented CEO John Donahoe.[5]

eBay's founder, Pierre Omidyar, envisioned a community built on commerce, sustained by trust, and inspired by opportunity. The company's mission was to "enable individual self-empowerment on a global scale" and employ "business as a tool for social good." Omidyar cited "trust between strangers" as the social impact tied to eBay's ability to remain profitable. The company's unique business model, which united buyers and sellers in an online marketplace, had attracted over 221 million registered users. eBay enabled e-commerce at multiple levels (local, national, and international) through an array of Web sites, including eBay Marketplaces, PayPal, Skype, *Rent.com*, and *Shopping.com*. The company's range of products and services had evolved from collectibles to household products, customer services, automobiles, and so on. The variety of products attracted a range of users that included students, small businesses, independent sellers, major corporations, and government agencies.

Despite eBay's outstanding growth performance, the company still faced a number of challenges in both domestic and international markets. The low entry barriers in the online marketplace attracted a number of large dot-com competitors, including Amazon, Yahoo, uBid, and Overstock. Historically, the company had acquired other online competitors, such as Stubhub (tickets), but established players such as Yahoo and Amazon posed a major threat to eBay's market share and ability to sustain profitability. Still, eBay's top management felt that the company would end up as a specialty business, an idea suggesting that it would face little threat from these major competitors:

> We have specialized in e-commerce, payment and voice communication. Google stands for search, Yahoo largely stands for content—so I think we may on the fringe compete, but I suspect that over time the businesses will become more specialized. (*Meg Whitman, February 8, 2006*)

The company had no plans for further big acquisitions but intended to expand and identify synergies within existing business lines.

eBay acknowledged its inability to grow and compete in certain international markets. The company localized sites in 24 countries and a presence in Latin America through its investment in *MercadoLibre.com*. However, eBay's numerous attempts to penetrate the Asia Pacific market, specifically China and Japan, ended in failure, with the company pulling out of Japan and buying out Chinese start-up Eachnet, essentially canceling years of invested work. According to many analysts,

* This case was prepared by Professor Alan B. Eisner and graduate student David J. Morates of Pace University. This case was solely based on library research and was developed for class discussion rather than to illustrate either effective or ineffective handling of an administrative situation. Copyright © 2007, 2009 Alan B. Eisner.

Exhibit 1 Income Statements (in thousands, except per-share amounts; year-end December 31)

	2004	2005	2006	2007	2008
Net revenues	$3,271,309	$4,552,401	$5,969,741	$7,672,329	$8,541,261
Cost of net revenues	614,415	818,104	1,256,792	1,762,972	2,228,069
Gross profit	2,656,894	3,734,297	4,712,949	5,909,357	6,313,192
Operating expenses:					
Sales and marketing	798,555	1,143,580	1,587,133	1,882,810	1,881,551
Product development	240,647	328,191	494,695	619,727	725,600
General and administrative	335,076	479,418	744,363	904,681	998,871
Provision for transaction and loan losses	157,447	212,460	266,724	293,917	347,453
Amortization of acquired intangible assets	65,927	128,941	197,078	204,104	234,916
Restructuring	—	—	—	—	49,119
Impairment of goodwill	—	—	—	1,390,938	—
Total operating expenses	1,597,652	2,292,590	3,289,993	5,296,177	4,237,510
Income from operations	1,059,242	1,441,707	1,422,956	613,180	2,075,682
Interest and other income, net	71,745	111,099	130,017	154,271	115,919
Interest expense	(8,879)	(3,478)	(5,916)	(16,600)	(8,037)
Income before income taxes	1,122,108	1,549,328	1,547,057	750,851	2,183,564
Provision for income taxes	(343,885)	(467,285)	(421,418)	(402,600)	(404,090)
Net income	$ 778,223	$1,082,043	$1,125,639	$ 348,251	$1,779,474
Net income per share:					
Basic	$ 0.59	$ 0.79	$ 0.80	$ 0.26	$ 1.37
Diluted	$ 0.57	$ 0.78	$ 0.79	$ 0.25	$ 1.36
Weighted average shares:					
Basic	1,319,458	1,361,708	1,399,251	1,358,797	1,303,454
Diluted	1,367,720	1,393,875	1,425,472	1,376,174	1,312,608

Source: eBay.

the company's recent interest in its South Korean rival Gmarket Inc. and joint venture with Beijing-based Tom Online were further indications that eBay couldn't compete in these countries. To remain successful and enjoy the same financial performance as it had in the past, eBay needed to develop an effective strategy to compete in major Asian markets and mitigate the risk of existing local competitors.

Evolution of Auctions

Traditional Auctions According to Greek scribes, the first known auctions occurred in Babylon in 500 BC. At that time, women were sold on the condition of marriage,

and it was considered illegal for daughters to be sold outside auctions. Auctions evolved during the French Revolution and throughout the American Civil War, where colonels auctioned goods that were seized by armies.[6] Although there were various types of auctions, they all provided a forum where sellers could find buyers or hobbyists who were looking to purchase rare items and collectibles. Auctions were considered one of the purest markets, since buyers paid what they were willing to spend for an item, thereby determining the true market value of the item. Over time, auction formats continued to evolve, and through technological advances and improved communication they found a new home—the Internet.

Online Auctions The primary difference between traditional and online auctions was that the online auction process occurred over the Internet as opposed to at a specific location where both buyers and sellers were present. Online auctions offered strategic advantages to both parties that were not typically available in traditional auctions. Buyers could select from millions of products and engage in multiple auctions simultaneously. Given the massive inventory of an online auction market, items were usually available in multiple auctions, allowing buyers to compare starting bid prices and search for better prices. Sellers were exposed to millions of buyers, since more buyers had access to the Internet and felt comfortable making purchases online. The net impact was increased price competition, since there were more buyers who were willing to purchase items at a higher price. Thus, the Internet gave buyers and sellers access to a marketplace that spanned the world.

Online auctions also offered the following strategic advantages:

1. *No time constraints.* A bid could be placed at any time.
2. *No geographic constraints.* Sellers and buyers could participate from any location with Internet access.
3. *Network economies.* The large number of bidders attracted more sellers, which attracted more bidders, and so on. This created a large system that had more value for both parties. Online auctions also allowed businesses to easily sell off excess inventory or discontinued items. This was done through either business-to-business (B2B) or business-to-consumer (B2C) auctions. Offering products and services in an online auction helped small businesses build their brand and reputation by establishing a devoted customer base. Finally, some businesses used the online marketplace as an inexpensive yet effective way to test-market for upcoming products.

E-Commerce

Although Vannevar Bush originally conceived the idea of the Internet in 1945, it wasn't until the 1990s that the Internet became overwhelmingly popular. According to Internet World Stats, in December 2008 there were over 1.5 billion Internet users in over 150 countries. Exhibit 2 shows Internet usage growth between 1995 and 2010.

As of December 19, 2008, North America was considered the region most penetrated by the Internet, with approximately 73.6 percent of the population already online. However, Internet usage growth between 2000 and 2008 was considerably less in North America than in other regions. The regions with the highest Internet usage growth were developing countries where penetration was low, such as Africa, Asia, Latin America, and the Middle East. Considering close to 80 percent of the world's population resides in these areas, it is inevitable that Internet usage growth will continue to increase dramatically in

these regions. Exhibit 3 shows the world Internet usage and population as of December 2008.

Although Asia constituted approximately 57 percent of the world's population, its penetration rate was only 15.3 percent. Compared to other regions with high usage growth rates such as Africa and the Middle East, Asia invested more in its technology infrastructure and contained by far the most current Internet users, making it a more attractive market. Exhibit 4 provides more detail on how Asia stacks against the rest of the world in terms of Internet usage.

As the usage growth of the Internet increased, so did the popularity of e-commerce. E-commerce, or electronic commerce, was the concept of conducting business transactions over the Internet. As in the case with online auctions, e-commerce eliminated boundaries such as time and geography, allowing businesses and customers to interact with one another constantly. As more users were exposed to the Internet, they became comfortable with the idea of conducting transactions online. In correlation with Internet growth usage, revenue generated through e-commerce increased dramatically since the 1990s. Exhibit 5 shows U.S. online retail revenues generated through e-commerce over the 2003–2008 period.

E-commerce grew rapidly in other regions as well, especially in Asia since China's admission into the World Trade Organization (WTO) on December 11, 2001. Induction in the WTO allowed China to conduct business with other nations more freely by reducing tariffs and eliminating market and government impediments.

Company Background

Computer programmer Pierre Omidyar founded the online auction Web site in San Jose, California, on September 3, 1995. Omidyar was born in Paris, France, and moved to Maryland with his family when his father took on a residency at Johns Hopkins University Medical Center. Omidyar became fascinated with computers and later graduated from Tufts University with a degree in computer science. While living and working in the San Francisco Bay area, he met his current wife, Pamela Wesley, a management consultant, who later became a driving force in launching the auction Web site. The couple's vision was to establish an online marketplace where people could share the same passion and interest as Pamela had for her hobby of collecting and trading Pez candy dispensers.[7] Omidyar also envisioned an online auction format that would create a fair and open marketplace, where the market truly determined an item's value. To ensure trust in the open forum, Omidyar based the site on five main values:

1. People are basically good.
2. Everyone has something to contribute.
3. An honest, open environment can bring out the best in people.
4. Everyone deserves recognition and respect as a unique individual.
5. You should treat others the way you want to be treated.

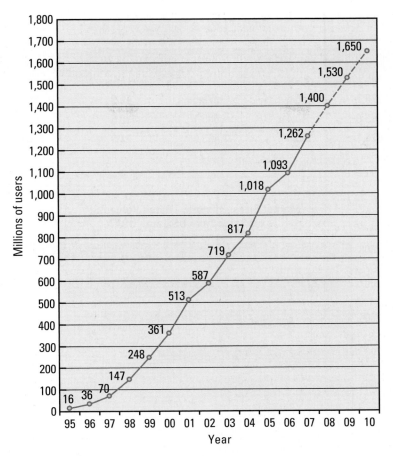

Exhibit 2 **Internet Usage Growth, 1995–2010**

Source: Internet World Stats—Global Village Online, 2008.

Exhibit 3 **World Internet Usage and Population Statistics, 2008**

World Regions	Population (millions)	Population (%)	Internet Usage (millions)	Percent Penetrated	Usage as % of World	Usage Growth, 2000–2008 (%)
Africa	955.2	14.3	51.1	5.3	3.5	1,031.2
Asia	3,776.2	56.6	578.5	15.3	39.5	406.1
Europe	800.4	12.0	384.6	48.1	26.3	266.0
Middle East	197.1	2.9	41.9	21.3	2.9	1,176.8
North America	337.2	5.1	248.2	73.6	17.0	129.6
Latin America	576.1	8.6	139.1	24.1	9.5	669.3
Australia	33.9	0.5	20.2	59.5	1.4	165.1
Total	**6,676.1**	**100.0**	**1,463.6**	**21.9**	**100.0**	**305.5**

Source: Internet World Stats—Usage and Population Statistics, 2008.

Exhibit 4 Internet Usage in Asia

Regions	Population (millions)	Internet %	Internet Users (millions)	Usage % Penetrated	Usage as % of World	Usage Growth, 2000–2008 (%)
Asia	3,776.2	56.6	578.5	15.3	39.5	406.1
Rest of world	2,899.9	43.4	885.1	30.5	60.5	258.8
Total	**6,676.1**	**100.0**	**1,463.6**	**21.9**	**100.0**	**305.5**

Source: Internet World Stats—Usage and Population Statistics, 2008.

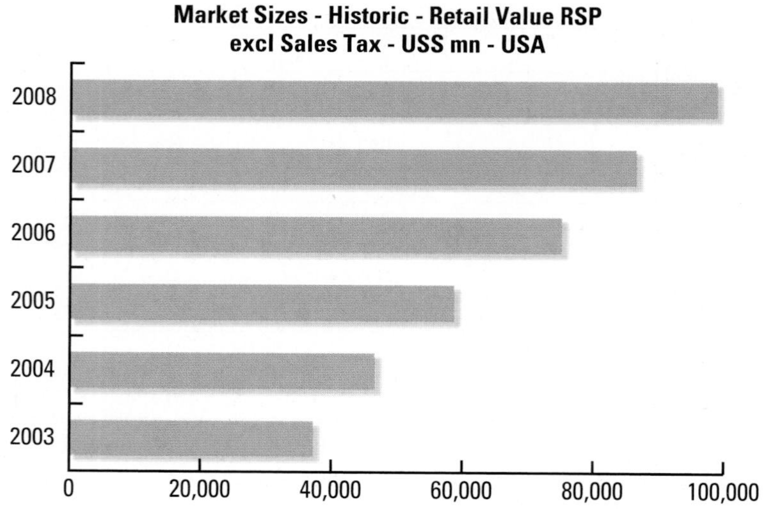

Market Sizes - Historic - Retail Value RSP excl Sales Tax - USS mn - USA

Exhibit 5 U.S. Online Retail Revenues

Source: Internet World Stats—E-Commerce Market Size and Trends, 2006.

On Labor Day weekend in 1995, Omidyar launched Auction Web, an online trading platform. After the business exploded, Omidyar decided to dedicate more attention to his new enterprise and work as a consultant under the name Echo Bay Technology Group. When he tried to register a Web site for his company, Omidyar discovered Echo Bay was unavailable, so he decided to use the abbreviated version *eBay,* which also stood for "electronic bay area." The company's name was also selected to attract San Francisco residents to the site and prompt them to buy and sell items.

Initially, the company did not charge fees to either buyers or sellers, but as traffic grew rapidly Omidyar was forced to charge buyers a listing fee to cover Internet service provider costs. When Omidyar noticed that the fees had no impact on the level of bids, he realized the potential for profitability of his business. To handle and manage the company's day-to-day operations, Omidyar hired Jeffrey Skoll (B.A.Sc. University of Toronto, MBA Stanford University). Skoll was hired as the company's first president, and he wrote the business plan that eBay later followed from its emergence as a start-up to its maturity as a financial

success. The two worked out of Skoll's living room and various Silicon Valley facilities until they eventually settled in the company's current location in San Jose, California.

By the middle of 1997, less than a year under the name eBay, the company was hosting nearly 800,000 auctions a day.[8] Although the rapid expansion of eBay's traffic caused the company to suffer a number of service interruptions, the site remained successful and continued to gain the confidence of its strong customer base. Skoll remained president until early 1998, when the company hired Meg Whitman as president and CEO. At the time, the company had only 30 employees and was solely located in the United States; in a decade the number of employees went up to over 15,000. In September 1998, eBay launched a successful public offering, making both Omidyar and Skoll instant billionaires. By the time eBay went public, less than three years after Omidyar had created the company, the site had more than a million registered users. The company grew exponentially in the late 1990s and, based on its 2008 performance, indicated no sign of stopping. Exhibit 6 highlights the company's recent growth performance by segments.

Exhibit 6 eBay Growth (in millions, year-end December 31)

	2006	2007	2008
Supplemental Operating Data:			
Marketplace Segment:			
Gross merchandise volume[1]	$52,474	$59,353	$59,650
Payments Segment:			
Net total payment volume[2]	$35,800	$47,470	$60,146
Communications Segment:			
Registered users[3]	171.2	276.3	405.3
SkypeOut minutes[4]	4,095	5,650	8,374

[1] Total value of all successfully closed items between users on eBay Marketplaces trading platforms during the period, regardless of whether the buyer and seller actually consummated the transaction.

[2] Total dollar volume of payments, net of payment reversals, successfully completed through our payments network or on Bill Me Later accounts during the period, excluding the payment gateway business.

[3] Cumulative number of unique user accounts, which includes users who may have registered via non-Skype based Web sites, as of the end of the period. Users may register more than once and, as a result, may have more than one account.

[4] Cumulative number of minutes that Skype users were connected with Skype's VoIP product to traditional fixed-line and mobile telephones.

Source: eBay.

Whitman stepped down as the president and CEO of the company on March 31, 2008. Through a decade of her successful leadership, Whitman had managed to build an increasingly diversified portfolio of businesses and transformed a company with just 30 employees and $4.7 million in revenue into one of the fastest-growing companies in history, with revenues of $8.5 billion. "With humor, smarts and unflappable determination, Meg took a small, barely known online auction site and helped it become an integral part of our lives," said Omidyar, chairman of the board, about Whitman, who remained on the board of directors.[9] Both Omidyar and Whitman were confident that the new CEO, John Donahoe, was a good choice to lead eBay. Donahoe joined the company in 2005 as president of eBay's largest division, Marketplaces, and within three years managed to double the revenues and profits for this business unit. Before joining eBay, Donahoe served as the CEO of Bain & Company, an international consulting firm based in Boston.[10] "I'm extremely confident in John's skills and the abilities of John's veteran management team," Meg Whitman commented on the transition.[11]

Shortly after his election, Donahoe announced fundamental changes targeted at improving the overall buying experience and protection for eBay users. The changes included lowering fees for listing items and raising minimum standards for the sellers, as well as offering incentives and discounts to reward sellers with the best buyer satisfaction ratings.[12] In addition, in June 2008, the company improved buyer and seller protection on eBay. First-time buyers were protected for 100 percent of an item's purchase price, while sellers would receive improved protection when items were paid for with PayPal.[13] Donahoe was confident that these changes would significantly reinforce healthy and frequent trading at eBay.

Year 2008 was also marked by eBay's increased commitment to social responsibility. On April 28, 2008, the eBay Foundation, the charitable division of eBay Inc., introduced an online fund-raising campaign, Community Gives. The new campaign aimed at generating funds for providing low-income families with children's books, caring for mistreated animals, and supplying water in poverty-stricken regions. "The mission of the initiative is to build on the positive impact of our businesses and make the most of our opportunity to be a force for good in the world," said Bill Barmeier, eBay's vice president of Global Citizenship.[14] By June 2008, eBay's Community raised $150 million for global causes through charity listings on eBay, an increase of $50 million since 2007.[15] In September 2008, eBay launched a new online marketplace, *WorldofGood.com*, offering products that had positive impact on people and the environment. "We created the *WorldofGood.com* marketplace to enable shoppers to purchase socially responsible products with confidence," commented Robert Chatwani, general manager of *WorldofGood.com*.[16]

eBay Platforms

eBay's overall strategy comprised three primary components: products, sense of community, and aggressive expansion. All three components evolved around the various geographic and specialty platforms the company introduced.

Product Categories   eBay had an array of product categories and trading platforms that offered a range of pricing formats, such as fixed pricing. Relatively new for the company, establishing a fixed-price format allowed eBay to compete directly with major competitors such as *Amazon.com* and penetrate new market space. Before fixed pricing, selling prices were solely determined by the highest auction bid, and this took days or weeks depending on the length of the auction. eBay's different trading platforms also offered distinct services and target-specific market niches, which allowed eBay to broaden its customer base. The platforms included:

- *PayPal:* Founded in 1998 and acquired by eBay in 2002, PayPal enabled individuals to securely send payments quickly and easily online. PayPal was considered the global leader in online payments, with tens of millions of registered users.
- *Rent.com:* Acquired by eBay in February 2005, *Rent.com* was the most visited online apartment listing service in the United States, with more than 20,000 properties listed.
- *Skype:* Acquired by eBay in October 2005, Skype was the world's fastest-growing online communication solution, allowing free video and audio communication between users of Skype software. By 2008, Skype connected more than 405 million registered users.[17]

eBay's acquisition of Skype was expected to enhance the customer experience by improving communication between buyers and sellers. According to former CEO Meg Whitman, "Communications is at the heart of e-commerce and community. By combining the two leading e-commerce franchises, eBay and PayPal, with the leader in Internet voice communications, we will create an extraordinary powerful environment for business on the Net." However, some analysts were confused by the hefty $2.6 billion acquisition and cited the move as being defensive and trying to acquire as much online traffic as possible. Still, eBay felt Skype would increase trade velocity in the marketplace, which was critical for categories that required more involved communications.

- *Shopping.com:* With thousands of merchants and millions of products and reviews, *Shopping.com* empowered consumers to make informed choices, which drove value for merchants. The company was acquired by eBay in August 2005.
- *Stubhub.com:* Acquired by eBay in January 2007, StubHub was an online marketplace for selling and purchasing tickets for sports events, concerts, and other live entertainment events.
- *Online classifieds:* By January 2009, eBay had the world-leading portfolio of online classifieds sites, including Intoko, Gumtree, *LoQUo.com*, and *mobile.de*, as well as Netherlands-based

Marktplaats.nl.[18] In 2007, eBay expanded its classifieds business through its acquisition of Kijiji.[19] In October 2008, eBay further diversified its classifieds portfolio by acquiring Den Bla Avis and BilBasen, providers of successful classifieds businesses in Denmark, for $390 million. "We are the global leader in classifieds with top positions in Canada, Australia, Germany, Japan and the United Kingdom, and sites in more than 1,000 cities across 20 countries," said CEO John Donahoe after the latest acquisition.[20]

- *eBay Express:* Introduced in April 2006, eBay Express behaved like a standard Internet shopping site but gave sellers access to over 200 million buyers worldwide. Sellers could design product categories within minutes and buyers could purchase from multiple sellers by using a single shopping cart.
- *eBay Motors:* This specialty site was considered the largest marketplace for automobile buyers and sellers. Buyers could purchase anything from automobile parts to new or antique vehicles.

The use of product categories such as eBay Express and eBay Motors provided further depth in eBay's product offerings and enabled the company to target a broader market.

Sense of Community   The underlying key to all eBay sites and trading platforms was creating trust between sellers and buyers. The company created "community values," and this was why eBay users were willing to send money to strangers across the country. The Feedback Forum was created in February 1996 and encouraged users to post comments about trading partners. Originally, Omidyar handled disputes between buyers and sellers via e-mail by putting the disputing parties in touch with each other to resolve the issue themselves. He soon realized that an open forum where users could post opinions and feedback about one another would create the trust and sense of community the site required. Buyers and sellers were encouraged to post comments (positive, negative, or neutral) about each other at the completion of each transaction. The individual feedback was recorded and amended to a user profile, which ultimately established a rating and reputation for each buyer and seller. eBay users could view this information before engaging in a transaction. The company believed that the feedback forum was critical for creating initial user acceptance for purchasing and selling over the Internet and that it contributed more than anything else to eBay's success.

Aggressive Expansion   To compete effectively and create a global trading platform, the company continued to develop in U.S. and international markets that utilized the Internet. With intense competition in the online auction industry, eBay aimed to increase market share and revenue through acquisitions and partnerships in related and unrelated businesses. For example:

- In June 2000, eBay acquired *Half.com* for $318 million.
- In August 2001, eBay acquired MercadoLibre, Lokau, and iBazar, Latin American auction sites.
- On August 13, 2004, eBay took a 25 percent stake in Craigslist, an online central network of urban communities.
- In September 2005, eBay invested $2 million in the Meetup social networking site.
- In August 2006, eBay announced international cooperation with Google.
- In January 2007, eBay acquired online ticket marketplace Stubhub for $310 million.

During this period, eBay also made a number of acquisitions and investments in international markets. In addition, in mid-2006, eBay announced an agreement to share services, such as advertising and online payments, with Yahoo in an attempt to minimize the intense competition of rival search-engine giant Google.[21]

Company Business Model

eBay's business model was based on a person-to-person marketplace on the Internet where sellers conveniently listed items for sale and interested buyers bid on these items. The objective was to create a forum that allowed buyers and sellers to come together in an efficient and effective manner. The business model overcame the inefficiencies of traditional fragmented marketplaces, which tended to offer a limited variety of goods. According to former CEO Meg Whitman, the company started with commerce and what grew out of that was a community, essentially creating a community-commerce model.[22] The company's success relied primarily on establishing a trustworthy environment that attracted a large number of buyers and sellers. As eBay's reputation grew, so did the number of buyers and sellers, keeping the company in line with Omidyar's original vision. However, as new competitors entered the online auction business and the popularity of the Internet increased, eBay tweaked its business model to accommodate the changes in the fast-paced environment.

The company was aggressively expanding globally and looking for new products and services to offer to customers. It was also looking closely at the kind of merchants who sold on eBay. In the beginning, eBay focused on a consumer-to-consumer business model, but since some of the individuals became small dealers, the model changed to a mix of consumer-to-consumer and business-to-consumer. The sellers wanted to maintain their business on eBay, since it was their most profitable distribution channel. eBay wanted new ways to generate revenue as a result of more small dealers and businesses selling their products through the company's Web site.

eBay generated revenue through three main channels: marketplaces, payments, and, most recently, communications.

Marketplaces, which generated revenue by charging sellers a fee for every item they sold, accounted for over 65 percent of the company's revenue. As of December 2008, marketplace revenue was approximately $5.6 billion of the company's $8.5 billion total revenue. Another $2.4 billion of the company's revenue came from fees charged through electronic payments made through the company Web site, primarily via PayPal. The newest source of revenue for eBay was communications (Skype), which produced $551 million of the company's revenue. Although free, eBay's communication software generated revenue through its premium offerings such as making and receiving calls to and from landline and mobile phones, as well as voice mail, ring tones, and call forwarding. Despite its small percentage of eBay's total revenue, the product was new and experienced the strongest growth between 2007 and 2008, when its revenue almost doubled. Exhibit 7 shows the company's recent revenue performance by type.

In addition to the primary revenue sources, there were specific elements of eBay's business model that made the company a success. eBay's dominance of the online auction market and the large number of buyers, sellers, and listed items were primary reasons for eBay's tremendous growth. The trust and safety programs, such as the Feedback Forum, continued to attract and retain new and current eBay users. The cost-effective and convenient trading, coupled with the strong sense of community, added further value to the company's business model. However, as the company continued to grow and new trends evolved, eBay had to continue to adjust its model to remain competitive. Exhibit 1 presents the company's consolidated income statement.

International Expansion

As competition intensified in the online auction industry, eBay expanded its international presence in an effort to create an online global marketplace. Gradually, eBay localized sites in the following countries:

- *Asia Pacific:* Australia, China, Hong Kong, India, Malaysia, New Zealand, Philippines, Singapore, South Korea, and Taiwan.
- *Europe:* Austria, Belgium, Denmark, France, Germany, Ireland, Italy, Netherlands, Poland, Spain, Sweden, Switzerland, and the United Kingdom.
- *North America:* Canada and the United States.

In many of the international Web sites, eBay provided local-language and -currency options to gain popularity and ensure the sense-of-community feeling. In most cases, eBay expanded its business by either acquiring or forming a partnership with a local company. This strategy helped eBay better understand local cultures and ensure that the company was meeting specific local needs. This approach proved successful with the company's equity investment in *MercadoLibre.com*, which targeted Argentina, Brazil, Chile, Colombia, Costa Rica, Dominican Republic, Ecuador, Mexico, Panama, Peru, Uruguay, and Venezuela. At the

Exhibit 7   Net Revenues by Type (in thousands, except percent changes)

	Year Ended December 31, 2006	Percent Change from 2006 to 2007	Year Ended December 31, 2007	Percent Change from 2007 to 2008	Year Ended December 31, 2008
Net Revenues by Type					
Net transaction revenues					
Marketplaces	$3,864,502	21%	$4,680,835	1%	$4,711,057
Payments	1,401,824	31%	1,838,539	26%	2,320,495
Communications	189,110	93%	364,564	44%	525,803
Total net transaction revenues	5,455,436	26%	6,883,938	10%	7,557,355
Marketing services and other revenues					
Marketplaces	469,788	45%	683,056	28%	875,694
Payments	38,706	128%	88,077	(6)%	83,174
Communications	5,811	197%	17,258	45%	25,038
Total marketing services and other revenues	514,305	53%	788,391	25%	983,906
Total net revenues	$5,969,741	29%	$7,672,329	11%	$8,541,261
Net Revenues by Segment:					
Marketplaces	$4,334,290	24%	$5,363,891	4%	$5,586,751
Payments	1,440,530	34%	1,926,616	25%	2,403,669
Communications	194,921	96%	381,822	44%	550,841
Total net revenues	$5,969,741	29%	$7,672,329	11%	$8,541,261
Net Revenues by Geography:					
U.S.	$3,108,986	20%	$3,742,670	6%	$3,969,482
International	2,860,755	37%	3,929,659	16%	4,571,779
Total net revenues	$5,969,741	29%	$7,672,329	11%	$8,541,261

Source: eBay.

end of 2006, *MercadoLibre.com* reported 18 million registered users who performed 15.8 million transactions worth $1.1 billion.[23] Other notable international growth acquisitions are listed below.

Asia Pacific

- *July 2003:* Acquired China-based Eachnet for approximately $150 million. eBay's failure to manage the company resulted in its recent partnership with communications company Tom Online.
- *June 2004:* Acquired all outstanding shares of India's *Baazee.com*, which later became eBay India.
- *September 2004:* Acquired Korean rival Internet Auction Co. by purchasing nearly 3 million shares.

Acquisition was not proved successful due to intense competition from top Korean auction site GMarket.

Europe

- *1999:* Acquired Alando auction house for $43 million, a company that later became eBay Germany. Alando was previously considered Germany's leading online trading company. Germany became eBay's second-largest market, accounting for 21 percent of the company's total listings.
- *November 2004:* Acquired Dutch competitor *Marktplaats.nl*, which had 80 percent of the Netherlands market share.

- *April 2006:* Acquired Sweden's leading online auction company, *Tradera.com*, for $48 million.
- *October 2008:* Acquired Denmark's leading online classifieds businesses, Den Bla Avis and BilBasen, for $390 million.[24]

For the most part, eBay was successful in expanding in Europe and Latin America, where it was able to quickly adapt to local needs through its partners. The company was also successful in countries it expanded to from the ground up, such as Canada and the United Kingdom. In 2007, the United Kingdom accounted for 15.5 percent of eBay's total listings. By engaging the local community in these countries, eBay customized its sites to meet specific local needs while providing access to the online global community.

eBay was considered the leader in each of its markets with the exception of Japan and China, in which it struggled repeatedly to gain market share. In 2002, eBay was forced to pull out of Japan due to rising costs and intense competition by rival Yahoo Japan. eBay also faced fierce competition in Korea, where GMarket, another investment of Yahoo, dominated the market.

Despite its lack of success in local Asian markets, eBay continued its attempts to expand into the region, recognizing the tremendous growth potential that was available. In June 2006, eBay formed a joint venture with PChome Online in Taiwan. PChome Online was an Internet service provider in Taiwan, with more than 10 million members.[25] The company offered services such as Internet portal, e-commerce platform, and telecommunications. The move was expected to provide eBay with the local e-commerce expertise it needed to launch a new trading Web site that catered to the needs of Taiwan's Internet users.

In 2006, eBay emphasized its commitment to the Chinese e-commerce market by announcing a new joint venture with Beijing-based Internet Company Tom Online Inc. Tom Online, which primarily sold cell phone add-on services, such as ring tones and avatars, put in $20 million for a 51 percent share and management control of eBay's online China site, Eachnet.[26] In 2002, eBay purchased a 30 percent stake in Eachnet and within a year bought out local investors. Central management control of Eachnet was maintained in eBay's San Jose, California, location. Many believed the move was a result of eBay's failure to adapt to local needs and successfully compete with China's online auction market leader Taobao, which controlled approximately 70 percent of the market. Jack Ma, the chief executive of *Alibaba.com*, Taobao's parent company, believed eBay's failure in China was due to an inability to build a community effect in the country, which according to Ma begins with customer satisfaction. Ma also felt that since eBay had to adhere to a global platform, meeting specific local needs was difficult because changes at a global level had to be approved in the United States, which further limited the company's ability to

produce a Web site tailored to the Chinese market.[27] In an Interview with *Internetnews* in 2005, Ma stated eBay's lack of success in China was predominantly due to the company's quickness to replace local management with foreigners and the mind-set to control the market through spending rather than building it from the ground up.[28] In 2008, eBay sought approval from South Korea's Fair Trade Commission to secure a stake in its successful competitor, Gmarket. This news suggested that eBay was once again struggling to compete in the Asian market.

Competitors

As eBay's product offerings and pricing formats evolved, so did its range of competitors. Originally, the company faced competition from alternative auctions or other venues for collectors, such as flea markets and garage sales. However, as the company grew and introduced fixed pricing, the range of competitors included large companies like Wal-Mart and Kmart that also had retail Web sites. eBay's product platforms, like eBay Motors, put the company in direct competition with auto dealers and other online auto sites such as Autobytes. Still, eBay faced the harshest competition from major online companies that included Yahoo and Amazon, which also had online auctions that rivaled eBay's.

Yahoo!   eBay's larger online competitor was Yahoo, which also had a strong global presence, particularly in Asian markets. Yahoo originally started as a search engine and quickly evolved to include additional products and services such as Yahoo! Mail, Yahoo! Maps, and Yahoo! Messenger. The company also offered e-commerce services through Yahoo! Shopping, Yahoo! Autos, Yahoo! Auctions, and Yahoo! Travel. Like eBay, Yahoo's e-commerce sites allowed users to obtain relevant information and make transactions and purchases online. However, Yahoo's business model primarily focused on generating revenue through search advertising. In the United States, in response to potential threats from Web giant Google, Yahoo and eBay formed an alliance in which Yahoo utilized eBay's payment system, PayPal, and eBay gained additional advertising through Yahoo searches. Still, Yahoo posed a major competitive threat in foreign markets, particularly Asia Pacific, through its partnerships with GMarket and Taobao.

GMarket   Yahoo's stake in Korean auction site GMarket proved successful, with more than 17.2 million unique visitors. Founded in 2000, GMarket was a Korean online auction and shopping-mall Web site that generated its revenue by charging a fee based on selling price.[29] Like Taobao, GMarket offered fixed prices and provided an option to negotiate prices with sellers on an exclusive basis. This allowed buyers to conduct deals instantly instead of waiting until bids were completed. GMarket also offered cheaper listings. These options along with constant new features allowed GMarket to dominate the Korean online auction industry.[30] GMarket frequently introduced new marketing initiatives to provide sellers with various options to attract new customers. GMarket grew financially powerful in 2006 when it launched its IPO and Yahoo purchased a 9 percent stake in the company. In 2008, eBay decided to secure an interest in its rival and was granted approval to purchase a combined 36.6 percent stake in Gmarket from Interpark Corp. and its chairman.[31]

Taobao   In 2005, Yahoo entered a strategic partnership with *Alibaba.com*, Taobao's parent company, which created an instant threat in the Chinese market. The move created one of the largest Internet companies in China, one with a leading position in business-to-business e-commerce, consumer e-commerce, and online payments. Like GMarket, Taobao offered buyers and sellers quick and convenient ways to conduct business. Its instant messaging and fixed price arrangements allowed transactions to be conducted quickly. In 2006, the company partnered with Intel to offer customers a wireless platform. This further improved communication and convenience when customers were conducting transactions. In 2009, Taobao was eBay's largest competitor in China, controlling over 70 percent of the Chinese online auction market.

Amazon   Despite not having a huge presence in the online auction industry, Amazon was still considered a fierce online global competitor. Amazon started as Earth's biggest bookstore and rapidly evolved to selling everything, including toys, electronics, home furnishings, apparel, health and beauty aids, groceries, and so on. Still, books, CDs, and DVDs accounted for more than 65 percent of the firm's sales. Although Amazon had a large international presence, the company's linkage to brick-and-mortar shops in the United States made it a greater threat locally than in foreign markets. Amazon's international local sites were in Canada, the United Kingdom, Germany, Japan, France, and China. Despite its large online presence, Amazon scaled back its online auction business, cutting staff and shutting down Livebid, as part of an overall corporate restructuring.

The Future of eBay

eBay had a number of opportunities in which it had already taken action. By 2009, eBay had made a number of strategic acquisitions that included *Rent.com*, international classified Web sites, *Stubhub.com*, *Shopping.com*, and Skype. These acquisitions added and complemented eBay's product offerings and further diversified the company's targeted market. With increased competition from Google and other major online companies, eBay had to continue to diversify and provide depth in its product offerings to remain competitive. Creating options and targeting distinct market niches would enable eBay to distinguish itself from competitors. This was particularly important because as e-commerce and Internet usage rates continued to grow, so would the market opportunity for eBay. Because of its market-leading brand, eBay was in a unique position to capture a significant share of the market at an early stage.

eBay could also expand its existing products and services, such as PayPal and Skype. Both products were relatively new and had the potential to grow and attract new customers, especially in international markets. Expanding PayPal into international markets would enable eBay to provide a simple way to conduct transactions across market borders. Considering the growth potential in developing markets such as those in Africa, Asia, and the Middle East, expanding PayPal would attract many new customers, thus increasing eBay's revenue base. In line with e-commerce growth, as more customers felt comfortable with conducting transactions online, PayPal had the potential to be the preferred form of payment over the Internet.

However, for eBay to capitalize on these opportunities, the company would have to overcome the challenges of expanding into large foreign markets such as China and Japan. With almost 70 percent of the North American population using the Internet and only a 15.3 percent usage rate in Asia Pacific, eBay had a tremendous opportunity to expand and gain new customers. Considering that the Asia Pacific region had more than 50 percent of the world's population and was experiencing some of the largest online usage growth percentages in the world, tapping into this market was critical for eBay to expand.

Endnotes

1. eBay. Meg Whitman to Step Down as President and CEO of eBay (press release). *http://news.ebay.com/releasedetail .cfm?ReleaseID=289314.*

2. eBay. eBay Announces Bold Changes Aimed at Improving Overall Customer Experience (press release). *http://news .ebay.com/releasedetail.cfm?ReleaseID=290446.*

3. South Korea OKs eBay's Purchase of Gmarket. August 15, 2008, *http://www.marketwatch.com/news/story/south-korea-oks-ebays-purchase/story.aspx?guid=% 7BBF3F40DB-7BD5-4E21-9715-3074575DC155%7D.*

4. F. Balfour. Tom Online: eBay's Last China Card. *Business-Week Online,* December 19, 2006.

5. eBay. Annual Report, 2008.

6. The History of Auction Method of Marketing. National Auctions Association, 2005, *www.onlyatauction.com.*

7. Pierre Omidyar—The Man behind eBay. Internet Based Moms, April 2007, *www.internetbasedmoms.com.*

8. Biography—Pierre Omidyar. Academy of Achievement, *www.achievement.org*, November 9, 2005.

9. eBay. Meg Whitman to Step Down.

10. eBay corporate Web site.

11. eBay. Meg Whitman to Step Down.

12. eBay. eBay Announces Bold Changes.

13. eBay. eBay and PayPal Increase Protections for Buyers and Sellers to Shop with Confidence (press Release). *http://news.ebay.com/releasedetail.cfm?ReleaseID= 317542.*

14. eBay. eBay Inc. and eBay Foundation Join Forces to Launch *Community Gives* (press release). *http://news.ebay .com/releasedetail.cfm?ReleaseID=306929.*

15. eBay. eBay Giving Works Celebrates Milestone of $150 Million Raised and Unveils New Program Enhancements (press release). *http://news.ebay.com/releasedetail .cfm?ReleaseID=317520.*

16. eBay. eBay Launches New Online Marketplace for Ethically Sourced and Eco-Friendly Products (press release). *http://news.ebay.com/releasedetail.cfm? ReleaseID=331792.*

17. eBay. Annual Report, 2008.

18. eBay. eBay Acquires Leading Classifieds Sites in Denmark (press release). *http://news.ebay.com/releasedetail.cfm? ReleaseID=338504.*

19. eBay corporate Web site.

20. eBay. eBay Inc. Buys Leading Payments and Classifieds Businesses, Streamlines Existing Organization to Improve Growth (press release). *http://news.ebay.com/releasedetail .cfm?ReleaseID=338505.*

21. Hoover's Company Records. In-Depth Records: eBay, Inc. February 13, 2007.

22. Q&A with eBay's Meg Whitman. *BusinessWeek Online,* May 31, 1999.

23. Argentina: MercadoLibre Has 18mil Registered Users. *IT Digest,* January 25, 2007, *www.infobae.com.*

24. eBay. eBay Acquires Leading Classifieds Sites in Denmark.

25. eBay. eBay and PChome Online to Form Joint Venture in Taiwan (press release). *www.ebay.com.*

26. Market Spotlight: Asia Internet strategy. LexisNexis, December 21, 2006.

27. Alibaba CEO Says Taobao Will Dominate China Online Auctions. *Forbes.com,* May 2005.

28. S. Kuchinskas. *Internetnews,* October 22, 2004, *www .internetnews.com.*

29. M. Ihlwan. Gmarket Eclipses eBay in Asia. *BusinessWeek Online,* June 28, 2006.

30. Out-eBaying eBay in Korea. *BusinessWeek Online,* July 17, 2006.

31. South Korea OKs eBay's Purchase of Gmarket. August 15, 2008, *http://www.marketwatch.com/news/story/ south-korea-oks-ebays-purchase/story.aspx?guid= %7BBF3F40DB-7BD5-4E21-9715-3074575DC155%7D.*

In January 2006, Google, the world-famous Internet giant, launched Google China (*www.google.cn*) in the belief that the benefits of a more open Internet and increased access to information for Chinese people could outweigh discomfort towards the Chinese government's regulation of partial censorship of search results (see Google in China (A) case[2]). In January 2010, however, Google officially announced that Google.cn experienced cyber attacks targeting the Gmail[3] accounts of several Chinese human rights activists. Google further announced that, as a result, it had decided to reconsider its approach to China, including the option of a complete exit from the Chinese market. By March 2010, the company had conducted a thorough evaluation of both the attack and its China operations, and much had been written in the media regarding Google's future in China. It was time to make a decision on what to do with the Chinese search engine—Google.cn—and the local operating functions such as research and development (R&D) and sales.

Google.com from 2006 to 2009

Google maintained strong growth in the period of 2006 to 2009: its revenue reached US$23 billion by 2009 (see Exhibit 1), nearly doubling its revenue from 2006. Google's legendary success was the result of a complex set of highly developed processes, in terms of both its ever-expanding innovative product offerings and its cutting-edge information technology infrastructure. In 2009, Google AdWords and AdSense dominated global online advertising: these technologies accounted for 97 percent of the company's total revenue[4] and enabled Google to enjoy two-thirds of the market share in the United States.[5] The strong presence of Google in the U.S. market even trigged a call by Consumer Watchdog for an antitrust probe against Google.[6]

Google's strong performance in online advertising provided a solid revenue base to finance the launch of a series of innovative products that reached a wide market and rapidly became popular. In 2006, Google launched the now-famous applications Picasa Web Album, Google Docs, Google Talk, Google Calendar and Google Checkout. In 2008, Google released its mobile operation system Android. Android was lauded as a possible competitor to Apple's iPhone platform. The same year witnessed the releases of Google Chrome, an open-source browser, and Google Translate.

These innovative products required unimaginable Internet-based computing power to operate. To support web search, video delivery, e-mail and image and document storage, Google spent billions of dollars creating this Internet-based operating infrastructure and developing proprietary technology. By 2008, Google was running over one million servers in parallel data centers around the world,[7] and processing over one billion search requests[8] and 20 petabytes[9] of user-generated data every day.[10] The investment in infrastructure allowed the company to guarantee required service levels and response times, as well as support rapid development and rollout of new Internet-based services.

China Internet Search Market Overview

The Internet search industry in China was rapidly evolving and highly competitive. It was estimated that Internet users in China reached 384 million by the end of 2009—more than the entire population of the United States, up from 45.8 million in 2002. In parallel to the rocketing growth of Internet users was the extent of Internet use in China. According to a survey conducted by McKinsey & Company in 2009, people in the 60 largest cities in China spent approximately 70 percent of their leisure time on the Internet. To grasp the commercial opportunity on the Internet in China, it was not surprising to see that online advertising had been growing at between 20 and 30 percent per year—twice the print media's growth rate, with a market size of approximately US$3 billion (RMB 20 billion) in 2009.[11]

Baidu, Google, Yahoo, Sohu and Sina were the major players in the Internet search industry in China. As the two largest search players, Baidu and Google dominated the market, accounting for over 90 percent of the searches since 2008 (see Exhibit 2). Sohu was more prominently used for MP3 and video searches, but lagged in web search. Yahoo had been struggling with its local partnering strategy and had failed to take advantage of large acquisitions locally, including the much-publicized Alibaba.

Google.cn   Google China was launched amid widespread criticism in 2006. It enabled Google to create a greater presence in the fast-growing Chinese search market. In return for being able to run a local Chinese service, Google agreed to block certain websites, utilizing a list of prohibited keywords maintained by the Chinese government. Due to this self-imposed censorship, people conducting Google.cn searches on the words included in this list would encounter the following message: "In

Exhibit 1 **Consolidated statements of income** (in thousands, except per share amount)

	Three Months Ending December 31		Twelve Months Ending December 31	
	2008	2009 (unaudited)	2008*	2009 (unaudited)
Revenue	$5,700,904	$6,673,825	$21,795,550	$23,650,563
Costs and expenses				
Cost of revenues	2,190,005	2,408,400	8,621,506	8,844,115
Research and development	733,342	736,234	2,793,192	2,843,027
Sales and marketing	505,993	583,149	1,946,244	1,983,941
General and administrative	411,360	465,059	1,802,639	1,667,294
Total costs and expenses	3,840,700	4,192,842	15,163,581	15,338,377
Income from operations	1,860,204	2,480,983	6,631,969	8,312,186
Impairment of equity investments	(1,094,757)	—	(1,094,757)	—
Interest income and other, net	69,899	87,688	316,384	69,003
Income before income taxes	835,346	2,568,671	5,853,596	8,381,189
Provision for income taxes	452,904	594,571	1,626,738	1,860,741
Net income	$382,442	$1,974,100	$4,226,858	$6,520,448
Net income per share —basic	$1.22	$6.22	$13.46	$20.62
Net income per share—diluted	$1.21	$6.13	$13.31	$20.41
Shares used in per share calculation—basic	314,651	317,237	313,959	316,221
Shares used in per share calculation—diluted	316,864	322,163	317,514	319,416

* Derived from audited financial statements.

Source: Google annual report 2009.

accordance with local laws, regulations and policies, part of the search result is not shown."[12]

Google had established R&D and sales functions to support its Internet search businesses in China. In 2005, it opened an R&D center in China to develop search engines specifically for the Chinese population, as well as take a part of the global R&D duties by collaborating with engineers in other Google offices. This center was one of the most desired places to work for Chinese information technology (IT) elites. By January 2010, the center hosted 600 engineers, with assignments ranging from localization for the Chinese Internet search market to participation in Google global R&D practice. Google also developed and expanded a competent sales and marketing team, numbering approximately 140 people by 2009, strategically based in three major first-tier cities: Beijing, Shanghai and Guangzhou.

With the establishment of the primary search product and the supporting functions, Google made significant progress in expanding its market share in China. After the launch of the Chinese website, market share went up from 16 to 31 percent in 2009. Revenue in the Chinese market rose to over US$300 million from $32 million in 2006 (see Exhibit 3). Google China had managed to grow by focusing on improving its Chinese-word search quality, expanding product lines and developing partnerships with local companies. Firstly, the R&D center mandated to customize Google.cn according to Chinese users' language conventions and specific local needs. Secondly, it launched a series of services to complement the search function, such as Google Earth, Google Hot List, Q&A and a free legal music download service—the latter launched in order to compete with its homegrown rival, Baidu. Thirdly, Google China developed a strategic partnership

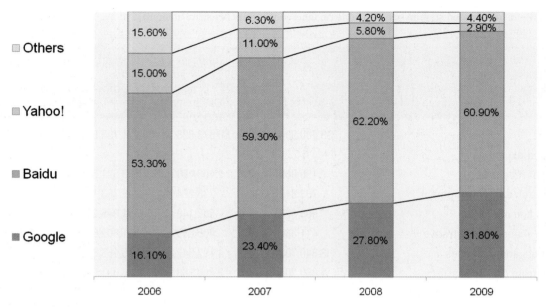

Exhibit 2 Market Share in China

Source: Estimates based on web search by the authors.

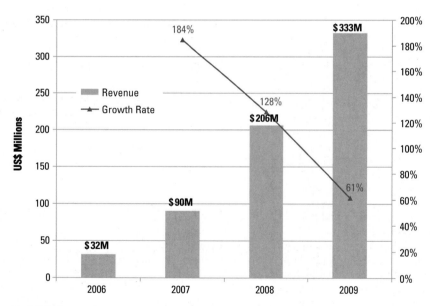

Exhibit 3 Google's Revenue Growth in China

Source: Estimates based on web search by the authors.

with China Mobile, China's largest telecom service operator, launching a customized smartphone based on Google's Android operating system.

Despite these advances, Google's journey in China was not without roadblocks. Due to a lengthy approval process demanded by the Chinese government, Google did not receive official license to operate its website in China until September 2007, more than 18 months after it set up Google.cn. In January 2009, Chinese regulators criticized Google—among other major players such as Baidu and Sina—for making pornography available through its search engine.[13] While Baidu and Sina formally apologized to the public, Google China seemed to express much less shame about the whole affair.[14] Consequently, in June 2009, Chinese regulators announced a suspension of both Google China's ability to search through foreign websites and its associative-word search function in punishment for failing to effectively respond to the government's criticism by removing pornographic content from its search results. This action drove existing Google users away, pushing them towards its rival, Baidu. In October 2009, Google was embroiled in a copyright dispute with Chinese authors whose works it had published in its online library, Google Books. The Chinese writers accused Google of copyright infringement, for which Google later apologized. In September 2009, amid the difficulties and debates over the Chinese government's censorship policies, Kai-Fu Lee, chief executive officer (CEO) of Google China, announced his resignation and his plans to start a venture fund.

Baidu.com Baidu was the leading Chinese-language search engine provider. The company name "Baidu" originated from a famous Chinese poem written over 800 years ago in the Chinese Song Dynasty: it literally means "hundreds of times," thus implying the persistent search for the ideal. In 2000, Baidu was established by two Chinese nationals, Robin Li and Eric Xu, who had studied and worked overseas before returning to China. Baidu announced its initial public offering on August 5, 2005, and was traded on the NASDAQ national market under the symbol "BIDU." It established three subsidiaries in China, with a sizeable workforce of over 7,000 employees. By 2006, when Google formally entered China, Baidu had occupied over 50 percent of China's online search market. Its leading position remained in 2009, with its market share increasing to 60 percent (Exhibit 2). Baidu implemented the international strategy of finding a Japanese subsidiary to provide Japanese search services at baidu.jp.[15]

Central to Baidu's strong position in China was its focus on developing the best Chinese-language search products and technologies to suit the needs and requirements of local search users and online marketers. For Chinese search users, Baidu exhibited strong competence in pinpointing queries in the Chinese language by tailoring its products and services according to Chinese users' needs and wants; for instance, it introduced "phonetic" or "pin-yin" searches, which allowed users to type in Chinese keywords based on their corresponding Chinese pronunciation, but using the English alphabet. This feature was designed to allow users to skip the process of switching from English alphabet inputting to Chinese character inputting, and to give confidence to users who were not certain of the accuracy of the written Chinese character keywords.

Similar to Google, Baidu's web search technology applied a combination of techniques to determine the importance of a web page independent of a particular search query, as well as the relevance of that page to a particular search query. These techniques included link analysis, information extraction, web crawling and Chinese-language processing. For Chinese-language processing, Baidu analyzed Chinese web pages by processing word segmentation and utilizing an encoding method based on Chinese-language characteristics; for example, it could identify Chinese names on a web page. When a user searched for a person based on the person's Chinese name, Baidu could display web pages that were specifically related to that person. It also mined user behavior and search interests from search query logs. These capabilities ensured a simple and reliable search experience for Chinese users.

Baidu's major revenue model was its media platform for online marketing clients. Its online marketing services included a pay-for-performance (P4P) platform and tailored solutions. The company's auction-based P4P platform enabled customers to place their website links and related descriptions on Baidu's search result list. The customers would bid to determine how much they were willing to pay for each time someone clicked on their listings in the Baidu search results. Unlike traditional online advertising services for which flat fees were charged, these marketing products and services were performance-based. Baidu was the first auction-based P4P model service provider in China. P4P took the market by storm because it was cost-effective and measurable.

Google Blog—"A New Approach to China"

On January 12, 2010, Google made an announcement on its official blog that it had detected several unusual security incidents in mid-December 2009:[16]

> Like many other well-known organizations, we face cyber attacks of varying degrees on a regular basis. In mid-December, we detected a highly sophisticated and targeted attack on our corporate infrastructure originating from China that resulted in the theft of intellectual property from Google. However, it soon became clear that what at first appeared to be solely a security incident—albeit a significant one—was something quite different.
>
> First, this attack was not just on Google. As part of our investigation we have discovered that at least twenty other large companies from a wide range of businesses—including the Internet, finance, technology, media, and chemical sectors—have been similarly targeted. We are currently in the process of notifying those companies, and we are also working with the relevant U.S. authorities.
>
> Second, we have evidence to suggest that a primary goal of the attackers was accessing the Gmail accounts of Chinese human rights activists. Based on our investigation to date, we believe their attack did not achieve

that objective. Only two Gmail accounts appear to have been accessed, and that activity was limited to account information (such as the date the account was created) and subject line, rather than the content of e-mails themselves.

Third, as part of this investigation but independent of the attack on Google, we have discovered that the accounts of dozens of U.S.-, China- and Europe-based Gmail users who are advocates of human rights in China appear to have been routinely accessed by third parties. These accounts have not been accessed through any security breach at Google, but most likely via phishing scams or malware placed on the users' computers.

We have already used information gained from this attack to make infrastructure and architectural improvements that enhance security for Google and for our users. In terms of individual users, we would advise people to deploy reputable anti-virus and anti-spyware programs on their computers, to install patches for their operating systems and to update their web browsers. Always be cautious when clicking on links appearing in instant messages and e-mails, or when asked to share personal information like passwords online.

We have taken the unusual step of sharing information about these attacks with a broad audience not just because of the security and human rights implications of what we have unearthed, but also because this information goes to the heart of a much bigger global debate about freedom of speech. In the last two decades, China's economic reform programs and its citizens' entrepreneurial flair have lifted hundreds of millions of Chinese people out of poverty. Indeed, this great nation is at the heart of much economic progress and development in the world today.

These attacks and the surveillance they have uncovered—combined with the attempts over the past year to further limit free speech on the web—have led us to conclude that we should review the feasibility of our business operations in China. We have decided we are no longer willing to continue censoring our results on Google.cn, and so over the next few weeks we will be discussing with the Chinese government the basis on which we could operate an unfiltered search engine within the law, if at all. We recognize that this may well mean having to shut down Google.cn, and potentially our offices in China.

The decision to review our business operations in China has been incredibly hard, and we know that it will have potentially far-reaching consequences. We want to make clear that this move was driven by our executives in the United States, without the knowledge or involvement of our employees in China who have worked incredibly hard to make Google.cn the success it is today. We are committed to working responsibly to resolve the very difficult issues raised.

Following this blog post, Google China turned off its search result filtering; however, the filtering was reactivated after five days without any acknowledgment, explanation or media coverage. Search queries in Chinese on the keywords "Tiananmen" or "June 4, 1989," for example, would deliver censored results with the standard censorship footnote.

The "Aurora" Attack

Two days after the attack (labeled "Operation Aurora") became public, McAfee, a world-renowned security software vendor, reported that the attackers had exploited zero-day vulnerabilities (i.e., taking advantage of a security vulnerability on the same day that the vulnerability becomes generally known[17]) in Internet Explorer. An analysis of the attack showed a complex package of programs that applied custom protocols and sophisticated infection techniques expressly designed to retrieve valuable files from compromised machines. Specifically, when a victim computer was compromised, a backdoor connection that linked the computer to several command and control servers would be established. The victim's machine would then begin exploring the protected corporate intranet. Using the intranet, the attack program would search for other vulnerable systems, as well as targeted information such as sources of intellectual property or e-mail user information, as in the case of the attack on Google China.[18] A week after the report by McAfee, Microsoft issued a fix for the issue and admitted that it had known about the security hole used since September 2009.[19]

According to an estimate by security vendor Isec Partners, the hackers who broke into Google went after more than 100 companies; moreover, researchers had been zooming in on the unidentified sources responsible for the attack. Some believed that the attacks originated from two educational institutions in China.[20] In the process, they uncovered another 68 command-and-control servers used to control the compromised computers.[21]

Aftermath Public Reactions

In the months following Google's announcement, a large number of comments from diverse standpoints had been aired. Privacy advocates applauded Google's move to disclose the cyber attacks and reverse its stand on censorship of its China search engine results: "Google has taken a bold and difficult step for Internet freedom in support of fundamental human rights," said Leslie Harris, president of the Center for Democracy and Technology. "No company should be forced to operate under government threat to its core values or to the rights and safety of its users."[22] Standing on the other side of the "privacy protection" perspective was Consumer Watchdog (*www .consumerwatchdog.com*), which interpreted Google's decision as "a diversionary tactic to draw attention away from its inability to provide adequate security for online data."[23] Others suspected that Google might have been using the attack as an excuse to set the stage for an exit from the Chinese market.

The fact that Google lagged behind Baidu in paid web search by a huge margin clearly demonstrated that Google did not enjoy the same success in China that it enjoyed elsewhere in the world. While closing down the operation in China could have potentially cost Google over US$300 million in annual revenue, this was but a small portion of Google's global revenue. Indeed, Google stock dropped by a mere half percent after Google made the announcement regarding the potential exit, indicating that this might not be a huge concern for the shareholders. Baidu's stock, on the other hand, soared by over 13 percent, showing that Google's move was probably more important to Baidu than Google in the short term.[24]

Other analysts suspected that Google's threat to exit from China might have been a strategy to pressure the Chinese government to renegotiate the rules of the game. While it was unlikely that the Chinese government would allow search results to be uncensored, "Google [was] probably hoping to win some concessions that [could] help it compete more effectively in the Chinese market," said Patricio Robles, an independent technology reporter. "Just as Google's original agreement to censor search results for the Chinese government was a calculated business decision, its decision to now turn on the Chinese government is a calculated business decision, too."[25] After all, China was one of the world's largest consumer markets and was important to most global companies, including Google.

In China, reactions on the web were critical of both the government and Google. One blogger said, "They [the government] had better cut the cable under the sea so that they don't have to worry at all."[26] Others predicted that, even if Google were to leave, any potential inconvenience caused by Google's exit would be short-lived: "The Internet is really big," said Wang Quiya, a 27-year-old worker in Beijing's financial district. "Something will take its place, right?"[27]

Some loyal users of Google, particularly many of the young, well-educated Chinese, were worried that the potential loss of access to Google.cn would make it difficult to obtain useful information, especially when most popular global Internet services such as Google.com, Facebook and Twitter were not available to users from within the geographic boundary of mainland China. Interviews held in Beijing's downtown and university districts by journalists from *The New York Times* showed that many young people viewed the possible loss of Google's maps, translation services, sketching software, access to scholarly papers and search function with distress. "How am I going to live without Google?" asked Wang Yuanyuan, a 29-year-old businessman in Beijing's business district.[28]

Next Step

While the public kept debating Google's next step in China, Google was behind the scenes discussing the future of Google China with the Chinese government. In late February, the company posted a number of articles advertising for new positions for its China business. Chinese local media speculated that "some consensus might have been achieved between Google and the Chinese government."[29] Google stated upon its entry into China that "we will carefully monitor conditions in China, including new laws and other restrictions on our services. If we determine that we are unable to achieve the objectives outlined, we will not hesitate to reconsider our approach to China." Has that time come?

Endnotes

1. This case has been written on the basis of published sources only. Consequently, the interpretation and perspectives presented in this case are not necessarily those of Google or any of its employees.
2. Ivey case 9B06E019.
3. An e-mail service provided by Google.
4. *Google Annual Report*, 2009.
5. "comScore releases November 2009 U.S. search engine rankings," *comScore*, December 16, 2009, accessed March 4, 2010. *http://www.comscore.com/Press_Events/ Press_Releases/2009/12/comScore_Releases_ November_2009_U.S._Search_Engine_Rankings,* accessed March 4, 2010.
6. Grant Gross, "Consumer group calls for antitrust probe against Google," itbusiness.ca, April 23, 2010, *www .itbusiness.ca/it/client/en/home/news.asp?id=57320,* accessed April 27, 2010.
7. "Google: One million servers and counting," *Pandia Search Engine News*, July 2, 2007, *www.pandia.com/sew/481- gartner.html,* accessed March 6, 2010.
8. Eric Kuhn, "Google unveils top political searches of 2009," Political Ticker Blog, December 18, 2009, *http://political ticker.blogs.cnn.com/2009/12/18/google-unveils-top- political-searches-of-2009/?fbid=3Su28m5jJux,* accessed March 6, 2010.
9. One petabyte = 1,000 terabytes or one million gigabytes.
10. Erick Schonfeld, "Google processing 20,000 terabytes a day and growing," *TechCrunch*, January 9, 2008, *http:// techcrunch.com/2008/01/09/google-processing-20000- terabytes-a-day-and-growing/,* accessed March 6, 2010.
11. Max Magni and Yuval Atsmon, "China's Internet obsession," *The Conversation – Harvard Business Review Blog*, February 24, 2010, *http://blogs.hbr.org/cs/2010/02/ chinas_internet_obsession.html,* accessed April 27, 2010.
12. *www.google.cn.*
13. Internet pornography has been outlawed in China since 2002. See *http://www.usatoday.com/tech/news/2002/01/18/ china-internet.htm,* accessed June 4, 2010.
14. Austin Modine, "Google China and Baidu apologize for porn links," The Register, January 7, 2009, *www .theregister.co.uk/2009/01/07/googlechina_baidu_sina_ apologize_for_pr0n_links/,* accessed April 27, 2010.
15. *http://ir.baidu.com/phoenix.zhtml?c=188488&p =irol-homeprofile.*
16. David Drummond, "A new approach to China," The Official Google Blog, January 12, 2010, *http://google blog.blogspot.com/2010/01/new-approach-to-china.html,* accessed February 6, 2010.

17. "Zero-day exploit," *SearchSecurity.com*, *http://search security.techtarget.com/sDefinition/0,,sid14_gci955554, 00.html,* accessed April 27, 2010.

18. "An insight into the Aurora communication protocol," McAfee Labs blog, *http://www.avertlabs.com/research/ blog/index.php/2010/01/18/an-insight-into-the-aurora-communication-protocol,* accessed June 15, 2010.

19. Ryan Naraine, "Microsoft knew of IE zero-day flaw since last September," *ZDNet*, January 21, 2010, *http://blogs .zdnet.com/security/?p=5324,* accessed March 3, 2010.

20. Owen Fletcher and Jaikumar Vijayan, "Don't blame us for Google hack, say indignant Chinese schools," *ITBusiness .ca*, February 24, 2010, *www.itbusiness.ca/it/client/en/ home/news.asp?id=56529,* accessed March 4, 2010.

21. Robert McMillan, "Google hackers broke into more than 100 companies' systems," *ITBusiness.ca*, March 2, 2010, *www.itbusiness.ca/it/client/en/home/News.asp? id=56617&PageMem=1,* accessed March 4, 2010.

22. Ellen Nakashima, Steven Mufson and John Pomfret, "Google threatens to leave China after attacks on activists' email," *The Washington Post*, January 13, 2010, *http://www .wired.com/threatlevel/2010/01/google-censorship-china/,* accessed June 4, 2010.

23. John M. Simpson, "Google does the right thing in China, but not necessarily for the right reason," *Consumer Watchdog*, March 22, 2010, *www.consumerwatchdog.org/ corporateering/articles/?storyId=33392,* accessed April 27, 2010.

24. Patricio Robles, "Is Google's China threat really a business maneuver?" *Econsultancy* (blog), January 14, 2010, *http:// econsultancy.com/blog/5244-is-google-s-china-threat-really-a-business-maneuver,* accessed March 4, 2010.

25. Ibid.

26. Ellen Nakashima, Steven Mufson and John Pomfret, "Google threatens to leave China after attacks on activists' email," *Washington Post*, January 13, 2010, *www .washingtonpost.com/wp-dyn/content/article/2010/01/12/ AR2010011203024.html,* accessed March 4, 2010.

27. Sharon LaFraniere, "China at odds with future in Internet fight," *The New York Times*, January 16, 2010, *www .nytimes.com/2010/01/17/world/asia/17china.html,* accessed March 4, 2010.

28. Ibid.

29. "Google China resumes recruiting," February 24, 2010, *http://www.sbs.com.au/news/article/1201707/headline,* accessed June 4, 2010.

Case 19 Pakistan: A Story of Technology, Entrepreneurs, and Global Networks*

In November 2007, Asad Jamal, founder of ePlanet Ventures, a technology fund based in Silicon Valley, faced a dilemma. A recent business plan submitted by an entrepreneur based in Lahore, Pakistan had rekindled nagging thoughts that Pakistan should be considered a "strategic play" for his venture fund. Although of Pakistani origin, Asad had spent the majority of his life away from the country, after getting his Bachelor's degree from the London School of Economics. He had developed a notable venture investment track record at ePlanet Ventures by demonstrating his ability to identify promising opportunities in the advertising, media, communications and wireless, computing software, consumer Internet, and other market spaces. As with any venture capitalist (VC), he was always on the lookout for new horizons. Asad was considering whether he wanted to be one of the first entrants in a nascent, largely untapped market. He once again turned his thoughts to the promising development he had witnessed in Pakistan during his visits over the previous 10 years.

History

Pakistan became an independent nation on August 14, 1947 when British India gained independence from British rule. Two countries were created, newly independent India and Pakistan. Although founded on democratic principles, Pakistan's political history had been tumultuous and the country had spent more than half its short life under military rule. A succession of military dictators, interspersed with ineffective and corrupt civilian regimes, failed to fully exploit the country's vast natural reserves and human assets.[1]

When Prime Minister Nawaz Sharif was deposed by General Musharraf in a 1999 military coup, Pakistan was on the verge of bankruptcy and in danger of becoming a failed state. The mood at that time was a mixture of apprehension and enthusiasm for the new beginning Musharraf had promised. By 2007, President Musharraf had restored some level of authority to parliamentary forces and still held a tenuous grip on power. Whatever his other achievements and failures, his supporters and detractors alike conceded that combined with his support for the war on terror, he reduced corruption and undertook wide-ranging

* This case was prepared by Sameer Sabir (MIT MBA '08), Tania Aidrus (MIT MBA '08) and Sarah Bird (MIT TPP '08) under the supervision of Kenneth P. Morse, Senior Lecturer, MIT Sloan School of Management, and Managing Director, MIT Entrepreneurship Center and Imran Sayeed, Lecturer, MIT Sloan School of Management.

and bold economic reforms with the aim of reinvigorating Pakistan's economy.[2] Between 2000 and 2007, Pakistan's per capita GNI (gross national income) grew from \$480 to \$800 (comparable to India's \$820) and the country's GDP (gross domestic product) growth rate went from 4.9% to 6.9%. Revenue as a percentage of GDP was greater than India's (13.5% vs. 12.6%). (See Exhibit 1 for more detailed economic data.) Despite Pakistan's uncertain political future, Musharraf's policies appeared to invigorate Pakistan's economy and stimulate entrepreneurship within the country.[3]

Pakistan's Large, Evolving Market

Pakistan was the sixth most populous country in the world with an increasingly empowered middle class whose needs were starting to resemble those of the West, from basic things such as access to satellite TV and the Internet. The U.S. venture capital community was realizing that many technologies that worked successfully in the West could be replicated in markets like Pakistan. For example the success of Baidu in China was based on a few smart entrepreneurs realizing, through local knowledge, that they could customize a search engine to meet the needs of the Chinese market and VCs such as ePlanet Ventures saw the same potential in Pakistan.

There were logical business considerations for investing in Pakistan, such as a large market, cost-base and talent, in addition to reasons based on cultural or family connections. Companies had already been outsourcing to Pakistan, particularly for call centers, but also more recently in the high-tech space. Even larger companies had been recently entering the market. En Pointe Technologies, a NASDAQ-listed provider of advisory services to SAP and information security–focused IT organizations, owned several subsidiaries in Pakistan employing over 700 people, as well as in India and other emerging countries.

The Economy and Regulatory Reform
Since 2002, Pakistan had seen strong GDP growth, averaging around 7% per year. Prior to this, GDP growth had been inhibited by a narrow production base, political instability, and poor and inconsistent policies synonymous with corruption. However, substantial remittances from Pakistanis working abroad, wide-ranging reforms (including an aggressive privatization program), aggressive tax policies, restructured public enterprise and banking sectors, the provision of basic services, and investment in the textiles sector, had stimulated growth and resulted in a consumer boom.[3]

As a country on the verge of bankruptcy prior to the September 11, 2001 terrorist attacks in the United States, Pakistan's fortunes had experienced a remarkable turnaround. Since 2001, as a result of the influx of billions

Exhibit 1   Demographic and Economic Statistics for Pakistan, India and China (2006)

World View	Pakistan	India	China
Population, total (millions)	159	1,109.81	1,311.80
Population growth (annual %)	2.1	1.4	0.6
Surface area (sq. km) (thousands)	796.1	3,287.30	9,598.10
GNI, Atlas method (current US$) (billions)	126.71	914.74	2,639.48
GNI per capita, Atlas method (current US$)	800	820	2,010
GNI, PPP (current international $) (billions)	382.81	2,742.82	6,168.66
GNI per capita, PPP (current international $)	2,410	2,470	4,700
People			
Life expectancy at birth, total (years)	65	64	72
Fertility rate, total (births per woman)	3.9	2.5	1.8
Adolescent fertility rate (births per 1,000 women ages 15–19)	33	63	7
Mortality rate, under 5 (per 1,000)	97	76	24
Immunization, measles (% of children ages 12–23 months)	80	59	93
Primary completion rate, total (% of relevant age group)	62	86	..
Ratio of girls to boys in primary and secondary education (%)	78	..	100
Environment			
Improved water source (% of population with access)	90	89	88
Improved sanitation facilities, urban (% of urban population with access)	90	52	74
Economy			
GDP (current US$) (billions)	126.87	916.25	2,657.87
GDP growth (annual %)	6.9	9.7	11.6
Inflation, GDP deflator (annual %)	9.3	5.6	3.3
Agriculture, value added (% of GDP)	19	18	12
Industry, value added (% of GDP)	27	29	48
Services, etc., value added (% of GDP)	53	52	40
Exports of goods and services (% of GDP)	15	22	40
Imports of goods and services (% of GDP)	23	25	32
Gross capital formation (% of GDP)	22	36	44
Revenue, excluding grants (% of GDP)	13.5	12.6	..
Cash surplus/deficit (% of GDP)	−4.2	−2.7	..
States and Markets			
Time required to start a business (days)	24	35	35
Market capitalization of listed companies (% of GDP)	35.9	89.4	91.3
Military expenditure (% of GDP)	3.8	2.7	2
Fixed line and mobile phone subscribers (per 100 people)	25	19	63

(continued)

Exhibit 1 Demographic and Economic Statistics for Pakistan, India and China (2006) (*continued*)

World View	Pakistan	India	China
Internet users (per 100 people)	7.5	10.8	10.4
High-technology exports (% of manufactured exports)	1	..	30
High-technology exports (% of manufactured exports)	1		30
Global Links			
Merchandise trade (% of GDP)	37	32	66
Net barter terms of trade (2000 = 100)	76		82
External debt, total (DOD, current US$) (millions)	35,909	153,075	322,845
Short-term debt outstanding (DOD, current US$) (millions)	1,230	11,971	173,377
Total debt service (% of exports of goods, services and income)	8.6	7.7	2.5
Foreign direct investment, net inflows (BoP, current US$) (millions)	4,273	17,453	78,095
Workers' remittances and compensation of employees, received (US$) (millions)	5,121	25,426	23,319
Official development assistance and official aid (current US$) (millions)	2,14	1,379	1,245

Source: *Pakistan Software Export Board.*

in U.S. aid in return for supporting the "War on Terror" combined with pro-reform government policies designed to stimulate the economy, Pakistan's business environment and investment climate was flourishing (Figure 1).

Pakistan's recent policy trends of liberalization and deregulation appeared to have had an impact, according to the World Bank's "Doing Business 2008" report, a business-specific index calculated from overall rankings

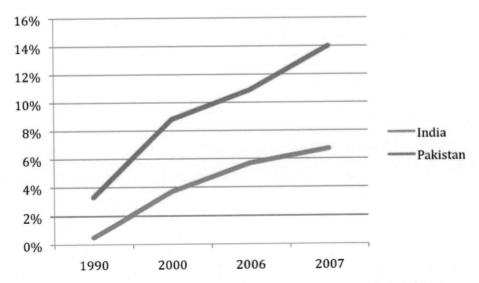

Figure 1 **Pakistan and India Foreign Direct Investment (Stock) as % of GDP**

Source: United Nations Conference on Trade and Development.

of over 150 countries on a scale of 1 (best) to 178 (worst). Pakistan was ranked #1 in South Asia for its "Ease of Doing Business" and #76 globally (India was #120). The country ranked highest in South Asia in categories such as "Starting a Business" (a study of the ease and simplicity of all procedures to start up and operate a commercial or industrial business) and "Protecting Investors" (a study of the strength of minority shareholder protections against directors misuse of corporate assets for personal gain). (See Figure 2). The introduction of the Private Equity and Venture Capital Funds Act of 2007 also provided an enabling regulatory environment for the capital markets, making it easier for funds outside of Pakistan to invest in the country with full protection as well as providing full tax exemption until 2014.

The Fear of Being First

Asad felt that things were looking up for Pakistan, but he still had a number of questions and doubts, which were giving him pause.

Politics Granted, Pakistan had been politically stable and even prosperous since 2000, albeit under a military dictatorship. Yet General Musharraf's grip on power was weakening, and Asad feared that political turmoil was around the corner. The question in his mind was whether the gains in the last eight years were permanent and whether enough had been done to make Pakistan's economy sustainable and able to weather any upheaval. History did not bode well in this regard. No Pakistani prime minister had ever served a full term in office, and although the recent military dictatorship had been benign and, in Asad's opinion, beneficial, there was no guarantee that the future was secure.

Scaling for Sustainable Growth Although Pakistan was starting to demonstrate a track record of entrepreneurship, all the individuals Asad had spoken to were primarily concerned with the ability to scale. Building a 30-person company was not the problem. Expanding it to a 300-person company was where the challenge lay.

The issue of being able to recruit a second layer of top-notch management was key. The common belief was that trusted management was hard to come by in Pakistan, and therefore the culture was still one of family-owned businesses with limited professional management. It would be impossible to scale new ventures without addressing this issue. The empowerment of a growing middle class and a trend for overseas Pakistanis to return home led Asad to believe that this problem could resolve itself, but how long would it take? Would the cost arbitrage in labor still remain if overseas Pakistanis had to be paid U.S. level salaries? The concept of equity and options were also new in Pakistan, yet were an integral part of the success of U.S. entrepreneurial ventures. Would Pakistani employees adapt to this model and would it be a sufficient motivator? Would Pakistani educational establishments continue to turn out highly-trained graduates? Would enough foreign-trained and foreign-educated executives return home?

Infrastructure Asad's next thought turned to infrastructure. Pakistan was becoming attractive not only because of its talent pool, but because this talent pool was generally 30–40% cheaper than its neighbors in India and China. The UAE and Saudi Arabia had already pumped billions of dollars of capital into the country. However, in terms of infrastructure, real estate was comparably expensive and, as in China and India, the main issue was the unreliable supply of electricity, water and other utilities, which meant companies had to build redundant systems into their infrastructure, which cost valuable dollars. Based on this, Asad wondered how real the cost advantage was. Was it enough to overcome these issues?

The Right Type of Business Asad wondered whether the developing skill-set in Pakistan was relevant for the type of investment ePlanet liked to make. According to his colleague Ayaz ul Haque, Managing Director in the Silicon Valley and New Delhi offices of ePlanet Ventures, "What we look for in a company in a country like

Figure 2   "Ease of Doing Business" Rankings for South Asian Countries

Country	Ease of Doing Business	Starting a Business	Employing Workers	Protecting Investors	Trading Across Borders	Enforcing Contracts
Pakistan	76	59	132	19	94	154
Sri Lanka	101	29	111	64	60	133
Bangladesh	107	92	129	83	155	19
India	120	111	85	33	79	177

Source: *World Bank 'Doing Business 2008' report.*

Pakistan is whether the business can survive and sustain itself in the local market. Given the political concerns in the country, if a business is based on outsourcing and 90% of its clientele is abroad, there is no knowing when those clients will yank their contracts away. Whereas if a business is domestically-focused, it can continue to thrive despite the political situation because life continues to move along regardless of who is in power."

Access to Markets   Asad reflected on why VCs were so often inclined to invest within a 15-minute drive of their geographic location. In his view this was an element of the shortsightedness that prevailed in the VC industry. The world was now a global village and, particularly in the consumer Internet/Web 2.0 space, this distance issue was now almost moot. He felt the same was almost true with regards to markets abroad. By promoting its product through YouTube, Scrybe demonstrated that it did not matter that it was located in a leafy suburb of Islamabad; it had wanted 5,000 users for its beta, yet it got close to 100,000. Naseeb Networks located in Lahore had hundreds of thousands of users.

With India, China and Dubai on Pakistan's doorstep, Asad was reassured somewhat. Pakistan traditionally had strong relations with China and the UAE, and his gut told him Pakistani businesses would be well received in those regions, as long as the product offerings were of high-enough quality.

However, in order for a business to survive, Asad agreed with Ayaz that it must also flourish in its home market, particularly if it was outside the consumer/Web 2.0 space. Here again, he wondered about the growing middle class. This came back around to the question of political stability and the continuation of liberalization and reforms to further economic development. Was the Pakistani economy strong enough at its current stage to continue the empowerment of the middle class?

Talent and Passion   As Asad thought back to his childhood in Pakistan, he remembered growing up wanting to get his higher education in the United Kingdom or the United States. However in the post-9/11 world where student visas and work authorizations in the United States were difficult to obtain for Pakistani citizens, the former "brain-drain" was fast becoming a "brain-gain" for Pakistan. In fact, in the technology space alone, Pakistani universities were producing upwards of 20,000 English-speaking graduates per year. Importantly, Pakistani educational establishments, particularly the missionary convent schools, instilled neutral English accents, enabling better communication with their Western counterparts.[4] Peter Lagerquist reported in the *Far Eastern Economic Review* as early as 2002 how companies such as Align Technologies, a Pasadena-based company, pioneered the use of Pakistani call centers and how the sitcom "Friends" was used as a training tool for employees with Master's degrees and who were fluent in English.

These young, technically trained graduates started turning to new horizons—namely setting up companies to target a global customer base in addition to the local market. Faizan Burdar, founder of Scrybe—an up-and-coming Pakistani Web 2.0 company—expressed different aspirations to Asad: "I realized that the Web would be hot and took a plunge with a shoestring budget and no formal investments. In fact, I didn't even have a U.S. visa so attracting funding from the U.S. sources, other than U.S-based Pakistanis, seemed impossible!"

Scrybe recently attracted funding from Adobe Systems and LMKR and was currently in beta testing. The software was referred to as "the most anticipated software" at the Museum of Modern Betas, a website that tracked emerging Web 2.0 projects.

Scrybe's success was not unique. Fuelled by a new breed of well-educated Pakistani entrepreneurs, there were numerous other home-grown IT start-ups in Pakistan making their mark on the global markets:

- **iTrango,** a game and 3D content studio, provided content for the wildly successful game Tomb Raider Legend, and also for high profile companies such as Nike, Lexus, Scion, and other global brands.
- **Trevor,** a software company, recently acquired by Bentley Motors, was one of the world's top providers of GIS/geospatial software solutions.
- **Post Amazors,** an animation house, provided content for the film, The Mask, and also the local character of Safe Guard for P&G, which was being used globally (Mexico).
- **EnterpriseDB** developed and supported EnterpriseDB Advanced Server, a leading Oracle-compatible relational database management system (RDBMS).
- **Ultimus** was one of the most widely deployed Business Process Management solutions in the world, enabling over 1800 companies to increase profitability by managing, automating, modelling and optimizing core business processes. Its customers included Microsoft, Lockheed Martin and others.
- **Sofizar** was a global marketplace for show tickets (with a call-center in Greenwich, Connecticut). Sofizar was the winner of the inaugural Business Acceleration Plan (BAP) sponsored by the MIT Enterprise Forum of Pakistan.
- **Sofcom** focused on products for human capital management, process monitoring and quality control with clients including GSK and Barclays. Sofcom was the winner of the second Business Acceleration Plan (BAP) sponsored by the MIT Enterprise Forum of Pakistan.
- **VioZar** was a global marketplace for unused telecom bandwidth whose customers included AT&T, Bell Canada, France Telecom and Orange. VioZar's CEO operated jointly from Toronto and Karachi.

Data from the Pakistan Software Export Board indicated that the "high-tech" industry had a solid presence in the three major economic centers, Karachi, Lahore and Islamabad, and that a number of overseas companies were setting up operations in the country (Figure 3).

Networks Bridging the Gap–OPEN

Asad reflected on his last visit to Boston, when he had met up with an old acquaintance, Tom O'Flannigan. Over lunch Asad had sat enthralled as he listened to Tom describe how the Irish immigrated en masse to the United States starting around the time of the Irish Potato Famine in 1850, up until the 1930s. The descendents of these individuals formed a highly-trained diaspora which played an instrumental role in Ireland's economic boom in the late 1990s. When they went home to start high-tech and other ventures, they took with them access to management, capital and markets. Asad wondered whether U.S.-based Pakistanis were starting to emulate this process.

The Organization for Pakistani Entrepreneurs (OPEN) was a voluntary non-profit organization formed by a group of U.S.-Pakistani entrepreneurs at MIT in 1998 to facilitate and encourage the growth of Pakistani entrepreneurs and professionals. The association's charter provided networking and enhanced business opportunities for entrepreneurs and professionals in the high-tech, energy and life sciences fields. From the first chapter in Massachusetts being incorporated in 2000, OPEN had grown to five chapters across the United States (Boston, New York, Washington D.C., Houston, Silicon Valley) as well as an international chapter in Dubai. According to Imran Sayeed, President of OPEN Global, OPEN enabled Pakistani-American entrepreneurs to get organized and develop an effective network.

That network had started to reach overseas. Monis Rahman (Naseeb Networks) and Zia Chishti (Align Technologies) were U.S.-based-and-trained Pakistani entrepreneurs who, amongst others, had taken all or parts of their

Figure 3 **Statistics of Pakistan IT Industry 2006**

Total number of Information Technology (IT) companies registered with Pakistan Software Export Board (PSEB)	1082
Number of substantial IT companies city-wise breakup	384 Karachi 276 Islamabad 353 Lahore 69 others
Total number of foreign IT and telecommunication companies working in Pakistan	60
Number of Capability Maturity Model Integration (CMMI)-assessed companies	One CMMI Level 5 company, one CMMI Level 5 company, three CMMI Level 3 companies and four CMMI Level 2 companies
Total industry size	US$ 2.8 billion (WTO-prescribed formula)
IT and IT-enabled services exports	US$ 1.4 billion (WTO-prescribed formula)
Percent growth in exports over the last year	61.18%
Number of IT graduates produced per year	Approximately 20,000
Export targets for the current fiscal year 2006-2007	US$ 108 million
Number of universities offering IT/ Computer Science (CS) programs	110
Number of IT professionals engaged in export-oriented activities (software development/call centers etc.)	More than 15,000
Total number of IT professionals employed in Pakistan	110,000
Total IT spending in the fiscal year 2005-2006	US$ 1.4 billion
Total space utilized in IT & Software Technology Parks	11 IT parks covering an area of 750,000 sq ft

Source: *Pakistan Software Export Board (www.pseb.com.pk)*.

businesses to Pakistan. In the other direction, Faizan Burdar, founder of Scrybe, had not even set foot in the United States and credited introductions to potential investors from OPEN members with starting the sequence of events that led them to receiving funding from a U.S. company.

Furthermore, OPEN, in collaboration with the MIT Entrepreneurship Center, had been taking an active role in educating Pakistani-based entrepreneurs. Workshops, seminars, and a recently concluded Business Acceleration Plan (BAP) competition, organized by the MIT Enterprise Forum of Pakistan, had resulted in increased mentorship provided to local entrepreneurs from their U.S. counterparts. Zafar Khan, CEO of Sofizar, and winner of the 2007 BAP Competition, said, "This program has helped me well beyond my extremely high expectations. I could not get this quality of help, even if I had employed a team of the highest-paid management-consultants. The mentors were sincere, and pushed me to improve. I didn't need to raise money . . . I just needed guidance and I got it."

The recent formation of the Karachi-based Tech Angels Network (TAN), led by 50 local business persons working with MIT faculty members and the president of the MIT Club of Pakistan, seemed to indicate that the start-up investment environment was becoming more attractive.

Success Stories This increasing entrepreneurial activity had not gone unnoticed by entrepreneurially-minded Pakistanis living in the United States. The Pakistani-American diaspora had started to recognize Pakistan as an attractive destination to locate elements of their U.S.-based ventures. As Faraz Hoodbhoy, co-founder of Silicon Valley-based PixSense, a firm which developed network sided software to improve cameraphone image sharing, said, "I knew I wanted to start a business and I had strong family connections in Pakistan. But I didn't choose to go to Pakistan because I wanted to do something great for the nation. I chose to do so simply for good business reasons." And so he moved parts of the business to Pakistan.

Similar moves were made by Umair Khan, an MIT graduate and serial entrepreneur based in Silicon Valley, with his first venture Clickmarks, an Internet content aggregation and distribution company; Zia Chishti of The Resource Group (TRG); and Sana Khan of TrueMRI. In each of these cases, these U.S.-based, Pakistani-born entrepreneurs saw the opportunity to compete effectively by harnessing Pakistan's strengths, namely an entrepreneur-friendly investment environment and talented, cost-effective workforce. Nadeem Elahi of TRG stated that he believed customer satisfaction for its portfolio companies had been approximately 50% better than companies with back-office operations in other South Asian countries.

Naseeb Networks was in some ways a model story regardless of its geographical location. Started in 2003 from offices in Lahore by Monis Rahman, an entrepreneur who had recently returned to his hometown after a 10-year stint in Silicon Valley, the company bootstrapped its way to positive cash flow in 2004, and successfully completed a series B investment round from ePlanet and DFJ Ventures. This deal was attractive to ePlanet in large part because Naseeb Networks' flagship website, Naseeb.com, a Muslim social and matchmaking site, held a huge market lead in a market which essentially incorporated all those of Muslim heritage and an Internet connection. Due to the nature of the business it successfully went global, and its physical location became irrelevant. Naseeb Networks' other sites, such as Rozee.pk, a recruitment site, handling job applications for all major multinationals operating in the country, were also market leaders in Pakistan.

Key to this success, however, was the ability of the CEO and founder to be able to straddle two continents effortlessly. By being able to access capital and corporate governance expertise in the United States and technical talent in Pakistan, Monis was able to take advantage of the best resources offered in each.

Exit Opportunities The million-dollar question was how to exit from investments. The Karachi Stock Exchange (KSE) was the biggest and most liquid exchange in Pakistan and was declared to be the "Best Performing Stock Market in the World" by BusinessWeek in the year 2002. As of June 29, 2007, 658 companies were listed with a combined market capitalization of approximately $66 billion and listed capital of $10.39 billion. The KSE 100 Index closed at 14,473 on December 7, 2007, up 40% for the year (Figure 4).

This was certainly encouraging. However, in the quest to build global companies, would companies based in Pakistan have the reach and opportunity to list on the major markets in the world? There were only three Pakistani companies listed on the London Stock Exchange, but none of them were technology companies (two banks and an oil and gas exploration company). No Pakistani companies as yet had listed on NASDAQ or any of the other U.S. exchanges. Asad thought about his experience with his investment in Baidu. Having no roots in the United States, this Chinese search engine became the most successful first-day foreign IPO in U.S. market history. With Dubai, Shanghai and India nearby, there appeared to be no reason why Pakistani companies could not list wherever they chose. Also, with the increase in M&A as a viable alternative exit route to IPOs in Europe and the United States, Asad cynically thought he could start 10 companies all of whom had a primary goal of being acquired by Google.

The key question in his mind was that given the overall situation, did Pakistani companies have the same potential?

Next Steps

Asad sat and considered the issues over a hot bowl of his favourite Boston speciality, clam chowder. His instincts told him that Pakistan was a seething cauldron of opportunity and potentially a next frontier for technology-based entrepreneurship. China had been done. India had been

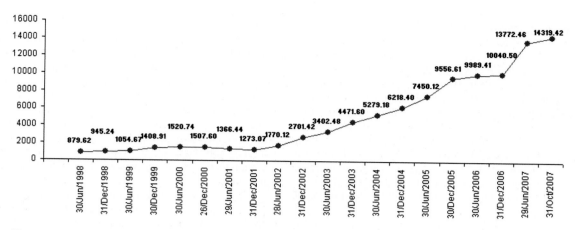

Figure 4 KSE 100 Index Market Performance

done. What was the next high-growth region, and was he willing to bet on his homeland? Keeping in mind that Pakistan was a mere 60 years old, would his limited partners give him the time to allow Pakistan to mature from the eastern equivalent of the Wild West, to a mature entrepreneurial community?

Adobe and Qualcomm had already invested in Pakistani companies, and ePlanet had the opportunity to make its first investment. Asad realized that most emerging economies had reached their current level of development from similar beginnings and Pakistan was no different. In risk there was reward. Did he want to learn from others'

mistakes or make those mistakes himself and learn from them? Should ePlanet be one of the first VC entrants into the Pakistani market?

Endnotes

1. Burki, Shahid. *Pakistan: 50 Years of Nationhood* (New York: Westview Press, 1999).
2. Louise Tillin, "Musharraf and the Economy," *www.bbc.co.uk*, April 22, 2002.
3. Ibid.
4. "Pakistan's Largest Call Center to Be Operative Today," *Pakistan Times*, August 15, 2005.

Case 20   The Best-Laid Incentive Plans*

Hiram Phillips finished tying his bow tie and glanced in the mirror. Frowning, he tugged on the left side, then caught sight of his watch in the mirror. Time to get going. Moments later, he was down the stairs, whistling cheerfully and heading toward the coffeemaker.

"You're in a good mood," his wife said, looking up from the newspaper and smiling. "What's that tune? 'Accentuate the Positive'?"

"Well done!" Hiram called out. "You know, I do believe you're picking up some pop culture in spite of yourself." It was a running joke with them. She was a classically trained cellist and on the board of the local symphony. He was the one with the Sinatra and Bing Crosby albums and the taste for standards. "You're getting better at naming that tune."

"Or else you're getting better at whistling." She looked over her reading glasses and met his eye. They let a beat pass before they said in unison: "Naaah." Then, with a wink, Hiram shrugged on his trench coat, grabbed his travel mug, and went out the door.

Fat and Happy

It was true. Hiram Phillips, CFO and chief administrative officer of Rainbarrel Products, a diversified consumer-durables manufacturer, was in a particularly good mood. He was heading into a breakfast meeting that would bring nothing but good news. Sally Hamilton and Frank Ormondy from Felding & Company would no doubt already be at the office when he arrived and would have with them the all-important numbers—the statistics that would demonstrate the positive results of the performance management system he'd put in place a year ago. Hiram had already seen many of the figures in bits and pieces. He'd retained the consultants to establish baselines on the metrics he wanted to watch and had seen various interim reports from them since. But today's meeting would be the impressive summation capping off a year's worth of effort. Merging into the congestion of Route 45, he thought about the upbeat presentation he would spend the rest of the morning preparing for tomorrow's meeting of the corporate executive council.

It was obvious enough what his introduction should be. He would start at the beginning—or, anyway, his own

beginning at Rainbarrel Products a year ago. At the time, the company had just come off a couple of awful quarters. It wasn't alone. The sudden slowdown in consumer spending, after a decade-long boom, had taken the whole industry by surprise. But what had quickly become clear was that Rainbarrel was adjusting to the new reality far less rapidly than its biggest competitors.

Keith Randall, CEO of Rainbarrel, was known for being an inspiring leader who focused on innovation. Even outside the industry, he had a name as a marketing visionary. But over the course of the ten-year economic boom, he had allowed his organization to become a little lax.

Take corporate budgeting. Hiram still smiled when he recalled his first day of interviews with Rainbarrel's executives. It immediately became obvious that the place had no budget integrity whatsoever. One unit head had said outright, "Look, none of us fights very hard at budget time, because after three or four months, nobody looks at the budget anyway." Barely concealing his shock, Hiram asked how that could be; what did they look at, then? The answer was that they operated according to one simple rule: "If it's a good idea, we say yes to it. If it's a bad idea, we say no."

"And what happens," Hiram had pressed, "when you run out of money halfway through the year?" The fellow rubbed his chin and took a moment to think before answering. "I guess we've always run out of good ideas before we've run out of money." Unbelievable!

"Fat and happy" was how Hiram characterized Rainbarrel in a conversation with the headhunter who had recruited him. Of course, he wouldn't use those words in the CEC meeting. That would sound too disparaging. In fact, he'd quickly fallen in love with Rainbarrel and the opportunities it presented. Here was a company that had the potential for greatness but that was held back by a lack of discipline. It was like a racehorse that had the potential to be a Secretariat but lacked a structured training regimen. Or a Ferrari engine that needed the touch of an expert mechanic to get it back in trim. In other words, the only thing Rainbarrel was missing was what someone like Hiram Phillips could bring to the table. The allure was irresistible; this was the assignment that would define his career. And now, a year later, he was ready to declare a turnaround.

Lean and Mean

Sure enough, as Hiram steered toward the entrance to the parking garage, he saw Sally and Frank in a visitor parking space, pulling their bulky file bags out of the trunk of Sally's sedan. He caught up to them at the security checkpoint in the lobby and took a heavy satchel from Sally's hand.

Moments later, they were at a conference table, each of them poring over a copy of the consultants' spiral-bound report. "This is great," Hiram said. "I can hand this out just as it is. But what I want to do while you're here is to really nail down what the highlights are. I have the floor for 40 minutes, but I guess I'd better leave ten for questions. There's no way I can plow through all of this."

"If I were you," Sally advised, "I would lead off with the best numbers. I mean, none of them are bad. You hit practically every target. But some of these, where you even exceeded the stretch goal. . . ."

Hiram glanced at the line Sally was underscoring with her fingernail. It was an impressive achievement: a reduction in labor costs. This had been one of the first moves he'd made, and he'd tried to do it gently. He'd come up with the idea of identifying the bottom quartile of performers throughout the company and offering them fairly generous buyout packages. But when that hadn't attracted enough takers, he'd gone the surer route. He'd imposed an across-the-board headcount reduction of 10% on all the units. In that round, the affected people were given no financial assistance beyond the normal severance.

"It made a big difference," he nodded. "But it wasn't exactly the world's most popular move." Hiram was well aware that a certain segment of the Rainbarrel workforce currently referred to him as "Fire 'em." He pointed to another number on the spreadsheet. "Now, that one tells a happier story: lower costs as a result of higher productivity."

"And better customer service to boot," Frank chimed in. They were talking about the transformation of Rainbarrel's call center—where phone representatives took orders and handled questions and complaints from both trade and retail customers. The spreadsheet indicated a dramatic uptick in productivity: The number of calls each service rep was handling per day had gone up 50%. A year earlier, reps were spending up to six minutes per call, whereas now the average was less than four minutes. "I guess you decided to go for that new automated switching system?" Frank asked.

"No!" Hiram answered. "That's the beauty of it. We got that improvement without any capital investment. You know what we did? We just announced the new targets, let everyone know we were going to monitor them, and put the names of the worst offenders on a great big 'wall of shame' right outside the cafeteria. Never underestimate the power of peer pressure!"

Sally, meanwhile, was already circling another banner achievement: an increase in on-time shipments. "You should talk about this, given that it's something that wasn't even being watched before you came."

It was true. As much as Rainbarrel liked to emphasize customer service in its values and mission statement, no reliable metric had been in place to track it. And getting a metric in place hadn't been as straightforward as it might've seemed—people had haggled about what constituted "on time" and even what constituted "shipped." Finally, Hiram had put his foot down and insisted on the most objective of measures. On time meant when the goods were promised to ship. And nothing was counted as shipped till it left company property. Period. "And once again," Hiram announced, "not a dollar of capital expenditure. I simply let people know that, from now on, if they made commitments and didn't keep them, we'd have their number."

"Seems to have done the trick," Sally observed. "The percentage of goods shipped by promise date has gone up steadily for the last six months. It's now at 92%."

Scanning the report, Hiram noticed another huge percentage gain, but he couldn't recall what the acronym stood for. "What's this? Looks like a good one: a 50% cost reduction?"

Sally studied the item. "Oh, that. It's a pretty small change, actually. Remember we separated out the commissions on sales to employees?" It came back to Hiram immediately. Rainbarrel had a policy that allowed current and retired employees to buy products at a substantial discount. But the salespeople who served them earned commissions based on the full retail value, not the actual price paid. So, in effect, employee purchases were jacking up the commission expenses. Hiram had created a new policy in which the commission reflected the actual purchase price. On its own, the change didn't amount to a lot, but it reminded Hiram of a larger point he wanted to make in his presentation: the importance of straightforward rules—and rewards—in driving superior performance.

"I know you guys don't have impact data for me, but I'm definitely going to talk about the changes to the commission structure and sales incentives. There's no question they must be making a difference."

"Right," Sally nodded. "A classic case of 'keep it simple,' isn't it?" She turned to Frank to explain. "The old way they calculated commissions was by using this really complicated formula that factored in, I can't remember, at least five different things."

"Including sales, I hope?" Frank smirked.

"I'm still not sure!" Hiram answered. "No, seriously, sales were the most important single variable, but they also mixed in all kinds of targets around mentoring, prospecting new clients, even keeping the account information current. It was all way too subjective, and salespeople were getting very mixed signals. I just clarified the message so they don't have to wonder what they're getting paid for. Same with the sales contests. It's simple now: If you sell the most product in a given quarter, you win."

With Sally and Frank nodding enthusiastically, Hiram again looked down at the report. Row after row of numbers attested to Rainbarrel's improved performance. It wouldn't be easy to choose the rest of the highlights, but what a problem to have! He invited the consultants to weigh in again and leaned back to bask in the superlatives. And his smile grew wider.

Cause for Concern

The next morning, a well-rested Hiram Phillips strode into the building, flashed his ID badge at Charlie, the guard, and joined the throng in the lobby. In the crowd waiting for the elevator, he recognized two young women from Rainbarrel, lattes in hand and headphones around their necks.

One was grimacing melodramatically as she turned to her friend. "I'm so dreading getting to my desk," she said. "Right when I was leaving last night, an e-mail showed up from the buyer at Sullivan. I just know it's going to be some big, hairy problem to sort out. I couldn't bring myself to open it, with the day I'd had. But I'm going to be sweating it today trying to respond by five o'clock. I can't rack up any more late responses, or my bonus is seriously history."

Her friend had slung her backpack onto the floor and was rooting through it, barely listening. But she glanced up to set her friend straight in the most casual way. "No, see, all they check is whether you responded to an e-mail within 24 hours of opening it. So that's the key. Just don't open it. You know, till you've got time to deal with it."

Then a belltone announced the arrival of the elevator, and they were gone.

More Cause for Concern

An hour later, Keith Randall was calling to order the quarterly meeting of the corporate executive council. First, he said, the group would hear the results of the annual employee survey, courtesy of human resources VP Lew Hart. Next would come a demonstration by the chief marketing officer of a practice the CEO hoped to incorporate into all future meetings. It was a "quick market intelligence," or QMI, scan, engaging a few of Rainbarrel's valued customers in a prearranged—but not predigested—conference call, to collect raw data on customer service concerns and ideas. "And finally," Keith concluded, "Hiram's going to give us some very good news about cost reductions and operating efficiencies, all due to the changes he's designed and implemented this past year."

Hiram nodded to acknowledge the compliment. He heard little of the next ten minutes' proceedings, thinking instead about how he should phrase certain points for maximum effect. Lew Hart had lost him in the first moments of his presentation on the "people survey" by beginning with an overview of "purpose, methodology, and historical trends." Deadly.

It was the phrase "mindlessly counting patents" that finally turned Hiram's attention back to his colleague. Lew, it seemed, was now into the "findings" section of his remarks. Hiram pieced together that he was reporting on an unprecedented level of negativity in the responses from Rainbarrel's R&D department and was quoting the complaints people had scribbled on their surveys. "Another one put it this way," Lew said. "We're now highly focused on who's getting the most patents, who's getting the most copyrights, who's submitting the most grant proposals, etc. But are we more creative? It's not that simple."

"You know," Rainbarrel's chief counsel noted, "I have thought lately that we're filing for a lot of patents for products that will never be commercially viable."

"But the thing that's really got these guys frustrated seems to be their 'Innovation X' project," Lew continued. "They're all saying it's the best thing since sliced bread, a generational leap on the product line, but they're getting no uptake."

Eyes in the room turned to the products division president, who promptly threw up his hands. "What can I say, gang? We never expected that breakthrough to happen in this fiscal year. It's not in the budget to bring it to market."

Lew Hart silenced the rising voices, reminding the group he had more findings to share. Unfortunately, it didn't get much better. Both current and retired employees were complaining about being treated poorly by sales personnel when they sought to place orders or obtain information about company products. There was a lot of residual unhappiness about the layoffs, and not simply because those who remained had more work to do. Some people had noted that, because the reduction was based on headcount, not costs, managers had tended to fire low-level people, crippling the company without saving much money. And because the reduction was across the board, the highest performing departments had been forced to lay off some of the company's best employees. Others had heard about inequities in the severance deals: "As far as I can tell, we gave our lowest performers a better package than our good ones," he quoted one employee as saying.

And then there was a chorus of complaints from the sales organization. "No role models." "No mentoring." "No chance to pick the veterans' brains." "No knowledge sharing about accounts." More than ever, salespeople were dissatisfied with their territories and clamoring for the more affluent, high-volume districts. "It didn't help that all the sales-contest winners this year were from places like Scarsdale, Shaker Heights, and Beverly Hills," a salesperson was quoted as saying. Lew concluded with a promise to look further into the apparent decline in morale to determine whether it was an aberration.

The Ugly Truth

But if the group thought the mood would improve in the meeting's next segment—the QMI chat with the folks at longtime customer Brenton Brothers—they soon found out otherwise. Booming out of the speakerphone in the middle of the table came the Southern-tinged voices of Billy Brenton and three of his employees representing various parts of his organization.

"What's up with your shipping department?" Billy called out. "My people are telling me it's taking forever to get the stock replenished."

Hiram sat up straight, then leaned toward the speakerphone. "Excuse me, Mr. Brenton. This is Hiram Phillips—I don't believe we've met. But are you saying we are not shipping by our promise date?"

A cough—or was it a guffaw?—came back across the wire. "Well, son. Let me tell you about that. First of all, what y'all promise is not always what we are saying we require—and what we believe we deserve. Annie, isn't that right?"

"Yes, Mr. Brenton," said the buyer. "In some cases, I've been told to take a late date or otherwise forgo the purchase. That becomes the promise date, I guess, but it's not the date I asked for."

"And second," Billy continued, "I can't figure out how you fellas define 'shipped.' We were told last Tuesday an order had been shipped, and come to find out, the stuff was sitting on a railroad siding across the street from your plant."

"That's an important order for us," another Brenton voice piped up. "I sent an e-mail to try to sort it out, but I haven't heard back about it." Hiram winced, recalling the conversation in the lobby that morning. The voice persisted: "I thought that might be the better way to contact your service people these days? They always seem in such an all-fired hurry to get off the phone when I call. Sometimes it takes two or three calls to get something squared away."

The call didn't end there—a few more shortcomings were discussed. Then Keith Randall, to his credit, pulled the conversation onto more positive ground by reaffirming the great regard Rainbarrel had for Brenton Brothers and the mutual value of that enduring relationship. Promises were made and hearty thanks extended for the frank feedback. Meanwhile, Hiram felt the eyes of his colleagues on him. Finally, the call ended and the CEO announced that he, for one, needed a break before the last agenda item.

Dazed and Confused

Hiram considered following his boss out of the room and asking him to table the whole discussion of the new metrics and incentives. The climate was suddenly bad for the news he had looked forward to sharing. But he knew that delaying the discussion would be weak and wrong. After all, he had plenty of evidence to show he was on the right track. The problems the group had just been hearing about were side effects, but surely they didn't outweigh the cure.

He moved to the side table and poured a glass of ice water, then leaned against the wall to collect his thoughts. Perhaps he should reframe his opening comments in light of the employee and customer feedback. As he considered how he might do so, Keith Randall appeared at his side.

"Looks like we have our work cut out for us, eh, Hiram?" he said quietly—and charitably enough. "Some of those metrics taking hold, um, a little too strongly?" Hiram started to object but saw the seriousness in his boss's eyes.

He lifted the stack of reports Felding & Company had prepared for him and turned to the conference table. "Well, I guess that's something for the group to talk about."

Should Rainbarrel revisit its approach to performance management?

Case 21   Building the New Bosco-Zeta Pharma (A)*

Markus Biennel was flustered. Having just announced Bosco Pharmaceutical's acquisition of Zeta AG (Zeta), the Bosco chairman was unsure about whether to follow his instinct to merge the two firms using only internal resources or whether he should accept the help of Deloitte Consulting.

John Powers, the Deloitte partner in charge of the project, advocated a complete overhaul of Bosco's organization in more than 100 countries to accommodate Zeta, which was one-fifth Bosco's size. But Biennel thought that because Zeta had so few complementarities with Bosco—primarily in the oncology sector—he was not sure whether Zeta's worldwide product structure should be adopted by Bosco or whether Zeta should be required to conform to Bosco's more geographic structure.

Bosco was a latecomer to the global M&A consolidation trend in the pharmaceutical industry, and, by

relying solely on in-house R&D to generate new products, the company had missed the window of opportunity for "in-licensing" new drugs from biotechnology start-ups. Biennel thought that the Zeta acquisition would provide a way to catch up.

Unfortunately, the market reaction to his announcement of the acquisition was not kind. As he gazed at the Rhine from his office on the 17th floor, he thought about the analysts' statements. Analyst A had said, "We are rather skeptical about the transaction, as the overlap of the therapeutic areas is rather small and because the cost reductions are predominantly planned in R&D, which should be retained to remain competitive." Analyst B had said, "The proposed deal is primarily targeting scale. Apart from the cost synergies, the fit between the two companies is limited." And Analyst C had said, "A choice to maintain their conglomerate structure despite better critical size in health care is negative for the investment case as investors willing to play the turnaround story in health care will be exposed to risks of downturn in material science."

Biennel understood the viewpoints of these analysts because Bosco's history had been bleak. In August 2005, the company had been forced to withdraw its major cholesterol-lowering drug from the market after it was linked to more than 220 deaths. Now, after several years of restructuring and on the heels of the Winthrough merger, the Zeta acquisition was the biggest in Bosco's 110-year history. The integration issues were not trivial, as the combined entity would have more than 40,000 employees in more than 100 countries. (See Exhibit 1 for both firms' financials.)

DARDEN ☷ **BUSINESS PUBLISHING**
UNIVERSITY *of* VIRGINIA

* This case was prepared by Nandini Bose (MBA '05), Yogesh Goswami, Sudeep Mathur, John Powers, all from Deloitte Consulting, and Paul M. Hammaker Research Professor L. J. Bourgeois III. It was written as a basis for class discussion rather than to illustrate effective or ineffective handling of an administrative situation. The contribution of Deloitte Consulting is gratefully acknowledged. Copyright © 2008 by the University of Virginia Darden School Foundation, Charlottesville, VA. All rights reserved. *To order copies, send an e-mail to sales@ dardenbusinesspublishing.com. No part of this publication may be reproduced, stored in a retrieval system, used in a spreadsheet, or transmitted in any form or by any means—electronic, mechanical, photocopying, recording, or otherwise—without the permission of the Darden School Foundation.*

Exhibit 1   Financial Metrics

	Bosco	Zeta
Key Metrics (in EUR millions)		
Total assets	35,000	6,000
Total revenue	25,000	5,000
Operating income	10,000	2,700
Total net income	+5,000	1,350
Margins (%)		
Operating margin	40	54
Net profit margin	20	27
Ratios		
Total debt to equity	0.75	0.08
Current ratio	1.8	2.3

Source: Bosco Investor Presentation.

Deal Background

Despite market reaction, the mood was upbeat at Bosco's headquarters in the industrial town of Weeze, Germany. "At the very least, the merger will restore some luster to Germany's pharma sector," observed Biennel. Bosco was an established, legendary name in the pharmaceutical industry as the discoverer of the pain-killing and fever-reducing wonder drug Colospirin in 1897, and as a leader in the modern drug industry. But Bosco had endured several setbacks during the last two decades of industry consolidation, as it was overshadowed by such companies as America's Pfizer, Britain's GlaxoSmithKline, and Switzerland's Novartis.

In the 1980s, Bosco had been one of the top five pharmaceutical and chemicals companies, but by the year 2000, it dropped to the second tier. Like a lot of companies, Bosco believed that sustainability was achieved through internal innovation by increasing its R&D expenditures rather than growing through acquisitions. As a result, when the industry began to consolidate, Bosco passed up some opportunities to participate. In addition, its focus on pharmaceuticals and its neglect of other businesses resulted in its having an unbalanced portfolio. Finally had Bosco's now-withdrawn cholesterol-lowering drug fulfilled its potential, it would have been a $4 billion to $5 billion asset. During the two years after its 2005 withdrawal, Bosco's market value plummeted.

In response, Bosco returned to its traditional, diversified, multimarket approach, participating in consumer and animal health and pharmaceuticals. Within the pharmaceutical sector, it focused on high-margin specialty products, efficient use of its sales force, and licensing as a source of new products.

Bosco also expanded in the consumer-health sector. Traditionally a lower-margin business than brand-name prescription drugs, consumer health had been growing rapidly and offered some often overlooked advantages. For example, there were limits on the synergies available for acquiring prescription pharmaceutical products. A pharmaceutical sales force could, at maximum, promote two products. After a merger, both legacy sales organizations were needed; however, a consumer business somewhat resembled a catalog business because new products could be added to existing sales and marketing organizations.

Driven by that logic, Bosco's consumer health-care division acquired Winthrough Consumer Health for $2 billion in August 2005. The deal brought Bosco pain relievers, antiseptic creams, and multivitamins, making Bosco the third-largest provider of nonprescription medicines. At the time, analysts thought Bosco had significantly overpaid for Winthrough. But compared with more recent acquisitions in the over-the-counter (OTC) consumer sector, Bosco actually got a bargain and the advantage of being in on the start of the OTC consolidation.

One particularly hard decision Bosco made was to exit a market that had been one of the richest in health care for decades: diagnostics. At the time, the market speculated that this was a high-risk strategy, and yet, 18 months later, just as with the Winthrough acquisition, it was considered a smart move. Letting go of diagnostics not only improved Bosco's profitability but also served as the catalyst that allowed the company to focus more closely on specialty products.

The Deal

On March 24, 2007, Hamburg-based Zeta accepted the (euro) EUR16 billion cash offer from Bosco. The deal merged Zeta, the world's largest maker of birth control pills and cancer drugs, and Bosco, Germany's last remaining pharmaceutical and chemical conglomerate.

The new company could boast a much richer pipeline—with two drugs filed with the U.S. Food and Drug Administration (FDA) and ten in late-stage testing. Investment bankers had predicted that the merger would lead to annual cost savings of EUR700 million by 2010. Biennel hoped to use Zeta's specialist sales force in the United States to market its own potential blockbuster, Nextvarian, which the FDA had approved at the end of 2006 as a treatment for kidney cancer. The drug was also being tested for treatment of liver, skin, and lung cancers.

Prescription drugs, along with OTC standbys such as Once Daily vitamins, accounted for 30% of Bosco's annual revenues of EUR25 billion in 2006. The new company could now focus on treatments for cancer and cardiovascular diseases and a select group of specialized therapeutic markets. Zeta brought Danielle, the world's top-selling contraceptive, and Alphaseron, a treatment for multiple sclerosis, which was expected to bring EUR100 million in annual sales.

After getting the approval of the management and supervisory boards, Bosco outlined the key points of the transaction:

- *Sites*: The headquarters of the consolidated pharmaceuticals business would be Hamburg. The key research locations were Duisburg and Cologne (Germany), as well as Gloucester, Minturn, and West Hartford (United States).
- *Employees*: Possible staff reductions would be equally and fairly allocated between the two companies.
- *Management*: The management of the combined pharmaceuticals business would be chosen on the basis of objective criteria and third-party advice.
- *Name*: To the extent legally possible, the new name for the combined pharmaceutical business would be Bosco-Zeta Pharma.
- *Corporate structure*: Management would report directly to Bosco Healthcare, one of Bosco's three business groups. Integration committees with equal representation of executives from both Zeta and Bosco would be established.

Pharmaceutical Industry[1]

In 2004, the global pharmaceuticals and biotechnology (P&B) industry was valued at EUR503 billion, having expanded at a compound annual growth rate (CAGR) of 9.9% since 2000. Although the pharmaceuticals segment generated revenues of EUR415 billion, the EUR88 billion biotechnology segment had outperformed pharmaceuticals consistently during the previous five years. And during the same period, governments in most of the world's major developed markets exerted significant downward pressure on pharmaceutical pricing. Generic competition had also created major downward price pressure since 2000.

During 2001–02, market growth slowed from 11% per year to 8%. By 2005, growth rates recovered, reflecting companies' efforts to restructure business models to emphasize product development and to improve efficiencies. The U.S. markets for P&B were the largest; U.S. sales were EUR238 billion or 47% of the global market. In comparison, Europe generated 23%, whereas the Asia/Pacific region accounted for a further 17%. By 2010, the global P&B industry was expected to reach a value of EUR807 billion for a CAGR of 9.9% from 2005.

The EUR88 billion biotechnology market was still relatively immature; none of the pure biotech firms were featured as leading players within the overall P&B industry. Instead, the top six players overall were all pharmaceutical giants. Collectively, these top six controlled 29% of the global market. Pfizer was the clear leader, with Sanofi-Aventis and GlaxoSmithKline closely matched for the number two position.

The pharmaceutical industry was one of the most research-intensive industries in the United States. On average, pharmaceutical firms invested as much as 17% to 22% of sales in R&D, compared with 3% for the average U.S. manufacturing firm.

In the last few years, the average return on investment for new drugs had fallen. In addition, spiraling R&D costs and the reduced likelihood of new drugs developing blockbuster status meant players had become more selective in their investments. Despite this, in 2007, there was a greater number of drug molecules approaching the market compared with the previous five years. As a result, companies focused on developing balanced portfolios, rather than on emphasizing blockbusters.

During that time, there had been a significant change in attitude toward private-label OTC products, which often mimicked their branded predecessors but at significantly discounted prices. It was particularly noticeable in Europe and North America, where consumers viewed certain OTC drugs as commodities. With leading brands struggling to differentiate their products in the face of this cheaper competition, companies needed to invest even more intensively in product R&D.

The United States was expected to maintain its position as the world's dominant market for biotechnology products with such players as Amgen, Biogen, and Genentech. Legislation providing a zero capital-gains tax rate for direct investment into the equities of entrepreneurial firms was likely to spur economic growth, create high-wage jobs, and ensure the future competitiveness of U.S. biotech entrepreneurial firms.

With several blockbuster biological products approaching patent expiry and the emergence of new approval pathways, the biotech-generics sector represented an attractive opportunity for companies looking to escape intensifying competition in the generic-pharmaceuticals sector. Despite strong opposition from the biotechnology industry, regulatory bodies were expected to establish approval pathways for generic biotech in the future, driven by the potential cost savings for governments and health care payers with access to lower-cost biotech generics.

Meanwhile, leading genomics[2] companies were restructuring their businesses in a push toward profitability. The market for technology agreements was becoming saturated, and genomics companies had been forced to develop products in-house in order to continue growth. Companies were increasingly investing in product development and marketing initiatives, reducing the number of in-licensing opportunities for pharmaceutical companies.

Bosco AG

Incorporated in 1902, Bosco Aktiengesellschaft (Bosco AG) offered a range of products, including ethical pharmaceuticals; health care products; agricultural products; and polymers. Bosco AG was the management holding company of the Bosco Group, which included approximately 280 consolidated subsidiaries (Exhibit 2). The business operations of the company were organized into the three groups:

- Bosco Healthcare: consumer care, animal health, and pharmaceuticals
- Bosco Crop Care: crop protection, environmental science, and bioscience segments
- Bosco Material Care: specialty materials for the polymers industry

Bosco Healthcare

Bosco Healthcare, in turn, consisted of three divisions: Consumer Care, Animal Care, and "Specialty Care" (pharmaceuticals) (Exhibit 3).

Consumer Care ranked among the largest marketers of OTC medications and nutritional supplements in the world. In January 2005, its acquisition of Winthrough Consumer Care placed Bosco among the top-three OTC consumer-health organizations in the world; it had a presence in more than 100 countries. Bosco Consumer Care operated in North America, Europe, Latin America, and Asia/Pacific. Some of its most recognized global brands were for analgesics for cough and cold, gastrointestinal products, dermatological/topical products, and multivitamins and dietary supplements.

Animal Care researched, developed, and marketed new products for animal health. Of the two business units—food-animal products and companion-animal products—the real growth driver was companion animals, particularly in the

Exhibit 2   Organizational Structure of Bosco AG

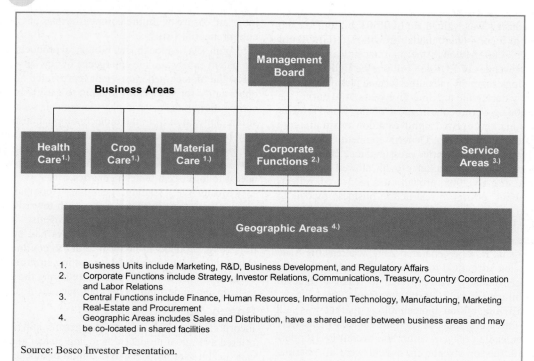

1. Business Units include Marketing, R&D, Business Development, and Regulatory Affairs
2. Corporate Functions include Strategy, Investor Relations, Communications, Treasury, Country Coordination and Labor Relations
3. Central Functions include Finance, Human Resources, Information Technology, Manufacturing, Marketing Real-Estate and Procurement
4. Geographic Areas includes Sales and Distribution, have a shared leader between business areas and may be co-located in shared facilities

Source: Bosco Investor Presentation.

Exhibit 3   Organizational Structure of Bosco Healthcare

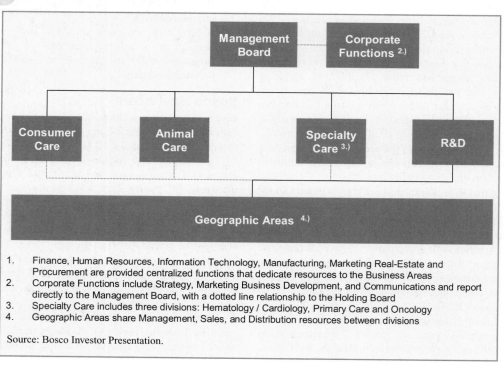

1. Finance, Human Resources, Information Technology, Manufacturing, Marketing Real-Estate and Procurement are provided centralized functions that dedicate resources to the Business Areas
2. Corporate Functions include Strategy, Marketing Business Development, and Communications and report directly to the Management Board, with a dotted line relationship to the Holding Board
3. Specialty Care includes three divisions: Hematology / Cardiology, Primary Care and Oncology
4. Geographic Areas share Management, Sales, and Distribution resources between divisions

Source: Bosco Investor Presentation.

Exhibit 4 Bosco-Pharma Product Portfolio

Therapeutic Area	Drug	Drug Description
Hematology/cardiology	Nabalat	Used to treat various types of angina (chest pain) and hypertension (high blood pressure).
	Ruetane	A recombinant factor VIII treatment indicated for the treatment of hemophilia.
	Tralysol	The only product approved by FDA for the prevention of perioperative blood loss and the need for blood transfusion among patients undergoing coronary-artery-bypass graft surgery.
Primary care	Flucoday	Established as the first step in diabetes therapy and reduces cardiovascular risks.
	Genitra	An ED medication that treats erectile dysfunction.
	Hypofloxacin	A prescription antibiotic effective against a broad range of bacteria. It is prescribed for prostatitis, cystitis, bacterial infections, and cancer.
	Ruetane	A recombinant factor VIII treatment indicated for the treatment of hemophilia.
Oncology	Nextvarian	Indicated for the treatment of patients with advanced renal cell carcinoma.
	Vader	Treats the symptoms of advanced prostate cancer.

Source: Bosco Investor Presentation.

United States. This business had above-average profitability in the industry and, in 2006, achieved almost double-digit growth in the United States. The animal health business covered worldwide markets, including China, Vietnam, and others in Southeast Asia.

Specialty Care (pharmaceuticals) focused on the development and marketing of ethical pharmaceuticals, with principal markets in North America, Western Europe, and Asia. A summary of Bosco's products and their therapeutic applications is shown in Exhibit 4. Specialty Care included three divisions:

1. Hematology/cardiology focused on the start of Phase II/Phase III of the formulation of long-acting Kogenate FS.

2. Primary care focused its R&D on maintaining current sales levels for key products, life-cycle management, and further in-licensing.

3. Oncology focused on further building outside the United States to push the launch of Nextvarian—the key product in the oncology area.

Within each division, Bosco was organized on a geographic basis. The distribution of pharmaceutical sales across global regions is shown in Table 1.

Within each region, marketing and distribution (sales) was organized on a country basis. The country's general manager reported to the region as a profit center. Each country was responsible for deciding which set of Bosco pharmaceuticals to promote.

Table 1 Distribution of Bosco Pharmaceutical Sales

Region	Europe, Middle East, Africa	North America	Latin America	Asia/Pacific
Sales % of total	50%	25%	10%	15%
Growth rates	5%	10%	20%	15%

Bosco M&A History

During the previous three years, Bosco made more than eight acquisitions and 11 divestitures, totaling revenues of more than EUR17.5 billion, including the successful integration of the EUR7 billion ACS acquisition and the EUR4.2 billion Winthrough OTC business in 2004.

Zeta AG

Incorporated in 1872, Zeta AG was a global research-based company engaged in the discovery, development, manufacturing, marketing, and sale of pharmaceutical products. The company operated eight R&D centers in Europe, Japan, and the United States. Its manufacturing facilities were located in Europe, the United States, Latin America, and Asia, and marketed and sold in more than 100 countries; Zeta had acquired 11 companies since 2004. Exhibit 5 shows Zeta's organizational structure.

Zeta concentrated its R&D and sales in four core business areas. Each business unit was responsible for sales and profits on a worldwide basis.

1. Gynecology and andrology (EUR2 billion sales in 2006, mostly in female contraception and menopause management)

2. Diagnostic imaging (EUR1.5 billion, primarily in X-ray media)

3. Specialized therapeutics (EUR1.2 billion, mostly in central nervous systems)

4. Oncology (EUR400 million, split between hematology and solid tumors)

Approximately 38% of Zeta's 2006 sales came from four key products: Alphaferon, sold in the United States and Canada under the Alphaseron trademark (16% of net sales); Danielle (11%); Angevit (6%); and U-vit (5%).

A list of Zeta's major products and therapeutic applications is shown in Exhibit 6. The global distribution of Zeta sales is shown in Table 2.

Deal Highlights

Bosco planned to merge Zeta into the Bosco Healthcare unit, whose name would be changed to Bosco-Zeta Pharma (BZP). Anticipated sales of this new unit were expected to be more than EUR9 billion, with increased total Healthcare division sales expected to reach EUR15 billion. The deal would allow Bosco to expand its footprint in the faster-growing specialty care business and reduce its

Exhibit 5   **Zeta's Organizational Structure**

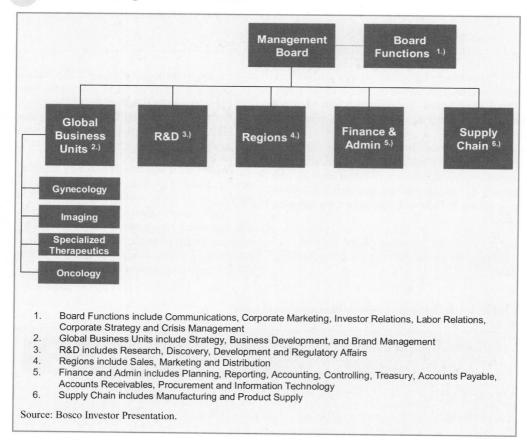

1. Board Functions include Communications, Corporate Marketing, Investor Relations, Labor Relations, Corporate Strategy and Crisis Management
2. Global Business Units include Strategy, Business Development, and Brand Management
3. R&D includes Research, Discovery, Development and Regulatory Affairs
4. Regions include Sales, Marketing and Distribution
5. Finance and Admin includes Planning, Reporting, Accounting, Controlling, Treasury, Accounts Payable, Accounts Receivables, Procurement and Information Technology
6. Supply Chain includes Manufacturing and Product Supply

Source: Bosco Investor Presentation.

Exhibit 6 Zeta Product Portfolio in 2006

Therapeutic Area	Drug	Drug Description
Gynecology	Belaniane	A hormonal birth control pill, a so-called oral contraceptive.
	Danielle	Oral contraceptive for women.
	Laine	Provides unique combined benefit of contraception and antiacne treatment.
	Macrogynine	A combined oral contraceptive pill.
	Meerina	An intrauterine contraception that offers a long-term birth control option without sterilization.
Oncology	Zodara	A chemotherapy drug that is given as a treatment for some types of cancer.
Specialized therapeutics	Alphaferon	A drug provided for treatment of multiple sclerosis.
Diagnostic imaging	U-vit	A nonionic iodinated radiological contrast agent.
	Angevit	A contrast agent used in magnetic resonance imaging (MRI).
	Ropamairion	An X-ray contrast agent.

Source: Bosco Investor Presentation.

Table 2 Distribution of Zeta Pharmaceutical Sales

Region	Europe	United States	Japan	Latin America/ Canada	Asia Pacific
Sales % of total	45%	25%	15%	20%	5%
Growth rates	5%	15%	0%	15%	10%

exposure to economic cycles. The Bosco Healthcare division would become the largest Bosco subgroup (almost 50% of the overall portfolio).

At a total value of EUR16 billion, this was Bosco's largest acquisition to date, representing a payout of $2.7 \times$ 2009E sales and $11.5 \times$ 2007E EBITDA. EPS would be dilutive for the first two years and accretive only by 2010. The deal was going to be financed through a mix of equity, term debt, and hybrid securities. Bosco would dispose of two noncore units from its other divisions to finance the deal in addition to approximately EUR7.6 billion in debt through Switzbank and Townbank. The rest was expected to come from EUR3 billion in marketable securities with Bosco.

Strategic Rationale

Boost to Health Care Business The merger would create a global health care company that would rank among the top 12 companies in the world (Exhibit 7). The combined pharmaceuticals business would be characterized by a balanced portfolio whose oncology, cardiology/hematology, and gynecology offerings would generate above-average growth. Bosco expected that the combined size of the future company would make it more attractive as a partner for in-licensing activities in pharmaceuticals.

A key role was envisaged for the future research platform produced by combining the R&D activities of the two companies. Following the acquisition, BZP would have two projects in registration, 10 in Phase III clinical testing, 10 undergoing Phase II trials, and an additional 20 in Phase I development.[3] After the acquisition, sales from the overall life sciences would rise to approximately 70% of total Bosco sales, up from approximately 60% before the deal. In addition, Bosco now could increase the Specialty Care products share of overall pharmaceutical sales from the current level of 25% to nearly 75%, giving the company a leadership position in this highly attractive market.

Exhibit 7   Top 20 Pharma Companies by Revenue in 2006

2006 Rank	Company	2006 Global Pharma Sales (in USD billions)
1	Company A	$44.0
2	Company B	$34.0
3	Company C	$32.0
4	Company D	$25.0
5	Company E	$24.0
6	Company F	$22.0
7	Company G	$22.0
8	Company H	$15.0
9	Company I	$15.0
10	Company J	$15.0
11	Company K	$14.70
12	**Bosco-Zeta Pharma**	**$14.0**
12	Company L	$14.0
13	Company M	$12.0
14	Company N	$10.0
15	Company O	$ 8.0
16	Company P	$ 8.0
17	Company Q	$ 7.0
18	**Bosco**	**$ 7.0**
19	Company R	$ 7.0
20	**Zeta AG**	**$ 6.0**

Source: Bosco Investor Presentation.

The combined biotech platform was expected to be the foundation for further growth. The products in this area included Alphaseron, Zeta's top-selling drug for the treatment of multiple sclerosis, and Leukinine, used to boost a patient's immune system during cancer therapy, together with Bosco's genetically engineered Factor VIII Ruetane. These biotech products generated sales of approximately EUR2 billion.

Synergy Potential

The merger of the Bosco and Zeta pharmaceuticals businesses would include the potential for significant revenue and cost synergies. As outlined in Table 3, Bosco anticipated synergy benefits of around EUR700 million annually, starting in year three.

Specific synergy items included:

- Global headcount reduction of approximately 6,000 people (10% of combined Healthcare business)
- Leveraging the combined oncology business
- Procurement and supply-chain optimization
- Production-site rationalization
- Integration of head office and central functions
- Rationalization of country platforms and commercial infrastructures
- Optimization of R&D activities

Units to Be Divested

Bosco planned to sell two subsidiaries of Bosco Material Science by the end of 2007 to finance the merger and narrow its strategic focus. The subsidiaries were deemed unfit for the core business of Bosco Material Science, which in the future would focus on expanding technology and market leadership in polycarbonate and isocyanate chemistries. The divestitures of these two units would reduce headcount by 4,400 and revenues by EUR1.25 billion.

Table 3   Sources of Synergy (in EUR millions)

		Year 1	Year 2	Year 3
Synergies:	% of total	250	450	700
• Procurement/manufacturing	10%–15%			
• Marketing and sales	20%–25%			
• R&D, approximately	25%–30%			
• General and administrative, approximately	25%–40%			
One-time costs		(500)	(500)	—
Net synergies		(250)	(50)	700

Source: Bosco Investor Presentation.

Organization of Bosco-Zeta Pharma

The new BZP organization was to be based primarily on the existing structure of Bosco Healthcare. The goal was to integrate Zeta functions into the respective "like" functions or divisions in Bosco, and in this way, preserve the Bosco Holding and Bosco Healthcare reporting and management. The proposed distribution of the Zeta Group into the Bosco organization is depicted in Exhibit 8.

Exhibit 8   Distribution of Zeta into the Bosco Organization

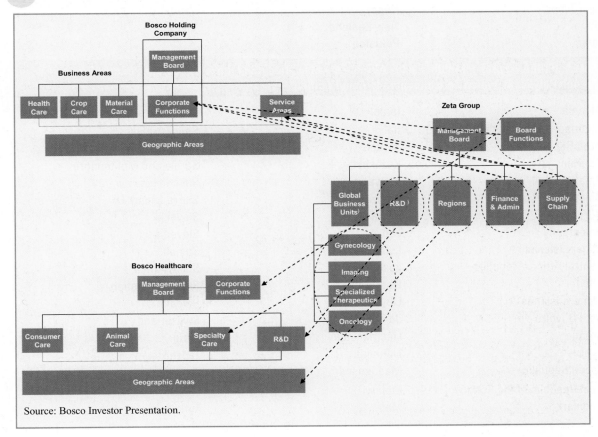

Source: Bosco Investor Presentation.

The Challenge Ahead

The German takeover code and corporate laws could potentially affect the timing, tone, and sequencing of certain integration activities. German takeover law allowed all shareholders, regardless of the percentage of shares owned, to hold up the close of a merger, pending a lengthy court review and could prevent synergy attainment for as long as a year.

Markus Biennel was aware that due diligence on the transaction was inadequate and that developing a new operating model would be crucial. His thoughts turned into questions: "Should I manage BZP as a regional organization with country managers in control of the entire portfolio of products? Or should I adopt Zeta's product structure throughout our own organization? Or, should we use a matrix structure? In what country or countries should I start the postmerger integration process?" (Exhibit 9) He wondered how the back-office functions of Bosco and Zeta would interact under the new operating model, and he asked himself: "How should I organize and staff

Exhibit 9   Country Operations Overlap

A. Countries where both firms had only marketing and distribution. (Regional designations were Bosco's; differences from Zeta's classification are noted.)

Asia/Pacific: (Bolded countries = Zeta classified as Europe)

Afghanistan	Indonesia	Palau
Bangladesh	Malaysia	Philippine Islands
Bhutan	**Maldive Islands**	Republic of Korea
Cambodia	Marshall Islands	Singapore
Dem Rep. of Korea	**Mongolia**	**Sri Lanka**
Dem Rep. of Laos	Myanmar (Burma)	Taiwan
East Timor	**Nepal**	Vanuatu
Guam	New Zealand	Vietnam
India	**Pakistan**	

EMEA: (EMEA = Europe, Middle East & Africa. Zeta classified all of these as "Europe" except for French Polynesia, which Zeta allocated to Asia/Pacific.)

Albania	Israel	Sao Tome and Principe
Algeria	Italy	Saudi Arabia
Arab Republic	Jordan	Senegal
Bahrain	Kazakhstan	Serbia and Montenegro
Belarus	Kenya	Seychelles
Botswana	Kirgiziya	Sierra Leone
Burundi	Kuwait	Slovakia
Cameroon	Latvia	Slovenia
Canary Islands	Lebanon	Somali
Central African Republic	Lesotho	South Africa
Chad	Liberia	Ssian Federation
Comoro Islands	Libyan Arab	Sweden
Cote D'Ivoire	Jamahiriya	Switzerland
Croatia	Liechtenstein	Syria
Cyprus	Lithuania	Tadzhikistan
Czech Republic	Madagascar	Tangier
Dem Republic of the Congo	Malawi	Tunisia
Denmark	Mali	Turkey

(*continued*)

Exhibit 9 **Country Operations Overlap** (*continued*)

EMEA: (EMEA = Europe, Middle East & Africa. Zeta classified all of these as "Europe" except for French Polynesia, which Zeta allocated to Asia/Pacific.)

Denmark	Mali	Turkey
Egypt	Malta	Turkmenistan
Estonia	Monaco	Uganda
Ethiopia	Mozambique	Ukraine
Faeroe Islands	Namibia	United Arab Emirates
Finland	Netherlands	United Kingdom
French Polynesia	Niger	United Rep. of Tanzania
Georgia	Norway	Uzbekistan
Ghana	Oman	Vatican City
Gibraltar	P. Armenia	West Bank (including Jerusalem)
Greenland	Palestinian Authority	Yemen
Iceland	Poland	Zambia
Iraq	Qatar	Zimbabwe
Ireland	Republic of the Congo	
Islamic Republic of Iran	San Marino	

Japan

Latin America: (Zeta classified these as Latin America and Canada)

Antigua and Barbuda Islands	Cuba	Nicaragua
Argentina	Dominican Republic	Paraguay
Aruba	Ecuador	Peru
Bolivia	El Salvador	Uruguay
Chile	Guatemala	Venezuela
Colombia	Haiti	

North America

Canada (Zeta = Latin America and Canada)

Puerto Rico (Zeta = United States)

B. Countries where either firm had additional facilities (in addition to marketing and distribution):

Region	Country	Bosco Operations	Zeta Operations
Asia/Pacific	Australia	Manufacturing	—
	Hong Kong	—	Manufacturing
	China	Manufacturing	—
EMEA	Belgium	—	Manufacturing
	France	R&D	Manufacturing
	Germany	R&D, manufacturing	R&D, manufacturing
	Hungary	R&D	—
	Portugal	Manufacturing	—
	Spain	R&D	Manufacturing
Latin America	Brazil	R&D, manufacturing	Manufacturing
	Mexico	Manufacturing	—
North America	USA	R&D, manufacturing	Manufacturing

Source: Bosco Investor Presentation.

the integration team? Have I overcommitted on synergies? What about cultural integration?" The big question, however, was whether he should integrate first and then change the culture or do it the other way around.

Endnotes

1. "Pharmaceuticals: Global Industry Guide," *Datamonitor*, M2 Communications Ltd., February 2008.
2. Genomics was the study of an organism's entire genome or hereditary information encoded in its DNA. Investigation of single genes, their functions, and roles had become very common in medical and biological research.
3. Clinical trials were conducted in phases. The trials at each phase have different purposes and help scientists answer different questions. In Phase I, researchers test an experimental drug or treatment for the first time in a small group of people (20–80) to evaluate its safety, determine a safe dosage range, and identify side effects. In Phase II, the experimental drug or treatment is given to a larger group of people (100–300) to see if it is effective and to further evaluate its safety. In Phase III, the experimental drug or treatment is given to large groups of people (1,000–3,000) to confirm its effectiveness, monitor side effects, compare it to commonly used treatments, and collect information that will allow the experimental drug or treatment to be used safely. In Phase IV, postmarketing studies delineate additional information, including the drug's risks, benefits, and optimal use.

Case 22 Procter & Gamble*

In January 2009, Procter & Gamble (P&G) announced that its revenues had declined by 3.2 percent during its previous quarter, with lower sales in nearly every business unit. Consumers were coping with the economic downturn by switching to P&G's lower-priced brands, choosing *Gain* over *Tide* detergent and *Luvs* over *Pampers* diapers. In spite of the lower revenue, CEO A. G. Lafley was pleased to report that his firm had managed to retain or gain market share in most of its product categories. At the same time, he did not expect to see much change in 2009. "We expect the environment will remain difficult and highly volatile, at least in the near term," he stated.[1]

These results suggested that the world's largest consumer products conglomerate could not maintain growth during a recession, even with million-dollar brands like Tide, Crest, Pampers, Gillette, and Right Guard. But the firm was still managing to post strong profits through the heavier use of discount coupons delivered as inserts in weekend newspapers. It also kept pushing on its premium-priced products by promoting their features. It claimed that Tide, for example, contained much less water and more cleaning agents than other, cheaper-priced detergents.

At the same time, Lafley has continued to take steps to position P&G for the longer term by focusing on speed and agility, both of which are likely to play a more significant role in the future. Since he took over the helm of P&G in June 2000, Lafley has been stripping away much of the bureaucracy in order to speed up the firm's product development and build on its well-known brands. He is trying to focus the firm on building a small number of "superbrands," each with annual sales of over $1 billion. Over the last decade, the firm has increased the number of such brands to 24 (see Exhibit 1).

During the past year, P&G has embarked on its most ambitious plan to expand into emerging markets despite the developing slowdown. "We just have a huge opportunity to service urban consumer households in developing markets who have plenty of income, even with an economic downturn," said Lafley.[2] Although emerging markets currently account for about 30 percent of P&G's annual sales, they have delivered more than 50 percent of its recent growth.

Lafley has many more ideas about how to make P&G relevant in the 21st century. He is trying to shift the focus of his firm away from its traditional reliance on household care. P&G has been making aggressive inroads into health and beauty products, making these areas account for the majority of the firm's sales and profits. Over the past year, the firm has even managed to establish itself as a major force in the luxury perfume business by partnering with various designer brands. In pushing for these changes, Lafley has been undertaking the most sweeping transformation of the company since it was founded by William Procter and James Gamble in 1837 as a maker of soap and candles.

An Attempted Turnaround

For most of its long history, P&G has been one of America's preeminent companies. The firm has developed several well-known brands such as Tide, one of the pioneers in laundry detergents, which was launched in 1946, and Pampers, the first disposable diaper, which was introduced in 1961. P&G built its brands through its innovative marketing techniques. In the 1880s, it was one of the first companies to advertise nationally. Later on, P&G invented the

Exhibit 1 **Business Segments**

Fabric Care and Home Care:
- *Key products:* Air care, batteries, dish care, fabric care, surface care
- *Billion-dollar brands:* Ariel, Dawn, Downy, Duracell, Gain, Tide

Baby Care and Family Care:
- *Key products:* Baby wipes, bath tissue, diapers, facial tissue, paper towels
- *Billion-dollar brands:* Bounty, Charmin, Pampers

Beauty:
- *Key products:* Cosmetics, deodorants, hair care, personal cleansing, prestige fragrances, skin care
- *Billion-dollar brands:* Head & Shoulders, Olay, Pantene, Wella

Grooming:
- *Key products:* Blades and razors, electric hair-removal devices, face and shave products, home appliances
- *Billion-dollar brands:* Braun, Fusion, Gillette, Mach 3

Health Care:
- *Key products:* Feminine care, oral care, personal health care, pharmaceuticals
- *Billion-dollar brands:* Actonel, Always, Crest, Oral B

Snacks, Coffee, and Pet Care:
- *Key products:* Coffee,* pet food, snacks
- *Billion-dollar brands:* Folgers,* Iams, Pringles

*Sold in 2008.

Source: P&G.

* This case was developed by Professor Jamal Shamsie, Michigan State University, with the assistance of Professor Alan B. Eisner, Pace University. Material has been drawn from published sources to be used for class discussion. Copyright © 2009 Jamal Shamsie and Alan B. Eisner.

soap opera by sponsoring *Ma Perkins* when radio caught on and *Guiding Light* when television took hold. In the 1930s, P&G was the first firm to develop the idea of brand management, setting up marketing teams for each brand and urging them to compete against each other.

By the 1990s, however, P&G was in danger of becoming another Eastman Kodak or Xerox, a once-great company that might have lost its way. Sales on most of its 18 top brands were slowing as it was being outhustled by more focused rivals such as Kimberly-Clark and Colgate-Palmolive. The only way P&G kept profits growing was by cutting costs, which would hardly work as a strategy for the long term. At the same time, the dynamics of the industry were changing as power shifted from manufacturers to massive retailers. Retailers such as Wal-Mart were starting to use their size to try to get better deals from P&G, further squeezing its profits.

In 1999, P&G decided to bring in Durk I. Jaeger to try to make the big changes that were obviously needed to get P&G back on track. But the moves that he made generally misfired, sinking the firm into deeper trouble. He introduced expensive new products that never caught on while letting existing brands drift. He also put in place a companywide reorganization that left many employees perplexed and preoccupied. During the fiscal year when he was in charge, earnings per share showed an anemic rise of just 3.5 percent, much lower than in previous years.

Also during that time, the share price slid 52 percent, cutting P&G's total market capitalization by $85 billion. The effects were widely felt within the firm, where employees and retirees hold about 20 percent of the stock (see Exhibits 2 to 5).

Jaeger's greatest failing was his scorn for the family. Jaeger, a Dutchman who had joined P&G overseas and worked his way to corporate headquarters, pitted himself against the P&G culture. Susan E. Arnold, president of P&G's previous beauty and feminine care division, said that Jaeger tried to make the employees turn against the prevailing culture, contending that it was burdensome and insufferable. Some go-ahead employees even wore buttons that read "Old World/New World" to express disdain for P&G's past.

A New Style of Leadership

On June 6, 2000, the day of his 30th wedding anniversary, Alan G. Lafley received a call from John Pepper, a former CEO who was now a board member. Lafley was asked to take the reins of P&G from Jaeger, a move representing a boardroom coup and unprecedented in the firm's history. In a sense, Lafley had been preparing for this job his entire adult life. He never hid the fact that he wanted to run P&G one day. Recruited as a brand assistant for Joy dish detergent in 1977, Lafley rose quickly to head P&G's soap and detergent business, where he introduced Liquid Tide in 1984. A decade later, he moved to

Exhibit 2   Income Statement (in thousands of dollars)

Period Ending:	2008	2007	2006
Total revenue	83,503,000	76,476,000	68,222,000
Cost of revenue	40,695,000	36,686,000	33,125,000
Gross profit	42,808,000	39,790,000	35,097,000
Operating expenses:			
Selling, general, and administrative	25,725,000	24,340,000	21,848,000
Operating income or loss	17,083,000	15,450,000	13,249,000
Income from continuing operations:			
Total other income/expenses net	462,000	564,000	283,000
Earnings before interest and taxes	17,545,000	16,014,000	13,532,000
Interest expense	1,467,000	1,304,000	1,119,000
Income before tax	16,078,000	14,710,000	12,413,000
Income tax expense	4,003,000	4,370,000	3,729,000
Net income from continuing ops	12,075,000	10,340,000	8,684,000
Net income	12,075,000	10,340,000	8,684,000

Source: P&G.

Exhibit 3 **Balance Sheet** (in thousands of dollars)

Period Ending:	2008	2007	2006
Assets			
Current assets:			
Cash and cash equivalents	3,313,000	5,354,000	6,693,000
Short-term investments	228,000	202,000	1,133,000
Net receivables	8,773,000	8,356,000	7,336,000
Inventory	8,416,000	6,819,000	6,291,000
Other current assets	3,785,000	3,300,000	2,876,000
Total current assets	**24,515,000**	**24,031,000**	**24,329,000**
Property, plant, and equipment	20,640,000	19,540,000	18,770,000
Goodwill	59,767,000	56,552,000	55,306,000
Intangible assets	34,233,000	33,626,000	33,721,000
Other assets	4,837,000	4,265,000	3,569,000
Total assets	**143,992,000**	**138,014,000**	**135,695,000**
Liabilities and Equity			
Current liabilities:			
Accounts payable	7,977,000	13,628,000	17,857,000
Short/current long-term debt	13,084,000	12,039,000	2,128,000
Other current liabilities	9,897,000	5,050,000	—
Total current liabilities	**30,958,000**	**30,717,000**	**19,985,000**
Long-term debt	23,581,000	23,375,000	35,976,000
Other liabilities	8,154,000	5,147,000	4,472,000
Deferred long-term liability charges	11,805,000	12,015,000	12,354,000
Total liabilities	**74,498,000**	**71,254,000**	**72,787,000**
Stockholders' equity:			
Preferred stock	1,366,000	1,406,000	1,451,000
Common stock	4,002,000	3,990,000	3,976,000
Retained earnings	48,986,000	41,797,000	35,666,000
Treasury stock	(47,588,000)	(38,772,000)	(34,235,000)
Capital surplus	60,307,000	59,030,000	57,856,000
Other stockholders' equity	2,421,000	(691,000)	(1,806,000)
Total stockholders' equity	**69,494,000**	**66,760,000**	**62,908,000**
Net tangible assets	**($24,506,000)**	**($23,418,000)**	**($26,119,000)**

Source: P&G.

Exhibit 4 **Financial Breakdown** (in billions of dollars)

Business Segment	Net Sales		Net Earnings	
	2008	2007	2008	2007
Fabric care and home care	23.8	21.5	3.4	3.1
Baby care and family care	13.9	12.7	1.7	1.4
Beauty	19.5	17.9	2.7	2.6
Grooming	8.3	7.4	1.7	1.4
Health care	14.6	13.4	2.5	2.2
Snacks, coffee, and pet care*	4.9	4.5	0.5	0.5

*Prior to sale of Folgers coffee in 2008.

Source: P&G.

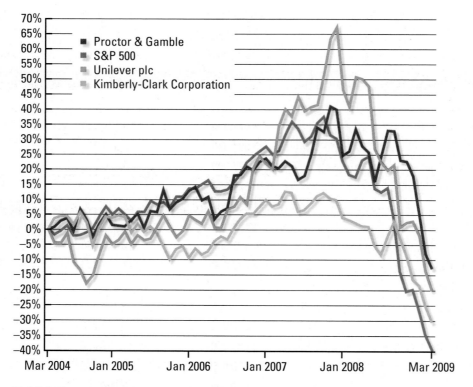

Exhibit 5 Stock Price History, March 2004–March 2009

Source: Data from *moneycentral.msn.com*.

Kobe, Japan, to head the Asian division. Lafley returned to Cincinnati in 1998 to run the company's entire North American operations.

By the time he had taken charge of P&G, Lafley had developed a reputation as a boss who steps back to give his staff plenty of responsibility and who helps shape decisions by asking a series of keen questions. As CEO, Lafley has refrained from making any grand pronouncements on the future of P&G. Instead, he has been spending an inordinate amount of time patiently communicating to his employees about the types of changes that he would like to see at P&G.

Lafley began his tenure by breaking down the walls between management and employees: Since the 1950s, all the senior executives at P&G had been located on the 11th floor at the firm's corporate headquarters. Lafley changed this setup, moving all five division presidents to the same floors as their staffs. Then he turned some of the emptied space into a leadership training center. On the rest of the floor, he knocked down the walls so that the remaining executives, including him, would share open offices.

Lafley chose to place his office next to the two people he talks to the most, who, in true P&G style, were officially identified by a flow study. They are the head of Human Resources, Ricard L. Antoine, and the vice chairman, Bruce Byrnes. In fact, Lafley has established a tradition of meeting with Antoine every Sunday evening to review the performance of the firm's 200 most senior executives. This reflects Lafley's determination to make sure the best people rise to the top. And Byrnes, whom Lafley refers to as "Yoda," the sagelike *Star Wars* character, gets a lot of face time because of his marketing expertise. As Lafley says, "The assets at P&G are what? Our people and our brands."[3]

Lafley's leadership style has been particularly visible in P&G's new conference room, where he and the firm's 12 other top executives meet every Monday at 8 a.m. to review results, plan strategy, and set the drumbeat for the week. The table is now round instead of rectangular. Instead of sitting where they were told, the executives now sit where they like. True to his character, Lafley maintains a low profile at most of these meetings. He occasionally joins in the discussion, but most of the time the executives talk as much to each other as to Lafley.

Indeed, Lafley's charm offensive has so disarmed most P&Gers that he has been able to make drastic changes within the company. He has replaced more than half of the company's top 30 officers (more replacements than made by any other P&G boss in memory) and trimmed its workforce by as many as 9,600 jobs. And he has moved more women into senior positions. In fact, Lafley skipped over 78 general managers with more seniority to name 42-year-old Deborah A. Henretta to head P&G's then-troubled North American baby care division. "The speed at which A. G. has gotten results is five years ahead of the time I expected," said Scott Cook, founder of software maker Intuit Incorporated, who joined P&G's board shortly after Lafley's appointment.[4]

A New Strategic Focus

Lafley has been intent on shifting the focus of P&G back to its consumers. At every opportunity that he gets, he tries to drill his managers and employees on not losing sight of the consumer. He feels that P&G has often let technology, rather than consumer needs, dictate its new products. He would like to see the firm work more closely with retail outlets, the places where consumers first see the product on the shelf. And he would like to see much more concern with the consumer's experience at home. At the end of a three-day leadership seminar, Lafley was thrilled when he heard the young marketing managers declare: "We are the voice of the consumer within P&G, and they are the heart of all we do."[5]

To better focus on serving the needs of P&G's consumers, Lafley has been putting a tremendous amount of emphasis on the firm's brands. In describing the P&G of the future, he said, "We're in the business of creating and building brands."[6] Since Lafley has taken over P&G, the firm has updated all of its 200 brands by adding innovative new products. It has begun to offer devices that build on its core brands, such as Tide StainBrush, a battery-powered brush for removing stains, and Mr. Clean AutoDry, a water-pressure-powered car cleaning system that dries without streaking.

Lafley has also pushed everyone at P&G to approach its brands more creatively (see Exhibit 6). Crest, for example, which used to be marketed as a toothpaste brand, is now defined as an oral care brand. The firm sells Crest-branded toothbrushes and tooth whiteners. There's even an electric toothbrush, SpinBrush, which was added to the Crest line after P&G acquired it in January 2001. The cheap, fun-to-use brush has created a new and positive vibe around the whole Crest brand. "People remember experiences," Lafley explained. "They don't remember attributes."[7]

A key element of Lafley's strategy, however, has been to move P&G away from basic consumer products such as laundry detergents, which can be knocked off by private labels, and shift the firm to higher-margin products. This has led him to focus more strongly on the firm's beauty and personal care business. Under Lafley, P&G made costly acquisitions of Clairol, Wella, and Gillette to complement its Cover Girl and Oil of Olay brands. His most

---

Exhibit 6 Significant Innovations

- Tide was the first heavy-duty laundry detergent.
- Crest was the first fluoride toothpaste clinically proved to help prevent tooth decay.
- Downy was the first ultra-concentrated rinse-add fabric softener.
- Pert Plus was the first 2-in-1 shampoo and conditioner.
- Head & Shoulders was the first pleasant-to-use shampoo effective against dandruff.
- Pampers was the first affordable, mass-marketed disposable diaper.
- Bounty was the first three-dimensional paper towel.
- Always was the first feminine protection pad with an innovative, dry-weave topsheet.
- Febreze was the first fabric and air care product that actually removes odors from fabrics and the air.
- Crest White Strips was the first patented in-home teeth-whitening technology.

Source: P&G.

dramatic innovation was that of moving his firm into prestige fragrances through licenses with Hugo Boss, Gucci, and Dolce & Gabbana. Over the past three years, prestige fragrances have become one of the fastest-growing segments of P&G's expanding beauty business.

P&G has also been considering moving out of some of its product categories. For a few years, it has been looking for potential buyers for its Pringles snacks and Iams pet foods. The firm completed a sale of its Folgers coffees late in 2008. In addition, Lafley has decided to move P&G out of the pharmaceuticals market, where it offers products such as Actonel for bone loss and Enablex for overactive bladders. He recently stated that the firm had already stopped investing in this business because of declining returns in prescription drugs. The firm would focus more on its health care products, which include Prilosec and Pepto-Bismol, which sell over the counter.

A Revolution Still in the Making

Although Lafley has given P&G a tremendous push toward rethinking its business model, it is quite clear that he has more revolutionary changes in mind. A confidential memo was circulated among P&G's top brass in late 2001 that drew a sharp response even from some of the firm's board members. The memo argued that P&G could be cut to 25,000 employees, less than one-quarter of its current size. Lafley admitted that the memo had drawn a strong reaction: "It terrified our organization."[8]

Even though Lafley did not write this infamous memo, it did reflect the central tenet of his vision: that P&G should do only what it does best and nothing more. He clearly wants a more outwardly focused, flexible company. This means that P&G does not have to do everything in-house. If no clear benefits stem from doing something within the firm, the work should be contracted out. Such a philosophy has serious implications for every facet of P&G's operations, from R&D to manufacturing.

Lafley has clearly challenged the supremacy of P&G's research and development operations. Confronting head-on the stubbornly held notion that everything must be invented within P&G, he has asserted that half of the firm's new products should come from the outside. Under his tenure, the percentage of new product ideas coming from outside the firm has increased from 10 percent, when he took over, to almost 50 percent.

A variety of other activities have also been driven out of the firm. In April 2003, Lafley turned over the manufacturing of all bar soaps, including Ivory, P&G's oldest surviving brand, to a Canadian contractor. Shortly afterward, he outsourced P&G's information-technology operation to the Hewlett-Packard Company. While Lafley shies away from saying just how much of P&G's factory and back-office operations he may eventually hand over to other firms, he does admit that facing up to the realities of the marketplace may force some hardships on its employees.

Such moves to outsource some activities may create more flexibility for the firm over the longer term. It could

decide how much it wants to invest in particular brands, products, or even lines of businesses. No one would dispute that these moves are clearly revolutionary for a firm such as P&G. "He's absolutely breaking many well-set molds at P&G," said eBay's CEO, Margaret C. "Meg" Whitman, whom Lafley had recently appointed to the board.[9]

Daunting Challenges

Lafley's bold moves to remake P&G into a company that is admired, imitated, and uncommonly profitable have garnered considerable attention. Since he took over the firm, he has addressed every aspect of the firm's strategy and organization. In so doing, he has made a wide range of changes that are expected to enable his firm to respond quickly and flexibly to emerging opportunities. John Pepper, a popular former boss who returned briefly as chairman when Jaeger left, stated, "It's now clear to me that A. G. is going to be one of the great CEOs in this company's history."[10]

Lafley's push into luxury perfumes represents one of his most radical moves. Analysts have questioned whether a firm that uses a very methodological approach to making and selling mass-market goods can be successful in a business that is known to be quirky and fickle. Most firms in the prestige-fragrance business keep trying to come up with new brands, as older one lose their cachet. P&G hopes to apply its brand development methods to sustaining its fragrance brands over time. "We need to find ways to do brand building," said Hartwig Langer, the firm's president of global prestige products.[11]

The reliance on external sources for new products could be another problematic area. As any scientist will attest, decisions to purchase a new product idea often tend to be extremely hard to make. The process of picking winners from other labs is likely to be both difficult and expensive. P&G already missed a big opportunity by passing up the chance to buy water-soluble strips that contain mouthwash. Listerine managed to grab the product and has profited handsomely from the deal.

The biggest risk, though, is that Lafley will lose the people at P&G. The firm's insular culture has been famously resistant to new ideas. Employees form a tightly knit family because most of them start out and grow up together at P&G, which promotes only from within. Over the years, these people have gradually adopted the culture of the firm and come to believe in it. Lafley is well aware of his predicament. He recently admitted, "I am worried that I will ask the organization to change ahead of its understanding, capability, and commitment."[12]

Finding new avenues of growth, however, could be the only way to balance P&G's increasing reliance on Wal-Mart. Former and current P&G employees say the discounter could account for one-third of P&G's global sales by the end of the decade. Meanwhile, the pressure from consumers and competitors to keep prices low will only increase. "P&G has improved its ability to take on those challenges, but those challenges are still there," said Lehman analyst Ann Gillin.[13]

Endnotes

1. Ellen Byron. Sales Fall across P&G's Units. *Wall Street Journal,* January 31, 2009, p. B5.
2. Jonathan Birchall. P&G Set to Expand in Emerging Markets. *Financial Times,* December 12, 2008, p. 22.
3. Robert Berner. P&G: New and Improved. *BusinessWeek,* July 7, 2003, p. 62.
4. *BusinessWeek,* July 7, 2003, p. 55.
5. Ibid., p. 62.
6. Ibid., p. 63.
7. Robert Berner and William C. Symonds. Welcome to Procter & Gadget. *BusinessWeek,* February 7, 2005, p. 77.
8. *BusinessWeek,* July 7, 2003, p. 55.
9. Ibid., p. 58.
10. Ibid., p. 55.
11. Ellen Byron. P&G's Push into Perfume Tests a Stodgy Marketer. *Wall Street Journal,* November 12, 2007, p. A15.
12. *BusinessWeek,* July 7, 2003, p. 58.
13. Ibid., p. 63.

Case 23   The Novartis Foundation for Sustainable Development: Tackling HIV/AIDS and Poverty in South Africa (A)*

In 1998, sociologist Kurt Madörin from the Swiss-based NGO *terre des hommes schweiz*[1] approached Klaus Leisinger and Karin Schmitt of the Novartis Foundation for Sustainable Development in Basel, Switzerland. There was an acute problem with orphans in sub-Saharan Africa, he told Leisinger, Novartis president and executive director, and Schmitt, director of foundation affairs and special projects. With one or both parents dying from AIDS, many African children were left vulnerable to homelessness, exploitation, abuse, violence, starvation, and other dangers. There were more than 8 million AIDS orphans in Africa, a number expected to reach 42 million by 2008.[2] Being an orphan often meant being a social outcast, and orphaned children were more likely to fall into greater poverty. At the time, there was no effective solution for dealing with the crisis; these parentless children were either put into orphanages, if available; lived on the streets; or were taken care of by an NGO (nongovernmental organization), which

gave them food, shelter, and clothing. The result often was deep psychosocial trauma for the orphans, which no group was equipped to handle. Madörin wanted to develop a program that would help the orphaned children of Africa deal with this psychosocial trauma. He wanted to start in Tanzania, where the number of orphans who had lost both parents had risen from 71,100 in 1992 to 174,400 in 1998.[3] A pilot program in Tanzania would help him assess the feasibility and effectiveness of such a program. But he needed financial and other assistance. Madörin asked Leisinger and Schmitt if the Novartis Foundation could help. They agreed to consider the proposal, although Novartis, one of the largest pharmaceutical companies in the world, did not manufacture or sell any HIV/AIDS-related products.

The HIV/AIDS Crisis

As the close of the 20th century approached, the 20-year-old AIDS crisis had ravaged many developing countries. Particularly hard-hit was sub-Saharan Africa, called by some the "global epicenter"[4] of the crisis. Of the estimated 33.4 million people living with HIV/AIDS worldwide in 1998, 22 million of them were in sub-Saharan Africa. Already, in this area, 12 million had died and life expectancy had plummeted from 62 years to 47. See Exhibit 1 for 1998 worldwide HIV/AIDS statistics and comparisons. Although the AIDS crisis was obviously a worldwide issue, the scale of the epidemic in Africa made "its repercussions qualitatively different from those in other parts of the world."[5] Because HIV transmission in African

Exhibit 1   **Worldwide AIDS Statistics—1998**

Region	Adults & Children Living with HIV/AIDS	Adults & Children Newly Infected with HIV	Adult Infection Rate
Sub-Saharan Africa	22.5 million	4.0 million	8.0%
North Africa & Middle East	210,000	19,000	0.13%
North America	890,000	44,000	0.56%
Latin America	1.4 million	160,000	0.57%
South & Southeast Asia	6.7 million	1.2 million	0.69%
East Asia & Pacific	560,000	200,000	0.068%
Australia & New Zealand	12,000	600	0.1%
Western Europe	500,000	30,000	0.25%
Caribbean	330,000	45,000	1.96%

Source: "AIDS Epidemic Update: December 1998," UNAIDS Joint United Nations Programme on HIV/AIDS.

countries occurred primarily through heterosexual contact, AIDS was considered a family disease.

Of particular concern, and cited in a sobering 1997 U.S. Agency for International Development (USAID) report called "Children on the Brink," was the number of orphans (or "children affected by AIDS," as the specialists preferred) the pandemic created. The statistics for Africa were deeply disturbing: AIDS had accounted for 16% of the deaths that orphaned African children in 1990, but estimates were that the proportion would be 68% by 2010.[6] The USAID report forecast that by the year 2010, 40 million to 42 million children worldwide, primarily in Africa, would be without one or both parents because of HIV/AIDS. The results of being orphaned, the report continued, would include severe emotional distress, malnutrition, no health care, and a lack of identity. These orphans also would face a variety of painful futures including child labor, no education, loss of inheritance, destitution, forced migration, and a vastly increased exposure to HIV infection. Historically, the worldwide percentage of orphans was around 2%, but predictions for 2010 were as high as 17% to 25%. In addition to the devastating physical effects (e.g., starvation and abuse), of great concern also was the psychosocial trauma these orphans were experiencing.

Previously, the "orphan" problem in African countries was mitigated by the fact that children who lost their parents were taken in by other family members: The extended family was the "safety net."[7] But AIDS had overburdened and weakened this informal social structure by increasing the number of orphans, reducing the number of caregivers, and damaging the overall safety net. Paradoxically, "the effectiveness of the traditional African social system in absorbing millions of vulnerable children has contributed to the complacency of governments and agencies in addressing the orphan crisis."[8]

Novartis

Novartis was the product of a record-breaking 1996 merger between "two Swiss giants of the pharmaceutical world"[9] and long-time competitors, Ciba-Geigy and Sandoz. The histories of the companies that formed Novartis in 1998 dated back to the 18th and 19th centuries. In addition to pharmaceutical products, Ciba-Geigy produced, among other things, pesticides, photographic products, eye care items, and synthetic plastics and resins. Sandoz specialized in pharmaceutical products, various industrial-use chemicals, infant and diet foods, and distribution of agricultural raw materials. Both companies had also acquired a number of U.S. biotech and genomics companies (Sandoz had a large stake in both Genetic Therapy and Systemix; Ciba-Geigy in Viagene and Chiron), although profits from these were not expected until at least 2006.[10] The merger, announced in early 1996 and officially sanctioned by the U.S. Federal Trade Commission in December of that year, was a seismic transaction, worth more than USD30 billion.[11] It took many people by surprise because the two companies had long been competitors, although

their physical locations being just across the Rhine River from each other allowed them to "stare into each other's labs from buildings on opposite banks of the river that flows through Basel."[12]

The merger made Novartis the second-largest drug company after Glaxo Wellcome. At the time, in the mid-1990s, mergers of large pharmaceuticals were understandable due to the difficult times for drug companies in general. Not only were the new drug pipelines "lackluster," but "[i]mportant drugs lose their profitability with age. Prices drop as similar, me-too drugs are approved."[13] And perhaps most importantly, "Patent protection for the original groundbreakers eventually runs out, and prices decline even further."[14] The patent on Voltaren, Ciba-Geigy's enormously popular and profitable antiarthritis drug, was on the verge of expiring.

The name Novartis was derived from *novae artes*, Latin for "new skills" and, according to the Novartis Web site, "reflects our commitment to bringing new health care products to patients and physicians worldwide."[15] In 1997, its first full year as a new company, Novartis did well: Total sales were up by 9% to (Swiss francs) CHF31.2. Net income had grown by 43% to CHF5.2 billion, and operating cash flow saw a 31% increase to CHF4.7 billion.[16] To reduce costs, the company had trimmed 9,100 employees, primarily through "natural fluctuation and early retirement" and, in the case of job redundancy, "offered severance packages that reflect our commitment to social responsibility."[17] The company had spun off some of its divisions, including Ciba-Geigy's specialty chemical unit (textile dyes, pigments, and polymers), choosing instead to focus on its Gerber products (Sandoz bought the baby-product business in 1994), pharmaceuticals, agricultural chemicals, and its over-the-counter medications such as Tavist, Ex-Lax, Gas-X, and Maalox. By the end of 1997, Novartis was competing "head-to-head" with Glaxo Wellcome, and had introduced five new products: Migranal, a migraine preventative nasal spray; Foradil, for asthma; Femara, a treatment for hormone-dependent cancer (e.g., breast cancer); Apligraf, a human skin regenerative biotechnology product; and Diovan, a hypertension drug.[18] Novartis was not involved in research and development of HIV/AIDS medicines, but its health care effort included fighting leprosy, malaria, and tuberculosis. See Exhibit 2 for company financial information and Exhibit 3 for the 1995 percentage of pharmaceutical world market share.

Origins of the Novartis Foundation for Sustainable Development

Development aid and humanitarian assistance had been a tradition of several Basel-based companies and started in a small Tanzanian location in 1949. At the request of the local bishop in Ifakara, zoologist Rudolf Geigy, an expert in pathogens and tropical diseases, visited Tanzania to see if he could devise a solution for the malaria, sleeping sickness, river blindness, and other diseases that ravaged the community. Using an improvised laboratory, Geigy

Exhibit 2 Novartis AG 1997 Financial Information (all figures in CHF millions)

Summarized Consolidated Income Statements		
For the Years Ended 31 December 1997 and 1996	1996	Pro forma 1997
Sales	31,180	26,144
Cost of goods sold	−9,847	−8,414
Operating expenses	−14,550	−12,803
Operating income	6,783	4,927
Financial income/expense, net	120	−83
Taxes and minority interests	−1,692	−1,207
Net Income	5,211	3,637

Summarized Consolidated Balance Sheets		
	31 Dec. 1997	1 Jan. 1997
Assets		
Long-Term Assets		
Tangible fixed assets	11,589	11,534
Other long-term assets	6,069	4,912
Total Long-Term Assets	**17,658**	**16,446**
Current Assets		
Inventories, trade accounts, receivables, and other current assets	15,684	15,273
Marketable securities, cash, and cash equivalents	18,486	18,527
Total Current Assets	**34,170**	**33,800**
Total Assets	**51,828**	**50,246**
Equity and Liabilities		
Equity		
Share capital, net	1,370	1,377
Reserves	25,431	22,187
Total Equity	**26,801**	**23,564**
Liabilities		
Long-Term Liabilities		
Financial debts	3,611	5,254
Deferred taxes, other long-term liabilities, and minority interests	4,360	3,892
Total Long-Term Liabilities and Minority Interests	**7,971**	**9,146**
Short-Term Liabilities		
Financial debts	7,465	6,722
Trade accounts payable and other short-term liabilities	9,591	10,814
Total Short-Term Liabilities	**17,056**	**17,536**
Total Liabilities and Minority Interests	**25,027**	**26,682**
Total Equity and Liabilities	**51,828**	**50,246**

Source: Novartis Operational Review, 1997, 29.

Exhibit 3 Percentage of Pharmaceutical World Market Share in 1995

Top 33%	
Glaxo Wellcome	4.7%
Novartis (Ciba and Geigy)	4.4%
Merck	3.5%
Hoechst Marion Roussel	3.5%
Bristol-Myers Squibb	3.1%
American Home Products	3.0%
Pfizer	2.9%
Johnson & Johnson	2.9%
Roche Pharmaceuticals	2.8%
SB	2.5%
Balance:	**66.7%**

Source: Reuters, "Sandoz-Ciba Merger Hailed as World's Biggest," *The Financial Post* (Toronto), 8 March 1996, 5.

studied ticks, fleas, and other regional insects. Eventually, the Rural Aid Centre was established in 1961, with financing by the Basel Foundation for Assistance to Developing Countries. This foundation was the creation of the former Ciba, Geigy, Sandoz, and companies based in Basel, which Geigy recruited for continued support. Geigy's firm belief was that "aid should have a sustainable impact and . . . be more than the distribution of charity,"[19] which became the credo of the Novartis Foundation.

In the early 1970s, the chairman of Ciba-Geigy, just recently formed from the merger of J. R. Geigy AG and Ciba, asked a young graduate student, Klaus Leisinger, to outline a working set of guidelines for an international company doing business in Africa. What Leisinger came up with, said Novartis's Karin Schmitt, was legendary for that time. "He had some very funny and courageous ideas," said Schmitt. "He felt you should Africanize the companies, that the local CEOs should be African."[20] In addition, Leisinger's paper emphasized selling solutions, not just products. The result was an "unequivocal" set of guidelines and obligations for doing business in a poor country. From Leisinger's paper emerged an Africa Policy, which then became a Corporate Policy for the Third World. At the same time, Novartis established a Third World Staff Unit, followed by a Third World Committee, which then, in 1979, became the Ciba-Geigy Foundation for Cooperation with Developing Countries on the basis that "the company did not content itself with declarations, but actually put its principles into practice."[21]

The purpose of the organization, according to its founding document, was to promote development of the poorest countries in the Third World, primarily by collaborating in agriculture, health care, and education, with the ultimate purpose of fostering self-help and providing aid in the event of a disaster. In 1990, this purpose was amended and "scientifically based analyses" and "consultations and information on development policy issues" were added to the list of resources to be made available. The objective of the foundation thus became three-pronged: consulting on development policy inside and outside the company, engaging in dialogue about development policy and human rights, and using its knowledge and insights in development projects.[22]

Schmitt emphasized that although the then Ciba-Geigy had a tradition of philanthropic work, the emphasis really was on achieving sustainable results. "You can give just money away," Schmitt said, "but that was never the purpose." Although Ciba-Geigy did give charitable donations, the company took development assistance very seriously. "You don't just throw money into things, make a nice publication, make photos, and make public relations with it, but you really build up something." The Novartis Foundation's charitable efforts were never designed to build markets where there are none because, as Schmitt said, that might lead to a conflict of interest between the company's commercial efforts and its interests in Third World country development. Its Leprosy Fund worked closely with governments, the World Health Organization (WHO), and nongovernmental leprosy organizations to address the sociocultural problems as well as medical needs of those suffering from leprosy in countries such as India, Sri Lanka, Madagascar, and Brazil.

The foundation staff was small, but its activities were wide and varied. There was, according to Schmitt, think tank and publication work.

> We work very much academically on issues like corporate citizenship and business ethics; but we were also greatly interested in green biotechnology, population policy "with a human face," and other broader issues of social and political relevance. We also take a scientific approach to our assistance programs, so that we really can disseminate knowledge in a form that is acceptable to the most different circles of stakeholders—to academia but also to lay people, but also to people who are working in development to governments to others.

Experimenting in Tanzania

What Madörin proposed doing in Tanzania had in a similar fashion already been tried out independently in Zimbabwe, where the HIV/AIDS orphan crisis was also severe. Stefan Germann, a Swiss aid worker who was at the time with the Swiss Salvation Army, had just founded the Massiye Camp, primarily to help develop the coping capacity of children affected by HIV/AIDS, and to focus on psychosocial support and life-skills development for orphans and other vulnerable children. Madörin wanted to do his work in a very remote rural area of Tanzania, where NGOs rarely go, because he thought if his concept could work there, it would work everywhere.

This type of project inevitably would have a modicum of controversy, with some questioning why an organization would focus on the psychosocial issues of children rather than their material needs. The answer, according to Madörin, was that giving children food and clothing was no longer enough. There was a "causal relationship between death, poverty, and alienation, resulting in grief, anger, and antisocial behavior."[23] If left unaddressed, Madörin contended, this "failure to support children to overcome this trauma will have very negative impact on society and might cause dysfunctional societies, jeopardizing years of investment in national development."[24] Nonetheless, Madörin's proposal was unusual and did not fit the normal profile of suggested programs to combat the effects of AIDS in Africa. Novartis also did not manufacture any HIV/AIDS medical products, leading some to question why the company would even consider addressing this particular problem. Novartis and its foundation did have the choice of many worthwhile opportunities to address crises in developing countries, whether or not related directly to its products. In addition to AIDS, there was leprosy, malaria, and tuberculosis, and although Novartis had addressed these health crises with various programs, in this case, the company decided to support a project that tried to approach, in an innovative way, a real socioeconomic need of vulnerable children. The idea was to develop "good practices," proof of the concept, and a sustainable program. Novartis also wanted to make all lessons learned in this process and implementation available to interested donors worldwide.

Endnotes

1. *terres des hommes schweiz* focused on the health, social care, and rights of children worldwide.
2. Benjamin F. Nelson, "Global Health: The U.S. and U.N. Response to the AIDS Crisis in Africa," *U.S. General Accounting Office Testimony* (February 2000): 2. *http://www.gao.gov/archive/2000/ns00099t.pdf* (accessed 12 September 2007).
3. "Number of AIDS Orphans Rapidly Increasing in Sub-Saharan Africa," *Reproductive Health Matters* 11, no. 22 (2003): 193.
4. *http://www.thebody.com/content/world/art33120.html* (accessed 25 April 2007).
5. Geoff Foster, "Supporting Community Efforts to Assist Orphans in Africa," *New England Journal of Medicine* 346, no. 24 (13 June 2002): 1907.
6. Foster, 1907.
7. Foster, 1907.
8. Foster, 1907.
9. Milt Freudenheim, "Merger of Drug Giants: A New Image for Corporate Switzerland," *The New York Times*, 8 March 1996, D1.
10. Stephen D. Moore, "Novartis Leaps Last Regulatory Hurdle," *The Wall Street Journal*, 18 December 1996, B11.
11. According to Freudenheim, this was the third-largest deal at that time, following Mitsubishi Bank's acquisition of the Bank of Tokyo for USD33.8 billion and Kohlberg Kravis Roberts's deal for RJR Nabisco for USD30.6 billion.
12. Stephen D. Moore and Philip Revzin, "Challenge for Novartis Lies in the Lab," *The Wall Street Journal*, 30 July 1996, B8.
13. Freudenheim
14. Freudenheim.
15. *http://www.novartis.com/about-novartis/company-history/index.shtml* (accessed 04 November 2007).
16. Novartis Operational Review 1997, 4.
17. Novartis Operational Review 1997, 4.
18. Bale Communications Inc., "Novartis Looking To Be the Biggest," *Adnews Online*, 18 December 1997.
19. "Success Through Perseverance and Patience: The History of the Novartis Foundation Is One of Continuity Over 25 Years," *http://www.novartisfoundation.org/platform/apps/Publication/getfmfile.asp?id=652&el=543&se=634215889&doc=14&dse=1* (accessed 17 July 2007).
20. Karin Schmitt (Novartis), interviewed by Jenny Mead, April 4, 2007, Darden Graduate School of Business Administration, Charlottesville, Virginia.
21. "Success Through Perseverance and Patience," 20.
22. "Success Through Perseverance and Patience," 21.
23. Stefan Germann, Kurt Madörin, and Ncazelo Ncube, "Psychosocial Support for Children Affected by AIDS: Tanzania, and Zimbabwe," *SAFAIDS* 9, no. 2 (June 2001): 11.
24. Germann et al., 11.

Case 24   Samsung Electronics*

In January 2009, Samsung Electronics began to slim down its operations into two divisions from the five separate ones that it had a year earlier. The sets division, called digital media and communications, will focus on consumer products such as television and mobile phones. The parts unit, called device solutions, will handle electronic components such as semiconductors and LCD panels. The firm had already merged its home appliance division, which made refrigerators and air conditioners, with its digital media section over the previous year.

The reorganization followed on the heels of a major shake-up of top executives at Samsung Electronics. In the aftermath of a tax evasion scandal involving the parent firm, Yun Jong Yong, the electronic firm's long-term CEO, was replaced in May 2008 by Lee Yoon Woo. In addition, the firm has begun to appoint several younger executives to its leadership team and reassign two-thirds of its executives to different positions. "There has been a sense of crisis in the company for more than one year," said one senior manager. "Radical change is in store."[1]

The moves represented a major effort to streamline operations to better address worsening economic conditions. Four years ago, the market value of Samsung had risen above $100 billion, making it one of only four Asian companies to move above that mark. Based in Suwon, South Korea, the firm moved past well-known rivals such as Sony, Nokia, and Motorola on the basis of its revolutionary products. Its feature-jammed gadgets have racked up numerous design awards, and the company has been rapidly muscling its way to the top of consumer brand-awareness surveys.

However, in spite of these advances, Samsung has not been able to deal with the growing impact of the global economic slowdown. Although the firm has been able to boast of having a lower cost structure than most of its rivals, it was expected to announce its first-ever quarterly loss, for the last quarter of 2008. (See Exhibits 1 and 2.) Much of the downturn could be attributed to an overcapacity in the global production of memory chips and liquid crystal displays, which has forced down prices. This may ease over the next couple of years as many of Samsung's smaller rivals are dropping their plans to expand capacity.

Among all the changes that Samsung has been making, analysts have paid particular attention to the appointment of Choi Gee Sung to head the newly formed digital media and communications unit. Choi's appointment signifies a break from the firm's tradition of picking top managers with backgrounds in engineering. In fact, Choi

---

* This case was developed by Professor Jamal Shamsie, Michigan State University, with the assistance of Professor Alan B. Eisner, Pace University. Material has been drawn from published sources to be used for class discussion. Copyright © 2009 Jamal Shamsie and Alan B. Eisner.

Exhibit 1   **Income Statement** (in trillions of Korean won, year-end December 31)

	2008	2007	2006	2005	2004
Net sales	121,294	98,508	85,426	80,630	81,963
Gross profit	31,532	27,627	25,779	25,378	29,010
Operating profit	6,031	8,973	9,008	7,575	11,761
Net income	5,525	7,421	7,926	7,640	10,790

Source: Samsung.

Exhibit 2   **Balance Sheet** (in trillions of Korean won, year-end December 31)

	2008	2007	2006	2005	2004
Total assets	105,301	93,375	81,366	74,462	69,005
Total liabilities	47,186	37,404	33,426	32,854	32,604
Total shareholders' equity	58,117	55,972	47,940	41,607	36,400

Source: Samsung.

is likely to take over as Samsung's next CEO when Lee relinquishes this post. Referring to the shift away from its heavy focus on technology, Kang Shin Woo, chief investment officer at fund manager Korea Investment Trust Management, said, "Samsung's benchmark is shifting from Japanese companies to innovators like Apple."[2]

Discarding a Failing Strategy

The transformation of Samsung into a premier brand can be attributed to the ceaseless efforts of Yun Jong Yong, who was appointed to the position of president and CEO in 1996. When Yun took charge, Samsung was still making most of its profits from lower-priced appliances that consumers were likely to pick up if they could not afford a higher-priced brand such as Sony or Mitsubishi. The firm had also become an established low-cost supplier of various components to larger and better-known manufacturers around the world.

Although Samsung was making profits, Yun was concerned about the future prospects of a firm that was relying on a strategy of competing on price with products that were based on technologies that had been developed by other firms. The success of this strategy was tied to the ability of Samsung to continually scout for locations that would allow it to keep its manufacturing costs down. At the same time, it would need to keep generating sufficient orders to maintain a high volume of production. In particular, Yun was concerned about the growing competition that the firm was likely to face from the many low-cost producers that were springing up in other countries such as China.

Yun's concerns were well founded. Within a year of his takeover, Samsung was facing serious financial problems that threatened its very survival. The company was left with huge debt as an economic crisis engulfed most of Asia in 1997, leading to a drop in demand and a crash in the prices of many electronic goods. In the face of such a deteriorating environment, Samsung continued to push for maintaining its production and sales records even as much of its output was ending up unsold in warehouses.

By July 1998, Samsung Electronics was losing millions of dollars each month. "If we continued, we would have gone belly-up within three or four years," Yun recalled.[3] He knew that he had to make some drastic moves in order to turn things around. Yun locked himself in a hotel room for a whole day with nine other senior managers to try and find a way out. They all wrote resignation letters and pledged to resign if they failed.

After much deliberation, Yun and his management team decided to take several steps to try to push Samsung out of its precarious financial position. To begin with, they decided to lay off about 30,000 employees, representing well over one-third of the firm's entire workforce. They also closed down many of Samsung's factories for two months so that they could get rid of its large inventory. Finally, they sold off about $2 billion worth of businesses like pagers and electric coffeemakers that were perceived to be of marginal significance for the firm's future.

Developing a Premium Brand

Having managed to stem the losses, Yun decided to move Samsung away from its strategy of competition based largely on the lower price of its offerings. Consequently, he began to push the firm to develop its own products rather than copying those that other firms had developed. (See Exhibit 3.) In particular, Yun placed considerable

Exhibit 3   **Revenue Breakdown** (in trillions of Korean won, year-end December 31)

	Year	Sales	Profits
Semiconductors Includes DRAMs, SRAMs & NAND flash chips	2007	22.3	2.3
	2006	22.8	5.1
	2005	20.3	5.4
	2004	20.2	7.8
Telecommunications Includes digital phones and handsets	2007	23.8	2.8
	2006	20.2	2.0
	2005	20.9	2.5
	2004	20.7	3.1
Digital media Includes plasma and projection displays and televisions	2007	26.5	1.1
	2006	20.7	0.7
	2005	17.7	0.2
	2004	17.6	0.4
LCD Includes panels for desktop and laptop computers	2007	17.1	2.1
	2006	13.9	0.8
	2005	8.7	0.6
	2004	7.8	1.9
Digital appliances Includes "intelligent" refrigerators, microwave ovens, air conditioners	2007	6.9	0.2
	2006	5.5	−0.1
	2005	5.6	−0.1
	2004	5.4	0.1

Source: Samsung.

emphasis on the development of products that would impress consumers with their attractive designs and their advanced technology. By focusing on such products, Yun hoped that he could develop Samsung into a premium brand that would allow him to charge higher prices.

To achieve this, Yun had to reorient the firm and help it to develop new capabilities. He recruited new managers and engineers, many of whom had developed considerable experience in the United States. Once they had been recruited, Yun got them into shape by putting them through a four-week boot camp that consisted of martial drills at the crack of dawn and mountain hikes that would last all day. To create incentives for this new talent, Yun discarded Samsung's rigid seniority-based system and replaced it with a merit-based system for advancement.

As a result of these efforts, Samsung began launching an array of products that were designed to make a big impression on consumers. They included the largest flat-panel televisions, cell phones with a variety of features such as cameras and PDAs, ever-thinner notebook computers, and speedier and richer semiconductors. (See Exhibit 4.) The firm calls them "wow products," and they are designed to elevate Samsung in the same way the Trinitron television and the Walkman had helped to plant Sony in the minds of consumers.

A large part of the success of Samsung's products can be tied to its efforts to focus on the specific needs of prospective customers. Mike Linton, executive vice president of Best Buy, stated that Samsung regularly gets information from retailers about the new features that customers want to see in their electronic devices. This close link with retailers helped Samsung to come up with two of its recent best-selling products: a combined DVD-VCR player and a cellular phone that also functions as a PDA. According to Graeme Bateman, head of research for Japanese investment bank Nomura Securities, "Samsung is no longer making poor equivalents of Sony products. It is making things people want."[4]

Finally, to help Samsung change its image among consumers, Yun hired a marketing whiz, Eric Kim, who has worked hard to create a more upscale image of the firm and its products. Kim moved Samsung's advertising away from 55 different advertising agencies around the world and placed it with one firm, Madison Avenue's Foote, Cone & Belding Worldwide, to create a consistent global brand image for its products. He also begun to pull Samsung out of big discount chains like Wal-Mart and Kmart and place more of its products into upscale specialty stores such as Best Buy and Circuit City.

Pushing for New Products

Yun took many steps to speed up Samsung's new product development process. He was well aware that Samsung would be able to maintain its higher margins only as long as his firm could keep introducing new products into the market well ahead of its established rivals. Samsung managers who have worked for big competitors say they have to go through far fewer layers of bureaucracy than they had to in the past to win approval for new products, budgets, and marketing plans, and this speeds up their ability to seize opportunities.

Apart from reducing the bureaucratic obstacles, Yun made heavy investments in key technologies ranging from semiconductors to LCD displays that could allow the firm to push out a wide variety of revolutionary digital products. Samsung has continuously invested more than any of its rivals in research and development, with the amount rising during the past couple of years to almost 9 percent of its revenue. It has a large force of designers and engineers working in 17 research centers located throughout the world. (See Exhibit 5.) Yun also forced the firm's own units to compete with outsiders in order to speed up the

Exhibit 4   **Global Market Ranking, 2007**

Product Category	Market Rank
Memory chips	1
Computer monitors	1
LCD panels	1
LCD TVs	1
Plasma TVs	1
DVD-VCR combos	1
Projection TVs	2
DVD players	2
MP3 players	2
Laser printers	2
Mobile phones	2
Microwave ovens	3
Camcorders	4

Source: Samsung.

Exhibit 5   **Designers Employed**

2006	550
2004	470
2002	310
2000	210
1998	170

Source: Samsung.

process of developing innovative new products. In the liquid-crystal-display business, Samsung bought half of its color filters from Sumitomo Chemical Company of Japan and sourced the other half internally, pitting the two teams against each other. "They really press these departments to compete," said Sumitomo President Hiromasa Yonekura.[5]

As a result of these steps, Samsung claims that the time it takes to go from new product concept to rollout is now as little as five months, compared to over a year that it used to take the firm just eight years ago. In large part, this has resulted from the effort of the firm's top managers, engineers, and designers, who work relentlessly in the five-story VIP center nestled amid the firm's industrial complex in Suwon. They work day and night in the center, which includes dormitories and showers for brief rests, to work out any problems that may hold back a product launch.

The progress made by teams that pursue new product designs in the VIP center makes it possible for Samsung to reduce complexity in the early stages of the design cycle. This allows the firm to move its products quickly to manufacturing with minimal problems and at the lowest possible cost. In turn, this can lead to a faster market launch of a product that is likely to be more innovative than all others. Kyunghan Jung, a senior manager of the center, explained: "Seventy to eighty percent of quality, cost and delivery time is determined in the initial stages of product development."[6] Such an emphasis on early design issues allowed Samsung to figure out how the D600, one of its latest music-playing camera phones, could be assembled in as little as eight seconds.

The speedier development process has allowed Samsung to introduce the first voice-activated phones, handsets with MP3 players, and digital camera phones that send photos over global systems for mobile communications networks. The firm has been just as fast in digital televisions, becoming the first to market projection TVs using new chips from Texas Instruments that employ digital-light processing. DLP chips contain 1.3 million micromirrors that flip at high speeds to create a sharper picture. Texas Instruments had given Japanese companies the technology early in 1999, but they never figured out how to make the TV sets economically. George Danko, Best Buy's senior vice president for consumer electronics, said of Samsung, "They'll get a product to market a lot faster than their counterparts."[7]

Designing for the Digital Home

Yun was hoping that Samsung's advances in digital technologies would increase its chances of dominating the digital home. He believed that his firm was in a better position to benefit from the day that all home appliances from handheld computers to intelligent refrigerators will be linked to one another and adapted to the personal needs of consumers. In particular, Samsung appears to be well placed to take advantage of its capabilities to design and manufacture a wide array of products that straddle traditional technology categories. "We have to combine computers, consumer electronics and communications as Koreans mix their rice with vegetables and meats," said Dae Je Chin, the head of Samsung's digital media division.[8]

Yun worked closely with Chin to summon engineers and designers from across the firm to mix wireless, semiconductor, and computer expertise in order to pursue its vision of domination of the digital home. One such product from the firm is NEXiO, a combined cell phone and handheld computer. The device has a 5-inch screen, large enough for a user to run a spreadsheet or to browse the Web. Another new offering is a refrigerator called Zipel that has a 15-inch flat-panel touch screen tucked into the door. The display can be used to surf the Internet and to send or receive e-mail.

In developing these products, Samsung has begun to place a lot of emphasis on the role of design in making its products irresistible in an increasingly competitive marketplace. Since 2000, the firm has opened or expanded design centers in San Francisco, London, Tokyo, Los Angeles, and Shanghai. (See Exhibit 6.) Inside these centers, designers observe the way that consumers actually use various products. They may watch, from behind a two-way mirror, how consumers stuff a refrigerator with bagfuls of groceries. Samsung has also begun to send its growing group of designers to various locations to spend a few months at fashion houses, furniture designers, and cosmetic specialists to stay current with trends in other industries.

Furthermore, Samsung created the post of chief design officer to make sure that designers can get their ideas to top managers. A successful rear-projection television was developed by a designer who pitched it to one of the heads of television production. Engineers are pushed to find ways to work with the designs that are presented to them. As a result of these efforts, Samsung has earned numerous citations at top design contests in the United States, Europe, and Asia. After winning 46 awards at a recent U.S. consumer electronics show, D. J. Oh, CEO of Samsung Electronics America, said, "Samsung strives to consistently lead the consumer electronics industry in product design and engineering innovation."[9]

Samsung has been relying on the attractiveness of its products to make them the centerpieces of a digital home. It has been displaying its version of a networked home in Seoul's Tower Palace apartment complex, where 2,400 families can operate appliances from washing machines to air conditioners by tapping on a wireless "Web pad" device, which doubles as a portable flat-screen TV. It may sound a bit futuristic, but when the digital home does become more realistic, Samsung will have a chance. "They've got the products, a growing reputation as the innovator, and production lines to back that up," said In-Stat/MDR consumer-electronics analyst Cindy Wolf.[10]

Exhibit 6 Samsung Milestones

1969	Samsung Electronics is established as a maker of televisions with technology borrowed from Sanyo.
1977	Samsung introduces its first color television.
1981	Samsung begins to focus on undercutting Japanese rivals with me-too products, with little emphasis on design.
1988	Samsung launches its first mobile phone.
1993	Samsung begins to reinvent the firm through design.
1994	Samsung hires design consultancy IDEO to help develop computer monitors.
1995	Samsung sets up its in-house design school, the Innovative Design Lab of Samsung.
1996	Yun Jong Yong takes over as CEO. He declares the "Year of Design Revolution," stressing that designers should lead in product planning.
1998	Asian financial crisis dents Samsung's ambitions, forcing it to cut design staff by 28%.
2000	Samsung once again focuses on design, and CEO Yun Jong Yong calls for design-led management.
2001	Yun initiates quarterly design meetings for top executives and opens design labs in Los Angeles and London.
2002	Samsung's "usability laboratory" is inaugurated in downtown Seoul.
2004	Market value of Samsung rises above $100 billion.
2008	Lee Yoon Woo takes over as CEO from Yun.
2009	Samsung is set to announce its first loss since 2000. The firm announces a major reorganization.

Source: Samsung.

Creating a Sustainable Model?

In spite of all the improvements that Samsung has made over the last decade, the firm is expected to announce its first quarterly loss since its brush with bankruptcy. With the sharp decline in demand, prices for most of the firm's products have been dropping, cutting into its profit margins. The divisional restructuring and the management changes were designed to streamline operations at Samsung to better address the worsening economic conditions. Recently, the firm stated that it hopes to eliminate bureaucracy and speed decision making at a time when flexibility is needed to deal with forces that threaten its existence.

To find new avenues for growth, Samsung recently made an unsuccessful bid to acquire SanDisk Corporation. The offer marked the first time that the firm had attempted a major acquisition. Samsung has mostly relied on organic growth to gain its status as a leading electronics firm. But the acquisition of SanDisk could have helped Samsung to expand its business into storage cards and other products that use advanced flash chips.

Given the failure to acquire SanDisk, Lee appears to be well aware of the challenges that lie ahead for Samsung. The life cycle of most electronics products can be brutally short, with prices tending to drop sharply over time. The profitability of a hardware firm rests on its ability to keep addressing new opportunities such as those offered by Microsoft's launch of the new Windows Vista operating systems. At the same time, it must keep seeking ways to reduce its costs in order to be competitive with lower-margin products.

Samsung has consistently refused to consider branching out like Sony or Apple into music, movies, and games. It has decided against such a move in spite of growing evidence that subscription-to-content can provide a firm with a more lucrative source of revenue. Instead, Yun chose to collaborate with various content and software providers such as Microsoft and Time Warner.

Lee understands that the future of Samsung lies in its ability to keep investing heavily in R&D and keep developing new factories in locations that offer lower costs. Critics point out that Samsung is still searching for a product that would be comparable to Apple's iPod or Sony's Walkman. But industry observers warn that the firm must not back off despite the current squeeze on profits. "It's critical for Samsung that the new leadership keep investing in new technologies and equipment," said Chang In Whan, chief executive at fund manager KTB Asset Management.[11]

Endnotes

1. Moon Ihlwan. Samsung Electronics: Same CEO, New Leadership Team. *BusinessWeek* online, January 19, 2009.
2. Ibid.
3. Frank Gibney, Jr. Samsung Moves Upmarket. *Time,* March 25, 2002, p. 49.
4. Cliff Edwards, Moon Ihlwan, and Pete Engardio. The Samsung Way. *BusinessWeek,* June 16, 2003, p. 60.
5. Peter Lewis. A Perpetual Crisis Machine. *Fortune,* September 19, 2005, p. 65.
6. Edwards, Ihlwan, and Engardio. The Samsung Way, p. 61.
7. Brad Stone. Samsung in Bloom. *Newsweek,* July 15, 2002, p. 34.
8. David Rocks and Moon Ihlwan. Samsung Design. *BusinessWeek,* December 6, 2004, p. 90.
9. Anonymous. Samsung Electronics Gets 46 CES Innovations Awards for 2009. *Wireless News,* November 24, 2008.
10. Jay Solomon. Seoul Survivors: Back from the Brink. *The Wall Street Journal,* June 13, 2002, p. A1.
11. Ihlwan. Samsung Electronics.

photo credits

company index

Mint.com, 338
MIT Enterprise Forum of Pakistan, C179
Mitsubishi, C66, C119, C211
Mitsui, C66
Mittal Steel, 263
mmO2, C129
Mobily, C48
Modern Engineering Inc., C104
Molson Companies, Ltd., 269
    product categories, C5
Money Auction, 330
Monsanto, 126, 175
Monster.com, 138, 169
MonsterTRAK, 169
Morgan Stanley, 209, 361
Morningstar, 65
Motorola, 68, 172, 191, 246n, 306, 457, 496,
    C48, C124, C128, C130, C131, C133,
    C211
    Iridium failure, 493
Mozilla Firefox, C46, C49
MRM Worldwide, 270
MSA Aircraft Interior Products, Inc., 369
MSX International Inc., C104
Museum of Modern Betas, C179
Music Genome Project, 336
MyC4, 330
My Docs Online, 104
MyNetwork TV, C98
MySimon, 105
MySpace, 126, C46, C50

n

Namdeb, C88
Napster, 191
Narayana Hrudayalaya Hospital, 292
NASCAR, 207
Naseeb Networks, C180, C181
National Association of Home-Based Businesses,
    325
National Automobile Dealers Association, C120
National Basketball Association, 360, 375
National Can Corporation, C8
    financial performance, C10
National Federation of Independent Business, 333
National Football League, 351
    and United Football League, 352
National Oil Corporation, C67
National Wildlife Federation, 59
Natural Resources Defense Council, 59
Nature Conservancy, 59
Naver, 346
NBC, C98
NCR, 245
NEC, 63, C25, C129
Nelco, C148
Nelito Systems, C148
Nestlé, 247, 251–252, 299, 306
Netflix, 210, 220, 344, 345
    crowdsourcing by, 212
Network Appliances, 215
New Alternatives, 65
NewPage Corporation, 169
News Corp., 348
    innovativeness ranking, C153

New York Times Company, 347
    challenged by Wall Street Journal, 348
NeXT Computer, C42
Nextel, 245
NeXT Software, C44
Nexx, 330
Nielsen Online, 104
Nike, Inc., 59, 131, 255, 290, 297, 349, 419–420
    external control mechanisms, 386
    innovativeness ranking, C153
Nikeid.com, 217
Nikon, 286
Niko Resources Ltd., 56
Nintendo Company, 107, 421, 477, C46, C49
    innovativeness ranking, C151
Nintendo Entertainment System, C25
Nintendo GameCube, C25
Nintendo of America, C28
Nintendo Wii, 478
Nintendo Wii, case
    balance sheet, C27
    company history, C25–C26
    competitors
        Microsoft Xbox 360, C30–C31
        Sony PlayStation 3, C31
    customer demographics, C29
    game developers, C29–C30
    game system comparisons, C30
    income statement, C26
    innovation, C25
    major competitors, C25
    online capabilities, C28–C29
    product features, C28
    production problems, C29
    product launch, C26–C27
    revenues in 2008, C25
    stock price performance, C28
    supply and demand problems, C31–C32
    technology development, C25
Nissan Japan Ltd., 86
Nissan Motors GB, 85, 110, 306, 424, C119, C121
    financial data, C102
    research and development expenditures, C102
    revenue and income, C105
    scenario planning, 86
Nivea, 82
Noba, 330
Nokia, C46, C48, C50, C128, C129, C130, C131,
    C133, C211
    innovativeness ranking, C151
Nokia chocolate phones, 209
Nokia Corporation, 80, 170, 191, 269, 306, 361
    problems at, 44–45
Nomura Securities, C213
Nordic Mobile Telephone, C124
Nordstrom, 126
Nortel, 269
North Face, 209
Novamont, 329
Novartis AG, 247, 260, C207, C209, C210
Novartis Foundation for Sustainable Develop-
        ment, case
    balance sheet, C208
    Corporate Policy for the Third World, C209
    experimenting in Tanzania, C209–C210
    and HIV/AIDS crisis, C206–C207, C209–C210
    income statement, C208
    Leprosy fund, C209
    origin of, C207–C209

    purpose, C209
    Third World Committee, C209
Novatek, C55
Novell, 81, 267, 351, 423
NPF Gazfund, C55
NTP, 192
NTT, C124
NTT DoCoMo, C127, C128, C131
Nucor Steel Company, 365, 412
Nutmeg Industries, 251
Nynex, 97

O

O. R. T. Technologies, 295
OC Oerlikon Corporation, 376
Oil of Olay, C203
Oklahoma City Thunder, 360
Olam International, 62
Oldsmobile, 403
Olympus, 527
Omega, 231
On Air, C80
ONGC Videsh, C67
OPEN Global, C180
Open Hand Alliance, C129
Oracle Corporation, 186, 273, 290, 301, 382, 445,
    533, C20, C179
Orange, C123, C128, C131, C133, C179
Orkut, 481
Otis Elevator, 84
O2, C123, C128
Overstock.com, 212, C156
Owens-Illinois, C7, C8
Oxford GlycoSciences, 299

p

Paccar, 215
Pacific Gas and Electric, 385
Palm Computing Inc., C123
Panasonic, 68, 341
Panda Restaurant Group, 249
Pandora, 335
    effect on music business, 336
Parker Pen, 250
Parmalat, 374, 384, 459
Parnasus Equity Income, 65
Partizipa, 330
Partner Brands, C36
Paychex, 105
PayPal, 158, 159, C156, C162, C163, C165, C166
PChomeOnline, C165
Pearl Meyer & Partners, 385
Pechiney International Group, C10, C19
Peermint, 330
Pennine Natural Gas, C61
Pentax, 286
PeopleSoft, 273
PepsiCo, 140, 171, 252, 286, 313, 417, 502, C4,
    C41
    in India, 314
    product categories, C5
Pepsi Cola Bottling Group, C8
Peterbilt, 215

name index

Page numbers followed by n refer to footnotes.

subject index

W

Z